Third Edition

OBSTETRICS
NORMAL & PROBLEM PREGNANCIES

Third Edition

OBSTETRICS
NORMAL & PROBLEM PREGNANCIES

Edited by

STEVEN G. GABBE, M.D.
Professor and Chairman
Department of Obstetrics and Gynecology
University of Washington School of Medicine
Seattle, Washington

JENNIFER R. NIEBYL, M.D.
Professor and Head
Department of Obstetrics and Gynecology
University of Iowa College of Medicine
Iowa City, IA

JOE LEIGH SIMPSON, M.D.
Ernst W. Bertner Professor and Chairman
Department of Obstetrics and Gynecology
Professor of Molecular and Human Genetics
Baylor College of Medicine
Houston, TX

WITH CONTRIBUTIONS BY

George J. Annas
Thomas J. Benedetti
Richard L. Berkowitz
Ira Bernstein
John Bissonnette
Watson A. Bowes, Jr.
D. Ware Branch
John E. Buster
Sandra Carson
Robert C. Cefalo
Frank A. Chervenak
David H. Chestnut

Usha Chitkara
Larry J. Copeland
Dwight P. Cruikshank
Richard Depp
Maurice L. Druzin
Patrick Duff
Sherman Elias
M. Gore Ervin
Roger K. Freeman
Anna-Riitta Fuchs
Fritz Fuchs
Charles P. Gibbs

Michael C. Gordon
Joy L. Hawkins
Patricia M. Hays
Jay D. Iams
Marc Jackson
Timothy R. B. Johnson
David C. Lagrew, Jr.
Mark B. Landon
William C. Mabie
Mary Ellen Mortensen
William F. O'Brien
Roy H. Petrie

Rosemary E. Reiss
Adam A. Rosenberg
Michael G. Ross
Philip Samuels
John W. Seeds
Lowell E. Sever
Baha M. Sibai
Phillip G. Stubblefield
Marlene A. Walker
Margaret Walsh
Thomas R. Wigton

Illustrated by Mikki Senkarik, M.S., A.M.I.

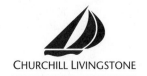

CHURCHILL LIVINGSTONE

New York, Edinburgh, London, Philadelphia, San Francisco

CHURCHILL LIVINGSTONE
A Division of Harcourt Brace & Company

Library of Congress Cataloging-in-Publication Data

Obstetrics : normal and problem pregnancies / edited by Steven G. Gabbe,
    Jennifer R. Niebyl, Joe Leigh Simpson ; with contributions by
    George J. Annas . . . [et al.] ; illustrated by Mikki Senkarik. — 3rd ed.
        p.   cm.
    Includes bibliographical references and index.
    ISBN 0–443–07690–1 (alk. paper)
    1. Obstetrics.   2. Pregnancy—Complications.   I. Gabbe, Steven G.
    II. Niebyl, Jennifer R.   III. Simpson, Joe Leigh.   IV. Annas George J.
    [DNLM: 1. Obstetrics. 2. Pregnancy. 3. Pregnancy Complications.
    WQ 100 O165 1996]
    RG524.03 1996
    618.2—dc20
    DNLM/DLC   96–20732

Distributed in the United Kingdom by Churchill Livingstone, Robert Stevenson House,
1–3 Baxter's Place, Leith Walk, Edinburgh EH1 3AF, and by associated companies,
branches, and representatives throughout the world.

Accurate indications, adverse reactions, and dosage schedules for drugs are provided in
this book, but it is possible that they may change. The reader is urged to review the
package information data of the manufacturers of the medications mentioned.

The Publishers have made every effort to trace the copyright holders for borrowed
material. If they have inadvertently overlooked any, they will be pleased to make the
necessary arrangements at the first opportunity.

Printed in the United States of America

Last digit is the print number: 7 6 5 4

The third edition of this textbook is dedicated to all of our contributors who have taken time from their busy schedules of patient care, teaching, research, and administrative responsibilities to craft so skillfully each of the chapters in our book. This book is also dedicated to three close friends who joined us for the first two editions, but who sadly passed away while this edition was in preparation: Dr. Fritz Fuchs, Dr. Patricia M. Hays, and Dr. Roy H. Petrie.

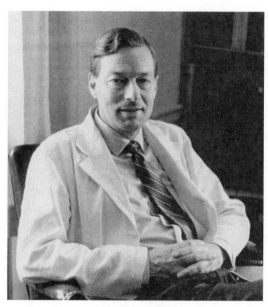

Dr. Fritz Fuchs

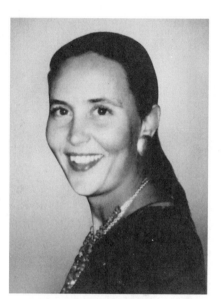

Dr. Patricia M. Hays

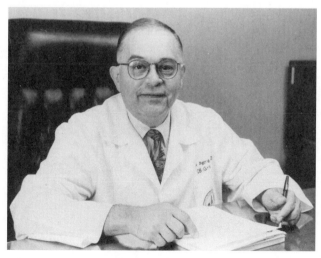

Dr. Roy H. Petrie

Contributors

GEORGE J. ANNAS, J.D., M.P.H.
Edward Utley Professor and Chair, Department of Health Law, Boston University Schools of Medicine and Public Health, Boston, Massachusetts

THOMAS J. BENEDETTI, M.D.
Professor and Director, Perinatal Medicine, Departments of Obstetrics and Gynecology, University of Washington School of Medicine, Seattle, Washington

RICHARD L. BERKOWITZ, M.D.
Professor and Chairman, Department of Obstetrics, Gynecology, and Reproductive Sciences, Mount Sinai School of Medicine of the City University of New York; Director of Obstetrics and Gynecology, Mount Sinai Hospital, New York, New York

IRA BERNSTEIN, M.D.
Assistant Professor, Department of Obstetrics and Gynecology, University of Vermont College of Medicine; Attending Physician, Women's Health Care Service, Fletcher Allen Health Care, Burlington, Vermont

JOHN BISSONNETTE, M.D.
Professor, Departments of Obstetrics and Gynecology and Cell Biology and Anatomy, Oregon Health Sciences University School of Medicine; Attending Physician, Department of Obstetrics and Gynecology, University Hospital, Portland, Oregon

WATSON A. BOWES, JR, M.D.
Professor, Department of Obstetrics and Gynecology, University of North Carolina at Chapel Hill School of Medicine, Chapel Hill, North Carolina

D. WARE BRANCH, M.D.
Associate Professor, Department of Obstetrics and Gynecology, University of Utah School of Medicine, Salt Lake City, Utah

JOHN E. BUSTER, M.D.
Professor and Director, Division of Reproductive Endocrinology and Fertility, Department of Obstetrics and Gynecology, Baylor College of Medicine, Houston, Texas

SANDRA A. CARSON, M.D.
Associate Professor, Division of Reproductive Endocrinology and Fertility, Department of Obstetrics and Gynecology, Baylor College of Medicine, Houston, Texas

ROBERT C. CEFALO, M.D., PH.D.
Professor, Department of Obstetrics and Gynecology, University of North Carolina at Chapel Hill School of Medicine, Chapel Hill, North Carolina

FRANK A. CHERVENAK, M.D.
Director of Obstetrics and Maternal–Fetal Medicine, Department of Obstetrics and Gynecology, Cornell University Medical College, The New York Hospital, New York, New York

DAVID H. CHESTNUT, M.D.
Alfred Habeeb Professor and Chairman of Anesthesiology, Professor of Obstetrics and Gynecology, University of Alabama School of Medicine, Birmingham, Alabama

USHA CHITKARA, M.D.

Associate Professor, Department of Gynecology and Obstetrics, Division of Maternal–Fetal Medicine, Stanford University School of Medicine; Director, Prenatal Diagnosis and Therapy, Department of Gynecology and Obstetrics, Stanford University Hospital, Stanford, California

LARRY J. COPELAND, M.D.

Professor of Obstetrics and Gynecology and Director, Division of Gynecologic Oncology, The Ohio State University College of Medicine, Columbus, Ohio

DWIGHT P. CRUIKSHANK, M.D.

Professor and Chairman, Department of Obstetrics and Gynecology, Medical College of Wisconsin, Milwaukee, Wisconsin

RICHARD DEPP, M.D.

Paul A. and Eloise Bowers Professor of Obstetrics and Gynecology, Chairman, Department of Obstetrics and Gynecology, Jefferson Medical College of Thomas Jefferson University, Philadelphia, Pennsylvania

MAURICE L. DRUZIN, M.D.

Professor and Chief, Division of Maternal-Fetal Medicine, Department of Gynecology and Obstetrics, Stanford University School of Medicine, Stanford, California

PATRICK DUFF, M.D.

Professor and Residency Program Director, Department of Obstetrics and Gynecology, University of Florida College of Medicine, Gainesville, Florida

SHERMAN ELIAS, M.D.

Professor of Obstetrics and Gynecology and Professor of Molecular and Human Genetics, Baylor College of Medicine, Houston, Texas

M. GORE ERVIN, PH. D.

Associate Professor, Department of Obstetrics and Gynecology, University of California, Los Angeles, School of Medicine, Los Angeles, California; Perinatal Research Laboratory, Department of Obstetrics and Gynecology, Harbor–UCLA Medical Center, Torrance, California

ROGER K. FREEMAN, M.D.

Professor, Department of Obstetrics and Gynecology, University of California, Irvine, College of Medicine, Irvine, California; Medical Director of Obstetrics and Gynecology, Women's Services, Long Beach Memorial Medical Center, Long Beach, California

ANNA-RIITTA FUCHS, D.SC.

Professor of Reproductive Physiology and Professor of Biophysics and Physiology, Department of Obstetrics and Gynecology, Cornell University Medical College; Department of Obstetrics and Gynecology, The New York Hospital, New York, New York

FRITZ FUCHS, M.D.

Emeritus Professor of Obstetrics and Gynecology, Cornell University Medical College; Honorary Attending Physician, Department of Obstetrics and Gynecology, The New York Hospital, New York, New York

STEVEN G. GABBE, M.D.

Professor and Chairman, Department of Obstetrics and Gynecology, University of Washington School of Medicine, Seattle, Washington

CHARLES P. GIBBS, M.D.

Professor and Chairman, Department of Anesthesiology, University of Colorado Health Sciences Center, Denver, Colorado

MICHAEL C. GORDON, M.D.

Staff Perinatologist, Chief, Outpatient Services, Department of Obstetrics and Gynecology, Wilford Hall Medical Center, Lackland AFB, TX

JOY L. HAWKINS, M.D.

Associate Professor, Department of Anesthesiology, University of Colorado Health Sciences Center; Director of Obstetric Anesthesia, University Hospital, Denver, Colorado

PATRICIA M. HAYS, M.D.

Associate Professor, Department of Obstetrics and Gynecology, Medical College of Virginia, Richmond, Virginia

JAY D. IAMS, M.D.
Frederick P. Zuspan Professor of Obstetrics and Gyne-
cology, The Ohio State University College of Medicine;
Director, Division of Maternal–Fetal Medicine, The
Ohio State University Medical Center, Columbus, Ohio

MARC JACKSON, M.D.
Assistant Professor, Department of Obstetrics and
Gynecology, University of Pennsylvania Medical Center,
Philadelphia, Pennsylvania

TIMOTHY R. B. JOHNSON, M.D.
Bates Professor of Diseases of Women and Children,
Research Scientist, Center for Human Growth and
Development, Professor of Women's Studies, Professor
and Chair, Department of Obstetrics and Gynecology,
University of Michigan Medical School, Ann Arbor,
Michigan

DAVID C. LAGREW, JR., M.D.
Assistant Professor, Department of Obstetrics and
Gynecology, University of California, Irvine, College of
Medicine, Irvine, California; Medical Director, Women's
Hospital, Saddleback Memorial Medical Center, Laguna
Hills, California

MARK B. LANDON, M.D.
Associate Professor, Division of Maternal–Fetal Medi-
cine, Department of Obstetrics and Gynecology, The
Ohio State University College of Medicine, Columbus,
Ohio

WILLIAM C. MABIE, M.D.
Professor, Division of Maternal–Fetal Medicine,
Department of Obstetrics and Gynecology, University
of Tennessee, Memphis College of Medicine; Director
of Obstetric Intensive Care Unit, Department of
Obstetrics and Gynecology, Regional Medical Center,
Memphis, Tennessee

MARY ELLEN MORTENSEN, M.D., M.S.
Clinical Associate Professor of Pediatrics and Preventive
Medicine, Division of Clinical Pharmacology/Toxicol-
ogy, Department of Pediatrics, The Ohio State Univer-
sity College of Medicine; Medical Director, Ohio Health
Operations, Nationwide Insurance, Columbus, OH

JENNIFER R. NIEBYL, M.D.
Professor and Head, Department of Obstetrics and
Gynecology, University of Iowa College of Medicine,
Iowa City, Iowa

WILLIAM F. O'BRIEN, M.D.
Professor, Department of Obstetrics and Gynecology,
University of South Florida College of Medicine,
Tampa, Florida

ROY H. PETRIE, M.D., SC.D.
Professor and Chairman, Department of Obstetrics
and Gynecology, St. Louis University School of
Medicine, St. Louis, Missouri

ROSEMARY E. REISS, M.D.
Associate Professor, Division of Maternal–Fetal
Medicine Department of Obstetrics and Gynecology,
The Ohio State University College of Medicine,
Columbus, Ohio

ADAM A. ROSENBERG, M.D.
Associate Professor of Pediatrics, Department of
Pediatrics, University of Colorado School of Medicine;
Director of Nurseries, University Hospital, Denver,
Colorado

MICHAEL G. ROSS, M.D., M.P.H.
Professor, Department of Obstetrics and Gynecology
and Public Health, University of California , Los Ange-
les, UCLA School of Medicine and UCLA School of
Public Health, Los Angeles, California; Acting Chair,
Department of Obstetrics and Gynecology, Harbor–
UCLA Medical Center, Torrance, California

PHILIP SAMUELS, M.D.
Associate Professor, Division of Maternal–Fetal Medi-
cine, Department of Obstetrics and Gynecology, The
Ohio State University College of Medicine, Columbus,
Ohio

JOHN W. SEEDS, M.D.
Professor, Department of Obstetrics and Gynecology,
Medical College of Virginia, Virginia Commonwealth
University, Richmond, Virginia

LOWELL E. SEVER, M.D.

Affiliate Professor, Departments of Epidemiology and Public Health, University of Washington School of Medicine; Program Manager, Centers for Public Health Research and Evaluation, Battelle Seattle Research Center, Seattle, Washington

BAHA M. SIBAI, M.D.

Professor and Chief, Division of Maternal–Fetal Medicine, Department of Obstetrics and Gynecology, University of Tennessee, Memphis, College of Medicine, Memphis, Tennessee

JOE LEIGH SIMPSON, M.D.

Ernst W. Bertner Professor and Chairman and Professor of Molecular and Human Genetics, Department of Obstetrics and Gynecology, Baylor College of Medicine, Houston, Texas

PHILLIP G. STUBBLEFIELD, M.D.

Professor, Department of Obstetrics and Gynecology, Boston University School of Medicine; Chairman, Department of Obstetrics and Gynecology, Boston City Hospital and Boston University Medical Center, Boston, Massachusetts

MARLENE A. WALKER, RNC, N.P.

Nurse Practitioner, Department of Obstetrics and Gynecology, The Johns Hopkins Hospital, Baltimore, Maryland

MARGARET WALSH, M.D.

Associate Professor, Department of Obstetrics and Gynecology, Medical College of Virginia, Virginia Commonwealth University, Richmond, Virginia

THOMAS R. WIGTON, M.D.

Assistant Professor, Department of Obstetrics and Gynecology, Medical College of Wisconsin, Milwaukee, Wisconsin

Preface to the Third Edition

More than a decade has passed since the publication of the first edition of *Obstetrics: Normal and Problem Pregnancies*. In the Preface to the second edition five years ago, we emphasized that change can bring not only uncertainty but the opportunity to learn and grow. As we are all aware, the rate of change has continued to accelerate. Every field of medicine has been affected by advances in technology and the restructuring of practice patterns. It could be argued that obstetrics and gynecology has experienced the greatest rate of change, both in information and clinical care. Each day seems to bring new information in genetics and prenatal diagnosis and in our understanding of infectious diseases, to name just two subjects that the obstetrician must apply to his or her practice. Our role as primary health care providers for women expands our responsibility to master a broad knowledge base in many areas, including pharmacology and medical complications of pregnancy.

The third edition of *Obstetrics: Normal and Problem Pregnancies* has been prepared to provide the reader with an effective resource to meet these challenges. Color has been added to headings, tables, and other key areas to emphasize important concepts. At the conclusion of each chapter, the reader will find a list of the key points on each subject. To allow us to include new information on the exciting advances in obstetrics, we have carefully edited and revised each chapter and, in some cases, combined chapters. Playing a key role in this process were not only authors who have contributed to the success of the first two editions of our textbook, but more than ten new contributors. Their collective efforts have helped us bring cutting-edge information to our readers, and we dedicate this edition to all of them.

Throughout the preparation and publication of the third edition of *Obstetrics: Normal and Problem Pregnancies*, we have received the support of a dedicated staff at Churchill Livingstone, and at our own offices. We are indebted to the guidance of Ms. Jennifer Mitchell and her staff, including Ann Ruzycka, Jennifer Hardy, and Dorothy Birch. Once again, Mikki Senkarik has contributed original illustrations for the textbook. Her unique ability to translate text to illustration and image to art is evident throughout the book. Helping us each step of the way was the secretarial and editorial support provided by Sally Bourne, Tracy Fox, Nancy Schaapveld, Patty Morris, and Lan Baumann.

In closing, it is our hope that the third edition of *Obstetrics: Normal and Problem Pregnancies* will prove to be as valuable a resource as the earlier editions of our textbook, as together we face the ever more demanding and rewarding practice of obstetrics.

Steven G. Gabbe, M.D.
Jennifer R. Niebyl, M.D.
Joe Leigh Simpson, M.D.

Preface to the First Edition

This book is written for a new generation of obstetricians and gynecologists. Today's obstetrician must not only be able to plot and interpret a labor curve and deliver a breech presentation but also must assess fetal heart rate tracings and scalp pH data. While doing so, he or she must also consider the legal and ethical ramifications for these actions. In the past decade, the practice of obstetrics has been altered by a technologic explosion. Antepartum and intrapartum fetal monitoring, diagnostic ultrasound, and a host of advances in prenatal genetic diagnosis have enabled obstetricians to identify and understand some of the most important disease processes. This information has already led to significant improvements in maternal and perinatal outcome. Yet, the practice of obstetrics and the applications of this technology must be built on a firm base of knowledge in anatomy, embryology, physiology, pathology, genetics, and teratology.

Obstetrics: Normal and Problem Pregnancies has been written to meet these needs. The first sections of the book provide the essential foundation for the practice of obstetrics. The reader can then proceed to discussions of the problems encountered in clinical practice and finally progress to the chapters devoted to high-risk obstetrics. Where does the information necessary to be a specialist end and that needed to be a subspecialist begin? This boundary is difficult to define. It is hoped that *Obstetrics: Normal and Problem Pregnancies* will serve as a reference source for the general practice of obstetrics and provide the necessary base of information for those in fellowship programs in maternal–fetal medicine.

The contributors to this book represent the vanguard in their areas of expertise. Each chapter has been written to stand on its own and, in general, can be read in one evening. As editors, we are most indebted to our collaborators for their excellent contributions and their willingness to create a new book with a new approach.

Our book could not have been written without the help of many special people. Toni M. Tracy, Editor-in-Chief at Churchill Livingstone, and Linda Panzarella, Sponsoring Editor, successfully guided us through this enormous but rewarding project. Lynne Herndon got us off to a good start. Mikki Senkarik prepared all of the original artwork for the book and, in doing so, showed her unique artistic skills and understanding. Dr. Gerald Lazarus, Chairman of the Department of Dermatology, Dr. Marshall Mintz of the Department of Radiology, and Dr. James Wheeler of the Department of Pathology, all at the Hospital of the University of Pennsylvania, provided guidance in the selection of illustrations for the chapters on infectious diseases, placental development, and antepartum fetal evaluation. Also, all of us owe so much to the secretarial support provided by Michele Simons and C. Winston Wisehart.

This is the first edition of *Obstetrics: Normal and Problem Pregnancies*. Now a neonate, it has completed its months and years of gestation. Hopefully, it will help those embarking on careers in obstetrics to enjoy the specialty as much as we have. We look forward to hearing comments, both positive and negative, from our readers.

Steven G. Gabbe, M.D.
Jennifer R. Niebyl, M.D.
Joe Leigh Simpson, M.D.

Contents

Anatomy and Physiology

Anatomy of the Pelvis*

The Bony Pelvis

The pelvis is surrounded by a bony girdle consisting of the sacrum and coccyx posteriorly and of the two hip bones (os coxae or innominate bones) laterally. The two hip bones curve anteriorly and are connected at the symphysis pubis; however, they are separated posteriorly by the sacrum and coccyx (Fig. 1-1). The innominate bone is composed of three bones—the ilium, ischium, and pubis—that are separate in the immature skeleton but are fused by cartilage in the adult. When the pelvis is in the sitting position, most of the weight of the trunk is supported by the ischium (ischial tuberosities); when the pelvis is erect, the weight of the trunk is transmitted by the pelvis to the lower limbs.

The *ilium* forms the broad upper portion of the bony pelvis. It extends downward and forms the upper part of the hip articulation. The curved upper margin forms the iliac crest; anterior and posterior limits form two projections termed the *anterosuperior iliac spine* and *posterosuperior iliac spine*. Various muscular attachments are derived from the lateral surface of the ilium: external and internal obliques, transversus abdominis, quadratus lumborum, erector spinae, sartorius, rectus femoris, gluteus maximus, gluteus medius, and gluteus minimus. The medial surface of the ilium is divided into a superior and inferior portion by the arcuate line. The superior portion is termed the *iliac fossa* to which is attached the iliacus muscle. The inferior portion forms a more flattened surface continuous with the medial

portions of the ischium and pubis. It is this inferior portion of the ilium and fused portions of the ischium and pubis that form the "true" or *minor pelvis*. That portion of the ilium above the arcuate line is called the "false" or *major pelvis*.

The *ischium* consists of a body and ramus, each portion of which forms the posterior aspect of the obturator foramen. The *ischial tuberosity* is a prominent projection of the lower part of the body of the ischium. The *ischial spine* is a sharp projection of the posterior aspect of the body of the ischium. The ischial spine and ischial tuberosity are separated by the lesser sciatic notch or foramen. Superior to the level of the ischial spine, the ischium forms a portion of the greater sciatic notch or foramen. The muscles of the levator ani and the coccygeus muscle derive, either in whole or in part, attachment from the medial surface of the ischium. The lateral aspect of the ischium provides attachments for the hamstrings, abductors, quadratus femoris, obturator externus, and gracilis muscles. The ischium also provides attachments to two important ligaments, the sacrospinous and sacrotuberous ligaments (Figs. 1-1 and 1-2).

The *pubis* consists of a body, a superior ramus, and an inferior ramus. The body is flattened anteriorly. The most medial end of the body of the pubis is covered with hyaline cartilage and meets its counterpart medially by uniting with a fibrocartilaginous joint called the *pubis symphysis*. The inner surface of the pubic body forms the anterior wall of the pelvic cavity and provides the anterior attachment for the levator ani. The superior and inferior rami form much of the boundaries of the obturator foramen.

At birth the three bones of the os coxae are separated by hyaline cartilage; the iliac crest and ischial tuberosi-

---

*This chapter was prepared by the editors, substantially reflecting the contribution in the two previous editions by Dr. Stanley F. Gould. The illustrations were prepared by Dr. Gould for use in the first edition.

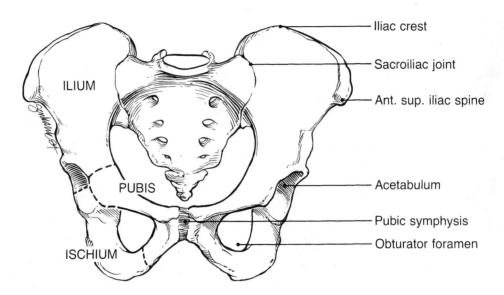

Fig. 1-1 Major components of the bony pelvis shown in a frontal superior view of the female pelvis. The plane of the pelvic brim faces forward and forms an angle of about 60 degrees to the horizontal. Features that most clearly distinguish the female from the male pelvis include a wider subpubic angle, wider sciatic notch, and greater distance from public symphysis and anterior edge of the acetabulum.

ties are cartilaginous. Growth occurs by addition of bone to the surfaces adjacent to the cartilage; the hip bone appears to grow interstitially. By age 7 to 9 years, the pubis and ischium fuse inferior to the obturator foramina. By contrast, superior fusion of the ilium, ischium, and pubis does not occur until puberty. Even after menarche, growth continues at the iliac crest, pubic symphysis, and ischial spines, ceasing only in young adult life. Not until age 25 years is the main mass of the hip bone finally fused with these cartilaginous portions of the iliac crest, pubic symphysis, and ischial tuberosity.

The opening of the true or minor pelvis is termed the *inlet* and is formed posteriorly by the upper anterior margin of the first sacral vertebra and and the anterior margin of the sacrum (promontory), laterally by the arcuate line of the ilium, and anteriorly by the pubic crest along the anterosuperior border of the body of the pubis. The pelvic cavity is surrounded by the ischium and pubis and by the ilium below the level of the arcuate line. The outlet of the true pelvis is bounded by the inferior margin of the symphysis pubis, the ischiopubic rami, the sacrotuberous ligaments, and the coccyx.

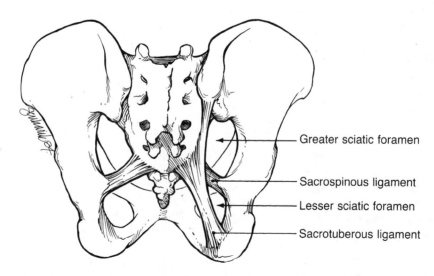

Fig. 1-2 Major ligaments and notches of the female pelvis, posterior view. During pregnancy, temporary changes take place in the ligaments that permit both movement of the joints and enlargement of the pelvic cavity. This becomes important during parturition.

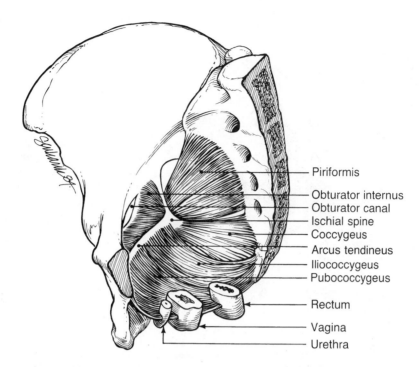

Fig. 1-3 Muscles of the pelvic diaphragm, oblique view. The pelvic diaphragm forms a muscular floor for the support of the pelvic organs. Note the location of the urethra, uterus, and rectum as they pierce the floor of the pelvic diaphragm.

In the standing, anatomic position, the plane of the pelvic inlet forms approximately a 60-degree angle with the horizontal. In the same position, the outlet forms an angle of approximately 10 degrees. In this position the anterosuperior iliac spines are in the same vertical plane as the pubic crests (Fig. 1-3).

Muscles and Fascia of the Pelvis

Because the pelvis is a curved basin, it is difficult to delineate the various walls clearly. There is no ambiguity, however, regarding those elements that form the floor of the pelvis. The posterior wall consists of the sacrum and the coccyx, with their associated muscles, the *piriformis* and *coccygeus*. The lateral walls are formed by the ischium and ilium, with the obturator internus forming the superior portion of the lateral wall and the levator ani forming the inferior limit of the lateral wall. The anterior surface is formed by the anterior aspect of the obturator internus muscle, by a portion of the pubic symphysis and pubes, and by the most anterior portion of the levator ani, which arises from the pubic bones. The floor of the pelvis is formed by the pelvic diaphragm of levator ani muscle.

Figure 3 shows the musculature of the pelvic wall as seen in sagittal section. The obturator internus arises from the pelvic surface of the obturator foramen and from the inner surface of the obturator membrane. The

obturator internus passes around the lesser sciatic notch and inserts in the greater trochanter. This muscle forms a major portion of the lateral wall of the pelvis and ischiorectal fossa but is actually classified as a muscle of the buttocks. It is covered by a heavy fascia (obturator fascia) that gives rise to the origin of the pelvic diaphragm, termed the *arcus tendineus* of the levator ani muscle. The other major muscle of the lateral pelvic wall is the *piriformis,* which arises primarily from the sacrum and through which course the sacral plexus and arteries to the buttocks. The piriformis is also a muscle of the buttocks, almost completely filling the greater sciatic foramen and inserting into the buttocks.

The *coccygeus,* also termed the *ischiococcygeus,* forms the most posterior portion of the pelvic diaphragm. It arises from the ischial spine, inserts onto the sacrum and coccyx, and lies immediately anterior to the sacrospinous ligament.

The pelvic viscera are largely supported by the levator ani, a tripartite muscle that forms most of the pelvic diaphragm (Figs. 1-4 and 1-5) and consists of the *iliococcygeus, pubococcygeus,* and *puborectalis muscles.* Not only does the levator ani form the major supporting structure for the pelvic viscera, but it provides the elasticity of the pelvic floor. It surrounds the urinary, vaginal, and rectal canals.

The *iliococcygeus* is the most broad and posterior portion of the levator ani, arising from the ischial spines and arcus tendineus. It inserts into the side and tip of

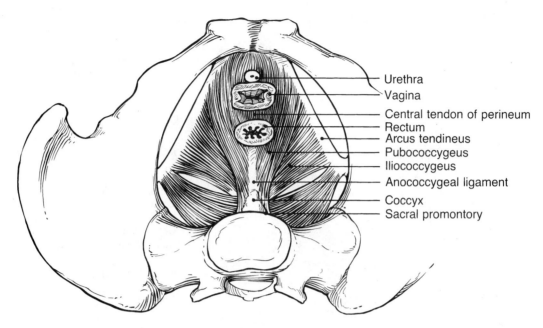

Fig. 1-4 Muscles of the pelvic diaphragm, superior view. As seen from above, the pelvic diaphragm consists of a number of different muscles and ligaments. The spaces between these muscles transmit a number of vessels and nerves as they leave the pelvis. Note the relationship of the central tendon of the perineum to the rectum and uterus.

the coccyx, while its more anterior fibers fuse in the midline with fibers from its counterpart on the opposite side. This fusion occurs between the anus and coccyx and is termed the *anococcygeal ligament*. The ilicococygeus is considered the most variable portion of the levator ani, highly developed in some women and largely fibrous in others.

The *pubococcygeus* forms the more anterior portion of the levator ani, arising from the posterior surface

of the pubis and arcus tendineus. Its medial fibers are directed posteriorly, while the more lateral aspects of the muscle course both posteriorly and medially. The dorsal vein of the clitoris is located between the muscles of the two sides. The more medial fibers of the pubococcygeus sweep around the vagina and the urethra to insert into the perineal body.

The third portion of the levator ani is formed by the *puborectalis muscle*. Although smaller in breadth than

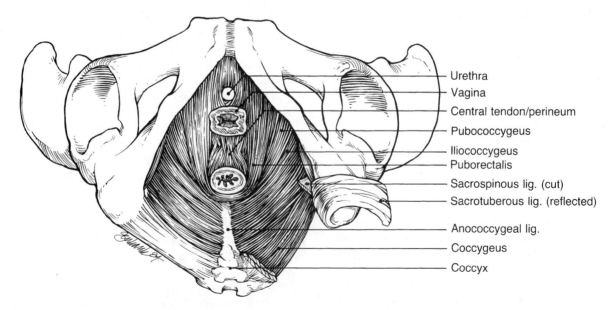

Fig. 1-5 Inferior view of muscles of the pelvic diaphragm. The pelvic diaphragm is bilaterally symmetric, with the perineal body (central tendon) and the anococcygeal ligament forming a strong median raphe. lig., ligament.

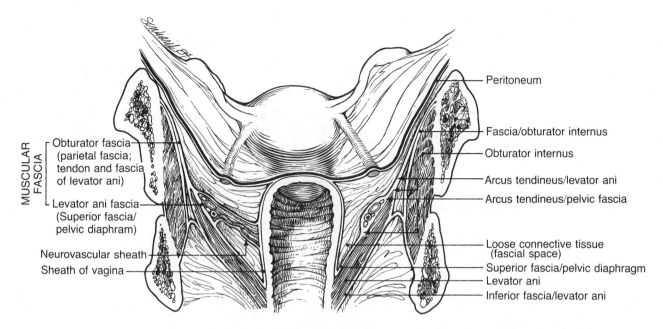

Fig. 1-6 Fascial and peritoneal relationships of the pelvic diaphragm. In this frontal view of the pelvis, the levator ani can be seen to slope downward and medially, surrounding the vagina. The loose connective tissue beneath the pelvic peritoneum is variable in thickness, depending on the general adiposity of the individual. Note also the continuity of the different fascias as they merge to form the neurovascular sheaths.

the pubococcygeus, this muscle is the most massive portion of the pelvic diaphragm. It arises in continuity with the most anterior portions of the pubococcygeus, but lies inferior to and is derived from the inferior surface of pubes. It courses posteriorly and fuses with fibers of the opposite side below the anococcygeal ligament to form a heavy muscular sling behind the rectum.

Each muscle within the pelvis is invested in a fascial sheath derived from the transversalis fascia of the more superior abdominal wall. This fascia is actually fused to the periosteum at the pelvic brim, but continues without interruption across the pelvis. Although division of this fascia is artificial, it is useful to think of the pelvic fascia in terms of a parietal fascia covering the muscles of the lateral walls, of a visceral (endopelvic) fascia covering the pelvic viscera, and of a fascia of the superior and inferior surfaces of the pelvic diaphragm (Fig. 1-6).

The *parietal* or *parietal-diaphragmatic fascia* is defined as that fascia lying over the piriformis and obturator internus muscles. The *obturator fascia* is the chief component of the parietal fascia, originating in the arcuate line of pubis and ilium. It is thick and consists of two parts: a thin outer layer, considered the fascia of the obturator internus, and a thick inner layer, considered the tendon of origin of the levator ani. This tendon of origin actually splits into three layers: an outer layer that follows the obturator internus into the ischiorectal fossa and an inner layer that splits into two layers that follow the surfaces of the levator ani, forming the supe-

rior and inferior fascias of the pelvic diaphragm. The *visceral* or *endopelvic fascias* are condensations of connective tissue around the pelvic organs, blending inferiorly with the fascia of the superior aspect of the pelvic diaphragm. It is this fascia that forms the "ligaments" of the pelvic viscera (uterosacral and cardinal), which are really perivascular condensations of subperitoneal tissue derived from the visceral pelvic fascia rather than true ligaments. Damage to these condensations of connective tissue and to their muscles of origin (levator ani) during parturition is of paramount concern in the development of pelvic relaxation and the development of cystocele, rectocele, and uterine procidentia.

The most anterior portion of the diaphragm is innervated by the pudendal nerve (S2 to S4). The levator ani forms the most significant supporting structure for the uterus. The pubococcygeus muscles provide support for the bladder; the puborectalis muscle is intricately involved in maintaining anal continence. Of considerable practical importance to obstetricians is that the levator ani is innervated by the third and fourth sacral nerves, with an overlapping distribution between these two roots.

The Perineum

From an anatomic viewpoint, the *perineum* is the area between the thighs that extends from coccyx to pubis—the inferior aspect of the pelvic outlet. Thus the lower or perineal surface of the levator ani forms the

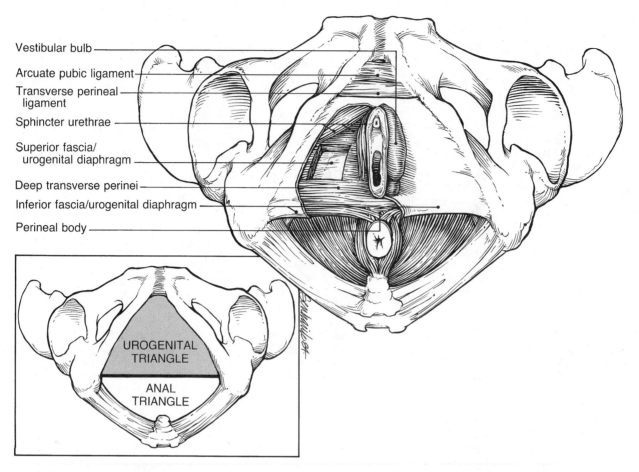

Vestibular bulb
Arcuate pubic ligament
Transverse perineal ligament
Sphincter urethrae
Superior fascia/ urogenital diaphragm
Deep transverse perinei
Inferior fascia/urogenital diaphragm
Perineal body

UROGENITAL TRIANGLE

ANAL TRIANGLE

Fig. 1-7 *Muscles of the deep perineal space, inferior view. As viewed with the patient in dorsal lithotomy position, the deep perineal space consists of smaller muscles than the superficial perineal space. Note that the vestibular bulb lies within the superficial perineal space. Inset: Division of the perineum into a urogenital (anterior) triangle and an anal (posterior) triangle.*

superior or upper boundary of the perineum, with the anal and urogenital canals piercing the levator ani and traversing the expanse of the perineum. Because the urogenital and anal canals traverse the perineum, the perineum may be divided into two distinct parts, each roughly triangular in shape and separated by a line drawn between and slightly anterior to the two ischial tuberosities: an anterior or *urogenital triangle* and a posterior or *anal triangle* (Fig. 1-7, inset). The urogenital triangle is further subdivided by the presence of a fibromuscular septum that extends across the anterior portion of the pelvic outlet below the levator ani, this septum being the urogenital diaphragm. Both triangles or regions share in common the levator ani as their superior boundary, and each triangle has a common sagittal midline attachment for its respective musculature. This common midline muscular attachment, which is roughly bisected by the interischial line described above, forms a fibromuscular mass called the central tendon of the perineum or perineal body. It is this fi-

bromuscular structure to which many obstetrician/gynecologists refer as the "perineum."

Regardless of its name, the central tendon of the perineum is interposed between the most anterior surface of the anal canal and the posterior surface of the vagina, anchoring the anterior surface of the anal canal and posterior surface of the vagina. Thus, expansion of the anal and vaginal canals occurs in a more lateral plane.

In both the urogenital and anal triangles, the most external or inferior boundaries of the perineum consist of the skin and superficial perineal fascia. This fascia is a continuation of the superficial fascia of the abdominal wall and follows the description of the fascia as seen superiorly: a superficial layer containing considerable adipose tissue known as the *fascia of Camper,* and a deeper, more fibrous layer, termed *Scarpa's fascia.* Unlike the well developed layers seen in the abdomen, however, the superficial perineal fascia is far less well delineated into these two distinct layers. The outer, more fatty portion of the superficial fascia in the perineum even lacks a specific name. This fatty portion of the superficial fascia is more highly developed around the vulva, giving form to the labia majora. It is continuous with the superficial fatty fascia of the thigh and blends posteriorly with the fat of the ischiorectal fossa. The more fibrous and deeper portion of the superficial perineal fascia, especially in the urogenital triangle, is also known as *Colles fascia.* Beneath Colles fascia there is another fascial layer, which is attached laterally to the ischiopubic rami and posteriorly to the posterior border of the urogenital diaphragm. This fascia is named the deep, inferior, or external perineal fascia and forms the true, most inferior boundary of the "spaces" of the perineum.

The anatomy of these fascial planes delineates the route and spread of cellulitis developing in an infected episiotomy. Initially, the skin and surrounding subcutaneous tissue, coalesced into the fascia of Camper in the labia, become infected. Deeper penetration of the infectious process to Colles fascia may be followed by spread to the vulva, medial thigh, and anterior abdominal wall into Scarpa's fascia. Necrosis of this layer results in so-called "necrotizing fasciitis." The muscles of the urogential diaphragm, along with its inferior fascia, may be involved in extensive cases. There may be spread to the levator ani fascia as well.

External Genialia

The *labia majora* are prominent folds of skin containing a well-developed fat pad derived from the fatty portion of the superficial fascia of the perineum. These fold are homologous to the scrotum of the male and surround a midline cleft containing the labia minora and vestibule. This cleft is termed the *pudendal cleft.* The labia majora are fused both anteriorly and posteriorly into anterior and posterior commissures.

The *labia minora* are smaller, thinner tissue folds that lie within the pudendal cleft and medial to the labia majora. These folds surround the vestibule of the vagina into which the vaginal and urethral orifices open. They are connected anteriorly and posteriorly as the anterior and posterior fourchette. The anterior fourchette is actually divided into two parts, a lateral portion where the labia minora fuse to form the prepuce of the clitoris just anterior to the glans clitoridis, and a medial portion that unites to form the frenulum of the clitoris.

The space between the labia minora is termed the *vaginal vestibule.* The vaginal orifice lies in the posterior portion of the vestibule. On either side of the vaginal orifice, slightly anterior to the commissure are the openings of the ducts of the greater vestibular glands (Bartholin's glands). The orifices of the paraurethral, or Skene's, glands are located on either side of the urethral meatus. Between the urethral and vaginal orifices, and within the vestibule, are the openings to the ducts of the lesser vestibular glands.

The homologue of the male penis, the *clitoris* lies just posterior to the pubic symphysis above the anterior commissure. It is composed of a *body* and *glans.* The body is formed by the union of the two corpora cavernosa, but, unlike the male, the corpus spongiosum surrounding the urethra is represented only by a slender thread of erectile tissue. The body of the clitoris is approximately 2.5 cm long and is covered by a small mass of erectile tissue called the *glans clitoridis* (clitoris). The homologue of the glans is the glans penis, which is provided with numerous sensory nerve endings. The prepuce and frenulum of the clitoris are derived from the labia minora.

Urogenital Triangle

The urogenital triangle is divided into a superficial space and a deep perineal space. Each space contains its own muscles, vessels, and nerves.

The superficial perineal space contains three sets or pairs of muscles: the *ischiocavernosae,* the *bulbocavernosae* (bulbospongiosae), and the *superficial transverse perinei* (Fig. 1-8). Included within this space are the greater vestibular glands (Bartholin's glands) and the vestibular bulbs. The superficial perineal space is bounded inferiorly by the deep perineal fascia. The superior boundary is the inferior fascia of the deep perineal space (Fig. 1-7).

The superficial transverse perinei muscles arise from the anterior portion of the ischial tuberosities and run transversely across the perineum, inserting in the central tendon. Many of the fibers of insertion merge imperceptibly with the external anal sphincter and the bulbocavernosus. Generally quite small and variably developed, the muscle can usually be seen during an episiotomy as distinct cross sections of muscle surrounded by a discrete circumferential fascia. It is important to recognize this muscle at the time of episiotomy repair, if the perineum is to be reopposed in the proper planes.

The ischiocavernosus muscles are associated with the crus of the clitoris; they arise from the medial surface of the ischial tuberosities, traverse the medial surface of the pubic rami, and insert into the pubic arch on each side of the crus of the clitoris.

The bulbocavernosus muscles arise posteriorly from the central tendon of the perineum. These muscles form the most medial boundaries of the superficial perineal spaces and are separated from each other by the vestibule of the vagina. They insert into the dorsum of the clitoris and into the inferior fascia of the urogenital diaphragm. Their origin shows continuity with the central tendon of the perineum.

The vestibular bulbs are the female homologue of the erectile components of the penile bulb in the male (Fig. 1-7). They lie on either side of the vestibule under cover of the bulbospongiosus muscles. They are com-

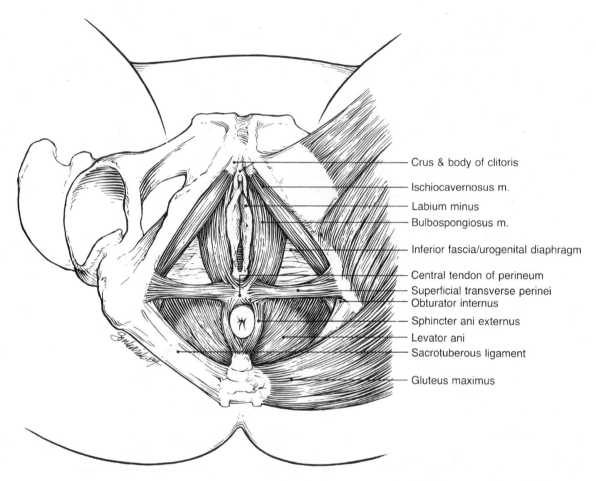

Fig. 1-8 Muscles of the superficial perineal space, from below. As viewed with the patient in dorsal lithotomy position, the muscles of the superficial perineal space of the urogenital triangle and the muscles of the anal triangle all converge in the midline. m., muscle.

Labels (top to bottom): Crus & body of clitoris; Ischiocavernosus m.; Labium minus; Bulbospongiosus m.; Inferior fascia/urogenital diaphragm; Central tendon of perineum; Superficial transverse perinei; Obturator internus; Sphincter ani externus; Levator ani; Sacrotuberous ligament; Gluteus maximus

pletely separated from each other by the vestibule and are far less vascular than their male counterpart. During sexual arousal, the vestibular bulbs become somewhat engorged. Immediately behind the vestibular bulb, although usually under cover by the bulbospongiosus, lies the greater vestibular gland. This gland is the homologue of the bulbourethral gland, which has a long, slender duct that opens into the vaginal vestibule.

The deep perineal space, also called the perineal membrane or triangular ligament, is a closed compartment that contains the urogenital diaphragm. Limited inferiorly by the inferior fascia of the urogenital diaphragm, it is bounded superiorly by the superior fascia to the ischiopubic rami. The muscles contained within this space include the deep perineal musculature, specifically the sphincter urethrae and deep transverse perineal muscles. This diaphragm is perforated by the urethra and the vagina (Fig. 1-7).

The sphincter urethrae arises from the rami of the ischium and pubis; it sends medially directed fibers toward the urethra. These fibers variably surround the distal urethra as well as the anterior portion of the vagina. The more posterior portion of the muscle sends transverse fibers across the deep perineal space, inserting into the sides of the vagina.

The deep transverse perinei are composed of transverse muscle fibers at the posterior border of the sphincter urethrae, inserting into the central tendon of the perineum. Unlike the situation in the male, the deep transverse perinei muscles play little or no role in maintaining urinary continence in the female.

Anal Triangle and the Ischiorectal Fossa

The anal triangle is traversed by the terminal portion of the anal canal and by the surrounding muscles forming the external anal sphincter. The *ischiorectal fossa* is the most significant space within this portion of the triangle; it lies laterally and posteriorly to the terminal portion of the anal canal.

Figure 1-9 depicts a frontal section through the ischiorectal fossa and the anal triangle. The ischiorectal

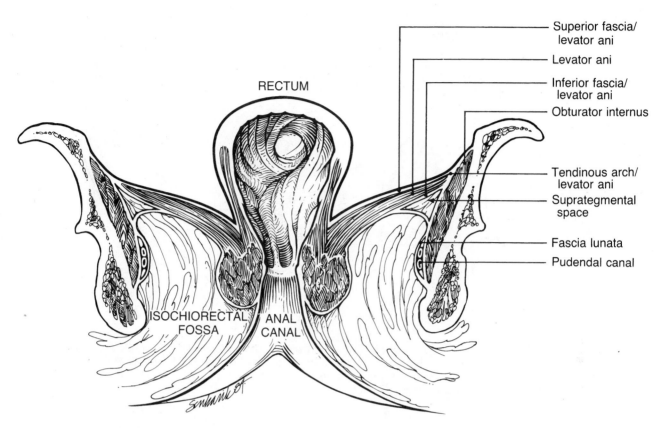

RECTUM

Superior fascia/
levator ani

Levator ani

Inferior fascia/
levator ani

Obturator internus

Tendinous arch/
levator ani

Suprategmental
space

Fascia lunata

Pudendal canal

ISCHIORECTAL
FOSSA

ANAL
CANAL

Fig. 1-9 Ischiorectal fossa, frontal section. The ischiorectal fossa surrounds the rectum and vagina and forms most of the potential space within the posterior triangle of the perineum. The fascia of the levator ani merges with the visceral sheath of the rectum and vagina to lend support.

fossa lies between the skin and levator ani and on each side of the anal canal. The fossa connects posteriorly with the fossa on the opposite side, thus making the two fossae continuous in the form of a horseshoe. Each fossa is bounded laterally by the obturator internus muscle and its fascia, while the medial walls are formed by the sloping inferior surface of the levator ani as it descends and surrounds the anal canal. Posterior to the anal canal, no medial wall exists, the levator ani forming the superior boundary of the ischiorectal fossa. The lateral walls and superior margin meet sharply at the origin of the levator ani from the obturator fascia.

The ischiorectal fossa is not confined to the anal triangle but extends both posteriorly beneath the lower edge of the gluteus maximus as far as the sacrotuberous ligament and anteriorly above the superior fascia of the urogenital diaphragm to the inferior surface of the levator ani (Fig. 1-10). The ischiorectal fossa is horseshoe-shaped, as the most anterior portions of the respective fossae are precluded from meeting in the midline structures of the urogenital system.

The ischiorectal fossa is fat-filled, for which reason it is termed a "potential" space. Connective tissue septa derived from the fascia lining the lateral walls of the fossa, as well as from Colles fascia, penetrate this fossal fat pad and provide support and shape to the adipose tissue. Presence of fat within the fossa permits distention of the anal canal during defecation and of the vaginal canal during the second stage of labor. This capacity for distention can also lead to significant accumulations of as much as 1 L of blood or pus. The ischiorectal fossa is therefore a prime location for concealed postpartum hemorrhage or infection. Ischiorectal fossa abscesses may push the levator ani superiorly and into contact with the wall of the lower portion of the rectum. These abscesses may cross to the other side of the pelvis, point, and drain through the anal canal or, more infrequently, rupture through the levator ani and produce severe intraperitoneal or retroperitoneal abdominal infection.

The fascia of the ischiorectal fossa consists of the tough fascia lining the obturator internus (obturator fascia) and of the inferior fascia of the levator ani. Along the lateral wall of the ischiorectal fossa, the fascia splits, forming the fascia lunata. In combination with the obturator fascia, this fascia forms a canal that carries the pudendal nerve and internal pudendal vessels. This canal is termed the *pudendal canal*, or *Alcock's canal* (Fig. 1-9).

The voluntary muscular sphincter, which accounts for fecal continence, is known as the external anal

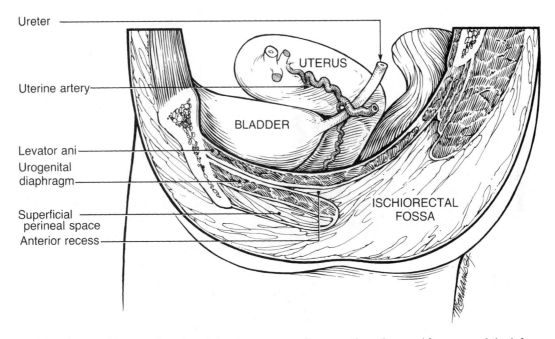

Ureter

UTERUS

Uterine artery

BLADDER

Levator ani

Urogenital diaphragm

ISCHIORECTAL FOSSA

Superficial perineal space

Anterior recess

Fig. 1-10 Ischiorectal fossa and urogenital diaphragm, sagittal section. The ischiorectal fossa extends both forward and backward from the anal triangle. The urogenital diaphragm subdivides the urogenital triangle, with the anterior recess of the ischiorectal fossa superior to it. The subcutaneous fat between the inferior aspect of the superficial perineal space and the skin varies among individuals.

sphincter, and is located within the anal triangle. This tripartite structure surrounds the anal canal and rectum from the inferior surface of the levator ani to the anal verge. Its total length is approximately 2 cm. The sphincter is composed of the joint effort of three muscles (Fig. 1-11): the subcutaneous, superficial, and deep components of the external anal sphincter. While there is no clear subdivision between these parts, their identification is possible in vivo. It is imperative that this anatomy be accurately restored should laceration or surgical incision occur at the time of parturition.

The superficial and deep portions of the external anal sphincter lie immediately deep to the perianal skin and run in a posterior to anterior direction to the anal triangle. These muscles originate in the coccyx and are often attached to the overlying skin. They run toward the perineal body and diverge around the sides of the anal canal and insert into the central tendon of the perineum. Surrounding the anal canal and running circumferentially around it is the third component of the external sphincter, the subcutaneous component.

Between the two bundles of the longitudinally directed superficial anal sphincter and posterior to the subcutaneous circumferential fibers is a triangular space termed *Minor's triangle*. This triangle is often the site of exit for anal fistulae. Through this subsphincteric potential space infection can gain entrance into the ischiorectal fossa.

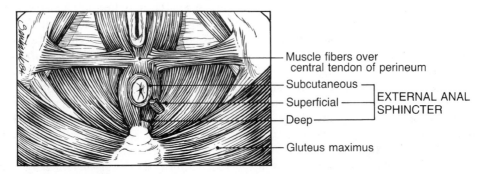

Muscle fibers over central tendon of perineum

Subcutaneous

Superficial

EXTERNAL ANAL SPHINCTER

Deep

Gluteus maximus

Fig. 1-11 External anal sphincter as viewed in dorsal lithotomy position. The external anal sphincter is composed of three muscles that arise from the coccyx and converge into the central tendon of the perineum. Midline or mediolateral episiotomy may damage this sphincter; proper reapproximation is essential for fecal continence.

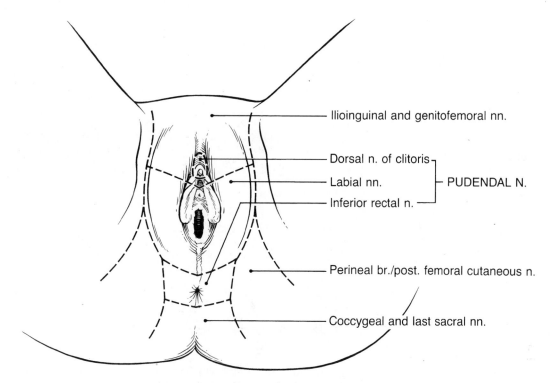

Fig. 1-12 Cutaneous nerve supply to the perineum. Most cutaneous innervation to the perineum comes from the pudendal nerve, but important regions are supplied by other sources. Pudendal block thus only anesthetizes a portion of the perineal surface. The exact limits of each specific nerve supply are variable. N, nerve; nn, nerves.

Nerve Supply to the Perineum

The cutaneous nerve supply to the perineum is derived from a number of different nerves. Local or regional anesthesia for surgical intervention demands a thorough understanding of the distribution of these nerves. The major nerves supplying the skin of the perineum are the *pudendal nerve* (S2 to S4), the coccygeal and last sacral nerve, *the perineal branch of the posterior femoral cutaneous nerve,* the ilioinguinal nerve (L1), and the genitofemoral nerve (L1,2) (Fig. 1-12). The area most laterally in the perineum is supplied by the posterior femoral cutaneous nerves, which innervate the perineal skin lateral to the anus and include the most posterior and lateral portions of the labia majora. The skin directly posterior to the anus, directly over the tip of the coccyx, is supplied by cutaneous twigs of the coccygeal and the fourth and fifth sacral nerves. The mons pubis and most anterior portions of the labia majora (except the clitoris) are innervated by the ilioinguinal and genitofemoral nerves derived from the lumbar plexus. These nerves descend from the anterior abdominal wall to supply this region of the perineum. The pudendal nerve is both motor and sensory to the perineum. The posterior two-thirds of the circumanal skin is innervated by the inferior rectal (hemorrhoidal or anal) branches of the pudendal nerve, while the anterior one-third of the perianal skin, most of the vulva, and most of the clitoris are supplied by the labial nerves and dorsal nerve of the clitoris. Given the overlap in the distribution among these nerves, one cannot rely on a singular nerve block to provide complete anesthesia. Consequently, pudendal block may not always yield the degree of anesthesia desired. Still, the pudendal nerve is the only large nerve in the anal portion of the perineum, traversing the area and giving off branches (inferior rectal nerves) as it courses toward the urogenital triangle (Fig. 1-13). These branches mainly innervate the external anal sphincter. The external anal sphincter may also be supplied by perineal branches of the fourth sacral nerve. The pudendal nerve leaves the pelvis below the piriformis muscle, courses through the buttocks where it crosses the ischial spine, and finally passes though the lesser sciatic foramen. After traversing the most posterior and lateral aspect of the perineum, it enters the pudendal canal and is joined by the internal pudendal vessels (Fig. 1-14). The nerve runs within the pudendal canal and quickly gives off the inferior rectal branches, which run medially and anteriorly toward the anal sphincter and perianal skin.

As the pudendal nerve continues beyond the origin of the inferior rectal nerves, it gives rise to the perineal nerve and dorsal nerve to the clitoris. These nerves continue within the pudendal canal in an anterior and medial direction. The perineal nerve then divides into

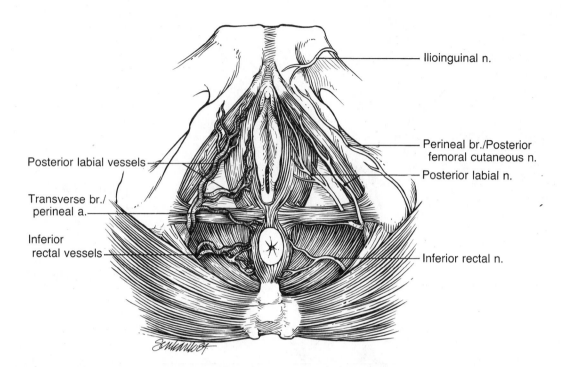

Fig. 1-13 Superficial perineal blood supply and nerves, as viewed with the patient in dorsal lithotomy position. The vessels and nerves to the superficial perineal space follow each other. The vasculature is markedly engorged during pregnancy, and there may be significant bleeding from these vessels because of laceration, trauma, or episiotomy. Note the transverse branch of the perineal artery, a vessel often encountered during routine midline or mediolateral episiotomy. br., branch; a., artery; n., nerve.

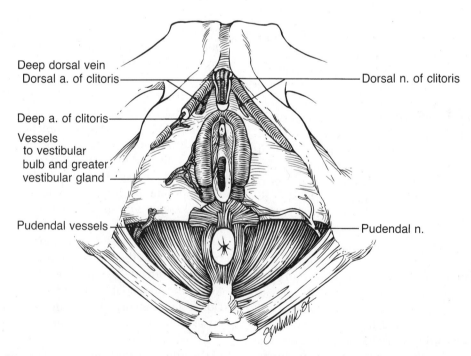

Fig. 1-14 Vessels and nerves of the deep perineal space. The vasculature and innervation to the deep perineal space enters the anterior triangle from superior to inferior, in contrast to the superficial perineal space vessels and nerves. Note that the blood supply and innervation to the vestibular bulb and greater vestibular gland (Bartholin's gland) are derived from the deep perineal vessels and nerves. a., artery; n, nerve.

superficial and deep branches just posterior to the posterior border of the urogenital diaphragm. At this point, branches course medially across the urogenital diaphragm and form the posterior labial branches, which supply the posterior, lateral, and anteroinferior portions of the vulva (Fig. 1-13). The superficial branches of the labial nerves supply the muscles of the superficial perineal space, while the deep branches innervate the musculature of the urogenital diaphragm.

The terminal portion of the pudendal nerve is the dorsal nerve to the clitoris (Fig. 1-14). At the anterior end of the pudendal canal, this nerve pierces the upper surface of the urogenital diaphragm, runs within the deep perineal space, and penetrates the inferior fascia of the urogenital diaphragm to provide innervation to the clitoris.

Vascular Supply to the Perineum

The major blood supply to the perineum is provided by the internal pudendal artery in a branching pattern like that of the pudendal nerve. The internal pudendal is the terminal branch of the internal iliac (hypogastric) artery and leaves the pelvis through the greater sciatic foramen between the piriformis and coccygeal muscles. It accompanies the pudendal nerve across the ischial spine, but lies lateral to the nerve and then enters the pudendal canal (Fig. 1-14). Almost immediately, the artery forms the inferior rectal arteries, which with corresponding nerves course through the ischiorectal fossa to supply the external anal sphincter and perianal skin (Fig. 1-13). After branching into the inferior rectal arteries, the internal pudendal artery gives off a transverse perineal branch that follows the superficial transverse perineal muscle. The artery continues anteriorly, following the pudendal nerve, and divides into posterior labial branches, which supply the muscles of the superficial and deep perineal spaces. The artery terminates as the dorsal artery to the clitoris, which enters the perineum through the ischiorectal fossa, penetrating the superior fascia of the urogenital diaphragm and supplying the anterior portion of the sphincter urethrae. The artery finally pierces the inferior fascia to vascularize the clitoris.

The veins of the perineum predictably follow the divisions of the artery and drain into the internal iliac vein. The only significant exception is the dorsal vein to the clitoris, which passes entirely into the pelvis, joining the vesicle plexus of veins. This anatomic consideration should be included in any evaluation of a spread of malignancy or infection involving the clitoris.

The Internal Genital Organs

The pelvic viscera include organs specific to the genital tract as well as organs that represent portions of the urinary and gastrointestinal systems. The organs of the female genital tract include the ovaries, fallopian tubes, uterus and cervix, and vagina. With the exception of the vagina, these organs are superior to the levator ani and are encased in whole or in part by the peritoneum, which is specialized to form specific quasimesenteric structures termed *ligaments*. The organs of the urinary system present within the pelvis include the bladder and lower parts of the ureters as well as a portion of the urethra. Organs representing the gastrointestinal tract include the lower end of the sigmoid colon, the rectum, and loops of small intestine (Fig. 1-15).

Ovaries

The ovaries are small, flattened, ovoid structures measuring about $4 \times 2 \times 1$ cm. Each ovary is described as having an upper and lower pole, an anterior and a posterior border, and a medial and a lateral surface. The anterior border is known as the *mesovarian border*.

The ovaries are located within the true pelvis, lying against the lateral pelvic wall just inferior to the bifurcation of the common iliac artery. They lie within the ovarian fossa, which is situated in the angle formed by the iliac vessels above, and by a ridge of peritoneum posteriorly, which is formed by the ureter as it passes the bifurcation of the common iliac artery (Fig. 1-15). The ovary lies posterior to a peritoneal reflection termed the broad ligament. The medial surface of the organ is covered in part by the fimbriated end of the fallopian tube.

Each ovary is suspended from the posterior layer of the broad ligament by a peritoneal reflection called the *mesovarium*. The vascular supply and innervation to the organ course through the mesovarium (Fig. 1-16). The surface of the ovary is covered by a modified peritoneum called the *germinal epithelium*, continuous with the mesovarium. A peritoneal "reflection" that attaches the upper pole of the ovary to the lateral pelvic wall is termed the *infundibulopelvic* or *suspensory "ligament"* of the ovary. The lower pole of the ovary is attached to the lateral wall of the uterus by the ovarian ligament proper.

The largest surface of the ovary, the lateral surface, is free and is often in contact with loops of small bowel within the pelvis. During pregnancy, the ovary not only enlarges but also leaves the pelvis as it follows the growing uterus into the upper abdomen. Immediately after parturition, the ovaries may be found at the level of the pelvic brim. They return to the true pelvis by the end of the puerperium.

Fallopian Tubes

The uterine, or fallopian, tubes represent the unfused portion of the paired paramesonephric (müllerian) ducts. The medial end of each tube joins with that portion of the paramesonephric duct that fuses to form the

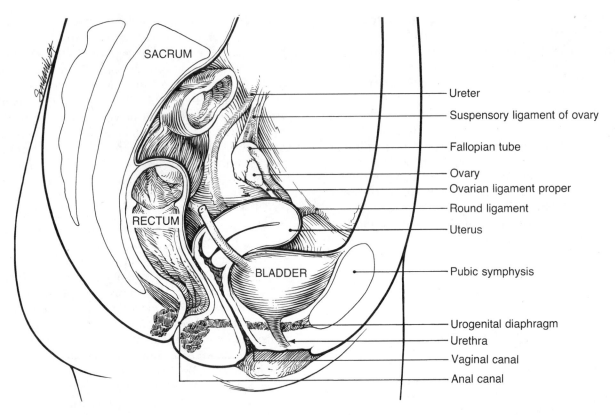

Fig. 1-15 Major organs of the pelvis, sagittal section. The internal organs of the pelvis are supported by the levator ani. Note how the anteverted, anteflexed uterus gains further support from both the urinary bladder and rectum. The ureter crosses the lateral aspect of the uterus at the level of the internal on its way to the bladder. The actual position of the ovary and fimbriated end of the tube is quite variable.

uterus, thereby opening into the endometrial cavity. Each fallopian tube is approximately 10 cm in length and is divided into four segments that can be distinguished on the basis of luminal diameter and histology. The area of the fallopian tube traversing the myome-

trium of the uterus and opening into the endometrial cavity is termed the *interstitial* or *intramural* portion. This section has a large muscular coat that merges imperceptibly with the adjacent and continuous myometrium. Moving laterally, the next region is termed the

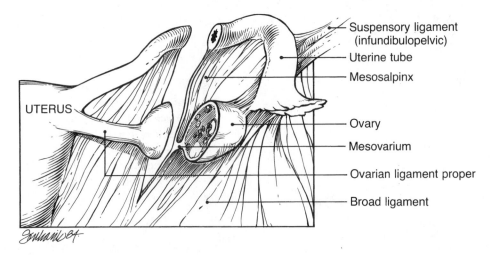

Fig. 1-16 Anatomy of the fallopian tube and ovary, posterior view. The ovary and tube are suspended by mesenteries derived as specialized portions of the broad ligament. The vasculature and nerves enter through the mesovarium and mesosalpinx.

isthmus. Here the lumen enlarges and the muscular coat thins. Lateral to the isthmus is the *ampulla,* which has the widest luminal diameter and in which fertilization occurs. The most lateral end of the fallopian tube is the fimbrial end, a flared or funnel-like opening into the pelvic portion of the peritoneal cavity. The clinical course of an ectopic pregnancy varies as a function of its specific location within the tube.

The fallopian tube is attached to the posterior aspect of the broad ligament by its own mesentery, called the *mesosalpinx* (Fig. 1-16). The mesosalpinx is reflected onto the hilus of the ovary as the mesovarium. The specific location of the tube within the pelvis will vary according to the phases of the menstrual cycle, as the fimbriated end of the tube is somewhat free to sweep the posterior aspect of the pelvis "in search" of the ovulated ovum.

Uterus

The uterus is the internal genital organ of nidation, formed by the fusion of the distal regions of both paramesonephric ducts. Actually only a continuation of the embryonic duct system, the uterus is highly modified by acquiring a substantial smooth muscle coat and by developing a highly differentiated and complex mucosa called the *endometrium.*

The uterus is a highly muscular, thick-walled, pear-shaped organ situated between the bladder and the rectum (Fig. 1-15). It is attached to the lateral pelvic side walls by a highly modified peritoneal mesentery, the broad ligaments, that both helps support the organ and serves as a supportive substrate for the vasculature and nervous innervation to the organ. The uterus is slightly flattened in its anteroposterior axis. It opens into the vagina inferiorly and is continuous with the fallopian tubes superiorly. The junction of the uterus with the vagina is termed the *cervix.*

The uterus is divided into a number of different anatomic regions that serve distinct functions during gestation and parturition (Fig. 1-17). The dome of the uterus is the fundus, which is superior to the ostia of the fallopian tubes. The greatest portion of the uterus is called the body or corpus. It is usually inclined somewhat anteriorly and forward. The junction between the cervix and the corpus is called the isthmus. This section is often referred to as the *internal os* because it is in this region that the histology abruptly changes between the simple columnar, mucus-secreting epithelium of the endocervix to the classic stratified mucosa of the endometrium. In the nonpregnant uterus, the isthmus appears to merge imperceptibly with the cervix. During pregnancy, however, specifically beginning around week 12, the isthmus enlarges and is added to the uterine corpus. During labor, this region thins and expands substantially and is termed the lower uterine segment. Scars produced by a low transverse cesarean delivery are no longer apparent following the puerperium, because the lower uterine segment again becomes part of the cervix.

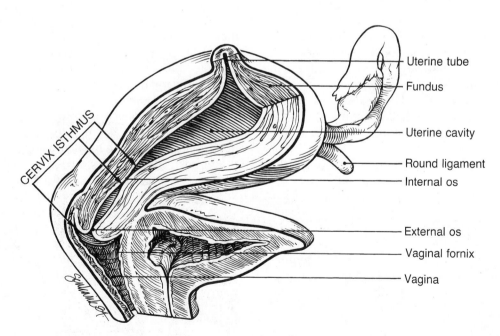

CERVIX ISTHMUS

- Uterine tube
- Fundus
- Uterine cavity
- Round ligament
- Internal os
- External os
- Vaginal fornix
- Vagina

Fig. 1-17 Anatomic regions of the uterus, lateral view. The uterus is composed of cervix, isthmus, corpus, and fundus. Because the regions of the uterus grow at different rates during pregnancy, the distance between cornual fallopian tube and fundus increases markedly with increasing gestation. Note that the peritoneal reflection of the bladder occurs at the level of the uterine isthmus.

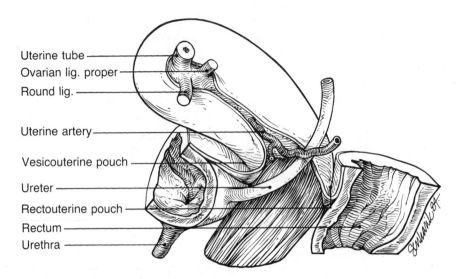

Uterine tube
Ovarian lig. proper
Round lig.

Uterine artery
Vesicouterine pouch
Ureter
Rectouterine pouch
Rectum
Urethra

Fig. 1-18 Anatomic relationships of the uterus, lateral view. The broad ligament contains the uterus and forms an anterior and posterior covering. The triangular space along the lateral uterine wall lies between the leaves of the broad ligament. Note the relationship of the ureter to the uterine artery. lig., ligament.

The uterus is covered by peritoneum on its anterior and posterior surfaces. The peritoneum on the posterior aspect of the uterus is carried past the cervix to the upper portion of the vagina, where it is reflected superiorly onto the anterior surface of the rectum. This reflection forms the rectouterine pouch, or *pouch of Douglas*. This pouch has also been termed the *posterior cul-de-sac* (Fig. 1-18). The peritoneum along the anterior surface of the uterus is reflected onto the bladder. This reflection forms the vesico-uterine pouch, or anterior cul-de-sac. The reflection begins at about the level of the uterine isthmus. The practical consequence of the above is that a surgical incision into the lower uterine segment during a cesarean delivery is actually retroperitoneal, lying inferior to the reflection of the anterior uterine peritoneum. The connective tissue adjacent to this peritoneal reflection becomes edematous during pregnancy, facilitating dissection at the time of surgery.

The *broad ligament,* the mesentery that suspends the uterus within the pelvis, is bilaminar and covers the uterus, tubes, and a portion of the ovary (Fig. 1-19). The mesosalpinx and mesovarium are only a portion of the broad ligament (Fig. 1-16). The portion of the broad ligament below the origin of the mesovarium is more accurately termed the mesometrium. The infundibulopelvic or suspensory ligament of the ovary is an extension of this broad ligament; the ovarian ligament proper lies within the anterior and posterior leaves of the broad ligament.

A highly specialized remnant of the gubernaculum of the fetal gonad, the *round ligament,* is also contained within the leaves of the broad ligament. This ligament attaches to the anterolateral aspect of the uterus, tra-

verses the broad ligament in its anteroinferior plane, and eventually enters the inguinal canal to insert into the labium majus. (Figs. 1-19 and 1-10). As the round ligament enters the inguinal canal, it may be accompanied by a peritoneal diverticulum termed the *processus vaginalis,* or *canal of Nuck.*

At the attachment of the broad ligament to the fundus of the uterus, the anterior and posterior layers are rather closely applied. As the broad ligament courses laterally and inferiorly, the anterior leaf expands forward and the posterior leaf diverges backward. Thus the broad ligament may be considered a quasipyramid with a broad attachment inferiorly. The base of this triangle resides near the pelvic floor (Fig. 1-19). Within this interligamentous space are found the uterine vasculature and ureters.

Perivascular connective tissue derived from the lateral pelvic walls lies between the leaves of the broad ligaments and swings medially to attach to the base of the uterus. This connective tissue is thickened at the base of the broad ligament and forms two ligaments known as the *uterosacral* and *cardinal* (or *lateral cervical*) *ligaments* (Fig. 1-20). The uterosacral ligaments are attached at their anterior ends to the lateral aspect of the cervix. They sweep posteriorly around the rectum and insert into the region of the second, third, and fourth foramina of the sacrum. As such, these ligaments form the rectouterine folds and thus limit the lateral aspect of the rectouterine pouch. The medial aspect of these ligaments is quite distinct, while the lateral aspect of the uterosacral ligaments merges with the cardinal ligaments.

The cardinal ligaments are situated at the base of the broad ligament and represent the condensed perivas-

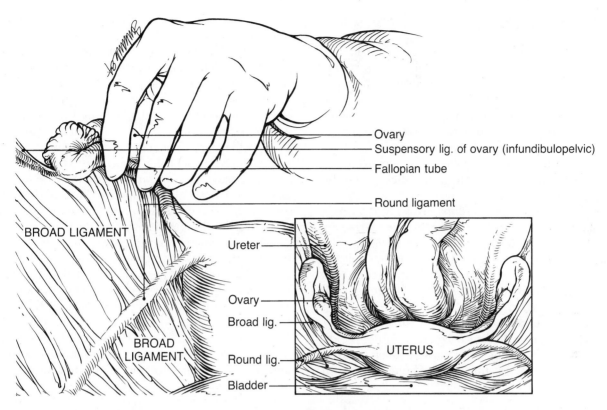

Fig. 1-19 Broad ligament and contained organs, frontal view. The round ligament runs within the anterior leaf of the broad ligament and inserts through the inguinal canal to the labium majus. *Inset:* The relationships as seen from an anterosuperior perspective. Note the rectovaginal pouch as seen from above and anteriorly. lig., ligament.

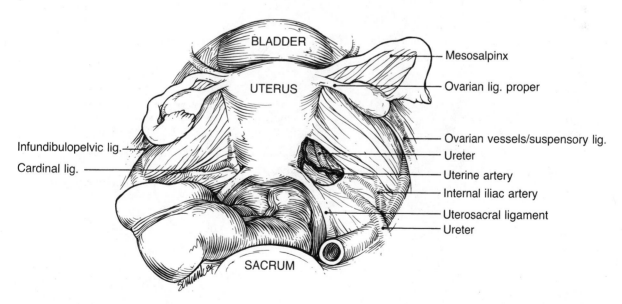

Fig. 1-20 Organs of the pelvis, posterior view. The rectouterine pouch is demarcated by the uterosacral ligaments. This pouch is often termed the *posterior cul-de-sac.* In this diagram a section of the posterior leaf of the broad ligament has been removed to show the relationship of the uterine artery to the ureter. Intraligamentous tumors, infection, endometriosis, or previous surgery can often alter this relationship. lig., ligament.

cular connective tissue anterior to the uterosacral ligaments. Thus this perivascular connective tissue is continuous with the connective tissue of the parametrium, no distinct differentiation between these two anatomic structures existing. Through continuity with the superior fascia of the levator ani, the vagina and uterus are thus attached to the pelvic diaphragm. Many other names have been given to these ligaments, including Mackenrodt's ligaments, the transverse cervical ligaments, the lateral pelvic ligaments, the cervicopelvic ligaments, the vascular or hypogastric sheath, and the parametrium.

Certain anatomic relationships involving the cardinal ligaments should be remembered. The uterine artery is located toward the upper border of the cardinal ligament running at a right angle to it. At the point at which the uterine artery makes an abrupt medial turn to course into the uterus (Fig. 1-21), the ureter may be found behind and beneath the artery. This relationship is of critical importance during surgical procedures that interrupt or violate the broad ligament in the region of the cardinal ligament. Care must be taken to avoid damaging the ureter at this point. Throughout much of its course within the pelvis, the ureter lies in direct relationship to the cardinal ligament.

Both the levator ani and the ligaments of the uterus have been given credit for providing the major support for the uterus within the pelvis. The uterosacral ligaments have been regarded as holding the cervix back toward the rectum, thereby keeping the uterus in an anteverted position. Their true role in providing support for the uterus is actually tenuous at best. Similarly, the cardinal ligaments have been vested with the function of uterine support, but because they are anatomically continuous with the superior fascia of the levator ani muscle, the major supportive role is more likely the pelvic diaphragm. The normal levator ani forms a relatively flat floor for the pelvis; the weight of the uterus is thus transmitted to the posterior aspect of the levator. If weakened by parturition or other trauma, the levator becomes more concave. Thus the weight of the uterus becomes directed more toward the genital hiatus than toward the posterior aspect of the pelvic diaphragm. The resultant shift in weight distribution would cause more and more funneling of the levator and result in uterine and/or vaginal descensus.

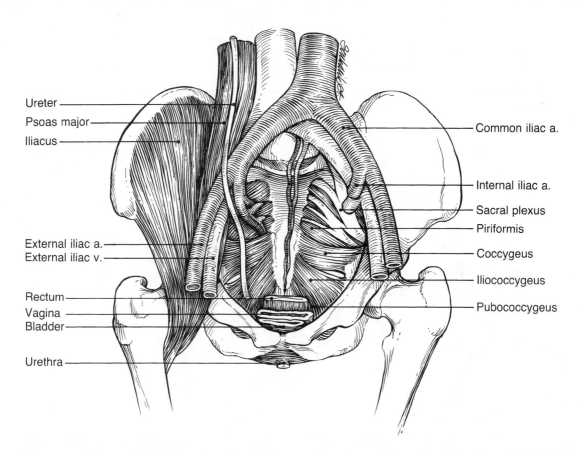

Ureter
Psoas major
Iliacus

Common iliac a.

Internal iliac a.
Sacral plexus
Piriformis

External iliac a.
External iliac v.

Coccygeus

Iliococcygeus

Rectum
Vagina
Bladder

Pubococcygeus

Urethra

Fig. 1-21 Major vessels of the pelvis, frontal view. The major vasculature of the pelvis is shown in relationship to the pelvic diaphragm. The proximity of the ureter to the internal iliac (hypogastric) artery is noteworthy. Ligation of the hypogastric artery may thus jeopardize the ureter unless care is taken. Note the anterior and posterior trunks of the internal iliac artery. a., artery; v., vein.

Vagina

The vagina extends from the vestibule of the perineum upward and backward to the cervix uteri. That region of the vagina immediately surrounding the cervix as it projects into the vagina is considered the vaginal vault, with the anterior and posterior divisions of this space and of the surrounding walls referred to as the *vaginal fornices*.

The vagina is a fibromuscular tube, the anterior wall of which is in close contact with the posterior surface of the bladder. The posterior vaginal wall adjoins the anterior wall of the rectum and the rectouterine pouch. The vagina is wider in its uppermost regions, with the lower end being the narrowest. In the empty condition, the anterior and posterior walls of the vagina are normally in contact with each other (Figs. 1-6 and 1-15).

The fascial sheath around the vagina merges with the fascia of the cardinal ligaments. Thus the support of the vagina is largely due to the superior fascia of the levator ani. A thin visceral fascia also surrounds the vagina. This sheath contains the vaginal plexus of veins. Between this visceral sheath and the visceral sheath of the bladder is a relatively loose and essentially bloodless cleavage plane. This plane permits dissection of the vaginal mucosa from the overlying bladder during anterior colporrhaphy. This is not the case around the urethra, where these sheaths are firmly fused together. Because the urethra is attached to the pubic arch, the vagina gains support from this attachment. Additional support for the vagina is derived from the urogenital diaphragm, through which the vagina traverses.

Vascular and Nervous Supply to the Pelvis and Pelvic Organs

Major Vessels of the Pelvis

The vascular supply of the pelvis and internal pelvic organs is derived from three sources: the *internal iliac, middle sacral,* and *superior rectal (hemorrhoidal) arteries* (Fig. 1-22).

The internal iliac artery, often called the hypogastric artery, is one of the terminal branches of the common iliac artery, arising approximately at the level of the lumbosacral articulation. The internal iliac artery is smaller than the external iliac and lies somewhat medial and posterior to it. The artery passes downward

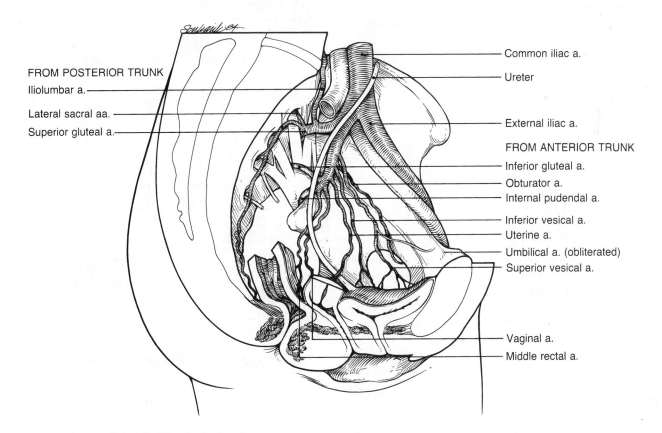

FROM POSTERIOR TRUNK
Iliolumbar a.
Lateral sacral aa.
Superior gluteal a.

Common iliac a.
Ureter
External iliac a.

FROM ANTERIOR TRUNK
Inferior gluteal a.
Obturator a.
Internal pudendal a.
Inferior vesical a.
Uterine a.
Umbilical a. (obliterated)
Superior vesical a.

Vaginal a.
Middle rectal a.

Fig. 1-22 Major vessels of the pelvis, lateral view. The major subdivisions of the anterior and posterior trunks are highly variable, and no singular branching pattern accounts for most patients. Note the relationship of the vessels to the sacral plexus. The uterus has been amputated at the level of the isthmus to permit a better view of the branching patterns of the anterior trunk. a., artery; aa., arteries.

into the pelvis, where it crosses the common (external) iliac vein. The common iliac vein lies lateral to the internal iliac artery. The ureter lies more superficially, either medial or slightly anterior to the artery.

At about the level of the piriformis muscle, the internal iliac artery divides variably into anterior and posterior divisions or trunks (Fig. 1-22). Somewhere between its derivation and the origin of the anterior and posterior trunks, the internal iliac artery gives off a branch to supply the pelvic portion of the ureter lying in relationship to the internal iliac artery.

The posterior trunk of the internal iliac artery gives rise to three major vessels: the *iliolumbar, lateral sacral,* and *superior gluteal arteries* (Fig. 1-22). The iliolumbar artery passes superiorly and laterally, deep into the obturator nerve and external iliac vessels, dividing into a lumbar and an iliac branch. The lumbar branch supplies the psoas major and quadratus lumborum muscles. The iliac branch runs across the iliacus muscle and supplies both the muscle and the ilium. The lateral sacral artery supplies contents of the vertebral column. This artery may form two or more branches, more commonly a superior and an inferior branch, which may be found along the ventral surface of the sacrum. The superior gluteal artery is derived most commonly from the posterior trunk. It leaves the pelvis through the greater sciatic foramen above the level of the piriformis, between the lumbosacral trunk and the first sacral nerve or between the first and second sacral nerves. This vessel is somatic in distribution, as are all of the branches of the posterior trunk, and supplies blood to the muscles of the buttocks. Anastomoses between the iliolumbar and superior gluteal vessels are not uncommon.

The anterior trunk of the internal iliac artery is the main visceral vasculature supply to the organs of the pelvis. The pattern of branching of the anterior trunk is highly variable. However, the major branches derived from the anterior trunk include the umbilical, vesical, middle rectal, uterine, vaginal, obturator, internal pudendal, and interior gluteal arteries (Fig. 1-22). The obturator, internal pudendal, and inferior gluteal vessels are somatic as well as genital in distribution.

The *internal pudendal artery* is considered by many to be the terminal branch of the anterior division of the internal iliac artery. Often sharing a common origin with the inferior gluteal artery, this branch passes downward along the ventral surface of the sacral plexus and exits the pelvis through the greater sciatic foramen. The internal pudendal is often smaller in caliber than the inferior gluteal artery and lies lateral to it. After leaving the pelvis, the inferior gluteal artery passes between the branches of the sacral plexus, supplying the gluteus maximus muscle, while the internal pudendal artery curves around the sacrospinous ligament (ischial spine), entering the ischiorectal fossa.

The *middle sacral artery* and *vein* (Fig. 1-21) are located in the midline of the pelvis. The artery is a direct branch of the aorta and passes down the front of the sacrum. It anastomoses with branches of the lateral sacral arteries. This vessel is important not only as a source of collateral supply to the pelvis, but also because it is easily damaged during such procedures as presacral neurectomy or sacrospinous vault fixation. The remainder of the vasculature will be discussed in relation to the organs supplied.

Blood Supply to the Ovary

The ovary receives a dual blood supply derived from two major vessels, the internal iliac artery and the aorta. The *ovarian artery* provides the superior blood supply and is a direct branch of the abdominal aorta. This artery descends to the pelvic brim and passes through the infundibulopelvic ligament (suspensory ligament), where it enters the mesovarium (Fig. 1-23). Here the artery anastomoses with the second major blood supply, the ovarian branch of the uterine artery. The ovarian artery becomes markedly enlarged during pregnancy and is thought by some to provide a major supply of blood to the fundus of the gravid uterus. It may also be of significant hemodynamic importance in the blood supply to the placenta. Surrounding each ovarian artery is a complex plexus of veins that drain into the vena cava on the right and into the renal vein on the left. This venous plexus likewise becomes significantly hypertrophied and engorged during pregnancy and is often the site of thrombus formation when intraperitoneal sepsis is present. Care must be exercised when performing a tubal ligation at the time of cesarean delivery because these veins are easily torn and can be the source of severe bleeding. Recall also that the infundibulopelvic ligament is extraperitoneal. Therefore, when large amounts of blood are lost into the infundibulopelvic ligament, hemodynamic compromise can result despite the absence of free intraperitoneal blood.

The *ovarian branch of the uterine artery* (Fig. 1-23) is the terminal branch of the uterine artery, and is the most superior and most lateral in position. It extends laterally in the broad ligament to reach the mesovarium, where it enters the ovarian hilus and anastomoses with the ovarian artery.

Blood Supply to the Fallopian Tube

The main blood supply to the fallopian tube is derived from the ovarian branch of the uterine artery (Fig. 1-23), called the *tubal branch*. This branch may also originate separately from the uterine artery and remain in the upper aspect of the broad ligament (mesosalpinx), where it will supply the tube. Alternatively, it may arise from a common point of origin with the ovarian branch

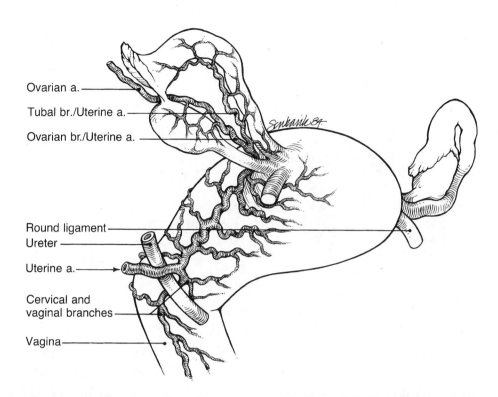

Ovarian a.

Tubal br./Uterine a.

Ovarian br./Uterine a.

Round ligament

Ureter

Uterine a.

Cervical and
vaginal branches

Vagina

Fig. 1-23 Blood supply to the uterus, tube, and ovary. The vasculature supply to the major pelvic organs is derived from the internal iliac (uterine) artery and the ovarian artery. Note the anastomotic plexuses of vessels along the lateral aspect of the uterus at the region of the cornu. Descending branches from the uterine artery supply the cervix and vagina. a., artery; br., branch.

of the uterine artery or from the most proximal end of the ovarian branch. Like the vasculature of the ovary, this artery and its vein become markedly engorged during pregnancy and must be carefully avoided when performing a tubal ligation.

Blood Supply to the Uterus

The uterus receives its blood supply from two major vessels: the uterine and ovarian arteries. In the nonpregnant state, the uterine artery is most important, but during pregnancy the vascular supply is derived from both the uterine and ovarian arteries.

The origin of the uterine artery off the internal iliac artery is quite variable, for which reason attempts at isolation and ligation during episodes of life-threatening postpartum hemorrhage are often fruitless if not dangerous. It often appears as an independent vessel from the internal iliac artery but has been described as arising from the inferior gluteal, internal pudendal, umbilical, and obturator arteries.

Once formed, the artery courses medially and anteriorly along the lateral pelvic wall (Fig. 1-23) in very close relationship to the ureter. As it reaches a position just lateral to the internal os of the cervix, the uterine artery makes an abrupt medial turn at the base of the cardinal ligament. At this point, the uterine artery is just in front

of and slightly above the ureter (Figs. 1-22 and 1-23). Here the uterine artery will give rise to small branches supplying the ureter.

Upon its approach to the cervix, the uterine artery bifurcates into ascending and descending trunks. The ascending branch is the largest, supplying the body and fundus of the uterus. The descending branch descends to supply cervical and often vaginal branches. The descending branch may on occasion provide branches to the urinary bladder. As the branches course within the substance of the uterus, the caliber of the vessels rapidly diminishes. For this reason incisions in the midline of the myometrium will produce less bleeding than will incisions that transversely incise the smooth muscle.

The uterine vein receives most of the venous effluent from the uterus and vagina and forms a complicated plexus above and below the uterine artery as it enters the uterus. These veins run laterally within the broad ligament to form one or two trunks that drain into the internal iliac vein. The connective tissue around these veins comprise a major portion of the cardinal ligament.

Blood Supply to the Vagina

The vagina is supplied by the *vaginal artery*, which is most often a branch of the internal iliac artery, either directly from a common trunk with the uterine artery

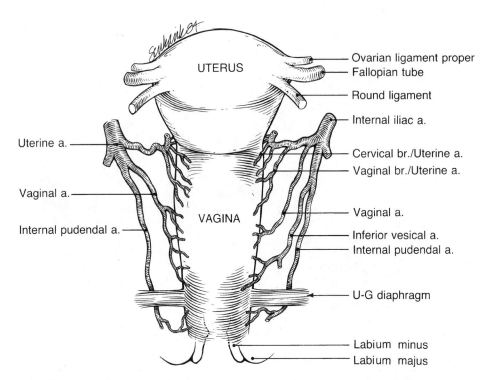

UTERUS

Ovarian ligament proper
Fallopian tube

Round ligament

Internal iliac a.

Cervical br./Uterine a.
Vaginal br./Uterine a.

Uterine a.

Vaginal a.

VAGINA

Vaginal a.

Internal pudendal a.

Inferior vesical a.
Internal pudendal a.

U-G diaphragm

Labium minus
Labium majus

Fig. 1-24 Blood supply to the vagina. Like the uterus, the vagina derives its blood supply from two major sources: the uterine and pudendal arteries. The internal pudendal artery supplies the vagina from inferior to superior. The vaginal artery, often a branch from the uterine artery, and the uterine artery itself supply the superior position of the vagina. a., artery; U-G, Urogenital; br., branch.

or directly from the uterine artery itself (Fig. 1-24). The vaginal artery may also arise from the internal pudendal artery. Irrespective, it supplies the upper portions of the vagina, whereas the lower portion of the vagina receives blood through branches from the internal pudendal and middle rectal arteries (Fig. 1-24).

The vessels cited above anastomose within the vaginal walls, and their anterior and posterior branches may join with each other on the anterior and posterior surfaces of the vagina. These vessels formed by the anastomoses on the anterior and posterior walls form unpaired arteries known as the *azygos* arteries of the vagina. The vaginal arteries also supply the fundus of the bladder and, according to some authorities, are the equivalent of the inferior vesical arteries of the male.

The veins of the vagina form a dense plexus within the walls and along the visceral sheath of the vagina. Blood drains into both the uterine and vesical venous plexuses. The venous drainage below the pelvic diaphragm drains chiefly into the pudendal veins.

Lymphatics of the Pelvis and Pelvic Organs

With a few notable exceptions, most lymphatic drainage from the pelvic viscera drains into the iliac plexus of nodes. The major node association is the internal iliac nodes from which lymph enters the periaortic or lumbar plexus of nodes (Fig. 1-25). The internal iliac nodes are subdivided into various groups, including the gluteal and obturator nodes, but their division is somewhat arbitrary. Lymphatic drainage directly into the superior rectal nodes or the inguinal nodes may occur as well.

Lymphatic drainage of the ovary and fallopian tube occurs directly into the lymph nodes about the aorta and vena cava, bypassing the iliac nodes. The lymphatic effluent from the uterus drains predominantly through either the periaortic nodes (fundus and upper body of the uterus) or laterally in the lower portion of the broad ligament to the internal and external iliac nodes along the lateral pelvic wall (lower part of the body). Some of the drainage from the fundus travels along the round ligament through the inguinal canals to end in the superficial inguinal nodes. The lymphatics of the cervix follow those of the vagina.

The lymphatic effluent of the vagina follows two directions. Approximately 75 percent of lymph drains upward and laterally, emptying into the internal iliac nodes or following the vaginal arteries to these nodes. The lowermost portion of the vagina drains downward to the vulva entering the superficial inguinal node chain.

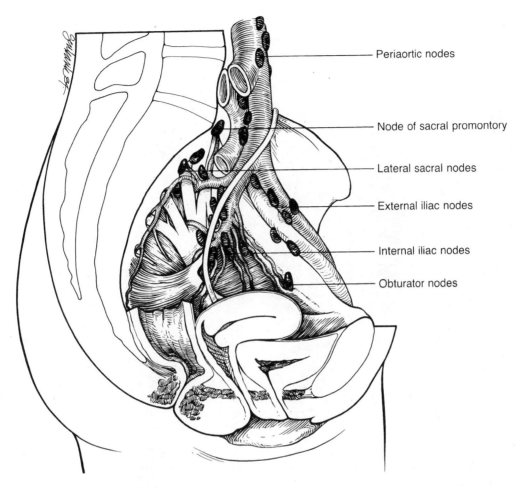

Periaortic nodes

Node of sacral promontory

Lateral sacral nodes

External iliac nodes

Internal iliac nodes

Obturator nodes

Fig. 1-25 Major lymphatics of the pelvis. The major lymph nodes of the pelvis follow the major vessels. Each group of nodes receives contributions from multiple organs. The groupings are somewhat arbitrary, for no distinct separation of individual node groups exists.

Collateral Circulation to the Pelvis

Worthy of comment is the highly developed architecture for collateral circulation within the pelvis. This collateral circulation is highly efficient, permitting almost instantaneous interruption of a major blood supply without producing significant ischemia.

The visceral branches of the internal iliac arteries anastomose with their counterparts on the opposite side, permitting collateral circulation between the two sides of the pelvis. Such significant collateral circulation exists between the somatic and visceral branches that bilateral hypogastric (internal iliac) artery ligation can be carried out without cessation of blood flow to pelvic organs. These parietal anastomotic bridges include connections between the gluteal arteries and the femoral circumflex arteries, anastomoses between the obturator artery and medial femoral circumflex artery, and anastomoses between iliac and lumbar branches of the iliolumbar artery and lumbar branches from the aorta. Anastomoses between the internal and external puden-

dal arteries are found in the perineum. Other important anastomoses include connections between the lateral and middle sacral arteries, between the middle and superior rectal (hemorrhoidal) vessels, and between vessels of the bladder and anterior abdominal wall.

Nerves of the Pelvis

The nerves and their plexuses within the pelvis are found along the lateral pelvic walls. From there they extend to the viscera through the special ligaments of the organs. Major plexuses include the sacral plexus and the pelvic portion of the autonomic plexus. The lumbar plexus is represented by the obturator nerve, which traverses the pelvis to reach the obturator canal. The major nerves of the pelvis are diagrammed in Figure 1-26.

The sacral plexus is formed on the anterior surface of the piriformis muscle lying between the muscle and the extraperitoneal pelvic connective tissue, which is often termed the *presacral fascia*. The uppermost contri-

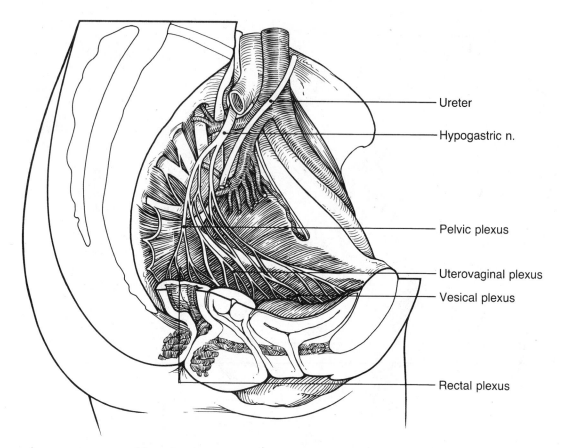

Fig. 1-26 Major nerves of the pelvis, lateral view. Few branches of the sacral plexus are evident as these nerves leave the pelvis even as the branches are forming. Most of the pelvic plexus lies medial to the vasculature. n., nerve.

bution to the sacral plexus is the lumbosacral trunk, which is composed of trunks from L4 and L5. The lumbosacral trunk is joined at the upper edge of the piriformis by the sacral portion of the plexus, which consists of the anterior rami of S1 to S3 and sometimes S4. The major branches of this plexus, which are almost impossible to identify in vivo without extensive dissection, include the superior gluteal nerve and the sciatic, inferior gluteal, posterior femoral cutaneous, and pudendal nerves. The pudendal nerve is considered the most caudal portion of the sacral plexus and represents S2, S3, and S4.

The sympathetic nervous system of the pelvis is derived from three major areas. These contributions include the sacral sympathetic trunks, the superior rectal (hemorrhoidal) plexus, and the hypogastric plexus. The sacral sympathetic trunks represent the continuation of the lumbar sympathetic trunks, which consist of a number of ganglia united by inferiorly and superiorly running fibers. These trunks lie medial to the sacral foramina but frequently communicate with each other across the front of the sacrum and coccyx. Although they may represent an additional afferent pathway that bypasses the superior hypogastric plexus, their functional significance is doubtful.

The superior rectal plexus is a continuation of the inferior mesenteric plexus and probably consists only of sympathetic fibers with connections to the hypogastric nerves. As with the sacral sympathetic plexus, it is not crucial to the pelvic viscera.

The superior hypogastric plexus or presacral nerve is the unpaired continuation of the lower end of the aortic plexus and is the major continuation of the sympathetic system. Located at about the level of the sacral promontory or slightly below, it divides into two plexuses or trunks that run along the lateral pelvic wall. These paired subdivisions have been termed the *hypogastric nerves.* Immediately lateral and to the right of the plexus is the right ureter, which traverses the lower aspect of the plexus. The ureter may be accidentally drawn into the operative field during a presacral neurectomy by medial displacement of the peritoneum covering the plexus.

The hypogastric nerves end in the pelvic plexus, an expanded network of fibers and ganglia on each side of the pelvic wall formed by the hypogastric nerves and pelvic splanchnic nerves. This pelvic plexus has also been termed the *inferior hypogastric plexus;* it contains sympathetic, parasympathetic, and afferent fibers from the definitive pelvic viscera. This plexus gives off the

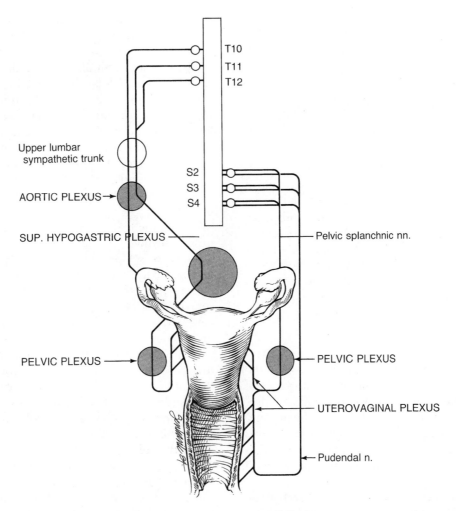

Fig. 1-27 Afferent innervation of the female genital tract. The left side of this diagram demonstrates the sympathetic nervous system. Fibers entering the spinal cord are illustrated on the right. The major afferent pain fibers for the uterus, tubes, and ovaries enter the cord at T10, T11, and T12. The afferent innervation of the vagina and external genitalia enter at S2, S3, and S4. sup., superior; n., nerve; nn., nerves.

rectal plexus and then continues forward to the recto-uterine fold, giving off the uterovaginal plexus, which courses medially and forward, joining the uterine vessels (Figs. 1-26 and 1-27). The plexus then continues forward and downward, passing along the posterior surface and then the base of the cardinal ligament until it reaches the bladder.

The innervation to the ovary is primarily derived from the abdomen, where branches of the renal plexus and upper part of the aortic plexus are found around the ovarian artery. Thus transection of the infundibulo-pelvic ligament interrupts the ovarian innervation while permitting the ovary to maintain a vascular supply through the ovarian branch of the uterine artery. Afferent fibers from the ovary enter the spinal cord at T10 (Fig. 1-27).

The nerves to the uterus and vagina form a dense plexus, termed the *uterovaginal plexus*. It is derived from

the pelvic plexus and consists of a mixture of sympathetic and afferent fibers. Parasympathetic fibers may also be represented. The plexus passes medially toward the cervix in the upper part of the cardinal ligament and meshes around the uterine vasculature within the cardinal ligament. This uterine plexus has often been referred to as *Frankenhauser's ganglion* (Fig. 1-27). At the level of the cervix, the plexus penetrates the walls and accompanies the vessels. A portion of the lower-most region of the plexus is directed toward the vagina and is designated the vaginal plexus.

The afferent supply from the uterine body and fundus travel with the hypogastric nerves and enter the spinal cord at T11 and T12. Pain fibers from the cervix run through the sacral nerves.

While the upper end of the vagina is supplied by simple extension of the uterovaginal plexus, the lower end of the vagina is innervated by the pudendal nerve.

The exact line of demarcation between these two distributions is poorly defined, but that region of the vagina closer to the perineum sends afferent fibers to S2, S3, and S4.

Anatomic Adaptations During Aging and Pregnancy

The female genital tract undergoes considerable change during pregnancy and the puerperium. These changes indicate that these organs are highly plastic in their anatomic structure and can adapt to both chronic and acute stimuli with remarkable ease. Anatomic changes that occur during aging and pregnancy underscore the fact that these are target organs for the sex steroids and that much of their adaption can be directly attributed to the changing hormonal milieu associated with puberty, pregnancy, and menopause.

Uterus

The uterus is a target organ for estrogen and progesterone; both steroid hormones play a decisive role in the remodeling that occurs during the different phases of a woman's life. Because the uterus is composed predominantly of smooth muscle and because the myometrial cell contains both estrogen and progesterone receptors, it is not surprising that the anatomy as well as the physiology of the uterus will change depending on a woman's hormonal status.

At birth, the uterus is composed of a relatively large cervix in comparison with the corpus and fundus. With puberty, the rising levels of estradiol initiate considerable growth and enlargement in the myometrial smooth muscle cells of the corpus and fundus. Although growth of the cervix occurs as well, it is outstripped by the more pronounced growth of the corpus and fundus, with the result being a markedly lower cervix to corpus ratio. Before puberty, the cervix occupies approximately 66 percent of the total uterine mass; after puberty, the cervix and corpus-fundus are approximately equal in size. The differential response in two seemingly identical smooth muscle cell populations is not unexpected, because the estrogen receptor of the cervix does not appear to be modulated with the same degree of sensitivity as are the steroid receptors of the corporeal and fundal myometrium. Should the woman become pregnant and subsequently parous, the enlarged corpus-fundus accounts for two-thirds of the uterine size, and the cervix is thus reduced to approximately one-third the total uterine mass (Fig. 1-28).

The nonpregnant parous uterus weighs approximately 70 g. During pregnancy, both hypertrophy and hyperplasia of the myometrial smooth muscle occur. This is due not only to the action of the steroid hormones but also to the marked distention of the uterus with the developing fetus. The body of the uterus at term weighs approximately 1,100 g, an almost 20-fold increase in mass. Similarly, the individual myometrial cell, through cellular hypertrophy, enlarges almost 100-fold to approximately 500 μm in length at term. Not only does the myometrium per se increase in cellular density and size during pregnancy, but there is a concomitant increase in the collagenous connective tissue and intercellular ground substance. Blood vessels, lymphatics, and nerves increase in number, length, and size; these changes occur as early as the first trimester.

During the first few months of pregnancy, the thickness of the myometrium in the corpus and fundus actually increases. However, the increased distention of the uterine cavity, because of the growing fetus, placenta, and amniotic fluid, causes the uterine wall to become remarkably thin by term. This thinning should not be confused with the softening that occurs because of the increasing levels of progesterone.

While the changes in the uterine cervix are not as dramatic as those of the uterine corpus and fundus, they are nevertheless highly significant. The cervix is composed primarily of collagenous connective tissue, with a relatively small amount of smooth muscle. Significant biochemical changes occur in the connective tissue that result in increased water content (see Ch. 5). Combined with a significant increase in vascularity, softening and cyanosis characterizing the cervix of the gravid woman results. The endocervical glands, under the influence of progesterone, secrete a thickened mucus that forms a cervical plug. Other changes in endocervical glandular histology include a relative basal cell hyperplasia caused by the increased levels of circulating estrogen. This is an interesting observation, considering that, unlike the myometrium, whose estrogen and progesterone receptors modulate with fluctuating levels of estradiol and progesterone, the steroid receptors of the cervix do not appear to change substantially in either quantity or distribution.

The changes in the anatomic regions of the uterus bear repetition here. During the antenatal period, a rather striking change occurs in the uterine wall, which becomes more pronounced during labor. The uterine isthmus is normally a small, almost nonexistent region of the uterus that lies between the cervix and the corpus. Under the influence of the steroid hormones of pregnancy and the distention of the growing products of conception, this isthmic region becomes demarcated from the cervix inferiorly and from the corpus superiorly (Fig. 1-29). As pregnancy progresses, the isthmus becomes increasingly prominent, with a thinner and thinner wall. This development of the isthmus culmi-

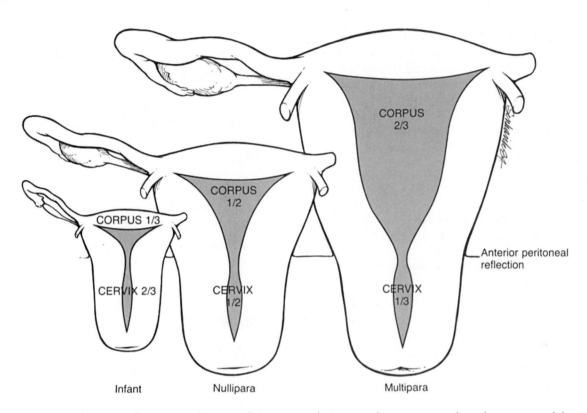

Fig. 1-28 Changes in the uterus with age and parity. At puberty, growth occurs primarily in the corpus and the fundus, although the cervix continues to grow as well. After menopause, the uterus regresses to a state more closely allied to that of the premenarcheal anatomy. During pregnancy the cervical portion is relatively greater than in the nonpregnant state.

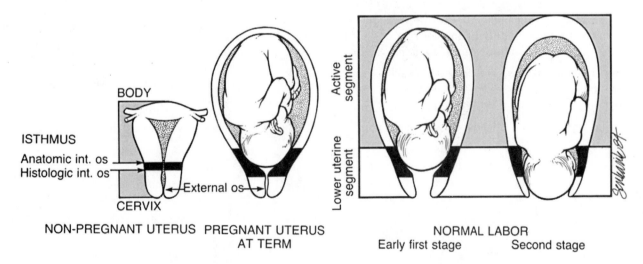

Fig. 1-29 Changes in the uterus caused by pregnancy and parturition. The hormonal changes of pregnancy as well as dynamic forces of labor cause the development of the lower uterine segment from the vestigial uterine isthmus. After parturition, these changes regress dramatically. Low transverse cesarean delivery inclusions are performed through this thinned isthmic region, known as the *lower uterine segment.*

nates during labor and is known as the lower uterine segment. This segment is very thin and contains little smooth muscle. As such, its contractility is markedly different from that of the corpus or fundus. Immediately after delivery, this stretched and thinned isthmus appears as a floppy region of myometrium immediately superior to the internal cervical os. By the end of the puerperium, the isthmus has become reincorporated into the cervical–corpus junction and is no longer visible.

10 Key Points

- To facilitate childbearing, the female pelvis—as opposed to the male pelvis—is characterized by a wider subpubic angle, increased width of the sciatic notch, and greater distance from the symphysis pubis to the anterior edge of the acetabulum.

- The levator ani, the major supporting structure for the pelvic viscera, is a tripartite muscle mass composed of the iliococcygeus, puboccygeus, and puborectalis; the iliococcygeus is the broadest and most posterior portion.

- Innervation of the levator ani is through the third and fourth sacral nerves.

- The major nerve supply of the perineum is derived from the pudendal. However, the ilioinguinal, genitofemoral, perineal branch of the posterior femoral cutaneous, coccygeal, and last sacral nerve also contribute; thus, a pudendal nerve block anesthetizes only a portion of the perineum.

- The internal iliac (hypogastric) artery arises at the level of lumbosacral articulation. It can be distinguished from the external iliac by its smaller size and by its more medial and more posterior position.

- The ureter lies more superficially and is either medial or slightly anterior to the internal iliac artery.

- The cardinal ligaments are located at the base of the broad ligament, are continuous with the connective tissue of the parametrium, and are attached to the pelvic diaphragm through continuity with the superficial superior fascia of the levator ani.

- Since the origin of the uterine artery is quite variable, its isolation and ligation for control of postpartum bleeding are often fruitless. The uterine artery usually arises as an independent vessel from the internal iliac artery, but it may also arise from the inferior gluteal, internal pudendal, umbilical, or obturator arteries.

- Afferent pain fibers for the uterus, tubes, and ovary enter the cord at T10, T11, T12; thus, spinal or epidural anesthesia must extend to these levels. Fortunately, efferent fibers to the uterus enter above these levels, thus not interfering with contractions.

- The body of the nonpregnant uterus weighs approximately 70 g, whereas at term it weighs approximately 1,100 g.

Suggested Readings

Embryology

Sadler TW: Langman's Medical Embryology. 6th Ed. Williams & Wilkins, Baltimore, 1990

Gross Anatomy

Agur, AMR: Grant's Atlas of Anatomy. 9th Ed. Williams & Wilkins, Baltimore, 1991

Gardner, ED: Gardner-Gray-O'Rahilly Anatomy: A Regional Study of Human Structure. 5th Ed. WB Saunders, Philadelphia, 1986

Hamilton WJ: Textbook of Human Anatomy. CV Mosby, St. Louis, 1976

Hollinshead WH: Anatomy for Surgeons. 3rd Ed. Vol. 3. Harper & Row, New York, 1982

Moore K: Clinically Oriented Anatomy. 3rd Ed. Williams & Wilkins, Baltmore, 1992

Snell RS: Clinical Anatomy for Medical Students. 5th Ed. Little, Brown, Boston, 1995

Williams PL, Bannister LL, Berry M et al: Gray's Anatomy. 38th Ed. Churchill Livingstone, Edinburgh, 1995

Chapter 2

Endocrinology and Diagnosis of Pregnancy

John E. Buster and Sandra A. Carson

The evolutionary advent of viviparity necessitated changes in the maternal metabolic, hormonal, and immunologic systems. To compensate for the increased and altered demands of an intracorporial pregnancy, a new organ—the placenta—and a series of proteins specific for and secreted only during pregnancy evolved. These proteins, aided by alterations in the already stimulated steroids, allow invasion of a half-foreign tissue into the maternal system that not only tolerates but actively nourishes and protects the growing fetus. The changes in the hormonal milieu also help to diagnose and monitor pregnancy, and they are the focus of this chapter.

Pregnancy Proteins

Ontogeny of Pregnancy Protein Production

From the moment of conception, proteins are released into the maternal system by the newly formed conceptus, presumably to alter the maternal immune metabolic, and hormonal responses to the advancing gestation. The production and secretion of these proteins mirror the demands that each developmental stage of gestation brings.

The Preimplantation Conceptus

Pregnancy proteins are present in the maternal circulation almost at the time of conception. Presumably released from the fertilized ovum after sperm penetration, a platelet activating factor (PAF)-like substance is evident almost immediately.[1–4] The conceptus remains in the tubal ampulla for approximately 80 hours after follicular rupture, travels through the isthmus for ap-

proximately 10 hours, and then enters the uterus as a 2- to 8-cell embryo.[5,6] The embryo develops into a blastocyst while freely floating in the endometrial cavity in the interval 90 to 150 hours after conception.[6] Although human chorionic gonadotropin (hCG) mRNA is detectable in the blastomeres of 6- to 8-cell embryos at 2 days, the hormone is not detectable until 6 days (blastocyst) in culture media.[7–9] Secretion into the maternal serum is limited by the absence of vascular communication.[10] Only after implantation is completed is hCG detectable in maternal serum 8 to 11 days after conception.[11–13]

The Implanted Conceptus

Blastomeres destined to form the placenta can be identified as trophectoderm lining the periphery of the blastocyst 5 days postconception (Fig. 2-1). By the tenth day, invading trophoblasts have formed 2 distinct layers: an inner layer composed of individual, well defined, and rapidly proliferating cells, the *cytotrophoblasts,* and an outer and thicker layer comprising continuous mass of cell plasma containing multiple nuclei with indistinct cell borders, the *syncytiotrophoblast* (Figs. 2-2 and 2-3). The syncytiotrophoblasts line the fetal side of the intervillous space opposite the decidualized endometrium on the maternal side (Fig. 2-3).

Cytotrophoblasts stain immunohistochemically for hypothalamic-like peptides: corticotropin releasing hormone (CRH), gonadotropin releasing hormone (GnRH), and thyrotropin releasing hormone (TRH).[14–26] The juxtaposed cytotrophoblasts stain immunohistochemically for corresponding pituitary-like peptides: adrenocorticotropic hormone (ACTH), hCG (analogous to pituitary luteinizing hormone or LH), and chorionic thyrotropin (hCT). This anatomic ar-

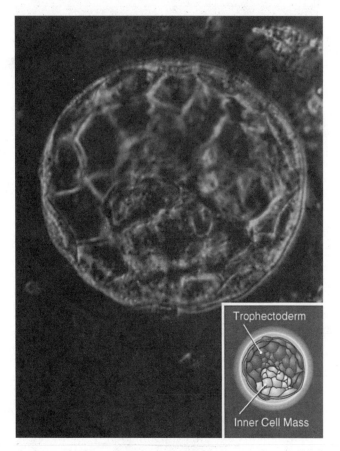

Fig. 2-1 The human preimplantation blastocyst. The inner cell mass, the cells destined to form embryonic structures, are seen between 3 and 6 o'clock. Trophectoderm, comprising the remainder, evolves into placenta and membranes.

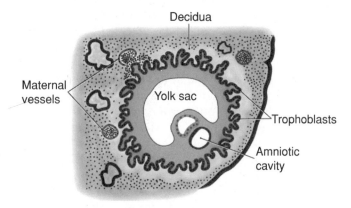

Fig. 2-2 Postimplantation embryo and placental structures. Trophoblasts are seen to invade maternal decidua, which contains blood-filled lacunar spaces. The embryo has evolved as a simple embryonic disc in association with a very large yolk sac and developing amniotic cavity.

rangement suggests that these two layers mirror the paracrine relationship of the hypothalamic-pituitary axis[14–26] (Table 2-1).

Syncytiotrophoblasts are the principal site of placental steroid and protein hormone biosynthesis. The cells have a large surface area and line the intervillous space, which exposes them directly to the maternal blood stream without the blood vessel endothelium and basement membrane which separates them from the fetal circulation. Thus, both cell types are ideal both for hormone secretion and nutrient exchange.[27] This anatomic arrangement also explains why placental proteins are secreted almost exclusively into the maternal circulation in concentrations much higher than those in the fetus.[27]

The syncytiotrophoblast cell layer contains abundant rough endoplasmic reticulum, golgi complexes, and mitochondria, the subcellular machinery that characterize hormone synthesis (Fig. 2-3). Prohormones are assembled from amino acids of maternal origin within the rough endoplasmic reticulum of the syncytiotrophoblast. Assembled into early secretory granules in the golgi complex, these prohormones are transferred across trophoblastic cell membranes as mature granules. The mature granules then become soluble as circulating hormones in maternal blood passing through the intervillous space[27] (Fig. 2-3).

Decidualized endometrium is a site of maternal steroid and protein biosynthesis that is related directly to the maintenance and protection of the pregnancy from immunologic rejection.

The Mature Placenta

Throughout the second and third trimester, the placenta adapts its structure to reflect its function. As fetomaternal exchange overwhelms hormone secretory functions, the relative numbers of trophoblasts decrease.[19] The villi near term (Figs. 2-3 and 2-4) consist largely of fetal capillaries with little or no stroma beyond that required for anatomic integrity. Cytotrophoblasts are sparse, and the remaining syncytium is thin, scarcely visible by light microscopy. In contrast to the early villus, in which the trophoblasts are present in abundance with a continuous basal cytotrophoblast layer and an overlying surface syncytium, the placenta's membranous interface between fetal and maternal circulation is extremely thin.[27] This villous structure facilitates specialized transport of compounds across the fetomaternal interface.[27]

Physiology of Pregnancy Proteins

The sequential appearance is characteristic for each protein, reflecting their various functions unique to pregnancy (Table 2-1).

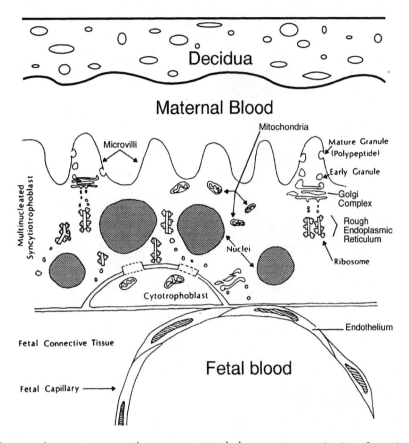

Fig. 2-3 The human placenta at term with a cross-sectional electron microscopic view. Syncytiotrophoblasts line the fetal surface of the intervillous space and interact directly with the maternal blood supply to secrete placental proteins directly into the circulation. Decidua lines the maternal surface of the intervillous space and secretes its own protein hormones into the maternal circulation.

Early Pregnancy Factor

Molecular Structure Early pregnancy factor (EPF) activity has been isolated from human pregnancy serum, placental extracts, and platelets.[28] EPF is an ill-defined immunosuppressive protein with a molecular weight somewhere between 10 to 21.5 kDa.[28-32] There is no specific assay for EPF, aside from a bioassay that assesses ability to bind to lymphocytes in vitro and to amplify the inhibition of rosette formation between lymphocytes and heterologous (sheep) red blood cells[1,2,33] (Fig. 2-5). This assay is lengthy, tedious, and highly variable.

Origin EPF is produced by the maternal ovaries as the result of stimulation by a platelet activation factor released from the conceptus at fertilization.[1,2] It is believed that sperm entry into the ovum releases a substance which, similar to PAF, activates platelets. In addition, this substance acts upon the ovary to stimulate EPF release.[1-4] EPF is also produced by the preimplanted blastocyst and may have a local endometrial function.[1-4] Because embryonic EPF probably does not reach the circulation until implantation, removal of the ovaries in experimental animals shortly after conception, but before implantation, produces immediate disappearance of EPF from the circulation.[1-4]

Normal Variation Serum EPF is the earliest known indication of fertilization. It is detectable in the circulation approximately 48 hours after conception with maximum levels in early first trimester and diminishes to almost undetectable levels at term[2] (Fig. 2-6). In early human studies, EPF was detected after intercourse in 18 of 28 ovulatory cycles, suggesting a fertilization rate of 67 percent. Embryonic loss was high (78 percent), because EPF disappeared from the circulation before the onset of menstruation in 14 of 18 cases.[34] In the remaining 4 cases, EPF remained detectable beyond 14 days with presence of a viable embryo.[35] EPF appears within 48 hours after successful in vitro fertilization embryo transfer.[1,2] It disappears within 24 hours after induced abortion and is undetectable in many spontaneous abortions and ectopic pregnancies.[36,37] Indeed, inability to detect EPF during pregnancy portends a poor diagnosis. Clinical application of EPF measure-

Table 2-1 Cytochemical Distribution of Pregnancy Proteins

Peptide	Abbreviation	Cytotrophoblast	Syncytiotrophoblast	Decidua	References
Hypothalamic-Like Hormones					
Corticotropin-releasing hormone	CRH	+		+	15, 52
Gonadotropin-releasing hormone	GnRH	+			16
Thyrotropin-releasing hormone	TRH	+			17, 77
Somatostatin	SRIF	+			26
Pituitary-Like Hormones					
Adrenocorticotropic hormone	ACTH		+		18
Human chorionic gonadotropin	hCG		+		19, 22–24
Human chorionic thyrotropin	hCT		?		20
Human placental lactogen	hPL		+		23, 24
Growth Factors					
Inhibin/activin	N/A		+		79
Transforming growth factor β	TGFβ		+		52, 87
Insulin-like growth factor 1 & 2	IGF-1; IGF-2		+		84
Epidermal growth factor	EGF		+		88
Other Pregnancy Proteins					
Pregnancy-specific β$_1$ glycoprotein	SP1		+		90
Placental protein 5	PP5		+		94
Pregnancy-associated plasma protein-A[a]	PAPP-A		+		93
Prolactin	PRL			+	25
Relaxin[a]	N/A			+	104, 106
IGF-1 binding protein	IGF-1BP, PP12			+	110, 111
Placental protein 14	PP14			+	109
Alpha-fetoprotein[b]	AFP				113

[a] Relaxin is secreted principally by the corpus luteum and secondarily from decidua.[110,111]
[b] AFP is fetal in origin.[113]

ments is promising but elusive because of difficulties in isolating the molecule and developing practical assays for it.[1–4]

Function EPF is believed to prevent rejection of an antigenically alien embryo. Binding to a specific lymphocyte population, it recruits suppressor cells, which in turn release soluble suppressor factors that are believed to protect the pregnancy.[1,2] In its association with dividing cells, EPF also has properties of a growth factor that regulates cell proliferation.[1,2]

Placental Proteins

Placental protein hormone synthesis may be a direct reflection of both trophoblastic mass and intervillous maternal blood flow.[27] Control of their release is poorly understood; one hypothesis suggests that placental hormone production is regulated by negative feedback to maintain a fixed intervillous hormone concentration. An alternative hypothesis suggests the hypothalamic-like placental peptides (CRH, GnRH, TRH, SRIF), located in the cytotrophoblasts stimulate the pituitary-like placental hormones (ACTH, hCG, hCT) located in the adjacent syncytiotrophoblasts.[14–27] The former hypothesis is only speculative, but does provide a convenient grouping of hormones which, for heuristic reasons, is used in this discussion.

Pituitary-like Hormones

Human Chorionic Gonadotropin
Molecular Structure HCG is a glycoprotein with structural similarity to follicle stimulating hormone (FSH), luteinizing (LH), and thyroid stimulating hormone (TSH). As are the other glycoprotein hormones, hCG is composed of two nonidentical subunits associated noncovalently[14,38] (Fig. 2-7). The α subunit consists of a 92-amino-acid sequence essentially identical and shared in common with the pituitary glycoprotein hormones. The β subunit, although structurally similar, differs just enough to confer specific biologic activity on the intact (dimer) hormones. The subunits differ primarily at the COOH terminus where the β subunit of hCG has a 30-amino-acid tailpiece that is not present in the hLH β subunit. Assuming an average carbohydrate content of 30 percent, the molecular weight of dimer hCG is approximately 36.7 kDa; the α-subunit contributes 14.5 kDa and the β subunit 22.2 kDa.[38]

Origin HCG mRNA is detectable in blastomeres of 6- to 8-cell embryos.[7] After implantation hormonal hCG is present in the outer syncytial layer.[19,22–24] α-hCG subunits are localized to the cytotrophoblasts with none in the syncytial layer.[19,22]

HCG secretion is related to mass of hCG-secreting trophoblastic tissues. Thus, the release of hCG in vivo

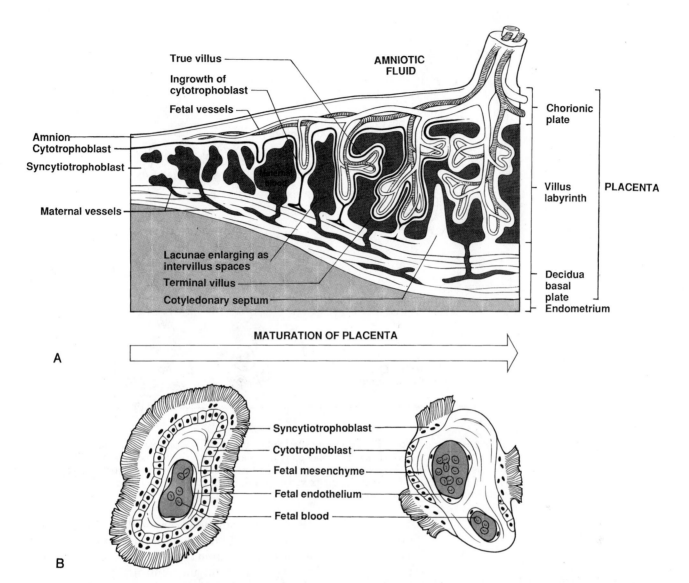

Fig. 2-4 **(A)** Gross morphology of the human placenta. The effects of advancing gestation on placental morphology evolves from left to right. Placental mass increases and hormonally active and invasive trophoblasts compose a lesser percentage of the total mass as the placenta evolves as an organ of transfer. (Modified from Willams and Warwick.[226] With permission) **(B)** Anatomic structure of early and late terminal villi. These transverse sections through terminal villi are from early (left) and term (right) pregnancy. Cytotrophoblastic cells become infrequent with placental maturity, and increasing fibrin deposits occur by term gestation as placental function adapts more to maternal fetal transfer and relatively less to hormone production. Fetal capillary endothelium is the only structure separating maternal fetal circulation in from the mature placenta. (Modified from Willams and Warwick.[226])

has been correlated with the respective trophoblast layer widths from weeks 4 through 20 and with placental weights from 20 to 38 weeks.[19] Between 3 and 9 weeks' gestation, rapidly rising hCG coincides with proliferation of immature trophoblastic villi and an extensive syncytial layer.[19] Between 10 and 18 weeks gestation, declining hCG is associated with a relative reduction in syncytiotrophoblasts and cytotrophoblast (Figs. 2-8A & B). From 20 weeks to term, a gradual increase in dimer hCG corresponds with a gradual increase in placental weight and villus volume.[19] In summary, rising hCG reflects the histology of a rapidly proliferating and invasive placenta. Falling hCG is associated with a relative reduction in trophoblasts and reflects a morphologic transformation of the placenta into an organ of transfer.[19]

HCG secretion is related to placental GnRH.[39] In an in vitro trophoblast perfusion system, hCG is released in 11 to 22 minute pulses where the pulse frequency and amplitude are believed entrained to the release of placental GnRH.[39] HCG production is stimulated by glucocorticoids and suppressed by DHEA-S.[40] Cyclic

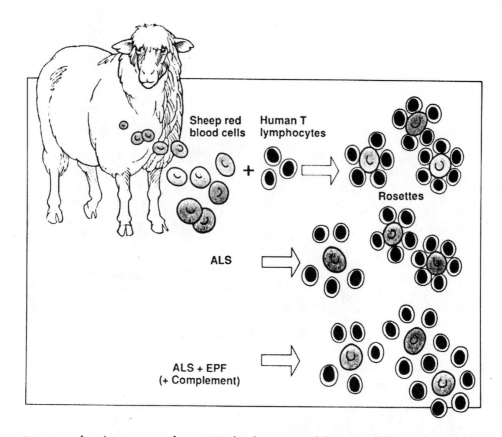

Fig. 2-5 Detection of early pregnancy factor (EPF) by the rosette inhibition test (RIT). Approximately 80 to 90 percent of human T-lymphocytes will bind spontaneously to sheep erythrocytes to form rosettes. Rosette formation is inhibited by antilymphocyte serum (ALS). Pregnancy serum contains a factor that reduces the amount of ALS required to produce inhibition, by binding to the receptors on the red cells. This factor is the *early pregnancy factor*. (Modified from Chard and Grudzinskas,[33] with permission.)

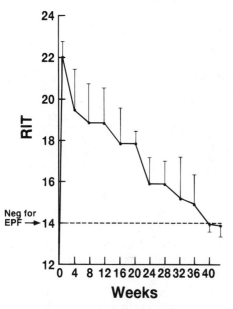

Fig. 2-6 Early pregnancy factor (EPF) activity in serum tested before and at various times througout pregnancy and after parturition. EPF activity is expressed as rosette inhibition titre (RIT; mean ± SEM). Broken lines indicate the RIT obtained with nonpregnant serum. (Modified from Morton et al.[1] with permission.)

AMP analogues augment secretion of hCG and α-hCG in vitro.[41] Finally, decidual inhibin and prolactin inhibit hCG production by term human trophoblasts while decidual activin augments it.[38,42]

Normal Variation Figures 2-8A–C depict maternal levels of dimer hCG, α-hCG subunit, and β-hCG subunits from 3 to 40 weeks gestational age.[19] At 4 weeks' gestation, mean doubling times of dimer hCG are 2.2 (SD ± 0.8) days falling to 3.5 (SD ± 1.2) days at 9 weeks.[19] The peak median level is 108,800 mlU/ml at 10 weeks.[19] Between 12 and 16 weeks, median dimer hCG decreases rapidly with a mean halving time of 2.5 (SD ± 1.1) days to 25 percent of first-trimester peak values. Levels continue to fall, from 16 to 22 weeks, at a slower mean halving rate of 4.1 (SD ± 1.8) days to become 10.7 percent of peak first trimester median hCG.[19] During the third trimester mean hCG rises gradually but significantly from 22 weeks until term.[19]

β-hCG subunit levels parallel dimer hCG (Fig. 2-8B). α-hCG, not detectable until about 6 weeks, rises in a sigmoid curve to reach peak levels in 36 weeks (Fig. 2-8C). Levels of subunit are very low relative to dimer hCG, approximately 2,000-fold to 150-fold less at 6 and 35 weeks, respectively[19] (Fig. 2-8C).

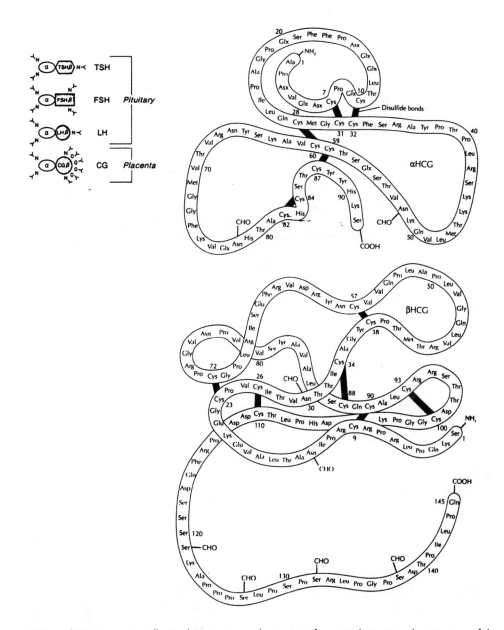

Fig. 2-7 HCG and LH are structurally similar to one another except for a "tailpiece" at the terminus of the β-side chain of hCG, which makes the latter structurally distinct. Disulfide bonds are marked with dark lines. Structural homology (insert) is shown for hCGs and three other pituitary glycoprotein hormones, LH, FSH, and TSH. The α-chain of hCG is biochemically and immunologically similar to the α-chain of the three pituitary glycoproteins. (Modified from Ren and Braunstein,[38] and from Walker,[56] with permission.)

Function HCG is believed to be the major factor in maintaining the corpus luteum.[43] It stimulates both adrenal and placental steroidogenesis,[44] it stimulates the fetal testes to secrete increasing testosterone to induce internal virilization.[45] HCG is immunosuppressive and may be involved in maternal lymphocyte function.[46] Finally, hCG possesses thyrotrophic activity.[47]

Adrenocorticotropin

Molecular Structure and Origin Placental ACTH is structurally similar to pituitary ACTH.[1–39] Under the para-crine influence of placental CRH from the juxtaposed cytotrophoblasts. Placental ACTH is produced by the syncytiotrophoblasts and secreted into the maternal circulation.[48–50]

Normal Variation and Function Circulating maternal ACTH is increased above nonpregnancy levels, but remains within the upper normal range.[51,52] Placental ACTH stimulates an increase in circulating maternal free cortisol resistant to dexamethasone suppression.[48,51] Thus, the relative hypercortisolism of preg-

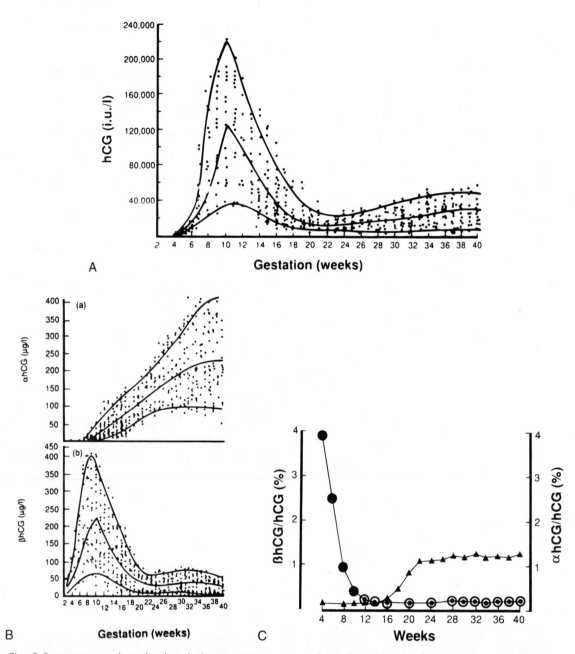

Fig. 2-8 **(A)** Dimeric hCG levels (mIU/ML)in 500 serum samples collected between 3 and 40 weeks' gestation (LMP) from 55 patients. The 5, 50, and 95 centiles are shown. **(B)** Subunits of serum α-hCG (a) and β-hCG (b) measured directly without correcting for hCG cross reaction; centiles 5, 50, and 95 are shown. **(C)** The mean percentage α-hCG/dimer (Δ) β-hCG/dimer (β) hCG ratios between 3 and 40 weeks' gestational age. (From Hay,[19] with permission.)

nancy occurs despite a high normal ACTH concentration. This regulation is possible by two differences in endocrine relationships during pregnancy. First, maternal ACTH response to exogenous CRH is blunted.[51] Second, a paradoxical relationship exists between placental ACTH and CRH and their end-organ product, cortisol: glucocorticoids augment placental CRH and ACTH secretion.[49,53] Teliologically, this positive feedback mechanism allows an increase in glucocorticoid

secretion in times of stress over and above the amount necessary if the mother was not pregnant.[53]

Human Sommatomammotrophin

Molecular Structure and Origin HCS or human placental lactogen (hPL) is a single chain polypeptide with two intramolecular disulfide bridges and a molecular weight of 22.3 kDa. Of the 191 amino acids, 167 (85 percent) are identical to human pituitary growth hormone and human pituitary prolactin.[54,55] Accordingly, hCS shares biologic properties with both growth hormone and prolactin.[54,55] The hCS gene belongs to a superfamily of five closely related genes localized contiguously on chromosome 17.[56] HCS is produced in the syncytiotrophoblast.

Normal Variation First detectable during the fifth week, hCS rises throughout pregnancy but maintains a constant hormone weight/placental weight relationship.[57] Concentrations reach their highest during the third trimester, from 3.3 μg/ml to 25 μg/ml at term[57] (Fig. 2-9). HCS levels rise and fall in response to fasting and glucose loading.[58]

Function HCS antagonizes insulin action, inducing glucose intolerance, lipolysis, and proteolysis in the maternal system, teliologically protecting transfer of glucose and amino acids to the fetus.[55] HCS is believed responsible for marked increases in maternal plasma insulin-like growth factor 1 (IGF-1) concentrations as pregnancies approach term.[57-59] It enhances insulin secretion, impairs glucose tolerance, and promotes nitrogen retention in pregnant and nonpregnant women[55-60] (Fig. 2-10). Surprisingly, women without the hCS gene have no detectable hCS but experience normal pregnancy outcome.[61]

Human Chorionic Thyrotropin HCT is structurally similar to pituitary TSH but does not have the common α subunit.[62] Placental content of hCT is very small.[20] HCG also has thyrotropic activity and probably experts more significant effects on maternal thyroid function than does hCT.[63]

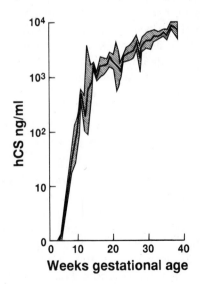

Fig. 2-9 Weekly concentrations of hCS (ng/ml) in maternal plasma throughout pregnancy. Solid dots represent the geometric mean; lines represent 95 percent confidence interval widths. LMP, last menstrual period. (Modified from Braunstein et al.[57] with permission).

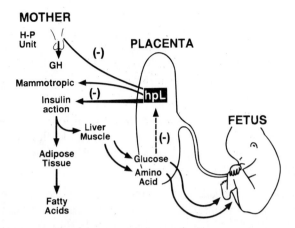

Fig. 2-10 Physiologic role of hCS during pregnancy. The current model of the functional role of hCS in maternal metabolism is that hCS preferentially increases glucose availability for the fetus by its lipolytic and insulin antagonist activity. (*), Inhibitory effect (Modified from Yen,[60] with permission.)

Hypothalamic-like Hormones

Gonadotropin Releasing Hormone
Molecular Structure and Origin Placental GnRH is biologically and immunologically similar to the hypothalamic decapeptide GnRH.[16]

Origin GnRH activity has been localized to the cytotrophoblastic cells along the outer surface layer of the syncytiotrophoblast. HCG is localized to adjacent syncytiotrophoblast.

Normal Variation GnRH histochemical activity peaks at 8 weeks and then decreases with advancing gestational age.[16-19] These changes parallel hCG concentration in both the placenta and maternal circulation.[19]

Function Placental GnRH stimulates hCG release through a dose dependent paracrine mechanism.[39] In first trimester placental tissue culture, there is little hCG augmentation by GnRH because hCG production is already close to maximum.[19] In mid-trimester, however, there is marked dose-dependent hCG augmentation of hCG release in vitro. This effect diminishes in the term placenta. In a superfusion system, 1-minute infusions of GnRH analog significantly increased pulse amplitude and frequency of hCG secretion.[39] GnRH administered intravenously during pregnancy does not increase serum hCG, presumably because placental GnRH receptors have low affinity and the GnRH is diluted in the maternal circulation. It is more likely that locally produced GnRH is the mechanism for stimulating of placental hCG.[39]

Corticotropin Releasing Hormone
Molecular Structure Placental CRH appears to be structurally similar to the 41 aminoacid hypothalamic CRH

peptide,[64,65] and is therefore readily measured by radioimmunoassay in amniotic fluid, fetal plasma, and maternal plasma. Both hypothalamic and placental CRH are products of the same gene, which is located on the long arm of chromosome 8.[66]

Origin Pro-CRH messenger RNA is present in the cytotrophoblast.[66] CRH activity is most intense in cytotrophoblasts during first trimester and diminishes toward term.[15] Also, there is intense CRH immunoreactivity in the decidua.[15]

Normal Variation CRH immunoreactivity has been measured in maternal plasma, fetal plasma and amniotic fluid.[67,68] Maternal CRH increases sharply beginning the twentieth week of gestation, reaching highest concentrations at term[67] (Fig. 2-11). Although concentrations in umbilical plasma are lower than in maternal plasma, there is a highly significant correlation between maternal and umbilical plasma CRH.[67] In amniotic fluid, there is an approximately 3-fold rise between second and third trimester.[67,68]

Function Placental CRH stimulates placental ACTH release in vitro in a dose dependent relationship.[40,53] Both CRH and ACTH are released into the fetal and maternal circulations, although their activity is moderated by a maternal CRH binding protein.[69] Placental CRH participates in the surge of fetal glucocorticoids associated with late third trimester fetal maturation.[40,67,69] Secretion of both CRH and ACTH increase when uterine blood flow is restricted. CRH is a potent uteroplacental vasodilator.[70,71] CRH is released into the fetal circulation in response to fetal stress and in conditions leading to growth restriction.[72–74] High circulating maternal CRH is believed responsible for the elevated plasma ACTH and cortisol in pregnant women, which renders them unresponsive to feedback suppression of plasma cortisol.[40,67–69,75] CRH stimulates prostaglandin synthesis in fetal membranes and placenta. Finally, CRH is frequently elevated in preeclampsia, fetal asphyxia and premature labor, and various conditions causing growth restriction.[72–74]

Somatostatin A substance similar to SRIF is identifiable in cytotrophoblasts and decidual stroma. Although it is logical to suggest that somatostatin is a hCS inhibiting factor, this cannot be confirmed in vitro.[76]

Thyrotropin Releasing Hormone TRH has been detected in the cytotrophoblast; however the molecule is chromatographically different from the hypothalamic TRH tripeptide.[77] Because the principal placental thyroid-stimulator is believed to be hCG, a significant role for placental TRH is tenuous.[78]

Growth Factors

Inhibin and Activin
Molecular Structure Inhibin and activin are heterodimeric glycoproteins each with α- and β-subunits.

Origin Inhibin and activin dimers have been localized to syncytiotrophoblast with their subunits detected in both cytotrophoblasts and syncytiotrophoblasts.[79] Inhibin is secreted by the corpus luteum and has been detected in decidua.[80,81]

Normal Variation Dimeric inhibin (α, β) in the maternal circulation begins to increase above nonpregnant levels by 12 days after conception, dramatically increasing at 5 gestational weeks to peak at 8 to 10 weeks. A subsequent decrease at 13 weeks, stabilizes until 30 weeks and then rises again with the approach of term[81] (Fig. 2-12). The early fluctuations in inhibin concentration probably reflect corpus luteum release, whereas the third trimester increase probably reflects inhibin originating from the placenta and decidua. Inhibin disappears to nondetectable levels after delivery. Inhibin α dimer has a similar pattern throughout pregnancy.[82]

Function Placental inhibin, functioning through a paracrine mechanism, is believed to inhibit the release of chorionic GnRH and hCG.[42,83] Activin stimulates release of GnRH and hCG. Decidual activin and inhibin probably have the same effects and appear to serve a role whereby maternal tissues modulate chorionic GnRH and hCG production. Potential immunosuppressive and mitogenic roles have been suggested.[83]

Insulin-like Growth Factor The placenta is an important site of intrauterine IGF-1 and IGF-2 synthesis.[84] Syncytiotrophoblasts from second-trimester placentas tran-

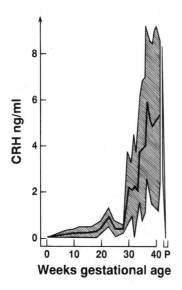

Fig. 2-11 Maternal serum concentrations of immunoreactive CRH in 256 individual pregnant women in relation to gestational age and at postpartum (mean ± SD). (Modified from Stalla et al.,[65] with permission.)

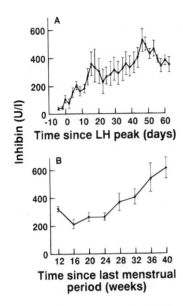

Fig. 2-12 Geometric mean (67 percent confidence intervals) plasma concentrations of inhibin. **(A)** Data plotted from four subjects in early pregnancy from whom three weekly samples were obtained before and after conception. **(B)** Data plotted from nine subjects in later pregnancy from whom samples were obtained at 4-week intervals starting at 12 weeks after the last menstrual period. (Modified from Tovanabutra et al.[81] with permission.)

scribe IGF-1 mRNA; IGF-2 mRNA is found in placental fibroblasts. Human placental tissues are rich in IGF receptors.[85,86] IGF-1 stimulates prolactin synthesis in human decidual cells and may affect steroidogenesis.[55]

Transforming Growth Factor β Transforming growth factor β (TGF-β) has been purified from placenta and is thought to be a paracrine regulator of mesenchymal-epithelial interactions.[52,87]

Epidermal Growth Factor Epidermal growth factor (EGF) is synthesized by the syncytiotrophoblast, and EGF receptors are observed on these same cells. EGF has been shown to increase release of hCG and hCS from in vitro studies of placental cells.[52,88]

Other Pregnancy-Related Peptides

Beside the chorionic glycoproteins, which are analogous to pituitary glycoprotein present in the non-pregnant state, the placenta secretes a host of proteins with no known analogue in the nonpregnant state. One group of these proteins was first identified by producing an antiserum to serum drawn in term pregnancy. Antiserum was then used to isolate and identify the pregnancy associated plasma proteins (PAPP) A through D. A second group was isolated by extraction of proteins from placental tissue that was later purified and characterized as pregnancy-specific β1-glycoprotein (Schwanger-schaftsspeziffische protein 1[SP-1]).

Pregnancy Specific β1-Glycoprotein SP-1 is a glycoprotein with a molecular weight of about 100 kDa. Secreted from trophoblastic cells, it is detected 18 to 23 days after ovulation.[89,90] Rising initially with an approximate 2- to 3-day doubling time, it reaches peak concentrations of 100 to 200 ng/ml at term. SP-1 is a potent immunosuppressivor of lymphocyte proliferation and may prevent rejection of the conceptus.[91]

Pregnancy Associated Plasma Protein-A PAPP-A, the largest of the pregnancy related glycoproteins, has a molecular weight of 750 kDa. It originates principally from placental syncytiotrophoblasts.[92,93] It is first detected at a mean time of 33 days after ovulation. It then rises initially with a 3-day doubling time and continues to rise until term.[92] PAPP-A may serve an immunosuppressive role during pregnancy.[93]

Placental Protein-5 A glycoprotein with a molecular weight of 36 kDa, placental protein 5 (PP5) is believed produced in the syncytiotrophoblasts. It is detected about 42 days after ovulation, with a continuous rise until term.[94] Because PP5 has antithrombin and antiplasmic activities, it is believed to be a natural blood coagulation inhibitor active at the implantation site.[95]

Decidual Proteins

Prolactin

Molecular Structure Decidual prolactin is a 197–199 amino acid peptide with chemical and biological properties identical to pituitary prolactin.[55]

Origin Prolactin, produced by decidualized endometrium, is first detectable in the endometrium cycle day 23, a time corresponding to implantation. Decidual prolactin secretion is thought to be induced by progesterone or a combination of estrogen and progesterone[96] with growth factors (e.g., IGF-1) and other polypeptide hormones (α-hCG) as co-regulators. Decidual prolactin is transported across intact amnion and chorion from adherent decidua and released into the amniotic fluid with little entering their fetal or maternal circulation.[97] Production, independent of dopaminergic control, is not affected by bromocryptine.[55] Circulating fetal prolactin is secreted by the fetal pituitary while circulating maternal prolactin is secreted by the maternal pituitary under the influence of estrogens. Both are suppressed by maternal ingestion of bromocryptine.

Normal Variation Decidual prolactin parallels the rapid rise in maternal serum prolactin until 10 weeks gestation, rises rapidly until 20 weeks, and then falls as term approaches[98] (Fig. 2-13).

Function Decidual prolactin regulates fluid and electrolyte flux through fetal membranes. Decidual prolac-

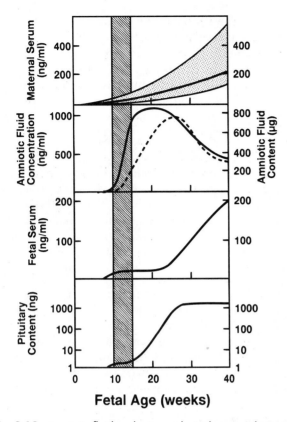

Fig. 2-13 Amniotic fluid prolactin peaks in the second trimester and declines toward term. In contrast, maternal and fetal prolactin increase to maximum level during the third trimester. (From Clements et al.,[98] with permission.)

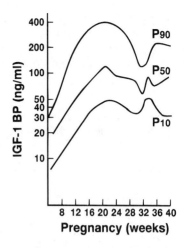

Fig. 2-14 Maternal serum IGF-1BP levels throughout pregnancy as measured by radioimmunoassay for PP12. (From Rutanen,[108] with permission.)

tin reduces permeability of the amnion in the fetal to maternal direction.[55,96,97,99–103]

Relaxin

Relaxin is a 6-kDa peptide hormone, structurally related to insulin, comprised of two short peptide chains which are linked by disulfide bridges.[104–106] It is believed that the corpus luteum is the major source of this hormone; however, relaxin has been identified in placenta and decidua. Relaxin is undetectable in women without ovaries and appears nonessential in normal pregnancy outcome.[104–106]

IGF-1 Binding Protein (IGF-1BP or PP12)

IGF-1 binding protein contains 234 amino acids with a molecular mass of approximately 25 kDa.[107] IGF-1BP is believed to originate from decidual stromal cells. In nonpregnant woman, circulating IGF-1BP does not change with the cyclicity of the endometrium. However, during pregnancy, there is a several fold increase in serum IGF-1BP levels that begins during the first trimester, peaks during second trimester, falls, and

then peaks' a second time before term[108] (Fig. 2-14). IGF-1BP inhibits the binding of IGF-1 to receptors in the decidua.[108]

Placental Protein

Placental protein (PP14) is a glycoprotein with 162 amino acids and a molecular weight of 28 kDA. It is synthesized in secretory and decidualized endometrium detectable on menstrual cycle day 24.[109] PP14 in serum rises sharply on approximately days 22 to 24 of the cycle, reaches peak values at the onset of menstruation, and is maintained at high levels if pregnancy occur.[110] In pregnant women, PP14 rises in parallel with hCG[111] (Fig. 2-15). PP14 levels are very low in patients with ectopic pregnancy, in which there is minimal decidual reaction. PP14 is thought to be an immunosuppressant.[109]

Fetal Proteins

Alpha-fetalprotein (AFP) is a glycoprotein with a molecular weight of about 69 kDa.[112]

AFP is believed to be synthesized sequentially in the yolk sac, gastrointestinal tract, and fetal liver.[113] It enters the fetal urine in abundance and is readily detected in the amniotic fluid. Concentrations of fetal plasma AFP, amniotic fluid AFP (AFAFP), and maternal serum AFP (MSAFP) are shown in Figure 2-16.[114] MSAFP peaks between 10 and 13 weeks' gestational age and then declines from 14 to 32 weeks. The rapid fall in fetal plasma AFP is believed due to increasing fetal blood volume and a decline in fetal production. AFP peaks at 12 and 14 weeks gestation and then steadily declines to term.[114] The concentration gradient between fetal plasma AFP and MSAFP is about 150- to 200-fold. Detectable as early as 7 weeks' gestation,

MSAFP reaches peak concentrations between 28 to 32 weeks.[114] The apparent paradoxical rise in MSAFP in association with decreasing AFAFP and fetal serum levels can be accounted for by increasing placental permeability to fetal plasma proteins that occurs with advancing gestation.[114]

Function AFP regulates fetal intravascular volume as an osmoregulator,[114] and may also be involved in immunoregulation.[115] AFAFP and MSAFP measurements are clinically important because they are elevated in associ-

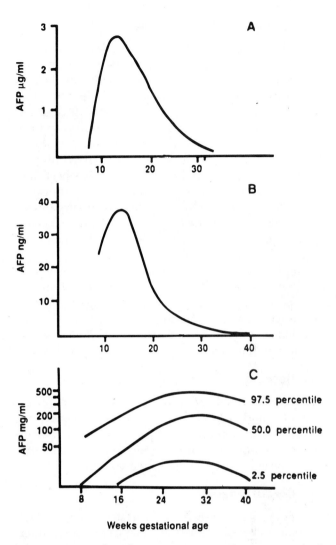

Fig. 2-16 Normal median concentrations of AFP in **(A)** fetal serum, **(B)** amniotic fluid, **(C)** maternal serum. Maternal serum is shown with 2.5 and 97.5 percentile limits. (From Habib,[114] with permission.)

ation with neural tube defects.[116] MSAFP is decreased in pregancies with Down syndrome (Ch. 9).[117]

Pregnancy Steroids

The novel pregnancy peptides described above are in part responsible for the altered steroid milieu in pregnancy. In addition to stimulation of maternal hormones, the fetus and placenta produce and secrete steroids into the maternal circulation. The changes in maternal hormone concentrations are integrally related to metabolic and immunologic changes vital to intracorporeal gestation.

Ontogeny of Fetoplacental Steroid Production

Origins and amounts of fetoplacental steroid shift dramatically during gestation.

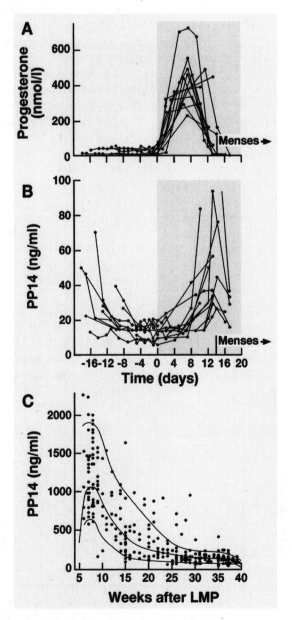

Fig. 2-15 **(A)** Serum progesterone and **(B)** PP14 concentrations in serum of normally ovulating women. PP14 rises approximately 8 days after the luteal phase rise of progesterone and remains elevated well into the next cycle. (From Seppala et al.,[109] with permission.) **(C)** PP14 concentrations in maternal serum throughout pregnancy (From Julkunen et al.,[110] with permission.)

The Preimplantation Conceptus

Estradiol and progesterone secretion by the conceptus and its cumulus is detectable in vitro well before implantation.[118,119] There is little information on the regulation of conceptus steroid production. Mechanical removal of the corona cells is associated with cessation of secretion, while return of corona cells in co-culture restores steroid secretion.[118] Steroid production, therefore, is likely negligible by the time the conceptus reaches the endometrial cavity, since it has been mechanically denuded of cumulus during transport through the oviduct. Once implantation occurs and secretion of trophoblastic hCG and other pregnancy-related peptides is established, steroid production by the conceptus resumes.[118–120]

Progesterone production by the preimplantation conceptus is believed important in tubal and uterine transport, because receptor sites for progesterone are highest in concentration in the mucosal layer of the distal one third of the fallopian tube. The ova and sperm are most likely to meet at this location.[121]

The Decidua

Cortisol is secreted by decidual tissues.[122,123] In concert with hCG and progesterone secreted by the conceptus, decidual cortisol probably suppresses the maternal immune rejection response, helping to confer immunologic "privilege" to the implanted conceptus.[122,123]

The Corpus Luteum

Progesterone, 17α-hydroxyprogesterone, estradiol, and androstenedione are the principal steroid products of the corpus luteum. Progesterone is considered the steroid of greatest importance because progesterone alone given to a lutectomized woman in early pregnancy will maintain a pregnancy that would otherwise abort.[124] Likewise, exogenous progesterone given to an agonadal woman pregnant with donated embryos sustains viability through the early first trimester until the pregnancy can be maintained with its own placental progesterone production.[125] Although the human corpus luteum secretes up to 40 mg of progesterone a day during the midluteal phase of the ovarian cycle and into early pregnancy, surprisingly small amounts of progesterone are required to maintain donor embryo pregnancies when no corpus luteum is present.[126–128]

Low density lipoprotein (LDL) cholesterol is the principal regulatory precursor of corpus luteum progesterone production.[129]

The Fetus and Placenta

The fetal adrenal cortex and placenta serve as incomplete but complementary steroidogenic organs, functioning in concert to become the principal sites of ste-roid production as gestation advances. After 7 weeks' gestational age, the placenta dominates steroid production. At this point pregnancy continues even if the corpus luteum is excised, for in its stead is the beginning of the fetoplacental unit.[130] At this time of gestation, pituitary basophilic cells are producing significant amounts of fetal ACTH and stimulate the fetal adrenal cortex, whose cells have been amassed for 4 weeks, awaiting trophic stimulation to synthesize steroids.[131] This corresponds to the time in gestation when estriol is first detectable in the maternal circulation. The intricate interdependence of the fetal and adrenal cortex and the placenta allow these two relatively small organs to exchange, metabolize, and secrete more steroids than any other human endocrine tissue.

Because the fetal adrenal and placenta contain incomplete but complementary steroidogenic enzyme systems, they constantly exchange circulating steroid precursors which produces the steroid profile that characterizes normal pregnancy. As one might expect, nature has also evolved an organ that exists only in pregnancy to handle this unique function—the fetal zone of the adrenal cortex.[132,133] This zone comprises 80 percent of the fetal cortical mass and grows with increasing steroid requirements of pregnancy. Between 32 and 36 weeks (Fig. 2-17), a marked increased in fetal adrenal cortex growth velocity reflects the acceleration of fetal maturation processes just before parturition.[134–137] This fetal zone then rapidly involutes postpartum.[132]

The anatomic distribution of key steroidogenic enzymes involved in the production of circulating intrauterine steroids is diagrammed in Figure 2-18.[137,138] The fetal adrenal cortex is functionally deficient in 3β-hydroxysteroid dehydrogenase, the enzyme that con-

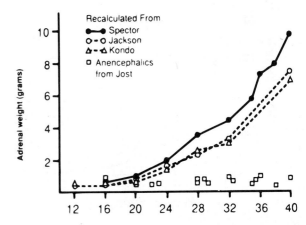

Fig. 2-17 Growth of the fetal adrenal cortex. Total fetal adrenal mass is shown as a function of gestational age. Rapid increase in growth velocity occurs between 32 and 36 weeks gestation. In anencephalic pregnancies, adrenal mass does not increase after the second trimester. (Data from Jost,[134] Kondo,[135] and Buster.[137])

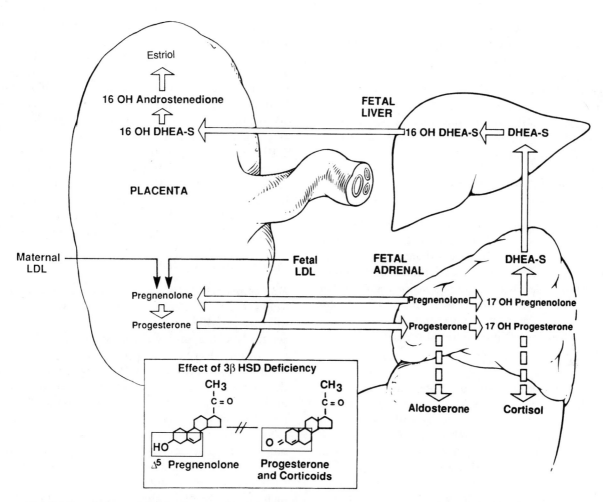

Fig. 2-18 Exchange of circulating steroid intermediates between fetal zone and placenta. Enzyme deficiencies of fetal zone are offset by enzyme activities of placenta enabling the two organs to work as a mutual cooperative to produce an extensive profile of steroids not otherwise possible. Although the bulk of fetal zone steroids are secreted as sulfoconjugates, the unconjugated counterparts are secreted in abundance as well. DHEA-S, dehydroepiandrosterone sulfate.

verts pregnenolone and DHEA to progesterone and androstenedione, respectively.[139] Therefore, the fetus cannot make progesterone or androstenedione, the immediate precursor to the sex steroids. The placenta, however, has an abundance of 3β-hydroxysteroid dehydrogenase. Therefore, the fetal adrenal cortex extracts LDL from the fetal circulation and converts it to pregnenolone sulfate and DHEAS.[137,140] Pregnenolone sulfate is delivered through the umbilical artery to the placenta. The placenta converts pregnenolone to progesterone and returns the latter to the fetus for synthesis into mineralocorticoids and glucocorticoids. Interestingly, the placenta contains a relative lack of 17α-hydroxylase.[138] Teleologically, this deficiency may exist to prevent placental metabolism of progesterone, which is the precursor of fetal adrenal cortex corticosteroids.[138] The placenta also has the enzymatic capability to extract LDL cholesterol and to convert it into

progesterone without relying on the fetal adrenal cortex.

The other fetal steroid precursor, DHEA-S, is first delivered to the fetal liver, where it is converted into 16α-hydroxydehydroepiandrosterone sulfate (16α-OH DHEAS) before being converted in the placenta first to 16α-hydroxyandrostenedione and then further aromatized into estriol.[138] The estrogens are subseqently secreted into the maternal and fetal circulations.[138]

Besides the obvious functional interdependence of these two organs, the placenta also acts as a structural stimulator of the fetal adrenal cortex. In the first 20 weeks of gestation placental hCG and progesterone play important roles in fetal adrenal cortex maintenance and regulation.[141] HCG stimulates fetal adrenal cortex production of DHEA-S in vivo. Atrophy of the fetal zone after delivery may be in part due to removal of the trophic effect of hCG, although hCG appears to be less important after week 20 of gestation.[141,142] Indeed, the fetal adrenal cortex acquires increasing sensitivity to circulating ACTH, with advancing gestational age during the second half of gestation being primarily influenced by ACTH.[143,144] In addition, prolactin receptors have also been demonstrated in the adrenal cortex, and prolactin may therefore act in association with ACTH and hCG to regulate fetal adrenal cortex steroid production.[145,148]

Regulation of Fetoplacental Steroidogenesis

Steroidogenic regulation has been investigated extensively in vitro by study of fetal placental tissue explants. In vivo, regulation has been investigated in catheterized primate models, particularly the rhesus monkey and baboon. Factors emerging as major regulators of fetoplacental steroidogenesis include 1) LDL cholesterol, 2) pituitary regulatory hormones, 3) intra-placental regulators, and 4) intra-adrenal regulators.[147-149]

LDL Cholesterol

LDL cholesterol, the principal lipoprotein utilized in fetal adrenal steroidogenesis, limits or augments steroid output by its availability. Between 50 to 70 percent of the cholesterol used for fetal adrenal steroidogenesis is extracted from circulating fetal LDL.[130,150,151] Fetal adrenal tissues contain high affinity, low capacity binding sites for LDL. In the presence of ACTH, adrenal binding capacity for LDL is increased.[150,152,153] Choles-

terol liberated from intra-adrenal hydrolysis of LDL is converted to steroids.

Simpson et al. proposed that fetal LDL cholesterol and the steroidogenic systems of the fetal adrenal and placenta may interact in a self-perpetuating positive feedback loop that becomes increasingly active with advancing gestation.[154] Most fetal LDL cholesterol arises de novo from synthesis in the fetal liver.[154] (Fig. 2-19). Fetal adrenal cortisol and placental estradiol (derived from fetal DHEA-S) augment de novo fetal liver biosynthesis of LDL. All of these interacting elements increase with advancing fetal maturity in a chain-like sequence of self perpetuating loops that increase steroid production to meet the needs of a growing fetus.[154]

Pituitary Regulatory Hormones

Fetal pituitary ACTH is detectable by the seventh week (9 weeks GA).[131,155] Plasma immunoreactive ACTH levels increase steadily until about 20 weeks. Levels remain relatively stable until approximately 34 weeks, when a significant decrement appears and persists until term.[153] Concentrations of ACTH over time therefore do not correlate with the increasing fetal adrenal mass or the increasing steroidogenic activities that characterize the third trimester.[153]

Fetal ACTH regulates steroidogenesis in both adrenal zones. ACTH receptor activity, expectedly present in both zones, is diminished somewhat in the fetal zone early during the second trimester when other trophic factors, such as hCG, are probably more important in

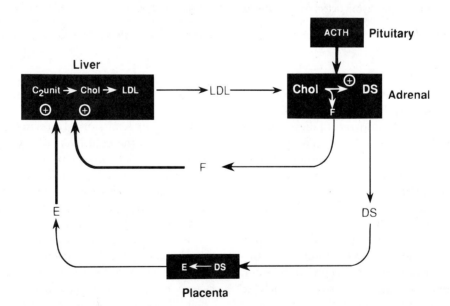

Fig. 2-19 Proposed scheme for the regulation of steroidogenesis in the human fetal placental unit. Fetal adrenal cortisol (F) and estradiol (E) are produced in the placenta from dehydroepiandrosterone sulfate (DS) of fetal adrenal origin, which regulates de novo fetal hepatic synthesis of cholesterol (Chol). Cholesterol bound to LDL is then provided to the fetal adrenal for F and DS production, which is enhanced by ACTH of fetal pituitary origin. (From Simpson et al.,[154] with permission.)

the maintenance of this structure.[154] In vitro superfusion system studies of human fetal adrenal tissue show that ACTH stimulates the release of Δ5 pregnenolone sulfate and DHEA-S, whereas isolated definitive zones secrete only cortisol when stimulated by ACTH.[154] ACTH, in addition to its effect on LDL binding, acts on its own adrenal cell membrane receptor subunit and then adenyl cyclase to express its direct stimulatory effect on steroidogenic enzymes.[154]

ACTH 1-19 and ACTH 1-38 have been extracted from human fetal pituitaries and have been shown in vitro to stimulate the production of DHEA-S and cortisol.[156,157] Although fetal ACTH is clearly a major fetal adrenotropic principle, its activity is modulated by other tropic factors such as CRH and prolactin.

Fetal pituitary prolactin is detectable at 10 weeks.[158] Cord prolactin concentrations increase with advancing gestation in parallel with increased adrenal mass.[159] With prolactin receptors demonstrated in the adrenal cortex, prolactin may act as a co-regulator with ACTH, hCG, and growth factors in fetal adrenal steroid production.[160,161] In fetal baboon experiments, both in vivo and in vitro, prolactin augments ACTH-stimulated adrenal androgen production.[149,162]

Intra-Placental Regulators

As the secretor of *hCG, placental CRH, progesterone,* and *estradiol,* the placenta is an important fetal zone co-regulator.[163]

HCG receptor activity is present in the fetal zone, and hCG stimulates fetal adrenal production of DHEA-S both in vitro and in vivo.[144,164] HCG appears to be less important after the 20th week when the fetal zone is primarily influenced by the ACTH. Fetal zone atrophy observed after delivery may be due to removal of placental hCG, but loss of other tropic factors is probably of similar importance.[154,156,161] Placental CRH, in a paracrine relationship with placental ACTH, probably participates with the fetal hypothalamus and pituitary in the surge of fetal glucocorticoids associated with the late third trimester.[165,166] This relationship was highlighted earlier in the chapter.

Placental progesterone inhibits the Δ5 to Δ4 steroid transformation in the fetal zone.[167,168] This effect is another explanation for the functional fetal adrenal 3βHSD deficiency. The fetal adrenal undergoes atrophy after delivery.

Placental estradiol modifies metabolism and production of corticoids and progesterone. In chronically catheterized baboons, the placenta regulates maternal cortisol-cortisone interconversion, and fetal pituitary production of ACTH.[148,165] This effect occurs by modulation of maternal cortisol across the placenta into the fetus.

Intra-Adrenal Regulators

The fetal adrenal becomes more sensitive to circulating ACTH with advancing gestational age.[149] At least three factors are involved:

Fetal adrenal mass increases between 32 and 36 weeks gestation.[134–136] The increase in cell numbers may be with increased numbers of ACTH receptors.[149] As such, becomes more responsive to ACTH.

Fetal adrenal blood flow, affected by arterial oxygen tension, tropic hormones, or intra-adrenal vascular changes, affects the exposure of fetal adrenal receptor subunits of differing numbers of tropic molecules.[149,165]

Growth factors modulate adrenal steroid pathway direction of the fetal adrenal as they do the the adult adrenal cortex. The fetal adrenal produces IGF-1 and IGF-2 with respective mRNAs stimulated by ACTH originating in the fetal pituitary or the placenta.[171,172]

Physiology of Fetoplacental Steroids and Pregnancy

Fetoplacental estrogens, progestogens and adrenocorticoids are secreted abundantly into both the both fetal and maternal circulation during pregnancy.

Estrogens

The origins and impact of estrogens in the maternal circulation vary with time in gestation and needs of the pregnancy.

Variation During Pregnancy

Estradiol originates almost exclusively from the maternal ovaries for the first five to six weeks gestation.[173] Later, the placenta secretes increasing quantities of estradiol, which it synthesizes from conversion of circulating maternal and fetal DHEA-S. After the first trimester, the placenta is the major source of circulating estradiol.[173] At term, approximately equal amounts of placental estradiol are converted from circulating maternal DHEA-S and fetal DHEA-S.[174,175] Estradiol concentrations are less than 0.1 ng/ml during the follicular phase and reach 0.4 ng/ml during the luteal phase of normal menstrual cycles.[176] Following conception, estradiol increases gradually to range from 6 to 30 ng/ml at term[177] (Fig. 2-20). In women with threatened first-trimester abortion, estradiol concentrations are abnormally low for gestational age. During the third trimester, low estradiol concentrations are associated with poor obstetrical outcome.

For the first four to six weeks of pregnancy,[173] estrone originates primarily from maternal sources (ovaries, adrenals, peripheral conversion). After this time, the placenta secretes increasing quantities of estrone

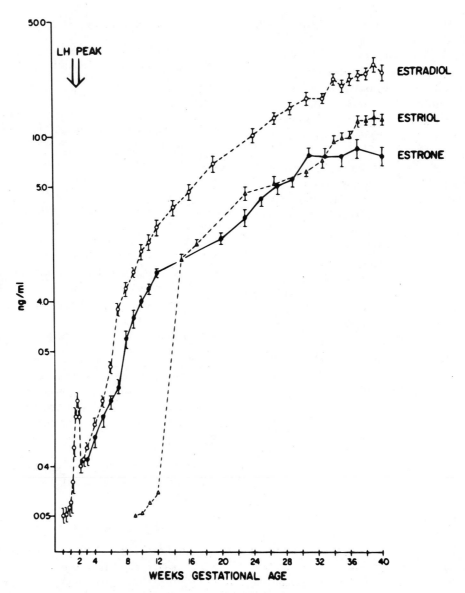

Fig. 2-20 Mean concentrations (± SEM) of estrone, estradiol, and estriol from conception to term. Unconjugated estriol is first detectable at about 9 weeks' gestational age. Gestational ages are calculated from the last menstrual flow.

from conversion of circulating maternal and fetal DHEA-S. For the remainder of pregnancy, the placenta remains the major source of circulating estrone.[173]

Estrone concentrations are less than 0.1 ng/ml during the follicular phase and may reach 0.3 ng/ml during the luteal phase of a normal menstrual cycle.[178] Following conception, estrone concentrations remain within the luteal phase range through weeks six to ten. Subsequently there is a gradual increase to a wide range of 2 to 30 ng/ml at term[173,177,178] (Fig. 2-20). Estrone concentrations probably reflect the same metabolic processes that are involved in the production of estradiol.

Estriol originates almost exclusively from the placenta and is produced principally from placental con-

version of fetal 16α-DHEA-S.[138,179] Estriol is first detectable in maternal serum at nine weeks.[173,174,180,181] This closely corresponds to the early steroidogenic evolution of the fetal adrenal cortex.[173] Its continued production is therefore dependent upon the presence of a living fetus. The concentration of estriol is less than 0.01 ng/ml in nonpregnant women. First detectable approximately 0.05 ng/ml at nine weeks,[173,178,180] estriol increases gradually to a range of approximately 10 to 30 ng/ml at term[179] (Fig. 2-20). Between 35 and 40 weeks gestational age, estriol concentrations increase sharply in a pattern that reflects a final surge of intrauterine steroidogenesis just prior to term.

Maternal concentrations of estriol may reflect abnormalities in fetal and placental development including fetal compromise, fetal anomalies, and hydatidiform mole.[180] Fetal death at any time during the second or third trimester produces a striking drop in estriol concentrations within 1 to 2 hours.[180] Within four to six hours, concentrations are consistently less than 1 ng/ml in the second trimester and less than 2.5 ng/ml in the third trimester.[180] Fetal anomalies associated with adrenal atrophy, such as anencephaly and Down syndrome, are associated with low concentrations.[180] For this reason, evaluation of unexplained low estriol in second and third trimesters should include ultrasonography and amniocentesis as appropriate. Hydatidiform moles are associated with low estriol.[180] Presumably this occurs because of the absence of a fetal adrenal and liver. The resultant deficiency of fetal 16α-hydroxylated sulfoconjugated precursors in molar pregnancy would account for the very low estriol values.[180]

Deteriorating fetoplacental health during the third trimester has long been associated with either falling or continuing low estriol concentrations.[180–183] Chronically compromised infants have markedly elevated cord LDL concentrations, low DHEA-S values, and decreased movement suggesting a depressed fetal CNS sleep state such that there is lowered metabolism and diminished oxygen consumption.[182,183] Diminished estriol production might be a consequence of this apparently protective state.[183]

Hormonal Functions During Pregnancy

Estrogens affect uterine vasculature, placenta steroidogenesis, and parturition.

Uterine Vasculature Estrogens augment uterine blood flow. In ovine models, direct estrogen injection into the uterine arteries through indwelling catheters produces striking increases in blood flow. Estradiol is the most potent estrogen in this role. Estrone and estriol, however, though less active, also produce the effect.[184] Because exposure of the uteroplacental bed to direct estriol secretion is massive, estriol may be the principal augmenter of uterine blood flow as described previously. This may be the dominant role of estriol in human pregnancy.[184]

Placental Steroidogenesis Estrogen regulated mechanisms may allow the fetus to govern production and secretion of progesterone during third trimester. In the baboon, estrogen regulates the biosynthesis of placental progesterone by regulating availability of LDL cholesterol for conversion to pregnenolone and to its downstream steroid products.[185] Thus in advanced pregnancy, the fetus may regulate placental progesterone production as it may require to control parturition and other progesterone related event.

Parturition Fetoplacental estrogens are closely linked to myometrial irritability, contractility, and labor. In primates, estrogens ripen the cervix, initiate uterine activity, and augment established labor.[186] Estrogens also increase the sensitivity of the myometrium to oxytocin by augmenting prostaglandin biosynthesis.[187,188] Because placental release of estrogens is linked to the fetal hypothalamus, pituitary, adrenals, and placenta,[186,188] the fetal pituitary adrenal axis appears to fine tune parturition timing in part through its effect on estrogen production. Thus, in human pregnancy in which the fetus is anencephalic, labor is either too early or too late. Similarly, surgical anencephaly in the fetal macaque disrupts the normal timing of parturition.[189] Parturition in humans is a precise event with a well-defined frequency distribution surrounding a mean gestational age of 270 days. In macaques, labor most often begins after a preparturitional increase of fetal adrenal steroids (DHEA-S) that is maximal between 2300 and 0300 hours.[188] A diurnal rhythm in uterine activity is also evident in which the maximal hourly values of intrauterine pressure and contraction frequency surround 2400 hours. In human studies, there is a similar entrainment of uterine activity with circulating maternal estrogens and progesterone as labor approaches.[190–192] There is firm evidence of increasing, rhythmical fetal adrenal and placental steroid output over the 5 weeks just before term that is important in preparing human pregnancy for the final cascade of oxytocin and prostaglandins that stimulate labor.[187–192]

The Progestogens

Progesterone and 17α-hydroxyprogesterone are the major progestogens in human pregnancy.

Variation During Pregnancy

Progesterone Progesterone originates almost entirely from the corpus luteum before six weeks gestational age but shifts more to the placenta after the seventh week. After 12 weeks the placenta is the major source of progesterone.[173,178] The placenta produces progesterone from circulating maternal LDL cholesterol and is minimally dependent upon fetal precursor.[129,138,173]

Progesterone concentrations are less than 1 ng/ml during the follicular phase of the normal menstrual cycle[176,177] (Fig. 2-21). In the luteal phase conceptual cycles, progesterone concentrations rise from 1 to 2 ng/ml on the day of the LH peak to a plateau of 10 to 35 ng/ml over the subsequent 7 days. Progesterone concentrations remain within this luteal range the tenth week (dated from last menstrual flow), and then show a sustained rise that continues until term. At term, progesterone concentrations range from 100 to 300 ng/ml.[173]

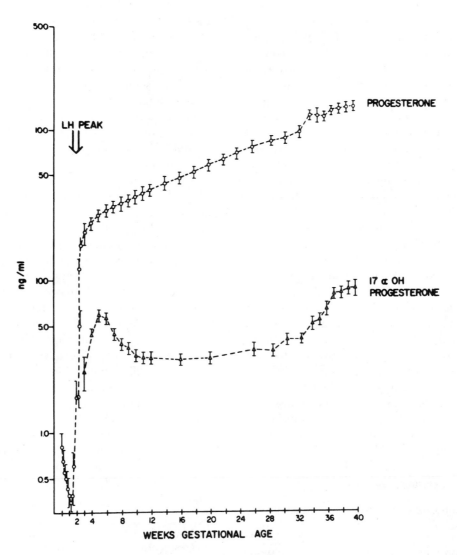

Fig. 2-21 Mean concentrations (±SEM) of progesterone and 17 α-hydroxyprogesterone from conception until term. Data are compiled from several reports. 17 α-hydroxyprogesterone shows a marked rise in concentrations beginning at 32 weeks until term. Gestational ages are calculated from the last menstrual flow.

Low progesterone levels are well tolerated in patients with no ovaries, carrying pregnancies with donor embryos.[126–128] In women with first-trimester threatened abortion, progesterone concentrations at the time of initial evaluation are predictive of ultimate outcome.[193] Abortion will occur in approximately 80 percent of those with progesterone concentrations under 10 ng/ml; viable pregnancies are virtually never observed at concentrations of <5.0 ng/ml.[194]

Conversely, in women with hydatidiform mole, progesterone concentrations are significantly elevated above the normal range.[195] In women whose pregnancies are complicated by Rh isoimmunization, progesterone concentrations are elevated approximately two fold above values for normal pregnancies of comparable gestational ages.[178] This elevation may be related to a twofold to threefold increase in placental mass associated with erythroblastosis.

Finally, progesterone concentrations are lower in women with ectopic pregnancy. Single serum progesterone levels have been widely used in diagnostic algorithms with serum β-hCG and ultrasound in diagnosis of ectopic pregnancy without laparoscopic surgery. Progesterone concentrations of less than 5 ng/ml are diagnostic of fetal death in the first trimester, thus, low progesterone levels prompt the performance of diagnostic curettage, which can distinguish between ectopic pregnancy and intrauterine fetal demise. Direct visualization of the ectopic implantation is not required.[194]

17α-hydroxyprogesterone 17α-hydroxyprogesterone originates predominantly from the corpus luteum during the first trimester of pregnancy.[196] The ovaries continue to be a significant source of 17α-hydroxyprogesterone throughout pregnancy. During the third trimester, however, the placenta uses fetal Δ5-sulfoconjugated precursors to secrete increasing amounts of 17α-hydroxyprogesterone. The placenta is probably the major source of this hormone at term.[196]

17α-hydroxyprogesterone concentrations are less than 0.5 ng/ml during the follicular phase of normal menstrual cycles. In conceptual cycles, 17α-hydroxyprogesterone concentrations rise to about 1 ng/ml on the day of the LH peak, fall slightly for about 1 day, rise again over the subsequent 4 to 5 days to a level of 1 to 2 ng/ml, and then increase gradually to a mean of approximately 2 ng/ml (luteal phase levels) at the end of 12 weeks. This level remains relatively stable until gestational age of about 32 weeks when there begins an abrupt sustained rise to a mean at 37 weeks of approximately 7 ng/ml, a level that persists until term[196] (Fig. 2-11). The rise beginning at 32 weeks is strongly correlated with the activity of fetal maturational processes known to begin at this time.

During the first 7 weeks gestation, through the time of the luteal-placental shift, 17α-hydroxyprogesterone concentrations reflect primarily the status of corpus luteum steroidogenesis.[196] In women undergoing spontaneous abortion, falling concentrations of 17α-hydroxyprogesterone parallel falling concentrations of progesterone.[196]

Hormonal Functions During Pregnancy

Progestogens affect tubal motility, the endometrium, uterine vasculature, and parturition.

Tubal Motility The preimplantation conceptus with its surrounding corona cells secretes progesterone long before implantation. Conceptus secreted progesterone may itself affect tubal motility as the conceptus is carried to the uterus.[121] Progesterone, by action mediated through catecholamines and prostaglandins, is believed to relax uterotubal musculature. Estradiol, also secreted by these structures, may balance the progesterone effect so as to maintain the desired level of tubal motility and tone.[121] Excess progesterone, as might occur from pharmacologically induced superovulation, may produce excessive relaxation of tubal musculature and could explain an apparent excess of ectopic pregnancies. Likewise, progesterone deficiency from blighted ova may cause accelerated oviduct transport with premature arrival of these ova to the uterus.

Endometrium Progesterone inhibits T lymphocyte-mediated tissue rejection and is believed to work in concert with hCG and decidual cortisol.[197,198] This inhibition of the rejection response may confer immunological privilege to the implanted conceptus and developing placenta. It has been suggested that placental progesterone protects the pregnancy by inhibiting T lymphocyte mediated tissue rejection responses.[197,198] In rodents, progesterone extends the survival of transplanted human trophoblasts,[198] and high local intervillous concentrations of progesterone are of major importance in blocking the cellular immune rejection of the foreign protein originating from the pregnancy.[198]

Uterine Vasculature Progesterone antagonizes estrogen-augmented uterine blood flow through depletion of cytoplasmic estrogen receptors.[199] Estrogen and progesterone appear to balance one another in the maintenance of blood flow at the implantation site.

Parturition Control Progesterone and the estrogens are antagonistic in the parturition process. Progesterone produces uterine relaxation,[189] stabilizing lysosomal membranes and inhibiting prostaglandin synthesis and release. By contrast, estrogens labilize lysosomal membranes and augment the synthesis of prostaglandins and their release.[188]

Although gradual increase in cord DHEA-S and maternal estriol occurs toward term, there is no corresponding drop in either fetal or maternal progesterone concentrations.[200] That progesterone is important in the maintenance of uterine quiescence is not doubted, however, because in the first trimester removal of the corpus luteum leads rapidly to myometrial contractions.[124] Likewise, labor ensues following administration of antiprogesterone compounds in the third trimester.[201] The antiprogesterone agents occupy progesterone receptors and inhibit the action of progesterone, which is clearly essential for maintenance of uterine quiescence. Yet, progesterone administration to women, except for very large doses, does not suppress human uterine contractions once begun.[201]

The ratios of estradiol and progesterone in various animals models are closely related to the stimulation of myometrial gap junction formation.[202]

Adrenocorticoids

Variation During Pregnancy

Fetal plasma cortisol and amniotic fluid cortisol and cortisol sulfate concentrations increase considerably with advancing gestational age and approaching parturition.[203,204] With the exception of the amniotic membranes and decidua, virtually all fetal organs convert cortisol to cortisone.[122,123] The intracellular mechanisms of cortisol-to-cortisone interconversion and its regulatory effect on the biological expression of cortisol are diagrammed in Figure 2-22. As parturition approaches, net conversion of cortisol to cortisone is decreased in many tissues such as fetal lung[204] (Fig. 2-23). As cortisol-to-cortisone conversion decreases, there

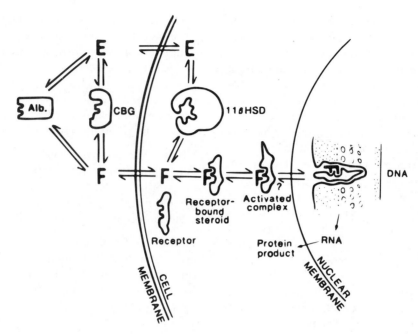

Fig. 2-22 Mechanism of intrauterine cortisol (F) modulation. Target organ cells autoregulate F interaction with corticoid receptors by diverting F to E (cortisone) through 11 β-HSD interconversion. (From Murphy,[122] with permission.)

is increasing circulating cortisol available to maturing fetal tissues.

Target Tissue Interaction During Pregnancy

The profile of circulating adrenocorticoids in the fetoplacental circulation is determined extensively by steroid interconversions between cortisol and cortisone. *The placenta* contains abundant 11-dehydrogenase activity. Although much of circulating fetal cortisol derives from transplacental passage of maternal cortisol, approximately 80 percent of maternal cortisol is converted to cortisone on entering the fetal circulation.[122,123] Corticoid measurements in placental tissues indicate a cortisol-cortisone ratio of far less than 1.0, thus reconfirming active intraplacental conversion of cortisol to cortisone.[122,123]

Chorionic membranes contain an abundance of 11-ketoreductase activity and therefore converts cortisone to cortisol. First detectable at approximately 18 weeks' gestational age, this activity continues through term.[122,123] Activity is also found in the adherent decidua and in the juxtaposed myometrium. As a result of chorionic membrane and uterine peripheral interconversion, the concentration of cortisol in uterine tissues is nine times that detectable in nonpregnant myometrium.[122,123] It is plausible that the maintenance of high cortisol concentrations in myometrium is part of the same immunosuppressive process of pregnancy maintenance that involves hCG and progesterone.[122,123]

Fetal lung contains predominantly 11-dehydrogenase activity and therefore predominantly converts cortisol to cortisone. With advancing gestation, the fetal lung cortisol-to-cortisone interconversion diminishes.[122,123] Lung tissue at birth shows no detectable cortisol-to-cortisone conversion. The net result of this transformation is increased pulmonary intracellular cortisol bioavailability, a process that may be related to maturation of the fetal lung, which is accelerating by 34 to 36 weeks' gestational age.[165]

Hormonal Functions During Pregnancy

Adrenocorticoids impact with particular relevance on regulation of intrauterine maturation. In normally progressing human pregnancy, multiple enzyme systems accelerate, beginning at approximately 32 weeks' gesta-

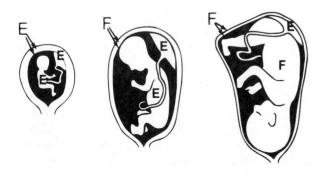

Fig. 2-23 Mechanism of intrauterine cortisol (F) modulation. Net conversion from E shifts toward F approaching term in fetal lung and membranes. (From Murphy,[122] with permission.)

tional age and finishing at approximately 37 weeks' gestational age.[165] Delivery at any time from 37 weeks to term generally produces newborn free of the hazards of prematurity. Although a variety of interdependent hormonal events are involved, the weight of available evidence indicates that fetal cortisol is the major effector in the induction of these final and essential maturational systems involving fetal lung and liver, the nervous system, and the adrenal medulla.[165]

Pregnancy Diagnosis and Monitoring

The novel hormones of pregnancy may be measured for diagnosis and detecting deviations from normal. A variety of assay techniques with varying sensitivities and specificities are available.

Human Chorionic Gonadotropin

There are four groups of hCG configuration that effect performance and interpretation of assays.

Dimeric hCG

Dimeric hCG and both subunits, α-hCG and β-hCG, rise sharply during the first trimester[19] (Figs. 2-7, 2-8A–C). The dimeric hCG is normally measured, either directly by sandwich-type assays or inferentially by detection of the β-subunit for diagnosis and monitoring of early pregnancy. HCG is detectable in serum in approximately 5 percent of patients by 8 days after conception, and in virtually all patients by day 11.[12] Deviation from the normal doubling patterns suggests that the pregnancy is either an ectopic gestation or is undergoing spontaneous abortion. Thus, if hCG fails to rise 66 percent in 2 days, ancillary procedures are necessary to differentiate between the two conditions.[205]

Dimeric and free subunit hCG are produced in the pituitary and released in association with pituitary LH.[206–208] Levels are much higher in postmenopausal women (110 pg/ml versus 10 pg/ml).[208] Nonpregnant levels of hCG are, however, well under the sensitivity (approximately 1 mIU/ml) detectable by the most sensitive clinical assays used in pregnancy monitoring.[208,209]

Free α- and β-hCG Subunits

Following in vitro fertilization and embryo transfer,[19] free β subunit of hCG may be detected as early as 7 days (1 day earlier than intact hCG). Free α-subunits are first detectable at gestational week 6 and rise in sigmoid fashion to peak at 36 weeks gestational age.[19] In general, α-hCG is used rarely for clinical interpretation, although the concentrations are elevated in persistent gestational trophoblastic neoplasia and are significantly lower in insulin-dependent diabetic women. Persistently elevated free β subunits in patients with trophoblastic disease may portend a poor prognosis.[210]

Beta-subunit Core Fragment (β-core)

β-core is a major component of the immunoreactive hCG in urine, particularly during second trimester.[38] β-core circulates in small amounts because of its very short half-life. With a molecular weight of approximately 10.0 kDa, β-core consists of two polypeptide chains, composed of residues 6–40 disulfide bridged to residues 55–92 of the β subunit.[38] β-core is detected by β subunit assays. Despite the conformational differences of hCG measured through the β subunit, assays in either serum or urine of the same patient produce very similar results quantitatively.[38]

Nicked hCG Subunits

Nicked hCG is an hCG subunit with deleted peptide linkages.[210] In the β-subunit these linkages are between residues 47–48 and between 44–45 or 46–47.[210] In the α-subunits, they are between 70–71. As nicking increases, receptor binding decreases.[38] For this reason, nicked hCG is biologically less active. Disparities in levels of nicked vs non-nicked hCG account for major discrepancies in the hormone levels observed with different assay methods.[210–212] Test results between commercial assays are not necessarily interconvertible. For this reason, investigators in this field believe that data involving hCG assay reporting should include information about assay interaction with nicked hCG, free β-subunit, and β-core fragment in this way standards, though not interconvertible, can be interpreted.[212]

HCG Standards

In comparing hCG measurements by different RIAs, the standard must be specified. Two standards are commonly encountered. The Third International Standard (3rd IS), which is the same as First International Reference Preparation, is less contaminated with free α and β subunits of hCG than the Second International Standard (2nd IS). The discrepancy is irrelevant in hCG assays specific for the intact hCG molecule (whole molecule or sandwich assays) because neither detects free β-subunits. However, the standards are important in interpreting results from radioimmunoassays that interact with the β subunit part of the molecule and are therefore unable to destinguish between free subunits and the intact molecule. Thus, the 3rd IS produces values approximately 1.5- to 2-fold greater for β subunit radioimmunoassay than does the 2nd IS.[38] This differ-

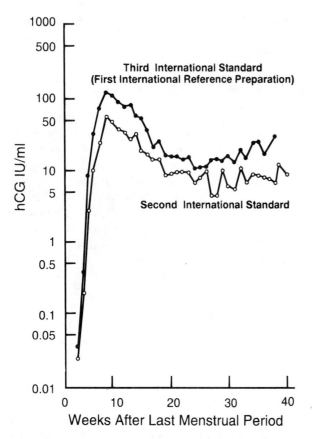

Fig. 2-24 Serum concentrations of hCG measured using the 2nd IS as the reference preparation versus results obtained using the 3rd IS (1st IRP) as the standard in hCG radioimmunoassays. Note the 1.5- to 2-fold greater concentrations of hCG measured using the 3rd IS relative to those obtained with the 2nd IS. (From Ren and Braunstein,[38] with permission.)

ence, more or less uniform throughout pregnancy, is illustrated in Figure 2-24.

HCG Assays

The choice of hCG assay from the variety available depends on the demands required of the test (Table 2-2).

Radioimmunoassay

The RIA is the traditional clinical laboratory technique for measuring hCG though its β subunit.[213] RIAs measure the combined concentrations of free β subunits plus dimeric hCG. HCG is labelled with a radioactive substance and is displaced from binding sites on an antibody directed against it by unlabelled hCG in the patient's serum. If none is displaced, there is no hCG in the patient's serum. If all is displaced, the patient's serum contains a high quantity of hCG. RIAs are quantitative and are useful in determining doubling times, as in the cases of ectopic pregnancy, spontaneous abortion, or gestational trophoblastic neoplasia. Although very precise, the RIA has limited sensitivity, requires hours to perform, and involves radioisotopes.[213] Thus, RIAs are being replaced by the technically simpler immunoradiometric assay (IRMA).

Immunoradiometric Assay

IRMA uses a sandwich principle to detect intact hCG (whole molecule assay). IRMA hCG assays require only about 30 minutes to complete and can detect very low concentrations of hCG.[214] IRMAs use a radioactive antibody to detect hCG in the serum. Briefly, anti-hCG antibodies are bound to a test tube, the patient's serum is added, and a second labelled antibody binds to the hCG-antibody complex already on the tube. The amount of labelled antibody bound to the tube is proportional to the amount of hCG in the patient's serum. The hCG molecule is thus "sandwiched" between two antibodies.[214] This "sandwich" assay is also the principle used in the nonradioactive enzyme linked immunosorbent assay (ELISA).

Enzyme Linked Immunosorbent Assay

ELISAs do not use radioisotopes.[215] The principle is the same as that of IRMA but instead of using a radiolabelled second antibody, the second antibody is labelled with a substance that can be detected by a color change after binding. Although not as precise, the assay is sensi-

Table 2-2 Commercial Assays Available for Detection and Measurements of hCG

Technique	Sensitivity (mIU/ml)	Time to Complete Test (Minutes)	Gestational Age When First Positive (Weeks)	Tests Available
RIA	5	4 hours	3–4	Many Products Available
IRMA	150	30	4	Neocept
	1500	2	5	Pregnosis
ELISA	25	80	3.5	Model
	<50	15	4	Sensichrome, Quest
	<50	5	4	Confidot, Test Pack, Icon
	175	20	4–5	Preganstick
FIA	1	2–3 hours	3.5	Opus hCG; Stratus hCG

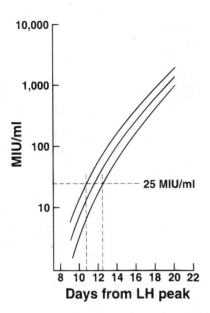

Fig. 2-25 Levels of circulating HCG in early pregnancy showing that an assay with a sensitivity of 25 mIU/ml would become positive in some subjects 10 to 11 days after the LH peak and in most subjects 12 to 13 days after the LH peak. (From Chard,[217] with permission.)

tive and quick, making it ideal for early pregnancy diagnosis. ELISAs can detect hCG at concentrations as low as 10 mIU/ml allowing for diagnosis up to 5 days before the first missed menses.[215] These assays are easily packaged for use in a physician's offices.

Fluoroimmunoassay

This technique is another "sandwich" assay, in which second antibody is tagged with a fluorescent label. The fluorescence emitted, proportional to the amount of hCG in the test serum, allows for detection of concentrations as low as 1 mIU/ml.[216] The technique takes 2 to 3 hours, uses no radioactivity, and is highly precise. FIA is used to detect and follow hCG concentrations.

Clinical Application of hCG Measurements

Pregnancy Diagnosis

HCG is first detectable in maternal blood at approximately 8 to 11 days after conception using very sensitive research assays (sensitivity 0.1 to 0.3 mIU/ml).[12,13,19] Most state-of-the-art pregnancy tests, however, have a sensitivity of 25 mIU/ml).[217] Time of detection is related to assay sensitivity[217] (Fig. 2-25).

False positive results occur in the range of 5 to 25 mIU/ml. False positive results can occur in perimenopausal and postmenopausal women because of endogenous pituitary hCG secretion, which occurs in synchrony with LH. For practical purposes, a level of less than 5 mIU/ml can be confidently stated as negative. A level exceeding 25 mIU/ml can be confidently stated as positive.[217] When there is uncertainty, repeating the test in 2 days normally confirms a trend upwards, which documents the existence of a pregnancy.

Ectopic Pregnancy

With rare exceptions, patients with ectopic pregnancy have hCG titers exceeding 20 mIU/ml (3rd IS standard); 98 percent titers exceeding 40 mIU/ml. Serial hCGs, in combination with vaginal ultrasound and serum progesterone measurements, are used widely for nonsurgical diagnosis of ectopic pregnancy.[217]

Spontaneous Abortion

Serum hCG fails to double or falls in patients with spontaneous abortion. Serial hCG showing an abnormally slow rise, or decrease may portend spontaneous abortion.

Screening for Fetal Down Syndrome

HCG concentrations are elevated in women carrying a fetus affected with Down syndrome.[218] This finding has been used in various calculations using maternal age, AFP levels, and hCG concentrations, with or without unconjugated estriol to estimate risk of carrying an affected fetus. Using serum analytes, one can identify approximately two thirds of affected fetuses with a 6 percent false positive (amniocentesis) rate.[38,218] β Subunits of hCG have been touted by some markers superior as to intact hCG measurements; however, this is contentious in the second trimester.[38,218,219]

Gestational Trophoblastic Disease

Serial hCG measurements are used to monitor therapy for gestational trophoblastic disease. Disappearance of hCG is used to predict the course of the disease.[220]

Early Pregnancy Factor

Pregnancy diagnosis before implantation may be possible through measurement of EPF, which is detectable 24 to 48 hours after fertilization. EPF cannot be detected 24 hours after delivery or termination of either an ectopic or intrauterine pregnancy[1-4] (Fig. 2-6).

Detection of EPF currently depends on a cumbersome biologic assay, the rosette inhibition test.[1-4] Although recently EPF has been isolated, identified, and sequenced, the exact nature of the molecular species is uncertain and clinical assays are not yet available.[1-4]

Diagnosis of conception before implantation will open possibilities for contraception, preimplantation genetics through uterine lavage, and highly accurate dating of intrauterine pregnancies.

Table 2-3 Gestational Age at Which Embryologic
Structures Are Detectable by Vaginal Ultrasound

Embryonic/Fetal Structure	Gestational Age of Detection
Gestational sac	4 weeks, 1–3 days
Yolk sac	5 weeks
Fetal heartbeats	5 weeks, 6 days
Limb buds	8 weeks
Head	8 weeks
Ventricles	8 weeks, 2–4 days
Choroid plexus	9 weeks
Hand, fingers	12 weeks

(Modified from Timor-Tritsch and Rottem,[224] with permission.)

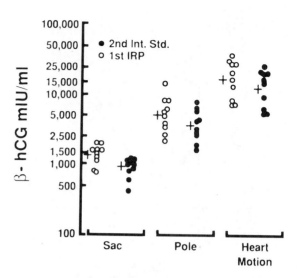

Fig. 2-26 Range of β-hCG titers (IRP) and predicted developmental landmarks detected by vaginal ultrasound. (From Jost,[134] with permission.)

Progesterone

Single progesterone measurements in the first trimester are useful in screening for ectopic pregnancy and spontaneous abortion. A single progesterone measurement of less than or equal to 5 ng/ml rules out a viable intrauterine pregnancy[194,221,222]; a progesterone value of less than or equal to 5 ng/ml thus, allows the physician to perform a dilatation and curettage without fear of interfering with a viable pregnancy.[194] If villi are found, the patient is unlikely to have an ectopic pregnancy.[144] A value 25 ng/ml or more rules out 98 percent of ectopic pregnancies.[194] Values between 5 and 25 ng/ml are problematic and require further investigation with ultrasound.[222]

RIAs are available to measure progesterone. Most require 3 to 4 hours. FIAs are also available to measure progesterone and offer the advantage of avoiding radioactivity. A rapid ELISA assay (dipstick) has recently been developed that allows quick identification in the office of pregnant women with progesterone levels of <15 ng/ml.[223] This type of test may be useful for screening large numbers of women at high risk for spontaneous abortion and ectopic pregnancy.

Combined Ultrasound and Hormone Measurements

Combined with hCG and progesterone, ultrasound is helpful in determining the viability and location of a pregnancy.[224,225] Transvaginal ultrasound allows detection of an intrauterine pregnancy as early as 4 weeks from the last menstrual period, when a gestational sac measures 4 to 5 mm[224] (Table 2-3). At 5 gestational weeks, the yolk sac becomes visible; at the end of the fifth week, transvaginal ultrasound detects all intrauterine pregnancies with a 95 percent confidence limit.[224,225] Fetal cardiac activity is detected just before 6 gestational weeks. In a well-timed pregnancy, these ultrasonic milestones are useful in detecting deviations from the norm. Table 2-4 lists the appearance of key embryologic findings associated with rising hCG.[225] When combined with serum measurements of hCG, ultrasonographic findings are vital in the diagnosis of an ectopic gestation and impending abortion.[224,225]

Using transabdominal ultrasound, all patients with a healthy intrauterine pregnancy whose hCG measured 6,500 mIU/ml had a gestational sac visible by ultrasound.[205] Similarly, transvaginal ultrasound visualizes all intrauterine pregnancies when the hCG exceeds 2,400 mIU/ml[225] (Fig. 2-26). When hCG levels exceed

Table 2-4 Appearance of Key Embryologic Structures in Association with Rising hCG Titers

Ultrasound Findings	Days from LMP	β-hCG (mIU/ml)	
		Third International Standard[a]	Second International Standard
Sac	34.8 ± 2.2	1,398 ± 155	914 ± 106
Fetal pole	40.3 ± 3.4[b]	5,113 ± 298[b]	3,783 ± 683
Fetal heart motion	46.9 ± 6.0[b]	17,208 ± 3,772[b]	13,178 ± 2,898[b]

Note: Failure to identify these structures in the uterus as hCG rises above these levels suggests ectopic pregnancy.
[a] Third International standard equal first international reference preparation.
[b] p < 0.05 when compared with sac.
(From Fossum et al.,[225] with permission.)

these concentrations and no intrauterine pregnancy is detectable by ultrasound, either uterine curettage to exclude villi or laparoscopy for visualization is necessary to diagnose an ectopic pregnancy.[225] Conversely, a heartbeat detected at 8 gestational weeks assures a patient that her chances of continuing her pregnancy is 98 percent.[225] Algorithms have been devised utilizing rapid progesterone assay, serial β-hCG, and ultrasound to diagnose ectopic pregnancy nonsurgically. This has been particularly important with the recent advancement of medical therapy for this condition; whereby laparoscopy is eschewed.[222]

Conclusions

No biological events can exceed the events considered in this chapter in the long-term importance to human development. Endocrine factors play important roles in the orchestration and outcome of these events. It is a privilege to detect, measure, observe, and occasionally assist nature in the nourishment and protection of the growing fetus in the otherwise invisible confines of the uterus.

10 Key Points

- Beginning with conception, a series of proteins specific for and secreted only during pregnancy evolve to facilitate invasion of half-foreign embryonic tissue into the uterine wall.

- Cytotrophoblasts, secreting hypothalamic peptides, function in juxtaposition to syncytiotrophoblast, secreting the corresponding pituitary-like peptides in an anatomic arrangement analogous to the hypothalamic–pituitary axis.

- Placental GnRH stimulates placental hCG production and release.

- Secretion of placental CRH and ACTH into the maternal circulation induces hypercortisolism mediated through the maternal hypothalamic–pituitary axis.

- hCG maintains the corpus luteum, stimulates adrenal and placental steroidogenesis, and modulates maternal immunologic response to the pregnancy.

- Human chorionic somatomammotropin antagonizes insulin action and induces maternal glucose intolerance, which promotes transfer of glucose and amino acids into the fetus.

- Decidual prolactin, a peptide similar to pituitary prolactin, regulates fluid and electrolyte flux through the fetal membranes; it is secreted independently of fetal or maternal dopaminergic control.

- Placental protein 14 (PP14), an immunosuppressive peptide, is synthesized in decidualized endometrium and may serve as a circulating marker of decidual growth.

- Progesterone secreted by the preimplantation conceptus modulates tubal motility in early pregnancy; progesterone secreted by the placenta inhibits maternal-fetal tissue rejection, antagonizes the effect of estrogen in augmenting uterine blood flow, and induces uterine relaxation before parturition.

- When pregnancy tests are set to high sensitivity (<1 mlU/ml) of hCG, false positives can occur because of endogenous pituitary hCG, which is released in synchrony with pituitary LH and is detected in the assay.

References

1. Morton H, Cavanagh AC, Athanasas-Platsis S, Quinn KA: Early pregnancy factor has immunosuppressive and growth factor properties. Reprod Fertil Dev 4:411, 1992
2. Morton H, Rolfe BE, Cavanagh AC: Pregnancy proteins: basic concepts and clinical applications. Sem Reprod Endocrinol 10:72, 1992
3. Cavanagh AC, Morton H, Rolfe BE, Gidley-Baird AA:

Ovum factor: a first signal of pregnancy? Am J Reprod Immuno 2:97, 1982

4. Morton H, Rolfe BE, Cavanagh AC: Ovum factor and early pregnancy factor. Curr Top Dev Biol 23:73, 1987

5. Croxatto HB, Ortiz ME, Diaz S et al: Studies on the duration of egg transport by the human oviduct, II: ovum location at various times following luteinizing hormone peak. Am J Obstet Gynecol 132:629, 1978

6. Buster JE, Bustillo M, Rodi IA et al: Biological and morphologic development of donated human ova recovered by nonsurgical uterine lavage. Am J Obstet Gynecol 153:211, 1985

7. Bonduelle ML, Liebaers DR, Van Steiteghem A et al: Chorionic gonadotrophin-beta mRNA, a trophoblast marker, is expressed in human 8-cell embryos derived from tripronucleate zygotes. Human Reprod 3:909, 1988

8. Lopata A, Hay DL: The surplus human embryo: its potential for growth, blastulation, hatching, and human chorionic gonadotropin production in culture. Fertil Steril 51:984, 1989

9. Hay DL, Lopata A: Chorionic gonadotropin secretion by human embryos in vitro. J Clin Endocrinol Metab 67:1322, 1988

10. Enders AC: Embryo implantation, with emphasis on the Rhesus monkey and the human. Reproduction 5:163, 1981

11. Navot D, Scott RT, Droesch K, Veeck LL et al: The window of embryo transfer and the efficiency of human conception in vitro. Fertil Steril 55:114, 1991

12. Lenton EA, Neal LM, Sulaiman R: Plasma concentrations of human chorionic gonadotropin from the time of implantation until the second week of pregnancy. Fertil Steril 37:773, 1982

13. Kosasa T, Levesque L, Goldstein DP, Taymor ML: Early detection of implantation using a radioimmunoassay specific for human chorionic gondotropin. J Clin Endocrinol Metab 36:622, 1973

14. Chard T: Proteins of the human placenta: some general concepts. p. 6. In Grudzinskas JG, Teisner BL, Sepala M (eds): Pregnancy Proteins: Biology, Chemistry and Clinical Application. Academic Press, San Diego, 1982

15. Saijonmaa O, Laatikaninen T, Wahlstrom T: Corticotrophin-releasing factor in human placenta: localization, concentration and release in vitro. Placenta 9:373, 1988

16. Khodr GS, Siler-Khodr TM: Placental luteinizing hormone-releasing factor and its synthesis. Science 207:315, 1980

17. Shambaugh G III, Kubek M, Wilber JF: Thyrotrophin-releasing hormone activity in the human placenta. J Clin Endocrinol Metab 48:483, 1979

18. Al-Timimi A, Fox H: Immunohistochemical localization of follicle-stimulating hormone, luteinizing hormone, growth hormone, adrenocorticotropic hormone and prolactin in the human placenta. Placenta 7:163, 1986

19. Hay DL: Placental histology and the production of human choriogonadotropin and its subunits in pregnancy. Brit Obstet Gynecol 95:1268, 1988

20. Harada A, Hershman JM: Extraction of human chori-

onic thyrotropin (hCT) from term placentas: failure to recover thyrotropic activity. J Clin Endocrinol Metab 47:681, 1978

21. Steiner DF: Peptide hormone precursors: biosynthesis, processing, and significance. p. 49. In Parson JA (ed): Peptide Hormones. University Park Press, Baltimore, 1976

22. Hoshina M, Hussa R, Pattillo R et al: The role of trophoblast differentiation in the control of the hCG and hPL genes. Adv Exp Med Biol 176:299, 1984

23. Hoshina M, Boime I, Mochizuki M: Cytological localization of hPL, hCG, and mRNA in chorionic tissue using in situ hybridization. Acta Obstet Gynecol Jpn 36:397, 1984

24. Kurman RJ, Young RH, Norris HJ et al: Immunocytochemical localization of placental lactogen and chorionic gonadotropin in the normal placenta and trophoblastic tumors, with emphasis on intermediate trophoblast and the placental site trophoblastic tumor. Int J Gynecol Pathol 3:101, 1984

25. Kasai K, Shik SS, Yoshida Y: Production and localization of human prolactin in placenta and decidua in early and at term normal pregnancy. Nippon Naibunpi Gakkai Zasshi 56:1574, 1980

26. Watkins WB, Yen SS: Somatostatin in cytotrophoblast of the immature human placenta: localization by immunoperoxidase cytochemistry. J Clin Endocrinol Metab 50:969, 1980

27. Chard T, Grudzinskas JG: Pregnancy protein secretion. Semin Reprod Endocrinol 10:61, 1992

28. Cavanagh AC, Morton H: The purification of early-pregnancy factor to homogeneity from human platelets and identification as chaperonin 10. Eur J Biochem 222:551, 1994

29. Di Trapani G, Orosco C, Perkins A, Clarke F: Isolation from human placental extracts of a preparation possessing 'early pregnancy factor' activity and identification of the polypeptide components. Hum Reprod 6:450, 1991

30. Zuo X, Su B, Wei D: Isolation and characterization of early pregnancy factor. Chin Med Sci J 9:34, 1994

31. Mehta AR, Eessalu TE, Aggarwal BB: Purification and characterization of early pregnancy factor from human pregnancy sera. J Biol Chem 264:2266, 1989

32. Clarke FM: Identification of molecules and mechanisms involved in the 'early pregnancy factor' system. Reprod Fertil Dev 4:423, 1992

33. Chard T, Grudzinskas JG: Early pregnancy factor. Biol Res Pregnancy 8:53, 1987

34. Mesrogli M, Schneider J, Maas DHA: Early pregnancy factor as a marker for the earliest stages of pregnancy in infertile women. Hum Reprod 3:113, 1988

35. Shahani SK, Moniz CL, Bordekar AD et al: Early pregnancy factor as a marker for assessing embryonic viability in threatened and missed abortions. Gynecol Obstet Invest 37:73, 1994

36. Straube W, Romer T, Zeenni L, Loh M: The early pregnancy factor (EPF) as an early marker of disorders in pregnancy. Zentralbl Gynakol 117:32, 1995

37. Hubel V, Straube W, Loh M et al: Human early preg-

nancy factor and early pregnancy associated protein before and after therapeutic abortion in comparison with beta-hCG, estradiol, progesterone and 17-hydroxyprogesterone. Exp Clin Endocrinol 94:171, 1989

38. Ren SG, Braunstein GD: Human chorionic gonadotropin. Semin Reprod Endocrinol 10:95, 1992

39. Barnea ER, Kaplan M: Spontaneous, gonadotropin-releasing hormone-induced, and progesterone-inhibited pulsatile secretion of human chorionic gonadotrophin in the first trimester placenta in vitro. J Clin Endocrinol Metab 69:215, 1989

40. Jones SA, Brooks AN, Challis JR: Steroids modulate corticotropin-releasing hormone production in human fetal membranes and placenta. J Clin Endocrinol Metab 68:825, 1989

41. Kato Y, Braunstein GD: Discordant secretion of placental protein hormones in differentiating trophoblasts in vitro. J Clin Endocrinol Metab 68:814, 1989

42. Mersol-Barg MS, Miller KF, Choi CM et al: Inhibin suppresses human chorionic gonadotropin secretion in term, but not first trimester, placenta. J Clin Endocrinol Metab 71:1294, 1990

43. Hanson FW, Powell JE, Stevens VC: Effects of hCG and human pituitary LH on steroid secretion and functional life of the human corpus luteum. J Clin Endocrinol Metab 32:211, 1971

44. Seron-Ferre M, Lawrence CC, Jaffee RB: Role of hCG in the regulation of the fetal adrenal gland. J Clin Endocrinol Metab 46:834, 1978

45. Huhtaniemi IT, Korenbrot CC, Jaffee RB: HCG binding and stimulation of testosterone biosynthesis in the human fetal testis. J Clin Endocrinol Metab 44:963, 1977

46. Adcock EW III, Teasdale F, August CS et al: Human chorionic gonadotropin: its possible role in maternal lymphoctye suppression. Science 181:845, 1973

47. Nisula BC, Ketelslegers JM: Thyroid stimulating activity and chorionic gonadotropin. J Clin Invest 54:494, 1974

48. Rees LH, Burke CW, Chard T et al: Possible placental origin of ACTH in normal human pregnancy. Nature 254:620, 1975

49. Genazzani AR, Fraioli F, Hurlimann J, Fioretti P, Felber JP: Immunoreactive ACTH and cortisol plasma levels during pregnancy. Detection and partial purification of corticotrophin-like placental hormone: the human chorionic corticotrophin (HCC). Clin Endocrinol 4:1, 1975

50. Petraglia F, Sawchenko PE, Rivier J, Vale W: Evidence for local stimulation of ACTH secretion by corticotropin-releasing factor in human placenta. Nature 328:717, 1987

51. Nolten WE, Reckert PA: Elevated free cortisol index in pregnancy: possible regulatory mechanism. Am J Obstet Gynecol 139:492, 1981

52. Prager D, Weber MM, Herman-Bonert V: Placental growth factors and releasing/inhibiting peptides. Semin Reprod Endocrinol 10:83, 1992

53. Robinson BG, Emanuel RL, Frim DM et al: Glucocorticoid stimulates expression of corticotropin-releasing hormone gene in human placenta. Proc Natl Acad Sci USA 85:5244, 1988

54. Niall HD, Hogan ML, Sauer R et al: Sequences of pituitary and placental lactogenic and growth hormones: evolution from a primordial peptide by gene reduplication. Proc Natl Acad Sci USA 68:866, 1971

55. Handwerger S, Brar A: Placental lactogen, placental growth horomone, and decidual prolactin. Sem Reprod Endocrinol 10:106, 1992

56. Walker WH, Fitzpatrick SL, Barrera-Saldana HA et al: The human placental lactogen genes: structure function, evolution and transcriptional regulation. Endo Soc 4:316, 1991

57. Braunstein GD, Rasor JL, Wade ME: Interrelationships of human chorionic gonadotropin, human placental lactogen, and pregnancy specific beta-1 glycoprotein throughout normal human gestation. Am J Obstet Gynecol 138:1205, 1980

58. Kim YJ, Felig P: Plasma human chorionic somatomammotropin levels during starvation in midpregnancy. J Clin Endocrinol Metab 32:864, 1971

59. Furlanetto RW, Underwood LE, Van Wyk JJ, Handwerger S: Serum immunoreactive somatomedin-C is elevated late in pregnancy. J Clin Endocrinol Metab 47:695, 1978

60. Yen SCC: Endocrinology of pregnancy. p. 382. In Creasy RK, Resnick R (eds.): Maternal–Fetal Medicine: Principles and Practice. Vol. 2. WB Saunders, Philadelphia, 1989

61. Simon P, Decoster C, Brocas H et al: Absence of human chorionic somatomammotropin during pregnancy associated with two types of gene deletion. Hum Genet 74:235, 1986

62. Youngblood WW, Humm J, Kizer S: Thyrotropin-releasing hormone-like bioactivity in placenta: evidence for the existence of substances other than Pyroglu-His-Pro-NH2 (TRH) capable of stimulating pituitary thyrotropin release. Endocrinol 106:541, 1980

63. Taliadourous GS, Canfield RE, Nisula BC: Thyroid-stimulating activity of chorionic gonadotropin and luteinizing hormone. J Clin Endocrinol Metab 47:855, 1978

64. Chrousos GP, Calabrese JR, Avgerinos P et al: Corticotropin releasing factor: basic studies and clinical applications. Prog Neuropsychopharmacol Biol Psychiatry 9:349, 1985

65. Stalla GK, Hartwimmer J, von-Werder K et al: Ovine (o) and human (h) corticotropin releasing factor (CRF) in man: CRF-stimulation and CRF-immunoreactivity. Acta Endocrinol (Copenh) 106:289, 1984

66. Shibahara S, Morimoto, Furutani Y et al: Isolation and sequence analysis of the human corticotropin-releasing factor precursor gene. EMBO J 2:775, 1983

67. Stalla GK, Bost H, Stalla J et al: Human corticotropin-releasing hormone during pregnancy. Gynecol Endocrinol 3:1, 1989

68. Laatikainen TJ, Raisanen IJ, Salminen KR: Corticotropin-releasing hormone in amniotic fluid during gestation and labor and in relation to fetal lung maturation. Am J Obstet Gynecol 159:891, 1988

69. Linton EA, Perkins AV, Woods RJ et al: Corticotropin releasing hormone-binding protein (CRH-BP): plasma levels decrease during the third trimester of normal human pregnancy. J Clin Endocrinol Metab 76:260, 1993

70. Sug-Tang A, Bocking AD, Brooks AN et al: Effects of restricting uterplacental blood flow on concentrations of corticotrophin-releasing hormone, adrenocortico-trophin, cortisol, and prostaglandin E2 in the sheep fetus during late pregnancy. Can J Physiol Pharmacol 70:1396, 1992

71. Clifton VL, Read MA, Leitch IM et al: Corticotrophin-releasing hormone-induced vasodilation in the human fetal placental circulation. J Clin Endocrinol Metab 79:666, 1994

72. Perkins AV, Linton EA, Eben F et al: Corticotrophin-releasing hormone and corticotrophin-releasing hormone binding protein in normal and pre-eclamptic human pregnancies. Br J Obstet Gynaecol 10:118, 1995

73. Goland RS, Jozak S, Warren WB et al: Elevated levels of umbilical cord plasma corticotropin-releasing hormone in growth-retarded fetuses. J Clin Endocrinol Metab 77:1174, 1993

74. Ruth V, Hallman M, Laatikainen T: Corticotropin-releasing hormone and cortisol in cord plasma in relation to gestational age, labor, and fetal distress. Am J Perinatol 10:115, 1993

75. Goland RS, Conwell IM, Warren WB, Wardlaw SL: Placental corticotropin-releasing hormone and pituitary-adrenal function during pregnancy. Neuroendocrinology 56:742, 1992

76. Macaron C, Kyncl M, Rutsky L et al: Failure of somatostatin to affect human chorionic somatomammotropin and human chorionic gonadotropin secretion in vitro. J Clin Endocrinol Metab 47:1141, 1978

77. Youngblood WW, Humm J, Kizer S: Thyrotropin-releasing hormone-like bioactivity in placenta: evidence for the existence of substances other than Pyroglu-His-Pro-NH2 (TRH) capable of stimulating pituitary thyrotropin release. Endocrinology 106:541, 1980

78. Taliadouros GS, Canfield RE, Nisula BC: Thyroid-stimulating activity of chorionic gonadotropin and luteinizing hormone. J Clin Endocrinol Metab 47:855, 1978

79. Petraglia F, Sawchenko P, Lim ATW et al: Localization, secretion, and action of inhibin in human placenta. Science 237:187, 1987

80. Abe Y, Hasegawa Y, Miyamoto K et al: High concentration of plasma immunoreactive inhibin during normal pregnancy in women. J Clin Endocrinol Metab 71:133, 1990

81. Tovanabutra S, Illingworth PJ, Ledger WL et al: The relationship between peripheral immunoactive inhibin, human chorionic gonadotrophin, oestradiol and progesterone during human pregnancy. Clin Endocrinol 38:101, 1993

82. Muttukrishna S, George L, Fowlert PA et al: Measurement of serum concentrations of inhibin-A (α-β_A dimer) during human pregnancy. Clin Endocrinol 42:391, 1995

83. Khong TY, Healy DL, Findlay JK, de Kretser DM: Inhibin and the human placenta: a critique. Reprod Fertil Dev 3:391, 1991

84. Mills NC, D'Ercole AJ, Underwood LE, Ilan J: Synthesis of somatomedin C/insulin-like growth factor I by human placenta. Molecular Biol Reports 11:231, 1986

85. Jonas HA, Harrison LC: The human placenta contains two distinct binding and immunoreactive species of insulin-like growth factor-I receptors. J Biol Chem 260:2288, 1985

86. Grizzard JD, D'Ercole AJ, Wilkins JR et al: Affinity-labeled somatomedin-C receptors and binding proteins from the human fetus. J Clin Endocrinol Metab 58:535, 1984

87. Altman DJ, Schneider SL, Thompson DA et al: A transforming growth factor beta 2 (TGF-beta 2)-like immunosuppressive factor in amniotic fluid and localization of TGF-beta 2 mRNA in the pregnant uterus. J Exp Med 172:1391, 1990

88. Brown MJ, Cook CL, Henry JL, Schultz GS: Levels of epidermal growth factor binding in third-trimester and term human placentas: elevated binding in term placentas of male fetuses. Amer J Obstet Gynecol 156:716, 1987

89. Lenton EA, Grudzinskas JG, Gordon YB et al: Pregnancy specific β_1-glycoprotein and chorionic gonadotropin in early pregnancy. Acta Obstet Gynecol Scand 60:489, 1981

90. Chou JY, Plouzek CA: Pregnancy-specific β_1-glycoprotein. Sem Reprod Endocrinol 10:116, 1992

91. Tatarinov YS: Trophoblast-specific beta-glycoprotein as a marker for pregnancy and malignancies. Gynecol Obstet Invest 9:65, 1978

92. Sinosich MJ, Teisner B, Folkersen J et al: Radioimmunoassay for pregnancy associated plasma protein. Clin Chem 28:50, 1982

93. Bischof Paul: Pregnancy-associated plasma protein-A. Sem Reprod Endcrinol 10:127, 1992

94. Obiekwe B, Pendlebury DJ, Gordon YB et al: The radioimmunoassay of placental protein 5 and circulating levels in maternal blood in the third trimester of normal pregnancy. Clin Chim Acta 95:509, 1979

95. Salem HT, Seppala M, Chard T: The effect of thrombin on serum placental protein 5 (PP5): is PP5 the naturally occurring antithrombin III of the human placenta? Placenta 2:205, 1981

96. Maslar IA, Ansbacher R: Effects of progesterone on decidual prolactin production by organ cultures of human endometrium. Endocrinol 118:2102, 1986

97. Raabe MA, MCoshen JA: Epithelial regulation of prolactin effect on amnionic premeability. Am J Obstet Gynecol 154:130, 1986

98. Clements JA, Reyes FI, Winter JS, Faiman C: Studies on human sexual development, IV: fetal pituitary and serum, and amniotic fluid concentrations of prolactin. J Clin Endocrinol Metab 44:408, 1977

99. Luciano AA, Varner MW: Decidual, amniotic fluid, maternal and fetal prolactin in normal and abnormal pregnancies. Obstet Gynecol 63:384, 1984

100. Pullano JG, Cohen-Addad N, Apuzzio JJ et al: Water and salt conservation in the human fetus and newborn,

I: evidence for a role of fetal prolactin. J Clin Endocrinol Metabl 69:1180, 1989

101. Golander A, Kopel R, Lazebnik N et al: Decreased prolactin secretion by decidual tissue of pre-eclampsia in vitro. Acta Endocrinol 108:111, 1985

102. Healy DL, Herington AC, O'Herlihy C: Chronic polyhydramnios is a syndrome with a lactogen receptor defect in the chorion laeve. Brit J Obstet Gynecol 92:461, 1985

103. McCoshen JA, Barc J: Prolactin bioactivity following decidual synthesis and transport by amniochorion. Am J Obstet Gynecol 153:217, 1985

104. Weiss G, O'Byrne EM, Hochman J et al: Distribution of relaxin in women during pregnancy. Obstet Gynecol 52:569, 1978

105. Fields PA, Larkin LH: Purification and immunohistochemical localization of relaxin in the human term placenta. J Clin Endocrinol Metab 52:79, 1981

106. Goldsmith LT, Weiss G, Steinetz BG: Relaxin and its role in pregnancy. Endocrinol Metab Clin North Am 24:171, 1995

107. Rutanen EM, Bohn H, Seppala M: Radioimmunoassay of placental protein 12: levels in amniotic fluid, cord blood, and serum of healthy adults, pregnant women, and patients with trophoblastic disease. Am J Obstet Gynecol 144:460, 1982

108. Rutanen E-M: Insulin-like growth factor binding protein-1. Sem Reprod Endocrinol 10:154, 1992

109. Seppala M, Riittinen L, Kamarainen M et al: Placental protein 14/progesterone-associated endometrial protein revisited. Sem Reprod Endocrinol 10:164, 1992

110. Julkunen M, Rutanen EM, Koskimies A et al: Distribution of placental protein 14 in tissues and body fluids during pregnancy. Br J Obstet Gynecol 92:1145, 1985

111. Seppala M, Julkunen M, Koistinen R et al: Proteins in the human endometrium. In: Naftolin F, DeChemey AH (eds): The Control of Follicle Development, Ovulation and Luteal Function: Lessons from In Vitro Fertilization. Serono Symposia publications, Raven Press 35:101, 1987

112. Alpert E, Drysdale JW, Isselbacher KJ et al: Human fetoprotein: isolation, characterization, and demonstration of microheterogeneity. J Biol Chem 247:3792, 1972

113. Gitlin D, Perricelli A, Gitlin GM: Synthesis of fetoprotein by liver, yolk sac, and gastrointestinal tract of the human conceptus. Cancer Res 32:979, 1972

114. Habib ZA: Maternal serum alpha-feto-protein: its value in antenatal diagnosis of genetic disease and in obstetrical-gynaecological care. Acta Obstet Gynecol Scand 61:1, 1977

115. Murgita RA, Tomasi TB Jr: Suppression of the immune response by alpha-fetoprotein on the primary and secondary antibody response. J Exp Med 141:269, 1975

116. Ferguson-Smith MA, May HM, Vince JD et al: Avoidance of anencephalic and spina bifida births by maternal serum-alphafetoprotein screening. Lancet 1:330, 1978

117. Wald N, Cuckle H: AFP and age screening for Down syndrome. Am J Med Genet 31:197, 1988

118. Shutt DA, Lopata A: The secretion of hormones during the culture of human preimplantation embryos with corona cells. Fertil Steril 35:413, 1981

119. Laufer N, DeCherney AH, Haseltine FP et al: Steriod secretion by the human egg—corona cumulus complex in culture. J Clin Endocrinol Metab 58:1153, 1984

120. Tulchinsky D, Hobel CJ: Plasma human chorionic gonadotropin, estrone, estradiol, estriol, progesterone, and 17-hydroxyprogesterone in human pregnancy, III: early normal pregnancy. Am J Obstet Gynecol 117:884, 1973

121. Punnonen R, Lukola A: Binding of estrogen and progestin in the human fallopian tube. Fertil Steril 36:610, 1981

122. Murphy BEP: Cortisol economy in the human fetus. p. 509. In James VHT, Serio M, Gusti G et al (eds): The Endocrine Function of the Human Adrenal Cortex. Academic Press, San Diego, 1978

123. Murphy BEP: Cortisol and cortisone in human fetal development J Steroid Biochem 11:509, 1979

124. Csapo AI, Pulkkinen MO, Wiest WG: Effects of luteectomy and progesterone replacement therapy in early pregnancy patients. Am J Obstet Gynecol 115:759, 1973

125. Sauer MV, Paulson RJ, Lobo RA: A preliminary report on oocyte donation extending reproductive potential to women over 40. N Engl J Med 323:1157, 1991

126. Sultan KM, Davis OK, Liu HC, Rosenwaks Z: Viable term pregnancy despite "subluteal" serum progesterone levels in the first trimester. Fertil Steril 60:363, 1993

127. Schneider MA, Davies MC, Honour JW: The timing of placental competence in pregnancy after oocyte donation. Fertil Steril 59:1059, 1993

128. Azuma K, Calderon I, Besanko M et al: Is the luteoplacental shift a myth? Analysis of low progesterone levels in successful art pregnancies. J Clin Endocrinol Metabl 77:195, 1993

129. Carr BR, MacDonald PC, Simpson ER: The role of lipoproteins in the regulation of progesterone secretion by the human corpus luteum. Fertil Steril 38:303, 1982

130. Carr BR, MacDonald PC, Simpson ER: The regulation of de novo synthesis of cholesterol in the human fetal adrenal gland by low desity lipoprotein and adrenocorticotropin. Endocrinol 107:1000, 1980

131. Baker BL, Jaffe RB: The genesis of cell types in the adenohypophysis of the human fetus as observed with immunocytochemistry. Am J Anat 143:137, 1975

132. Murphy BEP: Cortisol economy in the human fetus. p 509. In James VHT, Serio M, Gusti G et al (eds): The Endocrine Function of the Human Adrenal Cortex. Academic Press, New York, 1978

133. Johannison E: The foetal adrenal cortex in the human. Acta Endocrinol 58:130, 1968

134. Jost A: The fetal adrenal cortex. p. 426. In Greep RO, Astwood WB (eds): Handbook of Physiology. Vol. 6. Endocrinology Amer Physiol Soc, Washington, DC, 1975

135. Kondo S: Developmental studies on the Japanese human adrenals, I: ponderal growth. Bull Exp Biol 9:51, 1959

136. Spector WS: Handbook of Biological Data. WB Saunders, Philadelphia, 1956

137. Buster J: Fetal adrenal cortex. Clin Obstet Gynecol 23: 803, 1980

138. Dicztalusy E: Steroid metabolism in the feto-placental unit. In Pecile A, Finzi C (eds): The Feto-Placental Unit. Excerpta Medica, Amsterdam, 1969

139. Simpson ER, Carr BR, Parker CR et al: The role of serum lipoproteins in steroidogenesis by the human fetal adrenal cortex. J Clin Endocrinol Metal 49:146, 1979

140. Carr BR, Porter JC, MacDonald PC et al: Metabolism of low density lipoprotein by human fetal-adrenal tissue. Endocrinology 107:1034, 1980

141. Bloch E: Fetal adrenal cortex: function and steroidogensis. In Functions of the Adrenal Cortex. In McKerns KW (ed): Biochemical Endocrinology. Vol. 2. Appleton-Century-Crofts, East Norwalk, 1968

142. Seron-Ferre M, Lawrence CC, Siliteri PK et al: Steroid production by definitive and fetal zones of the human fetal adrenal gland. J Clin Endocrinol Metab 39:269, 1974

143. Winters AG, Oliver C, MacDonald JC et al: Plasma ACTH levels in the human fetus and neonate as related to age and parturition. J Clin Endocrinol Metab 39:269, 1974

144. Walsh SW, Norman RL, Novy MJ: In utero regulation of rhesus monkey fetal adrenals: effects of dexamethasone, adrenocorticotropin, thyrotropin-releasing hormone, prolactin, human chorionic gonadotropin and α-melanocyte stimulating hormone on fetal and maternal plasma steroids. Endocrinology 104:1805, 1979

145. Katikinem M, Davies TF, Catt KJ: Regulation of adrenal and testicular prolactin receptors by adrenocorticotropin and luteinizing hormone. Endocrinology 108: 2367, 1981

146. Winters AJ, Colston C, MacDonal PC et al: Fetal plasma prolactin levels. J Clin Endocrinol Metab 41:626, 1975

147. Pepe GJ, Waddell BJ, Albrecht ED: The effects of adrenocorticotropin and prolactin on adrenal dehydroepiandrosterone secretion in the baboon fetus. Endocrinology 122:646, 1988

148. Albrecht ED, Pepe GJ: Placental steroid horomone biosynthesis in primate pregnancy. Endocr Rev 11:124, 1990

149. Pepe GJ, Albrecht ED: Regulation of the primate fetal adrenal cortex. Endocr Rev 11:151, 1990

150. Carr BR, Porter JC, MacDonald PC et al: Metabolism of low density lipoprotein by human fetal adrenal tissue. Endocrinology 107:1034, 1980

151. Parker RC, Carr BR, Winkel CA et al: Hypercholesterolemia due to elevated low density lipoprotein-cholesterol in newborns with anencephaly and adrenal atrophy. J Clin Endocrinol Metab 57:37, 1983

152. Simpson ER, Carr BR, Parker CR et al: The role of serum lipoproteins in steroidogensis by the human fetal adrenal cortex. J Clin Endocrinol Metab 49:146, 1979

153. Winters AG, Oliver C, MacDonald JE et al: Plasma ACTH levels in the human fetus and neonate as related to age and parturition. J Clin Endocrinol Metab 39:269, 1974

154. Simpson ER, Parker CR, Carr BR: Role of lipoproteins in the regulation of steroidogenesis by the human fetal adrenal. In Jaffe RB, Dell ACqua S (eds): The Endocrine Physiology of Pregnancy and the Preipartal Period. Vol. 21. Serono Symposia Publications. Raven Press, New York, 1985

155. Begot M, Dubois MP, Dubois PM: Growth hormone and ACTH in the pituitary of normal and anencephalic human fetuses: immunocytochemical evidence for hypothalamic influences during development. Neuroendocrinology 24:208, 1977

156. Seron-Ferre M, Lawerence CC, Siliteri PK et al: Steroid production by definitive and fetal zones of the human fetal adrenal gland. J Clin Endocrinol Metab 47:603, 1978

157. Baird AC, Kan DW, Solomon S: Role of pro-opiomelanocortin-derived peptides in the regulation of steroid production of human fetal adrenal cells in culture. Endocrinology 97:357, 1983

158. Bugnon C, Lenys D, Bloch B et al: Cyto-immunologic study of early cell differentiation phenomena in the human fetal anterior pituitary gland. C R Seances Soc Biol Fil 168:460, 1974

159. Winters AJ, Colston C, MacDonald PC et al: Fetal plasma prolactin levels. J Clin Endocrinol Metab 41: 626, 1975

160. Katikineni M, Davies TF, Catt KJ: Regulation of adrenal and testicular prolactin receptors by adrenocorticotropin and luteinizing hormone. Endocrinology 108: 2367, 1981

161. Voutilaimem M, Miller WL: Coordinate tropic hormone regulation of mRNAs rinsulin-like growth factor II and the cholesterol side-chain-cleavage enzyme, P450scc, in human steroidogenic tissues. Pro Natl Acad Sci USA 84: 1590, 1987

162. Pepe GJ, Waddell BJ, Albrecht ED: The effects of adrenocorticotropin and prolactin on adrenal dehydroepiandrosterone secretion in the baboon fetus. Endocrinology 122:646, 1988

163. Johannisson E: The fetal adrenal cortex in the human. Acta Endocrinol 58:130, 1968

164. Seron-Ferre M, Lawrence CC, Jaffe RB: Role of HCG in regulation of the fetal zone of the human fetal adrenal gland. J Clin Endocrinol Metab 46:834, 1978

165. Liggins GC: Endocrinology of the foeto-maternal unit. In Sherman RP (ed): Human Reproductive Physiology. Blackwell Scientific Publications, Oxford, 1972

166. Laatikainen TJ, Raisanen IJ, Salminen KR: Corticotrophin-releasing hormone in amniotic fluid during gestion and labor and in relation to fetal lung maturation. Am J Obstet Gynecol 159:891, 1988

167. Bloch E: Fetal adrenal cortex: function and steroidogenesis. In Functions of the Adrenal Cortex. In Mckerns KW (ed): Biochemical Endocrinology. Vol. 2. Appleton-Century-Crofts, New York, 1968

168. Baggia S, Albrecht ED, Pepe GJ: Regulation of 11 beta-hydroxysteroid dehydrogenase activity in the baboon placenta by estrogen. Endocrinology 126:2742, 1990

169. Naaman E, Chatelain P, Saez JM et al: In vitro effect of insulin and insulin-like growth factor-I on cell multi-

plication and adrenocorticotropin responsiveness of fetal adrenal cells. Biol Reprod 40:570, 1989

170. Hotta M, Baird A: The inhibition of low density lipoprotein metabolism by transforming growth factor-beta mediates its effects on steroidogenesis in bovine adrenocortical cells in vitro. Endocrinology 121:150, 1987

171. Fant M, Munro H, Moses AC: An autocrine/paracrine role for insulin-like growth factors in the regulation of human placental growth. J Clin Endocrinol Metab 63:499, 1986

172. Han VK, Lund PK, Lee DC et al: Expression of somatomedin/insulin-like growth factors in the regulation of human placental growth. J Clin Endocrinol Metab 66:422, 1988

173. Tulchinsky D, Hobel CJ: Plasma human chorionic gonadotropin, estrone, estradiol, estriol, progesterone and 17-hydroxyprogesterone in human pregnancy. Am J Obstet Gynecol 117:884, 1973

174. Siiteri PK, MacDonald PC: Placental esrogen biosynthesis during human pregnancy. J Clin Endocrinol Metab 26:751, 1966

175. Tulchinsky D, Korenman SG: The plasma estradiol as an index of fetoplacental function. J Clin Invest 50:1490, 1971

176. Abraham GE, Odell WD, Swerdloff RS et al: Simultaneous radioimmunoassay of plasma FSH, LH, progesterone 17-hydroxyprogesterone, and estradiol-17β during the menstrual cycle. J Clin Endocrinol Metab 34:312, 1972

177. Lindbert BS, Johansson EDB, Nilsson BA: Plasma levels of nonconjugated oestrone, oestradiol-17β and oestriol during uncomplicated pregnancy. Acta Obstet Gynecol Scand 32:21, 1974

178. Tulchinsky D, Hobel CJ, Yeager E et al: Plasma estrone estradiol, estriol, progesterone, and 17-hydroxyprogesterone in human pregnancy, I: normal pregnancy. Am J Obstet Gynecol 112:1095, 1972

179. Klopper A, Masson G, Campbell D et al: Estriol in plasma: a compartmental study. Am J Obstet Gynecol 117:21, 1973

180. Tulchinsky D, Hobel CJ, Korenman SG: A radioligand assay for plasma unconjugated estriol in normal and abnormal pregnancies. Am J Obstet Gynecol 111:311, 1971

181. Landon MB, Gabbe SG: Fetal surveillance in the pregnancy complicated by diabetes mellitus. Clin Obstet Gynecol 34:535, 1991

182. Parker CR Jr, Simpson ER, Bilheimer DW et al: Inverse relationship between LDL-cholesterol and dehydroisoandrosterone sulfate in human fetal plasma. Science 208:512, 1980

183. Sadovsky E, Polshuk WZ: Fetal movements in utero. Obstet Gynecol 50:49, 1977

184. Resnik R, Killam AP, Battaglia FC et al: The stimulation of uterine blood flow by various estrogens. Endocrinology 94:1192, 1974

185. Henson MC, Pepe GJ, Albrecht ED: Regulation of placental low-density lipoprotein uptake in baboons by estrogen: dose-dependent effects of the anti-estrogen ethamoxytriphetol (MER-25). Biol Reprod 45:43, 1991

186. Novy MJ: Hormonal regulation of parturition in primates. In Sciara J (ed): Hormone Cell Interactions in Reproductive Tissues. Masson Publishing, New York, 1983

187. Hirst JJ, Chibbar R, Mitchell BF: Role of oxytocin in the regulation of uterine activity during pregnancy and in the initiation of labor. Sem Reprod Endocrinol 11:219

188. Olson DM, Zakar Tamas: Intrauterine tissue postaglandin synthesis: regulatory mechanisms. Sem Reprod Endocrinol 11:234, 1993

189. Haluska GJ, Novy MJ: Hormonal modulation of uterine activity during primate parturition. Sem Reprod Endocrinol 11:272, 1993

190. Ducsay CA, Seron-Ferre M, Germain AM, Valenzuela GJ: Endocrine and uterine activity rhythms in the perinatal period. Sem Reprod Endocrinol 11:285, 1993

191. Honnbier MB, Nathanielsz PW: Primate parturition and the role of the maternal circadian system. Eur J Obstet Gynecol Reprod Biol 55:193, 1994

192. Patrick J, Challis J, Campbell K et al: Circadian rhythms in maternal plasma cortisol and estriol concentrations at 30 to 31, 34 to 35, and 38 to 39 weeks' gestational age. Am J Obstet Gynecol 136:325, 1980

193. Nygren KG, Johansson ED, Wide L: Evaluation of the prognosis of threatened abortion from the peripheral plasma levels of progesterone, estradiol, and human chorionic gonadotropin. Am J Obstet Gynecol 116:916, 1973

194. Stovall TG, Ling FW, Carson SA, Buster JE: Serum progesterone and uterine curettage in differential diagnosis of ectopic pregnancy. Fertil Steril 57:456, 1992

195. Teoh ES, Das NP, Dawood MY et al: Serum progesterone and serum chorionic gonadotrophin in hydatidiform mole and choriocarcinoma. Acta Endocrinol 70:791, 1972

196. Tulchinsky D, Simmer H: Sources of plasma 17α-hydroxyprogesterone in human pregnancy. J Clin Endocrinol Metab 35:799, 1972

197. Siiteri PK, Febres F, Clemens LE et al: Progesterone and maintenance of pregnancy: is progesterone nature's immunosuppressant? Ann N Y Acad Sci 286:3384, 1977

198. Moriyama I, Sugawa T: Progesterone facilitates implantation of xenogenic cultured cells in hamster uterus. Nature 236:150, 1972

199. Hsueh AJW, Peck EJ, Clark JH: Progesterone antagonism of the estrogen receptor and estrogen-induced uterine growth. Nature 254:337, 1977

200. Parker CR, Leveno K, Carr BR et al: Umbilical cord plasma levels of dehydroepiandrosterone sulfate during human gestation. J Clin Endocrinol Metab 54:1216, 1982

201. Csapo AI: Antiprogesterones in fertility control. p. 16. In Zatuchni GI, Sciarra JJ, Speidel JJ (eds): Pregnancy Termination: Procedures, Safety and New Developments. Harper & Row, Hagerstown, 1979

202. Case ML, MacDonald PC: Human parturition: distinction between the initiation of parturition and the onset of labor. Sem Reprod Endocrinol 11:272, 1993

203. Fencl MD, Stillman RJ, Cohen J et al: Direct evidence of sudden rise in fetal corticoids late in human gestation. Nature 287:225, 1980

204. Murphy BEP: Human fetal serum cortisol levels related to gestational age: evidence of a midgestational fall and a steep late gestational rise, independent of sex or mode of delivery. Am J Obstet Gynecol 144:276, 1982

205. Kadar N, DeVore G, Romero R: Discriminatory hCG zone: its use in the sonographic evaluation for ectopic pregnancy. Obstet Gynecol 58:156, 1981

206. Odell WD, Griffin J: Pulsatile secretion of chorionic gonadotropin during the normal menstrual cycle. J Clin Endocrinol Metab 69:528, 1989

207. Odell WD, Griffin J, Bashey HM, Snyder PJ: Secretion of chorionic gonadotropin by cultured human pituitary cells. J Clin Endocrinol Metab 71:1318, 1990

208. Odell WD, Griffin J: Pulsatile secretion of human chorionic gonadotropin in normal adults. N Engl J Med 317:1688, 1987

209. Griffin J, Odell WD: Ultrasensitive immunoradiometric assay for chorionic gonadotropin which does not cross-react with luteinizing hormone nor free beta chain of hCG and which detects hCG in blood of non-pregnant humans. J Immunol Methods 103:275, 1987

210. Cole LA, Kardana A, Ying FC, Birken S: The biological and clinical significance of nicks in human chorionic gonadotropin and its free beta-subunit. Yale J Biol Med 64:627, 1991

211. Cole LA, Seifer DB, Kardana A, Braunstein GD: Selecting human chorionic gonadotropin immunoassays: consideration of cross-reacting moleculs in first-trimester pregnancy serum and urine. Am J Obstet Gynecol 168:1580, 1993

212. Kardana A, Cole LA: Polypeptide nicks cause erroneous results in assay of human chorionic gonadotropin free beta-subunit. Clin Chem 38:26, 1992

213. Rasor JL, Braunstein GD: A rapid modification of the beta-hCG radioimmunoassay: use as an aid in the diagnosis of ectopic pregnancy. Obstet Gynecol 50:553, 1977

214. Hales CN, Woodhead JS: Labelled antibodies and their use in the immunoradiomimetic assay. Methods Enzymol 70:334, 1980

215. Joshi UM, Roy R, Sheth AR et al: A simple and sensitive color test for the detection of human chorionic gonadotropin. Obstet Gynecol 57:252, 1981

216. Steenman UH, Alfthan H, Myllynen L et al: Ultrarapid and highly sensitive time-resolved fluoroimmunometric assay for chorionic gonadotropin. Lancet 2:647, 1983

217. Chard T: Pregnancy tests: a review. Human Reprod 7:701, 1992

218. Phillips OP, Shulman ES, Andersen RN, Morgan CD, Simpson JL: Maternal serum screening for fetal Down Syndrome in women less than 35 years of age using alpha-fetoprotein, hCG, and unconjugated estriol: a prospective 2-year study. Obstet Gynecol 80:353, 1992

219. Khazaeli MB, Buchina ES, Pattillo RA et al: Radioimmunoassay of free beta-subunit of human chorionic gonadotropin in diagnosis of high-risk and low-risk gestational trophoblastic disease. Am J Obstet Gynecol 160:444, 1989

220. Yedema KA, Verheijen RH, Kenemans P et al: Identification of patients with persistent trophoblastic disease by means of a normal human chorionic gonadotropin regression curve. Am J Obstet Gynecol 168:787, 1993

221. Stovall TG, Ling FW, Andersen RN, Buster JE: Improved sensitivity and specificity of a single measurement of serum progesterone over serial quantitative beta-human chorionic gonadotrophin in screening for ectopic pregnancy. Hum Reprod 7:723, 1992

222. Carson SA, Buster JE: Ectopic pregnancy. N Engl J Med 329:1174, 1993

223. Carson SA: Unpublished data

224. Timor-Tritsch IE, Rottem S (eds): Transvaginal Sonography. Elsevier Science, New York, 1988

225. Fossum GT, Davajan V, Kletzky OA: Early detection of pregnancy with transvaginal ultrasound. Fertil Steril 49:789, 1988

226. Williams L, Warwick L: Gray's Anatomy. 36th Ed. p. 125. WB Saunders, Philadelphia, 1980

227. Simpson ER, Parker CR, Carr BR: Role of lipoprotein in the regulation of steroidogenesis by the human fetal adrenal. In Jaffe RB, Dell Acqua S (eds): The Endocrine Physiology of Pregnancy and the Peripartal Period. Vol. 21. Raven Press, New York, 1985

Placental and Fetal Physiology

Michael G. Ross, M. Gore Ervin, and
John Bissonnette

Recognition of normal fetal growth, development, and behavior is an important part of obstetric practice. Should abnormalities in these parameters be identified, clinical strategies for fetal assessment, intervention, or both may be required. The basic concepts of placental and fetal physiology provide the building blocks necessary to understand pathophysiology, and thus the mechanisms of disease. Throughout this chapter, we attempt to review the essential tenets of placental and fetal physiology, while relating this information to normal and abnormal clinical conditions.

Much of our knowledge of placental and fetal physiology derives from observations made in mammals other than man. We have attempted to include only those observations reasonably applicable to the human placenta and fetus, and in most instances have not detailed the species from which the data were obtained. Should questions arise regarding the species studied, the reader is referred to the references at the end of this chapter.

Placental Physiology

The placenta provides the fetus with its essential nutrients, water and oxygen, a route for clearance of fetal excretory products, and produces a vast array of protein and steroid hormones and factors essential to the maintenance of pregnancy.

Placental Metabolism and Growth

This section focuses on the physiology of placental metabolism and growth and its influence on the fetus.

The critical function of the placenta is illustrated by its high metabolic demands. For example, placental ox-

ygen consumption equals that of the fetus and exceeds the fetal rate when expressed on a weight basis (10 ml/min/kg[1–3]). Between 22 to 36 weeks of gestation, the number of trophoblast nuclei[4] increases 4- to 5-fold, placing increased metabolic demands on the placenta. Glucose is the principal substrate for oxidative metabolism by placental tissue.[2,5] Of the total glucose leaving the maternal compartment to nourish the uterus and its contents, placental consumption may represent up to 70 percent.[2,6,7] In addition, a significant fraction of placental glucose uptake derives from the fetal circulation,[8] and reflects placental oxidative metabolism. Although one third of placental glucose may be converted to lactate,[2,4,5,9] placental metabolism is not anaerobic. Instead, placental lactate production represents a minor substrate for fetal brain. The factors regulating short-term changes in placental oxygen and glucose consumption have not been fully identified.

The regulation of placental growth is also an area of incomplete understanding. The increase in trophoblast number exceeds the increase in fetal placental capillary endothelial cells[4] during the second half of gestation. Whether trophoblast cell proliferation is the primary event, or is dependent upon endothelial cell growth is not known. Normal term placental weight averages 450 g, representing approximately one seventh (one-sixth with cord and membranes) of fetal weight. Large appearing placentas, either ultrasonographically or at delivery, may arise from a variety of etiologies. Several clinical observations suggest a link between decreased tissue oxygen content and increased placental growth. Thus, increased placental size is associated with maternal anemia,[10–12] fetal anemia due to erythrocyte isoimmunization, and hydrops fetalis secondary to fetal α-thalassemia with Bart's hemoglobin. The association of a large placenta with maternal diabetes also has been recognized, possibly a result of insulin stimulated mitogenic activity.

Receptors for growth promoting peptide hormones (factors) characterized in placental tissue[13] include the insulin receptor,[14–19] receptors for insulin like growth factors I and II (IGF-I, IGF-II), and epidermal growth factor (EGF).[20,21] IGF-I and IGF-II are polypeptides with a high degree of homology to human proinsulin.[22] Both IGF-I and IGF-II circulate bound to a carrier protein, and are 50 times more potent than insulin in stimulating cell growth.[22] EGF increases RNA and DNA synthesis and cell multiplication in a wide variety of cell types.[13] The observation that placental EGF binding is increased at term, relative to 8 to 18 weeks' gestation, led to a suggested role for EGF in the regulation of placental growth.[21] However, the integrated physiological role of these and other potential placental growth factors[23–25] remains to be defined.

Placental Transfer

General Considerations

In the hemochorial human placenta, maternal blood and solutes are separated from fetal blood by trophoblastic tissue and fetal endothelial cells. Thus, transit from the maternal intervillous space to the fetal capillary lumen takes place across a number of cellular structures (Fig. 3-1). The first step is transport across the microvillus plasma membrane of the syncytiotrophoblast. Since there are no lateral intercellular spaces in the syncytiotrophoblast, all solutes first interact with the placenta at this plasma membrane. The interior and basal (fetal) syncytiotrophoblast membranes may represent additional steps in the transport process. The discontinuous nature of the cytotrophoblast cell layer in later gestation suggest this layer should not limit maternal to fetal transfer. However, the presence of anionic sites on the glycoprotein backbone comprising the basal lamina[26] may potentially influence movement of large charged molecules. The fetal capillary endothelial cell imposes two additional plasma membrane surfaces. However, the presence of lateral intercellular spaces allows pericellular transport.

A number of specific mechanisms allow transit across the placental membranes, including passive diffusion, facilitated diffusion, active transport, and endocytosis/exocytosis. Solutes lacking specialized transport mechanisms cross by extracellular or transcellular diffusional transport pathways with permeability determined by size, lipid solubility, ionic charge and maternal serum protein binding. Lipid insoluble (hydrophilic) substances, which cross the trophoblast via extracellular pores, are restricted by molecular size in relation to the extracellular pore size. Up to a molecular weight of at

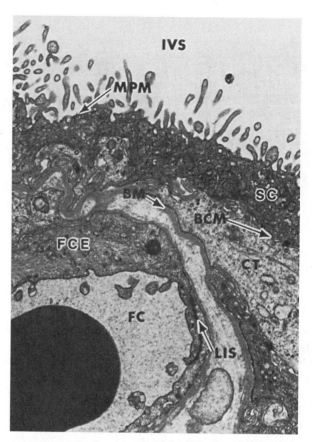

Fig. 3-1 Electron micrograph of human placenta demonstrating the cellular and extracellular components with which solutes must interact in moving from the maternal intervillous space (IVS) to the lumen of the fetal capillary (FC). MPM, microvillous plasma membrane of the syncytiotrophoblast; SC, syncytiotrophoblast; BMC, basal cell membrane of the syncytiotrophoblast; BM, basement membrane; CT, cytotrophoblast cell; FCE, fetal capillary endothelial cell; LIS, lateral intercellular space of fetal endothelial cell. (Courtesy of Kent L. Thornburg, Ph.D., Department of Physiology, Oregon Health Sciences University, Portland, OR.)

least 5000 daltons, placental permeability is proportional to the free diffusion of a molecule in water.[27] For example, urea (MW = 60) is at least 1,000 times more permeable than inulin (MW = 5,000).[27] Thus transfer of small solutes will be governed primarily by the maternal-fetal concentration gradient. Because transfer is relatively slow, and the extracellular pore surface area is limited, transfer of these molecules is referred to as "diffusion-limited." Conversely, highly lipid soluble (lipophilic) substances diffuse readily through the trophoblastic membrane. Thus molecular weight is relatively less important in restricting diffusion. Ethanol, a molecule similar in size to urea, is 500 times more lipid soluble and 10 times more permeable.[28] Because the entire trophoblast surface is available for diffusion and the permeability is high, transfer rates for lipophilic substances to the fetus are limited primarily by placental intervillous and umbilical blood flows ("flow-limited"). Both facilitated diffusion and active transport utilize carrier-mediated transport systems, with the latter requiring energy, either directly or indirectly linked with ionic pump mechanisms. Carrier transport systems are specifically limited to unique classes of molecules (e.g., neutral amino acids). In addition, substances may traverse the placenta via endocytosis (invagination of the cell membrane to form an intracellular vesicle containing extracellular fluids) and exocytosis (release of the vesicle to the extracellular space).

Transfer of Individual Solutes

Respiratory Gases

The exchange or transfer of the primary respiratory gases, oxygen and carbon dioxide, is likely "flow limited." Thus, the driving force for placental gas exchange is the partial pressure gradient between the maternal and fetal circulations. Estimates of human placental diffusing capacities[29] would predict that placental efficiency as an organ of respiratory gas exchange will allow equilibrium of oxygen and carbon dioxide tensions at the maternal intervillous space and fetal capillary. However, this prediction varies from the observed 10 mmHg difference in oxygen tension between the umbilical and uterine veins[30,31] and between the umbilical vein and intervillous[32] space. In addition, even though CO_2 is much more soluble than O_2 in water and tissues and will diffuse more readily than O_2, the P_{CO_2} difference from umbilical to uterine vein is small (3 mmHg).[33] P_{O_2} differences could be explained by areas of uneven distribution of maternal to fetal blood flows or shunting, limiting fetal and maternal blood exchange. The most important contribution is likely the high metabolic rate of the placental tissues themselves. Thus, trophoblast cell O_2 consumption and CO_2 production lower umbilical vein O_2 tension and increase uterine vein CO_2 tension to a greater degree than could be explained by an inert barrier for respiratory gas transfer.

The arteriovenous difference in the uterine circulation (and venoarterial difference in the umbilical circulation) widens during periods of lowered blood flow. Proportionate O_2 uptake increases and O_2 consumption remains unchanged over a fairly wide range of blood flows.[34] Thus, both uterine and umbilical blood flows can fall significantly without decreasing fetal O_2 consumption.[35,36]

Carbon dioxide is carried in the fetal blood both as dissolved CO_2 and as bicarbonate. Because of its charged nature, fetal-to-maternal bicarbonate transfer is limited. However, CO_2 likely diffuses from fetus to mother in its molecular form, and $[HCO_3]$ does not contribute significantly to fetal carbon dioxide elimination.[37] Thus, diffusion is not limiting, and the important variables for fetal O_2 uptake and CO_2 excretion reside with uterine and umbilical blood flows and carrying capacities of maternal and fetal bloods for O_2 and CO_2.

Glucose

Placental permeability for D-glucose is at least 50 times the value predicted on the basis of size and lipid solubility.[38] Thus specialized transport mechanisms must be available. Membrane proteins facilitating the translocation of molecules across cell membranes are termed transporters. The human placental glucose transporter has been identified as an approximately 55,000 MW component of the microvillous membrane.[39,40] In distinction to the adult kidney[41] and intestine, the placental glucose transporter is not sodium dependent, and in contrast to human adipocytes,[42] the transporter is not insulin sensitive.[43,44] The placental D-glucose transporter is saturable at high substrate concentrations; 50 percent saturation is observed at sugar levels of approximately 5 mM (90 mg/dl).[45] Thus, glucose transfer from mother to fetus is not linear, and transfer rates decrease as maternal glucose concentration increases. This effect is reflected in fetal blood glucose levels following maternal sugar loading.[46]

Amino Acids

Amino acid concentrations are higher in fetal umbilical cord blood than in maternal blood. Like monosaccharides, amino acids enter the syncytiotrophoblast via transport specific membrane proteins. However, in contrast to the glucose transporter, energy is indirectly required to transport amino acids from maternal blood into the trophoblast. Trophoblast cell amino acid uptake allows amino acids to move down their concentration gradient into fetal blood. Thus, amino acid transport is considered to be a "two-step" phenomenon.

Multiple systems mediate neutral and basic amino acid transport[47,48] (Table 3-1), and many of these systems are sodium dependent. Amino acid entry is coupled to sodium in a co-transport system located at the microvillous membrane which faces the maternal intervillous space.[49,50] So long as an inwardly directed sodium gradient is maintained, trophoblast cell amino acid concentrations will exceed maternal blood levels. The sodium gradient is maintained by Na^+-K^+ATPase located on the basal or fetal side of the syncytiotrophoblast.[51]

Transport of neutral amino acids with short polar or linear side chains is mediated by sodium-dependent System A (Table 3-1). Trophoblast cells have two mechanisms of regulating amino acid uptake using the A system. The absence of amino acids increases cellular amino acid uptake,[52-54] partly because of an increase in

Table 3-1 Placental Neutral Amino Acid Transport Systems

Transport	A	L	ASSC
Representative amino acids	Glycine, proline, alanine, serine, threonine, glutamine	Isoleucine, valine phenylalanine, alanine, serine, threonine, glutamine	Alanine, serine threonine, glutamine
Sodium dependency	+	−	+
Uptake increased by preincubation	+	−	+
Transinhibition	+	−	−

(Data from Enders et al.,[48] Smith et al.,[52,53] and Steel et al.[62])

carrier affinity.[52] Conversely, increases in trophoblast amino acid concentrations may suppress uptake (transinhibition). These mechanisms serve to maintain trophoblast cell amino acid levels constant during fluctuations in maternal plasma concentrations. The System L transporter is a sodium-independent system exhibiting high affinity for leucine and alanine while the sodium-dependent ASSC System remains controversial.[52,55] However, the systems are not exclusive, and a number of amino acids may be transported by multiple systems. Recently the molecular basis for a number of amino acid transport systems has been determined.[56] The acidic amino acids glutamate and aspartate are poorly transported from mother to fetus.[57–59] Glutamate, which shows a net loss to the placenta from the umbilical circulation,[60] is taken up at the fetal surface and converted into glutamine.[61] Controversy remains as to whether placental amino acid and/or glucose transport is regulated by fetal or maternal endocrine factors.[52–64] In diabetic pregnancies resulting in fetal macrosomia, the number of System A amino acid transporters in the brush border membrane is reduced compared with placentas from normal pregnancies and with placentas from pregnancies complicated by diabetes but resulting in infants of normal birth weight.[65]

Lipids

Although maternal lipids cross the placenta, the relatively low transfer rates[66,67] suggest fetal fatty acid accumulation in late pregnancy is not due to placental transfer.[66] Due to their hydrophobic nature, free fatty acids are relatively insoluble in plasma and circulate bound to albumin. Fatty acid transfer involves dissociation from maternal protein, and association with fetal plasma proteins. These protein binding steps are more important in determining mother to fetal fatty acid transfer than interaction with the lipid layers of the placenta.[68,69] Placental fatty acid transfer increases logarithmically with decreasing chain length (C16 to C8) and then declines somewhat for C6 and C4. This latter effect is due to a decrease in lipid solubility of the shorter chain molecules.[69] Placental uptake of choles-

terol is discussed in the section on receptor mediated endocytosis.

Water and Ions

Although water transfer across the placenta does not limit fetal water uptake during growth,[70] the factors regulating fetal water acquisition are poorly understood. Water transfer from mother to fetus is determined by a balance of osmotic, hydrostatic and colloid osmotic forces at the placental interface. Calculation of osmotic pressure from individual solute concentrations is unreliable because osmotic pressure forces depend upon the membrane permeability to each solute. Thus, sodium and chloride, the principal plasma solutes, are relatively permeable across the placenta[71] and would not be expected to contribute important osmotic effects.[72] As a result, although human fetal plasma osmolality is equal to or greater than maternal plasma osmolality,[73,74] these measured values do not reflect the actual osmotic force on either side of the membranes. Coupled with findings that hydrostatic pressure may be greater in the umbilical vein than the intervillous space,[75,76] these data do not explain mechanisms for fetal water accumulation. Alternatively, colloid osmotic pressure differences[77] and active solute transport probably represent the main determinants of water fluxes.

In comparison to other epithelia, the specialized placental mechanisms for ion transport are incompletely understood. Mechanisms for sodium transport in syncytiotrophoblast membranes are outlined in Figure 3-2. The maternal facing microvillous membrane contains an amino acid co-transporter,[50] a sodium phosphate co-transporter in which two sodium ions are transported with each phosphate radical,[78] and a sodium-hydrogen ion antiport which exchanges one proton for each sodium ion entering the cell.[79] A membrane potential with the inside negative (−30 MV) would promote sodium entry from the intervillous space.[80] The fetal directed basal side of the cell contains the Na,K-ATPase.[51] The microvillous or maternal facing trophoblast membrane also has a chloride bicarbonate exchanger whereby one chloride ion enters the

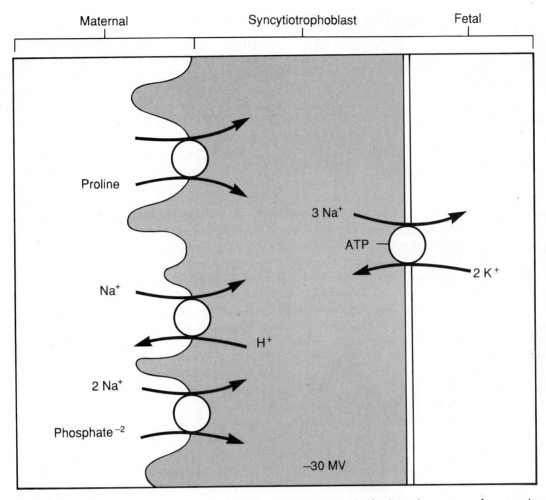

Fig. 3-2 Pathways for sodium entry into syncytiotrophoblast and exit to the fetal circulation. (Data from Boyd and Lund,[50] Whisett and Wallick,[51] Lajeunesse and Brunette,[78] and Bara et al.[80])

cell with the efflux of one bicarbonate radical.[81,82] In addition this membrane contains two Cl^- conductance pathways (ion channels) as determined by pharmacological inhibitors.[83] The integration of these various mechanisms for sodium and chloride transport from mother to fetus is not completely understood.

Calcium

Ionized calcium levels are higher in fetal than in maternal blood.[73,84] Higher fetal calcium levels are due to a syncytiotrophoblast basal membrane ATP-dependent Ca^{++} transport system[85] exhibiting high affinity (nanomolar range) for calcium. Calcium transport across the placenta is increased by the calcium-dependent regulatory protein calmodulin[85] and by 1,25-dihydroxycholecalciferol.[86] A calcium binding protein extracted from the placenta[87] differs from the human intestinal calcium binding protein[87] and may be an important regulator of maternal to fetal calcium transport.

Receptor Mediated Endocytosis/Exocytosis

The microvillous plasma membrane of the syncytiotrophoblast contains receptors specific for insulin,[14–18] low density lipoprotein (LDL),[88] immunoglobulin-G (IgG),[89] and transferrin.[90] While the precise steps for each protein-receptor complex are not yet defined, general mechanisms for post-ligand binding, cell entry and processing can be drawn from available data in other cell types.[91–94] Following ligand binding, the receptors aggregate on the cell surface and collect in specialized membrane structures termed coated pits (Fig. 3-3). These coated pits invaginate, pinch-off and enter the cell to form vesicles that fuse to form endosomes. The endosomes move deeper into the cytoplasm where the lower endosome pH facilitates ligand separation from its receptor.

The fate of ligand and receptor differs depending upon the specific substrate. While the insulin receptor is probably recycled to the cell surface, maternal insulin does not reach the fetal circulation due to lysosomal

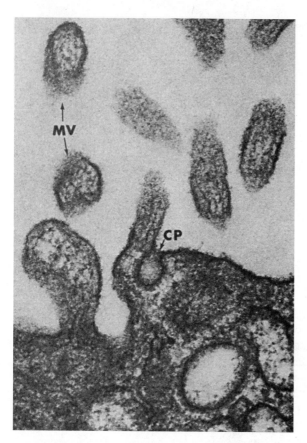

Fig. 3-3 Electron micrograph of human placental microvillous plasma membrane demonstrating presence of a coated pit (CP). Note the presence of cytoskeletal components extending into the microvillous space (MV). (Courtesy of Kent L. Thornburg, Ph.D., Department of Physiology, Oregon Health Sciences University, Portland, OR.)

degradation. Cholesterol enters with the LDL receptor and may be used for trophoblast pregnenolone/progesterone synthesis and/or is released into the fetal circulation.[95] IgG remains complexed to its receptor and is transferred to the fetus intact via exocytosis at the basal trophoblast membrane. Ferrotransferrin carries two ferric ions per molecule and is unique in that it does not separate from the transferrin receptor. Rather, the iron dissociates and binds to ferritin, a cytoplasmic iron-storing protein. Iron is then picked up at the basal side of the cell by fetal apotransferrin.

Placental Blood Flow

The transport characteristics of the placenta allow respiratory gases and many solutes to reach equal concentration between the maternal intervillous space blood (derived from uterine blood flow) and fetal capillary blood (derived from umbilical blood flow). Thus, the rate of blood flow in these two circulations is an important determinant of fetal oxygen and nutrient supply.

Uterine Blood Flow

Uterine blood flow during pregnancy supplies the myometrium, endometrium and placenta, with the latter receiving nearly 90 percent of total uterine blood flow near term. Thus, interest has focused primarily on regulation of uteroplacental blood flow. Over the course of a normal singleton ovine gestation, uterine blood flow increases more than 50-fold above nonpregnant values.[96] This long term increase in uterine blood flow is accompanied by a doubling of maternal cardiac output and a 40 percent increase in blood volume. Two primary factors contribute to this dramatic increase in uterine blood flow: placental growth and maternal arterial vasodilation. Along with fetal and placental growth, placental intervillous space volume almost triples between the 22nd and 36th weeks of gestation. Thus, the marked growth of the maternal placental vascular bed is consistent with the increase in placental diffusing capacity.[97,98] Secondly, the increase in blood flow is due in part to a direct estrogen-induced vasodilation of the uterine vasculature. These combined effects provide uterine blood flow rates at term of at least 750 ml/min,[99,100] or 10 to 15 percent of maternal cardiac output.

The uterine artery behaves as a nearly maximally dilated system. Still, uterine blood flow is subject to short term regulatory influences. Systemically administered vasodilator agents preferentially dilate systemic vessels, reducing uterine blood flow. Thus, concerns regarding administration of antihypertensive agents or regional anesthesia with sympathetic blockade are well founded. Although pregnant women display a refractoriness to infused pressor agents,[101] pressor agent-induced increases in uterine vascular resistance may exceed increases in systemic vascular resistance, reducing uteroplacental blood flow. Conversely, increased maternal plasma catecholamine levels during preeclampsia or pressor agents administered for treatment of maternal hypotension, may have adverse effects on uterine blood flow. Although respiratory gases are important regulators of blood flow in a number of organs, there is no indication that either oxygen or carbon dioxide are responsible for short term changes in uterine blood flow.[102] During uterine contractions the relationship between uterine arterial and venous pressures and blood flow no longer holds. Since intrauterine pressures are directly transmitted to the intervillous space,[103] increases in intrauterine pressure are reflected by decreases in placental blood flow.

Umbilical Blood Flow

Fetal blood flow to the umbilical circulation represents approximately 40 percent of the combined output of both fetal ventricles.[104,105] Over the last third of gestation increases in umbilical blood flow are proportional to fetal growth,[106] so that umbilical blood flow remains constant when normalized to fetal weight.[107] Although increases in villous capillary number represent the primary contributor to gestation dependent increases in umbilical blood flow, the factors which regulate this change are not known.

Short term changes in umbilical blood flow are primarily regulated by perfusion pressure. This relationship between flow and perfusion pressure is linear in the umbilical circulation.[107,108] As a result, small (2 to 3 mmHg) increases in umbilical vein pressure evoke proportional decreases in umbilical blood flow.[107,108] Since both the umbilical artery and vein are enclosed in the amniotic cavity, pressure changes due to increases in uterine tone are transmitted equally to these vessels without changes in umbilical blood flow. Relative to the utero-placental bed, the feto-placental circulation is resistant to vasoconstrictive effects of infused pressor agents, and umbilical blood flow is preserved unless cardiac output decreases. Thus, despite catecholamine-induced changes in blood flow distribution, and increases in blood pressure during acute hypoxia, umbilical blood flow is maintained over a relatively wide range of oxygen tensions.[109–112]

Immunologic Properties of the Placenta

The syncytiotrophoblast in contact with maternal blood in the intervillous space and the amniochorion in contact with maternal decidua represent the fetal tissues most prone to immunological reactions from maternal factors. The rejection of tissue grafts is under genetic control and the genes responsible for this phenomenon are termed histocompatibility genes. Their products at the cell surface-major histocompatibility antigens-are integral to the host's recognition of self and non-self. Neither β-2-microglobulin (which is tightly associated with HLA antigens) nor the HLA antigens A, B, C, DR or DC can be demonstrated on the surface of syncytiotrophoblast.[113,114] Recently invasive human cytotrophoblasts have been shown to express a trophoblast specific, nonclassical class 1b antigen, HLA-G. HLA-G has limited polymorphism, and antigen derived from paternal genes is not recognized as foreign by the maternal immune system.[115] However, the cytotrophoblast, which erodes into the maternal spiral arterioles, express an incomplete or truncated form of class I HLA antigens (reviewed in Beer[116]). The chorionic sac in the first trimester exhibits HLA-A, B and C antigens localized to non-villous trophoblast of the cytotrophoblast cell columns and cytotrophoblastic shell.[117] In addition, histocompatibility antigens can be demonstrated on fetal stromal cells such as fibroblasts and fetal endothelial cells within the placental villi.[118] While the normal syncytiotrophoblast at the hemochorial interface within the interstitial space lacks major histocompatibility antigens, the observation that transformed trophoblast in vitro can manifest these antigens suggests the genetic information is present but suppressed in normal tissues in vivo.[118] Neither the A, B or H blood group antigens[119] nor H-Y antigens[113] are thought to be present on the syncytiotrophoblast surface. The presence of antigens in fetal stroma cells and endothelium of placental villi also may be important to maintenance of the fetus. For example,[120] this area may act as an immunological sink to bind maternal antibodies so they do not reach the fetus.

The syncytiotrophoblast manifests unique antigens, termed trophoblast antigens and trophoblast-lymphocyte cross-reactive antigens.[118] Distinguishing the two groups is the latter's absorbtion by leukocytes. These trophoblast antigens are structural components of the plasma membrane and are distinct from soluble proteins produced by the placenta.[121] The trophoblast-lymphocyte cross-reactive antigens may be important for the induction of immunological blocking factors in maternal serum during the second and third trimester of normal pregnancy.[122] Antibodies against these antigens are thought to be important regulators of trophoblast growth.[116] The absence of trophoblast antigens, which the mother's immune system can recognize as non-self, may be related to a failure to produce these blocking factors, resulting in abortion.[116,118,123–125] Suppression of lymphocyte activation by local immunoregulatory responses in the decidua play an important role in preventing rejection of the trophoblast. However, these same responses may also contribute to localized infections at this site in the absence of systemic effects.[126] In addition to the placenta, both the mother and the fetus make important contributions to the immunological maintenance of pregnancy.[116,127]

Amniotic Fluid Volume

Mean amniotic fluid volume increases from 250 to 800 ml between 16 and 32 weeks' gestation. Despite considerable variability, the average volume remains stable up to 36 weeks and then declines to about 500 ml at term.[128] The origin of amniotic fluid during the first trimester of pregnancy is uncertain. Possible sources include a transudate of maternal plasma through the chorioamnion or a transudate of fetal plasma through the highly permeable fetal skin, prior to keratinization.[129] The origin and dynamics of amniotic fluid are better understood beginning in the second trimester, when the fetus becomes the primary determinant. Amniotic fluid volume is maintained by a balance of fetal fluid production (lung liquid and urine) and fluid resorption (fetal swallowing and flow across the amniotic and/or chorionic membranes to the fetal or maternal circulations).

The fetal lung secretes fluid at a rate of 300 to 400 ml/day near term.[130] Chloride is actively transferred from alveolar capillaries to lung lumen[131] and water follows the chloride gradient. Thus lung fluid represents a nearly protein free transudate with an osmolarity similar to that of fetal plasma.[132] Fetal lung fluid does not appear to regulate fetal body fluid homeostasis, as fetal intravenous volume loading does not increase lung fluid secretion. Rather, lung fluid likely serves to maintain lung expansion and facilitate pulmonary growth. Lung fluid must decrease at parturition to provide for the transition to respiratory ventilation. Notably, several hormones which increase in fetal plasma during labor [e.g., catecholamines, arginine vasopressin (AVP)] also decrease lung fluid production.[133–135] With the reduction of fluid secretion, the colloid osmotic gradient between fetal plasma and lung fluid results in lung fluid resorption across the pulmonary epithelium, and clearance via lymphatics. The absence of this process explains the increased incidence of transient tachypnea of the newborn, or "wet lung," in infants born by cesarean delivery in the absence of labor.

Fetal urine is the primary source of amniotic fluid, with outputs at term varying from 400 to 1,200 ml/day.[136,137] Between 20 and 40 weeks' gestation, in association with marked renal maturation, fetal urine production increases about 10-fold.[137] The urine is normally hypotonic[138] and the low osmolality of fetal urine accounts for the hypotonicity of amniotic fluid in late gestation[138] relative to maternal and fetal plasma. Numerous fetal endocrine factors, including AVP, atrial natriuretic factor (ANF), angiotensin II (AII), aldosterone and prostaglandins alter fetal renal blood flow, glomerular filtration rate, or urine flow rates.[139,140] In response to fetal stress, endocrine-mediated reductions in fetal urine flow may explain the association between fetal hypoxia and oligohydramnios. The regulation of fetal urine production is discussed further in the section on the fetal kidney.

Fetal swallowing is believed to be the major route of amniotic fluid resorption[141–144] though swallowed fluid contains a mixture of amniotic and tracheal fluids.[145] Human fetal swallowing has been demonstrated by 18 weeks' gestation,[146] with daily swallowed volumes of 200 to 500 ml near term.[142,143] Similar to fetal urine flow, daily fetal swallowed volumes (per body weight) are markedly greater than adult values. With the development of fetal neurobehavioral states, fetal swallowing occurs primarily during active sleep states associated with respiratory and eye movements.[146,147] Moderate increases in fetal plasma osmolality increase the number of swallowing episodes and volume swallowed,[148,149] indicating the presence of an intact thirst mechanism in the near term fetus.

Since amniotic fluid is hypotonic with respect to maternal plasma there is a potential for bulk water removal at the amniotic chorionic interface with maternal or fetal plasma. Although fluid resorption to the maternal plasma is likely minimal, intramembranous flow from amniotic fluid to fetal placental vessels may contribute importantly to amniotic fluid resorption.[150] Thus, intramembranous flow along with fetal swallowing may balance fetal urine and lung liquid production to maintain normal amniotic fluid volumes.

Fetal Physiology

Growth and Metabolism

Substrates

The caloric requirements of the growing fetus can be considered under two categories of metabolism: energy to sustain the existing organism (producing heat), and energy utilization for synthesis and accretion of new tissue. The metabolic rate reflects fetal oxygen consumption (approximately 8 ml/kg/min). Metabolic requirements for new tissue depend on the growth rate and the type of tissue acquired. Although the newborn infant has relatively increased body fat (16 percent),[151] fetal fat content is low at 26 weeks. Fat acquisition increases gradually up to 32 weeks, and rapidly thereafter—approximately 82 g (dry weight) of fat per week. In contrast, fetal acquisition of nonfat tissue is linear from 32 to 39 weeks, and averages half the fat acquisition rate in late gestation—approximately 43 g (dry weight) per week. The caloric requirements for both fat and nonfat tissue accretion are approximately 12 kcal/kg/day at 26 weeks[152,153] increasing to 40 kcal/kg/day in late gestation.

In addition to the caloric requirements for tissue growth, there are caloric requirements for fetal oxidative metabolism. Assuming both protein and carbohydrate serve as substrates for the fetal 8 ml/min/kg of oxygen consumption (the fatty acid contribution appears to be minimal), and 4.9 kcal are required per liter oxygen consumed, fetal oxygen consumption would require 56 kcal/kg/day. When combined with the 40 kcal/kg day required for tissue acquisition, the combined caloric requirements for a 3.0 kg fetus in late gestation would be on the order of 290 kcal/day. In terms of oxygen consumption, estimates suggest 20 percent is required to meet metabolic needs for acquiring new tissue, with the remainder used to sustain existing tissue.[154]

The exact partitioning of substrates for oxidative metabolism and tissue accretion in the fetus are not known.

Under normal conditions, glucose utilized by the fetus derives from the placenta rather than from endogenous glucose production.[155] Based on umbilical vein to umbilical artery glucose and oxygen concentration differences,[156] glucose alone cannot account for fetal oxidative metabolism. For example, assuming aerobic glucose metabolism, only 4.8 of the possible 6 moles of glucose are taken-up for each mole of oxygen.[156] In addition, the necessary enzymes for carbohydrate to lipid conversion are present in the fetus,[157] and glucose oxidation accounts for only two-thirds of fetal carbon dioxide production.[158] Thus, in addition to glucose, fetal oxidative metabolism depends upon other substrates. In fetal sheep, lactate is taken up by the umbilical circulation and oxidized to carbon dioxide.[158] The role of lactate in human fetal metabolism is not known.

In addition to protein synthesis, a large portion of the amino acids taken up by the umbilical circulation are used by the fetus for aerobic metabolism. While fetal uptake for a number of amino acids actually exceeds their accretion into fetal tissues,[159] glutamate is an exception. Placental-hepatic cycling also occurs for certain amino acids. For example, there is a net flux of glycine from the placenta to the fetal liver for uptake, while serine is released from the liver with little or no uptake by the placenta.[160,161]

Hormones

Fetal hormones influence fetal growth through both metabolic and mitogenic effects. Growth hormone and the insulin-like growth factors (IGF) are important for postnatal growth.[162] While the liver is a principle source of IGF-I, most, if not all tissues of the body produce IGF-I and IGF-II.[163,164] Thus, tissue IGF concentrations may be more important than plasma levels, and growth hormone effects may be mediated by localized IGF-I release. The correlation between small offspring and genetic manipulations resulting in only one allele and decreased IGF-II messenger RNA indicate IGF-II is important to fetal growth. While growth hormone has been thought to be less important to intrauterine than postnatal growth, changes in IGF, IGF-binding proteins or IGF-receptors may explain the apparent reduced role of growth hormone on fetal growth.[165–169] The fetal thyroid is also not important for overall fetal growth, but is important for central nervous system development.[165,166]

The importance of insulin for fetal growth is suggested from the increases in fetal weight, and heart and liver weights in infants of diabetic mothers.[170] Insulin levels within the high physiologic range increase fetal body weight,[171] and increases in endogenous fetal insulin significantly increase fetal glucose uptake.[172,173] In addition, fetal insulin secretion increases in response to

elevations in blood glucose, although the normal rapid insulin response phase is absent.[173] Plasma insulin levels sufficient to increase fetal growth[171] also may exert mitogenic effects,[164] perhaps through insulin-induced IGF-II receptor binding.[174] Separate receptors for insulin and IGF-II are expressed in fetal liver cells by the end of the first trimester.[175] Hepatic insulin receptor numbers (per gram tissue) triple by 28 weeks, while IGF-II receptor numbers remain constant.[175] The growth patterns of infants of diabetic mothers[176,177] indicate insulin levels may be most important in late gestation. Though less common, equally dramatically low birth weights are associated with the absence of fetal insulin.[166] Experimentally induced hypoinsulinemia causes a 30 percent decrease in fetal glucose utilization and decreases fetal growth.[178–180]

Fetal plasma IGF-I and IGF-II levels begin to increase by 32 to 34 weeks gestation.[181,182] However, IGF regulation in fetal life is not well understood. Embryonic fibroblast IGF-II synthesis can be induced by placental lactogen, suggesting placental lactogen may be important for fetal growth.[170] Placental lactogen receptors are present in human fetal liver and muscle in the second trimester, and hepatic binding capacity correlates with body weight.[183] However, undetectable placental lactogen levels may be observed in maternal or cord blood of normal birth weight newborns.[184]

The effect of endogenous insulin secretion on fetal glucose consumption has already been discussed. As in the adult, β-adrenergic receptor activation increases fetal insulin secretion, while α-adrenergic activation inhibits insulin secretion.[185,186] Fetal glucagon secretion also is modulated by the β-adrenergic system.[185] However, the fetal glycemic response to glucagon is blunted, probably due to a relative reduction in hepatic glucagon receptors.[187]

In addition to the insulin-like growth factors, other growth factors may be important to fetal organ growth. For example, epidermal growth factor has specific effects on lung growth and growth and differentiation of the secondary palate,[188] and normal sympathetic adrenergic system development is dependent on nerve growth factor.[188]

Fetal Circulation
Anatomy

The first step in understanding fetal cardiovascular physiology is to recognize the peculiarities unique to fetal circulatory anatomy. Beginning with well-oxygenated blood from the placenta (Fig. 3-4), the umbilical vein gives off branches to the left lobe of the liver and then continues as the ductus venosus. A major branch to the right then joins the portal vein to supply the right lobe of the liver. Approximately half of the estimated

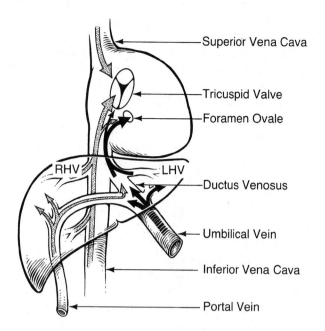

Fig. 3-4 Anatomy of the umbilical and hepatic circulation. RHV, right hepatic vein; LHV, left hepatic vein. (From Rudolph,[190] with permission.)

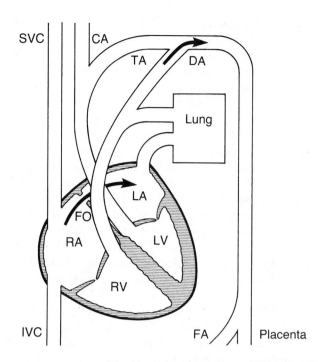

Fig. 3-5 Anatomy of fetal heart and central shunts, SVC, superior vena cava; CA, carotid artery; TA, thoracic aorta; DA, ductus arteriosus; RA, right atrium; FO, foramen ovale; LA, left atrium; RV, right ventricle; LV, left ventricle; IVC, inferior vena cava; FA, femoral artery. (From Anderson et al.,[191] with permission.)

umbilical blood flow (70 to 130 ml/min/kg fetal weight[189] after 30 weeks gestation) follows the ductus venosus.[190] Left hepatic vein blood combines with the well oxygenated ductus venosus flow in the inferior vena cava to form a stream which is preferentially directed across the foramen ovale into the left atrium (Figs. 3-4 and 3-5). As a result, blood with the highest oxygen content is delivered to the left ventricle, and ultimately supplies blood to the carotid circulation and upper body and brain. Flow across the foramen ovale is approximately one third of combined cardiac output.[191] Because blood from the ductus venosus to the right side of the liver combines with blood from the portal vein (only a small fraction of portal vein blood passes through the ductus venosus), right hepatic vein blood is less oxygenated than its counterpart on the left.[190] Right hepatic vein blood joins with inferior vena caval flow (which further lowers the oxygen content) to form a stream that is preferentially directed through the tricuspid valve (Fig. 3-4) into the right ventricle (Fig. 3-5). Superior vena cava blood flow also is preferentially directed through the tricuspid valve to the right ventricle. Thus, right ventricular output, representing about 60 percent of biventricular output,[191] is primarily directed through the ductus arteriosus to the descending aorta (Fig. 3-5). The high pulmonary vascular resistance and 2 to 3 mmHg higher mean pulmonary artery above aortic pressure directs flow to the ductus arteriosus, away from the pulmonary circulation,[191] (which receives only 5 to 10 percent of the combined ventricular output).

Fetal Heart

Estimates of fetal left ventricular output average 120 ml/min/kg body weight.[105] If left ventricular output is 40 percent of the combined biventricular output,[191] then total fetal cardiac output would be about 300 ml/min/kg. The distribution of the cardiac output to fetal organs is summarized in Table 3-2,[104,192] with fetal hepatic distribution reflecting only the portion supplied by the hepatic artery. In fact, hepatic blood flow derives principally from the umbilical vein and to a lesser extent the portal vein,[193] and represents about 25 percent of the total venous return to the heart.

Table 3-2 Distribution of Fetal Cardiac Output

Organ	Percentage of Biventricular Cardiac Output
Placenta	40.0
Brain	13.0
Heart	3.5
Lung	7.0
Liver	2.5 (hepatic artery)
Gastrointestinal tract	5.0
Adrenal glands	0.5
Kidney	2.5
Spleen	1.0
Body	25.0

(Data from Rudolph and Heymann[104] and Paton et al.[192])

Fetal ventricular output depends upon contractility, pulmonary artery and aortic pressures, and the heart rate. The relationship between mean right atrial pressure (the index often used for ventricular volume at the end of diastole) and stroke volume is depicted in Figure 3-6. The steep ascending limb represents the length-active tension relationship for cardiac muscle in the right ventricle.[194] Under normal conditions, fetal right atrial pressure resides at the break point in this ascending limb; increases in pressure do not increase stroke volume. Thus, the contribution of Starling mechanisms to increasing right heart output in the fetus is limited. In contrast, decreases in venous return and right atrial pressure will decrease stroke volume. Because the right ventricle is sensitive to afterload, a linear inverse relationship exists between stroke volume and pulmonary artery pressure.[194] Thus, the fall in pulmonary artery pressure at birth contributes to the increase in right heart output. Compared to the left, the fetal right ventricle has a greater anteroposterior dimension, increasing both volume and circumferential radius of curvature. This anatomic difference increases the radius to wall thickness ratio for the right ventricle, producing increased wall stress in systole and a decrease in stroke volume when afterload increases.[195]

The relationship between atrial pressure and stroke volume in the left ventricle is similar to that shown in Figure 3-6 for the right ventricle. Although the break point occurs near the normal value for left atrial pressure, there is a small amount of preload reserve.[196] In distinction to the fetal right ventricle, the left side is not sensitive to aortic pressure increases. Thus, postnatal increases in systemic blood pressure do not increase stroke volume. Late gestation fetal heart α-adrenergic receptor numbers are similar to the adult,[197] and increases in circulating catecholamine concentrations may increase stroke volume by 50 percent.[198] Blood flow to the myocardium reflects the greater stroke volume of the right side; right ventricular free wall and septal blood flows are higher than in the left ventricle.[199]

Glucose and lactate constitute the major substrates used for oxidative metabolism by the fetal heart. In contrast to the adult heart, free fatty acids are not metabolized in significant amounts by the myocardium in utero.[200] This may be a function of substrate availability, as palmitate can be oxidized by fetal heart muscle,[201] although to a lesser extent than in the neonate.

Fetal heart rate decreases during the last half of gestation, particularly between 20 to 30 weeks. If analysis is confined to episodes of low heart rate variability, mean heart rate decreases from 30 weeks to term. However, if all heart rate data are analyzed, mean heart rate is stable at 142 beats per minute over the last 10 weeks of gestation.[202] Variability in mean heart rate over 24 hours includes a nadir between 2 A.M. and 6 A.M. and a peak between 8 A.M. and 10 A.M.[203] Most fetal heart rate accelerations occur simultaneous with limb movement, primarily reflecting central neuronal brain stem output. Also, movement related decreases in venous return and a reflex tachycardia contribute.[204]

Because ventricular stroke volumes decrease with increasing heart rate, fetal cardiac output stays constant over a heart rate range of 120 to 180 beats per minute.[205–207] The major effect of this inverse relationship between heart rate and stroke volume is an alteration in end diastolic dimension. If end diastolic dimension

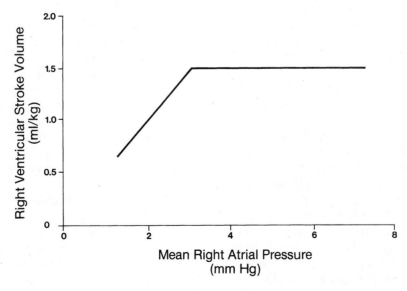

Fig. 3-6 Stroke volume of the fetal right ventricle as a function of mean right atrial pressure. (From Thornburg and Morton,[194] with permission.)

is kept constant, there is no fall in stroke volume and cardiac output goes up.[206,207]

Autonomic Regulation

Through reflex stimulation of peripheral baroreceptors, chemoreceptors and central mechanisms, the sympathetic and parasympathetic systems have important roles in the regulation of fetal heart rate, cardiac contractility and vascular tone. The fetal sympathetic system develops early, while the parasympathetic system develops somewhat later.[208-210] Nevertheless, in the third trimester parasympathetic tone is important to fetal heart rate regulation, as evidenced by the tachycardia observed in response to atropine.[211] Opposing sympathetic and parasympathetic inputs to the fetal heart contribute to R-R interval variability from one heart cycle to the next, and to basal heart rate variability over periods of a few minutes. However, even when sympathetic and parasympathetic inputs are removed, a level of variability remains.[211]

Fetal sympathetic innervation is not essential for blood pressure maintenance when circulating catecholamines are present.[212] Nevertheless, fine control of blood pressure and fetal heart rate requires an intact sympathetic system.[213] In the absence of functional adrenergic innervation, hypoxia-induced increases in peripheral, renal and splanchnic bed vascular resistances[109,111] and blood pressure are not seen.[214,215] However, hypoxia related changes in pulmonary, myocardial, adrenal and brain blood flows occur in the absence of sympathetic innervation, indicating that both local and endocrine effects contribute to regulation of blood flow in these organs.

Receptors in the carotid body and arch of the aorta respond to pressor or respiratory gas stimulation with afferent modulation of heart rate and vascular tone. Sensitivity of the fetal baroreflex response, in terms of the magnitude of decreases in heart rate per millimeter of mercury increase in blood pressure, is blunted relative to the adult.[216,217] However, fetal baroreflex sensitivity more than doubles in late gestation.[216] Although the set-point for fetal heart rate is not believed to depend on intact baroreceptors, fetal heart rate variability increases when functional arterial baroreceptors are absent.[218] The same observation has been made for fetal blood pressure. Thus, fetal arterial baroreceptors buffer variations in fetal blood pressure during body or breathing movements.[218,219] Changes in baroreceptor tone likely account for the increase in mean fetal blood pressure normally observed in late gestation.[219] In the absence of functional chemoreceptors, mean arterial pressure is maintained[218] while peripheral blood flow increases, suggesting peripheral arterial chemoreceptors are important to maintenance of resting peripheral vascular tone. Peripheral arterial chemoreceptors also are important components in fetal reflex responses to hypoxia; the initial bradycardia is not seen without functional chemoreceptors.[220]

Hormonal Regulation

Significant quantities of AVP are present in the human fetal neurohypophysis by the end of the first trimester.[221] Ovine fetal plasma AVP levels increase appropriately in response to changes in fetal plasma osmolality induced directly in the fetus[222,223] or via changes in maternal osmolality.[224,225] Due to functional high and low pressure baroreceptors and chemoreceptor afferents, decreases in fetal intravascular volume[226,227] or systemic blood pressure[228,229] also increase fetal AVP secretion. Thus, in the late gestation fetus as in the adult, both osmoreceptor and volume/baroreceptor pathways are integrated into a sensitive system regulating fetal AVP secretion. Hypoxia-induced AVP secretion can be demonstrated beyond mid-pregnancy of the ovine gestation,[230] and reductions in fetal Po_2 of 10 mmHg ($\simeq$50 percent) evoke profound increases in fetal plasma AVP levels (200 to 400 pg/ml or more).[231,232] Hypoxemia is the most potent stimulus known for fetal AVP secretion.[231]

The response pattern to AVP infusion includes dose dependent increases in fetal mean blood pressure and decreases in heart rate at plasma levels well below those required for similar effects in the adult.[232] Receptors distinct from those mediating antidiuretic effects in the kidney account for the role of AVP in fetal circulatory adjustments during hemorrhage,[233] hypotension,[234] and hypoxia.[235] The corticotropin releasing factor effects of AVP may contribute to hypoxia-induced increases in plasma ACTH and cortisol levels.[236-239] In addition to alterations in fetal heart rate, cardiac output, and arterial blood pressure, AVP-induced changes in peripheral, placental, myocardial and cerebral blood flows[240-243] directly parallel the cardiovascular changes associated with acute hypoxia. The effects of AVP on cardiac output distribution may serve to facilitate O_2 availability to the fetus during hypoxic challenges. However, other hypoxia related responses, including reductions in renal and pulmonary blood flows, and increased adrenal blood flow are not observed with infusion of AVP.[241]

Fetal plasma renin levels are elevated during late gestation.[244] The increase in fetal plasma renin activity may be attributed to changes in tubular sodium concentration,[245] a reduction in blood volume,[246] a fall in vascular pressure and renal perfusion pressure,[247] and hypoxemia.[248] The relationship between fetal renal perfusion pressure and log plasma renin activity is similar to that of adults.[249] Consistent with the effects of renal nerve activity on renin release in adults,[250] fetal renin gene expression is directly modulated by renal sympathetic nerve activity.[251]

Although fetal plasma angiotensin II (AII) levels increase in response to small changes in blood volume and hypoxemia,[252] fetal AII and aldosterone do not rise in relation to changes in plasma renin activity.[244] This apparent uncoupling of the fetal renin-angiotensin-aldosterone system and the subsequent increase in newborn AII levels may be due to the significant contribution of the placenta to plasma AII clearance in the fetus.[253] Limited angiotensin converting enzyme (ACE) availability due to reduced pulmonary blood flow and direct inhibition of aldosterone secretion by the normally high levels of atrial naturietic factor (ANF) may also contribute.

All infusion increases fetal mean arterial blood pressure. In contrast to AVP-induced bradycardia, fetal AII infusion increases heart rate (after an initial reflex bradycardia) apparently through a direct effect on the heart.[254] Both hormones increase fetal blood pressure similar to levels seen with hypoxemia. However, AII does not reduce peripheral blood flow, perhaps because circulation to muscle, skin and bone are always under maximum response to AII, thereby limiting increases in resting tone.[254] Angiotensin II infusions also decrease renal blood flow and increase umbilical vascular resistance, although absolute placental blood flow remains unchanged. While the adult kidney contains both AII receptor subtypes, the AT_2 subtype is the only form present in the human fetal kidney.[255] Maturational differences in the type of AII receptor expressed would be consistent with earlier studies demonstrating differing AII effects on fetal renal and peripheral vascular beds.[248] Thus, the receptors mediating AII responses in the renal and peripheral vascular beds differ during fetal life.

Available data suggest that fetal plasma AII levels are maintained within a narrow range and that this regulation may be important to overall fetal homeostasis. AII has the potential to decrease placental blood flow.[242] Furthermore, because AII infusion increases mean arterial pressure and renal and placental vascular resistances,[256] limiting fluctuations in fetal plasma AII levels may be of advantage to the regulation of fetal renal function.[257,258] The uncoupling of renin-induced angiotensin I production, limited ACE activity, and augmented placental AII clearance may all serve to protect the fetal cardiovascular system from large increases in plasma AII levels.

Fetal Hemoglobin

The fetus exists in a state of aerobic metabolism, with arterial blood P_{O_2} values in the 20 to 25 mmHg range. However, there is no evidence of metabolic acidosis.

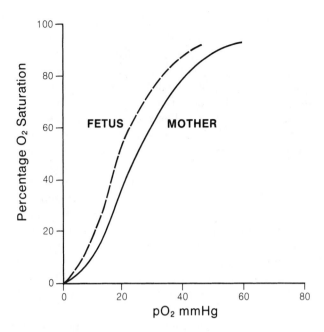

Fig. 3-7 Oxyhemoglobin dissociation curves of maternal and fetal human blood at pH 7.4 and 37°C. (Adapted from Hellegers and Schruefer,[259] with permission.)

Adequate fetal tissue oxygenation is achieved by several mechanisms. Of major importance are the higher fetal cardiac output and organ blood flows. A higher hemoglobin concentration (relative to the adult) and the greater oxygen carrying capacity of fetal hemoglobin also contribute. The resulting leftward shift in the fetal oxygen dissociation curve relative to the adult (Fig. 3-7) increases fetal blood oxygen saturation for any given oxygen tension. For example, at a partial pressure of 26.5 mmHg, adult blood oxygen saturation is 50 percent while fetal oxygen saturation is 70 percent. Thus, at a normal fetal PO_2 of 20 mmHg, fetal whole blood oxygen saturation may be 50 percent.[259]

The basis for increased oxygen affinity of fetal whole blood resides in the interaction of fetal hemoglobin with intracellular organic phosphate 2-3, diphosphoglycerate (2-3, DPG). The fetal hemoglobin (HgbF) tetramere is comprised of two α-chains (identical to adult) and two γ-chains. The latter differ from the β-chain of adult hemoglobin (HgbA) in 39 of 146 amino acid residues. Among these differences is the substitution of serine in the γ-chain of HgbF for histidine at the β-143 position of HgbA, which is located at the entrance to the central cavity of the hemoglobin tetramere. Due to a positively charged imidazole group, histidine can bind with the negatively charged 2-3, DPG. Binding of 2-3,DPG to deoxyhemoglobin stabilizes the tetramere in the reduced form. Because serine is nonionized and does not interact with 2-3,DPG to the same extent as histidine,[260] the oxygen affinity of HgbF is increased and the dissociation curve is shifted to the left. If HgbA or HgbF are removed from the erythrocyte and stripped of organic phosphates, the oxygen affinity for both hemoglobins is similar. However, addition of equal amounts of 2-3,DPG to the hemoglobins decreases the oxygen affinity of HgbA (dissociation curve shifts to the right) to a greater extent than for HgbF. Thus, even though overall oxygen affinities are similar, differences in 2-3,DPG interaction result in a higher oxygen affinity for HgbF. The proportion of HgbF to HgbA changes between 26 and 40 weeks of gestation. HgbF decreases linearly from 100 to about 70 percent, so that HgbA accounts for 30 percent of fetal hemoglobin.[261] This change in expression from γ to β-globulin synthesis takes place in erythroid progenitor cells.[262] Although the basis for this switching is not yet known, our understanding of human globin gene regulation has provided important insights into several fetal hemoglobin disorders such as the thalassemias and sickle cell anemia. Duplication of the α genes on chromosome 16 provides the normal fetus with four gene loci. The genes for the remaining globins are located on chromosome 11 and consist of Gγ, Aγ, δ, and β. The two γ genes differ only in that one codes for glycine at position 136 and the other for alanine. Hemoglobin A synthesis is dictated by the α- and β-genes, hemoglobin F by α and γ, and hemoglobin A_2 by α and δ. Sequences in the δ region may be responsible for the relative expression of the γ gene, such that fetal hemoglobin persists when these are absent.[263]

Fetal Kidney

The placenta maintains fetal water and ionic homeostasis. However, urine formation by the fetal kidney is important for amniotic fluid balance. Absolute glomerular filtration rate (GFR) increases during the third trimester. However, because GFR and fetal kidney weight increase in parallel, GFR per gram kidney weight does not change.[264] The genesis of new glomeruli is complete by about 36 weeks.[265] Therefore, subsequent increases in GFR must reflect increases in glomerular surface area for filtration, effective filtration pressure, and capillary filtration coefficient. Although glomerular filtration is related to hydrostatic pressure, and fetal blood pressure increases in the third trimester, both renal blood flow per gram of kidney weight and filtration fraction (GFR/renal plasma flow) remain constant.[264] Increases in filtration fraction in the neonate parallel increases in arterial pressure, suggesting the lower hydrostatic pressure within the glomerulus contributes to the relatively low filtration fraction and GFR of the fetal kidney.[264,266] Renal tubular sodium and chloride reabsorption increase in late gestation, such that glomerulotubular balance is maintained in the third trimester fetus.[266,267]

Although fetal GFR is low, approximately 20 percent of the filtered water is lost in the form of hypotonic urine. The positive free water clearance characterizing fetal renal function originally led to the hypothesis that the fetal kidney lacked AVP receptors. However, renal collecting duct responses to AVP can be demonstrated in the second trimester,[268] indicating diminished urine concentrating ability is not due to the absence of AVP receptors. Fetal renal V_2 receptors mediate AVP-induced tubular water reabsorption, and functional V_2 receptors are present in the fetal kidney by the beginning of the last third of gestation.[240,269] In addition, AVP-induced cyclic AMP production is not different from the adult.[270] Fetal infusion with a selective V_2 receptor agonist [deamino^1, D-Arg^8]-vasopressin (dDAVP) appropriately increases early and late gestation fetal renal water reabsorption without affecting blood pressure or heart rate.[234] Thus, V_2 receptors mediate AVP effects on fetal urine production and amniotic fluid volume.[234,240] The reduced concentrating ability of the fetal kidney primarily reflects the lower medullary interstitial urea concentrations and the relative short length of the Henle's loops.

ANF granules are present in the fetal heart, and fetal plasma ANF levels are elevated relative to the adult.[271] Fetal plasma ANF levels rise in response to volume expansion,[272] and ANF infusion increases ovine fetal renal sodium excretion, although this response is diminished during the last third of gestation.[273,274] Fetal ANF infusion also decreases fetal plasma volume, with minimal effect on blood pressure.[271] These observations suggest that the role of ANF in the fetus is primarily volume homeostasis, with minimal cardiovascular effects.

The ability of the fetal kidney to excrete titratable acid and ammonia is limited relative to the adult. In addition, the threshold for fetal renal bicarbonate excretion (defined as the excretion of a determined amount of bicarbonate per unit GFR) is much lower than in the adult. That is, fetal urine tends to be alkaline at relatively low plasma bicarbonate levels, despite the high fetal arterial P_{CO_2}.[275] Because fetal renal tubular glucose reabsorption is well developed, fetal renal glucose excretion is limited. In fact, the maximum ability of the fetal kidney to reabsorb glucose exceeds that of the adult when expressed as a function of GFR.[276]

Fetal Gastrointestinal System

Gastrointestinal Tract

Amniotic fluid contains measurable glucose, lactate and amino acid concentrations, raising the possibility that fetal swallowing could serve as a source of nutrient uptake. However, the normal amniotic fluid concentrations of these substrates are not sufficient to support significant uptake by the fetal intestines. In addition, the fetal gastrointestinal tract actually consumes small amounts of glucose, lactate and amino acids.[277]

Blood flow to the fetal intestine does not increase during moderate levels of hypoxemia. The artery to mesenteric vein difference in oxygen content is also unchanged so that at a constant blood flow intestinal oxygen consumption can remain the same during moderate hypoxemia. However, with more pronounced hypoxemia, fetal intestinal oxygen consumption falls as blood flow decreases and the oxygen content difference across the intestine fails to widen. The result is a metabolic acidosis in the blood draining the mesenteric system.[278]

Liver

Near term, the placenta is the major route for bilirubin elimination. Less than 10 percent of an administered bilirubin load is excreted in the fetal biliary tree over a 10 hour period; about 20 percent remains in plasma.[279] Thus, the fetal metabolic pathways for bilirubin and bile salts remain underdeveloped at term. The cholate pool size (normalized to body surface area) is one third and the synthetic rate one half adult levels. In premature infants, cholate pool size and synthesis rates represent less than half and one third, respectively of term infant values. In fact, intraluminal duodenal bile acid concentrations in the premature infant are near or below the level required to form lipid micelles.[279]

The unique attributes of the fetal hepatic circulation were detailed during the earlier discussion of fetal circulatory anatomy. Notably, the fetal hepatic blood supply is derived primarily from the umbilical vein. The left lobe of the liver receives its blood supply almost exclusively from the umbilical vein (there is a small contribution from the hepatic artery), while the right lobe receives blood from the portal vein as well. The fetal liver under normal conditions accounts for about 20 percent of total fetal oxygen consumption.[280] Because hepatic glucose uptake and release are balanced, net glucose removal by the liver is minimal under normal conditions.[280] During episodes of hypoxemia, α-adrenergic receptor-mediated increases in hepatic glucose release account for the hyperglycemia characteristic of short term fetal hypoxemia.[186] Hypoxia severe enough to decrease fetal oxygen consumption selectively reduces right hepatic lobe oxygen uptake, which exceeds that of the fetus as a whole. In contrast, oxygen uptake by the left lobe of the liver is unchanged.[280]

Fetal Adrenal and Thyroid Systems
Adrenal Glands

The fetal pituitary secretes ACTH in response to "stress", including hypoxemia.[281] The associated increase in cortisol exerts feedback inhibition of the continued ACTH response.[282] In the fetus and adult, proopiomelanocortin posttranslational processing yields ACTH, corticotropin-like intermediate lobe peptide (CLIP) and α-melanocyte stimulating hormone (α-MSH). The precursor peptide preproenkephalin is a distinct gene product giving rise to the enkephalins. Fetal proopiomelanocortin processing differs from the adult. For example, although ACTH is present in appreciable amounts, the fetal pituitary also contains large amounts of CLIP and α-MSH. The ratio of CLIP plus α-MSH to ACTH decreases from the end of the first trimester to term.[283] Because pituitary corticotropin (CRH) expression is relatively low until late gestation, AVP serves as the major corticotropin releasing factor in early gestation. With increasing gestational age, fetal cortisol levels progressively rise as a result of maturation of the fetal hypothalamic-pituitary axis. Cortisol is important to pituitary maturation (increasing the number of adult-type corticotrophs) and to adrenal maturation (increasing ACTH receptors).[284]

On a body weight basis, the fetal adrenal gland is an order of magnitude larger than in the adult. Cortisol is the major product of the fetal definitive zone, and fetal cortisol secretion is regulated by ACTH but not human chorionic gonadotrophin (hCG).[285,286] Unique to the fetal adrenal is the so-called fetal zone, which constitutes 85 percent of the adrenal at birth. Dehydroepiandrosterone sulfate (DHEAS) is the major product of the fetal zone. In mid-gestation DHEAS secretion is stimulated by both ACTH and hCG.[285,286] Corticosterone sulfate is a minor product of the maternal adrenal and is not metabolized during fetal to maternal transplacental passage,[287] making it an excellent index of fetal adrenal corticosteroid activity. Corticosterone sulfate levels increase in amniotic fluid after 30 weeks,[288] and in maternal plasma by late in the third trimester.[289] However, the late gestation increase in fetal adrenal cortisol production is not ACTH dependent. This apparent dissociation between fetal ACTH levels and cortisol secretion[287] may be explained by: (1) the large molecular weight precursors of ACTH may suppress ACTH action on the adrenal glands which are then allowed to express their full potential as the concentration of these precursors fall, or (2) the responsiveness of the fetal adrenal definitive zone to ACTH may increase. Low density lipoprotein bound cholesterol (see receptor mediated endocytosis above) is the major steroid precursor in the fetal adrenal.[290,291] Although influenced by the maternal diurnal pattern for cortisol secretion (morning greater than evening), the fetal adrenal diurnal pattern for secretion of DHEAS and cortisol (evening greater than morning) shows an appreciable lag phase relative to the maternal pattern.[285]

Resting fetal plasma norepinephrine levels exceed

epinephrine levels approximately 10-fold.[292,293] The fetal plasma levels of both catecholamines increase in response to hypoxemia, with norepinephrine levels invariably in excess of epinephrine levels.[293] Under basal conditions, norepinephrine is secreted at a higher rate than epinephrine, and this relationship persists during a hypoxemic stimulus.[294] Plasma norepinephrine levels increase in response to acute hypoxemia, but then decline after about five minutes of persistent hypoxemia. In contrast, adrenal epinephrine secretion begins gradually, but persists during thirty minutes of hypoxemia. These observations are consistent with independent sites of synthesis and regulation of the two catecholamines.[295] While the initial fetal blood pressure elevation during hypoxemia correlates with increases in norepinephrine, afterward, the response plateaus so that no further hypertension is seen with continued increases in norepinephrine.[293]

Thyroid Gland

The normal placenta is impermeable to thyroid-stimulating hormone (TSH), and triiodothyronine (T_3) transfer is minimal.[296] However, appreciable levels of maternal thyroxine (T_4) are seen in infants with congenital hypothyroidism.[297] By the 12th week of gestation, thyrotropin releasing hormone (TRH) is present in the fetal hypothalamus, and TRH secretion and/or pituitary sensitivity to TRH increases progressively during gestation. Extrahypothalamic sites including the pancreas also may contribute to the high fetal TRH levels.[296] By week 12 of gestation, TSH is detectable in the fetal pituitary and serum, and T_4 can be measured in fetal blood. Thyroid function is low until about 20 weeks, when T_4 levels increase gradually to term. TSH levels increase markedly between 20 and 24 weeks, then slowly fall until delivery. Fetal liver T_4 metabolism is immature, and T_3 levels are low until the 30th week. In constrast, reverse T_3 levels are high and decrease steadily in the last ten weeks of gestation.

Fetal Central Nervous System

Clinically relevant indicators of fetal central nervous system function are body movements and breathing movements. Fetal activity periods in late gestation are often termed active or reactive and quiet or nonreactive. The active cycle is characterized by clustering of gross fetal body movements, high heart rate variability, heart rate accelerations (often followed by decelerations) and fetal breathing movements. The quiet cycle is noted by absence of fetal body movements and a low variability in the fetal heart period.[298,299] Fetal heart period variability in this context refers to deviations about the model heart rate period averaged over short (seconds) periods,[300] and is distinct from beat to beat

variability. In the last six weeks of gestation, the fetus is in an active state 60 to 70 percent of total time. The average duration of quiet periods ranges from 15 to 23 minutes (see Table IV in Visser et al[300] for a review).

The fetal electrocorticogram shows two predominant patterns. Low voltage electrocortical activity is associated with bursts of rapid eye movements and fetal breathing movements.[301] Similar to rapid eye movement sleep in the adult, inhibition of skeletal muscle movement is most pronounced in muscle groups having a high percentage of spindles. Thus, the diaphragm, which is relatively spindle free, is not affected. Fetal body movements during low voltage electrocortical activity are reduced relative to the activity seen during high voltage electrocortical activity.[302] Polysynaptic reflexes elicited by stimulation of afferents from limb muscles are relatively suppressed when the fetus is in the low voltage state.[303] Short term hypoxia[302] or hypoxemia inhibit reflex limb movements, with the inhibitory neural activity arising in the midbrain area.[303] Fetal cardiovascular and behavioral responses to maternal cocaine use previously have been attributed to reductions in uteroplacental blood flow and resulting fetal hypoxia. However, recent fetal sheep studies indicate that acute fetal cocaine exposure evokes catecholamine, cardiovascular and neurobehavorial effects in the absence of changes in fetal oxygenation.[304] It is not yet clear whether cocaine-induced reductions in fetal low voltage electrocortical activity reflect alterations in cerebral blood flow, or a direct effect of cocaine on norepinephrine stimulation of central regulatory centers. However, these observations suggest that cocaine use during pregnancy may have significant neurological consequences for the fetus.

Fetal breathing patterns are rapid and irregular in nature, and are not associated with significant fluid movement into the lung.[301] The central medullary respiratory chemoreceptors are stimulated by carbon dioxide,[305] and fetal breathing is maintained only if central hydrogen ion concentrations remain in the physiologic range. That is, central (medullary cerebrospinal fluid) acidosis stimulates respiratory incidence and depth and alkalosis results in apnea.[306] Hypoxemia markedly decreases breathing activity, possibly due to inhibitory input from centers above the medulla.[307]

Under normal conditions, glucose is the principal substrate for oxidative metabolism in the fetal brain.[308] During low voltage electrocortical activity, cerebral blood flow and oxygen consumption are increased relative to high voltage values,[309] with an efflux of lactate. During high voltage activity, the fetal brain shows a net uptake of lactate.[310] The fetal cerebral circulation is sensitive to changes in arterial oxygen content. The marked increase in cerebral blood induced by hypoxemia maintains oxygen consumption without any widening of the arterial-venous oxygen content difference across the brain.[311] Increases in carbon dioxide also cause cerebral vasodilation. However, the response to hypercarbia is reduced relative to the adult.[312]

Summary

The fetus and placenta depend upon unique physiologic systems to provide an environment supporting fetal growth and development, in preparation for transition to extrauterine life. Because functions of the various physiological systems are often gestation specific, differences between the fetus and adult of one specie are often greater than are the adult differences between species. Thus, the clinician or investigator concerned with fetal life or neonatal transition must fully appreciate these aspects of fetal physiology and their application to patient care and/or research.

10 Key Points

- Pregnancy associated cardiovascular changes include a doubling of maternal cardiac output and a 40 percent increase in blood volume.
- Uterine blood flow at term averages 750 ml/min or 10 to 15 percent of maternal cardiac output.
- Normal term placental weight averages 450 grams, representing approximately one-seventh (one-sixth with cord and membranes) of fetal weight.
- Mean amniotic fluid volume increases from 250 to 800 ml between 16 and 32 weeks, and remains relatively stable thereafter until near term.
- Fetal urine production ranges from 400 to 1200 ml/day and is the primary source of amniotic fluid.
- The fetal umbilical circulation receives approximately 40 percent of fetal combined ventricular output (300 ml/min/kg).
- Umbilical blood flow is 70 to 130 ml/min after 30 weeks' gestation.
- Fetal cardiac output is constant over a heart rate range of 120 to 180 beats/min.
- The fetus exists in a state of aerobic metabolism, with arterial blood PO_2 values in the 20 to 25 mmHg range.
- Approximately 20 percent of the fetal oxygen consumption of 8 ml/kg/min is required in the acquisition of new tissue.

References

1. Chalier J, Schneider H, Dancis J: In vitro perfusion of human placenta, V: oxygen consumption. Am J Obstet Gynecol 126:261, 1976
2. Meschia G, Battaglia FC, Hay WW Jr, Sparks JW: Utilization of substrates by the ovine placenta in vivo. Fed Proc 39:245, 1980
3. Hauguel S, Chalier J, Cedard L, Olive G: Metabolism of the human placenta perfused in vitro: glucose transfer and utilization, O_2 consumption, lactate and ammonia production. Pediatr Res 17:792, 1983
4. Teasdale F: Gestational changes in the functional structure of the human placenta in relation to fetal growth: a morphometric study. Am J Obstet Gynecol 137:560, 1980
5. Holzman I, Phillips AF, Battaglia FC: Glucose metabolism, lactate and ammonia production by the human placenta in vitro. Pediat Res 13:117, 1979
6. Simmons MA, Battaglia FC, Meschia G: Placental transfer of glucose. J Devel Physiol 1:227, 1979
7. Hay WW Jr, Sparks JW, Wilkening RB et al: Partition of maternal glucose production between conceptus and maternal tissues in sheep. Am J Physiol 245:E347, 1983

8. Hay WW Jr, Sparks JW, Battaglia FC, Meschia G: Maternal-fetal glucose exchange: necessity of a three-pool model. Am J Physiol 246:E523, 1984

9. Sparks JW, Hay WW Jr, Bonds D et al: Simultaneous measurements of lactate turnover rate and umbilical lactate uptake in the fetal lamb. J Clin Invest 70:179, 1982

10. Beischer NA, Holsman M, Kitchen WH: Relation of various forms of anemia to placental weight. Am J Obstet Gynecol 101:80, 1968

11. Beischer NA, Sivasamboo R, Vohras S et al: Placental hypertrophy in severe pregnancy anaemia. J Obstet Gynaecol Brit Comm 77:398, 1970

12. Agboola A: Placental changes in patients with a low haematocrit. Brit J Obstet Gynaecol 82:225, 1975

13. Gospodarowicz D: Growth factors and their action in vivo and in vitro. J Pathol 141:201, 1983

14. Posner B: Insulin receptors in human and animal placental tissue. Diabetes 23:209, 1974

15. Nelson DM, Smith RM, Jarett L: Nonuniform distribution and grouping of insulin receptors on the surface of human placental syncytiotrophoblast. Diabetes 27:530, 1978

16. Whitsett JA, Lenard JL: Characteristics of the microvillus brush border of human placenta: insulin receptor localization in brush border membranes. Endocrinol 103:1458, 1978

17. Steel RB, Mosley JD, Smith CH: Insulin and placenta: degradation and stabilization, binding to microvillous membrane receptors, and amnio acid uptake. Am J Obstet Gynecol 135:522, 1979

18. Deal CL, Guyda HJ: Insulin receptors of human term placental cells and choriocarcinoma (JEG-3) cells: characteristics and regulation. Endocrinol 112:1512, 1983

19. Harrison LC, Itin A: Purification of the insulin receptor from human placenta by chromatography on immobilized wheat germ and receptor antibody. J Biol Chem 255:12066, 1980

20. Richards RC, Beardmore JM, Brown PJ et al: Epidermal growth factor receptors on isolated human placental syncytiotrophoblast plasma membrane. Placenta 4:133, 1983

21. Lai WH, Guyda HJ: Characterization and regulation of epidermal growth factor receptors in human placental cell cultures. J Clin Endocrinol Metab 58:344, 1984

22. Zapf J, Rinderknecht E, Humbel RE, Froesch ER: Non-supressible insulin-like activity (NSILA) from human serum: recent accomplishments and their physiologic implications. Metab Clin Exp 27:1803, 1978

23. Cooke NE, Ray J, Emery JG, Liebhaber SA: Two distinct species of human growth hormone-varient mRNA in the human placenta predict the expression of novel growth hormone proteins. J Biol Chem 263:9001, 1988

24. Eriksson L, Frankenne F, Eden S et al: Growth hormone secretion during termination of pregnancy. Further evidence of a placental variant. Acta Obstet Gynecol Scand 67:549, 1988

25. Frankenne F, Closset J, Gomez F: The physiology of growth hormones (GHs) in pregnant women and partial characterization of the placental GH variant. J Clin Endocrinol Metab 66:1171, 1988

26. King BF: Distribution and characterization of the anionic sites in trophoblast and capillary basal lamina of human placental villi. Anat Record 212:63, 1985

27. Thornburg KL, Faber JJ: Transfer of hydrophilic molecules by placenta and yolk sac of the guinea pig. Am J Physiol 233:C111, 1977

28. Bissonnette JM, Cronan JZ, Richards LL, Wickham WK: Placental transfer of water and nonelectrolytes during a single circulatory passage. Am J Physiol 236:C47, 1979

29. Delivoria-Papadopoulos M, Coburn RF, Forster RE II: The placental diffusing capacity for carbon monixide in pregnant women at term. p 259. In Longo LD, Bartles H (eds): Respiratory Gas Exchange and Blood Flow in the Placenta. US Dept of Health, Education, and Welfare, Bethesda, 1972

30. Rooth G, Sjostedt S: The placental transfer of gases and fixed acids. Arch Dis Child 37:366, 1962

31. Stenger V, Eitzman D, Anderson T et al: Observations on the placental exchange of the respiratory gases in pregnant women in cesarean section. Am J Obstet Gynecol 88:45, 1964

32. Sjostedt S, Rooth G, Caligara F: The oxygen tension of the blood in the umbilical cord and intervillous space. Arch Dis Child 35:529, 1960

33. Wulf H: Der Gasaustausch in der reifen Plazenta des Menschen. Z Geburtsh Gynak 158:117, 1962

34. Clapp JF III: The relationship between blood flow and oxygen uptake in the uterine and umbilical circulations. Am J Obstet Gynecol 132:410, 1978

35. Wilkening RB, Meschia G: Fetal oxygen uptake, oxygenations, and acid-base balance as a function of uterine blood flow. Am J Physiol 244:H749, 1983

36. Itskovitz J, LaGamma EF, Rudolph LAM: The effect of reducing umbilical blood flow on fetal oxygenation. Am J Obstet Gynecol 145:813, 1983

37. Longo LD, Delivoria-Papadopoulos M, Foster RE II: Placental CO_2 transfer after fetal carbonic anhydrase inhibition. Am J Physiol 226:703, 1974

38. Bissonnette JM: Studies in vivo of glucose transfer acorss the guinea-pig placenta. p 155. In Young M, Boyd RDH, Longo LD, Telegdy G (eds): Placental Transfer: Methods and Interpretations. WB Saunders, Philadelphia, 1981

39. Johnson LW, Smith CH: Identification of the glucose transport protein of the microvillous membrane of human placenta by photoaffinity labeling. Biochem Biophys Res Comm 109:408, 1982

40. Ingermann RL, Bissonnette JM, Koch PL: d-glucose-sensitive and -insensitive cytochalasin B binding proteins from microvillous plasma membranes of human placenta: identification of the d-glucose transporter. Biochim Biophys Acta 730:57, 1983

41. Turner RJ, Silverman M: Sugar uptake into brush border vesicles from normal human kidney. Proc Natl Acad Sci USA 74:2825, 1977

42. Ciaraldi TP, Kolterman OE, Siegel JA, Olefsky JM: Insulin-stimulated glucose transport in human adipocytes. Am J Physiol 236:E621, 1979

43. Johnson LW, Smith CH: Monosaccharide transport

across microvillous membrane of human placenta. Am J Physiol 236:E621, 1980

44. Bissonnette JM, Ingermann RL, Thronburg KL: Placental sugar transport. p 65. In Yudilevich DL, Mann GE (eds): Carrier-Mediated Transport of Solutes from Blood to Tissue. Longman, London, 1985

45. Ingermann RL, Bissonnette JM: Effect of temperature on kinetics of hexose uptake by human placental plasma membrane vesicles. Biochim Biophys Acta 734:329, 1983

46. Cordero L Jr, Yeh SY, Grunt JA, Anderson GG: Hypertonic glucose infusion during labor. Am J Obstet Gynecol 407:295, 1970

47. Christensin HN: Biological Transport. 2nd ed. Reading, MA, p. 175, 1975

48. Enders RH, Judd RM, Donohue TM, Smith CH: Placental amino acid uptake, III: transport systems for neutral amino acids. Am J Physiol 230:706, 1976

49. Ruzycki SM, Kelly LK, Smith CH: Placental amino acid uptake, IV: Transport by microvillous membrane vesicles. Am J Physiol 234:C27, 1978

50. Boyd CAR, Lund EK: l-Proline support by brush border membrane vesicles prepared from human placenta. J Physiol 315:9, 1981

51. Whitsett JA, Wallick ET: [3H] Oubain binding and Na⁺-K-ATPase activity in human placenta. Am J Physiol 238:E38, 1980

52. Smith CH, Adcock EW, Teasdale F et al: Placental amino acid uptake: tissue preparation, kinetics, and preincubation effect. Am J Physiol 224:558, 1973

53. Smith CH, Depper R: Placental amino acid uptake, II: tissue preincubation, fluid distribution and mechanisms of regulation. Pediatr Res 8:697, 1974

54. Longo LD, Yuen P, Gusseck DJ: Anaerobic glycogen-dependent transport of amnio acids by the placenta. Nature 243:531, 1973

55. Johnson LW, Smith CH: Neutral amino acid transport systems of microvillous membrane of human placenta. Am J Physiol 254:C773, 1988

56. Moe AJ: Placental amino acid transport. Am J Physiol. 268:C1321, 1995

57. Steglink LD, Pitkin RM, Reynolds WA et al: Placental transfer of glutamate and its metabolites in the primate. Am J Obstet Gynecol 122:70, 1975

58. Steglink LD, Pitkin RM, Brummel MC, Filer LJ Jr: Placental transfer of aspartate and its metabolites in the primate. Metabol 28:669, 1979

59. Schneider H, Mohlen K-H, Dancis J: Transfer of amino acids across the in vitro perfused human placenta. Pediatr Res 13:236, 1979

60. Hayashi S, Sanada K, Sagawa N et al: Umbilical vein–artery differences of plasma amino acids in the last trimester of human pregnancy. Biol Neonate 34:11, 1978

61. Schneider H, Mohlen K-H, Challier T-C, Dancis J: Transfer of glutamic acid across the human placenta perfused 'in vitro.' Br J Obstet Gynaecol 86:299, 1979

62. Steel RB, Smith CH, Kelly LK: Placental amino acid uptake, VI: regulation by intracellular substrate. Am J Physiol 243:C46, 1982

63. Dancis J, Money WL, Springer D, Levitz M: Transport of amino acids by placenta. Am J Obstet Gynecol 101:820, 1968

64. Karl PI, Alpy KL, Fisher SE: Amino acid transport by the cultured human palcental trophoblast: effect of insulin on AIB transport. Am J Physiol 262:C834, 1992

65. Kuruvilla AG, D'Souza SW, Glazier JD et al: Altered activity of the system A aminoacid transporter in microvillous membrane vesicles from placentas of macrosomic babies born to diabetic women. J Clin Invest 94:689, 1995

66. Dancis J, Jansen V, Kayden HJ et al: Transfer across perfused human placenta, II: free fatty acids. Pediat Res 7:192, 1973

67. Booth C, Elphick MC, Hentrickse W, Hull D: Investigation of [14C] linoleic acid conversion into [14C] arachidonic acid and placental transfer of linoleic and palmitic acids across the perfused human placenta. J Devel Physiol 3:177, 1981

68. Dancis J, Jansen V, Kayden HJ et al: Transfer across perfused human-placenta, III: effect of chain length on transfer of free fatty acids. Pediat Res 8:796, 1974

69. Dancis J, Jansen V, Levitz M: Transfer across perfused human placenta, IV: effect of protein binding on free fatty acids. Pediat Res 10:5, 1976

70. Faber JJ, Thornburg KL: Fetal homeostatis in relation to placental water exchange. Ann Rech Vet 8:353, 1977

71. Dancis J, Kammerman BS, Jansen V et al: Transfer of urea, sodium, and chloride across the perfused human placenta. Am J Obstet Gynecol 141:677, 1981

72. Faber JJ, Thornburg KL: Placental Physiology. p. 95. Raven Press, New York, 1983

73. Faber JJ, Thornburg KL: The forces that drive inert solutes and water across the epitheliochorial placentae of the sheep and the goat and the haemochorial placentae of the rabbit and the guinea pig. p. 203. In Young M, Boyd RDH, Longo LD, Teleydy G (eds): Placental Transfer: Methods and Interpretations. WB Saunders, Philadelphia, 1981

74. Battaglia F: Fetal blood studies, XIII: the effect of the administration of fluids intravenously to mothers upon the concentrations of water and electrolytes in plasma of human fetuses. Pediatrics 25:2, 1960

75. Reynolds SRM: Multiple simultaneous intervillous space pressures recorded in several regions of the hemochorial palcenta in relation to functional anatomy of the fetal cotyledon. Am J Obstet Gynecol 102:1128, 1968

76. Seeds AE: Water metabolism in the fetus. Am J Obstet Gynecol 92:727, 1965

77. Anderson DF, Faber JJ: Water flux due to colloid osmotic pressures across the haemochorial placenta of the guinea pig. J Physiol 332:521, 1982

78. Lajeunesse D, Brunette MG: Sodium gradient-dependent phosphate transport in placental brush border membrane vesicles. Placenta 9:117, 1988

79. Balkovetz DF, Leibach FH, Mahesh VB et al: Na⁺-H⁺ exchanger of human placental brush-border membrane: identification and characterization. Am J Physiol 251:C852, 1986

80. Bara M, Challier JC, Guit-Bara A: Membrane potential and input resistance in syncytiotrophoblast of human term placenta in vitro. Placenta 9:139, 1988

81. Shennan DB, Davis B, Boyd CAR: Chloride transport in human placental microvillous membrane vessicles, I: evidence for anion exchange. Pflugers Arch 406:60, 1986

82. Illsley NP, Glaubensklee C, Davis B, Verkman AS: Chloride transport across placental microvillous membranes measured by fluoresence. Am J Physiol 255:C789, 1988

83. Byrne S, Glazier JD, Greenwood SL et al: Chloride transport by human placental microvillous membrane vesicles. Biochim Biophys Acta 1153:122, 1993

84. Care AD, Ross R, Pickard DW et al: Calcium homeostasis in the fetal pig. J Devel Physiol 4:85, 1982

85. Fisher GJ, Kelly LK, Smith CH: ATP-dependent calcium transport across basal plasma membranes of human placental trophoblast. Am J Physiol 252:C38, 1987

86. Durand D, Barlet JP, Braithwaite GD: The influence of 1,25-dihydroxycholecalciferol on the mineral content of foetal guinea pigs. Reprod Nutr Dev 23:235, 1983

87. Tuan RS: Identification and characterization of a calcium-binding protein from human placenta. Placenta 3:145, 1982

88. Wild AE: Trophoblast cell surface receptors. In Loke YW, Whyte A (eds): Biology of the Trophoblast. Elsevier Biomedical Press, London, 1983

89. Johnson PM, Brown PJ: Fc receptors in the human placenta. Placenta 2:355, 1981

90. Loh TT, Higuchi DA, van Bockxmeer FM: Transferrin receptors on the human placental microvillus membrane. J Clin Invest 65:1182, 1980

91. Goldstein JL, Anderson RGW, Brown MS: Coated pits, coated vesicles and receptor-mediated endocytosis. Nature 279:679, 1979

92. Brown MA, Anderson RGW, Goldstein JL: Recycling receptors: The round trip itinerary of migrant membrane proteins. Cell 32:663 1983

93. Pastan IH, Willingham MC: Journey to the center of the cell: role of the receptosome. Science 214:504 1981

94. Dautry-Varsat A, Cierchanover A, Lodish HF: pH and the recycling of transferin during receptor-mediated endocytosis. Proc Natl Acad Sci USA 80:2258, 1983

95. Lin DS, Pitkin RM, Connor WE: Placental transfer of cholesterol into the human fetus. Am J Obstet Gynecol 128:735, 1977

96. Rosenfeld CR: Circulatory changes in the reproductive tissues of ewes during pregnancy. Gynecol Invest 5:252, 1974

97. Longo LD, Ching KS: Placental diffusing capacity for carbon monoxide and oxygen in unanesthetized sheep. J Appl Physiol 43:885, 1977

98. Bissonnette JM, Wickham WK: Placental diffusing capacity for carbon monoxide in unanesthetized guinea pigs. Respir Physiol 31:161, 1977

99. Assali NS, Douglas RA, Barid WW et al: Measurement of uterine blood flow and uterine metabolism. Am J Obstet Gynecol 66:248, 1953

100. Metcalfe J, Romney SL, Ramsey LH et al: Estimation of uterine blood flow and uterine metabolism. J Clin Invest 34:1632, 1995

101. Rosenfeld CR, Naden RP: Responses of uterine and nonuterine tissues to angiotensin II in ovine pregnancy. Am J Physiol 257:H17, 1995

102. Meschia G: Circulation to female reproductive organs. p. 241. In The Cardiovascular System: Peripheral Circulation and Organ Blood Flow. In Shepherd JT, Abboud FM (eds): Handbook of Physiology. Vol. 3. American Physiology Society, Bethesda, 1983

103. Hendricks CH, Quilligan EJ, Tyler CW, Tucker CJ: Pressure relationships between the intervillous space and the amniotic fluid in human term pregnancy. Am J Obstet Gynecol 77:1028, 1959

104. Rudolph AM, Heymann MA: Circulatory changes during growth in the fetal lamb. Circ Res 26:289, 1970

105. Wladimiroff JW, McGhie J: Ultrasonic assessment of cardiovascular geometry and function in the human fetus. Br J Obstet Gynaecol 88:870, 1981

106. Makowski EL, Meschia G, Droegemueller W, Battaglia FC: Measurement of umbilical arterial blood flow to the sheep placenta and fetus in utero. Circ Res 23:623, 1968

107. Berman W Jr, Goodlin RC, Heymann MA, Rudolph AM: Relationships between pressure and flow in the umbilical and uterine circulations of the sheep. Circ Res 38:262, 1976

108. Thornburg KL, Bissonnette JM, Faber JJ: Absence of fetal placental waterfall phenomenon in chronically prepared fetal lambs. Am J Physiol 230:886, 1976

109. Cohn HE, Sacks EJ, Heymann MA, Rudolph AM: Cardiovascular responses to hypoxemia and acidemia in fetal lambs. Am J Obstet Gynecol 120:817, 1974

110. Parer JT: Fetal oxygen uptake and umbilical circulation during maternal hypoxia in the chronically catheterized sheep. p. 231. In Longo LD, Reneau DD (eds): Fetal and Newborn Cardiovascular Physiology. Vol. 2. Garland STPM Press, New York, 1978

111. Peeters LLH, Sheldon RE, Jones MD Jr et al: Blood flow to fetal organs as a function of arterial oxygen content. Am J Obstet Gynecol 135:637, 1979

112. Cohn HE, Piasecki GJ, Jackson BT: The effect of fetal heart rate on cardiovascular function during hypoxemia. Am J Obstet Gynecol 138:1190, 1980

113. Galbraith RM, Kantor RRS, Ferra GB et al: Differential anatomical expression of transplantation antigens within the normal human placental chorionic villus. Am J Reprod Immunol 1:331, 1981

114. Sunderland CA, Naiem M, Mason DY et al: The expression of major histocompatibility antigens by human chorionic villi. J Reprod Immunol 3:323, 1981

115. Cross JC, Werb Z, Fisher SJ: Implantation and the placenta: key pieces of the development puzzle. Science 266:1508, 1994

116. Beer AE: Immunologic aspects of normal pregnancy and recurrent spontaneous abortion. Semin Reprod Endocinol 6:163, 1988

117. Sunderland CA, Redman CWG, Stirrat GM: HLA A,B,C antigens are expressed on nonvillous trophoblast of the early human placenta. J Immunol 127:2614, 1981

118. Faulk WP, Hsi B-L: Immunology of human trophoblast

membrane antigens. p. 535. In Loke YW, Whyte A (eds): Biology of Trophoblast. Elsevier, New York, 1983

119. Szulman AE: The ABH blood groups and development. Curr Top Dev Biol 14:127, 1980

120. Faulk WP: Immunobiology of human extraembryonic membranes. p. 253. In Wegman TG, Gill TJ (eds): Immunology of Reproduction. Oxford University Press, New York, 1983

121. Klopper A: The new placental proteins. Placenta 1:77, 1980

122. Rocklin RE, Kitzmiller JL, Farvoy MR: Maternal fetal relation, II: further characterization of an immunologic blocking factor that develops during pregnancy. Clin Immunol Immunopathol 22:305, 1982

123. Beer AE, Quebberman JF, Ayers JW, Haines RF: Major histocompatibility antigens maternal and paternal immune responses and chronic habitual abortion in humans. Am J Obstet Gynecol 141:987, 1981

124. Komlos L, Zamir R, Joshua H, Halbrecht I: Common HLA antigens in couples with repeated abortions. Clin Immunol Immunopathol 7:330, 1977

125. Taylor C, Faulk WP: Prevention of recurrent abortions with leukocyte transfusions. Lancet 2:68, 1980

126. Redline RW, Lu CY: Role of local immunosuppression in murine fetoplacental listerosis. J Clin Invest 79:1234, 1987

127. Jacoby DR, Olding LB, Oldstone MD: Immunologic regulation of fetal–maternal balance. Adv Immunol 35: 157, 1984

128. Brace RA, Wolf EJ: Normal amniotic fluid volume changes throughout pregnancy. Am J Obstet Gynecol 161:382, 1989

129. Anderson DF, Faber JJ, Parks CM: Extraplacental transfer of waters in the sheep. J Physiol 406:75, 1988

130. Mesher EJ, Platzker AC, Ballard PL et al: Ontogeny of tracheal fluid, pulmonary surfactant, and plasma corticoids in the fetal lamb. J Appl Physiol 39:1017, 1975

131. Olver RE, Schneeberger EE, Walters DV: Epithelial solute premeability, ion transport and tight junction morphology in the developing lung of the fetal lamb. J Physiol 315:395, 1981

132. Adamson TM, Boyd RDH, Platt HS, Strang LB: Composition of alveolar liquid in the foetal lamb. J Physiol 204:159, 1969

133. Walters DV, Olver RE: The role of catecholamines in lung fluid absorption at birth. Pediatr Res 12:239, 1978

134. Perks AM, Cassin S: The effects of arginine vasopressin on lung fluid secretion in chronic fetal sheep. p. 252. In Jones CT, Nathanielsz PW (eds): The Physiological Development of the Fetus and Newborn. Academic Press, London, 1985

135. Castro R, Ervin MG, Ross MG et al: Ovine fetal lung fluid response to atrial natriuretic factor. Am J Obstet Gynecol 161:1337, 1989

136. Gresham EL, Rankin JHG, Makowski EL et al: An evaluation of fetal renal function in a chronic sheep preparation. J Clin Invest 51:149, 1977

137. Rabinowitz R, Peters MT, Vyas S et al: Measurement of fetal urine production in normal pregnancy by real-time ultrasonography. Am J Obstet Gynecol 161:1264, 1989

138. Canning JF, Boyd RDH: Mineral and water exchange between mother and fetus. p. 481. In Beard RW, Nathanielsz PW (eds): Fetal Physiology and Medicine. Marcel Dekker, New York, 1984

139. Robillard JE, Weitzman RE: Developmental aspects of the fetal renal response to exogenous arginine vasopressin. Am J Physiol 238:F407, 1980

140. Lingwood B, Hardy KJ, Coghlan JP, Wintour EM: Effect of aldosterone on urine composition in the chronically cannulated ovine fetus. J Endocrinol 76:553, 1978

141. Harding R, Bocking AD, Sigger JN, Wickham PJD: Composition and volume of fluid swallowed by sheep. Q J Exp Physiol 69:487, 1984

142. Pritchard JA: Deglutition of normal and anencephalic fetuses. Obstet Gynecol 25:289, 1965

143. Pritchard JA: Fetal swallowing and amniotic fluid volume. Obstet Gynecol 28:606, 1966

144. Bradley RM, Mistretta CM: Swallowing in fetal sheep. Science 179:1016, 1973

145. Harding R, Bocking AD, Sigger JN, Wickham PJD: Composition and volume of fluid swallowed by fetal sheep. Quart J Exper Physiol 69:487, 1984

146. Abramovich DR: Fetal factors influencing the volume and composition of liquor amnii. Br J Obstet Gynecol 77:865, 1970

147. Harding R, Sigger JN, Poore ER, Johnson P: Ingestion in fetal sheep and its relation to sleep states and breathing movements. Q J Exp Physiol 69:477, 1984

148. Ross MG, Sherman DJ, Ervin MG et al: Stimuli for fetal swallowing: systemic factors. Am J Obstet Gynecol 161: 1559, 1989

149. Abramovich DR, Page KR, Jandial L: Bulk flows through human fetal membranes. Gynecol Invest 7:157, 1976

150. Gilbert WM, Brace RA: The missing link in amniotic fluid volume regulation: intramembranous flow. Obstet Gynecol 74:748, 1989

151. Widdowson EH, Spray CM: Chemical development in utero. Arch Dis Child 26:205, 1951

152. Sparks JW, Girand JR, Battaglia FC: An estimate of the calorie requirements of the human fetus. Biol Neonate 38:113, 1980

153. Battaglia FC: The comparative physiology of fetal nutrition. Am J Obstet Gynecol 148:850, 1984

154. Clapp JFI, Szeto HH, Larrow R et al: Fetal metabolic response to experimental placental vascular damage. Am J Obstet Gynecol 140:446, 1981

155. Kalhan SC, D'Angelo LJ, Savin SM, Adam PAJ: Glucose production in pregnant women at term gestation: sources of glucose for human fetus. J Clin Invest 63: 388, 1979

156. Morris FH Jr, Makowski EL, Meschia G, Battaglia FC: The glucose/oxygen quotient of the term human fetus. Biol Neonate 25:44, 1975

157. Warshaw JB: Fatty acid metabolism during development. Semin Perinataol 3:31, 1979

158. Hay WW Jr, Myers SA, Sparks JW et al: Glucose and lactate oxidation rates in the fetal lamb. Proc Soc Exp Biol Med 173:553, 1983

159. Lemons JA, Schreiner RL: Amino acid metabolism in the ovine fetus. Am J Physiol 244:E459, 1983

160. Battaglia FC: An update of fetal and placental metabolism: carbohydrates and amino acids. Biol Neonate 55: 347, 1989

161. Marconi AM, Sparks JW, Battaglia FC, Meschia G: A comparison of amino acid arteriovenous differences across the liver, hindlimb and placenta in the fetal lamb. Am J Physiol 257:E909, 1989

162. Schoenle E, Zopf J, Humbel RE, Groesch ER: Insulin-like growth factor I stimulates growth in hypophysectomized rats. Nature 296:252, 1982

163. D'Ercole AJ, Stiles AD, Underwood LE: Tissue concentration of somatomedin C: further evidence for multiple sites of synthesis and paracrine or autocrine mechanism of action. Proc Natl Acad Sci USA 81:935, 1984

164. King GL, Kahn CR, Rechler MM, Nissley SP: Direct demonstration of separate receptors for growth and metabolic activities of insulin and multiplication stimulating activity (an insulin-like growth factor) using antibodies to the insulin receptor. J Clin Invest 66:130, 1980

165. Jost A: Fetal hormones and fetal growth. Contrib Gynecol Obstet 5:1, 1979

166. Gluckman PD, Liggins GC: Regulation of fetal growth. p. 511. In Beard RW, Nathanielsz PW (eds): Fetal Physiology and Medicine. Marcel Dekker, New York, 1984

167. Gluckman PD: Functional maturation of the neuroendocrine system in the perinatal period: studies of the somatotrophic axis in the ovine fetus. J Develop Physiol 6:301, 1984

168. Palmiter RD, Norstedt G, Gelinas RE et al: Metallothionein–human GH fusion genes stimulate growth of mice. Science 222:809, 1983

169. Browne CA, Thorburn CA: Endocrine control of fetal growth. Biol Neonate 55:331, 1989

170. Hill DE: Fetal effects of insulin. Obstet Gynecol Ann 11:133, 1982

171. Susa JG, Gruppuso PA, Widness JA et al: Chronic hyperinsulinemia in the fetal rhesus monkey: effects of physiologic hyperinsulinemia on fetal substrates, hormones, and hepatic enzymes. Am J Obstet Gynecol 150:415, 1984

172. Philips AF, Dubin JW, Raye JR: Fetal metabolic responses to endogenous insulin release. Am J Obstet Gynecol 139:441, 1981

173. Hay WW, Meznarich HK, Sparks JW et al: Effect of insulin on glucose uptake in near-term fetal lambs. Proc Soc Exp Biol Med 178:557, 1985

174. Oppenheimer CL, Pessin JE, Massague J et al: Insulin action rapidly modulates the apparent affinity of the insulin-like growth factor II receptor. J Biol Chem 258: 4824, 1983

175. Sara VR, Hall K, Misaki M et al: Ontogenesis of somatomedin and insulin receptors in the human fetus. J Clin Invest 71:1084, 1983

176. Cardell BS: The infants of diabetic mothers: a morphological study. J Obst Gynecol Brit Comm 60:834, 1953

177. Siddiqi TA, Miodovnik M, Mimouni F et al: Biphasic intrauterine growth in insulin-dependent diabetic pregnancies. J Am Coll Nutr 8:225, 1989

178. Fowden AL, Comline RS: The effects of pancreatectomy on the sheep fetus in utero. Q J Exp Physiol 69:319, 1984

179. Fowden AL, Hay WW Jr: The effects of pancreatectomy on the rates of glucose utilization, oxidation and production in the sheep fetus. Q J Exp Physiol 73:973, 1988

180. Fowden AL: The role of insulin in fetal growth. J Develop Physiol 12:173, 1989

181. Bennett A, Wilson DM, Liu F et al: Levels of insulin-like growth factors I and II in human cord blood. J Clin Endocrinol Metab 57:609, 1983

182. Adams SO, Nissley SP, Handwerger S, Rechler MM: Developmental patterns of insulin-like growth factor I and II synthesis and regulation in rat fibroblasts. Nature 302:150, 1983

183. Hill DJ, Freemark M, Strain AJ et al: Placental lactogen and growth hormone receptors in human fetal tissues: relationship to fetal plasma human placental lactogen concentrations. J Clin Endocrinol Metab 66:1283, 1988

184. Nielsen PU, Pedersen H, Kampmann E-M: Absence of human placental lactogen in an otherwise uneventful pregnancy. Am J Obstet Gynecol 135:322, 1979

185. Sperling MA, Christensen RA, Ganguli S, Anand R: Adrenergic modulation of pancreatic hormone secretion in utero: studies in fetal sheep. Pediat Res 14:203, 1980

186. Jones CT, Ritchie JWK, Walker D: The effects of hypozia on glucose turnover in the fetal sheep. J Develop Physiol 5:223, 1983

187. Devaskar SU, Ganuli S, Styer D et al: Glucagon and glucose dynamics in sheep: evidence for glucagon resistance in the fetus. Am J Physiol 246:E256, 1984

188. Gospodarowicz D: Epidermal and nerve growth factors in mammalian development. Ann Rev Physiol 43:251, 1981

189. Jouppila P, Kirkinen P, Eik-Nes S, Koivula A: Fetal and intervillous blood flow measurements in late pregnancy. p. 226. In Kurjak A, Kratochwil A (eds): Recent Advances in Ultrasound Diagnosis. Excerpta Medica, Amsterdam, 1981

190. Rudolph AM: Hepatic and ductus venosus blood flows during fetal life. Hepatology 3:254, 1983

191. Anderson DF, Bissonnette JM, Faber JJ, Thornburg KL: Central shunt flows and pressures in the mature fetal lamb. Am J Physiol 241:H60, 1981

192. Paton JB, Fisher DE, Peterson EN: Cardiac output and organ blood flows in the baboon fetus. Biol Neonate 22: 50, 1973

193. Edelstone DI, Rudolph AM, Heymann MA: Liver and ductus venosus blood flows in fetal lambs in utero. Circ Res 42:426, 1978

194. Thornburg KL, Morton MJ: Filling and arterial pressures as determinants of RV stroke volume in the sheep fetus. Am J Physiol 244:H656, 1983

195. Pinson CW, Morton MJ, Thornburg KL: An anatomic basis for right ventricular dominance and arterial pressure sensitivity. J Dev Physiol 9:253, 1987

196. Thornburg KL, Morton MG: Filling and arterial pres-

sures as determinants of left ventricular stroke volume in fetal lambs. Am J Physiol 251:H961, 1986

197. Cheng JB, Goldfien A, Cornett LE, Roberts JM: Identification of B-adrenergic receptors using [3H] dihydroalprenolol in fetal sheep heart: direct evidence of qualitative similarity to the receptors in adult sheep heart. Pediatr Res 15:1083, 1981

198. Andersen PAW, Manning A, Glick KL, Crenshaw CC Jr: Biophysics of the developing heart, III: a comparison of the left ventricular dynamics of the fetal and neonatal heart. Am J Obstet Gynecol 143:195, 1982

199. Fisher DJ, Heymann MA, Rudolph AM: Regional myocardial blood flow and oxygen delivery in fetal, newborn and adult sheep. Am J Physiol 243:H729, 1982

200. Fisher DJ, Heymann MA, Rudolph AM: Myocardial oxygen and carbohydrate consumption in fetal lambs in utero and in adult sheep. Am J Physiol 238:H399, 1980

201. Werner JC, Sicard RE, Schuler HG: Palmitate oxidation by isolated working fetal and newborn hearts. Am J Physiol 256:E315, 1989

202. Visser GHA, Dawes GS, Redman CWG: Numerical analysis of the normal human antenatal fetal heart rate. Brit J Obstet Gynecol 88:792, 1981

203. Patrick J, Campbell K, Carmichael L, Probert C: Influence of maternal heart rate and gross fetal body movements on the daily pattern of fetal heart rate near term. Am J Obstet Gynecol 144:533, 1982

204. Bocking AD, Harding R, Wickham PJ: Relationship between accelerations and decelerations in heart rate and skeletal muscle activity in fetal sheep. J Develop Physiol 7:47, 1985

205. Kenny J, Plappert T, Doubilet P et al: Effects of heart rate on ventricular size, stroke volume, and output in the normal human fetus: a prospective Doppler echocardiographic study. Circulation 76:52, 1987

206. Anderson PAW, Glick KL, Killam AP, Mainwaring RD: The effect of heart rate on in utero left ventricular output in the fetal sheep. J Physiol 372:557, 1986

207. Anderson PAW, Killam AP, Mainwaring RD, Oakley AK: In utero right ventricular output in the fetal lamb: the effect of heart rate. J Physiol 387:297, 1987

208. Nuwayhid B, Brinkman CR III, Su C et al: Development of autonomic control of fetal circulation. Am J Physiol 228:337, 1975

209. Assali NS, Brinkman CR III, Woods JR et al: Development of neurohumoral control of fetal, neonatal, and adult cardiovascular functions. Am J Obstet Gynecol 129:748, 1977

210. Walker AM, Cannata J, Dowling MH et al: Sympathetic and parasympathetic control of heart rate in unanaesthetized fetal and newborn lambs. Biol Neonate 33:135, 1978

211. Dalton KJ, Dawes GS, Patrick JE: The autonomic nervous system and fetal heart rate variability. Am J Obstet Gynecol 146:456, 1983

212. Tabsh K, Nuwayhid B, Murad S et al: Circulatory effects of chemical sympathectomy in fetal, neonatal and adult sheep. Am J Physiol 243:H113, 1982

213. Jones CT, Roeback MM, Walker DW et al: Cardiovascular, metabolic and endocrine effects of chemical sympathectomy and of adrenal demedullation in fetal sheep. J Dev Physiol 9:347, 1987

214. Iwamoto HS, Rudolph AM, Miskin BL, Keil LC: Circulatory and humoral responses of sympathectomized fetal sheep to hypoxemia. Am J Physiol 245:H767, 1983

215. Schuijers JA, Walkere DW, Browne CA, Thorburn GD: Effect of hypoxemia on plasma catecholamines in intact and immunosympathectomized fetal lambs. Am J Physiol 251:R893, 1986

216. Shinebourne EA, Vapaavuori EK, Williams RL et al: Development of baroreflex activity in unanesthetized fetal and neonatal lambs. Circ Res 31:710, 1972

217. Dawes GS, Johnston BM, Walker DW: Relationship of arterial pressure and heart rate in fetal, newborn and adult sheep. J Physiol 309:405, 1980

218. Itskovitz J, LaGamma EF, Rudolph AM: Baroreflex control of the circulation in chronically instrumented fetal lambs. Circ Res 52:589, 1983

219. Yardley RW, Bowes G, Wilkinson M et al: Increased arterial pressure variability after arterial baroreceptor denervation in fetal lambs. Circ Res 52:580, 1983

220. Rudolph AM: The fetal circulation and its response to stress. J Develop Physiol 6:11, 1984

221. Skowsky WR, Fisher DA: Fetal neurohypophysial arginine vasopressin and arginine vasotocin in man and sheep. Pediatr Res 11:627, 1977

222. Weitzman RE, Fisher DA, Robillard JE et al: AVP response to an osmotic stimulus in the fetal sheep. Pediatr Res 121:35, 1978

223. Leake RD, Weitzman RE, Effros RM et al: Maternal fetal osmolar homeostasis: fetal posterior pituitary autonomy. Pediatr Res 13:841, 1978

224. Ervin MG, Ross MG, Youseff A et al: Renal effects of ovine fetal arginine vasopressin secretion in response to maternal hyperosmolality. Am J Obstet Gynecol 155:1341, 1986

225. Ross MG, Sherman DG, Ervin MG et al: Maternal dehydration/rehydration: fetal plasma and urinary responses. Am J Physiol 255:E674, 1988

226. Robillard JE, Weitzman RE, Fisher DA, Smith FG: The dynamics of AVP release and blood volume regulation during fetal hemorrhage in the lamb fetus. Ped Res 13:606, 1979

227. Rurak DW: Plasma vasopressin levels during hemorrhage in mature and immature fetal sheep. J Develop Physiol 1:91, 1979

228. Rose JE, Meis PJ, Morris M: Ontogeny of endocrine (ACTH, vasopressin, cortisol) responses to hypotension in lamb fetuses. Am J Physiol 240:E656, 1981

229. Ross MG, Ervin MG, Leake RD et al: Isovolemic hypotension in the ovine fetus: plasma AVP response and urinary effects. Am J Physiol 250:E564, 1986

230. Iwamoto HS, Kaufman TM, Rudolph AM: Response of young fetal sheep to acute hypoxemia. Soc Gynecol Invest 35:62, 1988

231. Stark R, Wardlow JL, Daniel SS et al: Vasopressin secretion induced by hypoxia in sheep: developmental changes and relationship to B-endorphin release. Am J Obstet Gynecol 143:204, 1982

232. Rurak DW: Plasma vasopressin levels during hypo-

xemia and the cardiovascular effects of exogenous vasopressin in foetal and adult sheep. J Physiol 277:341, 1978

233. Kelly RT, Rose JC, Meis PJ et al: Vasopressin is important for restoring cardiovascular homeostasis in fetal lambs subjected to hemorrhage. Am J Obstet Gynecol 146:807, 1983

234. Ervin MG, Terry KA, Calvario GC, Shaw S: Ovine fetal cardiovascular responses to acute hypotension during vasopressin V1 receptor blockade. Endocr Soc Abstract 75:789, 1993

235. Perez R, Espinoza M, Riquelme R et al: AVP mediates cardiovascular responses to hypoxemia in fetal sheep. Am J Physiol 256:R1011, 1989

236. Norman LJ, Lye SJ, Wlodek MD, Challis JRG: Changes in pituitary responses to synthetic ovine corticotropin releasisng factor in fetal sheep. Can J Pharmacol 63: 1398, 1985

237. Faucher DJ, Lowe TW, Magness RR et al: Vasopressin and catecholamine secretion during metabolic acidemia in the ovine fetus. Pediatr Res 21:38, 1987

238. Harper MA, Rose JC: Vasopressin-induced bradycardia in fetal and adult sheep is not dependent on an increase in blood pressure. Am J Obstet Gynecol 157:448, 1987

239. Apostolakis EM, Longo LD, Yellon SM: Regulation of basal adrenocorticotropin and cortisol secretion by arginine vasopressin in the fetal sheep during late gestation. Endocrinol 129:295, 1991

240. Ervin MG, Ross MG, Leake RD, Fisher DA: V1 and V2 receptor contributions to ovine fetal renal and cardiovascular responses to vasopressin. Am J Physiol 262: R636, 1992

241. Iwamoto HS, Rudolph AM, Keil LC, Heymann MA: Hemodynamic responses of the sheep fetus to vassopressin infusion. Circ Res 44:430, 1979

242. Irion GL, Mack CE, Clark KE: Fetal hemodynamic and fetoplacental vascular response to exogenous arginine vasopressin. Am J Obstet Gynecol 162:1115, 1990

243. Tomita H, Brace RA, Cheung CY, Longo LD: Vasopressin dose-response effects on fetal vascular pressures, heart rate and blood volume. Am J Physiol 249:H974, 1985

244. Robillard JR, Nakamura KT: Neurohormonal regulation of renal function during development. Am J Physiol 254:F771, 1988

245. Lumbers ER, Stevens AD: The effects of furosemide, saralasin and hypotension on fetal plasma renin activity and on fetal renal function. J Physiol 393:479, 1987

246. Gomez RA, Robillard JE: Developmental aspects of the renal response to hemorrhage during converting-enzyme inhibition in fetal lambs. Circ Res 54:301, 1984

247. Lumbers ER, Lee Lewes J: The actions of vasoactive drugs on fetal and maternal plasma renin activity. Biol Neonate 35:23, 1979

248. Nakamura KT, Ayres NA, Gomez A, Robillard JE: Renal responses to hypoxemia during renin-angiotensin system inhibition in fetal lambs. Am J Physiol 249:R116, 1985

249. Binder ND, Anderson DF: Plasma renin activity responses to graded decreases in renal perfusion pressure in fetal and newborn lambs. Am J Physiol 262:R524, 1992

250. Kopp UC, Dibona GF: Interaction between neural and nonneural mechanisms controlling renin secretion rate. Am J Physiol 246:F620, 1984

251. Page WV, Perlman VS, Smith FG et al: Renal nerves modulate kidney renin gene expression during the transition from fetal to newborn life. Am J Physiol 262: R459, 1992

252. Rudolph AM: Homeostasis of the fetal circulation and the part played by hormones. Ann Rech Vet 8:405, 1977

253. Gresores A, Rosenfeld CR, Magness RR, Roy T: Metabolic clearance rate of angiotensin II in fetal and pregnant sheep. Pediatr Res 31:60A, 1992

254. Iwamoto HS, Rudolph AM: Effects of angiotensin II on the blood flow and its distribution in fetal lambs. Cir. Res 48:183, 1981

255. Grone H-H, Simon M, Fuchs E: Autoradiographic characterization of angiotensin receptor subtypes in fetal and adult human kidney. Am J Physiol 262:F326, 1992

256. Iwamoto HS, Rudolph AM: Effects of angiotensin II on the blood flow and its distribution in fetal lambs. Circ Res 48:183, 1981

257. Robillard JE, Weismann RN, Gomez RA et al: Renal and adrenal responses to converting enzyme inhibition in fetal and newborn life. Am J Physiol 262:R249, 1983

258. Lumbers ER, Burrell JH, Menzies RI, Stevens AD: Effects of a converting enzyme inhibitor (captopril) and angiotensin II on fetal renal function. Br J Pharmacol 110:821, 1993

259. Hellegers AE, Schruefer JJP: Normograms and empirical equations relating oxygen tension, percentage saturation, and pH in maternal and fetal blood. Am J Obstet Gynecol 81:377, 1961

260. Bunn HF, Jandl JH: Control of hemoglobin function within the red cell. N Engl J Med 282:1414, 1970

261. Bard H, Makowski EL, Meschia G, Battaglia FC: The relative rates of synthesis of hemoglobins A and F in immature red cells of newborn infants. Pediatrics 45: 766, 1970

262. Alter BP, Jackson BT, Lipton JM et al: Control of the simian fetal hemoglobin switch at the progenitor cell level. J Clin Invest 67:458, 1981

263. Bank A, Mears JG, Ramirez F: Disorders of human hemoglobin. Science 207:486, 1980

264. Robillard JE, Weismann DN, Herin P: Ontogeny of single glomerular perfusion rate in fetal and newborn lambs. Pediatr Res 15:1248, 1981

265. Potter EL: Development of the human glomerulus. Arch Path 80:241, 1965

266. Lumbers ER: A brief review of fetal renal function. J Develop Physiol 6:1, 1984

267. Robillard JE, Sessions C, Kennedey RL et al: Interrelationship between glomerular filtration rate and renal transport of sodium and chloride during fetal life. Am J Obstet Gynecol 128:727, 1977

268. Abramow M, Dratwa M: Effect of vasopressin on the isolated human collecting duct. Nature 250:292, 1974

269. Kullama LK, Ross MG, Lam R et al: Ovine maternal and

fetal renal vasopressin receptor response to maternal dehydration. Am J Obstet Gynecol 167:1717, 1992

270. Strandhoy JW, Giammattei CE, Rose JC: Stimulation of renal medullary cAMP production by vasopressin (AVP) in fetal sheep. FASEB J 6:A1745, 1992

271. Smith FG, Sata T, Vasile VA, Robillard JE: Atrial natriuretic factor during fetal and postnatal life: a Review. J Develop Physiol 12:55, 1989

272. Robillard JE, Weiner C: Atrial natriuretic factor in the human fetus: effect of volume expansion. J Pediatr 113:552, 1988

273. Robillard JE, Nakamura KT, Varille VA et al: Ontogeny of the renal response to ANF in sheep. Am J Physiol 254:F634, 1988

274. Castro R, Ervin MG, Leake RD et al: Fetal renal response to ANF decreases with maturation. Am J Physiol 260:R346, 1991

275. Robillard JE, Sessions C, Burmeister L, Smith FG Jr: Influence of fetal extracellular volume contraction on renal reabsorption of bicarbonate in fetal lambs. Pediatr Res 11:649, 1977

276. Robillard JE, Sessions C, Kennedy RL, Smith FG Jr: Maturation of the glucose transport process by the fetal kidney. Pediatr Res 12:680, 1978

277. Charlton VE, Reis BL, Lofgren DJ: Consumption of carbohydrates, amino acids and oxygen across the intestinal circulation in the fetal sheep. J Develop Physiol 1:329, 1979

278. Edelstone DI, Holzman IR: Fetal intestinal oxygen consumption at various levels of oxygenation. Am J Physiol 242:H50, 1982

279. Lester R, Jackson BT, Smallwood RA et al: Fetal and neonatal hepatic function, II: birth defects 12:307, 1976

280. Bristow J, Rudolph AM, Itskovitz J, Barnes R: Hepatic oxygen and glucose metabolism in the fetal lamb. J Clin Invest 71:1047, 1983

281. Jones CT, Ritchie JWK: The effects of adrenergic blockage on fetal response to hypoxia. J Dev Physiol 5:211, 1983

282. Wood CE, Rudolph AM: Negative feedback regulation of adrenocorticotropin secretion by cortisol in ovine fetuses. Endocrinology 112:1930, 1983

283. Silman RE, Chard T, Lowry PJ et al: Human foetal pituitary peptide and parturition. Nature 260:716, 1976

284. Challis JRG, Brooks AN: Maturation and activation of hypothalemic pituitary adrenal function in fetal sheep. Endocr Rev 10:182, 1989

285. Challis JRG, Mitchell BF: Endocrinology of pregnancy and parturition. p. 106. In Warshaw JB (ed): The Biological Basis of Reproductive and Developmental Medicine. Elsevier, New York, 1983

286. Jaffe RB, Seron-Ferre M, Crickard K et al: Regulation and function of the primate fetal adrenal gland and gonad. Recent Prog Horm Res 37P:41, 1981

287. Challis JRG, Mitchell BR, Lye SJ: Activation of fetal adrenal function. J Dev Physiol 6:93, 1984

288. Murphy BEP: Conjugated glucocorticoids in amniotic fluid and fetal lung maturation. J Clin Endocrinol Metab 17:212, 1978

289. Fencl MD, Sillman RJ, Cohen J, Tulchinsky D: Direct evidence of sudden rise in fetal corticoids late in human gestation. Nature 287:225, 1980

290. Carr BR, Parker CRJ, Milewich L et al: The role of low density, high density and very low density lipoproteins in steroidogenesis by the human fetal adrenal gland. Endocrinology 106:1854, 1980

291. Simpson ER, Carr BR, Parker CR Jr et al: The role of serum lipoproteins in steroidogenesis by the human fetal adrenal cortex. J Clin Endocrinol Metab 49:146, 1979

292. Nylund L, Langercrantz H, Lunell N-O: Catecholamines in fetal blood during birth in man. J Dev Physiol 1:427, 1979

293. Cohen WR, Piasecki CJ, Jackson BT: Plasma catecholamines during hypoxemia in fetal lamb. Am J Physiol 243:R520, 1982

294. Cohen WR, Piasecki GJ, Cohn HE et al: Adrenal secretion of catecholamines during hypoxemia in fetal lambs. Endocrinol 114:383, 1984

295. Padbury J, Agata Y, Ludlow J et al: Effect of fetal adrenalectomy on catecholamine release and physiological adaptation at birth in sheep. J Clin Invest 80:1096, 1987

296. Fisher DA: Maternal–fetal thyroid function in pregnancy. Clin Perinatol 10:615, 1983

297. Vulsma T, Gons MH, De Vijlder JJ: Maternal–fetal transfer of thyroxine in congenital hypothyroidism due to a total organification defect of thyroid agenesis. N Engl J Med 321:13, 1989

298. Timor-Tritsch IE, Dierker LJ, Hertz RH et al: Studies of antepartum behavioral state in the human fetus at term. Am J Obstet Gynecol 132:524, 1978

299. Martin CB Jr: Behavioral states in the human fetus. J Reprod Med 132:524, 1978

300. Visser GHA, Goodman JDS, Levine DH, Dawes GS: Diurnal and other cyclic variations in human fetal heart rate near term. Am J Obstet Gynecol 142:535, 1982

301. Dawes GS, Fox HE, Leduc BM et al: Respiratory movements and rapid eye movement sleep in the foetal lamb. J Physiol 220:119, 1972

302. Natale R, Clewlow F, Dawes GS: Measurement of fetal forelimb movements in the lamb in utero. Am J Obstet Gynecol 140:545, 1981

303. Blanco CE, Dawes GS, Walker DW: Effect of hypoxia on polysynaptic hindlimb reflexes of unanesthetized foetal and newborn lambs. J Physiol 339:453, 1983

304. Chan K, Dodd PA, Day L et al: Fetal catecholamine, cardiovascular and neurobehavioral responses to cocaine. Am J Obstet Gynecol 167:1616, 1992

305. Connors G, Hunse C, Carmichal L et al: Control of fetal breathing in human fetus between 24 and 34 weeks gestation. Am J Obstet Gynecol 160:932, 1989

306. Hohimer AR, Bissonnette JM, Richardson BS, Machida CM: Central chemical regulation of breathing movements in fetal lambs. Respir Physiol 52:99, 1983

307. Dawes GS, Gardner WN, Johnson BM, Walker DW: Breathing activity in fetal lambs: the effect of brain stem section. J Physiol 335:535, 1983

308. Jones MD Jr, Burd LI, Makowski EL et al: Cerebral metabolism in sheep: a comparative study of the adult, the lamb, and the fetus. Am J Physiol 229:235, 1975

309. Richardson BS, Patrick JE, Abduljabbar H: Cerebral oxidative metabolism in the fetal lamb: relationship to electrocortical state. Am J Obstet Gynecol 153:426, 1985

310. Chao CR, Hohimer AR, Bissonnette JM: The effect of electrocortical state on cerebral carbohydrate metabolism in fetal sheep. Devel Brain Res 49:1, 1989

311. Jones MD, Sheldon RE, Peeters LL et al: Fetal cerebral oxygen consumption at different levels of oxygenation. J Appl Physiol 43:1080, 1977

312. Rosenberg AA, Jones MD Jr, Traystman RJ et al: Response of cerebral blood flow to changes in P_{co_2} in fetal, newborn, and adult sheep. Am J Physiol 242:H862, 1982

Chapter 4

Maternal Physiology in Pregnancy

Dwight P. Cruikshank, Thomas R. Wigton, and
Patricia M. Hays*

Many organs undergo physiologic changes during pregnancy. Understanding these changes is important in determining what is normal or abnormal in a pregnant woman.

Alimentary Tract

Appetite

Most women experience an increase in appetite beginning early in the first trimester and persisting throughout pregnancy. In the absence of nausea or "morning sickness," women eating according to appetite will increase their daily food intake by about 200 kcal by the end of the first trimester.[1] The recommended dietary allowance (RDA) calls for an additional 300 kcal/day during pregnancy.[2] Energy requirements vary, however, depending on the population studied,[3] and a greater increase may be necessary for adolescents, who are still growing themselves, and for women with high levels of physical activity.

There is extensive folklore about dietary cravings and aversions during pregnancy. Many of these are undoubtedly due to the individual woman's perception of which foods aggravate or ameliorate such symptoms as nausea and heartburn. The sense of taste may be blunted in some pregnant women, leading to an increased desire for highly seasoned food. Pica is not rare among pregnant women, and a history of such should be sought in those with poor weight gain or refractory

anemia. Among rural Southern black women the most common forms of pica involve consumption of clay or starch (either laundry or cornstarch), while in the United Kingdom the most common craving is for coal. Soap, toothpaste, and ice pica are also reported, and we have cared for one patient who consumed coffee grounds and another who ate newspaper during pregnancy.

Mouth

The pH of saliva is probably unchanged during pregnancy. Some investigators report a decline, and others a rise, in salivary pH; all of these studies suffer from methodologic deficiencies including failure to collect saliva anaerobically to prevent escape of CO_2 with a resultant change in pH.

The production of saliva is not altered in pregnancy. Kallander and Sonesson[4] catheterized the submandibular glands of pregnant women and found secretion rates of 0.10 ml/min compared with 0.15 ml/min in nonpregnant subjects. Ptyalism, an unusual complication of pregnancy, most often occurs in women suffering from nausea and may be associated with the loss of 1 to 2 L of saliva per day. It may be helped by decreased ingestion of starchy foods. Most authorities believe that ptyalism actually represents inability of the nauseated woman to swallow normal amounts of saliva rather than a true increase in the production of saliva.

There is no evidence that pregnancy causes or accelerates the course of dental caries. The gums, however, usually become edematous and soft and may bleed after tooth brushing. At times a tumorous gingivitis can occur during pregnancy, presenting as violaceous pedunculated lesions at the gum line that may bleed profusely. Called epulis gravidarum, these are the same

*This chapter is dedicated to the memory of Dr. Patty Hays, co-author of the first two editions of this chapter, who died unexpectedly and prematurely on December 17, 1994.

lesions dentists refer to as pyogenic granulomas. These changes usually regress 1 to 2 months after delivery; if they have not, or if these lesions bleed excessively during pregnancy, they should be excised.

Stomach

The tone and motility of the stomach are decreased during pregnancy, probably because of the smooth muscle-relaxing effects of progesterone. Decreased levels of motilin, a gut hormone that stimulates smooth muscle, have also been noted.[5] Nevertheless, scientific evidence regarding delayed gastric emptying is inconclusive. Davison et al[8] showed that during pregnancy, the half-time of stomach emptying after a 750-ml watery test meal was 17.8 minutes compared with 11.2 minutes in the nonpregnant state. Furthermore, the volume remaining in the stomach 30 minutes after such a meal was 186 ml in the nonpregnant state, 275 ml during pregnancy, and 393 ml during labor.[6] More recently, Maclie et al.,[7] using paracetamol absorption as an indirect measure of gastric emptying, could not demonstrate a delay in gastric emptying when comparing pregnant women to nonpregnant controls. Because the sensation of nausea does not occur without gastric relaxation, the decreased tone of the stomach may be in part responsible for nausea in pregnancy. In addition, the sphincter at the gastroesophageal junction shows reduced tone so that increases in intra-abdominal pressure lead to acid reflux into the esophagus, with resultant heartburn.

The reduced incidence and lessened symptoms of peptic ulcer disease during pregnancy are generally ascribed to reduced gastric acid secretion throughout pregnancy. While gastric acid secretion is reduced below nonpregnant values in the first and second trimesters, it is significantly greater in the third trimester both during fasting and after histamine stimulation.[8,9] The improvement in ulcer disease seen during pregnancy may be related to delayed gastric emptying, the normal increase in gastric mucous secretion, and a protective effect of prostaglandins on the gastric mucosa.

Small Bowel

The motility of the small bowel is reduced during pregnancy; transit time from stomach to cecum averages 58 $\pm$ 12 hours in the second trimester compared with 52 $\pm$ 10 hours in the nonpregnant state.[10] Wald et al.[11] measured both gastrointestinal transit time and levels of progesterone and estradiol during the third trimester and postpartum. These investigators confirmed that small bowel transit time is increased in pregnancy compared to the postpartum period. Absorption of nutrients from the small bowel, with the exception of iron,

is unchanged during pregnancy. The enhanced absorption of iron is not due to any alteration of small bowel function, but is rather a response to increased iron needs operating through the same mechanisms as in nonpregnant women.

Colon

Constipation, a common problem during pregnancy, results from several factors. These include mechanical obstruction by the uterus, reduced motility because of smooth muscle relaxation, and increased water absorption from the colon. Parry et al.[12] demonstrated a 59 percent increase in colonic water absorption and a 45 percent increase in sodium absorption during pregnancy, an effect perhaps caused in part by increased aldosterone levels.

Portal venous pressure is increased during pregnancy, leading to dilatation wherever there are portosystemic venous anastomoses. Dilatation of such vessels around the gastroesophageal junction is of no consequence unless the woman has preexisting esophageal varices, but similar dilatation of the hemorrhoidal veins results in the common complaint of hemorrhoids.

Gallbladder

The function of the gallbladder is markedly altered during pregnancy. In the second and third trimesters, fasting and residual volumes are twice as great as in nonpregnant controls, and the rate at which the gallbladder empties is much slower.[13]

The limited data on the composition of bile during human pregnancy are conflicting but, in pregnant nonhuman primates,[14] biliary cholesterol saturation is increased and the proportion of chenodeoxycholic acid is decreased. Similar results have also been observed in pregnant women.[15] As both predispose to gallstone formation, it appears that pregnancy does increase the likelihood of gallstone formation. The effect of more than one pregnancy appears to be additive.

Liver

Unlike the livers of many animals, the human liver does not enlarge during pregnancy.[16] Furthermore, despite a marked increase in cardiac output, hepatic blood flow is unchanged[17] or is only slightly increased so that the proportion of cardiac output flowing to the liver is decreased by about 35 percent. The histology of the liver is unchanged by normal pregnancy. Many of the clinical and laboratory signs usually associated with liver disease are present in normal pregnancy. Spider angiomata and palmar erythema, caused by elevated estrogen levels, are normal and disappear soon after delivery. Serum albumin levels fall progressively during

> ### Signs of Normal Pregnancy that may Mimic Liver Disease
>
> Spider angiomata
> Palmar erythema
> Reduced serum albumin concentration
> Elevated serum alkaline phosphatase activity
> Elevated serum cholesterol concentration

pregnancy and at term are 30 percent lower than non-pregnant values, averaging about 3.0 g/dl. Serum alkaline phosphatase activity rises progressively so that by term levels are two to four times those found in nonpregnant subjects. Most of this increase is due to placental production of the heat-stable isoenzyme, although there is probably some increase from hepatic sources as well, because nonpregnant women taking exogenous sex steroids also have increased alkaline phosphatase levels.[18] Serum cholesterol levels are elevated twofold by the end of pregnancy, as are those of most other lipids.

During pregnancy, the serum concentrations of many proteins produced by the liver increase in response to estrogen. Fibrinogen levels rise 50 percent by the end of the second trimester. The levels of ceruloplasmin and the binding proteins for corticosteroids, sex steroids, thyroid hormones and vitamin D are also increased.

Serum levels of bilirubin, aspartate aminotransferase (AST, formerly SGOT), alanine aminotransferase (ALT, formerly SGPT) and 5'-nucleotidase are unchanged in normal pregnancy, as is the prothrombin time. Whether levels of serum gamma-glutamyltranspeptidase (GGT) are altered in normal pregnancy is controversial; some investigators note normal values throughout pregnancy,[19,20] while others report a rise in the third trimester.[21]

Nausea and Vomiting of Pregnancy

Nausea and vomiting, or "morning sickness" complicate up to 70 percent of pregnancies.[22] Typical onset is between 4 and 8 weeks gestation, continuing to about 14 to 16 weeks. Although the symptoms often are quite distressing, morning sickness seldom leads to evidence of disturbed nutritional status such as weight loss, ketonemia, or electrolyte disturbances. The cause is not well understood, although relaxation of the smooth muscle of the stomach probably plays a role. There is some evidence that elevated levels of steroid hormones and human chorionic gonadotropin (hCG) may be involved. However, there does not appear to be good correlation between maternal serum hCG levels and

the degree of nausea and vomiting either in patients with normal pregnancies or in those with hydatidiform moles.[23] Interestingly, nonmolar pregnancies complicated by nausea and vomiting often have a more favorable outcome than do those without.[24,25]

Treatment is largely supportive, consisting of reassurance, psychological support, avoidance of foods found to trigger nausea, and frequent small meals. Until June 1983, the best pharmacologic treatment of this condition was a combination of doxylamine succinate, 10 mg, and pyridoxine, 10 mg (Bendectin, Merrell Dow).[26–30] Although Bendectin is no longer manufactured, doxylamine succinate and pyridoxine both remain available as over-the-counter preparations. A recent randomized, double blind placebo controlled trial of pyridoxine (25 mg orally three times daily for three days) decreased vomiting and improved symptoms in patients with severe nausea.[31]

Hyperemesis gravidarum, a more pernicious form of nausea and vomiting associated with weight loss, ketonemia, electrolyte imbalance, dehydration, and possible hepatic and renal damage, often persists throughout pregnancy. For these patients, one must rule out underlying diseases such as pyelonephritis, pancreatitis, cholecystitis, and hepatitis. Hospitalization with parenteral replacement of fluids, electrolytes, and calories is often necessary. Droperidol (Inapsine), a pregnancy category C neuroleptic used to decrease nausea and vomiting in postoperative patients, has also been used in hyperemesis gravidarum. Mild to moderate hypotension with tachycardia may limit its usefulness. We have found a continuous low-dose infusion of promethazine (Phenergan) helpful in hyperemesis gravidarum. To each liter of intravenous fluid, 25 mg promethazine is added, and the patient is given 5 to 6 L/day. The patient should be kept NPO and continued on parenteral therapy for at least 48 hours after all vomiting has ceased to prevent rapid reappearance of symptoms.

Respiratory System

Upper Respiratory Tract

During pregnancy, the mucosa of the nasopharynx becomes hyperemic and edematous, with hypersecretion of mucus secondary to increased estrogen. These changes often lead to marked nasal stuffiness, and epistaxis is common. Placement of nasogastric and nasotracheal tubes may cause excessive bleeding if significant lubrication is not used. Polyposis of the nose and nasal sinuses develops in some patients and then regresses after delivery. Because of all these changes, many patients complain of a chronic cold during pregnancy. The temptation to use nasal decongestant sprays should be avoided, because chronic use may lead to mucosal atrophy.

Mechanical Changes

The configuration of the thoracic cage changes early in pregnancy, much earlier than can be accounted for by mechanical pressure from the enlarging uterus. The subcostal angle increases from 68 to 103 degrees, the transverse diameter of the chest increases 2 cm, and the chest circumference increases 5 to 7 cm.[32] As pregnancy progresses, the level of the diaphragm is pushed up 4 cm; diaphragmatic excursion is not impeded by the enlarging uterus, but instead actually increases 1 to 2 cm. The old idea that diaphragmatic breathing is lessened in pregnancy is false; in fact, it is more diaphragmatic than costal, and all of the increased tidal volume seen in pregnancy can be accounted for by increased rib cage volume displacement.[33]

Lung Volume and Pulmonary Function

The most important change in lung volume during pregnancy is a 30 to 40 percent increase in tidal volume (V_t), which occurs at the expense of the expiratory reserve volume (ERV) (Fig. 4-1 and Table 4-1). Thus ERV falls approximately 20 percent (range 8 to 40 percent), while vital capacity and inspiratory reserve volume remain essentially stable. Because respiratory rate is unchanged, the 30 to 40 percent expansion of V_t is responsible for the entire 30 to 40 percent increase observed in minute ventilation.

The elevation of the diaphragm decreases the volume of the lungs in the resting state, thereby reducing total lung volume by 5 percent and residual volume (RV) by 20 percent. Since both ERV and RV are decreased approximately 20 percent, it follows that the sum of these two volumes, the functional residual capacity (FRC), is reduced by 20 percent as well.

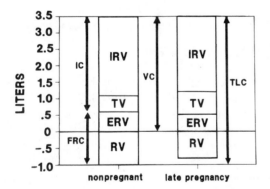

Fig. 4-1 Lung volumes in nonpregnant and pregnant women. TLC, total lung capacity; VC, vital capacity; IC, inspiratory capacity; FRC, functional residual capacity; IR, inspiratory reserve; TV, tidal volume; ERV, expiratory reserve; RV, residual volume.

The forced expiratory volume in 1 second (FEV_1) and the ratio of FEV_1 to forced vital capacity are both unchanged in pregnancy, suggesting that large airway function is unimpaired.[34] In fact, many studies demonstrate a reduction in airway resistance during pregnancy.[34]

Studies of small airway mechanics during pregnancy are limited. The data suggest, however, that small airway closure may occur above FRC or closer to FRC than in the nonpregnant state because of decreases in ERV and FRC in the face of unchanged closing volumes.[35,36] However, normal maximal expiratory flow-volume curves are obtained in pregnancy,[36] indicating that there is not significant small airway dysfunction.

Gas Exchange

Minute ventilation rises 30 to 40 percent by late pregnancy, although oxygen consumption increases only 15 to 29 percent.[37] This leads to higher alveolar (PAO_2) and arterial (PaO_2) PO_2 levels.[38] Normal PaO_2 levels in late pregnancy are 104 to 108 mmHg. That the PaO_2 does not further increase is probably due to the increased FRC in late pregnancy leading to small airway closure. A more significant result of the increased minute ventilation of pregnancy is a fall in $PACO_2$ and $PaCO_2$ levels. In the second half of pregnancy, normal $PaCO_2$ levels are 27 to 32 mmHg compared with 40 mmHg in the nonpregnant state. This change is important, for it increases the CO_2 gradient between fetus and mother and facilitates transfer of CO_2 from the fetus to the mother. Maternal arterial pH (pHa) is maintained at normal levels (7.40 to 7.45) during pregnancy, because the decreased $PaCO_2$ is compensated for by increased renal excretion of bicarbonate. Thus, during pregnancy, normal serum bicarbonate concentrations are 18 to 31 mEq/L, significantly below nonpregnant levels.

The increased minute ventilation of pregnancy, caused by increased V_t appears to be a result of higher progesterone levels. Although most studies suggest that progesterone increases the sensitivity of the repiratory center to CO_2,[39] there is some evidence that progesterone may act as a primary respiratory center stimulant.[40]

Dyspnea of Pregnancy

The sensation of dyspnea is a common complaint during pregnancy, occurring in 60 to 70 percent of normal subjects and usually beginning in the late first or early second trimester. The etiology is not understood. It is probably due to a combination of factors, including reduced $PaCO_2$ levels and an awareness of the increased V_t of normal pregnancy. As vital capacity does not change during pregnancy, serial measurements of V_c may help assess dyspnea during pregnancy.

Table 4-1   Lung Volumes and Capacities in Pregnancy

Measurement	Definition	Change in Pregnancy
Respiratory rate (RR)	Number of breaths per minute	Unchanged
Vital capacity (Vc)	Maximum amount of air that can be forcibly expired after maximum inspiration (IC + ERV)	Unchanged
Inspiratory capacity (IC)	Maximum amount of air that can be inspired from resting expiratory level (vt + IRV)	Increased 5%
Tidal volume (vt)	Amount of air inspired and expired with normal breath	Increased 30 to 40%
Inspiratory reserve volume (IRV)	Maximum amount of air that can be inspired at end of normal inspiration	Unchanged
Functional residual capacity (FRC)	Amount of air in lungs at resting expiratory level (ERV + RV)	Decreased 20%
Expiratory reserve volume (ERV)	Maximum amount of air that can be expired from resting expiratory level	Decreased 20%
Residual volume (RV)	Amount of air in lungs after maximum expiration	Decreased 20%
Total lung capacity (TLC)	Total amount of air in lungs at maximal inspiration (Vc + RV)	Decreased 5%

Skin

Vascular Changes

The elevated estrogen levels of pregnancy cause the frequent appearance of spider angiomata and palmar erythema.[41] Vascular spiders, red elevations with tiny vessels branching out from a central body, occur in 67 percent of white women and in 10 percent of black women. They are most common on the face, upper chest, and arms and regress completely after delivery. Diffuse or blotchy palmar erythema, identical to that seen in hepatic cirrhosis, occurs in 60 percent of pregnant subjects and regresses after delivery.

Connective Tissue

Striae gravidarum develop in approximately 50 percent of pregnant women. Initially pink or purple, they develop on the breasts, lower abdomen, and upper thighs; they eventually become white or silvery, but never completely disappear. The development of striae is not due to excessive weight gain, as they can become severe in women gaining as little as 10 to 15 lb, while others who gain enormously escape unscathed. The presence of striae appears to be solely due to the normal stretching of the skin in women whose connective tissue is genetically predisposed; unfortunately, no prophylactic skin treatment has proved effective in preventing them.

Sweat Glands

Eccrine sweating and the excretion rate of sebum are increased in normal pregnancy, while apocrine function appears to be decreased.

Pigmentation

Elevated levels of estrogen, progesterone, and α-melanocyte-stimulating hormone (α-MSH), a polypeptide similar to adrenocorticotropic hormone (ACTH), lead to hyperpigmentation in many pregnant women. This is usually most marked on the nipples and areolae, umbilicus, axillae, perineum, and in the midline of the lower abdomen, where the linea alba becomes the linea nigra.

Pregnancy-induced elevated levels of sex steroids, but apparently not α-MSH, also lead to the "mask of pregnancy" in many women. This condition was formerly referred to as chloasma, but the term melasma is now preferred. This blotchy, irregular hyperpigmentation of the forehead, cheeks, nose, and upper lip may also be seen in some women taking oral contraceptives. Both melasma and the other pigment changes described above occur more frequently in brunettes than in blondes, and, although they fade after delivery, may never disappear completely.

Pigmented nevi seem to be stimulated by pregnancy. Preexisting nevi may darken, enlarge, and show increased junctional activity on histologic examination, and new nevi may form. After pregnancy these changes tend to regress, and the junctional activity lessens. Nonetheless, excision of rapidly changing nevi in pregnancy remains a prudent course.

Hair

The anagen, or growth, phase of normal scalp hair lasts 2 to 6 years after which it enters the telogen, or resting, phase. After about 3 months of telogen, the old hair strand is lost and a new one grows to replace it. Normally 15 to 20 percent of hairs are in telogen at any one time, but in late pregnancy this falls to 10 percent or less. Then, after delivery, the number of hairs entering telogen increases remarkably so that by 2 months postpartum 30 percent are in that phase. It is normal, therefore, to see a marked increase in scalp hair loss 2 to 4 months after delivery. The often frantic patient should be reassured of the normality of this phenomenon and should be told that these hairs will all regrow within 6 to 12 months.

Masculinization of the skin, with facial hirsutism and perhaps acne, occurs rarely during pregnancy. In most cases, no cause can be found, and the patient should be reassured that the changes will regress after delivery. Occasionally, pelvic examination or ultrasound imaging will reveal large ovarian tumors in such women. These usually are luteomas of pregnancy, which represent exaggerated luteinization of normal ovaries rather than true neoplasms. These tumors regress after pregnancy so that surgical intervention during gestation is not indicated.

Urinary System

Anatomic Changes

The kidneys enlarge during pregnancy, their length as measured by intravenous pyelography increasing about 1 cm. This increase in size (and weight) is due to increased renal vascular and interstitial volume. The right kidney tends to enlarge more than the left. Pelvicalyceal dilatation by term averages 15 mm (range 5 to 25 mm) on the right and 5 mm (range 3 to 8 mm) on the left.[42]

The well-known dilatation of the ureters and renal pelves begins by the second month of pregnancy and becomes maximal by the middle of the second trimester, when ureteric diameter may be as much as 2 cm, and the volume of urine in each ureter 20 to 50 ml. The right ureter is almost invariably more dilated than the left, and the dilatation usually cannot be demonstrated below the pelvic brim. These findings have led some[43] to argue that the dilatation is entirely due to mechanical compression of the ureters by the enlarging uterus and the ovarian venous plexus. It would seem that mechanical factors are the most important cause of this dilatation, but the early onset of ureteral enlargement supports the hypothesis that smooth muscle relaxation caused by progesterone plays a role as well. However, at least one group of investigators[44] has in fact demonstrated increased ureteric tone during pregnancy; thus it seems that the role of progesterone is as yet unsettled.

The consequences of ureterocalyceal dilatation are obvious and include (1) increased incidence of pyelonephritis among gravidas with asymptomatic bacteriuria, (2) difficulty in interpreting urinary radiographs and in diagnosing urinary tract obstruction during pregnancy, and (3) interference with studies of renal blood flow, glomerular filtration, and tubular function, which, because of urinary stasis, must be done at high rates of urine flow.

Renal Hemodynamics

Renal plasma flow increases markedly and quite early in pregnancy. Dunlop[45] showed convincingly that effective renal plasma flow (ERPF) is increased 75 percent over nonpregnant levels, to a mean value of 840 ml/min, by 16 weeks gestation (Table 4-2). This increase is maintained until the late third trimester, when a small but significant decline in ERPF occurs. The late-pregnancy fall in ERPF has been well demonstrated in subjects studied serially, in both the sitting[45] and left lateral recumbent[46] positions.

Like ERPF, glomerular filtration rate (GFR) measured by inulin clearance increases early in pregnancy, with increases demonstrated by 5 to 7 weeks; by the end of the first trimester, GFR is 50 percent higher than in the nonpregnant state. This increase is maintained until the end of pregnancy; there is no late-pregnancy fall in GFR as there is in ERPF.

Because the ERPF increases 75 percent and the GFR 50 percent early in pregnancy, the filtration fraction falls significantly from nonpregnant levels until the late third trimester. At that time, when the ERPF falls but GFR does not, the filtration fraction returns to nonpregnant values of 20 to 21 percent.

Clinically, GFR is not determined by measuring the clearance of infused inulin (inulin is filtered by the glomerulus and is neither reabsorbed nor secreted by the tubules), but rather by measuring endogenous creatinine clearance. This test gives a less precise measure of GFR than does inulin clearance, because creatinine

Table 4-2 Serial Changes in Renal Hemodynamics

	Nonpregnant[a]	Seated Position (N = 25)[a]		Left Lateral Recumbent/Position (N = 17)[b]		
		16 wk	26 wk	36 wk	29 wk	37 wk
Effective renal plasma flow (ml/min)	480 ± 72	840 ± 145	891 ± 279	771 ± 175	748 ± 85	677 ± 82
Glomerular filtration rate (ml/min)	99 ± 18	149 ± 17	152 ± 18	150 ± 32	145 ± 19	138 ± 22
Filtration fraction	0.21	0.18	0.18	0.20	0.19	0.21

[a] Data from Dunlop.[45]
[b] Data from Equimokhai et al.[46]

is secreted by the tubules to a variable extent as well as being filtered by the glomerulus. Therefore, endogenous creatinine clearance is usually higher than the actual GFR. The endogenous creatinine clearance is greatly increased in pregnancy, and values of 150 to 200 ml/min are normal. As with GFR, the increase in creatinine clearance begins by 5 to 7 weeks gestation, is maximal by the end of the first trimester, and in normal subjects is maintained at peak levels until after delivery.

Blood Levels of Nitrogenous Metabolites

As a result of the increased GFR during pregnancy, serum urea and creatinine decline. The blood urea nitrogen (BUN) level falls about 25 percent in early pregnancy to 8 to 9 mg/dl by the end of the first trimester; these levels are maintained until delivery. Serum creatinine values likewise fall from a nonpregnant level of approximately 0.8 mg/dl to 0.7 mg/dl by the end of the first trimester and to 0.5 to 0.6 mg/dl by term.

Serum uric acid declines in early pregnancy, reaching a nadir by 24 weeks, at which time levels of 2.0 to 3.0 mg/dl are normal. After 24 weeks, uric acid begins to rise again[47] so that by the end of pregnancy the serum urate levels in most gravidas are essentially the same as in the nonpregnant state. This rise in serum urate levels appears to be due to increased renal tubular reabsorption of urate during the third trimester, the reason for which is unknown. Patients with preeclampsia have elevated plasma urate concentrations. However, because urate levels normally rise during late pregnancy, it is necessary to know a given subject's nonpregnant urate level before one can use third-trimester values in this clinical setting.[47]

Salt and Water Metabolism

Plasma osmolality begins to decline by 2 weeks after conception; by the fifth week of pregnancy, it is 10 mOsm/kg H_2O below normal nonpregnant values of 280 to 290 mOsm/kg H_2O. The fall is mainly due to a reduction in the serum concentration of sodium and associated anions. Thus, by early in gestation, plasma osmolality has decreased to 270 to 280 mOsm/kg, similar to the fall seen if a nonpregnant subject quickly drinks 1 L of water. Although the pregnant woman's response to either water loading or dehydration is either normal or enhanced, she does not respond to her lowered osmolality by a water diuresis. This suggests a resetting of the osmoreceptor system at a lower level during pregnancy.

Sodium metabolism is delicately balanced in normal pregnancy to permit a net accumulation of about 900 to 1,000 mEq sodium in the fetus, placenta, and maternal intravascular and interstitial fluids. The factors that tend to promote sodium loss during pregnancy include the 50 percent rise in GFR, which increases the filtered load of sodium by 50 percent. Furthermore, the elevated levels of progesterone promote natriuresis. To overcome these effects, the renal tubules must increase their reabsorption of sodium remarkably; in fact, the increase in tubular sodium reabsorption represents the largest renal readjustment that occurs during pregnancy.

Sodium reabsorption is promoted by the hormones aldosterone, estrogen, and deoxycorticosterone, all of which are increased in pregnancy. In fact, the rise in aldosterone production during pregnancy is most likely the key factor that prevents sodium diuresis from occurring despite the elevation in GFR and serum progesterone levels. Plasma aldosterone levels are 200 to 700 ng/L during late pregnancy compared with 100 to 200 ng/L in the nonpregnant state.[43] During normal pregnancy there is a diurnal variation to aldosterone secretion, with the peak (acrophase) at 10 A.M. to noon.[48]

Remarkable changes occur during pregnancy in the renin-angiotensin system. Plasma renin activity in pregnancy is 5 to 10 times the nonpregnant level. Likewise, renin substrate (angiotensinogen) and angiotensin levels are increased four-to fivefold. Although the normal pregnant woman has a reduced sensitivity to the hypertensive effects of angiotensin, the elevated levels in pregnancy lead to increased aldosterone production and preservation of sodium homeostasis. Atrial natriuretic peptide levels double by the third trimester of normal pregnancy, to a mean of 98 pg/ml from nonpregnant levels of about 44 pg/ml.[48] This is probably due to increased plasma volume leading to some atrial dilatation.

Excretion of Nutrients

Glucose excretion increases in almost all pregnant women. The urinary loss of glucose in the non pregnant state is less than 100 mg/day, but 90 percent of gravidas with a completely normal blood glucose level excrete 1 to 10 g glucose per day during pregnancy.[49] The major reason for the rise in glucose excretion is the 50 percent increase in GFR, presenting a much increased filtered load of glucose to the tubules. There may also be a change in the reabsorptive capacity of the proximal tubules themselves, but the old concept of a maximum tubular reabsorptive capacity for glucose (TmG) is almost certainly erroneous.[49,50] Two important consequences of increased glucose excretion during pregnancy are (1) inability to utilize urine glucose measurements in the management of the pregnant woman with diabetes mellitus because these values do not correlate with blood glucose levels and (2) increased susceptibility of pregnant women to urinary tract infections (UTI).

This susceptibility to UTI may also be enhanced by the normal increase in amino acid excretion during gestation. Hytten and Cheyne[51] found three distinct patterns of amino acid excretion during pregnancy. The excretion of glycine, histidine, threonine, serine, and alanine doubles by 16 weeks' gestation and is four to five times nonpregnant levels by term. The excretion of lysine, cystine, taurine, phenylalanine, valine, leucine, and tyrosine doubles by 16 weeks but then remains at this level or fall slightly as term approaches. The excretion of glutamic acid, methionine, ornithine, asparagine, and isoleucine does not rise during pregnancy, and the excretion of arginine actually falls.

No increase in protein loss in the urine occurs during normal pregnancy,[43] the nonpregnant range of 100 to 300 mg/24 hr being equally valid in pregnancy. Urinary loss of folate and vitamin B_{12} is increased in pregnancy, contributing to the decline in serum levels of these vitamins seen in normal gestation.

Cardiovascular System

Cardiac Output

Maternal cardiac output increases about 30 to 50 percent during pregnancy,[52] with the mean increase being about 33 percent, from a nonpregnant level of 4.5 L/min to a pregnancy maximum of approximately 6.0 L/min.[53] According to Hytten and Lind,[53] cardiac output is maximal by 10 weeks gestation. Other investigators[54] report that the rise in cardiac output is most rapid during the first trimester but that smaller increments continue with a peak at about 20 to 24 weeks. There is almost universal agreement now that cardiac output remains maximal until delivery, the previously described terminal decline being an artifact of testing in the supine position.

Cardiac output is the product of heart rate and stroke volume, both of which increase during normal pregnancy. The earliest rise in cardiac output appears to be due to an increase in stroke volume of from 5 to 10 ml to levels of 70 to 75 ml per stroke. As pregnancy progresses, there is a gradual increase in maternal heart rate so that by the beginning of the third trimester it has risen 15 to 20 bpm over nonpregnant levels. At this time, stroke volume declines to near-nonpregnant levels,[55] and the increase in heart rate is responsible for maintaining the elevated cardiac output.

Cardiac output in pregnancy depends on maternal position, being lower when the gravida lies supine. In the supine position, the enlarged uterus compresses the inferior vena cava, reducing venous return to the heart and in turn cardiac output. In fact, in late pregnancy there is probably complete occlusion of the inferior vena cava in the supine position,[56,57] with venous return from the lower extremities occurring through the dilated paravertebral collateral circulation. The effect of the supine position on cardiac output is most marked in late pregnancy; at 38 to 40 weeks, turning from the side to the back is associated with a 25 to 30 percent fall in cardiac output.[54] Although there does not seem to be an effect of the supine position on maernal cardiac output before 24 weeks gestation, between 24 to 28 weeks turning from the side to the back reduces cardiac output 8 percent, and between 28 to 32 weeks the associated drop is 14 percent. Using invasive methods, Clark et al observed a 9 percent decrease in cardiac output in the supine position between 36 to 38 weeks' gestation and an 18 percent decrease when standing compared to the left lateral decubitus position.[58]

Most pregnant women do not become hypotensive when lying supine, because the fall in cardiac output is compensated by a rise in peripheral vascular resistance. However, 1 to 10 percent of subjects manifest the supine hypotensive syndrome, with a fall in blood pressure associated with symptoms such as dizziness, lightheadedness, nausea, and even syncope. Some investigators[54] have proposed that such individuals have less well-developed paravertebral collateral circulation and perhaps a tendency toward vasovagal attacks as well.

The distribution of maternal cardiac output changes as pregnancy progresses. In the first trimester (as in the nonpregnant state), the uterus receives 2 to 3 percent of the cardiac output and the breasts less than 1 percent. By term the uterus is supplied with 17 percent of cardiac output and the breasts 2 percent, mostly at the expense of a reduction of the fraction of the cardiac output going to the splanchnic bed and skeletal muscle. The absolute blood flow to these latter areas is not reduced, however, because of the increase in cardiac output. The percentage of cardiac output going to the kidneys (20 percent), skin (10 percent), brain (10 percent), and coronary arteries (5 percent) is the same throughout pregnancy as when not pregnant.[59]

Arterial Blood Pressure

Blood pressure is highest when the pregnant woman is seated, somewhat lower when she lies supine, and lowest when she lies on her side. Furthermore, there is a 10 to 12 mmHg difference in blood pressure between the superior and inferior arms in the lateral recumbent position, the superior arm having the lower pressure. Clearly, consistency is important when measuring blood pressure serially throughout gestation.

Peripheral vascular resistance falls during pregnancy. The most obvious cause for this is the smooth muscle-relaxing effect of elevated progesterone levels, although heat production by the fetus may be responsible for some of the vasodilatation, especially in heat-losing areas of the skin. The reduction in resistance results in a progressive fall in systemic arterial blood pressure during the first 24 weeks of pregnancy, the systolic pressure falling an average of 5 to 10 mmHg and the diastolic pressure falling 10 to 15 mmHg.[60] Thus there is a slight increase in pulse pressure by 24 weeks' gestation. After 24 weeks, systolic and diastolic pressures gradually rise, retuning to nonpregnant levels by term. It is abnormal for arterial pressure during pregnancy to be greater than nonpregnant values.

Venous Pressure

Venous pressure in the upper extremities remains unchanged in pregnancy,[53] but there is a progressive rise in the lower extremities. Femoral venous pressure increases from values near 10 cmH$_2$O at 10 weeks' gestation to 25 cmH$_2$O near term[61] and is 2 to 3 cmH$_2$O higher on the side on which the placenta is implanted.[62] Central venous pressures are unchanged in pregnancy, averaging 10 cmH$_2$O in the third trimester.[63]

Left Ventricular Function

The preinjection period is the interval between the electrical stimulation of the left ventricle and the onset of blood flow through the aortic valve. Data regarding this interval in pregnancy are inconsistent, although most investigators find a prolongation in the third trimester.[54] Likewise, variable changes have been reported throughout gestation in the left ventricular ejection time (LVET), but there is agreement that in late pregnancy the LVET is shortened.[54]

Echocardiographic studies[40] have demonstrated that, despite increases in left ventricular dimensions and volume during pregnancy, most parameters of left ventricular function are the same as in the nonpregnant state. These include ejection fraction, rate of internal diameter shortening, percentage of fractional shortening, and ventricular wall thickness. Thus myocardial function is well preserved during gestation.

Central Hemodynamic Assessment

Clark et al.[64] studied 10 carefully selected normal patients at 36 to 38 weeks gestation and again at 11 to 13 weeks postpartum with arterial lines and Swan-Ganz catheterization to characterize the central hemodynamics of pregnancy (Table 4-3). During late pregnancy they found statistically significant increases in cardiac output and heart rate, accompanied by significant decreases in systemic vascular resistance (SVR) and

Table 4-3 Central Hemodynamic Assessment

	Nonpregnant	Pregnant
Cardiac output (L/min)	4.3	6.2
Heart rate (bpm)	71	83
Systemic vascular resistance (dyne·cm·sec^{-5})	1530	1210
Pulmonary vascular resistance (dyne·cm·sec^{-5})	119	78
Colloid oncotic pressure (mmHg)	21	18
Mean arterial pressure (mmHg)	86 (NS)	90
Pulmonary capillary wedge pressure (mmHg)	6.3 (NS)	7.5
Central venous pressure (mmHg)	3.7 (NS)	3.6
Left ventricular stroke work index (g·M·M^{-2})	41 (NS)	48

(From Clark et al.,[64] with permission.)

pulmonary vascular resistance (PVR) and colloid oncotic pressure. There were no significant changes in mean arterial pressure, pulmonary capillary wedge pressure (PCWP), central venous pressure, or left ventricular stroke work index during normal pregnancy.

They postulated that the higher stroke volume of pregnancy is not associated with increased end diastolic pressure (PCWP) because of ventricular dilatation. As a result of the marked fall in SVR and PVR, PCWP does not rise despite the increased blood volume. Their finding of a significantly decreased gradient between colloid oncotic pressure and PCWP explains why pregnant women have a greater propensity to pulmonary edema with changes in capillary permeability or cardiac preload.

Normal Changes That Mimic Heart Disease

Reduction in exercise tolerance is common during pregnancy, as is the sensation of tiredness. The normal hyperventilation of pregnancy may be mistaken as dyspnea by the woman and other observers.

Edema of the ankles is an almost universal finding in late pregnancy because of increased venous pressure in the legs, obstruction of lymphatic flow, and reduced plasma colloid osmotic pressure. After 20 weeks gestation, the jugular veins are usually somewhat distended, and their pulsations are more obvious. The higher position of the diaphragm during pregnancy makes the heart lie in a more horizontal plane, thereby displacing the point of maximal impulse on the chest wall laterally.

At the end of the first trimester, both components of the first heart sound become louder, and there is exaggerated splitting. The second heart sound usually

Signs and Symptoms of Normal Pregnancy that may Mimic Heart Disease

Symptoms
  Reduced exercise tolerance
  Dyspnea
Signs
  Peripheral edema
  Distended neck veins
  Point of maximal impulse displaced to left
Auscultation
  Increased splitting of first and second heart sounds
  Third heart sound (S3 gallop)
  Systolic ejection murmur along left sternal border
  Continuous murmurs
Chest x-ray
  Straightening of left heart border
  Heart position more horizontal
  Increased vascular markings in lungs
Electrocardiogram
  Left axis deviation
  Nonspecific ST-T wave changes

remains normal until the third trimester, when it becomes louder with persistent expiratory splitting. Up to 90 percent of normal pregnant women demonstrate a third heart sound or S3 gallop after midpregnancy.[65,66] Rarely a fourth heart sound may be auscultated in early pregnancy; phonocardiography detects an S4 in 10 to 15 percent of gravidas during the first half of pregnancy. Systolic ejection murmurs along the left sternal border occur in 96 percent of pregnant subjects[66] and are thought to be due to increased flow across the aortic and pulmonic valves. Diastolic murmurs are probably never normal in pregnancy, and their presence warrants evaluation by a cardiologist. A continuous murmur in the second, third, or fourth intercostal space, which may be heard bilaterally, is common in late pregnancy and early puerperium. Called the "mammary souffle," it is thought to be the result of increased flow through the vessels supplying the breasts.

Straightening of the left heart border is due to change in the position of the heart and prominence of the pulmonary conus. This, in addition to the more horizontal position of the heart caused by elevation of the diaphragm, give the appearance of cardiomegaly, but this is more apparent than real. The cardiothoracic ratio is unchanged in normal pregnancy.

Effect of Labor and the Immediate Puerperium

Hemodynamic measurements during labor, including periods between contractions, demonstrate a cumulative rise in cardiac output of about 40 percent above late-pregnancy levels. More recent data, obtained by echocardiographic Doppler methods, reveal a 12 percent increase in cardiac output during the first stage of labor with a mean increase of 34 percent by the initiation of the second stage.[67] Much of this increase appears to be due to pain and apprehension, however, because patients with caudal or epidural anesthesia demonstrate a much smaller rise.[68,69] The greater cardiac work of labor is not completely abolished by pain relief, because each contraction squeezes 300 to 500 ml blood out of the uterus into the circulation,[70] leading to enhanced venous return to the heart and a subsequent increase in cardiac output of 10 to 15 percent. Mean arterial blood pressure rises 10 mmHg during a contraction, although much of this increase is abolished by adequate pain relief.

The immediate puerperium is associated with a 10 to 20 percent rise in cardiac output[71] caused by release of the obstruction of venous return to the heart because the uterus is smaller and because of the rapid mobilization of extracellular fluid. The rise in cardiac output is accompanied by a reflex bradycardia, which means that the stroke volume is greatly increased. The bradycardia and increased stroke volume may persist for 1 to 2 weeks after delivery. These normal puerperal changes may be altered by excessive blood loss.

The Breasts

The breasts begin to change early in pregnancy; tenderness, tingling sensations, and a feeling of heaviness often occur within 4 weeks of the last menstrual period. The breasts rapidly enlarge in the first 8 weeks mostly because of vascular engorgement. Thereafter, the breasts enlarge progressively throughout pregnancy because of both ductal growth stimulated by estrogen and alveolar hypertrophy stimulated by progesterone. Little if any of the increase in breast size is attributable to the deposition of fat. The degree of breast enlargement is quite variable, ranging from 0 to 800 ml per breast, with an average value of about 200 ml per breast.[72] Therefore, total breast tissue increases an average of about 400 ml during pregnancy.

The nipples enlarge and become more mobile during pregnancy. The average increase in diameter is 2.0 to 2.5 mm, increasing from 9.5 to 11.5 mm in primigravidas and from 10.0 to 12.5 mm in parous women. Likewise, the areolae enlarge and become more deeply pigmented. The mean increase in the size of the areolae is 16 mm, from a nonpregnant size of 34 to 36 mm to about 50 to 52 mm in the early puerperium. Montgomery's glands (follicles, tubercles), small elevations throughout the areolae, enlarge and become more prominent. These are probably hypertrophic sebaceous glands, although histochemical studies suggest that they could be rudimentary mammary glands.[73]

In the latter half of pregnancy, colostrum, a thick yellow fluid, may leak or be expressed from the nipples. This normal finding is more common in parous women.

The interaction of numerous hormones, including estrogen, progesterone, prolactin, human placental lactogen (hPL), cortisol, and insulin are all necessary during pregnancy to prepare the breast for milk production. The profound drop in estrogen and progesterone levels after delivery seems to be the initiating stimulus for lactation.

The Skeleton

Postural Changes

Progressively increasing anterior convexity of the lumbar spine (lordosis) occurs during pregnancy. This compensatory mechanism keeps the woman's center of gravity over the legs, because the enlarging uterus would otherwise shift the center of gravity quite anteriorly. The unfortunate side effect of this necessary alteration is low back pain, an almost universal complaint during pregnancy.

The ligaments of the pubic symphysis and sacroiliac joints loosen during pregnancy, probably secondary to the effects of the hormone relaxin.[74] Marked widening of the pubic symphysis occurs by 28 to 32 weeks gestation, when its width has increased 3.0 to 4.0 mm,[75] from a nonpregnant mean of 4.10 mm in nulliparas and 4.60 in multiparas up to 7.70 to 7.90 mm. This mobility of the pelvic joints facilitates vaginal delivery but can lead to pelvic discomfort in late pregnancy. Relaxation of the joints coupled with the increased lordosis and protuberant abdomen also lead to unsteadiness of gait; trauma from falls is more common during pregnancy than at any other time in adult life.[76] Sturdy, supporting shoes should be recommended.

Calcium Metabolism

Maternal total serum calcium concentration declines throughout pregnancy until 34 to 36 weeks, after which there is a slight rise. At term, mean calcium levels are 4.52 ± 0.18 mEq/L, approximately 0.25 mEq/L below nonpregnant levels.[77] The decline in total calcium concentration parallels and is due to the fall in maternal serum albumin concentration; however, maternal

serum ionized calcium (Ca^{2+}) concentration is constant throughout pregnancy and unchanged from nonpregnant values.

Maternal ionized calcium levels remain unaltered despite several pregnancy-specific changes that should lower them; these include expanded extracellular fluid volume, increased GFR, elevated estrogen levels, and transfer of calcium to the fetus. That maternal ionized calcium levels are unchanged is attributable to the marked increase in maternal parathyroid hormone (PTH) levels during pregnancy; during the second half of pregnancy, maternal PTH levels increase progressively to about 135 percent of nonpregnant values at term.[78] The effect of this "physiologic hyperparathyroidism" is to maintain serum Ca^{2+} levels by increasing absorption from the gut and decreasing renal losses of calcium. Despite elevated levels of PTH in pregnancy, the skeleton is well maintained; studies of bone density demonstrate no loss because of current or past pregnancies.[79,80] This preservation of the skeleton may be due to the action of calcitonin, which counteracts the effects of PTH on the skeleton while permitting the effects of PTH on the gut and kidney to continue. Although the data are conflicting, calcitonin levels are either unchanged[78] or elevated[81] during normal pregnancy.

The rate of bone turnover and remodeling increases throughout pregnancy; thus at term it is twice as great as in nonpregnant subjects. The rate of turnover of the exchangeable calcium pool increases by 20 percent.

Hematologic Changes

Plasma Volume and Red Blood Cell Mass

In normal pregnancy, maternal plasma volume begins to increase at about 10 weeks gestation. Thereafter, it increases progressively until 30 to 34 weeks, after which time it plateaus. The mean increase in plasma volume by 30 to 34 weeks is 50 percent, although increases of 20 to 100 percent may be found in normal pregnancies.[82] Patients with multiple gestations have a greater increase in plasma volume than those with singletons. Likewise, larger babies are associated with a great expansion of maternal plasma volume, but it is not clear whether this is cause or effect.

Erythrocyte mass also begins to increase at about 10 weeks' gestation and thereafter increases progressively until term. The plateau seen in plasma volume after 30 to 34 weeks is not observed in red blood cell (RBC) mass. Without iron supplementation, RBC mass increases about 18 percent by term, from a mean nonpregnant level of 1,400 ml up to 1,650 ml at term. Women whose diet is supplemented with iron show a

Table 4-4 Hemoglobin Values in Pregnancy

Weeks Gestation	Mean Hemoglobin (g/dl)	Fifth Percentile Hemoglobin (g/dl)
12	12.2	11.0
16	11.8	10.6
20	11.6	10.5
24	11.6	10.5
28	11.8	10.7
32	12.1	11.0
36	12.5	11.4
40	12.9	11.9

(From U.S. Department of Health and Human Services.[84])

greater RBC mass increment, increasing about 400 to 450 ml, or 30 percent, by term.[83]

Because plasma volume increases 50 percent on the average while RBC mass increases only 18 to 30 percent, the hematocrit drops during a normal pregnancy. This so-called physiologic anemia of pregnancy reaches its nadir at 30 to 34 weeks. Thereafter, the hematocrit may rise somewhat, because RBC mass expansion continues but that of plasma volume does not.

The mean and fifth percentile hemoglobin concentrations of normal iron-supplemented pregnant women are listed in Table 4-4.[84] For patients living at altitudes below 3,000 feet, the fifth percentile value should be considered the cutoff for the diagnosis of anemia. For patients living at higher altitudes, this volume should be increased by 0.2 g/dl for every 1,000 feet above 3,000 and by 0.3 g/dl for every 1,000 feet above 7,000.

There are many reasons for the increased blood volume of pregnancy. Clearly, it protects the mother from the possibility of hemorrhage at the time of delivery. Furthermore, the increased plasma volume serves to dissipate fetal heat production and provide increased renal filtration, while the increased RBC mass is necessary to increase oxygen transport to meet the needs of the fetus.

Vaginal delivery of a singleton infant at term is associated with a mean blood loss of 500 ml, an uncomplicated cesarean birth about 1,000 ml, and cesarean hysterectomy 1,500 ml.[85-87] The vaginal delivery of twins results in a maternal blood loss of about 1,000 ml. In the normal situation, almost all the blood loss occurs within the first hour after delivery. Thereafter, only about 80 ml of blood is lost over the next 3 days.[85]

Leukocytes and Platelets

The peripheral white blood cell (WBC) count rises progressively during pregnancy. During the first trimester, the mean WBC count is 9,500/mm^3, with a normal range of 3,000 to 15,000/mm^3. During the second and third trimesters, the mean is 10,500/mm^3, with a range of 6,000 to 16,000/mm^3.[85] In labor, the count may rise to 20,000 to 30,000/mm^3, after which it gradually returns to nonpregnant levels by the end of the first week of the puerperium. The increase in WBC count during pregnancy and delivery is largely due to increased numbers of circulating neutrophil polymorphonuclear cells (granulocytes). In the last trimester and during labor, the peripheral smear of normal subjects may even demonstrate occasional myelocytes and metamyelocytes.

Investigations of platelet counts in pregnancy done before the availability of automated cell counters yielded conflicting results, with various workers reporting a decline, a rise, or no change in the platelet count during normal pregnancy. Most recent studies demonstrate a progressive decline in platelet count throughout pregnancy, although the healthy gravida's count will remain within the normal range for nonpregnant subjects.[88-90] Fay et al.[91] studied 2,114 pregnant women and reported a progressive fall from a mean platelet count of 275,000/mm^3 at less than 20 weeks to a mean of 260,000/mm^3 at more than 35 weeks, the drop being significant after 32 weeks. These investigators also demonstrated a progressive rise in mean platelet size (volume) after 28 weeks' gestation, indicating younger platelets; they concluded that the fall in platelet count in normal pregnancy is due to increased destruction in the periphery, a concept supported by the somewhat shorter average platelet life span in pregnancy (9.2 days) compared with the nonpregnant state (9.7 days).[92]

The Coagulation Mechanism

Pregnancy has long been called a hypercoagulable state, and indeed levels of fibrinogen (Factor I) increase during pregnancy to the range of 400 to 500 mg/dl. Furthermore, plasma levels of Factors VII through X rise progressively during pregnancy. By contrast, levels of prothrombin (Factor II) and Factors V and XII remain unchanged during pregnancy, while the platelet count and levels of Factors XI and XIII decline somewhat.[83,93]

Bleeding time and clotting time are unchanged during normal pregnancy, however. The "hypercoagulability" attributed to pregnancy does not seem to be due to changes in these parameters but rather to the perceived increase in the incidence of thromboembolism during pregnancy. The greatest risk of such complications is in the puerperium. If one assumes that the risk of thromboembolism in the nonpregnant state is 1.0, then during gestation this rises to 1.8, and during the puerperium to 5.5, demonstrating the importance of stasis and vessel wall injury in the genesis of thrombi.

Iron Metabolism in Pregnancy

Iron is absorbed from the duodenum only in the ferrous (divalent) state, its form in iron supplements. Ferric (trivalent) iron from vegetable food sources must be converted to the divalent state before it can be absorbed. If body iron stores are sufficient, only about 10 percent of ingested iron is absorbed, most of which remains in the mucosal cells of the duodenum until sloughing leads to excretion in the feces. Under conditions of increased iron needs, the fraction absorbed increases. The normal pregnant woman absorbs about 20 percent of ingested iron, while the iron-deficient gravida may absorb as much as 40 percent. Under these circumstances, iron is released from the mucosal cell into the circulation, where it is carried, bound to transferrin, to the liver, spleen, and bone marrow. In those sites it is freed from transferrin and is either incorporated into hemoglobin or myoglobin or stored as ferritin and hemosiderin.

The iron requirements of pregnancy are about 1,000 mg. This includes 500 mg used to increase the maternal RBC mass, 300 mg transported to the fetus, and 200 mg to compensate for normal daily iron losses by the mother (mainly from cells sloughed into the bowel). Thus the normal pregnant woman needs to absorb an average of about 3.5 mg/day of iron. In actuality, the iron requirements of pregnancy are not constant, but increase remarkably during the third trimester. The fetus receives almost all the iron transported to it during the last 12 weeks of pregnancy.

In the past it was controversial as to whether nonanemic pregnant women should receive routine iron supplementation. Most American obstetricians favored the practice, while those in Britain and Europe generally considered it unnecessary. With the availability of serum ferritin levels as a reflection of iron stores, it has become apparent that the unsupplemented patient, although not anemic, is significantly iron deficient at term.[94,95] Table 4-5, adapted from the work of Romslio et al.,[95] demonstrates that women who are not anemic at the beginning of pregnancy and who do not receive iron supplementation have a significant drop in hemoglobin concentration, serum iron, and serum ferritin levels by term, whereas such changes do not occur in women supplemented with iron.

It is important to remember that the purpose of iron supplementation during pregnancy is not to raise or even maintain the maternal hemoglobin concentration, nor to prevent iron deficiency in the fetus. Rather, the purpose of maternal supplementation is to prevent iron deficiency in the mother. Iron is actively transported to the fetus by the placenta against a high concentration gradient, and fetal hemoglobin levels do not correlate with maternal levels.[96] Maternal iron deficiency does not appear to lead to reduced fetal iron stores,[97] although this last point is still debated by some. It has been estimated that women who are iron sufficient at the beginning of pregnancy and who are not iron supplemented need about 2 years after delivery to replenish their iron stores from dietary sources. Because many women have a shorter interval than this between pregnancies and because many do not have an ideal diet, iron supplementation is recommended on a routine basis.

Table 4-5 Effect of Iron Supplementation During Pregnancy

	Iron Treated	Placebo Treated
Hemoglobin (g/dl)		
10 to 12 weeks	12.8	12.4
37 to 40 weeks	12.6	11.3[a]
Serum iron (μmol/L)		
10 to 12 weeks	19.2	20.4
37 to 40 weeks	21.9	9.5[a]
Serum ferritin (μg/L)		
10 to 12 weeks	28.0	27.0
37 to 40 weeks	24.0	6.0[a]
Serum iron-binding capacity		
(μm/dl)	58.1	64.1
10 to 12 weeks	75.4[a]	92.3[a]
37 to 40 weeks		

[a] Significant change between first trimester (10 to 12 weeks) and term (37 to 40 weeks). (Adapted from Romslo et al.,[95] with permission.)

Endocrine and Metabolic Changes

Thyroid

Despite alterations in thyroid morphology and histology and in laboratory indices of thyroid function, the normal pregnant woman is euthyroid. These changes are primarily due to the estrogen-induced increase in the thyroxine (T_4)-binding globulin (TBG) concentration and to the decrease in the size of the circulating pool of extrathyroidal iodide resulting from increased renal clearance of iodide. These alterations cause the thyroid to enlarge and to synthesize and secrete thyroid hormone actively.

During pregnancy, the thyroid gland increases in size but not as much as was commonly believed. Ultrasound studies show a 13 percent increase in the size of the gland during pregnancy, which is not enough to be detected by physical examination.[98] Histologically, there is increased vascularity and the follicles are larger with abundant colloid and frequent vacuolization. The depth of the follicular epithelium is increased, and papillary infolding may be seen, indicative of follicular hyperplasia.

Authorities generally agree that the fundamental hypothalamic-pituitary-thyroid relationships remain intact during pregnancy, although there are conflicting reports regarding the responsiveness of this axis. Although one study demonstrated a greater release of thyroid-stimulating hormone (TSH) in response to thyrotropin-releasing hormone (TRH) as pregnancy advanced,[99] most investigators have failed to confirm this finding.[100] The thyroidal uptake of iodide also appears to be normally responsive to thyroid hormone suppression and to TSH stimulation during pregnancy.[101]

Conflicting reports exist regarding the serum concentration of TSH during pregnancy. Some investigators have reported that TSH values do not change,[102] whereas others have reported a modest rise during the early trimesters.[103] With more sensitive assays, recent work suggests that serum TSH concentrations are in fact decreased during the early weeks of gestation and then rise to prepregnancy levels by the end of the first trimester.[104]

Although TSH levels decrease in early gestation, total T4(TT4) paradoxically increases.[105] Different investigators have suggested a role of human chorionic gonadotropin stimulation of the thyroid early in pregnancy. In addition, as a result of the estrogen-induced increase in TBG, the concentrations of thyroid hormones, total T4 and total triiodothyronine (TT3) rise sharply to a plateau that is maintained until after delivery. The concentration of TT4 increases from 5 to 12 μg/dl in nonpregnant euthyroid women to 9 to 16 μg/dl during pregnancy. Despite the elevation in the concentrations of TT4 and TT3, the concentrations of the active hormones free T4 (FT4) and free T3 (FT3) are unchanged during normal pregnancy and are within the normal range for nonpregnant female controls.[104]

Before the availability of FT4 determinations, the FT4 index (FTI), a calculated value derived from the serum TT4 and resin T3 uptake (RT3U) determinations, was used as an indirect approximation of FT4 concentration. During pregnancy, however, the FTI correlates poorly with the FT4 concentration measured directly. This lack of correlation has been attributed to the inability of the RT3U to determine accurately the thyroid-binding capacity at high concentrations of TBG.[106] Therefore, during pregnancy the FTI is not directly proportional to the FT4 and may be seriously misleading. Determination of FT4 concentration by equilibrium dialysis, although complex and expensive, is the only method that compensates for alterations in TBG, making it the most reliable method of evaluating thyroid function in pregnancy.[107] As a result of these methodologic problems, the ratio of TT4 to TBG has been proposed as a reasonable substitution when the accuracy of the particular FT4 assay being used is affected by high TBG levels.[106]

At physiologic maternal blood levels, little if any transplacental passage of thyroid hormones T4 and T3 occur.[108] Maternal TSH does not cross the placenta, but the thyroid-stimulating immunoglobulins and TRH cross readily.

Adrenal Glands

Although the combined weight of the adrenal glands does not increase significantly in pregnancy, expansion of the zona fasciculata, which primarily produces glucocorticoids, does occur. The plasma concentration of corticosteroid-binding globulin (CBG) rises significantly from values of 33 mg/dl in nonpregnant patients to a plateau of 70 mg/dl by the sixth month of pregnancy. This increase reflects enhanced hepatic synthesis, induced by the increased estrogen level associated with pregnancy.[109] The estrogen-mediated increase in CBG results in elevated plasma cortisol concentrations. The concentration of total plasma cortisol shows a twofold increase in the first trimester. By the end of the third trimester, the level is three times higher than the nonpregnant value.[110] No change in the affinity of cortisol to CBG is apparent. Thus the percentage distribution of cortisol among CBG-bound, albumin-bound, and the free compartments is unchanged during pregnancy.[110]

Only the fraction of cortisol that is not bound to CBG is metabolically active. Unlike thyroid hormone, the concentration of free plasma cortisol is elevated during pregnancy, increasing progressively from the first trimester until term, when levels are approximately 2.5 times higher than in the nonpregnant state.[110] The elevated free plasma cortisol concentration overlaps with values reported in Cushing syndrome, but the diurnal variation is preserved during pregnancy.[111] The increase in free cortisol during pregnancy is a result of a combination of increased production[111] and delayed plasma clearance.

Marked elevations in the maternal plasma concentration of deoxycorticosterone (DOC) are present by midgestation, reaching peak levels during the last trimester of pregnancy. In contrast to the nonpregnant state, plasma DOC levels during pregnancy do not respond either to ACTH stimulation or to dexamethasone suppression.[112] These findings suggest that an autonomous source of DOC, specifically the fetoplacental unit, may be responsible for the increased maternal plasma concentration of DOC, especially in late pregnancy.

Dehydroepiandrosterone sulfate (DHEAS) levels are decreased in pregnancy because of a marked rise in the metabolic clearance rate of this steroid.[104] Most studies have found a modest decline in circulating levels of DHEA as well. Maternal plasma levels of testosterone and androstenedione are slightly elevated during pregnancy, testosterone because of the estrogen-induced increase in sex hormone-binding protein and androstenedione because of an apparent small increase in its production rate.[113]

Pancreas and Fuel Metabolism

Pregnancy is characterized by hypertrophy and hyperplasia of the B-cells (insulin-producing cells) centrally located within the islets of Langerhans in the maternal pancreas. During normal pregnancy, maternal fasting is characterized by accelerated starvation. The fasting blood glucose level after a 12- to 14-hour fast is 15 to 20 mg/dl lower than that observed in the nonpregnant state.[114] This reduction in plasma glucose is evident even before 12 to 14 hours and is further exaggerated as the fasting period extends beyond 12 hours This exaggerated response is largely due to the constant drain on maternal glucose by the fetoplacental unit. The relative maternal hypoglycemia probably results in a decline in the fasting levels of insulin,[115,116] although some have reported unchanged[117] or increased[118] maternal fasting insulin levels. An exaggerated starvation ketosis is observed, with elevated blood levels of β-hydroxybutyric acid and acetoacetic acid after an overnight fast.[114] In summary, maternal hypoglycemia, hypoinsulinemia, and hyperketonemia characterize the maternal response to starvation.

By contrast, hyperglycemia, hyperinsulinemia, hypertriglyceridemia, and reduced tissue sensitivity to insulin characterize the maternal response to feeding. Despite postprandial hyperinsulinemia, the blood glucose response to the same carbohydrate load is greater during pregnancy than in the nonpregnant state,[119] indicating that there is peripheral resistance to the action of insulin, the so-called diabetogenic effect of pregnancy. In fact, tissue sensitivity to the effects of insulin may be reduced as much as 80 percent during normal pregnancy.[120]

The factors responsible for this diabetogenic effect include a variety of hormones secreted by the placenta, especially hPL. Carbohydrate metabolism is significantly altered by hPL. This hormone reduces the effectiveness of insulin by decreasing the sensitivity of peripheral tissues and of the liver to the effects of insulin. hPL secretion is proportional to total placental mass. Thus, insulin resistance increases as pregnancy advances, particularly during the second half of pregnancy. Elevated free cortisol concentrations may also contribute to the postprandial hyperglycemia characteristic of pregnancy.

The fetus is primarily dependent on glucose for its fuel requirements. The concentration of fetal plasma glucose is about 20 mg/dl less than maternal values. The rate of glucose delivery from the mother to the fetus is more rapid than can be accounted for by simple diffusion. This transfer occurs by facilitated diffusion, a carrier-mediated but not energy-dependent mechanism, resulting in the same fetal blood levels that would be achieved by simple diffusion, but at a faster rate. Maternal glucose levels are critically important in providing adequate glucose transfer to the fetus. However, hyperglycemia may alter embryogenesis (Ch. 31). The fetus does not depend on maternal insulin for for its utilization of glucose. In fact, maternal insulin and glucagon do not cross the placenta. Fetal insulin is present at 9 to 11 weeks' gestation and has a critical role in fetal growth.

Amino acids are actively transported by the placenta from the mother to the fetus, where they are used for protein synthesis and as an energy source. Free fatty acids are transferred from mother to fetus to a limited extent, providing only those essential fatty acids required for tissue synthesis. Ketones, however, freely diffuse across the placenta from mother to fetus and may in fact be hazardous to fetal health.

Pituitary Gland

The pituitary gland enlarges in normal pregnancy, principally because of proliferation of chromophobe cells in the anterior pituitary. Gonzalez et al.[121] recently studied pituitary size by magnetic resonance imaging in 32 normal gravidas and 20 nonpregnant controls. The mean pituitary volume in nonpregnant women was 300 ± 60 mm^3 compared with 437 ± 90 mm^3 by 12 weeks gestation (a 45 percent increase) and 708 ± 12 mm^3 at term (a 136 percent increase). They were unable to visualize the posterior pituitary in any third-trimester patient and speculated that it was compressed by growth of the anterior pituitary. The pituitary stalk remained in the midline in all patients.

The Eye

The two consistent and significant ocular changes during pregnancy are increased thickness of the cornea and decreased intraocular pressure. The corneas increase in thickness by about 3 percent, from a nonpregnant mean of 534 μm to a pregnant mean of 551 μm. This change is due to fluid retention, is apparent by 10 weeks' gestation, and regresses by the sixth week of the puerperium.[122] It is probably the reason for the contact lens intolerance reported by some women during gestation. Intraocular pressure falls by about 10 percent during pregnancy, from 16.1 mmHg in the nonpregnant state to 14.7 mmHg during pregnancy.

10 Key Points

- Pregnancy increases the risk of gallstone formation secondary to increased biliary cholesterol saturation.

- $PACO_2$ and $PaCO_2$ fall during pregnancy secondary to increased minute ventilation. This facilitates transfer of CO_2 from the fetus to the mother.

- The incidence of pyelonephritis is increased among pregnant women with asymptomatic bacteriuria.

- BUN and creatinine normally decrease during pregnancy as a result of the increased glomerular filtration rate.

- Plasma osmolality decreases during pregnancy due to a reduction in the serum concentration of sodium and associated anions.

- Cardiac output increases 30 to 50 percent during pregnancy. This is dependent on maternal position. Supine positioning and standing are both associated with a fall in cardiac output.

- Maternal plasma volume increases 50 percent during pregnancy. As RBC volume increases approximately 18 to 30 percent the hematocrit normally decreases during gestation.

- As a result of the marked fall in systemic vascular resistance and pulmonary vascular resistance, pulmonary capillary wedge pressure does not rise, despite an increase in blood volume.

- Nonanemic pregnant women, unsupplemented with iron, will be iron deficient at term. The purpose of iron supplementation is to prevent iron deficiency in the mother.

- Pregnancy is associated with a peripheral resistance to insulin, primarily mediated by human placental lactogen. Insulin resistance increases as pregnancy advances, especially in the third trimester.

References

1. Hytten FE, Lind T: Indices of alimentary function. p.13. In Hytten FE, Lind T (eds): Diagnostic Indices in Pregnancy. Documenta Geigy, Basel, 1973

2. Miller DF, Voris L: Chronologic change in the recommended dietary allowances. J Am Diet Assoc 54:2, 1969

3. Catalono PM, Hollenbeck C: Energy requirements in pregnancy: a review. Obstet Gynecol Surv 47:368, 1992

4. Kallendar D, Sonesson B: Studies on saliva in menstruating, pregnant and post-menopausal women. Acta Endocrinol (Copenh) 48:329, 1965

5. Christofides ND, Ghatei MA, Bloom SR et al: Decreased plasma motilin concentrations in pregnancy. Br Med J 285:1453, 1982

6. Davison JS, Davison MC, Hay DM: Gastric emptying time in late pregnancy and labour. J Obstet Gynaecol Br Commonw 77:37, 1970

7. Maclie AG, Magides AD, Richmond MN et al: Gastric emptying in pregnancy. Br J Anaesth 67:54, 1991

8. Murray FA, Eishine JP, Fielding J: Gastric secretion in pregnancy. J Obstet Gynaecol Br Emp 64:373, 1957

9. Hunt JN, Murray FA: Gastric function in pregnancy. J Obstet Gynaecol Br Emp 65:78, 1958

10. Parry E, Shields R, Turnbull AC: Transit time in the small intestine in pregnancy. J Obstet Gynaecol Br Commonw 77:900, 1970

11. Wald A, Van Thiel DH, Hoechstetter L et al: Effect of pregnancy on gastrointestinal transit. Dig Dis Sci 27:1015, 1982

12. Parry E, Shields R, Turnbull AC: The effect of pregnancy on the colonic absorption of sodium, potassium and water. J Obstet Gynaecol Br Commonw 77:616, 1970

13. Bracerman DZ, Johnson ML, Kern F: Effects of pregnancy and contraceptive steroids on gallbladder function. N Engl J Med 302:363, 1980

14. Deitrick JE, McSherry CK, Javitt NB: Bile salt kinetics in the pregnant baboon. A new model for the study of gallbladder function. Gastroenterology 65:536, 1973

15. Kem F Jr, Everson GT, Demark B et al: Biliary lipids, bile acids, and gallbladder function in the human female. J Clin Invest 68:1229, 1981

16. Combes B, Adams RH: Disorders of the liver in pregnancy. p. 297. In Assali NS (ed): Pathophysiology of Gestation. Academic Press, San Diego, 1971

17. Munnell EW, Taylor HC: Liver blood flow in pregnancy-hepatic vein catheterization. J Clin Invest 26:952, 1947

18. Song CS, Kappas A: The influence of estrogens, progestins, and pregnancy on the liver. Vitam Horm 26:147, 1968

19. Walker FB, Hobilt DL, Cunningham FG: Gamma glutamyl transpeptidase in normal pregnancies. Ostet Gynecol 43:745, 1974

20. Carter J: Liver function in normal pregnancy. Aust N Z J Obstet Gynaecol 30:296, 1990

21. Cerutti R, Ferrari S, Grella P: Behavior of serum enzymes in pregnancy. Clin Exp Obstet Gynecol 3:22, 1976

22. Jamfelt-Samsioe A, Veliner F-M: Nausea and vomiting in pregnancy—a contribution to its epidemiology. Gynecol Obstet Invest 16:221, 1983

23. Soules MR, Hughes CL, Garcia JA et al: Nausea and vomiting of pregnancy. Role of human chorionic gonadotropin and 17-hydroxyprogesterone. Obstet Gynecol 55:696, 1980

24. Yerushalmy J, Milkovich L: Evaluation of the teratogenic effect of meclizine in man. Am J Obstet Gynecol 93:553, 1965

25. Medalie JH: Relationship between nausea and/or vomiting in early pregnancy and abortion. lancet 2:117, 1957

26. Geiger CJ, Fahrenbach DM, Healey FJ: Bendectin in the treatment of nausea and vomiting in pregnancy. Obstet Gynecol 14:688, 1959

27. US Department of Health and Human Services: Indica-

tions for Bendectin narrowed. FDA Drug Bull 11:1, 1981

28. Kolata GB: How safe is Bendectin? Science 20:518, 1980
29. Cordero JF, Oakley GP, Greenberg F et al: Is Bendectin a teratogen? JAMA 245:2307, 1981
30. Shapiro S, Heinonen OP, Siskind V et al: Antenatal exposure to Bendectin in relation to congenital malformations, perinatal mortality rate, birth weight, and intelligence quotient score. Am J Obstet Gynecol 128:480, 1977
31. Sahakian V, Rouse D, Sipes S et al: Vitamin B6 is effective therapy for nausea and vomiting of pregnancy: a randomized double-blind placebo-controlled study. Obstet Gynecol 78:33, 1991
32. Thompson KJ, Cohen ME: Studies on the circulation in pregnancy, II: vital capacity observations in normal pregnant women. Surg Gynecol Obstet 66:591, 1938
33. Gilroy RJ, Mangura BT, Lavietes MH: Rib cage and abdominal volume displacement during breathing in pregnancy. Am Rev Respir Dis 137:668, 1988
34. Weinberger SE, Weiss ST, Cohen WR et al: Pregnancy and the lung. Am Rev Respir Dis 121:L559, 1980
35. Holdcroft A, Bevan DR, O'Sullivan JC et al: Airway closure and pregnancy. Anaesthesia 32:517, 1977
36. Baldwin GR, Moorthi DS, Whelton JA et al: New lung functions and pregnancy. Am J Obstet Gynecol 127:235, 1977
37. Hytten FE, Leitch I: The physiology of human pregnancy. 2nd Ed. Blackwell Scientific Publications, Oxford, 1971
38. Boutourline-Young H, Boutourline-Young E: Alveolar carbon dioxide levels in pregnant, parturient, and lactating subjects. J Obstet Gynaecol Br Emp 63:509, 1956
39. Lyons HA, Antonio R: The sensitivity of the respiratory center in pregnancy and after the administration of progesterone. Trans Assoc Am Physicians 72:173, 1959
40. Skatrud JB, Dempsey JA, Kaiser DG: Ventilatory response to medioxyprogesterone acetate in normal subjects: time course and mechanisms. J Appl Physiol 44:939, 1978
41. Bean WB, Cogswell R, Dexter M et al: Vascular changes of the skin in pregnancy. Vascular spiders and palmar erythema. Surg Gynecol Obstet 88:739, 1949
42. Fried A, Woodring JH, Thompson TJ: hydronephrosis of pregnancy. J Ultrasound Med 2:225, 1983
43. Hytten FE, Lind T: Indices of renal function. p. 18. In Hytten FE, Lind T (eds): Diagnostic Indices in Pregnancy. Documenta Geigy, Basel, 1973
44. Rubi RA, Sala NL: Ureteral functions in pregnant women, III: effect of different positions and of fetal delivery upon ureteral tonus. Am J Obstet Gynecol 101:230, 1968
45. Dunlop W: Serial changes in renal haemodynamics during normal human pregnancy. Br J Obstet Gynaecol 88:1, 1981
46. Equimokhai M, Davison JM, Philips PR, Dunlop W: Non-postural serial changes in renal function during the third trimester of normal human pregnancy. Br J Obstet Gynaecol 88:465, 1981
47. Lind T, Godfrey KA, Otun H: Changes in serum uric acid concentrations during normal pregnancy. Br J Obstet Gynaecol 91:128, 1984
48. Miyamoto S, Shimokawa H, Sumioki H et al: Circadian rhythm of plasma atrial natriuretic peptide, aldosterone, and blood pressure during the third trimester in normal and preeclamptic pregnancies. Am J Obstet Gynecol 158:393, 1988
49. Davison JM, Hytten FE: The effect of pregnancy on the renal handling of glucose. J Obstet Gynaecol Br Commonw 82:374, 1975
50. Kurtzman NA, Pillay VKG: Renal absorption of glucose in health and disease. Arch Intern Med 131:901, 1973
51. Hytten FE, Cheyne GA: The aminoaciduria of pregnancy. J Obstet Gynaecol Br Commonw 79:424, 1972
52. Katz R, Karliner JS, Resnik R: Effects of a natural volume overload state (pregnancy) on left ventricular performance in normal human subjects. Circulation 58:434, 1978
53. Hytten FE, Lind T: Indices of cardiovascular function. p. 30. In Hytten FE, Lind T (eds): Diagnostic Indices in Pregnancy. Documenta Geigy, Basel, 1973
54. Elkayam U, Gleicher N: Cardiovascular physiology of pregnancy. p. 5. In Elkayam U, Gleicher N (eds): Cardiac Problems in Pregnancy: Diagnosis and Management of Maternal and Fetal Disease. Alan R Liss, New York, 1982
55. Ueland K, Novy MJ, Peterson EN et al: Maternal cardiovascular dynamics, IV: the influence of gestational age on the maternal cardiovascular response to posture and exercise. Am J Obstet Gynecol 104:856, 1969
56. Clark SL, Cotton DB, Pivarnik JM et al: Position change and central hemodynamic profile during normal third-trimester pregnancy and postpartum. Am J Obstet Gynecol 164:883, 1991
57. Kerr MG: The mechanical effects of the gravid uterus in late pregnancy. J Obstet Gynaecol Br Commonw 72:513, 1965
58. Kerr MG, Scott DB, Samuel E: Studies of the inferior vena cava in late pregnancy. Br Med J 1:532, 1964
59. McAnolty JH, Metcalfe J, Ueland K: Heart disease and pregnancy. p. 1383. In Hurst JN (ed): The Heart. 6th Ed. McGraw-Hill, New York, 1985
60. MacGillivray I, Rose GA, Rowe B: Blood pressure survey in pregnancy. Clin Sci 37:395, 1969
61. McLennan CE: Antecubital and femoral venous pressure in normal and toxemia pregnancy. Am J Obstet Gynecol 45:568, 1943
62. Bickers W: The placenta: a modified arterio-venous fistula. South Med J 35:593, 1942
63. O'Driscoll K, McCarthy JR: Abruptio placentae and central venous pressures. J Obstet Gynaecol Br Commonw 73:923, 1966
64. Clark SL, Cotton DB, Lee W et al: Central hemodynamic assessment of normal term pregnancy. Am J Obstet Gynecol 161:1439, 1989
65. O'Rourke RA, Ewy GA, Marcus FI: Cardiac auscultation in pregnancy. Med Ann DC 39:92, 1970
66. Cutforth R, MacDonald MB: Heart sounds and murmurs in pregnancy. Am Heart J 71:741, 1966

67. Hunter D, Robson SC: Adaptation of the maternal heart in pregnancy. Br Heart J 68:540, 1992

68. Kerr MG: Cardiovascular dynamics in pregnancy and labour. Br Med Bull 24:19, 1968

69. Hendricks CH, Quilligan EJ: Cardiac output during labor. Am J Obstet Gynecol 71:953, 1956

70. Ueland K, Hansen JM: Maternal cardiovascular dynamics, III: labor and delivery under local and caudal analgesia. Am J Obstet Gynecol 103:8, 1969

71. Metcalfe J: The maternal heart in the postpartum period. Am J Caradiol 12:439, 1963

72. Hytten FE, Leitch I: Preparations for breast feeding. p. 234. In Hytten FE, Leitch I (eds): The Physiology of Human Pregnancy. Blackwell Scientific Publications, Oxford, 1971

73. Giacometi L, Montagna W: The nipple and the areola of the human female breast. Anat Rec 144:191, 1962

74. Hall K: Relaxin. J Reprod Fertil 1:368, 1960

75. Abramson D, Roberts SM, Wilson PD: Relaxation of the pelvic joints in pregnancy. Surg Gynecol Obstet 58:595, 1934

76. Fort AJ, Harlin RS: Pregnancy outcome after non-catastrophic maternal trauma during pregnancy. Obstet Gynecol 35:912, 1970

77. Pitkin RM, Gebhardt MP: Serum calcium concentrations in human pregnancy. Am J Obstet Gynecol 127:775, 1977

78. Pitkin RM, Reynolds WA, Williams GA, Hargis GK: Calcium metabolism in normal pregnancy: a longitudinal study. Am J Obstet Gynecol 133:781, 1979

79. Walker ARP, Richardson B, Walker F: The influence of numerous pregnancies and lactations on bone dimensions in South African Bantu and caucasian women. Clin Sci 42:189, 1972

80. Christianson C, Rodero P, Heinild B: Unchanged total body calcium in normal human pregnancy. Acta Bostet Gynecol Scand 55:141, 1976

81. Samaan NA, Anderson GD, Adam-Mayne ME: Immunoreactive calcitonin in mother, child and adult. Am J Obstet Gynecol 121:622, 1975

82. Pritchard JA: Changes in blood volume during pregnancy and delivery. Anesthesiology 26:393, 1965

83. Hytten FE, Lind T: Volume and composition of the blood. p. 36. In Hytten FE, Lind T (eds): Diagnostic Indices in Pregnancy. Documenta Geigy, Basel, 1973

84. US Department of Health and Human Services: MMWR 38:400, 1989

85. Pritchard JA, Baldwin RM, Dickey JC et al: Blood volume changes in pregnancy and the puerperium, II: red blood cell loss and changes in apparent blood volume during and following vaginal delivery, cesarean section, and cesarean section plus total hysterectomy. Am J Obstet Gynecol 84:1271, 1962

86. DeLeeuw NKM, Lowenstein L, Tucker EC et al: Correlation of red cell loss at delivery with changes in red cell mass. Am J Obstet Gynecol 100:1092, 1968

87. Euland K: Maternal cardiovascular dynamics, VII: Intrapartum blood volume changes. Am J Obstet Gynecol 126:671, 1976

88. Pitkin RM, Whitte DC: Platelet and leukocyte counts in normal pregnancy. JAMA 242:2696, 1979

89. Sejeny SA, Eastham RD, Baker SR: Platelet counts during normal pregnancy. J Clin Pathol 28:812, 1975

90. O'Brien JR: Platelet counts in normal pregnancy. J Clin Pathol 29:174, 1976

91. Fay RA, Hughes AO, Farron NT: Platelets in pregnancy: hyperdestruction in pregnancy. Obstet Gynecol 61:238, 1983

92. Wallenberg HCS, VanKessel PH: Platelet lifespan in normal pregnancy as determined by a nonradioisotope technique. Br J Obstet Gynaecol 85:33, 1978

93. Laros RK, Alger LS: Thromboembolism and pregnancy. Clin Obstet Gynecol 22:871, 1979

94. Taylor DJ, Mallen C, McDougall N, Lind T: Effect of iron supplementation on serum ferritin levels during and after pregnancy. Br J Obstet Gynaecol 89:1011, 1982

95. Romslo I, Haram K, Sagen N, Augensen K: Iron requirement in normal pregnancy as assessed by serum ferritin, serum transferrin saturation, and erythrocyte protoporphyrin determinations. Br J Obstet Gynaecol 90:101, 1983

96. McFee JG: Iron metabolism and iron deficiency during pregnancy. Clin Obstet Gynecol 22:799, 1979

97. Van Eijk HG, Kroos MJ, Hoogendoom GA et al: Serum ferritin and iron stores during pregnancy. Clin Chim Acta 83:81, 1978

98. Nelson M, Wickus GC, Caplan RH, Beguin EA: Thyroid gland size in pregnancy: an ultrasound and clinical study. J Reprod Med 32:888, 1987

99. Burrow FN, Polackwich R, Donabedian R: The hypothalamic-pituitary-thyroid axis in normal pregnancy. p. 1. In Fisher DA, Burrow GN (eds): Perinatal Thyroid Physiology and Disease. Raven Press, New York, 1975

100. Kanna V, Sinha MD, Deri PK, Pastogi GK: Plasma thyrotropin and its response to thyrotropin releasing hormone in pregnancy. Obstet Gynecol 42:547, 1973

101. Pochin EE: The iodine uptake of the human thyroid throughout the menstrual cycle and in pregnancy. Clin Sci 11:441, 1952

102. Fisher DA, Hobel CJ, Gazara R, Pierce CA: Thyroid function in the preterm fetus. Pediatrics 46:208, 1970

103. Malkasian GD, Mayberry WE: Serum total and free thyroxine in normal and pregnant women, neonates and women receiving progestogens. Am J Obstet Gynecol 108:1234, 1971

104. Harada A, Hershman JM, Reed AW et al: Comparison of thyroid stimulators and thyroid hormone concentrations in the sera of pregnant women. J Clin Endocrinol Metab 48:793, 1979

105. Ballabio M, Poshyachinda M, Ekins RP: Pregnancy-induced changes in thyroid function: role of human chorionic gonadotropin as putative regulator of maternal thyroid. J Clin Endocrinol Metab 73:824, 1991

106. Burr WA, Evans SE, Lee J et al: The ratio of thyroxine to thyroxine-binding globulin in assessment of thyroid function. Clin Endocrinol (Oxf) 11:333, 1979

107. Chopra IJ, Van Herle AJ, Chua Teco GN et al: Serum free thyroxine in thyroidal and nonthyroidal illnesses:

a comparison of measurements by radioimmunoassay, equilibrium dialysis, and free thyroxine index. J Clin Endocrinol Metab 51:135, 1980

108. Fisher DA, Lehman H, Lackey D: Placental transport of thyroxine. J Clin Endocrinol Metab 24:393, 1964

109. Doc RP, Fernandez R, Seal US: Measurements of corticosteroid-binding globulin in man. J Clin Endocrinol Metab 24:1029, 1964

110. Rosenthal HE, Slaunwhite WR Jr, Sandberg AA: Transcortin: a corticosteroid-binding protein of plasma, X: cortisol and progesterone interplay and unbound levels of these steroids in pregnancy. J Clin Endocrinol Metab 29:352, 1969

111. Nolten WE, Lindheimer MD, Rueckert PA et al: Diurnal patterns and regulation of cortisol secretion in pregnancy. J Clin Endocrinol Metab 51:466, 1980

112. Nolten WE, Lindheimer MD, Oparil S et al: Desoxycorticosterone in normal pregnancy, I: sequential studies of the secretory patterns of desoxycorticosterone, aldosterone, and cortisol. Am J Obstet Gynecol 132:414, 1978

113. Belisle S, Osathanondh R, Tulchinsky D: The effect of constant infusion of unlabelled dehydroepiandrosterone sulfate on maternal plasma androgens and estrogens. J Clin Endocrinol Metab 45:544, 1977

114. Felig P, Lynch V: Starvation in human pregnancy: hypoglycemia, hypoinsulinemia, and hyperketonemia. Science 170:990, 1970

115. Tson JE, Austin KL, Farinhold JW, Fiedler AJ: Endocrine metabolic response to acute starvation in human gestation. Am J Obstet Gynecol 125:1073, 1976

116. Felig P: Maternal and fetal fuel homeostasis in human pregnancy. Am J Clin Nutr 26:998, 1973

117. Taylor GO, Modie JA, Agbedana EO: Serum free fatty acids, insulin and blood glucose in pregnancy. Br J Obstet Gynaecol 85:592, 1978

118. Bleicher SJ, O'Sullivan JB, Freinkel N: Carbohydrate metabolism in pregnancy, V: the interrelations of glucose, insulin and free fatty acids in late pregnancy. N Engl J Med 271:866, 1964

119. O'Sullivan JB, Mahan CM: Criteria for the oral glucose tolerance test in pregnancy. Diabetes 13:278, 1964

120. Fisher PM, Sutherland HW, Bewsher PD: Insulin response to glucose infusion in normal human pregnancy. Diabetologia 19:15, 1980

121. Gonzalez JG, Elizondo G, Saldivar D et al: Pituitary gland growth during normal pregnancy: an in vivo study using magnetic resonance imaging. Am J Med 85:217, 1988

122. Weinreb RN, Lu A, Beeson C: Maternal corneal thickness during pregnancy. Am J Ophthalmol 105:258, 1988

Physiology and Endocrinology of Parturition

Anna-Riitta Fuchs and Fritz Fuchs

Successful transition from intrauterine to extrauterine life requires that the fetus be mature enough to adapt to the vastly different conditions outside the womb. The fetus is therefore vitally dependent on the timing of its birth, as evidenced by the fact that perinatal mortality is lowest at normal term and increases both before and after term. The mother also has a vital interest in the timing of parturition because her capacity to accommodate the fetus is limited and she must be able to expel it without endangering her life and the integrity of her reproductive organs.

Various species have developed different mechanisms for the orderly termination of pregnancy. The maternal endocrine adaptations to pregnancy and parturition are well known, whereas the fetal signals are still best known in various animal models, particularly sheep.[1] While animal studies are helpful, they do not permit conclusions with regard to the physiology of parturition in our own species because of the existing species variations.

The uterine transition from the state of pregnancy with sporadic contractions to the state of parturition with frequent rhythmic contractions is gradual and often cannot be indicated with precision. All parts of the uterus undergo preparation for parturition. They interact in the regulation of myometrial function either in a classic endocrine fashion with humoral mediators (the placenta, fetal, and maternal endocrine glands), or in a paracrine manner with direct tissue-to-tissue communication (myometrium, decidua, and fetal membranes), or with direct cell-to-cell communication, as between the resident leukocyte population and the surrounding cells, stromal cells in decidua, and cervical submucosa.

The following discussion covers the factors involved in this transition, but first, the function of the various parts of the uterus and the biomedical basis for myometrial contractions must be described.

Structure and Function of the Human Uterus

Structural Aspects

Myometrium

The human myometrium is composed of smooth muscle cells in a matrix consisting mainly of collagen and glycosaminoglycans. The muscle cells are arranged in a network of intricately interwoven bundles, most of which follow a spiral course. Since the human uterus is formed through fusion of the lower ends of the two müellerian tracts, two sets of spirals can be traced, forming angles with each other.[2] Some of the spirals continue into the cervix, where they thin out rapidly. This pattern provides exceptional wall strength and permits three-dimensional expansion without compromising the wall strength.

Myometrium, like all muscle cells, contains thick and thin filaments. It also contains intermediate filaments and dense bodies that serve as attachment sites for the contractile filaments they contain, a structural protein, α-actinin. The organization of filaments in smooth muscle has been the subject of controversy, but is believed to be as shown in Figure 5-1. This model accounts for the fact that smooth muscle contraction can result in a degree of shortening that is one order of magnitude greater than in skeletal muscle.

Growth of the uterus during gestation takes place both by cell division and by hypertrophy of individual cells. The growth is induced by the pregnancy hor-

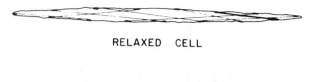

RELAXED CELL

FULL CONTRACTION

Fig. 5-1 Diagrammatic representation of a smooth muscle cell in the relaxed and contracted states, which shows the attachment of the contractile units to the cell surface. The densities along the cell membrane represent dense bodies and the lines between them the contractile units. One of the contractile units has been widened to emphasize the difference between the two contractile states. (From Fay and Delise,[174] with permission.)

mones estrogen and progesterone which in turn induce the synthesis of various growth factors that act alone or synergistically with the steroid hormones. The stimulus of distention also induces uterine growth. The uterus has a high degree of plasticity and can, if expanded gradually, greatly increase the intrauterine volume without any increase of the intrauterine tension, as seen in acute polyhydramnios.

The muscle cells are arranged in bundles but there are few cellular contacts between the individual cells until the end of pregnancy. The smooth muscle cells are surrounded by an intricate network of connective tissue elements; they are frequently connected end-to-end or attached side-by-side by fibrillar components of connective tissue. In late pregnancy, cellular contact zones, the so-called gap junctions (nexus), appear between adjacent myometrial cells as shown in several species.[3–5] Gap junctions (Fig. 5-2) are areas of specialized, intimate contacts between cells of the same type. They represent sites of exchange of ions and small molecules between adjacent cells and provide low resistance pathways for electrical impulses and chemical signals from one cell to the next. This increased electrical coupling facilitates synchronization of contractions which is required for the propagated activity of the organ. In the absence of gap junctions the spread of excitation is poor and contractions remain local and nonpropagated. During pregnancy the number of gap junctions was found to be low or absent in all animal species studied. In rat uterus, the formation of gap junctions in the myometrium is stimulated by estrogens and prostaglandins and inhibited by progesterone and prostaglandin synthetase inhibitors.[6] Their formation is also promoted by distension.[7] In the human the regulation of gap junction formation is still poorly understood. In early labor, both the number and area of gap junctions is increased. Still, considerable overlapping has been found between nonlaboring and laboring patients.[5] The gap junction protein within the myometrium is identical to the heart gap junction protein connexin-43 (Cx-43).[8,9] It is likely, although not proven, that gap junction formation also increases during labor.

Decidua

The decidua derives from the endometrium of the nonpregnant uterus, which undergoes characteristic structural changes under the influence of estrogen, progesterone, and probably relaxin, which is secreted by the corpus luteum in humans. The stromal cells enlarge and increase in number, resulting in thickening of the subepithelial layer. The glands and blood vessels also respond by increased growth. Subsequently, the decidua develops into a basal part beneath the placenta (*decidua basalis*), a capsular part covering the conceptus (*decidua capsularis*), and a parietal part covering the

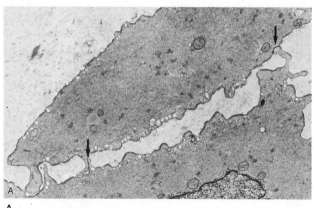

A

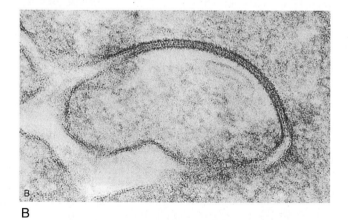

B

Fig. 5-2 (A) Two myometrial cells in the late pregnant human myometrium are connected by gap junctions (arrows) (×20,000). (B) Gap junction in larger magnification (×255,000), showing the close apposition of the cell membranes of the two cells, with a gap of about 2 to 3 nm between them. (Courtesy of Garfield RE, M.D., McMasters University, Hamilton, Ontario, Canada.)

Table 5-1 Cellular Sources of Paracrine Factors
in Decidual Parietalis (Vera) Capable of
Regulating Decidual
and Myometrial Function

Cell Type	Product	Target	Effect
Epithelial cells	PGF > PGE	Myometrium	Contraction
Stromal cells	PGE, PGF	Myometrium	Contraction
Mast cells	Histamine	Stromal cells	PG release
		Blood vessels	Vasodilation
Leukocytes	Cytokines	Stromal cells	PG release
	MPGF, PGE	Myometrium	Contraction
Endothelium and blood vessels	Endothelin	Myometrium blood vessels	Contraction Contraction
	EDRF/NO	Myometrium blood vessels	Relaxation Relaxtion

Abbreviations: PG, prostaglandin; EDRF, endothelium-derived relaxing factor, NO, nitric oxide.
(From Fuchs and Fuchs,[173] with permission.)

inner surface of the myometrium (*decidua vera*). By week 22, the capsular layer has disappeared owing to a reduced blood supply; the parietal decidua is then in direct contact with the fetal membranes, providing their closest vascular supply. A progressive degeneration of the endothelium takes place during pregnancy but a thin layer remains in certain portions until term.[10] Decidua contains many types of cells (Table 5-1). Many macrophages are found between the stromal cells at term, both before and after labor.[11–13]

Anatomically, the basal decidua separates the placenta from the myometrium and provides space not only for the coiling of the spiral arteries that supply each cotyledon but also for the large venous lakes that drain the blood from the intervillous space. The parietal decidua separating the conceptus and the myometrium is richly vascularized and at term contains some epithelial cells and several layers of the characteristic decidual cells of the stroma. Ultrastructurally the cells of decidua basalis and decidua parietalis differ, the former have a more developed Golgi and endoplasmic reticulum.[10]

Decidua plays an important part in the establishment of pregnancy by providing conditions that make implantation and early support of the embryo possible. It is believed to form an immunological barrier between the invading trophoblast and the myometrium, and has receptors for immunoglobins. The decidua also has an endocrine function. Decidual cells have the capacity to produce large amounts of prolactin[14] and small amounts of relaxin.[15] They also possess enzymes that metabolize steroid hormones and secrete pregnancy specific hormones.[16] Decidual cells,[17] particularly the macrophages,[18] have a great prostaglandin synthesiz-

ing capacity; both PGF$_{2\alpha}$ and PGE$_2$ are formed, PGF$_{2\alpha}$ in excess of about 4:1, and in some subsets of macrophages up to 12:1. Additionally, an important group of compounds, cytokines, that are released from cells and exert their functions in an intracrine, autocrine, paracrine or endocrine fashion are produced by decidual cells (see review in reference 19).

Cell membrane receptors for most cytokines have been found on decidual cells, in addition to receptors for immunoglobulins and peptide hormones such as prolactin, relaxin, oxytocin, and vasopressin. Steroid hormone receptors for estrogens, progesterone, and glucocorticoids are also present in decidua.

Cervix and Cervical Ripening

The uterine cervix is structured to protect the fetus during its development by remaining firmly closed and providing resistance to pressure from above that is created by the upright position and, in the last trimester, by the Braxton Hicks contractions, which occur with increasing frequency. While two-thirds or more of the myometrium is composed of smooth muscle cells, the muscular component tapers off in the cervix, constituting 25, 16 and 6 percent, respectively, in the upper, middle, and lower segments of the cervix. The muscular fibers are continuations of the spiral bundles from the corpus. The main components of the cervix are collagen and a ground substance rich in glycosaminoglycans, as well as some elastin fibers.

The collagen is synthesized in the connective tissue cells and laid down as fibers in the ground substance. The structural unit, tropocollagen, is a helix of three collagen chains of approximately 100,000 daltons each. The formation of the triple helix is intracellular; after extrusion of the helix, it is cleaved into its final length by peptidases. Crosslinks between the chains increase the tensile strength of the cervical tissue. Contributing to the consistency of the cervix is the composition of glycosaminoglycans in the ground substance of which dermatan is the most abundant. Dermatan binds tightly to collagen fibers, which provides cervix with a firm consistency during pregnancy.

The biochemical changes in the cervix, which we call cervical ripening, take place gradually over the last few weeks of gestation proving that the process of parturition begins days or weeks before the onset of labor. The collagen chains fracture and the fragments are solubilized by proteolytic enzymes. The glycosaminoglycans, dermatan and chondroitin, are to a large extent replaced by the more hydrophilic hyaluronic acid, increasing the water content of the ground substance. These processes change the consistency of the cervix which thereby becomes soft and distensible and its com-

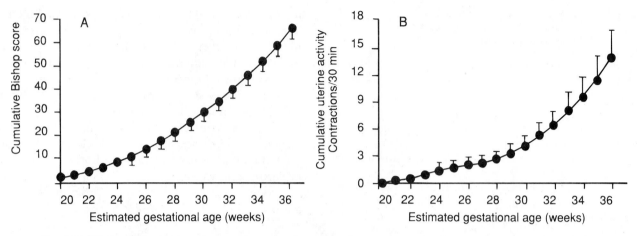

Fig. 5-3 (A) Cumulative Bishop score and estimated gestational age in a group of 13 women assessed at weekly or biweekly intervals. (B) Cumulative uterine activity and estimated gestational age in the same group of 13 women described in (A). Patients were monitored for 45 minutes before cervical assessment at each visit. Uterine activity recorded as contractions per 30 minutes. Values are means ± SE; the number of subjects at each point varied between 6 and 13. Changes in the slopes indicate a change in the score or uterine activity. There was an increase in Bishop scores from week 23 onward and an increase in uterine activity from week 28 of gestation onward. (Modified from Catalano et al.,[23] with permission.)

pliance to stretch increases.[20,21] For the clinical assessment of cervical changes various scoring systems have been developed, the most widely used is the score by Bishop.[22] This score begins to increase at a slow rate by the middle of gestation[23] (Fig. 5-3).

Cervical ripening is undoubtedly under hormonal control. In the rat it is promoted by relaxin and estrogens and is inhibited by progesterone. Ovarian hormones probably have similar effects on the human cervix. Yanaihara and co-workers[24] found ripened cervical tissue to contain higher concentrations of free estrone, conjugated estradiol, estriol, and dehydroepiandrosterone than the nonripened cervix, with further increases during labor. Administration of dehydroepiandrosterone, either systemically or locally in substantial doses, has been widely used in Japan for pharmacologic ripening of the cervix.[25] Studies in which the progesterone antagonist RU486 or other similar compounds were administered to monkeys, rats, and guinea pigs indicate that these antagonists have a marked ripening effect on the cervix.[26,27] Clinical trials in first trimester human pregnancy with mifepristone showed some softening of the cervix but less than that seen in experimental animals.[28] Since these antagonists cause a functional withdrawal of progesterone, these experiments provide strong evidence for the inhibitory action of progesterone on cervical ripening. It should be kept in mind, however, that mifepristone also cross reacts with the glucocorticoid receptor, although with lower affinity than with the progesterone receptor. Interestingly, labor did not occur spontaneously in any of the animals treated with these progesterone antagonists, but proceeded normally after administration of oxytocin.[26,27]

The role of relaxin in human cervical ripening is controversial.[29] Corpus luteum is the source of circulating relaxin in women. However, pregnant women with ovarian failure who have received a donated embryo undergo normal cervical ripening at parturition.[30] Whereas topical application of porcine relaxin suggested a ripening effect in pregnant women,[31] clinical trials with recombinant human relaxin did not show any ripening effect.[32]

Cervical ripening can be accelerated both by mechanical and pharmacologic factors. Laminaria rods that dilate the cervix by swelling with the uptake of water, and recently rods of a synthetic, hygroscopic polyvinyl alcohol sponge impregnated with magnesium sulfate, have been used. The dilation of the cervix caused by the slow swelling of the rod seems to act both mechanically and by acceleration of chemical changes, such as increased hydration of the tissues. These in turn may be due to an inflammatory reaction to the devices, because infiltrating leukocytes have been implicated in the cervical ripening process by providing a source of the collagenase involved in the cervical changes.[33]

Local application of prostaglandins, particularly PGE_2, has been the most successful method for cervical ripening; $PGF_{2\alpha}$ is less effective. In Europe, this method, introduced by British obstetricians,[34] has become the method of choice for induction of labor in high-risk pregnancies with an unripe cervix. As little as 0.4-mg PGE_2 injected into the cervical canal in a viscous gel, with a second dose 8 to 12 hours later if necessary, will induce labor in about one-half of such patients and facilitate induction with oxytocin or amniotomy, or both, in the remaining patients.[35] It is also very useful in patients with preterm rupture of membranes and an unripe cervix. The action of PGE_2 is not mediated by uterine contractions because cervical ripening proceeds even though uterine contractions, induced by the application of PGE_2 are abolished by prior administration of β-mimetics.[36] Prostaglandins may therefore have direct actions on cervical connective tissue.[37] The fact that relatively small doses of PGE_2 can accomplish rapid changes in the cervix suggests that endogenous PGE is involved in the physiologic mechanism of cervical ripening. Relevant in this regard is the fact that PGE content of cervical mucus of pregnant women increases significantly in the 2nd trimester.[38] Thus the slow gradual cervical ripening that begins around weeks 20 to 23 is associated with increased output of PGE from cervical mucosa.

The increased compliance to stretch that results from the ripening process does not in itself cause effacement and dilatation. As the cervix ripens, the cervical tissue is gradually pulled upward and effaced by incorporation into the lower segment of the corpus. It must be assumed that both effacement and dilatation are accomplished by the activity of the muscular component of the cervix and uterus. Thus, the Braxton Hicks contractions have an important role in the preparation of the birth canal in the prelabor phase of parturition.

Oxytocin and Cervical Function

Apart from indirect effects on cervical preparation for birth caused by oxytocin induced uterine contractions, oxytocin may have direct effects on cervical tissue as well. Cervical mucosa was recently found to be a target organ for oxytocin in the bovine.[38] In vitro, oxytocin significantly increased PGE_2 output from cervical tissues obtained from estrous cows but had no effect on PGE_2 output from tissues from cows in the luteal phase or pregnant cows. These results implicate oxytocin as a factor in the physiological ripening of the cervix at term and during parturition. Whether this applies to human cervix remains to be shown.[39]

Vascular Supply

The greatly enlarged uterine arteries provide the blood for the uterine tissues as well as for the conceptus, and the uterine veins drain both the uterus and the intervillous space. The vascular connections with the ovaries and the vagina are insignificant, although these vessels can become quite large in cervical pregnancies and placenta previa. About 70 percent of total uterine blood flow goes to the placenta near term. The uteroplacental vascular bed is a low resistance system which brings about a significant decrease in the total uterine vascular resistance and facilitates the marked increase in uterine blood flow during pregnancy.[40]

It has been proposed that the small blood vessels in the placenta and chorion may play a role in the putative inflammatory reactions in uterine tissues at term (see review in reference[41]). Mifepristone treatment was shown to induce PGHS-2 in these vessels which resulted in PGE_2 formation. PGE_2 is known to cause vasodilation and extravasation of fluid and cells, which in turn would stimulate leukocyte recruitment and activation. This could be relevant to cytokine-induced activation of prostaglandin synthesis in placenta, chorion, and decidua, and would provide support for the hypothesis that parturition is initiated by an inflammatory response.

Innervation

Uterine contractility is autonomous in the sense that the uterus can contract without an external nerve supply. However, even denervation does not rule out nervous influences, since the uterus itself contains adrenergic ganglionic cells. These cells can be visualized by special fluorescent staining methods.[42] In addition, autonomous nerves reach the uterus from the presacral ganglia, but they seem to contain mainly pain neurons. The uterine vascular bed has a sympathetic innervation; both α and β-receptors have been identified in the uterine blood vessels.

Adrenergic innervation of the uterus is under hormonal control; the content of neurotransmitters increases under the influence of estrogen but decreases under the influence of progesterone. A dramatic decrease occurs during pregnancy, especially in the body of the uterus,[43,44] which at term appears to be devoid of innervation. The uterus is also innervated by peptidergic nerves.[45]

Biochemical Aspects
Contractile Proteins

The contractile protein in the myometrium, as in all smooth and striated muscles, is actomyosin, formed by interaction of actin and myosin. Human myometrium contains from 1- to 5-mg myosin and from 16- to 60-mg actin per gram tissue with a ratio of actin to myosin about 14:1, which corresponds to the ratio of thin to the thick filaments observed in myometrial cells. In addition, tropomyosin (molecular weight [MW] 36,000) and a presumed structural protein, skeletin (MW 55,000), can be identified in protein extracts of human myometrium; α-actinin has been identified in the dense bodies. No difference in the concentration of actin and myosin is found between nonpregnant and pregnant myometria; the myosin purified from either source has identical adenosine triphosphatase (ATPase) activity and peptide pattern.[46]

Myosin forms the thick filaments, which are about 16 nm thick and 2.2 mm long, and with a molecular

GLOBULAR HEAD
2 Identical units each containing:
■ 1 site for ATP hydrolysis and actin binding
■ 2 light chains of ~20,000 & 17,000 daltons

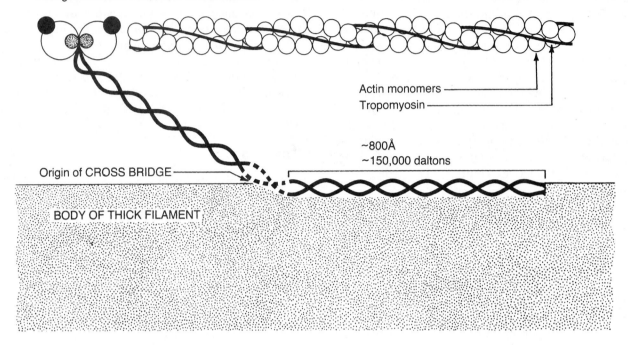

Actin monomers
Tropomyosin

~800Å
~150,000 daltons

Origin of CROSS BRIDGE

BODY OF THICK FILAMENT

Fig. 5-4 Diagrammatic representation of the myosin molecule, which is a hexamer consisting of one pair of heavy chains and two pairs of light chains. The molecule is very asymmetric, the carboxyl-terminal portion of the heavy chain being a fibrous, almost completely α-helically coiled structure that forms the thick filament. The amino-terminal portion is globular in shape and is associated with the light chains, although their precise position is unknown. The globular head binds to actin and exhibits ATPase activity. The light chain of MW 20,000 contains the phosphorylation site. The hinge region between head and tail is thought to be very flexible. (From Hartshorne and Gorecka,[175] with permission.).

weight of about 500,000. They consist of a helical tail and a globular head, formed by two heavy chains (MW 200,000, each). The head contains the ATPase enzymatic activity and the site for combination with actin. Two pairs of light chains of myosin of 20,000 and 27,000 MW, respectively, are attached to each globular head (MW≈240,000) (Fig. 5-4). The light chains are the sites of phosphorylation and of calcium binding.

Actin is a much smaller molecule, of about 42,000 MW. This protein polymerizes in physiologic solutions to form thin filaments, about 6 nm in diameter and much longer than the thick filaments. As in skeletal muscle, helically arranged strands of actin alternate with thin strands of tropomyosin (Fig. 5-4). Actomyosin is formed when actin activates the magnesium-dependent myosin ATPase, which provides the energy for the attachment of the globular head of myosin to the actin filament, forming cross bridges between thick and thin filaments. After attachment, the angle of the cross bridges changes, causing the filaments to slide past each other, thereby generating the contractile force. Detachment of the cross bridges results in relaxation.

Regulatory Proteins

The interaction of actin and myosin is a complex biochemical process regulated by calcium ions, the calcium-binding protein calmodulin, cAMP, and enzymes concerned with the phosphorylation and dephosphorylation of the myosin light chain. In the uterus, as in most other smooth muscles, myosin can react with actin and form actomyosin only when it is phosphorylated. Phosphorylation of the 20,000-MW light chain is mediated by an enzyme, myosin light-chain kinase (MLCK) (for references see reference 47), which is a key enzyme controlling smooth muscle cell contraction. MLCK is functionally dependent on calcium ions and the calcium-dependent regulatory protein, calmodulin. Calmodulin forms a complex with calcium when intracellular calcium rises from 10^{-7} to 10^{-6} M.[46] The kinase is activated by binding to the calcium-calmodulin complex; only the unphosphorylated form of MLCK can bind this complex with high affinity.

MLCK is inactivated by its own phosphorylation; this process is mediated by a cAMP-dependent protein kinase. When the MLCK is inactivated, a phosphatase will dephosphorylate the actomyosin, breaking the cross bridges and inducing relaxation. The levels of cAMP depend in turn on the relative activities of two enzymes: adenylate cyclase, which catalyzes the synthesis of cAMP and phosphodiesterase, which causes cAMP breakdown. An outline of the regulation of myometrial cell contraction by phosphorylation and intracellular calcium is depicted in Fig. 5-5.

Excitability of the Myometrial Cells

A key factor in the excitability of the contraction-relaxation process is the membrane potential, which is dependent on fluxes of ions—in particular, sodium, potassium, calcium, and chloride. These fluxes depend on the permeability of the cell membranes to each species of ions and the intrinsic metabolic processes that maintain ionic gradients across the cell membrane, including those that bind or liberate ions. The membrane potential determines the excitability of the cell.

Depolarization and subsequent repolarization provide the action potential. The normal excitation of the uterine muscle is tetanic, which means that the individual contraction is induced by a burst of rapid, repetitive potentials. The force of the contraction depends on the frequency of the tetanic potentials and the number of filaments involved. When gap junctions are present, the propagation of action potentials from cell to cell is facilitated. Random asynchronous cell contractions can maintain a baseline tonus of the organ, but simultaneous contractions of a majority of the cells are required for the development of significant increase in tension and the expulsive force. Synchronous contractions of the entire myometrium remain isometric as long as the membranes are intact and the cervix closed, thus maintaining a constant intrauterine volume. Braxton Hicks contractions may represent coincidental contractions of a large number of cells.

Extraction-Contraction Coupling

Calcium ion is vital not only for the contractile process in myometrial cells, but also for transmitting the signal of excitation from the cell membrane to the contractile machinery inside the cell.[48]

The level of intracellular free calcium is normally very low, less than 10^{-7}. It is controlled by specialized intracellular vesicles which sequester calcium avidly and by MgATPase dependent calcium extrusion pumps or by Na^+/Ca^{++} exchange mechanisms. The level of the free Ca^{++} can be raised by an influx of calcium through cell membranes either along a concentration gradient, through voltage dependent Ca^{++}-channels or receptor-operated calcium channels. Calcium can also be released from intracellular stores, a process that requires the participation of second messengers (Fig. 5-5).

Myometrial cells have a sparse sarcoplasmic reticulum so they depend largely on the influx of extracellular calcium to raise their intracellular free calcium levels. That is the basis for the effectiveness of calcium channel blockers as tocolytic agents.

Paracrine Interactions within the Uterus

In recent years it has become clear that the function of many tissues and organs are modulated not only by nervous and humoral factors from endocrine glands, but also by factors produced by nearby cells or tissues that reach their targets by diffusion. Such compounds are usually lipophilic and are rapidly metabolized in the tissues that secrete them, so that concentrations reaching the circulating blood are insignificant. The classical hormones probably also act to a certain degree in a paracrine manner; thus placental steroid hormones may also reach the adjoining decidua and myometrium by diffusion, and hormones produced in the decidua may likewise reach the adjoining myometrium and fetal membranes by a paracrine route. Examples of typical paracrine compounds are nitric oxide (NO), arachidonic acid metabolites (prostaglandins and leukotrienes), and the cytokines. Cytokines were originally believed to be products of lymphocytes activated by antigen, but it is now recognized that they are produced by virtually all cells of epithelial, endothelial, lymphoid, myeloid, and mesenchymal origin. Cytokines have numerous functions that are frequently shared by several of the compounds. They can also interact either synergistically or antagonistically. Cytokines that have been shown to participate in the regulation of endometrial/decidual function include interferon-γ, interleukin-1, interleukin-6, tumor necrosis factor-α, epidermal growth factor/transforming growth factor-α, transforming growth factor-β, colony-stimulating factor-1, and granulocyte-macrophage colony-stimulating factor, and probably others as well. Steroid hormones are major regulators of the concentrations of many, if not all, of the cytokines in the endometrium/decidua. In fact, many of the steroid actions in this tissue may be indirectly mediated by the cytokines which, according to current nomenclature, also comprise the growth factors.

Mechanism of Action of Oxytocin and Tocolytic Agents

All oxytocic agents exert their action by mobilizing calcium. The main endogenous oxytocic agents are the α-adrenergic agonists, the neurohypophyseal hormones, and the prostaglandins. Some biogenic amines (serotonin), other peptides (substance P, eloidosin), and leu-

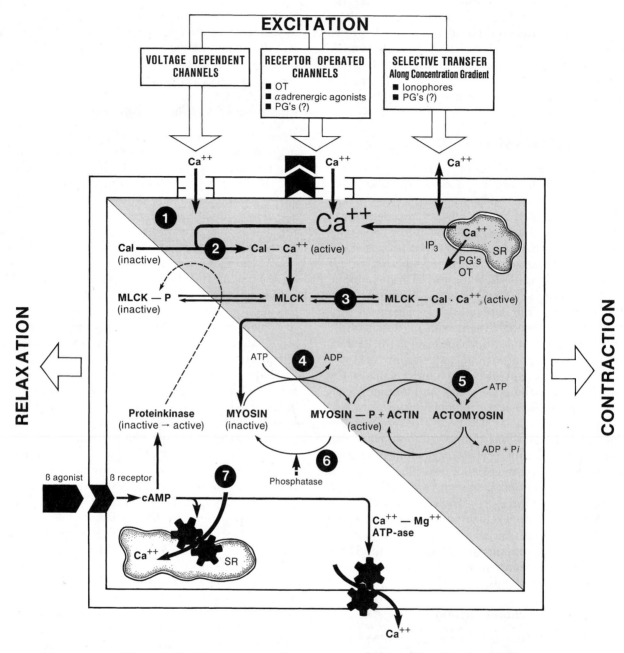

Fig. 5-5 The role of myosin light-chain (MLC) phosphorylation and calcium in uterine smooth muscle contraction. The diagonal separates the contracted state from relaxation. The numbers indicate the sequence of events thought to occur postexcitation: (1) intracellular calcium rises; (2) calmodulin binds to calcium to form an active complex; (3) the calmodulin-calcium complex interacts with MLCK to form an active complex; (4) this complex phosphorylates myosin, permitting activation of myosin ATPase activity by actin and (5) the formation of the actomyosin complex; (6) when the calcium level is reduced, MLCK is inactivated, phosphatase dephosphorylates myosin, and the muscle relaxes. (7) Calcium can enter the cell through voltage-dependent or receptor-operated channels. Activation of β-receptors results in a reduction of intracellular calcium through two possible mechanisms, both dependent on cAMP: (A) cAMP-dependent protein kinase is activated and phosphorylates MLCK, rendering it inactive, and (B) calcium is extruded from the cell by a cell membrane-associated, cAMP-activated calcium ATPase. Calcium can also be taken up and released by sarcoplasmic vesicles through a calcium-stimulated Mg-ATPase. Other organelles, particularly mitochondria, can also take up and release calcium. (Adapted from Braunwald[176] with permission.)

kotrienes can have an oxytocic action, but their importance for the in vivo regulation of human uterine function is not established.[49]

Tocolytic agonists cause relaxation by decreasing intracellular free calcium. This can be achieved in various ways. Calcium channel blockers decrease intracellular calcium by inhibiting influx from the extracellular space.[48] The β-adrenergic compounds act through receptors that are coupled to adenylcyclase and utilize cAMP as a second messenger. In the myometrial cells cAMP lowers intracellular free calcium by two mechanisms. It activates the uptake of Ca^{++} into intracellular vesicles and it activates a protein kinase that phosphorylates MLCK causing its inactivation and subsequent dissociation of the actomyosin complex.

Oxytocin antagonists block the effects of oxytocin initiated by receptor binding, including the opening of receptor operated Ca channels and stimulation of $PGF_{2\alpha}$ release.

Signal Transduction in Nonexcitable Cells and Arachidonic Acid Mobilization

All cells need a system whereby they can regulate cell function and coordinate organ function. Cells therefore possess various mechanisms for signal transduction. Cell membrane lipids and calcium have emerged as important participants in signal transduction also in tissues not having the capacity to elicit action potentials.

Nonexcitable cells do not have voltage dependent calcium channels, but they possess various cell membrane receptors that are coupled to the mobilization of calcium from intracellular stores. Occupation of these receptors by agonists activates phospholipase C (PLC), a membrane bound enzyme that hydrolyses phospholipids. The hydrolysis of membrane phospholipids by PLC can yield several second messengers including inositol triphosphate (IP_3) and diacylglycerol[50,51] IP_3 is water soluble and is released into the cytoplasm where it reacts with calcium storing vesicles to release free Ca^{++}. The reaction is extremely rapid and contains an amplification step, each IP_3 molecule releasing at least 20 Ca^{++} ions. The reaction is also rapidly extinguished. The other moiety of the phosphatidyl inositol molecule hydrolysed by PLC, diacylglycerol, is simultaneously split off but as a lipid it remains in the membrane. It can activate protein kinase C which has multifunctional catalytic activity and elicits a variety of cellular responses, including the liberation of arachidonic acid.[52]

Formation of diacylglycerol can, besides the activation of protein kinase C, lead directly to the mobilization of free arachidonic acid. Diacylglycerol contains the esterified arachidonic acid group of phosphatidylinositol in position 3 and is substrate for diacylglycerol lipase, which splits off the acyl group from position 2, and the subsequent action of a monoacylglycerol lipase yields free arachidonic acid. Decidual cells have the highest concentration of diacylglycerol lipase of all uterine tissues, but fetal membranes and placenta also have these lipases.[53]

Calcium mobilizing agonists can cause the liberation of free arachidonic acid also by the activation of phospholipase A_2 which is a Ca-dependent enzyme. Phospholipase A_2 is the most widely distributed enzyme involved in the liberation of arachidonic acid. Its substrates are phospholipids that have arachidonic acid in the number 2 position, such as phosphatidylethanolamine and phosphatidylcholine. All intrauterine tissues have high concentrations of these phospholipids, with amnion cells having the highest concentration of phosphatidylcholine.[54]

Physiology of Labor

Neural Mechanisms

There is ample evidence that the function of the uterus during parturition is controlled by humoral and not by neural factors. As already mentioned, the content of uterine neurotransmitters is regulated by the ovarian hormones, with estrogen increasing and progesterone decreasing the uterine content of norepinephrine. After an initial increase in early pregnancy, the histo-chemically demonstrable catecholamines virtually disappear from the corpus, while the cervix and vagina retain their neurotransmitter content.[43–45] It is therefore unlikely that neural activity can have much influence on myometrial function during parturition.

Does cervical innervation have a role in the ripening of the cervix and the initiation of labor? The dense sympathomimetic and peptidergic innervation of the cervix maintained throughout pregnancy could conceivably be of importance for cervical ripening.[45] The remarkable release of prostaglandins in response to cervical manipulation and stripping of the membranes[55] could perhaps be mediated by nervous activity, since catecholamines can release PGE_2 from nerve endings. The cervix and vagina have been implicated in the reflex release of oxytocin during labor, but the existence of such reflex (the so-called Ferguson reflex) has not been demonstrated in the human, nor in all animal species studied.[56]

Humoral and Paracrine Factors

The humoral factors affecting myometrial function include steroid hormones, oxytocic hormones, and relaxing hormones. Additionally, a number of cytokines that act in a paracrine manner belong to this group.

Steroids

The steroid hormones, estrogen and progesterone, have no direct effect on contractility but exert a regulatory influence through their action on protein synthesis and the synthesis of cell-surface receptors, phospholipids and other lipids, which are the determinants of membrane structure and the precursors for PG synthesis. It is well established that in contrast to most animal species, human parturition is not associated with any significant changes in the major steroid hormone levels nor in the ratio of estrogenic to progestational hormones.[57] However, marked diurnal variations in steroid levels have been observed in the rhesus monkey[58] and occur also in late pregnant women. In monkeys these variations coincide with diurnal variations in uterine contractility.[59] In late pregnant women uterine activity shows definite diurnal variations. The timing of the onset of parturition in women also has a significant diurnal distribution.[43] It is not unlikely that these circadian variations are causally related to the variations in uterine contractility. Their possible relationship to diurnal variations in maternal and fetal steroid secretion remains to be established, but it is of relevance that plasma oxytocin levels in late pregnant women exhibit nocturnal peaks which temporally correlate with increased nocturnal uterine activity. Plasma oxytocin was inversely correlated with plasma estradiol:progesterone ratio, which showed a significant nocturnal nadir.[60]

In several animal species fetal glucocorticoids, secreted in increasing amounts near term, direct the placental or luteal steroid synthesis to estrogens instead of progesterone and thereby initiate labor.[1] No such effect has been found for fetal glucocorticoids in the human, and their role in the initiation of human parturition, if any, is likely to be indirect via maturational changes in the fetus.

Relaxing Hormones

Catecholamines

Endogenous catecholamines exert their action through α and β-receptors, both of which are present in human pregnant myometrium.[61] Estrogens stimulate α-receptor formation; this is antagonized by progesterone which enhances β-receptor dominance. β-receptors are numerous in human pregnant uterus and their activation leads to myometrial relaxation as we have seen. Epinephrine is the main endogenous β-agonist. Since β-blockers have no significant effect on uterine contractility during pregnancy, endogenous β-agonists are of little significance for the function of the pregnant human uterus. During labor a considerable increase in maternal epinephrine secretion occurs which may have some significance for uterine relaxation between contractions and for the maintenance of low vascular tone in the uterine vessels.

Fetal catecholamines are excreted into the amniotic fluid in increased amounts during labor.[62] They may have an effect on the fetal membranes, on which binding sites for β-adrenergic agonists have been found.[53] Epinephrine stimulates $PGF_{2\alpha}$ release from the estrous rat uterus[63] and may have a similar effect on $PGF_{2\alpha}$ release from amniotic cells.

Relaxin

Relaxin is an ovarian hormone that is produced and secreted by the corpus luteum of pregnancy.[64] It is also synthesized in the decidua,[16] placenta,[16] and the breast tissue.[65] In many species relaxin has an important role in parturition through its effect on the pelvic ligaments. Relaxins inhibit spontaneous uterine contractions in many species[66] but has no effect on human nonpregnant or pregnant myometrium.[67] It is therefore doubtful whether relaxin is of any importance in human labor. Relaxin may play a role in the remodeling of myometrial and cervical connective tissue which takes place in early pregnancy and which is necessary for uterine growth; relaxin also induces decidualization of human endometrium.

Nitric Oxide

The endothelium-derived relaxing factor (EDRF) which causes vasodilation via stimulation of soluble guanylyl cyclase and subsequent elevation of the cyclic glucose monophosphate (GMP) concentration has been identified as nitric oxide (NO). It is enzymatically produced from L-arginine by nitric oxide synthase (NOS), which is found in many tissues, and exists as several isoforms. One major form is constitutionally expressed, another is inducible. NO stimulates cyclic GMP and mediates endothelial smooth muscle relaxation and macrophage activation, and functions in the central nervous system as a neurotransmitter. NOS is a Ca^{2+}/calmodulin dependent enzyme which is stimulated by elevated intracellular Ca^{2+}. Vascular endothelium and nervous tissues are the main sites of synthesis but NOS is also found in placenta and uterine tissues. It diffuses easily through cell membranes but is rapidly metabolically inactivated and is therefore the epitome of a paracrine factor acting on neighboring cells only. NO relaxes myometrium in vitro, and may promote uterine quiescence in vivo. The significance of placental NO synthesis may be the maintenance of low vascular tone in placental vessels and relaxation of the overlying myometrium. Data on labor related changes in NOS activity in the uterus is still too fragmentary and conflicting to draw conclusions in regard to its importance in the mechanism of labor.[68-70]

Oxytocic Hormones

The main endogenous oxytocic agents are the α-adrenergic neurotransmitters, the neurohypophysial hormones and prostaglandins E and F. In addition, a variety of other compounds that are oxytocic can be formed from arachidonic acid besides PGE and $PGF_{2\alpha}$ (Fig. 5-6). Thromboxane A synthesized in platelets and placenta is the most potent of the prostanoids[71] but is not formed by the myometrium and because of its rapid metabolism is unlikely to reach it from the vasculature or amniotic fluid. Arachidonic acid metabolites formed by the lipooxygenase pathway: the hydroperoxyeicosatetranoic acids (HPETEs) and their hydroxy analogs (HETEs), as well as the leukotrienes have been implicated in the mechanism of preterm labor, but only 5-HETE has a direct effect on myometrial contractions.[72,73] These compounds may perhaps affect uterine function indirectly.

Initiation of Labor

Withdrawal of Inhibitors or Release of Stimulators?

It was long believed that uterine quiescence during pregnancy is maintained by progesterone and that the uterus would contract spontaneously upon withdrawal of progesterone.[74,75] Evidence for withdrawal of progesterone at the end of human pregnancy has been elusive but even in species in which progesterone with-

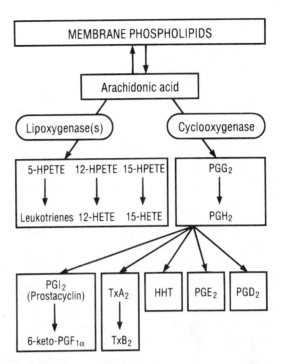

Fig. 5-6 Formation of eicosanoids from arachidonic acid by two enzymatic pathways, cyclo-oxygenase and lipo-oxygenase(s). Hydroperoxyeicosatetranoic acids (HPETEs) are formed by the incorporation of one mole of oxygen; the HPETEs are reduced to their hydroxy analogs (HETEs). The 5-HPETE can be converted to leukotrienes. The prostanoids are produced by the cyclo-oxygenase pathway. Nonenzymatic decomposition of arachidonic acid also occurs and can lead to species that affect cell function (e.g., as chemotactic factors).

drawal is a prerequisite for parturition the withdrawal plays a permissive role rather than a direct role on myometrial contractility.[76] Withdrawal of progesterone allows estrogenic effects such as the formation of cell membrane receptors and mobilization of arachidonic acid metabolism to dominate. Recently it has become possible by experimental means to produce progesterone withdrawal without affecting the production of other steroids by using progesterone antagonists. Administration of such antagonists to late pregnant monkeys and guinea pigs produced spontaneous contractions and cervical effacement but labor was not initiated unless oxytocin was administered,[25,26] confirming our earlier contention that participation of oxytocic hormones is essential for labor to proceed.[57,76,77]

Controversy exists, however, on the relative importance of the oxytocic hormones. According to some investigators the neuropeptide oxytocin has no physiological function in the initiation of spontaneous labor.[78] Instead, prostaglandins released from amnion were proposed as the stimulus for myometrial contractions during labor, the release of the prostaglandins being initiated by fetal factors. The following observations cannot, however, be accounted for by such a theory:

1. The onset of labor can be delayed and labor can be stopped in its early stages *either* by agents that inhibit oxytocin release (ethanol),[79] *or* by agents that inhibit prostaglandin synthesis (indomethacin, aspirin).[80,81]
2. The levels of PGE and PGF in the amniotic fluid are not raised at the onset of labor from levels observed in late pregnancy, they rise in the course of labor.[82,83]
3. Plasma oxytocin levels are increased in early labor and precede the rise in plasma $PGF_{2\alpha}$ metabolite levels, which occurs in the course of active labor.[84–87]
4. The uterine responsiveness to oxytocin undergoes a remarkable change during pregnancy and reaches a maximum at term, the optimal time of birth.[88] By contrast, the uterine responsiveness to prostaglandins undergoes only minor alterations during the course of pregnancy.[89]
5. Labor at term can be induced with oxytocin in doses that result in plasma oxytocin levels in the physiologic range[84,90]; by contrast, induction of labor with prostaglandins results in plasma levels that far exceed the physiologic range whether administered intravenously or intra-amniotically.[86,91,92]
6. Chorion has an active prostaglandin dehydrogenase system that permits only a small fraction of amniotic prostaglandins to pass through unaltered.[93,94]

We have proposed that initiation of labor depends on both maternal and fetal signals, both of which utilize oxytocin as a signal.[57,77] Additionally vasopressin, epidermal growth factor (EGF), platelet activating factor (PAF), and perhaps other cytokines may function as fetal signals. The signals from both mother and fetus are integrated in the decidua parietalis and transmitted to the myometrium using prostaglandins as second messenger. Evidence for this concept has accumulated in recent years and there is now agreement that decidua rather than amnion is the integrator of signals for the onset of labor.[95,96]

Regulation of Oxytocin Release and Action

Plasma Levels

It is important to recognize that oxytocin is so potent that the effective concentrations stimulating the uterus at term are in the picomolar range. For comparison the concentrations of PGE and PGF are in the nanomolar range. The great potency of oxytocin makes the measurement of plasma oxytocin difficult; this is compounded by the presence in pregnancy plasma of an enzyme, oxytocinase, that rapidly inactivates oxytocin after the sample is withdrawn. Moreover, the secretory pattern of oxytocin appears to be pulsatile, which makes frequent sampling necessary for accurate estimation of oxytocin secretion rates.

The pulsatile secretion pattern was confirmed when blood samples were collected every minute for 30 minutes from groups of normal, nonlaboring and laboring pregnant women,[85] using a sensitive and specific antibody.[97] Before the onset of labor the pulse frequency in 10 women was 1.3/min on the average. In the first stage of labor (cervix <4 cm) the pulse frequency was 3 to 4 times greater ($P < 0.001$), and in the second stage a further 3-fold increase ($P < 0.01$) was observed. In the third stage the pulse frequency decreased by about 60 percent but was much greater than before labor. Injections of 2 to 8 mU of oxytocin iv produced similar levels as the spontaneous pulses. This study proved conclusively that oxytocin secretion in pregnant women is increased during labor, including the early stages of labor. Additionally, oxytocin secretion in late pregnant women was found to exhibit a nocturnal peak[60].

Experimental and clinical trials indicate that pulsatile mode of administration of oxytocin is more effective than continuous infusion in stimulating uterine contractions.[98,99] It reduces the amount of oxytocin required for induction of labor or augmentation of dysfunctional labor significantly. The amount of oxytocin needed in an oxytocin challenge test to produce contractions was also significantly reduced when pulsatile rather than continuous infusion was used.[100]

The fetus also secretes oxytocin, as evidenced by the fact that the concentration is about twice as high in the umbilical artery as in the umbilical vein, which has about the same concentration as maternal venous blood.[101–103] Oxytocin is a relatively small molecule (MW 1,000) that is able to pass through the placenta. If the amount of oxytocin corresponding to the arteriovenous difference in the umbilical cord were passed to the mother, it would be equivalent to an infusion of 2 to 3 mU/min. This would almost double the amount of oxytocin reaching the uterus from the maternal circulation.

The placenta contains at least two aminopeptidases, which are capable of degrading oxytocin and vasopressin.[104] Oxytocin nevertheless is able to pass the placenta because injection of oxytocin on the maternal side reverses the arteriovenous difference in the umbilical cord.[31] Passage of oxytocin from fetus to mother has been demonstrated in baboons. Oxytocin is not the only substrate for the placental aminopeptidases which may be saturated by other aminopeptides present in higher concentrations than oxytocin during labor.

Oxytocin Receptor Concentrations

High-affinity, low-capacity oxytocin receptors are found in the uterus of premenopausal nonpregnant women in low concentrations.[105,106] Receptors are present both in the myometrium and endometrium. During pregnancy, the concentrations in both tissues rise dramatically, at 13 to 17 weeks they are about sixfold higher than the nonpregnant levels and at the end of pregnancy about 80- to 100-fold higher.[77,107,108] The highest concentrations of receptors are found in early labor when levels are two to three times higher than at term without labor (Fig. 5-7). In preterm labor, the levels are nearly as high as in term labor and again two to three times higher than the level in women at the same stage of gestation but not in labor. The results from ligand binding studies correlate well with oxytocin receptor gene expression in human uterus as demonstrated by Kimura et al. in a series of recent papers,[109,110] indicating that the regulation of oxytocin receptors occurs mainly at the transcriptional level.

The topographic distribution of oxytocin receptors in the fundus, corpus, and upper part of the lower segment is rather uniform, but in the lower part of the lower segment receptor concentrations taper off drastically and become very low in cervical tissue (Fig. 5-8).

The rise in myometrial receptor concentrations increases the response to oxytocin by two mechanisms: (1) lowering the threshold for stimulation of contractions by oxytocin, and (2) increasing the number of

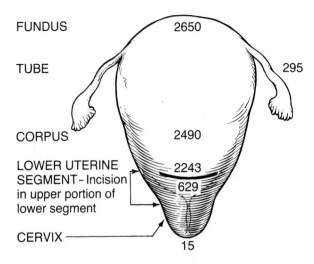

Fig. 5-8 Distribution of oxytocin receptors in a pregnant human uterus, removed in preterm labor at 34 weeks. Numerals denote OTR in fmol/mg DNA. (Adapted from Fuchs et al.,[107] with permission.)

contractile units recruited to contract simultaneously, thereby causing the tension developed by a given oxytocin concentration to rise. It is well documented that the uterine responsiveness to oxytocin increases throughout pregnancy,[88] which parallels the changes in the receptor concentrations. It has been a matter of controversy whether the responsiveness increases further in the last weeks before the onset of labor. Results from serial daily measurements indicate that there is a significant rise in oxytocin sensitivity during the last 5 to 7 days before the onset of spontaneous labor.[57,111] The threshold is lowered to the normally circulating oxytocin levels and labor begins. These events are schematically depicted in Fig. 5-9.

In late pregnancy so called Braxton Hicks contractions occur with increasing frequency. They are abolished by intake of ethanol, as are those of false labor.[79] Increased uterine activity declined significantly in comparison to controls during an infusion of an oxytocin antagonist.[112] The "spontaneous" contractions of the pregnant human uterus are therefore induced by endogenous oxytocin.

What controls oxytocin receptor concentrations in the human uterus? The answer is still shrouded in uncertainty. In experimental animals, estrogens induce the formation of oxytocin receptors and progesterone inhibits their formation,[113-115] mediated by suppression of estrogen receptors.[116] Estrogens probably have the same effect in the human, but the action of progesterone is clearly different, since oxytocin receptor levels increase in parallel with progesterone.[117,118] Another factor which affects oxytocin receptor concentrations is distention which acts synergistically with estrogen to increase oxytocin receptor density. Distention may be the cause for the increase during the last days of preg-

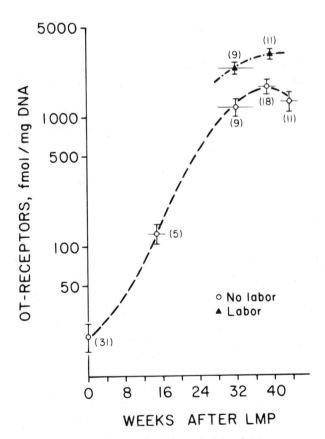

Fig. 5-7 Oxytocin receptor concentrations in human myometrium during pregnancy (O) and during preterm and term labor (▲). Note the logarithmic scale on the abscissa. Values are lognormal means; bars indicate SE. (From Fuchs and Fuchs,[57] with permission.)

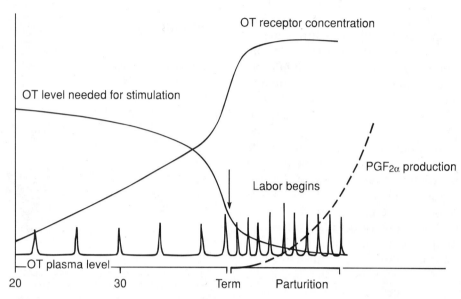

Fig. 5-9 Diagrammatic representation of the concentration of myometrial oxytocin, the level of oxytocin needed to elicit contractions, and maternal plasma oxytocin levels at the end of gestation and during labor. Oxytocin is secreted in pulses of low frequency. During labor, pulse frequency increases. Fetal secretion of oxytocin can be considerable and may contribute to the oxytocin level reaching the myometrium. $PGF_{2\alpha}$ production does not increase significantly until labor is in progress and then increases progressively throughout the third stage of labor. OT, oxytocin.

nancy because myometrial growth lags behind growth of the conceptus, particularly in multiple pregnancy.

Vasopressin

Vasopressin is more potent than oxytocin in nonpregnant women and retains its potency during pregnancy although the sensitivity to vasopressin increases less than that to oxytocin.[118] Vasopressin receptors are present in both nonpregnant[105,106,119] and pregnant uteri,[108,120] their concentrations increase in both myometrium and decidua during pregnancy. Vasopressin is bound with higher affinity than oxytocin to receptors in nonpregnant uteri, but in pregnant uteri the affinities are similar.

Maternal plasma levels of vasopressin remain low during pregnancy and labor, but the levels are considerably increased in patients who are carriers of familiar nephrogenic diabetes insipidus. The duration of labor in such patients is reported to be shorter than normal.[121] Vasopressin infusions have been used in the past to induce labor. High concentrations of vasopressin are found in the cord blood with a remarkably high arteriovenous difference.[102,122] Fetal hypoxia is a powerful stimulus for vasopressin release,[123] and vasopressin levels in cord blood are particularly high after fetal distress. Although the uterine sensitivity to vasopressin is somewhat lower than the oxytocin sensitivity, a high vasopressin level in the umbilical artery could add considerable oxytocic potency to that of the fetal oxytocin if vasopressin passes from the fetus to the mother. A significant amount of vasopressin is found in the amniotic fluid[123] and may diffuse through the membranes to reach the myometrium.

Both oxytocin and vasopressin stimulate phospholipase C and induce the hydrolysis of phosphatidylinositol in the decidua,[124] and can thereby mobilize free arachidonic acid and stimulate prostaglandin synthesis.[77]

Regulation of Prostanoid Release and Action

Oxytocic Potencies

Thromboxane (TX) is the most potent prostanoid in vivo, about 100 times as potent as $PGF_{2\alpha}$.[71] Prostacyclin (PGI_2) is a powerful vasodilator and relaxes various smooth muscles but has no effect on the human pregnant uterus in vivo.[71] PGI_2 has a transient oxytocic effect in rat uteri and potentiates the action of oxytocin.[125] The significance of PGI_2 for uterine physiology in pregnant women is due to its vasodilator activity.

PGE_2 is about ten times as potent as $PGF_{2\alpha}$ in the human uterus, but in contrast to $PGF_{2\alpha}$ has a biphasic effect. PGE_2 stimulates cAMP accumulation that causes relaxation and leads to desensitization of the uterus to the oxytocic actions of PGE_2.[126]

$PGF_{2\alpha}$ is the main prostanoid released during labor. $PGF_{2\alpha}$ has a similar action on the myometrium as oxytocin. It elevates intracellular free calcium both by opening calcium channels and by the release of calcium from intracellular vesicles. More important, $PGF_{2\alpha}$ has the capacity to increase the excitability of the myometrial cells at concentrations lower than those required for contraction, which results in an enhancement of the action of other oxytocics.[127] This could explain the remarkable sensitization of the uterus to oxytocin that occurs in the course of labor when $PGF_{2\alpha}$ secretion is increased.

Prostaglandin E and $F_{2\alpha}$ Receptors

Separate receptors exist for each of the natural prostanoids: PGE_2, $PGF_{2\alpha}$, PGD_2, PGI_2, and TXA_2.[120,129] Among these receptors extensive cross reactivity exists, which complicates the evaluation of their function. Human nonpregnant and pregnant myometrium contain all prostanoid receptors and subtypes. The control of prostaglandin receptors is poorly understood. Modulation by ovarian hormones is different than oxytocin receptors.[89] PGE_2 receptor concentrations in human myometrium are, in contrast to oxytocin, highest in nonpregnant women, and significantly lower in pregnant women.[130,131]

Prostanoid Concentrations in Uterine Tissues

All uterine tissues are capable of synthesizing prostaglandins from endogenous precursors.[17,54] Prostaglandin H synthase (PGHS) catalyzes the first steps of prostanoid biosynthesis. PGHS possesses two enzymatic activities, a cyclooxygenase activity that converts arachidonic acid to PGG_2 and a peroxidase activity that transforms PGG_2 to PGH_2 which is the precursor of the biologically active prostanoids (Fig. 5-6). Recent studies have shown the existence of two isoforms of PGHS. Type 1 (PGHS-1) is expressed constitutively in most types of tissue whereas type 2 (PGHS-2) is expressed only following cell activation by growth factors, cytokines, and mitogens (see review in reference 132). PGHS-1 and PGHS-2 are encoded by two-separate genes.[133] Reexamination of the production of prostanoids in light of this finding is currently being undertaken, and will probably clarify some of the contradictory findings reported in the past. The prostanoids produced by different tissues in vitro vary. Our understanding of the factors that direct the metabolism of arachidonic acid in different tissues in vivo is fragmentary.

There is general consensus that the *amnion* produces almost exclusively PGE_2, and a little $PGF_{2\alpha}$ and PGI_2, and has little or no metabolic capacity to inactivate them.[54,78,134] The large amounts of $PGF_{2\alpha}$ that accumulate in amniotic fluid during labor may therefore derive from other tissues, possibly the umbilical cord or chorion and decidua,[135] possibly also fetal urine.

Chorion produces both PGE_2 and $PGF_{2\alpha}$ but has a very active 15-ketodehydrogenase and 13, 14-reductase system that converts both prostanoids to inactive metabolites.[78,134,135] The transfer across the membranes from fetus to mother decreases during labor.[136] It is therefore doubtful how large a proportion of the prostanoids produced by amnion can pass through the chorion intact. For the induction of abortion by intra-amniotic instillation of PGE_2 or $PGF_{2\alpha}$ doses that far exceed those produced during spontaneous labor are required, milligram rather than microgram quantities.

Decidua parietalis (vera) produces both PGE_2, $PGF_{2\alpha}$ and PGI_2. It has the 15-ketodehydrogenase and 13,14-reductase enzyme complex but has considerably less activity than the chorion in this regard.[70,134] PGE_2 is metabolized more avidly than $PGF_{2\alpha}$ because PGE_2 is the preferred substrate for this enzyme. Furthermore, 9-ketoreductase activity has been demonstrated in human decidua.[137] This enzyme converts PGE_2 to $PGF_{2\alpha}$; and its activity is enhanced by oxytocin.[137] Decidua therefore releases predominantly $PGF_{2\alpha}$ and is considered to be the principal source of $PGF_{2\alpha}$ in the uterus.

Myometrium produces almost exclusively prostacyclin.[138] It is synthesized both in the vascular compartment and in the myometrium. The concentration of the endoperoxide and prostacyclin synthase increases during pregnancy about 3-fold from nonpregnant levels but no changes occur during the last trimester or in relation to labor.[138]

Placenta[17,139] and umbilical cord[135] have a great capacity to produce PGE_2 and TXA_2 and lesser amounts of PGI_2. However, TXA_2 production in the intact organ is blocked by an endogenous inhibitor.[139]

Mobilization of Arachidonic Acid during Labor

The cell membranes are the main source of the esterified arachidonic acid that serves as the precursor for prostanoid synthesis. Phospholipids are a major constituent of cell membranes. In the phospholipids of all intrauterine tissues,[53,54] arachidonic acid constitutes from 9 to 26 percent of the fatty acids. The most common mechanism by which arachidonic acid is released from membrane phospholipids is by cleavage from the 2 position of phospholipids by phospholipase A_2. PLC hydrolyzes the inositol phosphate bond of phosphatidylinositol, where arachidonic acid is the acyl group in the number 3 position. The release of arachidonic acid by the action of PLC therefore requires the subsequent action of diacylglycerol lipase and monoglycerol lipase. Although all uterine tissues possess the necessary lipases and phospholipases, decidua has the highest concentration of these lipases, whereas term amnion has the highest concentration of phospholipase A_2 and C.[54]

Free arachidonic acid can be converted to prostanoids or other eicosanoids along the pathways shown schematically in (Fig. 5-6). All arachidonic acid liberated by the action of the various lipases is not converted to prostanoids or lipooxygenase products in the cells. A considerable part is rapidly reesterified by acyltransferases or metabolized to produce energy. Prostanoid production depends on the balance of all these enzymatic activities.

No significant alterations have been detected in the phospholipid composition or lipase activities in relation to parturition with the exception of the phospholipase A_2 and C concentrations in amnion which are increased at term.[54] The content of arachidonic acid is lower and the concentration of prostaglandin E_2 and $F_{2\alpha}$ is higher in amnion tissue obtained after spontaneous vaginal delivery than in amnion tissue obtained at elective cesarean delivery suggesting that the mobilization of arachidonic acid from this tissue is increased during labor.[53,54] Usually liberation of arachidonic acid is the rate limiting step. Since free arachidonic acid

accumulates in amniotic fluid[78] during labor, precursor availability exceeds conversion to prostanoids.

As already mentioned, the tissue concentrations of prostanoids and the production rates measured in vitro do not necessarily reflect the situation in vivo, but merely indicate the capacity of the tissues to metabolize arachidonic acid.

Plasma Levels Plasma levels of the prostanoids themselves are poor indicators of production rates because of rapid metabolism in the lungs, kidney and liver. The measurement of stable metabolite levels has been helpful, particularly for $PGF_{2\alpha}$, whereas the corresponding metabolite for PGE_2 is very unstable. Technical difficulties regarding assay specificity have made measurements of plasma levels of 6-keto $PGF_{1\alpha}$, the nonenzymatic hydrolysis product of PGI_2, of questionable value.

The levels of the main metabolite of PGF_α, 15-keto, 13,14 dehydro-$PGF_{2\alpha}$ (PGFM), in maternal plasma increase slightly during pregnancy, reflecting the growth

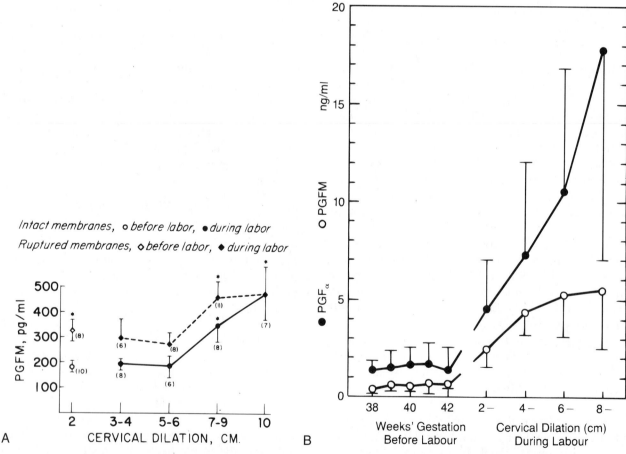

Fig. 5-10 (A) Plasma prostaglandin F metabolite levels in parturient women, measured in serial samples taken during the first stage of labor and arranged according to the cervical dilatation. Values for women with intact membranes (—) are shown separately from those with ruptured membranes (———). Prelabor values in women with premature rupture of membranes (◇) and intact membranes (○). (From Fuchs et al.,[84] with permission.) (B) $PGF_{2\alpha}$ (●) and its metabolite (○) levels in amniotic fluid in late gestation and during labor. Values are for samples obtained at amniotomy in individual patients (not serial samples). (From Keirse,[82] with permission.)

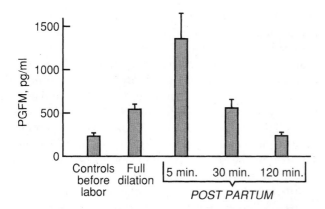

Fig. 5-11 Plasma levels of $PGF_{2\alpha}$ metabolite (PGFM) in parturient women measured in serial samples obtained at full dilatation and after delivery. Control levels were measured before the onset of labor. (Adapted from Fuchs et al.,[141] with permission.)

of the uterus. There is general agreement that during the active phase of labor, a rapid and progressive increase in plasma PGFM occurs but no significant changes have been observed before labor or in early labor (Fig. 5-10).[84,86,87,140] The increase in plasma PGFM parallels the increase in cervical dilation. Maximal levels occur after delivery of the baby, at the time of placental separation.[140–142] The concentrations of PGFM then fall rapidly suggesting that the peak production during the third stage originates in the placenta or fetal membranes. However, levels remain significantly increased at least one hour after delivery of the placenta and fetal membranes, indicating that decidua is a major source of uterine $PGF_{2\alpha}$ during labor (Fig. 5-11).

Conflicting results with regard to the PGEM metabolite have been reported, reflecting the instability of the compound and technical difficulties that have not yet been resolved.[143,144]

Urinary Excretion Excretion of stable urinary metabolites is a useful measure of the overall prostanoid production of the body. The production of PGE_2 and $PGF_{2\alpha}$ in men and nonpregnant women has been estimated to be in the range of 10 to 50 ug/24 g. During pregnancy the excretion of the metabolites of $PGF_{2\alpha}$ increases slightly[145] while the excretion of PGI_2 and TXA_2 metabolites rises considerably in the second trimester with a nonsignificant increase in the third trimester.[146,147] At term no significant increase is detected before the onset of labor but on the day of delivery excretion is higher. Of note, in the second trimester, the excretion of prostacyclin metabolites increases proportionately more than that of TXA_2 metabolites which supports the concept of relative dominance of PGI_2 over TXA_2 in normal pregnancies.[148]

Amniotic Fluid Levels Neither amnion cells nor amniotic fluid can inactivate prostanoids, and amniotic fluid

concentrations therefore reflect the production by amnion and the umbilical cord. PGE_2 and $PGF_{2\alpha}$ levels in human amniotic fluid remain low until the onset of labor provided that the membranes are intact and the cervix or internal os are not manipulated. During spontaneous and induced labor, a significant and progressive increase occurs (Fig. 5-10B). Stripping of the membranes, amniotomy, digital examination of the cervix, and spontaneous rupture of membranes result in rapid increases in prostanoid production that is reflected both in maternal plasma and amniotic fluid concentrations.[55,82,84,149] Puncture of the amniotic sac through the abdominal wall does not have the same effect, so the cervical pole of the fetal membranes and the area of the internal os of the cervix are more susceptible to traumatic release of prostanoids. During these procedures leukocytes from the cervix may gain access to the decidua and chorion and since activated leukocytes can initiate induction of PGHS synthesis quickly,[150] these infiltrating leukocytes might cause the elevation of amniotic fluid prostaglandin levels in this situation.

Initiation of Prostanoid Production at Parturition Because all intrauterine tissues have the capacity to generate prostaglandins throughout most of gestation, the release during labor is not regulated by substrate availability. Until the inducible isoform of prostaglandin synthase was discovered, no labor related change in the levels of this key enzyme were observed. Recently, however, the expression of PGHS-2 was shown to be increased in human amnion obtained after spontaneous vaginal delivery in comparison to amnion from elective cesarean delivery, whereas PGHS-1 levels were unaltered.[151] Whether this increase occurred as a consequence of labor or before the onset of labor cannot be decided on the basis of this report. The induction of PGHS-2 gene expression by bacterial products and activated macrophages in labor complicated by infection seems likely, since proinflammatory cytokines appear in amniotic fluid in such cases.[152] Whether or not induction of PGHS-2 synthesis in decidua and other uterine tissues precedes the onset of labor remains to be established, but it is an interesting concept.

The increased production of prostanoids during labor could ensue as a result of (1) withdrawal of inhibitory substances, or (2) increase in stimulators of synthesis.

Withdrawal of Endogenous Inhibitors Several likely compounds have been identified. Placenta contains a cytosolic inhibitor of TXA_2 synthesis.[139] Several phospholipase A_2 inhibitors have also been identified. The major group consists of lipocortins that are induced by glucocorticoids and are believed to be the basis for the anti-inflammatory action of glucocorticoids.[153] Lipocortins have been isolated from several organs, including the placenta. While glucocorticoids have been shown to inhibit prostanoid production in myometrial cells, their action in decidual or chorio-amnion cells is controversial.[78] Pregnancy serum contains inhibitory substances but no alteration in their concentration occurs at term and during labor.[154]

Gravidin, a PLA_2 inhibitor isolated from amniotic fluid,[155] has been identified as the secretory component of IgA.[156] The presence of other inhibitory compounds in the amniotic fluid which disappeared at term has also been reported.[157] However, when tested with slices of human uterine tissues instead of a system derived from sheep seminal vesicles, amniotic fluid from mid or late pregnancy had no inhibitory activity on basal prostaglandin output.[158] The presence of immunosuppressive cytokines in amniotic fluid and decidual cells has been demonstrated, including transforming growth factor-β and interleukin-4.[159] These cytokines decrease the production of PGE by amnion and decidual cells and increase the production of IL-1 receptor antagonist, which in turn inhibits IL-1 induced PGE production.[160] The relevance of these immunosuppressive cytokines for in vivo production of PGF_α in pregnant women has not been demonstrated yet. There is so far no conclusive evidence from these studies that a withdrawal of an inhibitory substance initiates the prostanoid production during labor.

It has been proposed that increased metabolism and elimination of the active prostaglandins could be responsible for the maintenance of low prostaglandin levels during pregnancy (see review in reference 161). Progesterone is thought to increase the synthesis of prostaglandin dehydrogenase enzyme (PGDH) because withdrawal of progesterone lowers PGDH activity causing a decline in prostaglandin inactivation.[161,162] Such a mechanism may be an equally important method of control of prostaglandin levels as inhibitors of synthesis.

Endogenous Stimulators of Prostanoid Synthesis Oxytocin was the first endogenous compound shown to stimulate PGE_2 and $PGF_{2\alpha}$ synthesis in decidua and amnion.[77] Because the fetus secretes oxytocin it was proposed as a fetal signal for parturition in women.[57] The stimulatory action of oxytocin has been confirmed by several authors. Oxytocin activates PLC in human decidua, thereby increasing $PGF_{2\alpha}$ production.[124] Oxytocin has been shown to be effective also in vivo. Other compounds have since been identified that stimulate prostanoid production in cultured amnion cells. They belong to the group now collectively called cytokines mentioned earlier (Table 5-1). EGF and platelet activating factor (PAF) have considerable activity and are found in amniotic fluid.[54,96] IL-1 and TNF-α, and prob-

ably other proinflammatory cytokines, are potent releasers of prostaglandin E and are expressed in human endometrium/decidua, placenta and placental membranes.[163] Any one of these compounds is therefore a potential signal for increased prostaglandin production and others will probably be found with similar action. Intrauterine infection is characterized by increased production of these proinflammatory cytokines by gestational tissues.[164,165] There is much evidence supporting the role of these factors in preterm labor in women with intrauterine infection, but the evidence for their participation in the initiation of normal labor is sparse, and no elevation of proinflammatory cytokines in amniotic fluid of women with normal pregnancy has been observed. Considering the importance of the process of parturition it is likely that both fetus and mother would utilize multiple signalling pathways to accomplish it.

Prostanoid production could also be initiated by a shift in the balance of the inhibitory and stimulatory substances. In cases of intrauterine inflammation the outcome of pregnancy may thus depend on the balance of activities of proinflammatory, contractility promoting cytokines and cytokines such as IL-4, TGF-1β, and IL-1 receptor antibody that suppress the activity of the proinflammatory cytokines. Such a shift need not be large at first, because once labor is in progress the production of prostanoids appears to be self perpetuating. $PGF_{2\alpha}$ can stimulate its own release, and myometrial contractions and intrauterine pressure changes can sustain $PGF_{2\alpha}$ release.[125]

Uterine Function During Labor

Having considered the functions of the various anatomic parts of the uterus at the cellular level, we shall now discuss the integrated function of the uterus as an organ during parturition. Essentially, this function is to develop sufficient expulsive force to propel the fetus through the birth canal against a varying degree of resistance. The work load is considerable and does require considerable energy. The uterine contractions must be intermittent to permit sufficient oxygen to be delivered to the fetus between contractions, and their force must progressively increase to enable the soft part of the birth canal to stretch gradually.

Many attempts have been made to quantitate uterine activity in labor. Two of the pioneers in uterine physiology, Alvarez and Caldeyro-Barcia,[166] devised the Montevideo unit to combine two variables: the amplitude and the frequency of the contraction. An alternative is the measurement of the active contraction area, described by Bourne and Burn as early as 1927,[167] which incorporates three variables: frequency, active pressure, and duration of contractions. Using modern electronic equipment for intrauterine pressure recording, the active contraction area is easy to measure by integrating the pressure above the baseline with time.

As reported by Steer et al.,[168] the active contraction area correlates better than any other measure with the rate of cervical dilatation in the active phase of labor. The mean value for uterine activity over the whole first stage of labor was found to be 1100 kiloPascal-seconds (kPas) per 15 minutes with an SD of 333 kPas/15 minutes in 22 consecutive patients in spontaneous labor. During the period of dilatation from 4 to 10 cm, the active contraction area increased from about 800 to 1,200 kPas/15 minutes, a 50 percent increase that occurred primarily between 7 and 9 cm of dilatation.

The rate of cervical dilatation achieved with a certain amount of uterine activity depends on the resistance of the cervix. Below 430 kPas/15 minutes, significant progress in labor is unlikely to occur, but even above 500 kPas/15 minutes some women will exhibit slow rates of cervical dilatation, due to increased cervical resistance. Augmentation of uterine activity in the presence of such resistance (slow progress in cervical dilatation) is not always advisable, especially if preaugmentation uterine activity is in the normal range. In these cases, hyperstimulation might occur with a risk for fetal compromise. The fact that the nulliparous cervix is more resistant than the multiparous cervix explains the difference in the average duration of labor in nulliparae and multiparae. According to Arulkumaran et al.,[169] less uterine work is required to dilate the cervix in multiparae than in nulliparae (Fig. 5-12), whereas in Steer's study there was no difference. However, the rate of cervical dilatation also depends on whether the expulsive forces are acting on the cervix. This may not be the case in certain forms of dystocia.

Friedman[170] has been influential in describing the temporal patterns of cervical dilatation and developing standard curves for nulliparous and multiparous women with which individual cases can be compared. An even better index of the efficiency of labor would be a combination of cumulative uterine activity and cervical dilatation with time.

To correlate the uterine activity with the total amount of oxytocic agents acting upon the uterus is impossible, since we cannot measure the amount of oxytocin and vasopressin reaching the myometrium from the fetus, nor the amount of prostaglandins generated within the uterus. During stimulation of the uterus with exogenous oxytocin, it is possible to correlate the uterine activity with the amount of oxytocin administered. Systems actually have been constructed that automatically regulate the infusion rate to provide a constant uterine activity. Amico et al.[171] and Seitchik et al.[90] have stud-

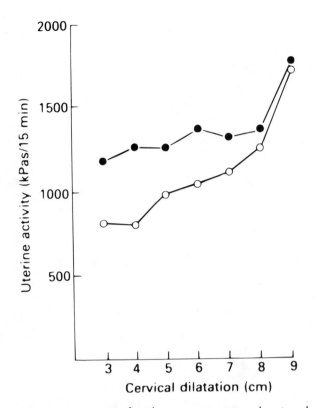

Fig. 5-12 Comparison of median uterine activity values in nulliparas (●) and multiparas (○) at each centimeter of cervical dilatation. (From Arulkumaran et al.,[169] with permission.)

ied amounts of oxytocin to be given and the blood concentrations obtained in cases of hypokinetic labor. Infusion rates of 1 to 5 mU/min were sufficient to give adequate activity in all but one of these 11 patients, and the concentration of oxytocin obtained was of the same order of magnitude as found in spontaneous labor, an observation that agrees with our own studies in oxytocin-induced labors.[85] The finding that uterine activity measured in kPas/15 min remains relatively stable at cervical dilations up to 4 to 6 cm and then increases, is compatible with the idea that oxytocin is the main driving force in the early part of labor, the mean levels of oxytocin remaining rather constant.[84] At cervical dilations over 4 to 6 cm, PGF generation increases rapidly, potentiating oxytocin-induced activity and perhaps becoming the major stimulant of uterine contractions.[84,86,87]

That it should be necessary to give an average dose of 75 mU/min to induce labor and obtain an activity of 1500 kPas/15 min in cases with an unripe cervix, as claimed by one group of investigators,[172] is unlikely and possibly dangerous. There is no doubt, however, that the dosage of oxytocin required to produce a certain level of uterine activity can vary considerably and is dependent on the uterine sensitivity to oxytocin, which again depends on the concentration of oxytocin receptors.

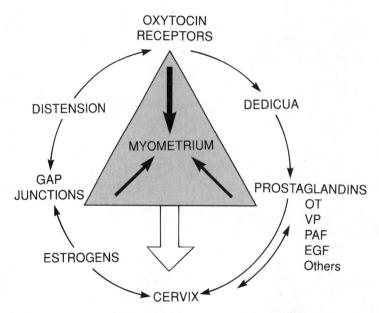

Fig. 5-13 Diagrammatic representation of the main factors involved in the control of uterine activity in pregnant women at term and during spontaneous labor. (From Fuchs,[177] with permission.)

A Model for Human Parturition

The preparation of the uterus for parturition begins in the third trimester and the initiation of labor is often a gradual process. It involves the following steps (Fig. 5-13):

1. Growth and remodeling of the cervix occurs under the influence of placental hormones and relaxin throughout gestation. The process accelerates during the last trimester when the circulating levels of estrogens and dehydroepiandrosterone increase. Release of PGE from cervical mucosa increases and acts synergistically with relaxin and placental estrogens to promote cervical remodeling and softening.

2. The increase in placental hormone secretion results in increased expression of oxytocin and vasopressin receptor genes and consequently the receptor concentrations in the myometrium and decidua increase steadily.

3. Oxytocin is secreted in pulses of low frequency throughout gestation. A variety of stimuli (from vagal afferents, food, stress, nipple stimulation, etc) also cause episodic release of oxytocin. In the last trimester the receptor concentration reaches a critical point when uterine contractions are elicited in response to the spontaneous pulses of oxytocin. These contractions exert pressure on the cervix and promote the progress of step 1.

4. Near term, distention of the uterus accelerates causing the formation of oxytocin receptors in myometrium and decidua to increase further. Distention and placental hormones also increases gap junction formation between myometrial cells, more units are recruited to contract in response to the oxytocin pulses, more tension is generated and more intrauterine pressure is developed accelerating the progress of step 1.

5. Intermittent uterine contractions cause transient hypoxic episodes that stimulate the release of fetal stress hormones, oxytocin, vasopressin, and ACTH. Maturational changes in the conceptus result in the excretion of substances that have the potential to stimulate prostaglandin synthesis such as EGF, PAF, and perhaps other cytokines. These substances are in direct contact with amnion but may also reach decidua through canaliculi in the amnion. Prostaglandin release is stimulated.

6. By mechanisms not yet fully understood, the frequency of oxytocin pulses increases, perhaps as a result of reflexes arising in the densely innervated cervical region which at term is under increasing pressure from above. Contractions are therefore elicited with increasing frequency. In the presence of gap junctions (see no. 5) the contractions become well propagated and labor begins. Decidual cells respond to oxytocin by the release of increasing amounts of $PGF_{2\alpha}$ which enhances the action of oxytocin, tension developed by the contractions increases and pressure on the cervix increases augmenting the release of prostaglandins from the decidua and the chorioamnion in the areas in apposition to the internal os. The myometrial response to oxytocin is further enhanced and labor becomes self-perpetuating.

Key Points

- The human myometrium is composed of smooth muscle cells and a matrix consisting mainly of glycogen and glycosaminoglycans. Uterine growth results from both cell division and hypertrophy of individual myometrial cells.

- Cervical ripening is under hormonal control, including estrogen and progesterone. Effacement and dilatation are accomplished by the activity of the muscular components of the cervix and uterus.

- The contractile protein of the myometrium, as in all smooth and striated muscle, is actomyosin, formed by interaction of actin and myosin. Myosin can react with actin and form actomyosin only when it is phorphorylated by the enzyme MLCK. This enzyme is functionally dependent on calcium ions and the calcium dependent regulatory protein, calmodulin, and is inactivated by its own phosphorylation.

- Tocolytic agonists cause uterine relaxation by decreasing intracellular free calcium. NO synthesized by the placenta may play a role in the maintenance of low vascular tone in placental vessels and relaxation of the overlying myometrium.

- The initiation of labor depends on oxytocin as the maternal signal and on oxytocin, vasopressin, and various cytokines as fetal signals.

- Oxytocin is secreted in a pulsatile pattern, approximately one pulse per minute before the onset of labor. The pulse frequency is to 3 to 4 times greater in the first stage of labor with a further threefold increase observed in the second stage of labor.

- Uterine responsiveness to oxytocin increases throughout pregnancy, paralleling changes in oxytocin receptor concentrations.

- All uterine tissues are capable of synthesizing prostaglandins from endogenous precursors. Two forms of prostaglandin H synthase which catalyzes the first steps of prostanoid biosynthesis have been identified, one that is expressed constitutively in most tissues, and a second that is inducible and is expressed only after cell activation by growth factors, cytokines, and mitogens. PGE_2 is about ten times as potent as $PGF_{2\alpha}$ in the human uterus. $PGF_{2\alpha}$ is the main prostanoid released during labor.

- Stripping of the membranes, amniotomy, digital examination of the cervix, and spontaneous rupture of the membranes result in rapid increases in prostanoid production, as reflected both in maternal plasma and amniotic fluid concentrations.

- With the onset of labor, the frequency of oxytocin pulses increases, resulting in more frequent contractions. $PGF_{2\alpha}$ is released in greater amounts, enhancing the action of oxytocin. With increased pressure on the cervix, the release of prostaglandins from the decidua and chorioamnion is augmented.

References

1. Liggins GC: Initiation of parturition. Br Med Bull 35: 145, 1979
2. Görttler K: Die Architektur der Muskelwand des menschlichen Uterus und ihre funktionelle Bedeutung. Gegenbaurs Morphol Jahrb 65:45, 1931
3. Garfield RE, Sims SM, Kannan MS, Daniel EE: Possible role of gap junctions in activation of myometrium during parturition. Am J Physiol 235:C168, 1978
4. Garfield RE, Hayashi RH: Appearance of gap junctions in the myometrium of women during labor. Am J Obstet Gynecol 140:254, 1981
5. Fuchs A-R, Fuchs F, Helmer H, Garfield RE: Lack of correlation between gap junction (GJ) and oxytocin (OT) receptor concentrations in pregnant and parturient human myometrium. Presented at the 39th Annual Meeting of the Society for Gynecological Investigation; San Antonio, TX, March 20–23, 1991
6. Garfield RE, Kannan MS, Daniel EE: Gap junction formation in myometrium: control by estrogens, progesterone and prostaglandins. Am J Physiol 238:C81, 1980
7. Wathes DC, Porter DG: Effect of uterine distension and estrogen treatment on gap junction formation in the myometrium of the rat. J Reprod Fertil 65:497, 1982
8. Tabb T, Thilander G, Grover A et al: An immunochemical and immunocytological study of the increase in myometrial gap junctions and connexin 43 in rats and humans during pregnancy. Am J Obstet Gynecol 167: 1267, 1992
9. Chow L, Lye SJ: Expression of the gap junction protein connexin-43 is increased in the human myometrium toward term and with the onset of labor. Am J Obstet Gynecol 170:788, 1994
10. Wynn RM: Histology and ultrastructure of the human endometrium. p. 341. In Wynn RM (ed): Biology of the Uterus. 2nd Ed. Plenum Press, New York, 1977
11. Nehemiah JC, Schnitzer JA, Schulman H, Novikoff AB: Human chorionic trophoblast, decidual cells and macrophages: a histochemical and electron microscopic study. Am J Obstet Gynecol 140:261, 1981
12. Bulmer JN, Morrison L, Smith JC: Expression of class II MHC gene products by macrophages in human uteroplacental tissue. Immunology 63:707, 1988
13. Vince GS, Starkey PM, Jackson MC et al: Flow cytometric characterization of cell populations in human pregnancy decidua and isolation of decidual macrophages. J Immunol Methods 132:181, 1990
14. Bischof P: Three pregnancy proteins (PP-12, PP-14 and PAPP-A): their biological and clinical relevance. Am J Perinatol 6:110, 1989
15. Riddick DH, Kusnick WF: Decidua: a possible source of amniotic fluid prolactin. Am J Obstet Gynecol 127: 187, 1977

16. Bigazzi M, Nardi E, Bruni P, Petrucci F: Relaxin in human decidua. J Clin Endocrinol Metab 51:939, 1980

17. Willman EA, Collins WP: The concentrations of prostaglandin E_1 and prostaglandin $F_{2\alpha}$ in tissues within the foetoplacental unit after spontaneous or induced labor. Br J Obstet Gynaecol 83:786, 1976

18. Norwitz ER, Starkey PM, Lopez Bernal A, Turnbull AC: J Endocrinol 131:327, 1991

19. Tabibzadeh S: Cytokines and the hypothalamic-pituitary-ovarian-endometrial axis. Hum Reprod Update 9:947, 1994

20. Danforth DN, Buckingham JC, Raddick JW: Connective tissue changes incident of cervical effacement. Am J Obstet Gynecol 80:939, 1960

21. McInnes DRA, Naftolin F, vander Rest M, Stubblefield PS: Cervical changes in pregnant women. p. 181. In: Dilation of the Uterine Cervix. Connective Tissue Biology and Clinical Management. Raven Press, New York, 1980

22. Bishop EH: Pelvic scoring for elective induction. Obstet Gynecol 24:266, 1964

23. Catalano PM, Ashikaga T, Mann LI: Cervical change and uterine activity as predictors of preterm delivery. Am J Perinatol 6:185, 1989

24. Nakayama T, Tahara K, Yanaihara T et al: Ripening human cervix. Steroid concentrations and proline hydroxylase activity in cervical tissue. Program of the Tenth World Congress on Obstetric Gynecology; October 17, 1982; San Francisco, Calif.

25. Ishikawa M, Shimizu T: Dehydroepiandrosterone sulfate and induction of labor. Am J Perinatol 6:173, 1989

26. Wolf JP, Sinosich M, Anderson TL et al: Progesterone antagonist (RU 486) for cervical dilatation, labor induction and delivery in monkeys: effectiveness in combination with oxytocin. Am J Obstet Gynecol 160:45, 1989

27. Elger W, Fähnrich M, Beier S et al: Endometrial and myometrial effects of progesterone antagonists in pregnant guinea pigs. Am J Obstet Gynecol 157:1065, 1987

28. WHO Task Force on Post Ovulatory Methods for Fertility Regulation. The use of mifepristone (RU486) for cervical preparation in first trimester pregnancy termination. Br J Obstet Gynaecol 97:260, 1990

29. Lao Guico-Lamm M, Sherwood OD: Monoclonal antibody specific for rat relaxin, II: passive immunization with monoclonal antibodies throughout the second half of pregnancy disrupts birth in intact rats. Endocrinology 123:2479, 1988

30. Eddie LW, Cameron IT, Leeton JF et al: Ovarian relaxin is not essential for the dilatation of the cervix. Lancet 336:243, 1990

31. MacLennan AH, Green RC, Grant P, Nicolson R: Ripening of the human cervix and induction of labor with intracervical purified porcine relaxin. Obstet Gynecol 68:598, 1986

32. Bell R, Permezel M, MacLennan A et al: Clinical trials of cervical ripening with human relaxin. p. 350. In MacLennan AH, Treager GW, Bryant-Greenwood G (eds): Progress in Relaxin Research. World Scientific Publishers, Singapore, 1995

33. Calder AA: Pharmacological management of the unripe cervix in the human. p. 317. In Naftolin F, Stubblefield PS (eds): Dilatation of the Uterine Cervix: Connective Tissue Biology and Clinical Management. Raven Press, New York, 1980

34. Goeschen K, Saling E: Induktion der Zervixreife mit Oxytocin versus PGF_2-alpha-Infusion versus PGE_2-Gel intrazervikal bei Risikoschwangeren mit unreifer Zervix. Geburtshilfe Frauenheilkd 42:810, 1982

35. Goeschen K, Fuchs A-R, Fuchs F et al: Effect of betamimetic tocolysis on cervical ripening and plasma prostaglandin $F_{2\alpha}$ metabolite levels after endocervical application of prostaglandin E_2. Obstet Gynecol 65:166, 1985

36. Uldbjerg N, Ekman G, Malmström A, Ulmsten U: Biochemical changes in human cervical connective tissue after local application of prostaglandin E_2. Gynecol Obstet Invest 15:291, 1983

37. Toth M, Rehnström J, Fuchs A-R: Prostaglandins E and F in cervical mucus of pregnant women. Am J Perinatol 6:145, 1989

38. Fuchs A-R, Ivell R, Freidman S et al: Oxytocin and the timing of parturition: influence of oxytocin receptor gene expression and stimulation of prostaglandin release. In Ivell R, Russell J (eds): Oxytocin: Molecular and Cellular Approaches in Medicine and Research. Plenum, London, 1995

39. Kubata Y, Kimura T, Takemura M et al: A novel method for detection of uterine oxytocin receptor in preparation for delivery using scraped endocervical cells. Horm Metab Res 26:442, 1994

40. Assali NS: Dynamics of the uteroplacental circulation in health and disease. Am J Perinatol 6:105, 1989

41. Kelly RW: Pregnancy maintenance and parturition: the role of prostaglandin in manipulating the immune and inflammatory response. Endoc Rev 15:684, 1994

42. Owman CH, Rosengren E, Sjöberg NO: Adrenergic innervation of the human female reproductive organs: a histochemical and chemical investigation. Obstet Gynecol 30:763, 1967

43. Sjöberg NO: Considerations of the cause for the disappearance of adrenergic transmitter in uterine nerves during pregnancy. Acta Physiol Scand 72:510, 1968

44. Sjöberg NO: Increase in transmitter content of adrenergic nerves in the reproductive tract of female rabbits after oestrogen treatment. Acta Endocrinol (Copenh) 57:405, 1968

45. Owman CH, Alm P, Sjöberg NO, Stiernqvist M: Structural, biochemical and pharmacological aspects of the uterine autonomous innervation and its remodeling during pregnancy. p. 6. In Huszar G (ed): The Physiology and Biochemistry of the Uterus in Pregnancy and Labor. CRC Press, Boca Raton, 1986

46. Cavaillé F, Legér JJ: Characterization and comparison of the contractile proteins from human gravid and nongravid myometrium. Gynecol Obstet Invest 16:341, 1983

47. Huszar G: Physiology of myometrial contractility and cervical dilation. p. 21. In Fuchs F, Stubblefield PS (eds): Preterm Birth: Causes, Prevention and Management. Macmillan, New York, 1984

48. Fleckenstein A, Tritthart H, Fleckenstein B et al: Selec-

tive inhibition of myocardial contractility by competitive calcium antagonists. Naunyn Schmiedebergs Arch Pharmacol 264:3, 1969

49. Fuchs AR: Plasma membrane receptors regulating myometrial contractility and their modulation by hormones. Semin Perinatol 19:15, 1995

50. Michell RH, Kirk GJ, Jones LM et al: The stimulation of inositol lipid metabolism that accompanies calcium mobilization in stimulated cells: defined characteristics and unanswered questions. Philos Trans R Soc Lond B Biol Sci 296:123, 1981

51. Berridge MJ, Irvine RF: Inositol triphosphate, a novel second messenger in cellular signal transduction. Nature 312:315, 1984

52. Nishizuka Y: The role of protein kinase C in cell surface signal transduction and tumor promotion. Nature 308:693, 1984

53. MacDonald OC, Porter JC, Schwarz BE, Johnson JN: Initiation of parturition in the human female. Semin Perinatol 2:273, 1978

54. Bleasdale JE, Johnston JM: Prostaglandins and human parturition: regulation of arachidonic acid mobilization. Rev Perinatol Med 5:151, 1984

55. Mitchell MD, Flint APF, Bibby J et al: Rapid increases in plasma prostaglandin concentrations after vaginal examination and amniotomy. BMJ 2:1183, 1977

56. Fuchs A-R, Olsen P, Petersen K: Effect of distension of uterus and vagina on uterine motility and oxytocin release in puerperal rabbits. Acta Endocr 50:239, 1965

57. Fuchs A-R, Fuchs F: Endocrinology of human parturition. Br J Obstet Gynaecol 91:948, 1984

58. Ducsay CA, McNutt CM: Circadian uterine activity in the pregnant rhesus macaque. Do prostaglandins play a role? Biol Reprod 38:988, 1989

59. Walsh SW, Ducsay CA, Novy MJ: Circadian hormonal interactions among the mother, fetus and amniotic fluid. Am J Obstet Gynecol 150:745, 1984

60. Fuchs A-R, Behrens O, Liu HC: Correlation of nocturnal increases in plasma oxytocin with a decrease in plasma estradiol:progesterone ratio in late pregnancy. Am J Obstet Gynecol 167:1559, 1992

61. Cooperstock M, England JE, Wolfe RA: Circadian incidence of labor onset hour in preterm birth and chorioamnionitis. Obstet Gynecol 70:1, 1987

61a. Roberts JS, Insel PA, Goldfien A: Regulation of myometrial andrenoreceptors and adrenergic response by sex steroids. Mol Pharmacol 20:52, 1981

62. Philippe M: Fetal catecholamines. Am J Obstet Gynecol 146:840, 1983

63. Ishikawa M, Fuchs A-R: Effects of epinephrine and oxytocin on the release of prostaglandin F from the rat uterus. Prostaglandins 15:89, 1978

64. Weiss GE, O'Byrne EM, Hochman JA et al: Secretion of progesterone and relaxin by the human corpus luteum at midpregnancy and at term. Obstet Gynecol 50:679, 1977

65. Tashima LS, Bryant-Greenwood G: H1/H2 relaxins in the breast. p. 556. In MacLennan AH, Treager GW, Bryant-Greenwood G (eds): Progress in Relaxin Research. World Scientific Publishing, Singapore, 1995

66. Porter DG: The myometrium and the relaxin enigma. Anim Reprod Sci 2:77, 1979

67. MacLennan A: The effect of relaxins on myometrial activity and cervical ripening. p. 63. In MacLennan AH, Treager GW, Bryant-Greenwood G (eds): Progress in Relaxin Research. World Scientific Publishing, Singapore, 1995

68. Yallampulli C, Garfield RE, Bryan-Smith M: Nitric oxide inhibits uterine contractility during pregnancy but not during delivery. Endocrinology 133:1899, 1993

69. Weiner CP, Knowles RG, Moncada S: Effect of pregnancy on myometrial NO synthase activity and cGMP in the guinea pig. Presented at the 41st Annual Meeting of the Society for Gynecological Investigation; March 22–26, 1994; Chicago, Ill.

70. Word RA, Cornwell TL: Roles of cyclic GMP and cGMP-dependent protein kinase in myometrial relaxation during pregnancy. Presented at the 41st Annual Meeting of the Society for Gynecological Investigation; March 22–26, 1994; Chicago, Ill.

71. Wilhelmsson L, Wikland M, Wiqvist N: PGF$_2$, TxA$_2$, and PGI$_2$ have potent and differentiated actions on human uterine contractility. Prostaglandins 21:277, 1981

72. Bennett PR, Elder MG, Myatt L: The effects of lipooxygenase metabolites of arachidonic acid on human myometrial contractility. Prostaglandins 33:837, 1987

73. Lopez Bernal A, Canette Soler R, Turnbull AC: Are leukotrienes involved in human uterine contractility? Br J Obstet Gynaecol 96:568, 1989

74. Csapo AI: Defense mechanism of pregnancy. Ciba Found Study Group 9:3, 1961

75. Knaus HH: Der Eintritt der Geburt. Zentralbl Gynäkol 90:77, 1968

76. Fuchs A-R: Hormonal control of myometrial function. Acta Endocrinol (Copenh) 89(suppl 221):9, 1978

77. Fuchs A-R, Fuchs F, Husslein P et al: Oxytocin receptors in the human uterus during pregnancy and parturition: a dual role for oxytocin in the initiation of labor. Science 215:1396, 1982

78. Casey ML, MacDonald PC: The initiation of labor in women: regulation of phospholipid and arachidonic acid metabolism and of prostaglandin production. Semin Perinatol 10:270, 1986

79. Fuchs A-R, Fuchs F: Ethanol for prevention of preterm birth. Semin Perinatol 5:236, 1981

80. Lewis RB, Schulman JD: Influence of acetylsalicylic acid, an inhibitor of PG synthesis, on the duration of human gestation and labor. Lancet 24:1159, 1973

81. Gamissans O, Balasch J: Prostaglandin synthetase inhibitors in the treatment of preterm labor. p. 223. In Fuchs F, Stubblefield PG (eds): Preterm Birth: Causes, Prevention, Management. Macmillan, New York, 1984

82. Keirse MJNC: Endogenous prostaglandins in human parturition. p. 101. In Keirse MJNC, Anderson ABM, Gravenhorst JB (eds): Human Parturition. Boerhave Series for Postgraduate Medical Education. Vol. 15. Leiden University Press, Leiden, 1979

83. Dray F, Frydman R: Primary prostaglandins in amniotic fluid in pregnancy and spontaneous labor. Am J Obstet Gynecol 126:13, 1976

84. Fuchs A-R, Goeschen K, Husslein P et al: Oxytocin and the initiation of human parturition, III: plasma concentrations of oxytocin and 13,14-dihydro-15-keto-prostaglandin F2-α in spontaneous and oxytocin-induced labor at term. Am J Obstet Gynecol 147:497, 1983

85. Fuchs A-R, Romero R, Parra M et al: Pulsatile release of oxytocin: significant increase in spontaneous labor. Am J Obstet Gynecol 165:1515, 1991

86. Ghodgaonkar RB, Dubin NH, Blake DA, King TM: The 13,14-dihydro 15-keto-prostaglandin concentrations in human plasma and amniotic fluid. Am J Obstet Gynecol 134:265, 1979

87. Dubin NH, Johnson JWC, Calhouin S et al: Plasma prostaglandin in pregnant women with term and pre-term deliveries. Obstet Gynecol 57:203, 1981

88. Caldeyro-Barcia R, Sereno JA: The response of human uterus to oxytocin throughout pregnancy. p. 177. In Caldeyro-Barcia R, Heller H (eds): Oxytocin. Pergamon Press, London, 1959

89. Fuchs A-R: The role of oxytocin in parturition. p. 163. In Huszar G (ed): The Physiology and Biochemistry of the Uterus in Pregnancy and Labor. CRC Press, Boca Raton, 1986

90. Seitchik J, Amico J, Robinson AG, Castillo M: Oxytocin augmentation of dysfunctional labor, IV: oxytocin pharmacokinetics. Am J Obstet Gynecol 150:225, 1984

91. Karim SMM: Prostaglandins and Reproduction. University Park Press, Baltimore, 1975

92. Rasmussen AB, Johannesen P, Allen J et al: Plasma prostaglandin$F_{2\alpha}$ and 13,14-dihydro-15keto-prostaglandin$F_{2\alpha}$ levels in women during induction of labor with iv infusion of $PGF_{2\alpha}$ in relation to uterine contractions. J Perinatol 13:15, 1985

93. McCoshen JA, Hoffman DR, Kredentser JV et al: The role of fetal membranes in regulating production, transport, and metabolism of prostaglandin E during labor. Am J Obstet Gynecol 163:1635, 1990

94. Mitchell BF, Rogers K, Wong S: The dynamics of prostaglandin metabolism in human fetal membranes and decidua around the time of parturition. J Clin Endocrinol Metab 77:759, 1993

95. MacDonald PC, Casey ML: The accumulation of prostaglandins (PG) in amniotic fluid is an after effect of labor and not indicative of a role for PGF_{α} or PGE in the initiation of human labor. J Clin Endocrinol Metab 76:133, 1993

96. MacDonald PC, Koga S, Casey ML: Decidual activation in parturition: examination of amniotic fluid for mediators of the immune response. Ann NY Acad Sci 6:315, 1993

97. Morris M, Stevens SW, Adams MR: Plasma oxytocin during pregnancy and lactation in the cynomolgus monkey. Biol Reprod 23:782, 1980

98. Randolph GW, Fuchs A-R: Pulsatile administration enhances the effect and reduces the dose of oxytocin required for induction of labor. Am J Perinatol 6:159, 1989

99. Dawood MY: Evolving concepts of oxytocin for induction of labor. Am J Perinatol 6:167, 1989

100. Perales AJ, Diago VJ, Monleon-Sancho J et al: Pulsatile versus continuous oxytocin infusion for oxytocin challenge test. Arch Gynecol Obstet 55:119, 1994

101. Chard T, Boyd NRH, Edwards CRW, Hudson CN: The release of oxytocin and vasopressin by the human fetus during labor. Nature 234:352, 1971

102. Dawood MY, Wang CF, Gupta R, Fuchs F: Fetal contribution to oxytocin in human labor. Obstet Gynecol 52:205, 1978

103. Chard T: Fetal and maternal oxytocin in human parturition. Am J Perinat 6:145, 1989

104. Lampelo S, Vanha-Perttula T: Fractionation and characterization of cystine aminopeptidase (oxytocinase) and arylamidase of the human placenta. J Reprod Fertil 56:285, 1979

105. Fuchs A-R, Fuchs F, Soloff MS: Oxytocin receptors in nonpregnant human uterus. J Clin Endocrinol Metab 60:37, 1985

106. Maggi M, Magini A, Fiscella A et al: Sex steroid modulation of neurohypophysial hormone receptors in human nonpregnant myometrium. J Clin Endocrinol Metab 74:385, 1992

107. Fuchs A-R, Fuchs F, Husslein P et al: Oxytocin receptors in the human uterus during pregnancy and parturition. Am J Obstet Gynecol 150:734, 1984

108. Maggi M, DelCarlo P, Fantoni G et al: Human myometrium during pregnancy contains and responds to V_1 vasopressin receptors as well as oxytocin receptors. J Clin Endocrin Metab 70:1142, 1990

109. Takemura M, Nokura S, Kimura T et al: Expression and localization of oxytocin receptor gene in human uterine endometrium in relation to the menstrual cycle. Endocrinology 132:1830, 1993

110. Takemura M, Kimura T, Nomura S et al: Expression and localization of human oxytocin receptor gene and its protein in chorion and decidua during parturition. J Clin Investig 93:2319, 1994

111. Kofler E, Husslein P, Langer M et al: Die Bedeutung der Oxytocinempfindlichkeit für den spontanen Wehenbeginn beim Menschen. Geburtshilfe Frauenheilkd 43:533, 1983

112. Goodwin TM, Paul R, Silver H et al: The effect of the oxytocin antagonist atosiban on preterm uterine activity in the human. Am J Obstet Gynecol 170:474, 1993

113. Soloff MS: Uterine receptor for oxytocin: effects of estrogen. Biochem Biophys Res Commun 65:205, 1975

114. Nissenson R, Flouret G, Hechter O: Opposing effects of estradiol and progesterone on oxytocin receptors in rabbit uterus. Proc Natl Acad Sci USA 75:2044, 1978

115. Fuchs A-R, Periyasami S, Alexandrova M, Soloff MS: Correlation between oxytocin receptor concentrations and responsiveness to oxytocin in pregnant rat myometrium: effect of ovarian steroids. Endocrinology 113:742, 1983

116. Clark JW, Peck EJ: Female Sex Steroids: Receptors and Functions. Monographs on Endocrinology. Springer-Verlag, Berlin, 1979

117. Fuchs A-R, Helmer H, Behrens O et al: A steep rise in oxytocin receptors precedes onset of labor. Biol Reprod 47:937, 1992

118. Embrey MP, Moir CJ: A comparison of the oxytocic

effects of synthetic vasopressin and oxytocin. J Obstet Gynaecol Br Commonw 74:648, 1967

119. Guillon G, Balestre MN, Roberts JM, Bottari SP: Oxytocin and vasopressin: distinct receptors in myometrium. J Clin Endocrin Metab 64:1129, 1987

120. Ivanisevic M, Behrens O, Helmer H, Fuchs A-R: Vasopressin receptors in human pregnant myometrium and decidua: interactions with oxytocin and vasopressin agonists and antagonists. Am J Obstet Gynecol 161:1639, 1989

121. Taslimi MM, Billedeaux LA, Ruiz AG, Herrick SN: Short labor in carriers of nephrogenic diabetes insipidus. Am J Gynecol Health 4:11, 1990

122. Pohjavuori M, Fyhrquist F: Hemodynamic significance of vasopressin in the newborn infant. J Pediatr Res 18:835, 1984

123. Stark RI, Daniel SS, Hussain MK et al: Vasopressin concentration in amniotic fluid as an index of fetal hypoxia: mechanism of release in sheep. Pediatr Res 18:835, 1984

124. Schrey MP, Reed AM, Steer PJ: Oxytocin and arginine vasopressin stimulate inositol phosphate production in human gestational myometrium and decidua cells. Biosci Rep 6:613, 1986

125. Williams KI: Prostaglandin synthesis and uterine contractility. p. 282. In Beltar S, Thomas JP, Vokaer A, Vokaer R (eds): Uterine Contractility. Masson, Paris, 1984

126. Krall JE, Barrett JD, Jamgotduan N, Korenman SG: Interaction of PGE_2 and β-adrenergic catecholamines in the regulation of uterine smooth muscle motility and adenylatecyclase in the rat. J Endocrinol 102:329, 1984

127. Coleman HA, Parkington H: Induction of prolonged excitability in myometrium of pregnant guinea pig by $PGF_{2\alpha}$. J Physiol (Lond) 399:33, 1988

128. Senior J, Sangha R, Baxter GS et al: In vitro characterization of prostanoid FP, DP, IP and TP receptors on the nonpregnant human myometrium. Br J Pharmacol 107:15, 1992

129. Senior J, Marshall K, Sangha R et al: In vitro characterization of prostanoid receptors on human myometrium at term pregnancy. Br J Pharmacol 108:501, 1993

130. Bauknecht T, Krake B, Rechenbach U et al: Distribution of PGE and $PGF_{2\alpha}$ receptors in human myometrium. Acta Endocr (Copenh) 98:446, 1981

131. Giannopoulos G, Jackson K, Kredentser J: Prostaglandin E and $F_{2\alpha}$ receptors in human myometrium during the menstrual cycle and in pregnancy and labor. Am J Obstet Gynecol 153:904, 1985

132. Jacobs A, Hwang D, Julian JA, Carson DD: Regulated expression of prostaglandin endoperoxide synthase-2 by uterine stroma. Endocrinology 135:1807, 1994

133. Tazawa R, Xu X-M, Wu KK, Wang L: Characterization of the genomic structure, chromosomal location and promoter of human prostaglandin H synthase-2 gene. Biochem Biophys Res Commun 103:190, 1994

134. Cheung PYC, Challis JRG: Prostaglandin E_2 metabolism in human fetal membranes. Am J Obstet Gynecol 161:1580, 1989

135. McCoshen JA, Tulloch HV, Johnson KA: Umbilical cord is the major source of prostaglandin E_2 in the gestational sac during term labor. Am J Obstet Gynecol 160:973, 1989

136. McCoshen JA, Johnson KA, Ghodkaongkar RB: PGE_2 release on the fetal and maternal sides of the amnion and chorion-decidua before and after term labor. Am J Obstet Gynecol 156:173, 1987

137. Schlegel W, Kruger S, Korte K: Purification of PGE_2-9-oxoreductase from human decidua vera. FEBS Letters 171:141, 1984

138. Moonen P, Klok G, Keirse MJNC: Increase in concentrations of prostaglandin endoperoxide synthase and prostacyclin synthase in human myometrium in late pregnancy. Prostaglandins 28:309, 1984

139. Dembelé-Duchesne MJ, Thaler-Dao H, Chairo C, Crastes de Paulet A: Some new prospects in the mechanism of control of arachidonate metabolism in human placenta and membranes. Prostaglandins 22:979, 1981

140. Granström E, Kindahl H, Swahn, ML: Profiles of prostaglandin metabolites in the human circulation: identification of late appearing, long-lived products. Biochim Biophys Acta 713:46, 1982

141. Fuchs A-R, Husslein P, Sumulong L, Fuchs F: The origin of circulating 13,14-dihydro-15-keto-$PGF_{2\alpha}$ during delivery. Prostaglandins 24:715, 1982

142. Noort WA, Van Bulck B, Vereecken A et al: Changes in plasma levels of $PGF_{2\alpha}$ and PGI_2 metabolites at and after delivery at term. Prostaglandins 37:3, 1989

143. Husslein P, Sinzinger H: Concentration of 13,14-dihydro-15-keto-prostaglandin E_2 in the maternal peripheral plasma during labour of spontaneous onset. Br J Obstet Gynaecol 91:228, 1984

144. Brennecke SP, Castle BM, Demers LM, Turnbull AC: Endogenous PGE_2 metabolite levels in the human during pregnancy as detected by a novel radioimmunoassay. Br J Obstet Gynaecol 92:345, 1985

145. Hamberg M: Quantitative studies on prostaglandin synthesis in man, III: excretion of the major urinary metabolite of $PGF_{1\alpha}$ and $F_{2\alpha}$ during pregnancy. Life Sci 14:247, 1974

146. Noort WA: Prostanoid Excretion in Human Term and Preterm Gestation. (Thesis.) p. 188. University of Leiden, Leiden, 1989

147. Noort WA, DeZwart FA, Keirse MJNC: Changes in urinary 6-keto-$PGF_{1\alpha}$ excretion during pregnancy and labor. Prostaglandins 35:573, 1988

148. Walsh SW: Preeclampsia: an imbalance in placental prostacyclin and the thromboxane production. Am J Obstet Gynecol 152:335, 1985

149. Husslein P, Kofler E, Rasmussen AB et al: Oxytocin and the initiation of human parturition, IV: plasma concentrations of oxytocin and 13,14-dihydro-15-keto $PGF_{2\alpha}$ during induction of labor by artificial rupture of membranes. Am J Obstet Gynecol 140:261, 1981

150. Maier JAM, Hla T, Macaig T: Cyclooxygenase is an immediate early gene induced by interleukin-1 in endothelial cells. J Biol Chem 65:10805, 1990

151. Hirst JJ, Teixera FJ, Zakar T, Olson DM: Prostaglandin endoperoxide-H synthase-1 and -2 messenger RNA lev-

els in human amnion with spontaneous labor onset. J Clin Endocrinol Metab 80:517, 1995

152. Mitchell MD, Branch DW, Lundin-Schiller S et al: Immunological aspects of preterm labor. Semin Perinatol 15:10, 1991

153. Hirata F: The regulation of lipomodulin, a phospholipase inhibitory protein, in rabbit neutrophils by phosphorylation. J Biol Chem 256:7730, 1981

154. Brennecke SP, Bryce RL, Turnbull AC: The prostaglandin synthase inhibiting ability of maternal plasma and the onset of human labour. Eur J Obstet Gynecol Reprod 14:81, 1982

155. Wilson T, Liggins GC: Purification and characterization of a uterine phospholipase inhibitor that loses activity after labor onset in women. Am J Obstet Gynecol 160:602, 1989

156. Wilson T, Christie DL: Gravidin, an endogenous inhibitor of phospholipase A_2 activity is a secretory component of IgA. Biochem Biophys Res Commun 176:447, 1991

157. Saeed SA, Strickland DM, Young DM et al: Inhibition of prostaglandin synthesis by human amniotic fluid: acute reduction in inhibitory activity of amniotic fluid obtained during labor. J Clin Endocrinol Metab 55:801, 1982

158. Rehnström J, Ishikawa M, Fuchs F, Fuchs A-R: Stimulation of myometrial and decidual prostaglandin production by amniotic fluid from term but not mid-trimester pregnancies. Prostaglandins 26:973, 1984

159. Altman DJ, Schneider SL, Thompson DA et al: A transforming growth factor β-like immunosuppressive factor in amniotic fluid and localization of TGF-β mRNA in the pregnant uterus. J Exp Med 17:1391, 1990

160. Bry K, Lappalainen U: Interleukin-4 and transforming growth factor-β1 modulate the production of interleukin-1 receptor antagonist and of prostaglandin E by decidual cells. Am J Obstet Gynecol 170:1194, 1994

161. Alam NA, Russell PT, Tabor MW, Moulton BC: Progesterone and estrogen control of uterine PG dehydrogenase activity during deciduomal growth. Endocrinology 98:859, 1975

162. Kelly RW, Bukman A: Antiprogestagenic inhibition of uterine prostaglandin inactivation: a passive mechanism for uterine stimulation. J Steroid Biochem 3:97, 1990

163. Kauma S, Matt D, Strom S et al: Interleukin-1β, human

leukocyte antigen HLA-DRalpha, and transforming growth factor-β expression in endometrium, placenta and placental membranes. Am J Obstet Gynecol 163:1430, 1990

164. Romero R, Avila C, Brekus CA, Morotti R: The role of systemic and intrauterine infection in preterm parturition. Ann NY Acad Sci 6:355, 1991

165. Morita I, Nakayama Y, Murota S: Characterization of the stimulatory effects of $PGF_{2\alpha}$ on the release of arachidonic acid. Prostaglandins 18:507, 1979

166. Alvarez H, Caldeyro-Barcia R: Contractility of the human uterus recorded by new methods. Surg Gynecol Obstet 91:1, 1950

167. Bourne AW, Burn JH: The dosage and action of pituitary extract and the ergot alkaloid on the uterus in labour, with a note on the action of adrenalin. J Obstet Gynaecol Br Emp 34:249, 1927

168. Steer PJ, Carter MC, Beard RW: Normal levels of active contraction area in spontaneous labor. Br J Obstet Gynaecol 91:211, 1984

169. Arulkumaran S, Gibb DMF, Lun KC et al: The effect of parity on uterine activity in labour. Br J Obstet Gynaecol 91:843, 1984

170. Friedman EA: Labor: Clinical Evaluation and Management. 2nd ed. Appleton-Century-Crofts, New York, 1978

171. Amico JA, Seitchik J, Robinson AG: Studies of oxytocin in plasma of women during hypocontractile labor. J Clin Endocrinol Metab 58:274, 1984

172. Jagani N, Schulman H, Fleischer A: Role of the cervix in the induction of labor. Obstet Gynecol 59:21, 1982

173. Fuchs A-R, Fuchs F: Endocrinology of term and preterm labor. p. 67. In Fuchs A-R, Fuchs F, Stubblefield PS (eds): Preterm Birth: Causes, Management and Prevention. 2nd Ed. McGraw-Hill, New York, 1993

174. Fay FS, Delise CM: Contraction of isolated smooth muscle cells: structural changes. Proc Natl Acad Sci USA 70:641, 1973

175. Hartshorne DJ, Gorecka A: Biochemistry of the contractile proteins of smooth muscle. p. 93. In Bohr DF, Samlyo AP, Sparkes HV Jr (eds): Handbook of Physiology. Vol. 3. American Physiological Society, Bethesda, 1983

176. Braunwald E: Mechanism of action of calcium-channel blocking drugs. N Engl J Med 207:1618, 1982

177. Fuchs AR: Oxytocin and oxytocin receptors: maternal signals for parturition. p. 177. In Garfield RE (ed): Uterine Contractility. Serono Symposia USA, Norwell, 1990

Chapter 6

Physiology and Endocrinology of Lactation

Anna-Riitta Fuchs

The Physiologic Significance of Breast Feeding

The mammary gland plays an essential role in the reproduction of most mammals. Failure to lactate means failure to reproduce because the young are too immature to ward off the invasion of environmental microbial agents and to feed on foreign food stuffs. At birth, the mammary gland takes over some of the functions fulfilled by the placenta during intrauterine life. It provides the neonate with a ready source of easily digested nutrients and with a variety of immunologic factors that protect against infection. The period of lactation provides a gradual transition from a total dependence on the maternal organism to an independent existence.

Technologic advances during the last century have made it possible to prepare formulas based on cow's milk or soy proteins that can provide acceptable substitutes for breast milk. Many mothers have found the use of such substitutes so convenient that breast feeding has drastically declined around the world. Where the standard of living and hygiene is high, bottle feeding has had less impact, but in developing countries the consequences have often been disastrous. The past 10 to 15 years have shown a marked increase in the motivation to breast feed, particularly among well-educated and affluent women in the United States and Europe. Unfortunately, large groups of disadvantaged mothers, both in the United States and abroad, whose infants would most benefit from breast feeding, are least likely to initiate it.

For the infant, the physical benefits of breast feeding include significant protection against infection, particularly diarrhea, and upper respiratory tract and ear infections. Breast feeding also affords protection against atopic disease (particularly when maintained for at least 6 months)[1] and intestinal parasitic disease.[2] Breast milk was superior to standard term formula when pooled milk from a milk bank was bottle-fed to preterm infants in a prospective, randomized, multicenter trial, thus eliminating confounding social and demographic differences between breast compared to formula feeding mothers.[3] The donor milk fed group had equally good outcome as a third group fed enriched preterm formula.

The benefits of breast feeding appear to be so well established that physicians should encourage prospective mothers to breast feed. Patients should be provided with sufficient information to permit a decision to breast feed or bottle feed made on a rational basis.

The decision whether to breast feed is influenced by many complex social and physiological factors. The prenatal care provider should discuss the benefits and perceived disadvantages of breast-feeding with the expectant mother during her prenatal care, and provide information and support. It is important to realize that in today's urban settings most mothers lack the social support system provided in earlier times by female relatives who themselves had breast-fed. The environment of the less privileged mothers tends to provide many negative and few positive inducements for breast-feeding, which should be taken into consideration when counseling such women on breast feeding. Hospital practices in the early postpartum period also have a significant effect on the subsequent infant feeding mode.[4] Unfortunately, in many institutions the routine practices still have a strong negative impact on breast-feeding.[5,6] Proper lactation counseling should be an essential part of every maternity ward.

The Mammary Gland and Its Secretory Function

The mammary gland undergoes remarkable proliferation and differentiation during pregnancy. After parturition, it synthesizes and secretes specific carbohydrates, proteins, and fats and selectively transfers minerals from plasma to milk in quantities sufficient to satisfy all the nutritional needs of the growing infant. In addition, it takes over an immunologic function, providing the infant with maternal antibiodies until its own immune system is established. Colostrum is the alveolar secretion before the production of milk.

Morphology of the Breast and the Mammary Gland

Gross Anatomy

The adult breast consists of glandular tissue embedded in stroma made up of connective tissue and adipose tissue. The stroma carries the blood vessels, nerves, and lymphatic vessels. In the resting state, the glandular tissue occupies only a small fraction of the total volume of the breast. The stromal elements give the mature breast its size and shape.

The glandular tissue is termed a compound tubular alveolar gland. It consists of an arborized duct system that drains clusters of sac-like structures called alveoli or acini. These alveoli form the basic unit of the secretory system (Fig. 6-1). Each alveolus is surrounded by a mesh of myoepithelial cells and by a capillary network. Each of the 15 to 20 lobes is drained by a single lactiferous duct. They converge toward the areola, beneath which they form the lactiferous sinuses that serve as small reservoirs of milk. Each lobe is separated by septa of connective tissue that merge imperceptibly with the fascia covering the anterior wall of the thorax.

The nipple is a condensation of epithelial tissue through which the lactiferous ducts pass to orifices at the surface. It is surrounded by specialized pigmented skin, the areola, which contains sweat glands and sebaceous glands (glands of Montgomery) that hypertrophy during pregnancy and serve to lubricate and protect the nipple during lactation. The sensory innervation of the peripheral skin appears to be influenced by the endocrine milieu. Thus, the tactile sensitivity as deter-

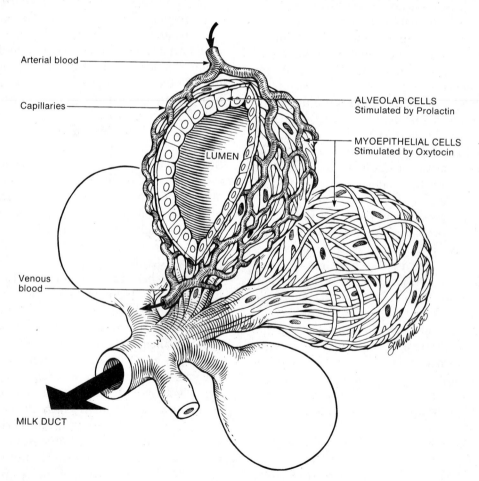

Fig. 6-1 Diagram of a cluster of alveoli, the basic units of the mammary gland. (Adapted from Cowie,[120] with permission.)

mined by a two-point discrimination test increases significantly in pregnant women within 24 hours of parturition.

The innervation of the nipple plays a vital role in lactation, mediating the reflex activation of the neurohumoral reflexes responsible for the removal of milk from the gland and the release of prolactin essential for the maintenance of lactation.

Microscopic Features of the Alveolar Cell

In the resting stage, the tubuloalveolar system is sparse, consisting of mostly ductal elements that are widely dispersed in the stroma. Two layers of epithelial cells line the alveoli, which are virtually indistinguishable from the simple cuboidal cells lining the ducts.[7] Myoepithelial cells, also small and cuboidal, form a distinct layer beneath the epithelial cells.[8]

The fully differentiated secretory epithelium of the lactating gland consists of a single layer of alveolar cells that are columnar and tall when the alveolar lumen is empty and that become flattened when the lumen is full (Fig. 6-2). During pregnancy, some of the junctional complexes are open or "leaky," permitting accumulation of cells, plasma proteins, and sodium chloride in the lumen. During lactation, the junctions are tight.[9–11]

Mechanisms of Secretion

Different pathways operate in parallel to transfer precursors into the alveolar cells and to transfer milk constituents from the cells to the alveolar lumina[10,12–14] (Fig. 6-3).

Exocytosis

Proteins and carbohydrates are secreted by exocytosis, whereby the membranes of the secretory vesicles fuse with the apical plasma membrane to expel their contents without the loss of membrane proteins. The proteins are synthesized in the endoplasmic reticulum and further processed and sorted in the Golgi apparatus, where calcium and phosphate combine with the milk protein casein to form aggregates, which are then packaged into secretory vesicles.

Lactose is also synthesized in the Golgi apparatus by lactose synthetase, an enzyme consisting of two parts: a protein, galactosyl transferase, bound to the Golgi membrane, and a soluble protein, α-lactalbumin, which also constitutes one of the secretory milk proteins. The Golgi membrane is impermeable to lactose. As lactose accumulates, water and ions are drawn osmotically into the Golgi system and into the alveolar lumen. At the apical end, lactose is packaged together with milk proteins into secretory vesicles from which they are released into the lumen by exocytosis.

Milk Fat Secretion

Lipids are secreted by an apocrine process in which the plasma membrane surrounds the droplets and is pinched off at the apex. Small amounts of cytoplasmic constituents are usually enclosed within the membrane providing a source of enzymes and lipases. The fatty acids in human milk are mostly long chain (over C-16) and originate both from dietary fat and adipose tissue,

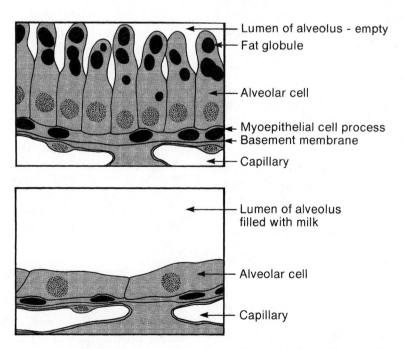

Fig. 6-2 Cells in the wall of an alveolus (A) just after milking and (B) just before milking. As the alveolus fills with milk, its walls are stretched and the shape of the cells is greatly altered. (Adopted from Cowie,[120] with permission.)

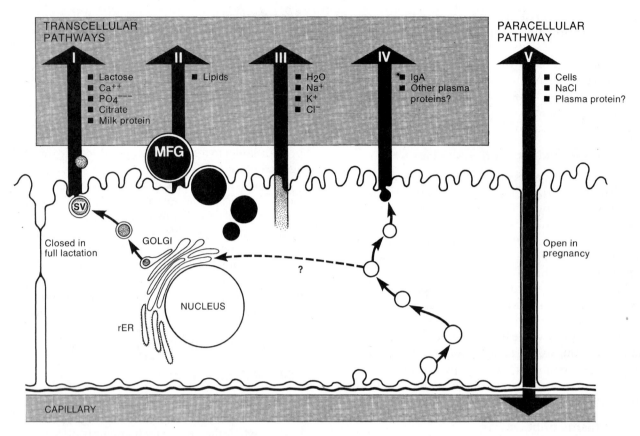

Fig. 6-3 The pathways for milk synthesis and secretion in the alveolar cell. (I) Exocytosis of milk protein and lactose in Golgi secretory vesicles. (II) Milk fat secretion in a plasma membrane-enclosed milk fat globule. (III) Diffusion of water and ions across the apical membrane. (IV) Pinocytosis-exocytosis of immunoglobulins. (V) The paracellular pathway for leukocytes and plasma components. SV, secretory vesicle; RER, rough endoplasmic reticulum; BM, basement membrane; MFG, milk fat globule. (Adapted from Neville et al.,[121] with permission.)

whereas shorter chain saturated fatty acids are synthesized de novo by the gland.

Diffusion

Monovalent cations and water are transported by diffusion. Water moves from the cell across these membranes in response to the osmotic gradient created by lactose, which accounts for about two-thirds of the osmotically active solutes in human milk. Sodium, potassium, and chloride concentrations are considerably lower in milk than in the cytoplasm and contribute about one-sixth the total osmolarity of milk. Equilibrium is attained at concentrations in milk that are lower than those in the cell.

Pinocytocis-Exocytosis

Immunoglobulins are transported through the alveolar cells by a receptor-mediated transcellular route.[15,16] The most abundant immunoglobulin found in human milk is secretory IgA, the major part of which is synthesized locally by plasma cells present in the breast.[17]

Small amounts of IgG, IgE, and IgM are also secreted into colostrum and milk.

Paracellular Pathway

Cellular elements, found in milk in great numbers, reach the lumen by a paracellular pathway.[12,18,19] These are mostly leukocytes, neutrophils, macrophages, and lymphocytes. The concentration of cells (but not their numbers) is reduced markedly during the first month of lactation. At that time, many of the cells are sloughed epithelial cells, although large numbers of leukocytes are found in mature milk.

Development of the Mammary Gland

The mammary gland develops in four distinct stages: (1) during embryonic and fetal life, (2) at puberty, (3) during pregnancy, and (4) in the early puerperium. Regression or atrophy may be considered a fifth stage seen after weaning or after the menopause.

Embryonic Development

The mammary gland can be identified from about the fifth gestational week onward. By week 20, the anlage for the lactiferous ducts (mammary bud) has invaded the mesodermal connective tissue, growing deeper with advancing gestation. The nipple and areola arise rather late in gestation. Thus, at birth, a rudimentary mammary gland is present, consisting of a nipple and a primitive duct system.[20,21]

Failure of proper proliferation of the mesenchyme underlying the mammary primordium results in a relatively common finding, inversion of the nipple. This condition often improves spontaneously during pregnancy.

Pubertal Development

Pubertal development, thelarche, normally starts between 8 and 14 years of age and is usually complete in about 4 years. At first, proliferation and branching of the duct system takes place, followed by the formation of the terminal bud system from which the alveoli and lobuli develop. In addition, a rapid deposition of fat and connective tissue in the stroma gives the mature breast its size and form. In nonpregnant adult women, no further glandular development takes place, unless pregnancy intervenes. The volume of the breast varies during the menstrual cycle, increasing by 15 to 30 cm^3 on the average in the premenstrual phase and returning to its initial volume during menstruation.[22] This change is mainly due to enhanced water retention in the stroma and infiltration of connective tissue with lymphoid and plasma cells.

Mammogenic Changes During Pregnancy

With the hormonal changes of pregnancy, both ductal and alveolar elements proliferate. This can be observed within 4 weeks of conception. In the early stages, ductal sprouting predominates, while from the third month on, lobuloalveolar multiplication dominates. There is a progressive increase in the size of the lobules throughout pregnancy, initially through cellular hyperplasia and later by hypertrophy. Stromal elements progressively diminish and at the end of gestation only thin septa of connective tissue separate the well-developed lobes of glandular tissue[8] (Fig. 6-4).

Around mid-gestation, the proliferation of the alveolar epithelium gradually ceases. Instead, the alveolar stem cells differentiate and begin to assume secretory characteristics. The alveoli are now lined with a single layer of epithelial cells, an appearance retained throughout late gestation and lactation. The myoepithelial cells hypertrophy, become flattened, and develop attenuated cytoplasmic processes that form an

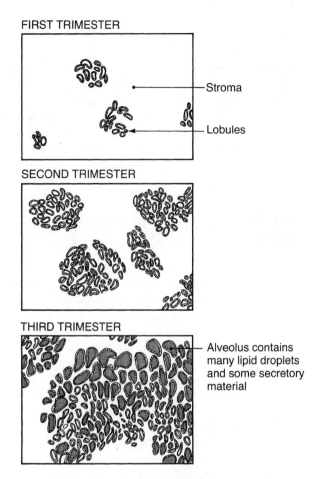

FIRST TRIMESTER

— Stroma

— Lobules

SECOND TRIMESTER

THIRD TRIMESTER

— Alveolus contains many lipid droplets and some secretory material

Fig. 6-4 Mammary gland development during pregnancy, illustrated by sections of the mammary gland of pregnant women. In early pregnancy the stroma is the dominant component, containing only scattered ducts. By mid-pregnancy the lobules of alveoli form lobes that are separated by stromal tissues. Secretion is present in some alveolar cells. In the last trimester the lobules of the alveoli are almost fully developed, with cells full of secretory material and the stromal tissue reduced to bands separating lobules and thicker strands between lobes.

open network around the epithelial cells. The glandular hypertrophy is associated with a conspicuous infiltration of the connective tissue and epithelium by a variety of leukocytes.[23] In late gestation, the alveoli begin to fill with a proteinaceous material composed of desquamated epithelial cells and a variety of leukocytes.

Postpartum Development

After parturition a rapid increase in cell size and in the number of secretory organelles occurs. The final differentiation of the mammary gland is completed during a few days. Within 48 hours the cells become tall, with abundant rough endoplasmic reticulum, well-developed Golgi, and numerous microvilli at their apical cell surface.[8,9,11] The alveoli distend with milk and, as they do, the epithelial cells become flattened and distorted. Unless the breast is emptied, necrotic changes quickly occur in the alveolar epithelium.[10]

Mammary blood flow rises markedly during pregnancy and increases further in early lactation. It appears to be closely correlated with the rate of milk secretion. In cows and goats, about 400 to 500 L of blood flow through the gland for each liter of milk produced. The mammary blood flow can be regulated by changes in cardiac output as well as by local factors that influence vasomotor tone.[24]

Endocrine Control of Mammary Gland Function

Ovarian and placental steroids, anterior pituitary hormones and placental polypeptide hormones, adrenal steroids, insulin, and thyroxine participate in mammary gland development and secretory function.

The initiation and maintenance of milk production depend on several processes, all of which are controlled by specific hormonal complexes: (1) mammogenesis, or the development of the mammary gland; (2) lactogenesis, or the initiation of milk secretion; (3) galactopoiesis, or the maintenance of established milk secretion; and (4) galactokinesis, or the removal of milk from the gland. Involution also plays a role in the maintenance of milk secretion because of the rapidity with which degenerative changes can occur in the mammary gland.

Mammogenic Hormones

Using hypophysectomized immature mice and rats, as well as animals subjected to hypophysectomy, ovariectomy, adrenalectomy, and given various hormonal replacement regimens, the minimal hormone milieu required for lactation has been established.[25,26] Our knowledge about the mammogenic hormones in humans is derived mostly from patients with genetic abnormalities in gonadal and pituitary function.

Ovarian hormones are clearly important, since they initiate breast development in agonadal patients or in animals ovariectomized before puberty. However, they are without effect in the absence of the pituitary. The sex steroids may therefore have an indirect action mediated by the anterior pituitary. Estrogen stimulates prolactin release and also sensitizes the mammary gland to the action of prolactin.[27] The mammogenic effects of relaxin require the presence of estrogen, and progesterone causes a further potentiation of relaxin effects.[28]

Normal mammary development has been reported in the congenital absence of growth hormone. Factors produced locally and in the liver, such as epidermal

---

MAMMOGENIC COMPLEX OF HORMONES

Ductal growth
    Estrogen
    Growth hormone
    Glucocorticoids
    Relaxin
Lobuloalveolar growth
    Estrogen
    Growth hormone
    Glucocorticoids
    Prolactin
    Progesterone

---

growth factor, somatomedin, and a specific mammary gland growth factor promote mammogenesis. Some of these factors are induced by estrogen.

Relaxin induces an estrogen dependent elongation and branching of the myoepithelial ducts including proliferation of the myoepithelial and epithelial cells lining the lumen of the ducts.[29] In rats relaxin has striking effect on the development of the nipple.[28] It also affects the stromal fat pad and connective tissue components in the stroma and parenchyma[29] in a similar manner as the connective tissue of the cervix. In the human the presence of relaxins H_1 and H_2 has recently been demonstrated; they are present in the cytoplasm of ductal and lobular epithelial cells as well as in myoepithelial cells.[30]

Breast stroma, particularly adipose tissue, appears to play an active role in the development of glandular tissue. An interaction of alveolar cells, ductal cells, and stromal cells may be necessary for normal growth. Adipose tissue from mammary glands supports the growth of mammary cells in culture and prevents individual ducts from fusing.[31,32] Because the mammary fat pad accumulates estrogen and possesses estrogen receptors, it may play a more active role in mammogenesis than previously suspected.[33] Relaxin induces growth of both the capillary bed and fat pad in rats.[28]

Lactogenic Hormones

Lactogenesis or the onset of milk secretion is usually measured by the output of milk sugar or the most abundant milk protein, casein.[25,26]

In pregnant women, placental lactogen can substitute for pituitary prolactin and growth hormone. Insulin and thyroxine are themselves without lactogenic effect but play a permissive role in this process.[34] Thyroid hormones selectively enhance the secretion of lactalbumin.[35] Prerequisites for lactogenesis are a fully devel-

REQUIREMENTS FOR LACTOGENESIS

Fully developed mammary gland
Prolactin
Glucocorticoids
Insulin
Thyroid hormones
Possibly growth hormone
Withdrawal of estrogen and progesterone

oped mammary gland and the withdrawal of estrogen and progesterone. While the sex steroids have a synergistic effect with prolactin on mammogenesis, they inhibit the lactogenic effects of prolactin.

Galactokinetic Hormones

Milk accumulating in the lumina of the alveoli cannot flow passively into the ducts. It must be squeezed out by the contraction of the surrounding myoepithelial cells, resulting in milk ejection. Oxytocin is the most powerful galactokinetic hormone, and is the physiologic stimulus that activates the myoepithelial cells and permits milk removal from the gland.[36] Vasopressin has about one-fifth to one-hundredth the potency of oxytocin in the human breast.[37]

The myoepithelial cells, like myometrial cells, have specific receptors for oxytocin.[38] In the rat mammary gland, the concentration of oxytocin receptors increases gradually during pregnancy, with a more marked increase after parturition. After delivery, a marked increase in the oxytocin sensitivity of the human myoepithelium occurs.[39–41]

Milk Ejection and the Suckling Stimulus

The release of oxytocin from the neurohypophysis is under neural control and the stimulus is provided by the suckling of the infant. The sensory nerve endings that mediate the afferent path of this neuroendocrine reflex lie beneath the areola and the nipple. The neurons that secrete oxytocin are located in the hypothalamus, concentrated mainly in the paraventricular and supraoptic nuclei. Long axons from these neurons extend into the posterior pituitary gland where the nerve terminals are located, abutting on a rich capillary network. The pathways of this neuroendocrine reflex are illustrated in Figure 6-5.

Oxytocin release is essential for milk removal. If local anesthesia is applied on the sensory nerve endings under the areola[36] or if the release of oxytocin is inhibited by high doses of ethyl alcohol, the young will be unable to obtain milk.[42,43] Only that fraction of milk that is stored in the lactiferous sinuses under the areola can be extracted by mechanical forces. Oxytocin and vasopressin are produced in separate neurons; therefore, oxytocin secretion is usually intact in patients who are unable to synthesize vasopressin, (i.e., women with diabetes insipidus).

Adequate milk ejection is essential for successful lactation. First, it makes the alveolar luminal milk available for the infant, and second, the removal of milk from the alveoli is necessary for the continuation of milk secretion. The flattened alveolar cells of distended alveoli cease their secretory activity and quickly begin to undergo degenerative changes.[10] Frequent suckling and adequate milk ejection therefore promote the production of milk. In the early puerperium, oxytocin treatment (e.g., buccal tablets) has been found to be helpful in women with very engorged breasts, probably because the distention of the breast makes it difficult for the newborn to apply proper pressure at the base of the nipple when suckling.

During a nursing period oxytocin is released over several minutes causing rhythmic intramammary pressure changes.[41] Plasma oxytocin levels rise rapidly after the onset of suckling, usually remain elevated while the infant is nursing and then drop.[44] In advanced lactation the increment in oxytocin levels in response to suckling increases.[45] This increase is seen only in mothers who exclusively breast feed and not in mothers who provide supplemental feeding.[46] (Fig. 6-6). This indicates that an infant that is accustomed to the bottle becomes a less effective sucker at the breast, and reflects the fact that feeding at the breast requires different coordination and movement of tongue and lips than feedings at the bottle.

In women, the reflex release of oxytocin often becomes conditioned. It is experienced as milk "let down" during the preparation for nursing the infant, or playing with the infant. After prolonged breast feeding, many mothers learn to decondition this reflex.

Oxytocin released during suckling also reaches the uterus, which it stimulates to contract.[43] The contractions are strong in the early puerperium and may be of significance for the expulsion of lochia and for the involution of the uterus.

Galactopoietic Hormones

In lactating women, prolactin appears to be the single most important galactopoietic hormone, since selective inhibition of prolactin secretion by bromocriptine inhibits lactation.[47,48] Ovarian hormones are not required for the maintenance of established milk production and have little effect on established lactation.

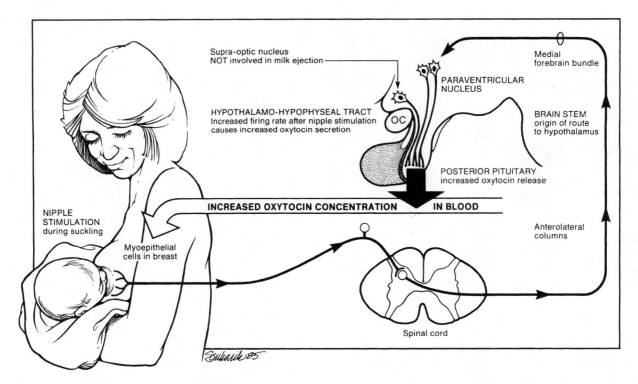

Fig. 6-5 The somatosensory pathways for the suckling-induced reflex release of oxytocin. (Adapted from Johnson and Everitt,[122] with permission.)

The Suckling Stimulus and Prolactin Release

Prolactin is secreted in increasing amounts during pregnancy, and during parturition a further increase is observed.[49] In pregnancy, high estradiol levels are

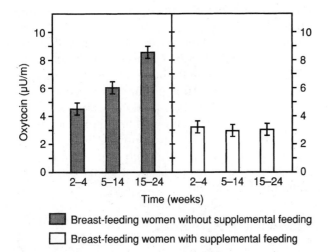

Fig. 6-6 Plasma oxytocin levels during suckling measured in four exclusively breast-feeding women (hatched columns) and in four women giving supplemental food (open columns) in early, middle, and late lactation. Values are mean ± SEM of averages for five measurements performed with 3-minute intervals at each suckling episode. (From Johnston et al.,[46] with permission.)

responsible for the rise in plasma prolactin, as estrogens stimulate the synthesis and release of prolactin from the pituitary lactotrophs. After delivery of the placenta, plasma estrogens decline; as a consequence, plasma prolactin levels also decline both in lactating and nonlactating women.

Suckling provides the continued stimulus that supports lactation,[50] and initiates both the milk ejection reflex and a reflex that releases prolactin (Fig. 6-7).

Prolactin release is controlled by hypothalamic dopaminergic neurons, which maintain a tonic release of dopamine from the median eminence into the portal vessels flowing into the capillary plexus of the anterior lobe. Dopamine inhibits prolactin release, while suckling removes this inhibitory influence.[27] Each suckling episode is associated with a rapid rise in plasma prolactin. Prolactin levels peak in 20 to 40 minutes and return to near baseline in about 3 to 4 hours.[49,51,52] Frequent nursing is required to maintain the elevated prolactin levels on which continued milk secretion depends. A significant decrease in the suckling-induced rise in plasma prolactin occurs if the nursing interval is prolonged to 16 to 24 hours. After delivery, a delay of 1 to 2 days in the initiation of nursing results in diminished responsiveness of the pituitary. To establish lactation, it is clearly important to put the baby to the breast as early as possible. This is especially important for mothers who have been delivered by cesarean delivery and

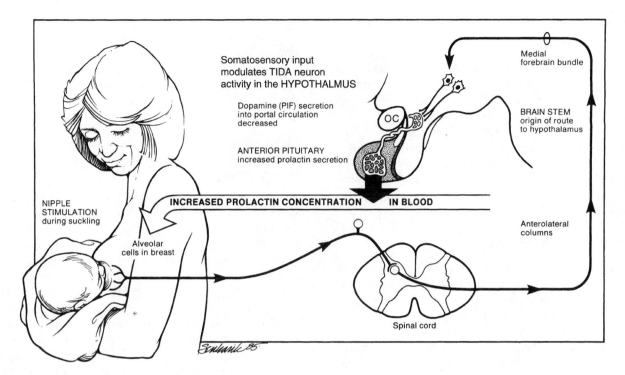

Fig. 6-7 Somatosensory pathways in the suckling-induced reflex release of prolactin. TIDA, tubuloinfundibular dopamine neuron activity; PIF, prolactin-inhibiting factor. (Adapted from Johnson and Everitt,[122] with permission.)

have not experienced the surge in prolactin and oxytocin associated with labor. Fever after delivery is not a contraindication, and the usual antibiotics given to the mother for infection are not a problem (Chapter 10).

The proper application of a breast pump also provides an adequate stimulus for both oxytocin and prolactin release. Therefore, a breast pump is useful when a sick infant is hospitalized or a preterm infant is unable to suck.

The suckling induced increment in plasma prolactin is quite variable even in the same individual. Like basal prolactin levels the suckling induced increment undergoes diurnal variations, the greatest increment occurring at night-time and the smallest in the morning.[53] Nighttime feeding should therefore be maintained if problems with insufficient milk occur. The suckling-induced increment in plasma prolactin diminishes with advancing lactation.[51] This change may be due to the decline in nursing frequency that usually takes place in the course of lactation. To maintain elevated plasma prolactin levels for prolonged periods, the mother must nurse at least six times each day.[54,56] A positive correlation between nursing frequency and the plasma prolactin levels after 8 to 10 months of lactation is observed.

Nicotine diminishes the amount of prolactin released in response to the suckling stimulus.[57] This may explain the decreased milk yield in smoking mothers, who lactate for a shorter time than comparable groups of nonsmoking mothers.

Other Neuroendocrine Responses to Suckling

Suckling also elicits the release of β-endorphin,[58] thyroid-stimulating hormone and cholecystokinin.[59] Inhibitory responses also occur, such as suppression of pulsatile luteinizing hormone (LH) release[60] and a selective inhibition of corticotrophin-release factor (CRF) release in certain stressful situations.[61] The suppression of LH release may be due to a marked decline in the expression of the luteinizing hormone-releasing hormone receptor gene during lactation, as demonstrated in rats.[62]

Reestablishing Lactation and Augmentation of Milk Yield

Reestablishment of lactation before the breast has undergone complete involution is possible after a period of abstinence from nursing. Frequent (e.g., every 2 hours) nursing or application of a breast pump is required to establish milk flow. The time needed for reestablishment is usually proportional to the duration of abstinence.

Drugs that stimulate prolactin release include reserpine, metoclopramide, sulpiride, and thyrotropin releasing hormone (TRH). These drugs have been employed to improve poor lactation with variable results.[63-66]

Augmentation of poor milk yield is usually best achieved by increasing the nursing frequency, including night time nursing, and, in instances of poor sucking activity, by application of a breast pump after each nursing episode to assure complete emptying of the breasts. Manual expression works as well but is more cumbersome. To relieve stress and anxiety, which inhibit the milk ejection reflex, gentle massage of the neck and shoulders by husband or friend is often helpful.

Lactational Insufficiency

Insufficient milk production is a poorly defined condition that can have many causes: inadequate mammogenesis, failure of lactogenesis, insufficient galactopoiesis, and impaired oxytocin secretion resulting in failure of lactokinesis. In a group of mothers attending a breast feeding center in Canada, the incidence of insufficient milk was 14 percent and a subgroup of these was diagnosed as having lactational insufficiency of unknown origin. A major feature of this subgroup was lack of mammogenesis.[67] The levels and bioactivity of prolactin were similar to controls. Oxytocin release in response to suckling was not evaluated. Absence of adequate milk ejection reflex can lead to insufficient milk production due to accumulation of local inhibitor peptides[68] as well as due to intramammary pressure-related alveolar epithelial cell necrosis. The failure of mammogenesis can indicate abnormalities at mammary gland receptors for mammogenic and lactogenic hormones.[69]

Involution

Involution of the mammary gland occurs in puerperal women who are not breast feeding. In lactating women, involution is more gradual as weaning is usually extended over a period of time. The reason for involution is in part hormonal, as prolactin secretion ceases when suckling is terminated. However, mechanical and local factors play an important role in this process, as indicated by the observation that an unsuckled breast undergoes involution, although prolactin secretion is maintained if the other breast is nursed. The flattened alveolar cells cease their secretory activity, and, within 24 hours, changes in the cellular organelles can be discerned, followed by autophagic activity by lysosomes within the epithelial cells, and infiltration of the tissue by leukocytes. The substantial engorgement that follows cessation of nursing also impedes blood flow, further stimulating the necrotic and autophagic changes. The reduction of glandular elements is followed by formation of connective tissue and deposition of adipose tissue that is completed in about 3 months. After cessation of lactation, the breast usually assumes its prepregnant size, although the glandular tissue does not regress completely,[10] and persistent alteration in the sensitivity of the mammary tissue to hormonal stimulation has been observed.[70]

Mammogenic and Lactogenic Hormones During Pregnancy and the Early Puerperium

At parturition, most mammogenic and lactogenic hormones are near maximal levels, with relaxin as the sole exception. In humans relaxin plasma levels parallel those of human chorionic gonadotrophin and are maximal in the first trimester, declining in midgestation to considerably lower levels that are maintained to term.[71]

Because mammary development is almost completed during the second trimester, lactogenesis also occurs in mothers who deliver preterm infants. The relative immaturity of the mammary epithelium is reflected in a somewhat different composition of the mother's milk in comparison to milk produced after a term delivery. The composition of preterm milk, discussed in greater detail later, corresponds to the somewhat different requirements for nutrients in preterm infants.

The Inhibitory Effect of Sex Steroids on Lactogenesis

Large doses of estrogen have been found to decrease the amount of prolactin incorporated into the alveolar epithelial cells and to prevent the rise in prolactin receptors that normally occurs in the course of lactation.[72-74]

The inhibitory effect of progesterone is more clearcut. It inhibits the induction of α-lactalbumin synthesis by prolactin, and consequently the synthesis and secretion of milk sugar.[74-77] Administration of prolactin cannot overcome this inhibitory effect of progesterone. The withdrawal of progesterone is therefore a critical step in lactogenesis. During lactation, progesterone receptors disappear from the mammary gland.[78] It is therefore not surprising that progesterone no longer has an inhibitory effect in established lactation[75] (Figs. 6-8 and 6-9).

Endocrine Consequences of Lactation

Postpartum Amenorrhea and Return of Ovulation

Postpartum amenorrhea is more prolonged, and the occurrence of first ovulation is delayed in lactating women when compared with those who do not breast feed. Lactational amenorrhea is one of the principal methods of birth spacing in much of the developing

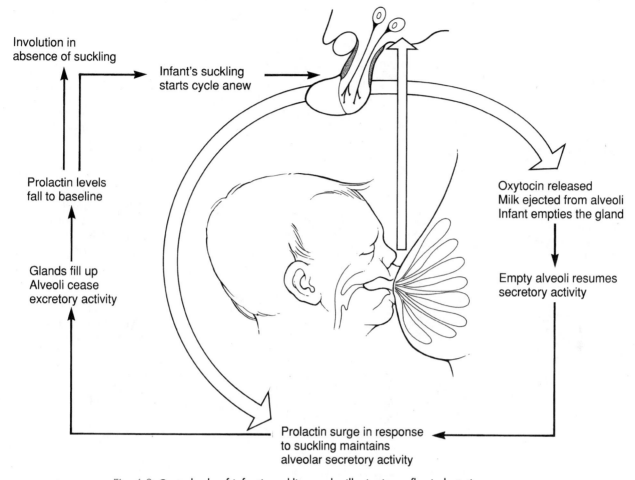

Involution in
absence of suckling

Infant's suckling
starts cycle anew

Prolactin levels
fall to baseline

Glands fill up
Alveoli cease
excretory activity

Oxytocin released
Milk ejected from alveoli
Infant empties the gland

Empty alveoli resumes
secretory activity

Prolactin surge in response
to suckling maintains
alveolar secretory activity

Fig. 6-8 Central role of infant's suckling and milk ejection reflex in lactation success.

world. Pregnancy rates during lactational amenorrhea vary somewhat in different countries but are always much lower than in nonlactating women and in lactating women in whom menstruation has resumed.

In nonlactating women ovulation usually occurs 7 to 10 weeks postpartum.[79,80] In lactating women, the anovulatory interval is quite variable and depends on the frequency of nursing episodes each day as well as on the nutritional status of the nursing woman. Those women with very poor nutrition resume ovulatory function much later than do well-nourished mothers. Ovulation precedes the first menstruation in more than one-half of lactating mothers.[79] With advancing lactation, anovulatory bleeding before the first ovulation becomes more prevalent.[81]

Is it safe for a lactating woman to wait for the first menstruation before beginning contraception? Studies in populations not using any contraception indicate that a significant number of women will become pregnant before the first menstruation, the percentages varying from 1.5 to 13 percent in different countries.[82] Women in the United States have the highest concep-

tion rates, 10 to 13 percent.[82] These data indicate that the first ovulation is associated with high fecundity and that it is advisable to begin contraception before resumption of menstruation.

Hormonal Basis for Lactational Amenorrhea

Several factors contribute to lactational amenorrhea: hypothalamic hypofunction, pituitary unresponsiveness, and ovarian refractoriness to gonadotropin stimulation.

In all women, both nursing and non-nursing, the pituitary response to gonadotropin-releasing hormone is suppressed during the early puerperium, returning gradually to normal levels over 6 weeks.[83,84] The positive feedback effect of estrogen on pituitary function is also suppressed. It returns to normal several weeks earlier in non-nursing than in nursing mothers.[85]

High plasma prolactin concentrations are responsible for ovarian hypoactivity in lactating women.[86,87] Estrogen levels remain low, in spite of normal follicle-stimulating hormone (FSH) levels, as long as plasma prolactin levels are elevated over the normal nonpreg-

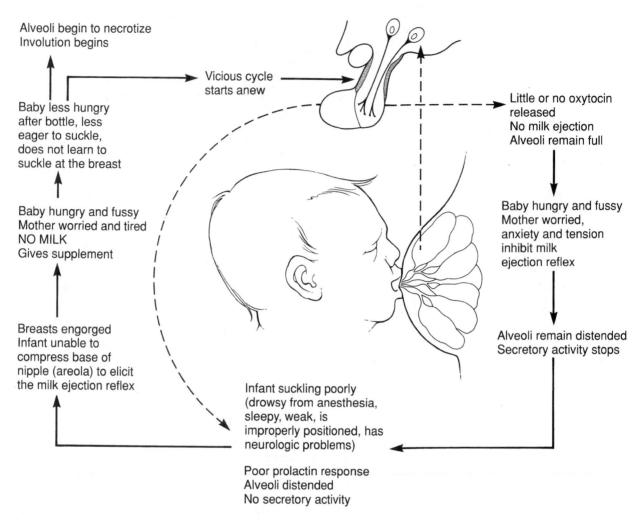

Fig. 6-9 Central role of poor suckling and failure to elicit milk ejection reflex in lactation failure. To break the vicious cycle (1) assure mother that she will have enough milk; (2) instruct proper positioning of baby so correct suckling is possible; (3) instruct mother in perioral stimulation of sleepy or lethargic infant; (4) instruct mother to express some milk manually if breast is very engorged so that infant can apply pressure on areola while suckling; (5) instruct mother to nurse frequently, including nighttime (prolactin surge greatest at night) if infant is poor feeder; (6) if all else fails, advise mother to use oxytocin nasal spray at each feeding; (7) if mother suffers fatigue, instruct other members of the family to help with chores.

nant range[88] (Fig. 6-10). At weaning plasma prolactin returns to the normal range, and plasma estrogen levels then rise. An ovulatory surge of estrogen usually occurs within 10 to 14 days, followed by an ovulatory surge of LH[88,89] (Fig. 6-11). When postpartum lactation is inhibited by bromocriptine, a dopaminergic drug that selectively inhibits prolactin release, plasma prolactin returns to baseline values within a few days, sooner than in nonlactating women who have used other methods of lactation suppression[90] (Fig. 6-10). Ovarian responsiveness to FSH is immediately restored in such women, and the first ovulation after delivery occurs within 3 to 4 weeks.

Besides the PRL plasma levels as such, the biochemical form (glycosylated or nonglycosylated) of PRL se-

creted in response to suckling is of significance for ovarian inhibition. A prospective study conducted in women who had indicated their wish for prolonged lactation, revealed that those who went on to breast-feed for over 6 months had a higher proportion of bioactive PRL than women who breast fed for less than 6 months. The levels measured by radioimmunoassay were similar in both groups.[91]

Effects of Lactation on Calcium Homeostasis

Low levels of circulating estrogens are characteristic for all lactating women. Lactation may increase osteoporosis because it also imposes an increased demand for calcium utilization. In the rat, the rate of calcium trans-

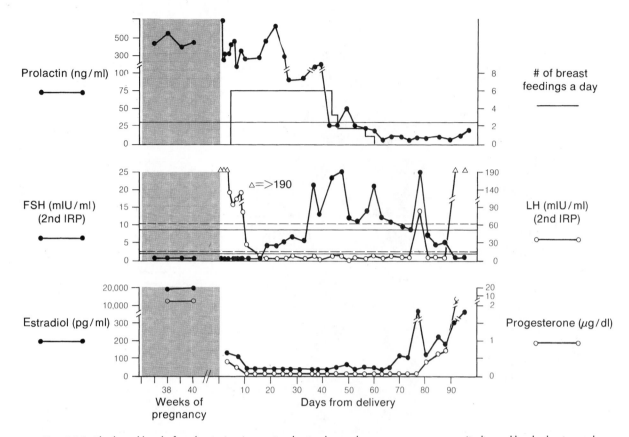

Fig. 6-10 The basal level of prolactin (top) remained raised over the nonpregnant range (indicated by the horizontal line in this and the middle panel) as long as suckling frequency was six per 24 hours but dropped to nonpregnant levels when suckling frequency decreased to two or less. The concentration of FSH returned to normal range within 3 weeks of delivery, while the concentration of LH remained low (middle). Estrogen levels were low (bottom) in spite of normal and even above-normal FSH levels but started to rise when prolactin levels fell to the normal nonpregnant range, and within 3 weeks a surge of estrogen was observed that initiated an ovulatory surge of LH. (From Rolland et al.,[90] with permission.)

fer into the milk exceeds the intestinal capacity to absorb calcium, and extensive demineralization of the skeleton occurs during lactation in this species. In women on a normal vitamin D-replete diet, increased intestinal absorption can meet the demands for calcium transfer into the milk, and little change takes place in the skeleton during pregnancy and lactation.[92–95] However, teenage mothers are at risk for bone demineralization because of their own increased need for calcium, and because they often have low dietary intakes of calcium and phosphorus.[96]

Under conditions of reduced dietary intake, including reduced dietary calcium, breast milk calcium concentration was found to depend on maternal calcium intake during pregnancy.[97]

The Composition of Human Milk

Colostrum and Mature Milk

During pregnancy a secretion called precolostrum is present in the alveolar lumina. It consists of cellular material and exudates of plasma, with a high concen-

tration of immunoglobulins, lactoferrin, serum albumin, and sodium and chloride ions, but very low levels of lactose.

After birth colostrum is secreted at a rate of about 40 ml/day for 3 to 4 days. The sudden increase in alveolar epithelial secretion following parturition results in a rapid increase in lactose, milk proteins, and the total volume of milk. The composition of breast milk therefore gradually changes during the first 1 to 2 weeks until mature milk is secreted. Average values for the major components in colostrum and in mature milk are given in Table 6-1.

The composition of human milk varies at different stages of lactation, at different times of day, during each feeding, and even between the breasts. It is therefore difficult to obtain true values for the composition of human milk. All these variations must be kept in mind in consulting the data presented in Table 6-2. The variations in fat content are most marked. Fat concentration rises steadily from the beginning to the end of each feeding,[98] and diurnal variations are considerable,

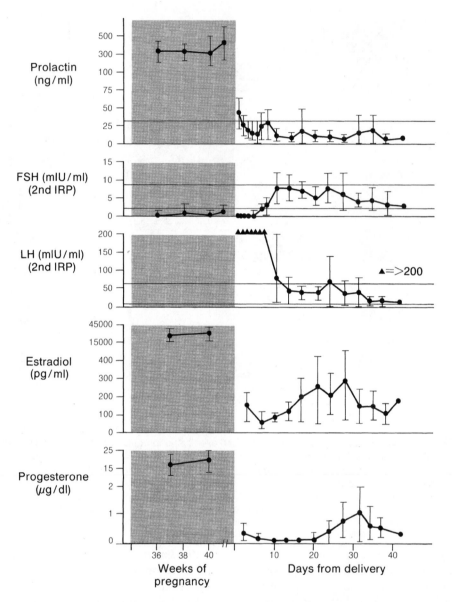

Fig. 6-11 Mean concentrations of prolactin, FSH, LH, estradiol, and progesterone in the puerperium during bromocriptine treatment in nine women. Horizontal lines indicate normal range in menstruating women. During treatment with bromocriptine plasma prolactin dropped immediately to nonpregnant levels, and the concentrations of FSH returned to normal range within 2 weeks. The ovaries responded immediately to the rise in FSH by an increase in estrogen production and subsequent ovulation. The low progesterone levels in these nine women suggest the formation of an inadequate corpus luteum. (From Rolland et al.,[88] with permission.)

with lowest concentrations around 6 A.M. and highest around 10 A.M. These differences can be as great as 15 to 30 g/L. The fat content of human milk increases with advancing lactation, at least up to 84 days postpartum, providing for the increasing caloric requirements of the growing infant. Intake of fat does influence the composition of milk fat, as up to 30 percent of fatty acids in milk can originate in dietary fat. The influence of dietary protein on the protein content of milk appears to be limited.

The stage of lactation influences the protein and car-

bohydrate content as well as mineral composition. Initially, protein and salt concentrations are high, but their levels decline during the first week as the secretion of milk is established and then decrease slowly with advancing lactation. The concentration of lactose increases rapidly during the first week and then more slowly to 6 months.

Preterm Milk

In women who deliver preterm infants, the protein and nonprotein nitrogen concentration of milk is higher

Table 6-1 The Concentration of the Major Milk Constituents in Colostrum and Mature Milk

Constituent (per dl)	Colostrum	Mature Milk
Total energy (kcal)	54	70
Milk sugar, lactose (g)	5.7	7.1
Fats (g)	2.9	4.5
Proteins (g)	2.3	0.86
Nonprotein nitrogen (g)	—	0.32
Minerals (ash) (mg)	30.8	20.2
Cells (macrophages, neutrophils, lymphocytes)	7–8×10^6	1–2×10^6

and the lactose concentration lower than in those women who deliver at term. This difference persists for 3 to 5 weeks[99–101] (Fig. 6-12). Since the protein requirement of the preterm infant is higher than of a term infant, its mother's milk is superior to pooled human milk.[102] However, pooled human milk is better than term formula.[3]

Preterm milk contains higher concentrations of essential long chain fatty acids and polyunsaturated fatty acids than term milk. The quantities are sufficient to maintain brain growth in preterm infants.[103] Preterm milk and mature milk contain a high concentration of nonprotein nitrogen, including all essential amino acids. Preterm milk also contains taurine, glycine, leucine, and cysteine which are considered essential for the preterm infant.

On the other hand, the calcium and phosphorus re-

Table 6-2 Composition of Mature Human Milk and Cow's Milk

Constituent (per dl)	Mature Milk[a] (30 days)	Cow's Milk[b]
Energy (kcal)	70	69
Total solids (g)	12.0	12.7
Lactose (g)	7.3	4.8
Total nitrogen (mg)	171	550
Protein nitrogen (mg)	129	512
Nonprotein nitrogen (mg)	42	32
Total protein (g)	0.9	3.3
Casein (g)	0.4	2.8
Whey protein[c] (g)	0.5	0.19
Lactalbumin (mg)	161	0.6
Lactoferrin (mg)	167	
IgA (mg)	142	
Total fat (g)	4.2	3.7
Unsaturated long-chain fatty acids (g)	2.9	1.0
Calcium (mg)	28	125
Phosphorus (mg)	15	96
Iron (ng)	40	100

[a] Data from Casey and Hambridge.[118]
[b] Data from National Research Council.[119]
[c] Whey protein includes β-lactoglobulin in cow's milk not present in human milk.

quirements of the preterm infant, whose relative growth rate is higher than that of the full term infant, are not always met with human milk. Rickets may develop in small infants despite addition of vitamin D. Supplementation of breast milk with calcium, phosphorus, and protein is therefore recommended for very low birth weight infants.[104]

Differences Between Human and Cow's Milk

Although the major constituents are the same in human milk and cow's milk, several significant differences exist both quantitatively and qualitatively (Table 6-2). In human milk, the caloric content is derived mainly from fats and carbohydrates, up to 99 percent of which is absorbed in the gut. In cow's milk and formulas, a greater proportion of calories is supplied by proteins that are less easily digested and may cause metabolic and amino acid imbalance. In human milk, 25 to 34 percent of nitrogen is present as nonprotein nitrogen, which provides an immediate source of all essential amino acids, including taurine, a sulfonated amino acid essential for brain development. A large proportion (75 percent) of the proteins in human milk are present as easily digested whey proteins, in contrast to cow's milk, in which casein is the main protein (80 percent). Moreover, the principal whey protein in cow's milk is β-lactoglobulin, a potent allergen. The high casein and butterfat concentration in cow's milk and many formulas leads to the formation of insoluble curds in the infant's gut. The curds bind calcium and inhibit its absorption. The high phosphorus: calcium ratio in cow's milk further decreases calcium absorption.

A much larger proportion of the fatty acids in human milk are unsaturated. Of the unsaturated fats, almost a third are long-chain polyunsaturated fatty acids, while they make up only one-sixth in cow's milk. Human milk also has a higher cholesterol content, which, together with polyunsaturated fatty acids, is needed for brain development.

In general, the bioavailability of all constituents in human milk is remarkably high and is superior to cow's milk or formulas. Even iron, present in concentrations 20 times lower in human milk than in formulas, is accumulated during the first months of life at the same rate as in formula-fed infants. A smaller volume of breast milk with a smaller caloric content will satisfy the requirements of an infant compared with the larger volume of formula needed.[105] Therefore, formula-fed infants often accumulate more body fat than do breast-fed infants. In addition, the last milk expressed at the end of nursing contains significantly more fat than does early milk.[98] This higher fat concentration may give the infant a sense of satiety. Breast-feeding alone can meet the nutritional requirements of the infant for periods from up to 15 months, depending on individual variations in milk yield.

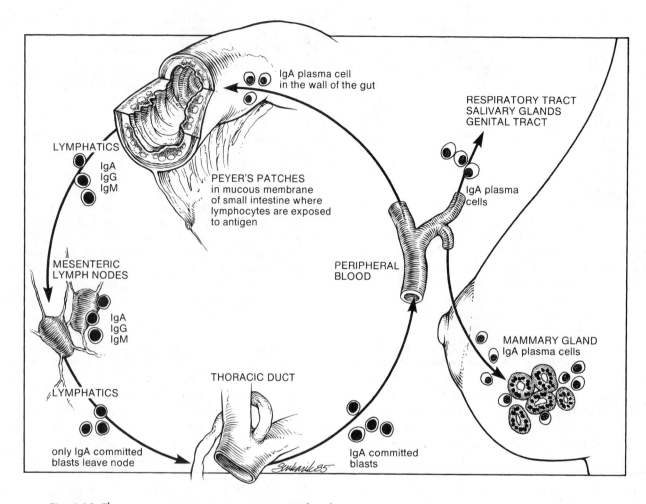

Fig. 6-12 The secretory immune system. Precursor B lymphocytes are exposed to antigens through the specialized epithelium of the Peyer's patches in the lumen of the gut. They are stimulated to divide and migrate into the mesenteric lymph nodes, where they again divide and differentiate into blasts. The IgA-committed lymphoblasts enter the bloodstream via the thoracic duct, where further differentiation takes place in contact with T cells. They "home" to sites of secretory antibody production in the gut, in the respiratory tract, and in the late-pregnancy or lactating mammary gland, where they mature into plasma cells that secrete antibody (IgA). Some of these cells and many macrophages migrate transepithelially into the alveolar lumen. (Adapted from Roux et al.,[112] with permission.)

Human milk contains significant amounts of epidermal growth factor throughout lactation, whereas bovine milk contains growth factors in the colostral stage only and bovine milk growth factors are different from those in human milk.[106] Human milk also contains trace elements, vitamins, and enzymes not present in cow's milk. Human milk also contains the sleep-inducing peptide and melatonin, which has a pronounced daily rhythm.[107]

Immunologic Aspects of Breast Feeding

Immunologic Significance of Colostrum and Milk

The mammary gland forms a part of an immune system that is specifically adapted to provide the newborn protection against gastrointestinal and respiratory tract infections.[17,108] Immunologic and maturational factors in colostrum may prevent atopic disease as well.[1]

The human infant at birth has acquired passive immunity against bacteria and their toxins, reflecting the accumulated experience of the mother. However, the predominant immunoglobulin present in mucosal secretions, secretory IgA, is not transmitted to the fetus in utero. The protection provided by the secretory IgA-rich colostrum and milk is of great importance for the establishment of an immune defense against microbial challenges. The mucosal epithelium of the newborn is capable of binding both IgA and IgM present in colostrum and milk.[109,110] The secretory IgA forms a protective coating that prevents the passage of infectious microorganisms into the systemic circulation.

Mucosal membranes of newborn infants and preterm infants in particular are permeable to antigens and mi-

Table 6-3 Immunologically Active Constituents and Resistance Factors in Human Milk and Colostrum

Soluble	Cellular	Other
Immunoglobulins (sIgA, IgA, IgG, IgM, IgE)	Monocytes	Bacterial antigens
Free secretory component	Macrophages	Hepatitis antigen
Immunosecretory mediators (complement, chemotactic factors)	Neutrophils	Rubella virus
Nonspecific factors (lactoferrin, lysozyme, lactoperoxidase, lipids, bifidus-factor)	Lymphocytes (B cells, plasma cells, T cells)	Cytomegalovirus
		Other viruses

croorganisms, facilitating access of intestinal antigens, particularly food allergens, into the systemic circulation. Binding of IgA antibodies to the mucosal surfaces prevents passage of such antigens through the epithelium. Feeding colostrum to preterm infants greatly diminishes infection rates and may protect against necrotizing enterocolitis.[105]

Immunologically Active Constituents in Human Milk and Colostrum

Human milk contains a number of immunologically active factors, as shown in Table 6-3. These include both soluble antigens and immunocompetent cells, as well as mediators of the immune response.[17–19,108,111] The bifidus factor together with the low buffering capacity of human milk, which results in an intestinal pH of 4 to 6, favor the growth of *Lactobacillus bifidus* and suppress the growth of pathogens. The predominant flora of breast-fed infants consists of *L. bifidus*, whereas that of bottle-fed infants consists of *streptococcus foecalis, E. coli,* and bacteroides.

The cells found in the mammary gland and its secretions are not a random collection of maternal leukocytes but represent a selected subpopulation of those cells that migrate from the gut-associated and bronchus-associated lymphoid tissues to other mucosa, where they secrete antibody independent of local antigen contact. They reflect the immunologic response of the mother to pathogens in her environment and, consequently, also to that of her newborn infant. (Fig. 6-12).[112]

Maternal Diet and Breast-Feeding

Energy Intake

During pregnancy the maternal organism stores 2 to 4 kg of fat that are mobilized during lactation, and this must be taken into account when calculating dietary allowances. About 50% of the fatty acids in milk originate in tissue stores in well-nourished women; women with little body fat must increase their energy intake correspondingly. A diet consisting on the average of 2,350 ± 250 kcal/day for a 60-kg woman has been found to provide adequate energy intake while allowing for a gradual reduction in weight to prepregnancy levels.[113,114]

Colic

Maternal diet has long been thought to be associated with the occurrence of infantile colic in breast-fed infants. A double blind placebo-controlled trial showed that the elimination of cow's milk from maternal diet had no beneficial effect. However, rates of colic were significantly more frequent on days when the mother ate certain foods (chocolate, fruits). The rates of colic also increased in proportion to the diversity of foods in the maternal diet showing that colic cannot be attributed to a single diet component.[115]

Atopic disease

The possible influence of maternal diet on the incidence of atopic disease has been the focus of considerable attention, but remains poorly understood. Breast feeding exclusively for the first 6 months provides considerable protection[1]; probably because the intake of foreign allergens is minimized. Allergens may also gain access to the infant through mother's milk from maternal diet. In a recent controlled study the presence or absence of two strong allergens, cow's milk and eggs, in maternal diet during the last 3 months of pregnancy and lactation had no significant effect on the development of atopic disease in the infant up to 18 months of age.[116] Genetic factors probably have a greater effect than maternal diet in the perinatal period. It seems prudent, however, to avoid allergens known to affect other family members in a family with a strong history of atopic disease.

Breast-feeding and Diabetes

Diabetic mothers are able to breast-feed and often have reduced insulin requirements during lactation because the uptake of glucose by the mammary gland is considerable. A group of breast-feeding insulin dependent diabetic mothers had at 6 weeks postpartum significantly lower fasting glucose levels than those who had stopped nursing or those who bottle fed.[117]

Key Points

- Breast feeding is protective against infant infection and atopic disease.

- Estrogen stimulates prolactin release, but inhibits the lactogenic effects of prolactin at the level of the breast. Estrogen withdrawal at delivery is important in the initiation of lactation.

- Progesterone stimulates glandular development but inhibits the secretion of milk by suppressing the syntheses of α-lactalbumin in the alveolar epithelial cells. In established lactation progesterone no longer has this effect.

- The release of oxytocin from the neurohypophysis is under neural control and the stimulus is provided by the suckling of the infant. Suckling also causes a rise in prolactin that is essential for galactopoiesis.

- Oxytocin stimulates the myoepithelial cells, resulting in milk ejection, and also stimulates uterine contractions.

- Increasing the frequency of suckling including night time nursing will increase milk production.

- In mothers who deliver preterm infants, the protein content of the milk is higher, but corresponds to the increased protein requirements of preterm infants.

- Postpartum amenorrhea is prolonged, the occurrence of first ovulation is delayed, and pregnancy rates are lower in lactating women compared to non-lactating women.

- Low levels of circulating estrogens occur in lactating women, causing vaginal dryness. Women who do not consume adequate calcium are at increased risk for osteoporosis.

- Colostrum is secreted for the first 2–3 days, after which the milk volume increases significantly.

- Secretory IgA is not transmitted to the fetus in utero, but is abundant in human milk, providing immune defense against infection.

References

1. Saarinen U, Kajosaari M, Backman A et al: Prolonged breast feeding as a prophylaxis for atopic disease. Lancet 2:163, 1979
2. Appleton JA, McGregor DO: Rapid expulsion of Trichinella spiralis in suckling rats. Science 226:70, 1984
3. Lucas A, Morley R, Cole TJ et al: A randomized multicentre study of human milk versus formula and later development in preterm infants. Arch Dis Childhood 70:F141, 1994
4. Bernard-Bonnin A-C, Statchenko S, Girard G: Hospital practices and breast-feeding duration: a meta-analysis of controlled trials. Birth 16:64, 1989
5. Winikoff B, Laukaran VA, Myers D, Stone R: Dynamics of infant feeding: mothers, professionals and the institutional context in a large urban hospital. Pediatrics 77:35, 1986
6. Venditelli F, Alain J, Dufetelle B et al: Maternal motivations for the choice of infant feeding. (In French.) J Clin Obstet Biol Reprod 23:323, 1994
7. Stirling JW, Chandler JA: The fine structure of normal resting terminal ductal lobular unit of the female breast. Virchows Arch Pathol Anat 372:205, 1976
8. Ferguson DJP, Anderson TJ: A morphological study of the changes which occur during pregnancy in the human breast. Virchows Arch Pathol Anat 401:163, 1983
9. Ferguson DJP, Anderson TJ: An ultrastructural study of lactation in the human breast. Anat Embryol 138:349, 1983
10. Helminen HJ, Ericsson JLE: Studies on mammary gland involution, I–III. J Ultrastruct Res 25:193, 214, 228, 1968
11. Tobon H, Salazar H: Ultrastructure of the human mammary gland, II: postpartum lactogenesis. J Clin Endocrinol Metab 40:334, 1975
12. Smith CW, Goldman AS: The cells of human colostrum: in vitro studies of morphology and functions. Pediatr Res 2:103, 1968
13. Smith JJ, Nickerson SC, Keenan TW: Metabolic energy and cytoskeletal requirements for synthesis and secretion by acini for rat mammary glands. Int J Biochem 14:87, 1982
14. Neville MC, Neifert MR: Lactation: Physiology, Nutrition, and Breast-Feeding. Plenum, New York, 1983
15. Brandtzaeg P: Structure, synthesis and external transfer of mucosa immunoglobulins. Ann Immunol (Paris) 124:C417, 1973
16. Lamm ME: Cellular aspects of immunoglobin A. Adv Immunol 22:223, 1976
17. Hanson LA, Winberg J: Breast milk and defense against infection in the newborn. Arch Dis Child 47:845, 1982
18. Goldman AS, Garza A, Nichols BL, Goldblum RM: Immunologic factors present in human milk during the first year of lactation. J Pediatr 100:563, 1982
19. Ogra SS, Ogra PL: Immunological aspects of human colostrum and milk, I: distribution characteristics and concentrations of immunoglobins. J Pediatr 92:546, 1978
20. Tobon H, Salazar H: Ultrastructure of the human mammary gland, I: development of the fetal gland throughout gestation. J Clin Endocrinol Metab 39:443, 1974
21. Raynaud A: Morphogenesis of the mammary gland. p. 3. In IR Falconer (ed): Lactation. University of Pennsylvania Press, Philadelphia, 1971
22. Milligan D, Drife JO, Short RV: Changes in breast volume during normal menstrual cycle and after oral contraceptives. BMJ 4:494, 1975
23. Weisz-Carrington P, Roux ME, Lamm ME: Plasma cells and epithelial immunoglobins in the mouse mammary

gland during pregnancy and lactation. J Immunol 199: 1036, 1977

24. Linzell JL: Mammary blood flow and methods of identifying and measuring precursors of milk. p. I: 143. In LB Larson, VR Smith (eds): Lactation: A Comprehensive Treatise. Vol. 1. Academic Press, San Diego, 1974

25. Lyons WR: Hormonal synergism in mammary growth. Proc R Soc Lond 149:303, 1958

26. Nandi S: Hormonal control of mammogenesis and lactogenesis in the C_3H/He Crgl mouse. Univ Calif (Berkeley) Publ Zool 65:4, 1959

27. Neill JD: Prolactin: its secretion and control. p. IV:469. In E Knobil, WH Sawyer (eds): Handbook of Physiology. Endocrinology. Vol. 4. American Physiological Society, Washington DC, 1974

28. Sherwood OD: Relaxin. p. I: 861. In: Knobil E, Niell JD (eds): The Physiology of Reproduction. 2nd Ed. Vol. 1. New York, Raven Press, 1994

29. Bigazzi M, Sacchi Bani T, Bani G: Relaxin and the human breast. p. 549. In: MacLennan AH, Treager GW, Bryant-Greenwood G (eds): Recent Progress in Relaxin Research. World Scientific Publications, Singapore, 1995

30. Tashima TT, Bryant-Greenwood G: H_1/H_2 relaxins in the human breast. p. 552. In MacLennan AH, Treager GW, Bryant-Greenwood G (eds): Recent Progress in Relaxin Research. World Scientific Publications, Singapore, 1995

31. Faulkin LJ, DeOme KB: Regulation of growth and spacing of gland elements in the mammary fat pad of the C3H mouse. J Natl Cancer Inst 24:953, 1960

32. Shyamala G, Ferenczy A: Mammary fat pad may be a potential site for initiation of estrogen action in normal mouse mammary glands. Endocrinology 115:1078, 1984

33. Haslam SZ, Gale JJ, Dachler SL: Estrogen receptor activation in normal mammary gland. Endocrinology 114: 1163, 1984

34. Topper YJ, Freeman CS: Multiple hormone interactions in the developmental biology of the mammary gland. Physiol Rev 60:1049, 1980

35. Battacharjee M, Vonderhaar BK: Thyroid hormones enhance the synthesis and secretion of lactalbumin by mouse mammary tissue in vitro. Endocrinology 115: 1070, 1984

36. Cross BA, Findlay ALR: Comparative and sensory aspects of milk ejection. p. 245. In M Reynolds, SJ Folley (eds): Lactogenesis: The Initiation of Milk Secretion at Parturition. University of Pennsylvania Press, Philadelphia, 1969

37. Sala NL: The milk ejecting effect induced by oxytocin and vasopressin during human pregnancy. Am J Obstet Gynecol 89:626, 1964

38. Soloff MS, Schroeder BT, Chakraborty J, Pearlmutter AF: Characterization of oxytocin receptors in the uterus and mammary gland. Fed Proc 36:1861, 1977

39. Sala NL, Althabe O: The milk ejecting effect induced by oxytocin during human lactation. Acta Physiol Latino Am 18:88, 1968

40. Wiederman J, Freund M, Stone ML: Oxytocin effect on myoepithelium of the breast throughout pregnancy. J Appl Physiol 19:310, 1964

41. Caldeyro-Barcia R: Milk ejection in women. p. 229. In M Reynolds, SJ Folley (eds): Lactogenesis: The Initiation of Milk Secretion at Parturition. University of Pennsylvania Press, Philadelphia, 1969

42. Fuchs AR, Wagner G: The effect of ethyl alcohol on the release of oxytocin (OT) in rabbits. Acta Endocrinol (Copenh) 44:593, 1963

43. Wagner G, Fuchs AR: Effect of ethanol on uterine activity during suckling in post partum women. Acta Endocrinol (Copenh) 58:133, 1968

44. Dawood MY, Khan-Dawood FS, Wahi RS, Fuchs F: Oxytocin release and plasma anterior pituitary and gonadal hormones in women during lactation. J Clin Endocrinol Metab 52:678, 1981

45. Fuchs AR, Dawood MY, Sumulong L et al: Release of oxytocin and prolactin by suckling in rabbits throughout lactation. Endocrinology 114:462, 1984

46. Johnston AM, Amico JA: A prospective longitudinal study of the release of oxytocin and prolactin in response to infant suckling in long term lactation. J Clin Endocrinol Metab 622:653, 1986

47. Del Pozo E, Brun del Re R, Varga L, Friesen HG: The inhibition of prolactin secretion in man by CB-154 (2-Br-alphaergocryptine). J Clin Endocrinol Metab 35: 768, 1972

48. Rolland R, Schellekens L: A new approach to the inhibition of puerperal lactation. J Obstet Gynocol Br Commonw 80:945, 1973

49. Tyson JE, Hwang P, Guyda H, Friesen HG: Studies of prolactin secretion in human pregnancy. Am J Obstet Gynecol 113:14, 1972

50. Selye H, Collip JB, Thomson DL: Nervous and hormonal factors in lactation. Endocrinology 18:237, 1934

51. Noel GL, Such HK, Frantz AG: Prolactin release during nursing and breast stimulation in postpartum and nonpostpartum subjects. J Clin Endocrinol Metab 38:413, 1974

52. Howie PW, McNeilly AS, McArdle T, Smart L: The relationship between suckling-induced prolactin response and lactogenesis. J Clin Endocrinol Metab 50:670, 1980

53. Diaz S, Seron-Ferre M, Cardenas H et al: Circadian variations of basal plasma prolactin, prolactin response to suckling and length of amenorrhea in nursing women. J Clin Endocrinol Metab 68:946, 1989

54. Delvoye P, Demaegd M, Delogne-Desnoeck J: The influence of the frequency of nursing and of previous lactation experience on serum prolactin in lactating mothers. J Biosoc Sci 9:447, 1977

55. Howie PW, McNeilly AS, Houston MJ et al: Effect of supplementary food on suckling patterns and ovarian activity. B M J 283:757, 1981

56. Stern JM, Konner M, Herman TN, Reichlin S: Nursing behaviour, prolactin and postpartum amenorrhoea during prolonged lactation in American and !Kung mothers. Clin Endocrinol 25:247, 1986

57. Andersen AN, Lund-Andersen C, Falck Larsen J et al: Suppressed prolactin but normal neurophysin levels in

cigarette smoking breast feeding mothers. Clin Endocrinol 17:363, 1982

58. Riskind PN, Millard WJ, Martin JB: Opiate modulation of the anterior pituitary hormone response during suckling in the rat. Endocrinology 114:1232, 1984

59. Uvnas-Moberg K: Release of gastrointestinal peptides in response to vagal activation induced by electrical stimulation, feeding and suckling. J Auton Nerv Syst 9:141, 1983

60. Fox S, Smith M: The suppression of pulsatile luteinizing hormone secretion during lactation in the rat. Endocrinology 115:2045, 1984

61. Lightman S, Young WS III: Lactation inhibits stress-mediated secretion of corticosteroid and oxytocin and hypothalamic accumulation of corticotropin releasing factor and encephalic messenger ribonucleic acids. Endocrinology 124:2358, 1989

62. Funabishi T, Brooks PJ, Weesner GD et al: Luteinizing hormone-releasing hormone receptor messenger RNA expression in the rat pituitary during lactation and the estrous cycle. J Neuroendocrinology 6:261, 1994

63. Kauppila A, Kivinen A, Ylikorkala O: Metoclopramide increases prolactin release and milk secretion in puerperium without stimulating the secretion of TSH or T_3 or T_4. J Clin Endocrinol Metab 52:436, 1981

64. Tyson JE, Perez A, Zanartu J: Human lactational response to oral thyrotropin releasing hormone. J Clin Endocrinol Metab 43:760, 1976

65. Zarate A, Villalobos H, Canales ES et al: The effect of oral administration of thyrotropin releasing hormone on lactation. J Clin Endocrinol Metab 43:301, 1976

66. Ylikorkala O, Kivinen S, Kauppila A: Oral administration of TRH in puerperal women: effects on insufficient lactation, thyroid hormones and prolactin to intravenous TRH. Acta Endocrinol (Copenh) 93:413, 1983

67. Livingstone V, Gout PW, Crickner SD et al: Serum lactogens possessed normal bioactivity in patients with lactation insufficiency. Clin Endocrinol 41:193, 1994

68. Prentice A, Addey C, Wild CJ: Evidence for local feedback control of human milk secretion. Biochem Soc Transact 17:122, 1989

69. Neifert MR, Seacat JM, Jobe WB: Lactation failure due to insufficient glandular development of the breast. Pediatrics 76:823, 1985

70. Bolander FF Jr: Persistent alterations in hormonal sensitivities of mammary glands from parous mice. Endocrinology 112:1796, 1983

71. Johnson MR: The regulation of circulating levels of relaxin during pregnancy and their importance during pregnancy and labour. p. 225. In: MacLennan AH, Treager GW, Bryant-Greenwood G. (eds): Recent Progress in Relaxin Research. World Scientific Publications, Singapore, 1995

72. Nolin JM, Bogdanove EM: Effects of estrogen on prolactin (PRL) incorporation by lutein and milk secretory cells and on pituitary PRL secretion in the postpartum rat: correlations with target cell responsiveness to PRL. Biol Reprod 22:393, 1980

73. Bohnet HG, Gomez F, Friesen HG: Prolactin and estrogen binding sites in the mammary gland of the lactating and nonlactating rat. Endocrinology 101:111, 1977

74. Hayden TJ, Bonney RC, Forsyth IA: Ontogeny and control of prolactin receptors in the mammary gland and liver on virgin, pregnant and lactating rats. J Endocrinol 80:259, 1979

75. Chatterton RT Jr, King WJ, Ward DA, Chien HL: Differential responses of prelactating and lactating mammary gland to similar tissue concentrations of progesterone. Endocrinology 96:861, 1975

76. Kuhn NJ: Progesterone withdrawal as the lactogenic trigger in the rat. J Endocrinol 44:39, 1969

77. Kuhn NJ: Specificity of progesterone inhibition of lactogenesis. J Endocrinol 45:615, 1969

78. Haslam SZ, Shyamala G: Effect of oestradiol on progesterone receptors in normal mammary gland and its relationship with lactation. Biochem J 182:127, 1979

79. Perez A, Vela P, Masnick GS, Potter RG: First ovulation after childbirth: the effect of breast feeding. Am J Obstet Gynecol 114:1041, 1972

80. Howie PW, McNeilly AS, Houston MJ et al: Fertility after childbirth: ovulation and menstruation in bottle and breast feeding mothers. Clin Endocrinol 17:323, 1982

81. Gray RH, Campbell OM, Zacur HA et al: Postpartum return of ovarian activity in non-breast-feeding women monitored by urinary assays. J Clin Endocrinol Metab 63:645, 1986

82. Simpson-Herbert M, Huffman S: The contraceptive effect of breast feeding. Stud Fam Plann 12:125, 1981

83. Tolis G, Guyda H, Pillorger R, Friesen HG: Breast feeding effects on the hypothalamic pituitary gonadal axis. Endocrine Res Comm 1:293, 1974

84. LeMaire WJ, Shapiro AG, Rigg ALT, Yang N: Temporary pituitary insensitivity to stimulation by synthetic LRH during the postpartum period. J Clin Endocrinol Metab 38:916, 1974

85. Baird DT, McNeilly AS, Sawers RS, Sharpe RM: Failure of estrogen-induced discharge of luteinizing hormone in lactating women. J Clin Endocrinol Metab 49:500, 1979

86. Dorrington J, Gore-Langton RE: Prolactin inhibits oestrogen synthesis in the ovary. Nature (Lond) 290:600, 1984

87. Wang C, Hsueh AJW, Erickson GF: Prolactin inhibition of estrogen production by cultured rat granulosa cells. Mol Cell Endocrin 20:135, 1980

88. Rolland R, Lequin RM, Schellekens LA: The role of prolactin in the restoration of ovarian function during the early postpartum period in the human female. Clin Endocrinol 4:15, 1975

89. Weinstein D, Ben-David M, Polishuk WZ: Serum prolactin and the suppression of lactation. Br J Obstet Gynaecol 83:679, 1976

90. Rolland R, DeJong FH, Schellekens LA, Leuqin RM: The role of prolactin in the restoration of ovarian function during the early postpartum period in the human: a study during inhibition of lactation by bromergocryptine. Clin Endocrinol 4:23, 1975

91. Capino C, Ampuero S, Diaz S et al: Prolactin bioactivity

and the duration of lactational amenorrhea. J Clin Endocrinol Metab 79:970, 1994

92. Lamke B, Brundin JM, Moberg D: Changes in bone mineral content during pregnancy and lactation. Acta Obstet Gynecol Scand 56:217, 1977

93. Lewis P, Rafferty B, Shelley B, Robinson CJ: A suggested physiological role of calcitonin: the protection of the skeleton during pregnancy and lactation. J Endocrinol 49:ix, 1971

94. Lund B, Selnes A: Plasma 1,25-dihydroxyvitamin D levels in pregnancy and lactation. Acta Endocrinol (Copenh) 92:330, 1979

95. Taylor TG, Lewis PE, Balderstone O: Role of calcitonin in protecting the skeleton during pregnancy and lactation. J Endocrinol 66:297, 1975

96. Chan GM, Slater P, Ronald N et al: Bone mineral status of lactating mothers of different ages. Am J Obstet Gynecol 144:438, 1982

97. Prentice A, Bibba B, Jarjou LMA et al: Is breast milk calcium concentration influenced by calcium intake during pregnancy. Lancet 344:411, 1994

98. Hytten FE: Clinical and chemical studies in human lactation, I–III. BMJ 2:175, 1954

99. Anderson GH, Atkinson SA, Bryan MH: Energy and macronutrient content of human milk during early lactation from mothers giving birth prematurely and at term. Am J Clin Nutr 34:258, 1981

100. Gross SJ, David RJ, Bauman L et al: Nutritional composition of milk produced by mothers delivering preterm. J Pediatr 96:41, 1980

101. Hohenauer L: Feeding of the mother's expressed breast milk to sick and premature babies: some aspects of practical interest. Eur J Obstet Gynecol Reprod Biol 15:385, 1983

102. Gross SJ: Growth and biochemical response of preterm infants fed human milk or modified infant formula. N Engl J Med 308:237, 1983

103. Clandini MT, Chappell JE, Hein T et al: Human milk as a source of long chain polyunsaturated fatty acids for preterm human infant neural tissues. Nutr Rev 42:247, 1984

104. Abrams SA, Schauler RJ, Garza G: Mineralization in former very low-birth-weight infants fed either with milk or commercial formula. J Pediatr 112:956, 1988

105. Jelliffe DB, Jelliffe EFP: The uniqueness of human milk. Am J Clin Nutr 24:967, 1977

106. Shing YW, Klagsbrun M: Human and bovine milk contain different sets of growth factors. Endocrinology 115:273, 1984

107. Illnerova H, Buresova M, Presl J: Melatonin rhythm in human milk. J Clin Endocrnol Metab 77:838, 1993

108. Beer AF, Billingham RE, Head JR: The immunologic significance of the mammary gland. J Invest Dermatol 63:65, 1974

109. Ogra SS, Ogra PL: Characteristics of lymphocyte reactivity and distribution of E-rosette forming cells at different times after the onset of lactation. J Pediatr 92:550, 1978

110. Crago SS, Kalkavy R, Prince SJ, Mesiecky J: Secretory component on epithelial cells is a surface receptor for polymeric immunoglobins. J Exp Med 147:1832, 1978

111. Goldblum RM, Ahlstedt S, Charlsson B et al: Anti body-forming cells in human colostrum after oral immunization. Nature 257:797, 1975

112. Roux ME, McWilliams M, Phillips-Quagliata JM: Origin of IgA secreting plasma cells in the mammary gland. J Exp Med 146:1311, 1977

113. Butte NF, Garza C, Stuff JE et al: Effects of maternal diet and body composition on lactational performance. Am J Clin Nutr 39:296, 1984

114. Strode MA, Dewey KG, Lonnerdal B: Effects of short-term caloric restriction on lactational performance of well-nourished women. Acta Pediatr Scand 75:222, 1986

115. Evans RW, Ferguson DW, Allardyce RA, Taylor B: Maternal diet and infantile colic in breast-fed infants. Lancet 1:1340, 1981

116. Lilza G, Dannaeus A, Foucard T, Graff-Lonnevig V: Effect of maternal diet during pregnancy and lactation on the development of atopic disease in infants up to 18 months of age. Clin Exp Allergy 19:473, 1989

117. Ferris AM, Davidowitz CK, Ingardia CM et al: Lactation outcome in insulin dependent diabetic women. J Am Dietetic Assoc 88:317, 1988

118. Casey CE, Hambridge KM: Nutritional aspects of breast-feeding. p. 204. In Neville MC, Meifert MR (eds): Lactation: Physiology, Nutrition, and Breast-Feeding. Plenum, New York, 1983

119. National Research Council: The composition of milks. Bull Natl Res Council: Wash. No. 254, 1953

120. Cowie AT: Lactation. p. 201. In Austin CR, Short RV (eds): Reproduction in Mammals. Book 3. Hormonal Control of Reproduction. 2nd Ed. Cambridge University Press, Cambridge, 1984

121. Neville MC, Allen JC, Walters C: The mechanisms of milk secretion. In Neville MC, Neifert MR (eds): Lactation: Physiology, Nutrition, and Breast-Feeding. Plenum, New York, 1983

122. Johnson M, Everitt B: Essentials of reproduction. p. 321. In Essentials of Reproduction. 2nd Ed. Blackwell Scientific, Oxford, 1984

Prenatal Care

<table>
<tr><td>Chapter
7</td><td># Preconception and Prenatal Care

Timothy R. B. Johnson, Marlene A. Walker, and Jennifer R. Niebyl</td></tr>
</table>

Definition of primary care:

> Integrated, accessible health care services by clinicians who are accountable for addressing a large majority of personal health care needs, developing a sustained partnership with patients, and practicing in the context of family and community.[1]

Prenatal care is an excellent example of preventive medicine and is very much a phenomenon of the twentieth century. In 1929, the Ministry of Health of Great Britain issued a memorandum on the conduct of prenatal clinics and provided guidelines for their organization that endure to this day.

During World War II, when wartime food rationing in England identified expectant and nursing mothers as persons having special dietary requirements, maternal mortality began to fall. In 1942, vitamin tablets were provided for all women in the last 6 months of pregnancy. Maternal mortality declined from 319 per 100,000 live births in 1936 to 15 in 1985. The decline in maternal mortality was partly attributed to prenatal care and partly to medical advances in availability of blood transfusions, antibiotics, and management of fluid and electrolyte balance.

Recent guidelines addressing the content and efficacy of prenatal care have focused on the medical and the psychosocial and educational aspects of the prenatal care system. Quality health care systems will use these maps in the development of their prenatal care programs. Prenatal care satisfies the definition of primary care from the Institute of Medicine, 1994. In fact, prenatal care services can be used by obstetricians/gynecologists and other primary care providers as a model for primary care. Prenatal care satisfies other criteria

for primary care in that it is comprehensive, continuous, and provides coordinated health care.[2] The paradigms for prenatal care and the guidelines that have been developed could easily be expanded to primary health care services for women.[3]

The prenatal care record describes in a consistent fashion the comprehensive care that is provided and allows for documentation of coordinated services.

The goal of prenatal care is to help the mother maintain her well-being and achieve a healthy outcome for herself and her infant. Education about pregnancy, childbearing, and childrearing is an important part of prenatal care, as are detection and treatment of abnormalities. This process is best realized when begun even before pregnancy. Two recent documents[4,5] addressing the content and efficacy of prenatal care have suggested changes in the current prenatal care system, and we believe that the next decade will see changes from current standards.[6-9] Many services provided traditionally during the intrapartum hospital stay will be provided at prenatal and postpartum outpatient visits.

Maternal Mortality

Maternal death is the demise of any woman from any pregnancy-related cause while pregnant or within 42 days of termination of pregnancy, irrespective of the duration and the site of pregnancy. A direct maternal death is an obstetric death resulting from obstetric complications of the pregnancy state, labor, or puerperium. An indirect maternal death is an obstetric death resulting from a disease previously existing or developing during the pregnancy, labor, or puerperium; death is not directly due to obstetric causes but may be aggravated by the physiologic effects of pregnancy. A nonmaternal death is an obstetric death resulting from accidental or incidental causes unrelated to the pregnancy or its management.

The maternal mortality rate is the number of maternal deaths (direct, indirect, or nonmaternal) per 100,000 women of reproductive age, but, since this denominator is difficult to determine precisely, the National Center for Health Statistics,[10] the World Health Organization, and others define the maternal mortality rate as the number of maternal deaths (indirect and direct) per 100,000 live births. Epidemiologists recognize this as the maternal mortality ratio.

In Georgia from 1990 to 1992 the maternal mortality rate was 21.9 per 100,000 live births.[11] The most frequent causes were hemorrhage (23 percent), embolism (22 percent), cardiac problems (21 percent), pulmonary problems (8 percent), pregnancy-induced hypertension (6 percent), and anesthesia complications (4 percent).

Pregnant women are still at increased risk of morbidity and mortality compared with women who are not pregnant. Ectopic pregnancy is more dangerous (38 deaths/100,000) than childbirth (9) or legal abortion (<1).[12]

Maternal mortality has been an underrecognized issue worldwide despite an estimated 500,000 maternal deaths per year from pregnancy-related causes.[13] Put in perspective, this is equivalent to six jumbo jet crashes per day with the deaths of all 250 passengers on board, all of them women in the reproductive years of life. There is also a marked inequity in geographic distribution, since 95 percent of these deaths occur in developing countries (Fig. 7-1). Unfortunately, the United States is seeing an increase in nonmaternal deaths of

pregnant women due to trauma and violence, many of these related to illegal drugs (Fig. 7-2).

The prenatal care provider can play a role in preventing these common causes of death in women by advocating use of seat belts and screening for alcohol, drug use, depression, and violence. Recent suggestions that the definition of maternal mortality include homicide and suicide is one way of focusing on the prevention of these important problems for pregnant women.[14]

Neonatal Mortality and Morbidity

Historically in developed countries, when decreased maternal mortality was achieved attention was then turned to fetal mortality and later to fetal morbidity. The stillbirth rate (fetal death rate) is the number of stillborn infants per 1,000 infants born. The neonatal mortality rate is the number of neonatal deaths (deaths in the first 28 days of life) per 1,000 live births. The perinatal mortality combines these two—the number of fetal deaths (stillbirths) plus neonatal deaths per 1,000 total births.

In 1990, the U.S. infant mortality rate was 9.2 per 1,000 live births, ranking the United States 19th internationally.[15] However, there are great international differences in the way live births are classified, as some countries exclude infants weighing less than 1 kg and those with fatal anomalies.

Prenatal Care

During the past 20 years, new technology has been introduced to assess the fetus antepartum, including electronic fetal monitoring, ultrasound, and amniocentesis,

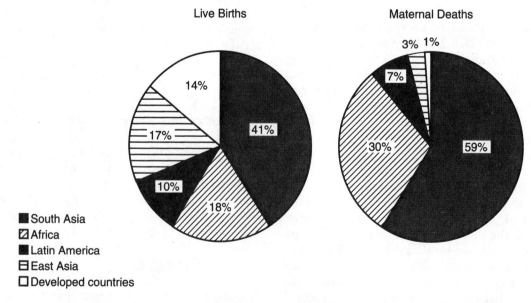

■ South Asia
▨ Africa
■ Latin America
⊟ East Asia
☐ Developed countries

Fig. 7-1 Worldwide distribution of live births and maternal deaths by region. (From WHO 861663.)

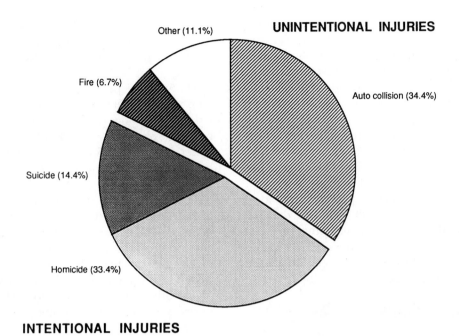

Other (11.1%)

UNINTENTIONAL INJURIES

Fire (6.7%)

Auto collision (34.4%)

Suicide (14.4%)

Homicide (33.4%)

INTENTIONAL INJURIES

Fig. 7-2 Distribution of deaths due to injury in the United States, 1980–1985 (N = 90). (From MMWR.[57])

with the fetus emerging as a patient in utero. Prevention of morbidity as well as mortality is now the goal. This has made the task of the prenatal clinic more complex, since mother and fetus now require an increasingly sophisticated level of care. At the same time, pregnancy is basically a physiologic process, and the normal pregnant patient may not benefit from this advanced technology. In this situation the pregnant woman's choices should be respected to ensure an optimal pregnancy outcome.

Prenatal care is provided at a variety of sites, ranging from the private office to the public health and county hospital clinics, to the patient's home. A variety of practitioners are involved, including the public health nurse, nurse practitioner, nurse-midwife, physician-in-training, family practitioner, obstetrician, and perinatologist. All have their own interests, experience, and expertise. Prenatal care requires a synthesis of knowledge and experience; in addition, it requires vigilance, compassion, and caring. To be utilized maximally, it must be available, affordable, accessible, and acceptable. Obstetricians must optimize their efforts by resourceful use of other professionals and support groups, including nutritionists, childbirth educators, and specialty medical consultants. Since most pregnant women are healthy, with normal pregnancies, they can be followed by an obstetric team including nurses, nurse practitioners, and nurse-midwives, with an obstetrician available for consultation. These women can be followed by practitioners who have adequate time to spend on patient education and parenting preparation,

while physicians can appropriately concentrate on complicated problems requiring their medical skills. This also provides for improved continuity of care, which is recognized as extremely important for patient satisfaction.

There have been no prospective controlled trials demonstrating efficacy of prenatal care overall. However, many individual components have been shown to be effective (e.g., treatment with corticosteroids to prevent respiratory distress syndrome and screening for and treating asymptomatic bacteriuria for prevention of pyelonephritis).[16] In retrospective studies, however, patients with increased numbers of visits have improved maternal and fetal outcomes. This may be because of self-selection of patients for care who are motivated to take care of themselves in other ways, as women with no prenatal care often come from underprivileged socioeconomic groups.

Efficacy of prenatal care also depends on the quality of care provided by the caretaker. If a blood pressure is recorded as elevated and no therapeutic maneuvers are recommended, this will not change the outcome. Recommendations must be made such as for bedrest to control blood pressure and must be carried out by the patient, whose compliance is essential to alter outcome.

Risk Assessment

The concept of risk in obstetrics can be examined at many levels. All the problems that arise in pregnancy, whether common complaints or more hazardous diseases, convey some risk to the pregnancy, depending on how they are managed by the patient and her care provider. Risk assessment has received detailed attention in recent years. It has been shown that most women and infants suffering morbidity and mortality will come from a small segment of women with high-risk factors; by reassessing risk factors before pregnancy, during pregnancy, and again in labor our ability to identify those at highest risk increases.[17] However, previous preterm birth is the most significant risk factor; thus risk scoring of primigravidas is of limited value.[18,19]

It is important to individualize patient care and to be thorough. The initial visit will include a detailed history and physical and laboratory examinations. The initial history requires that the patient be seen in an office setting. She should not be first seen undressed sitting on an examining table.

Preconceptional Education

We have reached a level in prenatal care where the optimal time to assess, manage, and treat many pregnancy conditions and complications is before pregnancy occurs.[20,21] The best time to see a woman for prenatal care is when she is considering pregnancy. At gynecologic visits, patients should be asked about their plans for pregnancy. At that time, much of the risk assessment described later in this chapter can be performed, as well as the basic physical and laboratory evaluations. If there are questions about the history, such as diethylstilbestrol (DES) exposure, family history of fetal anomaly, or previous cesarean delivery, further details can be obtained from family members or the appropriate medical facility. This is the time to draw a rubella titer and immunize the susceptible patient. Patients need to use contraception for 3 months thereafter (see Ch. 38). Toxoplasmosis screening may be indicated at this time. Patients who have negative screens are at risk for congenital toxoplasmosis and should be counseled to avoid risks such as contact with wild felines and ingestion of raw meat. Patients who screen positive can be reassured of lack of risk. Hepatitis B immunization can be given to appropriate patients and HIV testing offered.

Before pregnancy is the time to screen appropriate populations for genetic disease carrier states such as Tay Sachs disease or hemoglobinopathies. Resolution of these issues is much easier and less harried without the time limits placed by an advancing pregnancy. Medical conditions such as anemia, urinary tract infection, or hypothyroidism can be fully evaluated and the woman medically treated before pregnancy. If the patient is obese, weight reduction should be attempted before pregnancy. Patients in whom risks are very serious should be so counseled, and every attempt should be made to let them make a fully informed decision about pregnancy. Often significant risk factors can be treated or managed so as to reduce risk during pregnancy.

The value of prepregnancy counseling needs to be emphasized to all those who treat women at significant risk for pregnancy problems. Women who are followed by other physicians (family physicians, pediatricians, general internists) for such problems as diabetes, hypertension, or systemic lupus erythematosus should be seen, evaluated, and counseled before pregnancy.

There is evidence that for some conditions, such as diabetes mellitus and phenylketonuria, medical disease management before conception can positively influence pregnancy outcome. Medical management to normalize the biochemical environment should be discussed with the patient and appropriate management plans outlined before conception. This is also the time to review drug usage and other practices, such as alcohol ingestion and smoking (see Ch. 10). Advice can be given about avoiding medications in the first trimester, and general advice can be given concerning diet, exercise, and occupational exposures.

Periconceptional supplements with folic acid can reduce the incidence of neural tube defects. In a randomized prospective trial of women with a previously affected child, 4 mg folic acid daily lowered the recurrence risk of neural tube defects by 72 percent.[22] In a prospective trial of women planning their first pregnancy, 0.8 mg of folic acid daily prevented first occurrence neural tube defects and other defects.[23] The Centers for Disease Control and Prevention recommends that all women of childbearing age who are capable of becoming pregnant should consume 0.4 mg of folic acid daily, which is most easily achieved by taking a supplement. For women with a previously affected child, the recommendation is that the patient take 4 mg daily from 4 weeks before conception through the first 3 months of pregnancy.

The importance of gestational age dating can be discussed with the patient. Great precision can be achieved with an accurate menstrual calendar predating pregnancy. Women taking oral contraceptives may be advised to stop their pills at least 1 month before attempting pregnancy to help ascertain cycle length.

The Initial Preconceptional or Prenatal Visit

Social and Demographic Risks

Extremes of age are obstetric risk factors. The pregnant teenager has particular nutritional and emotional needs. She is at special risk for sexually transmitted diseases; it has been shown that she benefits particularly from education in areas of childbearing and contraception. The pregnant woman over age 35 is at increased risk for a chromosomally abnormal child,[24] and she must be so advised. Patients should be asked about family histories of Down syndrome, neural tube defects, hemophilia, hemoglobinopathies, and other birth defects, as well as mental retardation (see Ch. 9). Consultation for genetic counseling and genetic testing, if desired, may be appropriate. The age of the father may be important, as there may be genetic risks to the fetus when the father is older than 55 years.[25] Certain diseases may be race related. Black patients should be screened for sickle cell disease, those of Jewish and French Canadian heritage should be screened for Tay Sachs disease, and those of Mediterranean descent should be screened for β-thalassemia.

Low socioeconomic status should be identified and attempts to improve nutritional and hygienic measures undertaken. Appropriate referral to federal programs, such as that for women, infants, and children (WIC), and to public health nurses can have real benefits. If a patient has a history of previous neonatal death or stillbirth, records should be carefully reviewed so that the correct diagnosis is made and recurrence risk appropriately assessed. A history of drug abuse or recent blood transfusion should be elicited. The history of the patient's mother's reproductive record may lead to discovery of DES exposure. The history of medical illnesses should be detailed and records obtained if possible. A new rapid procedure for diagnosing prenatal disorders in primary care may be useful in pregnancy.[26]

Occupational hazards should be identified. If a patient works in a laboratory with chemicals, for example, she should be advised to limit her exposure. Patients whose occupations require heavy physical exercise or excess stress should be informed that they may need to decrease such activity.

Tobacco, alcohol, and recreational drug use can all adversely affect pregnancy and are a critical part of the history. Specific questions concerning smoking, alcohol, and drugs (prescriptive, over the counter, and illicit) should be asked.[27] Regular screening for alcohol and substance use should be carried out using such tools as the T-ACE questionnaire (Table 7-1)[28] or other simple screening tools, and appropriate directed therapy should be made available to those women who screen positive. Women should be urged to stop smoking prior to pregnancy and to drink not at all or minimally once they are pregnant. Drug addiction confers a particularly high risk, and addicted mothers require specialized care throughout pregnancy (see Ch. 10).

Violence against women is increasingly recognized as a problem that should be addressed, with reports suggesting that abuse occurs during 3 to 8 percent of pregnancies. Questions addressing personal safety and

Table 7-1 Alcohol Abuse Screening: the T-ACE Questionnaire[a]

T	How many drinks does it take to make you feel "high" (can you hold)? (*tolerance;* a positive response consists of two or more drinks)
A	Have people *annoyed* you by criticizing your drinking?
C	Have you ever felt you ought to *cut down* on your drinking?
E	Have you ever had a drink first thing in the morning to steady your nerves or to get rid of a hangover (*eye-opener*)?

Scoring: The tolerance question has substantially more weight (2 points) than the three other questions (1 point each).

[a] These questions were found to be significant identifiers of risk drinking in pregnancy (i.e., alcohol intake potentially sufficient to damage the embryo/fetus).

(From Sokol et al.,[28] with permission.)

violence should be included during the prenatal period and such tools as the Abuse Assessment Score (Fig. 7-3) are recommended.[29]

Medical Risk

Family history of diabetes, hypertension, tuberculosis, seizures, hematologic disorders, multiple pregnancies, congenital abnormalities, and reproductive wastage should be elicited. Often a family history of mental retardation, birth defect, or genetic trait is difficult to elicit; these areas should be emphasized at the initial history. A better history may be obtained if patients are asked to fill out a pre-interview questionnaire or history form. Any significant maternal cardiovascular, renal, or metabolic disease should be defined. Infectious diseases such as urinary tract disease, syphilis, tuberculosis, or herpes genitalis should be identified. Surgical history with special attention to any abdominal or pelvic operations should be noted. A history of previous cesarean birth should include indication, type of uterine incision, and any complications. A copy of the surgical report may be informative. Allergies, particularly drug allergies, should be prominent on the problem list.

Obstetric Risk

Previous obstetric and reproductive history are essential to care in subsequent pregnancy. The gravity and parity should be noted and the outcome for each prior pregnancy recorded in detail. Previous miscarriages confer not only risk and anxiety for another pregnancy loss but can increase the risk of genetic disease as well as preterm delivery.[30]

Previous preterm delivery is strongly associated with recurrence; it is important to delineate the events surrounding the preterm birth. Did the membranes rupture before labor? Were there painful uterine contractions? Was there bleeding? Were there fetal

---

Abuse Assessment Screen (Circle YES or NO for each question)

1. Have you ever been emotionally or physically abused by your partner or someone important to you? . . . . YES   NO

2. Within the last year, have you been hit, slapped, kicked, or otherwise physically hurt by someone? . . . . YES   NO

   If YES, by whom (circle all that apply)

   Husband   Ex-husband   Boyfriend   Stranger   Other   Multiple

   Total No. of times _____

3. Since you've been pregnant, have you been hit, slapped, kicked, or otherwise physically hurt by someone? . . . . YES   NO

   If YES, by whom (circle all that apply)

   Husband   Ex-husband   Boyfriend   Stranger   Other   Multiple

   Total No. of times _____

   Mark the area of injury on a body map

Score each incident according to the following scale:

   1 = Threats of abuse, including use of a weapon
   2 = Slapping, pushing; no injuries and/or lasting pain
   3 = Punching, kicking, bruises, cuts, and/or continuing pain
   4 = Beaten up, severe contusions, burns, broken bones
   5 = Head, internal, and/or permanent injury
   6 = Use of weapon, wound from weapon

(If any of the descriptions for the higher number apply, use the higher number)

4. Within the last year, has anyone forced you to have sexual activities? . . . YES   NO

   If YES, by whom (circle all that apply)

   Husband   Ex-husband   Boyfriend   Stranger   Other   Multiple

   Total No. of times _____

5. Are you afraid of your partner or anyone you listed above? . . . . YES   NO

Fig. 7-3 Determination of frequency and severity of physical abuse during pregnancy. (From McFarlane et al.[29] Used with permission of JAMA, 1992, 267(23):3176–3178. Copyright 1992, American Medical Association.)

abnormalities? What was the neonatal outcome? All these questions are vital in determining the etiology and prognosis of the condition, although specific recommendations will vary and the efficacy of routine prevention programs is not clear.[31] DES exposure, incompetent cervix, and uterine anomalies are all conditions that may be known from a previous pregnancy. Previous fetal macrosomia makes glucose screening essential.

After all the specific questions it is recommended to ask the patient a few simple questions: What important items haven't I asked? What else about you and your pregnancy do I need to know? What problems and questions do you have? Leaving time for open-ended questions is the best way to complete the initial visit.

Physical and Laboratory Evaluation

Physical examination should include a general physical examination as well as a pelvic examination. Baseline height and weight as well as prepregnancy weight are recorded. Special attention should be given to the initial vital signs, cardiac examination, and reflexes, since many healthy young women have not had a physical examination immediately before becoming pregnant. Any physical finding that might have an impact on pregnancy (e.g., DES changes in the cervix) or that might be affected by pregnancy (e.g., mitral valve prolapse) should be defined. Any factor that might become important later in pregnancy in assessing pathology or disease (e.g., reflexes) should be carefully noted. It is particularly important to perform and record a complete physical examination at this initial visit, since less emphasis will be placed on nonobstetric portions of the examination as pregnancy progresses in the absence of specific problems or complaints.

The pelvic examination should focus on the uterine size. Before 12 to 14 weeks, size can give a fairly accurate estimate of gestational age. Papanicolaou smear and culture for gonorrhea and chlamydia are done. The cervix should be carefully palpated, and any deviation from normal should be noted. Clinical pelvimetry should be performed and the clinical impression of adequacy noted. The pelvic examination is limited by examiner and patient variation as well as by obesity. If there is difficulty in examining the uterus, an ultrasound study is indicated.

Basic laboratory studies are routinely performed (Table 7-2). Some studies need not be repeated if recent normal values have been obtained, such as at an initial visit following a preconceptional visit or a recent gynecologic examination. Blood studies should include Rh type and screening for irregular antibodies, hemoglobin level, or hematocrit and serologic tests for syphilis and rubella. A urine sample should be obtained and tested for abnormal protein and glucose levels. Screening for asymptomatic bacteriuria has been traditionally done by urine culture, but screening may be simplified by testing for nitrites and leukocyte esterase.[32] Tuberculosis screening should also be performed in areas of disease prevalence.

The triple screen (α-fetoprotein, human chorionic gonadotropin [hCG], estriol) or maternal serum α-fetoprotein screening is offered at 15 to 16 weeks' gestation to screen for neural tube defects (see Ch. 9).

The laboratory evaluations outlined above are the minimum standard tests. Specific conditions will require further evaluation. A history of thyroid disease will lead to thyroid function testing. Anticonvulsant therapy requires blood level studies to determine adequacy of medication. Identification of problems on screening (e.g., anemia, abnormal glucose screen) will mandate further testing. Screening for varicella has been suggested for women with no known history of chicken pox.

The American College of Obstetricians and Gynecologists has recommended routine screening of all pregnant women for hepatitis B.[33] At minimum, patients at risk for hepatitis should be screened. This includes women of Asian origin, health care workers exposed to blood or blood products, women with previously undiagnosed jaundice or liver disease, parenteral drug abusers, prostitutes, women with tatoos, women with a history of blood transfusion, dialysis or renal transplant patients, women who work or reside in institutions for the retarded, and household contacts of persons infected with hepatitis B. HIV screening in high-risk populations should also be offered, since maternal therapy with AZT can reduce vertical transmission (see Ch. 38).

Recommendations of the Public Health Service Panel[4] for the content of prenatal care are summarized in Table 7-2.

Repeat Prenatal Visits

A plan of visits is outlined to the patient. This has been traditionally every 4 weeks for the first 28 weeks of pregnancy, every 2 to 3 weeks until 36 weeks, and weekly thereafter, if the pregnancy progresses normally.[34,35] The Public Health Service Panel[4] recently suggested that this number of visits can be decreased, especially in parous, healthy women, and a recent study[36] suggests that this can be done safely. If there are any complications, the intervals can be increased appropriately. For example, patients with hypertensive disease may require weekly visits. Fetal heart tones can be documented before the 12th week by Doppler devices and generally by the 20th week by Hillis-Delee stethoscope and this information used for gestational dating purposes.

At regular visits, the patient is weighed, the blood pressure is recorded, and the presence of edema is evaluated. Fundal height is regularly measured with a tape measure, fetal heart tones are recorded, and fetal position is noted. The goal of subsequent pregnancy visits is to assess fetal growth and maternal well-being. In addition, at each prenatal visit, time should be allowed for the following questions: Do you have any problems? Do you have any questions? Family members should be encouraged to come to prenatal visits, ask questions, and participate to the degree that the patient wishes.

A pelvic examination is usually only performed on the first visit. In patients at risk of prematurity or in those with a history of DES exposure, however, frequent cervical checks may reveal premature dilation or effacement.

Further laboratory evaluations are routinely performed at 28 weeks, when the hemoglobin or hematocrit and Rh type and the screen for antibodies, as well as the serologic test for syphilis and possibly HIV testing, can be repeated. If the patient is Rh negative and unsensitized, she should receive RhIg prophylaxis at this time. A glucose screening test for diabetes is also appropriately performed at this time (see Ch. 31), and routine fetal movement counting can begin using an organized system (Fig. 7-4).[37] At 36 weeks, a repeat hematocrit especially in those women with anemia or

Table 7-2   Recommendations for All Women for Prenatal Care

	Preconception or First Visit	Weeks								
		6–8[a]	14–16	24–28	32	36	38	39	40	41
History										
Medical, including genetic	X									
Psychosocial	X									
Update medical and psychosocial		X	X	X	X	X	X	X	X	X
Physical examination										
General	X									
Blood pressure	X	X	X	X	X	X	X	X	X	X
Height	X									
Weight	X	X	X	X	X	X	X	X	X	X
Height and weight profile	X									
Pelvic examination and pelvimetry	X	X								
Breast examination	X	X								
Fundal height			X	X	X	X	X	X	X	X
Fetal position and heart rate			X	X	X	X	X	X	X	X
Cervical examination	X									
Laboratory tests										
Hemoglobin or hematocrit	X	X		X		X				
Rh factor, type blood	X									
Antibody screen	X			X						
Pap smear	X									
Diabetic screen				X						
MSAFP			X							
Urine										
Dipstick	X									
Protein	X									
Sugar	X									
Culture		X								
Infections										
Rubella titer	X									
Syphilis test	X									
Gonococcal culture	X	X				X				
Hepatitis B	X									
HIV (offered)	X	X								
Toxoplasmosis	X									
Illicit drug screen (offered)	X									
Genetic screen	X									

[a] If preconception care has preceded.

at risk for peripartum hemorrhage (multipara, repeat cesarean) may be performed. Also appropriate cultures for sexually transmitted disease (gonorrhea, chlamydia) should be obtained as indicated in the third trimester.

After 41 weeks from the last menstrual period, the patient should be entered into a screening program for fetal well-being, which may include electronic monitoring tests or ultrasound evaluation (see Ch. 26).

Intercurrent Problems

It is the practice in prenatal care to evaluate the pregnant patient for the development of certain complications. Inherent in these checks is surveillance for intervening problems, an important one being preeclampsia. If a patient shows a tendency to blood pressure elevation at 28 weeks, for example, she should be seen again in a week, not a month. Blood pressure will change physiologically in response to pregnancy, but development of hypertension must be recognized and evaluation and hospitalization appropriately instituted.

Weight gain in pregnancy has been shown to be an important correlate of fetal weight gain and is therefore closely monitored. Too little weight gain should lead to an evaluation of nutritional factors and an assessment of associated fetal growth. Excess weight gain is one of the first signs of fluid retention, but it may also reflect increased dietary intake or decreased activity. Dependent edema is physiologic in pregnancy, but generalized or facial edema can be a first sign of disease. It is critical here, as in all areas, for the practitioner to understand the normal changes associated

Fetal Movement Record

HOLLISTER® maternal/newborn RECORD SYSTEM

PATIENT IDENTIFICATION

Patient's name ______________________

____

____

G	T	PT	A	L	LMP mo / day / yr	EDC mo / day / yr	QUICKENING DATE mo / day / yr	START DATE mo / day / yr	NO. OF WEEKS PREGNANT

PATIENT INSTRUCTIONS ON: mo / day / yr BY: BABY'S PHYSICIAN:

IMPORTANT TELEPHONE NUMBERS

DAY/OB CLINIC ______________________

FETAL ASSESSMENT CENTER ______________________

NIGHT/LABOR AND DELIVERY: ______________________

COMMENTS: ______________________

HOW TO USE THIS RECORD

Counting fetal movements is one way in which you may play an important role in checking the health of your baby. By counting and recording the number of movements made by your baby each day, you create a profile of your baby's activity during the final weeks of your pregnancy.

Instructions for completing this record:

Every day you will note on the record the time you start counting. Beginning at this time, you must keep a count of the number of times your baby kicks or moves until you reach a total of ___ kicks or movements. When you have counted ___ kicks or movements, note on the record the amount of time required for the baby to do this by filling in the square that matches this amount of time. For example, if you started counting Wednesday at 7:30 a.m., and your baby kicked or moved 10 times in 3 hours, fill in the square on the record as shown at the right. There can be a wide variation in the amount babies normally move and also in a woman's perception of those movements. If you experience less than ___ movements after ___ hours counting, simply fill in the actual number of kicks or movements in the shaded column 11.

TAKEN TO FEEL MOVEMENTS	M	T	W	T	F
START TIME			7:30		
1					
2					
3			■		
4					
5					

IMPORTANT

If you experience less than ___ kicks or movements per day for two days in a row, OR if your baby does not kick or move at all for ___ hours in any one day, IMMEDIATELY NOTIFY YOUR DOCTOR OR HOSPITAL LABOR AND DELIVERY STAFF at one of the above listed telephone numbers. This may be an indication that the baby is having a difficult time and needs further testing, but the only way to be certain is to check your baby at the hospital or clinic.

FOLD ON THIS LINE

BEGIN HERE

HOURS TAKEN TO FEEL ___ MOVEMENTS	WEEK #							WEEK #							WEEK #							WEEK #							WEEK #							WEEK #						
	M	T	W	T	F	S	S	M	T	W	T	F	S	S	M	T	W	T	F	S	S	M	T	W	T	F	S	S	M	T	W	T	F	S	S	M	T	W	T	F	S	S
START TIME																																										
1																																										
2																																										
3																																										
4																																										
5																																										
6																																										
7																																										
8																																										
9																																										
10																																										
11																																										

CONTINUE HERE

HOURS TAKEN TO FEEL ___ MOVEMENTS	WEEK #							WEEK #							WEEK #							WEEK #							WEEK #							WEEK #						
	M	T	W	T	F	S	S	M	T	W	T	F	S	S	M	T	W	T	F	S	S	M	T	W	T	F	S	S	M	T	W	T	F	S	S	M	T	W	T	F	S	S
START TIME																																										
1																																										
2																																										
3																																										
4																																										
5																																										
6																																										
7																																										
8																																										
9																																										
10																																										
11																																										

Hollister.
HOLLISTER INCORPORATED, 2000 HOLLISTER DR., LIBERTYVILLE, IL 60048
* TRADEMARK OF HOLLISTER INCORPORATED

5852 1088

Fig. 7-4 Fetal movement record. (Copyright 1988 Hollister Inc., Libertyville, IL. Reprinted with permission.)

with pregnancy in order to accept and explain the normal, but also to manage aggressively any abnormal changes.

Proteinuria reflects urinary tract disease, generally either infection or glomerular dysfunction, possibly the result of preeclampsia. Urinary tract infection should be looked for, and the degree of protein quantitated in a 24-hour urine collection.

Glycosuria, while common because of increased glucose filtered through the kidney in pregnancy, warrants evaluation for diabetes, if this is not being checked routinely.

Fetal abnormalities are usually first detected by deviation from the clinical expectation. In some conditions, risk of fetal anomaly will be so high as to prompt some kind of baseline screening or testing (e.g., amniocentesis, ultrasound, fetal echocardiography). At other times, risk only becomes evident during the course of prenatal care. Growth retardation and macrosomia can often be suspected clinically, usually on the basis of an abnormality in fundal growth. For the patient who has a history of these conditions or other predisposing factors, such as hypertension, renal disease, or diabetes, particular vigilance is in order. Excess amniotic fluid is another condition that can be clinically detected, and an etiology for the hydramnios should be sought. In addition to maternal conditions, hydramnios may be due to fetal disease that can also be defined using ultrasound and that may alter management of the pregnancy.

The Prenatal Record

Prenatal care should be documented by a prenatal record of good quality (Fig. 7-5). Many of the advances in risk assessment and in regionalization result directly from an improvement in this record. Technology allows sophisticated recording, display, and retrieval (often computer-based) of prenatal care records, but quality relies on accurate compiling and recording of the information. The record must be complete, yet simple; directive, but flexible; transmittable, legible, and able to display necessary data rapidly. European nations often have one record for uniform care; many states and regions have adopted records to permit internal consistency, and the American College of Obstetricians and Gynecologists has recently developed the record reproduced in Figure 7-5.

The commonly used records accurately reflect the following:

1. Demographic data, obstetric history
2. Medical and family history, including genetic screening
3. Baseline physical examination, with emphasis on gynecologic examination
4. Menstrual history, especially last normal menstrual period
5. Record of individual visits
6. Routine laboratory data
7. Problem list
8. Space for special notations and plans

These records must be made available to consultants, and they should be available at the facility where delivery is planned. If transfer is expected, a copy of the prenatal record should accompany the patient.

Prenatal Education

Patient education leads to better self-care. As maternal and neonatal outcomes improve, efforts become more sophisticated to improve understanding, involvement, and satisfaction with pregnancy and the perinatal period. In this area, more than any other, the options for paramedical support have expanded. Practitioners and patients have access to a vast array of support persons and groups to assist and advise in the pregnancy and subsequent parenthood. The wise practitioner stays abreast of these advances and integrates them into practice. Patients should be educated about care options and participate in decision-making.

Drugs and Teratogens

At the preconceptional or first prenatal visit, recommendations for nonpharmacologic remedies for common ailments can be given. This can often be integrated into a discussion of the common side effects of pregnancy. Because of widespread use of over-the-counter drugs, the patient should be warned to take only those drugs specifically approved or prescribed to her by her practitioner (see Ch. 10).

Radiologic Studies

Dental and radiologic diagnostic procedures should be performed during pregnancy when they are indicated. Dental restorative work especially should be performed to allow optimal maternal nutrition. Elective radiologic studies can safely be delayed until completion of the pregnancy.

Nutrition

One of the earliest purposes of prenatal care was to counsel and ensure that women received adequate nutrition for pregnancy. The health care provider may be influential in correcting inappropriate dietary habits. Strict vegetarians may need supplemental vitamin B_{12}.

Patient Addressograph

ACOG ANTEPARTUM RECORD

DATE _____

NAME _____
      LAST   FIRST   MIDDLE

ID # _____ HOSPITAL OF DELIVERY _____

NEWBORN'S PHYSICIAN _____ REFERRED BY _____

FINAL EDD_____

BIRTH DATE	AGE	RACE	MARITAL STATUS	ADDRESS:
MO DAY YR			S M W D SEP	

OCCUPATION	EDUCATION	ZIP: PHONE: (H) (O)
☐ HOMEMAKER	(LAST GRADE COMPLETED)	INSURANCE CARRIER/MEDICAID #
☐ OUTSIDE WORK		
☐ STUDENT Type of Work		

HUSBAND/FATHER OF BABY:	PHONE:	EMERGENCY CONTACT:	PHONE:

TOTAL PREG	FULL TERM	PREMATURE	AB, INDUCED	AB, SPONTANEOUS	ECTOPICS	MULTIPLE BIRTHS	LIVING

MENSTRUAL HISTORY

LMP ☐ DEFINITE ☐ APPROXIMATE (MONTH KNOWN)   MENSES MONTHLY ☐ YES ☐ NO   FREQUENCY: Q _____ DAYS   MENARCHE _____ (AGE ONSET)

☐ UNKNOWN ☐ NORMAL AMOUNT/DURATION   PRIOR MENSES _____ DATE   ON BCP'S AT CONCEPT. ☐ YES ☐ NO   hCG + _____ / _____ / _____

☐ FINAL _____

PAST PREGNANCIES (LAST SIX)

DATE MO / YR	GA WEEKS	LENGTH OF LABOR	BIRTH WEIGHT	SEX M/F	TYPE DELIVERY	ANES.	PLACE OF DELIVERY	PRETERM LABOR YES / NO	COMMENTS / COMPLICATIONS

PAST MEDICAL HISTORY

	O Neg + Pos.	DETAIL POSITIVE REMARKS INCLUDE DATE & TREATMENT		O Neg + Pos.	DETAIL POSITIVE REMARKS INCLUDE DATE & TREATMENT
1. DIABETES			16. D (Rh) SENSITIZED		
2. HYPERTENSION			17. PULMONARY (TB, ASTHMA)		
3. HEART DISEASE			18. ALLERGIES (DRUGS)		
4. AUTOIMMUNE DISORDER			19. BREAST		
5. KIDNEY DISEASE / UTI			20. GYN SURGERY		
6. NEUROLOGIC/EPILEPSY					
7. PSYCHIATRIC			21. OPERATIONS / HOSPITALIZATIONS (YEAR & REASON)		
8. HEPATITIS / LIVER DISEASE					
9. VARICOSITIES / PHLEBITIS					
10. THYROID DYSFUNCTION			22. ANESTHETIC COMPLICATIONS		
11. TRAUMA/VIOLENCE			23. HISTORY OF ABNORMAL PAP		
12. HISTORY OF BLOOD TRANSFUS.			24. UTERINE ANOMALY/DES		

	AMT/DAY PREPREG	AMT/DAY PREG	#YRS USE			
				25. INFERTILITY		
13. TOBACCO				26. RELEVANT FAMILY HISTORY		
14. ALCOHOL						
15. STREET DRUGS				27. OTHER		

COMMENTS: _____

_____

_____

Fig. 7-5 **ACOG antepartum record.** (Copyright 1994, The American College of Obstetricians and Gynecologists, Washington, DC. Reprinted with permission.) (*Figure continues.*)

Patient Addressograph

SYMPTOMS SINCE LMP

GENETICS SCREENING/TERATOLOGY COUNSELING
INCLUDES PATIENT, BABY'S FATHER, OR ANYONE IN EITHER FAMILY WITH:

	YES	NO			YES	NO
1. PATIENT'S AGE ≥ 35 YEARS				10. HUNTINGTON CHOREA		
2. THALASSEMIA (ITALIAN, GREEK, MEDITERRANEAN, OR ASIAN BACKGROUND): MCV < 80				11. MENTAL RETARDATION		
				IF YES, WAS PERSON TESTED FOR FRAGILE X?		
3. NEURAL TUBE DEFECT (MENINGOMYELOCELE, SPINA BIFIDA, OR ANENCEPHALY)				12. OTHER INHERITED GENETIC OR CHROMOSOMAL DISORDER		
4. DOWN SYNDROME				13. PATIENT OR BABY'S FATHER HAD A CHILD WITH BIRTH DEFECTS NOT LISTED ABOVE		
5. TAY–SACHS (EG, JEWISH, CAJUN, FR. CANADIAN)						
6. SICKLE CELL DISEASE OR TRAIT (AFRICAN)				14. ≥3 FIRST-TRIMESTER SPONTANEOUS ABORTIONS, OR A STILLBIRTH		
7. HEMOPHILIA				15. MEDICATIONS/STREET DRUGS/ALCOHOL SINCE LAST MENSTRUAL PERIOD		
8. MUSCULAR DYSTROPHY				IF YES, AGENT(S):		
9. CYSTIC FIBROSIS				16. ANY OTHER		

COMMENTS/COUNSELING: _____

_____

_____

_____

INFECTION HISTORY	YES	NO			YES	NO
1. HIGH RISK FOR HIV				4. PATIENT OR PARTNER HAS HISTORY OF GENITAL HERPES		
2. HIGH RISK HEPATITIS B/IMMUNIZED?				5. RASH OR VIRAL ILLNESS SINCE LAST MENSTRUAL PERIOD		
3. LIVE WITH SOMEONE WITH TB OR EXPOSED TO TB				6. HISTORY OF STD, GC, CHLAMYDIA, HPV, SYPHILIS		
				7. OTHER (SEE COMMENTS)		

COMMENTS: _____

_____

_____ INTERVIEWER'S SIGNATURE _____

INITIAL PHYSICAL EXAMINATION

DATE _____ / _____ / _____   PREPREGNANCY WEIGHT _____   HEIGHT _____   BP _____

1. HEENT	☐ NORMAL	☐ ABNORMAL	12. VULVA	☐ NORMAL	☐ CONDYLOMA	☐ LESIONS	
2. FUNDI	☐ NORMAL	☐ ABNORMAL	13. VAGINA	☐ NORMAL	☐ INFLAMMATION	☐ DISCHARGE	
3. TEETH	☐ NORMAL	☐ ABNORMAL	14. CERVIX	☐ NORMAL	☐ INFLAMMATION	☐ LESIONS	
4. THYROID	☐ NORMAL	☐ ABNORMAL	15. UTERUS SIZE	_____ WEEKS		☐ FIBROIDS	
5. BREASTS	☐ NORMAL	☐ ABNORMAL	16. ADNEXA	☐ NORMAL	☐ MASS		
6. LUNGS	☐ NORMAL	☐ ABNORMAL	17. RECTUM	☐ NORMAL	☐ ABNORMAL		
7. HEART	☐ NORMAL	☐ ABNORMAL	18. DIAGONAL CONJUGATE	☐ REACHED	☐ NO	_____ CM	
8. ABDOMEN	☐ NORMAL	☐ ABNORMAL	19. SPINES	☐ AVERAGE	☐ PROMINENT	☐ BLUNT	
9. EXTREMITIES	☐ NORMAL	☐ ABNORMAL	20. SACRUM	☐ CONCAVE	☐ STRAIGHT	☐ ANTERIOR	
10. SKIN	☐ NORMAL	☐ ABNORMAL	21. SUBPUBIC ARCH	☐ NORMAL	☐ WIDE	☐ NARROW	
11. LYMPH NODES	☐ NORMAL	☐ ABNORMAL	22. GYNECOID PELVIC TYPE	☐ YES	☐ NO		

COMMENTS (Number and explain abnormals): _____

_____

_____

_____ EXAM BY _____

Fig. 7-5 (Continued).

ACOG ANTEPARTUM RECORD

NAME _____
       LAST   FIRST   MIDDLE

DRUG ALLERGY:
ANESTHESIA CONSULT PLANNED   ☐ YES   ☐ NO

PROBLEMS/PLANS	MEDICATION LIST:	Start date	Stop date
1.	1.		
2.	2.		
3.	3.		
4.	4.		

EDD CONFIRMATION

INITIAL EDD:

LMP   ____ / ____ / ____   = EDD ____ / ____ / ____

INITIAL EXAM   ____ / ____ / ____ = ____ WKS = EDD ____ / ____ / ____

ULTRASOUND   ____ / ____ / ____ = ____ WKS = EDD ____ / ____ / ____

INITIAL EDD   ____ / ____ / ____   INITIALED BY _____

18–20-WEEK EDD UPDATE:

QUICKENING   ____ / ____ / ____ +22 WKS = ____ / ____ / ____

FUNDAL HT. AT UMBIL. ____ / ____ / ____ +20 WKS = ____ / ____ / ____

FHT W/ FETOSCOPE   ____ / ____ / ____ +20 WKS = ____ / ____ / ____

ULTRASOUND   ____ / ____ / ____ = ___ WKS = ____ / ____ / ____

FINAL EDD   ____ / ____ / ____   INITIALED BY _____

VISIT DATE
____
(YEAR)

Column headers (diagonal): WEEKS GEST. (BEST EST.) | FUNDAL HEIGHT (CM) | PRESENTATION | FHR | FETAL MOVEMENT | PRETERM LABOR SIGNS/SYMPTOMS: += PRESENT 0=ABSENT | CERVIX EXAM (DIL./EFF./STA.) | BLOOD PRESSURE | EDEMA | WEIGHT | URINE (GLUCOSE/ALBUMIN) | NEXT APPOINTMENT | PROVIDER (INITIALS)

8–18 WEEKS CVS/ AMNIO/ MSAFP

24–28 WEEKS GLUCOSE SCREEN/ RhIG

COMMENTS: _____
_____
_____
_____

Fig. 7-5 *(Continued)*.

LABORATORY AND EDUCATION

Patient Addressograph

INITIAL LABS	DATE	RESULT	REVIEWED
BLOOD TYPE	/ /	A　　B　　AB　　O	
D (Rh) TYPE	/ /		
ANTIBODY SCREEN	/ /		
HCT/HGB	/ /	_____ % _____ g/dl	
PAP SMEAR	/ /	NORMAL / ABNORMAL / _____	
RUBELLA	/ /		
VDRL	/ /		
URINE CULTURE/SCREEN	/ /		
HBsAg	/ /		

OPTIONAL LABS	DATE	RESULT	
HIV	/ /		
HGB ELECTROPHORESIS	/ /	AA　AS　SS　AC　SC　AF　↑A$_2$	
CHLAMYDIA	/ /		
PPD	/ /		
GC	/ /		
SICKLE CELL SCREEN	/ /		
TAY–SACHS	/ /		
OTHER			

COMMENTS/ADDITIONAL LABS

8–18-WEEK LABS (WHEN INDICATED/ELECTED)	DATE	RESULT	
ULTRASOUND	/ /		
MSAFP/MULTIPLE MARKERS	/ /		
DOWN SYNDROME	/ /		
AMNIO/CVS	/ /		
KARYOTYPE	/ /	46, XX OR 46, XY / OTHER_____	
AMNIOTIC FLUID (AFP)	/ /	NORMAL_____ ABNORMAL_____	

24–28-WEEK LABS (WHEN INDICATED)	DATE	RESULT	
HCT/HGB	/ /	_____ % _____ g/dl	
DIABETES SCREEN	/ /	1 HR_____	
GTT (IF SCREEN ABNORMAL)	/ /	_____FBS _____1 HR _____2 HR _____3 HR	
D (Rh) ANTIBODY SCREEN	/ /		
D IMMUNE GLOBULIN (RhIG) GIVEN (28 WKS)	/ /	SIGNATURE _____	

32–36-WEEK LABS (WHEN INDICATED)	DATE	RESULT	
ULTRASOUND	/ /		
VDRL	/ /		
GC	/ /		
HCT/HGB (RECOMMENDED)	/ /	_____ % _____ g/dl	
CHLAMYDIA	/ /		

PLANS/EDUCATION (COUNSELED ☐)

☐ ANESTHESIA PLANS _____

☐ TOXOPLASMOSIS PRECAUTIONS (CATS/RAW MEAT) _____

☐ CHILDBIRTH CLASSES _____

☐ PHYSICAL/SEXUAL ACTIVITY _____

☐ LABOR SIGNS _____

☐ NUTRITION COUNSELING _____

☐ BREAST OR BOTTLE FEEDING _____

☐ NEWBORN CAR SEAT _____

☐ POSTPARTUM BIRTH CONTROL _____

☐ ENVIRONMENTAL/WORK HAZARDS _____

☐ TUBAL STERILIZATION _____

☐ VBAC COUNSELING _____

☐ CIRCUMCISION _____

☐ TRAVEL _____

☐ LIFESTYLE, TOBACCO, ALCOHOL _____

REQUESTS _____

_____

TUBAL STERILIZATION　　DATE　　INITIALS

CONSENT SIGNED　_____ / _____ / _____　_____

AA128　12345/87654

Fig. 7-5 (Continued).

Occasionally, consultation with a registered dietitian may be necessary when there is poor compliance or a special medical need such as diabetes mellitus.

The U.S. Department of Agriculture has published the new food guide pyramid.[38] Americans are encouraged to eat 6 to 11 servings per day of bread, cereal, rice, and pasta; three to five servings per day of vegetables; two to four servings per day of fruit; two to three servings per day of milk, yogurt and cheese; and two to three servings per day of meat, poultry, fish, beans, eggs, and nuts. Fats, oils, and sweets should be used sparingly. Pregnant women need three servings per day of dairy products, a serving being a cup of milk or yogurt, 1 1/2 oz. of natural cheese, or 2 oz. processed cheese.

Dietary allowances for most substances increase during pregnancy. According to the 1989 RDAS, only the recommendations for iron, folic acid, and vitamin D double during gestation.[39] The RDA for calcium and phosphorus increase by one-half; the RDA for pyridoxine and thiamine increase by about one-third. The RDA for protein, zinc, and riboflavin increase by about one-fourth. The RDA for all other nutrients except vitamin A increase by less than 20 percent (Tables 7-3 & 7-4) and vitamin A not at all, as that is felt to be stored adequately. All of these nutrients, with the exception of iron, are supplied by a well-balanced diet.

The National Academy of Sciences currently recommends that 30 mg of ferrous iron supplements be given to pregnant women daily, since the iron content of the habitual American diet and the iron stores of many women are not sufficient to provide the increased iron required during pregnancy. For those at high nutritional risk, such as some adolescents, those with multiple gestation, heavy cigarette smokers, and drug and alcohol abusers, a vitamin/mineral supplement should be given. Increased iron is needed both for the fetal needs and the increased maternal blood volume. Thus, iron-containing foods should also be encouraged. Iron is found in liver, red meats, eggs, dried beans, leafy green vegetables, whole-grain enriched bread and cereal, and dried fruits. The 30 mg iron supplement is contained in approximately 150 mg of ferrous sulfate, 300 mg of ferrous gluconate, or 100 mg of ferrous fumarate. Taking iron between meals on an empty stomach will facilitate its absorption.

Since women of higher socioeconomic status have better reproductive performance and fewer low-birth-weight babies than do women of lower socioeconomic status, and since they also consume more protein, it is probably prudent to continue to recommend a generous amount of dietary protein. However, it has not been documented that protein supplementation will improve pregnancy outcome.[40] Acute caloric restriction in a well-nourished population such as occurred during the Dutch famine of 1944 to 1945 caused the average birth weight to drop about 250 g, yet no adverse effect on long-term outcome was observed. These mothers

Table 7-3   1989 Recommended Dietary Allowances

	Nonpregnant Women				Lactation (Months)	
	15–18	19–24	25–50	Pregnancy	1–6	7–12
Calories (kcal)						
Protein (g)	44	46	50	60	65	62
Vitamin A (μg RE)	800	800	800	800	1,300	1,200
Vitamin D (μg)	10	5	5	10	10	10
Vitamin E (mg TE)	8	8	8	10	12	11
Vitamin C (mg)	60	60	60	70	95	90
Thiamin (mg)	1.1	1.1	1.1	1.5	1.6	1.6
Riboflavin (mg)	1.3	1.3	1.3	1.6	1.8	1.7
Niacin (mg NE)	15	15	15	17	20	20
Vitamin B_6 (mg)	1.5	1.6	1.6	2.2	2.1	2.1
Folate (μg)	180	180	180	400	280	260
Vitamin B_{12} (μg)	2.0	2.0	2.0	2.2	2.6	2.6
Calcium (mg)	1,200	1,200	800	1,200	1,200	1,200
Phosphorus (mg)	1,200	1,200	800	1,200	1,200	1,200
Magnesium (mg)	300	280	280	320	355	340
Iron (mg)	15	15	15	30	15	15
Zinc (mg)	12	12	12	15	19	16
Iodine (μg)	150	150	150	175	200	200
Selenium μg	50	55	55	65	75	75

(Data from National Academy of Sciences.[39])

Table 7-4   Summary of Recommended Dietary Allowances for Women Aged ≥25–50 Years, Changes from Nonpregnant to Pregnant, and Food Sources

Nutrient	Nonpregnant	Pregnant	Percent Increase	Dietary Sources
Energy (kcal)	2,200	2,500	+13.6	Proteins, carbohydrates, fats
Protein (g)	50	60	+20	Meats, fish, poultry, dairy
Calcium (mg)	800	1,200	+50	Dairy products
Phosphorus (mg)	800	1,200	+50	Meats
Magnesium (mg)	280	320	+14.3	Seafood, legumes, grains
Iron (mg)	15	30	+100	Meats, eggs, grains
Zinc (mg)	12	15	+25	Meats, seafood, eggs
Iodine (μg)	150	175	+16.7	Iodized salt, seafood
Vitamin A (μg RE)	800	800	0	Dark green, yellow, or orange fruits and vegetables, liver
Vitamin D (IU)	200	400	+100	Fortified dairy products
Thiamin (mg)	1.1	1.5	+36.3	Enriched grains, pork
Riboflavin (mg)	1.3	1.6	+23	Meats, liver, enriched grains
Pyridoxine (mg)	1.6	2.2	+37.5	Meats, liver, enriched grains
Niacin (mg NE)	15	17	+13.3	Meats, nuts, legumes
Vitamin B_{12} (μg)	2.0	2.2	+10	Meats
Folic acid (μg)	180	400	+122	Leafy vegetables, liver
Vitamin C (mg)	60	70	+16.7	Citrus fruits, tomatoes
Selenium (μg)	55	65	+18.2	

(From National Academy of Sciences.[39])

ate a calorie-restricted balanced diet in their second and third trimesters.

Weight Gain

The total weight gain recommended in pregnancy is 25 to 35 lb for normal women.[41] Underweight women may gain up to 40 lb, and overweight women should limit weight gain to 15 to 25 lb. About 2 to 3 lb are from increased fluid volume, 3 to 4 lb from increased blood volume, 1 to 2 lb from breast enlargement, 2 lb from enlargement of the uterus, and 2 lb from amniotic fluid. At term, the infant weighs approximately 6 to 8 lb and the placenta 1 to 2 lb. A 4- to 6-lb increase in maternal stores of fat and protein are important for lactation. Usually 3 to 6 lb are gained in the first trimester and 1/2 to 1 lb/week in the last two trimesters of pregnancy.

If the patient does not show a 10-lb weight gain by midpregnancy, her nutritional status should be reviewed. Inadequate weight gain is associated with an increased risk of a low-birth-weight infant (Fig. 7-6). Inadequate weight gain seems to have its greatest effect in woman who are of low or normal weight before pregnancy. Underweight mothers must gain more weight during pregnancy to produce infants of normal weight. Patients should be cautioned against weight loss during pregnancy. Total weight gain in the obese can be modified downward to 15 lb, but less weight gain is associated with lack of expansion of plasma volume and the risk of intrauterine growth retardation.

When excess weight gain is noted, an assessment for fluid retention is also performed. In the assessment of edema, some dependent edema in the legs is normal as pregnancy advances because of venous compression by the weight of the uterus. Elevation of the feet and bedrest on the left side will help correct this problem. Turning the patient from her back to her left side increases venous return from the legs as the pressure on the vena cava is relieved. This maneuver increases the effective circulating blood volume, cardiac output, and thus the blood flow to the kidney. A diuresis will follow as well as increased blood flow to the uterus.

Limitation of fluids will neither prevent nor correct fluid retention. Salt is not restricted, although patients with hypertension may be advised to decrease salt load.

Rest

During the first trimester, patients are often more tired and should be advised to go to bed earlier or to try to take a nap during the day, if possible. Fatigue often lessens in the second trimester, but, in general, most patients need additional rest during pregnancy.

Activity and Employment

Most patients are able to maintain their normal activity levels in pregnancy. Mothers tolerate pregnancy with considerable physical activity, such as looking after small children, but heavy lifting and excessive physical activity should be avoided. Modification of activity level as the pregnancy progresses is seldom needed, except if the job involves physical danger. Recreational exercises

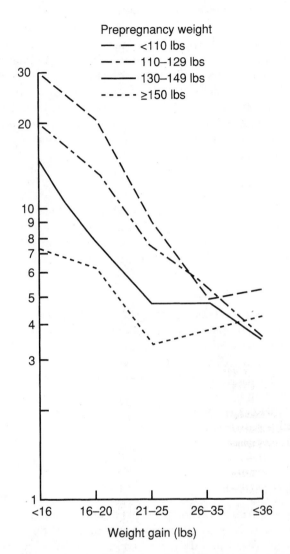

Prepregnancy weight
— — <110 lbs
—·— 110–129 lbs
——— 130–149 lbs
······ ≥150 lbs

Weight gain (lbs)

Fig. 7-6 Percentage of liveborn infants of low birth weight by maternal weight gain during pregnancy according to the mother's prepregnancy weight. Note: Low birth weight is defined as birth weight of less than 2,500 g or 5 pounds, 8 ounces. (From the 1980 National Natality Survey—United States.[58])

should be encouraged, such as those available in prenatal exercise classes. The patient should be counseled to discontinue activity whenever she experiences discomfort.

Healthy pregnant women may work until their delivery, if the job presents hazards no greater than those encountered in daily life. Strenuous physical exercise, standing for prolonged periods, and work on industrial machines as well as other adverse environmental factors may be associated with increased risk of poor pregnancy outcome, and these should be modified as necessary.[42,43]

Travel

The patient should be advised against prolonged sitting during car or airplane travel because of the risk of venous stasis and possible thromboembolism. The usual recommendation is a maximum of 6 hours per day driving, with stopping at least every 2 hours for 10 minutes to allow the patient to walk around and increase venous return from the legs. Support stockings are also recommended.

The patient should be instructed to wear her seatbelt during car travel, but under the abdomen as pregnancy advances. It may also be helpful to take pillows along in a car to increase comfort.

If the patient is traveling a significant distance, it might be helpful for her to carry a copy of her medical record with her in case an emergency arises in a strange city. She could also check into the medical facilities in the area or perhaps obtain the name of an obstetrician in the event of a problem.

Immunizations

Because of a theoretical risk to the fetus, pregnant women or women likely to become pregnant should not be given live, attenuated-virus vaccines. Yellow fever and oral polio may be given to women exposed to maternal infection. Despite theoretical risks, no evidence of congenital rubella syndrome in infants born to mothers inadvertently given rubella vaccine has been reported. Measles, mumps, and rubella viruses are not transmitted by those immunized and can be given to children of pregnant women. There is no evidence of fetal risk from inactivated virus vaccines, bacterial vaccines, toxoids, or tetanus immunoglobulin, which should be administered if appropriate.

Nausea and Vomiting in Pregnancy

Nonpharmacologic measures are usually recommended initially to treat nausea and vomiting in early pregnancy. Patients should avoid eating greasy or spicy foods. In addition, frequent small feedings in order to keep some food in the stomach at all times is helpful. A protein snack at night is advised, and the patient is instructed to keep crackers at her bedside so that she can have these before arising in the morning. Drug therapy for nausea in pregnancy is covered in Chapter 10.

Heartburn

Heartburn is a common complaint in pregnancy because of relaxation of the esophageal sphincter. Overeating contributes to this problem, as do spicy foods. The patient should be advised to save part of her meal for later if she is experiencing postprandial heartburn and also not to eat immediately before lying down. Pillows at bedtime may help. If necessary, antacids may be prescribed. Liquid antacids coat the esophageal lining more effectively than do tablets.

Hemorrhoids

Hemorrhoids are varicose veins of the rectum. Since straining during bowel movements contributes to their aggravation, avoidance of constipation is preventive, and prolonged sitting should also be avoided. Hemorrhoids will often regress after delivery but usually will not disappear completely.

Constipation

Constipation is physiologic during pregnancy with decreased bowel transit time, and the stool may be hardened. Dietary modification with increased bulk such as with fresh fruit and vegetables and plenty of water can usually help this problem significantly. Constipation is aggravated by the addition of iron supplementation; if dietary measures are inadequate, patients may require stool softeners. Additional dietary fibers such as Metamucil (psyllium hydrophilic muciloid) or surface-active agents such as Colace (docusate) are recommended. Laxatives are rarely necessary.

Urinary Frequency

Often during the first 3 months of pregnancy, the growing uterus places increased pressure on the bladder. Urinary frequency usually will improve as the uterus rises out of the pelvis by the second trimester. However, as the head engages near the time of delivery, urinary frequency may return as the head presses against the bladder. If the patient experiences pain with urination, it is appropriate to check for infection.

Round Ligament Pain

Frequently, patients will notice sharp groin pains due to spasm of the round ligaments associated with movement. This is more frequently felt on the right side due to the usual dextrorotation of the uterus. The pain may be helped by application of local heat such as with hot soaks or a heating pad. Patients may awaken at night with this pain after having suddenly rolled over in their sleep without realizing it. During the daytime, however, modification of activity with gradual rising and sitting down, as well as avoidance of sudden movement, will decrease problems with this type of pain. Analgesics are rarely necessary.

Syncope

Compression of the veins in the legs from the advancing size of the uterus places patients at risk of venous pooling associated with prolonged standing. This may lead to syncope. Measures to avoid this possibility include wearing support stockings and exercising the calves to increase venous return. In later pregnancy, patients may have problems with supine hypotension, a distinct problem when undergoing a medical evaluation or an ultrasound examination. A left lateral tilt position with wedging below the right hip will help keep the weight of the pregnancy off the inferior vena cava.

Backache

Backache can be prevented to a large degree by avoidance of excessive weight gain. Exercises to strengthen back muscles can also be helpful. Posture is important, and sensible shoes, not high heels, should be worn.

Sexual Activity

No restriction need generally be placed on sexual intercourse. The patient is instructed that pregnancy may cause changes in comfort and sexual desire. Frequently, increased uterine activity is noted after sexual intercourse; it is unclear whether this is due to breast stimulation, female orgasm, or prostaglandins in male ejaculate. For women at risk for preterm labor or with a history of previous pregnancy loss and who note such increased activity, use of a condom or avoidance of sexual activity may be recommended.

Circumcision

Newborn circumcision prevents phimosis and has been shown to decrease the incidence of cancer of the penis. It may result in a decreased incidence of urinary tract infections in children, but prospective studies have not confirmed this.[44] Education in good personal hygiene offers many of the advantages of circumcision without the risks.

Circumcision in the newborn is an elective procedure and should be performed only if the infant is stable and healthy. Local anesthesia reduces the observed physiologic response to newborn circumcision.[45]

Breast-Feeding

During prenatal visits, the patient should be encouraged to breast-feed her infant. Human milk is the most appropriate nutrient for human infants and also provides significant immunologic protection against infection. Infants who are breast-fed have a lower incidence of infection and require fewer hospitalizations than do infants who are fed formula exclusively.

Other advantages of lactation include economy, convenience, more rapid involution of the uterus, and natural child spacing. The reasons a woman decides to bottle-feed should be explored, as they may be based on a misconception. Encouragement will sometimes convince a hesitant mother who may then be able to nurse successfully.

Working outside the home need not be a contraindication to breast-feeding. Many women who previously would not have considered nursing an option, such as those with careers, are now finding time to breast-feed their infants. Nursing for only a few weeks or months is better than not nursing at all. Women should be aware that alternative ways of breast-feeding can be used to correspond with their work schedules. They can decrease the frequency of lactation to a few times a day in most cases and still continue to nurse. Other women may pump their breasts at work, leaving milk for the child's caretaker during the day and thus providing breast milk to the infant even more frequently. The milk may be collected in containers and, if refrigerated, is safe to use for 24 hours. For a longer duration, the milk should be frozen. Because freezing and thawing destroy the cellular content, fresh milk is preferred.

There is no need for specific nipple preparation during pregnancy. In one study, women prepared one nipple and not the other with a variety of techniques, including massage and breast creams, and found no difference in the two.[46] Soap and drying agents should not be used on the nipples, which should be washed only with water.

Preparation for Childbirth

The introduction of childbirth education and consumerism has had significant impact on the practice of obstetrics. The success of obstetric practice in preventing disasters has allowed interest to focus on the quality of the child and of the perinatal experience. Studies have shown that prepared childbirth can have a beneficial effect on performance in labor and delivery.[47] The prenatal period should be one in which the patient is exposed to information about pregnancy, normal labor and delivery, anesthesia and analgesia, obstetric complications, and obstetric operations (e.g., episiotomy, cesarean delivery, and forceps or vacuum delivery). The prenatal clinic is an appropriate place to obtain informed consent from the patient for her intrapartum care and management. Certainly, this affords a more dispassionate, quiet, and pain-free environment than the labor and delivery suite.

The education mentioned above is more than can be transmitted by the obstetrician at the initial or the shorter return visits, and patients expect more personal involvement than to be given a book or handout to read. The appropriate place for such education is a series of planned, structured prenatal education classes taught by informed, qualified individuals. These classes can be given in the physician's office, at the hospital, or in free-standing classes. National organizations such as the Childbirth Education Association and the American Society for Psychoprophylaxis in Obstetrics have recognized the need for such instruction and teach prepared childbirth. There are also advantages to office- and hospital-based programs, if the patient volume permits it, since specifics of management and alternatives offered by that practice or hospital can be discussed in these programs. On the other hand, free-standing classes offer the advantage of open-endedness and of presenting many options to the patient, who can then discuss them with her care provider. Many advances in family-centered practice (e.g., allowing fathers in the delivery room and operating room) have come from consumer requests and demands. A pregnant patient often makes a list of what she would like in the peripartum period to discuss with her practitioner. Thus, the care provider can understand her needs and desires, better address these needs and desires if labor and delivery do not proceed normally or as planned, and, finally, explain why certain requests are not possible or reasonable.

Signs of Labor

It is important to instruct the patient about certain warning signs that should trigger a call to her care provider or a visit to the hospital. All women should be informed of what to do if contractions become regular, if rupture of membranes is suspected, or if vaginal bleeding occurs. Patients should be given a number to call where assistance is available 24 hours a day.

Prepared Parenthood and Support Groups

As pregnancy progresses, special needs often arise; increasingly, educational support groups are being organized to assist in dealing with such needs. Support groups for families with Down syndrome infants, for mothers of twins or triplets, and for women who have had cesarean delivery have all shown that they can meet the special needs of these parents. Integration of parenting education in prenatal education has merit. Many parents are completely unprepared for the myriad of changes in their lives, and some idea of what to expect is beneficial.

Unsuccessful pregnancies lead to special problems and needs, for which social workers, clergy, and specialized support groups can be invaluable. Miscarriage, stillbirth, and infant death are particularly devastating events, best managed by a team approach with special attention to the grieving process. Referral to such groups as Compassionate Friends of Miscarriage, Infant Death, and Stillbirth is recommended.

Assessment of Gestational Age

During the course of the prenatal interview, assessment of gestational age begins with the question, "What was the first day of the last menstrual period?" From that point, the establishment of an estimated date of delivery and confirmation of that date by accumulation of supportive information remains one of the most important tasks of good prenatal care.

Human pregnancy has a duration of 280 days, measured from the first day of the last menstrual period (LMP) until delivery. The standard deviation is 14 days. It is important to remember that clinicians are measuring menstrual weeks (not conceptional weeks) with an assumption of ovulation and conception based on day 14 of a 28-day cycle. This gives pregnancy the 40-week gestational period in common clinical use. Much confusion exists among patients who try to measure pregnancy in terms of 9 months (40/4 = 10) or who try to measure in conceptional weeks. Another problem exists in women whose menstrual cycles do not follow a 28-day cycle and who therefore do not conceive on day 14 of the menstrual cycle.

It is often helpful to explain to patients and their families that their pregnancy will be described in terms of weeks, rather than months, and that the pregnancy can be broken into three trimesters lasting 1 to 14 weeks, 14 to 28 weeks, and 28 weeks to delivery. The commonly used term "4 months pregnant" has no meaning (one does not know whether this is 16 or 20 weeks) and has no place on a contemporary prenatal record. Every effort should be made to be consistent in usage to prevent confusion among patients and among clinicians who may assume care of the pregnancy.

Knowledge of gestational age is critical for obstetric decision-making. Generally, in a normal pregnancy, we can extrapolate from gestational age to estimate fetal weight. Throughout pregnancy, these, are the two most important determinants of fetal viability and survival. Without accurate knowledge of gestational age, diagnosis of such conditions as post-term pregnancy and intrauterine growth retardation is often impossible. Multiple gestation is most often detected early when the size of the uterine fundus is greater than expected for gestation. Appropriate management of preterm labor or a medically complicated pregnancy depends on an accurate estimate of fetal age and size. Within regional perinatal systems, records of gestational age are important for flow of information, and rapid access to consistent clear data is vital. In such situations, and during prolonged hospitalization, it is sometimes helpful to define gestational age further by using the notation of fractional weeks (27-4/7 weeks). It must be remembered, however, that we are describing a biologic system and that such precision is being used more for ease of communication and organization than for any ability to date the pregnancy with such a degree of accuracy.

Clinical Dating

The most reliable clinical estimator of gestational age is an accurate LMP. Using Naegele's rule, the estimated date of confinement is calculated by subtracting 3 months and adding 1 week from the first day of the LMP. A careful history must be taken from the patient verifying that the date given is the first day of the period as well as whether the period was normal, heavy, or light. The date of the previous menstrual period will help ascertain the length of the cycle. History should also be taken about previous use of oral contraceptives, which might influence ovulation.

Other clinical tools can be used to confirm and support LMP data, and, in cases in which the LMP is inaccurate or unknown, it has been shown that accumulated clinical information from early pregnancy can predict gestational age with an accuracy approaching that of menstrual dating.[48]

The size of the uterus on early pelvic examination, or by direct measurement of the abdomen from the pubic symphysis to the top of the uterine fundus (over the curve), provides useful information. Experienced practitioners can assess the early pregnancy with reproducibility before 12 to 14 weeks. Fundal height measurement in centimeters using the over-the-curve technique approximates the gestational age from 16 to 38 weeks within 3 cm (Fig. 7-7).

The uterus also tends to reach the umbilicus at about 20 weeks, and this too can be assessed when uterine fundal measurements are made.[48] The uterus may be elevated in early pregnancy in a patient with a previous cesarean delivery, making the fundal height appear abnormally high. Considerable variations in the level of the umbilicus and in the height of patients make this clinical marker variable. Quickening, the first perception of fetal movement by the mother, occurs at predictable times in gestation. In the first pregnancy, quickening is usually noted at about 19 weeks; in subsequent pregnancies, probably because of the experience of the observer, it tends to occur about 2 weeks earlier.[48] It is helpful to ask the woman to mark on a calendar the first time she feels the baby move and to report this date.

Audible fetal heart tones, in addition to being absolute evidence of pregnancy, are another marker of gestational age. Using an unamplified Hillis-DeLee fetoscope, they are generally audible at 19 to 20 weeks.[48] Observer experience, acuity, and the time spent listen-

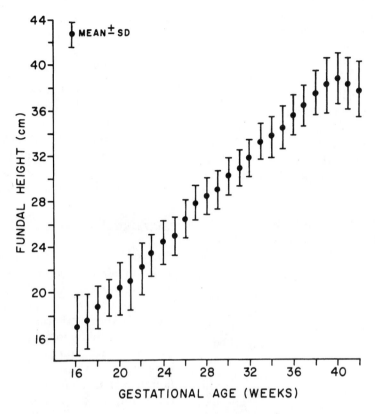

Fig. 7-7 Fundal height versus gestational age.

ing can all affect this number, so this guideline may need to be adapted individually.

Use of the electronic Doppler device is widespread and permits detection of the fetal heart by 11 to 12 weeks. Practitioners can set a standard individualized to their own equipment, which can be used as a gestational age marker. If fetal heart tones are not heard at the expected time, an ultrasound is appropriate to look for date/examination discrepancy, polyhydramnios, fetal viability, and twins.

The conversion of a negative urinary pregnancy test to a positive one may be helpful in assessing gestational age, but the sensitivity of the test used must be known in order to interpret the data accurately (see Ch. 2). These tests may be negative if they are performed too early.

Comparison of the various clinical estimators shows a known LMP date to be the most precise predictor. The clinical estimators can be ranked according to decreasing order of accuracy as follows: (1) last menstrual period, (2) the uterus reaching umbilicus, and (3) fetal heart tone documentation, fundal height measurements, and quickening. Because of inherent biologic variability and differences in the examiner acuity, the estimated date of confinement can be predicted with 90 percent certainty only within ±3 weeks by even the best single estimator.[49]

Ultrasound

Ultrasound plays a major role in assessment of size and duration of pregnancy. The NIH consensus conference in 1984 concluded that in a low-risk pregnancy followed from the first trimester, routine ultrasound examination was not justified for determining gestational age. However, a long list of indications justify an ultrasound examination.[50]

A randomized trial has shown that the risk of being called overdue was reduced from 8 to 2 percent for patients who received early ultrasound.[51] Also, twins were detected more often and perinatal mortality was reduced in the ultrasound group. The RADIUS (Routine Antenatal Diagnostic Imaging with Ultrasound) study reported no improvement in perinatal outcome with use of routine ultrasound in normal, low-risk women.[52,53] However, 61 percent of women were excluded for many reasons such as an uncertain menstrual history, and only 35 percent of anomalies were detected in the ultrasound-screened group (only 17 percent before 24 weeks). The meta-analysis by Bucher and Schmidt[54] indicated that routine scanning can detect many more anomalies, which can reduce perinatal mortality. The authors' practice is to perform ultrasound at 16 to 20 weeks for a baseline gestational age measurement and as a screening for fetal abnormality or multiple gestation. If ultrasound is not done routinely, the caregiver must be vigilant in detecting problems that are indications for a scan, and more frequent scans may be necessary.

Ultrasound is an accurate means of estimating gestational age in the first half of pregnancy.[55] The crown–rump length, biparietal diameter, and femur length in the first half of pregnancy correlate closely with age. As pregnancy progresses, fetal size varies considerably, and measurement of the fetus is a poor tool for estimation of gestational age, especially in the third trimester (see Ch. 11).

Assessment of Fetal Maturity Before Repeat Cesarean Delivery or Elective Induction of Labor

The American College of Obstetricians and Gynecologists—Committee on Obstetrics: Maternal Fetal Medicine[56] states that in a gestation in which 39 weeks have elapsed since the last menstrual period in a patient with normal menstrual cycles and no immediate antecedent use of oral contraceptives, fetal maturity can be assumed if one of the following clinical criteria for estimating gestational age is supported by at least one of the following laboratory determinations:

Clinical Criteria

1. Fetal heart tones have been documented for at least 20 weeks by nonelectronic fetoscope or at least 30 weeks by Doppler

2. Uterine size has been established by pelvic examination prior to 16 weeks of gestation

Laboratory Determinations

1. Thirty-six weeks have elapsed since a positive serum or urine hCG pregnancy test or
2. Ultrasound
   a. Measurement based on the crown–rump length obtained between 6 and 12 weeks of gestation or
   b. Other ultrasound confirmation of gestational age obtained before 24 weeks of gestation

Summary

Prenatal care is an effective, if incompletely understood and studied, intervention. It provides a model for primary care services for both obstetricians/gynecologists and other primary care providers. It satisfies the Institute of Medicine criteria for primary care as it is comprehensive, continuous, and provides coordinated services. Preconceptional care will introduce changes and improve it. Risk assessment, with subsequent elimination or management of risks, health education, advocacy, and disease prevention, as well as appropriate medical management of complications, remain the core of the process. Changes in number of visits and improved understanding of the successful components of prenatal care will improve services and efficiency without altering the substance of what has been developed and achieved.

Key Points

- Maternal mortality is the demise of any woman from any pregnancy-related cause while pregnant or within 42 days of termination of a pregnancy. The most frequent causes of maternal death are hemorrhage and embolism. The perinatal mortality combines the number of fetal deaths (stillbirths) plus neonatal deaths per 1,000 total births.

- Preconception evaluation should include rubella testing, hepatitis testing, and possibly toxoplasmosis testing, in addition to medical and family history. Further tests may be indicated depending on historical genetic risk factors identified.

- Preconception supplementation with folic acid can reduce the incidence of neural tube defects and other defects. All women of childbearing age should consume 0.4 mg of folic acid daily. Women who have had a child previously affected by a neural tube defect should take 4 mg daily from 4 weeks before conception through the first 3 months of pregnancy.

- The triple screen (α-fetoprotein, hCG, and estriol) can detect women younger than 35 years of age at increased risk for chromosomal abnormalities.

- The number of prenatal visits can be decreased in healthy parous women with safety.

- The total weight gain recommended for healthy women is 25 to 35 pounds. Underweight women may gain up to 40 pounds, and overweight women should limit weight gain to 15 to 25 pounds.

- Bedrest on the side increases venous return from the legs, as pressure on the vena cava is relieved. This maneuver increases the effective circulating blood volume, cardiac output, and, thus, the blood flow to the kidney. A diuresis follows, as well as increased blood flow to the uterus.

- The pregnant woman should be advised against prolonged sitting during car or airplane travel because of the risk of venous stasis and possible thromboembolism.

- Breast is best.

- Ultrasound evaluation between 16 and 20 weeks allows accurate assessment of gestational age and screening for fetal abnormality and multiple gestation.

References

1. Donaldson M, Yordy K, Vanselow N (eds): Defining Primary Care: An Interim Report. National Academy Press, Washington, DC, 1994
2. Starfield B: Primary Care: Concept, Evaluation, and Policy. Oxford University Press, New York, 1992
3. American College of Obstetricians and Gynecologists: The Obstetrician-Gynecologist and Primary-Preventive Health Care. ACOG, 1993
4. Public Health Service: Caring for Our Future: The Content of Prenatal Care—A Report of the Public Health Service Expert Panel on the Content of Prenatal Care. PHS-DHHS, Washington, DC, 1989
5. Chalmers I, Enkin M, Keirse M: Effective Care in Pregnancy and Childbirth. Oxford: Oxford University Press, 1989
6. Huntington J, Connell FA: For every dollar spent—The cost-savings argument for prenatal care. N Engl J Med 331:1303, 1994
7. Villar J, Garcia P, Walker G: Routine antenatal care. Curr Opin Obstet Gynecol 5:688, 1993
8. Peoples-Sheps MD, Kalsbeck WD, Siegal WC: Prenatal records: a national survey of content. Am J Obstet Gynecol 164:514, 1991
9. Baldwin LM, Raine T, Jenkins LD et al: Do providers adhere to ACOG standards? The case of prenatal care. Obstet Gynecol 84:549, 1994
10. Rochat RW, Koonin LM, Atrash HK, Jewett JF, and the Maternal Mortality Collaborative: Maternal mortality in the United States: Report from the Maternal Mortality Collaborative. Obstet Gynecol 72:91, 1988
11. CDC: Pregnancy-Related Mortality—Georgia, 1990–1992. MMWR 44:93, 1995
12. Grimes DA: The morbidity and mortality of pregnancy: still risky business. Am J Obstet Gynecol 170:1489, 1994
13. Rosenfield A: Maternal mortality in developing countries. An ongoing but neglected "epidemic." JAMA 262:376, 1989
14. Frautschi S, Cerulli A, Maine D: Suicide during pregnancy and its neglect as a component of maternal mortality. Int J Gynecol Obstet 47:275, 1994
15. Sachs BP, Fretts RC, Gardner R et al: The impact of extreme prematurity and congenital anomalies on the interpretation of international comparisons of infant mortality. Obstet Gynecol 85:941, 1995
16. Enkin MW: Randomized controlled trials in the evaluation of antenatal care. Int J Tech Assessment Health Care 8:(Suppl 1):40, 1992
17. Knox AJ, Sadler L, Pattison NS et al: An obstetric scoring system: its development and application in obstetric management. Obstet Gynecol 81:195, 1993
18. Mueller-Heubach E, Guzick DS: Evaluation of risk scoring in a preterm birth prevention study of indigent patients. Obstet Gynecol 160:829, 1989
19. Kogan MD, Alexander GR, Kotelchuck M, Nagey DA: Relation of the content of prenatal care to the risk of low birth weight. JAMA 271:134, 1994
20. Moos MK, Cefalo RC: Preconceptional health promotion: a focus for obstetric care. Am J Perinatol 4:63, 1987
21. Adams EM, Bruce C, Shulman MS et al: The PRAMS Working Group: Pregnancy planning and pre-conceptional counseling. Obstet Gynecol 82:955, 1993
22. MRC Vitamin Study Research Group: Prevention of neural tube defects: results of the Medical Research Council Vitamin Study. Lancet 338:131, 1991
23. Czeizel AE, Dudas I: Prevention of the first occurrence

of neural-tube defects by periconceptional vitamin supplementation. N Engl J Med 327:1832, 1992

24. Hook EB: Rates of chromosome abnormalities at different maternal ages. Obstet Gynecol 58:282, 1981

25. Stene J, Fischer G, Steve E et al: Paternal age effect in Down's syndrome. Am J Hum Genet 40:299, 1977

26. Spitzer RL, Williams JBW, Kroenke K et al: Utility of a new procedure for diagnosing mental disorders in primary care. JAMA 272:1749, 1994

27. Moore RD, Bone LR, Geller G et al: Prevalence detection and treatment of alcoholism in hospitalized patients. JAMA 261:403, 1989

28. Sokol RJ, Martier SS, Ager JW: The T-ACE questions: practical prenatal detection of risk-drinking. Am J Obstet Gynecol 160:863, 1989

29. McFarlane J, Parker B, Soeken K, Bullock L: Assessing for abuse during pregnancy. JAMA 267:3176, 1992

30. Creasy RC, Gummer BA, Liggins GC: System for predicting spontaneous preterm birth. Obstet Gynecol 55:692, 1980

31. Main D, Richardson DK, Hadley CB, Gabbe S: Controlled trial of a preterm labor detection program: efficacy and costs. Obstet Gynecol 74:823, 1989

32. Abbasi IA, Hess LW, Johnson TRB Jr et al: Leukocyte esterase activity in the rapid detection of urinary tract and lower genital tract infection in pregnancy. Am J Perinatol 2:311, 1985

33. American College of Obstetricians and Gynecologists Committee Opinion, Number 78, January 1990

34. American College of Obstetricians and Gynecologists: Standards for Obstetric and Gynecologic Services. 7th Ed. ACOG, Washington, DC, 1989

35. American Academy of Pediatrics/American College of Obstetricians and Gynecologists: Guidelines for Perinatal Care. 2nd Ed. Washington, DC, 1988

36. McDuffie R, Bischoff K, Cross J et al: An evaluation of risk-based prenatal care: a randomized controlled trial. Am J Obstet Gynecol 172:270, 1995

37. Grant A, Elbourne D, Valentin L, Alexander S: Routine fetal movement counting and risk of antepartum rate death in normally formed singletons. Lancet ii:345, 1989

38. U.S. Department of Agriculture: The Food Guide Pyramid. Home and Garden Bulletin. USDA, Washington, DC, 1992

39. National Academy of Sciences: Recommended Dietary Allowances. 10th Ed. National Academy Press, Washington, DC, 1989

40. Zlatnik FJ, Burmeister LF: Dietary protein in pregnancy: effect on anthropometric indices of the newborn infant. Am J Obstet Gynecol 146:199, 1983

41. Food and Nutrition Board Institute of Medicine, National Academy of Sciences: Nutrition During Pregnancy. p. 10. National Academy Press, Washington, DC, 1990

42. Mamelle N, Laumon B, Lazar P: Prematurity and occupational activity during pregnancy. Am J Epidemiol 119:309, 1984

43. Luke B, Mamelle N, Keith L et al: The association between occupational factors and preterm birth: a U.S. nurses' study. Am J Obstet Gynecol 173:849, 1995

44. American Academy of Pediatrics Task Force on Circumcision. Pediatrics 84:388, 1989

45. Maxwell LG, Yaster M, Wetzel RC et al: Penile nerve block for newborn circumcision. Obstet Gynecol 70:415, 1987

46. Brown MS, Hurloch JT: Preparation of the breast for breast feeding. Nurs Res 24:449, 1975

47. Scott JR, Rose NB: Effect of psychoprophylaxis (Lamaze preparation) on labor and delivery in primiparas. N Engl J Med 294:1205, 1976

48. Andersen HF, Johnson TRB, Flora JD et al: Gestational age assessment. II. Prediction from combined clinical observations. Am J Obstet Gynecol 140:770, 1981

49. Kramer MS, McLean FH, Boyd ME, Usher RH: The validity of gestational age estimation by menstrual dating in term, preterm and postterm gestations. JAMA 260:3306, 1988

50. U.S. Department of Health and Human Services: Ultrasound Imaging in Pregnancy. NIH Publ. No. 84-667. National Institutes of Health, Washington, DC, 1984

51. Eik-Nes SH, Okland O, Aure JC: Ultrasound screening in pregnancy: a randomized controlled trial. Lancet i:1347, 1984

52. Ewigman BG, Crane JP, Frigoletto FD et al: Effect of prenatal ultrasound screening on perinatal outcome. N Engl J Med 329:821, 1993

53. LeFevre ML, Bain RP, Ewigman BG et al: A randomized trial of prenatal ultrasonographic screening: impact on maternal management and outcome. Am J Obstet Gynecol 169:483, 1993

54. Bucher HC, Schmidt JG: Does routine ultrasound scanning improve outcome in pregnancy? Meta-analysis of various outcome measures. BMJ 307:13, 1993

55. Reece EA, Gabrielli S, Degennaro N, Hobbins JC: Dating through pregnancy: a measure of growing up. Obstet Gynecol Surv 44:544, 1989

56. American College of Obstetricians and Gynecologists: Committee Opinion, Number 77, Washington, DC, January 1990

57. MMWR 37 (SS5):26, 1988

58. National Natality Survey—United States. DHHS Pub. No. (PHS) 86-1922

Chapter 8

Teratology and the Epidemiology of Birth Defects: Occupational and Environmental Perspectives

Lowell E. Sever and Mary Ellen Mortensen

Pregnant women want to have a normal baby who develops into a healthy child and adult. Unfortunately, this wish is not always fulfilled. This chapter considers prenatal environmental influences acting maternally as potential causes of adverse development. The focus is on structural malformations (birth defects), but some attention is paid to aberrations in behavior and to other adverse reproductive outcomes. The importance of birth defects as a cause of infant mortality, the etiology of birth defects and basic concepts of teratology, epidemiologic methods used to evaluate possible adverse effects of environmental exposures on reproductive outcomes, and data about some specific environmental and occupational exposures are reviewed.

Importance of Birth Defects

A country's infant mortality rate is often used as a measure of the health of its children. In general, when the infant mortality rate is high (25 to 150 deaths before age 1 year per 1,000 live births), infectious diseases are a major contributor. When the rate is less than 25 per 1,000, birth defects, low birth-weight and prematurity-associated conditions such as respiratory distress syndrome, and sudden infant death syndrome (SIDS) are the leading causes, with infectious diseases becoming relatively unimportant. For example, in the United States in 1992 these three causes of infant mortality accounted for 53 percent of all infant deaths (Table 8-1).[1] Also in 1992, birth defects were the underlying cause of death for 7,449 infants under 1 year of age in the United States. This made birth defects the leading cause of infant mortality, responsible for 21.5 percent of infant deaths.

As part of the *Year 2000 Health Objectives,* an infant

mortality goal of 7 per 1,000 has been established.[2] To reach this goal, deaths due to birth defects must be reduced. An important strategy is to discover factors that may cause these adverse reproductive outcomes and reduce exposure to those that may be associated with chemicals and other agents in the environment.

Epidemiology of Birth Defects

Epidemiology is concerned with the distribution and determinants (causes) of diseases. Epidemiology seeks to identify associations that suggest disease etiology; a goal of such knowledge of causal mechanisms is to prevent and control disease. The etiologies of most birth defects are unknown. Even for defects that are considered to have polygenic or multifactorial causes (see Ch. 9), such as cardiac defects, the true etiology remains undetermined. Table 8-2, based on a recent review by Brent and Beckman,[3] shows the distribution of causes of birth defects in humans and the approximate percentages of defects attributable to each.

Table 8-1 Infant Mortality in the United States, 1992

Cause of Death	Number of Deaths	Percent
Birth defects	7,449	21.5
Prematurity, low birth weight, and respiratory distress syndrome	6,934	17.7
Sudden infant death syndrome	4,891	14.1
Subtotal	18,438	53.3
All other causes	16,190	46.7
Total	34,628	100.0

(Adapted from Centers for Disease Control and Prevention.[1])

Table 8-2 Causes of Human Malformations

Cause	Percent of Total
Genetic transmission	15–20
Chromosomal abnormalities	5
Environmental causes	
Maternal infections	3
Maternal conditions, including drug and substance addictions	4
Mechanical problems (deformations)	1–2
Drugs, chemicals, radiation, and hyperthermia	<1
Unknown	65

(Adapted from Brent and Beckman,[3] with permission.)

Etiology of Birth Defects

Genetic transmission accounts for about 15 to 20 percent of birth defects. The number of disorders known to have a genetic basis is increasing, as reference to successive editions of McKusick's catalogue of genetic disorders shows.[4,5] The overall percentage of defects attributable to genetic transmission, however, has not changed in any dramatic fashion. It is quite likely that information gained from the Human Genome Project will make major contributions to understanding the causes of some birth defects. Genetic disorders are considered in Chapter 9 and are not discussed further in this chapter.

Chromosomal aberrations, such as aneuploidies, translocations, and deletions, account for about 5 percent of defects. As with the simple genetic disorders, the number of identifiable chromosomally based defects is increasing with advances in cytogenetic methods. It is likely that additional malformation syndromes and cases of mental retardation are probably related to previously unrecognized chromosomal defects that will be understood better as the Human Genome Project progresses. Still, the percentage of all defects that can be attributed to chromosomal causes is small. Chromosomal defects are discussed in Chapter 9 and are not considered further here.

The general category of environmental causes, in Brent's categorization, includes both exogenous causes and those related to the maternal environment. Although exogenous factors are mediated by the mother, conditions intrinsic to her can adversely affect intrauterine development. For example, maternal diabetes,[6] maternal phenylketonuria (PKU),[7] and maternal thyroid disease[8] have all been associated with birth defects in the offspring.

Although much interest and concern focuses on the exogenous causes of birth defects, in terms of the recognized causes such factors are known to account for only a very small percentage of all birth defects. The known environmental causes of human birth defects include acute, high-dose ionizing radiation; maternal infections; drugs; and the organomercurial methylmercury. Some would also include polychlorinated biphenyls (PCBs) as developmental toxicants, although there are data to suggest that the impairments are reversible. Evidence is increasing for associations between some occupational exposures and birth defects.[9] For this discussion, the term *environmental* is restricted to those agents or chemical substances that may occur as contaminants in the ambient or occupational environment. The importance of the teratogenic effects of drugs in pregnancy is discussed in Chapter 10, and the teratogenic effects of infections during pregnancy are reviewed in Chapter 38.

Teratology: Basic Principles

To understand the etiology of birth defects, it is important to consider what is known about the principles of abnormal development (teratogenesis). Although only a small percentage of birth defects currently can be linked to environmental agents, the search for other agents is important.

Teratology has been defined as the study of abnormal development; it is directed at understanding the causes and mechanisms of maldevelopment. A teratogen is a substance, organism, or physical agent capable of causing abnormal development. A teratogen can cause abnormalities of structure or function, growth retardation, or death of the organism.

Traditionally, the identification and definition of teratogenic agents was based on the production of structural defects. More recently, the concept has been expanded to include agents acting during embryonic or fetal development that lead to deviation from normal morphology or function. There is growing interest in exploring the role of prenatal factors in more subtle or difficult-to-ascertain effects, such as growth retardation and functional abnormalities. Wilson's six general principles of teratogenesis[10] provide a framework for understanding how structural or functional teratogens may act. These principles provide a conceptual framework to understand and investigate maldevelopment.

Genotype and Interaction with Environmental Factors

The first of Wilson's principles is that susceptibility to a teratogen depends on the *genotype of the conceptus* and on the manner in which the genotype interacts with environmental factors. This is perhaps most clearly shown by experiments in which different genetic strains of mice have varied greatly in their susceptibility to teratogens that lead to oral clefts.[11] Some of the variability in responses to human teratogens, such as to anticonvulsant drugs such as valproic acid and hydantoin, probably relates to genotype of the embryo. The increasing complexity of these potential interactions is illustrated by a recent series of elegant studies by Musselman and colleagues.[12]

Timing of Exposure

The second of Wilson's principles is that susceptibility of the conceptus to teratogenic agents varies with the developmental stage at the time of exposure. This concept of *critical stages of development* is particularly applicable to alterations in structure. It is during the second to the eighth weeks of development after conception—the embryonic period—that most structural defects occur. For such defects, it is believed that there is a critical stage in the developmental process, after which abnormal embryogenesis cannot be initiated. For example, most investigators believe that the neural tube defects anencephaly and spina bifida result from the failure of the neural tube to close. Since this process occurs between 22 and 28 days postconception, any exogenous effect on development must be present at or before this time. Van Allen et al.[13] recently put forward convincing evidence that the neural tube has five distinct closure sites that may respond to different agents and that differ in their timing. Investigations of thalidomide teratogenicity have clearly shown that the effects of the drug differ as a function of the developmental stage at which the pregnant woman took it.[14]

Mechanisms

The third of Wilson's principles is that teratogenic agents act in specific ways (*mechanisms*) on developing cells and tissues in initiating abnormal embryogenesis (pathogenesis). Teratogenic mechanisms are considered separately below.

Manifestations

Wilson's fourth principle is that the *final manifestations* of abnormal development are death, malformation, growth retardation, and functional disorder. The manifestation is thought to depend largely on the stage of development at which exposure occurs; a teratogen may have one effect if exposure occurs during embryogenesis and another if the exposure is during the fetal period. Embryonic exposure is likely to lead to structural abnormalities or embryonic death; fetal exposure is likely to lead to functional deficits or growth retardation.

Agent

The fifth of Wilson's principles is that access of adverse environmental influences to developing tissues depends on the nature of the influence (*agent*). This principle relates to such pharmacologic factors as maternal metabolism and placental passage. While most clearly understood for chemical agents or drugs, the principle also applies to physical agents such as radiation or heat. For an adverse effect to occur, an agent must reach the conceptus, by being transmitted indirectly through maternal tissues or by directly traversing the maternal body.

Dose Effect

Wilson's sixth and final principle is that manifestations of abnormal development increase in degree from the no-effect to the lethal level as *dosage* increases. What this means is that the response (e.g., malformation, growth retardation) may be expected to vary according to the dose, duration, or amount of exposure. For most human teratogens, this dose-response is not clearly understood but, along with the principle of critical stages of development, these concepts are important in supporting causal inferences about human reproductive hazards. Data regarding in utero exposure to ionizing radiation clearly show the importance of dose on observed effects.[15] The potential complexity of relationships between dose and observed effects for teratogens has been discussed by Selevan and Lemasters.[16]

Mechanisms of Teratogenesis

In identifying human teratogens, it is important to consider the mechanisms of teratogenesis, Wilson's third principle. Wilson[10] suggested that a teratogenic insult can initiate changes in developing cells or tissues that can be categorized into nine mechanisms. Wilson proposed that an agent acts via a mechanism that alters normal cellular or biochemical processes; different alterations can produce similar defects through final common pathways. The proposed mechanisms are as follows: gene mutation, chromosomal abnormalities (e.g., breaks and nondysjunction), mitotic interference, altered nucleic acid integrity or function, lack of normal precursors or substrates, altered energy sources, changes in membrane characteristics, osmolar imbalance, and enzyme inhibition. With these mechanisms in mind, it may be easier to understand why such diverse etiologies for spina bifida as maternal hyperthermia, valproic acid exposure, and folic acid deficiency have been suggested.

In identifying reproductive hazards, relationships among teratogenesis, mutagenesis, and carcinogenesis should be considered, since these processes may occur through similar mechanisms.[16] Hemminki and associates[17] illustrated how various manifestations, classified as teratogenic, mutagenic, or carcinogenic, could result from alterations of DNA.

Considerations in Identifying Human Teratogens: Known and Suspected Human Teratogens and Reproductive Toxicants

The number of clearly demonstrated human teratogens and reproductive toxicants is limited. Known and suspected agents in three categories—infectious agents, drugs and chemicals, and physical agents—are listed in the box below.[18] This chapter focuses on chemicals and physical agents.

The complexity of the issues surrounding identifying and regulating teratogens and reproductive toxicants is illustrated by California's Safe Drinking Water and Toxics Enforcement Act of 1986 (Proposition 65), a law intended to protect California citizens from chemicals that cause cancer, birth defects, or other reproductive

---

Known and Suspected Human Teratogens

Infectious Agents
  Cytomegalovirus
  Herpes hominis type II virus
  Parvovirus B19
  Rubella virus
  Toxoplasma gondii
  Treponema pallidum
  Varicella virus
Drugs and Chemicals
  Alcohol
  Aminopterin, methylaminopterin (folate antagonists)
  Androgenic hormones
  Busulfan (alkylating agents)
  Coumarin anticoagulants
  Diethylstilbesterol
  Isotretinoin, etretinate, vitamin A excess
  Lead
  Organic mercury compounds
  Phenytoin
  Polybrominated biphenyls (PBBs)
  Polychlorinated biphenyls (PCBs)
  Tetracyclines
  Thalidomide
  Trimethadione
  Valproic acid
Physical Agents
  Hyperthermia
  High dose ionizing radiation

(Data from Shepard[18] and Brent and Beckman.[244])

effects.[19] A key initial step in the process is identifying those chemicals. To this end, a Governor's Scientific Advisory Panel was established to determine criteria for listing substances "known to cause developmental toxicity." In addition, a group of experts was assembled to review and comment on the criteria.[19] Other groups have attempted to describe the methods used to identify and regulate human reproductive and developmental toxicants.[20]

Animal Models for the Study of Human Teratogens

Premarket testing of drugs and food additives involves animal testing to determine potential teratogenicity. Although important in recognizing potential reproductive toxicants and teratogens, such studies have a number of significant limitations. Extrapolation from animal data may not be relevant to human exposures to an agent because of interspecies differences in metabolism, end-organ response, transport across the placenta, and sensitivity of fetal structures, to name a few. For example, humans and rabbits are sensitive to the teratogenic effect of thalidomide, but rats are relatively insensitive.[21] There are also problems extrapolating from high doses to low doses, as most teratologic experiments involve exposure at high doses. Since human exposures typically involve lower doses, effects must then be extrapolated. The assumption is often made that teratogenic risk is identical at high- and low-dose exposures (e.g., linearity of dose-response). This may not be true, and it is not surprising that there is little or no evidence for human teratogenicity at low doses for many substances teratogenic in animals at high doses (e.g., arsenic and some solvents).[22]

Among regulatory agencies there is increasing interest in the use of risk assessment methods for developmental toxicants. For example, the Environmental Protection Agency has published *Guidelines for the Health Assessment of Suspect Developmental Toxicants*.[23]

While teratologic testing of drugs and chemicals in animals serves an extremely important public health function, it does not necessarily prevent exposure of pregnant women to teratogens. Within the last 10 years, two drugs have been shown to be human teratogens: isotretinoin (Accutane) and valproic acid (Depakene). Although both agents were known to be teratogenic based on animal studies, it was only through human exposure that their teratogenicity in humans was established. In addition, tens of thousands of chemicals have never been tested for reproductive toxicity or teratogenicity.[16] The limitations of animal testing and the immense number of potentially hazardous substances underscore the need for human studies, the subject of the remainder of this chapter.

Contribution of Epidemiology

Environmental agents are of particular interest and concern because exposure of the conceptus to these factors is considered to be preventable by reducing or eliminating exposure of pregnant women. The combined forces of epidemiology and teratology are needed to study the effects of environmental exposures on reproductive outcomes.

Although most birth defects of public health significance probably involve the interaction of genetic and environmental factors (multifactorial etiology), the relative contributions and specific mechanisms of genetics and environmental agents remain unknown. By applying epidemiologic methods we attempt to determine the relative contributions of genetic and environmental factors to the etiology of these defects. Importantly, epidemiologic methods permit identification of specific agents associated with malformations or other adverse outcomes of pregnancy.[24]

Epidemiologic Concepts

Fundamental to epidemiology is the concept of variation between populations in the frequency of disease occurrence. Epidemiology is based on comparisons, determining what is occurring at one place compared with another place, what is going on at one time compared with another time, and what is going on with one group of people compared with another group of people. Rates of occurrence are compared; how these rates are determined is of major importance in epidemiology.

Occurrence rates for birth defects are usually expressed in terms of either rates of incidence or prevalence at birth. An incidence rate, calculated using cases occurring during a specified period of time, consists of a numerator, the number of new cases of a defect; and a denominator, the population at risk of developing the defect. Incidence rates are expressed in terms of some base population, such as per 1,000 births, and give a measure of the risk of the defect occurring within the population. Many investigators believe it is inappropriate to refer to birth defect rates as incidence rates, since the true population at risk, that is, the number of embryos, is unknown. Thus, there is an increasing tendency to refer to the occurrence of birth defects as prevalence at birth.[25] Prevalence requires knowing the number of cases that exist at a point in time, in this case defined as birth. Thus, we determine prevalence at birth since we can obtain information on the number of cases born in a population and the total number of births.

Examination of the occurrence rates for birth defects often shows geographic differences.[26] Such differences are found both between countries and between regions within countries. These differences are studied in an effort to identify possible etiologic factors. Detailed information on birth defect rates in the United States[27] and internationally[28,29] has recently been published.

Temporal variations in birth defect rates may occur within a population, and the interpretation of such variation may give insights into etiology. Two kinds of time-related changes are of particular interest: short-term increases that may be termed "epidemics" and long-term secular trends. Examples of the former are the epidemic of phocomelia in several European populations during the early 1960s[26] and a recent epidemic of anencephalus in South Texas.[30] An example of the latter is the recent decline in neural tube defect (NTD) rates in several areas of the world.[31] The increase in phocomelia was found to be associated with the introduction of the drug thalidomide. The decline in NTD rates has not been explained and is an example of a trend whose contributing factors need to be identified through epidemiologic study.

Epidemiologic Approaches to the Study of Birth Defects

Epidemiology is the study of the distribution and determinants of disease. Understanding disease distribution often provides insights into disease determinants. Understanding uneven distribution can lead to the identification of factors involved in disease etiology.[32] While epidemiologic studies usually are unable to establish causal relationships, such as can be done through animal experiments, associations between exposures and an outcome from well-conducted studies can provide strong, compelling evidence that the outcome results from the exposure.

Three major issues are involved in epidemiologic studies of birth defects that evaluate potential associations between exposures and outcomes: (1) the definition and ascertainment of outcomes of interest; (2) the definition, identification, and quantification of exposures or of other risk factors; and (3) the use of epidemiologic and statistical techniques to determine the strength of that association.[32]

Epidemiologic studies of birth defects and other adverse reproductive outcomes often present special challenges in terms of case definition and ascertainment (identification) and determination of exposure. The definition of what constitutes a case can present major problems in studies of birth defects. The completeness of ascertainment may vary by source and by defect. For example, one can argue that recent increases observed in the rates of patent ductus arteriosus (PDA) are due to increases in the incidence of the defect, better diagnosis, or increased survival of low-birth-weight infants in whom PDA frequently occurs. Even for defects that are readily recognizable at birth, such as NTDs, differences in sources of case ascertainment can lead to apparent differences in rates of occurrence,[33] which may be unrelated to differences in incidence.

There are three general categories of epidemiologic studies: descriptive, analytical, and experimental. The following discussion briefly considers some of the major features of these study designs, relating them to studies of birth defects and other adverse reproductive outcomes.

Descriptive Epidemiology

Case Reports

Most known teratogens and reproductive toxicants have been identified through case reports of an unusual number of cases or a constellation of abnormalities. These have often come from astute clinicians, who observed something out of the ordinary.[34-36] Although the importance of astute observations of abnormal aggregations of cases or patterns of malformations must be recognized, we cannot rely on such methods for identifying health hazards. Furthermore, etiologic speculations based on case reports or case series usually do not lead to a causal agent and are often false-positive speculations. Whereas case reports may identify a new teratogen, they can never provide an estimate of the risk of disease after exposure.

Descriptive Studies

Descriptive epidemiologic studies can be used to provide information about the distribution and frequency of some outcome of interest, resulting in rates of occurrence that can be compared among populations, places, or times. Defining the population at risk is the first step in a descriptive study. The population at risk can be defined geographically, such as residents within a state, or medically, such as being a patient at a particular hospital. Definition of the population at risk includes the time period under consideration. The population at risk constitutes the *denominator* for calculating rates of the occurrence of outcomes of interest.

The second step in a descriptive study is to determine the *numerator* for calculating rates for comparison. This involves two important concepts: (1) case definition (what defines a case to be counted?) and (2) case ascertainment (how are cases to be identified?).

Descriptive studies determine rates so that they can be compared. Possible differences in case ascertainment methods must be kept in mind. Some of the important issues associated with the determination of rates and their comparison have been discussed extensively by Borman and Cryer.[37]

Surveillance Programs

In surveillance programs, an at-risk population is identified and then followed over time to detect outcomes of interest. As they occur, cases are included in the database. Surveillance programs provide rates that can be examined for changes over time. They develop baseline data and subsequently permit early recognition of potential problems, based on ongoing data collection and analysis.

Birth defect surveillance (monitoring) systems (BDMS) are designed to identify cases occurring in a defined population, usually by reviewing vital records or hospital record abstracts or charts. The defined population often is a sociopolitical unit, such as a state, but some monitoring programs have been based on discharge data from particular groups of hospitals or births to women residing in a specified metropolitan area.

Two BDMS are operated by the Division of Birth Defects and Developmental Disabilities, National Center for Environmental Health, Centers for Disease Control and Prevention (CDC), Atlanta, Georgia. These two systems—the Birth Defects Monitoring Program (BDMP) and the Metropolitan Atlanta Congenital Defects Program (MACDP)—perform important surveillance functions.[38] The two systems follow populations defined differently and differ in sources of case ascertainment. Descriptions and comparisons of both systems are available.[39]

In the last 20 years, there has been a dramatic increase in the number of state-based birth defect surveillance systems. As of 1995, approximately half the states have some type of birth defect surveillance system.[40] These programs conduct routine reviews of occurrence rates of specific malformations and attempt to identify increases in rates or clusters of cases. Several of the states conducted case–control studies using cases from their surveillance program, and others have linked outcome data with environmental databases in an attempt to identify environmental reproductive hazards.[41-44] The use of cases from surveillance programs for hypothesis testing studies leads to a consideration of analytical epidemiology.

Analytical Epidemiology

Analytical epidemiologic studies are designed to generate or test hypotheses about associations between exposures and outcomes. The detection and quantification of such associations are major epidemiologic concerns. Such associations can be examined at either the group or individual level.

Ecologic Studies

Ecologic studies are important for generating hypotheses about the causes of an outcome such as a birth defect. In such studies, occurrence rates for an outcome are compared between groups thought to differ in terms of some exposure. Studies of this type do not collect information about exposures of individuals and are often used in environmental epidemiology, where residence in a particular area is used as an indicator of exposure. Lack of specific individual exposure data can be a critical limitation of this study design.

Examples of ecologic studies relevant to reproductive outcome include studies of congenital malformations in communities with vinyl chloride production facilities[45,46] and in communities with solvent-contaminated drinking water.[47] Ecologic studies often lead to hypotheses that can be tested using other study designs. Studies that allow associations between exposure and outcome to be assessed in particular individuals play a much more important role in epidemiologic research.

Case–Control Studies

The case–control study design, where groups of individuals with some outcome or disease of interest (cases), such as a congenital malformation, are compared to controls with regard to a history of one or more exposures, is the one most widely used in reproductive outcomes research. The controls are individuals as similar as possible to the cases, except that they are without the outcome of interest.

After cases and controls have been identified, the hypothesis to be tested is whether these two groups differ in exposure as well as outcome. How accurately exposure and its timing are determined may vary greatly among studies, but in any study the same methods must be used to establish the exposure of both cases and controls.[32]

Case–control studies are frequently used in epidemiology for several reasons. In testing etiologic hypotheses, they are applicable to outcomes of infrequent occurrence, and they can be conducted relatively rapidly and inexpensively. A disadvantage is that they have a potential for several important types of bias, including bias in recalling exposure, in selecting appropriate controls, and in ascertaining cases.

Most human studies of potential teratogens following descriptive studies have been case–control studies. After suspecting on the basis of case observations that thalidomide was teratogenic, Lenz[48] conducted a case–control study. Following ecologic studies of ambient exposure to vinyl chloride, the hypothesis of an association between vinyl chloride exposure and congenital malformations was tested using case–control studies.[46,49,50] The association between valproic acid use and spina bifida was verified by case–control studies.[51]

Cohort Studies

Cohort studies use the reverse approach from case–control studies; individuals who differ in exposure history are examined for differences in the occurrence of outcomes of interest. The groups are defined by the presence or absence of exposure to a given factor and then are followed over time and compared for rates of occurrence (i.e., incidence rates) of the outcome of interest.

Cohort studies have three advantages: (1) the cohort is classified by exposure before the outcome is determined, thereby eliminating the exposure recall bias; (2) incidence rates can be calculated among those exposed; and (3) multiple outcomes can be observed simultaneously.

Cohort studies, often called *prospective studies*, require that groups differing in exposure be followed through time, with outcomes observed. Therefore, these studies tend to be time-consuming and expensive. In addition, since occurrence rates for many adverse reproductive outcomes, such as congenital malformations, are low, large samples must be followed for long periods of time. Two main types of cohort studies have been developed: (1) those that identify a cohort and follow it into the future (concurrent cohort study) and (2) those that identify a cohort at some time in the past and follow it to the present (nonconcurrent cohort study).

In both cases, the risks of adverse outcomes are then compared between groups. Cohort studies enable investigators to calculate incidence rates that provide a measure of the risk of an outcome after the exposure. Risk in the exposed group can be compared with the risk in an unexposed group. Most frequently, the ratio of the incidence rate among the exposed to the rate among the unexposed is determined. This ratio, referred to as *relative risk*, is a measure of how much the presence of exposure increases the risk of the outcome.

Only a few large-scale concurrent cohort studies of problems of pregnancy outcome have been conducted. Probably the best known is the Collaborative Perinatal Project, conducted by the National Institute of Neurological and Communicative Disorders and Stroke. In this study, conducted between 1959 and 1966, about 55,000 women and their subsequently born children were studied extensively: the children were examined through age 8 years.[52] This study has provided considerable information on the use of drugs in pregnancy and birth defects and on many other topics (see Ch. 10).

Numerous studies of reproductive outcome have been conducted by the noncurrent cohort approach. These studies, also known as *historical prospective studies*, begin by identifying groups who differ in terms of some past exposure and follow them to the present and determine outcomes; exposure groups are defined before outcomes are known. A major advantage is that although the time frame is prospective, investigators do not have to follow the cohort into the future, waiting for events to occur. A disadvantage is that these studies require the ability to determine exposure status retrospectively.

A series of noncurrent cohort studies tested associations between smelters and spontaneous abortions.[53] Nordstrom and coworkers[54] compared histories of spontaneous abortions between women who differed in terms of occupational exposure to smelting processes. Later, Beckman and Nordstrom[55] surveyed exposed and unexposed male workers about their wives' histories of spontaneous abortions. In both instances, the findings supported a hypothesis of an association between the smelter and spontaneous abortions.

Experimental Epidemiology
Clinical Trials

The most common experimental study design in epidemiology is the clinical trial, in which the efficiency of a prevention or treatment regimen is evaluated. Ideally, subjects are randomly assigned to different treatment groups. The individuals must be as similar as possible in terms of unknown factors that may affect the response before they are randomly assigned to the treatment groups and receive the different regimens.[56]

The role of vitamin supplements taken during the periconception period in preventing NTDs has been evaluated in experimental studies. Smithells and coworkers[57,58] suggested that recurrence risks for NTDs were reduced in women who took the supplements during the period. In the original study, subjects were not randomized into different treatment groups, and because of this the conclusions have been criticized. More recent clinical trials of both NTD recurrence[59] and occurrence[60] have shown a protective effect of periconceptional folic acid supplementation, findings that have led to key public health recommendations regarding the use of folic acid to reduce the risk of these often devestating defects.[61]

In summary, experimental studies in epidemiology are unique in that they involve intervention as well as observation. In this way, they compare with approaches used in animal studies of teratology and other life sciences and yield results that can be analyzed like other experimental findings. They are limited, however, in what can be ethically tested, namely, treatment or preventive measures, rather than etiologic hypotheses.

Occupational and Environmental Hazards to Reproduction

Increasingly, attention has focused on the relationship between adverse reproductive outcomes and exposures to occupational and environmental hazards. Much of the concern about this relationship has grown not out of clearly demonstrated adverse effects but, rather, out of the possibility of such effects. Among the issues are those that relate to women's rights for equal employment opportunities and the problems of excluding women from some work situations because of potential effects of exposure on pregnancy outcomes.[62] While much of the concern has centered on the susceptibility of the embryo and fetus to teratogenic influences, interest has been expanding to embrace a whole gamut of factors in reproductive toxicology.

Adverse Reproductive Outcomes

Through a number of mechanisms, occupational or environmental exposures can produce adverse reproductive outcomes. Some of these outcomes include alterations in fertility caused by hormonal or gonadal effects and mutations at either the gene or chromosomal level. A variety of adverse outcomes result from direct effects of agents on the products of conception, ranging from death at various stages in the life span, to congenital malformations, to developmental disabilities, to cancers recognized in childhood. Another possible outcome is fetal death caused by effects on the intrauterine milieu and the maternal–fetal unit. This discussion focuses on the general outcome categories of sponta-

---

Reproductive Outcomes Potentially Associated With Maternal–Fetal Exposures

Altered fecundity
Increased time to pregnancy
Genetic defects
    Single-gene defects
    Chromosomal abnormalities
Reproductive wastage
    Early pregnancy loss
    Spontaneous abortions
Altered sex ratio
Congenital malformations
Low birth weight
    Intrauterine growth retardation
    Preterm delivery
Mortality
    Late fetal deaths
    Perinatal deaths
    Infant deaths
Functional disorders
    Developmental disabilities
    Behavioral disorders
Malignancies

neous abortions and congenital malformations; developmental disabilities, such as mental retardation, are mentioned briefly.

Exposure Assessment

As a prerequisite to evaluating the reproductive hazards associated with an occupational or environmental agent, one must be able to measure or estimate exposure to potential hazards. A number of investigators have recently addressed the problems associated with this exposure assessment.[32,63–66]

Considerations concerning occupational exposure can be categorized into three areas: defining and determining exposure, timing of exposure, and problems of mixed exposures.[32] In the first area, which can also be labeled exposure occurrence and measurement,[65] the problems relate to determining what a particular worker is exposed to and then determining the amount of exposure—if possible. Workers often may not be aware of the chemical substances to which they are exposed. If possible, determining exposure history should begin by questioning the worker and taking a job history. Ideally this should be augmented by reviewing the occupational and job history records that the employer maintains. The job history may make it possible for the investigator to determine the substances to which the worker was exposed. If so, the exposure records the employer maintains may include data from environmental monitoring.

Timing of exposure is crucial in studies of reproductive outcome. The critical stages in human development for teratogenesis were discussed earlier in this chapter. Except for exposures associated with mutational events, damage to the reproductive or endocrine systems, or storage of a substance for long periods in body tissues such as bone (lead) or fat (PCBs), exposures must occur within a limited period to produce teratogenic effects. For example, an agent suspected of causing an NTD could not be implicated as the cause of an infant's neural tube's failing to close if the mother had been exposed to the agent after the tube should have closed.

Employees may be exposed to a variety of potentially hazardous substances, leading to difficulty in demonstrating that a specific substance is a reproductive hazard. Most occupational exposures are to more than one substance, and it may not be possible to determine the reproductive effects of one agent—often occupational groups rather than specific exposures are studied. Studies of birth defects and other adverse reproductive outcomes associated with occupational groups have been reviewed recently.[9,67,68]

It is particularly difficult to determine exposures in studies of the ambient environment. There is growing interest and research activities in the use of biological markers of exposure in studies of adverse reproductive outcomes.[69–72]

An additional concern is confounding by nonoccupational exposure(s) and lifestyle factors, for example, alcohol and tobacco use. Family history also may affect risk of adverse outcomes.

Exposures That May Lead to Adverse Reproductive Outcomes

We shall now review what is known about the effects of prenatal exposure to certain occupational and environmental agents. Agents were selected on the basis of the availability of human data and on the authors' impressions of public concern that the agents may cause adverse reproductive effects.

Known human teratogens number about 30.[18] To date, only two have caused human maldevelopment (cerebral palsy and mental retardation) as a result of environmental contamination: high-dose ionizing radiation and methylmercury. Agents suspected of being teratogens on the basis of animal studies and limited epidemiologic studies are more numerous. When these agents are found to be polluting the environment, there is justifiable concern about potential prenatal exposure and adverse reproductive effects (Table 8-3). The difficulty of demonstrating an association between an environmental hazard and any adverse reproductive outcome must be appreciated.[73]

Several recent publications have addressed epidemiologic aspects of studying health effects of environmental contamination, including reproductive effects.[73–75] In a concise review, Heath[76] summarized some of the problems in epidemiologic studies of environmental hazards. Using as examples the childhood leukemia cluster in Woburn, Massachusetts, and the population exposure to waste chemicals at Love Canal, Heath identified three problems relevant to our discussion: low-dose, nonquantifiable exposures; the long and variable latency between exposure and outcome (disease); and the nonspecific nature of the outcome or disease. As a corollary to the last problem, Heath[76] pointed out that multiple factors probably play a causative role in most outcomes of interest including birth defects, low birth weight, spontaneous abortion, and cancer.

Ionizing Radiation

Acute High Dose

During the 1920s and 1930s ionizing radiation was used to treat women with pelvic disease; soon afterward, it was identified as the first known environmental human teratogen.[77] Systematic studies of atomic bomb survivors in Japan showed that in utero exposure to

Table 8-3 Occupational and Environmental Agents That May Be Associated With Human Adverse Reproductive Outcomes

Agent	Outcome
Ionizing radiation	
Acute high-dose	Microcephaly, mental retardation, growth retardaion
Chronic low-dose or before pregnancy	?Down syndrome
Methylmercury	Mental retardation, cerebral palsy, deafness, blindness, seizures (abnormal neuronal migration)
Mercury vapor	Cranial defects, spontaneous abortion, ?stillbirth
Lead	
High-dose	Infertility, spontaneous abortion, growth retardaton, psychomotor retardation, seizures, stillbirth
Chronic low-dose	Lower IQ, cognitive impairment in speech and language, attention deficit
Polychlorinated biphenyls	
High-dose	Spontaneous abortion, low birth weight, neuroectodermal dysplasia (skin staining, natal teeth, dysplastic nails, developmental and psychologic deficits), abnormal bone calcification
Chronic low-dose	Lower birth weight, smaller head circumference, ?cognitive impairment
Polybrominated biphenyls	
Chronic low-dose	?Lower birth weight, ?smaller head circumference, ?cognitive impairment
Anesthetic gases	
Chronic low-dose	Spontaneous abortion Birth defects
Organic solvents	
Chronic high-dose	Developmental impairment, facial dysmorphism, growth retardation (similar to fetal alcohol embryopathy)
Chronic low-dose	Spontaneous abortion, CNS malformations, orofacial clefts

high-dose radiation increased the risk of microcephaly and mental and growth retardation in the offspring.[15,78–81]

Studies of the Japanese survivors clearly show that distance from the hypocenter—the area directly beneath the detonated bomb—and the gestational age at the time of exposure were directly related to microcephaly and mental and growth retardation in the infant. Nine and 20 years after exposure, the greatest number of children with microcephaly and mental and growth retardation were in the group exposed at 15 weeks' gestation or earlier. These findings contrast with those of children exposed in utero during the third trimester and whose mothers were farthest from the hypocenter at the time of exposure. Of 55 such children evaluated 20 years later, only 1 was found to be microcephalic, and all were of normal intelligence.[79] Although teratogenic effects have been found in several organ systems of animals exposed to acute, high-dose radiation, no structural malformations other than those mentioned above have been reported among humans exposed prenatally.

Using data from animals and from outcomes of reported human exposures at various times during pregnancy, DeKaban[82] constructed a timetable for extrapolating acute, high-dose radiation (greater than 250 rads) to various reproductive outcomes in humans. Similarities between animal and known human effects support Dekaban's proposal.

Chronic Low Dose

Effects of chronic low-dose radiation on reproduction have not been identified in animals or humans. Increased risk of adverse outcomes was not detected among animals with continuous low-dose exposure (less than 5 rad) throughout pregnancy.[83]

The relationship between human structural malformations and background radiation has been examined in several epidemiologic studies in different geographic areas. Cosmic radiation was thought to be one factor that contributed to increased rates of anencephalus between 1950 and 1969 in several Canadian cities.[84] Using geologic estimates of natural radioactivity, some investigators have attributed increased malformation rates, including the rate for Down syndrome, to higher radioactivity levels.[85,86] Other studies of the association between estimated cosmic radiation exposure and congenital malformation rates have produced negative results.[87,88] Given that low-dose radiation could be one of a multitude of environmental factors that affect the risk of birth defects, perhaps it is not surprising that no consistent relationship is evident.

Mutagenesis

Children exposed in utero to radiation from the atomic bomb were studied over several years for evidence of genetic damage. No evidence for effects was found when six indicators were evaluated: congenital malformations, stillbirths and neonatal death rates, birth weight, sex ratio at birth, anthropomorphic measurements during the first year of life, and mortality in offspring (F1 generation).[77,89–91]

In contrast to the atomic bomb follow-up studies, other investigations have found that mutagenic effects may occur when women are exposed prenatally to diagnostic radiation. These effects include altered sex ratios among the offspring—slightly more females than expected[92]—and abnormal karyotypes in spontaneously aborted fetuses.[93]

Mutagenic effects in the offspring of irradiated women may be manifested years after the birth of the infant. Compared with nonradiated controls, the estimated risk of leukemia was increased 50 percent for children exposed in utero to radiation during maternal pelvimetry examinations.[94–96] Although this increase seems considerable, it translates into an approximate risk of 1 in 2,000 for exposed versus 1 in 3,000 for unexposed children. As Brent[83] points out, if one were to recommend that pregnancies be terminated whenever exposure from diagnostic radiation occurred because of the increased probability of leukemia in the offspring, 1,999 "exposed pregnancies" would have to be terminated to "prevent" a single case of leukemia.

Recently, questions have been raised about potential risks to children associated with parental (paternal) occupational exposure to low-dose radiation.[97] A case–control study by Gardner et al.[98,99] in the area around the Sellafield Nuclear Facility in the United Kingdom found a statistically significant association between paternal preconception radiation dose and childhood leukemia risk. A similar association had been observed between paternal preconception radiation and risk in workers at the Hanford Nuclear Facility in the United States.[100] The finding regarding childhood leukemia risk is a particularly contentious issue, contradicting studies of the children born to atomic bomb survivors who do not show genetic effects, such as increased risks of childhood cancers.[91] A study in the vicinity of nuclear facilities in Ontario also failed to demonstrate an association between childhood leukemia risk and paternal preconception dose (exposure).[101]

Video Display Terminals

Since the 1980s there has been concern about video display terminals (VDTs) linked to adverse reproductive outcomes. Much of the early concern grew out of reports of spontaneous abortion clusters among groups of women who used VDTs at work, and some of the reported clusters also included birth defects.[102] While it was suggested that these "unexpected" clusters were actually expected based on the frequency of occurrence of spontaneous abortions (10 to 15 percent of recognized pregnancies) and the extremely large number of women working with VDTs,[103] several large epidemiologic studies were carried out to examine the association.[104,105] Numerous papers have been published on this topic, along with a number of reviews.[68,102,103] Our interpretation of these studies is that VDT use does not increase the risk of adverse reproductive outcomes.

Organic Mercury—Methylmercury

Exposure to organic mercury compounds, such as methyl- or ethylmercury, is not common. In the United States, methylmercury was widely used as a fungicide until the 1960s, when U.S. production was halted because of the compound's toxicity and bioaccumulation. Today in the United States, exposure mainly occurs through the consumption of contaminated fish. Fish may become contaminated when organomercurials are present in water or when bacteria in water convert inorganic mercury to organic mercury, part of a complex environmental mercury cycle.[106]

Methylmercury effects were discovered in 1959 after an epidemic of poisoning in Minamata, Japan, that resulted in fetal neurologic damage with psychomotor retardation, seizures, cerebral palsy, blindness, and deafness.[107] In 1972, similar fetal effects were observed in Iraq after an epidemic of methylmercury poisoning.[108] In both epidemics, breast-fed infants had additional exposure through maternal milk.[107]

Unintentional human exposures have permitted a more thorough study of the reproductive effects of methylmercury than of any other environmental pollutant.[109–111] The persistence of organic mercury in the body (biological half-life about 70 days) and its accumulation in hair further make it possible to reconstruct prenatal exposure.[112] Methylmercury crosses the placenta easily and accumulates in embryonic and fetal tissues, particularly brain tissues, at concentrations exceeding those in the mother.[113,114] Methylmercury does not cause obvious structural malformations in humans; thus, the devastating effects are not apparent at birth and are manifested only as the child ages. The developing nervous system of the conceptus and infant is more sensitive to the toxic effects of organic mercury than that of the adult or older child,[107] and the infant of an asymptomatic mother can be affected severely.[108,111,115]

Little is known of the human effects of methylmercury at low levels of exposure. Minor neurologic differences, mainly brisker deep tendon reflexes, were found among native Quebec boys exposed in utero compared with boys who had no such exposure.[116] Low-level methylmercury exposure may be associated with an increased frequency of chromosomal abnormalities[117]; the significance of this finding for adverse health or reproductive effects is unknown.

Nonhuman primates chronically treated with low-dose methylmercury were more likely to experience reproductive failure (nonconception, spontaneous abortion) than nontreated controls.[118] Prenatal exposure of nonhuman primates resulted in offspring with impaired visual recognition that was consistent with developmental teratogenic effect.[119–121]

While there appears to be no association between congenital malformations and human environmental exposure, methylmercury is embryolethal in laboratory animals and causes various structural malformations (exencephaly, limb abnormalities) when high doses are given during critical periods in development.[122] Mattison et al[123] has reviewed experimental and human epidemiologic data regarding mercury and other metals, listing the site(s) of action or reproductive outcome studied. A recent review by Weiss[124] includes a quantitative risk assessment of the developmental neurotoxicology of methylmercury.

Elemental Mercury (Vapor)

Mercury is an unusual element. At room temperature it is liquid, with a high vapor pressure, and vapor concentrations can rise rapidly to toxic concentrations in closed or poorly ventilated areas. The vapor is odorless and colorless, making it virtually nondetectable without special equipment.

Women at risk for exposure work primarily in health-related occupations such as nursing, medicine, dentistry, and dental hygiene. Exposure may occur when dental amalgams are prepared and when thermometers or manometers are broken or mercury is spilled. In recent years, encapsulated amalgam preparation and electronic methods for measuring blood pressure and temperature have been developed. Consequently, mercury exposure in medicine and dentistry in the United States has probably decreased.

Given that large numbers of women of childbearing age may have been exposed occupationally to mercury vapor, there is a surprising dearth of animal and human epidemiologic studies of reproductive effects. In one study, mercury vapor exposure at 0.5 mg/m^3 throughout pregnancy resulted in cranial defects in 2 of 115 fetal rats.[125] Exposure during days 10 through 15 of gestation produced increased fetal resorption.[125] This vapor concentration is 10 times greater than the occupational limit of 0.05 mg/m^3 established by the Occupational Safety and Health Administration[126] and probably caused maternal toxicity that contributed to the observed fetal effects. To protect the developing conceptus, Koos and Longo[109] recommend that women of childbearing age should not be exposed to vapor concentrations exceeding 0.01 mg/m^3.

Animal studies demonstrate the ease with which elemental mercury crosses the placenta. Following mercury vapor exposure, fetal rat blood mercury concentrations were 65 times higher than the corresponding maternal values, and the highest mercury concentrations were found in the rat placenta.[127] Placental and fetal membranes from mercury-exposed dental workers contained two to three times more mercury than tissues taken from unexposed women.[128] The fetal and maternal blood mercury concentrations were similar in both groups, implying that the placenta and fetal tissues may act as a barrier at low levels of mercury vapor.[128]

Epidemiologic studies of reproductive effects have been conducted with dental assistants and female dentists. Radiation and anesthetic gases are potential confounding exposures overlooked in many studies. Other methodologic problems, such as nonverification of the outcome, absence of exposure data, and low survey response rates, often are not considered. The limited studies to date do not provide conclusive evidence that occupational exposure to mercury vapor is teratogenic or results in other adverse reproductive outcomes. The need for more animal and human studies of reproductive effects has been recognized.[129]

At least one case report has suggested a possible association between occupational exposure to mercury vapor and severe brain damage in a newborn.[130] A female dental surgeon, who worked in a surgery with mercury levels above the threshold limit value, gave birth to a small-for-dates baby with severe brain damage, not otherwise specified. The authors stress that a case report can only suggest an effect, but the finding is consistent with animal teratology.

Rowland[131] reviewed the reproductive effects of mercury vapor and presents data from studies of female dental assistants in California. Women who prepared 50 or more dental amalgams per week had a statistically insignificantly increased risk for spontaneous abortion. Women who prepared 30 or more amalgams a week in offices with poor mercury hygiene showed evidence of reduced fecundity. A detailed analysis of fecundity, assessed as time to pregnancy in this cohort of dental assistants, was published recently.[132] To our knowledge, there are no published data on congenital malformations among births to dental assistants in the United States.

Lead

Since the nineteenth century, exposure to high levels of lead has been known to cause embryotoxicity, growth and mental retardation, increased perinatal mortality, and developmental disability.[133] These adverse reproductive effects were seen when women in occupational settings were exposed to concentrations of lead in air that far exceeded levels allowable today. As a matter of historic interest, unscrupulous vendors sold pills containing lead as an abortifacient at the turn of the century.[134]

Sources of nonoccupational lead exposure commonly encountered by U.S. women are unlikely to result in detectable effects. Regulatory and public health efforts are directed at reducing preconceptional and prenatal exposure in order to reduce maternal-to-fetal lead transmission.

Because the nervous system may be more susceptible to the toxic effects during the embryonic and fetal periods than at any other time of life[114] and because maternal and cord blood lead concentrations are directly correlated,[135] lead concentrations in blood should not exceed 25 μg/dl in women of reproductive age.[136]

Ideally, the maternal blood lead level should be less than 10 μg/dl to ensure that a child begins life with minimal lead exposure. A dose-response relationship is strongly supported by numerous epidemiologic studies of children showing a reduction in IQ with increasing blood lead concentrations above 10 μg/dl. Of note, these studies measured blood lead concentrations over time (often 2 years or more) and reported averaged values. Other neurologic impairments associated with increased blood lead concentrations include attention deficit disorder ("hyperactivity"), hearing deficits, learning disabilities, and shorter stature. Thus, for public health purposes, childhood lead poisoning has been defined as a blood lead level of 10 μg/dl or higher.[137]

In occupational settings, federal standards mandate that women should not work in areas where air lead concentrations can reach 50 μg/cm^3, since this may result in blood concentrations above 25 to 30 μg/dl.[138] Subtle but permanent neurologic impairment in children may occur at lower blood lead concentrations.[139,140] Although controversial, such studies raise the possibility that the occupational standard may inadequately protect the fetus. Protection of fetuses from lead exposure was an important concern raised in the recent Johnson Controls case in the U.S. Supreme Court.[62] The issues of the neurodevelopmental effects of prenatal lead exposure have been discussed recently by Bellinger and Needleman.[141]

Lead screening of pregnant women is highly controversial and not presently recommended. In the absence of excessive exposure, most of the lead in blood comes from bone stores, and no intervention is available to reduce the blood lead.[142] Chelation therapy is potentially hazardous, and some agents are teratogenic.[143] On the other hand, screening could identify women who may benefit from environmental or other interventions to reduce their lead exposure. The CDC's Advisory Committee on Childhood Lead Poisoning Prevention may consider the pros and cons of prenatal lead screening during their deliberations in 1995 and 1996.

The Phenoxy Herbicide 2,4,5-T and Dioxins

These compounds are considered together because 2,3,7,8-tetrachlorodibenzodioxin (TCDD or dioxin) and other chlorinated dibenzodioxins were produced as contaminants during production of the herbicide 2,4,5-trichlorophenoxyacetic acid (2,4,5-T).[144] This herbicide is no longer marketed in the United States, largely because of concerns about possible teratogenic and fetotoxic effects (seen after high doses are administered to animals during critical periods of organogenesis).[145]

Agent Orange, a defoliant used in Vietnam, was a mixture of herbicides, including 2,4,5-T. During the later years of the Vietnam war, public opinion against the ecologic effects of Agent Orange was fueled by reports of birth defects in South Vietnamese babies born to mothers who lived in areas where Agent Orange had been sprayed. The ensuing debate about the potential human teratogenicity of Agent Orange involved numerous federal agencies, and the use of 2,4,5-T containing any chlorodioxin contaminants was cancelled in 1970.[146]

Because 2,4,5-T contained small amounts of TCDD and since long-term human effects were unknown, the U.S. Public Health Service began an immense follow-up of Vietnam veterans. One portion of the study evaluated Vietnam veterans' risks of fathering infants with birth defects. The investigators concluded that "Vietnam veterans who had greater estimated opportunities for Agent Orange exposure did not seem to be at greater risk for fathering babies with all types of defects combined."[147] Vietnam service was associated with a few defects, however; Agent Orange exposure, other Vietnam-related experience, or some unidentified risk factor may have been responsible for the associations.[147] In a subsequent follow-up study, Vietnam and non-Vietnam veterans were interviewed regarding congenital malformations in their offspring. Although Vietnam veterans were more likely to report birth defects in their offspring, hospital records showed similiar rates of birth defects for children born to both veteran groups.[148] In contrast, increased central nervous system, skeletal, and cardiovascular malformations and disease were reported among Australian Vietnam veterans.[149] This study was less rigorous than its American counterparts, since it was an unconventional case–control design and relatively few children had diagnoses confirmed by medical record review.

Concerns about the reproductive effects of dioxins continue to be expressed. The Environmental Protection Agency has included an extensive discussion of these issues in a recent reassessment of 2,3,7,8-TCDD.[150] Overall the data appear inadequate to support allegations of adverse reproductive outcomes following human exposure to the dioxin-contaminated herbicide, although this is a topic of continuing discussion.[146]

Polychlorinated Biphenyls

Polychlorinated biphenyls (PCBs) were widely used in industry because of their thermal stability and heat transfer properties.[151] PCBs are also extremely stable and resistant to metabolic or biologic degradation and have become ubiquitous in the environment because of past dumping or disposal in unregulated landfills and failure to recycle. PCBs are highly lipid soluble, accumulate in fat, and can be found at high concentrations in the breast milk of women despite low concentrations in their blood.[152] Details of PCB biochemistry and toxicology are available elsewhere.[153,154]

Two epidemics of cooking oil contamination are often cited as evidence that high-dose PCBs are hazardous to human reproduction. In these epidemics, adults consumed cooking oil tainted with thermally degraded PCBs and developed a disease termed "Yusho" (in Japan) and "Yu-cheng" (in Taiwan). The disease was characterized by chloracne (an acne-form rash), eyelid swelling and discharge, and skin hyperpigmentation.[155] Although PCBs alone are often blamed for these and subsequent health problems, it is clear that heat-degradation products of PCBs (polychlorodibenzofurans [PCDF] and polychlorinated quarterphenyls [PCQ]) contributed significantly to toxicity.[156,157]

High-dose transplacental exposure to the cooking oil resulted in congenital anomalies and low birth weight.[158] Skin and mucosal hyperpigmentation were the most often noted abnormalities.[158] Other anomalies included natal teeth, gingival hyperplasia, exophthalmos, skull calcifications, and delayed bone age.[158] Developmentally, exposed children demonstrated cognitive impairment that persisted up to age 7 years.[159]

In 1985 Rogan and coworkers[160] examined 117 children with prenatal and/or breast milk exposure to the PCB/PCDF/PCQ-contaminated oil. Compared with unexposed children, those exposed demonstrated delayed developmental milestones, psychologic deficits, and behavioral abnormalities. Physical abnormalities included shorter stature, lighter weight, and epidermal disorders such as acne, hyperpigmentation, deformed nails, gingival hypertrophy, and tooth chipping.[160] Together these findings suggest a neuroectodermal dysplasia due to combined effects of the PCBs and contaminants.[160]

In addition to the teratogenic effects, the contaminated oils led to excessive reproductive losses among exposed women. Increased risks for spontaneous abortion, stillbirth, and infant mortality were documented in follow-up study of a group of Taiwanese women.[161]

An unusual phenomenon has been noted with regard to low birth weight; in follow-up studies, "catch-up" growth occurred in most of the surviving infants, with attainment of normal body weight by 2 years of age.[153,161]

The effects of cooking oil contamination should be distinguished from those of ambient or low-level exposure to PCBs. Low-level PCB maternal exposure can occur throughout life by consumption of fish from PCB-contaminated waters as well as other dietary sources. While transplacental transfer of PCBs occurs,[162] the largest dose is delivered to the nursing infant via breast milk.[152,163] Maternal exposure and PCB transfer to nursing infants has resulted in justifiable concern about reproductive and developmental effects. Studies ongoing in the Great Lakes region are examining such effects. Presently, the benefits of nursing to an infant are believed to outweigh theoretical risks from possible PCB exposure via breast milk, except in an unusual situation in which the mother has a high body burden of PCBs.

Rhesus monkeys fed low levels of PCBs for prolonged periods demonstrate infertility, embryo resorption, spontaneous abortion, and intrauterine growth retardation.[164] This species seems to be exquisitely sensitive to PCBs, since these effects occur within a range of dietary PCB concentrations considered allowable in certain human foods. In laboratory animals, reproduction, immunologic response, and the liver (enzyme induction and tumor development) are the major areas affected by chronic low-level exposure.[165]

In human epidemiologic studies, maternal PCB exposure via fish consumption has been reported to be associated with a slight decrease in infant birth weight and head circumference, relative to unexposed controls.[166] Neonatal assessment of the same infants provides some evidence that at low concentrations, PCBs may be behavioral teratogens.[167] Short-term memory impairment noted in infancy persisted at 4 years of age only in those children whose cord blood PCB concentrations were in the top 5% of values for the cohort.[163]

A cohort of North Carolina children followed since birth appears to be representative of the general population, that is, without unusual PCB exposure. Periodic developmental evaluations, including standardized developmental tests, behavioral ratings, and school report card evaluations,[168] up to school age have not demonstrated a relationship between prenatal or postnatal (breast-feeding) PCB exposure.

The human epidemiologic studies of developmental effects of low-level PCB exposure have been reviewed recently by Rogan and Gladen[168] and Jacobson and Jacobson.[169] Additional studies of congener-specific effects on a variety of reproductive and developmental endpoints are being conducted currently. Presently, we agree with most who counsel that the benefits of breast-feeding outweigh theoretical risks to the infant from PCB exposure and that routine measurement of PCBs in breast milk is neither warranted nor feasible.[170]

Polybrominated Biphenyls

Polybrominated biphenyl (PBB) compounds are structurally similar to PCBs and share characteristics of high lipid solubility and resistance to metabolic or biologic degradation. Fortunately, PBBs are not as widespread environmental contaminants as PCBs because their use has been more limited.

PBBs were used as fire-retardants in the United States until 1974. In 1973 and 1974, cattle feed distributed in Michigan inadvertently became contaminated with PBBs. Before the contamination was recognized, people in the state consumed PBB-tainted meat and poultry. Reviews of the incident and subsequent health studies are available.[171-174]

Fetal mortality in high- versus low-exposure regions of Michigan was not appreciably different after the PBB contamination.[175] The study of fetal mortality is not conclusive because of potential inaccuracies in exposure estimates, the inability to control for confounding variables, and the possibility that fetal mortality may not be the best indicator of PBB reproductive effects. In addition, this study was based on fetal deaths occurring at greater than 20 weeks gestation, and risks for early fetal losses could be different than those for later deaths.[176]

Transplacental and breast milk exposure of infants was documented in the Michigan incident.[177] An early follow-up study reported that children with higher PBB body burdens scored lower on standardized tests of perceptual motor, attentional, and verbal abilities.[178] Later testing of these children showed that their overall developmental scores were within the normal range.[179]

Nitrates and Nitrite

Nitrate contamination of drinking water supplies may result from agricultural (fertilizer) run-off, sewerage, or industrial waste. Nitrates and nitrite appear not to be teratogenic in animals.[180,181] Administration of sodium nitrite to pregnant mice stimulated fetal erythropoiesis but did not affect fetal mortality, resorptions, average weight, number of offspring, or incidence of skeletal malformations.[182]

Although some results are suggestive, human epidemiologic studies provide no conclusive evidence that pregnant women who consume low levels of nitrates from drinking water are at increased risk for having a malformed baby. In South Australia an excess of birth defects prompted a case–control study examining the relationship between maternal drinking water source

(groundwater versus rainwater) and risk of malformations.[183] The risk of having a malformed infant was increased among women who drank groundwater. Risks for NTDs and oral clefts particularly were increased. Using estimated nitrate concentration, a dose-response relationship was found with a threefold increased risk at 5 to 15 mg/L nitrates and fourfold increased risk for greater than 15 mg/L nitrates. Study strengths include case ascertainment and monitoring of water nitrate concentrations during the study period; limitations include the assumption that water concentrations were constant during monitoring intervals and that subjects used the same source of drinking water throughout pregnancy. Most notable is the assumption that nitrates rather than some unmeasured drinking water contaminant was responsible. In fact, the seasonal variation in malformation risks suggests that dietary, nutritional, or other environmental factors may have contributed to the increased malformation rates.

A Canadian case–control study found that nitrate exposure from private wells was associated with an increased risk for delivering an infant with a CNS malformation. However, the opposite was found with drinking water obtained from other sources: increased nitrates were associated with a decrease in CNS malformations. To assess exposure, the investigators analyzed nitrates in water samples collected at addresses where study subjects lived at the time of delivery. Once again, the study is limited by the lack of information about other possible water contaminants. The contradictory risks associated with drinking water source, independent of nitrates concentration, also suggests that other factors contributed to the observed effects.[66]

Organic Solvents

Large numbers of women are employed in industries that use organic solvents, and women also may be exposed through use of household products or drinking water contamination. Not surprisingly, concerns have arisen that such exposures may cause any of several adverse reproductive outcomes.

Acute human health effects of high-dose solvent exposure are well known. Central nervous system effects including cortical atrophy, cerebellar degeneration, and loss of intellectual functioning have been documented as a result of chronic, high-dose solvent abuse ("sniffing" or "huffing").[184] Solvent intoxication is an established occupational hazard in such diverse groups as painters and rubber, semiconductor, and dry cleaning workers. Symptoms may follow inhalation, dermal, or ingestion exposure routes and may include headache, nausea, dizziness, and confusion progressing to CNS depression with loss of consciousness. Chronic exposure to low levels of solvents may lead to neuropsychiatric impairment and peripheral nerve damage.[185]

Analogous to the health effects described above, maternal solvent abuse by "sniffing" is reported to cause an embryopathy similar to the fetal alcohol syndrome (FAS). Hersch and associates[186] described three children with developmental and intellectual impairment, facial dysmorphism, and intrauterine growth retardation whose mothers abused spray paint throughout their pregnancies. Similar dysmorphic features and neurologic impairment have been described in other children born to mothers who chronically abused toluene or unnamed solvents during pregnancy.[187–189]

A fetal solvent syndrome and toluene embryopathy have been described that may be similar in pathogenesis to FAS.[190] Recently a pattern of structural and developmental anomalies similar to FAS has been reported in women who abused toluene during pregnancy.[191]

At lower levels of maternal exposure there is no clear evidence of embryopathic, fetal, or neurobehavioral adverse effects. Epidemiologic studies have examined reproductive outcomes of occupationally as well as environmentally exposed women.

Most occupational studies of this subject are case–control studies, with exposure status based on job descriptions and no actual exposure data available (air concentrations or duration of exposure, for example). Multiple solvent exposures often are likely.[192]

Holmberg and associates[193–195] used a compulsory birth defects registry in Finland to examine effects of maternal solvent exposure in a series of studies. The risk of CNS defects was 6 times more likely and the risk of orofacial clefts was 3.5 times more likely with first trimester maternal exposure. Upon reanalysis with additional data 3 years later, the association was no longer statistically significant and the authors concluded that still larger numbers of cases with these anomalies were needed for a conclusive study.[196]

Using occupational codes from birth certificates, Olsen[197] reported that mothers who were painters or worked in a laboratory were no more likely than unexposed mothers to have children with CNS, gastrointestinal, or congenital limb anomalies. Heidam[198] surveyed Danish women in selected occupations that could result in various chemical exposures. Compared with unexposed women, female painters had a slightly higher risk for spontaneous abortion. In a study of pregnancy outcomes among women employed at a semiconductor manufacturer, Pastides and associates[199] found an increased risk of spontaneous abortions for women working in the diffusion area. Materials used in the diffusion area include glycol ethers, toxic gases, and various solvents, providing potentially numerous and mixed exposures. Given the small number of pregnancies in exposed and unexposed groups, the authors consider their results as tentative, pointing out the need for larger prospective studies that include monitoring data to quantify exposure.[199]

Two subsequent studies have supported the earlier findings of associations between semiconductor manufacturing and spontaneous abortion risk. In a study of IBM employees, investigators from Johns Hopkins University reported an association between spontaneous abortion risk and working with ethylene glycol ethers in "clean rooms" (R.H. Gray, personal communication, 1993). Similarly, a study by investigators at the University of California, Davis, carried out for the Semiconductor Industry Association, found a significant increase in spontaneous abortion risk among fabrication workers. This increase was suggested to be associated with exposure to glycol ethers.[200]

On numerous occasions, drinking water contamination by organic solvents has resulted from storage tank leaks or hazardous waste leachate. Such contamination is a common "Superfund" issue confronting the public and the U.S. Environmental Protection Agency.[201] Affected communities may identify a temporal or geographic clustering of adverse reproductive effects, believing that the contamination has caused the epidemic. To date, there is no published evidence to support such a cause and effect relationship, but at least one study demonstrated an increased risk of spontaneous abortions among women during the time that their drinking water supply was contaminated with trichloroethane and other organic solvents.[47] A hospital-based study also was undertaken in response to community concerns that there were increased numbers of children born with congenital cardiac anomalies to women living in the contaminated area. The increased prevalence of cardiac anomalies was confirmed but found to be temporally unrelated to the drinking water contamination, making a causal relationship unlikely.[202]

In conclusion, toluene and possibly other organic solvents are probably teratogenic at high exposure levels seen with solvent abuse. The risk for the "fetal solvent syndrome" is unknown, and no exposure threshold for effect can be identified at this time. There is no conclusive evidence that low-level exposure increases the risk of congenital malformations or other adverse reproductive outcomes.

In a similar vein, when a pregnant woman asks if it is safe for her to paint the baby's nursery, Scialli[203] wisely advises counseling to minimize exposure without giving the impression that paint is an established developmental toxicant.

Anesthetic Gases

Large numbers of women working in medical and dental professions may be exposed occupationally to anesthetic gases, raising serious concerns about the reproductive hazards of such exposures. There is evidence that chronic first trimester exposure may increase the risk of spontaneous abortion.[204,205] Despite numerous studies, the question of whether or not a mother's exposure to anesthetic gas increases the risk of her bearing a congenitally malformed infant is still debated. One argument against a causal relationship is that no pattern of malformations has been found in studies reporting increased birth defect rates following maternal exposure during pregnancy.[206] On the other hand, animal studies have shown that anesthetic gases can be teratogenic at concentrations similar to those experienced by operating room personnel in the absence of gas scavenging systems.[207–209] Some investigators have found increased rates of birth defects in infants born to exposed women and have observed a dose-related effect.[204,209,210] In two studies, the rate of congenitally malformed infants was increased among female anesthetists who worked during the first 6 months of pregnancy compared with the rate among female anesthetists who did not work during pregnancy.[211,212] A criteria document prepared by the National Institute for Occupational Safety and Health (NIOSH) reviews animal data and epidemiologic studies published before 1977.[205] More recent reviews are also available.[213,214]

In a retrospective study of reproductive outcomes and anesthetic gas exposure in Ontario hospital personnel, Guirguis et al.[215] observed significantly more congenital malformations among female workers with anesthesia exposure than among a comparison group without such exposure. Increases were also observed in wives of exposed males. These findings were based on self reports, with an excess of minor malformations, and reporting bias is a potential problem. Statistically significantly increased risk of spontaneous abortion was also observed in the exposed cohort.

A recent study in France compared the rates of spontaneous abortions and birth defects in nurses who worked in operating rooms with those of nurses who worked in other departments of the same hospitals.[216] A total of 776 pregnancies was identified among 418 nurses. The rate of spontaneous abortions among nurses who worked in operating rooms during the pregnancy was significantly higher than among nurses working in other parts of the hospital. Self-reported first trimester exposures to anesthetics, ionizing radiation, formol, and all three were also significantly associated with increased risks of spontaneous abortion. While an increased risk following exposure to antineoplastic agents was reported, it was not statistically significant. The only significantly increased risk of birth defects was observed with formol exposure. Adjusted odds ratios based on logistic regression showed a significantly increased risk of birth defects associated with the combination exposure of anesthetics, ionizing radiation, and formol. The methods suggest that there may be potential recall bias associated with exposures to specific agents that do not apply to the general work location, such as the operating room.

Using a case–control approach, Matte et al.[217] studied potential associations between parental employment in health care occupations and birth defects. Cases for the study came from the Metropolitan Atlanta Congenital Defects Program registry and controls were randomly selected from live births without malformations occurring in the five-county metropolitan Atlanta area. A statistically significant association was observed between maternal employment as a nurse and congenital defects as a group. The risks for several specific birth defects were also significantly elevated for nurses. Of particular relevance to our discussion here, potential maternal exposure to anesthetic gases was significantly associated with risk of spina bifida, based on three exposed cases.

Virtually all epidemiologic studies of exposure to waste anesthetic gas and reproductive outcomes have design problems that affect the interpretation of reported results. Crude estimates of anesthetic gas exposure have been used because no actual measurements of gas concentrations were available. The specific gases were usually not identified, and exposure to mixtures of anesthetic agents is likely.[205] Many studies have been conducted by survey, with no validation of the responses and often, poor response rates. In such studies, selection bias cannot be evaluated because there is no information about nonresponders. Also not validating the reproductive history can lead to misleading results for several reasons. Study subjects may forget or inaccurately recall events that took place years before. Women who think they are exposed to an adverse environmental agent may be more likely to recall having a spontaneous abortion or a child with a minor malformation than are unexposed women.[218] One last problem pertains to the inherent difficulty of studying spontaneous abortions. To avoid the criticism that reported spontaneous abortions were not validated, investigators in one study considered only patients whose spontaneous abortions required for them to be hospitalized.[218] The problem with this approach is that women who have spontaneous abortions do not always require hospitalization, particularly if the abortion occurred during the first trimester or before pregnancy was diagnosed.

Data are accumulating regarding reproductive risks of occupational exposure to nitrous oxide. Rowland et al.[219] reported that exposure to 5 or more hours of unscavenged nitrous oxide per week among a cohort of female dental assistants was statistically significantly associated with reduced fertility. This was based on assessment of time to pregnancy and self-reported nitrous oxide exposure. In a subsequent report from the same cohort, Rowland et al.[220] observed an increased risk of spontaneous abortion among women in the cohort working with nitrous oxide 3 or more hours per week in offices not using scavenging equipment. This recent cohort study has not provided any information on malformation risks. The number of exposed births is too small (n = 98) to have sufficient statistical power to yield meaningful results for infrequent events.

Despite problems in study design, epidemiologic evidence supports the view that repeated maternal exposure to waste anesthetic gases during pregnancy should be minimized. Women who work in areas with a potential for repeated anesthetic gas exposure (no gas scavenger system in place) should be aware of the possibility of adverse reproductive effects and decide whether they want to continue to work in the same area during pregnancy or request to be transferred. In settings where anesthetic gases are administered, a gas scavenger system should be used, and particular attention must be given to maintaining that system. A properly functioning gas scavenging system should provide adequate protection from exposure.[205,221,222] Because there is always uncertainty about completely avoiding exposure to anesthetic gases, however, a woman with a history of pregnancy loss or having a child with congenital malformations may want to transfer to another work area.[210]

Environmental Contamination and Hazardous Waste Sites

What is the possible role of environmental contamination in causing birth defects? While the topic is controversial and the data are equivocal, there is some evidence that suggests that further study is warranted. Much of the concern focused around specific hazardous waste sites such as Love Canal, New York, and Woburn, Massachusetts. Studies at Love Canal showed an effect on birth weight[223–225] but no increased risk of congenital malformations. A study at Woburn suggested increased risks of selected birth defects associated with consumption of water from specific wells that had been contaminated with volatile organic compounds.[226] The original Woburn study has been criticized on methodologic grounds,[227] and recently completed studies by the Massachusetts Department of Public Health failed to show elevated birth defect risks.[228]

Three recent studies examined residential proximity to hazardous waste sites, as surrogates for exposure, and the risk of birth defects. Since one of the studies received considerable press coverage, it is worthwhile to examine this issue briefly.

Shaw et al.[44] carried out a case–control study using cases from the California Birth Defects Monitoring Program and controls randomly selected using birth certificate files. Cases and controls came from a five-county area in metropolitan San Francisco. Exposure was defined on the basis of various types of hazardous waste facilities found in the census tract of the mother's residence at the time of the birth of the case or control. It appeared that risk for cardiac/circulatory malformations was increased for women living near the facilities. When risks were examined by contaminant chemical class, the odds ratios for heart/circulatory malformations were elevated for each class except hydrocarbon solvents, with the odds ratio for cyanides being the highest. Gastrointestinal malformations were associated with hydrocarbon solvents and metals.

In a widely cited study, Geschwind et al.[43] examined birth defect cases from the New York State Congenital Malformation Registry based on proximity to hazardous waste sites. Cases and controls came from 20 counties in upstate New York and information on exposure to hazardous waste sites was based on geographic proximity to sites included in a large data base. Statistically significant associations were observed between hazardous waste sites and all birth defects combined and several groups of birth defects (nervous system, musculoskeletal system and skin). In addition, statistically significant associations were observed between specific types of contaminants and some types of birth defects: pesticides and musculoskeletal system; metals and nervous system; solvents and nervous system; and plastics and chromosomal anomalies. Notably, the observed increases in risk were for the most part small, control of confounding was minimal, there was considerable heterogeneity within the birth defect categories, and the methods used to assign exposure were subject to exposure misclassification.

The potential importance of some of these factors in influencing the results of the Geschwind et al. study is illustrated by a second study in upstate New York. As a follow up, Marshall et al.[229] studied musculoskeletal system and central nervous system malformations in 18 counties of upstate New York. Their cases included some of the cases studied by Geschwind et al.,[43] plus additional cases from 2 more recent years. Exposure assessment was based on residential proximity to hazardous waste sites using similar, but more precise, methods than those employed by Geschwind et al.[43] In contrast to the earlier study, Marshall et al.[229] failed to find significant associations between waste site proximity and either group of defects. They did, however, find a statistically significant association between central nervous system malformations and proximity to active industrial facilities. Marshall et al.[229] attribute the differences between their findings and those reported earlier to uncontrolled confounding, systematic misclassification, or chance. An important difference between the two studies is that the geographic data for the latter study were more refined, allowing for a more accurate determination of residential location.

The Obstetrician's Role in Evaluating Reproductive Risks in and Beyond the Workplace

Limitations of Available Reproductive Toxicity Information

Clinical questions about environmental or occupational exposures causing adverse reproductive outcomes are extremely difficult to answer, and the answers are seldom as helpful as they need to be. The difficulty occurs because the exposure for the patient and fetus is seldom known or measurable. If the exposure is known, there is almost never a study of similar exposure, with a sufficient sample size, that enables a physician to give a reliable estimate of risk or lack thereof.

For all the environmental exposures discussed in this chapter, no threshold is known below which no adverse reproductive outcome can be expected. Except for ionizing radiation and mercury, maximum recommended exposure levels are difficult to quantify.

Most diagnostic radiographs result in exposures of less than 5 rad, and the risk of congenital malformations or developmental delay in the infant probably is negligible at doses below 5 rad.[83] Therefore, under most circumstances, consultation to estimate dosage is not necessary, although it may provide some reassurance to the pregnant patient.

The most readily available data are usually from studies in laboratory animals. Although these data are useful in making judgments about setting standards or marketing an agent, they are seldom helpful in giving accurate risk information to a patient.

Human data usually consist of case reports, which seldom can establish a hazard and never can quantitate the magnitude of the risk. Epidemiologic studies, when available, often have limitations in design, execution, analysis, or interpretation. Thus, in most cases, the questions must be answered on the basis of reasoned judgments in the face of inadequate data.

Approach to Occupational Exposure Risk Assessment

The process by which a reasoned judgment can be made is summarized in Table 8-4 and the steps are described below. Paul and Himmelstein[63] provide a more detailed description of a similar evaluation process, and recent books[230,231] provide helpful guidance for clinicians.

Paul and Welch[232] have developed a number of recommendations relative to improving education and resources about occupational reproductive hazards. They identify problems in clinical risk evaluation and management and develop proposed solutions, including improving information resources for clinicians and improving education for health care providers.

Assessment of potential adverse health effects or toxicity from a chemical exposure begins with correct identification of the agent(s) (Table 8-4). As workers increasingly demanded their right to know the identity and toxicity of chemicals, the U.S. Occupational Safety and Health Administration (OSHA) drafted a regulation and state and local governments have passed so-called worker right-to-know laws.[233] One intent of the regulation and laws is to provide workers and physicians with toxicity information about each chemical used in a given workplace. An information sheet, the Material Safety Data Sheet (MSDS), is developed by the chemical manufacturer or distributer and includes basic identifying and specific toxicity information. Other details of the OSHA regulation and right-to-know laws are reviewed elsewhere.[233,234]

Obstetricians should be aware that copies of MSDSs are available upon request from an employer to any woman who may be occupationally exposed to a hazardous chemical. Unfortunately, these MSDs have been found to be of very limited usefulness for assessing reproductive hazards.[235] Supervisors, managers, and industrial hygienists may be able to provide additional identification, particularly when chemicals are mixed or modified through heating or industrial processes.

The next step is to characterize the extent to which the patient may be exposed. This can be relatively easy for substances such as lead and other heavy metals quantifiable in blood or urine. The radiation badge properly worn can provide exposure monitoring and should be checked frequently during pregnancy. OSHA has published occupational exposure standards for a large number of chemicals associated with adverse health effects.[126] These chemicals and agents must be monitored in the workplace, and such data may be helpful for exposure assessment.

Most often, however, no biologic or environmental data are available. Instead, the clinician must rely on a detailed description of the patient's job activities, precautions taken to avoid exposure (gloves, respirator, protective clothing, hand washing, etc.) and any clinical signs or symptoms suggesting excess exposure. All feasible routes of exposure should be considered, including ingestion (common if handwashing is not done before eating), inhalation (especially if hot vapors or odorless gases are produced), and dermal absorption (increased through irritated skin or prolonged contact

Table 8-4   Steps in Evaluating Exposures That May Result in Birth Defects or Other Adverse Reproductive Outcomes

Step/Action	Information Resources
1. Identify the exposure(s)	Material Safety Data Sheet (MSDS) Industry (supervisors, industrial hygienists)
2. Characterize extent of exposure(s)	Description of job activities Monitoring data (e.g., air sampling, radiation badge) Assess exposure routes Biologic sampling (e.g., lead, mercury)
3. Hazard evaluation	Health professionals (occupational/industrial physicians, medical toxicologists, geneticists) Regional poison control centers Teratology information services (National Institute for Occupational Safety and Health [NIOSH] Criteria Documents, Technical Bulletins) State Health Departments On-line databases (National Library of Medicine, Environmental Teratology Information Center, Environmental Mutagen, Carcinogen and Teratogen Department, ReproTox) Textbooks, periodicals
4. Risk assessment/judgment	Steps 1–2 Patient's family, medical, and reproductive history, other relevant exposures (e.g., alcohol, tobacco, drugs-of-abuse), background risk

with contaminated clothing). Similar considerations apply to nonoccupational exposures as well.

The third step is hazard evaluation. In this context, the physician must determine what is known of the reproductive effects of the chemicals or agents. Since no one can be all-knowing and no single information resource is sufficient for all patient questions, prudence dictates consulting a variety of sources. Physicians specializing in occupational or industrial medicine, medical toxicology, and genetics can be helpful. Such physicians may be affiliated with regional genetics centers or certified regional poison control centers. These centers may be able to recommend other helpful consultants as well. Numerous teratology information services (TIS) provide no-cost physician and patient telephone consultation. These services may vary considerably in how the consultation is provided, whether follow-up is done, nature of the staff qualifications, and the extent of medical supervision. Recently, the Council of Regional Networks for Genetic Services and the Organization of Teratology Information Services developed a framework for the provision of teratology information services.[236] This framework is seen as an important step toward the development of recommendations for strengthening existing programs and approaches to quality assurance.

Some TIS provide a written copy of the consultation to the referrring obstetrician. One university-affiliated TIS maintains and updates a reproductive toxicology data base (ReproTox) containing summaries of more than 3,000 chemicals and agents.[237] Obstetricians who choose to refer patients to any of these services should be familiar with the kinds of information and follow-up provided.

The National Library of Medicine in Bethesda,

Maryland, maintains several files on the TOXNET data base system, including reproductive and developmental toxicology information in bibliographic or text form. Examples include Developmental and Reproductive Toxicology (DART), GENE-TOX (genetic toxicology), and Environmental Mutagen Information Center (EMIC).

A variety of options are available for searching these data bases, including personal computer software (Grateful Med, commercial services) and CD-ROM copies in medical libraries or leased from commercial versions. Information is available from a TOXNET representative, National Library of Medicine, Specialized Information Services, 8600 Rockville Pike, Bethesda, MD 20894, (301)496-6531.

Another federal resource is the National Institute for Occupational Safety and Health (NIOSH), which publishes current recommendations for occupational exposure to a variety of agents or compounds. NIOSH also has a technical information service at its Cincinnati, Ohio, headquarters that may be able to provide in-house reports of investigations as well as NIOSH Technical Bulletins and Criteria Documents.

The American College of Obstetricians and Gynecologists publishes guidelines for several occupational exposures during pregnancy.[222] These guidelines include information about metals, solvents, and radiation—agents that also may be found as environmental contaminants.

Many state health or labor departments have a division responsible for occupational health issues. Staff may have expertise in industrial hygiene and safety, occupational medicine, and reproductive epidemiology and toxicology. Specific concerns about hazardous occupational exposures or adverse reproductive outcomes related to workplace exposures should be addressed to this division. In addition, state health departments may be helpful in evaluating associations between environmental exposures and adverse reproductive outcomes. Numerous off-the-shelf information resources include texts,[21,22,192,230,231,238–241] review articles,[3,20,63,83,242–244] and periodicals.

The final and most difficult step is formulating an assessment of risk. Chemical identity, extent of exposure, and the reproductive toxicity of the agent must be known. Unfortunately, all these necessary pieces of information are rarely available. If the exposure is known, available information rarely enables a physician to give a reliable estimate of risk. Thus, risk assessment is really a process of reasoned judgement as opposed to a quantitative estimate of risk. Formulating this judgement requires consideration of many factors, including the best estimate of the nature, extent, duration, and timing of exposure, the patient's medical, reproductive, and genetic history, lifestyle habits (especially tobacco, alcohol, and drugs-of-abuse), and, of course, reproductive toxicity information about the agent. Equally important, the patient should understand that with every pregnancy there is always a background risk for an adverse outcome. Birth defects and other adverse outcomes of pregnancy are relatively common events; approximately 12 to 15 percent of pregnancies result in a spontaneous abortion, and birth defects are observed in approximately 3 percent of all newborns. Frustrating though it is, the fact remains that it is usual not to know the cause for a given adverse outcome.

After completing this assessment process, the physician will be more familiar with and understand limitations of available information about a particular agent or chemical. The patient's exposure can be considered in the context of other relevant medical information, and this should be explained to the patient in nontechnical language. The physician may be able to recommend ways to decrease or minimize maternal exposure and determine if more close monitoring of the pregnancy is warranted.

Conclusion

Experimental studies in laboratory animals have identified a number of agents that are capable of causing abnormal development. While we know less about substances that are teratogenic in humans, a limited number of teratogenic drugs and chemicals have been identified. There is increasing evidence that some chemicals found in the occupational setting or in the ambient environment may be reproductive or developmental toxicants. While some of this evidence is for associations between exposures and congenital malformations, our interpretation is that there is more evidence for spontaneous abortions associated with occupational exposures than for congenital malformations. Since we believe that spontaneous abortion is one part of a spectrum of outcomes potentially associated with teratogenic exposures, agents that increase risks for spontaneous abortion are also likely to increase risks for congenital malformations.

It is important to refine exposure assessment and to improve outcome ascertainment to enhance epidemiologic studies that help determine the extent to which occupational and environmental exposures may contribute to birth defects and other adverse reproductive outcomes. This is particularly the case for studies of environmental contamination where residential location has commonly been used as a surrogate for exposure. Better exposure assessment and outcome ascertainment may also lead us to a better understanding of how such teratogens produce their effects so we can design and test intervention/prevention strategies. In the meantime, prenatal counseling about most occupational and environmental exposures requires a large measure of reasoned judgement and interpretation of imperfect/imprecise animal and epidemiologic data.

10 Key Points

- Birth defects are the single leading cause of infant mortality in the United States, accounting for over 21 percent of all deaths before 1 year of age.

- While causes for some types of birth defects are clearly established, for approximately two-thirds of all birth defects the causes are unknown.

- Teratogens have been shown to cause not only structural birth defects but intrauterine death, growth retardation, and functional abnormalities as well.

- Understanding the principles of teratogenesis can help in identifying and understanding the causes of abnormal development.

- Epidemiologic studies play an important role in increasing our knowledge about risk factors for birth defects.

- Exposure to high-dose ionizing radiation during gestation has been shown to cause microcephaly and mental retardation, but effects of low-dose exposures on the conceptus have not been identified.

- Prenatal exposure to metals, such as lead and mercury, have been shown to have adverse effects on the development and function of the central nervous system.

- Concerns about the reproductive and developmental effects of toxic waste sites and specific environmental contaminants, such as dioxins, polychlorinated biphenyls, and polybrominated biphenyls, have been raised but the data supporting such associations are inconsistent.

- Occupational exposures to organic solvents and anesthetic gases have been shown to be associated with increased risks for spontaneous abortions and birth defects in some studies.

- Obstetricians can play an important role in assessing risks of adverse reproductive outcomes associated with occupational exposures to their patients.

References

1. Centers for Disease Control and Prevention: Infant mortality—United States, 1992. MMWR 43:905, 1994
2. Public Health Service: Healthy People 2000: National Health Promotion and Disease Prevention Objectives. U.S. Department of Health and Human Services, Public Health Service, Washington, DC, 1991
3. Brent RL, Beckman DA: Environmental teratogens. Bull NY Acad Med 66:123, 1990
4. McKusick VA: Mendelian Inheritance in Man. Johns Hopkins University Press, Baltimore, 1966
5. McKusick VA: Mendelian Inheritance in Man: A Catalog of Human Genes and Genetic Disorders. Johns Hopkins University Press, Baltimore, 1994
6. Gabbe SG: Congenital malformations in infants of diabetic mothers. Obstet Gynecol Surv 32:125, 1977
7. Lenke RR, Levy HL: Maternal phenylketonuria and hyperphenylalaninemia: an international survey of the outcome of untreated and treated pregnancies. N Engl J Med 303:1202, 1980
8. Wilson JG: Environmental effects on development—teratology. p. 269. In NS Assali (ed): Pathophysiology of Gestation. Vol. 2. Academic Press, San Diego, 1972
9. Sever LE: Congenital malformations related to occupational reproductive hazards. Occup Med 9:471, 1994
10. Wilson JG: Current status of teratology—general principles and mechanisms derived from animal studies. p. 47. In Wilson JG, Fraser FC (eds): Handbook of Teratology. Vol. 1. Plenum, New York, 1977
11. Fraser FC: Relation of animal studies to the problem in man. p. 75. In Wilson JG, Fraser FC (eds): Handbook of Teratology. Vol. 1. Plenum, New York, 1977
12. Musselman AC, Bennett GD, Greer KA et al: Preliminary evidence of phenytoin-induced alterations in embryonic gene expression in a mouse model. Reprod Toxicol 8:383, 1994
13. Van Allen MI, Kalousek DK, Chernoff GF et al: Evidence for multi-site closure of the neural tube in humans. Am J Med Genet 47:723, 1993
14. Lenz W, Knapp K: Foetal malformations due to thalidomide. Geriatr Med Monthly 7:253, 1962
15. Sever LE: Neuroepidemiology of intrauterine radiation exposure. p. 241. In Molgaard C (ed): Neuroepidemiology: Theory and Method. Academic Press, San Diego, 1993
16. Selevan SG, Lemasters GK: The dose-response fallacy in human reproductive studies of toxic exposures. J Occup Med 29:451, 1987
17. Hemminki K, Sorsa M, Vainio H: Genetic risks caused by occupational chemicals. Scand J Work Environ Health 5:307, 1979
18. Shepard T: Human teratogenicity. Adv Pediatr 33:225, 1986
19. Mattison DR, Hanson JW, Kochar DM, Rao KS: Criteria for identifying and listing substances known to cause developmental toxicity under California's Proposition 65. Reprod Toxicol 3:3, 1989
20. U.S. General Accounting Office: Reproductive and Developmental Toxicants: Regulatory Actions Provide Uncertain Protection. GAO/PEMD-92-3, GAO, Washington, DC, 1991
21. Shepard TH (ed): Catalog of Teratogenic Agents. 5th Ed. p. 549. The Johns Hopkins University Press, Baltimore, 1986
22. Friedman JM, Prolifka JE: Teratogenic effects of drugs: A resource for clinicians (TERIS) Johns Hopkins University Press, Baltimore, 1994
23. Environmental Protection Agency: Guidelines for the health assessment of suspect developmental toxicants. Fed Reg 51:34028, 1986

24. Sever LE: Epidemiologic approaches to reproductive hazards of the workplace. Birth Defects 18:33, 1982

25. Sever LE: Incidence and prevalence as measures of the frequency of birth defects. Am J Epidemiol 118:608, 1983

26. Leck I: Correlations of malformation frequency with environmental and genetic attributes in man. p. 243. In Wilson JG, Fraser FC (eds): Handbook of Teratology. Vol. 3. Plenum, New York, 1977

27. Centers for Disease Control and Prevention: Congenital malformations surveillance. Teratology 48:545, 1993

28. A Report from the International Clearinghouse for Birth Defects Monitoring Systems: Congenital Malformations Worldwide. Elsevier, Amsterdam, 1990

29. EUROCAT Working Group: Surveillance of Congenital Anomalies 1980–1990. Institute of Hygiene and Epidemiology, Brussels, 1993

30. Sever LE: The conundrum of birth defect clusters. Health Environ Digest 7:10, 1994

31. Sever LE, Strassburg MA: Epidemiologic aspects of neural tube defects in the United States: changing concepts and their importance for screening and prenatal diagnostic programs. p. 243. In Mizejewski GJ, Porter IH (eds): Alpha-Fetoprotein and Congenital Disorders. Academic Press, San Diego, 1985

32. Sever LE, Hessol NA: Overall design considerations in male and female occupational reproductive studies. Prog Clin Biol Res 160:15, 1984

33. Sever LE, Sanders M, Monsen R: An epidemiologic study of neural tube defects in Los Angeles County. I. Prevalence at birth based on multiple sources of case ascertainment. Teratology 25:315, 1982

34. Gregg NM: Congenital cataract following German measles in the mother. Trans Ophthalmol Soc Aust 3:35, 1941

35. Lenz W: Discussion contribution by Dr. W. Lenz, Hamburg, on the lecture by Pfeiffer RA, Kosenow K: on the exogenous origin of malformations of the extremities. Tagung der Rheinisch-Westfälischen Kinderarztevereinigung in Dusseldonf, 1961

36. McBride WG: Thalidomide and congenital abnormalities. Lancet 2:1358, 1961

37. Borman B, Cryer C: Fallacies of international and national comparisons of disease occurrence in the epidemiology of neural tube defects. Teratology 42:405, 1990

38. Edmonds LD, Layde PM, James LM et al: Congenital malformation surveillance: two American systems. Int J Epidemiol 10:247, 1981

39. Lynberg MC, Edmonds LD: Surveillance of birth defects. p. 157. In Halperin W, Baker EL (eds): Public Health Surveillance. Van Nostrand Reinhold, New York, 1992

40. Lynberg MC, Edmonds LD: State use of birth defects surveillance. In Wilcox LS, Marks JS (eds): From Data to Action: CDC's Public Health Surveillance for Women, Infants, and Children. Public Health Service, Centers for Disease Control and Prevention (no date)

41. Bove F, Fulcomer M, Klotz J et al: Report on Phase IV-A: Public Drinking Water Contamination and Birthweight and Selected Birth Defects: A Cross-Sectional Study. New Jersey Department of Health, 1992

42. Bove F, Fulcomer M, Klotz J et al: Report on Phase IV-B: Public Drinking Water Contamination and Birthweight and Selected Birth Defects: A Case–Control Study. New Jersey Department of Health, 1992

43. Geschwind SA, Stolwijk AJ, Bracken M et al: Risk of congenital malformations associated with proximity to hazardous waste sites. Am J Epidemiol 135:1197, 1992

44. Shaw G, Schulman J, Frisch J et al: Congenital malformations and birthweight in areas with potential environmental contamination. Arch Environ Health 47:147, 1992

45. Infante PF: Oncogenic and mutagenic risks in communities with polyvinyl chloride production facilities. Ann NY Acad Sci 271:49, 1976

46. Theriault G, Iturra H, Gingras S: Evaluation of the association between birth defects and ambient vinyl chloride. Teratology 27:359, 1983

47. Deane M, Swan SH, Harris JA et al: Adverse pregnancy outcomes in relation to water contamination, Santa Clara County, California 1980–1981. Am J Epidemiol 129:894, 1989

48. Lenz W: Thalidomide and congenital abnormalities. Lancet 1:45, 1962

49. Edmonds LD, Falk H, Nissim JE: Congenital malformations and vinyl chloride. Lancet 2:1098, 1975

50. Edmonds LD, Anderson CE, Flynt JW Jr, James LM: Congenital central nervous system malformations and vinyl chloride monomer exposure: a community study. Teratology 17:137, 1978

51. Lammer EJ, Sever LE, Oakley GP: Teratogen update: valproic acid. Teratology 35:465, 1987

52. Sever LE, Olsen AR, Hinds NR et al: NINCDS Collaborative Perinatal Project: A User's Guide to the Project and Data. Vol. I. An Introduction to the History, Scope and Methodology of the Project. National Institute of Neurological and Communicative Disorders and Stroke, Contract NO1-NS-2-2311, 1983

53. Nordstrom S, Beckman L, Nordenson I: Occupational and environmental risks in and around a smelter in Northern Sweden. III. Frequencies of spontaneous abortion. Hereditas 88:41, 1978

54. Nordstrom S, Beckman I, Nordenson I: Occupational and environmental risks in and around a smelter in Northern Sweden. V. Spontaneous abortion among female employees and decreased birth weight in their offspring. Hereditas 90:291, 1979

55. Beckman L, Nordstrom S: Occupational and environmental risks in and around a smelter in Northern Sweden. IX. Fetal mortality among wives of smelter workers. Hereditas 97:1, 1982

56. Bracken MB: Design and conduct of randomized clinical trials in perinatal research. p 397. In Bracken MB (ed): Perinatal Epidemiology. Oxford University Press, New York, 1984

57. Smithells RW, Sheppard S, Schorah CJ et al: Apparent prevention of neural tube defects by periconceptional vitamin supplementation. Arch Dis Child 56:911, 1981

58. Smithells RW, Sheppard S, Schorah CJ et al: Possible

prevention of neural-tube defects by periconceptional vitamin supplementation Lancet 1:339, 1980

59. MRC Vitamin Study Research Group: Prevention of neural tube defects: results of the Medical Research Council Vitamin Study. Lancet 338:131, 1991

60. Czeizel AE, Dudas I: Prevention of the first occurrence of neural tube defects by periconceptional vitamin supplementation. N Engl J Med 327:1832, 1992

61. Centers for Disease Control and Prevention: Recommendations for the use of folic acid to reduce the number of cases of spina bifida and other neural tube defects. MMWR 41 (RR-14):1, 1992

62. Clauss CA, Berzon M, Bertin J: Litigating reproductive and developmental health in the aftermath of UAW versus Johnson Controls. Environ Health Perspect Suppl 2:205, 1993

63. Paul M, Himmelstein J: Reproductive hazards in the workplace: what the practitioner needs to know about chemical exposures. Obstet Gynecol 71:921, 1988

64. Lemasters GK, Selevan SG: Types of exposure models and advantages and disadvantages of sources of exposure data for use in occupational reproductive studies. Prog Clin Biol Res 160:67, 1984

65. Gordon JE: Assessment of occupational and environmental exposures. p. 450. In Bracken MB (ed): Perinatal Epidemiology. Oxford University Press, New York, 1984

66. Sever LE: Epidemiologic aspects of environmental hazards to reproduction. p. 63. In Talbott E, Craun G (eds): Introduction to Environmental Epidemiology. CRC Press, Boca Raton, FL, 1995

67. Gold EB, Sever LE: Childhood cancers associated with parental occupational exposures. Occup Med 9:495, 1994

68. Gold EB, Tomich E: Occupational hazards to fertility and pregnancy outcome. Occup Med 9:435, 1994

69. National Research Council Committee on Biological Markers: Biological Markers in Reproductive Toxicology. National Academy Press, Washington, DC, 1989

70. Hulka BS, Wilcosky T: Biological markers in epidemiologic research. Arch Environ Health 43:83, 1988

71. Lemasters GK, Schulte PA: Biologic markers in the epidemiology of reproduction. p. 385. In Schulte PA, Perara FP (eds): Molecular Epidemiology: Principles and Practices. Academic Press, San Diego, 1993

72. Lynberg MC, Khoury MJ: Interaction between epidemiology and laboratory sciences in the study of birth defects: design of birth defects risk factor surveillance in metropolitan Atlanta. J Toxicol Environ Health 40: 435, 1993

73. National Research Council: Environmental Epidemiology. National Academy Press, Washington, DC, 1991

74. Lybarger JA, Spengler RF, DeRosa CT: Priority Health Conditions: An Integrated Strategy to Evaluate the Relationship between Illness and Exposure to Hazardous Substances. ATSDR, Atlanta, 1993

75. Marsh GM, Caplan RJ: Evaluating health effects of exposure at hazardous waste sites: a review of state-of-the-art, with recommendations for future research. p. 3. In Andelman JB, Underhill DW (eds): Health Effects from Hazardous Waste Sites. Lewis Publishing, Chelsea, MI, 1987

76. Heath CW Jr: Epidemiology of dump exposures. p. 10. In Finberg L (ed): Chemical and Radiation Hazards to Children. Report of the 84th Ross Conference on Pediatric Research. Ross Laboratories, Columbus, OH, 1982

77. Miller RW: Measures of reproductive effects. p. 88. In Finberg L (ed): Chemical and Radiation Hazards to Children. Report of the 84th Ross Conference on Pediatric Research. Ross Laboratories, Columbus, OH, 1982

78. Miller RW: Effects of ionizing radiation from the atomic bomb on Japanese children. Pediatrics 41:257, 1968

79. Kirsch-Volders M (ed): Mutagenicity, Carcinogenicity, and Teratogenicity of Industrial Pollutants. Plenum, New York, 1984

80. Wood JW, Johnson KG, Omori Y et al: Mental retardation in children exposed in utero to the atomic bombs in Hiroshima and Nagasaki. Am J Public Health 57: 1381, 1967

81. Miller RW: Delayed effects occurring within the first decade after exposure of young individuals to the Hiroshima atomic bomb. Pediatrics 18:1, 1956

82. DeKaban AS: Abnormalities in children exposed to x-radiation during various stages of gestation: tentative timetable of radiation injury to the human fetus, part I. J Nucl Med 9:471, 1968

83. Brent RL: The effects of embryonic and fetal exposure to x-ray, microwaves, and ultrasound. Clin Perinatol 13: 615, 1986

84. Archer VE: Anencephalus, drinking water, geomagnetism and cosmic radiation. Am J Epidemiol 109:88, 1979

85. Gentry J, Parkhurst E, Bulin G: An epidemiologic study of congenital malformations in New York state. Am J Public Health 49:497, 1959

86. Kochupiluai N, Verma IC, Grewal MS, Ramalingaswami V: Down's syndrome and related abnormalities in an area of high background radiation in coastal Kenya. Nature 262:60, 1976

87. Brent RL: Radiations and other physical agents. p. 208. In Wilson JG, Fraser FC (eds): Handbook of Teratology. Vol. 1. Plenum, New York, 1977

88. Segall A, MacMahon B, Hannigan M: Congenital malformations and background radiation in northern New England. J Chronic Dis 17:915, 1964

89. Wood JW, Keehn RJ, Kawamoto S, Johnson KC: The growth and development of children exposed in utero to the atomic bombs in Hiroshima and Nagasaki. Am J Public Health 57:1374, 1967

90. Neel JV, Kato H, Schull WJ: Mortality in the children of atomic bomb survivors and controls. Genetics 76:311, 1974

91. Neel JV: Problem of "false positive" conclusions in genetic epidemiology: lessons from the leukemia cluster near the Sellafield nuclear installation. Genet Epidemiol 11:213, 1994

92. Meyer MB, Diamond EL, Merz T: Sex ratio of children born to mothers who had been exposed to x-rays in utero. Johns Hopkins Med J 123:123, 1968

93. Alberman E, Polani PE, Fraser-Roberts JA et al: Paren-

tal x-irradiation and chromosome constitution in their spontaneously aborted foetuses. Ann Hum Genet Lond 36:185, 1972

94. Stewart A, Kneale GW: Radiation dose effects in relation to obstetric x-rays and childhood cancers. Lancet 1:1185, 1970

95. Stewart A, Webb D, Giles D, Hewitt D: Malignant disease in childhood and diagnostic irradiation in utero. Lancet 2:447, 1956

96. Stewart A, Webb D, Hewitt D: A survey of childhood malignancies. BMJ 1:1495, 1958

97. Sever LE: Parental radiation exposure and children's health: are there effects on the second generation? Occup Med 6:613, 1991

98. Gardner MJ, Snee MP, Hall AJ et al: Results of case–control study of leukaemia and lymphoma among young people near Sellafield nuclear plant in West Cumbria. Br Med J 300:423, 1990

99. Gardner MJ, Hall AJ, Snee MP et al: Methods and basic data of case–control study of leukaemia and lymphoma among young people near Sellafield nuclear plant in West Cumbria. BMJ 300:429, 1990

100. Sever LE, Gilbert ES, Hessol NA, McIntyre JM: A case–control study of congenital malformations and occupational exposure to low-level ionizing radiation. Am J Epidemiol 127:226, 1988

101. McLaughlin JR, King WD, Anderson TW et al: Paternal radiation exposure and leukaemia in offspring: the Ontario case–control study. BMJ 307:959, 1993

102. Marcus M: Epidemiologic studies of VDT use and pregnancy outcome. Reprod Toxicol 4:51, 1990

103. Blackwell R, Chang A: Video display terminals and pregnancy. A review. Br J Obstet Gynaecol 95:446, 1988

104. Goldhaber MK, Polen MR, Hiatt RA: The risk of miscarriage and birth defects among women who use visual display terminals during pregnancy. Am J Indus Med 13:695, 1988

105. Schnorr TM, Grajewski BA, Hornung RW et al: Video display terminals and the risk of spontaneous abortion. N Engl J Med 324:727, 1991

106. World Health Organization: Environmental Health Criteria 1: Mercury. p. 48. WHO, Geneva, 1976

107. Harada M: Minamata disease: a medical report. p. 180. In Smith WE, Smith AM (eds): Minamata. Holt, Rinehart, New York, 1975

108. Bakir F, DamluJi SF, Amin-Zaki M et al: Methylmercury poisoning in Iraq. Science 181:230, 1973

109. Koos BJ, Longo LD: Mercury toxicity in the pregnant woman, fetus, and newborn infant. Am J Obstet Gynecol 126:390, 1976

110. Choi BH: Effects of prenatal methylmercury poisoning upon growth and development of fetal central nervous system. p. 473. In Clarkson TW, Nordberg GF, Sager PR (eds): Reproductive and Developmental Toxicology of Metals. Plenum, New York, 1983

111. Marsh DO, Myers GT, Clarkson TW et al: Fetal methylmercury poisoning: clinical and toxicologic data on 29 cases. Ann Neurol 7:348, 1980

112. Clarkson TW: The pharmacology of mercury compounds. Annu Rev Pharmacol 12:375, 1972

113. Tsuchiya H, Mitani K, Kodama K, Nakata T: Placental transfer of heavy metals in normal pregnant Japanese women. Arch Environ Health 39:11, 1984

114. Sandstead HH, Doherty RA, Mahaffey KA: Effects and metabolism of toxic trace metals in the neonatal period. p. 207. In Clarkson TW, Nordberg GF, Sager RP (eds): Reproductive and Developmental Toxicology of Metals. Plenum, New York, 1983

115. Pierce PE, Thompson JF, Likosky WH et al: Alkyl mercury poisoning in humans: report of an outbreak. JAMA 220:1439, 1972

116. McKeown-Eyssen G, Ruedy J, Neims A: Methylmercury exposure in northern Quebec. II. Neurologic findings in children. Am J Epidemiol 118:470, 1983

117. Skerfving S, Hansson K, Mangs C et al: Methylmercury-induced chromosome damage in man. Environ Res 7:83, 1974

118. Burbacher TM, Monnett C, Grant KS, Mottet NK: Methylmercury exposure and reproductive dysfunction in the nonhuman primate. Toxicol Appl Pharmacol 75:18, 1984

119. Gunderson VM, Grant KS, Burbacher TM et al: The effect of low-level prenatal methylmercury exposure on visual recognition memory in infant crab-eating macaques. Child Dev 57:1076, 1986

120. Mottet NK, Shaw CM, Burbacher TM: Health risks from increases in methylmercury exposure. Environ Health Perspect 63:133, 1985

121. Gunderson VM, Grant-Webster KS, Burbacher TM, Mottet NK: Visual recognition memory deficits in methylmercury-exposed *Macaca fascicularis* infants. Neurotoxicol Teratol 10:373, 1988

122. Gilani SH: Congenital abnormalities in methylmercury poisoning. Environ Res 9:128, 1975

123. Mattison DR: Female reproductive system. p. 43. In Clarkson TW, Nordberg GW, Sager PR (eds): Reproductive and Developmental Toxicology of Metals. Plenum, New York, 1983

124. Weiss B: The developmental neurotoxicity of methyl mercury. p. 112. In Needleman HL, Bellinger D (eds): Prenatal Exposure to Toxicants: Developmental Consequences. Johns Hopkins University Press, Baltimore, 1994

125. Steffek AJ, Clayton R, Siew C et al: Effects of elemental mercury vapor exposure on pregnant Sprague-Dawley rats. Teratology 35:59A, 1987

126. American Conference of Governmental Industrial Hygienists: Threshold Limit Values and Biological Exposure Indices for 1988–1989. ACGIH, Cincinnati, 1988

127. Clarkson TW, Magos L, Greenwood MR: The transport of elemental mercury into fetal tissues. Biol Neonate 21:239, 1972

128. Wannag A, Skjaerasen J: Mercury accumulation in placenta and foetal membranes. A study of dental workers and their babies. Environ Physiol Biochem 5:348, 1975

129. Agency for Toxic Substances and Disease Registry: Toxicological Profile for Mercury. p. 90. U.S. Public Health Service, ATSDR, Atlanta, GA, 1989

130. Gelbier S, Ingram J: Possible foetotoxic effects of mercury vapour: a case report. Public Health 103:35, 1989

131. Rowland AS: Reproductive effects of mercury vapor. Fund Appl Toxicol 19:326, 1992

132. Rowland AS, Baird DD, Weinberg CR et al: The effect of occupational exposure to mercury vapour on the fertility of female dental assistants. Occup Environ Med 51:28, 1994

133. Rom WN: Effects of lead on the female and reproduction: a review. Mount Sinai J Med 43:542, 1976

134. Hall A: The increasing use of lead as an abortifacient. BMJ 1:584, 1905

135. Creason JP, Svensgaard DJ, Baumgarner JE et al: Maternal-fetal tissue levels of sixteen trace elements in eight communities. U.S.E.P.A. Report EPA No. 600:1-78-033, 1978

136. Centers for Disease Control: Preventing lead poisoning in young children—United States. MMWR 34:66, 1985

137. Centers for Disease Control: Preventing lead poisoning in young children, pp. 7–15. U.S. Dept. of Health and Human Services, Public Health Service, Centers for Disease Control, Atlanta, 1991

138. Occupational Safety and Health Administration: Occupational exposure to lead. Final standard. Fed Reg 43: 52952, November 14, 1978

139. Needleman HL, Schell A, Bellinger D et al: The long term effects of exposure to low doses of lead in childhood. An 11-year follow-up report. N Engl J Med 322: 83, 1990

140. Bellinger D, Leviton A, Waternaux C et al: Longitudinal analyses of prenatal and postnatal lead exposure and early cognitive development. N Engl J Med 316:1037, 1987

141. Bellinger D, Needleman HL: The neurotoxicity of prenatal exposure to lead: kinetics, mechanisms, and expressions. p. 89. In Needleman HL, Bellinger D (eds): Prenatal Exposure to Toxicants: Developmental Consequences. Johns Hopkins University Press, Baltimore, 1994

142. Gulson BL, Mahaffey KR, Mizon K, Murray C: Contribution of tissue lead to blood lead in adult female subjects. J Lab Clin Med 125:703, 1995

143. Brownie CF, Brownie E, Noben D et al: Teratogenic effect of calcium edetate (CaEDTA) in rats and the protective effect of zinc. Toxicol Appl Pharmacol 82:426, 1986

144. Courtney KD, Gaylor DW, Hogan MD et al: Teratogenic evaluation of 2,4,5-T. Science 168:864, 1970

145. Kimbrough RD: Some fat-soluble stable industrial chemicals. p. 23. In Finberg L (ed): Chemical and Radiation Hazards to Children. Report of the 84th Ross Conference on Pediatric Research. Ross Laboratories, Columbus, OH, 1982

146. Institute of Medicine: Veterans and Agent Orange: Health Effects of Herbicides Used in Vietnam. National Academy Press, Washington, DC, 1993

147. Erickson JD, Mulinare J, McClain PW et al: Vietnam veterans risks for fathering babies with birth defects. JAMA 252:903, 1984

148. Centers for Disease Control: Centers for Disease Control Vietnam experience study: health status of Vietnam veterans. III. Reproductive outcomes and child health. JAMA 259:2715, 1988

149. Field B, Kerr C: Reproductive behavior and consistent patterns of abnormality in offspring of Vietnam veterans. J Med Genet 25:819, 1988

150. U.S. EPA: Health Assessment Document for 2,3,7,8-Tetrachlorodibenzo-P-Dioxin (TCDD) and Related Compounds (Review Draft). EPA, Washington, DC, 1994

151. Letz G: The toxicology of PCB's—an overview for clinicians. West J Med 138:534, 1983

152. Schwartz PM, Jacobson SW, Fein G et al: Lake Michigan fish consumption as a source of polychlorinated biphenyls in human cord serum, maternal serum, and milk. Am J Public Health 73:293, 1983

153. Safe S: Polychlorinated biphenyls (PCBs) and polybrominated biphenyls (PBBs): biochemistry, toxicology, and mechanism of action. CRC Crit Rev Toxicol 13: 319, 1985

154. Kimbrough RD: Human health effects of polychlorinated biphenyls (PCBs) and polybrominated biphenyls (PBBs). Annu Rev Pharmacol Toxicol 27:87, 1987

155. Kuratsune M, Yoshimura Y, Matsuzaka J, Yamagushi A: Epidmiologic study on yusho, a poisoning caused by ingestion of rice oil contaminated with a commercial brand of polychlorinated biphenyls. Environ Health Perspect 1:119, 1972

156. World Health Organization: Assessment of Health Risks in Infants Associated with Exposure to PCBs and PCDFs in Breast Milk. Report on a WHO Working Group. World Health Organization, Copenhagen, 1988

157. Buser HR: Polychlorinated dibenzofurans (PCDFs) found in yusho oil and used in Japanese PCB. Chemosphere 7:439, 1978

158. Yamashita F, Hayashi M: Fetal PCB syndrome: clinical features, intrauterine growth retardation and possible alteration in calcium metabolism. Environ Health Pespect 59:41, 1985

159. Chen Y-CJ, Guo Y-L, Hsu C-C, Rogan WJ: Cognitive development of Yu-Cheng ("oil disease") in children prenatally exposed to heat-degraded PCBs. JAMA 268: 3213, 1992

160. Rogan WJ, Gladen BC, Hung KL et al: Congenital poisoning by polychlorinated biphenyls and their contaminants in Taiwan. Science 241:334, 1988

161. Yen YY, Lan SJ, Ko YC, Chen CJ: Follow-up study of reproductive hazards of multiparous women consuming PCBs-contaminated rice oil. Bull Environ Contam Toxicol 43:647, 1989

162. Jacobson JL, Fein GG, Jacobson SW et al: The transfer of polychlorinated biphenyls and polybrominated biphenyls across the human placenta and into maternal milk. Am J Public Health 74:378, 1984

163. Jacobson JL, Jacobson SW, Humphrey HE: Effect of in utero exposure to polychlorinated biphenyls and related contaminants on cognitive functioning in young children. J Pediatr 116:38, 1990

164. Barsotti DA, Marler RJ, Allen JR: Reproductive dysfunction in rhesus monkeys exposed to low levels of polychlorinated biphenyls (Aroclor 1248). Food Cosmet Toxicol 14:99, 1976

165. Kimbrough RD: Laboratory and human studies on polychlorinated biphenyls (PCBs) and related compounds. Environ Health Perspect 59:99, 1985

166. Fein GG, Jacobson JL, Jacobson SW et al: Prenatal exposure to polychlorinated biphenyls: effects on birth size and gestational age. J Pediatr 105:315, 1984

167. Jacobson JL, Jacobson SW, Fein GG et al: Prenatal exposure to an environmental toxin: a test of the multiple effects model. Dev Psychol 20:523, 1984

168. Rogan WJ, Gladen BC: Neurotoxicity of PCBs and related compounds. Neurotoxicology 12:27, 1992

169. Jacobson JL, Jacobson SW: The effects of perinatal exposure to polychlorinated biphenyls and related contaminants. p. 130. In Needleman HL, Bellinger D (eds): Prenatal Exposure to Toxicants: Developmental Consequences. Johns Hopkins University Press, Baltimore, 1994

170. Frank JW, Newman J: Breast-feeding in a polluted world: uncertain risks, clear benefits. Can Med Assoc J 149:33, 1993

171. Fries GF: The PBB episode in Michigan: an overall appraisal. CRC Crit Rev Toxicol 16:105, 1985

172. Anderson HA, Lilis R, Selikoff IJ et al: Unanticipated prevalence of symptoms among dairy farmers in Michigan and Wisconsin. Environ Health Perspect 23:217, 1978

173. Bekesi JG, Roboz JP, Fischbein A, Mason P: Immunotoxicology: environmental contamination by polybrominated biphenyls and immune dysfunction among residents of the state of Michigan. Cancer Detect Prevent Suppl 1:29, 1987

174. Roboz J, Greaves J, Bekesi JG: Polybrominated biphenyls in model and environmentally contaminated human blood: protein binding and immunotoxicological studies. Environ Health Perspect 60:107, 1985

175. Humble CG, Speizer FE: Polybrominated biphenyls and fetal mortality in Michigan. Am J Public Health 74:1130, 1984

176. Sever LE: The state of the art and current issues regarding reproductive outcomes potentially associated with environmental exposures: reduced fertility, reproductive wastage, congenital malformations, and birth weight. U.S. E.P.A. Workshop on Reproductive and Developmental Epidemiology: Issues and Recommendations. U.S. E.P.A. 600/8-89-103, Cincinnati, 1989

177. Eyster JT, Humphrey HEB, Kimbrough RD: Partitioning of polybrominated biphenyls (PBBs) in serum, adipose tissue, breast milk, placenta, cord blood, biliary fluid, and feces. Arch Environ Health 38:47, 1983

178. Seagull EAW: Developmental abilities of children exposed to polybrominated biphenyls (PBB). Am J Public Health 73:281, 1983

179. Schwartz EM, Rae WA: Effect of polybrominated biphenyls (PBB) on developmental abilities in young children. Am J Public Health 73:277, 1983

180. Ema M, Kanoh S: Studies on the pharmacological bases of fetal toxicity of drugs. Fetal toxicity of potassium nitrate in two generations of rats. Folia Pharmacol Japan 81:469, 1983

181. Sleight SD, Sinha DP, Uzoukwu M: Effect of sodium nitrite on reproductive performance of pregnant sows. JAVMA 61:819, 1972

182. Globus M, Samuel D: Effect of maternally administered sodium nitrite on hepatic erythropoesis in fetal CD-1 mice. Teratology 18:367, 1978

183. Dorsch MM, Scragg RKR, McMichael AJ et al: Congenital malformations and maternal drinking water supply in rural South Australia: a case–control study. Am J Epidemiol 119:473, 1984

184. King MD: Neurological sequelae of toluene abuse. Hum Toxicol 1:281, 1982

185. Andrews LS, Snyder R: Toxic effects of solvents and vapors. p. 636. In Klaassen CD, Amdur MO, Doull J (eds): Casarett and Doull's Toxicology. The Basic Science of Poisons. 3rd Ed. Macmillan, New York, 1986

186. Hersh JH, Podruch PE, Rogers R, Weisskopf B: Toluene embryopathy. J Pediatr 106:922, 1985

187. Hersh JH: Toluene embryopathy: two new cases. J Med Genet 26:333, 1989

188. Toutant C, Lippmann S: Fetal solvents syndrome (letter). Lancet 1:1356, 1979

189. Goodwin TM: Toluene abuse and renal tubular acidosis in pregnancy. Obstet Gynecol 71:715, 1988

190. Pradhan S, Ghosh TK, Pradhan SN: Teratological effects of industrial solvents. Drug Dev Res 13:205, 1988

191. Pearson MA, Hoyme HE, Seaver LH, Rimsza ME: Toluene embryopathy: delineation of the phenotype and comparison with fetal alcohol syndrome. Pediatrics 93:211, 1994

192. Barlow SM, Sullivan FM: Reproductive Hazards of Industrial Chemicals. Academic Press, San Diego, 1982

193. Holmberg PC, Nurminen M: Congenital defects of the central nervous system and occupational factors during pregnancy. A case–referent study. Am J Ind Med 1:167, 1980

194. Holmberg PC: Central-nervous-system defects in children born to mothers exposed to organic solvents during pregnancy. Lancet 2:177, 1979

195. Holmberg PC, Hernberg S, Kurppa K et al: Oral clefts and organic solvent exposure during pregnancy. Int Arch Occup Environ Health 50:371, 1982

196. Kurppa K, Holmberg PC, Hernberg S et al: Screening for occupational exposures and congenital malformations. Scand J Work Environ Health 9:89, 1983

197. Olsen J: Risk of exposure to teratogens amongst laboratory staff and painters. Dan Med Bull 30:24, 1983

198. Heidam LZ: Spontaneous abortions among dental assistants, factory workers, painters, and gardening workers: a follow-up study. J Epidemiol Comm Health 38:149, 1984

199. Pastides H, Calabrese EJ, Hosmer DW, Harris DR: Spontaneous abortion and general illness symptoms among semiconductor manufacturers. J Occup Med 30:543, 1988

200. Schenker M, Beaumont J, Gold E et al: Epidemiologic Study of Reproductive and Other Health Effects Among Workers Employed in the Manufacture of Semiconductors: Final Report to the Semiconductor Industry Association. University of California, Davis, Davis, 1992

201. Agency for Toxic Substances and Disease Registry: Tox-

icological Profile for Trichloroethylene. U.S. Public Health Service, ATSDR, Atlanta, GA, October 1989

202. Swan SH, Shaw G, Harris JA, Neutra RR: Congenital cardiac anomalies in relation to water contamination, Santa Clara County, California, 1981–1983. Am J Epidemiol 129:885, 1989

203. Scialli AR: Who should paint the nursery? Reprod Toxicol 3:159, 1989

204. Spence AA, Cohen EN, Brown BW et al: Occupational hazards for operating room-based physicians. Analysis of data from the United States and the United Kingdom. JAMA 238:955, 1977

205. National Institute for Occupational Safety and Health: Criteria for a Recommended Standard: Occupational Exposure to Waste Anesthetic Gases and Vapors. DHEW Publ. No. 77–140. NIOSH, Washington, DC, 1977

206. Spence AA, Knill-Jones RP: Is there a health hazard in anaesthetic practice? Br J Anaesth 50:713, 1978

207. Mazze RE, Wilson AI, Rice SA, Baden JM: Reproduction and fetal development in rats exposed to nitrous oxide. Teratology 30:259, 1984

208. Corbett TH: Cancer and congenital anomalies associated with anesthetics. Ann NY Acad Sci 271:58, 1976

209. Edling C: Anesthetic gases as an occupational hazard—a review. Scand J Work Environ Health 6:85, 1980

210. Vessey MP, Nunn JF: Occupational hazards of anesthesia. BMJ 281:696, 1980

211. Corbett TH, Cornell RG, Endres JL, Lieding K: Birth defects among children of nurse-anesthetists. Anesthesiology 41:341, 1974

212. Knill-Jones RP, Moir DD, Rodrigues LV, Spence AA: Anesthetic practice and pregnancy—controlled survey of women anesthetists in the United Kingdom. Lancet 1:1326, 1972

213. Friedman JM: Teratogen update: anesthetic agents. Teratology 37:69, 1988

214. Infante PF, Tsongas TA: Anesthetic gases and pregnancy: a review of evidence for an occupational hazard. p. 287. In Hemminki K, Sorsa M, Vainio H (eds): Occupational Hazards and Reproduction. Hemisphere Publishing Corporation, Washington, 1985

215. Guirguis SS, Pelmear PL, Roy ML, Wong L: Health effects associated with exposure to anaesthetic gases in Ontario hospital personnel. Br J Indus Med 47:490, 1990

216. Saurel-Cubizolles MJ, Hays M, Estryn-Behar M: Work in operating rooms and pregnancy outcomes among nurses. Int Arch Occup Environ Health 66:235, 1994

217. Matte TD, Mulinare J, Erickson JD: Case–control study of congenital defects and parental employment in health care. Am J Indus Med 24:11, 1993

218. Axelsson GA, Rylander R: Exposure to anaesthetic gases and spontaneous abortion: response bias in a postal questionnaire study. Int J Epidemiol 11:250, 1982

219. Rowland AS, Baird DD, Weinberg CR et al: Reduced fertility among women employed as dental assistants exposed to high levels of nitrous oxide. N Engl J Med 327:993, 1992

220. Rowland AS, Baird DD, Shore DL et al: Nitrous oxide and spontaneous abortion in female dental assistants. Am J Epidemiol 141:531, 1995

221. Mattia MA: Anesthesia gases and methylmethacrylate. Am J Nurs 83:73, 1983

222. American College of Obstetricians and Gynecologists: Guidelines on Pregnancy and Work. The American College of Obstetricians and Gynecologists, Chicago, 1977

223. Curtiss JRB, Ginevan ME, Brown CD: Spatio/temporal analysis of human birth weight: an indicator of subtle environmental stress? p. 33. In: Health Impacts of Different Sources of Energy. International Atomic Energy Agency, Vienna, 1982

224. Goldman LR, Paigen B, Magnant MM, Highland JH: Low birth weight, prematurity and birth defects in children living near the hazardous waste site, Love Canal. Haz Waste Haz Mat 2:209, 1985

225. Vianna NJ, Polan AK: Incidence of low birth weight among Love Canal residents. Science 226:1217, 1984

226. Lagakos SW, Wessen BJ, Zelen M: An analysis of contaminated well water and health effects in Woburn, Massachusetts. J Am Stat Assoc 81:583, 1986

227. MacMahon B: Comment. J Am Stat Assoc 81:596, 1986

228. Massachusetts Department of Public Health: Woburn Environment and Birth Study, 1994

229. Marshall EG, Gensburg LJ, Geary NS et al: Analytic study to evaluate associations between hazardous waste sites and birth defects. Final Report for ATSDR grant H75/ATH 290110012. New York State Department of Health, Albany, NY, 1995

230. Paul M: Occupational and Environmental Reproductive Hazards: A Guide for Clinicians. Williams & Wilkins, Baltimore, 1993

231. Scialli AR: A Clinical Guide to Reproductive and Developmental Toxicology. CRC Press, Boca Raton, FL, 1992

232. Paul M, Welch L: Improving education and resources for health care providers. Environ Health Perspect Suppl 2:191, 1993

233. Occupational Safety and Health Administration: Hazard Communication Guidelines for Compliance. Publication No. OSHA 3111, U.S. Department of Labor. OSHA, Washington, DC, 1988

234. Himmelstein JS, Frumkin H: The right to know about toxic exposures. Implications for physicians. N Engl J Med 312:687, 1985

235. Paul M, Kurtz S: Analysis of reproductive health hazard information on material safety data sheets for lead and the ethylene glycol ethers. Am J Indus Med 25:403, 1994

236. Council of Regional Genetic Networks: Framework for provision of teratology information services. Reprod Toxicol 8:439, 1994

237. ReproTox Database, The Reproductive Toxicology Center, 2425 L Street, NW, Washington, DC, 20037

238. Richardson M: Reproductive Toxicology. VCH Publishers, New York, 1993

239. Sullivan FM, Watkins WJ, van der Venne MTR: Reproductive Toxicity. Vol. 1. Summary Reviews of the Scien-

tific Evidence. Office for Publications of the European Communities, Luxembourg, 1993

240. Koren G: Maternal–Fetal Toxicity, a Clinician's Guide. 2nd Ed. Marcel Dekker, New York, 1994

241. Schardein JL: Chemically Induced Birth Defects. 2nd Ed. Marcel Dekker, New York, 1993

242. Strobino B, Kline J, Stein ZA: Chemical and physical exposures of parents: effects on human reproduction and offspring. J Early Hum Dev 1:371, 1978

243. Council on Scientific Affairs: Effects of toxic chemicals on the reproductive system. JAMA 253:3431, 1985

244. Brent RL, Beckman DA: The contribution of environmental teratogens to embryonic and fetal loss. Clin Obstet Gynecol 37:646, 1994

Genetic Counseling and Prenatal Diagnosis

Joe Leigh Simpson

Approximately 3 percent of liveborn infants have a major congenital anomaly. About one-half of these anomalies are detected at birth; the remainder become evident later in childhood or, less often, adulthood. Although nongenetic factors may cause malformations, genetic factors are usually responsible. In addition, more than 50 percent of first trimester spontaneous abortions and at least 5 percent of stillborn infants show chromosomal abnormalities (see Ch 22). Given such an important role for genetic factors, knowledge of medical genetics clearly becomes integral to the practice of modern obstetrics.

This chapter first considers the principles of genetic counseling and genetic screening. Thereafter, disorders amenable to genetic screening and prenatal diagnosis are discussed.

Frequency of Genetic Disease

Phenotypic variation—normal or abnormal—may be considered in terms of several etiologic categories: (1) chromosomal abnormalities, numerical or structural; (2) single-gene or mendelian disorders; (3) polygenic and multifactorial disorders, polygenic implying an etiology resulting from cumulative effects of more than one gene and multifactorial implying interaction as well with environmental factors; and (4) teratogenic disorders, caused by exposure to exogenous factors (e.g., drugs) that deleteriously affect an embryo otherwise destined to develop normally. Principles of these mechanisms are reviewed elsewhere.[1]

Chromosomal Abnormalities

From surveys of more than 50,000 liveborn neonates, it has been established that the incidence of chromosomal aberrations is 1:160. Table 9-1 shows the incidences of individual abnormalities.[2]

Single-Gene Disorders

Approximately 1 percent of liveborns are phenotypically abnormal due to a single-gene mutation. Several thousand single-gene (mendelian) disorders have been recognized, and many more are suspected.[3] However, even the most common mendelian disorders (cystic fibrosis in whites, sickle cell anemia in blacks, β-thalassemia in Greeks and Italians, α-thalassemia in Southeast Asians, Tay-Sachs disease in Ashkenazi Jews) are individually rare. In aggregate, however, mendelian disorders account for 40% of the congenital defects seen in liveborn infants.

Polygenic/Multifactorial Disorders

Another 1 percent of neonates are abnormal, but possess a normal chromosomal complement and have not undergone mutation at a *single* genetic locus. As will be discussed below, it can be deduced that several different genes are involved (polygenic/multifactorial inheritance).[1] Disorders in this etiologic category include most common malformations limited to a single organ system. These include hydrocephaly, anencephaly, and spina bifida (neural tube defects), facial clefts (cleft lip and palate), cardiac defects, pyloric stenosis, omphalocele, hip dislocation, uterine fusion defects, and club foot. After the birth of one child with such anomalies, the recurrence risk in subsequent progeny is usually 1 to 5 percent.[1] This frequency is less than would be expected if only a single gene were responsible but greater than that for the general population. The recurrence risks for malformations are also 1 to 5 percent for offspring of affected parents. That recurrence risks are similar for both siblings and offspring diminishes the likelihood that environmental causes are the exclu-

Table 9-1 Chromosomal Abnormalities in Liveborn Infants[a]

Type of Abnormality	
Numerical aberrations	
Sex chromosomes	
47, XYY	1/1,000 MB
47, XXY	1/1,000 MB
Other (males)	1/1,350 MB
47, X	1/10,000 FB
47, XXX	1/1,000 FB
Other (females)	1/2,700 FB
Autosomes	
Trisomies	
13–15 (D group)	1/20,000 LB
16–18 (E group)	1/8,000 LB
21–22 (G group)	1/800 LB
Other	1/50,000 LB
Structural aberrations	
Balanced	
Robertsonian	
t(Dq;Dq)	1/1,500 LB
t(Dq;Gq)	1/5,000 LB
Reciprocal translocations and insertional inversions	1/7,000 LB
Unbalanced	
Robertsonian	1/14,000 LB
Reciprocal translocations and insertional inversions	1/8,000 LB
Inversions	1/50,000 LB
Deletions	1/10,000 LB
Supernumeraries	1/5,000 LB
Other	1/8,000 LB
Total	1/160 LB

[a] LB, live births; MB, male births; FB, female births
(Pooled data tabulated by Hook and Hamerton.[2])

Polygenic/Multifactorial Traits[a]

Hydrocephaly (excepting some forms of aqueductal stenosis and Dandy-Walker syndrome)
Neural tube defects (anencephaly, spina bifida, encephalocele)
Cleft lip, with or without cleft palate
Cleft lip (alone)
Cardiac anomalies (most types)
Diaphragmatic hernia
Omphalocele
Renal agenesis (unilateral or bilateral)
Ureteral anomalies
Posterior urethral values
Hypospadias
Müllerian fusion defects
Limb reduction defects
Talipes equinovarus (clubfoot)

---

[a]Relatively common traits considered to be inherited in polygenic/multifactorial fashion. For each, normal parents have recurrence risks of 1 to 5 percent after one affected child. After two affected offspring, the risk is higher.

---

sive etiologic factor because it is unlikely that households in different generations would be exposed to the same teratogen. Further excluding environmental factors as sole etiologic agents are observations that monozygotic twins are much more often concordant (similarly affected) than are dizygotic twins, despite both types of twins sharing a common intrauterine environment.

The above observations are best explained on the basis of polygenic/multifactorial inheritance. Although more than one gene is involved, only a few genes are necessary to produce the number of genotypes necessary to explain recurrence risks of 1 to 5 percent. That is, large numbers of genes and complex mechanisms need *not* be invoked. Polygenic/multifactorial etiology can thus plausibly be assumed responsible for most liveborns who have an anomaly of a single organ system and who have neither a chromosomal abnormality nor a mendelian mutation.

Teratogenic Disorders

Perhaps 15–20 proved teratogens are known, as reviewed in Chapter 10. Although many other agents are suspected teratogens, the quantitative combination of known teratogens to the incidence of anomalies seems relatively small (with the possible exception of alcohol).

Clinical Spectrum of Chromosomal Abnormalities

A few generalizations concerning chromosomal disorders can be offered that may prove helpful to the obstetrician, who may encounter such abnormalities during prenatal studies or in the delivery room. In this section we briefly review the clinical and cytogenetic features characteristic of the common chromosomal abnormalities. These and other disorders have been discussed in detail elsewhere, where complete references are provided.[1]

Autosomal Trisomy

Trisomy 21

Trisomy 21 (Down syndrome, mongolism) is the most frequent autosomal chromosomal syndrome, occurring in 1 of every 800 liveborn infants (Table 9-1). The relationship to advanced maternal age is well known. Characteristic craniofacial features include brachycephaly, oblique palpebral fissures, epicanthal folds, broad nasal bridge, a protruding tongue, and small, low-set ears with an overlapping helix and a prominent antihelix

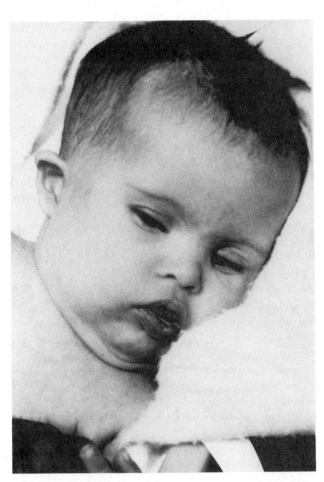

Fig. 9-1 An infant with trisomy 21. (From Simpson and Golbus,[1] with permission.)

(Fig. 9-1). The mean birth weight in Down syndrome, 2,900 g, is decreased but not so much as in some other autosomal syndromes. At birth, these infants are usually hypotonic. Other features include iridial Brushfield spots, broad short fingers (brachymesophalangia), clinodactyly (incurving deflections resulting from an abnormality of the middle phalanx), a single flexion crease on the fifth digit, and an unusually wide space between the first two toes. Contrary to widespread opinion, a single palmar crease (simian line) is not pathognomonic, being present in only 30 percent of individuals with trisomy 21 and in 5 percent of normal individuals. Relatively common internal anomalies include cardiac lesions and duodenal atresia. Cardiac anomalies and increased susceptibility to both respiratory infections and leukemia contribute to a reduced life expectancy. However, the mean survival is still into the fifth decade, and many affected individuals survive to older ages.

Patients with Down syndrome who survive beyond infancy invariably exhibit mental retardation. However, the degree of retardation is generally not as severe

as that of many other chromosomal aberrations. Mean IQ ranges approximately from 25 to 70. $46/47, +21$ mosaicism should be suspected if Down syndrome cases show IQs in the 70 to 80 range. Females are fertile. Although relatively few trisomic mothers have reproduced, about 30 percent of their offspring are also trisomic. Except possibly very exceptional cases, affected males are not fertile.

Several different cytogenetic mechanisms may be associated with Down syndrome, which is actually the result of triplication of a small portion of the No. 21 chromosome, namely, band q22. This triplication may be caused either by the presence of an entire additional No. 21 or by addition of only band q22. Of all cases of Down syndrome, 95 percent have primary trisomy (47 instead of the normal 46 chromosomes) (Fig. 9-2). These cases show the well-known relationship to maternal age.

By contrast, translocations show no definite relationship to parental age and may be either sporadic or familial. The translocation most commonly associated with Down syndrome involves chromosomes 14 and 21. With translocation Down syndrome [t(14q;21q)], one parent may have the same translocation chromosome, that is, 45,t(14q;21q). For parents with a translocation, the recurrence risk for a child with an unbalanced chromosome complement far exceeds the risk for recurrence of nondisjunction (1 percent). Empiric risks are approximately 10 percent for offspring of female translocation heterozygotes and 2 percent for offspring of male translocation heterozygotes.

Other structural rearrangements resulting in Down

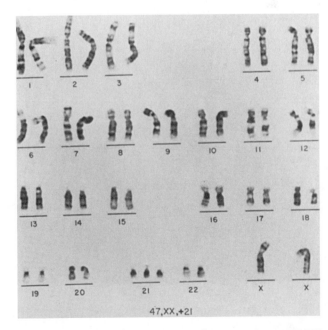

Fig. 9-2 Karyotype of a trisomy 21 cell. Trypsin-Giemsa (GTG) banding (From Simpson and Golbus,[1] with permission.)

syndrome include t(21q;21q), t(21q;21q), and translocations involving No. 21 and chromosomes other than a member of group D (Nos. 13 to 15) or G (Nos. 21 to 22). In t(21q;21q) no normal gametes can be formed. Thus, only trisomic or monosomic zygotes are produced, the latter presumably appearing as preclinical embryonic losses. Parents having the other translocations have a low empiric risk of having offspring with Down syndrome.

Trisomy 13

Trisomy 13 occurs in about 1 per 20,000 live births. Intrauterine and postnatal growth retardation are pronounced, and developmental retardation is severe. Nearly 50 percent of affected children die in the first month, and relatively few survive past 3 years of age. Characteristic anomalies include holoprosencephaly, eye anomalies (microphthalmia, anophthalmia, or coloboma), cleft lip and palate, polydactyly, cardiac defects, and low birth weight. Other relatively common features include cutaneous scalp defects, hemangiomata on the face or neck, low-set ears with an abnormal helix, and rocker-bottom feet (convex soles and protruding heels) (Fig. 9-3).

Trisomy 13 is usually associated with nondisjunctional (primary) trisomy (47, +13). As in trisomy 21, a maternal age effect exists. Translocations are responsible for less than 20 percent of cases, invariably associated with two group D (Nos. 13 to 15) chromosomes joining at their centromeric regions (Robertsonian translocation). If neither parent has such a rearrangement, the risk for subsequent progeny is not increased. If either parent has a balanced 13q;14q translocation, the recurrence risk for an affected offspring is increased but only to 1 to 2 percent. Homologous 13q;13q parental translocation carries the same dire prognosis as 21q;21q translocation.

Trisomy 18

Trisomy 18 occurs in 1 per 8,000 live births. Among liveborn infants, females are affected more often than males (3:1). Among stillborns and abortuses, however, the sex distribution is more equal.

Facial anomalies characteristic of trisomy 18 include microcephaly, prominent occiput, low-set and pointed "fawn-like" ears, and micrognathia. Skeletal anomalies include overlapping fingers (V over IV, II over III), short sternum, shield chest, narrow pelvis, limited thigh abduction or congenital hip dislocation, rocker-bottom feet with protrusion of the calcaneum, and a short dorsiflexed hallux ("hammer toe"). Cardiac and renal anomalies are common.

Mean birth weight (2,240 g) is below average. The mean survival time for these infants is only a few months. Those surviving show pronounced developmental and growth retardation. Fetal movement is feeble, and approximately 50 percent develop fetal distress during labor. Trisomy 18 is often detected among stillborn infants not clinically suspected of being trisomic.

Approximately 80 percent of trisomy 18 cases are caused by primary nondisjunction (47,XX,+18 or 47,XY,+18). In such cases, the recurrence risk is about 1 percent.

Other Trisomies

Although trisomies for several other autosomes have been observed in liveborns, such pregnancies more often terminate in abortuses. Trisomies for chromosomes 8, 9, and 14 and possibly other autosomies may exist in nonmosaic forms. Mosaic trisomy exists for No. 16 and other chromosomes. All trisomies show mental retardation, various somatic anomalies, and intrauterine growth retardation. The extent of retardation and the spectrum of anomalies vary. Recurrence risks can be assumed to be similar to trisomy 21, with differences, of course, for nonmosaic and mosaic cases.

Autosomal Deletions or Duplication

Deletions or duplications of portions of autosomes also exist. All are characterized by mental retardation and somatic anomalies, but their specific features vary. One example will suffice for illustrative purposes.

Deletion of a portion of the short arm of chromo-

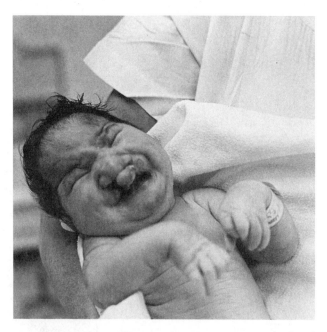

Fig. 9-3 An infant with trisomy 13. (From Simpson and Golbus,[1] with permission.)

some No. 5 (5p) produces the so-called cri-du-chat ("cat-cry") syndrome. These babies have a distinctive, monotonic, cat-like cry. During infancy, the facies become rounded ("moon-like") because of microcephaly, with hypertelorism, a broad nasal bridge, downward slanting of the palpebral fissures, and micrognathia. Ears are low set. As the child grows older, the facies become elongated, the philtrum shorter, and the cry more nonspecific in character. Despite severe mental retardation (mean IQ 20) and growth retardation, a few patients reach adulthood. The size of the deleted segment varies, but bands 5p14 and 5p15 are always deficient. The deletion is sporadic in 90 percent of cases, and the recurrence risk is no greater than that for any other couple of comparable parental ages. In 10 percent of these cases, unbalanced translocations or recombinants from inversions are present. In these instances, rearrangements are usually familial.

Sex Chromosomal Abnormalities

Monosomy X (45,X)

45,X individuals account for approximately 40 percent of gonadal dysgenesis cases ascertained by gynecologists. The incidence of 45,X in liveborn females is about 1 in 10,000. Because monosomy X accounts for 10 percent of all first trimester abortions, it can be calculated that more than 99 percent of 45,X conceptuses must end in early pregnancy loss.

Gonadal dysgenesis is usually associated with an abnormal sex chromosomal constitution. Associated complements include not only monosomy X but structural abnormalities of the X chromosome: (1) simple deletion of the short arm: 46,X,del(Xp); (2) simple deletion of the long arm: 46,X,del(Xq); (3) isochromosome for the long arm: 46,X,i(Xq); and (4) ring chromosomes: 46,X,r(X). Mosaicism is frequent, usually involving a coexisting 45,X cell line. Both the long arm and the short arm of the X chromosome contain determinants necessary for ovarian differentiation and for normal stature, as discussed in detail elsewhere.[4]

45,X individuals not only have streak gonads but invariably are short (less than 150 cm). Growth hormone treatment increases the final adult height 6 to 8 cm. Various somatic anomalies exist: renal and cardiac defects, skeletal abnormalities like cubitus valgus and clinodactyly, vertebral anomalies, pigmented nevi, nail hypoplasia, and a low posterior hairline. Performance IQ is lower than verbal IQ, but mentation should be considered normal. Adult-onset diseases include hypertension and diabetes mellitus.

Klinefelter syndrome

Males with two or more X chromosomes have small testes, azoospermia, elevated follicle-stimulating hormone (FSH) and luteinizing hormone (LH) levels, and decreased testosterone. The most frequent chromosomal complement associated with this phenotype—the Klinefelter syndrome—is 47,XXY. 48,XXXY and 49,XXXXY occur less often.

Mental retardation is uncommon in 47,XXY Klinefelter syndrome but is invariably associated with 48,XXXY and 49,XXXXY. Major skeletal, trunk, and craniofacial anomalies occur infrequently in 47,XXY but are commonly observed in 48,XXXY and 49,XXXXY. Regardless of the specific chromosomal complement, patients with Klinefelter syndrome all have unquestioned male phenotypes. Although the penis is hypoplastic, hypospadias is uncommon. Sterility has traditionally been considered a part of this syndrome, but with intracytoplasmic sperm injection (ICSI) and other assisted reproductive technologies (ART) the prognosis may become more hopeful.

Polysomy X in Females (47,XXX; 48,XXXX; 49,XXXXX)

About 1 per 800 liveborn females has a 47,XXX complement. 47,XXX individuals are seven to eight times more likely to show mental retardation than are individuals in the general population. However, the absolute risk for mental retardation is only 5 to 10 percent, and even then IQ is usually 60 to 80. Most 47,XXX patients have a normal reproductive system. The theoretical risk of 47,XXX women delivering an infant with an abnormal chromosomal complement is 50 percent, given one-half the maternal gametes carrying 24 chromosomes (24,XX). However, the empiric risk is much less. Somatic anomalies may or may not be more frequent in 47,XXX individuals than in 46,XX females. However, 48,XXXX and 49,XXXXX individuals are invariably retarded and more likely to have somatic malformations than 47,XXX individuals.

Polysomy Y in Males (47,XYY and 48,XXYY)

The presence of more than one Y chromosome is also a frequent chromosomal abnormality in liveborn males (1:1,000). Controversy notwithstanding, 47,XYY males seem more likely to be tall and display sociopathic behavior than are 46,XY males. The precise prevalence of these features is unknown, but one estimate is that 1 percent of 47,XYY males will be incarcerated compared with 0.1 percent of 46,XY males. 47,XYY males usually have normal male external genitalia.

Genetic History

All obstetrician/gynecologists must attempt to determine whether a couple, or anyone in their family, has a heritable disorder or is at increased risk for abnormal offspring. To address this question, some obstetricians find it helpful to elicit genetic information through the use of questionnaires or check lists that are often constructed in a manner that requires action only to positive responses. Figure 9-4 reproduces the form currently recommended by the American College of Obstetricians and Gynecologists (ACOG).

One should inquire into the health status of first-degree relatives (siblings, parents, offspring), second-degree relatives (nephews, nieces, aunts, uncles, grand-parents), and third-degree relatives (first cousins, especially maternal). Adverse reproductive outcomes such as repetitive spontaneous abortions, stillbirths, and anomalous liveborn infants should be pursued. Couples having such histories should undergo chromosomal studies in order to exclude balanced translocations. Genetic counseling may prove sufficiently complex to warrant referral to a clinical geneticist, or it may prove simple enough for the well-informed obstetrician to manage. If a birth defect exists in a second-

---

Prenatal Genetic Screen*

Name_____ Patient #_____ Date_____

1. Will you be 35 years or older when the baby is due?   Yes____ No____
2. Have you, the baby's father, or anyone in either of your families ever had any of the following disorders?
   Down syndrome (mongolism)   Yes____ No____
   Other chromosomal abnormality   Yes____ No____
   Neural tube defect, i.e., spina bifida (meningomyelocele or open spine), anencephaly Yes____ No____
   Hemophilia   Yes____ No____
   Muscular dystrophy   Yes____ No____
   Cystic fibrosis   Yes____ No____
   If yes, indicate the relationship of the affected person to you or to the baby's father:

   _____
3. Do you or the baby's father have a birth defect?   Yes____ No____
   If yes, who has the defect and what is it? _____
4. In any previous marriages, have you or the baby's father had a child born, dead or alive, with a birth
   defect not listed in question 2 above?   Yes____ No____
5. Do you or the baby's father have any close relatives with mental retardation?   Yes____ No____
   If yes, indicate the relationship of the affected person to you or to the baby's father:

   _____
   Indicate the cause, if known: _____
6. Do you, the baby's father, or a close relative in either of your families have a birth defect,
   any familial disorder, or a chromosomal abnormality not listed above?   Yes____ No____
   If yes, indicate the condition and the relationship of the affected person to you or to the baby's father:

   _____
7. In any previous marriage, have you or the baby's father had a stillborn child or three or
   more first-trimester spontaneous pregnancy losses?   Yes____ No____
   Have either of you had a chromosomal study?   Yes____ No____
8. If you or the baby's father are of Jewish ancestry, have either of you been screened for
   Tay-Sachs disease?   Yes____ No____
   If yes, indicate who and the results: _____
9. If you or the baby's father are black, have either of you been screened for sickle cell trait?
                                                                                                         Yes____ No____
   If yes, indicate who and the results: _____
10. If you or the baby's father are of Italian, Greek, or Mediterranean background, have either
    of you been tested for β-thalassemia?   Yes____ No____
    If yes, indicate who and the results: _____
11. If you or the baby's father are of Philippine or Southeast Asian ancestry, have either of
    you been tested for α-thalassemia?   Yes____ No____
    If yes, indicate who and the results: _____
12. Excluding iron and vitamins, have you taken any medications or recreational drugs since becoming
    pregnant or since your last menstrual period? (include nonprescription drugs)   Yes____ No____
    If yes, give name of medication and time taken during pregnancy: _____

Fig. 9-4 Questionnaire for identifying couples having increased risk for offspring with genetic disorders. (From American College of Obstetricians and Gynecologists,[102] with permission.)

degree relative (uncle, aunt, grandparent, nephew, niece) or third-degree relative (first cousin), the risk for that anomaly will usually not prove substantially increased over that in the general population. For example, identification of a second- or third-degree relative with an autosomal recessive trait places the couple at little increased risk for an affected offspring, an exception being if the patient and her husband are consanguineous. However, a maternal first cousin with an X-linked recessive disorder would identify a couple at increased risk for a similar occurrence.

Parental ages should also be recorded. Advanced maternal age (Table 9-2) warrants discussion irrespective of a physician's personal convictions regarding pregnancy termination, as knowledge of an abnormality may effect obstetric management. Ethnic origin should be recorded to exclude disorders noted in Table 9-3. Incidentally, the above applies for both gamete donors as well as couples achieving pregnancy by natural means.

Genetic Counseling

Although genetic counseling may require referral to a clinical geneticist, it is impractical for obstetricians to refer all patients with genetic inquiries. Indeed, obstetricians performing diagnostic procedures such as amniocentesis must counsel their patients before such a procedure. Salient principles of the genetic counseling process will therefore be described.

Communication

A first principle of counseling is to communicate in terms that are readily comprehensible to patients. It is useful to preface remarks with a few sentences recounting the major causes of genetic abnormalities—cytogenetic, single gene, polygenic/multifactorial (can be labeled "complex"), and environmental (teratogens). Writing unfamiliar words and using tables or diagrams to reinforce important concepts is helpful. Repetition is essential. Allow the couple not only to ask questions but to talk with one another to formulate their concerns.

Written information (letters or brochures) can serve as a couple's permanent record, allaying misunderstanding and assisting in dealing with relatives. Preprinted forms describing common problems (e.g., advanced maternal age) have the additional advantage of emphasizing that the couple's problem is not unique. More complicated scenarios require a letter.

Irrespective of how obvious a diagnosis may seem, confirmation is always obligatory. Accepting a patient's verbal recollection does not suffice, nor would accepting a diagnosis made by a physician not highly knowledgeable about the condition. The anomalous individual may need to be examined by the appropriate authority, and examining first-degree relatives may be required as well if the possibility of an autosomal dominant disorder (e.g., neurofibromatosis) exists. If a definitive diagnosis cannot be made, the physician should not hesitate to say so. Proper counseling requires proper diagnosis.

Nondirective Counseling

In genetic counseling one should provide accurate genetic information yet ideally dictate no particular course of action. Of course, completely nondirective counseling is probably unrealistic. For example, a

Table 9-2 Maternal Age and Chromosomal Abnormalities (Livebirths)[a]

Maternal Age	Risk for Down Syndrome	Risk for Any Chromosome Abnormalities[b]
20	1/1,667	1/526[b]
21	1/1,667	1/526[b]
22	1/1,429	1/500[b]
23	1/1,429	1/500[b]
24	1/1,250	1/476[b]
25	1/1,250	1/476[b]
26	1/1,176	1/476[b]
27	1/1,111	1/455[b]
28	1/1,053	1/435[b]
29	1/1,000	1/417[b]
30	1/952	1/384[b]
31	1/909	1/385[b]
32	1/769	1/322[b]
33	1/625	1/317[b]
34	1/500	1/260
35	1/385	1/204
36	1/294	1/164
37	1/227	1/130
38	1/175	1/103
39	1/137	1/82
40	1/106	1/65
41	1/82	1/51
42	1/64	1/40
43	1/50	1/32
44	1/38	1/25
45	1/30	1/20
46	1/23	1/15
47	1/18	1/12
48	1/14	1/10
49	1/11	1/7

[a] Because sample size for some intervals is relatively small, confidence limits are sometimes relatively large. Nonetheless, these figures are suitable for genetic counseling.
[b] 47, XXX excluded for ages 20–32 (data not available).
(Data from Hook[99] and Hook et al.[100])

Table 9-3 Genetic Screening in Various Ethnic Groups[a]

Ethnic Group	Disorder	Screening Test	Definitive Test
Ashkenazi Jews	Tay-Sachs disease	Decreased serum hexosamidase-A, possibly molecular analysis	Chorionic villus sampling (CVS) or amniocentesis for assay of hexosamidase-A or possibly direct molecular analysis
Blacks	Sickle cell anemia	Presence of sickle cell hemoglobin, confirmatory hemoglobin electrophoresis	CVS or amniocentesis for genotype determination (direct molecular analysis)
Mediterranean people	β-Thalassemia	Mean corpuscular volume (MCV) <80%, followed by hemoglobin electrophoresis	CVS or amniocentesis for genotype determination (direct molecular analysis or RFLP linkage analysis)
Southeast Asians and Chinese (Vietnamese, Laotian, Cambodian, Filipinos)	α-Thalassemia	MCV <80%, followed by hemoglobin electrophoresis	CVS or amniocentesis for genotype determination (direct molecular studies) (direct or RFLP linkage analysis)
Northern European whites	Cystic fibrosis (CF)	DNA analysis of CF gene for at least ΔF508 mutation and next 10 or more most common mutations	CVS or amniocentesis for genotype determination, definitive diagnosis on fetuses may not be possible

[a] Cystic fibrosis screening is recommended but not yet considered standard.

counselor's unwitting facial expressions may expose his or her unstated opinions. Merely offering antenatal diagnostic services implies approval. Despite the difficulties of remaining truly objective, one should attempt merely to provide information and then support the couple's decision.

Psychological Defenses

Psychological defenses permeate genetic counseling. If not appreciated, these defenses can impede the entire counseling process. Anxiety is low in couples counseled for advanced maternal age or for an abnormality in a distant relative. As long as the anxiety level remains low, comprehension of information is usually not impaired. However, couples who have experienced a stillborn infant, an anomalous child, or multiple repetitive abortions are more anxious. Their ability to retain information may be hindered.

Couples experiencing abnormal pregnancy outcomes manifest the same grief reactions that occur after the death of a loved one: denial, anger, guilt, bargaining, resolution. One should pay deference to this sequence by not attempting definitive counseling immediately after the birth of an abnormal neonate. Parents must be supported at that time, and the obstetrician should avoid discussing specific recurrence risks for fear of adding to the immediate burden. By 4 to 6 weeks the couple has begun to cope and is more receptive to counseling.

An additional psychological consideration is that of parental guilt. One naturally searches for exogenous factors that might have caused an abnormal outcome.

In the process of such a search, guilt may arise. Conversely, a tendency to blame the spouse may be seen. Usually guilt or blame is not justified, but occasionally the "blame" is realistic (e.g., in autosomal dominant traits). Fortunately, most couples can be assured that nothing could have prevented a given abnormal pregnancy.

Appreciating the psychological defenses described above helps one to understand the failure of ostensibly intelligent and well-counseled couples to comprehend genetic information.

Genetic Screening

Genetic screening implies routine monitoring for the presence or absence of a given condition in apparently normal individuals. Screening is now offered routinely for (1) all individuals of certain ethnic groups to identify those individuals heterozygous for a given autosomal recessive disorder (Table 9-3), (2) all pregnant women to detect elevated maternal serum α-fetoprotein for diagnosis of fetal neural tube defects, (3) all pregnant women 35 years of age and above to undergo invasive tests and to detect Down syndrome, and (4) all pregnant women *under* age of 35 years to undergo maternal serum screening to detect Down syndrome.

Neonatal Screening

One could theoretically screen neonates for many other genetic disorders. On the other hand, screening is actually recommended for relatively few disorders because prerequisites essential for initiating screening programs are not usually met. A first prerequisite is that widespread testing is ordinarily performed only if an abnormal finding would alter clinical management. Neonates are thus evaluated for those metabolic disorders (e.g., phenylketonuria, hypothyroidism) amenable to dietary or hormonal treatment. However, screening is not attempted for neonates with untreatable disorders. Thus, neonatal screening is not recommended for chromosomal abnormalities, Tay-Sachs disease, Duchenne muscular dystrophy, and cystic fibrosis.

Adult Screening

Adult population screening for Tay-Sachs disease, α- and β-thalassemia, and sickle cell anemia is reasonable in order to determine whether they are heterozygous for autosomal recessive disorders amenable to prenatal diagnosis. Table 9-3 lists disorders for which screening is currently recommended. The most well-known example in the United States is Tay-Sachs disease, an autosomal recessive disorder for which Ashkenazi Jews are at increased risk (heterozygote frequency 1/27). In the United States, Jewish individuals may be uncertain whether they are of Ashkenazic or Sephardic descent (90 percent are Ashkenazi); thus, obstetricians should screen all Jewish couples, and possibly also couples in which only one partner is Jewish. Increasing availability of prenatal diagnostic techniques also renders advisable routine heterozygote detection for β-thalassemia in Italians and Greeks, sickle cell anemia in blacks, and α-thalassemia in Southeast Asians and Philippines. Mean corpuscular volume (MCV) greater than 80 percent excludes heterozygosity for α- or β-thalassemia. Values less than 80 percent are more likely to reflect iron deficiency anemia than heterozygosity, but additional confirmatory tests are indicated to exclude heterozygosity for the thalassemias. Genes for all the above disorders have been isolated and cloned. However, mo-

lecular heterogeneity is enormous for all except sickle cell anemia (see below for further discussion). Thus, screening preferentially still utilizes the methods listed in Table 9-3. Possible exceptions include sickle cell anemia and Tay Sachs disease. In the latter molecular testing is equal but not superior to enzyme testing.

Population Screening for Cystic Fibrosis

Routine screening is not yet standard for cystic fibrosis, but there is much to recommend allowing individuals to avail themselves of genetic information. The salient finding is that about 75 percent of the cystic fibrosis mutations are due to deletion of amino acid 508 (ΔF508), resulting in loss of a phenylalanine residue[5] (Fig. 9-5). Should one screen the entire population for presence or absence of this mutation (ΔF508)? Indeed, about 50 percent of couples at risk for cystic fibrosis offspring can be identified by screening solely for this mutation, offering unequivocal prenatal diagnosis. However, managing the remaining couples at risk for cystic fibrosis is vexing. Included in this group are those couples in which one parent has the ΔF508 mutation but the other does not. If one parent has ΔF508 but the other does not, the actual risk of that couple having an affected child is 1 per 400.[6] If amniotic fluid analysis were possible for the cystic fibrosis gene product (protein), this would not matter so much. Unfortunately, no such assay exists, meaning prenatal diagnosis is not possible except to exclude the fetus who inherited the ΔF508 from the known heterozygous parent. Measuring microvillus intestinal enzymes in amniotic fluid is specifically not helpful, for a low value is more likely to connote a false-positive than a true-positive value.

The logical solution is to detect other mutations within the cystic fibrosis locus. Unfortunately, all other mutations are individually rated, the 10 to 15 most frequent after ΔF508 identifying an additional risk of only

NORMAL

DNA	..GAA	AAT	ATC	ATC	TTT	GGT	GTT	TCC..
PROTEIN	Glu	Asn	Ile	Ile	Phe	Gly	Val	Ser
POSITION	504	505	506	507	508	509	510	511

CYSTIC FIBROSIS

DNA	..GAA	AAT	ATC	AT-	--T	GGT	GTT	TCC..
PROTEIN	Glu	Asn	Ile	Ile		Gly	Val	Ser

Fig. 9-5 Schematic drawing illustrating ΔF508 mutation, which accounts for 75 percent of cystic fibrosis cases in of Northern European ancestry.

Table 9-4 Common Cystic Fibrosis Mutations in Northern Europeans and North Americans

Mutation	Population	
	Northern Europeans (N = 21,154)(100%)	North Americans (N = 10,438)(100%)
ΔF508	14,866 (70.27%)	6,900 (66.1)
G542X	439	234
N1303K	209	130
R553X	165	96
W1282X	120	245
621+1G→T	97	154
R117H	62	61
1078delT	53	1
R347P	55	26
1898+1G→A	41	2
R560T	40	24
3659delC	39	14
Other	780 (3.69%)	453 (4.34%)
Total detectable mutation	16,966 (80.2%)	8,340 (79.9%)
Nondetectable mutations	418 (19.8%)	2,098 (20.1%)

(Modified from The Cystic Fibrosis Genetic Analysis Consortium,[101] with permission.)

10 to 15 percent (Table 9-4). Nonetheless, multiplex PCR assays for the 10 to 15 most common mutations in Northern European populations allow approximately 85 to 90 percent of affected fetuses to be detected. In Ashkenazi Jews one particular mutation in addition to ΔF508 is especially frequent, facilitating screening in that population. In other populations screening is more difficult. Cystic fibrosis screening thus requires considerable patient education and follow through. For this reason such screening can be recommended but is not yet considered standard, unlike screening for the mendelian conditions cited in the previous section.

If a couple has had a child with cystic fibrosis, or has an affected relative, the discussion above is not germane. Such couples should be screened for the ΔF508 mutation and for all other cystic fibrosis mutations practical. If the mutation is not found, family studies to identify polymorphic loci informative for linkage analysis should be undertaken (see below Detection of Mendelian Disorders by Molecular Techniques).

MSAFP Screening for Neural Tube Defects

Relatively few (5 percent) NTDs occur in families who have had previously affected offspring. Thus, a method other than a positive family history is needed to identify couples in the general population at risk for a NTD. Maternal serum α-fetoprotein (MSAFP) serves this pur-

pose, identifying couples with a negative family history who nonetheless have sufficient risk to justify amniocentesis.

MSAFP is greater than 2.5 multiples of the median (MOM) in 80 to 90 percent of pregnancies in which the fetus has an NTD. Because considerable overlap exists between MSAFP in normal pregnancies and MSAFP in pregnancies characterized by a fetus with an NTD, systematic protocols for evaluating elevated MSAFP values are necessary. Elevated MSAFP occurs for reasons other than an NTD: (1) underestimation of gestational age, inasmuch as MSAFP increases as gestation progresses (Fig. 9-6); (2) multiple gestation (60 percent of twins and almost all triplets having MSAFP values that would be elevated if judged on the basis of singleton values); (3) fetal demise, presumably due to fetal blood extravasating into the maternal circulation; (4) Rh isoimmunization, cystic hygroma, and other conditions associated with fetal edema; and (5) anomalies other than NTD, usually characterized by edema or skin defects.

The initial MSAFP assay should be performed at 15 to 20 weeks gestation. Corrections for maternal weight and some other factors are necessary, using various algorithms. Obstetricians should expect their referring laboratory to have generated its own normal values and to provide a weight-adjusted MSAFP appropriate for gestational age. Without weight adjustment, dilutional effects can result in heavier women having a spuriously low value when in fact MSAFP might actually be elevated for women of their weight.

Values between 2.0 and 2.5 MOM are usually considered elevated. The precise value above which MSAFP is considered elevated is less important than setting a consistent policy per program. Values above 2.0 MOM are definitely considered elevated in insulin-dependent diabetic women, but in twin gestations MSAFP is judged abnormal only at 4.5 to 5.0 MOM or greater.

Approximately 5 percent of women will have an elevated MSAFP value. If gestational age assessment is determined accurately before MSAFP sampling, the number of women having an abnormal serum value will be lower (3 percent). A second MSAFP sample may or may not be necessary. There is virtue in reassaying MSAFP if the value lies between 2.50 and 2.99 MOM and if gestational age is 18 weeks or less. If not already performed, ultrasound is obviously required to exclude erroneous gestational age, multiple gestations, or fetal demise. Amniocentesis for AFP and acetylcholinesterase (ACHE) is necessary if no explanation for elevated MSAFP is evident on ultrasound. The presence of AChe indicates an open NTD or other anomalies.

MSAFP screening identifies 90 percent of anencephaly and 80 to 85 percent of spina bifida, albeit at the cost

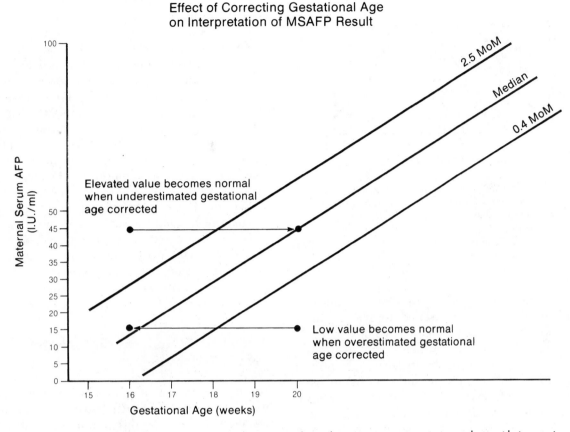

Effect of Correcting Gestational Age
on Interpretation of MSAFP Result

Fig. 9-6 Median maternal serum α-fetoprotein (MSAFP) throughout gestation. Increasing values with increasing gestational age require accurate dating to interpret low or high MSAFP.

of 1 to 2 percent of all pregnant women undergoing amniocentesis. Approximately 1 in 15 women having an unexplained elevated serum AFP will prove to have a fetus with an NTD (Table 9-5). Not well appreciated is that sensitivity of detecting an NTD in twin gestations is less than in singleton gestations, being only about 30 percent for spina bifida given a threshold of 4.5 MOM. The poor sensitivity exists because twins are usually discordant for an NTD. Liberal use of comprehensive ultrasound is recommended in twin gestations.

Some physicians prefer to utilize comprehensive ultrasound immediately after elevated MSAFP. Thus, am-

Table 9-5 Likelihood of Having a Fetus with NTD After Various Stages of an MSAFP Screening Program

Time	Risk
Before MSAFP	1/1,000
After one elevated MSAFP	1/50
Before sonogram	1/30
Before amniocentesis	1/15
Amniotic fluid AFP > 5 SD	1/2.2[a]
Acetylcholinesterase present	1/1.1

[a] Approximately equal number of other serious abnormalities or fetal demise.

niocentesis would not be performed in the absence of ultrasound evidence of an NTD. Although a logical approach, the sensitivity of NTD detection cannot be assumed to be as high as with MSAFP followed by amniocentesis.

Maternal Serum Screening for Detecting Fetal Trisomy

Several years after maternal serum screening for the detection of NTDs was introduced, it became clear that a low MSAFP level was associated with trisomy 21.[7] The possibility arose that maternal serum screening could be offered to women under the age of 35 for detection of Down syndrome. Low serum values could confer a risk sufficiently high that women who are not otherwise candidates for invasive procedures like amniocentesis or chorionic villus sampling (CVS) might wish to undergo such. This proposition is attractive because only 25 percent of infants with Down syndrome are born to women aged 35 and above. Thus, decreasing the population incidence requires identifying younger women at sufficient risk to justify an invasive procedure. However, screening for Down syndrome is more complicated than screening for NTDs because the risk of

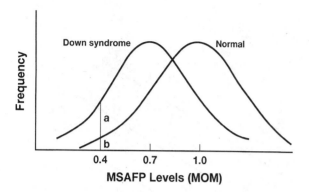

Fig. 9-7 Distribution MSAFP in the normal population and in the population of women carrying a Down syndrome infant with method of determining likelihood ratio. If MSAFP = 0.4 MOM, the likelihood ratio is 3.81. That is, the distance to the Down syndrome curve is 3.81 times greater than the distance to the unaffected curve. Thus, the midtrimester risk of Down syndrome for a 32-year-old woman increases from 1/563 to 1/148.

Down syndrome is age specific. An MSAFP value of, say, 0.4 easily raises the age-associated risk of a 34-year-old high enough to justify amniocentesis; however, the same value would not necessarily increase the risk similarly for a 25-year-old woman. For this reason the preferable way to identify couples with sufficient risk to justify invasive procedures is to utilize likelihood ratios (illustrated in Fig. 9-7). In the example given, a value of 0.4 MOM carries a likelihood ratio of 3.81 for having a child with Down syndrome: a + b/b = 3.81. If the a priori (age specific) risk is 1 in 581 (for a 25-year-old woman), the recalculated risk after taking into account serum analytes values is 1 in 148.

In addition to the association between low MSAFP and Down syndrome, an association exists for other analytes. The analyte having the greatest discriminatory value is human chorionic gonadotropin (hCG), which is elevated in Down syndrome pregnancies.[8] In the second trimester either intact hCG or free β-hCG will suffice for assay. Irrespective, the combination of hCG, AFP, and maternal age when analyzed with appropriate software allows detection of some 60 percent of cases of Down syndrome with an associated amniocentesis rate of no more than 5 percent.[9] Controversy exists concerning the usefulness of unconjugated serum estriol, an analyte that if present in low values is associated with Down syndrome. Using maternal serum estriol level should allow a slightly greater detection rate but with improved specificity, i.e., decreased number of false-positive serum values.

Worth emphasizing is that the sensitivity of detecting Down syndrome is age dependent. Detection rates are 90 percent for women aged 35 and above, but less than 25 percent for those in their early third decade. Moreover, utilization of this approach for the detection of Down syndrome in twin gestations is not standard.

Another caveat is that using a double or triple analyte screening program to identify Down syndrome would not detect trisomy 18. This circumstance arises because trisomy 18 is associated with low hCG. One solution is to offer an invasive procedure (amniocentesis) whenever the serum values are at or below each of these three thresholds: MSAFP ≤0.6 MOM, hCG ≤0.55 MOM, unconjugated estriol ≤0.5 MOM.[10]

The American College of Obstetricians and Gynecologists (ACOG) recently recommended women under the age of 35 years be counseled about maternal serum screening to detect Down syndrome.[11] Women aged 35 years and above should continue to be offered invasive procedures. If older women insist on maternal serum screening in lieu of an invasive procedure, they must appreciate that detection is not 100 percent but only 90 percent. Finally, early evidence appears quite strong that first trimester analytes will also detect Down syndrome. Associations exist between Down syndrome and low MSAFP, low PAPP-A, and elevated free β-hCG.[12]

Diagnostic Procedures for Prenatal Genetic Diagnosis

Prenatal genetic diagnosis usually requires obtaining fetal tissue, necessitating an invasive procedure like amniocentesis or CVS. In this section we shall consider common techniques and their safety.

Amniocentesis

Technique

In amniocentesis, amniotic fluid is aspirated, often for the purpose of genetic diagnosis at 15 to 16 weeks gestation (menstrual weeks). While the procedure has traditionally been performed at 15 to 16 weeks, it can be performed earlier (especially 12 to 14 weeks).[13] A 22-gauge spinal needle with stylet is usually employed. Ultrasound examination is obligatory in order to determine gestational age, placental position, location of amniotic fluid, and number of fetuses. Ultrasound should be performed concurrently with amniocentesis. Rh-immune globulin should be administered to the Rh-negative, Du-negative, unsensitized patient.

Bloody amniotic fluid is aspirated occasionally; however, this blood is almost always maternal in origin and does not adversely affect amniotic cell growth. By contrast, brown, dark red, or wine-colored amniotic fluid is associated with an increased likelihood of poor pregnancy outcome. The dark color indicates that intra-amniotic bleeding has occurred earlier in pregnancy, with hemoglobin breakdown products persisting; pregnancy loss eventually occurs in about one-third of such cases. If the abnormally colored fluid is characterized by elevated AFP, the outcome is almost always unfavorable (fetal demise or fetal abnormality). Greenish amniotic fluid is the result of meconium staining and is apparently not associated with poor pregnancy outcome.

In multiple gestations, amniocentesis can usually be performed on all fetuses. Following aspiration of amniotic fluid from the first sac, 2 to 3 ml of indigo carmine, diluted 1:10 in bacteriostatic water, is injected before the needle is withdrawn. A second amniocentesis is then performed at a site determined after visualizing the membranes separating the two sacs. It is important to note the locations of each sac in case selective termination is later required. Aspiration of clear fluid confirms that the second (new) sac was entered. Triplets and other multiple gestations can be managed similarly, sequentially injecting dye into successive sacs. Although cross-contamination of cells in multiple gestations appears to be rare, confusion may sometimes arise in interpreting amniotic fluid AChE or AFP results. Some obstetricians aspirate the second sac without dye injection or use a single puncture technique; however, I still prefers dye injection for confirmation.

After amniocentesis, the patient may resume all normal activities. Common sense dictates that strenuous exercise such as jogging or "aerobic" exercise be deferred for a day or so. The patient should report persistent uterine cramping, vaginal bleeding, leakage of amniotic fluid, or fever; however, physician intervention is almost never required, unless overt abortion occurs.

If only one fetus in a multiple gestation is abnormal, parents should be prepared to choose between aborting all fetuses or continuing the pregnancy with one or more normal and one abnormal fetus. Selective termination in the second trimester is possible, but success of this procedure is greater in the first trimester.[14]

Safety of Traditional Amniocentesis

Any procedure that involves entering the pregnant uterus logically carries risk to the fetus. Amniocentesis is no exception. Amniocentesis carries potential danger to both mother and fetus. Maternal risks are quite low, with symptomatic amnionitis occurring only rarely (0.1 percent). Minor maternal complications such as transient vaginal spotting or minimal amniotic fluid leakage occur in 1 percent or fewer of cases, but almost always these are self-limited in nature. Other very rare complications include intra-abdominal viscus injury or hemorrhage.

The safety of traditional amniocentesis has been addressed by several large collaborative studies. In 1976 the U.S. National Institute of Child Health and Human Development[15] published the first major prospective study of genetic amniocentesis, encompassing 1,040 subjects and 992 matched controls. Of all women who underwent amniocentesis, 3.5 percent experienced fetal loss between the time of the procedure and delivery compared with 3.2 percent of controls; the small difference was not statistically significant and disappeared completely when corrected for maternal age. In Canada a collaborative study did not include a concurrent control group,[16] assessing 1,223 amniocentesis performed during 1,020 pregnancies in 900 women. The pregnancy loss rate was 3.2 percent, similar to that reported in the U.S. collaborative study.

A British collaborative investigation later found that the rate of fetal loss following amniocentesis was significantly greater than in controls (2.6 percent versus 1 percent).[17] In the British study, however, a common indication for amniocentesis was elevated MSAFP, only later recognized as a factor associated with fetal loss and adverse perinatal outcome. Analysis after excluding subjects undergoing amniocentesis for that indication lowered the loss rates between subject and control groups to less than 1 percent, albeit still significantly different.[18]

None of the collaborative studies cited above was conducted with high-quality ultrasonography as defined by today's standards, nor was concurrent ultrasonography ever universally applied. A 1986 Danish study was a true randomized control study of 4,606 women aged 25 to 34 years who were without known risk factors for fetal genetic abnormalities[19]; a control group underwent no procedure. Women with three or more previous spontaneous abortions, diabetes mellitus, multiple gestation, or uterine anomalies or who used intrauterine contraceptive devices were excluded. Maternal age, social group, smoking history, number of previous induced and spontaneous abortions, stillbirths, livebirths, and low-birth-weight infants were comparable in the study and control groups, as was gestational age at time of entry into the study. Amniocentesis was performed under real-time ultrasound guidance with a 20-gauge needle by experienced operators. The spontaneous abortion rate after 16 weeks was 1.7 percent in the amniocentesis study group compared with 0.7 percent in controls (p <0.01); a 2.6-fold relative risk of spontaneous abortion was observed if the placenta was traversed. The frequency of fetal postural deformations did not differ between the two groups. However, respiratory distress syndrome was diagnosed more often (relative risk = 2.1) In the amniocentesis group, and more of these infants were treated for pneumonia (relative risk = 2.5).

In conclusion, it still seems wise to continue to counsel that the risk of pregnancy loss secondary to amniocentesis is 0.5 percent, or perhaps slightly less. At the author's medical center, serious maternal complications and fetal injuries are stated to be "remote" risks. Concurrent ultrasound is now recommended, but its utilization should not be assumed to decrease risks much below 0.5 percent.

Safety of Early Amniocentesis

The number of early amniocenteses reported to date is relatively small, and there are only limited data available from controlled studies. Thus, the safety and efficacy of the procedure is still unknown. Nonetheless, early experiences suggest early amniocenteses could be a promising technique. In 936 amniocenteses performed at ≤12.8 weeks gestation, Hanson and colleagues[20] reported loss rates of 0.7 percent (7/936) within 2 weeks of amniocentesis, an additional 2.2 percent before 28 weeks, and a final 0.5 percent stillbirths or neonatal deaths. Total losses (32/936 or 3.4 percent) were considered comparable to the 2.1 percent to 3.2 percent observed in ultrasonographically normal pregnancies not undergoing a procedure; however, maternal age and precise gestational age were not taken into account. Henry and Miller[21] also reported favorable results in amniocentesis at 12, 13, and 14 weeks gestation. Pregnancy losses prior to 28 weeks were 5/193 (2.6 percent), 5/426 (1.2 percent), and 18/1172 (1.5 percent), respectively.

Our group[22] compared our initial experience with 250 early amniocenteses (≤14 weeks) to our first 250 cases of transabdominal CVS (9.5 to 12.9 weeks). Loss rates for early amniocentesis and transabdominal CVS were 3.8 percent and 2.1 percent, respectively. We have also performed early amniocentesis in twin gestations, using a similar dye injection technique as described for traditional amniocentesis.[23]

Overall, amniocentesis at 12 to 14 weeks gestation should be a relatively safe and efficacious technique. However, reported data cannot yet support the claim that early amniocentesis is equal in safety to traditional amniocentesis. Contentions that procedure-related risks for early amniocentesis are comparable to traditional amniocentesis or even to CVS must be viewed with caution. Recently, Nicolaides et al.[24] compared amniocentesis and CVS at 10 to 13 weeks' gestation. Early amniocentesis was performed in 731 patients (493 by choice, 238 by randomization) and CVS in 570 (320 by choice, 250 by randomization). Both procedures were performed by transabdominal ultrasound-guided insertion of a 20-gauge needle. The spontaneous loss rate (intrauterine or neonatal death) was significantly higher after early amniocentesis (total group mean = 5.3 percent, 95 percent CI 3.8 to 7.2; randomized subgroup mean = 5.9 percent, CI 3.3 to 9.7) than after CVS (total group mean = 2.3 percent, CI 1.2 to 3.9; randomized subgroup mean = 1.2 percent, 0.3 to 3.5).

Chorionic Villus Sampling

CVS allows prenatal diagnosis in the first trimester to permit pregnancy termination early in gestation and also protect patient privacy. Both chorionic villi analysis and amniotic fluid cell analysis offer the same information concerning chromosomal status, enzyme levels, and DNA patterns. The one major difference is that assays requiring amniotic fluid, specifically AFP, necessitate amniocentesis.

Technique

CVS can be performed by transcervical, transabdominal, or transvaginal approaches. *Transcervical* CVS is usually performed with a flexible polyethylene catheter that encircles a metal obturator extending just distal to the catheter tip. The outer diameter is usually about 1.5 mm. Introduced transcervically under simultaneous ultrasonographic visualization (Fig. 9-8), the catheter/obturator is directed toward the trophoblastic tissue surrounding the gestational sac. After withdrawal of the obturator, 10 to 25 mg of villi are aspirated by negative pressure into a 20- or 30-cc syringe containing tissue culture media. The optimal time for transcervical sampling is 10 to 12 completed gestational weeks.

In *transabdominal* chorionic villus sampling (Fig. 9-9), concurrent ultrasound is used to direct an 18- or 20-gauge spinal needle into the long axis of the placenta. After removal of the stylet, villi are aspirated into a 20-cc syringe containing tissue culture media. Unlike transcervical CVS, transabdominal CVS can be performed throughout pregnancy, therefore serving as an alternative to cordocentesis (percutaneous umbilical blood sampling [PUBS]) later in pregnancy. If oligohydramnios is present, transabdominal CVS is preferable to PUBS.

A final technique is *transvaginal* CVS, using a spinal needle as in transabdominal CVS. This technique may be useful for a retroflexed uterus having a posterior placenta.

Facility to perform both transcervical and transabdominal CVS is crucial to optimal success. In about one-half to three-fourths of cases either approach is possible, but in the remaining cases either transabdominal or transcervical CVS is greatly preferable to the other approach. For example, cervical myomas or angulated uteri may preclude transcervical passage of the catheter, whereas transabdominal CVS would permit sampling. The transabdominal approach is obviously preferable in the presence of genital herpes, cervicitis, or bicornuate uteri. Sampling women sensitized to Rh(D) should probably be deferred until later in gestation. Sensitization following CVS is probably no greater than that following amniocentesis, but exacerbating the

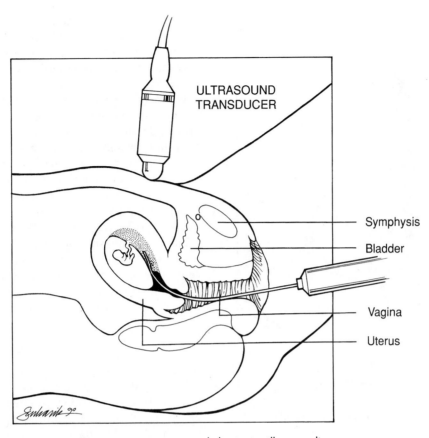

ULTRASOUND
TRANSDUCER

Symphysis

Bladder

Vagina

Uterus

Fig. 9-8 Transcervical chorionic villus sampling.

problem at 10 weeks compared with 16 weeks or later surely cannot be salutary.

Safety of Chorionic Villus Sampling

Pregnancy Losses

The U.S. Cooperative Clinical Comparison of Chorionic Villus Sampling and Amniocentesis study[25] and the Canadian Collaborative CVS-Amniocentesis Trial Group study[26] have reported that pregnancy loss rates after CVS are no different from loss rates after amniocentesis. In the U.S. study[25] 2,278 women self-selected transcervical CVS; 671 women similarly recruited in the first trimester selected amniocentesis. Randomization did not prove possible. The excess loss rate in the CVS group was 0.8 percent, not statistically significant. In a Canadian randomized study[26] 1,391 subjects were assigned to transcervical CVS and 1,396 to amniocentesis. The excess loss rate in the former was also 0.8 percent and again not statistically different. Variables shown to influence fetal loss rates adversely in CVS include fundal location of the placenta, number of catheter passages, small sample size, and prior bleeding during the current pregnancy. Almost all except the last are surrogates for technical difficulty. The frequency of intrauterine growth retardation, placental abruption, and

premature delivery are no higher in women undergoing CVS than expected in the general population.[27]

Transcervical CVS and transabdominal CVS appear to be equally safe procedures.[28] In another U.S. NICHD collaborative study, 1,194 patients were randomized to transcervical CVS and 1,929 patients to transabdominal CVS. The loss rates of cytogenetically normal pregnancies through 28 weeks were 2.5 percent and 2.3 percent, respectively.[29] Of considerable interest, the overall loss rate (i.e., background plus procedure-related) following CVS decreased by about 0.8 percent compared with rates observed during the earlier (1985 to 1987) transcervical versus amniocentesis self-selection study. This decrease in procedure-related loss rate probably reflects increasing operator experience as well as availability of both transcervical and transabdominal approaches. In a small randomized trial conducted in Italy, Brambati et al.[30] also found no difference between transabdominal and transcervical CVS. In contrast, in a Danish randomized comparison between amniocentesis, transabdominal CVS, and transcervical CVS, Smidt-Jensen et al.[31] reported similar fetal loss rates for transabdominal CVS and amniocentesis, but a significantly increased loss rate associated with transcervical CVS. However, Danish experience with transabdominal CVS is far greater than

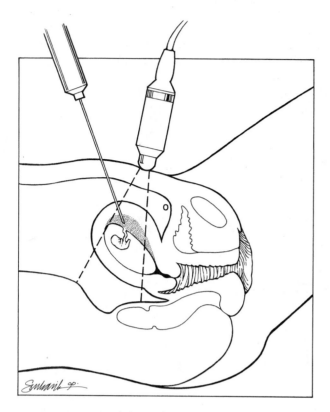

Fig. 9-9 Transabdominal chorionic villus sampling.

with transcervical CVS; thus, this comparison may have been biased.

The one major investigation substantively differing from all others is the United Kingdom Medical Research Council Study.[32] In this multicenter randomized study, comparison was made between second trimester amniocentesis and first trimester CVS performed in any fashion deemed suitable by the obstetrician. The outcome variable assessed was completed pregnancies. The 4.4 percent fewer completed pregnancies in the CVS cohort reflected both unintended and intended pregnancy terminations. The latter probably resulted from inexperience in cytogenetic interpretation, given the indication for some terminations seemingly being arguable in retrospect (i.e., confined placental mosaicism) (see below). The experience with CVS of the Medical Research Council Study operators was moreover considerably less than in the U.S. studies. For example, the only requirement for participation in the MRC study was 30 "practice" CVS procedures.

Overall, it appears reasonable to conclude that clinical judgement and ability to choose the optimal approach (transabdominal or transcervical) increases safety. For example, some technically difficult transcervical CVS procedures (e.g., fundal placentas) should be avoided in favor of a technically more straightforward transabdominal approach. Of course, the converse is

also true, a transcervical approach being favored over the transabdominal approach in a retroverted uterus with a posterior placenta. In experienced hands, the loss rates for CVS and amniocentesis appear comparable.[33]

No formal attempts to assess the safety of transvaginal CVS have been attempted. Both Sidranski et al.[34] and Shulman et al.[35] observed neither major complications nor obvious excessive fetal loss rates.

Finally, few data exist on the safety of CVS in multiple gestation. In a major U.S. study involving four medical centers, the total loss rate of chromosomally normal fetuses (spontaneous abortions, stillborns, neonatal deaths) was 5.0 percent,[36] only slightly higher than the 4.0 percent absolute rate observed for singleton pregnancies.[25] If the placental mass appears fused, amniocentesis is probably a preferred choice. However, CVS is appropriate in twin gestations when distinct placentas can be visualized by ultrasonography.

Limb Reduction Defects

Controversy about the safety of CVS has more recently shifted focus from concerns about the risk of fetal loss to its being the possible cause for congenital abnormalities. In 1991, Firth and colleagues[37] reported that 5 of 289 (1.7 percent or 17/1,000) infants exposed to CVS between 56 and 66 days of gestation (i.e., 42 to 50 days after fertilization) had severe limb reduction deformities (LRD). Four of the five infants had oromandibular-limb hypogenesis; the fifth had a terminal transverse limb reduction alone. There quickly followed a number of reports both supporting and refuting such an association.[38–41] In the United States, Burton et al.[42] reported a second cluster among 394 infants whose mothers had undergone CVS. Thirteen infants (3.3 percent) had major congenital abnormalities, including four with transverse LRD (10/1,000 or 1 percent). All four LRD were transverse distal defects involving hypoplasia or absence of the fingers and toes. Three of these cases followed transcervical sampling, using a device that in the hands of the reporting physicians was associated with an 11 percent fetal loss rate.

Teratogenic mechanisms by which CVS might cause LRD can be readily hypothesized. These include (1) decreased blood flow due to fetomaternal hemorrhage or pressor substances released by disturbance of villi or the chorion; (2) embolization of chorionic villus material or maternal clots into the fetal circulation; and (3) amniotic puncture and limb entrapment in exocoelomic gel.

Given this concern, the potential association of LRD with CVS has been explored through various registries. In the Italian Multicenter Birth Defects Registry,[43] eight cases of oromandibular-limb hypogenesis complex were entered into the registry from January 1988 through December 1991. Of 166 cases of transverse limb defects alone, 4 were exposed to CVS compared with 36 cases among 8,445 controls. A 1994 update of this study, based on 11 CVS-exposed cases, continued to reveal an association with transverse limb defects.[44] The greatest risk was associated with procedures performed at less than 70 days gestation (odds ratio 23.2; 95 percent 1.31 to 41.0); a lower, but still increased risk with procedures at 70 to 76 days (odds ratio 17.1; 95 percent CI 6.7 to 44.0); over 84 days there were no exposed cases, and the risk was interpreted as considerably lower. In contrast, analysis of other European registries in aggregate involving over 600,000 births showed that only 4 of 336 cases (1.2%) with limb reduction abnormalities had been exposed to CVS compared with 78 of 11,883 (0.66%) cases with other malformations (odds ratio 1.8; 95 percent CI 0.7 to 5.0).[45] A more recent report from Taiwan showed a number of LRD cases associated with CVS; however, no systematic population-based approach was performed. Almost all LRD cases were associated with CVS at less than 9 weeks.[46]

In 1994 the U.S. Centers for Disease Control and Prevention (CDC) held an open forum at which data were presented from a multistate case–control study conducted to quantify the risk for LRD associated with CVS.[47] The case subjects were 131 infants with nonsyndromic limb deficiency from seven population-based birth defects surveillance programs, born to women 34 years or older from 1988 through 1992. Controls were 131 infants with other birth defects matched to case subjects by the infant's year of birth, mother's age, race, and state of residence. Overall, the odds ratio for limb deficiency after CVS at 8 to 12 weeks gestation was 1.7 (95 percent CI 0.4 to 6.3). However, when analyzed for specific anatomic subtypes, there was an association for transverse digital deficiency (odds ratio 6.4; 95 percent CI 1.1 to 38.6). The absolute risk for such defects was said to be approximately 1 in 3,000.

On the other hand, a World Health Organization study group recently analyzed data collected through an international registry.[48] Among 138,000 infants born after CVS who were reported from 19 centers, 72 LRD cases were recorded. Pattern analysis of the types of limb defects and overall frequencies of specific LRD were compared with the background population study from British Columbia.[49] The pattern of defects showed the upper limb to be affected in 60 percent, the lower limb in 19 percent, and both upper and lower limbs in 21 percent; the general population frequencies were 68, 23, and 9 percent, respectively. Transverse limb defects occurred in 42 percent of infants in the cohort exposed to CVS compared with 42 percent in the general population. Longitudinal limb deficiencies were found in 53 percent of cases compared with 62

percent in the general population. It was concluded that both the types of limb defects and overall incidences were the same in the CVS group and the general population.

In summary, whether CVS is an etiologic factor in causing limb reduction defects remains arguable. At Baylor College of Medicine, we avoid performing CVS under 10 weeks' gestation and further consider it prudent to counsel patients about the LRD controversy. We state that the absolute risk at 10 to 12 weeks is believed to be very low, perhaps 1 in 3,000 if any increase risk exists. We also stress that the risk be placed in proper perspective, weighed against the substantial advantages that first trimester prenatal diagnosis with CVS offers.

Fetal Blood Sampling

Access to the fetal blood circulation was initially accomplished by fetoscopy, a method of directly visualizing the fetus, umbilical cord, and chorionic surface of the placenta using endoscopic instruments. Fetoscopy for this purpose has now been replaced by ultrasound-directed percutaneous umbilical blood sampling (PUBS), also termed cordocentesis or funipuncture.

Fetal blood chromosome analysis is used most commonly in genetics to help clarify chromosome mosaicism detected in cultured amniotic fluid cells or chorionic villi. Fetal blood sampling is used in the prenatal evaluation of many fetal hematologic abnormalities.[50] Fetal blood hematocrit level can be measured directly to assess hemolysis resulting from Rh or other blood antigen isoimmunization states. Fetal blood has been used for the diagnosis of blood factor abnormalities (gene products) like hemophilia A, hemophilia B or von Willebrand's disease. Recovery of fetal blood permits assessment of viral, bacterial or parasitic infections of the fetus. Serum studies of fetal blood permit quantification of antibody titers, and serum can be used to initiate viral, bacterial, or parasitic culture.

The technique most commonly used for fetal blood sampling is ultrasound-directed PUBS. The procedure can be safely undertaken from 18 weeks onward, although successful procedures have been reported as early as 12 weeks.[51] Due to its fixed position, the placental cord root is usually the site of choice whenever it is clearly visible. Alternatively, free loops of cord or the intrahepatic vein are possibilities.[50,51] The spinal needle is inserted into the fetal umbilical cord under direct ultrasound guidance, and a small amount of blood is aspirated. Presence of fetal blood in this initial sample is confirmed using a model ZBI Coulter counter and channelizer to differentiate fetal from maternal blood on the basis of the greater erythrocyte volume of fetal blood.

Fetal blood sampling appears to be relatively safe when performed by experienced physicians, albeit carrying more risk than CVS or amniocentesis. Maternal complications are rare, but include amnionitis and transplacental hemorrhage. Data from large perinatal centers estimate the risk of in utero death or spontaneous abortion to be 3 percent or less following PUBS.[52–54] Collaborative data from 14 North American centers, sampling 1,600 patients at varying gestational ages and for a variety of indications, revealed an uncorrected fetal loss rate of 1.6 percent.[51] However, no studies directly comparing loss rates in control and treated groups have been published. Assessment is also difficult because loss rates for fetuses subjected to PUBS vary greatly by the indication for the procedure. Loss rates for fetuses with ultrasound-detected anomalies are far greater than for fetuses being evaluated because of maternal blood group sensitization or for suspicion of chromosomal mosaicism. Thus, data regarding loss rates in matched control and treated groups are necessary to determine the true safety of PUBS. Estimating the risks associated with PUBS must take into account not only fetal and neonatal deaths but also risk of cesarean delivery for fetal distress, low Apgar scores, fetal anemia, and other indications of fetal and neonatal morbidity. Potential fetal complications that may lead to fetal death or iatrogenic premature delivery include infection, premature rupture of the membranes, hemorrhage, severe bradycardia, cord tamponade or thrombosis, and abruptio placenta.[50]

Indications for Prenatal Genetic Studies

Cytogenetic Disorders

Every chromosomal disorder is potentially detectable in utero. It is not appropriate, however, to perform amniocentesis or CVS in every pregnancy because for many couples the risk of an invasive procedure outweighs diagnostic benefits. In addition to couples tested as a result of positive findings in population screening programs (see above), certain indications are considered standard.

Advanced Maternal Age

The most common indication for antenatal cytogenetic studies is advanced maternal age. The incidence of trisomy 21 is 1 per 800 liveborn births in the United States, but the frequency increases with age (Table 9-2). Trisomy 13, trisomy 18, 47,XXX and 47,XXY also increase with advanced age.

For approximately 20 years it has been standard medical practice in the United States to offer invasive chromosomal diagnosis to all women who at their ex-

pected delivery date will be 35 years or older. The choice of age 35 is largely arbitrary, however, having been chosen during an interval when risk figures were available only in 5-year intervals (i.e., 30 to 34 years, 35 to 39 years, 40 to 44 years). Flexibility is thus appropriate when answering inquiries from women younger than 35 years, for indeed increasing numbers of women aged 33 or 34 years seek prenatal diagnosis.

The risk figures shown in Table 9-2 are applicable only for liveborns. The prevalence of abnormalities at the time when CVS or amniocentesis is performed is somewhat higher.[55,56] For example, the risk for a 35-year-old woman is 1/270 for Down syndrome at the time of amniocentesis (midtrimester). (Many maternal serum screenings for Down syndrome detection report risks at the time of screening, i.e., second trimester.) That the frequency of chromosomal abnormalities is lower in liveborn infants than in first or second trimester fetuses is due to the disproportionate likelihood that fetuses lost spontaneously have chromosomal abnormalities. That is, some abnormal fetuses would have died in utero had iatrogenic intervention not occurred in the second trimester. In fact, 5 percent of stillborn infants show chromosomal abnormalities. (see Ch. 22)

Maternal serum screening is now recommended for women under age 35 years to detect couples at sufficient risk for fetal trisomy to justify invasive procedures.[11] The logical corollary might be that a normal or slightly elevated MSAFP level decreases the risk of aneuploidy for older women to the extent that amniocentesis could be avoided. For this reason, British workers in particular recommend against amniocentesis in older women (35 to 37 years) having normal or slightly increased MSAFP values.[57] However, most U.S. authorities do not agree because of the potential legal hazard and because detection rates are not 100 percent but only 90 percent. In many other countries serum screening is offered to women of all ages.[58] If an older woman wishes to undergo maternal serum screening in lieu of an invasive test she should also be informed that sensitivity to detect abnormalities is even less by ultrasound screening.[59]

Previous Child With Chromosomal Abnormality

After the occurrence of one child or abortus with autosomal trisomy, the likelihood that subsequent progeny will also have autosomal trisomy is increased, even if parental chromosomal complements are normal. Recurrence risks are perhaps 1 percent.[60] The risk is not so high as once believed, but antenatal chromosomal studies should be offered for couples having a prior trisomic pregnancy.

Recurrence risk data following the birth of a liveborn

infant trisomic for a chromosome other than No. 21 are limited. Counseling that the risk is 1 percent for either the same or for a different chromosomal abnormality seems appropriate. Thus, antenatal studies will usually be necessary.

Parental Chromosomal Rearrangements

An uncommon but important indication for prenatal cytogenetic studies is the presence of a parental chromosomal abnormality. A balanced translocation is the usual indication, but inversions and other chromosomal abnormalities exist. As discussed above (see Spectrum and Principles of Genetic Disease—Chromosomal Abnormalities), empirical data invariably reveal that theoretical risks for abnormal (unbalanced) offspring are greater than empirical risks. Empirical risks approximate 12 percent for offspring of either male or female heterozygotes having reciprocal translocations.[61] For Robertsonian (centric fusion) translocations, risks vary according to the chromosomes involved. For t(14q;21q), risks are 10 percent for offspring of heterozygous mothers and 2 percent for offspring of heterozygous fathers (Fig. 9-10).[61] For other nonhomologous Robertsonian translocations, empirical risks for liveborns are less than 1 percent. For homologous translocations (e.g., 21q;21q), all liveborn offspring should have trisomy 21. For other homologous Robertsonian translocations (13q;13q or 22q; 22q), almost all pregnancies result in abortions.

Diagnostic Dilemmas in Prenatal Cytogenetic Diagnosis (Amniotic Fluid Cells or Chorionic Villi)

The obstetrician/gynecologist should be aware of the common pitfalls associated with the analysis of chorionic villi or amniotic fluid cells. An obvious problem is that cells may not grow, or growth may be insufficient for proper analysis. Analysis of maternal rather than fetal cells is another theoretical problem, which fortunately has proved uncommon in experienced hands. In amniocentesis, maternal cell contamination can be minimized by discarding the first few drops of aspirated amniotic fluid. In CVS, examination under a dissecting microscope allows one to distinguish villi from decidua.

A more vexing concern is the possibility that chromosomal abnormalities detected in villi or amniotic fluid

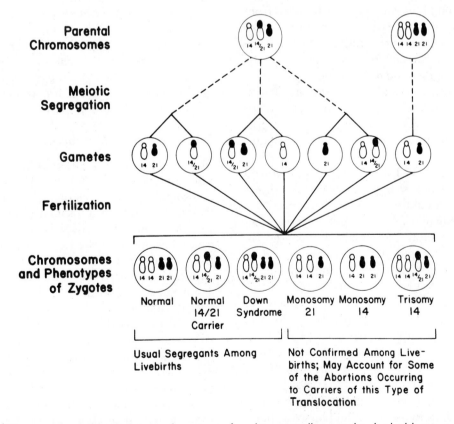

Fig. 9-10 Diagram of possible gametes and progeny of a phenotypically normal individual heterozygous for a Robertsonian translocation between chromosomes 14 and 21 (a form of D/G translocation). Three of the six possible gametes are incompatible with life. The likelihood that an individual with such a translocation would have a child with Down syndrome is theoretically 33 percent. However, the empirical risk is considerably less. (From Gerbie and Simpson,[98] with permission.)

may fail to reflect fetal status. One reason is that chromosomal aberrations may arise in culture (in vitro). This possibility should be suspected whenever an abnormality is restricted to only one of the several culture flasks or clones from a single amniotic fluid or CVS specimen. In fact, cells containing at least one additional structurally normal chromosome are detected in 1 to 2 percent of amniotic fluid or chorionic villus specimens.[62] If these abnormal cells are restricted to a single culture or clone, the phenomenon is termed *pseudomosaicism;* no clinical significance is attached. Defined by the presence of the same abnormality in more than one clone or culture flask, true fetal mosaicism is rarer in amniotic fluid and villi but clinically significant. True mosaicism can be confirmed by studies of the abortus or liveborn in at least 70 to 80 percent of cases[63] and cannot be truly excluded in the remainder because the abnormality could exist in a tissue not readily analyzable.

Chorionic villi divide more rapidly than amniotic fluid cells. Metaphases from trophoblasts derived from villi can be accumulated within hours of sampling. Analysis of these cells can provide rapid answers. However, discrepancies may arise between short-term trophoblast cultures and long-term cultures initiated from the mesenchymal core of the villi.[64] Discrepancies may further exist between CVS preparations of either type (short term or long term) and the embryo. Fortunately, it is possible to recognize and manage these discrepancies, usually by confirmatory amniocentesis and assessment of the expected interval growth. In most discrepancies, the fetus proves normal at amniocentesis, having shown normal interim growth between 10 and 16 weeks.

The U.S. NICHD Collaborative study involved 11,473 chorionic villus samples evaluated by direct methods, long-term culture, or both. There were no incorrect sex predictions.[64] No diagnostic errors occurred in 148 common autosomal trisomies ($+13$, $+18$, $+21$), 16 sex chromosomal aneuploidies, and 13 structural aberrations; a normal cytogenetic diagnosis with CVS was never followed by birth of a trisomic infant. The three triploids studied were confirmed; no confirmation was possible in the single tertraploid case. Not confirmed were several rare trisomies ($+16$, $+22$, $+7$), findings consistent with those in other investigations.[65] Overall, the accuracy of CVS is comparable to that of amniocentesis, but additional tests may be necessary before definitive establishment of nonmosaic rare trisomies and, as in amniotic fluid analysis, polyploidies. Of interest is that the U.S. NICHD study observed increased late loss rates (8.6 percent) in pregnancies showing confirmed placental mosaicism compared with 3.4 percent in pregnancies without mo-

saicism.[66] However, no increased frequency of pregnancy complications was observed.

The clinical significance of the above is that the obstetrician must realize that the neonatal phenotype cannot always be predicted on the basis of the amniotic fluid cells or chorionic villi complement. If a phenotypically normal parent carries the same balanced translocation as found in the fetus, reassurance usually suffices. On the other hand, if an ostensibly balanced translocation is detected in the fetus but in neither parent (a de novo translocation), the likelihood is 10 percent that the neonate will be phenotypically abnormal.[67] Presumably, the rearrangement is not truly balanced.

Mendelian Disorders

Increasing numbers of mendelian disorders are now detectable in utero. Initially only metabolic disorders were detectable on the basis of enzyme analysis. Antenatal diagnoses of hemoglobinopathies and hemophilia were later accomplished with fetal blood, originally obtainable only by fetoscopic sampling. DNA analysis now permits many diagnoses using any available nucleated cell (chorionic villi, amniotic fluid cells). The nature of the mutant or absent gene product need not necessarily even be known. We can predict confidently that in the foreseeable future all common mendelian disorders will be detectable. The rapid progress and increasing complexity required to diagnose mendelian traits dictate close liaison between the obstetrician/gynecologist and geneticist. Tabulated lists of detectable disorders should be considered suspect for timeliness.

Inborn Errors of Metabolism

Antenatal diagnosis is possible for approximately 100 inborn errors of metabolism. Most are transmitted in autosomal recessive fashion, although a few display X-linked recessive or autosomal dominant inheritance. Couples at increased risk will usually be identified because they previously had an affected child. Most metabolic disorders are so rare that it is unreasonable to expect obstetricians who are not geneticists to be fully cognizant of diagnostic possibilities.

Detection of a metabolic error requires that the enzyme be expressed in amniotic fluid cells or chorionic villi. This requirement is fulfilled by most metabolic disorders, a prominent exception being phenylketonuria (PKU). Fortunately, PKU can be detected by the molecular techniques described below. All metabolic disorders detectable in amniotic fluid have proved detectable as well in chorionic villi. Although cultured cells are usually necessary for diagnosis, occasionally one can arrive at a diagnosis on the basis of a product in amniotic fluid. The most prominent example is a 17α-hydroxyprogesterone, an elevated value of which indicates adrenal 21-hydroxylase deficiency (congenital adrenal hyperplasia). This disorder can also be detected by analysis of linked HLA markers in nuclei obtained by CVS or amniocentesis.[68]

Disorders Detectable Solely by Tissue Sampling

If a gene causing a given disorder is not expressed in amniotic fluid or chorionic villi, enzymatic analysis of such tissues will provide no information concerning presence or absence of the disorder. However, the gene might still be expressed in other tissues—blood, skin, muscle, or liver. Initially skin was obtained through fetoscopically directed biopsy, under direct vision; however, currently ultrasound-directed sampling permits use of smaller (14-gauge) instruments. Procedure-related losses following skin biopsy or other invasive procedures are presumed to be greater than that following CVS or amniocentesis; however, the severity of some disorders justifies tissue sampling if no other diagnostic method is available. Counseling a procedure-related loss of about 2 to 3 percent seems appropriate.[69]

Increasingly molecular advances will make tissue sampling obsolete. However, sampling fetal skin may be the only available method for diagnosing certain dermatologic abnormalities such as epidermolysis bullosa or congenital ichthyosis (harlequin ichthyosis).[69,70] Histologic and electron microscopic analyses of fetal skin are necessary. Muscle biopsy may be necessary to detect Duchenne muscular dystrophy if DNA markers are not informative.

Disorders Detectable by Molecular Methods

The power of molecular prenatal diagnosis is that any available nuclear cell can be utilized for diagnosis. All cells contain the same DNA, and the gene need not be

RESTRICTION ENDONUCLEASES

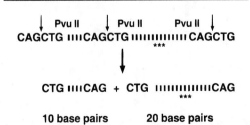

Fig. 9-11 Simplified diagram illustrating the manner in which a restriction endonuclease cuts DNA at a specific nucleotide sequence. PvuII recognizes the sequence CAGCTG and only that sequence. DNA is separated into fragments of different lengths on the basis of distances between restriction enzyme recognition sites. The further the distance between sites, the longer the length of intervening DNA (i.e., 20 versus 30 base pairs). Shorter DNA fragments (e.g., 20 base pairs show greater mobility and migrate further in an agarose cell).

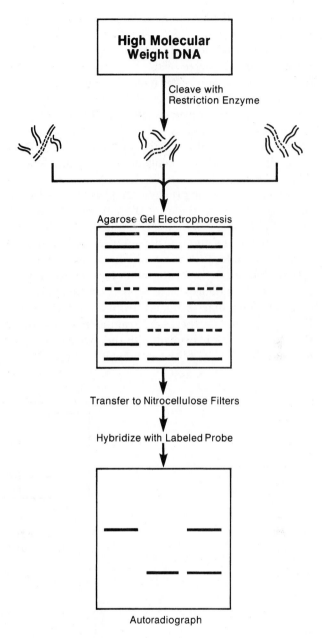

Fig. 9-12 Southern blotting cuts DNA at a specific sequence of nucleotides. After DNA is cleaved with restriction enzymes, the cleaved DNA is separated by size using agarose gel electrophoresis. The gel is then laid on a piece of nitrocellulose and buffer allowed to flow through the gel into the nitrocellulose. DNA fragments migrate out of the gel and bind to the filter. A replica of the gel's DNA fragment pattern is thus made on the filter. The filter can then be hybridized to a suitable radioactivity-labeled probe, with DNA fragments hybridizing to the probe identified after autoradiography.

expressed, unlike the situation when a gene product (enzyme protein) must be analyzed. Through molecular techniques developed within the last decade, Duchenne muscular dystrophy, cystic fibrosis, adult-onset polycystic kidney disease, Huntington's chorea, and most other undetectable disorders have become diagnosable.

To appreciate these advances, the obstetrician/gynecologist must be aware of the analytic techniques that made possible diagnosis by molecular methods. Pivotal was the discovery of *restriction endonucleases*. These bacterial enzymes recognize specific nucleotide sequences five to seven nucleotides in length and cut DNA only at those sites. Use of restriction enzymes permits DNA to be divided into fragments of reproducible lengths (Fig. 9-11).

In Southern blotting (Fig. 9-12), agarose gel electrophoresis is used to separate DNA fragments by size, after exposure to restriction endonucleases. The DNA is then denatured and transferred from the agarose gel to a nitrocellulose filter, on which specific fragments can be located by hybridization. Labeled strands of known DNA sequences act as probes, hybridizing a specific complementary sequence from among the many DNA fragments on the filter. Fragments that contain the sequence that hybridizes with the probe can be detected as bands. Use of size standards facilitates determining whether a particular-sized fragment is or is not present. This technique is called *Southern blotting*.

A modification of this approach involves use of synthetic oligonucleotides 15 to 18 in length, called *allele-specific oligonucleotides* (ASO). An ASO is designed to hybridize to an unknown sample if and only if the latter is characterized by all 15 to 18 nucleotides. ASOs that recognize normal DNA and any known mutant sequence can be designed and used for "dot-blot" DNA analysis or "slot-blot" analysis.

Integral to facile diagnosis was development of the *polymerized chain reaction* (PCR) procedure. In PCR, a target sequence can be amplified severalfold (10^5 to 10^6) (Fig. 9-13). For most purposes PCR amplification utilizes unique DNA primers that flank and are specific for the DNA region in question; thus, the sequence must be known. (Gene sequencing methodology now also utilizes PCR techniques to synthesize sequences whose nucleotide order can then be determined.) The region in question may consist of a portion of a gene containing a mutation, a polymorphic DNA sequence closely linked to a given locus, or a repetitive DNA se-

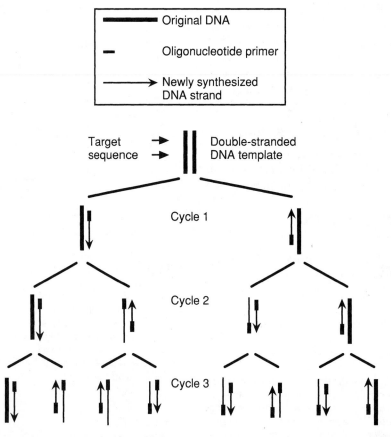

Fig. 9-13 Polymerized chain reaction (PCR). Placing the DNA in question, unique primers, and *Taq* polymerase together results in amplification (cycle 1). When the temperature is raised denaturation into single-stranded DNA occurs. Upon cooling a second amplification cycle continued. Continued amplification increases the amount of DNA located between primers in logarithmic fashion.

quence characteristic of a given chromosomal region. Irrespective, a heat-stable DNA polymerase extracted from *Thermas aquaticus* (*Taq* polymerase) is placed in a single tube with the DNA in question, excess deoxyribonucleoside triphosphates (adenine, thymine, guanine, cytosine), and the unique primers specific for the region being studied. DNA synthesis (amplification) is initiated (cycle 1 in Fig. 9-12). Raising the temperature denatures the newly amplified double-stranded DNA back into single-stranded DNA. Upon cooling, another amplification cycle can occur (cycle 2 in Fig. 9-12), this time with twice as many strands. The DNA sequence between primers amplifies in geometric fashion with each replication. In 3 to 4 hours 30 to 40 amplifications are achieved.

Diagnosis When the Molecular Basis Is Known

It is convenient for heuristic purposes to divide mendelian disorders into those in which the molecular basis (i.e., precise nucleotide abnormality) is known and those in which the gene is localized to a given chromosomal region but in which the molecular basis is not known. Known causes of mendelian disorders include absence of the gene or point mutations. If a disorder is known to be characterized by absence of DNA, one can determine whether a probe does or does not hybridize with the relevant sequence of DNA from an individual of unknown genotype. Again, failure of hybridization indicates that the individual lacks the DNA sequence in question; thus, the disorder is assumed present. This approach is currently used to diagnose all forms of α-thalassemia, many cases of Duchenne/Becker muscular dystrophy, some cases of β-thalassemia, and some forms of hemophilia.

A second general approach becomes applicable if the molecular basis involves a point mutation whose nucleotide sequence is known. The most straightforward example is sickle cell anemia, in which the triplet (codon) designating the sixth amino acid has undergone a mutation from adenine to guanine. As a result, codon 6 connotes valine rather than glutamic acid, leading to the abnormal protein ($β^s$). Fortunately, several restriction enzymes recognize the normal DNA sequence at codons 5, 6, and 7 (Fig. 9-14). One could also construct ASOs designed to hybridize only if every single nucleotide is present. Use of a $β^s$ oligonucleotide probe will confirm the specific mutant DNA sequence. Diagnosis with limited amounts of DNA can be achieved by the use of PCR amplification. A hybridized ASO usually appears as a "dot blot" (Fig. 9-15) or "slot blot."

Actually sickle cell anemia is very atypical for mendelian disorders in that its molecular basis is homogenous. Far more commonly many different molecular muta-

---

Selected Disorders Detectable by DNA Analysis

Direct
  α-Thalassemia
  β-Thalassemia (80%)
  Duchenne/Becker muscular dystrophy (80%)
  Hemophilia A and B (some forms)
  Sickle cell anemia (85–90%)
  Cystic fibrosis (whites of northern European ancestry)
Linkage analysis (restriction fragment length polymorphism or dinucleotide repeats)
  Adrenal 21-hydroxylase deficiency
  β-Thalassemia (20% worldwide; higher in United States)
  Cystic fibrosis (10–15% in whites northern European ancestry)
  Duchenne muscular dystrophy (20%)
  Hemophilia A and B (some forms)

---

tions are responsible (heterogeneity). We have already considered this concept with respect to cystic fibrosis, but analogous findings exist for almost all mendelian traits: hemophilia A and B, adult polycystic kidney disease, PKU, β-thalassemias, and others. Usually one molecular mutation is particularly common, a limited number considerably less so but in aggregate accounting for a respectable proportion (10 to 15 percent) of mutations; innumerable other mutations are very rare, some almost unique. A common approach is to amplify the unknown DNA and test with multiple ASOs (multiplex PCR). An important caveat is that a mutation not corresponding to one of the mutations tested will pass unrecognized. Various techniques facilitate identifying all mutations, but all of these procedures are laborious and still incomplete. Despite the molecular revolution, a place often still exists for analysis of the gene product (protein or enzyme).

Diagnosis When the Molecular Basis Is Not Known

The molecular approaches described above are applicable only when the precise molecular basis of a disorder is known. Unfortunately, this requirement is fulfilled less often than one would desire. One reason is that certain genes may not yet be cloned and isolated. Even if the chromosomal location is known, an interval passes before the sequence is determined. A second reason is the considerable heterogeneity noted previously to exist at the molecular level. Mutations at multiple nucleotide sites within the gene can all produce a dys-

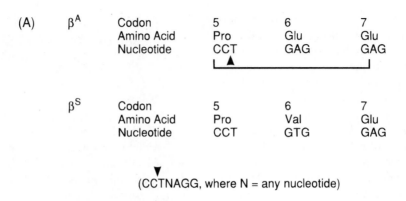

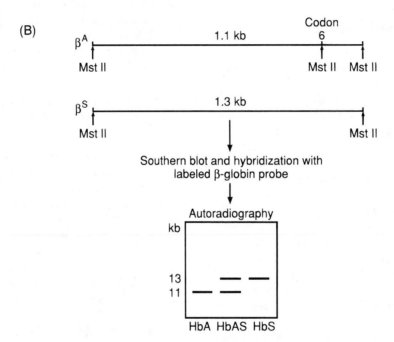

Fig. 9-14 Use of a radioactively labeled gene probe for β-globin for diagnosis of sickle cell anemia. The approach uses the choice of a specific restriction enzyme **(A)** followed by Southern blotting **(B)** to elicit differences on DNA lengths. A mutation from adenine (A) to thymine (T) results in loss of an MstII restriction recognition site (CCTNAGG, where N = any nucleotide).

OligoNucleotide Probe	Heterozygote (AS)	Heterozygote (AS)	Affected (SS)	Normal Genotype (AA)
β^S CCTG**T**GGAGAAGTCT			●	
β^A CCTG**A**GGAGAAGTCT				●

Fig. 9-15 Dot blot analysis. Oligonucleotides are constructed for sequences complementary to normal DNA (β^A) and mutant DNA (β^S). DNA challenged by the oligonucleotide probe will be hybridized if and only if the DNA contains all nucleotides connoted by the probe. Thus, AS individuals will respond to both β^A and β^S probes, whereas AA or SS individuals will respond only to one of the two probes (β^A and β^S, respectively). Homozygous individuals respond with a stronger (darker) signal than heterozygous individuals.

functional product. Given that genes are often very large, diagnostic complexities may be daunting. Sequencing the entire gene for every diagnostic situation is not practical, and even then the mutation might not be detected if it were located in a promoter region or involved in translation. If mutations occur in a more limited number of exons (coding sequences) within the gene, the problem is ameliorated but is not obviated.

The problem cited above can be addressed by linkage analysis, taking advantage of the ostensibly innocuous differences in DNA that exist among individuals in the general population. These differences are called *polymorphisms* and are analogous to such well-known polymorphisms as the ABO blood group locus. Clinically insignificant differences in DNA yield differences in DNA fragment lengths following exposure to a given restriction endonuclease. These differences are thus termed *restriction fragment length polymorphisms* (RFLPs). In linkage analysis a diagnosis is made not on the basis of analyzing the mutant gene per se but rather on the basis of presence or absence of a nearby marker. In RFLPs the marker is a DNA variant capable of being recognized following exposure to a given endonuclease. The marker could also be a dinucleotide or trinucleotide polymorphism. Throughout the genome there exist polymorphisms in which the number of nucleotide repeats (e.g., the dinucleotides cytosine and adenine, or CA) vary among individuals at a given locus. For example, some individuals may show 6 CA repeats, others 8, others 10 at a given locus. The almost innumerable number of such polymorphisms underlies the scientific basis of DNA analysis being used for forensic pathology.

To illustrate the principle of linkage analysis, let us assume that a given RFLP or nucleotide repeat is known to lie close to or preferably within the mutant gene of interest. One next needs to deduce the relationship of the mutant to the status of the marker. Starting with an individual of known genotype, usually an affected fetus or child, one determines on which parental chromosome a given DNA marker is located (cis-trans relationship). Is the marker located on the chromosome carrying the mutant gene, and is it located on the chromosome carrying the normal gene? Figure 9-16 illustrates a simple example.

There are pitfalls in linkage analysis using RFLP or nucleotide repeats. First, the marker may or may not be informative in a given family. If all family members show identical DNA fragment patterns at a given locus, that locus is obviously useless because affected and unaffected individuals cannot be distinguished from each other. If a given marker is uninformative, one searches for another marker that may prove informative. Fortunately, a potentially limitless number of markers exist. Second, the distance between the mutant gene and the

marker is crucial because the likelihood of meiotic recombination is inversely related to this distance. Recall that during meiosis I recombination can occur between homologous chromosomes. Genes are linked to one another if, after meiosis I, they remain together more often than expected by chance. Recombination can occur even between closely linked loci; thus, prenatal diagnosis based on linkage analysis is never 100% accurate. Using polymorphic markers on both sides of the mutant can minimize but not exclude the possibility of a recombinational event.

Despite these caveats, linkage analysis permits prenatal diagnosis in many situations not otherwise possible. Linkage analysis is particularly applicable to the increasing numbers of single-gene (mendelian) disorders with considerable molecular heterogeneity. These include Huntington's chorea, hemophilia A and B, adult onset polycystic kidney disease, and some forms of neufibromatosis, Duchenne/Becker muscular dystrophy, and β-thalassemia.

Polygenic/Multifactorial Disorders

Amniotic Fluid α-Fetoprotein

Failure of the neural tube to close during embryogenesis leads to anencephaly, spina bifida (myelomeningocele or meningocele), encephalocele, and other less common midline defects (e.g., lipomeningocele). Anencephaly is almost never compatible with long-term survival. Spina bifida is compatible with long-term survival, although it is frequently associated with hemiparesis, urinary incontinence, and hydrocephalus.

Anencephaly and spina bifida represent different manifestations of the same pathogenic process and reflect the same genetic etiology. Couples who have had a child with an NTD have approximately 1 percent risk for any subsequent offspring having spina bifida and 1 percent risk for subsequent offspring having anencephaly (2 percent for any NTD).[71] This holds true irrespective of the type of NTD present in the index case (proband). If a prospective parent has an NTD, the risk is also about 2 percent. Second-degree relatives (nieces, nephews, grandchildren) and third-degree relatives (first cousins) are less likely to be affected. A woman whose sister or brother had a child with an NTD carries a lower 0.5 to 1.0 percent risk for NTD offspring.[40] For reasons that are unclear, risks are slightly lower if the father's sibling had an NTD.

Antenatal diagnosis of an NTD is best accomplished by amniotic fluid α-fetoprotein (AF-AFP) assay. Through AF-AFP analysis, diagnosis of an NTD is possible in all anencephaly cases and in all of spina bifida cases except the 5 to 10 percent in which skin covers the lesion. Closed lesions are somewhat more common in encephaloceles. Ultrasonography by experienced

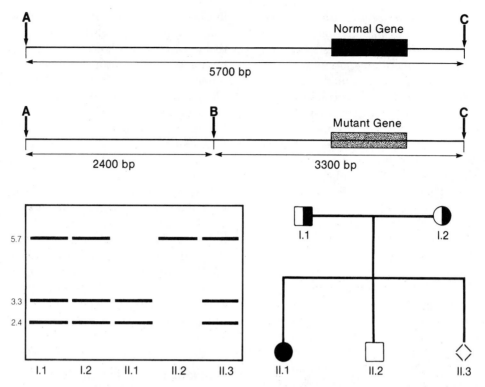

Fig. 9-16 Restriction fragment length polymorphisms (RFLPs), which are invaluable for certain prenatal diagnoses. Suppose one mutant gene is linked to another gene (B) that governs whether or not a restriction site (B) is present. If the restriction site is present, DNA is cut by a certain restriction enzyme (arrow) to produce 3,300- and 2,400-bp-long fragments. If the segment conferring the restriction site is not present, the total fragment is 5,700 bp long. The different lengths can serve as markers to allow genotypes to be deduced. Suppose two obligate heterozygotes 1.1 and 1.2 have one affected child. Suppose further that a probe for the gene hybridizes to the region A to C. The probe can thus identify three fragments (2,400, 3,300, and, 5,700 bp). If the affected child shows only the 2,400- and 3,300-bp fragments, it can be deduced that the mutant allele is in association (i.e., on the same chromosome) with the gene-conferring restriction site B and thus is producing both 2,400- and 3,300-bp fragments. The normal allele must be in association with the allele not conferring restriction B and thus is designated by the 5,700-bp fragment. Genotypes can thus be predicted from DNA analysis of chorionic villi and amniotic fluid cells. Fetus 11.3 can be assumed to be heterozygous because all three fragments (2,400, 3,300, and 5,700) are present.

physicians should readily exclude anencephaly, and spina bifida theoretically can be detected by serial views of the vertebral column shape of the cranium, ventricles, cerebellum, and cisternal magna. Unfortunately, few ultrasonographers know their sensitivity or specificity for detecting NTDs. Until such data are available, AF-AFP analysis should be considered the standard method for detecting an NTD despite frequent hopes and statements to the contrary.

AF-AFP may be spuriously elevated if the amniotic fluid is contaminated with fetal blood. This pitfall can be eliminated if AChE is assayed concurrently. AChE is present in the amniotic fluid of fetuses with open NTDs but is absent in normal amniotic fluid. If AChE is absent but fetal hemoglobin present, the elevated AFP is probably due to fetal blood. Some confusion may arise if amniocentesis is performed earlier than 13 weeks.

Elevated AFP is also associated with certain other polygenic/multifactorial anomalies (e.g., omphalocele,

gastroschisis, cystic hygroma). In these disorders, AChE may or may not be elevated. With certain mendelian traits (e.g., congenital nephrosis) AFP is elevated but AChE is not. Ultrasonographic studies should therefore be undertaken to corroborate elevated AF-AFP and to determine the nature of any defect present. On the other hand, failure to detect an anomaly by ultrasound does not necessarily indicate that elevated AF-AFP was spurious. If AF-AFP is elevated and AChE is present, the fetus should be considered abnormal irrespective of ultrasound findings.

Disorders Detectable Only by Ultrasound

Anomalies inherited in polygenic/multifactorial fashion usually carry recurrence risks of 1 to 5 percent for first-degree relatives (siblings, offspring, parent), a risk sufficiently high to justify prenatal diagnosis for many couples. The number of genes responsible for these defects is unknown, but presumably more than one;

thus, diagnosis on the basis of enzyme assays or DNA cannot seriously be entertained at present. Except for the few conditions amenable to AF-AFP analysis, the principal method of assessment involves visualization of fetal anatomy by ultrasound.

The typical couple at risk already has had a child with the anomaly in question, thus incurring a 1 to 5 percent risk for another affected child. To alter clinical management, a diagnosis should be made by 20 to 24 weeks gestation. This is sufficiently early to weigh the alternative options of termination, fetal surgery, or preterm delivery followed by neonatal surgery. PUBS and second trimester transabdominal CVS can exclude chromosomal abnormalities if either of the latter options are contemplated. A careful search for other defects is also necessary. For some anomalies (e.g., hydrocephaly) an isolated anomaly is rare, but for others (e.g., posterior urethral values) only a single malformation may be present.

Antenatal ultrasonography for anomaly detection should be performed only by highly experienced physicians. Physicians scanning obstetric patients only for fetal viability, multiple gestations, and placental location should explicitly inform their patients that anomaly assessment is not being attempted. Casual reassurance of fetal normalcy should be eschewed. It should further be realized that almost no individual has sufficient experience to calculate his or her own specificities or sensitivities.

Future Directions

Preimplantation Diagnosis

Despite the advantage CVS offers for first trimester prenatal diagnosis, even earlier diagnosis may be desirable. One reason is that one can envision certain treatment regimens (metabolic, gene insertion). A second reason is that some couples at risk for affected offspring may undergo repeated prenatal diagnosis and termination. Other couples strongly wish to avoid clinical terminations.

These disadvantages can be addressed by preimplantation genetic diagnosis, utilizing access to gametes (oocytes) or embryos before 6 days, the time at which implantation occurs. Potential approaches include (1) polar body biopsy, (2) aspiration of one to two cells from the six- to eight-cell embryo at 2 to 3 days, and (3) trophectoderm biopsy of the 5- to 6-day blastocyst.

Polar Body Biopsy

In the absence of recombination (crossing-over), a polar body showing a mutant allele should be complementary to a primary oocyte carrying the normal allele.

Thus, the normal oocyte could be allowed to fertilize in vitro and the resulting embryo transferred for potential implantation and pregnancy. Conversely, if the polar body were genetically normal, fertilization would not be permitted. The pitfall is that recombination can occur between homologous chromosomes. If crossing-over occurs, the single chromosome in the primary oocyte would have copies of both alleles. That is, the chromatids of a single chromosome would differ in genetic constitution. The genotype of the secondary oocyte could not be predicted without further testing, i.e., biopsy of either the second polar body or the embryo per se. Recombination especially becomes a problem for genes located near the telomeres because such genes show recombination frequencies approximating 50 percent. Nonetheless, this approach has been employed by Verlinsky et al.[72] in pregnancies at risk for ZZ α_1-antitrypsin deficiency, hemophilia A, ΔF508 cystic fibrosis and other disorders.

Polar body analysis and other forms of preimplantation genetic diagnosis would not be possible without PCR to amplify DNA. One pitfall is that although a signal is theoretically possible with a single cell, a signal is not always observed after PCR even when DNA of a known type is present. This may be due to either loss of DNA or failure of amplification. In the hands of the one group that has attempted human polar body analysis, PCR failed in 14 of 83 cases.[72] Worse, PCR failure may be allele specific. A further problem is that pressing PCR to its limits of its sensitivity greatly increases the risk of erroneous diagnosis due to contamination (e.g., from ambient normal cells).

Among 53 transfers by the same investigative group, there were four pregnancies. Two resulted in biochemical pregnancies, one in a clinical spontaneous abortion, and one in a viable pregnancy. Unfortunately, the latter proved at CVS to be affected, thereby constituting an erroneous polar biopsy diagnosis.

Biopsy of the Eight-Cell Embryo

The greatest experience in preimplantation genetic diagnosis involves the six- to eight-cell embryo. Biopsy at this stage requires obtaining cells contained within the zona pellucida. This can be obtained by direct aspiration with a pipette following mechanical or chemical dissociation. The sentinel work in this area has been conducted by Handyside and colleagues.[73,74] Using in vitro fertilization human embryos, a single cell is removed through a hole made in the zona pellucida by a drilling pipette (diameter 10 to 20 mm) containing acid Tyrode's solution. Only unaffected embryos are transferred. A recent report tabulated that 34 babies have been born worldwide following preimplantation diagnosis.[75] Both embryonic sex and mendelian muta-

Nested-Primer PCR: Cystic Fibrosis ΔF508

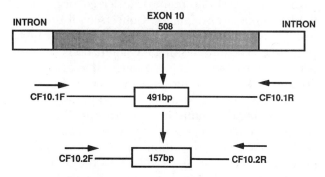

Fig. 9-17 Diagram illustrating nested-primer polymerase chain reaction (PCR), specifically of a type enabling one to detect ΔF508 cystic fibrosis on the basis of analysis of a single cell. Polymerase chain reaction is first initiated for a 491-bp fragment in exon 10, which contains the most common mutation in cystic fibrosis (ΔF508). After a given number of cycles (e.g., 30) with primers CD10.1F and CF10.1R, a 491-bp sequence is generated. A second set of primers (CF10.2F and CF10.2R), internal to the first, is then constructed to generate a 157-bp sequence. Nested-primer PCR allows far greater diagnostic sensitivity than possible on the basis of a traditional PCR. (From Simpson and Elias,[33] with permission.)

tions have been detected. For the latter special molecular approaches are necessary.

The first mendelian trait detected was ΔF508 cystic fibrosis.[74] This was achieved by first using nested primer PCR to amplify DNA (Fig. 9-17). Diagnosis was made by analyzing the presence or absence of the heteroduplex complex that forms only if nonidentical single-stranded DNA sequences anneal to one another (Fig. 9-18). Mixing DNA that is presumptively normal with known mutant ΔF508 DNA would produce a heteroduplex. Depending on diagnosis, a heteroduplex would or would not be expected. This approach was initially used in three couples, in which both parents were ΔF508 heterozygotes.[74] In one of the three couples one homozygous normal and one heterozygous embryo were transferred, resulting in one homozygous normal liveborn. Similar approaches have been used to detect Tay-Sachs disease and other mendelian disorders.[76]

A major worry is the risk of contamination from ambient cells. Failed PCR also occurs, but this is less catastrophic than contamination, for only the latter would ordinarily lead to a false-negative diagnosis. If in an autosomal recessive disorder the embryo were a heterozygote, failure to amplify the normal allele would erroneously indicate the embryo to be affected; therefore, no transfer would occur. The clinical consequence would be limited to a missed opportunity to achieve a pregnancy. Conversely, failing to amplify the abnormal allele would result in transfer of an embryo assumed erroneously to be homozygously normal but actually heterozygous. In either case allele-specific PCR failure would not result in a clinically significant error (i.e., false-negative diagnosis).

Heteroduplex Analysis
Diagnosis: ΔF508 (154bp)

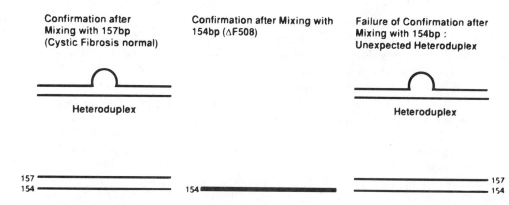

Confirmation after Mixing with 157bp (Cystic Fibrosis normal)

Confirmation after Mixing with 154bp (ΔF508)

Failure of Confirmation after Mixing with 154bp: Unexpected Heteroduplex

Heteroduplex

Heteroduplex

Fig. 9-18 Heteroduplex analysis illustrating approach necessary to diagnose ΔF508 cystic fibrosis on the analysis of a single cell, as would be accomplished for preimplantation genetics. Nested-primer PCR is first performed as shown in Figure 9-17. If the DNA fragment does not show ΔF508, a 157-bp fragment (normal) is generated. If ΔF508 is present, the lack of three nucleotides results in a fragment that is only 154-bp in length. Although distinguishing a 157-bp fragment from a 154-bp pair fragment is possible, this may be difficult. Determination is easier if the unknown sample is denatured and mixed with DNA from a normal individual (cystic fibrosis normal) or DNA from an individual known to show ΔF508. If DNA of the unknown individual (i.e., cell) is ΔF508, mixing with a 154-bp fragment results in a homoduplex (middle diagram). If the DNA ΔF508 is mixed with normal DNA (157-bp fragment), one observes not only the 157- and 154-bp fragments but also a heteroduplex resulting from incomplete reannealing when two dissimilar DNA fragments are placed together. The final figure (*right*) shows the presence of an unexpected heteroduplex, which would occur if the diagnosis of ΔF508 had been erroneous. (From Simpson and Elias,[33] with permission.)

The pregnancy rate per embryo following blastomere aspiration seems comparable to that observed with in vitro fertilization without biopsy. These data reassure us that removing a single cell from the eight cell human embryo is not necessarily deleterious.

Isolating Fetal Cells from Maternal Blood

Isolation and analysis of fetal cells in the maternal blood is being pursued as a noninvasive method of prenatal diagnosis.[77,78]

This idea has been considered seriously since Walknowska et al.[79] found XY metaphases in maternal blood of pregnant women carrying male fetuses. However, not all individuals carrying male fetuses showed XY metaphases, and XY metaphases were observed in some women carrying female fetuses. In the late 1970s, Herzenberg and colleagues[80] applied flow sorting technology to enrich sample content of fetal cells. In 1989, Lo et al.[81] showed conclusively that fetal cells existed in maternal blood. Women carrying a male fetus demonstrated a Y-specific signal. PCR-based studies show that fetal cells are present in maternal blood as early as 35 days gestation.[82] By the end of the first trimester, fetal DNA (Y sequences) are usually detectable.[83]

What Types of Fetal Cells Could Exist in Maternal Blood?

Trophoblasts are an obvious candidate cell, given their intimate relationship with the uterus. Syncytiotrophoblast buds and cytotrophoblasts are present in relatively high numbers in the maternal circulation early in pregnancy, the inevitable result of uterine invasion to establish the fetal circulation. However, these cells are believed to become trapped and sequestered by the lung at their first circulatory passage. A persistent difficulty in isolating trophoblasts has been obtaining monoclonal antibodies specific for placental antigens. Many antibodies have been generated but relatively few have proved useful. The greatest success has been achieved in Adelaide, where 6,000 monoclonal antibodies were produced from placental tissue to find 5 specific for fetal tissue.[84] In a pregnancy at risk for β-thalassemia, a mixture of three different monocolonal antibodies was used to recover cells that were then subjected to PCR to yield a correct diagnosis.[85]

Another potential cell type is the lymphocyte. Indeed, paternal HLA-DR sequences have been detected in maternal blood, presumably indicating the presence of fetal lymphocytes.[86,87] However, lymphocytes are not considered ideal candidate cells for isolation from maternal blood because this is the cell type most likely to persist from previous pregnancies.

Nucleated fetal red cells (erythroblasts) seem to be the most attractive cell type. Bianchi et al.[88] were the first to focus on these cells, using flow sorting on the basis of transferrin receptor (CD71) positivity and subjecting sorted cells to PCR for a Y sequence. Our group has applied different sorting criteria, followed by fluorescent in situ hybridization with chromosome-specific DNA probes (FISH); fetal trisomies were detected.[89–92] By 1993, we had studied 69 maternal blood samples and identified all by one of eight aneuploidies. Other groups have also detected fetal trisomies from the analysis of maternal blood.[93,94]

The US NICHD is currently involved in the evaluation of this technology for the detection of aneuploidy. The current study involving several collaborative centers will determine the sensitivity and specificity for diagnostic/chromosomal abnormalities and will require a study of at least 3,000 women. By 1997 data relevant to the propriety of introducing this technology into clinical practice will be available. Until then traditional invasive techniques like CVS or amniocentesis should be employed.

Mendelian Traits

Diagnosis of mendelian disorders has been accomplished by PCR analysis of fetal cells in maternal blood. Camaschella et al.[95] studied DNA obtained from maternal blood of three pregnancies at risk for β-thalassemia/hemoglobin Lepore$_{Boston}$ hemoglobin. Lepore$_{Boston}$ is a hybrid δ–β-globin gene, resulting from an unequal crossing-over between misaligned β and δ genes on chromosome 11. The abnormal gene is associated with a 7 kb deletion. PCR was used to amplify for hemoglobin Lepore$_{Boston}$-specific DNA in unsorted maternal blood of women with β-thalassemia trait whose partners carried the Lepore$_{Boston}$ mutation. This hemoglobin was correctly identified in two fetuses, whereas in a third the mutant gene was not present. Determination of fetal sex could be useful in couples at risk for X-linked recessive traits.

An exciting use of this technology lies in the management of Rh isoimmunization. The molecular basis of the Rh-negative genotype is gene deletion. Lo et al[96] determined fetal Rh(D) status in pregnancies of Rh-negative women known to be sensitized. Unsorted blood from 21 Rh(D) negative women were subjected to PCR for Rh(D) DNA sequences specific for the Rh(D) gene. Overall, 8 of the 10 women carrying an Rh(D) fetus showed a Rh(D) signal.

Conclusion

Few areas of obstetrics and gynecology have shown more rapid advances than prenatal diagnosis. Barely 20 years have passed since the initial amniocentesis and prenatal diagnosis, yet diagnosis and genetic screening are accepted as standard in our field. The next decade will bring further different advances, many alluded to in this chapter. Genes controlling all common monogenic disorders can be expected to become identified and sequenced. In addition to expanding the numbers of disorders amenable to prenatal diagnosis, information will be available for genetic screening, identifying more couples at risk before the birth of a first affected child.

Advances in noninvasive techniques can be expected, possibly through analysis of fetal cells in maternal blood.[78,97] Obstetricians can expect further breakthroughs in fetal treatment as well, including preimplantation gene therapy.

Key Points

- The frequency of major birth defects is 2 to 3 percent. Major etiologic categories include chromosomal abnormalities (1 per 160 live births), single-gene or mendelian disorders, polygenic/multifactorial disorders, and teratogenic disorders. Of the chromosomal abnormalities, approximately half represent autosomal trisomy and half sex chromosomal abnormalities.

- Principles of genetic counseling include adequate communication, appreciation of psychological defenses, and philosophy of non-directive counseling.

- Genetic screening in the nonpregnant population for heterozygote detection is appropriate for only selected autosomal recessive disorders: Tay Sachs disease in Jewish populations, α-thalassemia in Orientals, β-thalassemia in Mediterranean peoples (Greek and Italian), sickle cell in blacks.

- In all pregnancies, genetic screening should be performed for chromosomal abnormalities and NTDs. All women aged 35 years and above at delivery should be offered prenatal cytogenetic diagnosis. For younger women, maternal serum screening should be offered to detect autosomal trisomies. The profile of decreased MSAFP, elevated hCG, and decreased unconjugated serum estriol favors Down syndrome. Maternal serum analyte screening in combination with maternal age can detect 60 percent of Down syndrome cases, but the frequency varies according to maternal age (90 percent over age 35 but less than 25 percent in the early third decade). Screening for NTDs involves elevated MSAFP followed by amniotic fluid analysis; approximately 80 to 90 percent of NTDs can be detected at a cost of 5 percent amniocentesis.

- All invasive procedures carry risks. Amniocentesis at 15 weeks and above carries a procedure-related risk of approximately 0.5 percent loss. Amniocentesis before this time has not been subjected to rigorous trials to determine safety. CVS is considered, in experienced hands, equal to amniocentesis in terms of loss rates and diagnostic accuracy. Both transcervical and transabdominal CVS are equal in safety. Availability of both procedures allows the physician to choose the most appropriate technique.

- Controversy exists concerning LRDs associated with CVS. If a risk exists it appears to be greatest below 10 weeks of gestation, for which reason, in general, the procedure should generally be available at 10 weeks and beyond. A maximum limb reduction risk of 1 in 3,000 has been reported, and many believe that the risk is not greater than that of the general population. The rate of complications associated with fetal blood sampling is uncertain, but appears to be 1 to 2 percent. However, this varies according to the diagnosis being assessed. No studies have directly compared loss rates in control and tested pregnancies.

- Many single-gene disorders are detectable. Some can be detected by enzymatic analysis, whereas others can be recognized best or only through molecular methodologies.

- Two principal types of molecular analysis are employed. Direct analysis is possible if the gene sequence is known. Linkage analysis is necessary if the gene has been localized but not yet sequenced. Linkage analysis takes advantage of markers lying close to the gene in question; accuracy is not 100 percent because recombination can occur between the marker and the mutant gene.

- Preimplantation genetic diagnosis has been accomplished, principally by removing a single cell from the eight-cell embryo. Diagnosis requires special molecular techniques.

- Fetal cells have been recovered from maternal blood and fetal trisomies detected. Determining sensitivity and accuracy levels compared with amniocentesis and CVS is underway.

References

1. Simpson JL, Golbus MS: Genetics in Obstetrics and Gynecology. 2nd Ed. WB Saunders, Philadelphia, 1992
2. Hook EB, Hamerton JL: The frequency of chromosome abnormalities detected in consecutive newborn studies—differences between studies—results by sex and by severity of phenotypic involvement. p. 63. In Hook EB, Porter IH (eds): Population Cytogenetic Studies in Humans. Academic Press San Diego 1977
3. McKusick VA: Mendelian Inheritance in Man. 11th Ed. The Johns Hopkins University Press, Baltimore, 1994
4. Simpson JL: Disorders of Gonads and Internal Reproductive Ducts. In Rimoin DL, Connor JM, Pyeritz RE (eds): Emery & Rimoin's Principles and Practice of Medical Genetics. 3rd Ed. Churchill Livingstone, Edinburgh (in press)
5. Lemna WK, Feldman GL, Kerem BS et al: Mutation analysis for heterozygote detection and the prenatal diagnosis of cystic fibrosis. N Engl J Med 322:219, 1990
6. Elias S, Annas G, Simpson JL: Carrier screening for cystic fibrosis: implications for obstetrical and gynecological practice. Am J Obstet Gynecol 164:1077, 1991
7. Merkartz IR, Nitowsky HM, Macri JN et al: An association between low maternal serum alpha fetoprotein and fetal chromosome abnormalities. Am J Obstet Gynecol 148:886, 1984
8. Bogart MH, Pandiani MR, Jones OW: Abnormal maternal serum chorionic gonadotropin levels in pregnancies with fetal chromosome abnormalties. Prenat Diagn 7:623, 1987
9. Wald NJ et al: Maternal serum screening for Down syndrome in early pregnancy. Br Med J 297:883, 1988
10. Canick JA, Knight GJ, Palomaki GE et al: Low second trimester maternal serum unconjugated estriol in pregnancies with Down syndrome. Br J Obstet Gynecol 95:330, 1988
11. American College of Obstetricians and Gynecologists Committee Opinion. Down syndrome screening. ACOG Washington, DC, 141, 1994
12. Brambati B et al: First-trimester Down syndrome screening using nuchal translucency: a prospective study in patients undergoing chorionic villus sampling. Ultrasound Obstet Gynecol 5:9, 1995
13. Elias S, Simpson JL: Amniocentesis. p. 33. In Milunsky A (ed): Genetic Disorders and the Fetus. 3rd Ed: Plenum, New York, 1992
14. Evans MI, Dommergues M, Timor-Tritsch I et al: Transabdominal versus transcervical and transvaginal multifetal pregnancy reduction: international collaborative experience of more than one thousand cases. Am J Obstet Gynecol 170:902, 1994
15. National Institute of Child Health Development National Registry for Amniocentesis Study Group: Midtrimester amniocentesis for prenatal diagnosis: safety and accuracy. JAMA 236:1471, 1976
16. Simpson NE, Dellaire L, Miller JR et al: Prenatal diagnosis of genetic disease in Canada: report of a collaborative study. Can Med Assoc J 15:739, 1976
17. United Kingdom Medical Research Council: Working Party on amniocentesis. An assessment of the hazards of amniocentesis. Br J Obstet Gynaecol 85(suppl 21):1, 1978
18. National Institute of Child Health and Human Development Consensus Conference on Antenatal Diagnosis: NIH Publication No. 80-1973, December 1979
19. Tabor A, Philip J, Madsen MI et al: Randomized controlled trial of genetic amniocentesis in 4,606 low-risk women. Lancet 1:1287, 1986
20. Hanson FW, Tennant F, Hune S, Brookhyser K: Early amniocentesis: outcome, risks, and technical problems at ≤12.8 weeks. Am J Obstet Gynecol 166:1707, 1992
21. Henry GP, Miller WA: Early amniocentesis. J Reprod Med 37:396, 1992
22. Shulman LP, Elias S, Phillips OP, Grevengood C, Dungan JL, Simpson JL: Amniocentesis performed at 14 weeks gestation or earlier: comparison with first-trimester chorionic villus sampling. Obstet Gynecol 83:543, 1994
23. Shulman LP, Simpson JL, Elias S et al: Transvaginal chorionic villus sampling using transabdominal ultrasound guidance: a new technique for first-trimester prenatal diagnosis. Fetal Diagn Ther 8:144, 1993
24. Nicolaides K, Brizot ML, Patel F, Snijders R: Comparison of chorionic villus sampling and amniocentesis for fetal karyotyping at 10–13 weeks gestation. Lancet 344:435, 1994
25. Rhoads GG, Jackson LG, Schlesselman SE et al: The safety and efficacy of chorionic villus sampling for early

prenatal diagnosis of cytogenetic abnormalities. N Engl J Med 320:609, 1989

26. Canadian Collaborative CVS–Amniocentesis Clinical Trial Group: Multicentre randomized clinical trial of chorionic villus sampling. Lancet 337:1491, 1991

27. Golbus MS, Simpson JL, Fowler SE et al: Risk factors associated with transcervical CVS losses. Prenat Diagn 12:373, 1991

28. Jackson L, Wapner RJ: Chorionic villus sampling. p. 45. In Simpson JL, Elias S (eds): Essentials of Prenatal Diagnosis. Churchill Livingstone, New York, 1993

29. Jackson LG, Zachary JM, Desnik RJ et al: A randomized comparison of transcervical and transabdominal chorionic villus sampling. N Engl J Med 327:594, 1992

30. Brambati B, Lanzani A, Tului L: Transabdominal and transcervical chorionic villus sampling: efficiency and risk evaluation of 2,411 cases. Am J Med Genet 35:160, 1990

31. Smidt-Jensen S, Permin M, Philip J et al: Randomized comparison of amniocentesis and transabdominal and transcervical chorionic villus sampling. Lancet 340:1237, 1992

32. MRC Working Party on the Evaluation of Chorionic Villus Sampling: Medical Research Council European Trial of Chorion Villus Sampling. Lancet 337:1491, 1991

33. Simpson JL, Elias S: Prenatal diagnosis of genetic disorders. p. 61. In Creasy RK, Resnik R (eds): Maternal Fetal Medicine. 3rd Ed. WB Saunders, Philadelphia, 1994

34. Sidransky E, Black SH, Soenksen DM et al: Transvaginal chorionic villus sampling. Prenat Diagn 10:583, 1990

35. Shulman LP, Simpson JL, Elias S et al: Transvaginal chorionic villus sampling using transabdominal ultrasound guidance: a new technique for first-trimester prenatal diagnosis. Fetal Diagn Ther 8:144, 1993

36. Pergament E, Schulman JD, Copeland K et al: The risk and efficacy of chorionic villus sampling in multiple gestations. Prenat Diagn 12:377, 1992

37. Firth HV, Boyd PA, Chamberlin P et al: Severe limb abnormalities after chorion villus sampling at 55–66 days' gestation. Lancet 337:762, 1991

38. Mahoney MJ and USNICHD collaborators: Limb abnormalities and chorionic villus sampling. Lancet 337:1422, 1991

39. Jackson LG, Wapner RJ, Brambai B: Limb abnormalities and chorionic villus sampling. Lancet 337:1423, 1991

40. Mastroiacovo P, Cavalcanti DP: Limb reduction defects and chorion villus sampling. Lancet 337:1091, 1991

41. Hsieh F-J, Chen D, Tseng L-H et al: Limb-reduction defects and chorionic villus sampling. Lancet 337:1091, 1991

42. Burton BK, Schulz CJ, Burd L: Limb anomalies associated with chorionic villus sampling. Obstet Gynecol 79:726, 1992

43. Mastroiacovo P, Botto LD, Cavalcanti DP et al: Limb anomalies following chorionic villus sampling: a regis-

try based case–control study. Am J Med Genet 44:856, 1992

44. Mastroiacovo P, Botto LD: Chorionic villus sampling and limb deficiencies. Review of case control and cohort studies. p. 71. In Zakut H (ed): 7th International Conference on Early Prenatal Diagnosis of Genetic Disease. Jerusalem, Israel, 22–27 May 1994

45. Dolk H, Beatrand F, Lechat MF (Eurocat): Chorionic villus sampling and limb abnormalities. Lancet 339:876, 1992

46. Hsieh FJ, Shyu MK, Sheu BC et al: Limb defects after chorionic villus sampling. Obstet Gynecol 85:84, 1995

47. Olney RS, Khoury MJ, Alo CJ et al: Increased risk for transverse digital deficiency after chorionic villus sampling (CVS): results of the US multistate case-control study, 1988–1992, abstracted. Teratology 49:376, 1994

48. Froster UG, Jackson L: Safety of chorionic villus sampling: results from an International Registry, abstracted. Am J Hum Genet Suppl 55:1, 1994

49. Froster-Ikenius UG, Baird PA: Limb reduction defects in over one million consecutive live births. Teratology 39:127, 1989

50. Ryan G, Rodeck CH: Fetal blood sampling. p. 63. In Simpson JL, Elias S (eds): Essentials of Prenatal Diagnosis. Churchill Livingstone, New York, 1993

51. Nicolini U, Nicolaidis P, Fisk NM et al: Fetal blood sampling from the intrahepatic vein: analysis of safety and clinical experience with 214 procedures. Obstet Gynecol 76:47, 1990

52. Daffos F: Fetal blood sampling. Annu Rev Med 40:319, 1989

53. Ghidini A, Sepulvada W, Lockwood CJ, Romero R: Complications of fetal blood sampling. Am J Obstet Gynecol 168:1339, 1993

54. Wilson RD, Farquharson DF, Wittmann BK, Shaw D: Cordocentesis: overall pregnancy loss rate as important as procedure loss rate. Fetal Diagn Ther 9:142, 1994

55. Hook EB, Cross PK, Jackson L et al: Maternal age specific rates of 47, +21 and other cytogenetic abnormalities diagnosed in the first trimester of pregnancy of chorionic villus biopsy specimens: comparison with rates expected from observations at amniocentesis. Am J Hum Genet 42:797, 1988

56. Hook EB, Cross PK: Maternal age-specific rates of chromosome abnormalities at chorionic villus study: a revision (letter). Am J Hum Genet 45:474, 1989

57. Goodburn SF, Yates JRW, Raggatt PR et al: Second-trimester maternal serum screening using alpha-fetoprotein, human chorionic gonadotrophin, and unconjugated oestriol: experience of a regional programme. Prenat Diagn 14:391, 1994

58. Simpson JL: Non-invasive screening for prenatal genetic diagnosis. *WHO Bull* (in press)

59. Simpson JL: Prenatal cytogenetic screening (opinion): *Ultrasound Obstet Gynecol* 5:3, 1995

60. Stene J, Stene E, Mikkelsen M: Risk for chromosome abnormality at amniocentesis following a child with a non-inherited chromosome aberration. Prenat Diagn 4:81, 1984

61. Boué A, Gallano P: A collaborative study of the segrega-

tion of inherited chromosome structural rearrangements in 13356 prenatal diagnoses. Prenat Diagn 4:45, 1984

62. Simpson JL, Martin AO, Verp MS et al: Hypermodel cells in amniotic fluid cultures: frequency, interpretation, and clinical significance. Am J Obstet Gynecol 143: 250, 1982

63. Hsu LYF, Perlis TE: United States survey on chromosome mosaicism and pseudomosaicism in prenatal diagnosis. Prenat Diagn 4:97, 1980

64. Ledbetter DH, Zachary JM, Simpson JL et al: Cytogenetic results from the U.S. Collaborative Study on CVS: high diagnostic accuracy in over 11,000 cases. Prenat Diagn 12:317, 1992

65. Association of Clinical Cytogeneticists Working Party on Chorionic Villi in Prenatal Diagnosis: Cytogenetic analysis of chorionic villi for prenatal diagnosis: an acc collaborative study of U.K. data. Prenat Diagn 14:363, 1994

66. Wapner R, Simpson JL, Golbus MS et al: Confined chorionic mosaicism: association with fetal loss but not with adverse perinatal outcome. Prenat Diagn 12:357, 1992

67. Warburton D: Outcome of cases of de novo structural rearrangements diagnosed at amniocentesis. Prenat Diagn 4:69, 1984

68. Speiser PW, Laforgia N, Kato K et al: First trimester prenatal treatment and molecular genetic diagnosis of congenital hyperplasia (21-hydroxylase deficiency). J Clin Endocrinol Metab 70:838, 1990

69. Elias S, Easterly N: Prenatal diagnosis of hereditary skin disorders. Clin Obstet Gynecol 4:24:1069, 1981

70. Bakhavev VA, Aivazyan AA, Karetnikova NA et al: Fetal skin biopsy in prenatal diagnosis of some genodermatoses. Prenat Diagn 10:1, 1990

71. Milunsky A: Maternal serum screening for neural tube and other defects. p. 507. In Genetic Disorders and the Fetus. 3rd Ed. Plenum, New York, 1992

72. Verlinsky Y, Rechitsky S, Evsikov S et al: Preconception and preimplantation diagnosis for cystic fibrosis. Prenat Diagn 12:103, 1992

73. Handyside AH, Komtogianni EH, Hardy K, Winston RML: Pregnancies from biopsied human preimplantation embryos sexed by DNA amplification. Nature 344: 768, 1990

74. Handyside AH, Lesko JG, Tarin JJ et al: Birth of a normal girl after in vitro fertilization and preimplantation diagnostic testing for cystic fibrosis. N Engl J Med 327: 905, 1992

75. Verlinsky Y, Handyside A, Grifo J et al: Preimplantation diagnosis of genetic and chromosomal disorders. J Assist Reprod Genet 11:236, 1994

76. Liu J, Lissens W, Silber SJ et al: Birth after preimplantation diagnosis of the cystic fibrosis Δ508 mutation by polymerase chain reaction in human embryos resulting from intracytoplasmic sperm injection with epididymal sperm. JAMA 272:1858, 1994

77. Simpson JL, Elias S: Fetal cells in maternal blood: overview and historical perspective. p. 1. In Simpson JL, Elias S (eds): Fetal Cells in Maternal Blood: Prospects for Noninvasive Prenatal Diagnosis, New York: New York Academy of Science, 1994

78. Simpson JL, Elias S: Isolating fetal cells in the maternal circulation. *Hum Reprod Update* 1:409, 1995

79. Walknowska J, Conte FA, Grumbach MM: Practical and theoretical implications of fetal/maternal lymphocyte transfer. Lancet 1:119, 1969

80. Herzenberg LA, Bianchi DW, Schroder J et al: Fetal cells in the blood of pregnant women: detection and enrichment by fluorescence-activated cell sorting. Proc Natl Acad Sci USA 76:1453, 1979

81. Lo YMD, Wainscot JS, Gilmer MDG et al: Prenatal sex determination by DNA amplification from maternal peripheral blood. Lancet 2:1363, 1989

82. Thomas MR, Williamson R, Craft I et al: Y chromosome sequence DNA amplified from peripheral blood of women in early pregnancy, Lancet 343:413, 1994

83. Liou J-D, Pao CC, Hor JJ, Kao S-M: Fetal cells in the maternal circulation during first trimester in pregnancies. Hum Genet 92:309, 1993

84. Mueller UW, Hawes CD, Wright AE et al: Isolation of fetal trophoblast cells from peripheral blood of pregnant women. Lancet 336:197, 1990

85. Hawes CS, Suskin HA, Kalionis B et al: Detection of paternally inherited mutations for β-thalassemia in trophoblast isolated from peripheral maternal blood. p. 181. In Simpson JL, Elias S (eds): Fetal Cells in Maternal Blood: Prospects for Noninvasive Prenatal Diagnosis. New York: New York Academy of Sciences, 1994

86. Yeoh SC, Sargent IL, Redman CWG et al: Detection of fetal cells in maternal blood. Prenat Diagn 11:117, 1991

87. Sargent IL, Choo YS, Redman CWG: Isolating and analyzing fetal leukocytes in maternal blood. p. 147. In Simpson JL, Elias S (eds): Fetal Cells in Maternal Blood: Prospects for Noninvasive Diagnosis. New York: New York Academy of Science, 1994

88. Bianchi DW, Flint AF, Pizzimenti MF et al: Isolation of fetal DNA from nucleated erythrocytes in maternal blood. Proc Natl Acad Sci USA 87:3279, 1990

89. Wachtel SS, Elias S, Price J et al: Fetal cells in the maternal circulation: isolation by multiparameter flow cytometry and confirmation by PCR. Hum Reprod 6:1466, 1991

90. Price J, Elias S, Wachtel SS et al: Prenatal diagnosis using fetal cells isolated from maternal blood by multiparameter flow cytometry. Am J Obstet Gynecol 165: 1731, 1992

91. Elias S, Price J, Dockter M et al: First trimester prenatal diagnosis of trisomy 21 in fetal cells from maternal blood. Lancet 340:1033, 1992

92. Bianchi DW, Mahr A, Zickwolf GL et al: Detection of fetal cells with 47,XY, +21 karyotype in maternal peripheral blood. Hum Genet 90:368, 1992

93. Simpson JL, Elias S: Isolating fetal cells from maternal blood: advances in prenatal diagnosis through molecular technology, JAMA 270:2357, 1993

94. Gänshirt-Ahlert D, Börjesson-Stoll R, Burschyk M et al: Detection of fetal trisomies 21 and 18 from maternal blood using triple gradient and magnetic cell sorting. Am J Reprod Immun 30:194, 1994

95. Camaschella C, Alfarno A, Gottardi E et al: Prenatal diagnosis of fetal haemoglobin Lepore Boston disease on maternal peripheral blood. Blood 75:2102, 1990

96. Lo YMD, Bowell PJ, Selinger M et al: Prenatal determination of fetal RhD status by analysis of peripheral blood of rhesus negative mothers. Lancet 341:1147, 1993

97. Simpson JL, Elias S: Isolating fetal cells in maternal circulation for prenatal diagnosis. *Prenat Diagn* 14: 1229, 1994

98. Gerbie AT, Simpson JL: Antenatal diagnosis of genetic disorders. Postgrad Med 59:129, 1976

99. Hook EB: Rates of chromosomal abnormalities of different maternal ages. Obstet Gynecol 58:282, 1981

100. Hook EB, Cross PK, Schreinemachers DM et al: Chromosomal abnormality rates at amniocentesis and liveborn infants. JAMA 249:2043, 1983

101. The Cystic Fibrosis Genetic Analysis Consortium: Population variation of common cystic fibrosis mutations. Hum Mutat 4:167, 1994

102. American College of Obstetricians and Gynecologists: Antenatal Diagnosis of Genetic Disorders. Technical Bulletin No. 108. ACOG, Washington, DC, 1987

Chapter 10

Drugs in Pregnancy and Lactation

Jennifer R. Niebyl

Caution with regard to drug ingestion during pregnancy is usually advised. Until recently, the fetus was thought to rest in a privileged site with little exposure to the environment experienced by the mother. The term *placental barrier* has been in widespread use but is truly a contradiction, as the placenta allows the transfer of many drugs and dietary substances.

Lipid-soluble compounds readily cross the placenta, and water-soluble substances pass less well the greater their molecular weight. The degree to which a drug is bound to plasma protein also influences the amount of drug that is free to cross the placenta. Virtually all drugs cross the placenta to some degree, with the exception of large organic ions such as heparin and insulin.

Developmental defects in humans may be from genetic, environmental, or unknown causes. Approximately 25 percent are known to be genetic in origin; drug exposure accounts for only 2 to 3 percent of birth defects. Approximately 65 percent of defects are of unknown etiology but may be from combinations of genetic and environmental factors (see Ch. 9).

The incidence of major malformations in the general population is usually quoted as 2 to 3 percent.[1] A major malformation is defined as one that is incompatible with survival, such as anencephaly, or one requiring major surgery for correction, such as cleft palate or congenital heart disease, or one producing major dysfunction (e.g., mental retardation). If minor malformations are also included, such as ear tags or extra digits, the rate may be as high as 7 to 10 percent. The risk of malformation after exposure to a drug must be compared with this background rate.

There is a marked species specificity in drug teratogenesis.[2] For example, thalidomide was not found to be teratogenic in rats and mice but is a potent human teratogen. On the contrary, in certain strains of mice, corticosteroids produce a high percentage of offspring with cleft lip, although no studies have shown these drugs to be teratogenic in humans. The Food and Drug Administration (FDA) lists five categories of labeling for drug use in pregnancy:

A. Controlled studies in women fail to demonstrate a risk to the fetus in the first trimester, and the possibility of fetal harm appears remote.
B. Animal studies do not indicate a risk to the fetus; there are no controlled human studies, or animal studies do show an adverse effect on the fetus, but well-controlled studies in pregnant women have failed to demonstrate a risk to the fetus.
C. Studies have shown the drug to have animal teratogenic or embryocidal effects, but no controlled studies are available in women, or no studies are available in either animals or women.
D. Positive evidence of human fetal risk exists, but benefits in certain situations (e.g., life-threatening situations or serious diseases for which safer drugs cannot be used or are ineffective) may make use of the drug acceptable despite its risks.
X. Studies in animals or humans have demonstrated fetal abnormalities, or evidence demonstrates fetal risk based on human experience, or both, and the risk clearly outweighs any possible benefit.

The classic teratogenic period is from day 31 after the last menstrual period in a 28-day cycle to 71 days from the last period (Fig. 10-1). During this critical period, organs are forming, and teratogens may cause malformations that are usually overt at birth. The timing of exposure is important. Administration of drugs early in the period of organogenesis will affect the or-

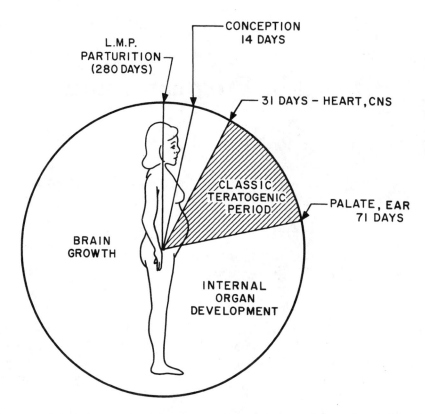

Fig. 10-1 Gestational clock showing the classic teratogenic period. (From Blake and Niebyl,[2] with permission.)

gans developing at that time, such as the heart or neural tube. Closer to the end of the classic teratogenic period, the ear and palate are forming and may be affected by a teratogen.

Before day 31, exposure to a teratogen produces an all-or-none effect. With exposure around conception, the conceptus usually either does not survive or survives without anomalies. Because so few cells exist in the early stages, irreparable damage to some may be lethal to the entire organism. If the organism remains viable, however, organ-specific anomalies are not manifested, because either repair or replacement will occur to permit normal development. A similar insult at a later stage may produce organ-specific defects.

Patients should be educated about avenues other than the use of drugs to cope with tension, aches and pains, and viral illnesses during pregnancy. Drugs should be used only when necessary. The risk-benefit ratio should justify the use of a particular drug, and the minimum effective dose should be employed. As long-term effects of drug exposure in utero may not be revealed for many years, caution with regard to the use of any drug in pregnancy is warranted.

Embryology

During the first 3 days after ovulation, development takes place in the fallopian tube. At the time of fertilization, a pronuclear stage exists during which the nuclei from the egg and the sperm retain their integrity within the egg cytoplasm. After the pronuclei fuse, the fertilized egg begins a series of mitotic cell divisions (cleavage). The two-cell stage is reached about 30 hours after fertilization. With continued division, the cells develop into a solid ball of cells (morula), which reaches the endometrial cavity about 3 days after fertilization. Thereafter, a fluid-filled cavity forms within the cell mass, at which time the conceptus is called a *blastocyst*. The number of cells increases from approximately 12 to 32 by the end of the third day to 250 by the sixth day.

Until approximately 3 days after conception, any cell is thought to be totipotential, that is, capable of initiating development of any organ system. For example, separation of cells during this period can give rise to monozygotic twins, each normal. At the blastocyst stage, cells first begin to differentiate. The blastocyst is located in the uterus, where implantation occurs 6 to 9 days after conception.

One group of cells forms the inner cell mass that will ultimately develop into the fetus. Different tissues will arise from each of the three cell layers. The brain, nerves, and skin will develop from the ectoderm; the lining of the digestive tract, respiratory tract, and part of the bladder, as well as the liver and pancreas from the endoderm, and connective tissue, cartilage, muscle, blood vessels, the heart, kidneys, and gonads develop from the mesoderm. The group of cells forming the periphery of the blastocyst is termed the *trophoblast*. The placenta and the fetal membranes will develop from this outer cell layer.

The trophoblast continues to grow, and lacunae form within the previously solid syncytiotrophoblast. The lacunae are the precursors of the intervillous spaces of the placenta, and by 2 weeks after conception maternal blood is found within them. Meanwhile, the cytotrophoblast is forming cell masses that will become chorionic villi.

From the third to the eighth week after conception, the embryonic disc undergoes major developments that lay the foundation for all organ systems. By 4 weeks after conception, the fertilized ovum has progressed from one cell to millions of cells. The rudiments of all major systems have differentiated, and the blueprints are set for developmental refinements. The embryo has been transformed into a curved tube approximately 6 mm long and isolated from the extraembryonic membranes.

At 5 weeks after conception, the embryo first begins to assume features of human appearance. The face is recognizable, with the formation of discernible eyes, nose, and ears. Limbs emerge from protruding buds; digits, cartilage, and muscles develop. The cerebral hemispheres begin to fill the brain area, and the optic stalk becomes apparent. Nerve connections are established between the retina and the brain. The digestive tract rotates from its prior tubular structure, and the liver starts to produce blood cells and bile. Two tubes emerge from the pharynx to become bronchi, and the lungs have lobes and bronchioles. The heart is beating at 5 weeks and is almost completely developed by 8 weeks after conception. The diaphragm begins to divide the heart and lungs from the abdominal cavity. The kidneys approach their final form at this time. The urogenital and rectal passages separate, and germ cells migrate toward the genital ridges for future transformation into ovaries or testes. Differentiation of internal ducts begins, with persistence of either müllerian or wolffian ducts. Virilization of external genitalia occurs in males. The embryo increases from approximately 6 to 33 mm in length and increases 50 times in weight.

Structurally, the fetus has become straighter, and the tubular neural canal along which the spinal cord develops becomes filled with nerve cells. Ears remain low on the sides of the head. Teeth are forming, and the two bony plates of the palate fuse in the midline. Disruptions during the latter part of the embryonic period lead to various forms of cleft lip and palate. By 10 weeks after the last menstrual period, all major organ systems have become established and integrated.

Development of other organs continues in the second and third trimesters of pregnancy. Therefore, we need to be concerned about drug use at this time in pregnancy, although the effects may not be recognized until later in life. Some of the uterine anomalies resulting from diethylstilbestrol (DES) occurred with exposure as late as 20 weeks but were not recognized until after puberty. The brain continues to develop throughout pregnancy and the neonatal period. Fetal alcohol syndrome may occur with chronic exposure to alcohol in the later stages of pregnancy.

Effects of Specific Drugs

Estrogens and Progestins

Oral contraceptives and other hormones given in the first trimester have been blamed in the past for a variety of birth defects, but recent studies have not confirmed any teratogenic risk for these drugs.

Data from the Collaborative Perinatal Project, a prospective study of 50,282 pregnancies between 1958 and 1965, initially supported the possibility of a risk of cardiac defects after first-trimester exposure to female hormones and oral contraceptives.[3] However, a reevaluation of these data has questioned this result.[4] Careful review of the records indicated that some patients had taken the medication too early or too late to affect the cardiovascular system. When infants with Down syndrome were excluded, no significant difference in the risk of cardiovascular anomalies remained. Another study of 2,754 infants born to mothers after bleeding in the first trimester suggested no increased risk associated with first trimester exposure to progestagens.[5] A meta-analysis of first trimester sex hormone exposure revealed no association between exposure and fetal genital malformations.[6] However, because of the medicolegal climate and the conflicting literature, it is wise to do a sensitive pregnancy test before refilling a prescription for pills or giving progestins to an amenorrheic patient.

Androgenic Steroids

Androgens may masculinize a developing female fetus. Progestational agents, most often the synthetic testosterone derivatives, may cause clitoromegaly and labial fusion if given before 13 weeks of pregnancy.[7] Danazol (Danocrine) has been reported to produce mild clitoral enlargement and labial fusion when given inadvertently for the first 10 to 12 weeks after conception (Fig. 10-2).[8] The abnormality was correctable by surgery.

Spermicides

Jick et al.[9] initially reported an increased risk of abnormal offspring in mothers who had used spermicides for contraception. In this study, however, women were

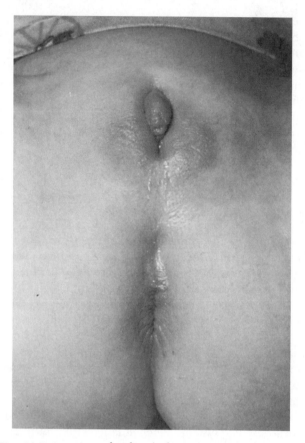

Fig. 10-2 Perineum of a female fetus exposed to danazol in utero. (From Duck and Katayama,[8] with permission.)

considered to be users if a prescription for spermicide had been filled within 600 days of delivery. There was no documentation that the women had ever used the spermicide, certainly not at the critical period for teratogenesis. Also, the medication is available over the counter and could have been used by controls.

Several studies later refuted this association. In the Collaborative Perinatal Project data,[10] 462 women reported spermicide use in the first 4 lunar months, with 438 also describing use during the month preceding the last menstrual period. The exposed women had 23 infants with anomalies (5 percent) compared with 4.5 percent in the nonexposed controls, not a significant difference.

In the study of Mills et al.,[11] the malformation rate in women using spermicides after their last menstrual period was 4.8/1,000 compared with 6.4/1,000 in the controls, not significantly different. The risk of preterm delivery, a low-birth-weight infant, and spontaneous abortion was no higher in the spermicide-exposed group. The study of Linn et al.[12] of 12,440 women found no relationship between contraceptive method and the occurrence of malformations. Clearly, the consensus of the scientific community is that vaginal spermicides are not associated with increased malforma-

tions when women use them either just before or during pregnancy.[13]

Anticonvulsants

Epileptic women taking anticonvulsants during pregnancy have approximately double the general population risk of malformations.[14] Compared with the general risk of 2 to 3 percent, the risk of major malformations in epileptic women on anticonvulsants is about 5 percent, especially cleft lip with or without cleft palate and congenital heart disease. Valproic acid (Depakene) carries approximately a 1 percent risk of neural tube defects and possibly other anomalies.[15] Valproic acid appears to cause spina bifida much more often than anencephaly, with a ratio of 5:1.[16]

Whenever a drug is claimed to be a teratogen, one always can raise the issue of whether the drug actually is a teratogen or the disease for which the drug was prescribed in some way contributed to the defect. Even when they take no anticonvulsant drug, women with a convulsive disorder have an increased risk of delivering infants with malformations; this information supports a role for the epilepsy itself rather than the anticonvulsant drug as a contributor to the birth defect.[14] Of infants born to 305 epileptic women on medication in the Collaborative Perinatal Project, 10.5 percent had a birth defect. Of the offspring of women who had a convulsive disorder and who had taken no phenytoin at all, 11.3 percent had a malformation. In contrast, the total malformation rate was 6.4 percent for the control group of women who did not have a convulsive disorder and who therefore did not take any antiepileptic drugs. The issue remains unresolved, as patients who take more drugs during pregnancy usually have more severe convulsive disorders than do those who do not take any anticonvulsants. A combination of more than three drugs or a high daily dose increases the chance of malformations.[17]

Possible causes of anomalies in epileptic women on anticonvulsants include the disease itself, a genetic predisposition to both epilepsy and malformations, genetic differences in drug metabolism, the specific drugs themselves, and deficiency states induced by drugs such as decreased serum folate. Phenytoin (Dilantin) decreases folate absorption and lowers the serum folate, which has been implicated in birth defects.[18] Therefore, folic acid supplementation should be given to these mothers, but may require adjustment of the anticonvulsant dose. Although epileptic women were not included in the Medical Research Council study, most authorities would recommend 4 mg/day folic acid for high-risk women.[19] (see Ch. 7).

Fewer than 10 percent of offspring show the fetal hydantoin syndrome,[20] which consists of microcephaly,

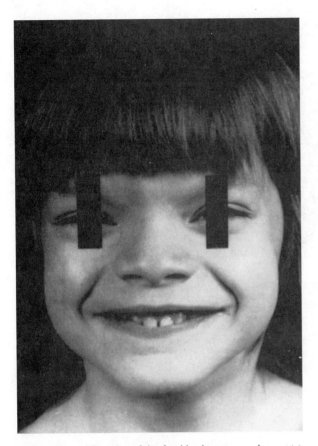

Fig. 10-3 Facial features of the fetal hydantoin syndrome. Note broad, flat nasal ridge, epicanthic folds, mild hypertelorism, and wide mouth with prominent upper Lip. (Courtesy of Dr. Thaddeus Kelly, Charlottesville, VA.)

growth deficiency, developmental delays, mental retardation, and dysmorphic craniofacial features (Fig. 10-3). In fact, the risk may be as low as 1 to 2 percent.[21] While several of these features are also found in other syndromes, such as fetal alcohol syndrome, more common in the fetal hydantoin syndrome are hypoplasia of the nails and distal phalanges (Fig. 10-4), and hyper-

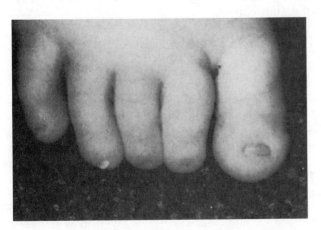

Fig. 10-4 Hypoplasia of toenails and distal phalanges. (From Hanson,[223] with permission.)

telorism. Trimethadione (Tridione) and carbamazepine (Tegretol) are also associated with an increased risk of a dysmorphic syndrome.[22] However, children exposed in utero to phenytoin scored 10 points lower on IQ tests than children exposed to carbamazepine or nonexposed controls.[23]

A genetic metabolic defect in arene oxide detoxification in the infant may increase the risk of a major birth defect.[24] Prenatal diagnosis of epoxide hydrolase deficiency may become available to indicate susceptibility to fetal hydantoin syndrome.[25]

In a follow-up study of long-term effects of antenatal exposure to phenobarbital and carbamazepine, anomalies were not related to specific maternal medication exposure. There were no neurologic or behavioral differences between the two groups.[26]

Some women may have taken anticonvulsant drugs for a long period without reevaluation of the need for continuation of the drugs. For patients with idiopathic epilepsy who have been seizure free for 2 years and who have a normal electroencephalogram (EEG), it may be safe to attempt a trial of withdrawal of the drug before pregnancy.[27]

Most authorities agree that the benefits of anticonvulsant therapy during pregnancy outweigh the risks of discontinuation of the drug if the patient is first seen during pregnancy. The blood level of drug should be monitored, monthly if possible, to ensure a therapeutic level but minimize the dosage. If the patient has not been taking her drug regularly, a low blood level may demonstrate her lack of compliance. Because the albumin concentration falls in pregnancy, the total amount of phenytoin measured is decreased as it is highly protein bound. However, the level of free phenytoin, which is the pharmacologically active portion, is unchanged. Neonatologists need to be notified when a patient is on anticonvulsants because this therapy can affect vitamin K-dependent clotting factors in the newborn. Vitamin K supplementation at 10 mg daily for these mothers has been recommended for the last month of pregnancy.[28,29]

Isotretinoin

Isotretinoin (Accutane) is a significant human teratogen. This drug is marketed for treatment of cystic acne and unfortunately has been taken inadvertently by women who were not planning pregnancy.[30] It is labeled as contraindicated in pregnancy (FDA category X) with appropriate warnings that a negative pregnancy test is required before therapy. Of 154 exposed human pregnancies to date, there have been 21 reported cases of birth defects, 12 spontaneous abortions, 95 elective abortions, and 26 normal infants in women who took isotretinoin during early pregnancy.[31] The

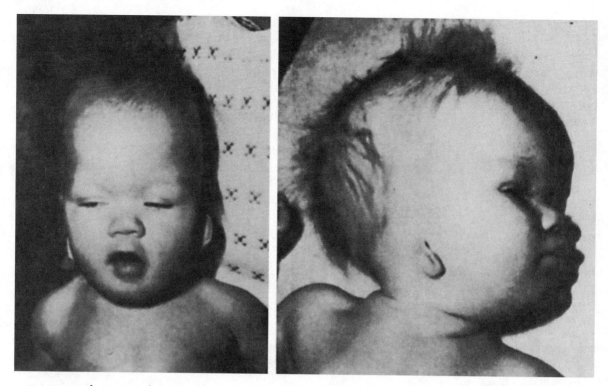

Fig. 10-5 Infant exposed to Accutane in utero. Note high forehead, hypoplastic nasal bridge, and abnormal ears. (From Lot et al.,[224] with permission.)

risk of structural anomalies in patients studied prospectively is now estimated to be about 25 percent. An additional 25 percent have mental retardation alone.[32] The malformed infants have a characteristic pattern of craniofacial, cardiac, thymic, and central nervous system anomalies. They include microtia/anotia (small/absent ears) (Fig. 10-5), micrognathia, cleft palate, heart defects, thymic defects, retinal or optic nerve anomalies, and central nervous system malformations including hydrocephalus.[31] Microtia is rare as an isolated anomaly yet appears commonly as part of the retinoic acid embryopathy. Cardiovascular defects include great vessel transposition and ventricular septal defects.

Unlike vitamin A, isotretinoin is not stored in tissue. Therefore, a pregnancy after discontinuation of isotretinoin is not a risk as the drug is no longer detectable in serum 5 days after its ingestion. In 88 pregnancies prospectively ascertained after discontinuation of isotretinoin, no increased risk of anomalies was noted, in contrast to etretinate (see below).[33]

Topical tretinoin (Retin-A) has not been associated with any teratogenic risk.[34]

Etretinate (Tegison)

This drug is marketed for use in psoriasis and may well have a teratogenic risk similar to that of isotretinoin. Case reports of malformation, especially central nervous system,[35] have appeared, but the absolute risk is

unknown. The half-life of several months makes levels cumulative, and the drug carries a warning to avoid pregnancy within 6 months of use.

Vitamin A

There is no evidence that vitamin A itself in normal doses is teratogenic. The levels in prenatal vitamins (5,000 IU/day orally) have not been associated with any documented risk. Eighteen cases of birth defects have been reported after exposure to levels of 25,000 IU of vitamin A or greater during pregnancy. Vitamin A in doses greater than 10,000 IU per day increases the risk of malformations.[35]

Psychoactive Drugs

There is no clear risk documented for most psychoactive drugs with respect to overt birth defects. However, effects of chronic use of these agents on the developing brain in humans is difficult to study, and so a conservative attitude is appropriate. Lack of overt defects does not exclude the possibility of behavioral teratology.

Tranquilizers

Conflicting reports of the possible teratogenicity of the various tranquilizers, including meprobamate (Miltown) and chlordiazepoxide (Librium), have appeared, but in prospective studies no risk of anomalies has been confirmed.[36,37] In most clinical situations, the risk-benefit ratio does not justify the use of benzodiazepines in pregnancy.

A fetal benzodiazepine syndrome has been reported in 7 infants of 36 mothers who regularly took benzodiazepines during pregnancy.[38] However, the high rate of abnormality occurred with concomitant alcohol and substance abuse and may not be due to the benzodiazepine exposure.[39] Perinatal use of diazepam (Valium) has been associated with hypotonia, hypothermia, and respiratory depression.

Lithium (Eskalith, Lithobid)

In the International Register of Lithium Babies,[40] 217 infants are listed as exposed at least during the first trimester of pregnancy, and 25 (11.5 percent) were malformed. Eighteen had cardiovascular anomalies, including six cases of the rare Ebstein anomaly, which occurs only once in 20,000 in the nonexposed population. Of 60 unaffected infants who were followed to age 5 years, no increased mental or physical abnormalities were noted compared with unexposed siblings.[41]

However, two other reports suggest that there was a bias of ascertainment in the registry and that the risk of anomalies is much lower than previously thought. A case–control study of 59 patients with Ebstein anomaly showed no difference in the rate of lithium exposure in pregnancy from a control group of 168 children with neuroblastoma.[42] A prospective study of 148 women exposed to lithium in the first trimester showed no difference in the incidence of major anomalies compared with controls.[43] One fetus in the lithium-exposed group had Ebstein anomaly, and one infant in the control group had a ventricular septal defect. The authors concluded that lithium is not a major human teratogen. Nevertheless, we do recommend that women exposed to lithium be offered ultrasound and fetal echocardiography.

Lithium is excreted more rapidly during pregnancy; thus, serum lithium levels should be monitored. Perinatal effects of lithium have been noted, including hypotonia, lethargy, and poor feeding in the infant. Also, complications similar to those seen in adults on lithium have been noted in newborns, including goiter and hypothyroidism.

Two cases of polyhydramnios associated with maternal lithium treatment have been reported.[44,45] Because nephrogenic diabetes insipidus has been reported in adults taking lithium, the presumed mechanism of this polyhydramnios is fetal diabetes insipidus. Polyhydramnios may be a sign of fetal lithium toxicity.

It is usually recommended that drug therapy be changed in pregnant women on lithium to avoid fetal drug exposure. Tapering over 10 days will delay the risk of relapse.[46] However, discontinuing lithium is associated with a 70 percent chance of relapse of the affective disorder in 1 year as opposed to 20 in percent those who remain on lithium. Discontinuation of lithium may pose an unacceptable risk of increased morbidity in women who have had multiple episodes of affective instability. These women should be offered appropriate prenatal diagnosis with ultrasound, including fetal echocardiography.

Antidepressants

Imipramine (Tofranil) was the original tricyclic antidepressant claimed to be associated with cardiovascular defects, but the number of patients studied remains small. Of 75 newborns exposed in the first trimester, 6 major defects were observed, 3 being cardiovascular.[47]

Amitriptyline (Elavil) has been more widely used. Although occasional reports have associated the use of this drug with birth defects, the majority of the evidence supports its safety. In the Michigan Medicaid study, 467 newborns had been exposed during the first trimester, with no increased risk of birth defects.[48]

Fluoxetine (Prozac) is being used with increasing frequency as an antidepressant. In two studies,[49,50] no increased risk of major malformations was found in 237 infants exposed in utero.

Anticoagulants

Warfarin (Coumadin) has been associated with chondrodysplasia punctata, which is similar to the genetic Conradi-Hunerman syndrome. This syndrome, occurring in about 5 percent of exposed pregnancies, includes nasal hypoplasia, bone stippling seen on radiologic examination, ophthalmologic abnormalities including bilateral optic atrophy, and mental retardation (Fig. 10-6). The ophthalmologic abnormalities and mental retardation may occur,[51] even with use only beyond the first trimester. Fetal and maternal hemorrhage have also been reported in pregnant women on warfarin, although the incidence can be lowered with careful control of the prothrombin time.

The alternative drug, heparin, does not cross the placenta, as it is a large molecule with a strong negative charge. Because heparin does not have an adverse effect on the fetus when given in pregnancy, it should be the drug of choice for patients requiring anticoagulation. Patients should be carefully taught subcutaneous administration of heparin. In one study, heparin treatment was associated with more thromboembolic complications and more bleeding complications than warfarin therapy.[52] Therapy with 20,000 units/day for greater than 20 weeks has also been associated with bone demineralization.[53] Thirty-six percent of patients had more than a 10 percent decrease from baseline

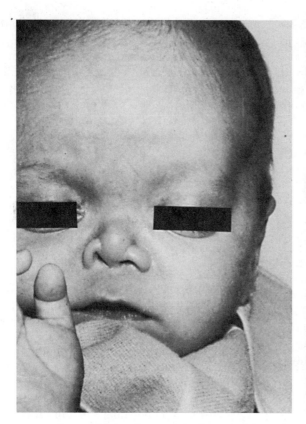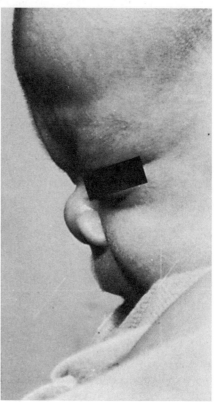

Fig. 10-6 Warfarin embryopathy. Note small nose with hypoplastic bridge. (From Shaul and Hall,[225] with permission.)

bone density to postpartum values.[54] The risk of spine fractures was 0.7 percent with low-dose heparin and 3 percent with a high-dose regimen.[55] Heparin can also cause thrombocytopenia.

The risks of heparin during pregnancy may not be justified in patients with only a single episode of thrombosis in the past.[56,57] Certainly conservative measures should be recommended, such as elastic stockings and avoidance of prolonged sitting or standing.

In patients with cardiac valve prostheses, full anticoagulation is necessary, as low-dose heparin resulted in three valve thromboses (two fatal) in 35 mothers so treated.[58]

Thyroid and Antithyroid Drugs

Propylthiouracil (PTU) and methimazole (Tapazole) both cross the placenta and may cause some degree of fetal goiter. In contrast, the thyroid hormones triiodothyronine (T3) and thyroxine (T4) cross the placenta poorly, so that fetal hypothyroidism produced by antithyroid drugs cannot be corrected satisfactorily by administration of thyroid hormone to the mother. Thus, the goal of such therapy during pregnancy is to keep the mother slightly hyperthyroid to minimize fetal drug exposure. As methimazole has been associated with scalp defects in infants,[59] as well as a higher incidence of maternal side effects, PTU is the drug of choice.

Radioactive iodine administered for thyroid ablation or for diagnostic studies is not concentrated by the fetal thyroid until after 12 weeks of pregnancy.[60] Thus, with inadvertent exposure, usually around the time of missed menses, there is no specific risk to the fetal thyroid from ^{131}I or ^{125}I administration.

The need for thyroxine increases in many women with primary hypothyroidism when they are pregnant, as reflected by an increase in serum thyrotropin (TSH) concentrations.[61] In one study, the mean thyroxine dose before pregnancy was 0.10 mg/day; it was increased to a mean dose of 0.25 mg/day during pregnancy. Although there are no known clinical effects of this modest level of hypothyroidism, it is prudent to monitor thyroid function throughout pregnancy and to adjust the thyroid dose to maintain a normal TSH level. Another study reported that although increased doses of T4 were required in pregnancy, the dose of desiccated thyroid did not need to be changed in two patients.[62] The need for change may reflect the degree of TSH suppression achieved in each patient before pregnancy.

Topical iodine preparations are readily absorbed

through the vagina during pregnancy, and transient hypothyroidism has been demonstrated in the newborn after exposure during labor.[63]

Digoxin (Lanoxin)

In 52 exposures, no teratogenicity of digoxin was noted.[64] Blood levels should be monitored in pregnancy to ensure adequate therapeutic maternal levels.

Digoxin-like immunoreactive substances may be mistaken in assays for fetal concentrations of digoxin. In one study of fetuses with cardiac anomalies,[65] there was no difference in the immunoreactive digoxin levels whether or not the mother had received digoxin. In hydropic fetuses, digoxin may not easily cross the placenta.[66]

Antihypertensive Drugs

α-Methyldopa (Aldomet) has been widely used for the treatment of chronic hypertension in pregnancy. Although postural hypotension may occur, no unusual fetal effects have been noted. Hydralazine (Apresoline) has also had widespread use in pregnancy, and no teratogenic effect has been observed (see also Ch. 28).

Sympathetic Blocking Agents

Propranolol (Inderal) is a β-adrenergic blocking agent in widespread use for a variety of indications. Theoretically, propranolol might increase uterine contractility. However, this has not been reported, presumably because the drug is not specific for β_2-receptors in the uterine wall. No evidence of teratogenicity has been found. Bradycardia has been reported in the newborn as a direct effect of a dose of the drug given to the mother within 2 hours of delivery of the infant.[67]

Several studies of propranolol use in pregnancy show an increased risk of intrauterine growth restriction or at least a skewing of the birth weight distribution toward the lower range.[68] Ultrasound monitoring of patients on this drug is prudent. Studies from Scotland suggest improved outcome with the use of atenolol (Tenormin) to treat chronic hypertension during pregnancy.[69]

Angiotensin-Converting Enzyme Inhibitors

Angiotensin-converting enzyme inhibitors (e.g., enalapril [Vasotec], captopril [Capoten]) can cause fetal renal failure in the second and third trimesters, leading to oligohydramnios, fetal limb contractures, craniofacial deformities, and hypoplastic lung development.[70] Fetal skull ossification defects have also been described.[71] For these reasons, pregnant women on these medications should be switched to other agents. Use during the first trimester has not been reported to be teratogenic.

Antineoplastic Drugs and Immunosuppressants

Methotrexate, a folic acid antagonist, appears to be a human teratogen, although experience with it is limited.[72] Infants of three women known to receive methotrexate in the first trimester of pregnancy had multiple congenital anomalies, including cranial defects and malformed extremities. Eight normal infants were delivered to seven women treated with methotrexate in combination with other agents after the first trimester. When low-dose oral methotrexate (7.5 mg/week) was used for rheumatoid disease in the first trimester, five full-term infants were normal, and three patients experienced spontaneous abortions.[73]

Azothioprine (Imuran) has been used by patients with renal transplants or systemic lupus erythematosus. The frequency of anomalies in 80 women treated in the first trimester was not increased.[72,74] Two infants had leukopenia, one was small for gestational age, and the others were normal.

Of 67 infants exposed to cyclosporine (Sandimmune) in utero, there was no increased risk of anomalies.[75,76] An increased rate of prematurity and growth restriction has also been noted, but it is difficult to separate the contributions of the underlying disease and the drugs given to these transplant patients.

Eight malformed infants have resulted from first-trimester exposure to cyclophosphamide (Cytoxan), but these infants were also exposed to other drugs or radiation.[77] Low birth weight may be associated with use after the first trimester, but this may also reflect the underlying medical problem.

Chloroquine (Aralen) is safe in doses used for malarial prophylaxis, and there was no increased incidence of birth defects among 169 infants exposed to 300 mg once weekly.[78] However, after exposure to larger anti-inflammatory doses (250 to 500 mg/day), two cases of cochleovestibular paresis were reported.[79] No abnormalities were noted in an additional 14 infants.[80]

When cancer chemotherapy is used during embryogenesis there is an increased rate of spontaneous abortion and major birth defects. Later in pregnancy there is a greater risk of stillbirth and intrauterine growth restriction, and myelosuppression is often present in the infant.[81]

Antiasthmatics

Theophylline (Theo-Dur, Slo-Bid) and Aminophylline

Both theophylline and aminophylline are safe for the treatment of asthma in pregnancy. No evidence of teratogenic risk was found in 76 exposures in the Collaborative Perinatal Project.[64] Because of increased renal clearance in pregnancy, dosages may need to be increased.

Epinephrine (Adrenalin)

Minor malformations have been reported with sympathomimetic amines as a group in 3,082 exposures in the first trimester, usually in commercial preparations used to treat upper respiratory infections.[64]

Terbutaline (Brethine)

Terbutaline has been widely used in the treatment of preterm labor (see Ch. 23). It is more rapid in onset and has a longer duration of action than epinephrine and is preferred for asthma in the pregnant patient. No risk of birth defects has been reported. Long-term use has been associated with an increased risk of glucose intolerance.[82]

Cromolyn Sodium (Intal)

Cromolyn sodium may be administered in pregnancy, and the systemic absorption is minimal. Teratogenicity has not been reported in humans.

Isoproterenol (Isuprel) and Metaproterenol (Alupent)

When isoproterenol and metaproterenol are given as topical aerosols for the treatment of asthma, the total dose absorbed is usually not significant. With oral or intravenous doses, however, the cardiovascular effects of the agents may result in decreased uterine blood flow. For this reason, they should be used with caution. No teratogenicity has been reported.[64]

Corticosteroids

All steroids cross the placenta to some degree, but prednisone (Deltasone) and prednisolone are inactivated by the placenta. When prednisone or prednisolone are maternally administered, the concentration of active compound in the fetus is less than 10 percent of that in the mother. Therefore, these agents are the drugs of choice for treating medical diseases such as asthma. Inhaled corticosteroids are also effective therapy, and very little drug is absorbed. When steroid effects are desired in the fetus, for example, to accelerate lung maturity, bethamethasone (Celestone) and dexamethasone (Decadron) are preferred, as these are minimally inactivated by the placenta. In several hundred infants exposed to corticosteroids in the first trimester, no increase in abnormalities was noted.[64,74,75]

Iodide

Iodide such as is found in a saturated solution of potassium iodide expectorant (SSKI) crosses the placenta and may produce a large fetal goiter, enough to produce respiratory obstruction in the newborn (Fig. 10-7).[60] Before a patient is advised to take a cough medicine, one should be sure to ascertain that it does not contain iodide.

Antiemetics

Remedies suggested to help nausea and vomiting in pregnancy without pharmacologic intervention include taking crackers at the bedside upon first awakening in the morning before getting out of bed, getting up very slowly, omitting the use of iron tablets, consuming frequent small meals, and eating protein snacks at night. Faced with a self-limited condition occurring at the time of organogenesis, the clinician is well advised to avoid the use of medications whenever possible and to encourage these supportive measures initially.

Vitamin B$_6$

Vitamin B$_6$ (pyridoxine) 25 mg tid has been reported in two randomized placebo controlled trials to be effective for treating the nausea and vomiting of pregnancy.[83,84] In several other controlled trials there was no evidence of teratogenicity.

Doxylamine

Doxylamine (Unisom) is an effective antihistamine for nausea in pregnancy and can be combined with vitamin B$_6$ to produce a therapy similar to the former preparation Bendectin. Vitamin B$_6$ (25 mg) and Unisom (25 mg) at bedtime, and one-half of each in the morning and afternoon, is an effective combination.

Ginger

Ginger has been used with success for treating hyperemesis,[85] when defined as vomiting during pregnancy that was severe enough to require hospital admission. A significantly greater relief of symptoms was found after ginger treatment than with placebo. Patients took 250 mg capsules containing ginger as powdered root four times a day, which is similar to the amount often used in recipes for cakes or cookies.

Although there are no teratogenic effects known for other antiemetics, much less information is available.

Meclizine (Bonine)

In one randomized placebo-controlled study, meclizine gave significantly better results than placebo.[86] Prospective clinical studies have provided no evidence that meclizine is teratogenic in humans. In 1,014 patients in the Collaborative Perinatal Project[64] and an additional 613 patients from the Kaiser Health Plan,[87] no teratogenic risk was found.

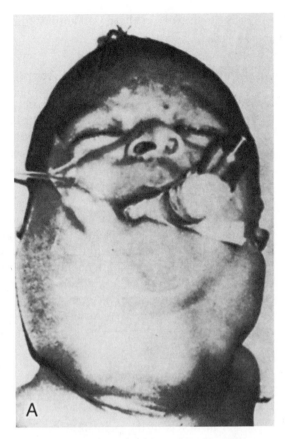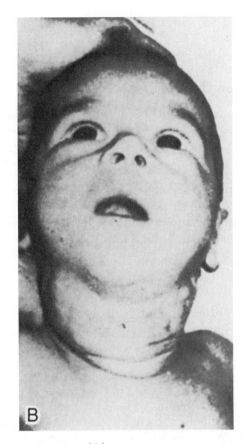

Fig. 10-7 Iodide-induced neonatal goiter. (A) Appearance on the first day of life. (B) Appearance at 2 months of age. (From Senior and Chernoff,[226] with permission.)

Dimenhydrinate (Dramamine)

No teratogenicity has been noted with dimenhydrinate, but a 29 percent failure rate and a significant incidence of side effects, especially drowsiness, has been reported.[88]

Diphenhydramine (Benadryl)

In 595 patients treated in the Collaborative Perinatal Project, no teratogenicity was noted with diphenhydramine.[64] Drowsiness can be a problem.

Trimethobenzamide (Tigan)

Trimethobenzamide, an antinauseant not classified as either an antihistamine or a phenothiazine, has been used for nausea and vomiting in pregnancy. The data collected from a small number of patients is conflicting. In 193 patients in the Kaiser Health Plan study[87] exposed to trimethobenzamide, there was a suggestion of increased congenital anomalies ($p < 0.05$); no concentration of specific anomalies was observed in these children, however, and some of the mothers took other drugs as well. In 340 patients in the Collaborative Peri-

natal Project,[64] no evidence for an association between this drug and malformations was found.

Phenothiazines

Because of the potential for severe side effects, the phenothiazines have not been used routinely in the treatment of mild or moderate nausea and vomiting, but have been reserved for the treatment of hyperemesis gravidarum. Chlorpromazine (Thorazine) has been shown to be effective in hyperemesis gravidarum, with the most important side effect being drowsiness.

Teratogenicity does not appear to be a problem with the phenothiazines when evaluated as a group. In the Kaiser Health Plan Study,[87] 976 patients were treated, and in the Collaborative Perinatal Project[64] 1,309 patients were treated; no evidence of association between these drugs and malformations was noted. Suspicion of an association between phenothiazines and cardiovascular malformations was observed, however, but this was considered of borderline significance and, in the context of multiple comparisons, of doubtful import. In one study,[89] chlorpromazine seemed to be associated with an increased risk of malformations in 141 exposed mothers. In 58 mothers treated with promethazine (Phenergan) and in 48 mothers given proclorperazine (Compazine), no increased risk of malformations was found.

Ondansetron (Zofran)

Ondansetron is no more effective than promethazine and has not been evaluated for terotogenicity.[90]

Emetrol

Emetrol is a phosphorylated carbohydrate solution that acts on the wall of the hyperactive gastrointestinal tract. It reduces smooth muscle contractions in direct proportion to the amount used and is relatively free from toxicity or side effects.

Acupressure

Acupressure is another modality that may be effective in reducing nausea but not vomiting in pregnant women.[91]

Antihistamines and Decongestants

No increased risk of anomalies has been associated with most of the commonly used antihistamines, such as chlorpheniramine (Chlortrimeton). However, in the Collaborative Perinatal Project,[64] the risk of malformations increased after exposure to brompheniramine (Dimetane) (10/65 infants), an effect that was not found for other antihistamines. Terfenadine (Seldane) has been associated in one study with an increased risk of polydactyly.[92]

An association between exposure during the last 2 weeks of pregnancy to antihistamines in general and retrolental fibroplasia in premature infants has been reported.[93]

In the Collaborative Perinatal Project[64] an increased risk of birth defects was noted with phenylpropanolamine (Entex LA) exposure in the first trimester. In one retrospective study, an increased risk of gastroschisis was associated with first trimester pseudoephedrine (Sudafed) use.[94] Although these findings have not been confirmed, use of these drugs for trivial indications should be discouraged as long-term effects are unknown. If decongestion is necessary, topical nasal sprays will result in a lower dose to the fetus than systemic medication.

Patients should be educated that antihistamines and decongestants are only symptomatic therapy for the common cold and have no influence on the course of the disease. Other remedies should be recommended, such as use of a humidifier, rest, and fluids. If medications are necessary, combinations with two drugs should not be used if only one drug is necessary. If the situation is truly an allergy, an antihistamine alone will suffice.

Antibiotics and Anti-infective Agents

As pregnant patients are particularly susceptible to vaginal yeast infections, antibiotics should only be used when clearly indicated. Therapy with antifungal agents may be necessary during or after the course of therapy.

Penicillins

Penicillin, ampicillin, and amoxicillin (Amoxil) are safe in pregnancy. In the Collaborative Perinatal Project,[64] 3,546 mothers took penicillin derivatives in the first trimester of pregnancy, with no increased risk of anomalies. There is little experience in pregnancy with the newer penicillins such as piperacillin (Pipracil) and mezlocillin (Mezlin). These drugs, therefore, should be used in pregnancy only when another better-studied antibiotic is not effective.

Most penicillins are primarily excreted unchanged in the urine, with only small amounts being inactivated in the liver. Patients with impaired renal function require a reduction in dosage.

Serum levels of the penicillins are lower and their renal clearance is higher throughout pregnancy than in the nonpregnant state.[95] The increase in renal blood flow and glomerular filtration rate results in increased excretion of these drugs. The expansion of the maternal intravascular volume during the late stages of pregnancy is another factor that affects antibiotic therapy. If the same dose of penicillin or ampicillin is given to both nonpregnant and pregnant women, lower serum levels are attained during pregnancy due to the distribution of the drug in a larger intravascular volume.

Transplacental passage of penicillin is by simple diffusion. The free circulating portion of the antibiotic crosses the placenta, resulting in a lower maternal serum level of the unbound portion of the drug. Administration of penicillins with high protein binding, e.g., oxacillin, cloxacillin (Cloxapen), dicloxacillin (Pathocil), and nafcillin (Unipen) to a pregnant woman leads to lower fetal tissue and amniotic fluid levels than the administration of poorly bound penicillins (e.g., penicillin G and ampicillin).[96]

The antibiotic is ultimately excreted in the fetal urine and thus into the amniotic fluid. The delay in appearance of different types of penicillins in the amniotic fluid depends primarily on the rate of transplacental diffusion, the amount of protein binding in fetal serum, and the adequacy of fetal enzymatic and renal function. A time delay may occur before effective levels of the antibiotic appear in the amniotic fluid.

Cephalosporins

In a study of 5,000 Michigan Medicaid recipients, there was a suggestion of possible teratogenicity (25 percent increased birth defects) with cefaclor, cephalexin, and cephradine, but not other cephalosporins.[97] Because other antibiotics that have been used extensively (e.g., penicillin, ampicillin, amoxicillin, erythromycin) have not been associated with an increased risk of congenital defects, they should be first-line therapy when such treatment is needed in the first trimester.

Maternal serum levels of cephalosporins are lower than in nonpregnant patients receiving equivalent dosages due to a shorter half-life in pregnancy, an increased volume of distribution, and increased renal elimination. They readily cross the placenta to the fetal bloodstream and ultimately the amniotic fluid.

Sulfonamides

Among 1,455 human infants exposed to sulfonamides during the first trimester, no teratogenic effects were noted.[64] However, the administration of sulfonamides should be avoided in women deficient in glucose-6-phosphate dehydrogenase, as a dose-related toxic reaction may occur resulting in red cell hemolysis. There is also a theoretical risk of hemolysis in the fetus if the drug is used near the time of delivery, as fetal red cells are normally relatively deficient in glutathione.[98]

Sulfonamides cause no known damage to the fetus in utero, as the fetus can clear free bilirubin through the placenta. These drugs might theoretically have deleterious effects if present in the blood of the neonate after birth, however. Sulfonamides compete with bilirubin for binding sites on albumin, thus raising the levels of free bilirubin in the serum and increasing the risk of hyperbilirubinemia in the neonate. For that reason, they are not the first choice in the third trimester. The sulfonamides are easily absorbed orally, and readily cross the placenta, achieving fetal plasma levels 50 to 90 percent of those attained in the mother.[99]

Sulfamethoxazole with Trimethoprim (Bactrim, Septra)

Sulfa is often given with trimethoprim to treat urinary tract infections. Two published trials have failed to show any increased risk of birth defects after first trimester exposure.[100,101] However, one unpublished study of 2,000 Michigan Medicaid recipients suggested an increased risk of cardiovascular defects after exposure in the first trimester.[102]

Sulfasalazine (Azulfidine)

Sulfasalizine is used for treatment of ulcerative colitis and Crohn's disease due to its relatively poor oral absorption. However, it does cross the placenta, leading to fetal drug concentrations approximately the same as those of the mother, although both are low. Neither kernicterus nor severe neonatal jaundice have been reported following maternal use of sulfasalazine even when the drug was given up to the time of delivery.[103]

Nitrofurantoin (Macrodantin)

Nitrofurantoin is used in the treatment of acute uncomplicated lower urinary tract infections as well as for long-term suppression in patients with chronic bacteriuria. Nitrofurantoin is capable of inducing hemolytic anemia in patients deficient in G6PD and theoretically in infants, whose red blood cells are deficient in gluthathione.[98] However, hemolytic anemia in the newborn as a result of in utero exposure to nitrofurantoin has not been reported.

No reports have linked the use of nitrofurantoin with congenital defects. In the Collaborative Perinatal Project,[64] 590 infants were exposed, 83 in the first trimester, with no increased risk of adverse effects. More recent studies have confirmed these findings.[104,105]

Nitrofurantoin absorption from the gastrointestinal tract varies with the form administered. The macrocrystalline form is absorbed more slowly than the crystalline and is associated with less gastrointestinal intolerance. Because of rapid elimination, the serum half-life is 20 to 60 minutes. Therapeutic serum levels are not achieved, and therefore this drug is not indicated when there is a possibility of bacteremia. Approximately one third of an oral dose appears in the active form in the urine.

Tetracyclines

The tetracyclines readily cross the placenta and are firmly bound by chelation to calcium in developing bone and tooth structures. This produces brown discoloration of the deciduous teeth, hypoplasia of the enamel, and inhibition of bone growth.[106] The staining of the teeth takes place in the second or third trimesters of pregnancy, while bone incorporation can occur earlier. Depression of skeletal growth was particularly common among premature infants treated with tetracycline. Alternate antibiotics are currently recommended during pregnancy.

Hepatotoxicity has been reported in pregnant women treated with tetracyclines in large doses, usually with intravenous administration for pyelonephritis. First-trimester exposure to tetracyclines has not been found to have any teratogenic risk in 341 women in the Collaborative Perinatal Project[64] or in 174 women in another study.[107]

Aminoglycosides

Streptomycin and kanamycin have been associated with congenital deafness in the offspring of mothers who took these drugs during pregnancy. Ototoxicity was reported with doses as low 1 g of streptomycin biweekly for 8 weeks during the first trimester.[108] Of 391 mothers who had received 50 mg/kg of kanamycin for prolonged periods during pregnancy, nine children (2.3 percent) were found to have hearing loss.[109]

Ototoxicity may be increased with simultaneous use of ethacrynic acid (Edecrin),[110] and nephrotoxicity may be greater when aminoglycosides are combined with cephalosporins. Neuromuscular blockade may be potentiated by the combined use of aminoglycosides and curariform drugs; therefore, the dosages should be reduced appropriately. Potentiation of magnesium-sulfate-induced neuromuscular weakness has also been reported in a neonate exposed to magnesium sulfate and gentamicin (Garamycin).[111]

No known teratogenic effect other than ototoxicity has been associated with the use of aminoglycosides in the first trimester. In 135 infants exposed to streptomycin in the Collaborative Perinatal Project,[64] no teratogenic effects were observed. In a group of 1,619 newborns whose mothers were treated for tuberculosis with multiple drugs, including streptomycin, the incidence of congenital defects was the same as in a healthy control group.[112]

Aminoglycosides are poorly absorbed after oral administration and are rapidly excreted by the normal kidney. Because the rate of clearance is related to the glomerular filtration rate, dosage must be reduced in the face of abnormal renal function. The serum aminoglycoside levels are usually lower in pregnant than in nonpregnant patients receiving equivalent doses because of more rapid elimination.[113,114] Thus, it is important to monitor levels to prevent subtherapeutic dosing.

Antituberculosis Drugs

There is no evidence of any teratogenic effect of isoniazid (INH), para-aminosalicylic acid (PAS), rifampin (Rifadin), or ethambutol (Myambutol).

Erythromycin

No teratogenic risk of erythromycin has been reported. In 79 patients in the Collaborative Perinatal Project[64] and 260 in another study,[107] no increase in birth defects was noted.

Erythromycin estolate (Ilosone) has been associated with subclinical reversible hepatotoxicity during pregnancy[115]; thus, other forms are usually recommended.

Erythromycin is not consistently absorbed from the gastrointestinal tract of pregnant women, and the transplacental passage is unpredictable. Both maternal and fetal plasma levels achieved after the administration of the drug in pregnancy are low and vary considerably, with fetal plasma concentrations being 5 to 20 percent of those in maternal plasma.[116,117] Thus, some authors have recommended that penicillin be administered to every newborn whose mother received erythromycin for the treatment of syphilis.[118] Fetal tissue levels increase after multiple doses.[117] The usual oral dose is 250 to 500 mg every 6 hours, but the higher dose may not be well tolerated in pregnant women who are susceptible to nausea and gastrointestinal symptoms.

Clindamycin (Cleocin)

Of 647 infants exposed to clindamycin in the first trimester, no increased risk of birth defects was noted.[119]

Clindamycin is nearly completely absorbed after oral administration; a small percentage is absorbed after topical application. The drug crosses the placenta, achieving maximum cord serum levels of about 50 percent of the maternal serum.[117] Clindamycin is 90 percent bound to serum protein, and fetal tissue levels increase following multiple dosing.[117] Maternal serum levels after dosing at various stages of pregnancy are similar to those of nonpregnant patients.[113]

Quinolones

The quinolones (e.g., ciprofloxacin [Cipro], norfloxacin [Noroxin]) have a high affinity for bone tissue and cartilage and may cause arthralgia in children. However, no malformations or musculo-skeletal problems were noted in 38 infants exposed in utero in the first trimester.[120]

Metronidazole (Flagyl)

Studies have failed to show any increase in the incidence of congenital defects among the newborns of mothers treated with metronidazole during early or late gestation. In a study of 1,387 prescriptions filled, no risk of birth defects could be determined.[121] A recent meta-analysis confirmed no teratogenic risk.[122]

Controversy regarding the use of metronidazole during pregnancy was stirred when metronidazole was shown to be mutagenic in bacteria by the Ames test, which correlates with carcinogenicity in animals. However, the doses used were much higher than those used clinically, and carcinogenicity in humans has not been confirmed.[123] As some have recommended against its use in pregnancy, metronidazole should still be given only for clear-cut indications and its use deferred until after the first trimester if possible.

Acyclovir (Zovirax)

The Acyclovir Registry has recorded 601 exposures during pregnancy, including 425 in the first trimester, with no increased risk of abnormalities in the infants.[124]

The Centers for Disease Control and Prevention recommends that pregnant women with disseminated infection (e.g., herpes encephalitis or hepatitis) or varicella pneumonia be treated with acyclovir.[125]

Lindane (Kwell)

After application of lindane to the skin, about 10 percent of the dose used can be recovered in the urine. Toxicity in humans after use of topical 1 percent lindane has been observed almost exclusively after misuse and overexposure to the agent. Although no evidence of specific fetal damage is attributable to lindane, the agent is a potent neurotoxin, and its use during pregnancy should be limited. Pregnant women should be cautioned about shampooing their children's hair, as absorption could easily occur across the skin of the hands of the mother. An alternate drug for lice is usually recommended, such as pyrethrins with piperonyl butoxide (RID).

Antifungal Agents

Nystatin (Mycostatin) is poorly absorbed from intact skin and mucous membranes, and topical use has not been associated with teratogenesis.[107]

The imidazoles are absorbed in only small amounts from the vagina. Chlotrimazole (Lotrimin) or miconazole (Monistat) in pregnancy is not known to be associated with congenital malformations. However, in one study a statistically significantly increased risk of first trimester abortion was noted after use of these drugs, but these findings were considered not to be definitive evidence of risk.[126] However, use of these drugs should be postponed until after the first trimester if possible for theoretical reasons.

Drugs for Induction of Ovulation

In more than 2,000 exposures, no evidence of teratogenic risk of clomiphene (Clomid) has been noted,[127] and the percentage of spontaneous abortions is close to the expected rate. Although infants are often exposed to bromocriptine (Parlodel) in early pregnancy, no teratogenic effects have been observed in more than 1,400 pregnancies.[128,129]

Mild Analgesics

Few pains during pregnancy justify the use of a mild analgesic. Pregnant patients should be encouraged to use nonpharmacologic remedies, such as local heat and rest.

Aspirin

There is no evidence of any teratogenic effect of aspirin taken in the first trimester.[64] Aspirin does have significant perinatal effects, however, as it inhibits prostaglandin synthesis. Uterine contractility is decreased, and patients taking aspirin in analgesic doses have delayed onset of labor, longer duration of labor, and an increased risk of a prolonged pregnancy.[130]

Aspirin also decreases platelet aggregation, which can increase the risk of bleeding before as well as at delivery. Platelet dysfunction has been described in newborns within 5 days of ingestion of aspirin by the mother.[131] Because aspirin causes permanent inhibition of prostaglandin synthetase in platelets, the only way for adequate clotting to occur is for more platelets to be produced.

Multiple organs may be affected by chronic aspirin use. Of note, prostaglandins mediate the neonatal closure of the ductus arteriosus. In one case report, maternal ingestion of aspirin close to the time of delivery was related to closure of the ductus arteriosus in utero.[132]

Low-dose aspirin (80 mg/day) may ultimately prove of benefit in prevention of preeclampsia and fetal wastage associated with autoimmune diseases. Wallenburg et al.[133] randomized patients who had positive angiotension II infusion tests to low-dose aspirin therapy or placebo and reduced the incidence of preeclampsia in the treated compared with the placebo group (see Ch. 28) Lubbe et al.[134] treated patients with lupus anticoagulant and fetal wastage with prednisone 40 to 60 mg/day and low-dose aspirin (75 mg/day) with improved fetal outcome (see Ch. 22). Cowchock et al.[135] have reported that in patients with antiphospholipid-associated fetal wastage, heparin is preferable to prednisone in combination with low-dose aspirin.

Acetaminophen (Tylenol, Datril)

Acetaminophen has also shown no evidence of teratogenicity. With acetaminophen, inhibition of prostaglandin synthesis is reversible so that, once the drug has cleared, platelet aggregation returns to normal. The bleeding time is not prolonged with acetaminophen in contrast to aspirin,[136] and the drug is not toxic to the newborn. Thus, if a mild analgesic or antipyretic is indicated, acetaminophen is preferred over aspirin. Absorption and disposition of acetaminophen in normal doses is not altered by pregnancy.[137]

Other Nonsteroidal Anti-inflammatory Agents

No evidence of teratogenicity has been reported for other nonsteroidal anti-inflammatory drugs (e.g., ibuprofen [Motrin, Advil], naproxen, [Naprosyn]), but limited information is available. Chronic use may lead to oligohydramnios, and constriction of the fetal ductus arteriosus or neonatal pulmonary hypertension as has been reported with indomethacin might occur.

Propoxyphene (Darvon)

Propoxyphene is an acceptable alternative mild analgesic with no known teratogenicity.[64] However, it should not be used for trivial indications as it carries potential for narcotic addiction. Evidence of risk in late pregnancy comes from case reports of infants of mothers who were addicted to propoxyphene and had typical narcotic withdrawal in the neonatal period.[138]

Codeine

In the Collaborative Perinatal Project, no increased relative risk of malformations was observed in 563 codeine users.[64] Codeine can cause addiction and newborn withdrawal symptoms if used to excess perinatally.

Smoking

Smoking has been associated with small size for gestational age as well as an increased prematurity rate.[139] The spontaneous abortion rate is up to twice that of nonsmokers. Abortions associated with maternal smoking tend to have a higher percentage of normal karyotypes and occur later than those with chromosomal aberrations[140] (see Ch. 22). The higher perinatal mortality rate associated with smoking is partly attributable to an increased risk of both abruptio placentae and placenta previa as well as premature and prolonged rupture of membranes. The risks of complications and of the associated perinatal loss rise with the number of cigarettes smoked. Discontinuation of smoking during pregnancy can reduce the risk of both pregnancy complications and perinatal mortality, especially in women at high risk for other reasons. Maternal passive smoking was also associated with a twofold risk of low birth weight at term in one study.[141]

There is also a positive association between smoking and sudden infant death syndrome (SIDS). In such reports, it is not possible to distinguish between apparent effects of maternal smoking during pregnancy and smoking after pregnancy, but both may play a role.

Alcohol

The fetal alcohol syndrome (FAS) has been reported in the offspring of alcoholic mothers and includes the features of gross physical retardation with onset prenatally and continuing after birth (Fig. 10-8).[142]

In 1980, the Fetal Alcohol Study Group of the Research Society on Alcoholism proposed strict criteria for the diagnosis of FAS.[143] At least one characteristic from each of the following three categories had to be present for a valid diagnosis of the syndrome:
1. Growth retardation before and/or after birth;
2. Facial anomalies, including small palpebral fissures, indistinct or absent philtrum, epicanthic folds, flattened nasal bridge, short length of nose, thin upper lip, low set, unparallel ears, and retarded midfacial development;
3. Central nervous system dysfunction including microcephaly, varying degrees of mental retardation, or other evidence of abnormal neurobehavioral development, such as attention deficit disorder with hyperactivity.

None of these features is individually pathognomonic for fetal alcohol exposure. Confirmatory evidence for this diagnosis is a history of heavy maternal drinking during pregnancy.

In the study of Jones et al.,[144] 23 chronically alcoholic women were matched with 46 controls and the pregnancy outcomes of the two groups compared.

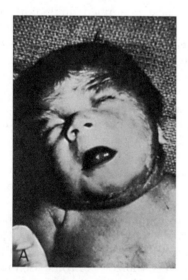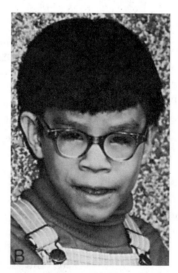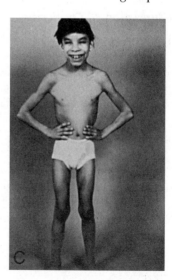

Fig. 10-8 Fetal alcohol syndrome. Patient photographed at (A) birth, (B) 5 years, and (C) 8 years. Note short palpebral fissures, short nose, hypoplastic philtrum, thinned upper lip vermilion, and falttened midface. (From Streissguth,[227] with permission.)

Among the alcoholic mothers, perinatal deaths were about eight times more frequent. Growth restriction, microcephaly, and IQ below 80 were considerably more frequent than among the controls. Overall outcome was abnormal in 43 percent of the offspring of the alcoholic mothers compared with 2 percent of the controls.

Ouellette et al.[145] addressed the risks of smaller amounts of alcohol. Nine percent of infants of abstinent or rare drinkers and 14 percent of infants of moderate drinkers were abnormal, not a significant difference. In heavy drinkers (average daily intake of 3 ounces of 100 proof liquor or more), 32 percent of the infants had anomalies. Overall, including anomalies, growth restriction, and an abnormal neurologic examination, 71 percent of the children of heavy drinkers were affected, twice the frequency of abnormality found in the moderate and rarely drinking groups. In this study, an increased frequency of abnormality was not found until 45 ml of ethanol (equivalent to three drinks) daily were exceeded. The study of Mills and Graubard[146] also showed that total malformation rates were not significantly higher among offspring of women who had an average of less than one drink per day (77.3/1,000) or one to two drinks per day (83.2/1,000) than among nondrinkers (78.1/1,000). Genitourinary malformations increased with increasing alcohol consumption, however, so the possibility remains that for some malformations no safe drinking level exists.

Heavy drinking remains a major risk to the fetus, and reduction even in midpregnancy can benefit the infant. An occasional drink during pregnancy carries no known risk, but no level of drinking is known to be safe.

Sokol et al.[147] have addressed history taking for prenatal detection of risk drinking. Four questions help differentiate patients drinking sufficiently to potentially damage the fetus (Table 10-1). The patient is considered at risk if more than two drinks are required to make her feel "high." The probability of "risk drinking" increases to 63% for those responding positively to all four questions.

Table 10-1   The T-ACE Questions Found To Identify Women Drinking Sufficiently To Potentially Damage the Fetus

T	How many drinks does it take to make you feel high (can you hold) (*Tolerance*)?
A	Have people *annoyed* you by criticizing your drinking?
C	Have you felt you ought to *cut down* on your drinking?
E	Have you ever had to drink first thing in the morning to steady your nerves or to get rid of a hangover (*eye-opener*)?

Two points are scored as a positive answer to the tolerance question and one each for the other three. A score of 2 or more correctly identified 69 percent of risk drinkers.
(From Sokol et al,[147] with permission.)

Marihuana

No teratogenic effect of marihuana has been documented. In a prospective study of 35 pregnancies,[148] infants born to marihuana users exhibited significantly more meconium staining (57 percent versus 25 percent in nonusers). However, users tended to come from lower socioeconomic backgrounds. Most adverse outcomes of pregnancy were too infrequent to permit reliable comparisons between the groups. Marihuana users had an increased incidence of precipitate labor (<3 hours total), 29 percent compared with 3 percent in the control group.[148]

In another population in which the users and nonusers of marihuana were similar in general health, ethnic background, nutritional habits, and use of tobacco, these differences were not confirmed (19 patients in each group).[149] In this same small group of patients, average use of marihuana six or more times per week during pregnancy was associated with a reduction of 0.8 weeks in the length of gestation, although no reduction in birth weight was noted. One study suggested a mean 73 g decrease in birth weight associated with marihuana use, when urine assays were performed rather than relying on self-reporting.[150]

Cocaine

A serious difficulty in determining the effects of cocaine on the infant is the frequent presence of many confounding variables in the population using cocaine. These mothers often abuse other drugs, smoke, have poor nutrition, fail to seek prenatal care, and live under poor socioeconomic conditions. These factors are difficult to take into account in comparison groups. Another difficulty is the choice of outcome measures for infants exposed in utero. The neural systems likely to be affected by cocaine are involved in neurologic and behavioral functions that are not easily quantitated by standard infant development tests.

Cocaine-using women have a higher rate of spontaneous abortion than controls.[151] Three studies have suggested an increased risk of congenital anomalies after first trimester cocaine use,[152–154] most frequently cardiac and central nervous system. In the study of Bingol et al.[153] the malformation rate was 10 percent in cocaine users, 4.5 percent in polydrug users, and 2 percent in controls. MacGregor et al.[154] reported a 6 percent anomaly rate compared with 1 percent for controls.

Cocaine is a central nervous system stimulant and has local anesthetic and marked vasoconstrictive effects. Abruptio placentae has been reported to occur immediately after nasal or intravenous administration.[151] Several studies have also noted increased still births, preterm labor, premature birth, and small for gestational age infants with cocaine use.[150–152,155,156]

The impairment of intrauterine brain growth as manifested by microcephaly is the most common brain abnormality in infants exposed to cocaine in utero.[157] In one study 16 percent of newborns had microcephaly compared with 6 percent of controls.[158] Somatic growth is also impaired, and so the growth restriction may be symmetric or characterized by a relatively low head circumference/abdominal circumference ratio.[159] Multiple other neurologic problems have been reported after cocaine exposure, as well as dysmorphic features and neurobehavioral abnormalities.[156]

Aside from causing congenital anomalies in the first trimester, cocaine has been reported to cause fetal disruption[160] presumably due to interruption of blood flow to various organs. Bowel infarction has been noted with unusual ileal atresia and bowel perforation. Limb infarction has resulted in missing fingers in a distribution different from the usual congenital limb anomalies. Central nervous system bleeding in utero may result in porencephalic cysts.

Narcotics

Menstrual abnormalities, especially amenorrhea, are common in heroin abusers, although they are not associated with the use of methadone. The goal of methadone maintenance is to bring the patient to a level of approximately 20 to 40 mg/day. The dose should be individualized at a level sufficient to minimize the use of supplemental illicit drugs, since they represent a greater risk to the fetus than do the higher doses of methadone required by some patients. Manipulation of the dose in women maintained on methadone should be avoided in the last trimester because of an association with increased fetal complications and in utero deaths attributed to fetal withdrawal in utero.[161] As management of narcotic addiction during pregnancy requires a host of social, nutritional, educational, and psychiatric interventions, these patients are best managed in specialized programs.

The infant of the narcotic addict is at increased risk of abortion, prematurity, and growth restriction. Withdrawl should be watched for carefully in the neonatal period.

Caffeine

There is no evidence of teratogenic effects of caffeine in humans. The Collaborative Perinatal Project[64] showed no increased incidence of congenital defects in 5,773 women taking caffeine in pregnancy, usually in a fixed-dose analgesic medication. There is still some conflicting evidence concerning the association between heavy ingestion of caffeine and increased pregnancy complications. Early studies suggested that the intake of greater than seven to eight cups of coffee per day (a cup of coffee contains about 100 mg of caffeine) was associated with low-birth-weight infants, spontaneous abortions, prematurity, and stillbirths.[162,163] However, these studies were not controlled for the concomitant use of tobacco and alcohol. In one report controlled for smoking, other habits, demographic characteristics, and medical history, no relationship was found between either low birth weight or short gestation and heavy coffee consumption.[164] Also, there was no excess of malformations among coffee drinkers. When pregnant women consumed over 300 mg per day caffeine, one study suggested an increase in term low birth weight infants,[165] less than 2,500 g at greater than 36 weeks.

Concomitant consumption of caffeine with cigarette smoking may increase the risk of low birth weight.[166] Maternal coffee intake decreases iron absorption and may contribute to maternal and fetal anemia.[167]

Two recent studies have shown conflicting results. One retrospective investigation reporting a higher risk of fetal loss was biased by ascertainment of the patients at the time of fetal loss, as these patients typically have less nausea and would be expected to drink more coffee.[168] A prospective cohort study found no evidence that moderate caffeine use increased the risk of spontaneous abortion or growth retardation.[169]

Aspartame (NutraSweet)

The major metabolite of aspartame is phenylalanine,[170] which is concentrated in the fetus by active placental transport. Sustained high blood levels of phenylalanine in the fetus as seen in maternal phenylketonuria (PKU) are associated with mental retardation in the infant. Within the usual range of aspartame ingestion, peak phenylalanine levels do not exceed normal postprandial levels, and even with high doses phenylalanine concentrations are still very far below those associated with mental retardation. These responses have also been studied in women known to be carriers of PKU, and the levels are still normal. Thus, it seems unlikely that use of aspartame in pregnancy would cause any fetal toxicity.

Drugs in Breast Milk

Many drugs can be detected in breast milk at low levels that are not usually of clinical significance to the infant. The rate of transfer into milk depends on the lipid solubility, molecular weight, degree of protein binding, degree of ionization of the drug, and the presence or absence of active secretion. Nonionized molecules of small molecular weight such as ethanol cross easily.[171]

If the mother has unusually high blood concentrations such as with increased dosage or decreased renal function, drugs may appear in higher concentrations in the milk.

The amount of drug in breast milk is a variable fraction of the maternal blood level which itself is proportional to the maternal oral dose. Thus, the dose to the infant is usually subtherapeutic, approximately 1 to 2 percent of the maternal dose on the average. This amount is usually so trivial that no adverse effects are noted. In the case of toxic drugs, however, any exposure may be inappropriate. Allergy may also be possible. Long-term effects of even small doses of drugs may yet be discovered. Also, drugs are eliminated more slowly in the infant with immature enzyme systems. Short-term effects of most maternal medications on breast-fed infants are mild and pose little risk to the infants.[172] As the benefits of breast-feeding are well known, the risk of drug exposure must be weighed against these benefits.

With respect to drug administration in the immediate few days postpartum before lactation is fully established, the infant receives only a small volume of colostrum, and thus little drug is excreted into the milk at this time. It is helpful to allay fears of patients undergoing cesarean deliveries that analgesics or other drugs administered at this time will have no known adverse effects on the infant. For drugs requiring daily dosing during lactation, knowledge of pharmacokinetics in breast milk may minimize the dose to the infant. For example, dosing after nursing will decrease the exposure as the blood level will be lowest before the next dose.

The American Academy of Pediatrics has reviewed drugs in lactation[173] and categorized the drugs as listed below.

Drugs Commonly Listed as Contraindicated During Breastfeeding

Cytotoxic Agents

Cyclosporine (Sandimmune), doxorubicin (Adriamycin), and cyclophosphamide (Cytoxan) might cause immune suppression in the infant, although data are limited with respect to these and other cytotoxic agents. In general, the potential risks of these drugs would outweigh the benefits of continuing nursing if these were required.

After oral administration to a lactating patient with choriocarcinoma, methotrexate was found in milk in low, but detectable levels (0.26 μg/100 ml). Most individuals would elect to avoid any exposure of the infant to this drug. However, in environments in which bottle feeding is rarely practiced and presents practical and cultural difficulties, therapy with this drug would not in

itself appear to constitute a contraindication to breast-feeding.[174]

Busulphan (Myleran) has been reported to cause no adverse effect in nursing infants.[175]

Bromocriptine (Parlodel)

This agent is an ergot alkaloid derivative which has an inhibitory effect on lactation. However, in one report a mother taking 5 mg/day for a pituitary tumor was able to nurse her infant.[176]

Ergotamine (Ergomar)

This medication has been reported to be associated with vomiting, diarrhea, and convulsions in the infant in doses used in migraine medications. However, short-term ergot therapy in the postpartum period for uterine contractility is not a contraindication to lactation.

Lithium (Eskalith, Lithobid)

Lithium reaches one-third to one-half the therapeutic blood concentration in infants, who might develop lithium toxicity, with hypotonia and lethargy.[177,178]

Amphetamines

One report of 103 cases of exposure to amphetamines in breast milk noted no insomnia or stimulation in the infants.[179] However, amphetamines are concentrated in breast milk.

Radioactive Compounds That Require Temporary Cessation of Breast Feeding

Radiopharmaceuticals require variable intervals of interruption of nursing to ensure that no radioactivity is detectable in the milk. Intervals generally quoted are, for gallium 67, 2 weeks;[131] I, 5 days; radioactive sodium, 4 days and ^{99}Tc, 24 hours. For reassurance, the milk may be counted for radioactivity before nursing is resumed.[180]

Drugs Whose Effects on Nursing Infants Are Unknown But May Be of Concern

Psychotropic drugs such as antianxiety, antidepressant, and antipsychotic agents are of special concern when given to nursing mothers for long periods. Although there are no data about adverse effects in infants exposed to these drugs via breast milk, they could theoretically alter central nervous system function.[173] Fluoxetine (Prozac) is excreted in breast milk at low levels.[181]

Temporary cessation of breast-feeding after a single dose of metronidazole (Flagyl) may be considered. Its half-life is such that interruption of lactation for 12 to

24 hours after single-dose therapy usually results in negligible exposure to the infant. It is excreted into breast milk with a milk–plasma ratio of about 1:0. Therefore, even if a woman continued to nurse, the infant would get a trivial dose.

Drugs Usually Compatible With Breast-Feeding

Narcotics, Sedatives, and Anticonvulsants

In general, no evidence of adverse effect is noted with most of the sedatives, narcotic analgesics, and anticonvulsants. Patients may be reassured that, in normal doses, carbamezapine (Tegretol),[182] phenytoin (Dilantin), magnesium sulfate, codeine, morphine, and meperidine (Demerol) do not cause any obvious adverse effects in the infants,[183] since the dose detectable in the breast milk is approximately 1 to 2 percent of the mother's dose, which is sufficiently low to have no significant pharmacologic activity.

With diazepam (Valium), the milk-plasma ratio at peak dose is 0.68, with only small amounts detected in the breast milk.[184] In two patients who took carbamazepine (Tegretol) while nursing, the concentration of the drug in breast milk at 4 and 5 weeks postpartum was similar, about 60 percent of the maternal serum level. Accumulation does not seem to occur, and no adverse effects were noted in either infant.[185]

In studies in which phenobarbital[186] and phenytoin (Dilantin) levels were measured, only small amounts of these drugs were detected in breast milk. Phenobarbital and diazepam (Valium) are slowly eliminated by the infant, however, and so accumulation may occur. Women consuming barbiturates or benzodiazepines should observe the infants for sedation.

In 10 preeclamptic patients receiving magnesium sulfate 1 g/h intravenously for 24 hours after delivery, magnesium levels in breast milk were 64 μg/ml compared with 48 μg/ml in controls.[187] Breast milk calcium levels were not affected by magnesium sulfate therapy.

Analgesics

Aspirin is transferred into breast milk in small amounts. Since acids exist primarily in the ionized form, salicylate transport from plasma into milk is not favored. The risk is related to high dosages (e.g., greater than 16 300-mg tablets per day in the mother, when the infant may get sufficiently high serum levels to affect platelet aggregation or even cause metabolic acidosis). No harmful effects of acetaminophen (Tylenol, Datril) have been noted. In one patient taking propoxyphene (Darvon) in a suicide attempt, the level in breast milk was half that of the serum. A breast-feeding infant could theoretically receive up to 1 mg of propoxyphene a day if the mother were to consume the maximum dose continually.[188] One infant was reported to have poor muscle tone when the mother was taking propoxyphene every 4 hours.

Antihistamines and Phenothiazines

Although studies are not extensive, no harmful effects have been noted from antihistamines or phenothiazines, and they have not been found to affect milk supply. Decongestants should be avoided in women who are having trouble with milk supply.

Aminophylline

Maximum milk concentrations of aminophylline are achieved between 1 and 3 hours after an oral dose. The nursing infant has been calculated to receive less than 1 percent of the maternal dose with no noted adverse effects. To minimize neonatal drug exposure, however, a nursing mother should try to breast-feed her infant immediately before her doses of the drug.[189]

Antihypertensives

After a single 500-mg oral dose of chlorothiazide (Diuril), no drug was detected in breast milk at a sensitivity of 1 μg/ml.[190] In one mother taking 50 mg of hydrochlorothiazide (Hydrodiuril) daily, peak milk levels were about 25 percent of maternal blood levels. The drug was not detectable in the nursing infant's serum, and the infant's electrolytes were normal.[191] Thiazide diuretics may decrease milk production in the first month of lactation.[173]

Propranolol (Inderal) is excreted in breast milk, with milk concentrations after a single 40-mg dose less than 40 percent of peak plasma concentrations. In one patient on a continuous dosage of 40 mg four times daily, plasma and breast milk concentrations peaked 3 hours after dosing and the peak breast milk concentration of 42 ng/ml was 64 percent of the corresponding plasma concentration. After a 30-day regimen of 240 mg/day of propranolol, the predose and 3-hour postdose propranolol concentrations in breast milk were 26 and 64 ng/ml, respectively. Thus, an infant consuming 500 ml/day of milk would ingest a maximum of 21 μg in 24 hours at a maternal dose of 160 mg/day and a maximum of 32 μg in 24 hours at a maternal dose of 240 mg/day. This amount represents approximately 1 percent of a therapeutic dose. This amount of drug is unlikely to cause any adverse effect.[192–194]

Atenolol (Tenormin) is concentrated in breast milk to about three times the plasma level.[195] One case has been reported in which a 5-day-old term infant had signs of β-adrenergic blockade with bradycardia (80 bpm) with the breast milk dose calculated to be 9 percent of the maternal dose.[196] Adverse effects in other infants have not been reported, with most infants receiving about 1 percent of the maternal dose.

Clonidine (Catapres) concentrations in milk are almost twice maternal serum levels.[197] Neurologic and laboratory parameters in the infants of treated mothers are similar to those of controls.

Anticoagulants

Most mothers requiring anticoagulation may continue to nurse their infants with no problems. Heparin does not cross into milk and is not active orally.

At a maternal dose of warfarin (Coumadin) of 5 to 12 mg/day in seven patients with maternal plasma concentrations of 0.5 to 2.6 µg/ml, no warfarin was detected in infant breast milk or plasma at a sensitivity of 0.025 µg/ml. This low concentration is probably due to the fact that warfarin is 98 percent protein bound. Thus, 1 L of milk would contain 20 µg of the drug at maximum, an insignificant amount to have an anticoagulant effect.[198] Another report confirms that warfarin appears only in insignificant quantities in breast milk.[199] The oral anticoagulant bishydroxycourmarin (Dicumarol) has been given to 125 nursing mothers with no effect on the infants' prothrombin times and no hemorrhages.[200] Thus, with careful monitoring of maternal prothrombin time so that the dosage is minimized and of neonatal prothrombin times to ensure lack of drug accumulation, warfarin may be safely administered to nursing mothers.

This safety does not apply to all oral anticoagulant drugs, however. Phenindione,[201] a drug not used in the United States, has caused infant bleeding.

Corticosteroids

In one patient requiring corticosteroids, breast milk was obtained 2 hours after an oral dose of 10 mg of prednisone (Deltasone). The levels in the milk were 0.1 µg/100 ml of prednisolone and 2.67 µg/100 ml of prednisone. Thus, an infant taking 1 L of milk would obtain 28.3 µg of the two steroids, an amount not likely to have any deleterious effect.[202]

Mackenzie et al.[203] administered 5 mg of radioactive prednisolone to seven patients and found 0.14 percent of the sample to be secreted in the milk in the subsequent 60 hours, a negligible quantity. Thus, breastfeeding is allowed in mothers taking corticosteroids. Even at 80 mg/day, the nursing infant would ingest less than 0.1 percent of the dose, less than 10 percent of its endogenous cortisol.[204]

Digoxin (Lanoxin)

After a maternal dose of 0.25 mg, peak breast milk levels of 0.6 to 1 ng/ml occur, and the milk–plasma ratio at the 4-hour peak is 0.8 to 0.9. This represents a small amount due to significant maternal protein binding. In 24 hours, an infant would receive about 1 percent of the maternal dose.[205] No adverse effects in nursing infants have been reported.

Antibiotics

Penicillin derivatives are safe in nursing mothers. In the usual therapeutic doses of penicillin or ampicillin (Amoxil), the mother's milk–plasma ratios are only up to 0.2, and no adverse effects are noted in the infants. In susceptible individuals or with prolonged therapy, diarrhea and candidiasis are theoretical concerns.

Dicloxicillin (Pathocil) is 98 percent protein bound. If this drug is used to treat breast infections, very little will get into the breast milk, and nursing may be continued.

Cephalosporins appear only in trace amounts in milk. In one study after cefazolin 500 mg IM three times a day (Ancef, Kefzol), no drug was detected in breast milk.[206] After 2 g of cefazolin IV, 1.51 µg/ml was detected, for a milk–plasma ratio of 0.023 at the 3-hour peak level. Thus, the infant was exposed to only 0.075 percent of the maternal dose.

Tooth staining or delayed bone growth from tetracyclines have not been reported after the drug was taken by a breast-feeding mother. This finding is probably due to the high binding of the drug to calcium and protein, limiting its absorption from the milk. The amount in the milk is about half the level in the mother's plasma. Therefore, the amount of free tetracycline available is too small to be significant.

Sulfonamides only appear in small amounts in breast milk and are ordinarily not contraindicated during nursing. However, the drug is best avoided during the first 5 days of life or in premature infants when hyperbilirubinemia may be a problem, as the drug may displace bilirubin from binding sites on albumin. In one study of sulphapyridine, the drug and its metabolites were detected in plasma and milk at levels of 4 to 7 µg/ml. Thus, the infant would receive less than 1 percent of the maternal dose. When a mother took sulfasalazine (Azulfidine) 500 mg every 6 hours, the drug was undetectable in all milk samples.

Gentamicin (Garamycin) is transferred into breast milk, and half of nursing newborn infants have the drug detectable in their serum. The low levels detected would not be expected to cause clinical effects.[207]

Nitrofurantoin (Macrodantin) is excreted into breast milk in very low concentrations. In one study the drug could not be detected in 20 samples from mothers receiving 100 mg four times a day.[208]

Erythromycin is excreted into breast milk in small amounts, with milk–plasma ratios of about 0.5. No reports of adverse effects on infants exposed to erythromycin in breast milk have been noted. Azithromycin (Zithromax) also appears in breast milk in low concentrations.[209] Clindamycin (Cleocin) is excreted into breast milk in low levels, and nursing is usually continued during administration of this drug.

There are no reported adverse effects on the infant of isoniazid (INH) administered to nursing mothers, and its use is considered compatible with breast-feeding.[173] Acyclovir (Zovirax) is excreted in breast milk in low concentrations.[210]

Oral Contraceptives

Estrogen and progestin combination oral contraceptives cause a dose-related suppression of the quantity of milk produced. The use of oral contraceptives containing 50 μg and more of estrogen during lactation has been associated with shortened duration of lactation, decreased milk production, decreased infant weight gain, and decreased composition of nitrogen and protein content of the milk. However, the composition and volume of breast milk may vary considerably even in the absence of birth control pills. Lactation is inhibited to a lesser degree if the pill is started about 3 weeks postpartum and with lower doses of estrogen than 50 μg. Although the magnitude of the changes is low, the changes may be of nutritional importance, particularly in malnourished mothers. However, if the patient persists in taking birth control pills while nursing, there is no documented adverse effect of this practice.

An infant consuming 600 ml of breast milk daily from a mother using an oral contraceptive containing 50 μg of the ethinylestradiol receives a daily dose in the range of 10 ng of the estrogen.[211] The amount of natural estradiol received by infants who consume a similar volume of milk from mothers not using oral contraceptives is estimated at 3 to 6 ng during anovulatory cycles and 6 to 12 ng during ovulatory cycles. No consistent long-term adverse effects on children's growth and development have been described. Evidence indicates that norgestrel (Ovrette) is metabolized rather than accumulated by the infants, and, to date, no adverse effects have been identified as a result of progestational agents taken by the mother. Progestin-only contraceptives do not cause alteration of breast milk composition or volume,[212] making them ideal in the breast-feeding mother.

Alcohol

Alcohol levels in breast milk are similar to those in maternal blood. One report has appeared of intoxication in an infant whose mother ingested 750 mg of port wine in 24 hours.[213]

If a moderate social drinker had two cocktails and had a blood alcohol concentration of 50 mg/100 ml, the nursing infant would receive about 82 mg of alcohol, which would produce insignificant blood concentrations.[214] There is no evidence that occasional ingestion of alcohol by a mother is harmful to the infant. However, one study showed that ethanol ingested chronically through breast milk might have a detrimental effect on motor development, but not mental development, in the infant.[215] Also, alcohol in breast milk has an immediate effect on the odor of the milk, and this may decrease the amount of milk the infant consumes.[216]

Propylthiouracil

Propylthiouracil (PTU) is found in breast milk in small amounts.[217] If the mother takes 200 mg PTU three times a day, the child would receive 149 μg daily, or the equivalent of a 70-kg adult receiving 3 mg/day. Several infants have been studied up to 5 months of age with no changes in thyroid parameters, including TSH. Lactating mothers on PTU can continue nursing with close supervision of the infant.[217,218] PTU is preferred over methimazole (Tapazole) due to its high protein binding (80 percent) and lower breast milk concentrations.[219]

Caffeine

Caffeine has been reported to have no adverse effects on the nursing infant, even after the mother consumes several cups of strong coffee.[219] In one study, the milk level contained 1 percent of the total dose 6 hours after coffee ingestion, which is not enough to affect the infant. In another report, no significant difference in 24-hour heart rate or sleep time was observed in nursing infants when their mothers drank coffee for 5 days or abstained for 5 days.[220] If a mother drinks excessive amounts of caffeine and caffeine accumulates in the infant, the child might show signs of wakefulness.

Smoking

Nicotine and its metabolite cotinine enter breast milk. Infants of smoking mothers achieve significant serum concentrations of nicotine even if they are not exposed to passive smoking, and exposure to passive smoking further raises the levels of nicotine.[221] Women who smoke should be encouraged to stop smoking during lactation as well as during pregnancy.[222]

Conclusions

Many medical conditions during pregnancy and lactation are best treated initially with nonpharmacologic remedies. Before a drug is administered in pregnancy, the indications should be clear and the risk/benefit ratio should justify drug use. If possible, therapy should be postponed until after the first trimester. In addition, patients should be cautioned about the risks of social drug use such as smoking, alcohol, and cocaine during pregnancy. Most drug therapy does not require cessation of lactation, as the amount excreted into breast milk is sufficiently small to be pharmacologically insignificant.

10 Key Points

- Infants of epileptic women taking anticonvulsants have double the rate of malformations of unexposed infants; the risk of fetal hydantoin syndrome is less than 10 percent.

- The risk of malformations after in utero exposure to isotretinoin is 25 percent, and an additional 25 percent of infants have mental retardation.

- Heparin is the drug of choice for anticoagulation during pregnancy, although there is some risk of osteoporosis from its use.

- Angiotensin-converting enzyme inhibitors can cause fetal renal failure in the second and third trimesters, leading to oligohydramnios, craniofacial deformities, and hypoplastic lungs.

- Vitamin B_6 25 mg tid is a safe and effective therapy for first trimester nausea and vomiting; doxylamine (Unisom) is also effective in combination with B_6.

- Most antibiotics are generally safe in pregnancy. Cephalosporins and trimethoprim may carry an increased risk in the first trimester, and tetracyclines cause tooth discoloration in the second and third trimesters. Aminoglycosides can cause fetal ototoxicity.

- Aspirin in analgesic doses inhibits platelet function and prolongs bleeding time; thus, alternate analgesics are preferred in pregnancy.

- Fetal alcohol syndrome occurs in infants of mothers drinking heavily during pregnancy. A safe level of alcohol intake during pregnancy has not been determined.

- Cocaine has been associated with increased risk of spontaneous abortions, abruptio placentae, and congenital malformations, in particular, microcephaly.

- Most drugs are safe during lactation, as subtherapeutic amounts appear in breast milk, approximately 1 to 2 percent of the maternal dose.

References

1. Wilson JG, Fraser FC (eds): Handbook of Teratology. Plenum, New York, 1979
2. Blake DA, Niebyl JR: Requirements and limitations in reproductive and teratogenic risk assessment. p. 1. In Niebyl JR (ed): Drug Use in Pregnancy. 2nd Ed. Lea & Febiger, Philadelphia, 1988
3. Heinonen OP, Slone D, Monson RR et al: Cardiovascular birth defects and antenatal exposure to female sex hormones. N Engl J Med 296:67, 1977
4. Wiseman RA, Dodds-Smith IC: Cardiovascular birth defects and antenatal exposure to female sex hormones:

a reevaluation of some base data. Teratology 30:359, 1984

5. Katz Z, Lancet M, Skornik J et al: Teratogenicity of progestagens given during the first trimester of pregnancy. Obstet Gynecol 65:775, 1985

6. Raman-Wilms L, Tseng AL, Wighardt S et al: Fetal genital effects of first-trimester sex hormone exposure: a meta-analysis. Obstet Gynecol 85:141, 1995

7. Wilkins L: Masculinization of female fetus due to use of orally given progestins. JAMA 172:1028, 1960

8. Duck SC, Katayama KP: Danazol may cause female pseudohermaphroditism. Fertil Steril 35:230, 1981

9. Jick H, Walker AM, Rothman KJ et al: Vaginal spermicides and congenital disorders. JAMA 245:1329, 1981

10. Shapiro S, Slone D, Heinonen OP et al: Birth defects and vaginal spermicides. JAMA 247:2381, 1982

11. Mills JL, Reed GF, Nugent RP et al: Are there adverse effects of periconceptional spermicide use? Fertil Steril 43:442, 1985

12. Linn S, Schoenbaum SC, Monson RR et al: Lack of association between contraceptive usage and congenital malformations in offspring. Am J Obstet Gynecol 147:923, 1983

13. Simpson JL, Phillips OP: Spermicides, hormonal contraception and congenital malformations. Adv Contracept 6:141, 1990

14. Shapiro S, Hartz SC, Siskind V et al: Anticonvulsants and parental epilepsy in the development of birth defects. Lancet 1:272, 1976

15. Robert E, Guibaud P: Maternal valproic acid and congenital neural tube defects. Lancet 2:937, 1982

16. Lindhout D, Schmidt D: In utero exposure to valproate and neural tube defect. Lancet i:1392, 1986

17. Nakane Y, Okuma T, Takashashi R et al: Multi-institutional study on the teratogenicity and fetal toxicity of antiepileptic drugs: a report of a collaborative study group in Japan. Epilepsia 21:663, 1980

18. Dansky LV, Rosenblatt DS, Andermann E: Mechanisms of teratogenesis: folic acid and antiepileptic therapy. Neurology 42:32, 1992

19. Centers for Disease Control: Recommendations for the use of folic acid to reduce the number of cases of spina bifida and other neural tube defects. MMWR 41:1, 1992

20. Hanson JW, Smith DW: The fetal hydantoin syndrome. J Pediatr 87:285, 1975

21. Gaily E, Granstrom M-L, Hiilesmaa V et al: Minor anomalies in offspring of epileptic mothers. J Pediatr 112:520, 1988

22. Jones KL, Lacro RV, Johnson KA et al: Pattern of malformations in the children of women treated with carbamazepine during pregnancy. N Engl J Med 320:1661, 1989

23. Scolnik D, Nulman I, Rovet J et al: Neurodevelopment of children exposed in utero to phenytoin and carbamazepine monotherapy. JAMA 271:767, 1994

24. Strickler SM, Miller MA, Andermann E et al: Genetic predisposition to phenytoin-induced birth defects. Lancet ii:746, 1985

25. Buehler BA, Delimont D, VanWaes M et al: Prenatal prediction of risk of the fetal hydantoin syndrome. N Engl J Med 322:1567, 1990

26. Van der Pol MC, Hadders-Algra M, Huisjes JH et al: Antiepileptic medication in pregnancy: late effects on the children's central nervous system development. Am J Obstet Gynecol 164:121, 1991

27. Callaghan N, Garrett A, Goggin T: Withdrawal of anticonvulsant drugs in patients free of seizures for two years. N Engl J Med 318:942, 1988

28. Davies VA, Argent AC, Staub H et al: Precursor prothrombin status in patients receiving anticonvulsant drugs. Lancet i:126, 1985

29. Deblay MF, Vert P, Andre M et al: Transplacental vitamin K prevents haemorrhagic disease of infant of epileptic mother. Lancet i:1247, 1982

30. Rosa F: JAMA 251:3208, 1984

31. Lammer EJ, Chen DT, Hoar RM et al: Retinoic acid embryopathy. N Engl J Med 313:837, 1985

32. Adams J: High incidence of intellectual deficits in 5 year old children exposed to isotretinoin "in utero." Teratology 41:614, 1990

33. Dai WS, Hsu M-A, Itri L: Safety of pregnancy after discontinuation of isotretinoin. Arch Dermatol 125:362, 1989

34. Jick SS, Terris BZ, Jick H: First trimester topical tretinoin and congenital disorders. Lancet 341:1181, 1993

35. Rothman KJ, Moore LL, Singer MR et al: Teratogenicity of high vitamin A intake. N Engl J Med 333:1369, 1995

36. Rosenberg L, Mitchell AA, Parsella JL et al: Lack of relation of oral clefts to diazepam use during pregnancy. N Engl J Med 309:1282, 1983

37. Czeizel A: Lack of evidence of teratogenicity of benzodiazepine drugs in Hungary. Reprod Toxicol 3:183, 1988

38. Laegreid L, Olegard R, Wahlstrom J et al: Abnormalities in children exposed to benzodiazepines in utero. Lancet i:108, 1987

39. Bergman V, Rosa F, Baum C et al: Effects of exposure to benzodiazepine during fetal life. Lancet 340:694, 1992

40. Linden S, Rich CL: The use of lithium during pregnancy and lactation. J Clin Psychiatry 44:358, 1983

41. Weinstein MR, Goldfield MD: Cardiovascular malformations with lithium use during pregnancy. Am J Psychiatry 132:529, 1975

42. Zalzstein E, Koren G, Einarson T et al: A case–control study on the association between first trimest exposure to lithium and Ebstein's anomaly. Am J Cardiol 65:817, 1990

43. Jacobson SJ, Jones K, Johnson K et al: Prospective multi-centre study of pregnancy outcome after lithium exposure during first trimester. Lancet 339:530, 1992

44. Krause S, Ebbesen F, Lange AP: Polyhydramnios with maternal lithium treatment. Obstet Gynecol 75:504, 1990

45. Ang MS, Thorp JA, Parisi, VM: Maternal lithium therapy and polyhydramnios. Obstet Gynecol 76:517, 1990

46. Cohen LS, Friedman MJ, Jefferson JW: A reevaluation of risk of in utero exposure to lithium. JAMA 271:146, 1994

47. Briggs GC, Freeman RK, Jaffe SJ: p. 435. Drugs in Preg-

nancy and Lactation. Williams & Wilkins, Baltimore, 1994

48. Briggs GC, Freeman RK, Yaffe SJ: p. 38. Drugs in Pregnancy and Lactation. Williams and Wilkins, Baltimore, 1994

49. Pastuszak A, Schick-Boschetto B, Zuber C et al: Pregnancy outcome following first-trimester exposure to fluoxetine (Prozac). JAMA 269:2446, 1993

50. Briggs GC, Freeman K, Yaffe SJ: p. 374. Drugs in pregnancy and lactation. Williams & Wilkins, Baltimore, 1994

51. Hill RM, Stern L: Drugs in pregnancy: effects on the fetus and newborn. Drugs 17:182, 1979

52. Sbarouni E, Oakley CM: Outcome of pregnancy in women with valve prostheses. Br Heart J 71:196, 1994

53. deSwiet M, Ward PD, Fidler J et al: Prolonged heparin therapy in pregnancy causes bone demineralization. Br J Obstet Gynaecol 90:1129, 1983

54. Barbour LA, Kick SD, Steiner JF et al: A prospective study of heparin-induced osteoporosis in pregnancy using bone densitometry. Am J Obstet Gynecol 170:862, 1994

55. Dahlman TC: Osteoporotic fractures and the recurrence of thromboembolism during pregnancy and the puerperium in 184 women undergoing thromboprophylaxis with heparin. Am J Obstet Gynecol 168:1265, 1993

56. Tengborn L, Bergqvist D, Matzsch T et al: Recurrent thromboembolism in pregnancy and puerperium: is there a need for thromboprophylaxis? Am J Obstet Gynecol 160:90, 1989

57. Lao TT, deSwiet M, Letsky E et al: Prophylaxis of thromboembolism in pregnancy: an alternative. Br J Obstet Gynaecol 92:202, 1985

58. Iturbe-Alessio I, del Carmen Fonseca M, Mutchinik O et al: Risks of anticoagulant therapy in pregnant women with artificial heart valves. N Engl J Med 315:1390, 1986

59. Mujtaba Q, Burrow GN: Treatment of hyperthyroidism in pregnancy with propylthiouracil and methimazole. Obstet Gynecol 46:282, 1975

60. Burrow GN: Thyroid diseases. p. 229. In Burrow GN, Ferris TF (eds): Medical Complications During Pregnancy. WB Saunders, Philadelphia, 1988

61. Mandel SJ, Larsen PR, Seely EW et al: Increased need for thyroxine during pregnancy in women with primary hypothyroidism. N Engl J Med 323:91, 1990

62. Tamaki H, Amino N, Takeoka K et al: Thyroxine requirement during pregnancy for replacement therapy of hypothyroidism. Obstet Gynecol 76:230, 1990

63. l'Allemand D, Gruters A, Heidemann P et al: Iodine-induced alterations of thyroid function in newborn infants after prenatal and perinatal exposure to povidone iodine. J Pediatr 102:935, 1983

64. Heinonen OP, Slone S, Shapiro S: Birth Defects and Drugs in Pregnancy. Publishing Sciences Group, Littleton, MA, 1977

65. Weiner CP, Landas S, Persoon TJ: Digoxin-like immunoreactive substance in fetuses with and without cardiac pathology. Am J Obstet Gynecol 157:368, 1987

66. Weiner CP, Thompson MIB: Direct treatment of fetal supraventricular tachycardia after failed transplacental therapy. Am J Obstet Gynecol 158:570, 1988

67. Pruyn SC, Phelan JP, Buchanan GC: Long-term propranolol therapy in pregnancy: maternal and fetal outcome. Am J Obstet Gynecol 135:485, 1979

68. Redmond GP: Propranolol and fetal growth retardation. Semin Perinatol 6:142, 1982

69. Rubin PC, Clark DM, Sumner DJ: Placebo-controlled trial of atenolol in treatment of pregnancy-associated hypertension. Lancet 1:431, 1983

70. Hanssens M, Keirse MJNC, Vankelecom F et al: Fetal and neonatal effects of treatment with angiotensin-converting enzyme inhibitors in pregnancy. Obstet Gynecol 78:128, 1991

71. Piper JM, Ray WA, Rosa FW: Pregnancy outcome following exposure to angiotensin-converting enzyme inhibitors. Obstet Gynecol 80:429, 1992

72. Buscema J, Stern JL, Johnson TRB Jr: Antineoplastic drugs in pregnancy. p. 89. In JR Niebyl (ed): Drug Use in Pregnancy. 2nd Ed. Lea & Febiger, Philadelphia, 1988

73. Kozlowski RD, Steinbrunner JV, MacKenzie AH et al: Outcome of first-trimester exposure to low-dose methotrexate in eight patients with rheumatic disease. Am J Med 88:589, 1990

74. Haugen G, Fauchald P, Sodal G et al: Pregnancy outcome in renal allograft recipients: influence of ciclosporin A. Eur J Obstet Gynecol Reprod Biol 39:25, 1991

75. Hou S: Pregnancy in organ transplant recipients. Med Clin North Am 73:667, 1989

76. Pickrell MD, Sawers R, Michael J: Pregnancy after renal transplantation: severe intrauterine growth retardation during treatment with cyclosporin A. Br Med J 296:825, 1988

77. Briggs GC, Freeman RK, Yaffe SJ: p. 233. Drugs in Pregnancy and Lactation. Williams & Wilkins, Baltimore, 1994

78. Wolfe MS, Cordero JF: Safety of chloroquine in chemosuppression of malaria during pregnancy. BMJ 290:1466, 1985

79. Hart CW, Naunton RF: The ototoxicity of chloroquine phosphate. Arch Otolaryngol 80:407, 1964

80. Levy M, Buskila D, Gladman DD et al: Pregnancy outcome following first trimester exposure to chloroquine. Am J Perinatol 8:174, 1991

81. Zemlickis D, Lishner M, Degendorfer P et al: Fetal outcome after in utero exposure to cancer chemotherapy. Arch Intern Med 152:573, 1992

82. Main EK, Main DM, Gabbe SG: Chronic oral terbutaline therapy is associated with maternal glucose intolerance. Obstet Gynecol 157:644, 1987

83. Sahakian V, Rouse D, Sipes S et al: Vitamin B$_6$ is effective therapy for nausea and vomiting of pregnancy: a randomized double-blind, placebo-controlled study. Obstet Gynecol 78:33, 1991

84. Vutyavanich T, Wongtra-Rjan S, Ruangsri R: Pyridoxine for nausea and vomiting of pregnancy: a random-

ized double-blind placebo-controlled trial. Am J Obstet Gynecol 173:881, 1995

85. Fischer-Rasmussen W, Kjaer SK, Dahl C, et al: Ginger treatment of hyperemesis gravidarum. Eur J Obstet Gynecol Reprod Biol 38:19, 1990

86. Diggory PLC, Tomkinson JS: Nausea and vomiting in pregnancy: a trial of meclozine dihydrochloride with and without pyridoxine. Lancet 2:370, 1962

87. Milkovich L, Van Den Berg BJ: An evaluation of the teratogenicity of certain antinauseant drugs. Am J Obstet Gynecol 125:244, 1976

88. Cartwright EW: Dramamine in nausea and vomiting of pregnancy. West J Surg Obstet Gynecol 59:216, 1951

89. Rumeau-Rouquette C, Goujard J, Huel G: Possible teratogenic effect of phenothiazines in human beings. Teratology 15:57, 1977

90. Sullivan CA, Johnson CA, Roach H et al: A prospective randomized, double-blind comparison of the serotonin antagonist ondansetron to a standardized regimen of promethazine for hyperemesis gravidarum. A preliminary investigation. Am J Obstet Gynecol 172:299, 1995

91. Belluomini J, Litt RC, Lee KA et al: Acupressure for nausea and vomiting of pregnancy: a randomized, blinded study. Obstet Gynecol 84:145, 1994

92. Briggs GG, Freeman RK, Yaffe SJ: p. 807. Drugs in pregnancy and lactation. 4th Ed. Williams & Wilkins, Baltimore, 1994

93. Zierler S, Purohit D: Prenatal antihistamine exposure and retrolental fibroplasia. Am J Epidemiol 123:192, 1986

94. Werler MM, Mitchell AA, Shapiro S: First trimester maternal medication use in relation to gastroschisis. Teratology 45:361, 1992

95. Philipson A: Pharmacokinetics of antibiotics in pregnancy and labour. Clin Pharmacokinet 4:297, 1979

96. Kunin CM: Clinical pharmacology of the new penicillins. I. The importance of serum protein binding in determining antimicrobial activity and concentration in serum. Clin Pharmacol Ther 7:166, 1966

97. Briggs GG, Freeman RK, Yaffe SJ: p. 148. Drugs in Pregnancy and Lactation. 4th Ed. Williams & Wilkins, Baltimore, 1994

98. Briggs GG, Freeman RK, Yaffe SJ: p. 625. Drugs in Pregnancy and Lactation. 4th Ed. Williams & Wilkins, Baltimore, 1994

99. Monif GFG: Infectious Diseases in Obstetrics and Gynecology. Harper & Row, New York, 1974

100. Ochoa AG: Trimethoprim and sulfamethoxazole in pregnancy. JAMA 217:1244, 1971

101. Brumfitt W, Pursell R: Double-blind trial to compare ampicillin, cephalexin, co-trimoxazole, and trimethoprim in treatment of urinary infection. BMJ 2:673, 1972

102. Briggs GG, Freeman RK, Yaffe SJ: p. 847. Drugs in Pregnancy and lactation. 4th Ed. Williams & Wilkins, Baltimore, 1994

103. Jarnerot G, Into-Malmberg MB, Esbjorner E: Placental transfer of sulphasalazine and sulphapyridine and some of its metabolites. Scand J Gastroenterol 16:693, 1981

104. Hailey FJ, Fort H, Williams JR et al: Foetal safety of nitrofurantoin macrocrystals therapy during pregnancy: a retrospective analysis. J Int Med Res 11:364, 1983

105. Lenke RR, VanDorsten JP, Schifrin BS: Pyelonephritis in pregnancy: a prospective randomized trial to prevent recurrent disease evaluating suppressive therapy with nitrofurantoin and close surveillance. Am J Obstet Gynecol 146:953, 1983

106. Cohlan SQU, Bevelander G, Tiamsic T: Growth inhibition of prematures receiving tetracycline. Am J Dis Child 105:453, 1963

107. Aselton P, Jick H, Mulnsky A et al: First-trimester drug use and congenital disorders. Obstet Gynecol 65:451, 1985

108. Robinson GC, Cambon KG: Hearing loss in infants of tuberculous mothers treated with streptomycin during pregnancy. N Engl J Med 271:949, 1964

109. Nishimura H, Tanimura T: Clinical Aspects of the Teratogenicity of Drugs. Excerpta Medica, Amsterdam, 1976

110. Jones HC: Intrauterine ototoxicity: a case report and review of literature. J Natl Med Assoc 65:201, 1973

111. L'Hommedieu CS, Nicholas D, Armes DA et al: Potentiation of magnesium sulfate-induced neuromuscular weakness by gentamicin, tobramycin, and amikacin. J Pediatr 102:629, 1983

112. Marynowski A, Sianozecka E: Comparison of the incidence of congenital malformations in neonates from healthy mothers and from patients treated because of tuberculosis. Ginekol Pol 43:713, 1972

113. Weinstein AJ, Gibbs RS, Gallagher M: Placental transfer of clindamycin and gentamicin in term pregnancy. Am J Obstet Gynecol 124:688, 1976

114. Zaske DE et al: Rapid gentamicin elimination in obstetric patients. Obstet Gynecol 56:559, 1980

115. McCormack WM, George H, Donner A et al: Hepatotoxicity of erythromycin estolate during pregnancy. Antimicrob Agents Chemother 12:630, 1977

116. Philipson A, Sabath LD, Charles D: Erythromycin and clindamycin absorption and elimination in pregnant women. Clin Pharmacol Ther 19:68, 1976

117. Philipson A, Sabath LD, Charles D: Transplacental passage of erythromycin and clindamycin. N Engl J Med 288:1219, 1973

118. South MA, Short DH, Knox JM: Failure of erythromycin estolate therapy in in utero syphilis. JAMA 190:70, 1964

119. Briggs GC, Freeman RK, Jaffe SJ: p. 187. Drugs in Pregnancy and Lactation. Baltimore: Williams and Wilkins, 1994

120. Berkovitch M, Pastuszak A, Gazarian M et al: Safety of the new quinolones in pregnancy. Obstet Gynecol 84:535, 1994

121. Piper JM, Mitchel EF, Ray WA: Prenatal use of metronidazole and birth defects: no association. Obstet Gynecol 82:348, 1993

122. Burtin P, Taddio A, Ariburnu O et al: Safety of metronidazole in pregnancy: a meta-analysis. Am J Obstet Gynecol 172:525, 1995

123. Beard CM, Noller KL, O'Fallon WM et al: Lack of evidence for cancer due to use of metronidazole. N Engl J Med 301:519, 1979

124. Centers for Disease Control: Pregnancy outcomes following systemic prenatal acyclovir exposure—June 1, 1984–June 30, 1993. MMWR 42:806, 1993

125. Andrews EB, Yankaskas BC, Cordero JF et al: Acyclovir in pregnancy registry: six years' experience. Obstet Gynecol 79:7, 1992

126. Rosa FW, Baum C, Shaw M: Pregnancy outcomes after first trimester vaginitis drug therapy. Obstet Gynecol 69:751, 1987

127. Asch RH, Greenblatt RB: Update on the safety and efficacy of clomiphene citrate as a therapeutic agent. J Reprod Med 17:175, 1976

128. Riuz-Velasco V, Tolis G: Pregnancy in hyperprolactinemic women. Fertil Steril 41:793, 1984

129. Turkalj I, Braun P, Krupp P: Surveillance of bromocriptine in pregnancy. JAMA 247:1589, 1982

130. Collins E, Turner G: Salicylates and pregnancy. Lancet 2:1494, 1973

131. Stuart JJ, Gross SJ, Elrad H et al: Effects of acetylsalicyclic acid ingestion on maternal and neonatal hemostasis. N Engl J Med 307:909, 1982

132. Areilla RA, Thilenius OB, Ranniger K: Congestive heart failure from suspected ductal closure in utero. J Pediatr 75:74, 1969

133. Wallenburg HCS, Dekker GA, Makovitz JW et al: Low-dose aspirin prevents pregnancy-induced hypertension and pre-eclampsia in angiotensin-sensitive primigravidae. Lancet i:1, 1986

134. Lubbe WF, Butler WS, Palmer SJ et al: Lupus anticoagulant in pregnancy. Br J Obstet Gynaecol 91:357, 1984

135. Cowchock FS, Reece EA, Balaban D et al: Repeated fetal losses associated with antiphospholipid antibodies: a collaborative randomized trial comparing prednisone with low-dose heparin treatment. Am J Obstet Gynecol 166:1318, 1992

136. Waltman T, Tricomi V, Tavakoli FM: Effect of aspirin on bleeding time during elective abortion. Obstet Gynecol 48:108, 1976

137. Rayburn W, Shukla U, Stetson P et al: Acetaminophen pharmacokinetics: comparison between pregnant and nonpregnant women. Obstet Gynecol 155:1353, 1986

138. Tyson HK: Neonatal withdrawal symptoms associated with maternal use of propoxyphene hydrochloride (Darvon). J Pediatr 85:684, 1974

139. Berkowitz GS: Smoking and pregnancy. p. 173. In JR Niebyl (ed): Drug Use in Pregnancy. 2nd Ed. Lea & Febiger, Philadelphia, 1988

140. Alberman E, Creasy M, Elliott M et al: Maternal factors associated with fetal chromosomal anomalies in spontaneous abortions. J Obstet Gynecol 83:621, 1976

141. Martin TR, Bracken MB: Association of low birth weight with passive smoke exposure in pregnancy. Am J Epidemiol 124:633, 1986

142. Jones KL, Smith DW, Ulleland CN et al: Patterns of malformation in offspring of chronic alcoholic mothers. Lancet 2:1267, 1973

143. Rosett HL: A clinical perspective of the fetal alcohol syndrome. Alcoholism Clin Exp Res 4:119, 1980

144. Jones KL, Smith DW, Streissguth AP et al: Outcome of offspring of chronic alcoholic women. Lancet 2:1076, 1974

145. Ouellette EM, Rosett HL, Rosman NP et al: Adverse effects on offspring of maternal alcohol abuse during pregnancy. N Engl J Med 297:528, 1977

146. Mills JL, Graubard BI: Is moderate drinking during pregnancy associated with an increased risk of malformations? Pediatrics 80:309, 1987

147. Sokol RJ, Martier SS, Ager JW: The T-ACE questions: practical prenatal detection of risk-drinking. Am J Obstet Gynecol 160:863, 1989

148. Greenland S, Staisch KJ, Brown N et al: The effects of marijuana use during pregnancy: part 1—a preliminary epidemiologic study. Am J Obstet Gynecol 143:408, 1982

149. Fried PA, Buckingham M, Von Kulmiz P: Marijuana use during pregnancy and perinatal risk factors. Am J Obstet Gynecol 146:992, 1983

150. Zuckerman B, Frank DA, Hingson R et al: Effects of maternal marijuana and cocaine use on fetal growth. N Engl J Med 320:762, 1989

151. Acker D, Sachs BP, Tracey KJ et al: Abruptio placentae associated with cocaine use. Am J Obstet Gynecol 146:220, 1983

152. Little BB, Snell LM, Klein VR et al: Cocaine abuse during pregnancy: maternal and fetal implications. Obstet Gynecol 73:157, 1989

153. Bingol N, Fuchs M, Diaz V et al: Teratogenicity of cocaine in humans. J Pediatr 110:93, 1987

154. MacGregor SN, Keith LG, Chasnoff IJ et al: Cocaine use during pregnancy: adverse perinatal outcome. Am J Obstet Gynecol 157:686, 1987

155. Keith LG, MacGregor S, Friedell S et al: Substance abuse in pregnant women: recent experience at the perinatal center for chemical dependence of Northwestern Memorial Hospital. Obstet Gynecol 73:715, 1989

156. Chasnoff IJ, Griffith DR, MacGregor S et al: Temporal patterns of cocaine use in pregnancy. JAMA 261:1741, 1989

157. Volpe JJ: Effect of cocaine use on the fetus. N Engl J Med 327:399, 1992

158. Handler A, Kistin N, Davis F et al: Cocaine use during pregnancy: perinatal outcomes. Am J Epidemiol 133:818, 1991

159. Little BB, Snell LM: Brain growth among fetuses exposed to cocaine in utero: asymmetrical growth retardation. Obstet Gynecol 77:361, 1991

160. Chasnoff IJ, Chisum GM, Kaplan WE: Maternal cocaine use and genitourinary tract malformations. Teratology 37:201, 1988

161. Finnegan LP, Wapner RJ: Narcotic addiction in pregnancy. p. 203. In Niebyl JR (ed): Drug Use in Pregnancy. Lea & Febiger, Philadelphia, 1988

162. Mau G, Netter P: Kaffee- und alkoholkonsum-risikofaktoren in der schwangerschaft? Geburtsch Frauenheilkd 34:1018, 1974

163. Van den Berg BJ: Epidemiologic observations of prematurity: effects of tobacco, coffee and alcohol. In Reed DM, Stanley FJ (eds): The Epidemiology of Prematurity. Urban and Schwarzenberg, Baltimore, 1977

164. Linn S, Schoenbaum SC, Monson RR et al: No association between coffee consumption and adverse outcomes of pregnancy. N Engl J Med 306:141, 1982

165. Martin TR, Bracken MB: The association between low birth weight and caffeine consumption during pregnancy. Am J Epidemiol 126:813, 1987

166. Beaulac-Baillargeon L, Desrosiers C: Caffeine–cigarette interaction on fetal growth. Am J Obstet Gynecol 157:1236, 1987

167. Munoz LM, Lonnerdal B, Keen CL et al: Coffee consumption as a factor in iron deficiency anemia among pregnant women and their infants in Costa Rica. Am J Clin Nutr 48:645, 1988

168. Infante-Rivard C, Fernandez A, Gauthier R et al: Fetal loss associated with caffeine intake before and during pregnancy. JAMA 270:2940, 1993

169. Mills JL, Holmes LB, Aarons JH et al: Moderate caffeine use and the risk of spontaneous abortion and intrauterine growth retardation. JAMA 269:593, 1993

170. Sturtevant FM: Use of aspartame in pregnancy. Int J Fertil 30:85, 1985

171. Kesaniema YA: Ethanol and acetaldehyde in the milk and peripheral blood of lactating women after ethanol administration. J Obstet Gynaecol Br Commonw 81:84, 1974

172. Ito S, Blajchman A, Stephenson M et al: Prospective follow-up of adverse reactions in breast-fed infants exposed to maternal medication. Am J Obstet Gynecol 168:1393, 1993

173. American Academy of Pediatrics: Committee on Drugs. The transfer of drugs and other chemicals into human milk. Pediatrics 93:137, 1994

174. Johns BG, Rutherford CD, Laighton RC et al: Secretion of methotrexate into human milk. Am J Obstet Gynecol 112:978, 1972

175. Bounaneaux Y, Duren J: Busulphan in nursing infants. Ann Soc Belg Med Trop 44:381, 1964

176. Canales ES, Garcia IC, Ruiz JE et al: Bromocriptine as prophylactic therapy in prolactinoma during pregnancy. Fertil Steril 36:524, 1981

177. Sykes PA, Quarrie J, Alexander FW: Lithium carbonate and breast feeding. Br Med J 2:1299, 1976

178. Linden S, Rich CL: The use of lithium during pregnancy and lactation. J Clin Psychiatry 44:358, 1983

179. Ayd FJ Jr: Excretion of psychotropic drugs in human breast milk. Int Drug Ther News Bull 8:33, 1973

180. Berlin CM: The excretion of drugs in human milk. p. 125. In Schwartz RH, Yaffe SJ (eds): Drug and Chemical Risks to the Fetus and Newborn. Alan R Liss, New York, 1980

181. Burch KJ, Wells BG: Fluoxetine/norfluoxetine concentrations in human milk. Pediatrics 89:676, 1992

182. Niebyl JR, Blake DA, Freeman JM et al: Carbamezapine levels in pregnancy and lactation. Obstet Gynecol 53:139, 1979

183. Briggs GG, Freeman RK, Yaffe SJ: p. 126. Drugs in Pregnancy and Lactation. 4th Ed. Williams and Wilkins, Baltimore, 1994

184. Cole AP, Hailey DM: Diazepam and active metabolite in breast milk and their transfer to the neonate. Arch Dis Child 50:741, 1975

185. Pynnonen S, Sillanpaa M: Carbamazepine and mother's milk. Lancet 2:563, 1975

186. Nau H, Rating D, Hauser I et al: Placental transfer and pharmacokinetics of primidone and its metabolites phenobarbital, PEMA and hydroxypphenobarbital in neonates and infants of epileptic mothers. Eur J Clin Pharmacol 18:31, 1980

187. Cruikshank DP, Varner MW, Pitkin RM: Breast milk magnesium and calcium concentrations following magnesium sulfate treatment. Am J Obstet Gynecol 143:685, 1982

188. Ananth J: Side effects in the neonate from psychotrophic agents excreted through breastfeeding. Am J Psychiatry 135:801, 1978

189. Yurchak AM, Jusko NJ: Theophylline secretion into breast milk. Pediatrics 57:518, 1976

190. Weithmann MW, Krees SV: Excretion of chlorothiazide in human breast milk. J Pediatr 81:781, 1972

191. Miller ME, Cohn RD, Burghart PH: Hydrochlorothiazide disposition in a mother and her breast-fed infant. J Pediatr 101:789, 1982

192. Bauer JH, Pope B, Zajicek J et al: Propranolol in human plasma and breast milk. Am J Cardiol 43:860, 1979

193. Leviton AA, Marion JC: Propranolol therapy during pregnancy and lactation. Am J Cardiol 32:247, 1973

194. Anderson PO, Salter FJ: Propranolol therapy during pregnancy and lactation. Am J Cardiol 37:325, 1976

195. White WB, Andreoli JW, Wong SH et al: Atenolol in human plasma and breast milk. Obstet. Gynecol 63:42S1, 1984

196. Schmimmel MS, Eidelman AJ, Wilschanski MA et al: Toxic effects of atenolol consumed during breast feeding. J Pediatr 114:476, 1989

197. Hartikainen-Sorri AL, Heikkinen JE, Koivisto M: Pharmacokinetics of clonidine during pregnancy and nursing. Obstet Gynecol 69:598, 1987

198. Orme ME, Lewis PJ, deSwiet M et al: May mothers given warfarin breastfeed their infants? Br Med J 1:1564, 1977

199. deSwiet M, Lewis PJ: Excretion of anticoagulants in human milk. N Engl J Med 297:1471, 1977

200. Brambel CE, Hunter RE: Effect of Dicumarol on the nursing infant. Am J Obstet Gynecol 59:1153, 1950

201. Eckstein HB, Jack B: Breastfeeding and anticoagulant therapy. Lancet 1:672, 1970

202. Katz FH, Duncan BR: Entry of prednisone into human milk. N Engl J Med 293:1154, 1975

203. MacKenzie SA, Seeley JA, Agnew JE: Secretion of prednisolone into breast milk. Arch Dis Child 50:894, 1975

204. Ost L, Wettrell G, Bjorkhem I et al: Prednisolone excretion in human milk. J Pediatr 106:1008, 1985

205. Loughnan PM: Digoxin excretion in human breast milk. J Pediatr 92:1019, 1978

206. Yoshioka H, Cho K, Takimoto M et al: Transfer of Cefazolin into human milk. J Pediatr 94:151, 1979

207. Celiloglu M, Celiker S, Guven H et al: Gentamicin excretion and uptake from breast milk by nursing infants. Obstet Gynecol 84:263, 1994

208. Hosbach RE, Foster RB: Absence of nitrofurantoin from human milk. JAMA 202:1057, 1967

209. Kelsey JJ, Moser LR, Jenning JC et al: Presence of azithromycin breast milk concentrations: a case report. Am J Obstet Gynecol 170:1375, 1994

210. Meyer LJ, de Miranda, P, Sheth N et al: Acyclovir in human breast milk. Am J Obstet Gynecol 158:586, 1988

211. Nilsson S, Nygren KG, Johansson EDB: Transfer of estradiol to human milk. Am J Obstet Gynecol 132:653, 1978

212. Committee on Drugs, American Academy of Pediatrics. Breast-feeding and contraception. Pediatrics 68:138, 1981

213. Wyckerheld-Bisdom CJ: Alcohol and nicotine poisoning in nurslings due to mother's milk. Maandschr v Kindergeneesk 6:332, 1937

214. Wilson JT, Brown RD, Cherek DR et al: Drug excretion in human breast milk: principles of pharmacokinetics and projected consequences. Clin Pharmacokinet 5:1, 1980

215. Little RE, Anderson KW, Ervin CH et al: Maternal alcohol use during breastfeeding and infant mental and motor development at one year. N Engl J Med 321:425, 1989

216. Mennella JA, Beauchamp GK: The transfer of alcohol to human milk. Effects on flavor and the infant's behavior. N Engl J Med 325:981, 1991

217. Kampmann JP, Hansen JM, Johansen K et al: Propylthiouracil in human milk. Lancet 1:736, 1980

218. Cooper DS: Antithyroid drugs: to breast-feed or not to breast-feed. Am J Obstet Gynecol 157:234, 1987

219. Illingsworth RS: Abnormal substances excreted in human milk. Practitioner 171:533, 153

220. Ryu JE: Effect of maternal caffeine consumption on heart rate and sleep time of breast-fed infants. Dev Pharmacol Ther 8:355, 1985

221. Luck W, Nau H: Nicotine and cotinine concentrations in serum and urine of infants exposed via passive smoking or milk from smoking mothers. J Pediatr 107:816, 1985

222. Labrecque M, Marcoux S, Weber J-P et al: Feeding and urine cotinine values in babies whose mothers smoke. Pediatrics 83:93, 1989

223. Hanson JWM: Fetal hydantoin syndrome. Teratology 13:186, 1976

224. Lot IT, Bocian M, Pribam HW, Leitner M: Fetal hydrocephalus and ear anomalies associated with use of isotretinoin. J Pediatr 105:598, 1984

225. Shaul W, Hall JG: Multiple congenital anomalies associated with oral anticoagulants. Am J Obstet Gynecol 127:191, 1977

226. Senior B, Chernoff HL: Iodide goiter in the newborn. Pediatrics 47:510, 1971

227. Streissguth AP: CIBA Foundation Monograph 105. Pitman, London, 1984

Chapter 11

Obstetric Ultrasound: Assessment of Fetal Growth and Anatomy

Frank A. Chervenak and Steven G. Gabbe

Diagnostic ultrasound has emerged as an important tool for antepartum fetal surveillance. This technology has permitted the most accurate assessment of gestational age and has enabled the obstetrician to follow fetal growth serially and to detect fetal growth disorders. In addition, ultrasound has become an essential aid in the safe performance of a variety of diagnostic procedures, including amniocentesis, chorionic villus sampling, and cordocentesis. Finally, the use of real-time ultrasound has permitted the obstetrician to assess fetal well-being through the evaluation of fetal movements, breathing activity, tone, and the volume of amniotic fluid.

Biophysics of Ultrasound

To use ultrasound most effectively, the obstetrician must understand the basic biophysics of the technique.[1] Sound is a waveform of energy that causes small particles in a medium to oscillate. The frequency of sound refers to the number of peaks or waves that traverse a given point per unit of time and is expressed in hertz. Sound with a frequency of one cycle or one peak per second would have a frequency of 1 Hz. Ultrasound applies to high-frequency sound waves exceeding 20,000 Hz. Diagnostic ultrasound instruments operate in a higher range of frequencies, varying from 2 to 10 million Hz, or 2 to 10 MHz.

Ultrasound energy is produced by a transducer containing crystal structures that convert electrical energy to ultrasound waves and the returning echoes to electrical energy. Therefore, each crystal in the transducer acts as both a transmitter and a receiver. The power of ultrasound refers to the amount of work being done by the ultrasound field as it interacts with the medium in which the sound waves are propagating and is expressed in terms of watts. Most therapeutic equipment operates in the range of 1 to 50 W, while diagnostic and monitoring units use 0.1 to 100 mW. The standard unit used to define the power of ultrasound equipment is watts per square centimeter which describes the amount of energy delivered per given surface area.

The safety of diagnostic ultrasound has been questioned. Diagnostic ultrasound equipment generates a sound pulse every 1 msec, and the duration of the pulse is 1 μs. The time the sound pulse is off is 1,000 times greater than the time it is on. Therefore, the duty factor of diagnostic ultrasound, defined as the ratio between the emission of a sound wave and the reception of the sound wave, is 1:1,000 or 0.001. During a 15-minute diagnostic evaluation, the fetus is exposed to only 1 second of ultrasound energy. The safety of diagnostic ultrasound is discussed later in more detail.

Principles of Imaging

A two-dimensional picture is created when the returning ultrasound echoes are displayed on an oscilloscope screen.[1] The ultrasound signal returning to the transducer is converted to an electrical impulse, and the strength of that electrical impulse is directly proportional to the strength of the returning echo. The density of the medium into which the sound wave has been transmitted and through which it is reflected will determine the strength of the signal. The velocity of the reflected sound wave will be faster and its signal on the oscilloscope brighter after reflection off bone than off tissues that are less dense, such as muscle, fat, brain, or water. Air greatly decreases the transmission of sound waves. For this reason, a coupling medium or gel is applied between the surface of the transducer and the skin. A full maternal bladder provides an important window for diagnostic obstetric ultrasound. The bladder displaces gas-filled loops of bowel that would obstruct the propagation of sound, thereby providing a medium that enhances the transmission of the ultrasound waves.

Ultrasound can be used to produce diagnostic images in several ways. With M mode (motion mode), the reflected echo is displayed as a spot that generates a horizontal line on a moving display. In this way, one can examine the motion of structures against time. This technique has been widely applied in the assessment of cardiac anatomy, including the dimensions of the cardiac chambers, ventricular wall thickness, and valvular motion. B mode (brightness modulation) converts the strength of the returning echoes into signals of varying brightness that are proportional to the amplitude of the returning echo. A storage oscilloscope is used to create a compounded image of the target and, in this way, produce a two-dimensional picture. Real-time array transducer systems create these images within a fraction of a second. When the image of the fetus is compounded at a rate faster than the flicker fusion rate of the eye, the fetus will appear to be moving in real time. In a linear array transducer, a series of crystals are aligned along the transducer. The standard transducer used in these systems is 3.5 MHz. The higher the frequency of the sound, the better the reproduction and resolution, but the shallower the depth of penetration. B-mode sector scanning uses a moving transducer head containing the crystals or a wheel containing multiple transducers that moves through a prescribed sector. Sector scanning facilitates the visualization of structures behind the symphysis pubis. The obstetrician will often use a curvilinear transducer, incorporating the advantages of both the linear array and the sector transducers.

Doppler ultrasound differs significantly from the imaging techniques that have been described. In this application of ultrasound, employed in Doppler velocimetry (Ch. 12) and antepartum and intrapartum fetal heart rate monitoring (Chs. 12 and 14), the receiver detects shifts in the frequency of the returning sound waves rather than in the amplitude of these reflected echoes. Targets moving toward the receiving transducer produce an increase in the frequency of the echo, while objects moving away decrease the frequency. Doppler ultrasound uses a continuous beam of sound rather than intermittent transmission, which characterizes real-time ultrasound.

Safety of Ultrasound

Concern has been expressed by basic scientists, physicians, and consumers about the safety of diagnostic ultrasound.[2,3] The dissipation of energy from ultrasound can produce heating of the exposed tissues.[4] Ultrasound may also create cavitation or the formation of bubbles and microstreaming, the flow of liquid around these oscillating bubbles. In experimental systems, exposure to high-intensity ultrasound has been associated with alterations in immune response, increases in sister chromatid exchange frequencies,[5] fetal malformations, and growth restriction. However, these effects have *not* been seen with diagnostic ultrasound.

The total ultrasound exposure for a fetus will depend on the number of ultrasound examinations performed, the type of equipment used, and the amount of energy received, which is dependent on the duration of the examination. It has been recommended that the length of each ultrasound study and the type of equipment used be recorded.[3]

The amount of ultrasound energy received by the fetus varies directly with the intensity of the ultrasound signal and is inversely related to the square of its distance from the emitting source. If one is using a 3.5-MHz transducer, which focuses at approximately 8 cm, exposed tissues will receive only 1/64th of the energy originally emitted from the transducer. Thus far, the safe level of ultrasound intensity has been defined as less than 100 mW/cm^2 for unfocused ultrasound and below 1 W/cm^2 for focused ultrasound. Most instruments in use today produce maximum power levels less than 50 mW/cm^2 in a standard scan mode.[6]

Studies of clinical outcomes of infants exposed to ultrasound have failed to demonstrate any significant effects. No effect on neurologic function, including speech, hearing, and vision, or on school performance has been observed.[7,8] In 1993, the American Institute of Ultrasound in Medicine (AIUM) Bioeffects Committee concluded[6]:

> Diagnostic ultrasound has been in use since the late 1950s. Given its known benefits and recognized efficacy for medical diagnosis, including use during human pregnancy, the American Institute of Ultrasound in Medicine (AIUM) herein addresses the clinical safety of such use:
>
> No confirmed biological effects on patients or instrument operators caused by exposure at intensities typical of the present diagnostic ultrasound instruments have ever been reported. Although the possibility exists that such biological effects may be identified in the future, current data indicate that the benefits to patients of the prudent use of diagnostic ultrasound outweigh the risks, if any, that may be present.

In considering the safety of any diagnostic procedure, one must also consider the skill with which the examination is conducted and the way in which the results are interpreted and utilized. False-positive and false-negative diagnoses appear to be the greatest risk for the patient undergoing an obstetric ultrasound examination. What guidelines should be followed to ensure that an obstetrician is adequately trained in the application of ultrasound? AIUM has published guidelines for training in diagnostic ultrasound.[9] These recommendations call for completion of an approved residency program, fellowship, or postgraduate training with a minimum of 3 months supervised experience. The guidelines also specify involvement in the evaluation and interpretation of at least 500 diagnostic ultrasound examinations.

Transvaginal Ultrasound

Transvaginal ultrasound with its ability to use higher frequency transducers can result in better visualization of the early pregnancy.[10–14] The gestational sac, yolk sac, and embryo can be seen earlier and with more detail than transabdominal ultrasound. Extrauterine pathology, such as an ectopic pregnancy or an ovarian mass, can be better evaluated. This enhanced visualization with vaginal ultrasound is especially important in the obese patient and when there is a retroverted or myomatous uterus.

A gestational sac can be seen with transvaginal ultrasound as early as 4.5 menstrual weeks[15] (see Table 2-4). This sac is surrounded by an echogenic ring that represents trophoblastic tissue. The normal gestational sac is located in the upper uterine body and has a smooth contour and a round shape. Once seen, the gestational sac grows at a fairly constant rate of 1 mm in mean diameter per day.[16]

The yolk sac is visualized when the gestational sac is 10 mm or larger. Visualization of a yolk sac documents that an anechoic area in the uterus represents a true gestational sac and not the pseudogestational sac seen in ectopic pregnancy. Between the seventh and the thirteenth menstrual weeks the yolk sac gradually increases in diameter from about 3 to 6 mm (Figs. 11-1, 11-2).[17,18]

The amnion develops about the same time as the yolk sac, but, because it is thinner, the amnion is more difficult to visualize. It surrounds the embryo and is opposite the yolk sac. The amnion grows rapidly during early pregnancy, and fusion with the chorion is usually complete by the sixteenth week. At that time, the extra-embryonic coelom is obliterated.

Cardiac activity is usually the first manifestation of the embryo at about 6 menstrual weeks. Once the embryo is 5 mm, cardiac activity should be present; its absence is indicative of early demise.[19–21] When cardiac activity is not present and the embryo is less than 5 mm, the findings are not conclusive. The normal heart rate can be as low as 90 beats per minute at 6 menstrual weeks and increases during the first trimester.[22] Embryonic movements can be seen between 7 and 8 menstrual weeks.

Although the gestational sac can be used to date an early pregnancy, the most accurate sonographic mea-

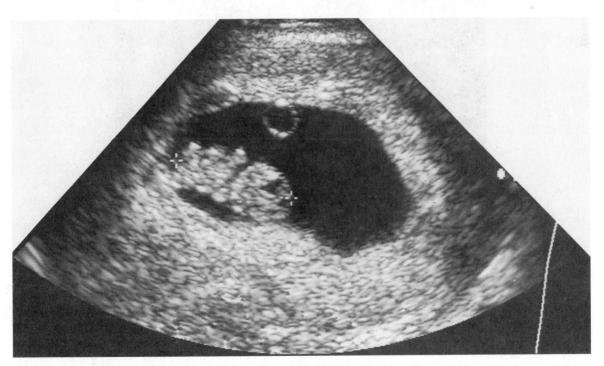

Fig. 11-1 Sonogram demonstrating crown–rump length (between crosses) of 8-week fetus. Yolk sac is in the near field.

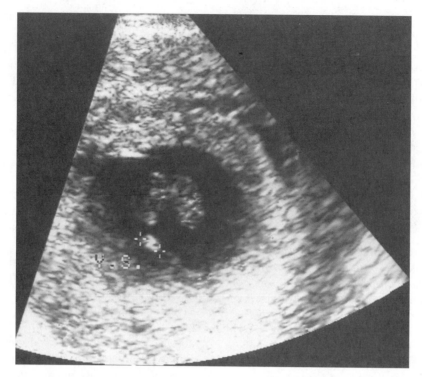

Fig. 11-2 Sonogram demonstrating embryonic demise in 7-week embryo. No heart activity was present. Calcified yolk sac is outlined by crosses.

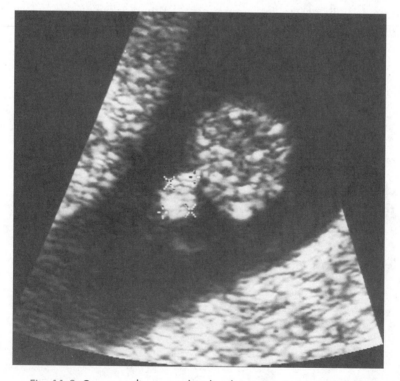

Fig. 11-3 Crosses outline normal midgut herniation in 10-week fetus.

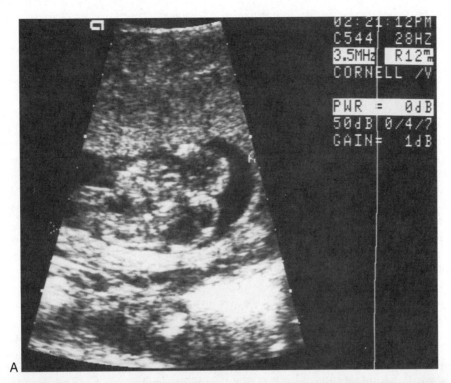

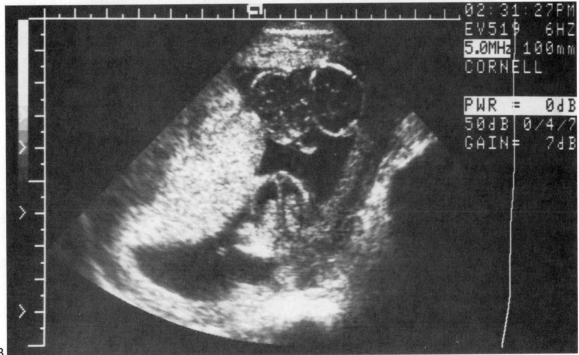

Fig. 11-4 (A) Sonogram at 11 weeks demonstrating conjoined twins. (B) Sonogram showing conjoined twins in near field and normal triplet in far field.

sure is the crown–rump length.[23] During the first trimester, this method is accurate to within 4 to 5 days. As this is the single best tool to assess gestational age at any time in pregnancy, it should be considered for patients at risk for growth restriction and other complications of pregnancy.

The embryonic pole, a flat, echogenic structure, can be visualized when it is 2 to 4 mm during the seventh menstrual week. During the eighth week a large head with a posterior cystic space, representing the rhombencephalon, can be visualized, together with the spinal column and the lower and upper extremities. By the ninth week, the falx cerebri and the choroid plexus can be seen, and, by the eleventh week, the echogenic choroid plexus fills the prominent ventricles. The cerebellum may not be visualized until after 12 weeks.[10–14]

Between the eighth and twelfth weeks, there is a normal midgut herniation (Fig. 11-3).[24] This should not be confused with an omphalocele, which can be diagnosed with certainty after that time. The liver can be seen at 9 to 10 weeks; the stomach, at 10 to 12 weeks; the bladder, at 11 to 13 weeks; and the four chambers of the heart, at about 12 weeks.[10–14]

Many of the fetal anomalies identified during a transabdominal anatomic survey at 18 to 20 weeks can be diagnosed earlier with transvaginal ultrasound. The anomalies with the most serious disruptions of anatomy, such as anencephaly, holoprosencephaly, cystic hygroma, and conjoined twins, may be detected (Fig. 11-4).[10–14] However, at this time, first trimester vaginal ultrasound is not as accurate in detecting anomalies. This is because some structures, such as the brain, are not as well developed and other structures, such as the heart, are too small to be adequately evaluated. Therefore, first trimester ultrasound should not be used as a substitute for a second trimester evaluation of anatomy.[25]

An important aspect of first trimester vaginal ultrasound is the evaluation of nuchal thickness to predict chromosomal aberrations. Nicolaides[26] has shown that a nuchal translucency of 3 mm or greater (Fig. 11-5) at 10 to 13 mm weeks of gestation occurs in 86 percent of trisomic and 4.5 percent of chromosomally normal fetuses. In addition, the observed number of trisomies when the nuchal translucency was less than 3 mm was five times less than the number expected on the basis of maternal age. This simple sonographic sign can therefore discriminate between high- and low-risk groups for trisomy and may be of great value to patients when deciding either for or against invasive testing to determine the fetal karyotype.

Although the main value of vaginal ultrasound is in early pregnancy, it may be of clinical use later in gestation. Vaginal ultrasound permits direct visualization of the internal cervical os and therefore permits accurate assessment of the location of the placenta and its distance from the internal os. The diagnosis or exclusion

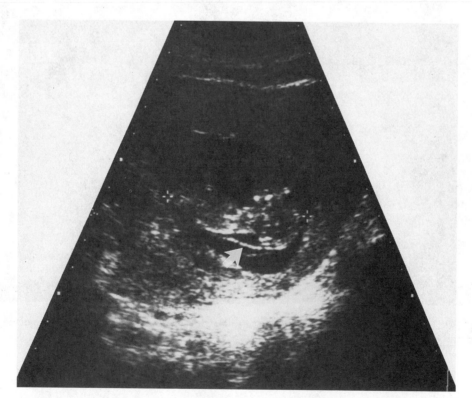

Fig. 11-5 Sonogram demonstrating nuchal translucency (arrow) greater than 3 mm in 10-week embryo.

of placenta previa is therefore facilitated.[27] In addition, because the cervix can be accurately visualized, vaginal ultrasound may identify early signs of preterm labor or incompetent cervix, such as funneling or shortening of the cervical length,[28] and thereby directly aid in patient care (Ch. 23). Lastly, vaginal ultrasound can improve visualization of intracranial anatomy when the head is engaged and permits enhanced views of cranial structures in coronal and sagittal planes.[29]

Second Trimester

Assessment of Gestational Age

When performed during the first 18 weeks of gestation, ultrasound permits an extremely accurate assessment of gestational age. The early studies of Robinson and Fleming[23] demonstrated that a fetal crown–rump length, a measurement from the top of the fetal head to its rump, could define gestational ages between 6 and 10 weeks with an error of ± 3 to 5 days (Table 11-1). In general, the gestational age of the pregnancy in weeks is equal to 6.5 plus the crown–rump length of the fetus in centimeters. When performing a crown–rump length measurement, care must be taken to avoid confusing the yolk sac with the fetal head. Beyond 12 weeks, the fetus begins to curve and the crown–rump length loses its accuracy.

The biparietal diameter (BPD) is the measurement most often used for establishing fetal gestational age. Campbell et al.[31] found the BPD to be the most accurate predictor of the estimated date of confinement (EDC) when performed between 12 and 18 weeks' gestation. In their study, the crown–rump length was as predictive of the EDC as an excellent menstrual history. The transaxial or transverse BPD is best obtained at the level of the thalami and cavum septum pellucidum (Fig. 11-6). The strong midline echo, once thought to be the falx, has now been shown to result from the apposition of the two sides of the brain. The BPD measurement is made from the outer edge of the skull to the inner edge of the opposite side.

Table 11-1 Ultrasonographic Assessment of Fetal Age

Measurement	Gestational Age (Menstrual Weeks)	Range (Days)
Crown–rump length	5–12	±3
Biparietal diameter	12–20	±8
	20–24	±12
	24–32	±15
	>32	±21
Femur length	12–20	±7
	20–36	±11
	>36	±16

(From Gabbe and Iams,[30] with permission.)

From 12 to 28 weeks' gestation, the relationship between BPD and gestational age is linear.[32] The error when measuring the BPD using a 3.5-MHz transducer is ± 1 to 1.5 min. This error will be least significant early in gestation when the fetal head is growing rapidly (Table 11-1). However, late in gestation, growth of the fetal head slows, and errors of several weeks may be made in estimating gestational age. In addition, later in gestation, the fetal head becomes more elongated in its anterior posterior plane. Such dolichocephaly may be assessed by measuring the cephalic index, the ratio of the BPD divided by the occipital frontal diameter. This ratio should normally be 0.75 to 0.85. If the ratio falls outside this range, the BPD should not be used to estimate gestational age. Femur length may be applied in such cases. At a given gestational age, a group of fetuses will vary in their BPD. This biologic variation is another source of error in estimating gestational age with advancing gestation. Sabbagha and Hughey[33] used serial determinations of BPD in the second and early third trimesters to determine a growth-adjusted sonographic age. With this technique, the significance of biologic variation can be reduced by determining the normal growth rate for a given fetus.

Assessment of Fetal Viability

Real-time ultrasound can be used to confirm the presence of fetal death in utero. The absence of fetal cardiac motion as well as the presence of fetal scalp edema and overlapping of the fetal cranial bones confirms fetal death.

Third Trimester

Evaluation of Fetal Growth

When establishing gestational age and evaluating fetal growth, it is best to evaluate a variety of parameters, including the BPD, long bones, especially the femur and humerus, as well as the abdominal circumference (AC) (Fig. 11-7), outer and inner orbital diameters, and transcerebellar diameter. The uniformity of fetal growth that characterizes early gestation is lost after 20 weeks. Therefore, a single ultrasound study performed late in pregnancy cannot accurately establish gestational age (Table 11-1). Fetal AC or perimeter measured at the level of the umbilical vein has been used not only to assess gestational age, but to detect the presence of intrauterine growth restriction (IUGR) and macrosomia (Fig. 11-7). Composite tables estimating fetal weight have been constructed by several authors and are usually based on a combination of (1) head size, as measured by BPD or head circumference (HC); (2) femur length (FL); and (3) AC. Tables by Hadlock et

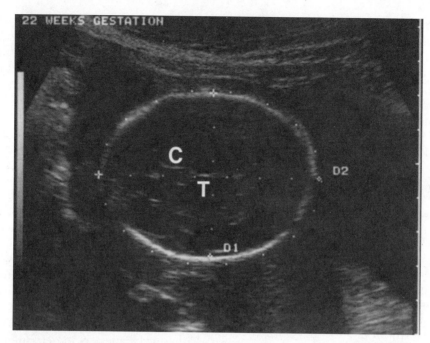

Fig. 11-6 A determination of the BPD at the level of the thalami (T) and cavum septum pellucidum (C). The BPD measurement is made from the outer edge of the skull to the opposite inner edge (D1) and on a line perpendicular to the midline. The occipitofrontal diameter (D2) is also shown. The electronic calipers (dots) have been placed to obtain a measurement of the HC.

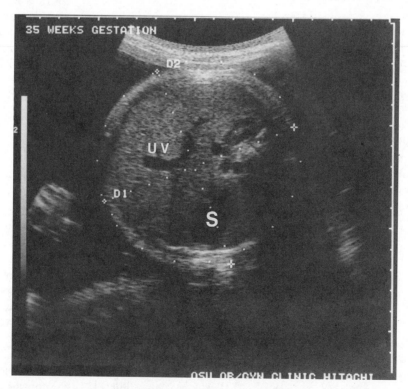

Fig. 11-7 Transverse or axial view of the abdomen demonstrates the fetal stomach (S) and umbilical vein (uv). Note that the abdomen is round and the umbilical vein is well within the substance of the liver. This is the proper level for determination of the fetal AC; electronic calipers (dots) have been placed to make this measurement. The AC may also be calculated using measurements of the anteroposterior (D1) and transverse (D2) abdominal diameters using the following formula: AC = D1 + D2 × 1.57.

al.[34] and Shepard et al.[35] are currently in most common use. Shepard et al. demonstrated that the BPD and fetal AC may be combined to calculate estimates of fetal weight that are likely to be within 10 percent of actual weight.

Abnormal Fetal Growth

Fetal growth restriction is discussed in Chapter 25.

Fetal Macrosomia

Macrosomia has been defined by some investigators as a birth weight in excess of 4,000 to 4,500 g.[36] Other studies, utilizing population-specific growth curves, categorize infants with a birth weight above the 90th percentile as large for gestational age (LGA). Excessive fetal growth resulting in macrosomia has long been recognized as an important cause of perinatal morbidity and mortality, especially in the pregnancy complicated by diabetes mellitus. At delivery, the macrosomic fetus is more likely to suffer shoulder dystocia, traumatic injury, and asphyxia.

Macrosomia in the infant of the diabetic mother (IDM) is characterized by selected organomegaly, with increases in both fat and muscle mass resulting in a disproportionate increase in the size of the abdomen and shoulders. However, brain growth is not altered, and, therefore, the HC is usually normal. Thus, the macrosomia of the IDM is asymmetric. The macrosomic infant of an obese woman without glucose intolerance will demonstrate excessive growth of *both* the AC and HC, or symmetric macrosomia.

Antenatal sonographic detection of the LGA fetus could allow optimal selection of the route of delivery to reduce the likelihood of birth trauma. Unfortunately, our clinical ability to evaluate fetal size at term remains poor, with only 35 percent of large infants being identified by excessive symphysis–fundal height measurements.[37]

Sonographic estimation of fetal weight has been employed to improve the detection of excessive growth. Using Shepard's formula, Ott and Doyle[38] determined fetal weight in 595 patients undergoing real-time ultrasound estimation within 72 hours of delivery. Overall, almost 75 percent of LGA infants were detected using an estimated fetal weight (EFW) above the 90th percentile as the cut-off for diagnosis. There were a significant number of false positives, as the predictive value of a positive test was only 63.2 percent. An EFW below the 90th percentile predicted a normally grown fetus in 96 percent of cases. Tamura et al.[39] also applied Shepard's formula in a study of 147 diabetic women during the last 2 weeks of the third trimester and reported a sensitivity of 77 percent in detecting infants with birth weights exceeding the 90th percentile.

Several studies have emphasized the limited predictive value of ultrasound to identify the macrosomic fetus.[40-43] Overall, both the sensitivity and positive predictive value in these reports range between 50 and 60 percent. It must be remembered that formulas for estimation of fetal weight are associated with a 95 percent confidence range of at least 10 to 15 percent.[34] Thus, the predicted weight using ultrasonography would have to exceed 4,700 g for all fetuses with weights in excess of 4,000 g to be accurately identified!

Measurement of the AC is probably the most reliable sonographic parameter for the detection of macrosomia. Using an AC above the 90th percentile obtained within 2 weeks of delivery, Tamura et al.[39] correctly identified 78 percent of LGA fetuses. When both the AC and EFW exceeded the 90th percentile, an LGA infant was correctly diagnosed in 88.8 percent of cases. Bochner et al.[44] used early third trimester ultrasound measurements of the AC to determine the risk for both macrosomia and birth trauma at term. In a series of 201 women with gestational diabetes mellitus, 36 of 41 cases of macrosomia were identified by the presence of an AC above the 90th percentile at 30 to 33 weeks' gestation. The false-positive rate was high, with 28 normally grown fetuses having large AC measurements. Of note, the risk for shoulder dystocia was 9.3 percent in the suspected LGA group versus 0.8 percent in the group with a normal AC measurement at 30 to 33 weeks.

Although the HC to AC ratio has been used for the detection of asymmetric IUGR (Ch. 25), this index has not been well evaluated as a predictor of macrosomia. The HC/AC ratio should be reduced in cases of asymmetric macrosomia, since abdominal size is disproportionately large compared with head growth (Fig. 11-8).[45] The HC/AC ratio does require an accurate knowledge of gestational age, since the ratio varies throughout pregnancy.

The FL/AC ratio, which is gestational age independent after 21 weeks, has also been evaluated as an indicator of fetal macrosomia. A low FL/AC ratio should reflect increased AC growth. Using a cut-off of less than 20.5 percent, representing the 10th percentile, Hadlock et al.[46] were able to detect only 63 percent of LGA fetuses. Even with a less stringent cut-off of less than 21.0 percent, Landon et al.[47] could identify only 58 percent of LGA fetuses of diabetic women studied late in the third trimester.

In summary, detection of the macrosomic infant using both clinical *and* ultrasonographic techniques remains challenging. In patients at risk for fetal macrosomia—women who have diabetes mellitus, are obese, or whose pregnancies go beyond 42 weeks—a "growth profile" including ultrasound measurements of estimated fetal weight and HC/AC and FL/AC ratios may

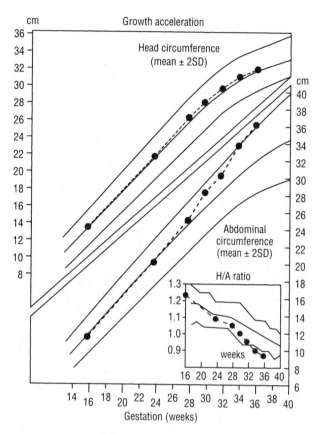

Fig. 11-8 Growth chart in a case of asymmetric macrosomia. While HC growth is preserved, AC growth is accelerated in the third trimester. For this reason, the HC/AC or H/A ratio shown in the lower right corner of the graph is reduced. This growth pattern is characteristic of the accelerated growth of the fetus of the diabetic mother. (From Chudleigh and Pearce,[45] with permission.)

improve the identification of excessive fetal growth.[48] In patients at low risk for macrosomia, a fundal height measurement of 4 cm or more than expected for gestational age should signal the need for an ultrasound study.

Assessment of Amniotic Fluid Volume

Ultrasound has proved valuable in the evaluation of amniotic fluid volume. Early application of this technology included measurements of the largest vertical pocket of fluid. Oligohydramnios, a reduction in amniotic fluid volume, was diagnosed when the largest pocket of amniotic fluid measured in two perpendicular planes was less than 1 cm. Chamberlain et al.[49] reported this degree of oligohydramnios in 0.85 percent of more than 7,500 patients evaluated. When defined in this way, oligohydramnios was associated with a 40-fold increase in perinatal mortality (187.5/1,000); a 17-fold increase in lethal congenital anomalies such as renal agenesis, polycystic kidney disease, or complete

obstruction of the genitourinary system (9.4 percent); and an 8-fold increase in growth restriction (39 percent). Hydramnios or excessive amniotic fluid was diagnosed when the largest pocket of amniotic fluid exceeded 8 cm in two perpendicular planes.[50]

Several investigators have questioned the diagnostic accuracy of the largest or maximum vertical pocket concept as an index of overall amniotic fluid volume and perinatal outcome. Bottom et al.[51] reported that subjective assessment of amniotic fluid volume was as valuable as measurements of the maximum vertical pocket. They did note that suspected fetal growth restriction and suspected post-term gestation were negatively correlated with the maximum vertical pocket, while suspected fetal growth acceleration and increasing birth weight were positively correlated. Hoddick et al.[52] reported poor sensitivity when applying the 1-cm vertical pocket as an index of oligohydramnios for the detection of IUGR.

In an effort to find a more reproducible and quantitative technique to assess amniotic fluid volume, Phelan and colleagues[53,54] developed the amniotic fluid index (AFI). The AFI measurement is performed with the pa-

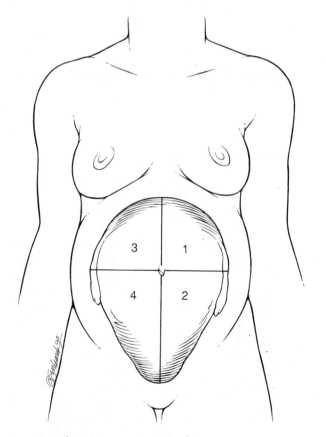

Fig. 11-9 The AFI measurement utilizes ultrasound to assess the depth of fluid pockets in each quadrant of the uterus. Note that the umbilicus divides the uterus into upper and lower halves, and the linea nigra divides the uterus into right and left halves.

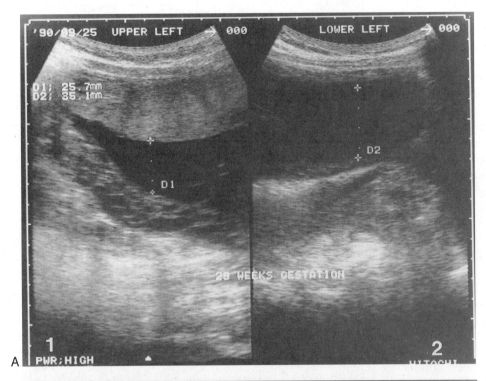

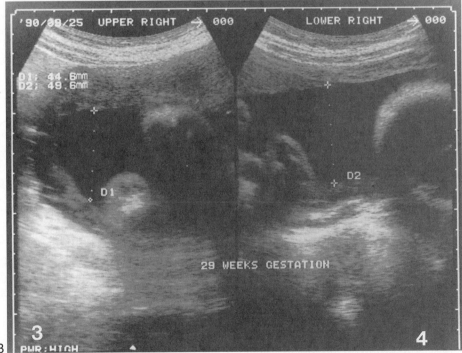

Fig. 11-10 (A & B) Ultrasound determination of the AFI at 29 weeks' gestation. The numbers in the corner of each ultrasound section correspond to those in Figure 11-9. The AFI was 15.6 cm, which is normal at this gestational age (see Table 11-2).

tient in the supine or semi-Fowler positive position. The maternal abdomen is divided into quadrants (Fig. 11-9 and 11-10). The umbilicus is used as one reference point to divide the uterus into upper and lower halves, and the linea nigra is used as the midline to divide the uterus into right and left halves. The ultrasound transducer head is then placed on the maternal abdomen along the longitudinal axis. The transducer head is maintained perpendicular to the floor, and the vertical diameter of the largest amniotic fluid pocket in each quadrant is identified and measured. The total of each of these measurements is summed to obtain the AFI in centimeters. If a fetal extremity or portion of the umbilical cord is observed in the quadrant to be measured, the transducer head is moved slightly to exclude these structures. A linear array, sector, or curvilinear transducer may be used to determine the AFI.[55] Care must be taken to avoid excessive pressure on the transducer, as this might decrease the AFI.[56] Moore and Cayle[57] have modified this approach by measuring only those amniotic fluid pockets completely clear of cord or extremities. The technique is extremely reproducible, with intraobserver and interobserver variations averaging 1.0 and 2.0 cm, respectively.[57–59] When the AFI is determined in a patient at 20 weeks' gestation or lower, the uterus is divided into halves using the linea nigra, and the largest pocket identified in each half is added to produce an AFI.

Using this technique, Phelan et al.[53] found that the mean AFI in over 350 pregnancies at 36 to 42 weeks was 12.9 ± 4.6 cm. Patients with an AFI less than 5.0 cm at term were considered to have oligohydramnios, while those with an AFI of 20 cm or greater were considered to have polyhydramnios. When the AFI fell below 5 cm, Rutherford et al.[58] noted that the frequency of nonreactive nonstress tests, fetal heart rate decelerations, meconium staining, cesarean sections for fetal distress, and low Apgar scores increased. Based on a maximum vertical pocket of 8 cm or more to define polyhydramnios, fetal structural anomalies have been observed in 36 to 63 percent of cases with polyhydramnios.[60,61]

Moore and his colleagues have demonstrated the validity of the AFI and established normative values for this measurement. In a pregnant sheep model, Moore and Brace[62] first found that the AFI demonstrated a close linear relationship to the actual amount of amniotic fluid and was 88 percent accurate in quantitating amniotic fluid volume. Moore and Cayle[57] next studied 791 uncomplicated pregnancies prospectively to establish normal values for the AFI (Table 11-2). At term, the mean AFI was 11.5 cm, while the 5th and 95th percentiles were 6.8 and 19.6 cm, respectively. These values are similar to those reported by Phelan and coworkers. Moore[63] has also demonstrated the superiority of

Table 11-2 Amniotic Fluid Index Percentile Values (mm)

| Week | Percentile | | | | | n |
	2.5th	5th	50th	95th	97.5th	
16	73	79	121	185	201	32
17	77	83	127	194	211	26
18	80	87	133	202	220	17
19	83	90	137	207	225	14
20	86	93	141	212	230	25
21	88	95	143	214	233	14
22	89	97	145	216	235	14
23	90	98	146	218	237	14
24	90	98	147	219	238	23
25	89	97	147	221	240	12
26	89	97	147	223	242	11
27	85	95	146	226	245	17
28	86	94	146	228	249	25
29	84	92	145	231	254	12
30	82	90	145	234	258	17
31	79	88	144	238	263	26
32	77	86	144	242	269	25
33	74	83	143	245	274	30
34	72	81	142	248	278	31
35	70	79	140	249	279	27
36	68	77	138	249	279	39
37	66	75	135	244	275	36
38	65	73	132	239	269	27
39	64	72	127	226	255	12
40	63	71	123	214	240	64
41	63	70	116	194	216	162
42	63	69	110	175	192	30

(From Moore and Cayle,[57] with permission.)

the AFI over the maximum vertical pocket in detecting abnormalities of amniotic fluid volume. In this study of 1,178 high-risk patients, oligohydramnios was defined as an AFI less than the 5th percentile for gestational age, while hydramnios was defined as an AFI greater than the 95th percentile for gestational age. The ability of a maximum vertical pocket of 3 cm or less to identify cases with oligohydramnios by AFI was poor, with a sensitivity of only 42 percent and a positive predictive value of 51 percent. Moore[63] noted that 58 percent of cases with oligohydramnios by AFI had normal values when using the largest vertical pocket technique. The detection of polyhydramnios, defined as a maximum vertical pocket of 8.0 cm or greater, was also limited in cases identified to have excessive amniotic fluid by AFI.

In summary, while there is reasonably good correlation between quantitation of amniotic fluid volume using subjective assessment of amniotic fluid volume, measurements of the maximum vertical pocket, and AFI, the AFI appears to have significant advantages.

This index appears highly reproducible and may, therefore, be more uniformly utilized by a number of different examiners. Furthermore, the AFI may be applied with greater reliability at each gestational age using the normative values that have been developed by Moore and Cayle.[57] Finally, the AFI has greater sensitivity and predictive value in evaluating the pregnancy at risk for oligohydramnios and polyhydramnios.

Sonographic Evaluation of Fetal and Placental Anatomy

Evaluation of fetal and placental anatomy is an integral part of ultrasound examinations during the second and third trimesters. A basic ultrasound examination that documents fetal life, fetal number, fetal presentation, gestational age and growth, amniotic fluid volume, and placental localization without an evaluation of fetal anatomy, therefore, should be considered incomplete. The following is meant to represent the examination of fetal anatomy that should be part of the basic study. A comprehensive sonographic examination of fetal anatomy is often more detailed when it is targeted to look for a certain anomaly.[64-73]

The fetal skull should be elliptical with the cranium ossified and intact. The ventricular system should be evaluated by assessment of the width of the atrium (Fig. 11-11), and the cerebellum should be visualized (Fig. 11-12) and nuchal thickness measured. An attempt should be made to visualize the face, especially to rule

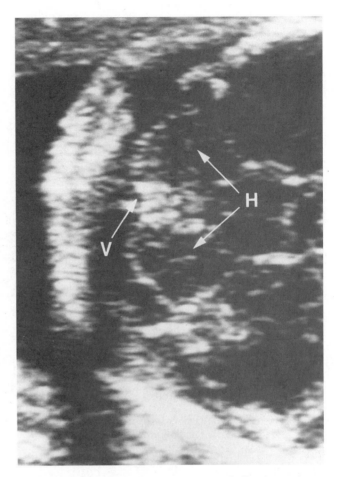

Fig. 11-12 Sonogram demonstrating cerebellar hemispheres (H). V, cerebellar vermis.

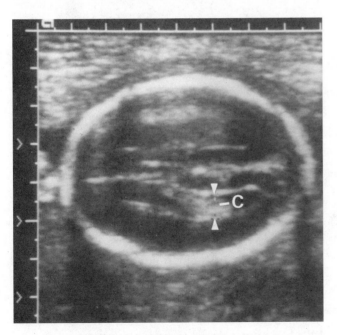

Fig. 11-11 Transverse sonogram of fetal skull demonstrating normal ovoid contour. Arrows define width of the atrium of the lateral ventricle. C, choroid plexus.

out a facial cleft (Fig. 11-13). The spine is easier to evaluate in its entirety in the second trimester than in the third. A sagittal sonogram should be complemented by a series of transverse sonograms to identify normal anterior and normal posterior ossification elements (Figs. 11-14 and 11-15). A four-chambered view of the heart should be obtained. Ventricles and atria of equal and appropriate sizes and an intact ventricular septum should be observed (Fig. 11-16). Evaluation of outflow tracts should be attempted (Fig. 11-17). The fetal bladder (Fig. 11-18), stomach (Fig. 11-19), and kidneys (Fig. 11-20) should be visualized. The abdominal wall should be intact (Fig. 11-21). The long bones of at least the lower extremities should be visualized (Figs. 11-22, 11-23). Although fetal gender often may be identified in the second and third trimesters, this should not be considered an integral part of the examination[64-73] (Figs. 11-24 and 11-25).

In addition to the assessment of placental location, ultrasound can provide an evaluation of placental anatomy[25-26] (Fig. 11-26; see also Fig. 2-4). Although difficult during the first trimester, the location of the pla-

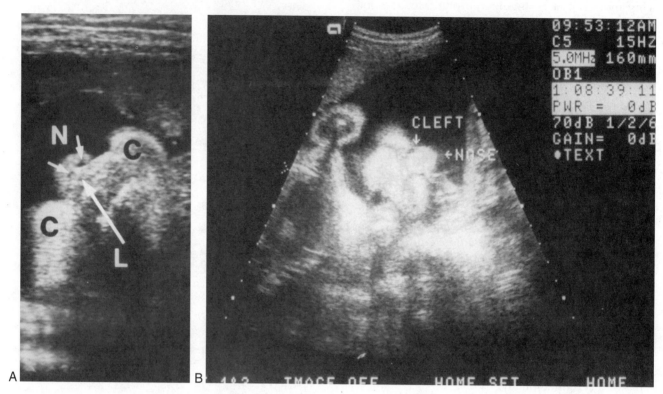

Fig. 11-13 (A) Sonogram of normal fetal face demonstrating upper lip (L), cheeks (C), and nostril (N). (B) Sonogram demonstrating cleft lip (arrow).

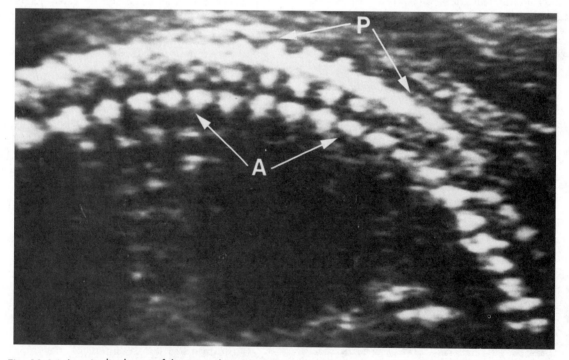

Fig. 11-14 Longitudinal view of the spine demonstrating anterior (A) and posterior (P) ossification elements.

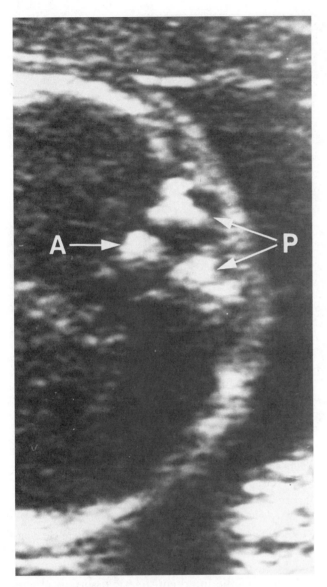

Fig. 11-15 Ttransverse view of the spine demonstrating anterior (A) and posterior (P) ossification elements.

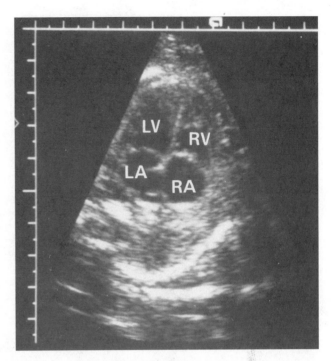

Fig. 11-16 Four-chamber view of the heart. LA, left atrium; LV, left ventricle; RA, right atrium; RV, right ventricle.

centa can be clearly established by the second trimester. Early in gestation, the placental substance is homogeneous, but, as pregnancy advances, echospared areas corresponding to flow of blood from the maternal spiral arterioles and calcium deposition can be seen. The chorionic plate, the fetal surface of the placenta, is initially straight and well defined, but develops indentations as gestation progresses. The basal layer of the placenta is characterized by a hypoechoic area representing venous blood flow. As gestation advances, the basal layer reveals more calcifications. A system of placental grading based on the characteristics of the chorionic plate, placental substance, and basal layer has been utilized to predict fetal pulmonary maturity (Ch. 12).

Placental thickness can be directly related to gesta-

tional age, with the thickness of the placenta in millimeters corresponding approximately to the weeks of gestation. For example, at 20 weeks' gestation, the placenta will be approximately 20 mm thick. Placentomegaly, a placenta of greater than normal thickness, has been associated with maternal diabetes mellitus, fetal hydrops, placental hemorrhage, intrauterine infection including syphilis, chromosomal abnormalities, and hydatidiform mole (Fig. 11-27), or a placental chorioangioma (Fig. 11-28).

Ultrasound Diagnosis of Fetal Anomalies

Antenatal ultrasound scanning at about 18 to 20 weeks of gestation permits the detection of most major fetal structural anomalies.[64,65,71,77-79] It is important to appreciate, however, that even a thorough ultrasound evaluation during the second trimester will not detect all structural malformations. Anomalies such as hydrocephalus, duodenal atresia, microcephaly, achondroplasia, and polycystic kidneys may not manifest until the third trimester, when the degree of anatomic distortion is sufficient to be sonographically detectable.

What fetal malformations should be identified during a basic ultrasound examination? Nelson et al.[80] surveyed 27 radiologists and 15 obstetricians with expertise in this field who were told that the patient was referred for a dating scan between 20 and 24 weeks' gestation and had no complicating obstetric problems.

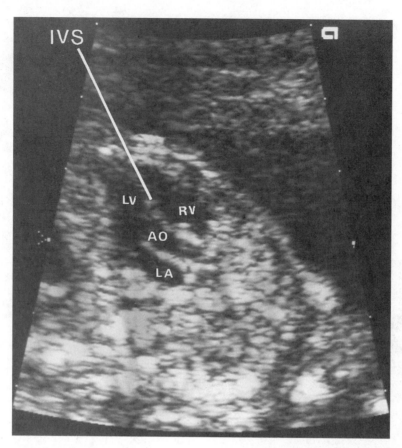

Fig. 11-17 Sonogram demonstrating outflow tract (AO), left ventricle (LV), left atrium (LA), and right ventricle (RV). The anterior wall of the aortic outflow tract is contiguous with the interventricular septum (IVS).

The anomalies believed to be observable in the majority of cases included anencephaly, hydranencephaly, ventriculomegaly of greater than 15 mm, alobar holoprosencephaly, open spina bifida, a large amount of ascites, bilateral hydronephrosis greater than 20 mm, omphalocele, gastroschisis, and hydrothorax with a mediastinal shift. A useful classification of fetal anomalies is based on the nature of the dysmorphology that permits sonographic detection.

Absence of a Normally Present Structure

A dramatic example of the absence of a structure normally detected by ultrasound is anencephaly, the absence of calvaria and forebrain (Fig. 11-29). Ultrasound clearly reveals the absence of echogenic skull bones and the presence of a heterogeneous mass of cystic tissue, called the area cerebrovasculosa, which replaces well-defined cerebral structures. In 1972, anencephaly was the first fetal anomaly to be diagnosed with sufficient certainty to support a decision to terminate a pregnancy.[81]

Alobar holoprosencephaly is the absence of midline cerebral structures, resulting from incomplete cleavage of the primitive forebrain. The "midline echo" of the fetal head, normally generated by acoustic interfaces in the area of the interhemispheric fissure, is absent. However, absence of a midline echo is not specific to alobar holoprosencephaly; an additional sonographic sign should be sought to confirm a diagnosis, which may include hypotelorism, nasal anomalies, and facial clefts. The detection of the facial aberration helps to confirm the diagnosis of alobar holoprosencephaly (Fig. 11-30).[82]

The kidneys are normally visualized as bilateral, ovoid, paraspinal masses with echospared renal pelves. When not visualized, the diagnosis of renal agenesis should be suspected. Severe oligohydramnios and the inability to visualize the bladder support the diagnosis of renal agenesis. Although antenatal diagnosis of renal agenesis is possible, false-positive and false-negative diagnoses occur from inadequate visualization due to the presence of oligohydramnios and simulation of the sonographic appearance of kidneys by the ovoid-shaped adrenal glands.[83]

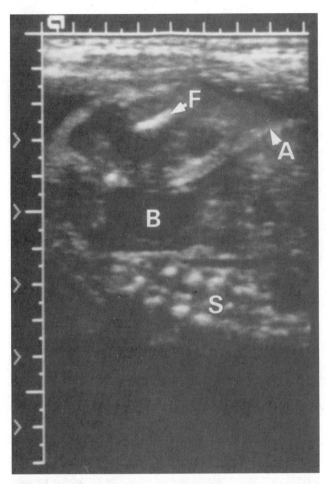

Fig. 11-18 Sonogram demonstrating fetal bladder (B), spine (S), abdominal wall (A), and femur (F).

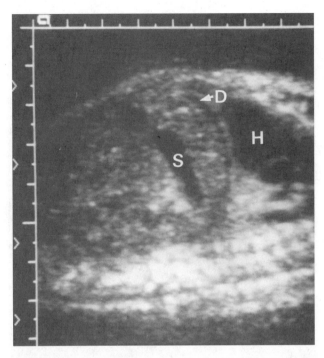

Fig. 11-19 Sonogram demonstrating fetal stomach (S), diaphragm (D), and heart (H).

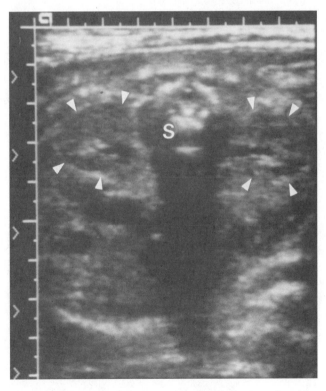

Fig. 11-20 Sonogram demonstrating fetal kidneys outlined by arrows. S, fetal spine.

Presence of an Additional Structure

Masses that distort normal fetal anatomy can be readily identified with ultrasound. Teratomas are the most common neoplasms of fetuses. They are derived from pluripotent cells and are composed of a diversity of tissue foreign to the anatomic site from which they arise. They may be visualized as distortions of fetal contour, often in the sacrococcygeal area or along the fetal midline. The internal sonographic appearance, characterized by irregular cystic and solid areas and occasional calcifications, helps to identify the lesion (Fig. 11-31).[84]

Fetal cystic hygromas are fluid-filled masses of the fetal neck that arise from abnormal lymphatic development. They are generally anechoic, with scattered septations and the presence of a midline septum arising from the nuchal ligament. If the lymphatic disorder causing the hygromas is widespread, it may produce fetal hydrops and intrauterine death[85,86] (Fig. 11-32).

Fetal hydrops or fetal anasarca may be identified by the distortion of the normal fetal surface by skin edema.

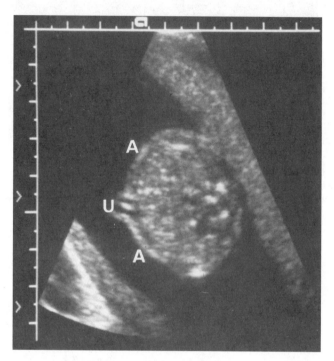

Fig. 11-21 Sonogram demonstrating intact abdominal wall (A) and umbilical cord insertion (U).

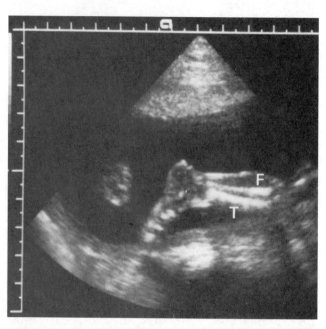

Fig. 11-23 Sonogram demonstrating tibia (T) and fibula (F).

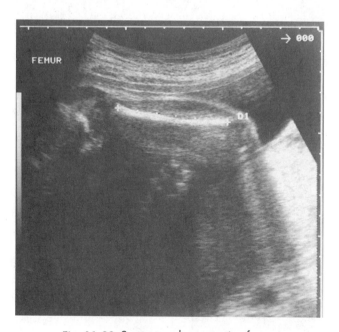

Fig. 11-22 Sonogram demonstrating femur.

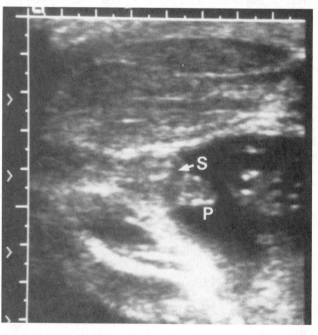

Fig. 11-24 Sonogram demonstrating male genitalia, P, penis; S, scrotum.

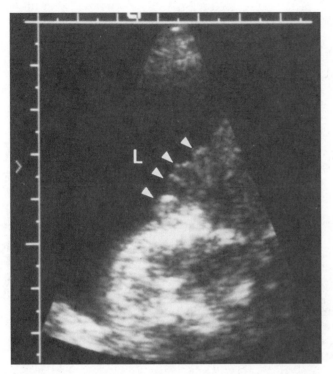

Fig. 11-25 Sonogram demonstrating female genitalia. L, labia.

Ascites, pleural effusions, and pericardial effusions also may be identified. The etiologies of fetal hydrops are many and varied[87–89] (Fig. 11-33).

Herniation Through Structural Defects

A common theme in the development of the fetus is the formation of compartments containing vital structures by folding and midline fusion. Incomplete fusion in a variety of locations can lead to defects and herniations of contained structures.[90]

The neural tube and overlying mesoderm begin their closure in the region of the fourth somite, with fusion extending both rostrally and caudally during the fourth week of fetal life.[90] Incomplete closure at the rostral end produces cephaloceles, with herniations of meninges and, frequently, of brain substance through a defect in the cranium (Fig. 11-34).[91] Failed fusion at the caudal end produces spina bifida with protruding meningoceles and meningomyeloceles (Fig. 11-35). Sonographic diagnosis of each of these anomalies depends on the demonstration of a defect in the normal structure of the cranium or spine and of a protruding sac, often containing tissue.[92,93]

The Arnold-Chiari malformation is an anomaly of the hindbrain that has two components. The first is a variable displacement of a tongue of spinal canal. The second is a similar caudal dislocation of the medulla

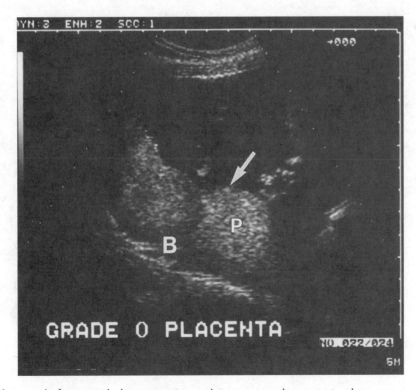

Fig. 11-26 Ultrasound of a normal placenta at 24 weeks' gestation, demonstrating homogeneous placenta substance (P), smooth chorionic plate (arrow), and hypoechoic basal layer (B).

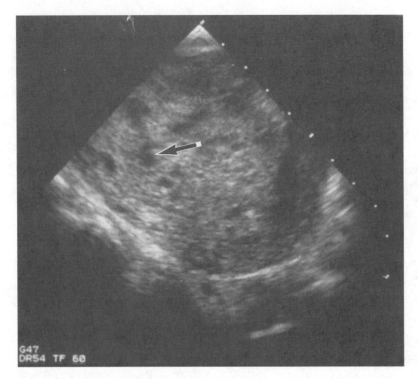

Fig. 11-27 On ultrasound, a hydatidiform mole reveals hypoechoic structures (arrow) corresponding to enlarged, hydropic villi.

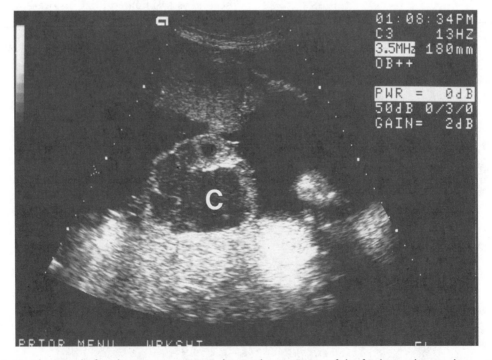

Fig. 11-28 Ultrasound of a chorioangioma (C), a benign hemangioma of the fetal vasculature, demonstrates a large, hypoechoic mass. Large chorioangiomas, those greater than 5 cm in diameter, may be associated with hydramnios and preterm labor.

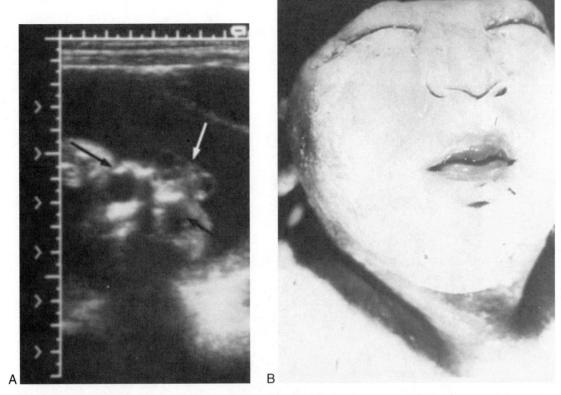

Fig. 11-29 (A) Coronal sonogram of fetal head demonstrating anencephaly. Black arrows point to orbits. White arrow points to area cerebrovasculosa. (B) Postmortem photograph of infant with anencephaly demonstrating prominent area cerebrovasculosa.

and fourth ventricle. Most, if not all, cases of spina bifida are complicated by the Arnold-Chiari malformation.[94] The Arnold-Chiari malformation can serve, therefore, as an important marker for spina bifida. Two characteristic sonographic signs (the "lemon" and the "banana") of the Arnold-Chiari malformation have been described.[95] A scalloping of the frontal bones can give a lemon-like configuration, in axial section, to the skull of an affected fetus during the second trimester. The caudal displacement of the cranial contents within a pliable skull is thought to produce this scalloping effect. Similarly, as the cerebellar hemispheres are displaced into the cervical canal, they are flattened rostrocaudally, and the cisterna magna is obliterated, thus producing a flattened, centrally curved, banana-like sonographic appearance. In extreme instances, the cerebellar hemispheres may be absent from view during fetal head scanning. These characteristic cranial signs are valuable adjuncts to the sonographer in the search for spina bifida (Fig. 11-36).[95]

Omphaloceles result from failure of the intestines to retract from their temporary location in the umbilical cord and the subsequent herniation of other abdominal contents, including both hollow and solid structures contained within a peritoneal sac. Insertion of the umbilical cord into the sac helps to differentiate an omphalocele from gastroschisis, which has no covering membrane. Nonetheless, distinguishing these two entities may be difficult[96] (Figs. 11-37, 11-38).

The diaphragm forms from four separate structures that fuse to separate the pleural and peritoneal cavities. When a diaphragmatic hernia is present, abdominal contents may be visualized within the chest on transverse sonographic scanning. A disruption in this development of the diaphragm may be seen in the sagittal plane.[97,98]

Dilatation Behind an Obstruction

In this class of anomalies, the structural defect itself is rarely seen. Rather, what is observed is the distention of structures behind a defect. Such dilatation is caused by obstruction to the normal flow of cerebrospinal fluid, urine, or swallowed amniotic fluid.

Hydrocephalus is characterized by a relative enlargement of the cerebroventricular system with an accompanying increase of pressure of the cerebrospinal fluid within the fetal head. Hydrocephalus is suggested by a lateral ventricular atrial width greater than 1 cm,[99–101] a dangling choroid plexus,[102] and an asymmetric ap-

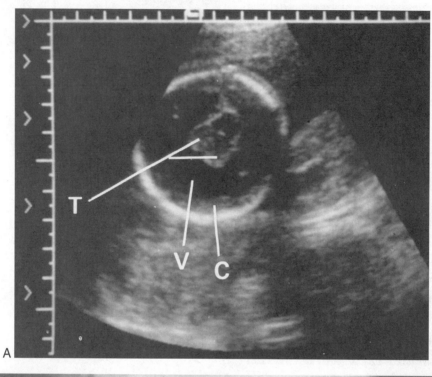

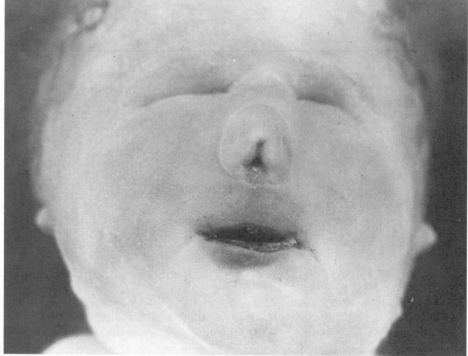

Fig. 11-30 (A) Cranial sonogram demonstrating alobar holoprosencephaly. V, common ventricle; T, prominent fused thalamus; C, compressed cerebral cortex. (B) Cebocephaly with hypotelorism and normally placed nose with a single nostril. (From Chervenak et al.,[82] with permission.)

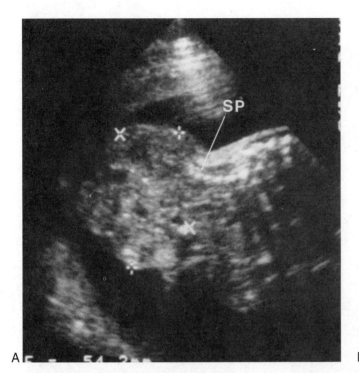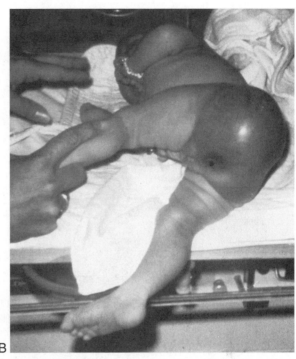

Fig. 11-31 (A) Sonogram of sacrococcygeal teratoma outlined by Xs protruding beneath fetal spine (SP). (B) Neonate with sacrococcygeal teratoma. (From Chervenak et al.,[84] with permission.)

pearance of the choroid plexus.[101,102] The location of the obstruction may be determined by observing which portions of the ventricular system are enlarged (Fig. 11-39). There is a frequent association of fetal hydrocephalus with other anomalies, especially spina bifida.[103]

Fetal small bowel obstruction may cause dilatation proximal to the area of obstruction. Duodenal atresia has been observed to produce its characteristic "double bubble" sign, consisting of enlarged duodenum and stomach with narrowing at the pylorus and duodenum and is commonly associated with Down syndrome[104] (Fig. 11-40). Obstruction in the lower gastrointestinal tract (e.g., imperforate anus) is generally not detected on antenatal ultrasound unless there is an associated lesion.

Obstructions to urinary flow with proximal dilatation can occur at the uteropelvic and uterovesicular junctions (Fig. 11-41). These are commonly unilateral defects, whereas obstruction at the urethra from posterior urethral valves characteristically produces bilateral dilatation of the ureters and renal pelves.[106–108] When a posterior urethral valve produces a complete obstruction, renal dysplasia and pulmonary hypoplasia may result.

Abnormal Fetal Biometry

Several fetal anomalies are best diagnosed not by observing alterations in shape or consistency, but by determining abnormalities in size. The science of fetal biometry has generated many nomograms defining normal values for parts of the fetal anatomy at various gestational ages.[109]

Fetal microcephaly is usually the result of an underdeveloped brain. Although commonly associated with cerebral structural malformations, microcephaly may be produced by a brain that is normal in configuration but merely small. The accurate diagnosis of microcephaly has proved challenging because compressive forces within the uterus may distort the shape of the fetal head. The best correlation between microcephaly diagnosed in utero and neonatal microcephaly is made when multiple parameters are measured and suggest a small head.[110,111]

A variety of skeletal dysplasias may affect the growth of long bones. Measurement may suggest a particular skeletal dysplasia, depending on which bones are foreshortened. The shape of these bones, their density, the presence of fractures, or the absence of specific bones may aid in differentiating the various bony abnormalities.[112]

When interorbital distances are inconsistent with gestational age, hypotelorism or hypertelorism may be suggested. Abnormal distance between the orbits may serve as a clue to several malformation syndromes (e.g., alobar holoprosencephaly[82] and median cleft face syndrome[113]) (Fig. 11-42).

The internal architecture of the kidneys may be difficult to assess in the presence of oligohydramnios. The

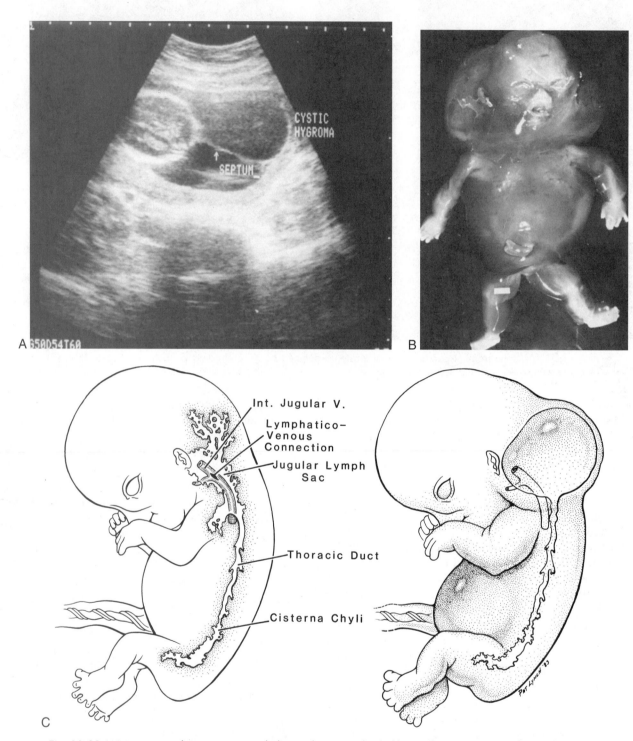

Fig. 11-32 (A) Sonogram demonstrating nuchal cystic hygroma divided by midline septum. (B) Postmortem photograph demonstrating fetus with cystic hygroma protruding from posterolateral neck. (C) Lymphatic system in normal fetus with patent connection between jugular lymph sac and internal jugular vein (left), and fetus with cystic hygroma and hydrops from failed lymphaticovenous connection (right). (Fig. B is from Chervenak et al.,[67] with permission; Fig. C is from Chervenak et al.,[85] with permission.)

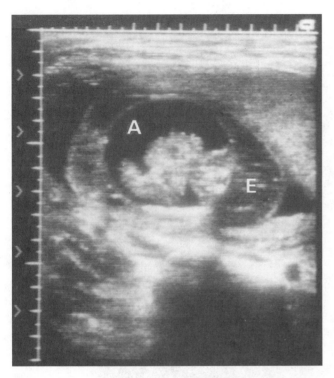

Fig. 11-33 Transverse sonogram through fetal abdomen demonstrating fetal hydrops. E, edema of abdominal wall; A, ascites.

diagnosis of polycystic kidneys thus is aided by renal measurement. In addition to being echogenic, polycystic kidneys usually are enlarged and display an abnormally increased kidney circumference/abdominal circumference ratio.[114,115]

Absent or Abnormal Fetal Motion

Abnormalities in fetal motion may suggest a malformation that cannot itself be seen. Although the fetus normally can assume contorted positions in utero, the persistence of such an unusual posture over time may suggest an orthopedic or neurologic anomaly such as clubfoot (Fig. 11-43)[116] or arthrogryposis.[117]

The fetal heart is the most conspicuously dynamic part of the fetus. Real-time ultrasound is invaluable in diagnosing most fetal cardiac anomalies (Fig. 11-44). A four-chamber view of the heart should be obtained in any obstetric ultrasound examination in which fetal anatomy is surveyed. Examination of the fetal outflow tracts increases the detection of heart anomalies. In cases of a suspected fetal arrhythmia, atrial and ventricular rates can be determined.[118–123]

Ultrasound Detection of Chromosomal Abnormalities

Ultrasound examination can suggest a chromosomal aberration. Sonographic markers for the most serious karyotype abnormalities are often present. Holopro-

sencephaly, facial clefts, hypotelorism, omphalocele, polydactyly, and heart defects are associated with trisomy 13, while growth restriction, micrognathus, overlapping fingers, omphalocele, horseshoe kidney, and heart defects are associated with trisomy 18. Early onset severe growth restriction, large head, syndactyly, and heart defects suggest triploidy. Turner syndrome (45X) is classically associated with nuchal cystic hygroma, but this ultrasound finding can occur in a wide variety of genetic disorders.[64,68]

Major structural malformations, including hydrops, duodenal atresia, and heart defects, are associated with trisomy 21 but are detected sonographically in only about 30 percent of cases.[126,127] Nuchal skin thickness, defined as 6 mm or more, is a useful screening tool for trisomy 21 and other chromosomal malformations (Fig. 11-45).[123,128,129] Other sonographic signs used to screen for Down syndrome include short femur, short humerus, pyelectasis, mild cerebral ventriculomegaly, clinodactyly with hypoplastic middle phalanx of the fifth digit, widely spaced first and second toes, low set ears, echogenic bowel, and a single palmar crease.[126,127,130]

Choroid plexus cysts can occur in about 1 percent of fetuses and, while most are closely associated with trisomy 18, can be a marker for other chromosomal abnormalities[131,132] (Fig. 11-46). The need for a karyotype determination when the only structural abnormality seen is a choroid plexus cyst remains controversial.[133,134] Benaceraff et al.[133] have calculated that the performance of amniocentesis for choroid plexus cysts would result in more fetal loss than in detection of unsuspected chromosomal aberrations. In the authors' view, when a choroid plexus cyst is identified with ultrasound, it should be disclosed to the pregnant woman and amniocentesis offered, but not recommended.

In summary, if a major structural malformation is detected with ultrasound, karyotype determination should be considered by the pregnant woman. At the present time, nuchal thickness is a most clinically useful ultrasound marker for trisomy, with the relative value of other ultrasound markers under investigation.

Management of a Pregnancy Complicated By an Ultrasonically Diagnosed Fetal Anomaly

If a fetal anomaly is diagnosed by obstetric ultrasound, the fetus should be carefully evaluated for other anomalies before management options can be considered. Echocardiography and karyotype determination should usually be part of this evaluation. Copel et al.[135] have shown that 23 percent of fetuses referred for echocardiography because of an extracardiac anomaly had

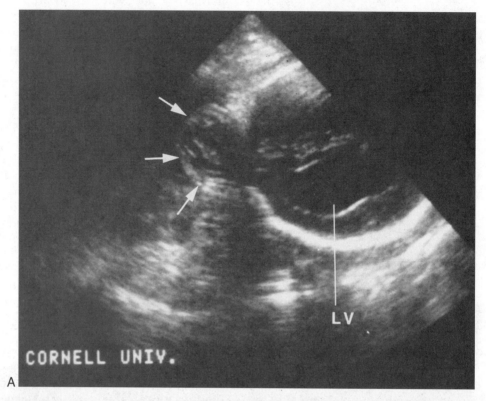

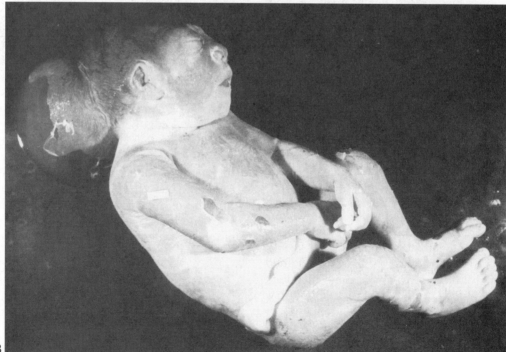

Fig. 11-34 (A) Occipital encephalocele (outlined by arrows). LV, dilated lateral ventricle. (B) Large encephalocele with resultant microcephaly. (From Chervenak et al.,[91] with permission.)

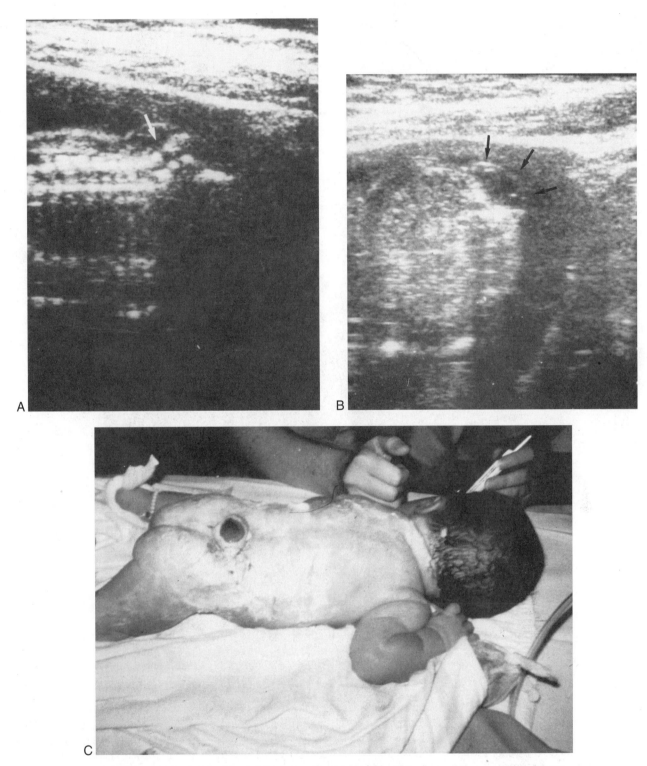

Fig. 11-35 (A) Longitudinal sonogram of fetal spine with arrows pointing to meningomyelocele. (B) Transverse sonogram through fetal spine with arrow pointing to meningomyelocele. (C) Intact lumbosacral meningomyelocele in neonate. (From Chervenak et al.,[67] with permission.)

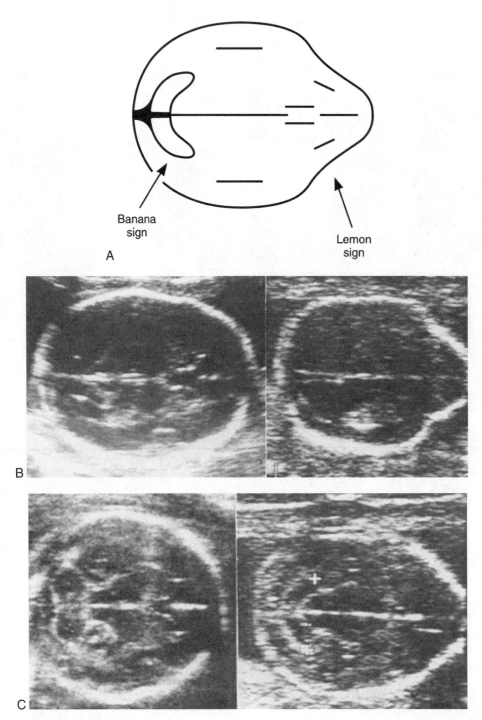

Fig. 11-36 (A) Diagrammatic representation of "banana" and "lemon" signs in fetus with spina bifida. (B) Transverse section of normal fetal head in an 18-week fetus at level of cavum septi pellucidi (left). Transverse section of fetal head at level of cavum septi pellucidi in an 18-week fetus with open spina bifida showing "lemon" and "banana" sign (right). (C) Suboccipital bregmatic view of fetal head in an 18-week fetus with normal cerebellum and cisterna magna (left). Suboccipital bregmatic view of fetal head in an 18-week fetus with open spina bifida, demonstrating "banana" sign (+). (From Nicolaides et al.,[95] with permission.)

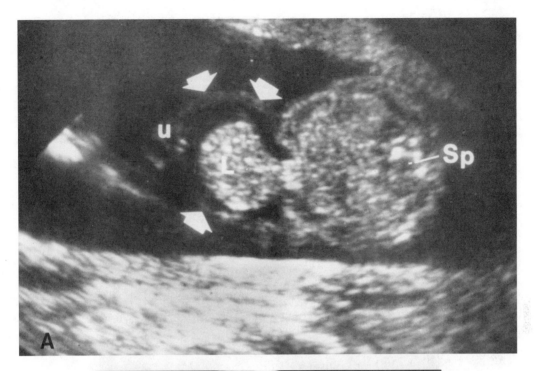

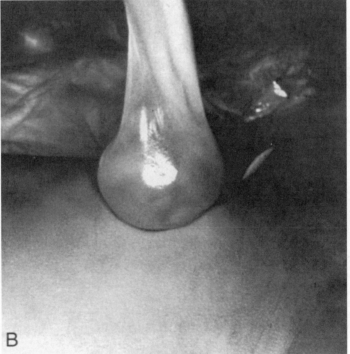

Fig. 11-37 Omphalocele. (A) The surrounding membrane (arrowheads), cord insertion into the apex of the omphalocele (u), liver (L) herniated into the omphalocele sac, and spine (Sp) can be seen. (B) Gross picture of an omphalocele, although smaller than that illustrated in the accompanying ultrasound. Note that the abdominal contents are surrounded by a membrane and protrude into the base of the umbilical cord. (Courtesy of Dr. Harbhajan Chawla.)

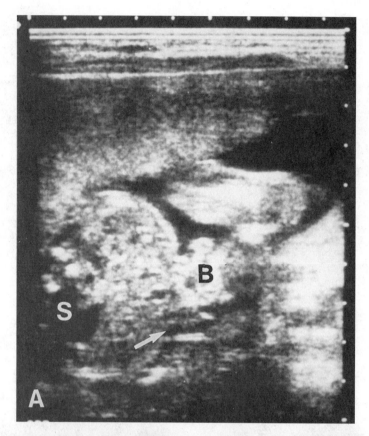

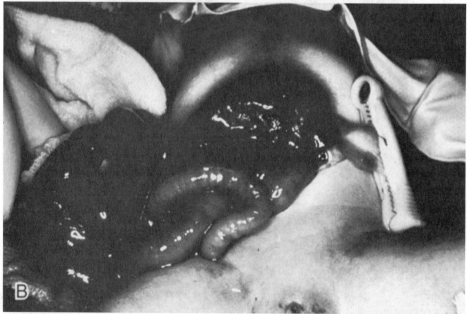

Fig. 11-38 (A) Loops of bowel (B) without a surrounding membrane are characteristic of gastroschisis. The arrow points to the insertion of the umbilical cord. Since the stomach (S) is on the left of the fetus, the site of the bowel herniation is to the right of the umbilical cord. (B) Matted loops of bowel in a neonate with gastroschisis. Note the absence of a surrounding membrane. As in the ultrasound, the abdominal contents are seen to the right of the umbilical cord. (Courtesy of Dr. Harbhajan Chawla.)

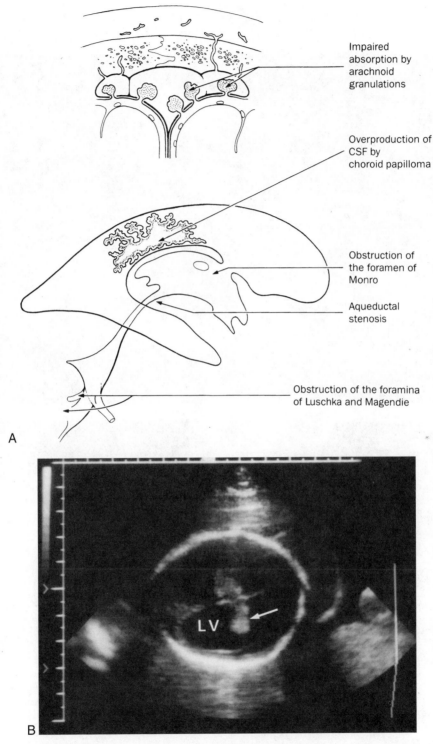

Impaired
absorption by
arachnoid
granulations

Overproduction of
CSF by
choroid papilloma

Obstruction of
the foramen of
Monro

Aqueductal
stenosis

Obstruction of the foramina
of Luschka and Magendie

A

LV

B

Fig. 11-39 (A) Common sites of obstruction of cerebrospinal fluid flow resulting in ventriculomegaly. (B) Transverse sonogram of fetal head demonstrating hydrocephalus. LV, dilated lateral ventricle; arrow points to dangling choroid plexus. (Fig. A is from Chervenak et al.,[67] with permission.)

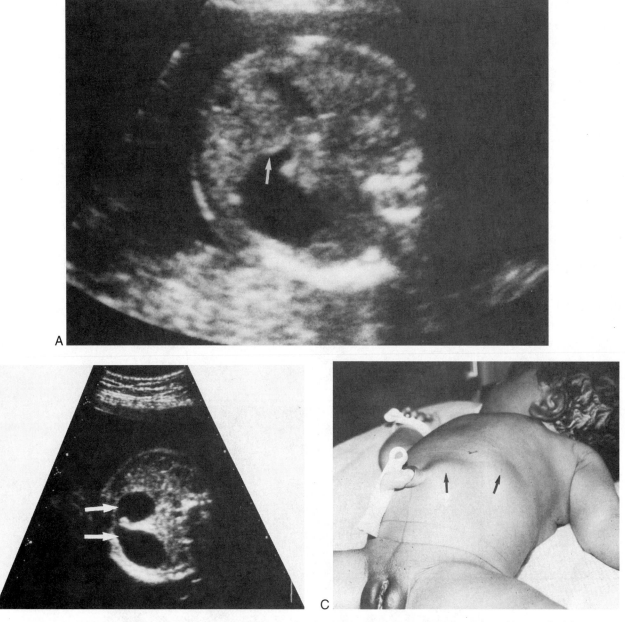

Fig. 11-40 (A) Sonogram demonstrating normal duodenum (arrow). (B) Sonogram illustrating classic "double bubble" sign. The two echo-free areas (arrows) represent the stomach and proximal duodenum. (C) Infant with "double bubble" sign (arrows) and duodenal atresia.

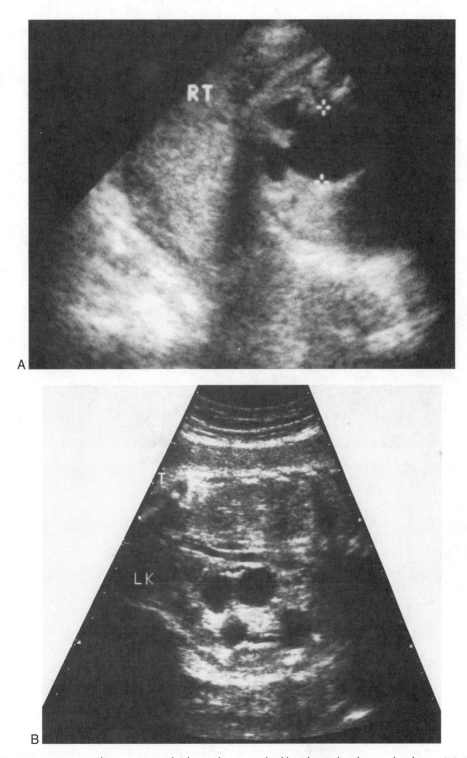

Fig. 11-41 (A) Sonogram demonstrating hydronephrosis with dilated renal pelvis and calyces. (B) Sonogram demonstrating dysplastic left kidney with noncommunicating cysts (proximal) and normal right kidney (distal).

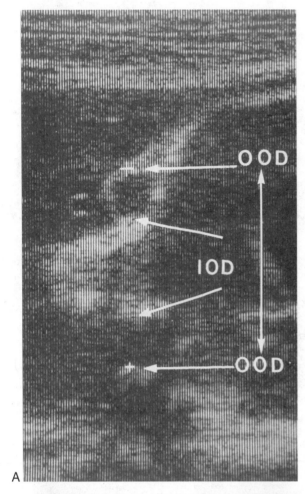

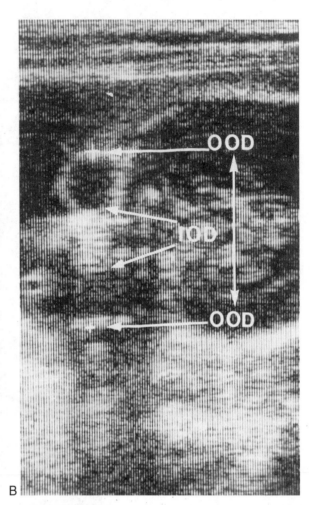

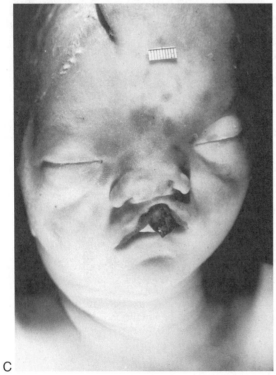

Fig. 11-42 (A) Transverse scan through orbits of fetus affected with median cleft face syndrome demonstrates hypertelorism. Inner orbital distance (IOD) and outer orbital distance (OOD) are increased for gestational age of 31 weeks. (B) Transverse scan through orbits of normal fetus at 37 weeks of gestation demonstrates normal IOD and OOD. (C) Infant with median cleft face syndrome at postmortem examination. Severe hydrocephalus, collapsed cranial bones, flattened nose, and cleft lip with protruding mass are demonstrated. (From Chervenak et al.,[113] with permission.)

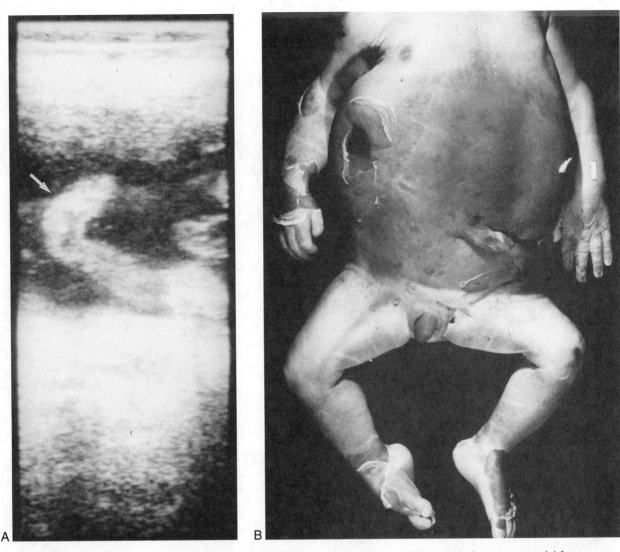

Fig. 11-43 (A) Sonogram demonstrating clubfoot (arrow). (B) Postmortem photograph demonstrating clubfoot.

congenital heart disease. Approximately one-third of fetuses with structural anomalies have a chromosomal disorder.[136–139] This additional information is invaluable to define fetal prognosis. For example, the prognosis for isolated hydrocephalus is substantially better than that for hydrocephalus associated with alobar holoprosencephaly and trisomy 13. Amniocentesis is the most widely utilized technique for determination of fetal karyotype when an ultrasonically diagnosed anomaly is detected, but fetal blood sampling or placental biopsy may be necessary if a rapid result is required.

After the fetal evaluation is completed, the certainties and uncertainties of fetal prognosis should be explained to the pregnant woman and her partner. The disclosure requirements of the informed consent process require the physician to present information about the range of available management options: aggressive

management, termination of pregnancy, non-aggressive management, and cephalocentesis.[140] These disclosure requirements obligate the physician to be objective when presenting this information. That is, the physician is not justified in withholding information about available management options to which he or she might object for reasons of personal conscience.[141]

Aggressive Management

To optimize fetal outcome, there should be an interdisciplinary approach, including specialists in maternal–fetal medicine, neonatology, genetics, pediatric surgery, and pediatric cardiology.[142–144] Social work services may provide important support to the family before as well as after birth. Such a team approach is best equipped to address the important questions of where, when, and how the infant should be delivered, as well as the role of invasive fetal therapy.

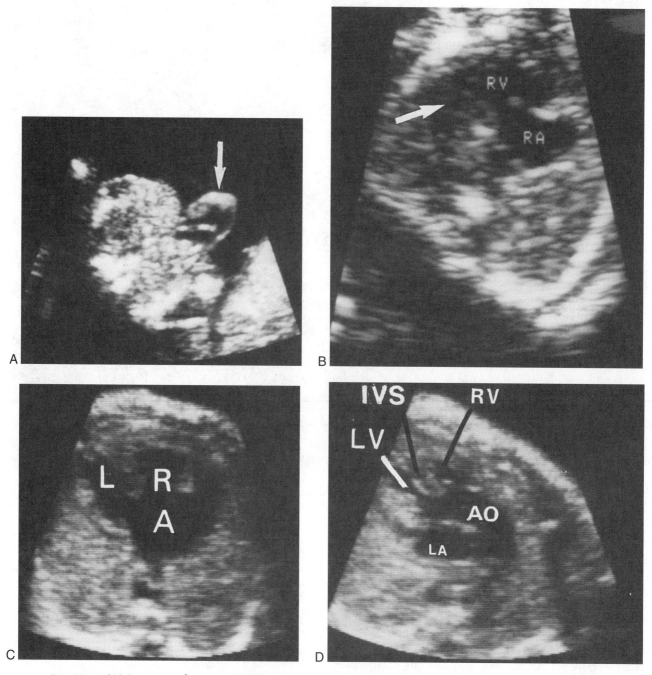

Fig. 11-44 (A) Sonogram demonstrating ectopic cordis with arrow pointing to heart outside the chest. (B) Sonogram demonstrating hypoplastic left heart. RV, right ventricle; RA, right atrium. Arrow points to region of hyplastic left ventricle. (C) Sonogram demonstrating A-V canal in fetus with Down syndrome. L, left ventricle; R, right ventricle; A, common atrium. (D) Sonogram of fetus with tetralogy of Fallot demonstrating enlarged aortic outflow tract (AO). Its anterior wall overrides the interventricular septum (IVS). RV, right ventricle; LV, left ventricle; LA, left atrium.

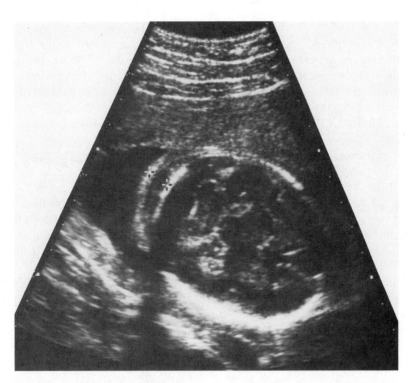

Fig. 11-45 Sonogram demonstrating nuchal skin thickness greater than 6 mm.

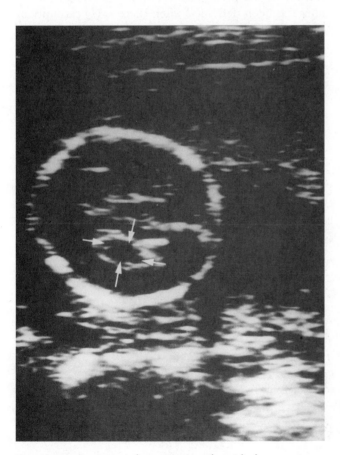

Fig. 11-46 Sonogram demonstrating choroid plexus cyst outlined by arrows.

Most infants with anomalies are best delivered in a referral center with a neonatal intensive care unit experienced in caring for such infants. In such a setting there is immediate access to diagnostic and therapeutic medical and surgical interventions.

Delivery at term is optimal for most fetal anomalies. For some malformations, however, such as hydrocephalus, delivery as soon as fetal lung maturation has occurred may be advisable in order to expedite corrective neonatal surgery.[145] Rarely, because of the risk of imminent fetal death, an anomaly such as progressive fetal hydrops may necessitate delivery prior to fetal lung maturity.[143]

Most fetuses with anomalies can be delivered vaginally. Cesarean delivery may be necessary to avoid dystocia if conditions such as a sacrococcygeal teratoma or conjoined twins are present. For other anomalies, such as spina bifida, cesarean delivery may be recommended in order to minimize trauma to fetal tissues.

Rarely, an invasive approach such as shunt placement may be considered to optimize outcome during the antenatal period. This strategy should only be considered when the natural history of the anomaly diagnosed is dismal and a relatively simple intrauterine correction is possible. The sonographic and karyotypic evaluations described above are especially important before an invasive approach can be considered. The disclosure requirements of the informed consent process necessitate that the experimental nature of invasive fetal therapy and the potential harms to the fetus and the mother be carefully explained. In addition, it is generally agreed that after 32 weeks of gestation such efforts offer no clear advantage over delivery and neonatal treatment. Given the risk of iatrogenic premature delivery as well as the experimental nature of these procedures, a normal coincident twin is considered to be a contraindication to this approach.[142,143,147]

The most common form of invasive fetal therapy has been intrauterine shunt placement. The purpose of such a shunt is to drain fluid under high pressure in a fetal organ to the lower pressure of the amniotic fluid. Such a shunt may have a role in the treatment of a complete bladder outlet obstruction that would be expected to result eventually in renal failure and pulmonary hypoplasia.[147–149] Analysis of fetal urine after bladder aspiration may help to define which fetuses are candidates for this vesiculoamniotic shunt.[149,150] Intrauterine aspiration or shunt placement may also be of value in cases of isolated pleural effusions[151–153] (Fig. 11-47). In fetal hydrocephalus, however, current experience does not demonstrate a clear benefit, and ventriculoamniotic shunt placement should be avoided.[147,154,155]

A group of investigators in San Francisco has pioneered open fetal surgery to manage such conditions as congenital diaphragmatic hernia and complete bladder obstruction. In such cases, hysterotomy and exteri-

orization of the fetus is followed by repair of the abnormality, replacement of the fetus, and continuation of the pregnancy.[142,156] At this time it is not possible to make a final judgment concerning the place of this fascinating modality in fetal therapy. More clinical experience is needed to better define the benefits to the fetus and the harms to the mother.

Termination of Pregnancy

Prior to fetal viability, abortion of any pregnancy is a woman's right as established by *Roe v. Wade*.[157] The option of abortion prior to fetal viability is, therefore, available to a pregnant woman when *any* fetal anomaly is diagnosed by ultrasound. Ethically, this option is supported by an approach that holds that all of obstetric ethics is essentially a function of the pregnant woman's autonomy[158,159] as well as an approach that holds that autonomous-based obligations to the pregnant woman should be balanced against beneficence-based obligations to her and the fetus she is carrying.[141]

After fetal viability, there is limited legal access in the United States to termination of pregnancy because of a fetal anomaly. Ethically, the option of terminating third trimester pregnancies complicated by fetal anomalies has been defended when there is (1) certainty of diagnosis and (2) either (a) certainty of death as an

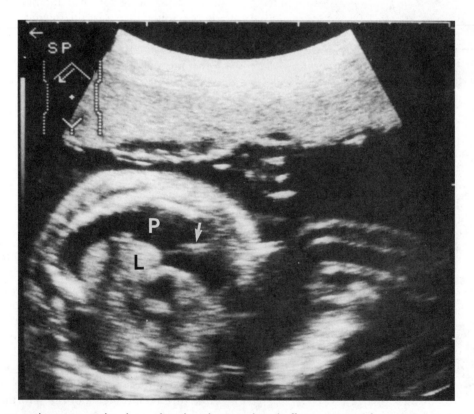

Fig. 11-47 A shunt (arrow) has been placed to drain a pleural effusion (P) in a fetus at 24 weeks' gestation. Note the compressed lung (L).

outcome of the anomaly diagnosed or (b) certainty of the absence of cognitive developmental capacity as a result of the anomaly diagnosed in some cases of short-term survival. Anencephaly is a clear example of a sonographically diagnosed anomaly that meets these criteria.[160] Trisomy 21 is a clear example of an anomaly that does not meet these criteria.[161]

Nonaggressive Management

The above-mentioned criteria for termination of pregnancy for fetal anomalies during the third trimester are quite restrictive. In addition, even if ethical criteria for third trimester termination of pregnancy were met, it may not be possible to perform termination in some situations because of legal concerns. Nonaggressive management is the noninclusion of obstetric interventions to benefit the fetus, such as fetal surveillance, tocolysis, cesarean delivery, or delivery in a referral center. Ethically, the option of nonaggressive management for third trimester pregnancies complicated by fetal anomalies has been defended when there is (1) a very high probability of a correct diagnosis and (2) either (a) a very high probability of death as an outcome of the anomaly diagnosed or (b) a very high probability of severe irreversible deficit of cognitive developmental capacity as a result of the anomaly diagnosed.

Cephalocentesis

When a pregnancy is complicated by fetal hydrocephalus with macrocephaly, there may be a role for cephalocentesis, which is the transabdominal or transvaginal aspiration of cerebrospinal fluid to avoid cesarean delivery. Ethical justification for this procedure can be based on an analysis of beneficence-based and autonomy-based obligations to the pregnant woman and the fetus she is carrying. Such an analysis needs to respect the heterogeneity of fetal hydrocephalus: isolated fetal hydrocephalus, hydrocephalus with severe associated anomalies (such as alobar holoprosencephaly), and hydrocephalus with other associated anomalies (such as an arachnoid cyst)[163,164] (Fig. 11-48).

Who Should Have an Obstetric Ultrasound Examination?

In 1984, the Consensus Development Conference, sponsored by the National Institute of Child Health and Human Development (NICHHD),[3] supported ultrasound examinations in the following clinical situations:

1. Estimation of gestational age for patients with uncertain clinical dates or verification of dates for patients who are to undergo scheduled elective repeat cesarean delivery, indicated induction of labor, or other elective termination of pregnancy
2. Evaluation of fetal growth
3. Vaginal bleeding of undetermined etiology in pregnancy
4. Determination of fetal presentation
5. Suspected multiple gestation
6. Adjunct to amniocentesis
7. Significant uterine size/clinical dates discrepancy
8. Pelvic mass
9. Suspected hydatidiform mole
10. Adjunct to cervical cerclage placement
11. Suspected ectopic pregnancy
12. Adjunct to special procedures, such as fetoscopy, intrauterine transfusion, shunt placement, in vitro fertilization, embryo transfer, or chorionic villi sampling

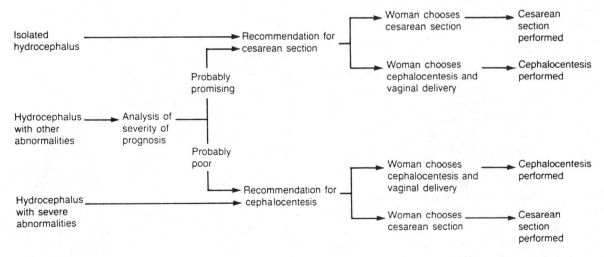

Fig. 11-48 Resolution strategies for conflicts in the intrapartum management of hydrocephalus with macrocephaly. (From Chervenak and McCullough,[163] with permission.)

13. Suspected fetal death
14. Suspected uterine abnormality
15. Intrauterine contraceptive device location
16. Ovarian follicle development surveillance
17. Biophysical evaluation for fetal well-being
18. Observation of intrapartum events
19. Suspected polyhydramnios or oligohydramnios
20. Suspected abruptio placenta
21. Adjunct to external version from breech to vertex presentation
22. Estimation of fetal weight or presentation in premature rupture of membranes or vertex presentation
23. Abnormal serum α-fetoprotein value
24. Follow-up observation of identified fetal anomaly
25. Follow-up evaluation of placenta localization for identified placenta previa
26. History of previous congenital anomaly
27. Serial evaluation of fetal growth in multiple gestation
28. Evaluation of fetal condition in late registrants for prenatal care

Although the above indications are widely accepted, routine performance of obstetric ultrasound examinations, the performance of an ultrasound study on every obstetric patient at approximately 18 weeks' gestation remains controversial.

A routine obstetric ultrasound examination describes what the American College of Obstetricians and Gynecologists (ACOG) has called a *basic* ultrasound examination, which would include the following information: fetal number, fetal presentation, documentation of fetal life, placental location, assessment of amniotic fluid volume, assessment of gestational age, survey of fetal anatomy for gross malformations, and an evaluation for maternal pelvic masses.[68,165] When the findings of a basic ultrasound examination suggest a fetal abnormality or in patients at greater risk of a fetal abnormality, a comprehensive ultrasound examination may be indicated. As noted by ACOG, the comprehensive ultrasound study should be conducted by an individual experienced in these evaluations.

At the present time, routine obstetric ultrasound is practiced in many European countries. In West Germany, the German National Health Insurance Institute has recommended that two routine ultrasound examinations be performed on each pregnant woman. Failure to do these studies would render the obstetrician libel to litigation should complications that could have been detected develop during the pregnancy. The Royal College of Obstetricians and Gynaecologists has concluded that a routine obstetric ultrasound examination is justifiable.[2]

Routine obstetric ultrasound is not widely practiced in the United States. The 1988 National Maternal and Infant Health Survey revealed that 58 percent of women in the United States had at least one ultrasound, most often performed to evaluate gestational age (37 percent) and placental location (10 percent), determine fetal position (8 percent), and confirm fetal life (6 percent), as well as for a variety of other indications.[166] A survey of obstetricians in Iowa, representing the physicians responsible for more than 70 percent of all deliveries in that state, revealed that 31 percent recommended routine ultrasound.[167] In a survey of Fellows of ACOG from the southeastern part of the United States (District IV), two-thirds reported that they did have ultrasound equipment in their offices.[168] However, of the 429 Fellows questioned, only 15 percent scanned every pregnancy.

Routine obstetric ultrasound offers at least six advantages: accurate dating of all pregnancies; accurate evaluation of maternal serum levels of α-fetoprotein, human chorionic gonadotropin, and unconjugated estriol (triple screening); early detection of multiple pregnancies; placental localization to rule out placenta previa; detection of structural abnormalities of the fetus; and psychological benefit to the parents.[169,170]

The ideal timing for a routine ultrasound study would appear to be approximately 18 weeks' gestation. At this gestational age, the pregnancy can be accurately dated and fetal anatomy well visualized. Should a fetal abnormality be identified, sufficient time is available to perform a comprehensive ultrasound, obtain a fetal karyotype if necessary, and counsel the patient and her partner.

A large number of clinical studies support the value of routine obstetric ultrasound. In an investigation of 11,045 women for whom an ultrasound at 16 to 18 weeks was used as the standard for dating a pregnancy, Kramer et al.[171] found that obstetric dating based on the patient's last menstrual period was most likely to be in error in identifying a preterm or post-term pregnancy. Kramer et al.[171] concluded that the mistakes made in dating using menstrual gestational age "support the argument for routine gestational dating with an early ultrasound examination," particularly when one considers the clinical consequences of poor dating. Reviewing their experience with maternal serum markers to screen for Down syndrome in over 25,000 women, Haddow et al.[172] noted that "Universal dating by ultrasonography before screening would greatly lessen the number of women who are wrongly told that their pregnancies are high risk, and it would allow subsequent diagnostic steps to be taken more expeditiously."

Routine ultrasound performed at 18 weeks' gestation will detect nearly all multiple pregnancies.[173–175] Clinical experience gained in Sweden as well as in the United States indicates that earlier identification of a twin gestation can reduce perinatal mortality and morbidity, perhaps by allowing more close observation and intervention.

An ultrasound performed at 18 weeks' gestation will reveal that approximately 10 percent of placentas overlie the cervical os, allowing the obstetrician to exclude placenta previa in the remaining 90 percent of cases. Of patients with a low-lying placenta at 18 weeks, only those women in whom the placenta completely covers the os are at risk for a placenta previa in the third trimester. A repeat ultrasound evaluation should be performed in these cases.[165,176]

One of the most important benefits of routine ultrasound appears to be the identification of major congenital malformations. Major anomalies occur in 2 to 3 percent of all births, and data from the Centers for Disease Control and Prevention demonstrate that birth defects are a leading cause of infant mortality, accounting for more than 20 percent of all infant deaths (see Ch. 12). Cardiac abnormalities result in nearly one-third of infant deaths due to birth defects, with respiratory, central nervous system, and chromosomal abnormalities each responsible for approximately 13 percent of these losses. Systematic examination of fetal structure as part of the basic ultrasound study outlined by ACOG can identify a significant proportion of these abnormalities. Data from six European studies, including 52,295 patients scanned between 1980 and 1991, demonstrate that routine ultrasound has a sensitivity of 52.9 percent and a positive predictive value of 95.9 percent in identifying major structural anomalies.[177] The specificity and negative predictive value were 99.9 and 99.2 percent, respectively.

Several investigations have confirmed the psychological benefit of routine ultrasound, revealing that women who have undergone a scan are more likely to follow the recommendations of their health care providers to stop smoking and drinking alcohol.[178,179]

Until recently, the proposed benefits of routine ultrasound had not been evaluated in large, prospective, randomized studies. Six small studies did reveal that routine ultrasound was associated with fewer inductions for suspected prolonged pregnancy, less morbidity in postdate infants, greater birth weight in twins, and fewer cases of unexpected bleeding from placenta previa.[180–185]

In 1990, Saari-Kemppainen et al.[186] reported the results of a prospective, randomized investigation of routine ultrasonography performed in the early second trimester including 9,000 Finnish women. The study compared routine ultrasound screening between 16 and 20 weeks, with selective screening performed for usual practice standards. Routine ultrasonography was associated with fewer outpatient clinic visits and antenatal hospitalizations, improved early detection of twins, and identification of patients at risk for placenta previa.

There were no differences in the number of labor inductions or mean birth weights in the two groups. Perinatal mortality was significantly lower in the screened than in the control group (4.6/1,000 vs. 9.0/1,000). This reduction by almost one-half was due primarily to early detection of major malformations that led to induced abortion. Additional benefits were correction of the expected date of delivery by 10 or more days in over 11 percent of the screened group and a decrease in the rate of prolonged pregnancy. The authors concluded that their findings justified routine ultrasound screening of all pregnancies at 16 to 20 weeks for the detection of major congenital abnormalities under circumstances in which induced abortion was acceptable.

The RADIUS study, the Routine Antenatal Diagnostic Imaging with Ultrasound trial, is the largest prospective randomized investigation evaluating the efficacy of routine ultrasound screening.[187–189] To determine if routine ultrasound could improve the detection of congenital malformations, pregnancies with multiple gestations, abnormal fetal growth, placental abnormalities, and errors in the estimation of gestational age and reduce the frequency of adverse perinatal outcomes, Ewigman and his colleagues[187] studied 15,151 low-risk patients recruited from 92 obstetric and 17 family medicine practices in six states. Ultrasound screening was performed twice in 7,812 study subjects, first at 15 to 22 weeks and again at 31 to 35 weeks, while the 7,718 women in the control group had an ultrasound only if medically indicated. The adverse outcomes evaluated included fetal or neonatal deaths, severe morbidity such as the need for mechanical ventilation for more than 48 hours, a stay of more than 30 days in the special care nursery, and moderate morbidity including a brachial-plexus injury.

Women in the experimental group had an average of 2.2 ultrasound studies. Forty-five percent of control subjects also had an ultrasound, for an average of 0.6 studies per control patient. No statistically significant difference was noted in the rate of adverse perinatal outcomes in this investigation: 5.0 percent in the experimental group and 4.9 percent for the control subjects.[187] No difference was observed in the rate of preterm births or in birth weight distribution. Of 187 major anomalies in the infants of ultrasound-screened patients, 65 (34.8 percent) were detected. Of these, 31 (16.6 percent) were identified before 24 weeks' gestation. In the control group, only 18 of 163 major malformations (11 percent) were recognized, 8 (4.9 percent) before 24 weeks' gestation.[189] When outcomes were examined in subgroups of patients with postdate pregnancies, multiple gestations, or infants with a birth weight below the 10th percentile, no differences were noted. In an analysis of data on maternal management and outcome, LeFevre et al.[188] noted no significant differences in the rates of induced abortion, amniocentesis, tests of fetal well-being, external version, induction, cesarean delivery, and the distribution of total hospital days. However, the use of tocolytics and the rate of postdate pregnancy were both slightly lower in the screened group. These investigators concluded that screening ultrasonography did not improve perinatal outcome compared with ultrasonography performed only for medical indications.

While the RADIUS trial is an important study, a number of significant concerns have been raised in applying the results to general obstetric practice.[177,190] The adverse perinatal outcomes studied were due primarily to prematurity or birth trauma. Clearly, prematurity cannot be reduced by routine ultrasound, nor will a second ultrasound examination performed as early as 31 to 35 weeks help to identify the macrosomic fetus at risk for birth trauma. As noted by Berkowitz[190] in an accompanying editorial, the study population was at extremely low risk for perinatal problems. Women who were eligible for the study had to be at least 18 years of age and speak English. Only 13 percent of them smoked, and more than 40 percent of them had graduated from college.[187] When O'Day et al.[191] applied these criteria to 1,000 Medicaid patients at the University of Texas, Houston, only 78 women met the eligibility criteria for the RADIUS trial. Accurate dating of all pregnancies has been cited as an advantage of routine ultrasound. Yet, in the RADIUS trial, women had to know their last menstrual period within 1 week. Not surprisingly, gestational age was reassigned in only 11 percent of the study subjects.[187] Even in those women assigned to the routine ultrasound group, the detection of major anomalies was poor, only 34.8 percent, and of the 65 malformations identified, only 31 were recognized before 24 weeks.

Why do these results differ from the large clinical experiences of many centers? The answer may be that there is nothing "routine" about a routine ultrasound examination. A basic ultrasound study must be carefully performed by an experienced sonographer. Of note, the rate of detection of fetal malformations at tertiary centers in the RADIUS trial was 37 percent (21/57), but only 12 percent (6/65) in nontertiary centers. Few women in the RADIUS trial who had a fetal malformation identified elected to terminate their pregnancies.[187] This choice may be based on cultural differences compared with the study in Helsinki,[186] to the severity of the anomalies recognized, or, perhaps, lack of confidence in the diagnosis.[177] Unforturnately, the RADIUS trial did not evaluate the psychological benefits of routine ultrasound screening, which have been recognized in other prospective studies. Clinicians caring for patients in the routine ultrasound arm of the RADIUS trial, while having the results of the ultra-

sound studies available, did not follow established protocols in their management of pregnancies complicated by growth restriction, prolonged pregnancy, or multiple gestations.[188] Furthermore, the number of cases in each of these high-risk groups was limited. These shortcomings make it difficult to evaluate whether routine ultrasound is useful in the care of such patients. Finally, it is important to point out that ultrasound screening did not *increase* the risk of adverse perinatal outcomes.

In their discussion of the results of the RADIUS trial, the authors note that the cost of screening more than 4 million pregnant women annually in the United States at $200 per ultrasound scan would be more than 1 billion dollars. This figure could be reduced to 500 million dollars since only 40 percent of all pregnancies screened were eligible for the study. However, several other factors should be considered in calculating this cost. Barrett and Brinson[192] found that a routine ultrasound performed at the first prenatal visit is the most cost-effective of all prenatal laboratory assessments performed. DeVore[193] has examined the cost of detecting a malformed fetus in the RADIUS trial compared with the California MSAFP screening program. For tertiary centers in the RADIUS trial with a detection rate for fetal anomalies of 6.8/1,000, the cost was $29,533 compared with a detection rate of 1.7/1,000 and a cost of $115,575 for nontertiary centers. The detection rate in the California MSAFP program is 1.3/1,000, yielding a cost of $40,338 for each identified malformed ferns. One must compare this expense to those of caring for a severely malformed infant.

In its most recent technical bulletin, ACOG[165] offered the following recommendations concerning routine ultrasound:

> Routine ultrasonography in early pregnancy can help to reduce the incidence of labor induction for suspected postdatism, and decrease the frequency of undiagnosed major fetal anomalies and undiagnosed twins. However, significant effects on infant outcome are not confirmed by randomized, controlled trials. Although obstetric ultrasound studies are performed routinely in many European countries, in the United States the routine use of ultrasonography cannot be supported from a cost-benefit standpoint.

While the debate concerning routine obstetric ultrasound continues, a reasonable strategy for this dilemma is the concept that prenatal informed consent for sonogram be considered.[194] Shortly after the pregnancy is diagnosed, the woman should be provided with information about the actual and theoretical benefits and harms of a routine ultrasound examination. Because the sonographic detection of fetal anomalies has been recognized as a benefit of routine ultrasound, withholding this information from the pregnant patient would not appear to be justified. Thus, a routine obstetric ultrasound examination is *offered*, but not necessarily recommended.

Conclusions

In summary, studies of routine ultrasound have failed to demonstrate any associated adverse effects on the mother or fetus. Routine ultrasound has a high positive predictive value for conditions known to be associated with poor perinatal outcome such as twins, placenta previa, and congenital malformations. To date, two large prospective randomized studies have evaluated the benefits of routine ultrasound in obstetric practice.[186–189] One, performed in Finland,[186] demonstrated a reduction in perinatal mortality, resulting from the identification of major fetal anomalies. The second, the RADIUS trial,[187–189] performed in the United States, failed to show an improvement in perinatal outcome. Nevertheless, a large clinical experience from several centers both in the United States and Europe has repeatedly found that routine ultrasound screening at 18 weeks can improve gestational dating in approximately 10 to 25 percent of patients, detect nearly all multiple gestations, exclude placenta previa in most patients and recognize those at greatest risk for this condition, detect one-third to one-half of major fetal malformations, and reduce parental anxiety and increase compliance with the recommendations of health care providers. The cost of routine ultrasound screening must be compared with the costs created by false-positive diagnoses, which may lead to unnecessary patient anxiety and further intervention, and to the cost savings resulting from reduction in the rate of inductions for suspected prolonged pregnancy, a decrease in the rate of preterm delivery for twins, and the identification of a fetus with an anomaly likely to survive but with a poor quality of life. Finally, like any analytic technique, the value of ultrasound screening is dependent on the skill with which the study is performed and the manner in which the results are interpreted and utilized in clinical care.[170]

Key Points

- Ultrasound energy is produced by a transducer containing crystal structures that convert electrical energy to ultrasound waves and the returning echoes to electrical energy.

- No deleterious effects on the pregnant woman or fetus caused by exposure to ultrasound at the intensities used for imaging have ever been reported.

- Although the gestational sac can be used to date an early pregnancy, measurement of the crown–rump length is the single best method to assess gestational age at any time in pregnancy.

- From 12 to 28 weeks' gestation, the relationship between the biparietal diameter and gestational age is linear.

- Formulas for estimation of fetal weight are associated with a 95 percent confidence range of at least 10 to 15 percent.

- Measurement of the fetal abdominal circumference is probably the most reliable sonographic parameter for the detection of macrosomia.

- At term, an AFI less than 5.0 cm indicates oligohydramnios and greater than 20 cm polyhydramnios.

- The thickness of the placenta in millimeters corresponds to the number of weeks gestation.

- The "lemon" and "banana" signs are important cranial markers for spina bifida.

- Major structural malformations, including hydrops, duodenal atresia, and cardiac anomalies, are observed in 30 percent of cases of Down syndrome (trisomy 21).

References

1. Manning F: Ultrasound in perinatal medicine. p. 195. In Creasy RK, Resnik R (eds): Maternal–Fetal Medicine: Principles and Practice. WB Saunders, Philadelphia, 1989
2. Report of the Royal College of Obstetricians and Gynaecologists Working Party on Routine Ultrasound Examination in Pregnancy, December 1984
3. U.S. Department of Health and Human Services: Diagnostic Ultrasound in Pregnancy. NIH Publ. No. 84-667. National Institutes of Health, Washington, DC, 1984
4. Maulik D: Biologic effects of ultrasound. Clin Obstet Gynecol 32:645, 1989
5. Porfirio B, Dallapiccola B, Cittanti C et al: Sister chromatid exchanges in cultured amniocytes exposed to diagnostic ultrasound in vitro. Acta Radiol 35:58, 1994
6. American Institute of Ultrasound in Medicine: Bioeffects & Safety of Diagnostic Ultrasound, 1993
7. Salvesen KA, Vatten LJ, Jacobsen G et al: Routine ultra-

sonography in utero and subsequent vision and hearing at primary school age. Ultrasound Obstet Gynecol 2: 243, 1992

8. Salvesen KA, Vatten LJ, Bakketeig LS, Eik-Nes SH: Routine ultrasonography in utero and speech development. Ultrasound Obstet Gynecol 4:101, 1994

9. Nelson LH III, Kurtz AB, Hissong SL, Lawrence H: Training guidelines for physicians who interpret diagnostic ultrasound examinations. AIUM Reporter, May 1993

10. Timor-Tritsch IE, Rottem S (eds): Transvaginal Sonography. 2nd Ed. Elsevier Science, New York, 1991

11. Fleischer AC, Kepple DM: Transvaginal Sonography. A Clinical Atlas. JB Lippincott, Philadelphia, 1992

12. Nyberg DA, Hill LM, Bohm-Veley M, Mendelson EB: Transvaginal Ultrasound. Mosby Year Book, Saint Louis, 1992

13. Dodson MG: Transvaginal Ultrasound. Churchill Livingstone, New York, 1991

14. Timor-Tritsch IE, Rottem S: Normal and abnormal fetal anatomy in the first fifteen weeks. p. 353. In Timor-Tritsch IE, Rottem S (eds): Diagnostic Ultrasound Applied to Obstetrics and Gynecology. 3rd Ed. JB Lippincott, Philadelphia, 1994

15. Fossum GT, Davajan V, Kletzky OA: Early detection of pregnancy with transvaginal ultrasound. Fertil Steril 49: 788, 1988

16. Nyberg DA, Mack LA, Laing FC, Palten RM: Distinguishing normal from abnormal gestational sac growth in early pregnancy. J Ultrasound Med 6:23, 1987

17. Reece EA, Scioscia A, Pinta E et al: Prognostic significance of the human yolk sac assessed by ultrasonography. Am J Obstet Gynecol 159:1191, 1988

18. Lindsay DJ, Lyons EA, Levi CS et al: Yolk sac diameter and shape at endovaginal US: predictors of pregnancy outcome. Radiology 183:115, 1992

19. Levi CS, Lyons EA, Zheng XH: Endovaginal ultrasound: demonstration of cardiac activity in embryos of less than 5 mm in crown–rump length. Radiology 176: 71, 1990

20. Brown DL, Emerson DS, Felker RE: Diagnosis of early embryonic demise by endovaginal sonography. J Ultrasound Med 9:631, 1990

21. Simpson JL, Mills JL, Holmes LB et al: Low fetal loss rates after ultrasound-proved viability in early pregnancy. JAMA 258:2555, 1987

22. Howe RS, Isaacson HJ, Albert JL, Contiforis CB: Embryonic heart rate in human pregnancy. J Ultrasound Med 10:367, 1991

23. Robinson HP, Fleming JEE: A critical evaluation of sonar crown–rump length measurement. Br J Obstet Gynaecol 82:702, 1975

24. Timor-Tritsch IE, Warner WB, Peisner DB, Pirrone E: First trimester midgut herniation: a high-frequency transvaginal sonographic study. Am J Obstet Gynecol 161:831, 1989

25. Philips J: Sensitivity and specificity in ultrasonographic screening. p. 141. In Simpson JL, Elias S (eds): Essentials of Prenatal Diagnosis. Churchill Livingstone, New York, 1993

26. Nicolaides KM: Fetal nuchal translucency: ultrasound screening for fetal trisomy in the first trimester of pregnancy. Br J Obstet Gynaecol 101:782, 1994

27. Farine D, Fox HE, Timor-Tritsch IE: Vaginal approach to the ultrasound diagnosis of placenta previa. p. 1503. In Chervenak FA, Isaacson G, Campbell S (eds): Ultrasound in Obstetrics and Gynecology. Little, Brown, Philadelphia, 1993

28. Gome ZR, Galasso M, Romero R et al: Ultrasonographic examination of the uterine cervix is better than cervical digital examination as a predictor of the likelihood of premature delivery in patients with preterm labor and intact membranes. Am J Obstet Gynecol 171:956, 1994

29. Monteagudo A, Reuss ML, Timor-Tritsch IE: Imaging the fetal brain in the second trimester using transvaginal sonography. Obstet Gynecol 77:27, 1991

30. Gabbe SG, Iams JD: Intrauterine growth retardation. p. 169. In Iams JD, Zuspan FP (eds): Manual of Obstetrics and Gynecology. CV Mosby, St. Louis, 1990

31. Campbell S, Warsof S, Little D et al: Routine ultrasound screening for the prediction of gestational age. Obstet Gynecol 65:613, 1985

32. Kurtz A, Wapner R, Kurtz R et al: Analysis of biparietal diameter as an accurate indicator of gestational age. J Clin Ultrasound 8:319, 1980

33. Sabbagha R, Hughey M: Standardization of sonar cephalometry and gestational age. Obstet Gynecol 52:402, 1978

34. Hadlock EP, Harrist RB, Carpenter RJ et al: Sonographic estimation of fetal weight. Radiology 150:535, 1984

35. Shepard M, Richard V, Berkowitz R et al: An evaluation of two equations for predicting fetal weight by ultrasound. Am J Obstet Gynecol 142:47, 1982

36. Macrosomia: American College of Obstetricians and Gynecologists, Technical Bulletin, Number 159, 1991

37. Persson B, Stangenberg M, Lunnell NO et al: Prediction of size of infants at birth by measurement of symphysis fundus height. Br J Obstet Gynaecol 93:206, 1986

38. Ott WJ, Doyle S: Ultrasonic diagnosis of altered fetal growth by use of a normal ultrasound fetal weight curve. Obstet Gynecol 63:201, 1984

39. Tamura RK, Sabbagha RE, Depp R et al: Diabetic macrosomia: accuracy of third trimester ultrasound. Obstet Gynecol 67:828, 1986

40. Chervenak JL, Divon MY, Hirsch J et al: Macrosomia in the postdate pregnancy: is routine ultrasonographic screening indicated? Am J Obstet Gynecol 161:753, 1989

41. Pollack RN, Hauer-Pollack G, Divon MY: Macrosomia in postdates pregnancies: the accuracy of routine ultrasonographic screening. Am J Obstet Gynecol 167:7, 1992

42. Delpapa EH, Mueller-Heubach E: Pregnancy outcome following ultrasound diagnosis of macrosomia. Obstet Gynecol 78:340, 1991

43. Sandmire HF: Whither ultrasonic prediction of fetal macrosomia? Obstet Gynecol 82:860, 1993

44. Bochner CJ, Medearis AL, Williams J et al: Early third-trimester ultrasound screening in gestational diabetes to determine the risk of macrosomia and labor dystocia at term. Am J Obstet Gynecol 157:703, 1987

45. Chudleigh P, Pearce JM (eds): Obstetric Ultrasound. Churchill Livingstone, Edinburgh, 1986

46. Hadlock FP, Harrist RB, Fearneyhough TC et al: Use of femur length/abdominal circumference ratio in detecting the macrosomic fetus. Radiology 154:503, 1985

47. Landon MB, Mintz MC, Gabbe SG: Sonographic evaluation of fetal abdominal growth: predictor of the LGA infant in pregnancies complicated by diabetes mellitus. Am J Obstet Gynecol 160:115, 1989

48. Deter RL, Hadlock FP: Use of ultrasound in the detection of macrosomia: a review. J Clin Ultrasound 13:519, 1985

49. Chamberlain P, Manning F, Morrison I et al: Ultrasound evaluation of amniotic fluid volume. I. The relationship of marginal and decreased amniotic fluid volumes to perinatal outcome. Am J Obstet Gynecol 150: 245, 1984

50. Chamberlain P, Manning F, Morrison I et al: Ultrasound evaluation of amniotic fluid volume. II. The relationship of increased amniotic fluid volume to perinatal outcome. Am J Obstet Gynecol 150:250, 1984

51. Bottoms SF, Welch RA, Zador IE et al: Limitations of using maximum vertical pocket and other sonographic evaluations of amniotic fluid volume to predict fetal growth: technical or physiologic? Am J Obstet Gynecol 155:154, 1986

52. Hoddick WK, Callen PW, Filly RA et al: Ultrasonographic determination of qualitative amniotic fluid volume in intrauterine growth retardation: reassessment of the 1 cm rule. Am J Obstet Gynecol 149:758, 1984

53. Phelan JP, Smith CV, Broussard P, Small M: Amniotic fluid volume assessment using the four-quadrant technique in the pregnancy between 36 and 42 weeks' gestation. J Reprod Med 32:540, 1987

54. Phelan FP, Ahn MO, Smith CV et al: Amniotic fluid index measurements during pregnancy. J Reprod Med 32:601, 1987

55. Del Valle GO, Bateman L, Gaudier FL, Sanchez-Ramos L: Comparison of three types of ultrasound transducers in evaluating the amniotic fluid index. J Reprod Med 39:869, 1994

56. Flack NJ, Dore C, Southwell D et al: The influence of operator transducer pressure on ultrasonographic measurements of amniotic fluid volume. Am J Obstet Gynecol 171:218, 1994

57. Moore TR, Cayle JE: The amniotic fluid index in normal human pregnancy. Am J Obstet Gynecol 162:1168, 1990

58. Rutherford SE, Smith CV, Phelan JP et al: Four-quadrant assessment of amniotic fluid volume. J Reprod Med 32:587, 1987

59. Bruner JP, Reed GW, Sarno AP et al: Intraobserver and interobserver variability of the amniotic fluid index. Am J Obstet Gynecol 168:1309, 1993

60. Carlson DE, Platt LD, Medearis AL et al: Quantifiable polyhydramnios: diagnosis and management. Obstet Gynecol 75:989, 1990

61. Damato N, Filly RA, Goldstein RB et al: Frequency of fetal anomalies in sonographically detected polyhydramnios. J Ultrasound Med 12:11, 1993

62. Moore TR, Brace RA: Amniotic fluid index (AFI) in the term ovine pregnancy: a predictable relationship between AFI and amniotic fluid volume. In: Proceedings of the 35th Annual Meeting of the Society for Gynecologic Investigation, Baltimore, Maryland, March 1988

63. Moore TR: Superiority of the four-quadrant sum over the single-deepest-pocket technique in ultrasonographic identification of abnormal amniotic fluid volumes. Am J Obstet Gynecol 163:762, 1990

64. Nyberg DA, Mahony BS, Pretorius DH: Diagnostic Ultrasound and Fetal Anomalies: Text and Atlas. Year Book Medical Publishers, Chicago, 1990

65. Romero R, Pilu G, Jeanty P et al: Prenatal Diagnosis of Congenital Anomalies. Appleton & Lange, Norwalk, CT, 1988

66. Seeds JS, Azizkhan RG: Congenital Malformations: Antenatal Diagnosis, Perinatal Management, and Counseling. Aspen Publishers, Rockville, MD, 1990

67. Chervenak FA, Isaacson G, Lorber J: Anomalies of the Fetal Head, Neck and Spine: Ultrasound Diagnosis and Management. WB Saunders, Philadelphia, 1988

68. Ultrasound in Pregnancy. ACOG Technical Bulletin 116. American College of Obstetricians and Gynecologists, Washington, DC, 1988

69. Leopold GR: Antepartum obstetrical ultrasound examination guidelines. J Ultrasound Med 5:241, 1986

70. Filly RA: Level 1, level 2, level 3 obstetric sonography: I'll see your level and raise you one. Radiology 172:312, 1989

71. Callen PN: Ultrasonography in Obstetrics and Gynecology. p. 1. WB Saunders, Philadelphia, 1994

72. Sabbagha RE, Kamel EM: Standard Ultrasound Obstetric Examination in Diagnostic Ultrasound Applied to Obstetrics and Gynecology. p. 59. JP Lippincott, Philadelphia, 1994

73. Campbell S: The obstetric ultrasound examination. p. 187. In Chervenak FA, Isaacson G, Campbell S (eds): Ultrasound in Obstetrics and Gynecology. Little, Brown, Philadelphia, 1993

74. Jauniaux E, Campbell S: Ultrasonographic assessment of placental abnormalities. Am J Obstet Gynecol 163: 1650, 1990

75. Jauniaux E, Ramsay B, Campbell S: Ultrasonographic investigation of placental morphologic characteristics and size during the second trimester of pregnancy. Am J Obstet Gynecol 170:130, 1994

76. Nelson LH III: Ultrasonography of the Placenta—A Review. American Institute of Ultrasound in Medicine, 1994

77. Sabbagha R (ed): Diagnostic Ultrasound Applied to Obstetrics and Gynecology. JP Lippincott, Philadelphia, 1994

78. Chervenak FA, Isaacson G, Campbell S (eds): Ultrasound in Obstetrics and Gynecology. Little, Brown, Philadelphia, 1993

79. Manning FA: The anomalous fetus. p. 451. In: In Fetal Medicine. Principles and Practice. Appleton & Lange, Norwalk, 1995

80. Nelson NL, Filly RA, Goldstein RB, Callen PW: The AIUM/ACR antepartum obstetrical sonographic guide-

lines: expectations for detection of anomalies. J Ultrasound Med 4:189, 1993

81. Campbell S, Johnstone FD, Hold EM et al: Anencephaly: early ultrasonic diagnosis and active management. Lancet 2:1226, 1972

82. Chervenak FA, Isaacson G, Mahoney MJ et al: The obstetric significance of holoprosencephaly. Obstet Gynecol 63:115, 1984

83. Romero R, Cullen M, Grannum P et al: Antenatal diagnosis of renal anomalies with ultrasound. III. Bilateral renal agenesis. Am J Obstet Gynecol 151:38, 1985

84. Chervenak FA, Isaacson G, Touloukian R et al: The diagnosis and management of fetal teratomas. Obstet Gynecol 66:666, 1985

85. Chervenak FA, Isaacson G, Blakemore KJ et al: Fetal cystic hygroma: cause and natural history. N Engl J Med 309:822, 1984

86. Johnson MP, Johnson A, Holzgreve W et al: First trimester cystic hygromas: cause and outcome. Am J Obstet Gynecol 168:156, 1993

87. Holzgreve W, Curry CJR, Golbus MS: Investigation of nonimmune hydrops fetalis. Am J Obstet Gynecol 150:805, 1984

88. Machin GA: Hydrops revisited: literature review of 1414 cases published in the 1980s. Am J Med Gen 34:366, 1989

89. Santolaya J, Alley D, Jaffe R, Warsof SL: Antenatal classification of hydrops fetalis. Obstet Gynecol 79:256, 1992

90. Arey LB: Developmental Anatomy. pp. 245, 465. WB Saunders, Philadelphia, 1974

91. Chervenak FA, Isaacson G, Mahoney MJ et al: The diagnosis and management of fetal cephalocele. Obstet Gynecol 64:86, 1984

92. Hobbins JC, Venus I, Tortora M et al: Stage II ultrasound examination for the diagnosis of fetal abnormalities with an elevated amniotic fluid alpha-fetoprotein concentration. Am J Obstet Gynecol 142:1026, 1982

93. Platt LD, Feuchtbaum L, Filly R et al: The California maternal serum alpha-fetoprotein screening program: the role of ultrasonography in the detection of spina bifida. Obstet Gynecol 166:1328, 1992

94. McIntosh R: The incidence of congenital malformations: a study of 5964 pregnancies. Pediatrics 14:505, 1954

95. Nicolaides KM, Campbell S, Gabbe SG, Guidetti R: Ultrasound screening for spina bifida: cranial and cerebellar signs. Lancet 2:72, 1986

96. Nakayama DK, Harrison RM, Gross BH et al: Management of the fetus with an abdominal wall defect. J Pediatr Surg 19:408, 1984

97. Marwood RP, Dawson MR, Gross BH et al: Antenatal diagnosis of diaphragmatic hernias. Br J Obstet Gynaecol 88:71, 1981

98. Sharlane GK, Lockhart SM, Heward AJ, Allan P: Prognosis in fetal diaphragmatic hernia. Am J Obstet Gynecol 166:9, 1992

99. Cardoza JD, Goldstein RB, Filly RA: Exclusion of fetal ventriculomegaly with a single measurement: the width of the lateral ventricular atrium. Radiology 169:711, 1988

100. Cardoza JD, Filly RA, Podarsky AE: The dangling choroid plexus: a sonographic observation of value in excluding ventriculomegaly. Am J Radiol 151:767, 1988

101. Benaceraff BR, Birnholz JC: The diagnosis of fetal hydrocephalus prior to 22 weeks. J Clin Ultrasound 15:531, 1987

102. Benaceraff BR: Fetal hydrocephalus: diagnosis and significance. Radiology 169:858, 1988

103. Chervenak FA, Duncan C, Ment LR et al: The outcome of fetal ventriculomegaly. Lancet 2:179, 1984

104. Lees RF, Alford BA, Brenbridge NAG et al: Sonographic appearance of duodenal atresia in utero. Am J Roentgenol 131:701, 1978

105. Romero R, Jeanty P, Pilu G et al: The prenatal diagnosis of duodenal atresia. Does it make any difference? Obstet Gynecol 71:739, 1988

106. Hobbins JC, Romero R, Grannum P et al: Antenatal diagnosis of renal anomalies with ultrasound. I. Obstructive uropathy. Am J Obstet Gynecol 148:868, 1984

107. Corteville JE, Gray DL, Crane JP: Congenital hydronephrosis: correlation of fetal ultrasonographic findings with infant outcome. Am J Obstet Gynecol 165:384, 1991

108. Mandell J, Blyth B, Peters CA et al: Structural genitourinary defects detected in utero. Radiology 178:193, 1991

109. Deter RL, Harrist RB, Birnholz JC, Hadlock FP: Quantitative Obstetrical Ultrasonography. Churchill Livingstone, New York, 1986

110. Chervenak FA, Jeanty P, Cantraine F et al: The diagnosis of fetal microcephaly. Am J Obstet Gynecol 149:512, 1984

111. Chervenak FA, Rosenberg J, Brigthman RC et al: A prospective study of the accuracy of ultrasound in predicting fetal microcephaly. Obstet Gynecol 69:908, 1987

112. Romero R, Pilu G, Jeanty P et al: Prenatal Diagnosis of Congenital Anomalies. p. 311. Appleton & Lange, Norwalk, CT, 1988

113. Chervenak FA, Tortora M, Mayden K et al: Antenatal diagnosis of median cleft face syndrome: sonographic demonstration of cleft lip and hypotelorism. Am J Obstet Gynecol 149:94, 1984

114. Grannum P, Bracken M, Silverman R et al: Assessment of fetal kidney size in normal gestation by comparison of ratio of kidney circumference to abdominal circumference. Am J Obstet Gynecol 136:249, 1980

115. Romero R, Cullen M, Jeanty P et al: The diagnosis of congenital renal anomalies with ultrasound. II. Infantile polycystic kidney disease. Am J Obstet Gynecol 150:259, 1984

116. Chervenak FA, Tortora MN, Hobbins JC: Antenatal sonographic diagnosis of clubfoot. J Ultrasound Med 4:49, 1985

117. Goldberg JD, Chervenak FA, Lipman RA et al: Antenatal sonographic diagnosis of arthrogryposis multiplex congenita. Prenat Diagn 6:45, 1986

118. Allan LD, Crawford DC, Anderson RH et al: Echocardiographic and anatomical correlation in fetal congenital heart disease. Br Heart J 52:542, 1984

119. Copel JA, Pilu G, Green J et al: Fetal echocardiographic screening for congenital heart disease: the importance

of the four-chamber view. Am J Obstet Gynecol 157: 648, 1987

120. Gertgesell HP (ed): Symposium of fetal echocardiography. J Clin Ultrasound 13:227, 1985

121. Devore G: Fetal echocardiography. p. 199. In Chervenak FA, Isaacson G, Campbell S (eds): Ultrasound in Obstetrics and Gynecology. Little, Brown, Boston, 1994

122. Reed KL, Anderson CF, Shenker L: Fetal Echocardiography: An Atlas. Alan R. Liss, New York, 1988

123. Kleinman CS, Copel JA: Fetal cardiac dysrhythmias: diagnosis and therapy. p. 195. In Chervenak FA, Isaacson G, Campbell S (eds): Ultrasound in Obstetrics and Gynecology. Little, Brown, Boston, 1993

124. Hill LM: Chromosomal abnormalities. p. 449. In McGahan JP, Porto M (eds): Diagnostic Ultrasound. JP Lippincott, Philadelphia, 1994

125. Kalousek DK, Fitch N, Paradice BA: Pathology of the Human Embryo and Previable Fetus: An Atlas. p. 188. Springer-Verlag, New York, 1990

126. Benaceraff BR, Gelman R, Frigoletto FD: Sonographic identification of second-trimester fetuses with Down syndrome. N Engl J Med 317:1371, 1987

127. Nyberg DA, Resta RG, Luthy DA et al: Prenatal sonographic findings of Down syndrome: review of 94 cases. Obstet Gynecol 76:370, 1990

128. Crome JP, Gray DL: Sonographically measured nuchal skinfold as a screening tool for Down syndrome: results of a prospective clinical trial. Obstet Gynecol 77:533, 1991

129. Benaceraff BR, Neuberg D, Bromley B, Frigoletto FD: Sonographic scoring index for prenatal detection of chromosomal abnormalities. J Ultrasound Med 11:449, 1992

130. Hill LM, Gurzevich D, Belfar ML et al: The current role of sonography in the detection of Down syndrome. Obstet Gynecol 74:620, 1989

131. Rotmensch S, Luo JS, Nores JA et al: Bilateral choroid plexus cysts in trisomy 21. Am J Obstet Gynecol 166: 591, 1992

132. Platt LD, Carlson DE, Medearis AL et al: Fetal choroid plexus cysts in the second trimester of pregnancy. A cause for concern. Am J Obstet Gynecol 64:1652, 1991

133. Benacerraf BR, Hanlon B, Frigoletto F: Are choroid plexus cysts an indication for second-trimester amniocentesis? Am J Obstet Gynecol 162:1001, 1990

134. Gupta JK, Cave M, Lilford RJ et al: Clinical significance of fetal choroid plexus cysts. Lancet 346:724, 1995

135. Copel JA, Pilu G, Kleinmann CS: Congenital heart disease and extracardiac anomalies: associations and indications for fetal echocardiography. Am J Obstet Gynecol 154:1121, 1986

136. Palmer CG, Miles JH, Howard-Peebles PN et al: Fetal karyotype following ascertainment of fetal anomalies by ultrasound. Prenat Diagn 7:551, 1987

137. Platt LD, DeVore GR, Lopez E et al: Role of amniocentesis in ultrasound-detected fetal malformations. Obstet Gynecol 68:153, 1986

138. Williamson RA, Weiner CP, Patil S et al: Abnormal pregnancy sonogram: selective indication for fetal karyotype. Obstet Gynecol 69:15, 1987

139. Nicolaides K, Shawwa L, Brizot M, Snijders R: Ultrasonographically detectable markers of fetal chromosomal defects. Ultrasound Obstet Gynecol 3:56, 1993

140. Chervenak FA, McCullough LB: An ethically justified, clinically comprehensive management strategy for third-trimester pregnancies complicated by fetal anomalies. Obstet Gynecol 75:311, 1990

141. Chervenak FA, McCullough LB: Does obstetric ethics have any role in the obstetrician's response to the abortion controversy? Am J Obstet Gynecol 163:1425, 1990

142. Harrison M, Golbus M, Filly R: The Unborn Patient. Grune & Stratton, New York, 1984

143. Seeds JW, Azizkhan RG: Congenital Malformations. Antenatal Diagnosis, Perinatal Management, and Counseling. Aspen Publishers, Rockville, MD, 1990

144. Romero R, Oyarzun E, Sirtori M, Hobbins JC: Detection and management of anatomic congenital anomalies. Obstet Gynecol Clin North Am 15:215, 1988

145. Chervenak FA, Berkowitz RL, Tortora M et al: The management of fetal hydrocephalus. Am J Obstet Gynecol 151:933, 1985

146. Luthy DA, Wardinsky T, Shurtleff DB et al: Cesarean section before the onset of labor and subsequent motor function in infants with open spina bifida. N Engl J Med 162:662, 1991

147. Manning FA, Harrison MR, Rodeck C et al: Catheter shunts for fetal hydronephrosis and hydrocephalus: special report. N Engl J Med 315:336, 1986

148. Manning FA: The anomalous fetus. p. 451. In Manning FA (ed): Fetal Medicine. Principles and Practice. Appleton & Lange, Norwalk, CT, 1995

149. Albar H, Manning FA, Harman CR: Treatment of urinary tract and CNS obstruction. p. 259. In Harman CR (ed): Invasive Fetal Testing and Treatment. Blackwell Scientific, Cambridge, 1995

150. Anderson RL, Golbus MS: Bladder aspiration. In Chervenak FA, Isaacson G, Campbell S (eds): Textbook of Ultrasound in Obstetrics and Gynecology. Little, Brown, Boston, 1993

151. Rodeck CH, Fisk NM, Fraser DI, Nicolini U: Long-term in utero drainage of fetal hydrothorax. N Engl J Med 319:1135, 1988

152. Nicolaides KH, Azar G: Thoracoamniotic shunting. p. 1289. In Chervenak FA, Isaacson G, Campbell S (eds): Textbook of Ultrasound in Obstetrics and Gynecology. Little, Brown, Boston, 1993

153. Vaughn JI, Fisk NM, Rodeck CM: Fetal pleural effusions. p. 219. In Harman CR (ed): Fetal Testing and Treatment. Blackwell Scientific, Cambridge, 1995

154. Clewell WH, Johnson ML, Meier PR et al: A surgical approach to the treatment of fetal hydrocephalus. N Engl J Med 306:1320, 1982

155. Clewell W: Current status of ventriculo-amniotic shunt placement. In Kurjak A, Comstock C, Chervenak FA (ed): Ultrasound and the Fetal Brain. Parthenon, Carnforth, 1996

156. Harrison MR, Adzick NS, Longaker MT et al: Successful repair in utero of a fetal diaphragmatic hernia after removal of herniated viscera from the left thorax. N Engl J Med 322:1582, 1990

157. *Roe v. Wade*, 410 US 113, 1973

158. Elias S, Annas GJ: Reproductive Genetics and the Law. Year Book Medical Publishers, Chicago, 1987

159. Annas GJ: Protecting the liberty of pregnant patients. N Engl J Med 316:1213, 1987

160. Chervenak FA, Farley MA, Walters L et al: When is termination of pregnancy during the third trimester morally justifiable? N Engl J Med 310:501, 1984

161. Chervenak FA, McCullough LB, Campbell S: Is third trimester abortion justified? Br J Obstet Gynaecol 102:434, 1995

162. Chervenak FA, McCullough LB: Nonaggressive obstetric management. An option for some fetal anomalies during the third trimester. JAMA 261:3439, 1989

163. Chervenak FA, McCullough LB: Ethical challenges in perinatal medicine: The intrapartum management of pregnancy complicated by fetal hydrocephalus with macrocephaly. Semin Perinatol 11:232, 1987

164. Chervenak FA, McCullough LB: Fetal destructive procedures in operative obstetrics. p. 354. In O'Grady JP, Gimovsky ML, McIlhargie LJ (eds): Operative Obstetrics. Williams & Wilkins, Baltimore, 1995

165. Ultrasonography in Pregnancy. ACOG Technical Bulletin, No. 187. American College of Obstetricians and Gynecologists, Washington, DC, 1993

166. Marinac-Dabic D, Moore RM Jr, Bright RA et al: Use of prenatal ultrasound in the United States: the results from the 1988 National Maternal and Infant Health Survey. J Perinatol 13:169, 1993

167. Ewigman B, Cornelison S, Horman D, LeFevre M: Use of routine prenatal ultrasound by private practice obstetricians in Iowa. J Ultrasound Med 10:427, 1991

168. Horger EO, Tsai CC: Ultrasound and the prenatal diagnosis of congenital anomalies: a medicolegal perspective. Obstet Gynecol 74:617, 1989

169. Warsof SL, Pearce JM, Campbell S: The present place of routine ultrasound screening. Clin Obstet Gynaecol 10:445, 1985

170. Gabbe SG: Routine versus indicated scans. p. 67. In Sabbagha RE (ed): Diagnostic Ultrasound Applied to Obstetrics and Gynecology. 3rd Ed. JB Lippincott Company, Philadelphia, 1994

171. Kramer MS, McLean FH, Boyd ME, Usher RH: The validity of gestational age estimation by menstrual dating in term, preterm, and postterm gestations. JAMA 260:3306, 1988

172. Haddow JE, Palomaki GE, Knight GJ et al: Prenatal screening for Down's syndrome with use of maternal serum markers. N Engl J Med 327:588, 1992

173. Grennert L, Persson P-H, Gennser G: Benefits of ultrasonic screening of a pregnant population. Acta Obstet Gynecol Scand 78(suppl):5, 1978

174. Persson P-H, Kullander S: Long-term experience of general ultrasound screening in pregnancy. Am J Obstet Gynecol 146:942, 1983

175. Hughey MJ, Olive DL: Routine ultrasound scanning for detection and management of twin pregnancy. J Reprod Med 30:427, 1985

176. Sanderson DA, Milton PJD: The effectiveness of ultrasound screening at 18–20 weeks gestational age for pre-

177. Romero R: Routine obstetric ultrasound. Utrasound Obstet Gynecol 3:303, 1993

178. Reading AE, Campbell S, Cox DN, Sledmere CM: Health beliefs and health care behaviour in pregnancy. Psychological Med 12:379, 1982

179. Waldenstrom U, Nilsson S, Fall O et al: Effects of routine one-stage ultrasound screening in pregnancy: a randomised controlled trial. Lancet 2:585, 1988

180. Bennett MJ, Little G, Dewhurst SJ, Chamberlain G: Predictive value of ultrasound measurement in early pregnancy: a randomized controlled trial. Br J Obstet Gynaecol 89:338, 1982

181. Eik-Nes SH, Okland O, Aure JC, Ulstein M: Ultrasound screening in pregnancy: a randomised controlled trial. Lancet 1:1347, 1984

182. Bakketeig LS, Jacobsen G, Brodtkorb CJ et al: Randomised controlled trial of ultrasonographic screening in pregnancy. Lancet 2:207, 1984

183. Neilson JP, Munjanja SP, Whitfield CR: Screening for small for dates fetuses: a controlled trial. BMJ 289:1179, 1984

184. Belfrage P, Fernstrom I, Hallenberg G: Routine or selective ultrasound examinations in early pregnancy. Obstet Gynecol 69:747, 1987

185. Ewigman B, LeFevre M, Hesser J: A randomized trial of routine prenatal ultrasound. Obstet Gynecol 76:189, 1990

186. Saari-Kemppainen A, Karjalainen O, Ylostalo P et al: Ultrasound screening and perinatal mortality: controlled trial of systematic one-stage screening in pregnancy. Lancet 336:387, 1990

187. Ewigman BG, Crane JP, Frigoletto FD et al: Effect of prenatal ultrasound screening on perinatal outcome. N Engl J Med 329:821, 1993

188. LeFevre ML, Bain RP, Ewigman BG et al: A randomized trial of prenatal ultrasonographic screening: impact on maternal management and outcome. Am J Obstet Gynecol 169:483, 1993

189. Crane JP, LeFevre ML, Winborn RC et al: A randomized trial of prenatal ultrasonographic screening: impact on the detection, management, and outcome of anomalous fetuses. Am J Obstet Gynecol 171:392, 1994

190. Berkowitz RL: Should every pregnant woman undergo ultrasonography? N Eng J Med 329:874, 1993

191. O'Day M, Ivey T, Bianchi A, Wilkins I: Application of RADIUS study criteria to a low-income obstetric population. SPO Abstract 305. Am J Obstet Gynecol 172:345

192. Barrett JM, Brinson J: Evaluation of obstetric ultrasonography at the first prenatal visit. Am J Obstet Gynecol 165:1002, 1991

193. DeVore GR: The routine antenatal diagnostic imaging with ultrasound study: another perspective. Obstet Gynecol 84:622, 1994

194. Chervenak FA, McCullough LB, Chervenak JL: Prenatal informed consent for sonogram: an indication for obstetric ultrasonography. Am J Obstet Gynecol 161:857, 1989

diction of placenta praevia. J Obstet Gynecol 11:320, 1991

Chapter 12

Antepartum Fetal Evaluation

Maurice L. Druzin and Steven G. Gabbe

Not too long ago, the first aim of obstetric care was to prevent maternal death due to tuberculosis, syphilis, difficult deliveries, and haemorrhage. When this battle was won, at least in developed countries, and when perinatal mortality had dropped spectacularly, more time and interest could be focused on the fetus.[1]

Antepartum fetal deaths now account for nearly 40 percent of all perinatal mortality in the United States. The obstetrician must be concerned not only with prevention of this mortality, but with the detection of fetal compromise and the timely delivery of such infants in an effort to maximize their future potential.[2] This chapter reviews the definition and causes of perinatal mortality, the techniques available for assessing fetal condition, how one may evaluate their diagnostic accuracy, and the clinical application of these techniques to obstetric practice.

The Etiology of Perinatal Mortality

The perinatal mortality rate (PMR) has been defined by the National Center for Health Statistics (NCHS) as the number of late fetal deaths (fetal deaths of 28 weeks' gestation or more) plus early neonatal deaths (deaths of infants 0 to 6 days of age) per 1,000 live births plus fetal deaths.[3] A live birth is the complete expulsion or extraction of a product of conception from its mother, irrespective of the duration of the pregnancy, that, after separation, breathes or shows any evidence of life, such as beating of the heart, pulsation of the umbilical cord, or definite movement of voluntary muscles, whether or not the umbilical cord has been cut or the placenta is attached; each product of such a birth is considered liveborn. According to the NCHS, the neonatal mortality rate is defined as the number of neonatal deaths

(deaths of infants 0 to 27 days of age) per 1,000 live births; the postneonatal mortality rate, the number of postneonatal deaths (the number of infants 28 to 365 days of age) per 1,000 live births; and the infant mortality rate, the number of infant deaths (deaths of infants under 1 year of age) per 1,000 live births. The definition of PMR provided by the World Health Organization (WHO) is somewhat different, including the number of fetuses and live births weighing at least 500 g or, when birth weight is unavailable, the corresponding gestational age (22 weeks) or body length (25 cm crown–heel) dying before day 7 of life per 1,000 such fetuses and infants. The American College of Obstetricians and Gynecologists (ACOG) has recently recommended that only deaths of fetuses and infants weighing 500 g or more at delivery be used to compare data among states in the United States.[4] For international comparisons, only deaths of fetuses and infants weighing 1,000 g or more at delivery should be included.[4]

Since 1965, the PMR in the United States has fallen steadily. Using the NCHS definition, the PMR reported in 1991 was 8.7/1,000.[5] The overall neonatal mortality rate was 5.6/1,000, with fetal deaths at 3.1/1,000. The PMR for blacks, 15.7/1,000, was more than twice that of whites, 7.4/1,000. The significantly greater PMR in blacks results from higher rates of *both* neonatal and fetal deaths.

While the majority of fetal deaths occur before 32 weeks' gestation, Grant and Elbourne[6] have emphasized that, in planning a strategy for antepartum fetal monitoring, one must examine the risk of fetal death in the population of women who are still pregnant at that point in pregnancy. When this approach is taken, one finds that fetuses at 40 to 41 weeks are at a 3-fold greater risk and those at 42 or more weeks are at a 12-

fold greater risk for intrauterine death than fetuses at 28 to 31 weeks.

The overall pattern of perinatal deaths in the United States has changed considerably during the past 30 years. Data collected between 1959 and 1966 by the Collaborative Perinatal Project revealed that 30 percent of perinatal deaths could be attributed to complications of the cord and placenta.[7] Other major causes of perinatal loss were maternal and fetal infections (17 percent), prematurity (10 percent), congenital anomalies (8 percent), and erythroblastosis fetalis (4 percent). In this series, 21 percent of the deaths were of unknown causes. In 1982, the major cause of early neonatal death was attributed to conditions originating in the perinatal period, such as infections, intraventricular hemorrhage, hydrops, meconium aspiration, and maternal complications such as diabetes mellitus and hypertension.[2] Congenital anomalies were the second leading cause of early neonatal death, accounting for 23 percent of such losses, while intrauterine hypoxia and birth asphyxia were responsible for 5 percent.

The infant mortality rate has fallen progressively from 47.0/1,000 in 1940 to 26.0/1,000 in 1960, 12.6/1,000 in 1980, 9.2/1,000 in 1990, and 7.9/1,000 in 1994.[8] While the infant mortality rate includes all deaths of infants under 1 year of age, 50 percent of all infant deaths occur in the first week of life, and 50 percent of these losses result in the first day of life.[4] Clearly, perinatal events play an important role in infant mortality. In 1994, the leading cause of infant mortality reported by the NCHS was "perinatal conditions not separately listed," including maternal complications such as hypertension and substance abuse, multiple pregnancy, placenta previa and abruption, breech delivery, prolonged pregnancy and macrosomia, congenital pneumonia and viral infections, meconium aspiration, and Rh isoimmunization. This diverse category accounted for 25.4 percent of infant mortality, while congenital anomalies and sudden infant death syndrome were responsible for 20.3 and 14.8 percent, respectively. Short gestation and low birth weight contributed 12.3 percent and respiratory distress syndrome 6.7 percent. Only 2.1 percent of infant mortality was attributed to intrauterine hypoxia–birth asphyxia.

Fetal deaths may be divided into those that occur during the antepartum period and those that occur during labor, intrapartum stillbirths. From 70 to almost 90 percent of fetal deaths occurred before the onset of labor.[9] Manning et al.[10] point out that antepartum deaths may be divided into four broad categories: (1) chronic asphyxia of diverse origin; (2) congenital malformations; (3) superimposed complications of pregnancy, such as Rh isoimmunization, placental abruption, and fetal infection; and (4) deaths of unexplained cause. If it is to succeed, a program of antenatal surveillance must identify malformed fetuses (Ch. 11) and recognize those at risk for asphyxia.

Recent data describing the etiology of fetal deaths in the United States are not available. Lammer and colleagues[9] reviewed the causes of 574 fetal deaths in Massachusetts during 1982. For the first time, the fetal mortality rate in that state exceeded the neonatal mortality rate, emphasizing that if further decreases in the PMR are to be achieved, they will need to come from reductions in fetal as well as neonatal mortality. Fetal mortality was higher among women who were black, unmarried, over age 34, under age 20, of parity 5 or higher, and received no prenatal care or care only in the third trimester. Ten percent of all fetal deaths occurred in multiple gestations, for a fetal mortality rate of 50/1,000, or a rate seven times that of women with singleton pregnancies. More than half of all fetal deaths were assigned to either asphyxia or maternal conditions, including hypertension and placenta abruption and infarction. Overall, 30 percent of the fetal deaths were attributed to maternal causes, 28 percent to hypoxia, 12 percent to congenital anomalies, and 4 percent to infection. In almost 25 percent, no cause could be identified. Of note, when autopsy data were reviewed, there was disagreement between the fetal death record and autopsy findings in 55 percent of cases.

Fretts and colleagues[11,12] recently analyzed the causes of deaths in fetuses weighing more than 500 g in 94,346 births at the Royal Victoria Hospital in Montreal from 1961 to 1993. The population studied was predominantly white and included patients from all socioeconomic groups. Approximately 95 percent made four or more prenatal visits. Overall, the fetal death rate declined by 70 percent, from 11.5/1,000 in the 1960s to 3.2/1,000 during 1990 to 1993.[12] The decline in the fetal death rate may be attributed to the prevention of Rh sensitization, antepartum fetal surveillance, improved detection of intrauterine growth restriction (IUGR) and fetal anomalies with ultrasound, and improved care of maternal diabetes mellitus and preeclampsia. Fetal deaths due to intrapartum asphyxia and Rh isoimmunization fell dramatically, from 13.1 to 1.2/1,000 for intrapartum asphyxia and 4.3 to 0.7/1,000 for Rh disease.[11] Deaths due to lethal anomalies declined by 50 percent, 10.8 to 5.4/1,000, because early terminations of pregnancy were performed for anencephaly. While fetal mortality resulting from IUGR fell 60 percent, 17.9 to 7.0/1,000 births, the growth-restricted fetus still had a more than 10-fold greater risk for fetal death than an appropriately grown fetus. Fretts et al. noted that most of these deaths occurred between 28 and 36 weeks' gestation and that the diagnosis of IUGR was rarely identified before death. In addition to IUGR, leading causes of fetal death after 28 weeks' gestation included abruption and unexplained antepartum losses. Despite a marked fall in unexplained fetal deaths, 38.1 to 13.6/1,000, these losses were still responsible for more than 25 percent of all stillbirths. Fetal–maternal hemorrhage may occur in 10 to 15 percent of cases of unexplained fetal deaths. Fetal deaths due to infection, most often associated with premature rupture of the membranes before 28 weeks' gestation, did not decline over the 30 years of the study. Fretts et al.[11] also noted that, after controlling for risk factors such as multiple gestation, hypertension, diabetes mellitus, placenta previa and abruption, previous abortion, and prior fetal death, women 35 years of age or older had a nearly twofold greater risk for fetal death than women under 30.

Schauer et al.[13] summarized data from seven studies evaluating the causes of fetal death after 20 weeks. The largest group was unexplained, mostly asphyxial intrauterine deaths, 9 to 50 percent; major anomalies, 7 to 21 percent; antepartum hemorrhage with or without verified abruption (as in the Fretts et al. data the single largest known cause of fetal death), 12 to 17 percent; IUGR, 7 to 15 percent; hypertension, 1.9 to 15.7 percent; isoimmunization, 2.3 to 7.7 percent; diabetes mellitus, less than 1 to 4.8 percent; and infection, 2.1 to 6.1 percent. In a prospective study of 107 late fetal deaths, all of which had a full autopsy, Schauer et al.[13] observed a similar distribution of causes: asphyxia, 66 percent; multiple anomalies, 6 percent; chromosomal disorders, 6 percent; infection, 3 percent, and unknown, 19 percent. The chromosomal abnormalities included trisomy 21, trisomy 18, and 45,XO.

In summary, based on available data, approximately 30 percent of antepartum fetal deaths may be attributed to asphyxia; 30 percent to maternal complications, especially placenta abruption, hypertension, and preeclampsia; 15 percent to congenital malformations and chromosomal abnormalities; and 5 percent to infection. At least 20 percent of stillbirths will have no obvious etiology.

Can these antepartum fetal deaths be prevented? Grant and Elbourne[6] have noted that "antepartum late fetal death is the component of perinatal mortality that has shown greatest resistance to change over recent years. In part, this reflects its relative unpredictability; in part, it reflects the relatively long period of time over which it can occur." Obstetric and pediatric assessors reviewed the circumstances surrounding each case of perinatal death in the Mersey region of England to identify any avoidable factors contributing to the death.[14] There were 309 perinatal deaths in this population, consisting of 157 stillbirths and 152 deaths in the first week of life. Of the 309 perinatal deaths, 182 (58.9 percent) were considered to have had avoidable factors. Most avoidable factors were found to be obstetric rather than pediatric or maternal and social. A high proportion (73.8 percent) of normal-birth-weight infants with no fetal abnormalities and no maternal complications had avoidable factors. The failure to respond appropriately to abnormalities during pregnancy and labor, including results from the monitoring of fetal growth or intrapartum fetal well-being, significant maternal weight loss, or reported reductions in fetal movement, constituted the largest groups of avoidable factors. Kirkup and Welch[15] confirmed these results in an analysis of avoidable factors contributing to fetal death in nonmalformed infants weighing 2,500 g or more. Patients at highest risk for fetal death included women of a parity of 3 or more and those who had no prenatal care before 20 weeks. The Mersey Region Working Party on Perinatal Mortality concluded that, in light of increasing public awareness about obstetric management and, in some instances, an antipathy toward modern procedures, the failure to act on abnormalities discovered during monitoring would assume greater importance.[14] These workers found that in no case was the induction of labor as a result of such monitoring considered an avoidable factor.

A large clinical experience has demonstrated that antepartum fetal assessment can have a significant impact on the frequency and causes of antenatal fetal deaths. Schneider and colleagues[16] reviewed a decade of experience with antepartum fetal heart rate monitoring from 1974 through 1983. The contraction stress test was used primarily during the first 2 years of the study, followed by the nonstress test. Overall, the perinatal mortality rate was found to be 22.4/1,000 in the nontested population and 11.8/1,000 in the tested high-risk population, a highly significant difference. The stillbirth rate in the nontested population, 11.1/1,000, was twice that of patients who were followed with antepartum surveillance. When corrected for congenital anomalies, the stillbirth rate in the tested high-risk population was only 2.2/1,000. Of 18 stillbirths within 7 days of testing, the majority were due to congenital anomalies and placental abruption.

In a carefully performed study, Stubblefield and Berek[17] reviewed the causes of perinatal death in term and post-term births at the Boston Hospital for Women. The most frequent cause of death of a term or post-term infant was extrinsic perinatal hypoxia, and the second most common cause was a lethal malformation. Overall, extrinsic perinatal hypoxia accounted for 56.1 percent of the deaths of term infants and 71.4 percent of the deaths of post-term infants. Major malformations were implicated in 26.3 percent of the deaths of term infants. Twenty-nine of the 32 antenatal deaths occurred between 37 and 42 weeks' gestation. The authors concluded that two-thirds of the antenatal deaths were associated with chronic processes such as placental infarction that might have been detected had routine antepartum fetal surveillance been used. In obstetric populations in which high-risk patients are monitored, the majority of stillbirths now occur in what had previously been considered normal pregnancies.

Application of Antepartum Fetal Testing

Before using antepartum fetal testing, the obstetrician must ask several important questions[18]:

1. Does the test provide information not already known by the patient's clinical status?
2. Can the information be helpful in managing the patient?
3. Should an abnormality be detected, is there a treatment available for the problem?
4. Could an abnormal test result lead to increased risk for the mother or fetus?
5. Will the test ultimately decrease perinatal morbidity and mortality?

Unfortunately, few of the tests commonly employed today in clinical practice have been subjected to prospective and randomized evaluations that can answer these questions.[19,20] In most cases when the test has been applied and good perinatal outcomes were observed, the test has gained further acceptance and has been used more widely. In such cases, one cannot be sure whether it is actually the information provided by the test that has led to the improved outcomes or whether it is the total program of care that has made the difference. When prospective randomized investigations are conducted, large numbers of patients must be studied since many adverse outcomes such as intrauterine death are uncommon even in high-risk populations.[20] While several controlled trials have failed to demonstrate improved outcomes with nonstress testing, the study populations ranged from only 300 to 530 subjects.[21–24]

The first box below lists the information one might predict from an antepartum fetal test. Although one would want to detect IUGR or discover the presence of a significant congenital malformation, the most valuable information provided by antepartum fetal assessment may be that the fetus is well and requires no intervention. In this way, the pregnancy may be safely prolonged and the fetus allowed to gain further maturity. The second box below lists those aspects of obstetric management that might be influenced by antepartum testing. Certainly, one would not want to begin a program of testing unless one were prepared to use the information.

Using the information has invariably meant prompt intervention by delivery that may not be indicated and could lead to potentially avoidable complications of

prematurity. A more current approach is to use the term *intervention* to describe other types of procedures short of premature delivery. This strategy would include using combinations of antepartum tests in an organized sequence to evaluate the fetus further, administration of antenatal steroids, bedrest, prolonged oxygen therapy, and correction of maternal metabolic, cardiopulmonary, or other medical disorders. *Intervention* may also refer to fetal therapy such as intrauterine transfusion for anemia, removal of fluid from body cavities, diagnostic procedures, and direct administration of medication to the fetus. Testing can be initiated at

---

Aspects of Fetal Condition that Might Be Predicted by Antepartum Testing

Perinatal death

Intrauterine growth restriction (IUGR)

Nonreassuring fetal status, intrapartum

Neonatal asphyxia

Postnatal motor and intellectual impairment

Premature delivery

Congenital abnormalities

Need for specific therapy

(Adapted from Chard and Klopper,[2] with permission.)

Obstetric Management That Might Be Influenced by Antepartum Testing

Preterm delivery

Route of delivery

Bedrest

Observation

Drug therapy

Operative intervention in labor

Neonatal intensive care

Termination of pregnancy for a congenital anomaly

(Adapted from Chard and Klopper,[2] with permission.)

1. Patients at high risk of uteroplacental insufficiency
   Prolonged pregnancy
   Diabetes mellitus
   Hypertension
   Previous stillbirth
   Suspected IUGR
   Advanced maternal age
2. When other tests suggest fetal compromise
   Suspected IUGR
   Decreased fetal movement
3. Routine antepartum surveillance

early gestational ages, 25 to 26 weeks, to identify the fetus at risk. Maternal and fetal interventions can then be considered. Obviously, prolongation of intrauterine life is the primary goal, and better understanding of the pathophysiology of the premature fetus and the use of combinations of tests will allow this to be accomplished. In the event of impending in utero death or severe compromise, premature delivery, while the last resort, is a reasonable option, given the remarkable survival statistics being reported in modern neonatal intensive care units. The use of postnatal surfactant and improved mechanical ventilators are only some of the advances leading to survival and intact neurologic survival statistics that would have been incomprehensible a decade ago.[25-27]

In selecting the population of patients for antepartum fetal evaluation, one would certainly include those pregnancies known to be at high risk of uteroplacental insufficiency (Table 12-1).

The question of routine antepartum fetal surveillance must be carefully examined. Antepartum fetal testing can more accurately predict fetal outcome than antenatal risk assessment using an established scoring system.[28] Patients judged to be at high risk based on known medical factors but whose fetuses demonstrated normal antepartum fetal evaluation had a lower PMR than did patients considered at low risk whose fetuses had abnormal antepartum testing results. Routine antepartum fetal evaluation would be necessary to detect most infants dying in utero as the result of hypoxia and asphyxia.[17] It would seem reasonable, therefore, to consider extending some form of antepartum fetal surveillance to all obstetric patients. As described below, assessment of fetal activity by the mother may be an ideal technique for this purpose.

Statistical Assessment of Antepartum Testing

To determine the clinical application of antepartum diagnostic testing, the predictive value of the tests must be considered.[29,30] This information can most easily be presented in a 2 × 2 matrix. Table 12-2 presents this matrix using the contraction stress test (CST) and intrauterine fetal death as examples. The sensitivity of the test is the probability that the test will be positive or abnormal when the disease is present. The specificity of the test is the probability that the test result will be negative when the disease is not present. Note that the sensitivity and specificity refer not to the actual numbers of patients with a positive or abnormal result, but to the proportion or probability of these test results. The predictive value of an abnormal test would be that fraction of patients with an abnormal test result who have the abnormal condition, while the predictive value of a normal test would be the fraction of patients with a normal test result who are normal (Table 12-2).

Antepartum fetal tests may be used to screen a large obstetric population to detect fetal disease. In this setting, a test of high sensitivity is preferable, since one would not want to miss patients whose fetuses might be compromised. One would be willing to overdiagnose the problem, that is, accept some false-positive diagnoses. In further evaluating the patient whose fetus may be at risk and when attempting to confirm the presence of disease, one would want a test of high specificity. One would not want to intervene unnecessarily and deliver a fetus that was doing well. In this setting, multiple tests may be helpful. When multiple test results are normal, they tend to exclude disease. When all are abnormal, however, they tend to support the diagnosis of fetal disease.

The prevalence of the abnormal condition has great impact on the predictive value of antepartum fetal tests. Table 12-3 presents data for a population of 1,000 patients in whom the prevalence of the disease is 50 percent. The sensitivity of the test being evaluated is 75 percent, and its specificity is 98 percent. These figures are similar to those observed for several antepartum tests now in use. In this setting, an abnormal test result is likely to be associated with a true fetal abnormality.

Table 12-2   Two-by-Two Matrix of Possible Results for the CST

Test Result	Perinatal Outcome	
	Normal (Normal Newborn)	Abnormal (Intrauterine Fetal Death)
Normal (negative CST)	A True negative	B False negative
Abnormal (positive CST)	C False positive	D True positive

Sensitivity = D/(D + B).
Specificity = A/(A + C).
Predictive value of a positive test = D/(C + D).
Predictive value of a negative test = A/(A + B).

Table 12-3   Fifty Percent Prevalence

	Perinatal Outcome	
Test Result	Normal	Abnormal
Normal	490 True negative	125 False negative
Abnormal	10 False positive	375 True positive

Sensitivity = 75%.
Specificity = 98%.
Predictive value of a positive test = 97.4% (375/385).
Predictive value of a negative test = 79.6% (490/615).

Table 12-4   Two Percent Prevalence

	Perinatal Outcome	
Test Result	Normal	Abnormal
Normal	960 True negative	5 False negative
Abnormal	20 False positive	15 True positive

Sensitivity = 75%.
Specificity = 98%.
Predictive value of a positive test = 42.8% (15/35).
Predictive value of a negative test = 99.4% (960/965).

The predictive value of a positive test is 97.4 percent. However, when the prevalence of the disease falls to 2 percent, as it may be for intrauterine fetal deaths, even tests with a high sensitivity and specificity are associated with many false predictions (Table 12-4). In this circumstance, an abnormal test is more likely to indicate a false-positive diagnosis (n = 20) than it is a true positive diagnosis (n = 15).

In interpreting the results of studies of antepartum testing, the obstetrician must consider the application of that test to his or her own population. If the study has been done in a population of patients at great risk, it is more likely that an abnormal test will be associated with an abnormal fetus. If the obstetrician is practicing in a community with patients who are, in general, at

low risk, however, an abnormal test result would more likely be associated with a false-positive diagnosis.

For most antepartum diagnostic tests, a cut-off point used to define an abnormal result must be arbitrarily established.[31] The cut-off point is selected to maximize the separation between the normal and diseased populations (Fig. 12-1). Changing the cut-off will have a great impact on the predictive value of the test. For example, suppose that 10 accelerations in 10 minutes were required for a fetus to have a reactive nonstress test (threshold A). The fetus who fulfilled this rigid definition would almost certainly be in good condition. However, many fetuses who failed to achieve 10 accelerations in 10 minutes would also be in good condition, but would be judged to be abnormal by this cut-off. In

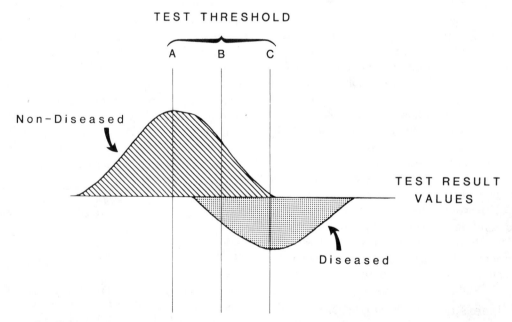

Fig. 12-1 Hypothetical distribution of test results in a normal and diseased population, demonstrating the differences in test sensitivity and specificity with a change in test threshold. Making it more difficult for the fetus to pass the test by raising the test threshold (A) will increase the sensitivity, but decrease the specificity, of the test. On the other hand, making the test easier to pass by decreasing the test threshold (C) will increase the specificity of the test, but decrease the sensitivity. (Adapted from Carpenter and Coustan,[31] with permission.)

this instance, the test would have many abnormal results. It would be highly sensitive and capture all of the abnormal fetuses, but it would have a low specificity. If the number of accelerations required to pass a nonstress test were lowered to 1 in 10 minutes, it would decrease the sensitivity of the test (threshold C). That is, one might miss a truly sick fetus. At the same time, however, one would improve the specificity of the test or its ability to predict that percentage of the patients who are normal. Using the criteria of 2 accelerations of the fetal heart rate in 20 minutes for a reactive nonstress test (threshold B), one hopes to have a test with both high sensitivity and high specificity.

Biophysical Techniques of Fetal Evaluation

Fetal State

When interpreting tests that monitor fetal biophysical characteristics, one must appreciate that, during the third trimester, the normal fetus may exhibit marked changes in its neurologic state.[32,33] Four fetal states have been identified. The near-term fetus spends approximately 25 percent of its time in a quiet sleep state (state 1F) and 60 to 70 percent in an active sleep state (state 2F). Active sleep is associated with rapid eye movements (REM). In fetal lambs, electrocortical activity during REM sleep is characterized by low-voltage, high-frequency waves. The fetus exhibits regular breathing movements and intermittent abrupt movements of its head, limbs, and trunk. The fetal heart rate in active sleep (state 2F) exhibits increased variability and frequent accelerations with movement. During quiet, or non-REM, sleep, the fetal heart rate slows and heart rate variability is reduced. The fetus may make infrequent breathing movements and startled movements. Electrocortical activity recordings at this time reveal high-voltage, low-frequency waves. Near term, periods of quiet sleep may last 20 minutes, and those of active sleep approximately 40 minutes.[33] The mechanisms that control these periods of rest and activity in the fetus are not well established. External factors such as the mother's activity, her ingestion of drugs, and her nutrition may all play a role.

When evaluating fetal condition using the nonstress test or the biophysical profile, one must ask whether a fetus that is not making breathing movements or shows no accelerations of its baseline heart rate is in a quiet sleep state or is neurologically compromised. In such circumstances, prolonging the period of evaluation will usually allow a change in fetal state, and more normal parameters of fetal well-being will appear.

Maternal Assessment of Fetal Activity

Maternal assessment of fetal activity is a simple yet valuable method for monitoring fetal condition. Most patients can understand and follow protocols for counting fetal activity, and this method is obviously inexpensive. Therefore, maternal assessment of fetal activity may be ideal for routine antepartum fetal surveillance.

Studies performed using real-time ultrasonography have demonstrated that during the third trimester the human fetus spends 10 percent of its time making gross fetal body movements and that 30 such movements are made each hour.[34] Periods of active fetal body movement last approximately 40 minutes, while quiet periods last about 20 minutes. Patrick et al.[34] noted that the longest period without fetal movements in a normal fetus was approximately 75 minutes. The mother is able to appreciate about 70 to 80 percent of gross fetal movements. The fetus does make fine body movements such as limb flexion and extension, hand grasping, and sucking, which probably reflect more coordinated central nervous system (CNS) function. However, the mother is generally unable to perceive these fine movements. Fetal movement appears to peak between 9:00 p.m. and 1:00 a.m., a time when maternal glucose levels are falling.[34] In a study in which maternal glucose levels were carefully controlled with an artificial pancreas, Holden et al.,[35] found that hypoglycemia was associated with increased fetal movement. Fetal activity does not increase after meals or after maternal glucose administration.[36,37]

Maternal evaluation of fetal activity may reduce fetal deaths due to asphyxia. Using a sheep model, Natale et al.[38] demonstrated that fetal activity is extremely sensitive to a decrease in fetal oxygenation. A small fall in fetal P_{O_2} was associated with a cessation of limb movements in the fetal lamb.

Several methods have been used to monitor fetal activity in clinical practice. In general, the presence of fetal movements is a reassuring sign of fetal health. However, the absence of fetal activity requires further assessment before one can conclude that fetal compromise exists. Sadovsky et al.[39] recommended that mothers count fetal activity for 30 to 60 minutes each day, two or three times daily. If the mother has fewer than three movements in 1 hour, or if she appreciates no movements for 12 hours, the movement alarm signal, further evaluation of fetal condition must be made. Rayburn et al.[40] suggested that patients count fetal activity at least 60 minutes each day. Fewer than three movements an hour for 2 consecutive days may be a sign of fetal compromise. Pearson and Weaver[41] advocated the use of the Cardiff Count-to-Ten chart. They found that only 2.5 percent of 1,654 daily movement counts recorded by 61 women who subsequently delivered healthy infants fell below 10 movements per 12 hours. Therefore, they accepted 10 movements as the minimum amount of fetal activity the patient should perceive in a 12-hour period. The patient is asked to start counting the movements in the morning and to record the time of day at which the tenth movement has been perceived. Should the patient not have 10 movements during 12 hours, or should it take longer each day to reach 10 movements, the patient is told to contact her obstetrician. Sadovsky et al.[42] found that, of those techniques currently used in clinical management, the movement alarm signal and the technique of Pearson and Weaver are the most valuable.

Whatever technique is used must be carefully explained to the patient. While most women are reassured by keeping a fetal activity chart and maternal–fetal attachment may be enhanced, some patients do become more anxious.[43,44] Women who were concerned about monitoring fetal movement complained that they were not given adequate information about variations in fetal activity patterns and maternal perception of movement.

While there will be a wide but normal range in fetal activity, with fetal movement counting, each mother and her fetus serve as their own control.[6] Fetal and placental factors that influence maternal assessment of fetal activity include placental location, the length of fetal movements, the amniotic fluid volume, and fetal anomalies.[45] If the placenta is anterior, maternal perception of fetal movements may be decreased. Movements lasting 20 to 60 seconds are most likely to be felt by the mother.[46] Hydramnios will reduce the mother's appreciation of fetal activity. Hydramnios may be associated with a fetal anomaly and should be further evaluated using ultrasonography. Rayburn and Barr[47] reported that 26 percent of fetuses with major malformations show decreased fetal activity compared with only 4 percent of normal fetuses. Anomalies of the CNS are most commonly associated with decreased activity. Approximately 80 percent of all mothers will be able to comply with a program of counting fetal activity.[6,48] Maternal factors that influence the evaluation of fetal movement include maternal activity, obesity, and medications. Mothers appear to appreciate fetal movements best when resting in the left lateral recumbent position. Patients should therefore be told to lie down when counting fetal movement, an additional benefit of this approach to fetal evaluation. Obesity decreases maternal appreciation of fetal activity. Maternal medications such as narcotics or barbiturates may depress fetal movement.

Several large clinical studies have demonstrated the efficacy of maternal assessment of fetal activity in preventing unexplained fetal deaths. In a prospective randomized study, Neldam[48] asked one group of 1,562

pregnant patients at 32 weeks' gestation to count fetal activity three times each week for 2 hours after their main meals. Fewer than three fetal movements each hour was regarded as a sign of potential fetal compromise and was further evaluated with an ultrasound examination and a nonstress test. In the monitored group of patients, only one stillbirth occurred. Ten stillbirths were noted in a control population of 1,549 women. Overall, 4 percent of patients in the monitored group reported their baby was not moving adequately, a low figure but one similar to that observed in other studies. Of these 60 patients, almost 25 percent were found to have a fetus in distress based on further antepartum testing. Neldam[48] attributed the prevention of 14 fetal deaths to the use of maternal assessment of fetal activity.

Rayburn[49] found that in the 5 percent of his patients who reported decreased fetal activity the incidence of stillbirths was 60 times higher, the risk of fetal distress in labor two to three times higher, the incidence of low Apgar scores at delivery 10 times greater, and the incidence of severe growth restriction 10 times higher. Rayburn also observed that the normal fetus does *not* decrease activity in the week before delivery.

Using the Cardiff Count-to-Ten chart, Liston et al.[50] noted that 11 of 150 high-risk patients (7.3 percent) reported fewer than 10 movements in a 12-hour period. Two of these patients suffered perinatal deaths, and 33 percent experienced fetal distress in labor. Overall, 60 percent of patients who reported decreased fetal activity did exhibit evidence of fetal compromise. The number of false alarms was quite manageable.

Two prospective studies have yielded conflicting results regarding the efficacy of fetal movement counting as a technique for preventing fetal deaths. Grant and coworkers[51] recruited 68,000 European women who were randomly allocated within 33 pairs of clusters to either routine fetal movement counting using the Cardiff Count-to-Ten method or to standard care. Women counted for an average of almost 3 hours per day, and about 7 percent of the charts showed at least one alarm. Of concern, the rate of compliance for reporting decreased fetal movement was only 46 percent. Furthermore, compliance for charting movements and reporting alarms was lower among women who had a late fetal death. The antepartum death rates for nonmalformed singleton fetuses were equal in both experimental groups. However, in none of the 17 cases in which reduced movements were recognized and the fetus was still alive when the patient arrived at the hospital was an emergency delivery attempted. Why? Grant et al.[51] conclude that intervention was not undertaken because of false reassurance from follow-up testing, especially heart rate monitoring, and because of errors in clinical judgment. One might conclude that this large prospec-

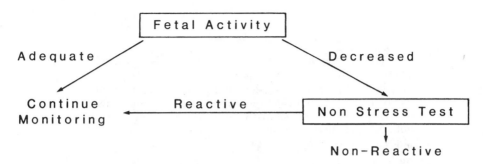

Fig. 12-2 Maternal assessment of fetal activity is a valuable screening test for fetal condition. Should the mother report decreased fetal activity, a NST is performed. In this situation most NSTs will be reactive.

tive study failed to demonstrate a reduction in the antepartum fetal death rate as a result of fetal movement counting. However, what it seems to prove most clearly is that patient compliance is an essential part of this program as is appropriate evaluation of the patient who presents with decreased fetal activity.

In contrast to the study by Grant and coworkers, an investigation by Moore and Piacquadio[52] demonstrated an impressive reduction in fetal deaths resulting from a formal program of fetal movement counting. Patients used the Count-to-Ten approach but were told to monitor fetal activity in the evening, a time of increased fetal movement. Most women observed 10 movements in an average of 21 minutes, and compliance was greater than 90 percent. Patients who did not perceive 10 movements in 2 hours, a level of fetal activity slightly more than five standard deviations below the mean, were told to report immediately for further evaluation. During a 7-month control period, a fetal mortality rate of 8.7/1,000 was observed in 2,519 patients, and 11 of 247 women who came to the hospital with a complaint of decreased fetal movement had already suffered an intrauterine death. During the study period, the fetal death rate fell to 2.1/1,000, and only 1 of 290 patients with decreased fetal movement presented after fetal death had occurred. The number of antepartum tests required to assess patients with decreased fetal activity rose 13 percent during the study period. This investigation has been expanded to include almost 6,000 patients, and a fetal death rate of 3.6/1,000, less than half that found in the control period, has been achieved.[53]

In conclusion, there appears to be a clearly established relationship between decreased fetal activity and fetal death. Therefore, it would seem prudent to request that *all* pregnant patients, regardless of their risk status, monitor fetal activity starting at 28 weeks' gestation (Fig. 12-2). The Count-to-Ten approach developed by Moore and Piacquadio[53] seems ideal.

Contraction Stress Test

The CST, also known as the oxytocin challenge test (OCT), was the first biophysical technique widely applied for antepartum fetal surveillance. It was well known that uterine contractions produced a reduction in blood flow to the intervillous space. Analyses of intrapartum fetal heart rate monitoring had demonstrated that a fetus with inadequate placental respiratory reserve would demonstrate late decelerations in response to hypoxia (see Ch. 14). The CST extended these observations to the antepartum period. The response of the fetus at risk for uteroplacental insufficiency to uterine contractions formed the basis for this test.

Performing the CST

The CST may be conducted in the labor and delivery suite or in an adjacent area, although the likelihood of fetal distress requiring immediate delivery in response to uterine contractions or hyperstimulation is extremely small. The CST should be performed by staff familiar with the principles and technique of such testing. In many institutions, an antenatal diagnostic unit has been developed for this purpose. The patient is placed in the semi-Fowler's position at a 30- to 45-degree angle with a slight left tilt to avoid the supine hypotensive syndrome. The fetal heart rate is recorded using a Doppler ultrasound transducer, while uterine contractions are monitored with the tocodynamometer. Maternal blood pressure is determined every 5 to 10 minutes to detect maternal hypotension.[54] Baseline fetal heart rate and uterine tone are first recorded for a period of approximately 10 to 20 minutes. In some cases, adequate uterine activity will occur spontaneously, and additional uterine stimulation will not be necessary. An adequate CST requires uterine contractions of moderate intensity lasting approximately 40 to 60 seconds with a frequency of three in 10 minutes. These criteria were selected to approximate the stress experienced by the fetus during the first stage of labor. If uterine activity is absent or inadequate, nipple stimulation is used to initiate contractions or intravenous oxytocin is begun. Oxytocin is administered by an infusion pump at 0.5 mU/min. The infusion rate is doubled every 20 minutes until adequate uterine contractions

Table 12-5 Interpretation of the Contraction Stress Test

Interpretation	Description	Incidence (%)
Negative	No late decelerations appearing anywhere on the tracing with adequate uterine contractions (three in 10 minutes)	80
Positive	Late decelerations that are consistent and persistent, present with the majority (>50 percent) of contractions without excessive uterine activity; if persistent late decelerations seen before the frequency of contractions is adequate, test interpreted as positive	3–5
Suspicious	Inconsistent late decelerations	5
Hyperstimulation	Uterine contractions closer than every 2 minutes or lasting >90 seconds, or five uterine contractions in 10 minutes; if no late decelerations seen, test interpreted as negative	5
Unsatisfactory	Quality of the tracing inadequate for interpretation or adequate uterine activity cannot be achieved	5

have been achieved.[55] One does not usually need to exceed 10 mU/min to produce adequate uterine activity. After the CST has been completed, the patient should be observed until uterine activity has returned to its baseline level. With nipple stimulation, the test may take approximately 30 minutes. If oxytocin is needed, 90 minutes may be required to perform the CST.

Contraindications to the test include those patients at high risk for premature labor, such as patients with premature rupture of the membranes, multiple gestation, and cervical incompetence, although the CST has not been associated with an increased incidence of premature labor.[56] The CST should also be avoided in conditions in which uterine contractions may be dangerous, such as placenta previa and a previous classical cesarean section or uterine surgery.

Interpreting the CST

Most clinicians utilize the definitions proposed by Freeman to interpret the CST[56,57] (Table 12-5). In an attempt to decrease the frequency of suspicious tests that would require further evaluation, Martin and Schifrin[58] developed the "10-minute window" concept. A positive test would be any 10-minute segment of the tracing that includes three contractions, all showing late decelerations. A negative test is one in which no positive window is seen and there is at least one negative window, three uterine contractions in 10 minutes with no late decelerations (Figs. 12-3, 12-4). The CST would be read as negative and not suspicious if an occasional late deceleration were seen, but a negative window was also present. They used the term *equivocal* rather than *suspicious* for a CST with an occasional late deceleration but no negative window. Equivocal implies that one is unable to make a determination of fetal condition based on the available information. A CST with both a positive and negative window would be interpreted as positive.

Variable decelerations that occur during the CST may indicate cord compression often associated with oligohydramnios. In such cases, ultrasonography should be performed to assess amniotic fluid volume. However, even if the amniotic fluid volume is demonstrated to be adequate, cord compression patterns need careful follow-up, because cord accidents with subsequent fetal death may occur in the presence of normal amounts of amniotic fluid on sonography. What ap-

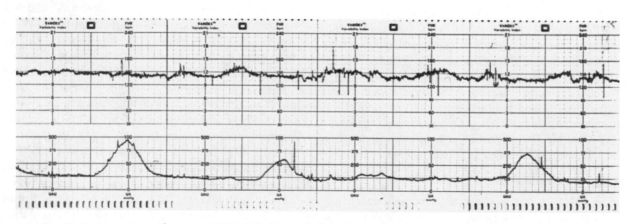

Fig. 12-3 A reactive and negative CST. With this result, the CST would ordinarily be repeated in 1 week.

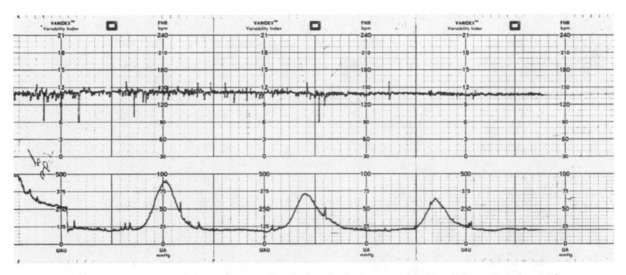

Fig. 12-4 A nonreactive and negative CST. After this result, the test would ordinarily be repeated in 24 hours.

pears to be a normal volume of amniotic fluid may contain meconium, which has a specific gravity different from clear amniotic fluid and therefore does not allow the cord to float freely. In cases of early placental insufficiency, the amount of Wharton's jelly in the umbilical cord may be diminished prior to the clinical appearance of oligohydramnios. The loss of the protective Wharton's jelly may make the umbilical vessels vulnerable to compression and lead to diminished blood flow.

A negative CST has been consistently associated with good fetal outcome. A negative result therefore permits the obstetrician to prolong a high-risk pregnancy safely. Nageotte et al.[59] reported only one preventable fetal death in 1,337 high-risk patients within 7 days after a negative CST. In a series of 679 pregnancies complicated by a prolonged gestation, Freeman et al.[60] observed no perinatal deaths when the CST was used as the primary method of surveillance. Of 337 women with a previous intrauterine fetal death, none had a stillbirth during a pregnancy in which they were followed with CSTs.[61] Druzin et al[61a] reported no antepartum deaths in a series of 819 patients tested at 280 days or more gestation, using both the NST and attempted ripple stimulation CST. There were no differences in perinatal outcome in the group with a reactive NST, irrespective of the CST result. Similarly, Gabbe et al.[62] and Lagrew et al.[63] have reported only one fetal death within 1 week of a negative CST in 811 pregnancies complicated by insulin-dependent diabetes. Other studies have shown the incidence of perinatal death within 1 week of a negative CST to be less then 1/1,000.[64–66] Many of these deaths, however, can be attributed to cord accidents, malformations, placental abruption, and acute deterioration of glucose control in patients with diabetes mellitus. Thus, the CST, like most methods of antepartum fetal surveillance, cannot predict acute fetal compromise. If the CST is negative,

a repeat study is usually scheduled in 1 week. While testing patients with a weekly CST is practical, it is also arbitrary. Changes in the patient's clinical condition may warrant more frequent studies.

A positive CST has been associated with an increased incidence of intrauterine death, late decelerations in labor, low 5-minute Apgar scores, IUGR, and meconium-stained amniotic fluid (Fig. 12-5).[66] In a prospective and blinded study, Ray et al.[67] observed three fetal deaths in 15 patients with positive CSTs. The incidence of low Apgar scores in this group was 53 percent. Overall, the likelihood of perinatal death after a positive CST has ranged from 7 to 15 percent. On the other hand, there has been a significant incidence of false-positive CSTs that, depending on the end point used, will average approximately 30 percent.[54] The positive CST is more likely to be associated with fetal compromise if the baseline heart rate lacks accelerations or "reactivity" and the latency period between the onset of the uterine contractions and the onset of the late deceleration is less than 45 seconds.[68,69]

There is no doubt that the high incidence of false-positive CSTs is one of the greatest limitations of this test, as such results could lead to unnecessary premature intervention. False-positive CSTs may be due to misinterpretation of the tracing; supine hypotension, which decreases uterine perfusion; uterine hyperstimulation, which is not appreciated using the tocodynamometer; or an improvement in fetal condition after the CST has been performed. The high false-positive rate also indicates that a patient with a positive CST need not necessarily require an elective cesarean delivery. If a trial of labor is to be undertaken after a positive CST, the cervix should be favorable for induction so that direct fetal heart rate monitoring and careful assessment of uterine contractility with an intrauterine pressure catheter can be performed. False-positive re-

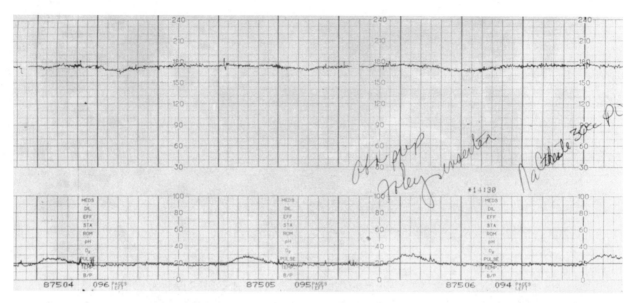

Fig. 12-5 A nonreactive and positive CST with fetal tachycardia. At 34 weeks, the patient, a poorly compliant insulin-dependent diabetic, reported decreased fetal activity. The NST revealed a fetal tachycardia of 170 bpm and was nonreactive. The CST was positive, and a BPP score was 2. The patient's cervix was unfavorable for induction. The patient underwent a low transverse cesarean delivery of a 2,200-g male infant with Apgar scores of 1 and 3. The umbilical arterial pH was 7.21.

sults are not increased when the CST is used early in the third trimester.[70] A negative or positive CST obtained between 28 and 33 weeks' gestation appears to have the same diagnostic significance as it would later in gestation. Merrill et al.[71] reported prolongation of pregnancy for up to 13 days in the presence of a nonreactive nonstress test and a positive CST test if the biophysical profile (BPP) score was six or greater.[71] This approach should only be used in the premature fetus and when careful follow-up with daily fetal assessment, using the nonstress test, CST, and BPP can be reliably performed.

A suspicious or equivocal CST should be repeated in 24 hours. Most of these tests will become negative. Bruce et al.[72] did observe that 5 of 67 patients (7.5 percent) with an initially suspicious CST exhibited positive tests on further evaluation. In 36 patients the CST became negative, whereas in 26 patients it remained suspicious. Like the suspicious CST, a test that is unsatisfactory or shows hyperstimulation should be repeated in 24 hours.

Several investigators have performed follow-up studies of children who demonstrated a positive CST. Scanlon et al.[73] found that infants delivered within 24 hours of a positive CST showed poor state organization and reflexive performance. In contrast, Crane and coworkers[74] evaluated 12 children 5.5 months to 4.75 years after a positive CST and observed that most had grossly normal neurologic and psychologic development. Beischer et al.[75] assessed 45 children ranging in age from 2 months to 8 years, 9 months whose antenatal

heart rate tests exhibited "critical fetal reserve," fetal heart rate baseline variability of less than 5 bpm, absence of accelerations, and late decelerations in response to Braxton Hicks contractions. In only four cases was significant neurologic impairment detected. An important determinant in the long-term outcome for these children would be the early recognition of nonreassuring fetal heart rate patterns and the prevention of intrapartum compromise.

The Nipple Stimulation CST

At the present time, many centers utilize nipple stimulation to produce the uterine contractions needed for the CST. With nipple stimulation, the CST can generally be completed in less time, and an intravenous infusion is not required. Therefore, this approach would appear to be an ideal first step in performing a CST.

Several methods have been used to induce adequate uterine activity.[55,76,77] The patient may first apply a warm moist towel to each breast for 5 minutes. If uterine activity is not adequate, the patient is asked to massage one nipple for 10 minutes. Using this protocol, Oki et al.,[76] achieved adequate uterine contractions in 30 minutes or less in 87.5 percent of 657 patients tested. The incidence of negative tests (72 percent) and positive tests (2 percent) was not different from that seen with the oxytocin-induced CST. Huddleston et al.[78] reported great success using intermittent nipple stimulation. The patient gently strokes the nipple of one breast with the palmar surface of her fingers through her clothes for 2 minutes and then stops for 5 minutes. This cycle is repeated only as necessary to achieve adequate uterine activity. In a series of 193 patients and 345 CSTs, 97 percent of the tests required only three cycles of stimulation. The average time for a CST performed in this way was 45 minutes, and 67.5 percent of the patients completed their tests in 40 minutes or less. The nipple stimulation CST was negative in 80.3 percent of patients and positive in 2.6 percent of patients. All the patients in the Huddleston et al.[78] series were able to achieve adequate uterine contractions with nipple stimulation, and none required an oxytocin infusion. Intermittent rather than continuous nipple stimulation is important in avoiding hyperstimulation. Defined as contractions lasting more than 90 seconds or five or more contractions in 10 minutes, hyperstimulation has been reported in approximately 2 percent of tests when intermittent nipple stimulation is employed.[79,80]

The Nonstress Test

In 1969, Hammacher[81] noted that "the fetus can be regarded as safe, especially if reflex movements are accompanied by an obvious increase in the amplitude of oscillations in the basal fetal heart rate." This observation that accelerations of the fetal heart rate in response to fetal activity, uterine contractions, or stimulation reflect fetal well-being has formed the basis for the nonstress test (NST), the most widely applied technique for antepartum fetal evaluation.

In late gestation, the healthy fetus exhibits an average of 34 accelerations above the baseline fetal heart rate each hour.[82] These accelerations, which average 20 to 25 bpm in amplitude and approximately 40 seconds in duration, require intact neurologic coupling between the fetal CNS and the fetal heart.[82] Fetal hypoxia will disrupt this pathway. At term, fetal accelerations are associated with fetal movement more than 85 percent of the time, and more than 90 percent of gross movements are accompanied by accelerations. Fetal heart rate accelerations may be absent during periods of quiet fetal sleep. Studies by Patrick et al.[82] demonstrated that the longest time between successive accelerations in the healthy term fetus is approximately 40 minutes. However, the fetus may fail to exhibit heart rate accelerations for up to 80 minutes and still be normal.

While an absence of fetal heart rate accelerations is most often due to a quiet fetal sleep state, CNS depressants such as narcotics and phenobarbital, as well as the β-blocker propranolol, can reduce heart rate reactivity.[83,84] Chronic smoking is known to decrease fetal oxygenation through an increase in fetal carboxyhemoglobin and a decrease in uterine blood flow. Fetal heart rate accelerations are also decreased in smokers.[85]

The NST is usually performed in an outpatient setting. In most cases, only 10 to 15 minutes are required to complete the test. It has virtually no contraindications, and few equivocal test results are observed. The patient may be seated in a reclining chair, with care being taken to ensure that she is tilted to the left to avoid the supine hypotensive syndrome.[55,86] The patient's blood pressure should be recorded before the test is begun and then repeated at 5- to 10-minutes intervals. Fetal heart rate is monitored using the Doppler ultrasound transducer, and the tocodynamometer is applied to detect uterine contractions or fetal move-

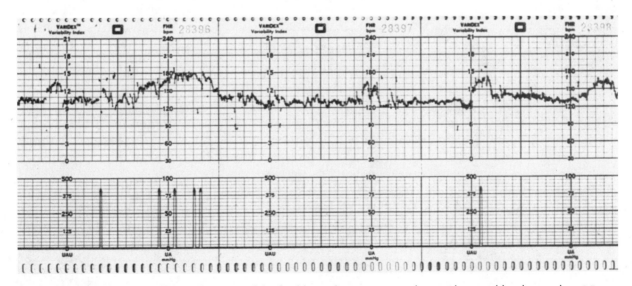

Fig. 12-6 A reactive NST. Accelerations of the fetal heart that are greater than 15 bpm and last longer than 15 seconds can be identified. When the patient appreciates a fetal movement, she presses an event marker on the monitor, creating the arrows on the lower portion of the tracing.

ment. Fetal activity may be recorded by the patient using an event marker or noted by the staff performing the test. The most widely applied definition of a reactive test requires that at least two accelerations of the fetal heart rate of 15 bpm amplitude and 15 seconds duration be observed in 20 minutes of monitoring (Fig. 12-6).[86] Since almost all accelerations are accompanied by fetal movement, fetal movement need not be recorded with the accelerations for the test to be considered reactive. However, fetal movements do provide another index of fetal well-being.

If the criteria for reactivity are not met, the test is considered nonreactive (Fig. 12-7). The most common cause for a nonreactive test will be a period of fetal inactivity or quiet sleep. Therefore, the test may be extended for an additional 20 minutes with the expectation that fetal state will change and reactivity will appear. Keegan et al.[87] noted that approximately 80 percent of tests that were nonreactive in the morning became reactive when repeated later the same day. In an effort to change fetal-state, some clinicians have manually stimulated the fetus or attempted to increase fetal glucose levels by giving the mother orange juice. There is no evidence that such efforts will increase fetal activity.[88,89] If the test has been extended for 40 minutes, and reactivity has not been seen, a CST or BPP should be performed. Of those fetuses that exhibit a nonreactive NST, approximately 25 percent will have a positive CST on further evaluation.[86,90,91] Reactivity that occurs during preparations for the CST has proved to be a reliable index of fetal well-being.

Overall, on initial testing, 85 percent of NSTs will be reactive and 15 percent will be nonreactive (Fig. 12-

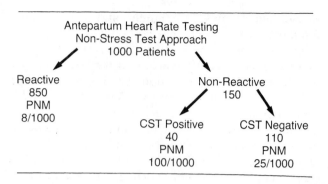

Fig. 12-8 Results of nonstress testing in 1,000 high-risk patients. In general, 85 percent of the NSTs will be reactive and 15 percent nonreactive. Of those patients with a nonreactive NST approximately 25 percent will have a positive CST on further evaluation. The highest perinatal mortality (PNM) will be observed in patients with a nonreactive NST and positive CST. Patients with a nonreactive NST and negative CST will have a perinatal mortality rate higher than that found in patients whose NST is initially reactive. (PNM rates based on data from Evertson et al.[91])

8).[86] Fewer than 1 percent of NSTs will prove unsatisfactory because of inadequately recorded fetal heart rate data. On rare occasions, a sinusoidal heart rate pattern may be observed as described in Chapter 14. This undulating heart rate pattern with virtually absent variability has been associated with fetal anemia, fetal asphyxia, congenital malformations, and medications such as narcotics. In one of the earlier reports on the use of NST, Rochard et al.[92] described a sinusoidal pattern in 20 of 50 pregnancies complicated by Rh isoimmunization. One-half of these pregnancies ended in a perinatal death, and 40 percent of the surviving infants required prolonged hospitalization. Only 10 percent of

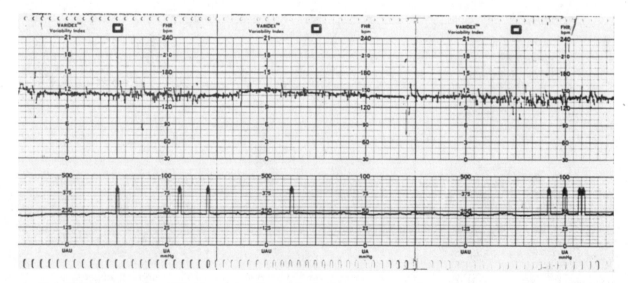

Fig. 12-7 A nonreactive NST. No accelerations of the fetal heart rate are observed. The patient has perceived fetal activity as indicated by the arrows in the lower portion of the tracing.

the babies with a sinusoidal pattern had an uncomplicated course.

The NST is most predictive when normal or reactive. Overall, a reactive NST has been associated with a perinatal mortality of approximately 5/1,000.[86,93] At least one-half of the deaths of babies dying within 1 week of a reactive test may be attributed to placental abruption or cord accidents. The perinatal mortality rate associated with a nonreactive NST, 30 to 40/1,000, is significantly higher, for this group includes those fetuses who are truly asphyxiated. On the other hand, when considering perinatal asphyxia and death as endpoints, a nonreactive NST has a considerable false-positive rate. Most fetuses exhibiting a nonreactive NST will not be compromised but will simply fail to exhibit heart rate reactivity during the 40-minute period of testing. Malformed fetuses also exhibit a significantly higher incidence of nonreactive NSTs.[94] Overall, the false-positive rate associated with the nonreactive NST is approximately 75 to 90 percent.[86]

The likelihood of a nonreactive test is substantially increased early in the third trimester.[95] Between 24 and 28 weeks' gestation, approximately 50 percent of NSTs are nonreactive.[96] Both Lavin et al.[97] and Druzin et al.[98] have reported that 15 percent of NSTs remain nonreactive between 28 and 32 weeks. After 32 weeks, the incidences of reactive and nonreactive tests are comparable to those seen at term. In summary, when accelerations of the baseline heart rate are seen during monitoring in the late second and early third trimester, the NST has been associated with fetal well-being.

Before 27 weeks' gestation, the normal fetal heart rate response to fetal movement may in fact be a bradycardia.[99] However, in some settings such as IUGR associated with antiphospholipid syndrome, bradycardia at a gestational age of 26 to 28 weeks may be a predictor of fetal compromise and impending fetal death. Druzin et al.[100] reported three cases in which antenatal steroid administration and elective premature delivery led to good perinatal outcome. In these challenging cases, the entire clinical situation needs to be evaluated, and a full discussion with the patient, including neonatal consultation, should be initiated prior to intervention and delivery of the very preterm fetus exhibiting fetal heart rate decelerations.

When nonreactive, the NST is extended in an attempt to separate the fetus in a period of prolonged quiet sleep from those who are hypoxemic or asphyxiated.[101–103] In three studies, approximately 3 percent of fetuses tested remained nonreactive after 80 to 90 minutes of evaluation. Brown and Patrick[101] noted that all NSTs that were to become reactive did so by 80 minutes or remained nonreactive for up to 120 minutes. Two stillbirths and one neonatal death occurred in seven cases with prolonged absence of reactivity. The mean arterial cord pH at delivery in this group was

6.95! In 27 pregnancies in which the fetus failed to exhibit accelerations during 80 minutes of monitoring, Leveno et al.[102] reported 11 perinatal deaths. In this study, IUGR was documented in 74 percent of cases, oligohydramnios in 81 percent, fetal acidosis in 41 percent, meconium staining of the amniotic fluid in 30 percent, and placental infarction in 93 percent. Therefore, if the NST is extended and a persistent absence of reactivity is observed, the fetus is likely to be severely compromised.

Vibroacoustic stimulation (VAS) may be utilized to change fetal state from quiet to active sleep and shorten the length of the NST (Fig. 12-9). Most studies have employed an electronic artificial larynx which generates sound pressure levels measured at 1 m in air of 82 dB with a frequency of 80 Hz and a harmonic of 20 to 9,000 Hz.[104] Whether it is the acoustic or vibratory component of this stimulus that alters fetal state is unclear. Gagnon et al.[105] reported that a low-frequency vibratory stimulus applied at term changed fetal state within 3 minutes and was associated with an immediate and sustained increase in long-term fetal heart rate variability, heart rate accelerations, and gross fetal body movements. VAS may produce a significant increase in the mean duration of heart rate accelerations, the mean amplitude of accelerations, and the total time spent in accelerations.[106] Using VAS, the incidence of nonreactive NSTs was reduced from 12.6 to 6.1 percent in a retrospective study and from 14 to 9 percent in a prospective investigation.[107,108] A reactive NST after VAS stimulation appears to be as reliable an index of fetal well-being as spontaneous reactivity. However, those fetuses that remain nonreactive even after VAS may be at increased risk for poor perinatal outcome.[109] In a study conducted by Trudinger and Boylan,[110] intrapartum fetal distress, growth restriction, and low Apgar scores were increased in fetuses that were nonreactive after acoustic stimulation. Kuhlman and Depp[109] have reported that the auditory brainstem response in the fetus is functional at 26 to 28 weeks' gestation, and Druzin et al.[111] noted that the incidence of reactive NSTs after VAS was significantly increased after 26 weeks' gestation. Therefore, VAS may be helpful after 26 weeks.

In most centers that use VAS, the baseline fetal heart rate is first observed for 5 minutes.[104] If the pattern is nonreactive, a stimulus of 3 seconds or less is applied near the fetal head. If the NST remains nonreactive, the stimulus is repeated at 1-minute intervals up to three times. If there continues to be no response to VAS, further evaluation should be carried out with a CST or BPP. In summary, VAS may be helpful in shortening the time required to perform an NST and may be especially useful in centers where large numbers of NSTs are done.

Could the sound generated by an electronic artificial larynx damage the fetal ear? Using intrauterine micro-

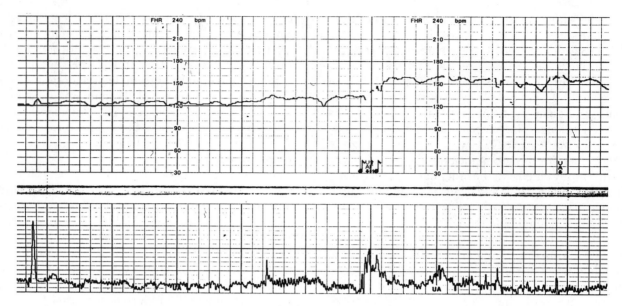

Fig. 12-9 Reactive NST after VAS. The stimulus was applied in panel 54042 at the point marked by the musical notes. A sustained fetal heart rate acceleration was produced.

phones, Smith and colleagues[112] documented baseline intrauterine sound levels of up to 88 dB during labor. Transabdominal stimulation with an electronic artificial larynx increased these levels minimally, up to 91 to 111 dB. In studies by Arulkumaran et al.[113] sound vibrations and sound intensity were noted to be attenuated by amniotic fluid. Therefore, a 90 dB sound pressure produced by VAS in air resulted in exposure of the fetal ear to the equivalent of 40 dB, the level of normal conversation at about 3 feet. Arulkumaran et al.[113] concluded that intrauterine sound levels from VAS were not hazardous to the fetal ear. Two other studies have confirmed the safety of VAS use during pregnancy. Arulkumaran et al.[114] and Ohel et al.[115] reported no long-term evidence of hearing loss in children followed in the neonatal period and up to 4 years of age.

Significant fetal heart rate bradycardias have been observed in 1 to 2 percent of all NSTs.[116-120] Druzin et al.[116] defined such bradycardias as a fetal heart rate of 90 bpm or a fall in the fetal heart rate of 40 bpm below the baseline for 1 minute or longer (Fig. 12-10). This definition has been most widely applied. In a review of 121 cases, bradycardia was associated with increased perinatal morbidity and mortality, particularly antepartum fetal death, cord compression, IUGR, and fetal malformations.[121] Although about one-half of the NSTs associated with bradycardia were reactive, the incidence of a nonreassuring fetal heart rate pattern in labor leading to emergency delivery in this group was identical to that of patients exhibiting nonreactive NSTs. Clinical management decisions should be based on the finding of bradycardia, *not* on the presence or

absence of reactivity. Bradycardia has the higher positive predictive value for fetal compromise (fetal death or fetal intolerance of labor) than does the nonreactive NST. In this setting, antepartum fetal death is most likely due to a cord accident.[116,119,120]

If a bradycardia is observed, an ultrasound examination should be performed to assess amniotic fluid volume and to detect the presence of anomalies such as renal agenesis. When expectant management has been followed, such bradycardias have been associated with a perinatal mortality rate of 25 percent. Several reports have therefore recommended that delivery be undertaken if the fetus is mature. When the fetus is premature, one might elect to administer corticosteroids to accelerate fetal lung maturation before delivery. Continuous fetal heart rate monitoring is necessary if expectant management is followed.

In most cases, mild variable decelerations are not associated with poor perinatal outcome. Meis et al.[122] reported that variable decelerations of 20 bpm or more below the baseline heart rate but lasting less than 10 seconds were noted in 50.7 percent of patients having an NST. While these decelerations were more often associated with a nuchal cord, they were not predictive of IUGR or a nonreassuring fetal heart rate pattern, or more severe variable decelerations during labor. Phelan[104] has added, however, that when mild variable decelerations are observed, even if the NST is reactive, an ultrasound examination should be done to rule out oligohydramnios. A low amniotic fluid index and mild variable decelerations increase the likelihood of a cord accident.

In selected high-risk pregnancies, the false-negative

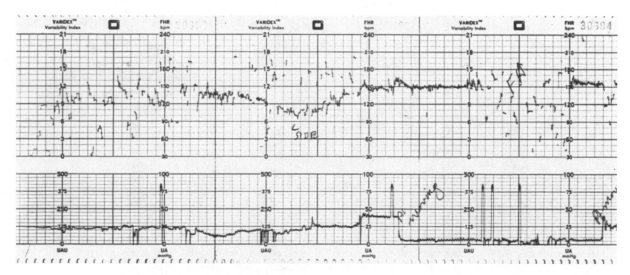

Fig. 12-10 A NST in this primigravid patient of 43 weeks' gestation reveals a spontaneous bradycardia (panel 30692). The fetal heart rate has fallen from a baseline of 150 to 100 bpm. Upon induction of labor, the patient required cesarean delivery for fetal distress associated with severe variable decelerations. The amniotic fluid was decreased in amount and was meconium stained.

rate associated with a weekly NST may be unacceptably high.[123,124] Boehm et al.[125] reported a reduction in the fetal death rate in their high-risk population from 6.1 to 1.9/1,000 when the frequency of the NST was increased from once to twice weekly. Barrett et al.[123] have emphasized that in pregnancies complicated by IUGR and diabetes mellitus, twice-weekly testing should be utilized. In reviewing the literature, they noted that the fetal death rate within 1 week after a nonreactive NST was significantly increased in both diabetes mellitus (14/1,000) and IUGR (20/1,000). Miyazaki and Miyazaki,[126] reported an 8 percent false-negative rate in 125 prolonged gestations evaluated with the NST. In the prolonged pregnancy and IUGR, oligohydramnios may occur, leading to cord compression and fetal demise. The assessment of amniotic fluid volume has clearly proved important in such cases. Barss and coworkers[127] reviewed the incidence of stillbirths within 1 week of a reactive test in patients with a prolonged gestation. For the general high-risk population, a false-negative rate of 2.7/1,000 was reported. Although the incidence in pregnancies complicated by a prolonged gestation was not higher (2.8/1,000), Barss et al.[127] noted that even this low rate can be considered excessively high in view of the fact that these fetuses are otherwise normal and mature. In summary, it appears that the frequency of the NST should be increased to twice weekly in pregnancies complicated by diabetes mellitus, prolonged gestation, and IUGR.[125]

Which antepartum heart rate test is best? The NST has proved to be an ideal screening test and remains the primary method for antepartum fetal evaluation at most centers. It can be quickly performed in an outpatient setting and is easily interpreted. In contrast, the CST is usually performed near the labor and delivery suite, may require an intravenous infusion of oxytocin, and may be more difficult to interpret. In initial studies, a reactive NST appeared to be as predictive of good outcome as a negative CST. Nevertheless, as more data have been gathered, it appears that the ability of the CST to stress the fetus and evaluate its response to intermittent interruptions in intervillous blood flow provides an earlier warning of fetal compromise. Murata et al.[128] found that, in the dying fetal rhesus monkey, the fetal pH at which late decelerations appear is significantly higher (7.32) than the pH at which fetal heart rate accelerations disappear (7.22). In a large collaborative project in which 1,542 patients were evaluated primarily with the NST and 4,626 with the CST, Freeman et al.[129] observed that the corrected perinatal mortality associated with a reactive NST, 3.2/1,000 was significantly higher than that observed with a negative CST, 1.4/1,000. While both fetal death rates are extremely low for a high-risk population, that associated with the CST is clearly better.

The healthy fetus should exhibit a reactive baseline heart rate with no late decelerations when a CST is performed. However, as the fetus deteriorates, one will first observe late decelerations, and, finally, the most ominous fetal heart rate pattern, the nonreactive NST and positive CST[64,69,130] (Fig. 12-5). When a nonreactive NST is followed by a positive CST, the positive incidence of perinatal mortality has been approximately 10 percent, a nonreassuring fetal heart rate pattern has occurred in most laboring patients, and IUGR has been reported in 25 percent of cases. The unusual combination of a reactive NST and a positive CST has been associated with a higher incidence of IUGR and

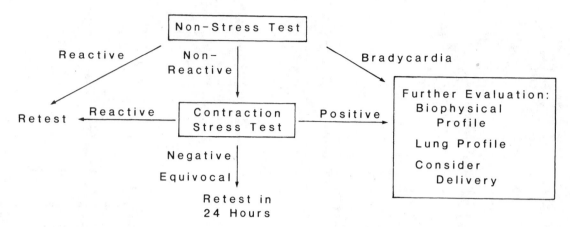

Fig. 12-11 A branched testing scheme using the NST, CST, and BPP. Delivery is considered when the NST is nonreactive and the CST is positive. Delivery is also considered when a bradycardia is observed during the NST. The fetal BPP may be used to decrease the incidence of unnecessary premature intervention.

late decelerations in labor than that seen with a negative CST.[131] The likelihood of fetal death is increased in patients demonstrating a nonreactive NST followed by a negative CST.[65,132,133] Consequently, repeating the NST in 24 hours appears the prudent course in such cases (Fig. 12-11).

Finally, arguments about the "best test" are counterproductive. Each test has its strengths and weaknesses, and a thorough understanding of the nature of the antepartum test, taking into consideration its advantages and disadvantages, is essential. The type of test and its application should be "condition" or diagnosis specific in which a similar basic screening approach is used, adding different types of evaluation and increased frequency of testing as appropriate for the clinical situation.

Fetal Biophysical Profile

The use of real-time ultrasonography to assess antepartum fetal condition has enabled the obstetrician to perform an in utero physical examination and evaluate dynamic functions reflecting the integrity of the fetal CNS.[134] As emphasized by Manning et al.,[135] "fetal biophysical scoring rests on the principle that the more complete the examination of the fetus, its activities, and its environment, the more accurate may be the differentiation of fetal health from disease states."

Fetal breathing movements were the first biophysical parameter to be assessed using real-time ultrasonography. It is thought that the fetus exercises its breathing muscles in utero in preparation for postdelivery respiratory function. With real-time ultrasonography, fetal breathing movement (FBM) is evidenced by downward movement of the diaphragm and abdominal contents and by an inward collapsing of the chest. Fetal breathing movements become regular at 20 to 21 weeks and are controlled by centers on the ventral surface of the

fourth ventricle of the fetus.[136] They are observed approximately 30 percent of the time, are seen more often during REM sleep, and, when present, demonstrate intact neurologic control. While the absence of FBM may reflect fetal asphyxia, this finding may also indicate that the fetus is in a period of quiet sleep.[32,33]

Several factors other than fetal state and hypoxia can influence the presence of FBM. As maternal glucose levels rise, FBM becomes more frequent, and, during periods of maternal hypoglycemia, FBM decreases. Maternal smoking will also reduce FBM, probably as a result of fetal hypoxemia.[137] Narcotics that depress the fetal CNS will also decrease FBM.

Platt and colleagues[138] were among the first to examine the ability of FBM to predict perinatal outcome. Using real-time ultrasonography, they judged FBM to be present if at least one episode of FBM of at least 60 seconds duration was observed within any 30-minute period of observation. Of 136 fetuses studied, 116 (85 percent) exhibited FBM. The incidence of fetal distress was significantly higher in fetuses without FBM, 60 percent (12/20), as was the incidence of low Apgar scores at 5 minutes, 50 percent (10/20). The comparable figures for fetuses demonstrating FBM were 3 percent (4/116) for a nonreassuring fetal heart rate pattern and 4 percent (5/116) for low Apgar scores.

Further research demonstrated that the evaluation of FBM could be used to distinguish the truly positive CST from a false-positive CST. Those fetuses that displayed FBM but had a positive CST were unlikely to exhibit fetal distress in labor. However, when a fetus failed to show FBM and demonstrated late decelerations during the CST, the likelihood of fetal compromise was great. A pattern emerged from these studies that as long as one antepartum biophysical test was normal, the likelihood that the fetus would have a normal outcome was high.[139,140] As the number of abnormal

Table 12-6 Technique of Biophysical Profile Scoring

Biophysical Variable	Normal (Score = 2)	Abnormal (Score = 0)
Fetal breathing movements	At least one episode of > 30 seconds duration in 30 minutes observation	Absent or no episode of ≥30 seconds duration in 30 minutes
Gross body movement	At least three discrete body/limb movements in 30 minutes (episodes of active continuous movement considered a single movement)	Up to two episodes of body/limb movements in 30 minutes
Fetal tone	At least one episode of active extension with return to flexion of fetal limb(s) or trunk; opening and closing of hand considered normal tone	Either slow extension with return to partial flexion or movement of limb in full extension or absent fetal movement
Reactive fetal heart rate	At least two episodes of acceleration of ≥15 bpm and 15 seconds duration associated with fetal movement in 30 minutes	Fewer than two accelerations or acceleration <15 bpm in 30 minutes
Qualitative amniotic fluid volume	At least one pocket of amniotic fluid measuring 2 cm in two perpendicular planes	Either no amniotic fluid pockets or a pocket <2 cm in two perpendicular planes

(Adapted from Manning et al.,[146] with permission.)

tests increased, however, the likelihood that fetal asphyxia was present increased as well.

Using these principles, Manning et al.[141] developed the concept of the fetal BPP score. These workers elected to combine the NST with four parameters that could be assessed using real-time ultrasonography: FBM, fetal movement, fetal tone, and amniotic fluid volume. FBMs, fetal movement, and fetal tone are mediated by complex neurologic pathways and should reflect the function of the fetal CNS at the time of the examination. On the other hand, amniotic fluid volume should provide information about the presence of chronic fetal asphyxia. One additional parameter, placental grading, has been added by some investigators.[136,142] Finally, the ultrasound examination performed for the BPP has the added advantage of detecting previously unrecognized major fetal anomalies.

Vintzileos et al.[136] stressed that those fetal biophysical activities that are present earliest in fetal development are the last to disappear with fetal hypoxia. The fetal tone center in the cortex begins to function at 7.5 to 8.5 weeks. Fetal tone would therefore be the last fetal parameter to be lost with worsening fetal condition. The fetal movement center in the cortex-nuclei is functional at 9 weeks and would be more sensitive than fetal tone. As noted above, FBM becomes regular at 20 to 21 weeks. Finally, fetal heart rate control, residing within the posterior hypothalamus and medulla, becomes functional at the end of the second trimester and early in the third trimester. An alteration in fetal heart rate would theoretically be the earliest sign of fetal compromise.

A BPP score was developed that is similar to the Apgar score used to assess the condition of the newborn.[141] The presence of a normal parameter, such as a reactive NST, was awarded two points, while the absence of that parameter was scored as zero. The highest score a fetus can receive is 10, while the lowest score is zero. The BPP may be used as early as 26 to 28 weeks' gestation. Twice weekly testing is recommended in pregnancies complicated by IUGR, diabetes mellitus,

Table 12-7 Management Based on Biophysical Profile

Score	Interpretation	Management
10	Normal infant; low risk of chronic asphyxia	Repeat testing at weekly intervals; repeat twice weekly in diabetic patients and patients at ≥42 weeks gestation
8	Normal infant; low risk of chronic asphyxia	Repeat testing at weekly intervals; repeat testing twice weekly in diabetics and patients at ≥42 weeks gestation; oligohydramnios is an indication for delivery
6	Suspect chronic asphyxia	If ≥36 weeks gestation and conditions are favorable, deliver; if at <36 weeks and L/S <2.0, repeat test in 4–6 hours; deliver if oligohydramnios is present
4	Suspect chronic asphyxia	If ≥36 weeks gestation, deliver; if <32 weeks, repeat score
0–2	Strongly suspect chronic asphyxia	Extend testing time to 120 minutes; if persistent score ≥4, deliver, regardless of gestation age

(Adapted from Manning et al.,[143,146] with permission.)

prolonged gestation, and hypertension with proteinuria. The criteria proposed by Manning et al.,[141] and the clinical actions recommended in response to these scores are presented in Tables 12-6 and 12-7. Regardless of a low score on the BPP, Manning et al. have emphasized that vaginal delivery is attempted if other obstetric factors are favorable.

In a prospective blinded study of 216 high-risk patients, Manning and colleagues[141] found no perinatal deaths when all five variables described above were normal, but a perinatal mortality rate of 60 percent in fetuses with a score of zero. Fetal deaths were increased 14-fold with the absence of fetal movement, and the perinatal mortality rate was increased 18-fold if FBM were absent. Any single test was associated with a significant false-positive rate ranging from 50 to 79 percent.

However, combining abnormal variables significantly decreased the false-positive rate to as low as 20 percent. The false-negative rate, that is, the incidence of babies who were compromised but who had normal testing, was quite low, ranging from a perinatal mortality rate of 6.9/1,000 for infants with normal amniotic fluid volume to 12.8/1,000 for fetuses demonstrating a reactive NST. These investigators found that, in most cases, the ultrasound-derived BPP parameters and NST could be completed within a relatively short time, each requiring approximately 10 minutes.

Manning[143] has presented his experience with 26,780 high-risk pregnancies followed with the BPP. It should be noted that since 1984, a routine NST has not been performed if all of the ultrasound parameters were found to be normal for a score of 8.[144] An NST

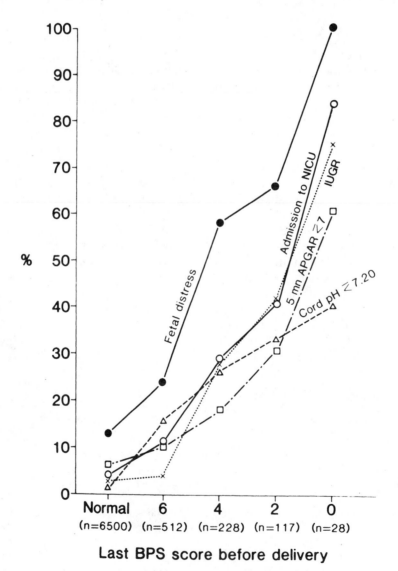

Last BPS score before delivery

Fig. 12-12 The relationship between five indices of perinatal morbidity and last biophysical profile score before delivery. A significant inverse linear correlation is observed for each variable. (From Manning et al.,[143] with permission.)

is done when one ultrasound finding is abnormal. The corrected PMR in this series was 1.9/1,000, with less than 1 fetal death per 1,000 patients within 1 week of a normal profile. Of all patients tested, almost 97 percent had a score of 8, which means that only 3 percent required further evaluation for scores of 6 or less. In a study of 525 patients with scores of 6 or less, poor perinatal outcome was most often associated with either a nonreactive NST and absent fetal tone or a nonreactive NST and absent FBM.[145] A significant inverse linear relationship was observed between the last BPP score and both perinatal morbidity and mortality (Figs. 12-12, 12-13).[143] The false-positive rate, depending on the endpoint used, ranges from 75 percent for a score of 6 to less than 20 percent for a score of 0. Manning[146] has recently summarized the data reported in eight investigations using the BPP for fetal evaluation. Overall, 23,780 patients and 54,337 tests were reviewed. The corrected perinatal mortality rate, excluding lethal anomalies, was 0.77/1,000.

The BPP correlates well with fetal acid-base status.

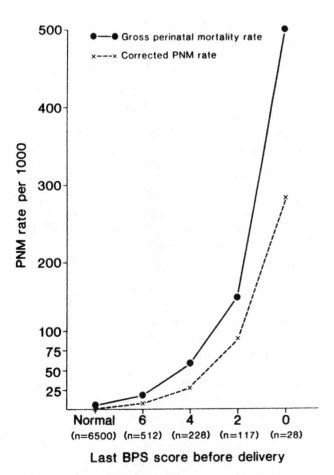

Fig. 12-13 The relationship between perinatal mortality, both total and corrected for major anomalies, and the last BPP score before delivery. A highly significant inverse and exponential relationship is observed. (From Manning et al.,[143] with permission.)

Vintzileos et al.[147] studied 124 patients undergoing cesarean birth *before* the onset of labor. Deliveries were undertaken for severe preeclampsia, elective repeat cesarean section, growth restriction, breech presentation, placenta previa, and fetal macrosomia. Acidosis was defined as an umbilical cord arterial pH less than 7.20. The earliest manifestations of fetal acidosis were a nonreactive NST and loss of FBM. With scores of 8 or more, the mean arterial pH was 7.28, and only 2 of 102 fetuses were acidotic. For 13 fetuses with scores of 5 to 7, the mean pH was 7.19, and 69 percent were acidotic. Nine fetuses with scores of 4 or less had a mean pH of 6.99, and all were acidotic.

Is an NST needed if all ultrasound parameters of the BPP are normal? Prospective and blinded studies by Platt et al.[148] and Manning et al.[149] using both the BPP and NST have demonstrated that each of these tests is a valuable predictor of normal outcome. In the experience of Manning et al., an NST was needed in less than 5 percent of tests. As emphasized by Eden et al.,[150] however, the NST will allow the detection of fetal heart rate decelerations. In the presence of reduced amniotic fluid, these decelerations may be associated with a cord accident. Eden et al. reported that when spontaneous fetal heart rate decelerations lasting at least 30 seconds with a decrease of at least 15 bpm are seen in the presence of normal amniotic fluid, there is an increased likelihood of late decelerations in labor and cesarean delivery for fetal distress.

Several drawbacks of the BPP should be considered. Unlike the NST and CST, unless the BPP is videotaped it cannot be reviewed. If the fetus is in a quiet sleep state, the BPP can require a long period of observation. The present scoring system does not consider the impact of hydramnios. In a pregnancy complicated by diabetes mellitus, the presence of excessive amniotic fluid is of great concern.

The false-positive (false abnormal) rate of a particular test has always been of concern because of the possibility of unnecessary intervention (usually delivery) and subsequent iatrogenic complications. The BPP was developed in part to address the issue of the high false abnormal rate of the CST and the NST. There has been little attention paid to the possible false-positive rate of the abnormal or equivocal BPP. This is particularly relevant because the BPP is most commonly used as the final backup test in the NST and CST sequence of testing and is critically important when dealing with the premature fetus. As noted above, the false-positive rate of a score of zero is less than 20 percent, but for a score of six is up to 75 percent. Inglis et al.[151] used VAS to define fetal condition with BPP scores of six or less in 81 patients at 28 to 42 weeks. Obstetric and neonatal outcomes of 41 patients whose score improved to normal after VAS were compared with those of 238 patients who had normal scores without VAS. The obstetric and neonatal outcomes were not significantly different between the two groups. VAS improved the BPP in about 80 percent of cases. Use of VAS for an equivocal BPP did not increase the false-negative rate and may reduce the likelihood of unnecessary obstetric intervention.[151]

Doppler Velocimetry

For decades, obstetricians have attempted to measure blood flow in the fetal and uteroplacental circulations. The techniques applied have usually been invasive or have required the use of radioactive tracers. Most recently, the principle of Doppler ultrasound has been utilized to measure blood flow in the uterine and fetal vessels.

The Doppler effect is the key principle upon which flow studies are based.[152] We have all noted that the frequency of sound produced by an ambulance siren changes as the ambulance approaches us and then passes. The pitch of the siren becomes higher as the ambulance comes closer and lower after it has passed. Similarly, a moving column of red blood cells will scatter and reflect a beam of ultrasound with a frequency shift proportional to the velocity of the blood flow. In other words, the frequency of the reflected sound is proportional to the speed of the moving red blood cells. Determining blood flow velocity will provide an indirect assessment of changes in blood flow. Calculation of flow velocity is derived from the equation

$$f_d = 2 f_0 \frac{V\cos\theta}{2},$$

where f_d is the change in ultrasound frequency or Doppler shift; f_0 is the transmitted frequency of the incident ultrasound; V is the velocity of the reflector or red blood cells; θ is the angle between the beam and the direction of movement of the reflector or red blood cells; and c is the velocity of sound in the medium (Fig. 12-14). The speed of sound in tissues is 1,540 m/sec. The number 2 in the equation accounts for the time spent from the transmission of the sound signal at its origin to its return. The value for cosine θ approaches 1 as θ approaches 0. Volume flow may be calculated by multiplying the mean velocity by the cross-sectional area of the vessel as measured by ultrasound. The velocity of sound in tissues is constant, and the frequency of the incident ultrasound is fixed by the transducer. Therefore, if the angle between the blood vessel studied and the ultrasound beam remains constant, the Doppler shift frequency, f_d, will be directly proportional to the flow velocity, V. The frequency of ultrasound used in Doppler velocimetry studies is 3 to 5 MHz. Velocities are measured in meters per second.

Duplex systems to assess blood flow combine real-time imaging with pulsed wave Doppler. The vessel to be insonated can be identified, and the ultrasound beam generated from a single piezoelectric crystal placed across that vessel using range gating. Duplex systems have been applied to study blood flow in the fetal aorta and cerebral circulation.

Technical and practical problems must be considered when utilizing a duplex Doppler system.[152] Theta, the angle of the beam to the vessel insonated, should ideally be kept below 30 degrees and should not exceed 55 degrees. As this angle increases, large errors may be made in estimating flow velocity. One must accurately measure the diameter of the vessel studied to calculate its cross-sectional area. Since the radius is squared to calculate the area of the blood vessel, a small error in this measurement can produce a major error in estimating volume flow. The beam must be placed uniformly across the vessel so that the flow of all red blood cells is in the same direction and with the same velocity. The high pass or thump filter used to remove low-frequency signals generated from the vessel wall also eliminates low flow velocities and may lead to an overestimation of mean blood flow velocity. If the thump filter is set too high, low-frequency end-diastolic velocities may be eliminated. Since blood flow is usually expressed in milliliters per kilogram per minute, one must also accurately estimate the fetal weight. Finally, duplex Doppler systems are quite expensive.

For the above reasons, continuous wave Doppler systems have been more widely applied.[152,153] These units, which are considerably less expensive, use both an emitting crystal and a receiving crystal at frequencies of 2 to 10 MHz. They also employ considerably less power (less than 25 mW/cm^2) than the pulsed Doppler systems (100 to 1,000 mW/cm^2). Continuous wave systems do not allow one to image the vessel to be insonated. Rather, one must depend on the identification of characteristic waveforms produced by maternal and fetal vessels.

Continuous wave Doppler systems generate flow velocity waveforms that reflect the distribution and intensities of the Doppler frequency shifts over time.[152,153] As long as the angle of insonation and the transmitted frequency of the ultrasound beam are constant, these frequency shifts are directly proportional to changes in flow velocity within the vessel. The upswing of the frequency shift reflects stroke volume or cardiac contractility, while the downswing reflects vessel compliance and indicates peripheral resistance.

A variety of angle-independent indices have been developed to quantify the flow velocity waveforms produced.[153,154] It must be emphasized that these indices do not measure blood flow itself. Most commonly used is the peak systolic (S)/diastolic (D) ratio, the S/D ratio, also know as the A/B ratio (Figs. 12-15, 12-16). The

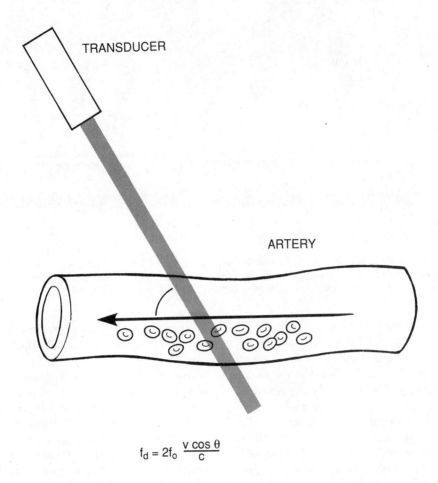

$$f_d = 2f_o \frac{v \cos \theta}{c}$$

Fig. 12-14 Application of the Doppler principle to determine blood flow velocity. The frequency (f_o) of the ultrasound beam directed at a moving column of red blood cells with velocity V will be increased to f_d in proportion to V and the cosine of the angle of intersection of the vessel by the beam (θ).

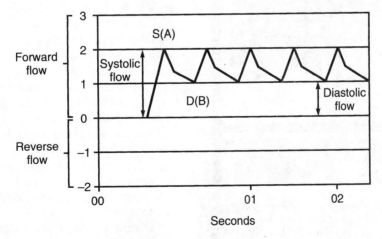

Fig. 12-15 Diagram of a normal umbilical artery flow velocity waveform. Note the forward flow during both systole and diastole, the latter indicating low resistance in the placental bed. (Adapted from Warsof and Levy,[153] with permission.)

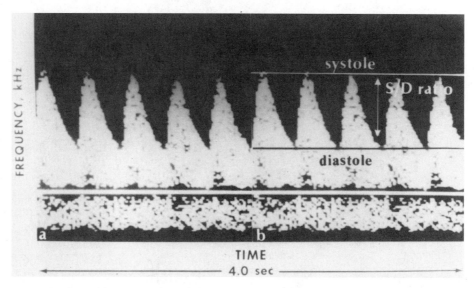

Fig. 12-16 Doppler flow velocity waveforms of the normal umbilical artery. Note that umbilical arterial flow velocities are recorded above the baseline, while nonpulsatile umbilical vein flow in the opposite direction is found below the baseline (A). Measurement of the S/D ratio is also illustrated (B). (From Bruner et al.,[235] with permission.)

greater the diastolic flow, the lower the ratio. As peripheral resistance increases, diastolic flow falls, and the S/D ratio increases. The pulsatility index is calculated as the systolic minus diastolic values divided by the mean of the velocity waveform profile (S − D/mean). An additional ratio, the resistance index, or Pourcelot ratio, is expressed as S − D/S. The latter two ratios are useful when the diastolic flow is absent or reversed. Maulik et al.[154] have found that the resistance index has the best diagnostic efficacy in predicting perinatal compromise.

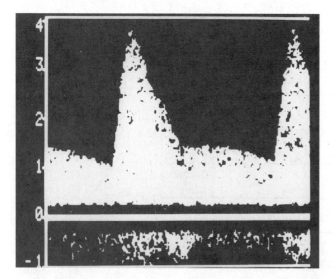

Fig. 12-17 Flow velocity waveform of the uterine artery early in the second trimester. Note the high pulsatility as demonstrated by systolic flow followed by reduced diastolic flow. While this pattern is normal at this time in gestation, during the third trimester this finding would represent an abnormal uterine artery flow velocity waveform.

As noted above, vessels within the maternal circulation and fetoplacental unit produce characteristic waveforms.[155] In addition, waveforms generated from maternal vessels can obviously be distinguished from waveforms in the fetal circulation by the slower heart rate. During the first trimester, the uterine artery normally demonstrates high pulsatility, as demonstrated by systolic flow followed by reduced diastolic flow (Fig. 12-17).[155] This pattern results from high downstream resistance in the uterine vessels, which causes reflection of the incident pressure pulse and dampens the diastolic portion of that pulse. A diastolic notch can also be identified early in gestation. By the end of the second trimester, flow velocity waveforms in the normal uterine artery demonstrate a systolic peak associated with a large diastolic component, indicating decreased resistance in the placental bed (Fig. 12-18).[155,156] Increased resistance or vascular impedance in the placental bed has been associated with IUGR and is reflected by a reduction in end-diastolic flow.

The normal umbilical artery demonstrates a peak in systole with a large amount of end-diastolic flow, reflecting decreased placental resistance (Figs. 12-15 and 12-16).[153] There is a progressive reduction in pulsatility and increase in diastolic flow throughout gestation. Abnormal umbilical artery flow shows decreased end-diastolic flow or, in extreme situations, absent or reversed end-diastolic flow (Figs. 12-19 and 12-20).[153,157]

When evaluating flow velocity waveforms, it is important that at least three to five waveforms be obtained at different angles of insonation. The fetus should be in a quiet state. Fetal breathing movements shorten the cardiac cycle, increasing end-diastolic frequencies and decreasing the S/D ratio. When studying the umbilical

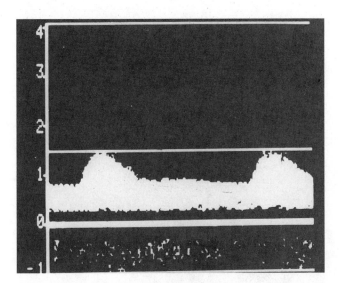

Fig. 12-18 Flow velocity waveform in the normal uterine artery during the third trimester. Note the systolic peak associated with a large diastolic component, indicating decreased resistance in the placental bed.

artery, it is important to demonstrate flow in the umbilical vein in the opposite direction to verify that the umbilical artery has been insonated. Umbilical vein velocities can be seen as a continuous band across the lower portion of the umbilical artery flow waveform.

The criteria for normal flow velocity waveforms in both the maternal and fetal circulations have been reported by many investigators.[155,158,159] Umbilical artery waveforms are characterized by a progressive decline in S/D ratio from early pregnancy until term. This change reflects growth of small muscular arteries in the tertiary stem villi of the placenta. By 30 weeks' gestation, the S/D ratio in the umbilical artery should be below 3 (Fig. 12-21).[158] In the uterine artery, increased diastolic flow is noted at 14 to 20 weeks, reflecting trophoblastic invasion of the spiral arterioles. Thereafter, there is minimal decline in the S/D ratio. The uterine artery S/D ratio should fall below 2.6 by 26 weeks' gestation.[155] Furthermore, the diastolic notch seen early in gestation should disappear. Abnormal uterine artery waveforms in the second trimester may herald the subsequent development of preeclampsia (Fig. 12-22).

The broadest application of Doppler flow has been the study of the pregnancy at risk for or demonstrating IUGR. This subject is discussed in Chapter 25. In summary, an elevation in the S/D ratio in the umbilical artery may precede the onset of growth restriction. When IUGR has been identified, an abnormal umbilical S/D ratio may be more predictive of neonatal morbidity than the NST.[160] The absence of end-diastolic flow in the pregnancy complicated by growth restriction has been associated with nonreassuring intrapartum fetal heart rate patterns and an increased perinatal mortality rate.

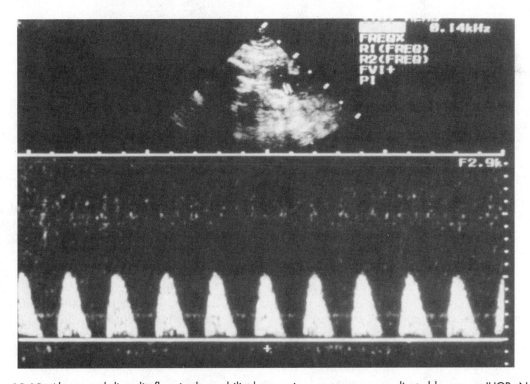

Fig. 12-19 Absent end-diastolic flow in the umbilical artery in a pregnancy complicated by severe IUGR. Note the systolic peak without evidence of diastolic flow. The real-time ultrasound image that allows visualization of the vessel to be studied, in this case the umbilical artery, can be seen in the upper portion of the figure.

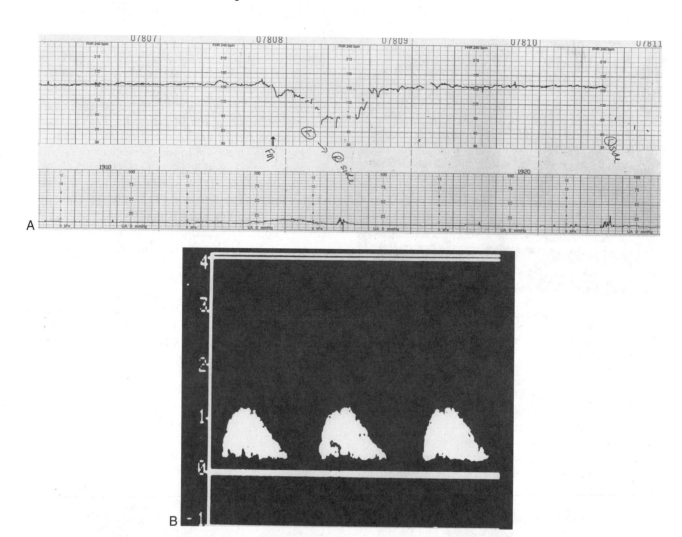

Fig. 12-20 The patient, a 27-year-old, primigravid, class C diabetic, was hospitalized for preeclampsia at 32 weeks' gestation. Her NST was nonreactive. The fetal BPP at this time was 6. The following day, the patient's NST remained nonreactive and revealed spontaneous fetal heart rate decelerations with uterine contractions (A). The BPP score at this time was 2. Prior to delivery by primary cesarean section, a Doppler flow study was performed that revealed absent end diastolic flow (B). A normally grown, 1,650-g, female infant was delivered with Apgar scores of 8 at 1 minute and 8 at 5 minutes. The umbilical arterial pH was 7.23, with a base excess of −.6. The placenta was small and calcified. The baby required oxygen by hood for 24 hours but had no significant morbidity.

How accurately do changes in umbilical artery flow velocity waveform indices reflect alterations in fetal blood flow? Using a sheep model, Trudinger et al.[161] embolized the umbilical placental circulation with microspheres each day for 9 days in late gestation. The umbilical artery S/D ratio rose at 4 days, reflecting increased vascular resistance in the placental bed. Umbilical blood flow did not fall significantly until the end of the study period. Morrow and Ritchie,[162] using a similar experimental model, reported a progressive increase in the S/D ratio leading to absent and then reversed diastolic flow. These changes produced by embolization of the umbilical artery are similar to those seen in the human fetus with IUGR. Increasing the fetal hematocrit and blood viscosity by 100 percent had little effect on the S/D ratio. These investigators also observed that hypoxia did not alter the S/D ratio and concluded that abnormalities in the umbilical artery flow velocity waveform reflect placental pathology and *not* asphyxial changes. Copel et al.[163] has made similar observations using a sheep model in which umbilical blood flow and S/D ratio were measured shortly after embolization. In this study, normal umbilical artery S/D ratios were found even in the presence of fetal acidosis. It appears, then, that while the umbilical artery S/D ratio can provide an approximation of umbilical artery flow, it best reflects changes in placental vascular resistance. How the fetus has responded to this placental abnormality and whether it is hypoxemic cannot be judged by flow velocity waveform indices.

How do Doppler studies compare with other techniques for antepartum fetal surveillance? Devoe and

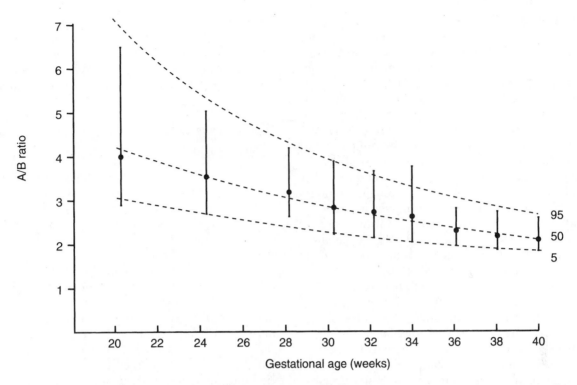

Fig. 12-21 Normal reference values for the S/D or A/B ratio in the umbilical artery throughout gestation. The 95th, 50th, and 5th percentiles are shown at each gestational age. Note that the ratio falls below 3 after 30 weeks' gestation. (From Thompson et al.[158] with permission.)

colleagues[164] evaluated 1,000 consecutive high-risk pregnancies using the NST, a measurement of amniotic fluid volume, and umbilical artery velocimetry. The PMR associated with this approach was 2.1/1,000. Using perinatal mortality, fetal distress, low 5-minute Apgar score, and neonatal acidosis as end points, each method had a specificity over 90 percent. Sensitivities ranged from 69 percent for the NST to 21 percent for the S/D ratio. The positive predictive value for any abnormal test was 54 percent, but increased to 100 per-

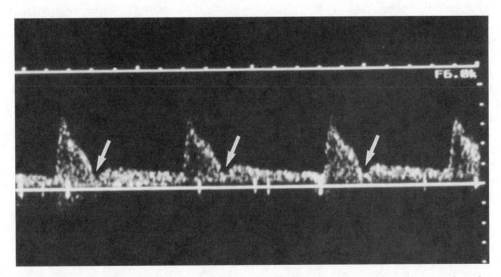

Fig. 12-22 The patient, a 30-year-old primigravida at 30 weeks' gestation, had an ultrasound performed for lagging uterine growth. Estimated fetal weight was 910 g, and the amniotic fluid volume was reduced. A Doppler flow study demonstrated notching of the uterine artery. Within 12 hours, the patient developed hypertension with a blood pressure of 180/110 mmHg, proteinuria, hyperreflexia, and a headache. She underwent primary cesarean delivery of a 975-g infant who did well in the nursery.

cent when *all* of the tests were abnormal. The best predictive values for Doppler studies were found in pregnancies complicated by hypertension and IUGR. Overall, however, the NST was the single test with the best predictive accuracy. Most recently, Alfirevic and Neilson performed a meta-analysis of 12 randomized controlled trials of umbilical and uterine artery velocimetry in high-risk pregnancies. The use of Doppler studies was associated with a decrease in perinatal deaths and cesarean deliveries for fetal distress.[165]

The absence or reversal of umbilical end-diastolic frequencies has been considered an extremely ominous finding, and recommendations for immediate delivery to avoid fetal death or irreversible compromise have been made by many investigators.[166–168] It has also been suggested that reverse flow is more predictive of poor perinatal outcome than absent diastolic flow because it implies virtual cessation of effective uteroplacental circulation.[169] The relatively high frequency of congenital malformations, including chromosomal abnormalities, in patients with markedly abnormal Doppler studies should lead to further evaluation of the fetus. Many of these anomalies are incompatible with life, and this knowledge may lead to alteration of obstetric management.

Thornton and Lilford,[20] summarizing the data from seven studies, found that absent or reversed end-diastolic flow had a sensitivity of 67 percent (20/30) in predicting perinatal death. Fairlie et al.[170] studied cases complicated by pregnancy-induced hypertension and evaluated patients exhibiting both absent umbilical artery end-diastolic frequencies and reversal of umbilical artery end-diastolic frequencies in terms of perinatal outcome. All patients were delivered based on findings of the NST and the BPP. There was a 1- to 14-day duration between abnormal Doppler findings and delivery, which was based on evaluation of fetal condition using the NST and BPP. Johnstone et al.[168] and Divon et al.[171] reported similar outcomes in small numbers of patients in whom abnormal Doppler findings were noted but not used as the final indication for delivery. All of these studies stress that absent and reversal of end-diastolic flow are predictors of adverse perinatal outcome and that these pregnancies require close, intensive, ongoing surveillance, but they conclude that decisions concerning the timing of delivery can be made reliably based on results of the NST and BPP.

Doppler velocimetry seems to be most reliable in conditions predisposing to IUGR such as chronic hypertension, pregnancy-induced hypertension, collagen vascular disorders, and other diseases in which vasospasm plays a major role. This technique is also valuable in the follow-up of pregnancies with a diagnosis of IUGR or growth discordancy, such as in discordant twins (see Ch. 24). In other common obstetric conditions requiring fetal surveillance such as prolonged

pregnancy and diabetes mellitus, Doppler velocimetry offers no advantage over conventional techniques. In addition, use of umbilical artery Doppler velocity for screening in low-risk pregnancies has not been shown to be either predictive of poor perinatal outcome or cost effective.[172]

The Assessment of Fetal Pulmonary Maturation

This section reviews those techniques that enable the obstetrician to predict accurately the risks of respiratory distress syndrome (RDS) for the infant requiring premature delivery and to avoid the unnecessary tragedy of iatrogenic prematurity.

RDS is caused by a deficiency of pulmonary surfactant, an anti-atelectasis factor that is able to maintain a low stable surface tension at the air–water interface within alveoli. Surfactant decreases the pressure needed to distend the lung and prevents alveolar collapse (see Ch. 20). The type II alveolar cell is the major site of surfactant synthesis. Surfactant is packaged in lamellar bodies, discharged into the alveoli, and carried into the amniotic cavity with pulmonary fluid.

Phospholipids account for more than 80 percent of the surface active material within the lung, and more than 50 percent of this phospholipid is dipalmitoyl lecithin. The latter is a derivative of glycerol phosphate and contains two fatty acids as well as the nitrogenous base choline. Other phospholipids contained in the surfactant complex include phosphatidylglycerol (PG), phosphatidylinositol (PI), phosphatidylserine (PS), phosphatidylethanolamine (PE), sphingomyelin, and lysolecithin. PG is the second most abundant lipid in surfactant and significantly improves its properties.

An accurate assessment of gestational age and fetal maturity is essential before an elective induction of labor or cesarean delivery or before the delivery of a patient whose fetus may not have matured normally such as a growth-restricted fetus or the fetus of a poorly controlled diabetic mother. Many of the techniques used in clinical practice in the past not only failed to predict gestational age, but provided little information about fetal pulmonary maturation.[173]

Prior to the now common practice of using ultrasound to establish gestational age and amniotic fluid studies to assess fetal pulmonary maturation, iatrogenic prematurity was an important clinical problem. In 1975, Goldenberg and Nelson[174] concluded that untimely or unwarranted intervention was responsible for 15 percent of their cases of RDS. In a similar study, Hack et al.[175] observed that 12 percent of all infants with RDS in their neonatal intensive care unit were born after elective deliveries. None of these infants had had documentation of pulmonary maturation before delivery. In 1977, Maisels et al.[176] reported their experience with 18 cases of RDS in neonates born after elective intervention. The lecithin:sphingomyelin (L/S) ratio was used in only one case and ultrasound dating in three.

Several changes in clinical practice appear to have decreased the incidence of RDS due to iatrogenic prematurity. Patients who have had a previous low transverse cesarean delivery are now being encouraged to attempt a vaginal birth. In such cases, since the onset of spontaneous labor is awaited, documentation of fetal pulmonary maturation prior to elective intervention is not required. Berkowitz et al.[177] noted a marked reduction in cases of iatrogenic RDS at their institution. Between 1970 and 1973, elective delivery without adequate documentation of fetal maturity occurred in 11 of 63 pregnancies (11.1 percent) resulting in RDS. In contrast, from 1980 to 1983, only 1 of 71 pregnancies (1.4 percent) delivered electively resulted in RDS. Berkowitz et al. concluded that this decline in iatrogenic RDS presumably reflects increased availability of ultrasound and fetal lung maturity studies and advances in the application and interpretation of these diagnostic procedures.

Assessment of Fetal Pulmonary Maturity

Available methods for evaluating fetal pulmonary maturity can be divided into four categories: (1) quantitation of pulmonary surfactant, such as the L/S ratio; (2) measurement of surfactant function including the shake test; (3) evaluation of amniotic fluid turbidity; and (4) association with placental grade and cephalometry using ultrasonography.

Quantitation of Pulmonary Surfactant

Lecithin/Sphingomyelin Ratio

The L/S ratio developed by Gluck and associates[178] and Kulovich et al.[179] has proved the most valuable assay for the assessment of fetal pulmonary maturity. The amniotic fluid concentration of lecithin increases markedly at approximately 35 weeks' gestation, while sphingomyelin levels remain stable or decrease. Rather than determine the concentration of lecithin that could be altered by variations in amniotic fluid volume, Gluck and coworkers used sphingomyelin as an internal standard and compared the amount of lecithin to that of sphingomyelin. Amniotic fluid sphingomyelin exceeds lecithin until 31 to 32 weeks, when the L/S ratio reaches 1. Lecithin then rises rapidly, and an L/S ratio of 2.0 is observed at approximately 35 weeks. Wide variation in the L/S ratio at each gestational age has been noted. Nevertheless, a ratio of 2.0 or greater has repeatedly been associated with pulmonary maturity. In more than 2,100 cases, a mature L/S ratio predicted the absence

of RDS in 98 percent of neonates.[180] With a ratio of 1.5 to 1.9, approximately 50 percent of infants will develop RDS. Below 1.5, the risk of subsequent RDS increases to 73 percent. Thus, the L/S ratio, like most indices of fetal pulmonary maturation, rarely errs when predicting fetal pulmonary maturity, but is frequently incorrect when predicting subsequent RDS.[181] Many neonates with an immature L/S ratio will not develop RDS.

Several important variables must be considered in interpreting the predictive accuracy of the L/S ratio. A prolonged interval between the determination of an immature L/S ratio and delivery will necessarily increase the number of falsely immature results. It is probably best to discard amniotic fluid samples heavily contaminated by blood or meconium, because the effects of these compounds on the determination of the L/S ratio are quite unpredictable.[182,183] Blood has been reported to both increase and decrease the ratio, while meconium can produce falsely mature results. The presence of PG in a bloody or meconium-stained amniotic fluid sample remains a reliable indicator of pulmonary maturity.[184] PG is not normally found in blood, and meconium generally does not interfere with the identification of PG.[185,186] Finally, it is essential that the obstetrician know the analytic technique used and the predictive value of a mature L/S ratio in his or her laboratory.

Many perinatal processes alter the final interpretation of the L/S ratio. Surfactant deficiency, immaturity, and intrapartum complications are the prime factors in determining the pathogenesis of RDS.[187] Birth asphyxia may lead to RDS in many infants despite an L/S ratio greater than 2.0. In earlier studies, infants with severe Rh disease and infants of diabetic mothers were reported to have developed RDS despite mature L/S ratios. More recent data indicate that the L/S ratio is reliable in both high-risk conditions.[188,189] Kjos and colleagues[189] found no cases of RDS due to surfactant deficiency in a study of 54 pregestational and 472 gestational diabetics.

In subsequent studies, Kulovich and associates[179,190] emphasized that full assessment of fetal pulmonary maturity, the lung profile, requires determination of the L/S ratio, percent precipitable lecithin, and the acidic phospholipids PI and PG. A rapid L/S ratio may be performed in approximately 1 hour. Determinations of the L/S ratio and lung profile require approximately 5-ml amniotic fluid and take one-half to 3 hours to complete. PI appears at 26 to 30 weeks' gestation, increases in parallel with the rise in L/S ratio at 35 to 36 weeks, and then decreases. PG, which does not appear until 35 weeks' gestation and increases rapidly between 37 to 40 weeks, is a marker of completed pulmonary maturation. Most infants who lack PG but who have a mature L/S ratio fail to develop RDS. However, PG may provide further insurance against the onset of RDS despite intrapartum complications. Using the total lung profile can significantly reduce the number of falsely mature L/S ratios, as some infants with L/S ratios below 2.0 do demonstrate PG.[191] While some investigators have reported accelerated pulmonary maturation in pregnancies complicated by preeclampsia or twins, others have not confirmed these findings.[192,193] PG can be produced by some bacteria such as *Gardnerella vaginalis*, *Listeria*, and *Escherichia coli*, and false-positive results have been reported in amniotic fluid specimens collected from the vagina.[194]

Slide Agglutination Test for PG

A rapid immunologic semiquantitative agglutination test (Amniostat-FLM) can be used to determine the presence of PG.[195] This assay can detect PG at a concentration greater than 0.5 μg/ml of amniotic fluid. The test takes 20 to 30 minutes to perform and requires only 1.5 ml of amniotic fluid. Besides being highly sensitive, several studies have found a positive Amniostat-FLM to correlate well with the presence of PG by thin-layer chromatography and the absence of subsequent RDS. In a study evaluating samples from the vaginal pool and those obtained by amniocentesis, the overall concordance for the Amniostat-FLM and thin-layer chromatography results was 89 percent.[195] No cases of RDS were observed when the Amniostat-FLM assay demonstrated PG. This technique can be applied to samples contaminated by blood and meconium.

Microviscosimeter

The relative lipid content of amniotic fluid may be evaluated by fluorescence depolarization analysis.[196] A lipid-soluble dye is incubated for 30 minutes with the amniotic fluid specimen, and the amount of dye absorbed into the phospholipid membrane structures within the fluid is determined by measuring the fluorescence of polarized light with the microviscosimeter (Felma, Elscint). The fluorescence polarization, or P value, falls as the L/S ratio rises. Few falsely mature results have been reported with P values ranging from less than 0.310 to 0.336. Specimens contaminated with blood cannot be used for this analysis. One disadvantage of this technique is the high cost of the microviscosimeter. The test is technically easier and faster than the L/S ratio, but, because of the financial considerations mentioned above, is not widely used in this country.

TDx Test (Surfactant Albumin Ratio)

The TDx analyzer, an automated fluorescence polarimeter, has been utilized to assess surfactant content in amniotic fluid.[197–199] The test requires 1 ml of amniotic fluid and can be run in less than 1 hour. The surfactant

albumin ratio (SAR) is determined with amniotic fluid albumin used as an internal reference. A ratio of 50 to 70 mg surfactant per gram of albumin has been considered mature. The TDx test correlates well with the L/S ratio and has few falsely mature results, making it an excellent screening test. Approximately 50 percent of infants with an immature TDx result will develop RDS.

Measurement of Surfactant Function

Shake Test

In 1972, Clements and colleagues[200] described the shake test, an assay of surfactant function that evaluates the ability of pulmonary surfactant to generate a stable foam in the presence of ethanol. Ethanol, a nonfoaming competitive surfactant, eliminates the contributions of protein, bile salts, and salts of free fatty acids to the formation of a stable foam. At an ethanol concentration of 47.5 percent, stable bubbles that form after shaking are due to amniotic fluid lecithin. Positive tests, a complete ring of bubbles at the meniscus with a 1:2 dilution of amniotic fluid, are rarely associated with neonatal RDS. The shake test must be regarded as a screening procedure that yields useful information if mature.

Foam Stability Index

The test is based on the manual foam stability index (FSI), a variation of the shake test designed by Sher and Statland.[201] The kit currently available contains test wells with a predispensed volume of ethanol. The addition of 0.5-ml amniotic fluid to each test well in the kit produces final ethanol volumes of 44 to 50 percent. A control well contains sufficient surfactant in 50 percent ethanol to produce an example of the stable foam end point. The amniotic fluid:ethanol mixture is first shaken, and the FSI value is read as the highest value well in which a ring of stable foam persists.[202]

This test appears to be a reliable predictor of fetal lung maturity.[203] Subsequent RDS is very unlikely with an FSI value of 47 or higher. The methodology is simple, and the test can be performed at any time of day by persons who have had only minimal instruction. The assay appears to be extremely sensitive, with a high proportion of immature results being associated with RDS, as well as moderately specific, with a high proportion of mature results predicting the absence of RDS. Contamination of the amniotic fluid specimen by blood or meconium invalidates the FSI results. The FSI can function well as a screening test.

Tap Test

This recently developed test provides a rapid semiquantitative measurement of surfactant function.[204–206] The test is performed by mixing 1 ml of amniotic fluid with 1 drop of 6N hydrochloric acid and then adding approximately 1.5 ml of diethyl ether. A 6 × 150 mm test tube is briskly tapped three or four times, creating an estimated 200 to 300 bubbles in the ether or top layer. In amniotic fluid from the mature fetus, the bubbles quickly rise from the bottom layer of the amniotic fluid to the surface and break down, while in amniotic fluid from an immature fetus the bubbles are stable or break down slowly. Note that these end points are opposite those used in the FSI or shake test. The cut-off for maturity has been set at five bubbles. If no more than five bubbles persist in the ether layer, the test is considered mature. The test is read at 2, 5, and 10 minutes. Fluid obtained from both amniocentesis or a freely flowing vaginal pool may be used. Amniotic fluid contaminated by blood, meconium, or vaginal mucus should be centrifuged before the assay is performed.

Several studies report excellent predictive values for mature tests that were greater than 95 percent, while the predictive value for immature tests ranged from 40 to 60 percent.[204–207] These results were comparable to those obtained with phospholipid profiles. Fluid contaminated by blood or meconium or obtained from the vaginal pool did not demonstrate an increased incidence of falsely mature tests.

The tap test may be a valuable screening test, particularly if a phospholipid profile is not available.

Evaluation of Amniotic Fluid Turbidity

Visual Inspection

During the first and second trimesters, amniotic fluid is yellow and clear. It becomes colorless in the third trimester. By 33 to 34 weeks' gestation, cloudiness and flocculation are noted, and, as term approaches, vernix appears. Amniotic fluid with obvious vernix or fluid so turbid it does not permit the reading of newsprint through it will usually have a mature L/S ratio.[208]

Optical Density

Sbarra and coworkers[209] and Cetrulo and coworkers[210] assessed the relationship between the optical density (OD) of fresh amniotic fluid at 650 nm and the L/S ratio. This method is thought to evaluate the turbidity changes in amniotic fluid that are dependent on the total amniotic fluid phospholipid concentration. Although a wavelength of 400 nm was originally used, interference by pigments from meconium, bilirubin, and hemolyzed blood led to a choice of 650 nm. An OD of 0.15 or greater at this wavelength correlates extremely well with a mature L/S ratio and the absence of RDS.[211,212] Falsely immature results were observed in 6 to 8 percent of the patients of Sbarra et al.,[209] but have exceeded 30 percent in other studies.[213] Hy-

dramnios may decrease amniotic fluid turbidity and could contribute to these findings. Because the test requires only a spectrophotometer and can be performed rapidly, the OD is a useful screening test. The test must be performed on a clear amniotic fluid specimen, as contamination with blood or meconium invalidates the results.

Lamellar Body Counts

Lamellar bodies are the storage form of surfactant released by fetal type II pneumocytes into the amniotic fluid. Because they have the same size as platelets, the amniotic fluid concentration of lamellar bodies may be determined using a commercial cell counter.[214–217] The test requires less than 1 ml of amniotic fluid and takes only 15 minutes to perform. A lamellar body count greater than 30,000 to 55,000/μl is highly predictive of pulmonary maturity, while a count below 10,000/μl suggests a significant risk for RDS. The cut-off used to predict fetal pulmonary status will depend on the type of cell counter used and the speed of centrifugation of the amniotic fluid specimen. Neither meconium nor lysed blood has a significant effect on the lamellar body count.

Placental Grading and Cephalometry

With the exception of amniotic fluid specimens obtained from the vaginal pool, the evaluation of fetal pulmonary maturation requires that a sample of amniotic fluid be obtained by amniocentesis. In the past, third trimester amniocentesis was associated with significant fetal and maternal risks. Fetal complications have included fetal bleeding from laceration of the placenta or umbilical cord, fetomaternal bleeding, premature labor and premature rupture of the membranes, placental abruption, and fetal injury. Maternal complications, though rare, have included hemorrhage, in some cases from perforation of the uterine vessels, abdominal wall hematomas, Rh sensitization, and infection.

Ultrasound guidance for third trimester amniocentesis has significantly decreased the risks of the procedure. In a review of seven studies that included 4,115 third trimester amniocenteses, the frequency of complications was 3 percent for rupture of the membranes within 24 hours, 7 percent for a bloody tap, 4.4 percent for failed amniocentesis, 3.3 percent for labor within 24 hours, 1 percent for fetal trauma, and 0.05 percent for fetal death.[218]

Golde and Platt[219] have stressed that a bloody tap warrants careful observation. At term, the fetal blood volume is relatively small, and fetal bleeding may have disastrous consequences. These investigators recommend that when a bloody tap occurs the patient be monitored continuously with electronic fetal heart rate monitoring until an Apt test or Kleihauer-Betke test confirms that the blood is of maternal origin and the fetus has demonstrated no evidence of compromise. Should a nonreassuring fetal heart rate pattern be observed, cesarean delivery is performed. When fetal blood is recovered, the fetus is delivered if its pulmonary status is mature even if is has not exhibited fetal distress. For those fetuses with pulmonary immaturity, Golde and Platt[219] recommend treatment with corticosteroids and delivery thereafter.

In an effort to avoid the traumatic complications of amniocentesis, several investigators have examined the correlation between placental morphology on ultrasonography and fetal pulmonary maturation. In 1979, Grannum et al.[220] described four stages of placental maturation based on the appearance of the basal and chorionic plates of the placenta and the placental substance. With progression from the least mature placenta, grade 0, to the most mature placenta, grade 3, one observes increasing deposition of calcium within the placental septa. Grannum noted an excellent correlation between the presence of a grade 3 placenta and a mature L/S ratio. This parallel maturation between the fetal lung and placenta has been confirmed by several examiners. Harman et al.[221] reported that 93 percent of grade 3 placentas were associated with a mature L/S ratio and 75 percent with the presence of PG. Kazzi et al.[222] have attempted to refine this classification by describing as mature only those placentas that are entirely grade 3. Placentas that have a grade 3 appearance in one portion, but that are less mature in other areas, are judged intermediate. In this series, no fetus with a mature or entirely grade 3 placenta developed RDS. Unfortunately, at term, only approximately 18 percent of patients will demonstrate a grade 3 placenta. Furthermore, the observation of a grade 3 placenta in pregnancies complicated by maternal hypertension, diabetes mellitus, IUGR, and Rh isoimmunization cannot reliably be associated with a mature L/S ratio.[223] In summary, it appears that the presence of a grade 3 placenta in an uncomplicated pregnancy at term strongly suggests fetal pulmonary maturation.[224]

Other investigators have assessed the correlation between the BPD and fetal pulmonary maturation. Gross et al.[225] reported that in 294 pregnancies the presence of a BPD of 9.0 cm or more was associated with a gestational age of at least 38 weeks in 97 percent of cases, with the presence of PG in 87 percent of patients and with the absence of RDS in all infants. These workers estimated that more than one-third of all amniocenteses in their series could have been eliminated using the predictive value of the BPD. Several investigators have now confirmed that a BPD of at least 9.2 cm will reliably predict the absence of RDS in uncomplicated

pregnancies.[226] This approach should not be used for patients with diabetes mellitus.

In summary, ultrasound parameters that correlate with fetal pulmonary maturation may be helpful when the risk of amniocentesis is increased, as with an anterior placenta. However, as emphasized by Hadlock et al.,[227] the most appropriate use of ultrasound in predicting fetal lung maturity is early documentation of gestational age so that elective delivery later in pregnancy can be safely undertaken.

Determination of Fetal Pulmonary Maturation in Clinical Practice

A large number of techniques are now available to assess fetal pulmonary maturation. Several rapid screening tests, including the TDx test, FSI, OD_{650}, and Amniostat-FLM appear to be highly reliable when mature. In an uncomplicated pregnancy, when a screening test such as the TDx demonstrates fetal pulmonary maturation, one can safely proceed with delivery. This approach is also extremely cost effective.[228,229] However, when the screening test is immature, the L/S ratio and lung profile should be used. Similarly, in complicated pregnancies such as those with diabetes mellitus, IUGR, and Rh isoimmunization, the L/S ratio and lung profile should be determined to assess fetal pulmonary maturation. As noted above, in an uncomplicated pregnancy at term, when an amniocentesis would be difficult because of placental or fetal location, placental grade and fetal BPD may be used as an indirect measure of fetal pulmonary maturation.

Summary

How can one most efficiently use all the techniques available for antepartum fetal surveillance? Obstetricians should take a "diagnosis-specific" approach to testing. That is, they must consider the pathophysiology of the disease process that will be evaluated and then select the best method or methods of testing for that problem. For example, in the pregnancy complicated by significant Rh isoimmunization, one might want to use serial evaluations of fetal hemoglobin. In a pregnancy complicated by diabetes mellitus, careful monitoring of maternal glucose levels should accompany antepartum heart rate testing. In contrast, in a pregnancy complicated by suspected growth restriction, one would want to make serial evaluations of amniotic fluid volume with ultrasound to detect oligohydramnios.

In a prolonged pregnancy, one would use a parallel testing scheme. In this situation, the obstetrician is not concerned with fetal maturity, but rather with fetal well-being. Several tests are performed at the same time, such as antepartum fetal heart rate testing and the BPP. It is acceptable in this high-risk situation to intervene when a single test is abnormal. One is willing to accept a false-positive test result to avoid the intrauterine death of a mature and otherwise healthy fetus.

On the other hand, in most other high-risk pregnancies, such as those complicated by diabetes mellitus or hypertension, it is preferable to allow the fetus to remain in utero as long as possible. In these situations, a branched testing scheme is used. To decrease the likelihood of unnecessary premature intervention, the obstetrician uses a series of tests and, under most circumstances, would only deliver a premature infant when all parameters suggest fetal compromise. In this situation, one must consider the likelihood of neonatal RDS as predicted by the evaluation of amniotic fluid indices and review these risks with colleagues in neonatology.

Maternal assessment of fetal activity would appear to be an ideal first-line screening test for both high-risk and low-risk patients. The use of this approach may decrease the number of unexpected intrauterine deaths in so-called normal pregnancies. Although a negative CST has been associated with fewer intrauter-

ine deaths than a reactive NST, the NST appears to have significant advantages in screening high-risk patients. It can be easily and rapidly performed in an outpatient setting. The nipple stimulation CST provides an excellent alternative for those who favor primary use of the CST, particularly in the prolonged pregnancy and those cases complicated by diabetes mellitus and IUGR. Most clinicians, however, use the BPP or CST to assess fetal condition further in patients exhibiting a persistently nonreactive NST. This sequential approach may be particularly valuable in avoiding unnecessary premature intervention.

Figure 12-23 presents a practical testing scheme that has been utilized successfully by several centers.[104,134,230,231] The NST, an indicator of present fetal condition, may be combined with the amniotic fluid index (AFI) (Ch. 10), a marker of long-term status, in a modified BPP. VAS may be used to shorten the time required to achieve a reactive NST. While most patients are evaluated weekly, patients with diabetes mellitus, IUGR, or a prolonged gestation are tested twice weekly. If the NST is nonreactive despite VAS or extended monitoring, or if the AFI is abnormal, either a CST or

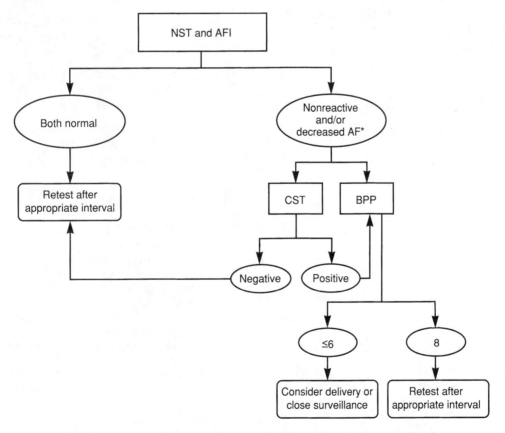

Fig. 12-23 Flow chart for antepartum fetal surveillance in which the NST and AFI are used as the primary methods for fetal evaluation. A nonreactive NST decreased AF are further evaluated using either the CST or the BPP. Further details regarding the use of the BPP are provided in Table 12-7. *If the fetus is mature and amniotic fluid volume is reduced, delivery should be considered before further testing is undertaken. (Adapted from Finberg et al.,[134] with permission.)

full BPP is performed. Using this approach, Clark et al.[230] found no unexpected antepartum fetal deaths in a series of 2,628 high-risk pregnancies. VAS shortened the mean testing time to 10 minutes. Only 2 percent of all NSTs were nonreactive. However, 17 percent of these were followed by a positive CST or biophysical profile score of 4 or less. Clark et al. have extended their experience with this technique to include an additional 3,005 tests. One fetus died 2 days after a reactive NST due to a cord accident. Therefore, only one fetal death has been observed in almost 9,000 tests after a reactive NST and normal AFI! In a series of 6,543 fetuses, Vintzileos et al.[232] reported no fetal deaths due to hypoxia within 1 week of a reactive NST and an ultrasound study demonstrating normal amniotic fluid. Most recently, Nageotte et al.[233] demonstrated that the modified BPP was as good a predictor of adverse fetal outcome as a negative CST. Furthermore, the CST as a backup test was associated with a higher rate of intervention for an abnormal test than the use of a complete BPP as a backup test.

Finally, tests of any kind can only do so much. As emphasized by Wilson and Schifrin[234]: "improvement does not lie with tests alone. It is axiomatic that informed and interested personnel must translate test results into meaningful clinical activity and communicate thoroughly with the patient."

Key Points

- The prevalence of an abnormal condition (i.e., fetal death) has great impact on the predictive value of antepartum fetal tests.

- The near-term fetus spends approximately 25 percent of its time in a quiet sleep state (state 1F) and 60 to 70 percent in an active sleep state (state 2F).

- Approximately 5 percent of women monitoring fetal movement will report decreased fetal activity.

- The incidence of perinatal death within 1 week of a negative CST is less than 1/1,000.

- The observation that accelerations of the fetal heart rate in response to fetal activity, uterine contractions, or stimulation reflect fetal well-being is the basis for the NST.

- The frequency of the NST should be increased to twice weekly in pregnancies complicated by diabetes mellitus, prolonged gestation, and IUGR.

- Use of VAS for an equivocal BPP does not increase the false-negative rate and may reduce the likelihood of unnecessary obstetric intervention.

- The absence of end-diastolic flow in the umbilical artery flow velocity waveform has been associated with an increased perinatal mortality rate.

- Most amniotic fluid indices of fetal pulmonary maturation rarely err when predicting maturity, but are frequently incorrect when predicting subsequent RDS.

- The NST, an indicator of present fetal condition, and the amniotic fluid index, a marker of long-term fetal status, have been combined in the modified BPP.

References

1. Eskes TKAB: Introduction. p. xv. In Nijhuis J (ed): Fetal Behaviour. Oxford University Press, New York, 1992

2. Chard T, Klopper A: Introduction. p. 1. In Placental Function Tests. Springer-Verlag, New York, 1982

3. Friede A, Rochat R: Maternal mortality and perinatal mortality: definitions, data, and epidemiology. p. 35 In Sachs B (ed): Obstetric Epidemiology. PSG Publishing Company, Littleton, MA, 1985

4. American College of Obstetricians and Gynecologists: Perinatal and infant mortality statistics. Committee Opinion 167, December, 1995

5. U.S. Department of Health and Human Services: ChildHealth USA '94. U.S. Government Printing Office, Washington, DC, 1995

6. Grant A, Elbourne D: Fetal movement counting to assess fetal well-being. p. 440. In Chalmers I, Enkin M, Keirse MJNC (eds): Effective Care in Pregnancy and Childbirth. Oxford University Press, Oxford, 1989

7. Naeye RL: Causes of perinatal mortality in the United

States Collaborative Perinatal Project. JAMA 238:228, 1977

8. Guyer B, Strobino DM, Ventura SJ, Singh GK: Annual summary of vital statistics—1994. Pediatrics 96:1029, 1995

9. Lammer EJ, Brown LE, Anderka MT, Guyer B: Classification and analysis of fetal deaths in Massachusetts. JAMA 261:1757, 1989

10. Manning FA, Lange IR, Morrison I, Harman CR: Determination of fetal health: methods for antepartum and intrapartum fetal assessment. p. 6. In Leventhal J (ed): Current Problems in Obstetrics and Gynecology, Year Book Medical Publishers, Inc., Chicago, 1983

11. Fretts RC, Boyd ME, Usher RH, Usher H: The changing pattern of fetal death, 1961–1988. Obstet Gynecol 79:35, 1992

12. Fretts RC, Schmittdiel J, McLean FH et al: Increased maternal age and the risk of fetal death. N Engl J Med 333:953, 1995

13. Schauer GM, Kalousek DK, Magee JF: Genetic causes of stillbirth. Semin Perinatol 16:341, 1992

14. Mersey Region Working Party on Perinatal Mortality. Perinatal health. Lancet 1:491, 1982

15. Kirkup B, Welch G: "Normal but dead": perinatal mortality in the non-malformed babies of birthweight 2–5 kg and over in the Northern Region in 1983. Br J Obstet Gynaecol 97:381, 1990

16. Schneider EP, Hutson JM, Petrie RH: An assessment of the first decade's experience with antepartum fetal heart rate testing. Am J Perinatol 5:134, 1988

17. Stubblefield P, Berek J: Perinatal mortality in term and postterm births. Obstet Gynecol 56:676, 1980

18. Duenhoelter J, Whalley P, MacDonald P: An analysis of the utility of plasma immunoreactive estrogen measurements in determining delivery time of gravidas with a fetus considered at high risk. Am J Obstet Gynecol 125:889, 1976

19. Mohide P, Keirse MJNC: Biophysical assessment of fetal well-being. p. 477. In Chalmers I, Enkin M, Keirse MJNC (eds): Effective Care in Pregnancy and Childbirth, Oxford University Press, Oxford, 1989

20. Thornton JG, Lilford RJ: Do we need randomised trials of antenatal tests of fetal wellbeing? Br J Obstet Gynaecol 100:197, 1993

21. Flynn AM, Kelly J, Mansfield H et al: A randomized controlled trial of non-stress antepartum cardiotocography. Br J Obstet Gynaecol 89:427, 1982

22. Brown VA, Sawers RS, Parsons RJ et al: The value of antenatal cardiotocography in the management of high-risk pregnancy: a randomized controlled trial. Br J Obstet Gynaecol 89:716, 1982

23. Lumley J, Lester A, Anderson I et al: A randomized trial of weekly cardiotocography in high-risk obstetric patients. Br J Obstet Gynaecol 90:1018, 1983

24. Kidd LC, Patel NB, Smith R: Non-stress antenatal cardiotocography—a prospective randomized clinical trial. Br J Obstet Gynaecol 92:1156, 1985

25. Ferrera TB, Hoekstra RF, Couser RJ et al: Survival and follow-up of infants born at 23–26 weeks gestational age: effects of surfactant therapy. J Pediatr 124:119, 1994

26. Allen M, Donohue P, Dushman A: The limit of viability—neonatal outcome of infants born at 22–25 weeks gestation. N Engl J Med 329:1597, 1993

27. Schwartz RM, Luby AM, Scanlon JW, Kellog RJ: Effect of surfactant on morbidity, mortality and resource use in newborn infants weighing 500–1500 grams. N Engl J Med 330:1476, 1994

28. Schifrin B, Foye G, Amato J et al: Routine fetal heart rate monitoring in the antepartum period. Obstet Gynecol 54:21, 1979

29. Stempel L: Eenie, meenie, minie, mo . . . what do the data really show? Obstet Gynecol 144:745, 1982

30. Peipert JF, Sweeney PJ: Diagnostic testing in obstetrics and gynecology: a clinician's guide. Obstet Gynecol 82:619, 1993

31. Carpenter M, Coustan D: Criteria for screening tests for gestational diabetes. Am J Obstet Gynecol 144:768, 1982

32. Manning FA: Assessment of fetal condition and risk: analysis of single and combined biophysical variable monitoring. Semin Perinatol 9:168, 1985

33. Van Woerden EE, VanGeijn HP: Heart-rate patterns and fetal movements. p. 41. In Nijhuis J (ed): Fetal Behaviour. Oxford University Press, New York, 1992

34. Patrick J, Campbell K, Carmichael L et al: Patterns of gross fetal body movements over 24-hour observation intervals during the last 10 weeks of pregnancy. Am J Obstet Gynecol 142:363, 1982

35. Holden K, Jovanovic L, Druzin M, Peterson C: Increased fetal activity with low maternal blood glucose levels in pregnancies complicated by diabetes. Am J Perinatol 1:161, 1984

36. Phelan JP, Kester R, Labudovich ML: Nonstress test and maternal glucose determinations. Obstet Gynecol 67:4, 1982

37. Druzin ML, Foodim J: Effect of maternal glucose ingestion compared with maternal water ingestion on the nonstress test. Obstet Gynecol 67:4, 1982

38. Natale R, Clewlow F, Dawes G: Measurement of fetal forelimb movements in the lamb in utero. Am J Obstet Gynecol 140:545, 1981

39. Sadovsky E, Yaffe H, Polishuk W: Fetal movement monitoring in normal and pathologic pregnancy. Int J Gynaecol Obstet 12:75, 1974

40. Rayburn W, Zuspan F, Motley M, Donaldson M: An alternative to antepartum fetal heart rate testing. Am J Obstet Gynecol 138:223, 1980

41. Pearson J, Weaver J: Fetal activity and fetal well being: an evaluation. BMJ 1:1305, 1976

42. Sadovsky E, Ohel G, Havazeleth H et al: The definition and the significance of decreased fetal movements. Acta Obstet Gynecol Scand 62:409, 1983

43. Draper J, Field S, Thomas H: Women's views on keeping fetal movement charts. Br J Obstet Gynaecol 93:334, 1986

44. Mikhail MS, Freda MC, Merkatz RB et al: The effect of fetal movement counting on maternal attachment to fetus. Am J Obstet Gynecol 165:988, 1991

45. Sorokin Y, Kierker L: Fetal movement. Clin Obstet Gynecol 25:719, 1982

46. Johnson TRB, Jordan ET, Paine LL: Doppler recordings of fetal movement: II. Comparison with maternal perception. Obstet Gynecol 76:42, 1990

47. Rayburn W, Barr M: Activity patterns in malformed fetuses. Am J Obstet Gynecol 142:1045, 1982

48. Neldam S: Fetal movements as an indicator of fetal well being. Lancet 1:1222, 1980

49. Rayburn W: Antepartum fetal assessment. Clin Perinatol 9:231, 1982

50. Liston R, Cohen A, Mennuti M, Gabbe S: Antepartum fetal evaluation by maternal perception of fetal movement. Obstet Gynecol 60:424, 1982

51. Grant A, Valentin L, Elbourne D, Alexander S: Routine formal fetal movement counting and risk of antepartum late death in normally formed singletons. Lancet 2:345, 1989

52. Moore TR, Piacquadio K: A prospective evaluation of fetal movement screening to reduce the incidence of antepartum fetal death. Am J Obstet Gynecol 160:1075, 1989

53. Moore TR, Piacquadio K: Study results vary in count-to-10 method of fetal movement screening. Am J Obstet Gynecol 163:264, 1990

54. Collea J, Holls W: The contraction stress test. Clin Obstet Gynecol 25:707, 1982

55. Antepartum Fetal Surveillance. American College of Obstetricians and Gynecologists Technical Bulletin 188, January 1994

56. Braly P, Freeman R, Garite T et al: Incidence of premature delivery following the oxytocin challenge test. Am J Obstet Gynecol 141:5, 1981

57. Freeman R: The use of the oxytocin challenge test for antepartum clinical evaluation of uteroplacental respiratory function. Am J Obstet Gynecol 121:481, 1975

58. Martin C, Schifrin B: Prenatal fetal monitoring. p. 155. In Aladjem S, Brown A (eds): Perinatal Intensive Care. CV Mosby, St. Louis, MO 1977

59. Nageotte MP, Towers CV, Asrat T et al: The value of a negative antepartum test: contraction stress test and modified biophysical profile. Obstet Gynecol 84:231, 1994

60. Freeman R, Garite T, Modanlou H et al: Postdate pregnancy: utilization of contraction stress testing for primary fetal surveillance. Am J Obstet Gynecol 140:128, 1981

61. Freeman RK, Dorchester W, Anderson G, Garite TJ: The significance of a previous stillbirth. Am J Obstet Gynecol 151:7, 1985

61a. Druzin ML, Karver ML, Wagner W et al: Prospective evaluation of the contraction stress test and non stress tests in the management of post-term pregnancy. Surg Gynecol Obstet 174:507, 1992

62. Gabbe SG, Mestman JH, Freeman RK et al: Management and outcome of diabetes mellitus, classes B–R. Am J Obstet Gynecol 129:723, 1977

63. Lagrew DC, Pircon RA, Towers CV et al: Antepartum fetal surveillance in patients with diabetes: when to start? Am J Obstet Gynecol 168:1820, 1993

64. Evertson L, Gauthier R, Collea J: Fetal demise following negative contraction stress tests. Obstet Gynecol 51:671, 1978

65. Grundy H, Freeman RK, Lederman S, Dorchester W: Nonreactive contraction stress test: clinical significance. Obstet Gynecol 64:337, 1984

66. Freeman R, Anderson G, Dorchester W: A prospective multi-institutional study of antepartum fetal heart rate monitoring. I. Risk of perinatal mortality and morbidity according to antepartum fetal heart rate test results. Am J Obstet Gynecol 143:771, 1982

67. Ray M, Freeman R, Pine S et al: Clinical experience with the oxytocin challenge test. Am J Obstet Gynecol 114:1, 1972

68. Bissonnette J, Johnson K, Toomey C: The role of a trial of labor with a positive contraction stress test. Am J Obstet Gynecol 135:292, 1979

69. Braly P, Freeman R: The significance of fetal heart rate reactivity with a positive oxytocin challenge test. Obstet Gynecol 50:689, 1977

70. Gabbe S, Freeman R, Goebelsmann U: Evaluation of the contraction stress test before 33 weeks' gestation. Obstet Gynecol 52:649, 1978

71. Merrill PM, Porto M, Lovett SM et al: Evaluation of the non-reactive positive contraction stress test prior to 32 weeks: the role of the biophysical profile. Presented at the Society of Perinatal Obstetricians, Sixth Annual Meeting, San Antonio, 1986

72. Bruce S, Petrie R, Yeh S-Y: The suspicious contraction stress test. Obstet Gynecol 51:415, 1978

73. Scanlon J, Suzuki K, Shea E, Tronick E: A prospective study of the oxytocin challenge test and newborn neurobehavioral outcome. Obstet Gynecol 54:6, 1979

74. Crane J, Anderson B, Marshall R, Harvey P: Subsequent physical and mental development in infants with positive contraction stress tests. J Reprod Med 26:113, 1981

75. Beischer N, Drew J, Ashton P et al: Quality of survival of infants with critical fetal reserve detected by antenatal cardiotocography. Am J Obstet Gynecol 146:662, 1983

76. Oki EY, Keegan KA, Freeman RD, Dorchester W: The breast-stimulated contraction stress test. J Reprod Med 32:919, 1987

77. Keegan KA, Helm DA, Porto M et al: A prospective evaluation of nipple stimulation techniques for contraction stress testing. Am J Obstet Gynecol 157:121, 1987

78. Huddleston J, Sutliff G, Robinson D: Contraction stress test by intermittent nipple stimulation. Obstet Gynecol 63:669, 1984

79. Curtis P, Evens S, Resnick J et al: Patterns of uterine contractions and prolonged uterine activity using three methods of breast stimulation for contraction stress tests. Obstet Gynecol 73:631, 1989

80. Devoe LD, Morrison J, Martin J et al: A prospective comparative study of the extended nonstress test and the nipple stimulation contraction stress test. Am J Obstet Gynecol 157:531, 1987

81. Hammacher K: The clinical significance of cardiotocography. p. 80. In Huntingford P, Huter K, Saling E (eds): Perinatal Medicine. 1st European Congress, Berlin. Academic, San Diego, 1969

82. Patrick J, Carmichael L, Chess L, Staples C: Accelerations of the human fetal heart rate at 38 to 40 weeks' gestational age. Am J Obstet Gynecol 148:35, 1984

83. Margulis E, Binder D, Cohen A: The effect of propranolol on the nonstress test. Am J Obstet Gynecol 148:340, 1984

84. Keegan K, Paul R, Broussard P et al: Antepartum fetal heart rate testing. III. The effect of phenobarbital on the nonstress test. Am J Obstet Gynecol 133:579, 1979

85. Phelan J: Diminished fetal reactivity with smoking. Am J Obstet Gynecol 136:230, 1980

86. Lavery J: Nonstress fetal heart rate testing. Clin Obstet Gynecol 25:689, 1982

87. Keegan K, Paul R, Broussard P et al: Antepartum fetal heart rate testing. V. The nonstress test—an outpatient approach. Am J Obstet Gynecol 136:81, 1980

88. Druzin M, Gratacos J, Paul R et al: Antepartum fetal heart rate testing. XII. The effect of manual manipulation of the fetus on the nonstress test. Am J Obstet Gynecol 151:61, 1985

89. Eglinton G, Paul R, Broussard P et al: Antepartum fetal heart rate testing. XI. Stimulation with orange juice. Am J Obstet Gynecol 150:97, 1984

90. Keegan K, Paul R: Antepartum fetal heart rate testing. IV. The nonstress test as a primary approach. Am J Obstet Gynecol 136:75, 1980

91. Evertson L, Gauthier R, Schifrin B et al: Antepartum fetal heart rate testing. I. Evolution of the nonstress test. Am J Obstet Gynecol 133:29, 1979

92. Rochard F, Schifrin B, Goupil F et al: Nonstressed fetal heart rate monitoring in the antepartum period. Am J Obstet Gynecol 126:699, 1976

93. Phelan J: The nonstress test: a review of 3,000 tests. Am J Obstet Gynecol 139:7, 1981

94. Phillips W, Towell M: Abnormal fetal heart rate associated with congenital abnormalities. Br J Obstet Gynaecol 87:270, 1980

95. Natale R, Nasello C, Turliuk R: The relationship between movements and accelerations in fetal heart rate at twenty-four to thirty-two weeks' gestation. Am J Obstet Gynecol 148:591, 1984

96. Bishop E: Fetal acceleration test. Am J Obstet Gynecol 141:905, 1981

97. Lavin J, Miodovnik M, Barden T: Relationship of nonstress test reactivity and gestational age. Obstet Gynecol 63:338, 1984

98. Druzin ML, Fox A, Kogut E et al: The relationship of the nonstress test to gestational age. Am J Obstet Gynecol 153:386, 1985

99. Aladjem S, Vuolo K, Pazos R et al: Antepartum fetal testing: evaluation and redefinition of criteria for clinical interpretation. Semin Perinatol 5:145, 1981

100. Druzin ML, Lockshin M, Edersheim T et al: Second trimester fetal monitoring and preterm delivery in pregnancies with systematic lupus erythematosus and/or circulating anticoagulant. Am J Obstet Gynecol 157:1503, 1987

101. Brown R, Patrick J: The nonstress test: how long is enough? Am J Obstet Gynecol 141:646, 1981

102. Leveno K, Williams M, DePalma R et al: Perinatal outcome in the absence of antepartum fetal heart rate acceleration. Obstet Gynecol 61:347, 1983

103. DeVoe L, McKenzie J, Searle N et al: Clinical sequelae of the extended nonstress test. Am J Obstet Gynecol 151:1074, 1985

104. Phelan JP: Antepartum fetal assessment—new techniques. Semin Perinatol 12:57, 1988

105. Gagnon R, Foreman J, Hunse C et al: Effects of low-frequency vibration on human germ fetuses. Am J Obstet Gynecol 161:1479, 1989

106. Gagnon R, Hunse C, Foreman J: Human fetal behavioral states after vibratory stimulation. Am J Obstet Gynecol 161:1470, 1989

107. Smith CV, Phelan JP, Paul RH et al: Fetal acoustic stimulation testing: a retrospective experience with the fetal acoustic stimulation test. Am J Obstet Gynecol 153:567, 1985

108. Smith CV, Phelan JP, Platt LD et al: Fetal acoustic stimulation testing. II. A randomized clinical comparison with the nonstress test. Am J Obstet Gynecol 155:131, 1986

109. Kuhlman KA, Depp R: Acoustic stimulation testing. Obstet Gynecol Clin North Am 15:303, 1988

110. Trudinger BJ, Boylan P: Antepartum fetal heart rate monitoring: value of sound stimulation. Obstet Gynecol 55:265, 1980

111. Druzin ML, Edersheim TG, Hutson JM et al: The effect of vibroacoustic stimulation on the nonstress test at gestational ages of thirty-two weeks or less. Am J Obstet Gynecol 1661:1476, 1989

112. Smith CV, Satt B, Phelan JP et al: Intrauterine sound levels: intrapartum assessment with an intrauterine microphone. Am J Perinatol 7:312, 1990

113. Arulkumaran S, Talbert D, Hsu TS et al: In-utero sound levels when vibroacoustic stimulation is applied to the maternal abdomen: an assessment of the possibility of cochlea damage in the fetus. Br J Obstet Gynaecol 99:43, 1992

114. Arulkumaran S, Mircog B, Skurr BA et al: No evidence of hearing loss due to fetal acoustic stimulation test. Obstet Gynecol 78:2, 1991

115. Ohel G, Horowitz E, Linder N et al: Neonatal auditory acuity following in utero vibratory acoustic stimulation. Am J Obstet Gynecol 157:440, 1987

116. Druzin M, Gratacos J, Keegan K et al: Antepartum fetal heart rate testing. VII. The significance of fetal bradycardia. Am J Obstet Gynecol 139:194, 1981

117. Phelan J, Lewis P: Fetal heart rate decelerations during a nonstress test. Obstet Gynecol 57:288, 1981

118. Pazos R, Vuolo K, Aladjem S et al: Association of spontaneous fetal heart rate decelerations during antepartum nonstress testing and intrauterine growth retardation. Am J Obstet Gynecol 144:574, 1982

119. Dashow E, Read J: Significant fetal bradycardia during antepartum heart rate testing. Am J Obstet Gynecol 148:187, 1984

120. Bourgeois F, Thiagarajah S, Harbert G: The significance of fetal heart rate decelerations during nonstress testing. Am J Obstet Gynecol 150:215, 1984

121. Druzin ML: Fetal bradycardia during antepartum testing, further observations. J Reprod Med 34:47, 1989

122. Meis P, Ureda J, Swain M et al: Variable decelerations during non-stress tests (NST): a sign of fetal compromise? Presented at the Society of Perinatal Obstetricians, Fourth Annual Meeting, San Antonio, TX, 1984

123. Barrett J, Salyer S, Boehm F: The nonstress test: an evaluation of 1,000 patients. Am J Obstet Gynecol 141: 153, 1981

124. Miller JM Jr, Horger EO III: Antepartum heart rate testing in diabetic pregnancy. J Reprod Med 30:515, 1985

125. Boehm FH, Salyer S, Shah DM et al: Improved outcome of twice weekly nonstress testing. Obstet Gynecol 67: 566, 1986

126. Miyazaki F, Miyazaki B: False reactive nonstress tests in postterm pregnancies. Am J Obstet Gynecol 140:269, 1981

127. Barss V, Frigoletto F, Diamond F: Stillbirth after nonstress testing. Obstet Gynecol 65:541, 1985

128. Murata Y, Martin C, Ikenoue T et al: Fetal heart rate accelerations and late decelerations during the course of intrauterine death in chronically catheterized rhesus monkeys. Am J Obstet Gynecol 144:218, 1982

129. Freeman R, Anderson G, Dorchester W: A prospective multi-institutional study of antepartum fetal heart rate monitoring. II. Contraction stress test versus nonstress test for primary surveillance. Am J Obstet Gynecol 143: 778, 1982

130. Slomka C, Phelan J: Pregnancy outcome in the patient with a nonreactive nonstress test and a positive contraction stress test. Am J Obstet Gynecol 139:11, 1981

131. Devoe L: Clinical features of the reactive positive contraction stress test. Obstet Gynecol 63:523, 1984

132. Druzin M, Gratacos J, Paul R: Antepartum fetal heart rate testing. VI. Predictive reliability of "normal" tests in the prevention of antepartum death. Am J Obstet Gynecol 137:746, 1980

133. Kadar N: Perinatal mortality related to nonstress and contraction stress tests. Am J Obstet Gynecol 142:931, 1982

134. Finberg HJ, Kurtz AB, Johnson RL et al: The biophysical profile: a literature review and reassessment of its usefulness in the evaluation of fetal well-being. J Ultrasound Med 9:583, 1990

135. Manning FA, Morrison I, Lange IR et al: Fetal assessment based on fetal biophysical profile scoring: experience in 12,620 referred high-risk pregnancies. Am J Obstet Gynecol 151:343, 1985

136. Vintzileos A, Campbell W, Ingardia C, Nochimson D: The fetal biophysical profile and its predictive value. Obstet Gynecol 62:271, 1983

137. Gennser G, Marsal K, Brantmark B: Maternal smoking and fetal breathing movements. Am J Obstet Gynecol 123:861, 1975

138. Platt L, Manning F, Lemay M, Sipos L: Human fetal breathing: relationship to fetal condition. Am J Obstet Gynecol 132:514, 1978

139. Manning F, Platt L, Sipos L, Keegan K: Fetal breathing movements and the nonstress test in high-risk pregnancies. Am J Obstet Gynecol 135:511, 1979

140. Schifrin B, Guntes V, Gergely R et al: The role of real-time scanning in antenatal fetal surveillance. Am J Obstet Gynecol 140:525, 1981

141. Manning F, Platt L, Sipos L: Antepartum fetal evaluation: development of a fetal biophysical profile. Am J Obstet Gynecol 136:787, 1980

142. Vintzileos AM, Campbell WA, Feinstein SJ et al: The fetal biophysical profile in pregnancies with grade III placentas. Am J Perinatol 4:90, 1987

143. Manning FA, Harman CR, Morrison I et al: Fetal assessment based on fetal biophysical profile scoring. Am J Obstet Gynecol 162:703, 1990

144. Manning FA, Morrison I, Lange IR et al: Fetal biophysical profile scoring: selective use of the nonstress test. Am J Obstet Gynecol 156:709, 1987

145. Manning FA, Morrison I, Harman CR et al: The abnormal fetal biophysical profile score. V. Predictive accuracy according to score composition. Am J Obstet Gynecol 162:918, 1990

146. Manning FA: Biophysical profile scoring. p. 241. In Nijhuis J (ed): Fetal Behaviour. Oxford University Press, New York, 1992

147. Vintzileos AM, Gaffney SE, Salinger LM et al: The relationship between fetal biophysical profile and cord pH in patients undergoing cesarean section before the onset of labor. Obstet Gynecol 70:196, 1987

148. Platt L, Eglinton G, Sipos L et al: Further experience with the fetal biophysical profile. Obstet Gynecol 61: 480, 1983

149. Manning F, Lange I, Morrison I et al: Fetal biophysical profile score and the nonstress test: a comparative trial. Obstet Gynecol 64:326, 1984

150. Eden RD, Seifert LS, Kodack LD et al: A modified biophysical profile for antenatal fetal surveillance. Obstet Gynecol 71:365, 1988

151. Inglis SR, Druzin ML, Wagner WE, Kogut E: The use of vibroacoustic stimulation during the abnormal or equivocal biophysical profile. Obstet Gynecol 82:371, 1993

152. Burns PN: Doppler flow estimations in the fetal and maternal circulations: principles, techniques and some limitations. p. 43. In Maulik D, McNellis D (eds): Reproductive & Perinatal Medicine (VIII): Doppler Ultrasound Measurement of Maternal–Fetal Hemodynamics. Perinatology Press, Ithaca, NY, 1987

153. Warsof SL, Levy DL: Doppler blood flow and fetal growth retardation. p. 158. In Gross TL, Sokol RJ (ed): Intrauterine Growth Retardation, A Practical Approach. Year Book, Chicago, 1989

154. Maulik D, Yarlagadda P, Youngblood J, Ciston P: Comparative efficacy of umbilical arterial Doppler indices for predicting adverse perinatal outcome. Am J Obstet Gynecol 164:434, 1991

155. Fleischer A, Schulman H, Farmakides G et al: Uterine artery Doppler velocimetry in pregnant women with hypertension. Am J Obstet Gynecol 154:806, 1986

156. Ducey J, Schulman H, Farmakides G et al: A classifica-

tion of hypertension in pregnancy based on Doppler velocimetry. Am J Obstet Gynecol 157:680, 1987

157. Reed KL, Anderson CF, Shenker L: Changes in intracardiac Doppler blood flow velocities in fetuses with absent umbilical artery diastolic flow. Am J Obstet Gynecol 157:774, 1987

158. Thompson RS, Trudinger BJ, Cook CM et al: Umbilical artery velocity waveforms: normal reference values for A/B ratio and Pourcelot ratio. Br J Obstet Gynaecol 95: 589, 1988

159. Hendricks SK, Sorensen TK, Wang KY et al: Doppler umbilical artery waveform indices—normal values from fourteen to forty-two weeks. Am J Obstet Gynecol 161: 761, 1989

160. Trudinger BJ, Cook CM, Jones L et al: A comparison of fetal heart rate monitoring and umbilical artery waveforms in the recognition of fetal compromise. Br J Obstet Gynaecol 93:171, 1986

161. Trudinger BJ, Stevens D, Connelly A et al: Umbilical artery flow velocity waveforms and placental resistance: the effects of embolization of the umbilical circulation. Am J Obstet Gynecol 157:1443, 1987

162. Morrow R, Ritchie K: Doppler ultrasound fetal velocimetry and its role in obstetrics. Clin Perinatol 16:771, 1989

163. Copel JA, Schlafer D, Wentworth R et al: Does the umbilical artery systolic/diastolic ratio reflect flow or acidosis? Am J Obstet Gynecol 163:751, 1990

164. Devoe LD, Gardner P, Dear C et al: The diagnostic values of concurrent nonstress testing, amniotic fluid measurement, and Doppler velocimetry in screening a general high-risk population. Am J Obstet Gynecol 163: 1040, 1990

165. Alfirevic Z, Neilson JP: Doppler ultrasonography in high-risk pregnancies: systematic review with meta-analysis. Am J Obstet Gynecol 172:1379, 1995

166. Rochelson BL, Schulman H, Farmakides G: The significance of absent end-diastolic velocity in umbilical artery waveforms. Am J Obstet Gynecol 156:1213, 1987

167. Woo JSK, Liang ST, Lo RLS: Significance of absent or reversed end diastolic flow in Doppler umbilical artery waveforms. J Ultrasound Med 6:291, 1987

168. Johnstone FD, Haddad NG, Hoskins P et al: Umbilical artery Doppler flow velocity waveform: the outcome of pregnancies with absent end diastolic flow. Eur J Obstet Gynecol Reprod Biol 28:171, 1988

169. Brar HS, Platt LD: Reverse end-diastolic flow velocity on umbilical artery velocimetry in high-risk pregnancies: an ominous finding with adverse outcome. Am J Obstet Gynecol 159:559, 1988

170. Fairlie F, Moretti M, Walker J, Sibai B: Determinations of perinatal outcome in pregnancy-induced hypertension with absence of umbilical artery end-diastolic frequencies. Am J Obstet Gynecol 164:1084, 1991

171. Divon MY, Girz BA, Lieblich R, Langer O: Clinical management of the fetus with markedly diminished umbilical artery end-diastolic flow. Am J Obstet Gynecol 161: 1523, 1989

172. Mason GC, Lilford RJ, Porter J, Tyrell S: Randomized comparison of routine versus highly selective use of Doppler ultrasound in low risk pregnancies. Br J Obstet Gynaecol 100:130, 1993

173. Strassner H, Nochimson D: Determination of fetal maturity. Clin Perinatol 9:297, 1982

174. Goldenberg R, Nelson K: Iatrogenic respiratory distress syndrome. Am J Obstet Gynecol 123:617, 1975

175. Hack M, Fanaroff A, Klaus M et al: Neonatal respiratory distress following elective delivery: a preventable disease? Am J Obstet Gynecol 126:43, 1976

176. Maisels M, Rees R, Marks K et al: Elective delivery of the "term" fetus—an obstetrical hazard. JAMA 238:2036, 1977

177. Berkowitz GS, Chang K, Chervenak FA et al: Decreasing frequency of iatrogenic neonatal respiratory distress syndrome. Am J Perinatol 3:205, 1986

178. Gluck L, Kulovich M, Borer R et al: The interpretation and significance of the lecithin/sphingomyelin ratio in amniotic fluid. Am J Obstet Gynecol 120:142, 1974

179. Kulovich M, Hallman M, Gluck L: The lung profile. Am J Obstet Gynecol 135:57, 1979

180. Harvey D, Parkinson C, Campbell S: Risk of respiratory distress syndrome. Lancet 1:42, 1975

181. Creasy G, Simon N: Sensitivity and specificity of the L/ S ratio in relation to gestational age. Am J Perinatol 1: 302, 1984

182. Buhi W, Spellacy W: Effects of blood or meconium on the determination of the amniotic fluid lecithin/sphingomyelin ratio. Am J Obstet Gynecol 121:321, 1975

183. Tabsh K, Brinkman C, Bashore R: Effect of meconium contamination on amniotic fluid lecithin:sphingomyelin ratio. Obstet Gynecol 58:605, 1981

184. Stedman C, Crawford S, Staten E et al: Management of preterm premature rupture of membranes: assessing amniotic fluid in the vagina for phosphatidylglycerol. Am J Obstet Gynecol 140:34, 1981

185. Strassner H, Golde S, Mosley G et al: Effect of blood in amniotic fluid on the detection of phosphatidylglycerol. Am J Obstet Gynecol 138:697, 1980

186. Hill L, Ellefson R: Variable interference of meconium in the determination of phosphatidylglycerol. Am J Obstet Gynecol 147:339, 1983

187. Thibeault D, Hobel C: The interrelationship of the foam stability test, immaturity, and intrapartum complications in the respiratory distress syndrome. Am J Obstet Gynecol 118:56, 1974

188. Horenstein J, Golde SH, Platt LD: Lung profiles in the isoimmunized pregnancy. Am J Obstet Gynecol 153: 443, 1985

189. Kjos SL, Walther FJ, Montoro M et al: Prevalence and etiology of respiratory distress in infants of diabetic mothers: predictive value of fetal lung maturation tests. Am J Obstet Gynecol 163:898, 1990

190. Kulovich M, Gluck L: The lung profile. II. Complicated pregnancy. Am J Obstet Gynecol 135:64, 1979

191. Hallman M, Teramo K: Measurement of the lecithin/ sphingomyelin ratio and phosphatidylgylcerol in amniotic fluid: an accurate method for the assessment of fetal lung maturity. Br J Obstet Gynaecol 88:806, 1981

192. Winn HN, Romero R, Roberts A et al: Comparison of

fetal lung maturation in preterm singleton and twin pregnancies. Am J Perinatol 9:326, 1992

193. Schiff E, Friedman SA, Mercer BM, Sibai BM: Fetal lung maturity is not accelerated in preeclamptic pregnancies. Am J Obstet Gynecol 169:1096, 1993

194. Lambers DS, Brady K, Leist PA et al: Ability of normal vaginal flora to produce detectable phosphatidylglycerol in amniotic fluid in vitro. Obstet Gynecol 85:651, 1995

195. Towers CV, Garite TJ: Evaluation of the new Amniostat-FLM test for the detection of phosphatidylglycerol in contaminated fluids. Am J Obstet Gynecol 160:298, 1989

196. Barkai G, Mashiach S, Lanzer D et al: Determination of fetal lung maturity from amniotic microviscosity in high-risk pregnancy. Obstet Gynecol 59:615, 1982

197. Steinfeld JD, Samuels P, Bulley MA et al: The utility of the TDx test in the assessment of fetal lung maturity. Obstet Gynecol 79:460, 1992

198. Bayer-Zwirello LA, Jertson J, Rosenbaum J et al: Amniotic fluid surfactant-albumin ratio as a screening test for fetal lung maturity—two years of clinical experience. J Perinatol XIII:354, 1993

199. Apple FS, Bilodeau L, Preese LM, Benson P: Clinical implementation of a rapid, automated assay for assessing fetal lung maturity. J Reprod Med 39:883, 1994

200. Clements JA, Platzker A, Tierney D et al: Assessment of the risk of the respiratory-distress syndrome by a rapid test for surfactant in amniotic fluid. N Engl J Med 286:1081, 1972

201. Sher G, Statland B, Freer D, Hisley J: Performance of the amniotic fluid foam stability–50 percent test. A bedside procedure for the prenatal detection of hyaline membrane disease. Am J Obstet Gynecol 134:705, 1979

202. Sher G, Statland B: Assessment of fetal pulmonary maturity by the Lumadex Foam Stability Index Test. Obstet Gynecol 61:444, 1983

203. Lockitch G, Wittmann BK, Snow BE et al: Prediction of fetal lung maturity by use of the Lumadex-FSI test. Clin Chem 32:361, 1986

204. Socol ML: The tap test: confirmation of a simple, rapid, inexpensive, and reliable indicator of fetal pulmonary maturity. Am J Obstet Gynecol 162:218, 1990

205. Guidozzi F, Gobetz L: The tap test—a rapid bedside indicator of fetal lung maturity. Br J Obstet Gynaecol 98:479, 1991

206. Kassanos D, Botsis D, Gregoriou O et al: The tap test: a simple and inexpensive method for the diagnosis of fetal pulmonary maturity. Int J Gynecol Obstet 41:135, 1993

207. Yapar EG, Gökmen O: Comparison of two tests and absorbance at 650 nm for assessing fetal lung maturity. J Reprod Med 40:423, 1995

208. Strong TH Jr, Hayes AS, Sawyer AT et al: Amniotic fluid turbidity: a useful adjunct for assessing fetal pulmonary maturity status. Int J Gynecol Obstet 38:97, 1992

209. Sbarra A, Selvaraj R, Cetrulo C et al: Positive correlation of optical density at 650 nm with lecithin/sphingomyelin ratios in amniotic fluid. Am J Obstet Gynecol 130:788, 1978

210. Cetrulo C, Sbarra S, Selvaraj R et al: Amniotic fluid optical density and neonatal respiratory outcome. Obstet Gynecol 55:262, 1980

211. Turner R, Read J: Practical use and efficiency of amniotic fluid OD 650 as a predictor of fetal pulmonary maturity. Obstet Gynecol 61:551, 1983

212. Khouzami V, Beck J, Sullivant H et al: Amniotic fluid absorbance at 650 nm: its relationship to the lecithin/sphingomyelin ratio and neonatal pulmonary sufficiency. Am J Obstet Gynecol 147:552, 1983

213. Plauche W, Faro S, Wycheck J: Amniotic fluid optical density: relationship to L/S ratio, phospholipid content, and desquamation of fetal cells. Obstet Gynecol 58:309, 1981

214. Ashwood ER, Palmer SE, Taylor JS, Pingree SS: Lamellar body counts for rapid fetal lung maturity testing. Obstet Gynecol 81:619, 1993

215. Fakhoury G, Daikoku NH, Benser J, Dubin NH: Lamellar body concentrations and the prediction of fetal pulmonary maturity. Am J Obstet Gynecol 170:72, 1994

216. Greenspoon JS, Rosen DJD, Roll K, Dubin SB: Evaluation of lamellar body number density as the initial assessment in a fetal lung maturity test cascade. J Reprod Med 40:260, 1995

217. Dalence CR, Bowie LJ, Dohnal JC et al: Amniotic fluid lamellar body count: a rapid and reliable fetal lung maturity test. Obstet Gynecol 86:235, 1995

218. Newton ER, Cetrulo CL, Kosa DJ: Biparietal diameter as a predictor of fetal lung maturity. J Reprod Med 28:480, 1983

219. Golde S, Platt L: The use of ultrasound in the diagnosis of fetal lung maturity. Clin Obstet Gynecol 27:391, 1984

220. Grannum P, Berkowitz R, Hobbins J: The ultrasonic changes in the maturing placenta and their relation to fetal pulmonic maturity. Am J Obstet Gynecol 133:915, 1979

221. Harman C, Manning R, Stearns E et al: The correlation of ultrasonic placental grading and fetal pulmonary maturation in five hundred sixty-three pregnancies. Am J Obstet Gynecol 143:941, 1982

222. Kazzi G, Gross T, Sokol R et al: Noninvasive prediction of hyaline membrane disease: an optimized classification of sonographic placental maturation. Am J Obstet Gynecol 152:213, 1985

223. Gast MJ, Ott W: Failure of ultrasonic placental grading to predict severe respiratory distress in a neonate. Am J Obstet Gynecol 146:464, 1983

224. Shah YG, Graham D: Relationship of placental grade to fetal pulmonary maturity and respiratory distress syndrome. Am J Perinatol 3:53, 1986

225. Gross T, Sokol R, Kazzi G et al: When is an amniocentesis for fetal maturity unnecessary in nondiabetic pregnancies at risk? Am J Obstet Gynecol 149:311, 1984

226. Slocum WA, Martin JN Jr, Martin RW et al: third-trimester biparietal diameter as a predictor of fetal lung maturity. Am J Perinatol 4:266, 1987

227. Hadlock FP, Irvin JF, Roecker et al: Ultrasound prediction of fetal lung maturity. Radiology 155:469, 1985

228. Garite TJ, Freeman RK, Nageotte MP: Fetal maturity cascade: a rapid and cost-effective method for fetal lung maturity testing. Obstet Gynecol 67:619, 1986

229. Herbert WNP, Chapman JF: Clinical and economic

considerations associated with testing for fetal lung maturity. Am J Obstet Gynecol 155:820, 1986

230. Clark SL, Sabey P, Jolley K: Nonstress testing with acoustic stimulation and amniotic fluid volume assessment: 5973 tests without unexpected fetal death. Am J Obstet Gynecol 160:694, 1989

231. Mills MS, James KD, Slade S: Two-tier approach to biophysical assessment of the fetus. Am J Obstet Gynecol 163:12, 1990

232. Vintzileos AM, Campbell WA, Nochimson DJ et al: The use and misuse of the fetal biophysical profile. Am J Obstet Gynecol 156:527, 1987

233. Nageotte MP, Towers CV, Asrat T, Freeman RK: Perinatal outcome with the modified biophysical profile. Am J Obstet Gynecol 170:1672, 1994

234. Wilson R, Schifrin B: Is any pregnancy low risk? Obstet Gynecol 55:653, 1980

235. Bruner JP, Gabbe SG, Levy DW et al: Doppler ultrasonography of the umbilical cord in normal pregnancy. J Southern Med Assoc 86:52, 1993

SECTION 3

Intrapartum Care

Chapter 13

Labor and Delivery

William F. O'Brien and Robert C. Cefalo

Management of Labor and Delivery

Definitions

Labor can be defined as progressive dilatation of the uterine cervix in association with repetitive uterine contractions. This definition serves to exclude instances in which cervical dilatation occurs without uterine contractions such as an incompetent cervix. Also excluded are uterine contractions that occur without true progressive dilatation, as is common in the latter stage of pregnancy. Labor can either be spontaneous or induced, either term or preterm. The physiology of labor is reviewed in Chapter 12.

Normal Mechanisms of Labor

Stages and Phases of Labor

Normal labor is a continuous process, but for reasons of study it has been divided into three stages, with the first stage further subdivided into three phases. The first stage of labor is the interval between the onset of labor and full cervical dilatation. The second stage of labor is the interval between full cervical dilatation and the delivery of the infant. The third stage of labor encompasses the period between the delivery of the infant and delivery of the placenta.

The first stage of labor has been subdivided by Friedman[1] in his classic studies on the course of labor. Analyzing the progress of spontaneous labor by graphically plotting cervical dilatation against time, he described three phases. A latent phase of variable duration was defined as the period between the onset of labor and a point at which a change in the slope of cervical dilatation is noted. A phase of maximal dilatation was defined as that period of labor when the rate of cervical dilata-

tion was maximal. This phase usually began at 2 to 3 cm dilatation. A short deceleration phase followed the acceleration phase and was terminated at full cervical dilatation. It should be noted that not all investigators have accepted the validity of a separate deceleration phase. A descent phase was described that usually coincides with the second stage of labor. Investigators examining various ethnic groups have demonstrated that, fortunately, the parameters of progression in labor do not differ among these populations.[2] A listing of the average and fifth percentile limits of progression in labor is given in Table 13-1.

The Mechanisms of Labor

The usual presentation of the fetus to the birth canal is the vertex presentation wherein the occiput of the fetus is the lowermost part with regard to the longitudinal axis of the mother. This presentation occurs in approximately 95 percent of all term labors. The mechanisms of labor, also known as the cardinal mechanisms, refer to the changes in the position of the fetal head during passage through the birth canal. Because of the asymmetry of the shape of both the fetal head and the maternal bony pelvis, such rotations are required for the average size fetus to accomplish passage through the birth canal. These rotations of the fetal head are accomplished by the propulsive force of uterine activity occurring during labor. The cardinal movements of labor are usually described as (1) engagement, (2) descent, (3) flexion, (4) internal rotation, (5) extension, (6) external rotation, and (7) expulsion. As noted above, a division into distinct movements occurring at separate times is artificial. Obviously, descent occurs throughout the passage through the birth canal as does flexion of the fetal head.

Table 13-1 Progression of Spontaneous Labor Parameter

Parameter	Mean or Median	5th Centile
Nulliparas		
Total duration	10.1 hr	25.8 hr
Stages		
First	9.7 hr	24.7 hr
Second	33.0 min	117.5 min
Third	5.0 min	30 min
Latent Phase (duration)	6.4 hr	20.6 hr
Maximal dilation (rate)	3.0 cm/hr	1.2 cm/hr
Descent (rate)	3.3 cm/hr	1.0 cm/hr
Multiparas		
Total duration	6.2 hr	19.5 hr
Stages		
First	8.0 hr	18.8 hr
Second	8.5 min	46.5 min
Third	5.0 min	30 min
Latent phase (duration)	4.8 hr	13.6 hr
Maximal dilation (rate)	5.7 cm/hr	1.5 cm/hr
Descent (rate)	6.6 cm/hr	2.1 cm/hr

Engagement

In the normal flexed position, the largest transverse diameter of the fetal head is the biparietal diameter (Fig. 13-1). Engagement is the descent of the biparietal diameter of the fetal head to a level below the plane of the pelvic inlet. When this has occurred, the head is said to be engaged. Clinically, engagement is usually measured by palpation of the presenting part of the occiput. If the lowest portion of the occiput is at or below the level of the maternal ischial spines, engagement has usually taken place. This is because the average distance between the plane of the pelvic inlet and the ischial spines is approximately 5 cm, while the distance between the biparietal plane and the lowermost part of the occiput averages 3 to 4 cm. Engagement is

considered an important clinical parameter, as it demonstrates that, at least at the level of the pelvic inlet, the maternal bony pelvis is sufficiently large to allow the descent of the fetal head. It should be noted that, although engagement is classically listed as one of the cardinal movements of labor, engagement often occurs before the onset of true labor, especially in nulliparas.

Descent

Since the obvious purpose of labor is the expulsion of the fetus through the birth canal, descent is the most important component of labor. Descent of the fetus is not continuous, however, but usually occurs in a discontinuous fashion, with the greatest rate of descent in the deceleration phase of the first stage of labor and during the second stage of labor.

Flexion

Flexion of the fetal head is a passive motion whereby the presenting diameters of the fetal head to the maternal pelvis are optimized (Fig. 13-2). Although flexion of the fetal head onto the chest is present, to some degree, in most fetuses before labor, complete flexion with the placement of the fetal chin on the thorax usually occurs only during the course of labor.

Internal Rotation

During internal rotation, the fetal occiput gradually rotates from its original position (usually transverse with regard to the birth canal) toward the symphysis pubis or, less commonly, toward the hollow of the sacrum. As in flexion, this rotation is passive with regard to the fetus and again facilitates the presentation of the smallest possible diameters of the fetal head to the birth canal. As the musculature of the pelvic floor, including the coccygeus and ileococcygeus muscles, form a V-

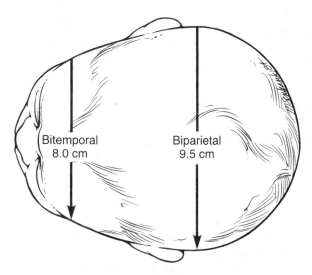

Fig. 13-1 Average transverse diameters of the term fetal skull.

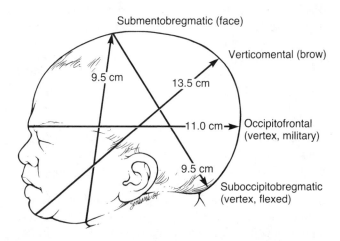

Fig. 13-2 Possible presenting diameters of the average term fetal skull.

shaped hammock diverging anteriorly, the occiput of the fetus (the widest portion of the presenting part) rotates toward the symphysis pubis, allowing the widest portion of the fetus to transverse the birth canal at its area of greatest dimension.

Extension

Extension occurs after the fetus has descended to the level of the maternal vulva. This descent brings the base of the occiput into contact with the inferior margin of the symphysis pubis. At this point the birth canal curves upward. The fetal head is delivered by extension from the flexed to the extended position, rotating around the symphysis pubis. The forces responsible for this motion are the downward force exerted on the fetus by the uterine contractions associated with the upward forces exerted by the muscles of the pelvic floor. In combination, these forces form a diagonal vector resulting in extension of the fetal head.

External Rotation

After delivery of the head, the forces exerted on the head by the maternal bony pelvis and its musculature are relieved. At this point, the unopposed forces of the fetal musculature assume precedence and the fetus resumes its normal "face-forward" position with the occiput and spine lying in the same plane.

Expulsion

After external rotation of the fetal head, further descent brings the anterior shoulder to the level of the symphysis pubis. The shoulder is delivered in much the same manner as the head, with rotation of the anterior shoulder under the symphysis pubis. After the shoulders, the rest of the body is usually quickly delivered.

Management of Normal Labor and Delivery

Initial Assessment

As in all patient care encounters, initial management of labor should include an appropriate history, physical examination, and necessary laboratory testing. At 36 weeks' gestation (or earlier if premature labor is likely), the patient's prenatal record should be available to the personnel in the labor area. When the patient is admitted, prenatal data should be reviewed, with pertinent information transferred to the labor record. Besides updating the history in the prenatal chart, significant new data that have accrued since the last antepartum visit should be obtained. Of special interest are time of onset of contractions, status of fetal membranes, presence or absence of vaginal bleeding, a notation of fetal activity, history of allergies, time and content of last

ingestion of food or fluids, and use of any medications. An admitting physical examination should include the patient's vital signs, notation of fetal position and presentation, reporting of the fetal heart rate, as well as frequency, duration, and quality of uterine contractions. If no contraindications exist to pelvic examination, the degree of cervical dilatation, effacement, status of the membranes, and type and station of the presenting part should be noted.

An important aspect of the initial assessment is estimation of fetal weight. Although this has traditionally been accomplished via clinical estimation based on Leopold's maneuvers, the availability of immediate access to sonography has led to the use of sonographic estimations by many. This approach may be quite helpful if the fetus is preterm or apparently small for gestational age. In the apparently normal sized, term fetus, however, estimation of fetal weight by the physician, and even the mother, is at least as good as sonographic estimations.

Risk Status Assignment

Using information available from the prenatal record as well as information gleaned from the initial assessment of the patient, an assignment of her risk status should be made. Identification of the high-risk patient is critical in the proper management of labor and delivery. Approximately 20 percent of pregnant women who can be identified antenatally as high risk account for 55 percent of poor pregnancy outcomes. In addition, 5 to 10 percent of pregnant women are identified as high risk only during the course of labor, and these patients result in 20 to 25 percent of poor pregnancy outcomes. It is important to realize, however, that approximately 20 percent of perinatal morbidity and mortality arise from a group of patients who are assessed to be at low risk. Therefore, all women require adequate surveillance throughout labor and delivery.

Standard Procedures

Over the course of the last decade, significant changes in the policies of institutions and physicians regarding once routinely recommended procedures such as shaving of perineal hair, enemas, showers, intravenous catheters, and positioning during labor and delivery have occurred. Modern management methods include the involvement of the patient and her family in these decisions with informed and prudent guidelines formulated by the health care team.

Emotional support of the patient during the birthing process leads to a lower incidence of intrapartum complications and postpartum emotional problems.[4] Patients who have had no prenatal care should undergo a complete history and physical examination, blood count, blood typing, Rh determination, and urine testing upon admission. Those patients who have had antepartum care require only a urine sample to be tested for the presence of protein and glucose, a determination of hematocrit, blood count, and submission to the laboratory of a specimen of blood to be available in the event of subsequent need for cross-matching.

Management of Labor and Patients Without Identifiable Risks

After the patient has been admitted, she should be introduced to the members of the health care team who will be responsible for her care. An assessment of the quality of the uterine contractions as well as cervical examinations at appropriate intervals should be performed in order to detect evidence of any abnormality of the labor. Vaginal examinations should be kept to the minimum required for the evaluation of the labor pattern. Cleansing of the perineum with an antiseptic and the use of a sterile lubricant may decrease potential contamination. The fetal heart rate should be recorded at least every 30 minutes or more during the first stage of labor. The heart rate should be auscultated immediately after uterine contractions.

During the second stage of labor, the fetal heart rate should be auscultated at least every 15 minutes, and preferably after each uterine contraction. Because inhalation anesthesia may be needed for cesarean delivery or for management of complications of the third stage of labor, most hospitals in the United States limit oral intake to small sips of water, ice chips, or hard candies. This contrasts with the general policy in British hospitals, where oral intake of fluids is almost universal and solids are often allowed as well.[5] Aspiration pneumonitis, a major cause of anesthetic-associated maternal mortality, is related to the acidity of gastric contents. The use of a clear antacid such as 0.3-M sodium citrate during the course of labor has been recommended by many authors.

Preparation for delivery should be started with consideration given to the patient's parity, the progression of labor, presentation of the fetus, and complications of the labor. For patients without identifiable risks, delivery may be conducted either in birthing rooms or in traditional delivery areas. Although the lithotomy position is often used for vaginal delivery in the United States, many patients and physicians prefer the lateral or Sims position or the partial sitting position. During delivery, the maternal blood pressure and pulse should be evaluated and recorded every 10 minutes. Since automated blood pressure recording has become popular at many centers, it should be kept in mind that these recordings will have higher systolic and lower diastolic readings then those obtained manually.[6]

Management of Labor in High-Risk Patients

Continuous electronic fetal monitoring is recommended for patients identified as high risk. Internal uterine pressure monitoring provides important information regarding the quality and quantity of contractions. Abnormal findings by electronic fetal monitoring should be described and interpreted by qualified obstetric personnel. An assessment of fetal scalp capillary pH can be performed in situations of potential fetal distress and may clarify suspicious or confusing fetal heart rate patterns. In patients at high risk, if no specific problems have been identified during the course of labor, management should proceed in a manner similar to that recommended for low-risk patients.

Assisted Spontaneous Delivery

The goals of assisted spontaneous delivery are the reduction of maternal trauma, prevention of fetal injury, and initial support of the newborn.

Episiotomy

An episiotomy is an incision into the perineal body made before delivery in order to enlarge the area of the outlet and thereby facilitate delivery. Although there is general agreement that episiotomy is indicated in cases of arrested or protracted descent or accompanying forceps or vacuum delivery, the role of prophylactic episiotomy is widely debated. Cited advantages include the substitution of a straight surgical incision for ragged spontaneous lacerations, reduction in the duration of the second stage, and reduction of trauma to the pelvic floor musculature. Although elective episiotomy has been advocated principally as a method to reduce the likelihood of subsequent pelvic relaxation,[7] this association has never been proven.[8]

Disadvantages of episiotomy include increased blood loss, especially if the incision is made too early, and possibly an increase in trauma over that which would have occurred spontaneously. Although a mediolateral episiotomy may serve to reduce the likelihood of third-degree lacerations, this procedure is considerably more painful than a median episiotomy and is performed less frequently than in the past.

In view of the lack of objective evidence on the value of prophylactic episiotomy and the often emotional nature of the issue, the decision to perform an episiotomy is best left to the individual physician and the patient.

In the absence of complicating factors such as rectal or perineal lesions, a medial episiotomy is preferred. The incision should be performed when the fetal head has distended the vulva to 2 to 3 cm unless earlier delivery is indicated. Care should be taken to displace the perineum from the fetal head. The size of the incision will depend on the length of the perineum but is generally one-half the length of the perineum.

Although an episiotomy may be performed with a scalpel, incisions are usually made with a straight Mayo scissors. The incision should be placed vertically into the midline of the perineal body and be of sufficient size to increase the area of the introitus without compromise of the anal sphincter.

Mediolateral episiotomies are less likely to be associated with damage to the anal sphincter or the rectal mucosa. This advantage is usually offset by greater difficulty in repair, increased blood loss, and a more painful postpartum course.

Although proper repair of rectal damage due to extension of a median episiotomy rarely results in long-term morbidity, abnormalities in this area such as inflammatory bowel disease or prior surgery may indicate mediolateral episiotomy as the procedure of choice. Mediolateral episiotomy is performed by incision at a 45 degree angle from the inferior portion of the hymeneal ring. The length of the incision is less critical than with median episiotomy, but longer incisions require more lengthy repair. The side to which the episiotomy is performed is usually dictated by the dominant hand of the obstetrician, as a right-sided episiotomy is more easily performed by a right-handed individual. For both median and mediolateral episiotomies, the incision should be extended vertically up the vaginal mucosa for a distance of approximately 2 to 3 cm.

Delivery of the Head

In the vertex presentation, the fetal head is delivered by extension. The goal of assisted delivery of the head is the prevention of rapid delivery. If extension does not occur with ease, assistance in the form of a modified Ritgen's maneuver may be provided. The hand, protected by a sterile towel, is placed on the perineum and the fetal chin palpated. The chin is then gently pressed upward, effecting extension of the fetal head.

After expulsion of the head, external rotation is allowed. If the cord is palpable around the neck, it should be looped over the head or, if not reducible, doubly clamped and cut. Mucus should be aspirated from the fetal mouth, oropharynx, and nares. Although usually performed with a bulb syringe, in the presence of meconium thorough aspiration with a DeLee suction catheter reduces the risk of meconium aspiration syndrome.

Delivery of the Shoulders and Body

Once the fetal airway has been cleared, the physician places his or her hands along the parietal bones of the fetus, and the mother is asked to bear down gently. The fetus is directed posteriorly until the anterior shoulder has passed beneath the symphysis.

After delivery of the anterior shoulder, the mother should be asked to pant. The fetus is slowly directed anteriorly until the posterior shoulder passes the perineum.

After delivery of the shoulders, the fetus should be grasped with the palm of one hand above the shoulders and the other hand along the spine. The infant should be cradled as delivery is completed either spontaneously or with a gentle maternal push. Once delivered, the infant should be held securely and wiped dry with a sterile towel, while any mucus remaining in the airway is suctioned.

Cord Clamping

After delivery, there is a net transfer of blood from the placenta to the infant. Spasm of the umbilical artery occurs within approximately 1 minute of birth. However, the remaining communication between the neonate and placenta, the umbilical vein, permits passage of blood for up to 3 minutes after birth. The pressure gradient for the flow in the umbilical vein is dependent on intrauterine pressure and neonatal venous pressure. Since these pressures are usually fairly low during the immediate postdelivery period, gravitational effects are important. The physician can therefore influence the degree of postnatal placental transfusion by both the interval between delivery and cord clamping and by altering the height at which the infant is held after delivery. In most instances, the volume of this transfusion is not important, and the timing of the cord clamping is dictated by convenience. Since intentional manipulation of the volume of transfusion can result in either relative hypervolemia or hypovolemia of the neonate, such procedures should be reserved for unusual situations.[9]

Pelvimetry and Labor

Pelvic Shapes, Planes, and Diameters

It is intuitively obvious that successful vaginal delivery is dependent on the relative size of the fetus and the maternal pelvis. Not surprisingly, therefore, a great deal of information has accumulated about the size and shape of the female pelvis. Measurements of great precision have been made directly in cadavers and using x-ray techniques in large numbers of women. In general, these measurements have divided the pelvis into a series of planes that must be traversed by the fetus during passage through the birth canal. It should be kept in mind, however, that these planes describe the bony limits of the pelvis, and consideration of the influence of the soft tissues of the birth canal has been rare.

Table 13-2 Pelvic Types and Characteristics

Type	Shape	Posterior Sagittal Diameter	Prognosis
Gynecoid	Round	Average	Good
Anthropoid	Long, oval	Long	Good
Android	Heart shaped	Short	Poor
Platypelloid	Flat, oval	Short	Poor

The bony pelvis is a bowl-shaped structure open at the anterior inferior margin. It is bounded anteriorly by the pubic portion of the innominate-bones, which are joined in the midline at the symphysis pubis. The lateral margins are the innominate bones that are joined by synchondroses to the sacrum, which, along with the coccyx, forms the posterior margin. The true pelvis lies below the linea terminalis, which demarcates the line of fusion between the iliac and ischial portion of the innominate bones.

The most commonly measured planes are the pelvic inlet and the midplane. The pelvic inlet (obstetric conjugate) is bounded anteriorly by the posterior border of the symphysis pubis, posteriorly by the sacral promontory, and laterally by the linea terminalis. As the shape of this plane varies considerably, the measurement of its transverse diameter is conventially made at the widest point. The midpelvic plane is bounded laterally by the inferior margins of the ischial spines, anteriorly by the lower margin of the symphysis pubis, and posteriorly by the sacrum (usually S4 or S5).

Pelves have been classified into four basic types based on the shape of the inlet. This classification, based on the x-ray studies reported by Caldwell et al.,[10] separates those with favorable characteristics (gynecoid, anthropoid) from those with less efficient utilization of space within the pelvis (android, platypelloid). The differing types are usually described according to their shapes, as demonstrated in Table 13-2. The distinguishing feature between favorable and unfavorable types is the amount of space posterior to the greatest transverse diameter. This space is most easily characterized by the posterior sagittal diameter extending from the sacral promontory to the greatest transverse diameter. Unfortunately, this simple characterization of pelvic types does not completely characterize the pelvis, since in reality many women fall into intermediate classes and distinctions become arbitrary.

Clinical Pelvimetry

Although many external measurements of the female pelvis have been advocated as predictive of pelvic size, only a few such measurements enjoy current usage. The most commonly used is the diagonal conjugate. This important measurement is the distance from the inferior border of the symphysis pubis to the sacral promontory. It is an easily obtainable index of the obstetric conjugate and therefore the anteroposterior (AP) diameter of the pelvic inlet.

The measurement is made by positioning the tip of the middle finger at the sacral promontory and noting the point on the hand that contacts the symphysis pubis. The diagonal conjugate is generally 1.5 to 2.0 cm longer than the obstetric conjugate.

The second clinical measurement still in use is the bisischial diameter. With the patient in the lithotomy position, the ischial tuberosities are palpated and the distance between them measured. A value of greater than 8 cm is considered adequate. A small measurement may imply a generally small pelvis or convergence of the pelvic sidewalls.

Other characteristics of the pelvis may be noted on digital examination but only described qualitatively (small, average, large). These include the angulation of the pubic rami beneath the pubic arch, the apparent size of the ischial spines, the size of the sacrospinous notch, and the degree of curvature of the sacrum and coccyx. Although the qualitative nature of these measurements detracts from their general utility, they may supply significant information about the overall shape of the pelvis.

X-Ray Pelvimetry

Although pelvic measurement has been accepted for centuries as an adjunct for the management of labor, precision in pelvic measurements was not achieved prior to the advent of x-ray pelvimetry. Initial enthusiasm for the use of this technique, however, was later tempered by an increasing appreciation of the potential hazards of radiation to the fetus. Although used much less frequently today, x-ray pelvimetry still plays an important role in the management of some patients, especially those with breech presentation.

Systems of x-ray pelvimetry rely primarily on AP and transverse (T) views of the pelvis. These systems compensate for magnification by inclusion of a metallic ruler to which measurements are compared or by calculation of film object distances.

The systems developed by Thoms or Colcher and Sussman depend on comparisons between the diameters measured to tables of average and critical limits. The most commonly used measurements are the AP and T diameters and their totals at the pelvic inlet and at the pelvic midplane. Commonly used values for these measurements are listed in Table 13-3. It should be noted that the critical limits cited imply that a high likelihood of cephalopelvic disproportion may exist. A popular modification of this technique is a calculation of areas as popularized by Mengert.[11] He demonstrated that below a critical limit (85 percent of the

Table 13-3 Average and Critical Limit Values for Pelvic Measurements by X-ray Pelvimetry

Diameter	Average Value	Critical Limit
Inlet		
AP (cm)	12.5	10
T (cm)	13.0	12
Total (cm)	25.5	22.0
Area (cm^2)	145.0	123.0
Midplane		
AP (cm)	11.5	10.0
T (cm)	10.5	9.5
Total (cm)	22.0	20
Area (cm^2)	125.0	106.0

mean value) labor was associated with a high rate of cesarean or difficult deliveries.

A major disadvantage of these systems is the lack of information on fetal size. This deficiency is addressed by the technique originally described by Friedman.[12] In this system, corrected values for the diameters of the planes are used to calculate spheres to which the calculated volume of the fetal cranium is compared. The criteria for disproportion rely on the deficit between the calculated capacities of the pelvic planes and the volume of the fetal cranium. More recently, Morgan and Thurman[13] have utilized the fetal-pelvic index, combining ultrasound measurements of the fetus with x-ray pelvimetry. This technique has proven valuable in identifying women at risk for fetal–pelvic disproportion (see Ch. 26).

Risks of X-Ray Pelvimetry

The primary concern governing the use of x-ray pelvimetry is exposure of the fetus to ionizing radiation. This concern has been based on several retrospective studies that have demonstrated a higher incidence of childhood malignancy in infants exposed to x-ray in utero.[14,15] Although these studies suffer from serious methodologic flaws with respect to scientific proof and a number of reports have failed to detect such an association, they are supported by firm theoretical considerations, and it is prudent to consider antenatal pelvimetry potentially carcinogenic for the fetus.

Allowing for this potential hazard, the risks and benefits of the procedure must be carefully weighed. The likelihood of childhood malignancy based on these retrospective studies is approximately 1 cancer per 5,000 infants exposed. This risk is quite small in comparison to the hazard of perinatal mortality associated with cephalopelvic disproportion. Data from the Collaborative Perinatal Study[16] document a perinatal death rate of 17.9 per 1,000 in the presence of maternal dystocia. This potentially favorable risk benefit ratio, however, must be considered in light of the real benefits derived. In most recent reports, the results of x-ray pelvimetry were not used to guide clinical management, and the

fetus therefore gained little benefit from the study.[17] Clearly, a potentially hazardous procedure with results that are not likely to influence management has little place in sound medical practice.

On the other hand, x-ray pelvimetry may be helpful in labors complicated by breech presentations. Most authorities agree that the hazards of breech presentation are sufficient to warrant x-ray pelvimetry for cases in which vaginal delivery is contemplated. Perinatal mortality for vaginal breech delivery in the presence of abnormal pelvimetry findings ranges from 2.2 to 8.5 percent.[18] Recognizing these hazards as well as the potential limitations of x-ray pelvimetry, most modern authors have recommended that women with pelvic diameters of less than average size are best managed by cesarean delivery.[9,20] Although these stringent criteria serve to exclude approximately half the candidates for vaginal delivery, they have achieved acceptable levels of perinatal morbidity in this hazardous setting.

Computer Tomography

Computer tomography has the potential for high quality measurements of the bony pelvis with a substantial reduction in fetal radiation exposure. This has led to use of this technique as the primary method of pelvic mensuration in some institutions.[21] Despite this potential, however, decisions regarding adoption of computer tomography must include cost and the observation that similar reductions in fetal radiation exposure are possible with modification of traditional techniques.[22]

Obstetric Palpation—Leopold's Maneuvers

Although abdominal palpation of the gravid uterus for the diagnosis of fetal lie and presentation dates back to antiquity, a codified method of examination was first described by Leopold and Sporlin in 1894. Palpation is divided into four separate maneuvers that can identify fetal landmarks and reveal fetomaternal relationships. Although abdominal examination has several limitations (small fetus, obese mother, polyhydramnios, multiple gestation), and ascertainment of fetal position and station are less precise than vaginal examination, the procedure is safe, well tolerated, and may add valuable information in the management of labor.

Leopold's maneuvers consist of a series of four palpations of the uterus. Over the years the numerical sequence has varied, but the objectives remain the same. Basically, the Leopold's maneuvers answer four questions:

1. *What is at the fundus?* With the patient lying supine and her knees comfortably flexed, the examiner stands at her side facing her head. The examiner

places his or her hands (it is hoped, warm) at the fundus of the uterus. Palpation with the tips of the fingers ascertains the presence or absence of a fetal pole (vertical vs. transverse lie) and the nature of the fetal pole. The fetal breech is larger, less well defined, and less ballottable than the cranium.

2. *Where are the spine and small parts?* After examination of the fundus, the lateral walls of the uterus are examined. In vertical lies, the sides will usually be occupied by the fetal back and small parts (extremities). The location of the fetal spine is determined by the characteristic properties of the spine, a long, firm, linear structure. The small parts are characterized by their different contours and occasionally by rapid movement. The fingers of one hand are used for palpation, while the other hand fixes the fetus.

3. *What is presenting in the pelvis?* The examiner now turns toward the feet of the patient. The fingertips are placed laterally above the symphysis and brought toward the midline. When the fetus is encountered, the characteristics of the fetal pole are noted. In addition, the degree of descent of the fetal pole beneath the symphysis is noted as an indication of the station of the presenting part.

4. *Where is the cephalic prominence?* In cephalic presentations, a point of the fetal head may be noted as a protuberance that arrests the hand outlining the fetus. As the hands are moved along the lateral walls of the fetus toward the pelvis, either the occiput or the chin will be encountered if the head is not deep within the pelvis. If the head is neither flexed nor extended, the chin (located on the same side as the small parts) will be prominent. In deflexed attitudes (face presentation), the occiput will be encountered below the fetal spine. If the head is well flexed, neither structure will be prominent.

In most patients, the information gleaned from Leopold's maneuvers will be sufficient for the diagnosis of position and station. Rather than being considered an alternative, abdominal palpation should be viewed as a valuable adjunct to vaginal examination.

Disorders of Labor

Abnormal Patterns

Abnormal patterns of labor are defined by deviation from the norms for the phases of labor as defined earlier in this chapter. For all phases, except the latent phase, the abnormality may be either protraction or arrest (an arrested latent phase implies that labor has not truly begun). Since these disorders differ considerably in implication and management, they will be considered separately.

Prolonged Latent Phase

The latent phase of labor is defined as the period of time starting with the onset of regular uterine contractions and terminated by the onset of the active phase. Using the criteria listed in Table 13-1, this phase is considered prolonged if it exceeds approximately 20 hours in nulliparas or 14 hours in multiparas. Although the duration of this phase of labor apparently has little direct implication on perinatal mortality, prolongation can certainly be taxing to the mother and her attendants. In many women, cervical effacement during the latent phase, especially in nulliparas entering labor prior to significant effacement, presents a problem.

The basis for management of prolonged latent phase consists of recognition of possible etiologies and individualized treatment.[23] Although less frequently encountered today than when Friedman originally studied this group, oversedation must be considered. Most patients will simply be those who have entered labor without substantial cervical effacement. For these women the process that normally occurs over weeks must be compressed into hours.

Unless there is a maternal or fetal indication for expeditious delivery, most authorities agree that the management of choice consists of therapeutic rest. This allows the patient a respite from the physical and emotional rigors of labor and can aid in the distinction between true and false labor. Since this therapeutic rest is generally induced with a rather large dose of morphine (15 to 20 mg), it is essential that an evaluation of the myometrial contraction pattern and cervical examination be made to exclude those patients entering into the active phase.

After several hours of rest (usually sleep), approximately 85 percent of patients so treated will progress to the active phase. Approximately 10 percent will cease to have contractions, and the diagnosis of false labor may be made. For the approximately 5 percent of patients in whom therapeutic rest fails and in patients for whom expeditious delivery is indicated, oxytocin infusion may be used.

Two other methods of management must be condemned. Amniotomy holds little benefit for the patient with prolonged latent phase and may serve only to increase the risk of intrauterine infection or cord prolapse. Finally, cesarean delivery for this indication alone benefits neither the fetus nor the mother.

Disorders of the Active Phase
Cervicographic and Manometric Analysis of Labor

The major classification of abnormalities of the active phase of labor is based on the cervicographic analysis of labor. According to this classification, abnormalities are defined by their departure from the normal pattern of cervical dilatation.[24] In addition to this system, a number of investigators have proposed a classification based on the electromechanical state of the uterus.[25,26] Inefficient uterine activity is divided into hypertonic and hypotonic dysfunction. Hypotonic dysfunction reflects an insufficient generation of action potentials from the myometrial pacemaker, inadequate propagation of the signal throughout the myometrium, or lack of mechanical response to the signal. Hypertonic dysfunction includes a group of disorders associated with contractions that are generated in the lower pole of the uterus or in multiple sites. In either circumstance, the contraction pattern fails to result in cervical effacement and dilatation.

In the clinical setting, the distinction between hypotonic and hypertonic dysfunction is made on the basis of clinical and manometric criteria. Hypotonic dysfunction occurs in both nulliparas and multiparas and may be seen at any point during labor. It is often an indication of relative cephalopelvic disproportion, malposition, or maternal fatigue. Uterine contractions are infrequent, of low amplitude, and accompanied by low or normal baseline pressures. Maternal discomfort is minimal. Hypertonic dysfunction is primarily a condition of nulliparas and is usually associated with early labor. Frequent contractions of low amplitude are often associated with an elevated baseline pressure. Maternal discomfort is significant and backache frequent. In addition to hypertonic and hypotonic dysfunction, cervicographic abnormalities of labor may be eutonic in which manometric parameters of uterine activity are normal.

Primary Dysfunctional Labor

Primary dysfunctional labor is defined as active-phase dilatation that occurs at a rate less than the 5th percentile. This value is 1.2 cm/hr in nulliparas and 1.5 cm/hr in multiparas (Fig. 13-3). An example of this disorder is shown in Figure 13-4.

Optimal management of primary dysfunctional labor is a major distinction between the American and British schools of labor management. The American approach is based on the studies of Friedman and Sachtleben.[27] in which amniotomy, oxytocin, or sedation had little effect, while physiologic support and further observation seemed to provide the best course. The British approach, exemplified by the reports from the National Maternity Hospital in Dublin, includes prompt amniotomy and oxytocin infusion.[28]

Despite these major differences in approach, several important similarities exist. Both groups acknowledge the importance of recognition of primary dysfunctional labor as a frequent predecessor of secondary arrest of labor and as a risk factor for perinatal mortality. Gravidas exhibiting this disorder require careful maternal and fetal surveillance. In addition, both groups agree that primary dysfunctional labor alone is not an indication for cesarean delivery.

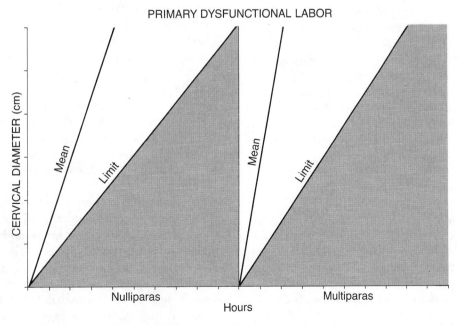

Fig. 13-3 Mean and lower limit for rate of cervical dilatation in nulliparas and multiparas. Rates below the 5th percentile signify primary dysfunctional labor.

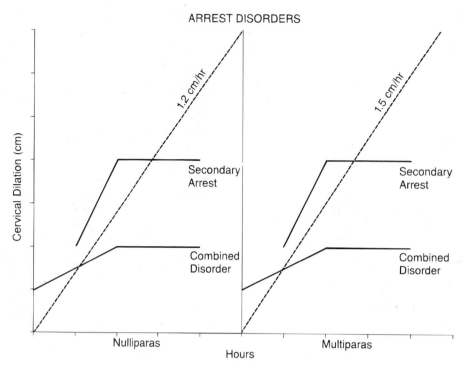

Fig. 13-4 Active phase-arrest disorders. Combined disorder implies an arrest in a gravida previously exhibiting primary dysfunctional labor.

Secondary Arrest of Cervical Dilatation and Combined Disorders of Active Phase

Secondary arrest was defined by Friedman and Sachtleben[29] as cessation of a previously normal dilatation for a period of 2 hours. An example of this disorder is shown in Figure 13-4. It should be noted that this definition is somewhat artificial, and arrests of 1 hour have been associated with an increase in second-stage abnormalities and fetal morbidity.

A combined disorder of active phase dilatation is defined as arrest of dilatation occurring when the patient has previously exhibited primary dysfunctional labor. This pattern is demonstrated in Figure 13-4. In Friedman and Sachtleben's series,[29] this group had a less favorable outcome with regard to vaginal delivery than did patients with secondary arrest alone.

Although less controversial than primary dysfunctional labor, management of arrest in the active phase varies considerably. As noted elsewhere in this chapter, x-ray pelvimetry is advocated by some but is generally considered of little value in the treatment of this disorder. Ambulation has been reported to be beneficial, but the number of patients managed by this method has been quite limited. Although a trial of labor is advocated universally, a uniform definition of such a trial is lacking.

Realizing these difficulties, a generally accepted management program would consist of a careful examination followed by amniotomy and initiation of intrauterine monitoring if indicated. The examination should include an assessment for signs of fetal distress, maternal fatigue, or excessive fetal size. A detailed vaginal examination should be performed to verify cervical dilatation, fetal station, presentation, and position. Clinical pelvimetry should be performed with notation of overall pelvic capacity and pelvic type. Unusual causes of dystocia such as uterine leiomyomata, ovarian tumors, vaginal cysts, or septae as well as fetal malformations should be considered.

If the uterine activity is noted to be optimal, then further stimulation of the myometrium by oxytocin infusion should be undertaken only with extreme caution, if at all. If, however, hypotonic uterine dysfunction exists and no other cause of arrest has been noted, oxytocin infusion may be used with a high degree of success and safety.

The optimum duration of this "trial of labor" is poorly defined. Fortunately, the large majority of patients (70 to 80 percent in Friedman's series) respond successfully and resume progression of cervical dilatation. Although precise information is difficult to obtain, most authorities cite continued arrest over 2 to 4 hours as an indication for cesarean delivery. It must be noted, however, that even in the group in which progress is noted there is an increased frequency of second stage abnormalities and operative deliveries.

Abnormalities of the Second Stage

The second stage of labor is the interval between full cervical dilatation and delivery of the infant. Abnormalities of the second stage may either be a protraction or arrest of descent. A less frequently utilized term, *failure of descent*, describes a phenomenon that occurs rarely in normal presentations.

Protraction of descent has been defined as descent occurring at less than 1 cm/hr in nulliparas and 2 cm/hr in multiparas.[31] This definition, however, suffers from two major flaws. First, the accuracy and precision of estimation of fetal station is considerably less than the estimation of cervical dilatation. Second, the location of the presenting part within the birth canal is noted in terms of station with the pelvis divided into six equal parts. Since the length of the birth canal varies considerably and is generally between 11 and 15 cm, conversion of change in station to descent in centimeters per hour is difficult if not impossible.

These problems notwithstanding, it is clear that gravidas may exhibit protracted descent with etiologies similar to those seen for primary dysfunctional labor. The potential fetal risk inherent in prolonged second stage has been known for some time. Studies from the early 1950s documented increasing infant mortality correlating with the length of the second stage.[32] Reviews of electronic fetal heart rate tracings obtained during this phase have documented a high incidence of variable decelerations and prolonged decelerations.[33] The gradual fall in fetal scalp capillary pH that occurs throughout labor is accelerated during the second stage.[34]

Until recently, these factors led to a policy of intervention whenever the second stage exceeded 2 hours in length. Subsequent experience, however, has demonstrated that when electronic fetal monitoring is reassuring, operative intervention may be avoided provided that descent is progressive.[35]

Arrest of descent, on the other hand, is more accurately diagnosed (at least when both examinations are conducted by a single examiner) and more urgent. As in arrest of dilatation, this disorder requires prompt re-evaluation of uterine contractility, maternal and fetal well being, and cephalopelvic relationships. Obvious problems such as hypotonic dysfunction, overdistended bladder, strong perineal resistance, conduction anesthesia, or ineffectual bearing down should be treated appropriately with a high expectation of success. In the absence of such factors, however, very careful judgment is required. Estimation of fetopelvic relationships, including station, caput formation, moulding, palpation of the fetal head above the symphysis, and malrotation, is mandatory. For patients in whom low forceps delivery is possible, this is the procedure of choice. When a low forceps delivery is not possible, the choice among midforceps delivery, vacuum extraction, oxytocin infusion, or cesarean delivery is extremely difficult and controversial. In view of the emotional problems in making such decisions, consultation is often helpful.

Stimulation of Uterine Activity

Measurements of Uterine Activity

Parameters of uterine activity usually measured during labor include the frequency, duration, and intensity of contractions. In addition, with the use of direct pressure monitors, baseline tone may be determined. Three major techniques for the measurement of uterine contractions are commonly employed. The oldest of these is palpation, performed by resting a hand on the uterine fundus. The examiner notes the frequency, apparent duration, and relative intensity of contractions (subjectively rated as +1 to +3). The major advantages of palpation include simplicity and the direct contact between patient and examiner. Disadvantages include the inability to measure intensity or duration of contractions accurately, lack of information concerning baseline tone, difficulty in measurement in the obese patient, and inability to correlate fetal heart rate patterns with uterine contractions.

External tocodynamometry measures the change in shape of the abdominal wall as a function of uterine contractions. Although sharing most of the disadvantages of palpation, this method does permit graphic display of uterine activity in relationship to fetal heart rate patterns.

The most precise method for determination of uterine activity is the direct method. Direct measurements require the insertion of a fluid-filled catheter directly into the uterine cavity, usually through the cervix after rupture of the membranes.

The quantification of uterine activity has received a considerable amount of attention since the pioneering studies of Caldeyro-Barcia and Posiero[25] during the 1950s. These studies demonstrated that cervical dilatation can be considered as an exponential function of uterine work (uterine pressure time).[36] The most commonly used units of uterine activity are the Montevideo Unit (average intensity frequency/10 min) and the Uterine Activity Unit (1 mm Hg/min).[37] Although on-line computer analysis of uterine activity has been achieved, there is no evidence that this aids in labor management.[38]

Clinically, all measurements of uterine activity demonstrate marked interpatient and intrapatient variations. Although some definitions of "active management" include augmentation of all patients with suboptimal uterine activity, current policies in the United States indicate that intervention is not required unless an abnormality in the progression of labor is documented. When such an abnormality is noted and uterine activity is not optimal (i.e., contractions of less than 50 mmHg every 3 minutes, or below 250 Montevideo Units),[39] administration of an oxytocic agent is recommended.

Oxytocic Agents

Oxytocin is a peptide hormone that is stored and released from the posterior pituitary gland. It consists of eight amino acids, six of which it shares with the neuropeptide vasopressin. Oxytocin was first successfully purified in 1951 and was identified and synthetically prepared in 1953. Only intravenous solutions of oxytocin are approved for induction and augmentation of labor.

Commercial solutions contain 10 IU/ml oxytocin (1 mg of synthetic oxytocin is equivalent to 450 IU). Oxytocin infusions have as their most important mechanism of action the stimulation of myometrial contractions. This action is dependent on the degree of responsiveness of the myometrium. Sensitivity of the uterus to oxytocin varies with the hormonal milieu in gestation and increases between the 20th and 40th weeks of pregnancy. Stimulation of myometrial activity appears to be dependent on an increase in the permeability of myometrial cells to sodium ions. Very high infusion rates of oxytocin have been associated with hypertension, and bolus injections may cause hypotension. When administered intravenously as dilute solutions at recommended rates, few cardiovascular side effects are noted, however.

Oxytocin in the form of crude pituitary extracts has been used in clinical obstetrics since the early 1900s. Because of the extreme variability in myometrial stimulation associated with these crude extracts, early enthusiasm was tempered by disastrous results from uterine hyperactivity with fetal compromise and maternal damage. With standardization of synthetic preparations and an understanding of the importance of strict control of the infusion rate, oxytocin infusion has become an accepted and effective form of therapy.

The recommended rate of administration for oxytocin is usually that which simulates normal labor. This rate may vary from 0.5; mIU/min to greater than 30 mIU/min, although some authorities recommend a maximal rate of 20 mIU/min.[40,41] Even at low infusion rates, however, contractions associated with oxytocin do not truly mimic spontaneous uterine contractions as the rate of rise in intrauterine pressure appears to be greater than that seen in spontaneous labor.[42] Recent studies have demonstrated that, when used in patients demonstrating a protraction disorder, oxytocin infu-

sion rates greater than 6 mIU/min are rarely required.[43] Approximately 30 to 40 minutes are needed for the full effect of an increase in dosage to be evident in the contraction pattern.

Despite the frequent use of oxytocin in clinical obstetrics, considerable debate still exists as to its proper utilization. Some authorities recommend the use of oxytocin only following x-ray pelvimetry or when uterine contractions are infrequent, of low amplitude, or both. Other investigators recommend oxytocin infusion whenever a protraction disorder of labor has been documented, despite apparently adequate uterine contractility. Regardless of these variations, it is clear that the use of an oxytocin infusion is associated with a high rate of success. Overall, approximately 80 percent of patients with documented disorders of labor respond to oxytocin infusion with subsequent progression of labor and vaginal delivery.[29]

Prostaglandins

Prostaglandins are a group of 20 carbon compounds derived from unsaturated fatty acids that possess high degrees of biologic activity. In the human, the major precursor for prostaglandis is arachidonic acid. Prostaglandin synthesis depends on the release of arachidonic acid from triglyceride esters and subsequent conversion by a group of enzymes collectively known as *prostaglandin synthetases*.

Although a large number of prostaglandins and prostaglandin-like substances exist, most obstetric interest has centered on prostaglandin F_2 (PGF_2) and prostaglandin E_2 (PGE_2). Both prostaglandins are potent stimulators of myometrial activity.

Myometrial contractility in response to prostaglandins, unlike that with oxytocin, is not greatly dependent on the duration of pregnancy. This activity has led to the widespread use of prostaglandins midtrimester abortion and following intrauterine death.

Prostaglandins have been compared with oxytocin for the term patient for both induction and augmentation of labor. These studies have generally failed to demonstrate a superiority of prostaglandins over oxytocin in terms of efficacy.[44] It is unlikely that prostaglandins will replace oxytocin for these indications.

Active Management of Labor

The increasing incidence of cesarean deliveries noted in the United States during the 1970s has prompted an examination of the methods used for labor management. Considerable interest has been directed toward the disparity in the incidences of cesarean delivery between the United States and Ireland. O'Driscoll et al.[45] have maintained that the low rate of cesarean delivery at the National Maternity Hospital in Dublin is due to a philosophy of labor management known as active management. The basic principles of active management include

1. Strict criteria for admission to the labor suite
2. Early amniotomy
3. Hourly cervical examinations.
4. Oxytocin administration for dilatation rates less than 1 cm/hr
5. High (by American standards) concentrations of oxytocin in patients requiring augmentation
6. Expected durations of less than 12 hours for the first stage of labor and 2 hours for the second stage

Adherence to these principles at the National Maternity Hospital in Dublin has been associated with a primary cesarean delivery rate of 5 to 6 percent. Direct comparison of cesarean delivery rates between countries is difficult, however. As demonstrated by Levens et al.,[46] the rate of cesarean deliveries is dependent on a number of demographic factors, including age and race, in addition to the method of management. Despite these difficulties, trials of active management in several hospitals have met with favorable results.[47]

In a study of active management in a large public hospital, institution of this policy led to a reduction in the rate of cesarean deliveries in nulliparas from 23 to 25 percent to 18 to 20 percents with the reduction being confined to cesareans for dystocia.[48] In a randomized, controlled trial of over 700 nulliparas, the rate of cesarean delivery was 10.5 percent in the active management group versus 14.1 percent in the control group.[49] In neither of these studies was active management associated with an increase in perinatal morbidity. It would therefore seem that active management offers the potential for the safe reduction in the rate of caesarean delivery due to dystocia.

Forceps Delivery and Vacuum Extraction

Types and Specialized Functions

Although obstetric forceps vary greatly in design, all types consist of two separate portions that are inserted into the vagina sequentially. Each blade is moved into the correct position opposing the fetal head prior to the joining (locking) of the blades.

Each half consists of the blade proper (which is applied to the fetal head), a shank, and a handle. The halves are joined by a lock usually located at the junction of the shanks and the handles. The overall architecture of a forceps is determined by two curves, the cephalic curve, which allows for the area of the fetal head, and the pelvic curve, compensating for the curvature of the birth canal.

The blades may be either solid or fenestrated, and most forceps designs are available in either type. The most commonly used forceps types utilize either the "English" lock, in which the articulation is fixed, or the "sliding" lock, which permits movement between the forceps halves along the longitudinal axis of the shanks. The shanks may be either separated or overlapping. Instruments are illustrated in Figures 13-5 and 13-6.

Forceps may be divided into major groups according to their intended use. Most instruments fall into the "classic" category. These forceps have a fixed lock and a pelvic curve yielding a concave longitudinal axis. Three commonly used instruments are the Simpson forceps (fenestrated blade, separated shanks), the Elliot forceps (fenestrated blade, overlapping shanks), and the Tucker-McLane forceps (solid blade, overlapping shanks). The forceps in this category are primarily intended for use when the fetal head does not require rotation prior to delivery.

The second major category includes the "specialized" forceps. These instruments have been designed to facilitate delivery in cases requiring rotation of the fetal head (Kielland, Barton) or for breech delivery (Piper). Kielland's forceps differ from classic instruments in that the pelvic curve has been modified such that the blades lie below rather than above the plane

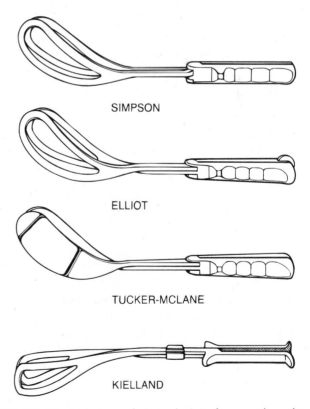

SIMPSON

ELLIOT

TUCKER-McLANE

KIELLAND

Fig. 13-5 Lateral views of some obstetric forceps. The pelvic curve, a prominent feature of classic instruments, is lacking in the Kielland forceps.

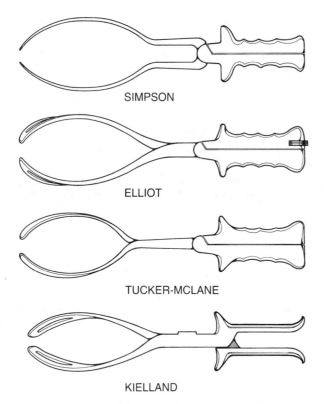

SIMPSON

ELLIOT

TUCKER-MCLANE

KIELLAND

Fig. 13-6 AP view of some forceps. Note the difference between the separated shanks of the Simpson forceps and the overlapping shanks of the Elliot forceps.

of the shanks. This modification facilitates rotation of the forceps about a point rather than around a circle as is required with the classic instruments. Second, these forceps use a sliding lock, enabling the user to adjust for asynclitism of the fetal head.

Barton's forceps have decreased in popularity over the past 20 years. Designed for use in a platypelloid pelvis, these forceps allow traction with the fetal head in a transverse position until the introitus has been reached. Piper's forceps have blades below the plane of elongated shanks. These modifications are designed to facilitate application to the aftercoming head in breech delivery.

Classification of Forceps Delivery

Forceps deliveries are classified according to the station of the fetal head at the time of application. Although all systems of classification use station as the primary criterion, the number of divisions included vary. The Committee on Obstetrics, Maternal and Fetal Medicine of the American College of Obstetricians and Gynecologists,[50] has offered the following classification:

1. Outlet forceps: application of forceps when the scalp is visible at the introitus without separating the labia, the fetal skull has reached the pelvic floor, the fetal head is at or on the perineum, and the angle between the AP line and the sagittal suture does not exceed 45 degrees.
2. Low forceps: application when the leading point of the skull is at station +2 or more, subclassified as to whether the angle between the sagittal suture and AP exceeds 45 degrees
3. Mid-forceps: application of forceps when the head is engaged but the presenting part is above station +2

Evaluation of this classification has indicated that it yields better correlation with short-term maternal and neonatal morbidity than do older classifications.[50]

One older classification was "high forceps," which has been abandoned due to fetal risk. This was forceps to the unengaged head, in which the fetal head is floating and ballottable above the brim of the true pelvis. "Low-mid-forceps" was that in which the fetal biparietal diameter was at or below the level of the ischial spines, with the presenting part within a fingerbreadth of the perineum between contractions.

Indications and Contraindications

Few areas in obstetrics have been surrounded with as much controversy as the use of obstetric forceps. Low forceps delivery, once considered optimal management in the United States,[7] is now often considered meddlesome and unnecessary and has decreased considerably in popularity.

The major controversy, however, surrounds the mid-forceps delivery. As a group, infants delivered by this method demonstrate an increased incidence of perinatal mortality, perinatal morbidity, and long-term neurologic defects.[50,51] Opponents of the continued use of this technique argue that these data suggest that mid-forceps delivery should be abandoned in a manner similar to high forceps.[52,53] Proponents of the continued usage of mid-forceps believe that the great majority of infants with poor outcome after mid-forceps delivery result from deliveries that are considered difficult.[54] Since current terminology does not permit distinction among the varying degrees of fetal hazard involved with the procedure, all mid-forceps deliveries have been condemned. Studies in which mid-forceps have been associated with poor outcome, moreover, are retrospective in nature and subject to the problems of multiple confounding variables that may have significantly biased the outcome.[55] The Committee on Obstetrics, Maternal and Fetal Medicine of the American College of Obstetricians and Gynecologists has suggested that outlet forceps may be used to shorten the second stage of labor when it is in the best interests of the mother or fetus. More difficult forceps delivery (low or midforceps) may be considered when the second stage is prolonged, for fetal distress, or for maternal indications such as cardiac disease or exhaustion. In a recent survey of residency programs in the United States and Canada, outlet and low forceps were used at all institutions, but 14 percent of the programs had abandoned the use of midforceps delivery.[56]

Although it is unlikely that this controversy will be resolved in the near future, all authorities agree that mid-forceps deliveries should be reserved for competent operators following careful consideration of the potential fetal risks.

Prerequisites for Forceps Delivery

All forceps deliveries require that several criteria be met before the application of the forceps. These include

1. The membranes must be ruptured.
2. The cervix must be fully dilated.
3. The operator must be fully acquainted with the use of the instrument.
4. The position and station of the fetal head must be known with certainty.
5. Adequate maternal anesthesia for proper application of the forceps must be present.
6. The maternal pelvis must be adequate in size for atraumatic delivery.
7. The characteristics of the maternal pelvis must be appropriate for the type of delivery being considered.
8. The fetal head must be engaged.

Midforceps deliveries require that strong consideration be given to alternative approaches such as administration of oxytocin, cesarean delivery, or simply expectant management. Cases in which instrumental rotation is considered may prove amenable to digital or manual rotation. Specifically hazardous are mid-forceps deliveries in which the fetus is less than 2,500 g or greater than 4,500 g, or when there has been an abnormality in the progression of labor.

Technique of Application and Delivery

Before attempted forceps application, the patient should be properly prepared and positioned. The patient should be placed in the modified lithotomy position and cleansed and draped in the usual manner. The bladder, if full, should be emptied by catheterization. Adequate anesthesia is mandatory for both maternal and fetal safety. Although little anesthesia may be required for easily performed outlet forceps, low and mid-forceps procedures require properly administered and monitored conduction or general anesthesia.

A thorough examination of the fetal position and characteristics of the maternal pelvis is mandatory. Exact knowledge of fetal position, station, and degree of asynclitism is essential to proper application. If the maternal pelvis appears to be inadequate in size or to possess unfavorable characteristics for the proposed procedure (e.g., rotation in an android or platypelloid pelvis), the procedure should be reconsidered.

Before application of the forceps, the operator should perform a "phantom application" by positioning the forceps in front of the perineum in the correct position of the final application. This phantom application aids in the evaluation of proper placement.

Outlet Forceps

Since, by definition, an outlet forceps delivery always requires the sagittal suture of the fetal skull to be directly AP, no correction for fetal position is required. In the occiput anterior (OA) position, following separation of the blades of the forceps, the left blade is held by the right hand of the operator. The handle is held loosely in the left hand so that the position of the forceps is essentially vertical. The blade is then introduced directly posteriorly and guided in an arc by the right (intravaginal) hand along the left side of the maternal pelvis to the correct position along the left parietal bone of the fetus. The hand of the operator is then removed from the vagina, allowing the blade of the forceps to remain in place. The remaining half of the forceps is then inserted in a similar manner, except the right blade is held in the left hand and guided to the right parietal bone of the fetus.

Following the application, the handles are brought together and locked. Before the initiation of traction, it is mandatory that the application be checked for correct positioning.

Checking the Application

Safe use of obstetric forceps requires proper application to the fetus. Proper application involves a true cephalic placement (biparietal, bimalar). The application of compressive or tractive forces to any other area of the fetal skull may result in serious cranial or neurologic damage. Proper application must be determined by assessing the position of the forceps in relation to three landmarks on the fetal skull. The first check determines the position of the plane of the shanks with regard to the posterior fontanelle. The median angle of the fontanelle should be located halfway between the blades of the forceps and approximately 1 to 1.5 cm above the plane of the shanks. The second check requires that the sagittal suture be perpendicular to the plane of the shanks throughout its length. The third check is to ensure that the blades of the forceps are sufficiently ap-

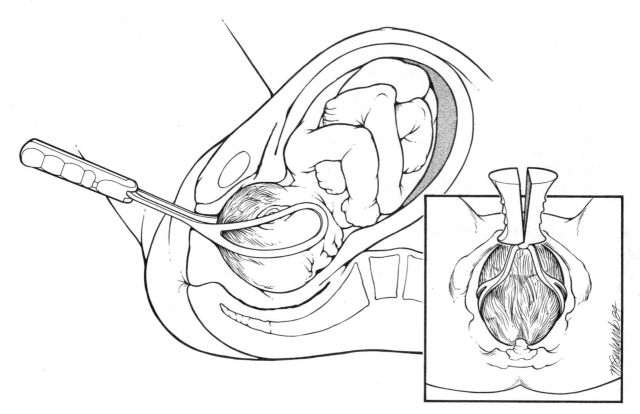

Fig. 13-7 Proper application of obstetric forceps.

plied to the parietal bones. Only 1 to 1.5 cm of the blades should be palpable beyond the fetal skull (if the blades are fenestrated, no more than a fingertip should be able to be inserted). If not all criteria for proper application are met, readjustment must be made before attempts at traction or rotation. An illustration of proper application is shown in Figure 13-7.

Low Forceps and Mid-Forceps

Application of the forceps for low forceps and mid-forceps deliveries when the fetal head is directly OA or occiput posterior (OP) is identical to that for low forceps. In cases where fetal position is rotated slightly (ROA, LOA, ROP, LOP), attempts at manual or digital rotation should be made before instrumental rotation. If this fails, following a phantom application the forceps should be applied such that the posterior blade is inserted first. For the LOA and ROP positions, this is the left blade; for ROA and LOP, this is the right blade. The blades are inserted according to the same principles as for low forceps, remembering that the proper location of the shanks is dictated by the position of the fetal skull, not the axis of the maternal pelvis. Thus, after application, the shanks of the forceps will point toward either the left (LOA, ROP) or right (ROA, LOP) shoulder of the operator. In cases in which the right blade is the posterior blade, the shanks of the forceps must

be rotated around each other (left under right) for locking to take place. After application, the three checks of proper application are made and, if necessary, the blades are adjusted.

If the fetal head is not flexed, flexion is accomplished before rotation. Since forceps of the classic type include a prominent pelvic curve, rotation of the handles of the forceps must be about an arc. This rotation is carried out until the sagittal suture rests in the direct antero-posterior position. After rotation, the position of the forceps should be rechecked before traction.

Occiput Transverse Positions

Forceps delivery from the occiput transverse position is best accomplished with the use of specialized forceps. These instruments (Kielland, Barton) require considerable skill and experience, and their use has decreased greatly in recent years. The design and use of these instruments differs significantly from the classic forceps.

In the gynecoid or anthropoid pelvis, the Kielland forceps permits the rotational axis of the forceps to be in line with the plane of the fetus. Thus, the rotation can be accomplished without the need for a large sweeping motion of the handles of the forceps during rotation. Two main methods of application of the Kielland forceps have come into popular usage. The "classic" or "inversion" method entails the application of the anterior blade of the forceps beneath the symphysis pubis with the cephalic curve of the blade following the curve of the undersurface of the symphysis pubis. The application is carried on until the forceps have been applied in apposition to the anterior surface of the fetal head. This blade is rotated at 180 degrees so that the cephalic curve of the blade corresponds with the cephalic curve of the fetus. The second blade is then applied directly to the posterior parietal region of the fetus.

The "wandering" application of the anterior blade is made in a manner similar to that of a classic forceps with insertion posteriorly and rotation about either the frontal or occipital region of the fetus to lie eventually in apposition to the anterior ear of the fetus. The second or posterior blade is then applied as in the classic application. After application and checks of proper positioning, the head is flexed and rotation is accomplished so that the head comes into the OA position. At this point, delivery is accomplished by traction either with the Kielland forceps or by reapplication of a classic type of forceps. If the Kielland forceps are used for traction, care must be taken to protect the posterior wall of the vagina. If the handles are raised as the head is delivered, lacerations of the posterior vaginal wall may result.

Barton's forceps are used when there is a transverse arrest of the fetus within a pelvis of the platypelloid type. The anterior blade is hinged and is applied in a wandering maneuver similar to that described for the Kielland forceps. The posterior blade, which has a sharp cephalic curve, is applied directly. After a check for proper application, traction is applied without rotation using a traction handle. Rotation to the OA position is not accomplished until the fetus is at the outlet.

Traction

After the application of forceps, delivery is accomplished according to the principle of axis traction; force is applied in a plane perpendicular to the plane of the pelvis at which the fetal head lies. The pelvis is curved in a reversed J shape, and it is in this direction that the series of force vectors should be applied. When the fetal head lies at the mid-pelvis, traction is directed posteriorly; at the pelvic floor, horizontally; and before expulsion, anteriorly.

To produce traction according to these changing vectors, axis traction may be accomplished either manually or via axis-traction attachments. Manual traction is applied via the Saxtorph-Pajot maneuver. The vector is generated by force applied downward or upward on the shanks with one hand while the other hand pulls outward on the handles. Although this method is adequate for delivery from low stations, axis traction is best accomplished via the use of attachments that guide the operator continuously throughout the proper path of traction. The most commonly used axis-traction attachment is fastened at the finger guards of classic instruments.

The Use of Vacuum Extraction

First popularized by Malmstrom[59] during the mid-1950s, the use of vacuum extraction-assisted delivery has become widespread in Europe. The classic instrument consists of a disk-shaped cup through which a vacuum of up to 0.8 kg/cc^2 is applied to the fetal scalp. This suction induces a caput succedaneum (chignon) within the cup to which tractional force is applied during uterine contractions. Randomized studies comparing forceps with vacuum have not shown a significant difference in success rate or complications, and the choice of instrument appears to remain one of operator preference.[60]

The indications and contraindications to vacuum extraction are essentially the same as those for forceps delivery. An advantage of vacuum extraction, however, is that delivery may be accomplished with minimal maternal analgesia.

Currently available instruments include metal cups in three sizes (40, 50, 60 mm) and Silastic cups, which are cone shaped. Manually or electrically operated vacuum sources are available, but the latter are preferred.

The cup should be applied to the fetal head away from the fontanelles, with care being taken that no maternal tissue is entrapped within the cup. After application, a vacuum is established at 0.2 kg/cc^2 as the cup is held in place. The vacuum is raised every 2 minutes by intervals of 0.2 kg/cc^2 until a final vacuum of 0.7 to 0.8 kg/cc^2 is reached. These slow increments in vacuum are necessary for the proper development of the chignon.

Once a proper vacuum has been reached, traction may begin. One hand is used for traction, while the other maintains the fetal head in flexion and confirms that the cup has remained in place. Traction is applied in conjunction with uterine contractions only. The vacuum should not be maintained for longer than 30 minutes.

The Third Stage of Labor

The interval between delivery of the infant and delivery of the placenta with attached umbilical cord and fetal membranes lasts less than 10 minutes in most women and occurs within 15 minutes in approximately 95 percent of all deliveries.

Separation of the placenta is a consequence of continued uterine contractions following expulsion of the fetus. These contractions reduce the area of the uterine placental bed with subsequent disruption of the placental attachment along a plane in the spongiosa layer of the decidua vera. Continued powerful and prolonged contractions serve to control blood loss from the spiral arteries through compression and transport the placenta from the fundus into the lower uterine segment.

Since placental separation relies solely on uterine contractions, interference with this process by techniques such as fundal compression or traction on the umbilical cord can increase the incidence of complications such as hemorrhage or uterine inversion. During this interval, proper management requires only gentle palpation of the uterine fundus for uterine contractions and observation for excessive blood loss.

Although most authorities agree that the use of oxytocic agents are valuable in the reduction of blood loss during the third stage, the timing of administration varies between institutions. On the basis of controlled trials, dilute intravenous oxytocin appears to be superior to intravenous or intramuscular ergometrine.[61] Timing of administration, however, is controversial. Administration immediately following delivery may reduce total blood loss but can hamper management in cases involving an undiagnosed second twin or placenta accreta. In the United States, administration after delivery of the placenta appears to be the most common practice. During the interval between delivery of the infant and separation of the placenta, the physician should conduct a careful and thorough examination of the cervix, vagina, and perineum unless his or her assistance is required with neonatal resuscitation. The uterine fundus should be examined transabdominally to ensure that it is firm and that the uterine size is appropriate.

In the absence of anesthesia, intravaginal exploration for obstetric trauma can be quite uncomfortable, and the mother should be notified in advance of the procedures to be performed. Three or four fingers of one hand placed against the posterior vaginal wall and depressed will provide excellent visualization of the vagina and cervix in most cases. Using a sponge forceps, the obstetrician should grasp the anterior lip of the cervix and visualize the entire rim of the cervix either simultaneously or sequentially. If a laceration is seen, its length and position should be noted for subsequent repair.

After cervical inspection, a surgical sponge should be rolled and placed in the forceps. The instrument is then placed in the vagina and the sponge used to elevate the vaginal apex. This will permit complete visualization of both vaginal sidewalls for evidence of lacerations or hematoma formation.

Perineal inspection involves examination of the AP fourchette, the vaginal vestibule, hymenal ring, perineal body, external rectal sphincter, and the rectal mucosa. Examination of the rectal sphincter and mucosa is especially important, as failure to recognize injuries to these structures can result in serious morbidity.

Separation of the placenta is usually rapidly followed by its passage into the lower uterine segment. This event can usually be detected by the occurrence of the classic signs of placental detachment. These include (1) a gush of blood from the vagina, (2) descent of the umbilical cord, (3) a change in shape of the uterine fundus from discoid to globular, and (4) an increase in the height of the fundus as the lower uterine segment is distended by the placenta. After separation, the placenta, cord, and membranes should be delivered by maternal expulsive efforts along with gentle traction on the umbilical cord. Excessive traction will only serve to increase the likelihood of tearing of the membranes.

After passage of the placenta through the vulva, membranes that are still adherent to the decidua are usually separated simply by the weight of the placenta. If this does not occur, gentle traction on the membranes with a ring forceps may be required.

After delivery, the placenta, cord, and membranes should be examined. Inspection of the placenta should include the fetal (shiny) and maternal (dull) surfaces, umbilical cord, and fetal membranes. Macroscopic examination of the placenta disk itself can be quite rewarding. The weight of the placenta, excluding the cord and membranes, varies with fetal weight with a ratio of approximately 1:6. Abnormally large placentas are associated with fetal hydrops or congenital syphilis.

Abnormalities of lobulation, including bilobate placentas and physical separation of one or more placental lobes (succenturiate placenta) are fairly common and important to note. Although one of the major complications associated with abnormal lobulation, bleeding from vessels coursing between the different sections of placenta, occurs prior to delivery, retention of a portion of placenta can lead to postpartum hemorrhage or infection.

Inspection and palpation of the placenta may reveal areas of fibrosis, infarction, or calcification. Although each of these conditions may be seen in the normal, term placenta, excessive loss of surface area can result in impairment of exchange between mother and fetus.

The classic hallmark of placental abruption is a depressed area on the maternal side of the placenta with an attached blood clot. These findings, however, may not be present if the event is recent or sufficiently remote from delivery to allow organization of the clot.

The umbilical cord averages about 50 to 60 cm in length, but there is a broad range in otherwise normal pregnancies. Extremes of length have been associated with a variety of problems, including oligohydramnios and cord compression. The insertion of the cord into the placenta should be noted. Abnormal insertions include marginal insertions in which the cord is located at the edge of the placenta, and membranous insertions, in which the vessels of the umbilical cord course through the membranes prior to attachment to the placental disk. The latter is associated with risk of vasa previa. The cord itself should be inspected for the correct number of vessels, true knots, hematomas, and strictures. A single umbilical artery is associated with other anomalies in about 20 percent of infants.

The fetal membranes may also provide clues to abnormalities of labor. The most common finding is meconium staining, which occurs within a few hours of meconium passage. Opaque membranes usually indicate chorioamnionitis, which may or may not be associated with other findings of intrauterine infection. Occasionally, small 1 to 5 mm beads of vermix and fetal skin are found on the membranes following prolonged oligohydramnios, a condition know as amnion nodosum.

The placenta and membranes should be examined for signs of tearing or missing pieces. A vessel coursing along the membranes should arouse suspicion of an accessory lobe.

The need for manual intrauterine exploration is controversial. Although some authorities believe that manual exploration is indicated in all deliveries,[62] in the absence of adequate anesthesia this may be quite difficult and uncomfortable to the patient. Intrauterine exploration is required when there is suspicion of retained tissue, when there is excessive uterine bleeding, and in cases of premature delivery or vaginal birth after caesarean (VBAC).[63]

Induction of Labor

Induction of labor is the initiation of uterine contractions before the spontaneous onset of labor by medical and/or surgical means for the purpose of delivery. It may be categorized as elective or indicated. Before the decision to induce labor, the physician should document the type of induction and that the patient had been informed and accepts the indications, the methods, and potential complications, including the possibility of cesarean delivery.

Indicated Induction

In general, induction of labor may be indicated when the benefit of delivery to the mother or fetus outweighs the potential problem if the pregnancy continues. There may be maternal or fetal indications. These conditions may arise if the maternal medical or surgical condition worsens under expectant therapy or if there is evidence of impaired intrauterine existence. If obstetric data confirm that the pregnancy is at term or if fetal pulmonary maturity has been documented, the decision to induce labor is not difficult. At times, however, the benefit of a premature delivery of a fetus from a hostile intrauterine environment may outweigh the potential problems associated with prematurity.

Before induction, a thorough evaluation of the patient is indicated. This process, as well as the indications for the induction, should be documented on the chart. The pediatricians should be notified of the induction so that they can make specific plans for management of the neonate.

The maternal pelvis should be assessed as to its adequacy for vaginal delivery. This assessment may be performed by clinical rather than x-ray pelvimetry. The fetal presentation should be vertex and the fetus should not be macrosomic. In 1964, Bishop[64] evaluated multiparous patients for elective induction of labor and developed a score for different variables found from the vaginal exam. This scoring system has provided valid parameters for evaluating all patients prior to the induction of labor.[65,66] Table 13-4 represents a modification of Bishop's method for predicting the ease of inductibility in which a score of 0, 1, 2, or 3 is given for dilatation, effacement, consistency, and position of the cervix and for station of the vertex. A total score of 9 or above indicates that induction of labor should be successful. Ideally, the best results are obtained when prelabor contractions have contributed to the formation of the lower uterine segment and the cervix is soft in consistency, 50 percent effaced, dilated 2 cm or more, anterior in position, and vertex engaged in the pelvis. If spontaneous prelabor has not occurred and the cervix is not favorable, it may take 10 to 12 hours of good uterine contractility to "ripen" the cervix. It should be recognized that the induction process attempts to accomplish in hours what may take several days of spontaneous prelabor.

Indications

The following are accepted, but not all inclusive, maternal or fetal indications for induction of labor: preeclampsia, eclampsia, premature rupture of membranes, chorioamnionitis, abruptio placenta, fetal death, suspected fetal distress as evidenced by biochemical or biophysical indicators, prolonged gestation, diabetes mellitus, chronic hypertension, renal disease, or isoimmunization.

Contraindications

In general, any contraindication to spontaneous labor and delivery per vagina should be a contraindication to induced labor. Contraindications may include, but are not limited to, the following: previous uterine incision secondary to metroplasty, extensive myomectomy, cephalopelvic disproportion resulting from abnormali-

Table 13-4 Bishop Prelabor Scoring System

Factor	Score			
	0	1	2	3
Dilation (cm)	Closed	1–2	3–4	5 or more
Effacement (%)	0–30	40–50	60–70	80 or more
Station	−3	−2	−1–0	+1, +2
Consistency	Firm	Medium	Soft	
Position of cervix	Posterior	Mid-position	Anterior	

ties of pelvic bones or malpresentation of fetus (e.g., shoulder, complete or footling breech), invasive cervical carcinoma, central or total placenta previa, or an active or culture-proven genital herpes infection. Grand multiparity and uterine overdistention secondary to multiple gestation or hydramnios and previous cesarean delivery are relative contraindications.

Methodology

Surgical

Stripping of Membranes

Digitally separating the chorioamniotic membrane from the wall of the cervix and lower uterine segment appears to release prostaglandins produced locally from the membranes and adjacent decidua.[67,68] Prostaglandins may be involved in stimulating myometrial contractions and the onset of labor. In addition, the method may excite an autonomic neural reflex or cause the release of maternal oxytocin from the posterior pituitary, which may initiate labor.[69] In order for stripping or sweeping of the membranes to be successful, the vertex should be well applied to the cervix. Risks of this technique include the potential for introducing uterine infection, bleeding from an unsuspected placenta previa, and accidental rupture of the membranes. As the effects of membrane stripping are not predictable and the efficacy of this method has not been proven, it should not be used alone or as a routine practice for induction.

Amniotomy

In patients with a high Bishop score, artificial rupture of the membranes has been reported to be 88 percent successful in inducing labor.[70] The technique of amniotomy involves perforation of the chorioamniotic membranes, which are palpable through the cervix and digitally retracting the membranes over the vertex. In addition to retracting the membranes, the amniotic fluid should be released without dislodging the vertex. The amount and character of the fluid should be noted and documented.

Advantages of amniotomy are (1) high success rate; (2) observation of the amniotic fluid for blood or meconium; and (3) ready access for an intrauterine pressure catheter, a direct fetal scalp electrode, and for fetal scalp blood sampling. Risks include (1) umbilical cord prolapse, (2) adverse change in fetal position, (3) prolonged rupture of membranes and increased risk of ascending uterine or fetal infection, (4) fetal injury, and (5) rupture of vasa previa and subsequent fetal hemorrhage. With due caution and attention, many of the risks can be avoided. Amniotomy has been associated with greater frequency of disalignment of fetal cranial bones.[71] The significance of these findings on fetal outcome is yet to be determined. In a prospective, randomized study of nulliparas, early amniotomy reduced the incidence of dystocia and the length of labor, but did not affect the incidence of cesarean delivery.[72]

Before amniotomy, the vertex should be well applied to the cervix and engaged in the pelvis to prevent prolapse of the umbilical cord. Amniotomy may be performed with a toothed clamp (Allis) or a plastic hook (Amnihook, Hollister, Chicago). Vaginal examination is first performed to evaluate the cervix and station of the vertex. One or two fingers of the examining hand are introduced into the cervix, and the membranes are swept away from the cervix. The membranes are then ruptured by passing the instrument through the cervical canal across the examining hand usually aside the examining finger or in the groove formed between two examining fingers. Whether an Amnihook or Allis clamp is chosen, it is gently applied to the membranes and turned, hooking or scratching the membranes. The opening in the membranes is widened and the membranes retracted over the vertex by blunt dissection with the examining finger. The time of the amniotomy and the presence of meconium or blood in the fluid must be documented in the chart. Bleeding may occur and, if persistent, should be investigated for a maternal or fetal source. The application of a fetal scalp electrode or introduction of an intrauterine pressure catheter should be completed prior to removing the examining fingers.

After amniotomy, a thorough cervical examination

should attempt to uncover prolapse of the cord. The fetal heart rate should be carefully monitored electronically or by auscultation for evidence of fetal distress. The fetal heart rate may increase transiently postamniotomy. However, decelerations or bradycardia of the fetal heart rate are rare without overt or occult umbilical cord prolapse.

Stripping of the membranes and/or amniotomy may initiate labor through the release of arachidonic acid and the subsequent formation of prostaglandins. Maternal plasma levels of 13, 14-dihydro-15-keto-prostaglandin F have increased markedly within a short time after amniotomy.[66] If the vertex is well engaged and the leaking of the fluid minimal, ambulation may further facilitate the onset of labor. If uterine contractions do not ensue after 2 to 4 hours, then intravenous oxytocin should be initiated.

Medical: Oxytocin

In 1948 Theobald et al.[73] initiated the use of oxytocin given by intravenous drip for the induction of labor. Synthetic oxytocin is available as a solution for intravenous or intramuscular use and as a nasal spray. In the United States, only the intravenous solution has been approved by the Food and Drug Administration (FDA) for medically indicated induction of labor when fetal viability is expected. Oxytocin will stimulate myometrial contractions. However, variability in patient sensitivity and response to oxytocin is the rule rather than the exception. The safest method and the most predictable results are obtained with a properly regulated continuous intravenous infusion of a dilute solution.

During the first stage of spontaneous labor, endogenous oxytocin from the posterior pituitary is released in spurts: initially at low levels and with increasing levels during the second stage.[74] With continuous intravenous oxytocin infusion, plasma oxytocin concentration increases during the first 20 minutes. After 20 minutes, the concentration of plasma oxytocin does not change significantly. The amount of oxytocin being metabolized by placental oxytocinase appears to be equal to the amount infused. The mean plasma oxytocin half-life is 3 to 4 minutes, with a range of 2 to 7 minutes. A rapid fall in plasma levels occurs after the intravenous infusion is discontinued.

A primary intravenous line of an electrolyte-containing solution with a large-bore catheter or needle is started and administered at a rate sufficient to keep the vein open. A stock solution containing 10 USP units (1 ml) of synthetic oxytocin is added to 500 ml of 5 percent dextrose in water. A large syringe (usually 60 ml) is filled from the diluted oxytocin stock solution, and the syringe is placed in a controlled infusion pump. The prepared solution from the syringe is next connected or piggybacked into the primary line through a sidearm near the intravenous insertion site in the patient's arm. The 500-ml standard stock solution containing the oxytocin should never be connected directly to the patient.

The rate of administration is usually recommended as that which produces contractions every 2 to 3 minutes, lasting 60 to 90 seconds with 50 to 60 mmHg intrauterine pressure and a resting uterine tone of 10 to 15 mmHg if intrauterine pressure monitoring is used. Dosage may vary from 0.5 to 30 to 40 mU/min of oxytocin. Induction is started with 0.5 mU/min, and the rate is doubled every 15 to 20 minutes until uterine activity that simulates normal labor in both quality and quantity of contractions is obtained. It is unusual for a patient to require more than 20 to 40 mU/min of oxytocin to achieve myometrial contractions that mimic spontaneous labor and to achieve satisfactory changes in cervical dilatation. As labor progresses, the frequency and intensity of contractions may increase. The infusion rate of oxytocin can then be reduced to prevent hyperstimulation.

Control of the intravenous dose is best achieved by using a constant infusion pump. If a pump is not available, the dosage of oxytocin may be regulated by a manually controlled infusion of a dilute solution of 10 USP units in 1,000 ml or 5 percent dextrose/normal saline infusion. Monitoring of uterine contractions and fetal heart rate is recommended throughout the induction and is best accomplished with continuous electronic monitoring. Constant surveillance of uterine activity is recommended to avoid uterine hyperstimulation. Electronic fetal heart rate monitoring may facilitate the detection of fetal distress by documenting fetal heart rate decelerations in response to uterine contractions.

A thorough knowledge of the pharmacologic and physiologic actions of oxytocin and of appropriate techniques for monitoring the mother and fetus are mandatory for all personnel administering oxytocin. They must be qualified to identify complications and be able to take immediate action when problems arise. A written protocol for oxytocin administration that has been approved by the appropriate hospital staff should be available on the labor and delivery floor.

Complications

Hypercontractility

The most frequently encountered complication of intravenously administered oxytocin is uterine hyperstimulation. Hyperstimulation refers to excessive frequency of contractions (polysystole) or increased uterine tone (hypertonias), which may produce fetal distress, abruptio placentae, or uterine rupture. The use of electronic monitoring has increased the early detection of these potentially lethal maternal or fetal complications.

Oxytocin-induced uterine activity appears to be more frequently associated with uterine hypertonia and hyperactivity than spontaneous labor.[75] If the uterus is overstimulated, placental gas exchange may be jeopardized, leading to fetal acidosis or hypoxemia. Since intravenous oxytocin has a short half-life, one can expect uterine relaxation with improved intervillous blood flow and gas exchange to follow soon after the infusion has been discontinued. In the presence of hyperstimulation, the patient should also be turned to her side and oxygen administered.

Water Intoxication

Oxytocin is related structurally and functionally to vasopressin. As such, it shares the effects of vasopressin, or antidiuretic hormone (ADH). The use of regulatory infusion pumps and electrolyte-containing solutions can help to prevent water intoxication, which can lead to hyponatremia, confusion, convulsions, coma, congestive heart failure, and death. The ADH effect is rarely seen when the dosage of oxytocin remains below 20 mU/min. Fluid overload and hyponatremia may be prevented by strict intake and output recordings, use of balanced salt infusions, and avoiding prolonged administration of an oxytocin infusion of 20 to 40 mU/min.

Hypertension

A constant intravenous infusion of dilute oxytocin not exceeding 20 mU/min usually has no effect on blood pressure. However, in the presence of preeclampsia or with an infusion rate of 20 to 40 mU/min, slight elevation of blood pressure can occur.

Uterine Rupture

Uterine rupture may occur with the use of oxytocin. This obstetric disaster is more common in grand multiparous patients, in women who have undergone prior uterine surgery, with fetal malpresentations, and with a markedly overdistended uterus. These conditions are relative contraindications to the use of oxytocin. After uterine rupture, contractions may cease even if the oxytocin infusion is continued.

Amniotic Fluid Embolism

Amniotic fluid embolism has been seen in patients undergoing an oxytocin-induced labor, especially if the indication for the induction is fetal demise and the membranes are artificially ruptured.

Elective Induction

In a strict sense, elective induction of labor may be defined as a termination of pregnancy without an indication. In a broader sense, elective induction of labor refers to the initiation of labor when control over the timing of labor may be beneficial, such as in patients who live a great distance from the hospital or have a history of rapid labors. Elective induction of labor should not be attempted for the convenience of the patient or physician. Two major problems associated with elective induction are iatrogenic prematurity and increased cesarean delivery due to failed induction. In the event of a bad outcome that developed as a result of an elective induction of labor, the burden of proof must demonstrate that the risk of allowing the pregnancy to continue exceeded that of the induction. Prerequisites for the technique of elective induction include all that has been outlined above for an indicated induction. It must be noted that, in 1978, the FDA ruled that injectable oxytocin not be used for elective induction of labor.

To avoid iatrogenic prematurity, a detailed assessment of fetal maturity as outlined in the Guidelines for Perinatal Care[76] must be made: Fetal maturity can be assumed if at least two of the following clinical criteria for estimating gestational age are present and supported by at least one of the following laboratory determinations:

Clinical Criteria

1. 39 weeks have elapsed since the last menstrual period of a patient with normal menstrual cycles and no immediate antecedent use of oral contraceptives.
2. Fetal heart tones have been documented for 20 weeks by nonelectronic fetoscope or for 30 weeks by Doppler ultrasound.

Laboratory Determinations

1. 36 weeks have elapsed since a positive serum human chorionic gonadotrophin pregnancy test.
2. Ultrasound
   a. Measurements based on a crown–rump length obtained between 6 and 11 weeks' gestation.
   b. Measurements based on the biparietal diameter obtained before 20 weeks' gestation.

If these criteria are not met, amniotic fluid analysis for lecithin/sphingomyelin (L/S) ratio or phosphatidylglycerol may provide satisfactory evidence of fetal lung maturity.

Combined Medical–Surgical Methods

A combination of the above methods is frequently employed for the induction of labor. A constant infusion of dilute intravenous oxytocin and artificial rupture of the membranes after the initiation of labor appears to be a successful technique. Other clinicians prefer to rupture the membranes first, and, if labor has not ensued in several hours, they then begin intravenous oxytocin administration.

The Future

Investigations have focused on the use of the synthetic PGE_2 and PGF_2 to ripen the cervix before amniotomy or oxytocin induction. These prostaglandin preparations are not used to induce labor in a viable pregnancy at term.

Such compounds as ergot derivatives, quinine, sparteine sulfate, subcutaneous or intramuscular oxytocin, or nasal oxytocin spray are listed only for historical interest and should not be used for the induction of labor.

Glossary

Asynclitism: When the biparietal diameter of the fetal head is parallel to the planes of the pelvis, the head is in synclitism. The sagittal suture is midway between the front and back of the pelvis. When either the anterior or posterior parietal bone precedes the sagittal suture, asynclitism is present.

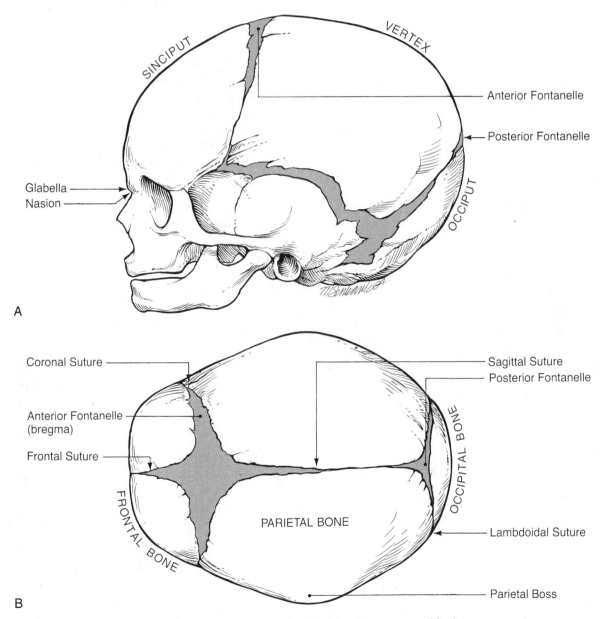

Fig. 13-8 (A & B) Landmarks on the fetal skull for determination of fetal position.

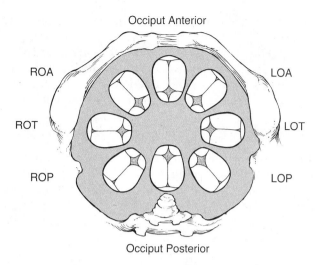

Occiput Anterior

ROA   LOA

ROT   LOT

ROP   LOP

Occiput Posterior

Fig. 13-9 Possible positions for a fetus with a vertex presentation.

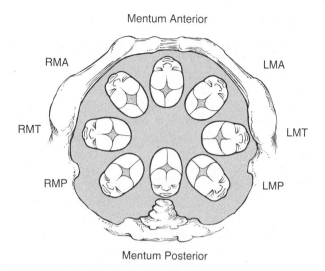

Mentum Anterior

RMA   LMA

RMT   LMT

RMP   LMP

Mentum Posterior

Fig. 13-10 Possible positions for a fetus with a face presentation.

Attitude: The relationship of the fetal parts to each other. This usually refers to the position of the head with regard to the trunk.

Dilatation: Also referred to as dilation. The degree of patency, expressed in centimeters of diameter, of the internal os of the cervix.

Denominator: A reference point on the fetus used to determine position. These points include landmarks in the fetal skull (Fig. 13-8), the fetal chin, the sacrum, and the acromion.

Effacement: A process that occurs in the latter part of pregnancy and labor by which the cervix is drawn intra-abdominally by the uterine corpus. This process is demonstrable by a shortening and thinning of the remaining intravaginal portion of the cervix. Effacement is expressed as the percentage by which the length of the cervix has been reduced and ranges from 0 (no reduction in length) to 100 percent (no cervix palpable below the fetal presenting part). It is sometimes described in centimeters of cervical length.

Engagement: Engagement occurs when the largest transverse diameter of the presenting part has descended past the plane of the pelvic inlet.

Labor: Repetitive uterine contractions associated with progressive cervical dilatation. Labor may be spontaneous or induced, term or preterm.

Lie: Relationship between the long axis of the fetus and that of the mother.

Position: Relationship between the denominator of the fetus (occiput in cephalic presentations) and the vertical (anterior, posterior) and horizontal (right, left) planes of the birth canal. Examples for cephalic and face presentations are shown in Figures 13-9 and 13-10.

Presentation: The fetal part that lies closest to the pelvic inlet. The three main presentations are cephalic (vertex), breech, and shoulder.

Station: A measure of the degree of descent of the presenting part of the fetus through the birth canal. Divided into seven stations (−3 to +3), with the midpoint (zero station) at the plane of the maternal ischial spines.

Key Points

- β Identification of the high-risk patient is critical in the proper management of labor and delivery.

- β The hazards of breech delivery are sufficient to warrant radiographic pelvimetry for cases in which vaginal delivery is contemplated.

- β The duration of the latent phase of labor has no direct impact on perinatal mortality.

- β The classification of abnormalities of the active phase of labor is based on the cervicographic analysis of labor.

- β In some settings, application of the principles of active management of labor has led to a reduction in the rate of cesarean delivery, with no change in perinatal mortality.

- β Prior to forceps delivery, fetal position and the characteristics of maternal pelvis must be known with certainty.

- β Examination of the placenta, umbilical cord, and membranes is an important part of delivery management.

- β Induction of labor may be indicated when the benefit of delivery to the mother or fetus outweighs the potential problems if the pregnancy continues.

- β The induction process attempts to accomplish in hours what may take several days of spontaneous prelabor.

- β Variability in patient sensitivity and response to oxytocin is the rule rather than the exception.

References

1. Friedman EA: Labor: Clinical Evaluation and Management. Appleton-Century-Crofts, New York, 1967

2. Duignan NM, Studd JWW, Hughes AO: Characteristics of normal labour in different racial groups. Br J Obstet Gynaecol 82:593, 1975

3. Chauhan SP, Lutton PM, Bailey KJ et al: Intrapartum clinical, sonographic, and parous patients' estimates of newborn birth weight. Obstet Gynecol 79:956, 1992

4. Kennell J, Klaus M, McGrath S et al: Continuous emotional support during labor in a US hospital. A randomized controlled trial. JAMA 265:2197, 1991

5. Michael S, Reilly CS, Caunt JA: Policies for oral intake during labour. A survey of maternity units in England and Wales. Anaesthesia 46:1071, 1991

6. Wolman WL, Chalmers B, Hofmeyr GJ, Nikodem VC: Postpartum depression and companionship in the clinical birth environment: a randomized, controlled study. Am J Obstet Gynecol 168:1388, 1993

7. DeLee JB: The prophylactic forceps operation. Am J Obstet Gynecol 1:34, 1920

8. Goodlin RC: On protection of the maternal perineum during birth. Obstet Gynecol 62:393, 1983

9. Yao AC, Lind J: Placental transfusion. Am J Dis Child 127:128, 1974

10. Caldwell WE, Moloy HC, D'Esposo DA: Studies on pelvic arrests. Am J Obstet Gynecol 36:928, 1938

11. Mengert WF: Estimation of pelvic capacity. JAMA 138:169, 1948

12. Friedman EA: The therapeutic dilemma of arrested labor. Contemp Obstet Gynecol 11:34, 1978

13. Morgan MA, Thurman GR: Efficacy of the fetal–pelvic index in nulliparous women at high risk for fetal–pelvic disproportion. Am J Obstet Gynecol 166:810, 1992

14. Diamond EL, Schnierler H, Lillienfeld AM: The ratio of intrauterine radiation to subsequent mortality and development of leukemia in children: a prospective study. Am J Epidemiol 97:283, 1973

15. Harvey EB, Boice JD, Honeyman M, Flannery JT: Prenatal x-ray exposure and childhood cancer in twins. N Engl J Med 312:541, 1985

16. Niswander K, Gordon M, Berendes H et al: The women and their pregnancies: the collaborative perinatal study of the National Institute of Neurological Disease and Stroke. Washington DC, US Dept of Health Education and Welfare, 1972

17. O'Brien WF, Cefalo RC: Evaluation of x-ray pelvimetry and abnormal labor. Clin Obstet Gynecol 25:157, 1982

18. Benson WL, Boyce DC, Vaughn DL: Breech delivery in the primigravida. Obstet Gynecol 40:417, 1972

19. Joyce DN, Giva-Osagie F, Stevenson GW: Role of pelvimetry in active management of labour. BMJ 4:405, 1975

20. Collea JV, Chen C, Quilligan EJ: The randomized management of frank breech presentation: a study of 208 cases. Am J Obstet Gynecol 137:235, 1980

21. Morris CW, Heggie JC, Acton CM: Computed tomography pelvimetry: accuracy and radiation dose compared with conventional pelvimetry. Austral Radiol 37:186, May 1993

22. Christian SS, Brady K, Read JA, Kopelman JN: Vaginal breech delivery: a five-year prospective evaluation of a protocol using computed tomographic pelvimetry. Am J Obstet Gynecol 163:848, 1990

23. Friedman EA, Sachtleben MR: Dysfunctional labor. I. Prolonged latent phase in the nullipara. Obstet Gynecol 17:135, 1961

24. Friedman EA: The functional divisions of labor. Am J Obstet Gynecol 109:274, 1971

25. Caldeyro-Barcia R, Posiero JJ: Physiology of uterine contractions. Clin Obstet Gynecol 3:386, 1960

26. Jocoate TN, Baker K, Martin RB: Inefficient uterine action. Surg Gynecol Obstet 95:257, 1952

27. Friedman EA, Sachtleben MR: Dysfunctional labor. II. Protracted active phase dilatation in the nullipara. Obstet Gynecol 17:566, 1961

28. O'Driscoll K, Meagher P: Active Management of Labor. WB Saunders, Philadelphia, 1980

29. Friedman EA, Sachtleben MR: Dysfunctional labor. III. Secondary arrest of dilatation in the nullipara. Obstet Gynecol 19:576, 1962

30. Read JA, Miller FC, Paul RH: Randomized trial of ambulation versus oxytocin for labor enhancement: a preliminary report. Am J Obstet Gynecol 139:699, 1981

31. Friedman EA, Satchtleben MR: Station of the fetal presenting part. V. Protracted descent patterns. Obstet Gynecol 36:558, 1970

32. Hellman LM, Prystowski H: The duration of the second stage of labor. Am J Obstet Gynecol 63:1223, 1952

33. Gaziano EP, Freeman DW, Bendel RP: FHR variability and other heart rate observations during second stage labor. Obstet Gynecol 56:42, 1980

34. Jacobson L, Rooth G: Interpretative aspects on the acid base composition and its variation in fetal scalp blood and maternal blood during labour. J Obstet Gynaecol Br Commonw 78:971, 1971

35. Cohen W: Influence of the duration of the second stage of labor on perinatal outcome and puerperal morbidity. Obstet Gynecol 49:266, 1977

36. Harbert GM: Uterine contractions. Clin Obstet Gynecol 25:177, 1980

37. Huey JR, Miller FC: The evaluation of uterine activity: a comparative analysis. Am J Obstet Gynecol 135:2, 1979

38. Jacobson JD, Gregerson GN, Dale PS, Valenzuela GJ: Real-time microcomputer-based analysis of spontaneous and augmented labor. Obstet Gynecol 76:755, 1990

39. Miller FC: Uterine activity, labor management, and perinatal outcome. Sem Perinatol 2:181, 1978

40. Turnbull AC, Anderson ABM: Induction of labour. J Obstet Gynaecol Br Commonw 5:32, 1968

41. Toaff ME, Herzoni J, Toaff R: Induction of labour by pharmacological and physiological doses of intravenous oxytocin. Br J Obstet Gynaecol 85:101, 1978

42. Seitchick J, Chatkoff ML: Intrauterine pressure waveform characteristics in hypocontractile labor before and after oxytocin administration. Am J Obstet Gynecol 123:426, 1975

43. Seitchick J, Castillo M: Oxytocin augmentation of dysfunctional labor. I. Clinical data. Am J Obstet Gynecol 144:899, 1982

44. Simons CL: Prostaglandins and labor: problems and benefits. Contemp Obstet Gynecol 12:91, 1978

45. O'Driscoll K, Foley M, MacDonald D: Active management of labor as an alternative to cesarean section for dystocia. Obstet Gynecol 63:485, 1984

46. Levens K, Cunningham C, Pritchard J: Cesarean section: an answer to the house of Horne. Am J Obstet Gynecol 153:838, 1985

47. Akoury HA, Brodie G, Caddick R et al: Active management of labor and operative delivery in nulliparous women. Am J Obstet Gynecol 158:255, 1988

48. Boylan PC, Parisi VM: Effect of active management on latent phase labor. Am J Perinatol 7:363, 1990

49. Lopez-Zeno JA, Peaceman AM, Adashek JA, Socol ML: A controlled trial of a program for the active management of labor. N Engl J Med 326:450, 1992

50. Hagadorn-Freathy AS, Yeomans ER, Hankins GDV: Validation of the 1988 ACOG forceps classification system. Obstet Gynecol 77:356, 1991

51. Friedman EA, Niswander KR, Sachtleben MR, Naftaly N: Dysfunctional labor. X. Immediate results to the infant. Obstet Gynecol 106:776, 1969

52. Friedman EA, Sachtleben MR, Bresky PA: Dysfunctional labor. XII. Long-term effects on the infant. Am J Obstet Gynecol 127:779, 1977

53. Bowes WA, Bowes C: Current role of the midforceps operation. Clin Obstet Gynecol 23:549, 1980

54. Chez RA: Midforceps delivery: is it an anachronism? Contemp Obstet Gynecol 15:82, 1980

55. Dudley AG, Markham SM, McNil O: Elective versus indicated midforceps delivery: a comparative study. Obstet Gynecol 37:19, 1971

56. Ramin SM, Little BB, Gilstrap LC: Survey of forceps delivery in North America in 1990. Obstet Gynecol 81:307, 1993

57. Richardson DA, Evans MI, Cibils LA: Midforceps delivery: a critical review. Am J Obstet Gynecol 145:621, 1983

58. Hughey MJ, McElin TW, Lussky R: Midforceps operations in perspective. I. Midforceps rotation operations. J Reprod Med 20:253, 1978

59. Malmstrom T: Vacuum extractor: an obstetrical instrument. Acta Obstet Gynecol Scand 33:1, 1954

60. Williams MC, Knuppel RA, O'Brien WF et al: A randomized comparison of assisted vaginal delivery by obstetric forceps and polyethylene vacuum cup. Obstet Gynecol 78:789–94, 1991

61. Sorbe B: Active pharmacologic management of the third stage of labor. Obstet Gynecol 52:694, 1978

62. Thierstein ST, Jahn HC, Lange K: Routine third-stage exploration of the uterus. Obstet Gynecol 10:269, 1957

63. Blanchette H: Elective manual exploration of the uterus after delivery: a study and review. J Reprod Med 19:13, 1977

64. Bishop EH: Pelvic scoring for elective induction. Obstet Gynecol 24:260, 1964

65. Friedman EA, Niswander KR, Bayonet-Rivera NP, Sachtleben MR: Relation of pre-labor evaluation to inductibility and the course of labor. Obstet Gynecol 29:539, 1966

66. Friedman EA, Niswander KR, Bayonet-Rivera NP, Sachtleben MR: Prelabor status evaluation. II. Weighted score. Obstet Gynecol 29:539, 1967

67. Liggins GC: Initiation of parturition. Br Med Bull 35:145, 1979

68. Seilers SM, Hodgson HT, Mitchell MD et al: Release of prostaglandins after amniotomy is not mediated by oxytocin. Br J Obstet Gynaecol 87:43, 1980

69. Chard T: The physiology of labor and its initiation. In T Chard, M Richards (eds): Benefits and Hazards of the New Obstetrics. JB Lippincott, Philadelphia, 1977

70. Booth JH, Kurdizak VB: Elective induction of labor: a controlled study. Can Med Assoc J 103:245, 1970

71. Fraser WD, Marcoux S, Moutquin JM et al: Effect of early amniotomy on the risk of dystocia in nulliparous women. N Engl J Med 328:1145, 1993

72. Baumgarten K: Advantages and disadvantages of low amniotomy. J Perinatal Med 4:2, 1976

73. Theobald GW, Graham A, Campbell J et al: The use of posterior pituitary extract in physiological amounts in obstetrics. BMJ 2:123, 1948

74. Dawood YM: Oxytocin: new data may help establish the ideal dose. Contemp Obstet Gynecol 13:181, 1979

75. Seitchek J, Castillo M: Oxytocin augmentation of dysfunctional labor. I. Clinical data. Am J Obstet Gynecol 144:899, 1982

76. Freeman RK, Poland RL (eds): Guidelines for Perinatal Care. American College of Obstetricians & Gynecologists, American Academy of Pediatrics, 1992

Intrapartum Fetal Evaluation

Rosemary E. Reiss, Steven G. Gabbe,
and Roy H. Petrie

More than any other recent development, changes in the methods of intrapartum fetal evaluation introduced during the past two to three decades have altered the theory and practice of obstetrics. Between 1960 and 1970, sophisticated fetal surveillance systems, including intermittent fetal blood acid–base determinations and continuous electronic fetal heart rate monitoring, were introduced with the expectation that stillbirths and neonatal neurologic injury caused by intrapartum hypoxemia could be significantly reduced or eliminated. Indeed, some centers with knowledgeable and dedicated personnel have realized some or all of these expectations. However, in most prospective randomized studies, the incidence of neurologic damage and perinatal death associated with the use of electronic fetal heart rate monitoring is not significantly lower than that documented with older methods of fetal surveillance, including intermittent fetal heart rate auscultation by stethoscope or Doppler. Moreover, in several trials electronic fetal heart rate monitoring was associated with an increased incidence of cesarean delivery. Consequently, the routine use of electronic fetal monitoring for intrapartum fetal evaluation has been disparaged by some.

Despite this controversy, there has been little interest among obstetricians in reverting to the more traditional fetal monitoring techniques, especially in those patients judged to be at high risk. The reasons for this reluctance to return to the older and simpler fetal surveillance techniques are multiple, but chief among them include (1) the undisputed reliability and assurance (greater than 98 percent) that a good fetal/neonatal outcome is associated with normal continuous fetal heart rate data and/or acid–base measure-

ment, which safely allows continuation of labor; (2) the unacceptably great expense involved in providing the one-on-one nursing that is mandatory to perform adequate intermittent fetal heart rate auscultation; and (3) the knowledge that, although nonreassuring continuous fetal heart rate data may not be uniformly associated with poor perinatal outcome, it does provide a warning of potential problems and a gauge of fetal response to actions undertaken to improve fetal condition.

With the introduction of continuous fetal heart rate monitoring, the term *fetal distress* came into wide use to describe situations of abnormal fetal heart rate patterns. However, growing experience with fetal assessment techniques has also brought awareness that these tests have many false-positive results and that abnormalities do not necessarily indicate the fetus is jeopardized. The American College of Obstetrics and Gynecology (ACOG) in 1994 issued a Committee Opinion[1] recommending that the term *nonreassuring fetal status* replace *fetal distress*. In this chapter, both terms are used, but *fetal distress* is restricted to indicate fetal hypoxia and acidosis.

Historical Perspective

It was not until the 1940s and 1950s that serious attention was directed to the rate of neonatal morbidity and fetal mortality. It had long been known that many fetuses died in utero before the onset of labor. A significant number of fetuses entered labor alive but were stillborn at delivery. That labor was a risk factor for neonatal morbidity and fetal mortality was well accepted. Infection, trauma, fetopelvic disproportion, abnormalities in placentation, and asphyxia were all recognized as risk factors that could compromise fetal condition.

Despite their appreciation of these dangers, before the mid-1900s, obstetricians could do little to change the poor perinatal outcomes. Few diagnostic techniques were available for antepartum evaluation of fetal well-being. Even if fetal jeopardy had been recognized, except at full dilatation and with reasonable descent into the pelvis, it was impossible to expedite delivery without the expectation of marked maternal morbidity and mortality. The introduction of antibiotics, blood typing, and safe pharmacologic agents to stimulate uterine contractions, coupled with the recognition of normal and abnormal patterns of labor, made it feasible to terminate a gestation or labor safely using oxytocin stimulation, early forceps delivery, or cesarean delivery. Once pregnancy and labor could be interrupted safely, information about the antepartum and intrapartum conditions of the fetus became vital if improvement in perinatal outcome was to be accomplished.

The early investigative efforts of such researchers as Barcroft,[2] Barron,[3] Apgar,[4] Freda,[5] and James et al[6] described fetal physiology in response to the stresses of the labor process. Their observations included the potential for contractions to reduce blood flow from mother to placenta and from the placenta to the fetus. The mechanism for fetal damage and death in such cases was identified as an insufficient supply of oxygen to the fetus secondary to a reduction in blood flow from the mother to the intervillous space or from the placenta to the fetus. Inadequate fetal oxygenation decreases or eliminates the supply of adenosine triphosphate (ATP) derived from the Krebs cycle and mandates that ATP be obtained from the Embden-Meyerhoff pathway. This process not only yields significantly less ATP, but also creates lactic acid as a byproduct. As lactate accumulates, it causes fetal brain cells to swell and finally to rupture. With sufficient brain cell necrosis, fetal damage or death can occur.[7]

By the mid-1960s to early 1970s, an understanding of fetal respiratory physiology was developed that provided a basis for diagnostic techniques to detect fetal compromise. Saling,[8] Hammacher et al,[9] Hon and Quilligan,[10] Caldeyro-Barcia et al,[11] and others developed technologies during the 1950s and early 1960s that allowed the clinician, for the first time, to monitor fetal status during labor. By the late 1960s and early 1970s, equipment for intrapartum fetal evaluation had become commercially available.

One last change was needed before significant improvement in fetal outcome could be attempted. This change was related to the philosophy of management for mother and fetus. Through the mid to late 1960s, the obstetrician was primarily concerned with the well-being of the mother. The guiding philosophy was that, if the perinatal outcome was unsatisfactory, the mother and father could try again. With a better understanding of fetal physiology and an appreciation that clinical management could change fetal condition, it became apparent that improved perinatal outcomes required deliveries with less hypoxia, less anesthesia and analgesia, and less trauma.

Therefore, an increasing number of cesarean deliveries was performed to reduce the potential for fetal damage or death from asphyxia. During the past decade and a half, the cesarean delivery rate has risen from 3 to 4 percent to 15 to 25 percent. Obviously, not all these operative deliveries are performed because of concern that the fetus is in jeopardy. But the clinical lesson has been learned that with improved effort relating to diagnosis and management, fetal morbidity and mortality, especially related to asphyxia, could be reduced. Accordingly, many institutions over the past two decades have shown dramatic reductions in perinatal mortality from 30 in 1,000 to 6 to 8 in 1,000. Many believe that a considerable portion of this improvement has been due to skilled intrapartum fetal surveillance. However, contrary to expectation, the incidence of cerebral palsy has not declined since the introduction of monitoring. Analysis of fetal heart rate tracings in infants developing cerebral tracing has shown that only a small proportion of this disorder can be related to intrapartum events.

Methodologies for Intrapartum Fetal Evaluation

In an effort to determine which fetus is likely to experience a reduction in oxygenation and to develop acidosis during labor, obstetricians looked at a number of potential indicators of fetal jeopardy. The presence of meconium in the amniotic fluid, fetal movement, acid–base balance, heart rate, and respirations have been evaluated as indicators of fetal condition.

Before the routine clinical use of fetal heart rate and acid–base monitoring during labor, Fenton and Steer[12] reviewed the steps by which fetal heart rate and meconium have come to be regarded as indicators of fetal stress during labor. They believe that fetal heart rate was probably first described by Marsac in 1650 and subsequently by Mayor in 1815 and Kergaradec in 1822. In 1843, Kennedy reported with considerable detail the changes in the fetal heart rate noted during pregnancy and labor, as did Bodson, who described signs of fetal distress in which there was "excessive frequency, great irregularity, or marked slowing of the fetal heart rate." In 1903, von Winckel suggested that a fetal heart rate above 160 or below 100 bpm should be regarded as evidence of distress. Subsequently, obstetricians of the present generation have noted increased perinatal mortality and morbidity with a fetal heart rate greater than 160 to 180 bpm or below 100 to 120 bpm. We now understand that fetal heart rate is under central nervous system (CNS) control and modified by increased vagal discharge in response to hypoxia and hypotension. Hypoxia can also directly depress the myocardium. Thus, fetal heart rate changes can be sensitive indicators of hypoxia.

In patients with thick meconium, the incidence of fetal and neonatal morbidity is increased. Fenton and Steer[12] ascribe the recognition of meconium passage during labor as an indicator of fetal distress to Schwartz in 1858. Later observers reported patients with meconium but without changes in fetal heart rate whose newborns were in good condition at birth. To determine the significance of meconium and heart rate as indicators of fetal distress, Fenton and Steer examined almost 8,000 deliveries over a 2-year interval. Fetal distress was present in 9.9 percent of these cases. These investigators found that the combination of thick meconium and a fetal heart rate under 100 bpm was associated with a perinatal mortality of 22.2 percent. They also noted that meconium alone, or the slowing of the heart rate alone, was not a sufficient indicator of fetal distress to warrant intervention and found that fetal survival was directly correlated with the interval between discovery of the signs of fetal distress and delivery. They concluded that 30 minutes was a critical interval.

In a paper written after the institution of routine clinical utilization of both continuous fetal heart rate and intermittent acid–base evaluation, Miller et al,[13] substantiated the earlier findings of Fenton and Steer.[12] They noted that the incidence of Apgar scores below 7 at 5 minutes was 3.5 times higher when meconium was present. They also confirmed earlier evidence that meconium alone was a relatively poor indicator of fetal and neonatal jeopardy unless an abnormal fetal heart rate or other risk factor was present.

During the late 1950s and 1960s, a number of investigators made attempts to correlate fetal condition with fetal heart rate.[14–16] It was soon appreciated that fetal heart rate counted over a period of time and expressed as a mean (e.g., 150 bpm averaged over 4 to 5 minutes) was an inadequate measurement. A number of investigators[17,18] demonstrated that the use of a stethoscope was also inadequate for the evaluation of fetal heart rate response to stress. Seasoned clinicians using stethoscopically derived fetal heart rate data were wrong at least one-third of the time in their evaluation of heart rate information.

To understand the responses of the fetal heart rate to labor, the clinician needed a continuous record of heart rate. Beginning in 1958 an electronic system, the current fetal heart rate monitor, was developed by Hon[16] and others to detect and plot heart rate automatically in a continuous fashion. The fetal heart rate tracing could then be correlated with continuously recorded uterine activity data.

In 1961, Saling[8] introduced the first direct assessment of fetal well-being during labor. Relying on the biochemical principles by which a decrease in fetal oxygenation would diminish the production of ATP by the Krebs cycle and cause the Embden-Meyerhoff pathway to be utilized, Saling proposed that the production of H+ ion in the form of lactate would cause the pH of the fetus to drop. Reviewing the biochemical responses during hypoxia, Saling chose to look at fetal pH rather than the Po_2 level for two reasons: (1) the level of Po_2 fluctuated quite rapidly during labor and the drift in readings of the Po_2 electrode did not permit precise monitoring and (2) pH values provided a good overall representative evaluation of fetal acid–base balance. Investigators around the world have substantiated Saling's original work and advocated the use of pH and base deficit measurements to differentiate between chronic and acute fetal distress.[18–20].

Intermittent Fetal Heart Rate Monitoring

Low-Risk Patients

When using a stethoscope, a fetoscope, or a portable Doppler device, the fetal heart rate is generally monitored and recorded during a contraction and for 30 seconds following the contraction. There are no studies to provide data regarding optimal intervals for monitoring low-risk patients. The current ACOG recommendations[21] suggest auscultation after contractions every 30 minutes during the first stage of labor and at least every 15 minutes in second stage for low-risk patients. In most of the randomized trials in which the safety of intermittent monitoring by auscultation was studied, nurses auscultated the fetal heart rate every 15 minutes during the first stage of labor and every 5 minutes in second stage.[22–25] If the patient is in the hospital during early latent phase labor, intermittent fetal heart rate monitoring during ambulation is frequently performed at intervals of 45 to 60 minutes until contractions become regular at 3- to 4-minute intervals.

High-Risk Patients

In a higher risk patients, the fetal heart rate is intermittently obtained and recorded every 15 minutes during the first stage of labor and every 5 minutes during the second stage of labor. The heart rate is preferably obtained during and 30 seconds following a uterine contraction. Using auscultation, abnormalities related to basal rate, long-term variability, and postcontraction slowing may be identified. When these changes are noted, additional fetal surveillance is warranted. Continuous internal fetal heart rate monitoring with appropriate fetal blood acid–base determination should be used to clarify an abnormality of the auscultated fetal heart rate.

Continuous Fetal Heart Rate Monitoring

To evaluate the effects of intrapartum events on the fetus continuously, it is necessary to determine the fetal heart rate on a beat-to-beat basis. With each beat of the fetal heart, a new calculation of rate is made based on what the fetal heart rate would be if all temporal intervals between beats were (1) the same as that between the last two heart beats and (2) uniform during 1 minute. Ideally, there should be no averaging of heart rate over a given interval or a given number of beats. The data collected should also be displayed continuously. This type of calculation is impossible to achieve with a stethoscope, because the heart rate auscultated by the human ear must be averaged over a given number of beats in seconds or minutes, and this averaging destroys the physiologic detail.

To record the fetal heart rate continuously and instantaneously, a signal must be obtained each time the heart beats, and some mechanical or electronic device must measure the interval between two successive heart beats, calculate the fetal heart rate, and plot each successive rate that is calculated. In clinical practice, the utilization of either an ultrasound transducer on the maternal abdominal wall or an electrode attached to the fetal scalp has become the standard technique for collecting fetal heart rate data. With the scalp electrode, the R wave of the fetal QRS complex initiates counting by the cardiotachometer of the monitor. The cardiotachometer determines the time between each R wave (the R-R interval), and a rate in beats per minute is generated. For example, an R-R interval difference of 500 msec or 0.5 second would produce an instantaneous rate of 120 bpm.

By convention, instantaneously calculated fetal heart rate and uterine activity are recorded on graph paper driven at a uniform speed. The paper speed is usually 3 cm/min, although 1 cm/min may be employed to save paper. The vertical scaling is 30 to 240 bpm over 7 cm and 0 to 100 mmHg (torr) over 4 cm. Thick vertical lines are placed at 1-minute intervals (Fig. 14-1). The heart rate tracing should be clearly labeled with the date, the patient's name, her identification number, and important clinical information. The tracing should be kept as a permanent part of the patient's medical record.

To evaluate uterine contractions or uterine activity, two methods have been developed. A tocodynamometer may be placed on the maternal abdomen overlying the gravid uterus and secured with a belt encircling the midsection of the body. The tocodynamometer detects alterations in the curvature of the abdomen resulting from changes in the configuration of the contracting uterus. Because no direct measurements are obtained, this system will not provide quantitative data on the strength or amplitude of contractions. However, the tocodynamometer will accurately record the frequency of contractions and show with reasonable accuracy the duration of the contractions. The second system for collecting information about uterine contractility requires the insertion of a small catheter filled with sterile water into the chorioamniotic sac after rupture of the membranes. The fluid-filled catheter is attached to a strain gauge and placed at a level that corresponds to the midpoint of the vertical axis of the uterus. Accurate pressure readings can then be obtained that indicate the onset, strength or amplitude, and duration of uterine contractions.

External Monitoring

In some cases, it may be clinically undesirable or impossible to rupture the membranes. Similarly, the obstetrician may not wish to use a fetal electrode or intrauterine pressure catheter. In these situations, the external form of fetal monitoring utilizing a tocodynamometer and

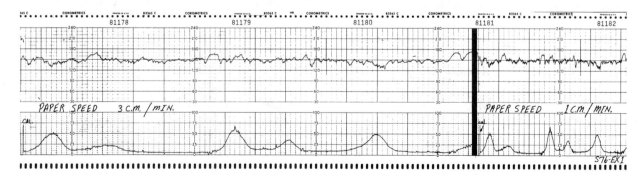

Fig. 14-1 Internal fetal heart rate data gathered at the standard recording speed of 3 cm/min for the first portion. The same data are being recorded at a speed of 1 cm/min in the last segment. Normal long-term and short-term variabilities are present. Note that the uterine activity channel has been calibrated so that the intrauterine pressure readings can be measured correctly.

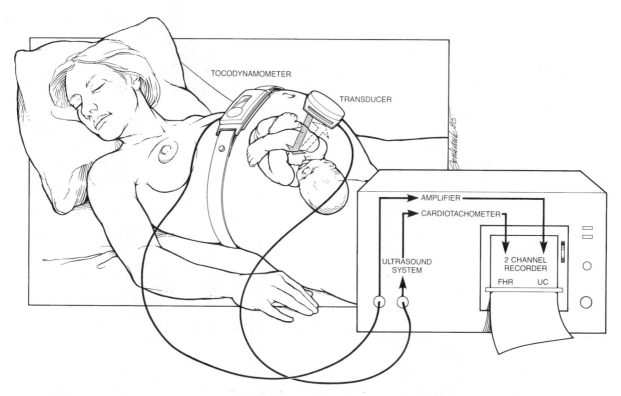

Fig. 14-2 Instrumentation for external monitoring. Contractions are detected by the pressure-sensitive tocodynamom-eter, amplified, and then recorded. Fetal heart rate is monitored using the Doppler ultrasound transducer, which both emits and receives the reflected ultrasound signal that is then counted and recorded.

ultrasound transducer can be applied (Fig. 14-2). An ultrasound transducer is affixed to the maternal abdomen at a position overlying the fetal heart so that sound waves can be transmitted toward the fetal heart valves. As the valves move, the reflected sound waves return to the transducer, permitting an accurate assessment of fetal heart rate activity.

The mitral and aortic valves generally provide four events during each systole: mitral opening, mitral closure, aortic opening, and aortic closure. With four different signals, the electronic counting device of the fetal monitor, the cardiotachometer, will, at random, pick one of these four signals to count. This process introduces a certain amount of "false" heart rate variability into the calculation of fetal heart rate when one considers that the first event may be used for one beat, the last event for the next beat, one of the two intermediate events for subsequent beats, and so forth. Systems have been developed that use a directional depth-range Doppler system, permitting continuous monitoring of only one of these signals.

There are few complications or side effects of external monitoring, although difficulty may be encountered in interpreting heart rate and uterine activity data if the recording is of poor quality. As the fetus moves in utero, the ultrasound transducer must be adjusted to maintain a good signal. This may be especially true in the obese

patient. Similarly, the external tocodynamometer transducer may need adjustment in position or in tension to obtain a good recording of uterine contractions. Until very recently, the use of continuous external fetal monitoring confined the parturient to bed. Newly available cordless transducers permit ambulation.

Internal Monitoring

Internal monitoring requires the spontaneous or artificial rupture of the chorioamnion (Fig. 14-3). Usually, the cervix needs to be dilated 1 to 2 cm before the uterine pressure catheter can be inserted and the fetal electrode attached. The electrode is placed during a vaginal examination. With the examiner's finger inserted through the cervical os against the fetal scalp, a cartilaginous plate is first identified. The obstetrician must be certain the electrode will not be placed over the fetal face or fontanel. An electrode introducer is next inserted along the finger to come to rest against the fetal vertex. Rotating the introducer 90 to 360 degrees will attach the spiral electrode to the fetal scalp. The introducer is removed, and the ends of the wires from the electrode are connected to a maternal leg plate that contains a ground lead and is attached to the fetal monitor. The fetal electrode is composed of two parts (Fig. 14-4). The spiral electrode itself is attached

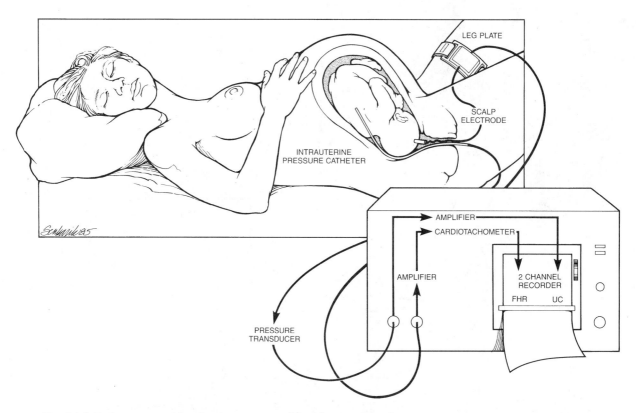

LEG PLATE

SCALP ELECTRODE

INTRAUTERINE PRESSURE CATHETER

AMPLIFIER

CARDIOTACHOMETER

AMPLIFIER

2 CHANNEL RECORDER

FHR   UC

PRESSURE TRANSDUCER

Fig. 14-3 Techniques used for direct monitoring of fetal heart rate and uterine contractions. Uterine contractions are assessed with an intrauterine pressure catheter connected to a pressure transducer. This signal is then amplified and recorded. The fetal electrocardiogram is obtained by direct application of the scalp electrode, which is then attached to a leg plate on the mother's thigh. The signal is transmitted to the monitor, where it is amplified, counted by the cardiotachometer, and then recorded.

to the fetus and the circuit closed when a second, or reference, electrode comes in contact with electrolyte-containing secretions in the maternal vagina. It is also possible for the maternal electrocardiographic (ECG) signal to be conducted through a dead fetus to the fetal electrode and be amplified and counted by the fetal monitor's cardiotachometer. The use of real-time ultrasonography to evaluate fetal cardiac valvular action can resolve this question quickly and perhaps avoid an unnecessary operative delivery. The scalp electrode allows the patient more freedom of movement than does the ultrasound transducer, because maternal or fetal movement will not alter the quality of the signal. During placement of the internal monitoring apparatus, the patient should remain in a lateral position to avoid hypotension secondary to vena caval compression.

Internal fetal heart rate monitoring involves breaking the skin or scalp to attach the electrode. In rare cases, a small pustule may form at the electrode site. The incidence of this infectious problem has been reported to be between 1 in 500 and 1 in 2,000 cases.[26] These lesions can generally be treated by drainage and

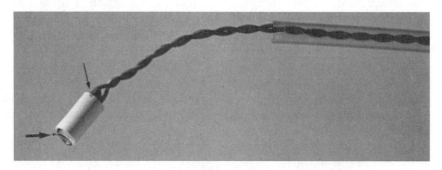

Fig. 14-4 Fetal spiral electrode used for direct monitoring of the fetal heart rate. The thick arrow points to the stainless steel spiral; the thin arrow designates the reference electrode.

topical antibiotics. No complications from scalp electrodes were reported in infants born to 6,474 women in the monitored arm of a randomized trial of electonic fetal monitoring.[23]

After the electrode has been attached, a catheter for the determination of uterine activity can be inserted. The soft plastic intrauterine catheter is filled with sterile water to avoid corrosion of the pressure strain gauge, which may occur with dextrose and water or saline. The catheter should be filled with fluid before it is introduced to avoid the possibility of an air embolus. The soft, fluid-filled catheter is inserted through a stiffer plastic guide. The guide is moved along the examiner's finger, which has been positioned just inside the cervix between the fetal presenting part and the cervix. To prevent perforation of the uterus, the guide must be passed no further than the examiner's fingers. The intrauterine pressure catheter is then manually pushed through the guide until it is halfway up the uterine cavity, a distance of approximately 18 inches from the tip of the catheter to the labia minora. (Most commercial manufacturers now place a marker at the 18-inch level.) The guide is then removed, and the catheter is attached to the strain gauge. Utilizing a three-way stopcock, the catheter is flushed to removed any vernix or air, and the strain gauge is calibrated.

Occasionally, when inserting the intrauterine pressure catheter, the stiff plastic guide may penetrate the myometrium or disrupt the placental site. Accordingly, the obstetrician must guard against this complication and avoid extending the guide beyond his or her finger. It is exceedingly uncommon for the soft plastic intrauterine pressure catheter to penetrate the myometrium.

Many clinicians believe that an internal pressure catheter will increase the risk of chorioamnionitis and postpartum endomyometritis. Most studies have failed to confirm this suspicion. There is no doubt, however, that the longer an intrauterine catheter and electrode are in situ before a cesarean delivery is performed, the greater the likelihood of postpartum febrile morbidity.[27,28]

Physiologic Control of Fetal Heart Rate (see Ch. 3)

Baseline Heart Rate

The human mean fetal heart rate varies between 120 and 160 bpm; however, rates as low as 90 or as high as 180 are not uncommon or necessarily abnormal, especially if they are transient. With advancing gestation there is a gradual slowing of the baseline fetal heart rate due to increasing parasympathetic tone.[29] Persistent periods (10 minutes or longer) of heart rate above 160 bpm are classified as a baseline tachycardia. Persistent fetal heart rate below 120 bpm are known as fetal bradycardia. Persistent intervals of tachycardia or bradycardia are more likely to be associated with hypoxia than is a normal heart rate (Figs. 14-5 and 14-6). Fetal tachycardia has also been identified in cases complicated by maternal fever, fetal infection, maternal thyrotoxicosis, fetal anemia, and fetal tachyarrhythmias. If the patient has received β-sympathomimetric drugs or parasympatholytic agents such as atropine, fetal tachycardia may also be observed.[29] Fetal bradycardia can be seen in patients treated with β-blockers such as propranolol. Damage to the conduction system of the fetal heart causing congenital heart block and a rate of 50 to 70 bpm can result from congenital heart malformation or maternal autoimmune disease.

Heart Rate Variability

Perhaps the most reliable indicator of fetal well-being available to the obstetrician is the finding of normal beat-to-beat heart rate variability. Fetal heart rate variability can only be appreciated when it is continuously and instantaneously calculated and recorded on a beat-by-beat basis. Heart rate variability represents the interplay between the cardioinhibitory and cardioaccelerator centers in the fetal brain stem. It is unusual for a heart rate under normal nervous system control to be constant. Rather, there is considerable variation or

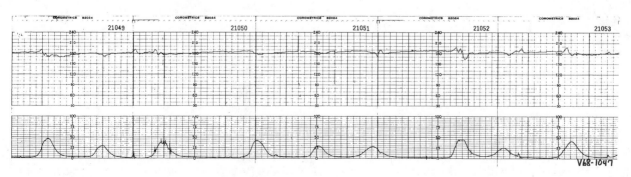

Fig. 14-5 Internal monitoring. A baseline tachycardia is noted at a rate of 180 to 190 bpm. Uterine activity is occurring every 2 to 3 minutes, with an intensity of 30 to 45 mmHg and a normal resting tone of 5 mmHg.

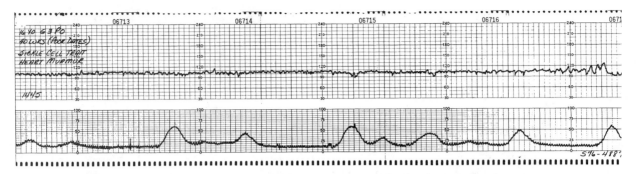

Fig. 14-6 Internal heart rate monitoring and an external tocodynamometer are being utilized. A fetal heart rate bradycardia at 100 to 110 bpm with good variability over the 20-minute interval is displayed. The small undulating aspects of the uterine pressure recording represent maternal respiration.

short-term variability on a beat-to-beat basis, usually ranging from 3 to 5 bpm around an imaginary average heart rate. Long-term variability occurs as well, with fluctuations with amplitude 5 to 20 bpm occurring at three to five cycles per minute.[30] (Fig. 14-7). The presence of normal fetal heart rate variability is one of the best indicators of intact integration between the CNS and heart of the fetus. By the time a fetus reaches 28 weeks' gestation or more the CNS should be sufficiently mature to produce normal variability. The loss of heart rate variability often suggests fetal hypoxia, but other factors may be responsible, including a fetal sleep state, drugs that depress the CNS, a fetal tachycardia of more than 180 bpm, and anomalies of the heart and CNS.[31] When evaluating beat-to-beat variability, an external fetal heart rate monitor cannot be utilized as a precise indicator of variability with one exception. When a flat heart rate is observed with ultrasound techniques, close correlation between the external and internal systems can be anticipated (Figs. 14-8 and 14-9). The external system, when working properly, can permit adequate evaluation of long-term variability.

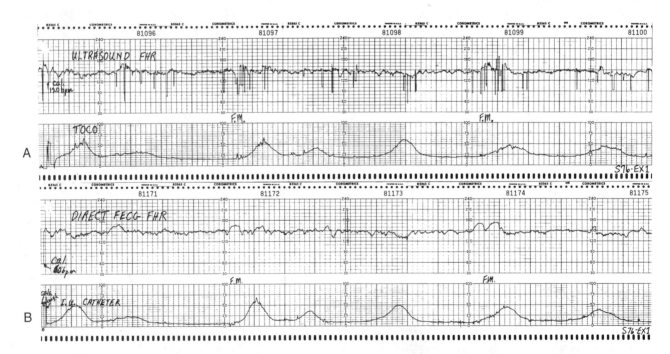

Fig. 14-7 The use of external monitoring with ultrasound and a tocodynamometer (A), with the same data being recorded using an internal system with a fetal electrode and an intrauterine pressure catheter (B). Note that the characteristics of the heart rate channel are similar but with considerable noise or increased variability (A), reflecting the recording characteristics of the ultrasound system. Nevertheless, long-term variability with its cyclicity can still be appreciated. The tocodynamometer is positioned to approximate the calibrated intrauterine pressure reading. However, by turning the calibration knob on the tocodynamometer, one can position uterine activity information anywhere on the vertical scale for uterine activity.

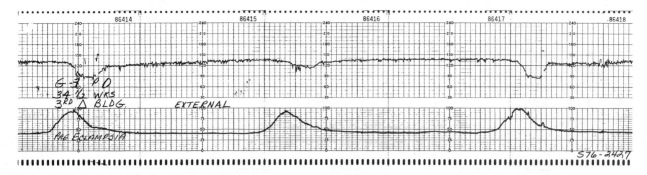

Fig. 14-8 A case complicated by third-trimester bleeding in which external heart rate and uterine activity data are collected. Note the presence of persistent late decelerations with only three contractions in 20 minutes as well as the apparent loss of variability of the fetal heart rate. The rise in baseline tone on the uterine activity channel cannot be evaluated with the external system.

The clinical significance of short-term variability or beat-to-beat variability has been assessed for a number of years. Wherever there is good beat-to-beat variability present on a heart rate tracing without other indicators of loss of fetal well-being, the likelihood of delivering a significantly jeopardized fetus is exceedingly low. Even when other parameters suggest fetal distress, the presence of good beat-to-beat variability is generally a reassuring finding.[32]

Exaggerated or increased fetal heart rate variability (more than 25 bpm) may be representative of a shifting Po_2 and Pco_2 relationship mediated by the baro- and chemoreceptors. Unless repetitive decelerations are also present, there is generally no significant change in fetal oxygenation or fetal status (Fig. 14-10).[33] The presence of increased fetal heart rate variability that is followed by loss of beat-to-beat variability can be ominous.

Although it occurs infrequently, a sinusoidal heart rate (Fig. 14-11) may have great clinical importance. This baseline heart rate is usually within a normal range of 120 to 160 bpm. However, it has a somewhat smooth, undulating pattern of uniform long-term variability with an amplitude of 5 to 20 bpm that resembles a sine wave. There is an absence of short-term variability. The sinusoidal heart rate has often been associated with fetal anemia, as in Rh isoimmunization. The physiologic mechanism for this pattern is unknown. Some investigators believe that it represents aberrant neurologic control of the heart rate that may result from anemia or hypoxia. Sinusoidal-like heart rate patterns can be seen following the administration of some narcotic analgesics and related agents. Whenever a persistent sinusoidal baseline heart rate pattern is noted, it is advisable to collect fetal scalp capillary blood for an acid–base determination. The possibility of fetal anemia due to fetomaternal hemorrhage or hemolysis should also be considered.

Fetal Arrhythmias

As long as the fetal QRS wave is clear and regular, the fetal heart rate will be instantaneously counted and expressed in beats per minute for each fetal heart rate. However, occasional electrical and/or mechanical interference from external and internal sources may be in-

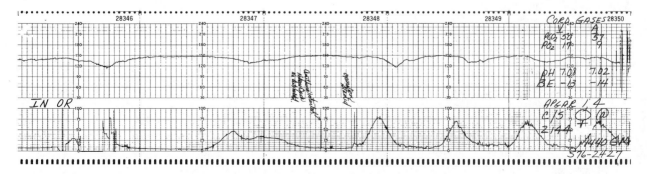

Fig. 14-9 The same patient described in Figure 14-8 following a double set-up examination that ruled out a placenta previa and allowed placement of an internal monitoring system. Note that the flat heart rate demonstrated in Figure 14-8 is indeed found when internal monitoring is used. After cesarean delivery, the attending staff have listed all pertinent data, including Apgar scores, weight, sex, cord pH, and respiratory gases for cord vein and artery.

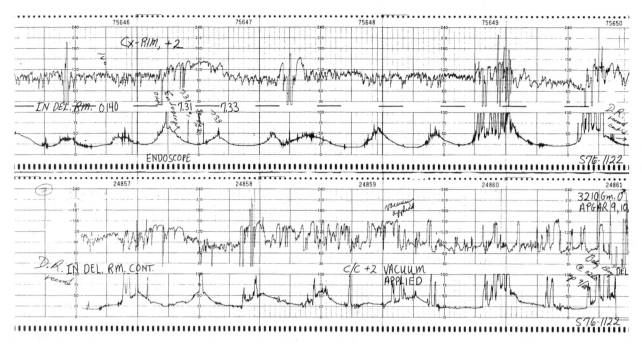

Fig. 14-10 Exaggerated variability with a baseline bradycardia of 90 to 110 bpm. Note accelerations. Concern about this tracing led to evaluation of the fetal scalp pH, which was found to be normal (7.31, 7.33). When the baseline fell further, it was elected to deliver the infant using the vacuum extractor (panel 24859). The 3,210-g male had Apgar scores of 9 and 10, consistent with accelerations, exaggerated variability, and the fetal capillary pH values.

troduced, and the clarity and reliability of the fetal heart rate tracing can be lost. Such interference has often been referred to as "noise" or "artifact." Interference caused by mechanical sources usually creates a pattern of artifact that is random. In evaluating this problem, one should confirm that all electrical connections are secure. The obstetrician should be certain that the scalp electrode is firmly fastened and that the wires to the leg plate have not loosened. To evaluate a fetal arrhythmia one can obtain a continuous tracing from an ECG monitor attached directly to the fetal heart rate monitor. In this way, the obstetrician can evaluate the presence of the P, QRS, and T waves of the fetal

signal. M-mode fetal echocardiography can also be useful.

While many fetal cardiac arrhythmias are transient and of little clinical significance, some have been associated with fetal compromise. Sustained fetal tachycardia at a rate above 200 bpm warrants investigation, and may lead to heart failure and hydrops (Fig. 14-12). Atrial supraventricular tachycardia (rate 220 to 240) is most common, with atrial fibrillation or flutter seen less often. Ventricular tachycardias are exceedingly rare. The fetus with complete heart block will usually demonstrate a rate of 50 to 70 bpm. Approximately 40 percent of these infants will have congenital heart disease, par-

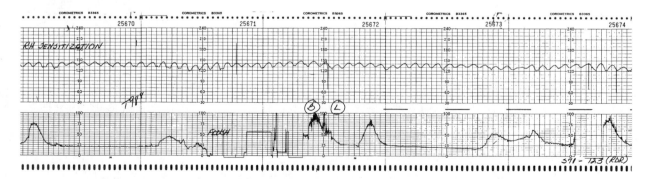

Fig. 14-11 The sinusoidal heart rate pattern with its even undulations is demonstrated. Internal monitoring shows the absence of beat-to-beat variability characteristic of true sinusoidal patterns.

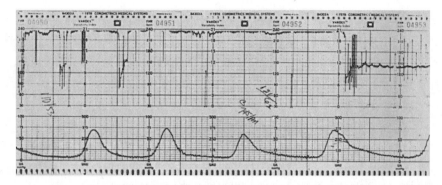

Fig. 14-12 The patient, a 26-year-old, gravida 6, para 3, aborta 2, entered spontaneous labor at 37 weeks' gestation. Monitoring with a scalp electrode and an external tocodynamometer demonstrates a fetal supraventricular tachycardia approaching 240 bpm in panels 04950 through 04952. In panel 04953, the fetal heart returns to a normal baseline rate of 140 bpm. The patient was delivered vaginally of a 3,300-g male infant with Apgar scores of 9 and 9. The infant required digitalization for a persistent tachycardia during the neonatal period. The conversion of the heart rate from the supraventricular tachycardia to a normal rate at the end of this tracing may have been due to vagal stimulation secondary to pressure on the fetal head. Antenatal treatment of the fetus with a supraventricular tachycardia has included maternal therapy with propranolol, verapamil, and digitalis. Fewer than 10 percent of fetuses with a supraventricular tachycardia will demonstrate a cardiac malformation. (From Bergmans et al,[95] with permission.)

ticularly a ventricular septal defect. Maternal autoantibodies associated with systemic lupus erythematosus or Sjøgren syndrome (antiRo or antiLa antibodies), which cross the placenta and cause inflammation and fibrosis in the conducting system, are found in most of the others. Fetal heart failure and hydrops have also been associated with congenital heart block.

Periodic Changes

Important periodic changes in fetal heart rate have been observed in association with uterine contractions. Transient slowing of the fetal heart rate is known as a *deceleration*, while a transient increase is known as an *acceleration*. The four patterns of clinical significance are accelerations and early, variable, and late decelerations. Only two mechanisms alter fetal heart rate: (1) a reflex response secondary to the nervous control of the heart by direct nervous innervation or by humoral control of the autonomic nervous system and (2) transient slowing of the heart when fetal myocardial hypoxia is present.

Early Deceleration

With an early deceleration, the fetal heart rate demonstrates a slowing or deceleration as a contraction begins, reaching its lowest point just as the acme of the contraction is reached and returning to baseline levels just as the contraction is finished. The heart rate never falls below 100 bpm (Fig. 14-13). This deceleration is known as an *early deceleration* because it starts early in the contraction. The early deceleration is thought to be due to pressure on the fetal head as it moves down the birth canal, and the mechanism is one of reflex

slowing mediated by the vagus nerve with release of acetylcholine at the sinoatrial node commensurate with the pressure applied to the fetal vertex. Accordingly, this pattern can be blocked by the use of a vagolytic drug such as atropine. These early decelerative changes are innocuous and can be observed throughout labor without alteration in fetal condition, acid–base status, or neonatal or long-term outcome.

Variable Deceleration

The variable deceleration is a reflex-mediated change in fetal heart rate, again mediated by the vagus nerve,[2] but generally caused by umbilical cord compression that may occur as a result of the cord being around the fetus's neck, under its arm, or between some part of the fetus and the uterine wall (Fig. 14-14). This pattern is often seen in association with oligohydramnios. As the umbilical cord is compressed, fetal peripheral resistance increases. Fetal P_{O_2} falls and P_{CO_2} rises. Baroreceptors and chemoreceptors fire, causing a swift and somewhat erratic release of acetylcholine at the sinoatrial node with a sharp angular drop in heart rate, usually to a range below 100 bpm. The variable deceleration may begin before the onset of a contraction, with the onset of a contraction, or following the onset of a contraction. This change in fetal heart rate can be blocked to some degree by the administration of atropine, but is not affected by the administration of oxygen. The variable deceleration is the most common periodic pattern noted during labor and generally can be corrected by changing maternal position to alleviate cord compression.

If the fetal heart rate does not fall below 80 bpm and

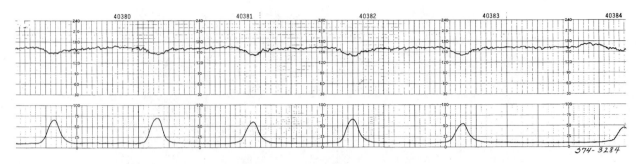

Fig. 14-13 Internal monitoring demonstrates a baseline heart rate of approximately 160 bpm, minimal to moderate short-term variability, and persistent early decelerations with each contraction.

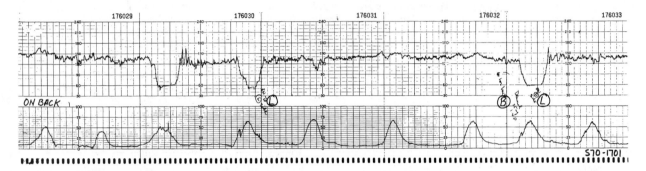

Fig. 14-14 Internal monitoring reveals uterine contractions every 2 to 3 minutes of 50- to 60-mmHg intensity and a baseline of 5 to 10 mmHg. Variable decelerations occur intermittently, providing adequate intervals between contractions for CO_2 and O_2 exchange and fetal recovery.

the deceleration is brief, cord compression is usually of minimal clinical significance. However, with prolonged or deep variable decelerations (Table 14-1), a significant reduction in respiratory gas exchange may occur. Carbon dioxide accumulates in the fetal compartment, causing a transient respiratory acidosis. If the decelerations are severe and repetitive, hypoxia and metabolic acidosis may result. Fetal myocardial hypoxemia may then produce a delayed recovery to baseline. If this occurs, great care must be taken to eliminate this stress. If severe variables cannot be alleviated the fetus may require early delivery. When the fetal heart rate falls below 60 bpm, loss of nodal control of the heart resulting in momentary "cardiac arrest" may occur.

Late Deceleration

A transient, but repetitive deceleration of the fetal heart rate noted to begin well after the contraction is under way is known as a *late deceleration* (Figs. 14-9 and 14-

Table 14-1 Grading of Variable Decelerations

Grade	Nadir (bpm)	Duration (sec)
Mild	Any	<30
Moderate	70–80 bpm	>60
	<70 bpm	>30–<60
Severe	<70 bpm	>60

(Modified from Kubli et al.,[40] with permission.)

15). It reaches its lowest point after the acme of the contraction has been achieved and does not return to the baseline rate until after the contraction is over. Late decelerations indicate uteroplacental insufficiency and decreased intervillous exchange between mother and fetus with intermittent fetal hypoxia. As the uterine contraction peaks, limiting intervillous blood flow, fetal oxygenation is impaired, hence the late timing of the deceleration. In a setting of mild transient hypoxia, late decelerations represent a reflex vagally mediated response and are associated with normal heart rate variability. Laboratory investigations in a sheep model have demonstrated that late decelerations initially result from fetal nonacidemic hypoxia that triggers a chemoreceptor response leading to vagal discharge, and from transient fetal hypertension that stimulates fetal baroreceptors.[34] However, when hypoxia is prolonged and severe enough to produce acidemia, direct myocardial depression results in decelerations following contractions even in animals with pharmacologic sympathetic and parasympathetic blockade of reflex arcs.

Late decelerations may occur with placental abruption, excessive uterine activity of either a spontaneous or pharmacologically induced nature, and maternal hypotension, anemia, or ketoacidosis. In fetuses with intrauterine growth restriction (IUGR), even normal contractions may reveal the lack of reserve for respiratory exchange in the placental vascular tree. Shallow, repeti-

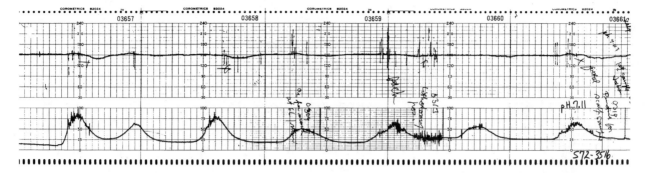

Fig. 14-15 With internal monitoring, very shallow late decelerations are noted with loss of variability. Note the fetal capillary pH of 7.11, indicative of a rather marked acidosis. Not surprisingly, scalp puncture did not produce a fetal heart rate acceleration.

tive late decelerations of only 5 to 10 bpm below baseline, especially in a setting of reduced beat-to-beat variability, are at least as ominous as deep ones (see Fig. 14-15). In fact, as the fetus becomes more acidemic, late decelerations tend to be shallower as vagal reflexes are abolished and only myocardial depression persists. Such cases may be characterized by late decelerations with absent heart rate variability. In the dying fetus, late decelerations give way to a marked bradycardia.

Mixed Patterns

Occasionally, two decelerative fetal heart rate patterns may be seen together. This combination has been called a *mixed pattern* (Fig. 14-16). In managing such cases, clinical decisions should be based on the worst component of the mixed pattern. Whatever the origin of the fetal hypoxia with late deceleration, it must be corrected, or the infant must be delivered to avoid damage.

Accelerations

Transient increases in fetal heart rate associated with uterine contractions or fetal movement are known as *accelerations* and are usually indicators of a fetus that

is adequately oxygenated (Fig. 14-17). In some cases, accelerations result from partial cord occlusion. With mild cord compression, only the umbilical vein may be compressed, producing fetal hypotension and a baroreceptor-mediated increase in heart rate. Acid–base determinations during accelerations almost uniformly demonstrate a normal fetal pH.

Summary

A healthy fetus is characterized by a normal heart rate with normal heart rate variability and by the absence of significant repetitive late heart rate decelerations. The presence of fetal heart rate accelerations strengthens the diagnosis of fetal well-being. In a potentially compromised fetus, the heart rate pattern is characterized by significant repetitive decelerations and by an abnormal baseline fetal heart rate. Other nonreassuring characteristics include the absence of fetal heart rate accelerations and the loss of fetal heart rate variability. The presence of repetitive late decelerations, repetitive moderate to severe variable decelerations, a sinusoidal pattern, or a baseline tachycardia, particularly when associated with diminished fetal heart rate variability, all indicate the need to evaluate fetal status

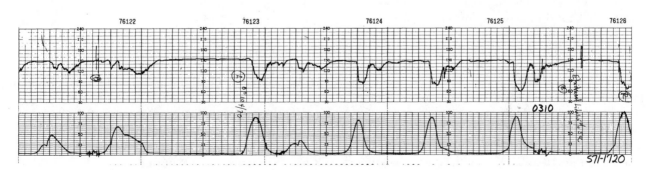

Fig. 14-16 Using internal monitoring, a mixed variable–late pattern is noted. Generally the periodic pattern begins as a variable deceleration with a slow return to baseline, indicative of a late deceleration. The potential fetal compromise associated with the fetal heart rate pattern should be judged by the worst component of the pattern, the late deceleration.

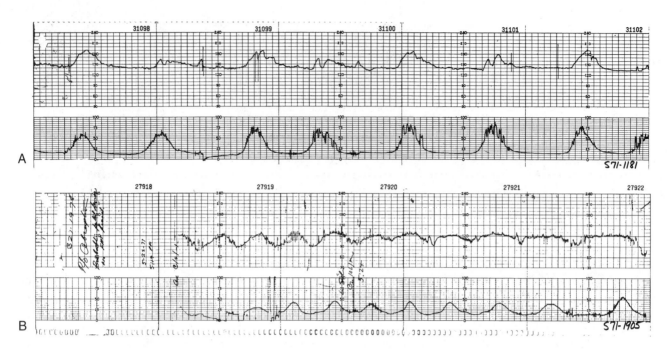

Fig. 14-17 (A) Internal monitoring is used, and accelerations are noted with each contraction. (B) It is difficult to judge the baseline heart rate, making it difficult to determine whether there are persistent repetitive accelerations or persistent repetitive late decelerations. This differential may be critical; if the baseline heart rate cannot be established, a measurement of fetal capillary pH or base deficit can be most helpful.

further. This sometimes involves the collection of fetal scalp capillary blood for the determination of fetal acid–base balance.

Fetal Acid–Base Evaluation

Blood Collection for Respiratory Gases

In the early 1960s, Saling,[8,35] a German obstetrician, introduced an innovative technique for obtaining fetal blood for the determination of acid–base status. For the first time, the obstetrician could assess fetal pH and oxygenation during labor. Over the next 15 years, fetal blood sampling became an integral aspect of intrapartum surveillance in many institutions.

Over the three decades since fetal surveillance by acid–base determinations of capillary blood was introduced, a number of studies have been performed that have verified the validity of this form of monitoring. The supporting data have come from animal models in which central blood values have been correlated with capillary scalp pH,[32] studies comparing cord acid–base[34–36] data with capillary values, and studies relating both cord and fetal capillary acid–base determinations to neonatal performance and outcome.[37,38] Since the introduction of fetal heart rate monitoring, a number of investigators have demonstrated the linear correlation between the severity of heart rate patterns and the degree of acidosis present (Table 14-2.[39–43] During labor, fetal acidosis may result from impaired fetomaternal exchange. A transient fall in fetal pH may be due to acute umbilical cord compression that leads to the rapid accumulation of carbon dioxide and a respiratory acidosis. Of greater concern is inadequate fetal oxygenation because of impaired respiratory gas exchange in the intervillous space. When there is inadequate fetal oxygenation for energy production and the aerobic processes for generating ATP fail, the anaerobic pathway of energy production is used. Lactic acidosis results, and fetal pH falls. Accordingly, if sufficient hypoxia and acidosis develop, brain damage or death from asphyxia may occur. The collection of fetal blood for pH and respiratory gas evaluation, when performed at the appropriate time, may alert the obstetrician to impending fetal jeopardy and permit correction of the underlying problem or delivery by whatever route is safest for mother and fetus.

Normal fetal capillary and umbilical blood pH and respiratory gas values are given in Tables 14-3 and 14-4. The fetal capillary scalp pH value will normally decline in early labor from approximately 7.30 to 7.25 at delivery. Traditionally a pH value of 7.25 or greater has been considered normal for the fetus during labor.[8,31] The pH range of 7.20 to 7.24 has been referred to as a preacidotic range. Many believe a fetal capillary pH value of 7.19 or less indicates potential fetal acidosis and, if substantiated on two collections 5

Table 14-2   Relationship of Fetal Heart Rate Pattern, Fetal Acid–Base Level, and 5-Minute Apgar Score

	Fetal Scalp pH		5-Minute Apgar Score ≥7 (%)	
Cord pH Pattern	Kubli[40]	Tejani[42]	pH ≥7[a]	pH ≥7.25[a]
Normal tracing	7.30 ± .04	7.33 ± .01	92	91
Accelerations		7.34 ± .01	91	97
Early decelerations	7.30 ± .04	7.33 ± .01	92	93
Variable decelerations (all)		7.30 ± .01	78	77
Moderate	7.26 ± .04			
Severe	7.15 ± .07			
Late decelerations (all)		7.29 ± .01	63	66
Moderate	7.21 ± .05			
Severe	7.12 ± .07			

[a] Data from Tejani et al.[43]

Table 14-3   Normal Umbilical Cord Blood-Gas Values

	Vein	Artery
pH	7.34 ± 0.15	7.28 ± 0.15
P_{O_2}	30 ± 15	15 ± 10
P_{CO_2}	35 ± 8	45 ± 15
Base deficit	5 ± 4	7 ± 4

Table 14-4   Fetal Capillary Blood Respiratory Gas Values

Normal	Respiratory Acidosis	Metabolic Acidosis
pH 7.25–7.40	Decreased	Decreased
P_{O_2} 18–22	Usually stable	Decreased
P_{CO_2} 40–50	Increased	Usually stable
Base deficit 0–11	Usually stable	Increased

Table 14-5   Base Deficit (Excess)[a] in Fetal Capillary Blood

Base (mEq/L)	Indication
0–9	Normal
9–11	Borderline
>11	Potential metabolic acidosis

[a] Base deficit and base excess have the same numerical value; however, a positive value is used for base deficit and a negative value for base excess (i.e., a base deficit of 6 is the same as a base excess of −6).

to 10 minutes apart, represents sufficient acidosis to warrant termination of labor. However, a number of investigators have demonstrated that it is uncommon to find significant neonatal sequelae until a pH range of less than 7.10 is noted, and this value may be as low at 7.00.[45–47]

To maintain the pH at a relatively constant level, fetal blood and tissues contain buffers, chiefly plasma bicarbonate and hemoglobin. The base excess or deficit is an indication of fetal buffer reserves available to neutralize H + ions or fixed acids (see Table 14-5). A large base deficit when pH values are satisfactory or borderline suggests impending loss of fetal well-being. A normal base deficit in the setting of a low pH suggests a respiratory acidosis from which the fetus may recover rapidly. The longer the fetus is exposed to recurrent hypoxemia, necessitating anaerobic metabolism, the more buffer is consumed and the more likely the pH will fall suddenly. With recurrent stress and a growing base deficit, the temporal interval before deterioration

of fetal condition becomes progressively shorter despite apparently stable pH values.

In clinical practice, a trend of serial pH determinations correlated with the clinical setting is of greater importance than the absolute value of a single pH determination. The evaluation of base deficit as well as pH helps to distinguish between respiratory and metabolic acidosis and gives an indication of the duration of hypoxemia. It should be remembered that heart rate variability provides an important commentary on the severity of ominous periodic patterns. The fetus with normal heart rate variability and late decelerations will have a significantly higher scalp pH than will the fetus with decreased variability and late decelerations.

Maternal acidosis may occasionally cause fetal acidosis secondary to equilibration of H + ions across the placenta. When maternal acidosis is associated with fetal acidosis, the comparison of maternal and fetal base deficit can be used to distinguish the truly hypoxic fetus. A freely flowing maternal venous blood sample can be used for these analyses. In a normally oxygenated fetus, capillary pH is usually about 0.1 pH unit below the maternal value. When maternal acidosis is observed, every effort should be made to determine the etiology (e.g., sepsis, ketoacidosis, or dehydration) and appropriate correction undertaken. Maternal respiratory alkalosis associated with hyperventilation has been reported to elevate fetal pH falsely.

To collect fetal blood, the chorioamnion must be ruptured and the cervix must be sufficiently dilated, approximately 2 to 3 cm, to provide exposure to the fetal scalp. The presenting part must be sufficiently low in the pelvis to remain reasonably immobile. When the fetus is presenting as a breech, fetal blood can be obtained from the buttocks. A conical vaginal endoscope is passed through the vagina and cervix so that the small end of the endoscope comes to rest against the fetal scalp at a site not overlying a suture line or fontanel. Amniotic fluid, blood, mucus, and meconium are removed by the use of sponges on a long holder. Once the scalp is cleaned, a small amount of silicone is spread over the exposed area. The layer of silicone has two purposes: it smooths the fetal hair for easier visualization of the scalp, and it provides a smooth surface on which a globule of fetal capillary blood can form. Using a microscalpel set in a plastic guard, the fetal scalp is punctured. To aid in the collection of blood, this puncture should be performed just at the beginning of a contraction so that scalp blood flow is facilitated. A long glass heparinized capillary tube is then introduced into the endoscope, and, using gravity and capillary action, the fetal blood is collected into the capillary tube. The tube holds approximately 250 μl of blood when full. Newer instruments require only 25 to 40 μl of fetal blood for determination of pH and respiratory gases. A pH value alone may be determined with as little as 20 μl of blood.

Fetal blood sampling can be performed with the mother in the conventional dorsal lithotomy position. It can also be performed with the mother in the lateral Sims position on a flat bed. After the fetal blood sample has been collected, pressure should be applied to the puncture site by a sponge on a long holder. Pressure is continued through the completion of two contractions and the puncture site then observed through a third contraction. If there is no bleeding from the puncture site, the endoscope can be removed. However, if bleeding continues, additional pressure may be required. Rarely, pressure alone will not provide adequate hemostasis, and a metal clip may be applied across the puncture site. Cases have been reported in which an emergency cesarean delivery was required because of continued fetal hemorrhage. Such fetuses often have an unrecognized genetic or pharmacologically induced bleeding disorder.[48,49] Sampling an area of fetal scalp that has been traumatized may give a falsely low pH. Caput formation should not alter the pH.

Unless the fetal blood sample will be processed immediately, one end of the capillary tube should be stopped with sealing clay, and a small metal rod or "flea" introduced into the other end of the capillary tube. Using a magnet, the fetal blood sample should then be mixed with the heparin by moving the metal rod from one end of the tube to the other. The second end of the capillary tube should be sealed with clay and the tube placed on ice until the pH and acid–base determinations can be performed. Ideally, the equipment for these determinations should be present in a laboratory near the obstetric suite.

Until the introduction of continuous fetal heart rate monitoring during the early 1970s, fetal scalp sampling alone was used to monitor fetal well-being in known high-risk situations, including IUGR and prolonged pregnancy. Because of the intermittent nature of this technique, many fetal blood samples were needed to assess fetal condition. With the introduction of continuous fetal heart rate monitoring, fetal acid–base surveillance in labor is used mainly when the heart rate patterns are unclear or confusing or to gauge whether it is safe to continue to observe a fetus with a nonreassuring tracing whose delivery is expected to occur within a relatively short time.

Correlation of Stimulated Fetal Accelerations and Fetal pH/Buffer Evaluation

Clark et al[50] investigated the predictive value of fetal heart rate accelerations evoked by scalp stimulation at the collection of fetal capillary blood. These investigators found that during the scalp blood sampling process, when the scalp was stimulated and an acceleration of 15 bpm lasting 15 seconds occurred, the fetal pH value was almost always 7.22 or greater. Unfortunately, the reverse does not hold true, and several normal fetuses did not accelerate with scalp stimulation. Firm pressure on the fetal scalp during digital examination may be used in place of scalp blood sampling to evoke accelerations in normal fetuses.

A number of investigators have used vibro-acoustic fetal stimulation to evoke a fetal heart rate acceleration. An artificial larynx, generating 80 dB of mixed noise and vibration, is placed on the maternal abdomen approximately one-third the distance from the symphysis pubis to the xiphoid process. A stimulation interval of 2 to 5 seconds is used. This may produce a fetal heart rate acceleration. Such fetal heart rate accelerations have been associated with a fetus that is in good condition physiologically. Polzin et al[51] have demonstrated, using continuous internal fetal heart rate monitoring, that a 5-second vibro-acoustic stimulation to the fetus resulting in either a 10-bpm acceleration lasting 10 seconds or a 15-bpm acceleration lasting 15 seconds will correlate with a mean pH value of 7.29 ± 0.07. However, about 50 percent of healthy fetuses will not respond with an acceleration to this stimulation. These findings have been corroborated by several investigators.[52,53]

Thus the use of scalp or acoustic stimulation can reduce the need for more intrusive testing with scalp pH. These techniques can be used earlier in labor than scalp sampling, since they do not require rupture of the membranes. In the presence of an ambiguous fetal heart rate tracing, a scalp pH is usually unnecessary if the fetus responds to scalp or acoustic stimulation with accelerations. Scalp stimulation is especially useful to differentiate fetal sleep from acidosis when a fetal tracing shows reduced variability but no decelerations.

A recent retrospective study has suggested that the introduction of fetal stimulation tests and our current appreciation of the significance of fetal heart rate variability now obviates the need for intrapartum fetal blood sampling.[54] No increase in cesarean delivery rates, low 5-minute Apgar scores, or perinatal asphyxia was observed in a large teaching hospital with more than 14,000 deliveries annually, despite a decline in the usage of scalp pH assessment from 1.43 percent of deliveries in 1986 to 0.03 percent of births in 1992. This study had only historical controls and made no analysis of changes in other practices influencing perinatal outcome over the same time period. Since earlier demonstrations that fetal pH assessment reduces cesarean delivery rates have been made in randomized controlled trials,[22,23] caution is warranted before concluding that fetal blood sampling no longer has a role in intrapartum fetal assessment.

Fetal Pulse Oximetry

Because fetal scalp sampling is uncomfortable for the laboring patient (and presumably for the fetus) and provides only intermittent data, the possibility of a less invasive modality for monitoring fetal blood gases is intriguing. Pulse oximetry, a technique that exploits the principle that arterial oxygen saturation can be determined based on the difference in photometric characteristics of oxyhemoglobin and deoxyhemoglobin, is now widely used to monitor adults and newborns on labor floors and intensive care nurseries to decrease the need for arterial blood gases.[55] Though such a tool might be very attractive for intrapartum assessment of the fetus and is actively being investigated, there have been many technical obstacles. Because the shape of the presenting fetal part makes transmission pulse oximetry impossible, reflectance probes must be used. These instruments measure back-scattered instead of transmitted light. Obtaining good continuous contact with fetal skin is also problematic. Meconium and fetal hair make oximetry monitoring from the fetal scalp difficult. Clinical trials are in progress using a probe that is held against the fetal face or neck by the uterine

wall.[56–58] The accuracy of pulse oximetry in predicting fetal asphyxia remains to be studied. Since the oxygen content of the fetal blood fluctuates more rapidly than pH and may be less reflective of fetal status, this tool may prove clinically unwieldy.

Fetal ECG

In addition to the fetal heart rate, a fetal ECG waveform can be obtained from the fetal scalp electrode used for internal fetal monitoring, albeit with much electrical noise. Recent innovations in signal processing and filtering that improve the signal-to-noise ratio now allow meaningful information to be extracted from the fetal ECG waveform more readily. Based on animal studies showing fetal ST segment and T wave changes with hypoxia,[59,60] the incorporation of fetal ECG analysis into intrapartum fetal monitoring schemes has been proposed. Recently a large randomized trial (n = 1,200), comparing fetal heart rate monitoring alone with monitoring plus fetal ECG, found a reduction in the rate of operative deliveries for fetal distress in the ECG group.[61] No differences in neonatal outcome were observed. More extended research trials will be necessary to evaluate the clinical utility of this new fetal monitoring modality.

Umbilical Cord Acid–Base Analysis

Umbilical blood gas values are often used to relate intrapartum fetal heart rate data to acid-base status and neonatal condition at birth.[39] These data help to establish the state of fetal oxygenation at birth.[62,63] A doubly clamped, 10- to 30-cm segment of umbilical cord is obtained and, using preheparinized 1- to 2-ml syringes, samples of blood can be collected from the umbilical artery or vein. When obtainable, the umbilical artery blood gas is preferable since it more closely reflects fetal status. Samples are then analyzed for respiratory gases (see Table 14-3). Some investigators have advocated obtaining cord blood gas measurements after all deliveries.[63] These data will confirm normal acid–base status in 98 percent of vigorous newborns and nearly 80 percent of infants judged to be depressed at birth. Cord blood gas studies are most helpful when a delivery is performed for fetal distress, when the newborn is depressed, and when one delivers an infant at greater risk for subsequent neurologic handicap, for example, a premature or growth-restricted infant.

Fetal Therapy

Amnioinfusion

Amnioinfusion, the transcervical instillation of fluid into the amnioinic sac, is now widely used intrapartum to improve the intrauterine environment in settings of oligohydramnios. Amniotic fluid plays an important role in cushioning the umbilical cord from compression by contractions and fetal parts. In 1976, Gabbe et al[64] first demonstrated that oligohydramnios produced by amniotomy caused variable decelerations due to umbilical cord compression in a rhesus monkey model. Cord compression could be alleviated by infusing normal saline to restore intrauterine volume. A technique for amnioinfusion during human labor was first described in 1983 by Miyazaki and Taylor.[65] Miyazaki and Nevarez[66] later randomized laboring patients with repetitive variable decelerations to a treatment group who received amnioinfusion, and a control group managed by traditional methods of intrauterine resuscitation. Intrauterine infusion of saline eliminated the decelerations in 51 percent of treated patients, while decelerations resolved in only 4 percent of uninfused controls. The incidence of cesarean delivery for fetal distress was significantly lower in nulliparous patients who received amnioinfusion, 14.8 percent (n = 27) versus 47.6 percent (n = 21). Though the rate of cesarean delivery was also lower in infused multiparas, the difference did not reach statistical significance. These authors suggested that amnioinfusion might benefit the fetus by diluting meconium, in addition to reducing cord compression.

Several studies of amnioinfusion in patients with meconium support this hypothesis. Wenstrom and Parsons[67] randomized laboring patients with thick meconium but normal fetal pH to amnioinfusion and control groups. They found less meconium below the vocal cords and a lower incidence of operative delivery following amnioinfusion. In a similar study Sadovsky et al[68] reported that amnioinfusion reduced the incidence of umbilical artery pH less than 7.2; it also reduced the number of infants with meconium below the cords or requiring positive pressure ventilation. Reduction in neonatal morbidity in pregnancies complicated by meconium has since been confirmed by several groups of investigators.[69–72] Other studies suggest that intrapartum amnioinfusion may be of benefit when oligohydramnios is diagnosed even before variable decelerations or thick meconium are noted.[73–75] In the largest investigation of prophylactic amnioinfusion, Schrimmer et al[75] randomized 305 patients with a low amniotic fluid index (less than 5 cm) to amnioinfusion or routine care. The treated patients had fewer operative interventions for fetal distress, fewer cesarean deliveries, and higher umbilical artery pHs than the control patients.

Protocols used for amnioinfusion vary in detail, but differences are probably not of great clinical significance. Normal saline is the fluid most commonly used, though one investigation using sheep fetuses found that lactated Ringers produced less change in fetal sodium and chloride concentrations than normal saline infusion,[76] Nageotte et al[74] did not find any disturbance of electrolytes in human fetuses exposed to normal saline amnioinfusion. Initially 250 to 1,000 ml of fluid is infused at a rate of 10 to 15 ml/min via an intrauterine pressure catheter. Though some investigators assessed amniotic fluid index by ultrasound to judge the adequacy of volume replacement, in clinical practice a predetermined volume or the resolution of variable decelerations is usually used as the endpoint. The initial fluid volume is followed by a continuous infusion of 100 to 200 ml/h by pump or by gravity drainage to replace fluid leaking out during contractions. If fluid is administered more rapidly than 15 ml per minute, it should be warmed to body temperature. Intrauterine pressure can be monitored via the same intrauterine pressure catheter,[66] a second one, or a double lumen catheter.

Complications of amnioinfusion appear to be very rare and have recently been surveyed by Wenstrom et al[77] Uterine tone may increase with amnioinfusion, and hypertonus has been reported, illustrating the importance of monitoring intrauterine pressure, volume infused, and volume leaking out. Prolonged fetal bradycardia has been reported following rapid infusion (50 ml/min) of unwarmed fluid. Maternal respiratory failure and amniotic fluid embolism have been described in patients receiving amnioinfusion, but it is not clear whether these were the result of the infusion per se or other risk factors. A statistically nonsignificant trend toward increased amnionitis or neonatal sepsis has been reported in some studies,[73,75] though most report reduced risk of endometritis, probably because of reduced rates of cesarean delivery. It is not clear whether increased risk of amniotic fluid embolus or amnionitis should be attributed to amnioinfusion or to other risk factors, including the placement of an intrauterine pressure catheter per se.

Tocolysis

The primary stress that the fetus must tolerate during labor is the contraction itself, because it decreases perfusion of the intervillous space and compresses the uterine contents. Excessive uterine activity can produce hypoxic or reflex fetal heart rate decelerations, loss of variability, or baseline changes. When possible, resuscitation of the fetus in utero by reducing uterine activity to a level that the fetus is able to tolerate is preferable to operative delivery at a time when the pH may be low and the P_{CO_2} elevated. One or two parenteral injections of tocolytic agents such as 0.25 mg of subcutaneous terbutaline or 4 to 6 g of intravenous magnesium sulfate[78] can be used for this purpose. Although the response of the worrisome fetal heart rate pattern to this therapy may be used to judge fetal status, assessment of fetal acid–base status may be advisable especially if normal heart rate variability is not fully restored. Using tocolysis in this manner, a significant number of cesarean deliveries can be avoided. Even when it has been decided to proceed to cesarean delivery for fetal distress, a single injection of a tocolytic agent will frequently reduce uterine activity, thereby allowing some recovery before delivery occurs.

Management of Nonreassuring Fetal Heart Rate Patterns

In an effort to reduce intrapartum hypoxia, it seems reasonable to use and integrate all available fetal data-collecting systems. Because the diagnostic accuracy of continuous fetal heart rate monitoring in confirming fetal well-being is no less than 98 percent, it is logical to use this as the primary system. However, since fetal heart rate monitoring is less able to identify the fetus that is truly in distress, it also appears reasonable to add intermittent fetal capillary blood collection for acid–base values to supplement fetal heart rate monitoring. Using both systems, the diagnostic accuracy for *fetal compromise* approaches that for the diagnosis of well-being using fetal heart rate only. In the ideal setting, the obstetrician should be intimately familiar with both techniques. A protocol for intrapartum monitoring with fetal heart rate evaluation supplemented by acid–base determinations is given below. Although in some instances conservative, it is within the ability of most obstetric units. When followed, this protocol has the potential to reduce the number of fetuses born in an asphyxiated condition without significantly increasing unnecessary intervention.

General Principles

1. Patients at high risk for uteroplacental insufficiency (e.g., in settings of prolonged pregnancy, IUGR, oligohydramnios, meconium-stained fluid) should be monitored continuously. After rupture of the membranes, a fetal scalp electrode should be placed to assess fetal heart rate variability more accurately.
2. If an external technique is in use and there is flattening of the baseline or decelerations, an internal electrode should be placed to assess true heart rate variability and to better correlate the timing of decelerations with uterine contractions.
3. For a mixed fetal heart rate pattern, the patient should be managed according to the most ominous pattern.
4. If there is an abnormal fetal heart rate pattern, such as a confusing pattern, late or severe variable decelerations, a baseline tachycardia, or loss of variability, a fetal stimulation test should be done. If the fetus

does not respond with an acceleration or the abnormal pattern persists, a fetal scalp capillary blood sample should be obtained for acid–base determination. (Figs. 14-18 and 14-19)
5. In the presence of maternal fever, a satisfactory fetal capillary blood determination should not be relied on solely as an indication of fetal well-being. Sepsis may cause fetal compromise despite a normal pH.

Management of Fetal Heart Rate Patterns

Early Deceleration

In the vast majority of patients with early decelerations, the deceleration's nadir does not fall below 100 bpm. This pattern is usually associated with uncomplicated labor and delivery, and thus no intervention is in order. If the maximal deceleration falls below 100 bpm and is repetitive, a vaginal examination should be performed to check for a prolapsed cord. In the absence of cord prolapse this fetal heart rate pattern may be observed with subsequent contractions and managed expectantly in a fashion similar to a variable pattern.

Late Deceleration

With repetitive late decelerations, the following steps to improve delivery of oxygen to the intervillous space should be initiated:

1. If oxytocin is in use, discontinue it. After appropriate reevaluation, if the pattern has corrected, oxytocin may be restarted.
2. Start oxygen at 6 to 8 L/min with a tight-fitting face mask.
3. Change the maternal position (e.g., supine to left or right lateral, elevate legs, knee-chest).
4. Check maternal blood pressure; if the mother is hypotensive, correct the hypotension as follows:
   a. Increase the rate of administration of electrolyte-containing intravenous fluids.
   b. If the hypotension is thought to be secondary to regional anesthesia, consult with an obstetric anesthesiologist regarding the possible use of a vasopressive agent (e.g., ephedrine 15 mg IV).
5. If the late decelerations are attributable to other maternal problems that adversely affect the fetus, such as maternal hypoxia, ketoacidosis, or sickle cell crisis, measures to correct the underlying condition should also be taken. If these are not promptly remediable, delivery may be indicated (when safe for the mother) even if fetal pH proves normal.

The heart rate tracing should be assessed for variability during and between late decelerations. If variability

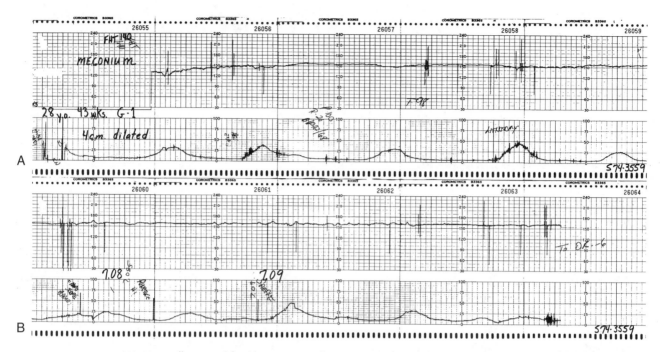

Fig. 14-18 (A) Essentially normal fetal heart rate and uterine activity are noted in this nullipara at 43 weeks with meconium. No periodic patterns are noted, but minimal heart rate variability is seen. (B) Because of the fetal metabolic acidosis that may occur in this setting, a baseline fetal capillary pH was obtained on two occasions (panels 26060 and 26061). The values were 7.08 and 7.09. Thereafter, this patient was quickly delivered by cesarean section. In this case, fetal capillary scalp sampling clearly benefited the fetus.

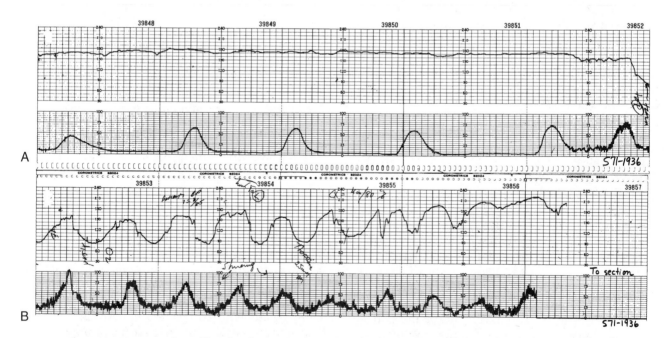

Fig. 14-19 (A) Unexplained baseline fetal tachycardia. Heart rate variability is poor. The patient suffered a shaking chill (panel 39852), as reflected in the "jitteriness" of the uterine activity tracing. (B) With the chill, and presumably with increased maternal oxygen consumption, severe late decelerations occurred. A baseline fetal scalp pH performed earlier may have been helpful in the management of this case.

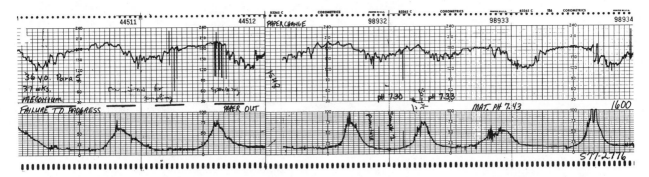

Fig. 14-20 Internal monitoring shows baseline tachycardia with persistent late decelerations. Good variability is present, and uterine activity is not excessive. Since the fetal capillary pH is still reassuring (7.30 and 7.33, panel 98932) it is reasonable to attempt to correct the pattern before delivery.

is normal and accelerations are present or can be stimulated, the fetus is unlikely to be acidotic and time may be allowed for recovery of the tracing following the conservative maneuvers described above (Fig. 14-20.) If the fetal heart rate pattern does not normalize, or if there is poor variability, fetal capillary blood should be collected to assess fetal acid–base status. Fetal samples may be collected using maternal positions other than the dorsolithotomy position, to avoid supine hypotension and decreased uterine perfusion.

1. If the fetal pH is in the pathologic range (less than 7.20), prompt delivery should be undertaken by the method that is quickest and safest for both mother and fetus.
2. If the fetal pH is in the prepathologic range (7.20 to 7.24) but the late deceleration pattern persists, another pH should be obtained in 15 to 20 minutes. If the pH is falling or the base deficit is large, the patient should be delivered promptly.
3. If the late deceleration pattern persists, but fetal acid-base status is satisfactory and it is decided to allow labor to continue, confirmation of satisfactory fetal acid-base status must be determined at 20-minute intervals as long as late decelerations are observed and scalp or acoustic stimulation does not produce accelerations. If repetitive scalp sampling cannot be done, delivery of the fetus is in order (Figs. 14-20 and 14-21). The use of a tocolytic agent such as intravenous ritodrine or subcutaneous terbutaline to arrest labor and allow recovery of the fetus before delivery is often useful.

Variable Deceleration

When variable decelerations are mild and not repetitive, the pattern is usually associated with good fetal outcome. However, variable decelerations may worsen as labor progresses. Amnioinfusion should be initiated

if variables are recurrent. It is preferable to begin an amnioinfusion before variables are severe because 20 to 30 minutes are needed to instill adequate fluid. If decelerations become repetitive, fall below 90 bpm at their nadir, and last longer than 60 seconds, fetal condition can deteriorate. This type of pattern most often occurs during the late first and the second stages of labor. When an ominous variable deceleration pattern is present, the following steps should be initiated:

1. If oxytocin is in use, discontinue it. When the pattern has been corrected and after appropriate reevaluation, oxytocin may be restarted.
2. Unless clinically contraindicated (e.g., suspected placenta previa), a vaginal examination should be performed immediately to check for a prolapsed cord and to determine the progress of labor.
3. Maternal hypotension should be identified and corrected.
4. Maternal position should be changed (consider left lateral, right lateral, Trendelenburg, reverse Trendelenburg, or knee-chest).
5. Oxygen is started at 6 to 8 L/min with a tight-fitting face mask.
6. If uterine activity is excessive, the use of intravenous tocolysis with terbutaline or magnesium sulfate may be considered.
7. If the patient is in the second stage, postponing pushing for a few contractions may give the fetus a chance to recover.

If these management measures do not correct the pattern and if the variable decelerations worsen, the obstetrician should:

1. Prepare for delivery by the method that is quickest and safest for both mother and fetus (i.e., alert the operating room, shave the abdomen, and so forth).
2. Assess fetal acid–base status by a stimulation test or

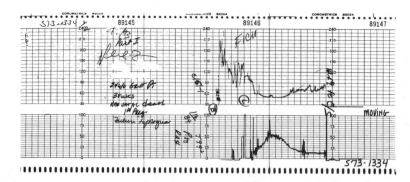

Fig. 14-21 In preparation for oxytocin augmentation of labor for failure to progress, an internal pressure catheter was placed and an electrode attached to the fetal scalp. Note that with the attachment of the fetal electrode the fetal heart rate suddenly decelerates to approximately 50 bpm, with a slow and irregular return. Some fetuses are very sensitive to manipulation of the scalp and can have a sudden prolonged deceleration mediated by the vagus nerve. This patient was taken to the operating room and observed. The fetal heart rate returned to a normal level in a few minutes, and subsequently the patient was vaginally delivered of a healthy baby.

by analysis of fetal capillary blood. Care should be exercised to obtain the fetal capillary blood sample *after* the deceleration has returned to the baseline and just before the next contraction. There is rapid diffusion of CO_2 across the placenta. With the alleviation of cord compression, wide variations in fetal pH values may occur, depending on the timing of scalp sampling. Caution must therefore be taken in interpreting the values. Because the initial respiratory acidosis of variable decelerations may shortly progress to a metabolic acidosis unless cord compression is corrected, pH, P_{CO_2}, and a base deficit represent useful fetal blood determinations in the management of these cases.

3. If the fetus does not have a metabolic acidemia, immediate delivery can be delayed if a safe vaginal delivery is expected within 20 to 30 minutes, unless the fetal heart rate pattern worsens acutely.

Prolonged Sudden Deceleration

Occasionally, an unexpected and often unexplained prolonged deceleration may occur. The fetal heart rate will drop below 80 bpm, and the deceleration can last several minutes. Though occasionally triggered by a vagal discharge in response to fetal manipulation (Fig. 14-21), such sudden prolonged decelerations usually result from a mechanism that can cause fetal hypoxia, notably:

1. Uterine hyperactivity, usually oxytocin related (Fig. 14-22)
2. Conduction anesthesia with hypotension (Fig. 14-23)
3. Supine hypotension
4. Unrelieved cord compression
5. Maternal respiratory arrest (convulsions, high spinal anesthesia, intravenous narcotics) (Fig. 14-24)

Should a prolonged sudden deceleration occur, the following steps should be instituted:

1. Consider the causes of prolonged decelerations and attempt to correct them, including using tocolytic therapy for excessive uterine activity.
2. Change maternal position until an effective position is found.
3. Perform a vaginal examination, unless contraindicated, to check for cord prolapse and the progress of labor.
4. Institute oxygen at 6 to 8 L/min with a tight-fitting face mask.
5. Increase the infusion of intravenous fluids.

If these measures do not resolve the problem and vaginal delivery is not imminent after 5 minutes of a fetal heart rate at 60 bpm, cesarean delivery is indicated. If these steps do alleviate the deceleration, assessment of fetal acid–base status by a fetal stimulation test or by fetal and maternal acid–base determinations should be obtained 10 to 15 minutes after the fetal heart rate has recovered. If the fetal pH is below 7.25, a second sample should be obtained within 15 minutes or until the pH is above 7.25.

After recovery careful observation of the fetal heart rate should be maintained. If the deceleration should occur a second or third time, corrective measures need to be instituted and preparation for immediate delivery undertaken. If at all possible, delivery should be accomplished 10 to 15 minutes into the recovery period to allow the fetus to benefit from intrauterine resuscitation.

Sinusoidal Fetal Heart Rate Pattern

If a sinusoidal pattern occurs and is unrelated to the administration of narcotics, a fetal blood sample for acid–base determination should be obtained. A fetal

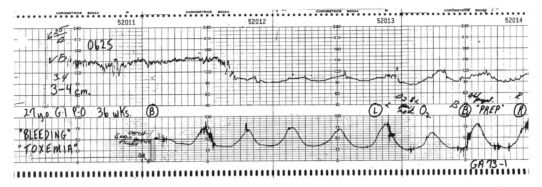

Fig. 14-22 Internal monitoring is used for this nullipara at 36 weeks with pregnancy-induced hypertension and bleeding. Internal monitoring demonstrates good heart rate variability. The intrauterine pressure catheter, following appropriate calibration (panel 52011), demonstrates an elevated resting tone (30 mmHg) and frequent contractions, suggesting placental abruption. Note that the heart rate falls in panel 52012, and the patient is taken to the operating room for cesarean delivery, where a "total abruption" was found.

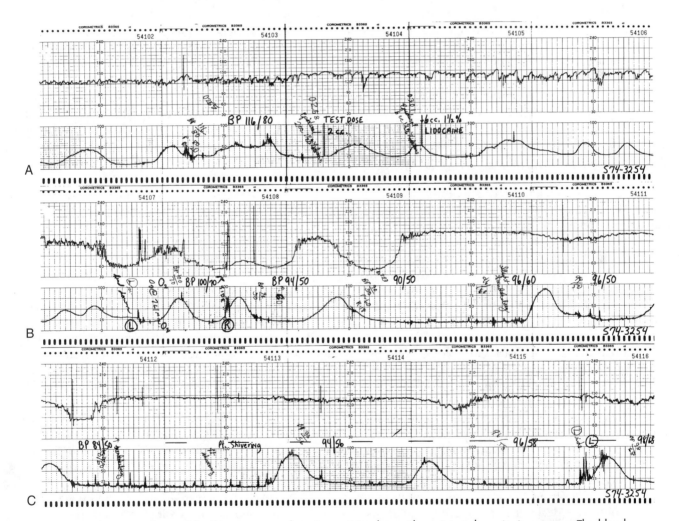

Fig. 14-23 (A) Normal fetal heart rate and uterine activity data with an internal monitoring system. The blood pressure is normal, and a test dose of a local anesthetic agent is used in preparation for epidural anesthesia. Approximately 3.5 minutes after the test dose, additional local anesthetic is administered. (B) Heart rate decelerations are noted (panels 54107 to 54109), along with a fall in maternal blood pressure. These decelerations appear to be of both reflex and hypoxic etiologies. Heart rate variability is reduced in panel 54110 and remains so throughout the remainder of the tracing. (C) Late decelerations are seen in panels 54111 to 54116. Similar heart rate changes may be noted after administration of a paracervical block.

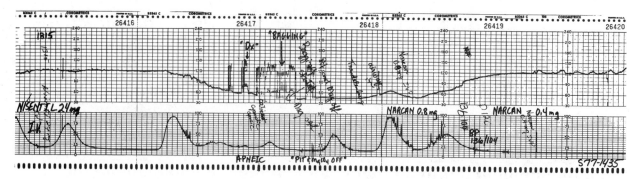

Fig. 14-24 Before this recording, the patient had received the narcotic analgesic Nisentil. An additional dose of 24 mg was given intravenously at the onset of this tracing, followed by a marked fall in fetal heart rate in panel 26417. The patient had suffered a respiratory arrest because of the Nisentil, and the change in fetal heart rate can be attributed to hypoxia. The mother was intubated and "bagged" to reestablish respiration. The narcotic antagonist Narcan was administered, and, with the establishment of normal maternal respiration, the fetal heart rate returned to a normal level.

hematocrit may also be performed to detect the presence of fetal anemia. If abnormal values are found, immediate delivery should be considered. The neonatal staff should also be informed of the fetal blood values, so that they can prepare for immediate newborn resuscitation and/or transfusion.

Risk Versus Benefit of Continuous Electronic Fetal Monitoring

While there is ample scientific data indicating that cord compression, fetal hypoxia, and acidosis can produce characteristic fetal heart rate patterns (variable decelerations, late decelerations, and decreased variability) and that these patterns can be more readily appreciated using continuous electronic monitoring rather than intermittent auscultation, it remains hotly debated whether the clinical application of continuous electronic fetal monitoring improves neonatal outcome. Transient episodes of fetal hypoxia, often associated with nonreassuring fetal heart rate tracing patterns, occur commonly during labor and are usually well tolerated by the fetus. Normal labor is associated with a gradual decline in pH, often to levels that would indicate profound acidosis in an older infant. Determining when to interrupt a labor based on the fetal heart rate tracing is not just a question of acknowledging a nonreassuring pattern. Despite the enormous expectations for improvement in perinatal outcomes following the introduction of electronic fetal heart rate monitoring, and the observed decline of intrapartum stillbirths since that time, only 1 trial[25] of 12 randomized controlled trials[22–25,79–86] published over the past 20 years has shown a statistically significant reduction in perinatal mortality, and only a few have shown a reduction in neonatal morbidity in patients monitored continuously.

The largest well-randomized trial, performed at Dublin's National Maternity Hospital between 1981 and 1983, compared continuous internal monitoring with auscultation every 15 minutes in the first stage of labor and after each contraction in the second stage.[23] More than 6,000 patients were enrolled in each arm of the trial. No differences were found in intrapartum or neonatal death rates or in low Apgar scores. A twofold higher rate of neonatal seizures and abnormal neonatal neurologic examinations were observed in the auscultation group. However, in a 4-year follow-up study there were no differences between the groups in the incidence of cerebral palsy.[87] Poor correlation between nonreassuring fetal heart rate patterns and cerebral palsy has been documented in a number of other studies.[88–90] In a recent study, Nelson and colleagues found that the odds ratio was 3.6 (CI 1.9–6.7) for moderate to severe cerebral palsy in patients with an abnormal fetal heart rate tracing in labor. In this study, an abnormal tracing was defined as one in which late decelerations or decreased variability was documented in the chart by the obstetrician caring for the patient. However, only 0.19 percent of term infants with abnormal heart rate patterns in labor developed cerebral palsy.[91]

Thacker and colleagues[92] have recently published an excellent meta-analysis of randomized trials of monitoring techniques, scoring them for quality, and discussing their clinical relevance. Overall they found significantly fewer 1-minute Apgar scores below 4 (relative risk [RR] is 0.82; 95 percent confidence interval [CI] is 0.65 to 0.98) and neonates with early seizures (RR is 0.50; 95 percent CI is 0.30 to 0.82) in the monitored groups. While continuous monitoring had no significant effect on risk for perinatal death, there was a significant protective effect in trials conducted outside the United States. (RR is 21, 95 percent CI is 0.12 to 0.29).

An increase in the frequency of cesarean delivery due

to the introduction of fetal monitoring has been frequently cited in the lay as well as the scientific press. This has been attributed to the immobilization of the parturient imposed by the monitor, as well as to overzealous interventions in response to abnormal heart rate tracings. Though cesarean delivery rates have been higher in the monitored arm of several randomized controlled trials,[22,25,80,82,83] more detailed scrutiny suggests this is not an inevitable result of electronic monitoring. Comparing cesarean delivery and monitoring with cesarean delivery and auscultation, Thacker et al[92] found a relative risk of only 1.22 (CI is 1.04 to 1.39) in data from all nine applicable trials. They noted that no difference was found in the best designed studies. In their cumulative meta-analysis, the relative risk declined as newer studies were added. Furthermore, there was no difference in trials in which fetal scalp sampling was combined with monitoring.

The inability of randomized controlled trials to show statistically significant reduction in perinatal mortality does not adequately tell the story of electronic fetal monitoring's impact. Over the two decades since electronic monitoring became widely applied, perinatal mortality has fallen due to many changes in intrapartum and neonatal care.[92–95] Therefore, further reduction in the already low rates of death due to asphyxia will be difficult to achieve. It is interesting that perinatal outcomes were improved with electronic fetal monitoring in recent randomized controlled trials in less-developed nations.

Electronic fetal monitoring has altered our training of physicians and nurses and the staffing patterns of our labor floors. Though frequent intermittent auscultation performed well in many randomized controlled trials, nursing and midwifery support was also optimized in these studies. Thus, the studies document the potential efficacy of intermittent auscultation, but may overestimate its effectiveness in clinical practice. It is interesting that the intrapartum death rate was lower in both monitored and unmonitored groups during the period of the Dublin study[23] than during the period immediately preceding the trial, and it was lower not only than the rates in patients excluded from the study because of oligohydramnios and meconium (11.4/1,000) but also lower than in those excluded because of rapid labors (3.5/1,000). Similarly, in the study performed in Zimbabwe,[85] the introduction of research midwives on the labor floor appeared to improve outcomes independently of the monitoring mode. These data suggest a possible improvement of overall care due to participation in a study itself, which may have obscured the potential benefits from external fetal monitoring as used in clinical practice. We should therefore proceed cautiously if we wish to reverse the trend toward universal electronic fetal monitoring.

We have learned an enormous amount about fetal pathophysiology by the introduction of electronic fetal monitoring. The importance of fetal heart rate variability was previously unknown. The recognition of different types of decelerative patterns and our understanding of their etiologies has greatly improved as a result of continuous monitoring. Studies of the correlation between fetal heart rate patterns and blood gases have decreased the need for fetal scalp sampling. This knowledge permeates our current management of the conduct of labor, and knowledge about fetal heart patterns gleaned from electronic fetal monitoring now influences our interpretation of auscultated heart rate. We have learned that the prevention of intrapartum stillbirths and depressed neonates is a reasonable goal for intrapartum monitoring of whatever type, but that the eradication of cerebral palsy is not. If we apply what has been discovered carefully, we should be able to use electronic monitoring in a selective and intelligent manner, minimizing unnecessary interventions, while identifying most fetuses in jeopardy.

Key Points

- Normal fetal heart rate is between 120 and 160 bpm. The fetal heart rate is under CNS control through sympathetic and parasympathetic reflexes mediated through the vagus.

- Normal fetal heart rate variability consists of a beat-to-beat variation in rate of 3 to 5 bpm (short-term variability) and longer term fluctuations of 5 to 20 bpm with three to five cycles per minute.

- Labor presents a challenge to fetoplacental oxygen and carbon dioxide exchange because contractions reduce intervillous flow and may compress the umbilical cord.

- Normal fetal capillary pH is 7.25 to 7.40. During the course of normal labor there is a gradual decline in fetal pH.

- Loss of fetal heart rate variability can indicate hypoxia but may also be produced by fetal sleep, drugs that depress the CNS, fetal arrhythmias, and cardiac or CNS anomalies.

- In the presence of normal heart rate variability with spontaneous or induced accelerations of more than 15 bpm lasting at least 15 seconds, fetal acidemia is extremely unlikely regardless of the presence of decelerations.

- External fetal monitors use ultrasound detection of valve movement to assess fetal heart rate and may give a false impression of beat-to-beat (short-term) variability when little is present. The absence of variability in a tracing from an external monitor is reliable.

- In the presence of oligohydramnios or meconium, intrapartum amnioinfusion (instillation of fluid into the amniotic sac via an intrauterine pressure catheter) has been shown to reduce the rates of cesarean delivery for fetal distress and of meconium aspiration syndrome.

- Late decelerations are indicative of hypoxia produced by decreased intervillous exchange of respiratory gases during contractions. Variable decelerations are drops in fetal heart rate caused by umbilical cord compression that increases vagal discharge. They are characterized by abrupt onset and resolution. If they are prolonged, a mixed pattern combining features of late deceleration with those of variables may be produced.

- Though there is correlation between abnormal fetal heart rate patterns and neurologic depression at birth, fetal heart rate patterns are poor predictors of long-term neurologic sequelae.

References

1. American College of Obstetricians and Gynecologists: Fetal distress and birth asphyxia. Committee Opinion 137, ACOG, Washington DC, 1994

2. Barcroft J: Researches on Pre-natal Life. Charles C Thomas, Springfield IL, 1947

3. Barron DH: The exchange of the respiratory gases in the placenta. Neonatal Stud 1:3, 1952

4. Apgar V: A proposal for a new method of evaluation of the newborn infant. Curr Res Anesth Analg 32:260, 1953

5. Freda V: Hemolytic disease. Clin Obstet Gynecol 16:72, 1973

6. James LS, Weisbrot IM, Prince CE et al: The acid–base status of human infants in relation to birth asphyxia and the onset of respiration. J Pediatr 52:379, 1958

7. Myers RE: Two patterns of perinatal brain damage and their conditions of occurrence. Am J Obstet Gynecol 112: 246, 1972

8. Saling E: Neues Vorgehen zur Untersuchung des Kindes unter der Gebrut. Arch Gynakol 197:108, 1961

9. Hammacher K, Huter KA, Bokelmann J et al: Foetal heart frequency and perinatal condition of foetus and newborn. Gynaecologia (Basel) 166:348, 1968

10. Hon EH, Quilligan EJ: The classification of fetal heart rate. II. A revised working classification. Conn Med 31: 779, 1967

11. Caldeyro-Barcia R, Casacuberta C, Busros R et al: Correlation of intrapartum changes in fetal heart rate with fetal blood oxygen and acid–base balance. p. 205. In Adamsons K (ed): Diagnosis and Treatment of Fetal Disorders. Springer-Verlag, New York, 1968

12. Fenton AN, Steer CM: Fetal distress. Am J Obstet Gynecol 83:354, 1962

13. Miller FC, Sacks DA, Yeh S-Y: Significance of meconium during labor. Am J Obstet Gynecol 130:473, 1978

14. Dawes GS, Handler JJ, Mott JC: Some cardiovascular responses in foetal, newborn and adult rabbits. J Physiol (Lond) 139:123, 1957

15. Assali NS, Holm L, Parker H: Regional blood flow and vascular resistance in response to oxytocin in the pregnant sheep and dog. J Appl Physiol 16:1087, 1961

16. Hon EH: The electronic evaluation of the fetal heart rate. Am J Obstet Gynecol 75:1215, 1958

17. Miller FC, Pearse KE, Paul RH: Fetal heart rate pattern recognition by the method of auscultation. Obstet Gynecol 64:332, 1984

18. Wood C, Lumbley J, Renou P: A clinical assessment of foetal diagnostic methods. J Obstet Br Commonw 74: 823, 1967

19. Beard RW: Fetal blood sampling. Br J Hosp Med 3:523, 1970

20. Hon EH, Khazin AF: Biochemical studies of the fetus. II. Fetal pH and Apgar scores. Obstet Gynecol 33:237, 1969

21. American College of Obstetricians and Gynecologists: Fetal Heart Rate Patterns: Monitoring, Interpretation, and Management. Technical Bulletin 207. Washington, DC, ACOG, 1995

22. Haverkamp AD, Orleans M, Langendoerfer S et al: A

controlled trial of the differential effects of intrapartum fetal monitoring. Am J Obstet Gynecol 134:399, 1979

23. MacDonald D, Grant A, Sheridan-Pereira M et al: The Dublin randomized controlled trial of intrapartum fetal heart rate monitoring. Am J Obstet Gynecol 152:524, 1985

24. Luthy DA, Shy KK, van Belle G et al: A randomized trial of electronic fetal monitoring in preterm labor. Obstet Gynecol 69:687, 1987

25. Vintzileos AM, Antsaklis A, Varvarigos IV et al: A randomized trial of intrapartum electronic fetal heart rate monitoring versus intermittent auscultation. Obstet Gynecol 81:899, 1993

26. Ledger WJ: Complications associated with invasive monitoring. Semin Perinatol 2:187, 1978

27. Gassner CB, Ledger WJ: The relationship of hospital acquired infection to invasive intrapartum monitoring techniques. Obstet Gynecol 126:33, 1976

28. Gibbs RS, Listwa HM, Read JA: The effect of internal fetal monitoring on maternal infection following cesarean section. Obstet Gynecol 48:653, 1976

29. Schifferli P, Caldeyro-Barcia R: Effects of atropine and beta adrenergic drugs on the heart rate of the human fetus. p. 264. In Boreus L (ed): Fetal Pharmacology. Raven Press, New York, 1973

30. Martin CB: Physiology and clinical use of fetal heart rate variability. Clin Perinatol 9:339, 1982

31. Zalar RW Jr, Quilligan EJ: The influence of scalp sampling on the cesarean section rate for fetal distress. Am J Obstet Gynecol 123:206, 1975

32. Paul RH, Suidan AK, Yeh SY et al: Clinical fetal monitoring. VII. The evaluation and significance of intrapartum baseline fetal heart rate variability. Am J Obstet Gynecol 123:206, 1975

33. Hutson JM, Mueller-Heubach E: Diagnosis and management of intrapartum reflex fetal heart rate changes. Clin Perinatol 9:325, 1982

34. Martin CB, de Haan J, van der Wildt B et al. Mechanisms of late deceleration in the fetal heart rate, a study with autonomic blocking agents in fetal lambs. Eur J Obstet Gynecol Reprod Biol 9:361, 1979

35. Saling E: Technik der endoskopischen microblutentnahme am feten. Geburtshilfe Frauenheilkd 24:464, 1964

36. Adamsons K, Beard RW, Cosmi EV et al: The validity of capillary blood in the assessment of the acid–base state of the fetus. p. 175. In Adamsons K (ed): Diagnosis and Treatment of Fetal Disorders. Springer-Verlag, New York, 1968

37. Bowe ET, Beard RT, Finster M et al: Reliability of fetal blood sampling. Am J Obstet Gynecol 107:279, 1970

38. Beard RW, Morris ED, Clayton SG: pH of fetal capillary blood as an indication of the condition of the fetus. J Obstet Gynaecol Br Commonw 74:812, 1967

39. Wilble JL, Petrie RH, Koons A et al: The clinical use of umbilical cord acid–base determinations in perinatal surveillance and management. Clin Perinatol 9:387, 1982

40. Kubli FW, Hon EH, Khazin AF et al: Observations on heart rate and pH in the human fetus during labor. Am J Obstet Gynecol 104:1190, 1969

41. Low JA, Cox MJ, Karchmar EJ et al: The prediction of intrapartum fetal metabolic acidosis by fetal heart rate monitoring. Am J Obstet Gynecol 139:299, 1981

42. Tejani N, Mann N, Bhakthavathsalan A, Weiss R: Correlation of fetal heart rate–uterine contraction patterns with fetal scalp blood pH. Obstet Gynecol 46:392, 1975

43. Tejani N, Mann L, Bhakthavathsalan A: Correlation of fetal heart rate patterns and fetal pH with neonatal outcome. Obstet Gynecol 48:460, 1976

44. Beard RW, Filshie GM, Knight CA et al: The significance of the changes in the continuous fetal heart rate in the first stage of labor. J Obstet Gynaecol Br Commonw 78:865, 1971

45. Nelson KB: Perspective on the role of perinatal asphyxia in neurologic outcome; its role in developmental deficits in children. Can Med Assoc J, suppl 141:3, 1989

46. Goldaber KG, Gilstrap LC, Leveno KJ et al: Pathologic fetal acidemia. Obstet Gynecol 78:1103, 1991

47. Winkler CL, Hauth JC, Tucker JM et al: Neonatal complications at term as related to the degree of umbilical artery acidemia. Am J Obstet Gynecol 164:637, 1991

48. Mountain KR, Hirsh J, Gallus AS: Neonatal coagulation defect due to anticonvulsant drug treatment in pregnancy. Lancet 1:265, 1970

49. Webb MT, Petrie RH, Pippenger CE: Fetal circulatory collapse during induction of labor in pregnant patient with epilepsy. Am J Obstet Gynecol 130:727, 1978

50. Clark SL, Gimovsky ML, Miller FC: Fetal heart rate response to scalp blood sampling. Am J Obstet Gynecol 114:706, 1982

51. Polzin GB, Blakemore KJ, Petrie RH, Amon E: Fetal vibro-acoustic stimulation: magnitude and duration of fetal heart rate accelerations as a marker of fetal health. Obstet Gynecol 72:621, 1988

52. Smith CV, Nguyen HN, Phelan JP, Paul RH: Intrapartum assessment of fetal well-being: a comparison of fetal acoustic stimulation with acid–base determination. Am J Obstet Gynecol 155:726, 1986

53. Umstad M, Bailey C, Permezel M: Intrapartum fetal stimulation testing. Aus NZJ Obstet Gynecol 32:222, 1992

54. Goodwin TM, Milner-Masterson L, Paul RH: Elimination of fetal scalp blood sampling on a large clinical service. Obstet Gynecol 83:971, 1994

55. Bowes WA, Corke BC, Hulka J: Pulse oximetry: a review of the theory, accuracy, and clinical applications. Obstet Gynecol 74:546, 1989

56. Dildy GA, Van den Berg PP, Katz M et al: Intrapartum fetal pulse oximetry: fetal oxygen saturation trends during labor and relation to delivery outcome. Am J Obstet Gynecol 171:679, 1994

57. Luttkus A, Fengler TW, Friedmann W, Dudenhausen JW: Continuous monitoring of fetal oxygen saturation by pulse oximetry. Obstet Gynecol 85:183, 1995

58. van den Berg, Dildy GA, Luttkus A, Mason GC et al: The validity of monitoring fetal arterial oxygen saturation with pulse oximetry during labor, abstract O153. J Soc Gynecol Invest 2:213, 1995

59. Rosen KG, Kjellmer J: Changes in the fetal heart rate and ECG during hypoxia. Acta Physiol Scand 93:59, 1975

60. Greene KR, Dawes GS, Lilja H, Rosen KG: Changes in the ST waveform of the fetal lamb with hypoxemia. Am J Obstet Gynecol 144:950, 1982

61. Westgate JH, Harris M, Curnow JSH, Greene KR: Randomized trial of cardiotocography alone or with ST waveform analysis for intrapartum monitoring. Lancet 340: 194, 1992

62. Gilstrap LC, Leveno KJ, Burris J et al: Diagnosis of birth asphyxia on the basis of fetal pH, Apgar score, and newborn cerebral dysfunction. Am J Obstet Gynecol 161:825, 1989

63. Thorp JA, Sampson JE, Parisi VM, Creasy RK: Routine umbilical cord blood gas determinations? Am J Obstet Gynecol 161:600, 1989

64. Gabbe SG, Ettinger BB, Freeman RK, Martin CB: Umbilical cord compression associated with amniotomy: laboratory observations. Am J Obstet Gynecol 126:353, 1976

65. Miyazaki FS, Taylor NA: Saline amnioinfusion for relief of variable or prolonged decelerations. Am J Obstet Gynecol 146:670, 1983

66. Miyazaki FS, Nevarez F: Saline amnioinfusion for relief of repetitive variable decelerations: a prospective randomized study. Am J Obstet Gynecol 153:301, 1985

67. Wenstrom KD, Parsons MT: The prevention of meconium aspiration in labor using amnioinfusion. Obstet Gynecol 73:647, 1989

68. Sadovsky Y, Amon E, Bade M, Petrie RH: Prophylactic amnioinfusion during labor complicated by meconium: a preliminary report. Am J Obstet Gynecol 161:613, 1989

69. Cialone PR, Shere DM, Ryan RM et al: Amnioinfusion during labor complicated by particulate meconium stained fluid decreases neonatal morbidity. Am J Obstet Gynecol 170:842, 1994

70. Spong CY, Ogundipe OA, Ross MG: Prophylactic amnioinfusion for meconium stained amniotic fluid. Am J Obstet Gynecol 171:931, 1994

71. Eriksen NL, Hosteffer M, Parisi VM: Prophylactic amnioinfusion in pregnancies complicated by thick meconium. Am J Obstet Gynecol 171:1026, 1994

72. Dye T, Aubry R, Gross S, Artal R: Amnioinfusion and intrauterine prevention of meconium aspiration. Am J Obstet Gynecol 171:1601, 1994

73. Owen J, Henson BV, Hauth JC: A prospective randomized study of saline solution amnioinfusion. Am J Obstet Gynecol 162:1146, 1990

74. Nageotte MP, Bertucci L, Towers CV et al: Prophylactic amnioinfusion in pregnancies complicated by oligohydramnios: a prospective study. Obstet Gynecol 77:677, 1991

75. Schrimmer DB, Macri CJ, Paul RH: Prophylactic amnioinfusion as a treatment for oligohydramnios in laboring patients: a prospective, randomized trial. Am J Obstet Gynecol 165:972, 1991

76. Shields LE, Brace RA: Fetal electrolyte and acid–base responses to amnioinfusion: lactated Ringers versus normal saline. Proc 13th Annun Meeting SPO, February 1993

77. Wenstrom K, Andrews WW, Maher JE: Amnioinfusion survey: prevalence, protocols, and complications. Obstet Gynecol 86:572, 1995

78. Reece EA, Chervenak FA, Romero R, Hobbins JC: Magnesium sulfate in the management of acute intrapartum fetal distress. Am J Obstet Gynecol 148:104, 1984

79. Renou P, Chang A, Anderson I et al: Controlled trial of fetal intensive care. Am J Obstet Gynecol 126:470, 1976

80. Haverkamp AD, Thompson HE, McFee JG et al: The evaluation of continuous fetal heart rate monitoring in high risk pregnancy. Am J Obstet Gynecol 125:310, 1976

81. Kelso IM, Parsons RJ, Lawrence GF et al: An assessment of continuous fetal heart rate monitoring in labor: a randomized trial. Am J Obstet Gynecol 131:526, 1978

82. Wood C, Renou, Oats J et al: A controlled trial of fetal heart rate monitoring in a low-risk obstetric population. Am J Obstet Gynecol

83. Neldam S, Osler M, Hansen PK et al: Intrapartum fetal heart rate monitoring in a combined low- and high-risk population: a controlled clinical trial. Eur J Obstet Gynecol Reprod Biol 23:1, 1986

84. Leveno KJ, Cunningham FG, Nelson S et al: A prospective comparison of selective and universal electronic fetal heart rate monitoring in 34,995 pregnancies. N Engl J Med 315:615, 1986

85. Mahomed K, Nyoni R, Mulambo T et al: Randomized controlled trial of intrapartum fetal heart rate monitoring. BMJ 308:497, 1994

86. Herbst A, Ingermarsson I: Intermittent vs continuous electronic fetal monitoring in labour: a randomized study. Br J Obstet Gynaecol 101:663, 1994

87. Grant A, O'Brien N, Joy M-T et al: Cerebral palsy among children born during the Dublin randomized trial of intrapartum monitoring. Lancet II:1233, 1989

88. Editorial: Cerebral palsy, intrapartum care, and a shot in the foot. Lancet II:1251, 1989

89. Keegan KA, Waffarn F, Quilligan EJ: Obstetric characteristics and fetal heart rate patterns of infants who convulse during the newborn period. Am J Obstet Gynecol 153: 732, 1985

90. Painter MJ, Scott M, Hirsch RP et al: Fetal heart rate patterns during labor: neurologic and cognitive development at six to nine years of age. Am J Obstet Gynecol 159:854, 1988

91. Nelson KB, Dambrosia JN, Tina TY, Grether JK: Uncertain value of electronic fetal monitoring in predicting cerebral palsy. N Engl J Med 334:613, 1996

92. Thacker SB, Stroup DF, Peterson HB: Efficacy and safety of intrapartum electronic fetal monitoring: an update. Obstet Gynecol 86:613, 1995

93. Shamsi HH, Petrie RH, Steer CM: Changing obstetrical practices and amelioration of the perinatal outcome in a university hospital. Am J Obstet Gynecol 133:855, 1979

94. Rosen MG: Consensus report by the Task Force on Cesarean Childbirth. NIH, Hyattsville, MD US Department of Health and Human Services, Public Health Service, National Institutes of Health, NIH Publ 82–2067, 1981

95. Bergmans MG, Jonker GJ, Kock CLV: Fetal supraventricular tachycardia: review of the literature. Obstet Gynecol Surv 40:61, 1985

Chapter 15

Obstetric Anesthesia

Joy L. Hawkins, David H. Chestnut, and Charles P. Gibbs

The word *anesthesia* encompasses all techniques used by anesthesiologists: general anesthesia, regional anesthesia, local anesthesia, and analgesia. Traditionally, general anesthesia includes four stages during which not only sensation but also consciousness and motor and reflex activities are gradually lost. During stage I, termed *analgesia,* memory and sensitivity to pain fade, yet consciousness and protective reflexes such as swallowing and laryngeal closure persist. Inhalation analgesia may be used for vaginal delivery, commonly in combination with local infiltration or pudendal block. Alone, this degree of anesthesia is not sufficient for even minor surgical incisions, including episiotomy. Stage II, the excitement stage, borders consciousness and unconsciousness. The patient may be agitated and uncooperative. Protective laryngeal reflexes may be either hyperactive or obtunded. Anesthesiologists avoid the second stage by keeping the patient in stage I or by rapidly inducing stage III with the aid of fast-acting barbiturates and muscle relaxants. The patient must also pass through this stage on awakening. Induction of and emergence from general anesthesia are usually the most dangerous times for the patient, because marked cardiovascular, respiratory, and laryngeal reflex changes occur.

Stage III, which is used for most surgical procedures, has four planes. As anesthesia deepens, it progressively depresses the central nervous, cardiovascular, and respiratory systems. Laryngeal reflexes nearly disappear; thus vomiting or regurgitation render the patient particularly susceptible to aspiration unless her airway is protected by an endotracheal tube. Stage IV terminates in death.

Anesthesiologists can produce all stages of general anesthesia. With the proper dose, concentration, and combination of agents, a specific anesthetic technique is matched to the requirements of a given procedure. The requirements for general anesthesia for cesarean delivery differ considerably from those for craniotomy, cholecystectomy, or exploratory laparotomy for a ruptured ectopic pregnancy, yet all these patients will be rendered unconscious, immobile, and pain free.

Balanced general anesthesia is the type of general anesthesia employed for obstetrics; it usually refers to various combinations of barbiturates, inhalation agents, opioids, and muscle relaxants as opposed to high concentrations of potent inhalation agents alone. General anesthesia is used in obstetrics mainly for cesarean delivery and rarely is required for vaginal delivery.

Regional analgesia/anesthesia uses local anesthetics to provide sensory as well as various degrees of motor blockade over a specific region of the body. In obstetrics, regional techniques include major blocks, such as spinal and lumbar or caudal epidural, as well as minor blocks, such as paracervical, pudendal, and local infiltration (Fig. 15-1). In some cases, the anesthesiologist may combine a local anesthetic and opioid for epidural or spinal administration.

Pain Pathways

Pain during the first stage of labor results primarily from cervical dilatation and secondarily from uterine contractions themselves. Painful sensations travel from the uterus via visceral afferent (sympathetic) nerves that enter the spinal cord through the posterior segments of thoracic spinal nerves 10, 11, and 12 (Fig. 15-1). Pain during the second stage of labor results primarily from distention of the pelvic floor, vagina, and perineum by the presenting part of the fetus. (Some physicians contend that uterine contractions themselves may also contribute to pain during the second stage.) The sensory fibers of sacral nerves 2, 3, and 4 (i.e., the pudendal nerve) transmit painful impulses from the perineum to the spinal cord (Fig. 15-1).

Personnel

An anesthesiologist is a physician who has completed 4 years of postgraduate residency training in anesthesia. A nurse anesthetist is a registered nurse (with variable background and training) who has completed a 2-

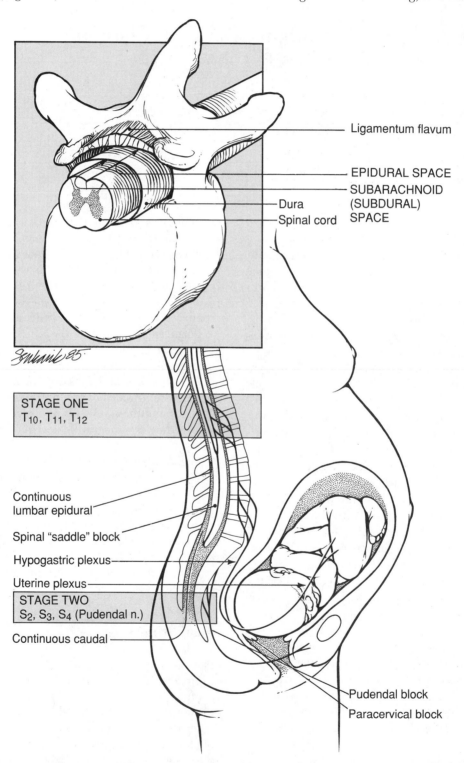

Ligamentum flavum

EPIDURAL SPACE
SUBARACHNOID (SUBDURAL) SPACE

Dura
Spinal cord

STAGE ONE
T_{10}, T_{11}, T_{12}

Continuous lumbar epidural

Spinal "saddle" block

Hypogastric plexus

Uterine plexus

STAGE TWO
S_2, S_3, S_4 (Pudendal n.)

Continuous caudal

Pudendal block
Paracervical block

Fig. 15-1 Pain pathways of labor and delivery and nerves blocked by various anesthetic techniques.

to 3-year training program sponsored by the American Association of Nurse Anesthetists. Most states require that nurse anesthetists be supervised or directed by a physician. Ideally, an anesthesiologist assumes this role, which results in an efficient anesthesiologist/anesthetist team. Such an anesthesiologist/anesthetist team provides anesthesia for 62.3 percent of operations in the United States. Anesthesiologists working independently provide anesthesia for 23.3 percent of operations. Nurse anesthetists, independent of anesthesiologists, provide anesthesia for 7.6 percent of operations, usually in smaller hospitals.[1] Almost all hospitals with more than 300 beds will have an anesthesiologist on the medical staff, while only 16 percent of hospitals with less than 50 beds will have a physician anesthesiologist available.[2] In this situation, the operating surgeon or obstetrician will, or must, assume the role of supervisor. When anesthetic-related untoward events occur, the nonanesthesiologist supervising a nurse anesthetist often will be ultimately responsible for the treatment and outcome of those events. The American Society of Anesthesiologists and the American College of Obstetricians and Gynecologists (ACOG) issued the Joint Statement on the Optimal Goals for Anesthesia Care in Obstetrics.[3] That statement recommends that there be a qualified anesthesiologist responsible for all anesthetics in every hospital providing obstetric care. The statement notes: "The administration of general or regional anesthesia requires numerous medical judgments and technical skills. Nurse anesthetists are not trained as physicians and cannot be expected to make medical decisions. Obstetricians seldom have sufficient training or experience in anesthesia to allow them to properly supervise nurse anesthetists."[3]

Pain and Stress

When considering obstetric anesthesia, reasonable questions include the following: How painful is labor? How stressful is labor? What are the effects of pain and stress? What role does anesthesia play? Melzack and colleagues[4] provided perhaps the most sophisticated, enlightened, and in-depth study of labor pain. Using the McGill Pain Questionnaire, which measures intensity and quality of pain, these investigators quantified and described the reaction of 87 nulliparous and 54 parous patients to labor pain. When pain rating index scores were assigned to each parturient's description of labor pain and compared with those of other patients suffering different kinds of pain, 59 percent of nulliparous and 43 percent of parous patients described their labor pain in terms more severe than did those suffering back and cancer pain. More than 50 percent of the obstetric patients described their pain as sharp, cramping, and intense; more than 33 percent as ach-

ing, throbbing, stabbing, shooting, heavy, and exhaustive; and 25 percent of nulliparous patients and 9 percent of parous patients as horrible or excruciating. In contrast, only 24 percent of parous patients and 9 percent of nulliparous patients described the pain as relatively minor. Although those with childbirth training reported less pain than those without such training, the differences were small. Eighty-one percent of trained patients requested epidural anesthesia compared with 82 percent of those without training. The most substantial predictors of pain intensity proved to be socioeconomic status and prior menstrual difficulties.

How does the body respond to the pain and stress of labor? Does the response affect mother, fetus, or both? Most investigators have described and quantified the body's response to stress in terms of the release of certain hormones, namely, adrenocorticotropic hormone (ACTH), cortisol, catecholamines, and β-endorphins (Fig. 15-2).

What kind of responses does labor invoke? The following have been reported: prolonged increases of plasma cortisol levels in early labor,[5] increases of both ACTH and cortisol during labor and immediately postpartum,[6] and increases in epinephrine, norepinephrine, and β-endorphins throughout labor.[7-10] These are the same responses described during other types of pain,[11] surgical stress,[12] and even hypoxia.[13,14] Thus many of the hormones associated with stress are elevated during labor.

What are the effects of these hormones on pregnancy? Elevated epinephrine levels are found in patients with anxiety and prolonged labor, which is not surprising, considering the well-known uterine relaxant effects of β-adrenergic agents.[15] Animal studies indicate that both epinephrine and norepinephrine can decrease uterine blood flow and cause fetal asphyxia.[16-18] Furthermore, these alterations may occur without clinical signs, because uteroplacental blood flow can change in the absence of heart rate and blood pressure change.[17] Maternal psychological stress can detrimentally affect the fetal cardiovascular system and acid-base status as demonstrated in baboons and monkeys.[19-21] In pregnant sheep, catecholamines increase and uterine blood flow decreases after both painful and nonpainful stimuli (Fig. 15-3). In humans, sudden noise and flashing lights predictably increase maternal heart rate. Not so predictably, fetal heart rate responds similarly within 45 seconds.[22] Fear produces similar effects.[22]

If one accepts that anxiety, pain, and labor are forms of stress and that stress may be harmful, can anesthesia, by alleviating pain, minimize the effects of that stress? Postpartum women suffer objective deficits in cognitive and memory function.[23] Intrapartum analgesia does not exacerbate, but rather *lessens* the defect compared

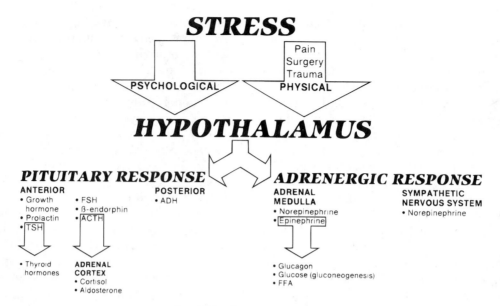

Fig. 15-2 The stress response.

with unmedicated parturients. Presumably, cognitive function is adversely affected by the stress of labor, which is mitigated by judicious use of analgesics. Epidural anesthesia prevents increases in both cortisol and 11-hydroxycorticosteroid levels during labor,[24,25] but systemically administered opioids do not.[26] Epidural anesthesia also attenuates elevations of epinephrine,[7] norepinephrine,[8] and endorphin[27] levels. Presumably, regional anesthesia blocks afferent stimuli to the hypothalamus and thus inhibits the body's response to stress[28] (Fig. 15-4).

What of the fetus? There is convincing evidence that

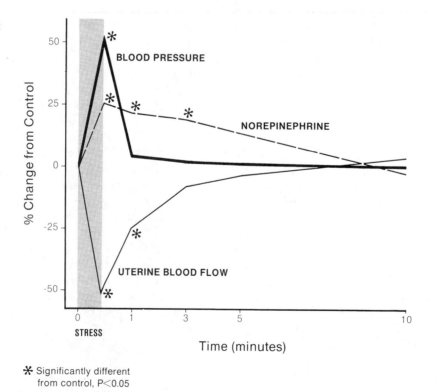

✳ Significantly different from control, P<0.05

Fig. 15-3 Effects of electrically induced stress (30 to 60 seconds) on maternal mean arterial blood pressure, plasma norepinephrine levels, and uterine blood flow. (Modified from Shnider et al.,[274] with permission.)

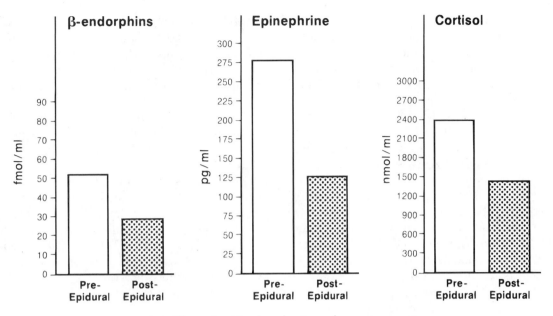

Fig. 15-4 Effects of epidural analgesia on the response to stress.

anesthesia, sedation, or both effectively decrease asphyxia-inducing effects of psychologically induced stress in monkey and baboon fetuses.[20,21,29] Furthermore, the acid-base status of human infants whose mothers receive epidural anesthesia during the first stage of labor is altered less than in infants of mothers who do not receive regional anesthesia. During the second stage of labor, the salutary effects of anesthesia may be limited to the mother.[30,31]

Anesthesia for Labor

Psychoprophylaxis

Psychoprophylaxis is a nonpharmacologic method of minimizing the perception of painful uterine contractions. Relaxation, concentration on breathing, gentle massage (effleurage), and partner participation contribute to its effectiveness. One of the method's most valuable contributions is that it is often taught in prepared childbirth classes where patients learn about the physiology of pregnancy and the normal processes of labor and delivery. In many instances, husband and wife may even visit the hospital and the labor and delivery suites before labor. Thus the fear of the unknown is largely mitigated.

Although psychoprophylactic techniques may discourage the use of drugs, not all patients are alike and not all will be satisfied with psychoprophylaxis.[32] The greatest disadvantage is the potential for believing the use of drug-induced pain relief is a sign of failure and will harm the child. Those who believe that accepting analgesia is a sign of failure do not understand that some labors are longer than others or more painful than others and that some patients have lower pain thresholds then others. Furthermore, there are times when anesthesia will be *required* for vaginal or cesarean delivery. In these instances, both mother and fetus should benefit from all that modern medicine can provide. Anyone who doubts that modern anesthetic techniques can be applied to the pregnant patient without harm to her or to her unborn child need only reflect that approximately 25 percent of all births in the United States today are cesarean births. All these patients receive anesthesia, yet few believe that such anesthesia results in harm to the fetus, and no one would suggest that these patients avoid anesthesia. If a mother is led to believe that she is a failure by "giving in" to anesthesia, which may have been indicated for forceps delivery or cesarean delivery, and her infant has a deficit resulting from an unrelated etiology, both she and her husband could believe that the anesthesia caused the problem and live the rest of their lives bearing a tragic and unnecessary sense of guilt.

Systemic Opioid Analgesia

Opioids (also known as narcotics) are drugs possessing morphine-like pharmacologic actions.[33] Morphine and codeine are natural alkaloids derived from opium, which is obtained from unripe seed capsules of the poppy plant. Opioids such as hydromorphone and heroin are semisynthetic compounds made by a simple alteration of the morphine molecule. Meperidine, alphaprodine, and fentanyl are synthetic compounds resembling morphine.[34] All opioids provide pain relief and a sense of euphoria, hence their use in obstetrics.

However, opioids also produce respiratory depression, the degree of which is usually comparable for equipotent analgesic doses. Also, all opioids freely cross the placenta to the newborn.[35-37] Therefore, the risk associated with opioids for obstetrics is obvious—all can produce respiratory depression in both mother and newborn.[38-40] Nevertheless, when used properly, they can be safe and effective.

In the past, because large doses of the long-acting opioids (e.g., morphine) were given intramuscularly throughout labor, depressant effects on the infant were observed.[41,42] Currently, morphine is rarely used for pain relief during labor. Instead, smaller doses of other opioids are used and are administered via the more predictable intravenous route. Therefore, recent reports detail little neonatal depression.[43-46] In addition, anesthesiologists recently have begun to give opioids (with or without local anesthetics) via the epidural or subarachnoid (i.e., spinal) space. Opioids may then bind to opioid receptors in the spinal cord and thereby produce segmental analgesia.

The immediate treatment for respiratory depression caused by opioids is ventilation. Infants depressed by opioids may be sleepy and may not breathe adequately. Initially they typically are not hypoxic, hypercarbic, or acidotic; however, if they are not ventilated, then hypoxia, hypercarbia, and acidosis will result. Hypoxia and acidosis (not opioids per se) may cause neonatal injury. If properly cared for, infants with opioid-induced depression will suffer no ill effects. Proper care includes ventilation, oxygenation, gentle stimulation, and the judicious use of the opioid antagonist naloxone. Positive-pressure ventilation is the single most effective measure and can be provided via face mask or intubation. Without ventilation, other measures are fruitless.

Naloxone, 0.1 mg/kg, should be given intravenously if possible, but it can be given intramuscularly or subcutaneously. This dose (i.e., 0.1 mg/kg) is higher than that previously recommended and should ensure an increased likelihood of effectiveness.[47] It may be repeated in 3 to 5 minutes if there is no immediate response. If there is no response after two or three doses, the depression is most likely not due to opioid effect.[48] Nursery personnel should be advised when naloxone has been given because it has a short duration of action, and therefore repeat administration may be necessary in the nursery. Naloxone should not be used prophylactically. Specifically, it should not be given to the mother just before delivery. Pain relief afforded the mother by the opioid will be antagonized. Furthermore, because of the unpredictability of placental transfer, it is difficult to estimate how much naloxone would get to the infant. Indeed, naloxone may not be necessary at all. It should not be given routinely to all opioid-exposed newborns.[48] Finally, naloxone should not be given to infants of opioid-dependent mothers, because this may precipitate withdrawal in the physically dependent newborn infant.[48] Naloxone is a useful drug that should be available whenever opioids are used. However, it is an adjunct to ventilation, not a substitute for it.

Opioids also may produce neurobehavioral changes in the newborn, and these changes may persist for as long as 2 to 4 days.[49-51] Although some have indicated that the effects may persist and be influential in later life, such has not been proved true.[52] In fact, the significance of neurobehavioral changes in general is open to question.

An important and significant disadvantage of opioid analgesia is the prolonged effect of these agents on gastric emptying. When parenteral or epidural opioids are used, gastric emptying is prolonged, and if general anesthesia becomes necessary, the risk of aspiration is increased.[53-55]

Morphine

Morphine is now primarily used to provide sedation and rest during the latent phase of labor. With intramuscular administration, the onset of analgesia occurs in 10 to 20 minutes and lasts for approximately 2.5 to 4 hours. With intravenous administration, the onset of analgesia is less than 3 to 5 minutes and lasts approximately 1.5 to 2 hours.[34] Occasionally, bradycardia will follow an injection of morphine. Also, histamine release may occur and result in orthostatic hypotension. One of the more frequent and bothersome side effects of morphine is nausea and vomiting. Urinary retention is also common. As with most opioids, a small amount of morphine is eliminated in the urine unchanged. The remainder is gradually detoxified by the liver.

Meperidine

Meperidine is perhaps the most commonly used opioid intrapartum; 100 mg is roughly equianalgesic to 10-mg morphine, but purportedly it has a less depressive effect on respiration.[39] Usually, 25 mg is administered intravenously, or 50 to 75 mg is given intramuscularly. Shnider and Moya[38] showed that both timing and dosage influence neonatal depression. When administered within 1 hour of delivery, little depression of Apgar scores or time to sustained respiration occurs. With a 50-mg intramuscular dose, the greatest depression occurs during the second hour; when 75 to 100 mg is administered, the depression extends through the second and third hours. Notably, when secobarbital, 100 mg, is added, depression extends even further to the fourth hour after administration.[38] The peculiar metabolism of meperidine may partially explain the lack of depression in the first hour. Part of meperidine is metabolized to an active metabolite, normeperidine. Thus, although the increase and decrease of meperidine concentrations take place immediately in both mother and fetus, the increase of the active metabolite normeperidine is slow and thereby exerts its effect on the newborn during the second hour after administration.[36,56] Furthermore, Kuhnert and colleagues[57,58] observed that multiple doses of meperidine result in greater accumulation of both meperidine and normeperidine in fetal tissues.

Intramuscularly the analgesic action of meperidine begins in approximately 10 to 20 minutes and persists for 2 to 3 hours. Lazebnik and colleagues[59] recently noted that plasma concentrations of meperidine are higher after deltoid injection than after gluteus muscle injection. They suggested that the deltoid muscle might be the preferred intramuscular site during labor. Intravenously, the onset of analgesia begins almost immediately and lasts approximately 1.5 to 2 hours. Side effects are similar to those of morphine except that tachycardia occasionally results rather than bradycardia. As with morphine, nausea and vomiting are frequent, and there is considerable delay in gastric emptying. Slightly less urinary retention occurs with meperidine than with morphine.[34]

Fentanyl

Fentanyl is a short-acting synthetic opioid with rapid pharmacokinetics and no active metabolites. In a randomized comparison with meperidine, fentanyl 50 to 100 µg every hour provided equivalent analgesia with fewer neonatal effects and less maternal sedation and nausea.[60] The main drawback of fentanyl is its short duration of action, requiring frequent redosing or the use of a patient-controlled intravenous infusion pump.[61,62]

Butorphanol

Butorphanol is a synthetic agonist/antagonist opioid analgesic drug. One to 2 mg is administered intravenously and compares favorably with 40 to 80 mg of meperidine.[43,44,63] Nausea and vomiting appear to occur less with butorphanol than with other opioids.[43,44] The major advantage is a ceiling effect for respiratory depression; that is, respiratory depression from multiple doses appears to plateau.[64,65] The major side effects are somnolence and dizziness.

Nalbuphine

Nalbuphine is another synthetic agonist/antagonist opioid. Its analgesic potency is similar to that of morphine when compared on a milligram per milligram basis. As with butorphanol, a purported advantage of nalbuphine is its ceiling effect for respiratory depression.[66] It may cause less maternal nausea and vomiting than meperidine, but it tends to produce more maternal sedation and dizziness.[67]

Patient-Controlled Opioid Analgesia

In some centers opioids are administered by patient-controlled intravenous infusion. The infusion pump is programmed to give a predetermined dose of drug upon patient demand. The physician may program the pump to include a lock-out interval (that is, there is a minimum interval between doses of drug). Thus the physician may limit the total dose administered per hour. Advantages of this method include the fact that some patients appreciate the sense of autonomy, as well as the fact that one avoids lengthy delays between doses. There are conflicting data as to whether this practice results in a decreased or increased total dose of opioid during labor.[68-70]

Sedatives

Sedatives do not possess analgesic qualities and are most often used early in labor to relieve anxiety or to augment the analgesic qualities and reduce the nausea associated with opioids. All sedatives and hypnotics cross the placenta freely. Perhaps the most important aspect of these drugs is that except for the benzodiazepines they have no known antagonists. Those most frequently used are barbiturates, phenothiazines, and benzodiazepines.

Barbiturates

Because barbiturates and other sedatives are not analgesic, patients may be less able to cope with pain than if they had received no pharmacologic assistance at all; that is, normal coping mechanisms may be blunted.[71,72] Although barbiturates can depress both cardiovascular and respiratory functions in mother and newborn, low doses have little effect. The combination of barbiturate (100 mg secobarbital) with opioid (50 to 100 mg meperidine) increases the degree of newborn depression.[38] In addition, effects that do occur may persist for a prolonged time. For example, attention span can be depressed for as long as 2 to 4 days.[73] Thus these drugs should rarely be used during labor.

Phenothiazines

Promethazine is perhaps the most widely used phenothiazine. However, propiomazine, promazine, and hydroxyzine are also commonly administered. When given in small doses in combination with an opioid, these drugs do not seem to produce additional neonatal depression.[74-76] However, like the barbiturates, these agents rapidly cross the placenta and, in large doses, can depress the fetus for a significant period. Also like the barbiturates, they have no known antagonist.

Benzodiazepines

Diazepam was the first widely used benzodiazepine. A major disadvantage of diazepam is that it disrupts temperature regulation in newborns, which renders them less able to maintain body temperature.[77] The drug may persist in the fetal circulation for as long as 1 week.[78] As with many drugs, beat-to-beat variability of the fetal heart rate is reduced markedly even with a single intravenous dose (i.e., 5 to 10 mg).[79] However, these doses have little effect on acid-base or clinical status of the newborn.[80] Sodium benzoate, a buffer in the injectable form of diazepam, competes with bilirubin binding to albumin. Thus unbound bilirubin is increased and could be a threat to infants susceptible to kernicterus.[81] Unlike diazepam, midazolam is water soluble, and it is shorter acting than diazepam.[82] There are conflicting data regarding its effects on the fetus and neonate.[83,84]

A disadvantage of all the benzodiazepines is their tendency to cause maternal amnesia. This can be a significant disadvantage if the drug is given near the time of delivery.[85] Flumazenil, a specific benzodiazepine antagonist, can reliably reverse benzodiazepine-induced sedation and ventilatory depression.[86]

Scopolamine

An anticholinergic sedative that also has amnesic effects, scopolamine has no analgesic effects and often results in total amnesia of the event. It must be used in association with sedation, usually with both narcotics and barbiturates, or bizarre behavior may result. The only place in modern obstetrics for such a regimen is in association with midtrimester loss or stillbirth when the patient requests amnesia.

Placental Transfer

Essentially, all analgesic and anesthetic agents except muscle relaxants cross the placenta readily,[87–90] and small amounts of a dose of muscle relaxant will cross. That muscle relaxants do not generally cross the placenta is one of the major factors that enables anesthesiologists to utilize general anesthesia for cesarean delivery without causing fetal paralysis.

Placental transfer of any agent begins with uptake of the agent into the bloodstream of the mother and thus distribution to all internal organs, one of which is the uterus. The distribution of uterine blood flow determines the final common pathway to the uterus and placenta. Eighty percent of uterine blood flow goes to the area of the placenta, while 20 percent goes to the myometrium and thus never comes into contact with either placenta or fetus.[91] The intermittent spurting character of the maternal spiral arterioles also prevents a portion of the drug in blood distributed to the uterus from reaching the placental circulation and fetus. Because not all of these spiral arterioles are functioning at the same time, some of the anesthetic bypasses the area of exchange and remains in the maternal circulation.

Once in the fetal circulation, a part of the drug will travel directly to the liver, where some will be "soaked up," some will be metabolized, and some will eventually reach the inferior vena cava. The other part will be shunted directly across the ductus venosus into the inferior vena cava. That portion of drug reaching the inferior vena cava will proceed to the right atrium, where some will enter the right ventricle, and hence to the pulmonary artery, where all but 10 percent will be shunted directly across the ductus arteriosus to the lower part of the systemic circulation, bypassing the cerebral circulation. The remainder of the drug that reaches the right atrium will be shunted across the foramen ovale into the left atrium, left ventricle, and out the aorta into the upper part of the fetal circulation, which includes the brain, where the greatest effect occurs. Thus, even with this very brief description of the fetal circulation, it is easy to see how the mother can be affected by a certain concentration of drug without the fetus being affected.

Factors Influencing Placental Transfer From Mother to Fetus

Drug
- Molecular weight
- Lipid solubility
- Ionization, pH of blood
- Spatial configuration

Maternal
- Uptake into bloodstream
- Distribution via circulation
- Uterine blood flow
  - Amount
  - Distribution (myometrium versus placenta)

Placental
- Circulation: intermittent spurting arterioles
- Lipoid membrane: Fick's law of simple diffusion

Fetal
- Circulation: ductus venosus, foramen ovale, ductus arteriosus

Because the placenta has the properties of a lipid membrane, most drugs and all anesthetic agents cross by a mechanism called *simple diffusion*. The physico-chemical factors governing transfer across a lipid membrane by simple diffusion is described by Fick's law.[87]

$$Q/T = [K \, A(C_m - C_f)] \, /X$$

where Q/T is the rate of diffusion, K is the diffusion constant of the drug, A is the available area, C_m is the maternal blood concentration, C_1 is the fetal blood concentration, and X is the thickness of the membrane. Thus the amount of drug that crosses the placenta increases as concentrations in the maternal circulation and total area of the membrane increase and decreases as the thickness of the membrane increases. The effective surface area of the human placenta is approximately 11 m², and its thickness is approximately 3.5 μm. The diffusion constant, K, accounts for the properties of the drug itself, including molecular weight, spatial configuration, degree of ionization, lipid solubility, and protein binding. For example, bupivacaine is highly protein bound, a characteristic that some believe explains why fetal blood concentrations of it are so much lower than with other local anesthetics. On the other hand, bupivacaine is also highly lipid soluble, and the more lipid soluble a drug is, the more freely it passes through a lipid membrane. Furthermore, once in the fetal system, lipid solubility enables the drug to be taken up by fetal tissues rapidly, which again contributes to the lower blood concentration of the agent.

The degree of ionization of a drug is also important. Most drugs exist in both an ionized and nonionized state. It is the nonionized state that freely crosses lipid membranes. Drugs such as muscle relaxants are highly ionized; thus very little crosses to the fetus. The degree of ionization is influenced by the pH of the medium. For example, local anesthetics are more ionized at lower pH values. Such factors become clinically relevant in obstetrics, because occasionally the pH of the mother's blood will be 7.4, while that of the fetus will be 7.0 or less. In this instance, the nonionized portion of the drug in the maternal circulation crosses to the fetus, becomes ionized, and thus remains in the fetus (Fig. 15-5).[92]

Lumbar Epidural Analgesia/Anesthesia

Epidural blockade is a major regional anesthetic technique in which local anesthetic is injected into the epidural space. Epidural blockade may be used to provide *analgesia* during labor or surgical *anesthesia* for vaginal or cesarean delivery. A large-bore needle (16-, 17-, or 18-gauge) is used to locate the epidural space. Next, a catheter is inserted through the needle, and the needle is removed over the catheter. Local anesthetic is in-

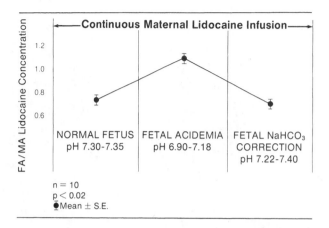

Fig. 15-5 Fetal-maternal arterial (FA/MA) lidocaine ratios were significantly higher ($p < 0.02$) during fetal acidemia than during control or when pH was corrected with bicarbonate. N = 10; mean ± SE. (From Biehl et al.,[92] with permission.)

jected through the catheter, which remains taped in place to the mother's back to enable subsequent injections throughout labor (Figs. 15-1 and 15-6). Thus it is often called *continuous epidural analgesia*. A test dose of local anesthetic is given first to check for the possibility that the catheter was unintentionally placed in the sub-arachnoid (spinal) space or in a blood vessel. Single-dose techniques are occasionally used for vaginal delivery or for cesarean delivery when the duration of pain is expected to be brief. For the single-dose technique, the catheter is omitted.

Two forms of epidural analgesia are used for labor: lumbar and caudal. The catheter is placed via a lumbar interspace in the former and via the sacral hiatus in the latter (Fig. 15-1). More local anesthetic is necessary for the caudal technique, because the local anesthetic must fill the entire sacral canal before filling the epidural space up to T10; 15 to 20 ml of local anesthetic is required. In contrast, for the lumbar technique, 8 to 10 ml (and often less) suffices, because the local anesthetic is injected much closer to its site of action.

For the caudal approach, because the local anesthetic is injected at the sacral area, sacral nerves 2, 3, and 4 are always affected. Because these nerves innervate the pelvic floor, the muscles of the pelvic floor will become insensitive and relaxed throughout labor. Moreover, the patient's legs will be affected and occasionally will be rendered immobile, depending on the strength of the local anesthetic. Pressure exerted on the pelvic floor by the descending vertex plays a major role in ensuring proper rotation of the fetal head to the occiput anterior position, and resistance may not be adequate to rotate the head when muscles of the pelvic floor are relaxed. Thus an increase in occiput transverse or occiput posterior positions may result with the caudal technique. Also, because the patient's percep-

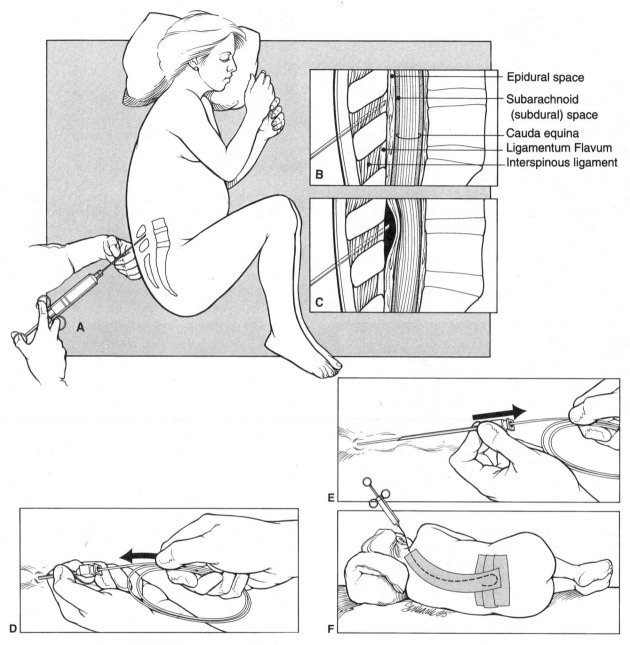

Fig. 15-6 Technique of lumbar epidural puncture by the midline approach. (A) This side view shows left hand held against patient's back, with thumb and index finger grasping hub. Attempts to inject solution while point of needle is in the interspinous ligament meet resistance. (B) Point of needle is in the ligamentum flavum, which offers marked resistance and makes it almost impossible to inject solution. (C) Entrance of the needle's point into epidural space is discerned by sudden lack of resistance to injection of saline. Force of injected solution pushes dura-arachnoid away from point of needle. (D) Catheter is introduced through needle. Note that hub of needle is pulled caudad toward the patient, increasing the angle between the shaft of the needle and the epidural space. Also note technique of holding the tubing: it is wound around the right hand. (E) Needle is withdrawn over tubing and held steady with the right hand. (F) Catheter is immobilized with adhesive tape. Note the large loop made by the catheter to decrease risk of kinking at the point where the tube exits from the skin. (From Bonica,[34] with permission.)

tion of pressure on the perineum by the presenting part is a stimulus for her to increase voluntary effort, blocking or minimizing this perception may prolong the second stage. For these reasons, the caudal approach is less favorable for labor, although it may be useful when anesthesia is needed for perineal procedures. A rare but serious complication of caudal anesthesia is accidental injection of local anesthetic into the fetal head, leading to newborn apnea, bradycardia, and convulsions.[93]

Most anesthesiologists now prefer the lumbar approach and use a technique described as *segmental epidural analgesia* (Fig. 15-7). Because nerves that carry painful impulses during the first stage of labor are small sympathetic nerves and because they are easily blocked, only the smallest amount and the weakest effective concentration of local anesthetic is injected via the L2-L3, L3-L4, or L4-L5 interspace. Thus both sensation and motor function of the perineum and lower extremities remain mostly intact. The patient can move about and perceive the impact of the presenting part on the perineum. If perineal anesthesia is needed for delivery, a larger concentration and dose of local anesthetic can be administered at that time through the catheter (Fig. 15-7). Alternatively, for perineal anesthesia, the obstetrician can perform a pudendal block or local infiltration of the perineum.

The segmental epidural technique, when performed properly, is effective and safe for both mother and fetus. In most instances, total or near total pain relief is accomplished without resorting to depressant and sometimes disorienting drugs. The mother remains awake, alert, and aware of her surroundings. She can communicate with her husband, her physician, and the nursing personnel. She will remember and appreciate her entire labor and delivery. Finally, because anesthesia can be extended to the perineum at the time of delivery, the obstetrician can accomplish whatever kind of delivery is necessary, spontaneous or instrumental, with or without an episiotomy.

A new technique of labor analgesia involves passing a small-gauge pencil-point spinal needle through the epidural needle prior to catheter placement. This combined spinal-epidural or coaxial technique provides rapid onset of analgesia using a very small dose of opioid or a local anesthetic and opioid combination.[94,95] Because the dose of drug used in the subarachnoid space is much smaller than that used for epidural analgesia, the risks of local anesthetic toxicity or high spinal block are avoided. Side effects are usually mild and include pruritus and nausea. The risk of postdural puncture headache is no different from that with epidural analgesia alone.[96] Some practitioners have used this technique to allow parturients to ambulate during labor since there is little or no interference with motor function.[94]

Even though the advantages would seem to make epidural or combined spinal epidural analgesia the ideal analgesic technique, and many believe it to be so, there are disadvantages. These include hypotension,

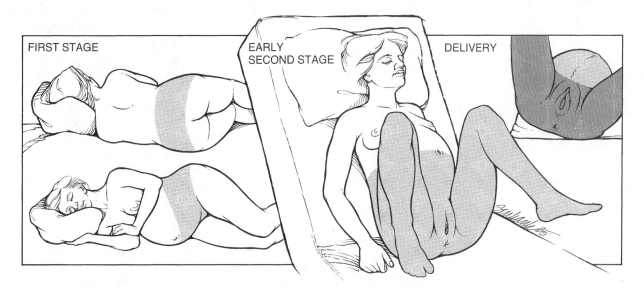

Fig. 15-7 Segmented epidural analgesia for labor and delivery. A single catheter is introduced into the epidural space to advanced so that its tip is at L2. Initially, small volumes of low concentrations of local anesthetic are used to produce segmental analgesia. For the second stage, the analgesia is extended to the sacral segments by injecting a larger amount of the same concentration of local anesthetic, with the patient in the semirecumbent position. After internal rotation, a higher concentration of local anesthetic is injected to produce motor block of the sacral segments and thus achieve perineal relaxation and anesthesia. The wedge under the right buttock causes the uterus to displace to the left. (from Bonica,[275] with permission.)

local anesthetic toxicity, allergic reaction, high or total spinal anesthesia, neurologic injury, spinal headache, and, in some cases, adverse effects on progress of labor.

Hypotension

Hypotension is defined variably, but most often it is defined as a systolic blood pressure less than 100 mmHg or a 20 percent decrease from control values. It occurs after approximately 10 percent of epidural blocks given during labor, but the incidence has been reported to be as low as 1.4 percent in some large series.[97–101] Hypotension occurs primarily as a result of sympathetic blockade. Local anesthetics block not only pain fibers but sympathetic fibers as well, which normally maintain blood vessel tone. When these fibers are blocked, vasodilation results and blood pools in the lower extremities, decreasing the return of blood to the right side of the heart. Cardiac output then decreases, and hypotension results. Hypotension threatens the fetus by decreasing uterine blood flow and threatens the mother by decreasing cerebral blood flow. When hypotension is recognized promptly and treated effectively, very little, if any, untoward effects accrue to either (Table 15-1).[102–104] However, in the acutely or chronically compromised fetus, hypotension can result in further compromise if not treated immediately.[105]

Treatment of hypotension begins with prophylaxis, which demands an intravenous catheter and an infusion of 500 to 1,000-ml isotonic crystalloid solution. The infusion fills the expanded vascular space caused by vasodilatation. Glucose is easily transported across the placenta; therefore, dextrose-containing solutions are avoided for this purpose because they can cause neonatal hypoglycemia.[106] Left uterine displacement must be maintained during the block because compression of the inferior vena cava and aorta may decrease

cardiac output and/or uteroplacental perfusion. Proper treatment depends on immediate diagnosis. To diagnose hypotension the person administering the anesthesia must be present and attentive, which means not being involved in anything else that cannot be abandoned. Once diagnosed, hypotension is corrected by increasing the rate of intravenous fluid infusion and exaggerating left uterine displacement. If these simple measures do not suffice, a vasopressor is indicated, and the vasopressor of choice is ephedrine, given in 5- to 10-mg doses. Ephedrine is a mixed α- and β-agonist, and it is less likely to compromise uteroplacental perfusion than the pure α-agonists.[107] α-Adrenergic agents such as methoxamine or phenylephrine are avoided in most cases (Fig. 15-8), although they may be useful when a parturient is excessively tachycardic in association with hypotension, or if tachycardia associated with ephedrine may be detrimental. Clinical studies have suggested that phenylephrine in small doses may be given safely to treat hypotension during regional anesthesia for cesarean delivery.[108]

Local Anesthetic Toxicity

The incidence of systemic local anesthetic toxicity (high blood concentrations of local anesthetic) after lumbar epidural analgesia is less than 0.5 percent.[109] However, convulsions due to local anesthetic toxicity were the most common damaging event in the obstetric anesthesia Closed Claims Project database, and 83 percent resulted in neurologic injury or death to the mother, newborn, or both.[110] Most often, toxicity occurs when the local anesthetic is injected into a vessel rather than into the epidural space or when too much is administered even though injected properly. Occasionally, the dosage can be miscalculated: 1 ml of 1 percent lidocaine contains 10 mg of lidocaine, not 1 mg. All local anesthetics have maximal recommended doses that should not be exceeded. For example, the maximum recommended dose of lidocaine is 4 mg/kg when used without epinephrine and 7 mg/kg when used with epinephrine. (Epinephrine delays and decreases the uptake of local anesthetic into the bloodstream.) Package inserts for all local anesthetics contain dose information (Table 15-2).

Local anesthetic reactions have two components, central nervous system (CNS) and cardiovascular. Usually, the CNS component precedes the cardiovascular component. Prodromal symptoms of the CNS reaction include excitation, bizarre behavior, ringing in the ears, and disorientation. These symptoms may culminate in convulsions, which are usually brief. After the convulsions, depression follows and manifests predominantly by the postictal state. The cardiovascular component of the local anesthetic reaction usually begins

Table 15-1   Epidural Analgesia: Hypotension Versus No Hypotension[a]

	Hypotension[b] (N = 5)	No Hypotension (N = 20)
Umbilical artery		
pH	7.269	7.311
BE (mEQ/L)	−1.4	−1.3
Po₂ (mmHg)	23.6	23.2
SaO₂ (%)	48.2	50.2
Umbilical vein		
pH	7.344	7.366
BE (mEq/L)	−1.8	−1.5
Po₂ (mmHg)	41.0	33.7
SvO₂ (%)	84.6	72.0

[a] Values are means; they indicate that properly treated hypotension need not result in a compromised fetus.

[b] Hypotension was severe enough to be treated with the vasopressor ephedrine.

(Modified from James et al,[207] with permission.)

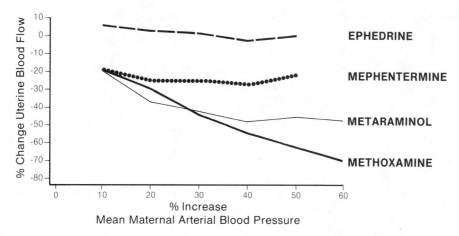

Fig. 15-8 Changes in uterine blood flow at equal elevations of mean arterial blood pressure after vasopressor administration (pregnant ewes). (From Ralston et al.,[107] with permission.)

with hypertension and tachycardia but is soon followed by hypotension, arrhythmias, and in some instances cardiac arrest. Thus the cardiovascular component also has excitant and depressant characteristics. Usually the CNS and cardiovascular components are widely separated, because it takes a significantly higher blood concentration of local anesthetic to cause the cardiovascular symptoms than it does the CNS symptoms. Thus one frequently sees the CNS component without the more serious cardiovascular component. Bupivacaine may represent an exception to this principle.[111,112] There are reports of several patients who experienced serious arrhythmias and marked cardiovascular depression after administration of 0.75 percent bupivacaine, and most physicians now believe that there is little difference in the doses required to cause the two types of reactions to bupivacaine. Moreover, resuscitation of these patients was difficult or impossible, probably because of the drug's prolonged blocking effect on sodium channels.[113] Indeed there now is laboratory evidence that bupivacaine is more cardiotoxic than equianalgesic doses of other amide local anesthetics and that

pregnancy may enhance that cardiotoxicity.[114] Several manufacturers of bupivacaine have recommended that the 0.75 percent concentration not be used in obstetric patients and that the drug not be used for paracervical block.[115] Of course, it is possible to give the same total dose of bupivacaine by giving a larger volume of 0.5 percent bupivacaine. In other words, use of a more dilute concentration of drug does not guarantee safety. Thus it is important that the physician give bupivacaine, or any other local anesthetic, by slow, incremental injection.[116]

The bupivacaine controversy has resulted in greater emphasis on the administration of a safe and effective test dose (to exclude unintentional intravenous or subarachnoid injection of local anesthetic) before injection of a therapeutic dose of local anesthetic. Many anesthesiologists give a test dose that includes 15 μg of epinephrine.[117,118] An increase in heart rate of at least 25 to 30 bpm would signal intravascular injection. Others have questioned whether an epinephrine-containing test dose is the best choice in obstetric patients.[119]

Treatment of a local anesthetic reaction depends on recognizing the signs and symptoms as they occur. Again, to recognize the signs and symptoms, the anesthesia-care provider must be present. If possible, once prodromal symptoms arise, the injection of local anesthetic should be stopped. However, if convulsions have already occurred, treatment is aimed at maintaining proper oxygenation and preventing the patient from harming herself. Convulsions use considerable amounts of oxygen, which results in hypoxia and acidosis (Table 15-3).[120] Adequate oxygenation is essential for both mother and fetus, because a hypoxic mother results in a hypoxic and acidotic fetus. Should the convulsions continue for more than a brief period, small intravenous doses of thiopental (25 to 50 mg) or diazepam (5 to 10 mg) are useful. In obstetrics, because of the

Table 15-2 Maximal Recommended Doses of Common Local Anesthetics

| Local Anesthetic | Without Epinephrine | | With Epinephrine[a] | |
	mg/kg	Dose (mg/70 kg)	mg/kg	Total (mg/70 kg)
Bupivacaine	2.5	175	3.0	225
Chloroprocaine	11.0	800	14.0	1,000
Etidocaine	4.0	300	5.5	400
Lidocaine	4.0	300	7.0	500
Mepivacaine	5.0	400	—	—
Tetracaine	1.5	100	—	—

[a] All epinephrine concentrations 1:200,000.

Table 15-3 Blood-Gas Determinations During and After Local Anesthetic-Induced Convulsions

Convulsion	Time	Oxygen (L/min)	Blood-Gas Values				
			pH	P_{CO_2} (mmHg)	P_{O_2} (mmHg)	HCO_3 (mEq/L)	Base Excess (mEq/L)
Patient 1							
1st	9:50:00	10[a]	—	—	—	—	—
2nd	9:50:30		7.27	48	48	21.5	−4
3rd	9:51:00		—	—	—	—	—
4th	9:53:00		7.09	59	33	17.1	−10
Cessation	9:54:00		—	—	—	—	—
	9:55:30		7.01	71	210	17.2	−11
	10:22:00	6[b]	7.25	48	99	20.5	−5
		Room air	7.56	25	106	22.5	0
Patient 2							
1st	9:47:00		—	—	—	—	—
2nd	9:47:30		6.99	76	87	17.4	−10.2
3rd	9:48:00		—	—	—	—	—
Cessation	9:50:00		—	—	—	—	—
	10:02:00	10[a]	7.16	54	140	18.5	−6.9

[a] Bog and mask with oral Guedel airway and artificial respiration.
[b] Nasal prongs.
(Modified from Moore et al,[120] with permission.)

adverse effects of diazepam on the neonate, thiopental would be the agent of choice. Occasionally succinylcholine is used for paralysis to prevent the muscular activity associated with the convulsions and to facilitate ventilation and perhaps intubation. Before using thiopental, diazepam, or succinylcholine, consideration must be given to the depressant effects that these agents will add to the depressant phase of the local anesthetic reaction. Therefore, appropriate equipment and personnel must be available to maintain oxygenation, a patent airway, and cardiovascular support. Resuscitation of the pregnant patient is essentially the same as that of the nonpregnant patient except that left uterine displacement must be maintained. Usually this means that the uterus will have to be lifted off the inferior vena cava manually for resuscitation with the patient supine.

Allergy to Local Anesthetics

There are two classes of local anesthetics: amides and esters. A true allergic reaction to an amide-type local anesthetic (e.g., lidocaine, bupivacaine, mepivacaine, etidocaine) is extremely rare. Allergic reactions to the esters (2-chloroprocaine, procaine, tetracaine) are also rare but occur more often. Generally, when a patient says she is "allergic" to local anesthetics, she is referring to what is perhaps a normal reaction to the epinephrine that is occasionally added to local anesthetics, particularly by dentists. Epinephrine can cause increased heart rate, pounding in the ears, and nausea, symptoms that may be interpreted as an allergy. It is therefore important to document any history of allergy. Was there a rash?

Hives? Difficulty breathing? If so, which local anesthetic was used? If a specific local anesthetic can be identified, choosing one from the other class should be safe.

High Spinal or "Total Spinal" Anesthetic

This complication occurs when the level of anesthesia rises dangerously high, resulting in paralysis of the respiratory muscles, including the diaphragm. The incidence of total spinal anesthesia after epidural anesthesia is less than 0.03 percent and after spinal anesthesia is 0.1 percent.[109] Total spinal anesthesia can result from a miscalculated dose of drug, unintentional subarachnoid injection during an epidural block, or improper positioning of a patient after spinal block with hyperbaric local anesthetic solutions. Motor nerves to the diaphragm, the major respiratory muscle, emanate from C3 to C5; therefore, the anesthetic must be at this level before phrenic nerve paralysis results. Moreover, the phrenic nerve is a large motor nerve, which requires considerable local anesthetic for complete block. Because the accessory muscles of respiration are paralyzed earlier, their paralysis may result in apprehension and anxiety. The patient usually can breathe adequately as long as the diaphragm is not paralyzed. However, treatment must be individualized, and dyspnea, real or imagined, should always be considered an effect of paralysis until proved otherwise. In addition to respiratory symptoms, cardiovascular components, including hypotension and even cardiovascular collapse, may occur.

Treatment of total spinal anesthesia includes rapidly assessing the true level of anesthesia. Therefore, to de-

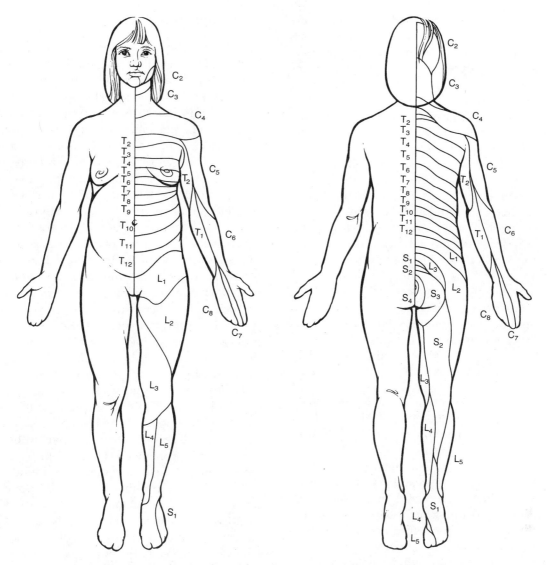

Fig. 15-9 Dermatome chart. (Adapted from Haymaker and Woodhall,[276] with permission.)

termine the precise level of anesthesia, persons who perform major regional anesthesia should be thoroughly familiar with dermatome charts (Fig. 15-9). Furthermore, these persons should also recognize what a certain sensory level of anesthesia means in regard to innervation of other organs or systems. For example, a T4 sensory level may represent total sympathetic nervous system blockade. Numbness and weakness of the fingers and hands indicate that the level of anesthesia has reached the cervical level (C6 to C8), which is dangerously close to the innervation of the diaphragm. If the diaphragm is not paralyzed, the patient is breathing adequately, and cardiovascular stability is maintained, administration of oxygen and assurance that things will eventually be better may suffice. If the patient continues to be anxious or if the level of anesthesia seems to be involving the diaphragm, then assisted ventilation is indicated. Occasionally, this can be accomplished with

a bag and face mask without rendering the patient unconscious. Most often, however, endotracheal intubation will be necessary. If so, induction of general anesthesia will facilitate the process. Cardiovascular support is provided as necessary. If the person administering regional anesthesia is well acquainted with the signs and symptoms of high spinal anesthesia and its treatment, serious sequelae should be extremely rare. The onset is easy to diagnose, and the treatment is relatively simple. However, the same admonition applies as with hypotension and local anesthetic toxicity: early symptoms cannot be diagnosed if the person administering the block is not present and attentive.

Paralysis and Nerve Injury

Paralysis after either epidural or spinal anesthesia is extremely rare; even minor injuries such as foot-drop and segmental loss of sensation are rare. All forms of nerve injury occur in less than 1 in 10,000 applications of regional anesthesia.[121] More serious injuries are even less frequent. Today, commercially prepared drugs, ampules, and disposable needles make infection and caustic injury nearly unheard of. Several years ago there were several cases of neurologic deficit after use of 2-chloroprocaine, primarily after unintentional subarachnoid (i.e., spinal) injection of large volumes of the drug.[122–124] These cases prompted performance of several laboratory studies to evaluate any potential neurotoxicity of 2-chloroprocaine. The earlier formulation of 2-chloroprocaine contained the antioxidant 0.2 percent sodium bisulfite. Currently the consensus is that 2-chloroprocaine itself is not neurotoxic, but that the low pH of the local anesthetic solution and the inclusion of the sodium bisulfite together may produce neurologic dysfunction.[125] The current formulation of 2-chloroprocaine does not contain sodium bisulfite. Curiously, there have been recent reports of transient back pain after epidural use of the new formulation of 2-chloroprocaine in nonpregnant patients.[126,127]

When nerve damage follows regional analgesia during obstetric or surgical procedures, the anesthetic technique must be suspect. Nerve damage can result from other causes, however. For example, incorrectly positioned stirrups may cause nerve injury after both gynecologic and obstetric procedures.[128–130] Also, nerve damage can be secondary to a difficult forceps application.[128–130] During abdominal procedures, overzealous or prolonged application of pressure with retractors on sensitive nerve tissues may result in injury.[128–130] Fortunately, most neurologic deficits after labor and delivery are minor and transient.[131] Nonetheless, one should consider consultation with a neurologist or neurosurgeon. Although patients are often concerned about the development of back pain following epidural anesthesia, the incidence of back pain in postpartum women is the same with or without the use of regional anesthesia. The incidence of back pain after childbirth is 44 percent at 1 to 2 months postpartum[132] and 49 percent at 12 to 18 months postpartum[133] again, unrelated to the use of epidural anesthesia.

One of the more dramatic and correctable forms of nerve damage follows compression of the spinal cord by a hematoma that has formed during the administration of spinal or epidural anesthesia, presumably from accidental puncture of an epidural vessel. If the condition is diagnosed early, usually with the aid of a neurologist or neurosurgeon, the hematoma can be removed by laminectomy and the problem resolved without permanent damage. Fortunately, this is a very rare complication. Nonetheless, spinal and epidural blocks are contraindicated if clotting is abnormal. Any prolonged motor or sensory deficit after regional anesthesia should be investigated immediately and thoroughly.

Spinal Headache

Spinal headache may follow uncomplicated spinal anesthesia. This complication can also occur when, during the process of administering an epidural block, the dura is punctured and spinal fluid leaks out (i.e., "wet tap"). The incidence of this complication varies between 1 and 3 percent, and its occurrence depends on the experience of the person performing the epidural block.[134] Once a "wet tap" occurs, a spinal headache results in as many as 70 percent of patients. (The incidence is much less following spinal anesthesia, because smaller needles are used.) Characteristically, the headache is more severe in the upright position and is relieved by the prone position. The headache is thought to be caused by loss of cerebral spinal fluid, which allows the brain to settle and thus meninges and vessels to stretch. Hydration, abdominal binders, and the prone position have all been advocated as prophylactic measures. However, most anesthesiologists now agree that these actions are of little value.[135] In some hands, epidural saline injected through the catheter has proven to be an effective prophylactic measure.[136]

Treatment of the headache, once it has occurred, may be initiated with oral analgesics, caffeine,[137] and continued hydration. If these simple measures do not prove immediately effective, an epidural blood patch is placed. Approximately 15 ml of the patient's own blood is placed aseptically into the epidural space; the blood coagulates over the hole in the dura and prevents further leakage.[138] Patients can be released within 1 to 2 hours.[139] Patients should be instructed to avoid coughing or straining at stool for the first several days after performance of the blood patch; a stool softener is recommended. The epidural blood patch has been found to be remarkably effective and nearly complication free.[140–142] There remains controversy whether one should perform a prophylactic blood patch before the onset of spinal headache.[143–146]

Because epidural anesthesia is associated with these side effects and complications, those who administer it must be thoroughly familiar not only with the technical aspects of its administration but also with the signs and symptoms of complications and their treatment. Specifically, the American Society of Anesthesiologists and ACOG stated: "Persons administering or supervising obstetric anesthesia should be qualified to manage the infrequent but occasionally life-threatening complications of major regional anesthesia such as respiratory and cardiovascular failure, toxic local anesthetic convulsions, or vomiting and aspiration. Mastering and retaining the skills and knowledge necessary to manage these complications require adequate training and frequent application."[3]

Effects on Labor and Method of Delivery

One of the more controversial aspects of regional anesthesia for obstetrics is the question of whether these techniques influence the length and pattern of labor, the incidence of malposition, the use of forceps, and the rate of cesarean delivery. The perspectives of the anesthesiologist and the obstetrician differ when trying to answer these questions. The anesthesiologist is concerned primarily with relieving pain and sees regional anesthesia as the ideal method because it depresses neither mother nor fetus, provides exceptional pain relief, and even optimal operating conditions for the obstetrician. The obstetrician, although concerned with pain relief, is also concerned with the progress of labor and the method of delivery. Reports on the effects of epidural analgesia on labor are numerous and conflicting.

Study Design

Most published studies of the effect of epidural analgesia on progress of labor are retrospective and, if prospective, are nonrandomized. Studies that compare patients who received epidural analgesia versus those who did not are typically biased in favor of the nonepidural group of patients. Specifically, patients who have rapid, uncomplicated labor are less likely to ask for, and even if they ask for it are less likely actually to receive, epidural analgesia. In other words, the epidural group will include more patients with dysfunctional, difficult, and complicated labors. In fact, it is possible that the very reason why some, but not all, parturients request and receive epidural analgesia may relate to a greater likelihood of abnormal labor. For example, prolonged latent phase is associated with an increased need for cesarean delivery,[147] and rupture of membranes prior to the onset of labor increases the likelihood of operative delivery.[148] In both of these situations labor may be prolonged, oxytocin use is more common, and epidural analgesia may be requested more often. On the other hand, it is also problematic when one attempts to evaluate the influence of epidural analgesia on labor by use of historical controls. For example, if one compares the incidence of midforceps delivery after the introduction of epidural analgesia to a hospital (e.g., in 1989) versus the incidence of midforceps delivery before the use of epidural analgesia in that hospital (e.g., in 1979), one might note no change in the incidence of midforceps delivery and therefore conclude that the introduction of epidural analgesia did not affect the incidence of midforceps delivery. The problem with that approach is that other changes in obstetric practice may have occurred during that 10-year interval. For example, some obstetricians are less willing to perform difficult midforceps delivery today than they were a decade ago. Therefore, it would be inappropriate to conclude that epidural analgesia did not influence the incidence of midforceps delivery in that hospital.

Variation in Epidural Technique

A second difficulty with interpretation of existing studies is that epidural analgesia is not a generic procedure. The influence of epidural analgesia on the progress of labor may vary according to the choice and dose of the local anesthetic administered. In general, anesthesiologists today use more dilute solutions of local anesthetic for epidural anesthesia than were used a decade ago. The use of low-dose intrathecal opioids and ambulation during early labor is increasing. There is greater attention to titrating the dose of the local anesthetic to the specific needs of the patient. For example, Naulty and colleagues[149] made an abrupt change in their epidural analgesia technique in June 1987. Specifically, they had been providing epidural analgesia during labor with either 1.5 percent lidocaine or 0.25 to 0.5 percent bupivacaine, but they changed their technique to include 0.125 to 0.25 percent bupivacaine with fentanyl. They then compared the results during the 9 months before the change versus those during the 9 months after the change. They noted a significant decrease in the percentage of patients admitted for labor who eventually underwent cesarean delivery. Specifically, during the 9 months before the change, 19.6 percent of patients in labor had cesarean delivery, whereas after the change 15.1 percent required cesarean delivery. Furthermore, there was a significant decrease in the percentage of patients who received epidural analgesia and who subsequently underwent cesarean delivery. Finally, the incidence of forceps deliveries decreased from 17.3 percent before the change to 6.3 percent after the change.

Another potential source of variation in management and outcome is the timing of administration of epidural analgesia. Although controversial, many physicians believe that institution of analgesia during the latent phase of the first stage of labor is more likely to delay the progress of labor. Friedman[150] stated:

> Spinal anesthesia given prior to the onset of the phase of dilatation in the first stage of labor will impede progress of the latent phase, and forestall the normal progressive changes of late labor. It would seem that spinal block given after the latent phase has ended, in a patient whose labor is otherwise normal, and to a level which does not exceed that necessary for uterine pain relief (tenth thoracic) should not influence labor. The general impression of caudal or epidural anesthesia as it affects labor is that of negligible influence unless misused.

The Committee on Obstetrics: Maternal and Fetal Medicine of ACOG issued a statement about dystocia.

Regarding the latent phase of labor, they stated: "The latent phase may be prolonged by excessive medication and inappropriate timing of conduction anesthesia." Regarding the active phase, they stated: "The normal active phase tends to be resistant to the inhibitory effects of the usual amounts of analgesia. At times, further sedation or epidural anesthesia, hydration, or ambulation may be advantageous." Furthermore, the Committee stated: "A hypertonic pattern may be observed in the active phase. Prolongation of a hypertonic pattern may result in maternal exhaustion, marked pain, and decreased uteroplacental blood flow. The combination of sedation, epidural anesthesia and oxytocin infusion may prove effective."[151]

The problem with delaying institution of epidural analgesia until the onset of the active phase of labor is that it is often difficult to make that diagnosis prospectively. Furthermore, it is also inappropriate to delay institution of epidural analgesia until the patient has reached an arbitrary cervical dilatation.[152] For example, approximately 50 percent of patients will enter the active phase of labor by 4-cm cervical dilatation, but a minority will not enter active labor until more than 5 cm cervical dilatation. If one delays institution of epidural analgesia until the patient reaches an arbitrary dilatation (e.g., 5-cm cervical dilatation), one will subject some patients to unnecessary periods of severe pain. On the other hand, earlier institution of epidural analgesia may slow labor in some patients. This can usually be corrected with the use of oxytocin.

Management of the Second Stage

A third problem with interpretation of studies of epidural anesthesia and progress of labor relates to the indication for performance of instrumental delivery. In general, an obstetrician is more likely to perform elective forceps delivery in a comfortable patient with effective epidural anesthesia than in an uncomfortable patient with no anesthesia. Furthermore, heretofore some obstetricians have arbitrarily terminated the second stage at 2 hours in nulliparous patients and at 1 hour in parous patients. There is evidence that effective epidural analgesia may slightly prolong the second stage of labor.[153,154] However, a delay in the second stage is not necessarily harmful to infant or to mother, provided there is normal electronic fetal heart rate monitoring and adequate maternal hydration and analgesia.[153,155-157] Indeed, ACOG has defined a prolonged second stage as more than 3 hours in nulliparous patients *with* regional anesthesia as compared with more than 2 hours in nulliparous patients without regional anesthesia.[158]

Prospective Studies of Epidural Anesthesia and Progress of Labor

Unfortunately, there are few prospective, randomized studies of the effect of epidural analgesia on the progress of labor. The fact that epidural analgesia provides analgesia superior to other techniques causes physicians to be reluctant to randomize patients to a nonepidural group. Robinson and colleagues[159] randomized 386 parturients to receive either epidural anesthesia or systemic analgesia (i.e., meperidine with inhalation analgesia) during labor. They noted that "epidural block was more effective than systemic analgesia in the relief of pain and discomfort in all stages of labor." They also noted that there was a significant increase in the incidence of instrumental delivery in the epidural group. Unfortunately, the randomization occurred before final consent was obtained. Patients were free to withdraw from the study after they learned their group assignment, and many did. Only 93 of the original patients completed the study. One can suspect that more patients with a long, difficult labor dropped out of the systemic analgesia group. This suspicion is confirmed when one notes that there was a threefold increase in the incidence of induction of labor in the epidural group. Furthermore, patients in the epidural group received 0.5 percent bupivacaine, a concentration higher than that used by most anesthesiologists today. Finally, the authors did not report the incidence of cesarean delivery in either group.

Philipsen and Jensen[160] reported the second published study in which patients were randomized to receive either epidural analgesia or systemic opioid during the first stage of labor. Patients in the epidural group received 0.375 percent bupivacaine, although the authors noted that they attempted to produce a segmental block from T10 to L1. They also stated: "In an attempt to retain the bearing-down reflex and to allow the mother to take active part in the second stage of labor, the analgesic effect was allowed to wear off at the beginning of the second stage and a top-up dose was not given if the cervix was dilated beyond 8 cm." There was no significant difference between groups in the method of delivery. Thirty-three of 57 (58 percent) women in the epidural group versus 34 of 54 (63 percent) women in the meperidine group had spontaneous delivery. Fourteen of 57 (25 percent) women in the epidural group versus 14 of 54 (26 percent) women in the meperidine group underwent instrumental vaginal delivery.

There are several studies in which nulliparous patients already receiving epidural anesthesia were randomized with respect to management of epidural anesthesia during the second stage.[153,161-163] Phillips and Thomas[161] reported no increase in duration of the second stage, and a nonsignificant decrease in the incidence of instrumental delivery, in 28 nulliparous women who received additional epidural bupivacaine (i.e., 0.25 percent) at complete cervical dilatation compared with 28 women who received no additional bupivacaine. However, this study was randomized but nonblinded, and it is unclear as to how the two groups actually differed, as there was no significant difference between groups in total dosage of bupivacaine or in mean number of doses of bupivacaine (i.e., four doses per patient in each group).

Chestnut and colleagues[162] performed a study in which nulliparous patients already receiving a continuous epidural infusion of 0.75 percent lidocaine were randomized to receive either additional 0.75 percent lidocaine or saline placebo after 8-cm cervical dilatation. The epidural infusion of lidocaine or saline placebo was continued in all patients until delivery. Maintenance of the epidural infusion of 0.75 percent lidocaine until delivery did not prolong the second stage or increase the frequency of instrumental delivery, but it also did not reliably provide second-stage analgesia or perineal anesthesia. Specifically, women who continued to receive epidural lidocaine until delivery did not clearly perceive that they had better analgesia than did women who received saline placebo.

Subsequently, Chestnut and colleagues[153] performed a study in which nulliparous women already receiving a continuous epidural infusion of 0.125 percent bupivacaine were randomized to receive either additional 0.125 percent bupivacaine or saline placebo beyond 8 cm cervical dilatation. Patients continued to receive the epidural infusion of bupivacaine or saline placebo until delivery. Maintenance of the epidural infusion of bupivacaine until delivery resulted in a second-stage analgesia that was clearly superior to that provided by replacement of the bupivacaine with placebo. Infusion of bupivacaine until delivery prolonged the second stage of labor approximately 30 minutes, and it also increased the incidence of instrumental delivery. However, maintenance of epidural bupivacaine analgesia did not result in an increased incidence of abnormal position of the vertex, and it did not result in a more frequent performance of cesarean delivery. Furthermore, there were nonsignificant tendencies toward better neonatal condition in the bupivacaine group as evaluated by umbilical cord blood acid-base status and Apgar scores.

Cesarean Delivery Rate

Does the use of epidural analgesia for labor influence the cesarean delivery rate? Gribble and Meier[164] found no difference in the cesarean delivery rates before and after the availability of "on-demand" epidural analgesia for labor. The patients were managed by the same group of obstetricians using the same management techniques in both time intervals. When use of epidural labor analgesia was 0 percent the cesarean delivery rate was 9.0 percent, while after the use of epidural analgesia had risen to 48 percent, the cesarean delivery rate was 8.6 percent. A number of other authors have also shown that cesarean rates can actually decrease while the use of epidural analgesia increases. Larson[165] found the cesarean delivery rate actually decreased from 27.6 to 22.9 percent ($p = 0.0007$) after a 24-hour in-house obstetric anesthesiology service was established. The use of epidural analgesia rose from 0 to 31.6 percent during the same time period.[165] Iglesias et al.[166] and Socol et al.[167] assessed the impact of changes in obstetric management on decreasing the incidence of cesarean delivery Both groups found they could decrease the cesarean delivery rate at the same time the use of epidural analgesia was increasing in their hospitals.

The decline in cesarean delivery rates in these studies is achieved primarily by increasing the use of vaginal birth after cesarean (VBAC), active management of labor, and oxytocin use. The availability of epidural analgesia may be an important factor in patient acceptance of VBAC and in the obstetrician's willingness to aggressively manage labor and use oxytocin. This active management of labor is exemplified by the National Maternity Hospital in Dublin. At that institution, the epidural rate increased from 10 percent in 1987 to 45 percent in 1992 while the cesarean delivery rate remained unchanged at 4 to 5 percent.[168] The practitioners in Dublin note that "epidural analgesia may be of major benefit in labor and need not reduce the chance of spontaneous vaginal delivery if the passive phase of second stage of labor is lengthened."

Other work has also shown that obstetric management influences outcome independent of the type of labor analgesia utilized. In a retrospective review of epidural analgesia *managed by obstetricians*, women having epidural analgesia for labor actually had a *decreased* risk of cesarean delivery (odds ratio 0.31).[169] Epidural analgesia was used in 60 percent of their patients during the final 6 years. Neuhoff and colleagues[170] retrospectively investigated cesarean deliveries for failed progress in labor at their hospital, comparing the clinic and private services to determine the importance of different management strategies. The cesarean birth rate on the clinic service was 5 percent versus 17 percent on the private service, while the use of epidural analgesia was comparable on both services (41.6 versus 41.7 percent). Cesarean births were increased on the private service when epidural analgesia was used, but cesarean delivery rates remained stable on the clinic service whether or not epidural analgesia was employed.

A series of articles by Thorp and colleagues[171–173] on the relationship between epidural analgesia and cesarean delivery have caused great concern among obstetricians, parturients, and anesthesiologists. This group has published both retrospective and prospective studies of the effects of epidural use on cesarean section rates for dystocia. The first publication was a retrospective review of 711 consecutive nulliparous women at term in spontaneous labor.[171] They found that women who received epidural analgesia had a longer duration of labor, were more likely to receive oxytocin, and had a 10.3 percent cesarean delivery rate for dystocia versus 3.8 percent in the nonepidural group. A subsequent retrospective study of 500 consecutive patients again showed an increased cesarean delivery rate in the epidural versus nonepidural group (11.4 vs 2.4 percent) and noted that nulliparous women who had epidural analgesia administered before 5 cm of cervical dilatation seemed to have the greatest effect on the incidence of cesarean delivery.[172] The authors concluded that "epidural analgesia in first labors may have contributed significantly to the cesarean epidemic". Most recently, Thorp and colleagues[173] published a prospective study in which nulliparous women were randomized to receive intravenous meperidine or epidural bupivacaine. There was a significant slowing of cervical delitation the epidural group, as well as a 25 percent incidence of cesarean delivery (n = 12) versus a 2.2 percent cesarean delivery rate in the nonepidural group (n = 1). Neonatal outcome was similar in both groups, and pain relief was rated superior in the epidural group by nurses and patients. Eleven of the 12 cesarean deliveries in the epidural group were of women who had received the epidural before 5 cm dilatation. The authors suggested that nulliparous women offered epidural analgesia for labor should be warned their potential for cesarean delivery is markedly increased.

These results contrast sharply with two subsequent prospective studies reported by Chestnut et al.[174,175] The first followed nulliparous women *already* receiving oxytocin for induction or augmentation of labor.[174] When patients were dilated 3 or more cm but less than 5 cm, they were randomized to receive intravenous nalbuphine or epidural bupivacaine. Patients in the nalbuphine group could receive an epidural anesthetic once they were 5 cm or more or 1 hour after a second dose of nalbuphine (as a rescue alternative). Attempts were made to minimize motor block in the epidural group. Early administration of epidural analgesia did not prolong the first stage of labor or increase the incidence of malposition of the vertex, instrumental vaginal delivery, or cesarean delivery. The incidence of cesarean delivery was 18 percent in the early epidural group (12 percent for dystocia) and 19 percent in the late epidural group (16 percent for dystocia). Umbilical cord blood pH values were lower in the late epidural group.

Chestnut et al.[175] used a similar study design to determine whether early use of epidural analgesia affected obstetric outcome in nulliparous women in *spontaneous* labor. Early use of epidural analgesia did not increase the use of oxytocin augmentation, prolong the first stage of labor, or increase the incidence of malposition or instrumental delivery. There was no increase in cesarean delivery rate in the early epidural group (10 percent) versus the late epidural group (8 percent). Umbilical cord blood pH levels were again lower in the late epidural group. The overall higher cesarean delivery rates in women requiring induction or augmentation of labor again supports the idea that these parturients are already at higher risk for cesarean delivery and should be considered as a separate category.[147,148]

What might cause the difference in outcomes[176] between the prospective works of Thorp et al. and Chestnut et al.? In the work of Chestnut et al., all patients ultimately received epidural analgesia, while in the study by Thorp et al., only one patient in the meperidine group ultimately received epidural analgesia. In the prospective study by Thorp et al., the authors took responsibility for the obstetric management decisions and obviously were not blinded to the anesthetic group. Their study patients were limited to an indigent population, while those of Chestnut et al. were evenly divided between indigent and private patients. Chestnut et al. adjusted the epidural infusion to minimize the degree of motor block, but the Thorp et al. group did not indicate the degree of maternal motor block or whether epidural analgesia was managed in such a way as to minimize excessive motor block.

Recommendations

What can be concluded from these studies of epidural analgesia and the progress of labor? *First*, it is probably preferable to avoid institution of epidural analgesia during early, latent-phase labor in most patients. In general, epidural analgesia should not be instituted until the obstetrician is satisfied that the labor is established, that is, until the patient is having regular contractions and the cervix is dilating progressively. However, it is difficult to assign a specific cervical dilatation as indicating the time to administer epidural analgesia; for some it will be 3 to 4 cm and for others, 4 to 6 cm. Psychoprophylactic techniques are probably most effective during the latent phase of labor and will allow many patients to forego supplemental analgesia during that period. However, physicians should recognize that some patients experience severe pain during latent-phase labor. This is especially true if the patient is receiving intravenous oxytocin. It is best to individualize decisions regarding timing of epidural analgesia. Thus, in some patients, early institution of epidural analgesia may be appropriate. In these situations, it may be possible to utilize intrathecal or epidural opioids and allow the patient to ambulate until labor has become more active. The American Society of Anesthesiology and ACOG have written a joint statement on pain relief in labor that notes in part, "There is no other circumstance where it is considered acceptable for a person to experience severe pain, amenable to safe intervention, while under a physician's care."[177]

Second, it is preferable to use dilute solutions of local anesthetic rather than more concentrated solutions. For example, 0.25 percent bupivacaine will provide satisfactory analgesia in most patients, and it is rarely necessary to give a more concentrated solution of bupivacaine for analgesia during labor. If a patient develops motor block, the local anesthetic solution can be made more dilute and supplemented with opioids as needed.

Third, the obstetrician should recognize that a brief period of decreased uterine activity often follows the institution of epidural analgesia. In some patients, there is a brief period of decreased uterine activity followed by reestablishment of the contraction pattern and resumption of normal labor (Fig. 15-10).[178] This may actually be due to the intravenous hydration given prior to epidural analgesia.[179] In one study a 1,000-ml fluid load decreased uterine activity for a short period of time, while an epidural block without fluid load was associated with increased uterine activity. In some patients, epidural analgesia may accelerate labor, perhaps by decreasing maternal concentrations of catecholamines. At least one study has documented a favorable influence of epidural analgesia in patients with discoordinate uterine contractions and prolonged labor.[180] However, in other patients, analgesia may seem to slow or to stop labor for more than a brief period. In such patients, the obstetrician should be willing to augment labor by giving oxytocin intravenously.

Fourth, there remains disagreement regarding whether it is advisable to add epinephrine to the therapeutic dose of local anesthetic. Some anesthesiologists

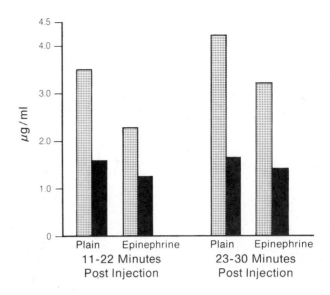

Maternal concentration
Cord concentration

Fig. 15-11 Histogram of mean maternal and cord plasma concentrations of lidocaine, 20-ml 2 percent solution with or without the addition of 1:250,000 epinephrine, in patients who were delivered 11 to 22 minutes or 23 to 30 minutes after administration of lidocaine by the lumbar epidural route. (From Thomas et al.,[277] with permission.)

add epinephrine to local anesthetic solutions to produce vasoconstriction in the area where the local anesthetic is injected. In this way, the blood absorbs smaller amounts of anesthetic over a longer time period. Thus there is a decreased concentration of local anesthetic in the maternal blood, and less local anesthetic crosses the placenta to the fetus (Fig. 15-11). Also, the addition of epinephrine may result in a more solid block, especially if one is administering lidocaine. On the other hand, some studies have demonstrated that the addition of epinephrine to local anesthetic solution is more likely to decrease uterine activity than administration of local anesthetic without epinephrine. In one study,

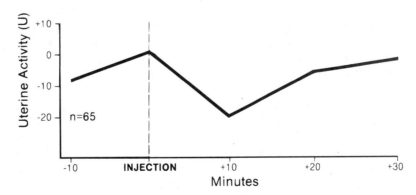

Fig. 15-10 Effect of epidural injections of lidocaine with epinephrine on uterine activity levels in 65 cases. (From Lowensohn et al.,[178] with permission.)

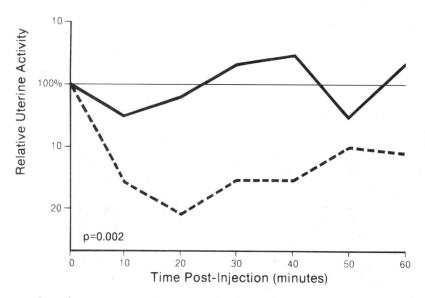

Fig. 15-12 Mean values of uterine activity after epidural administration of lidocaine (solid line) or lidocaine with epinephrine (dotted line). (From Matadial and Cibils,[101] with permission.)

plain lidocaine decreased uterine activity briefly in 16 patients but increased it in 14 patients. In contrast, lidocaine with epinephrine (1:200,000) decreased uterine activity in 39 patients and increased it in only 12. Furthermore, mean uterine activity (Montevideo Units) decreased much more when epinephrine was used (Fig. 15-12). Another study reported similar results in uterine activity but no significant effect of epinephrine on the length and progression of labor.[181] Recently other studies have also suggested that the addition of epinephrine to local anesthetic does not prolong the duration of labor.[182–185] This is especially likely to be true if a very dilute concentration of epinephrine is administered.[182–185]

Fifth, should epidural analgesia be continued or discontinued during the second stage of labor? We believe that it is inappropriate to withhold analgesia routinely during the second stage. Johnson et al.[186] concluded: "Voluntary effort is decreased in some patients in the second stage of labor with spinal and peridural analgesia. Since this is not a consistent finding, and some patients actually exhibited increased capability for bearing down after the anesthesia, it must be an individual reaction without the actual loss of ability." It is important to understand that epidural analgesia during labor is not a generic procedure. For example, in one study[162] maintenance of the infusion of local anesthetic until delivery did not prolong the second stage or increase the incidence of instrumental delivery, but it also did not reliably provide second-stage analgesia. In a similar study[153] performed at the same institution, infusion of a different local anesthetic until delivery provided excellent second-stage analgesia, but it prolonged the second stage and increased the incidence

of instrumental delivery. In the first study,[162] the block during the second stage was clearly inadequate in most patients, while in the second study[153] the block was probably excessive in some patients. Clearly, a dense epidural block may decrease the ability of some patients to push effectively. On the other hand, other patients will push more effectively in the presence of analgesia. In clinical practice, it seems best to individualize patient management. If the block is too dense and the patient cannot push effectively, then there should be diminution of the level and/or intensity of analgesia. In other patients, the block should be maintained or strengthened. The optimal approach is to provide a reasonable level of analgesia consistent with the parturient's ability to push effectively. Of course, it is also important that patients be actively coached in pushing.

Sixth, one should avoid arbitrary termination of the second stage. As noted earlier, the ACOG has redefined the "normal" limits of the duration of the second stage in patients with and without regional anesthesia.[158] Indeed, in some patients with effective epidural analgesia, it may be appropriate to allow a second stage of more than 3 hours provided that there is continued progress in descent of the vertex.

Seventh, it is important to recognize that risk to mother and infant of instrumental delivery performed under the ideal conditions provided by spinal or epidural anesthesia may differ from the risk of instrumental delivery performed without adequate anesthesia. Indeed, regional anesthesia may well allow for more complete cooperation by the patient, a more accurate application of the forceps, and a more gentle birth.

Eighth, there remains controversy whether there is a cause-and-effect relationship between the use of epidural analgesia and prolonged labor or operative delivery. Epidural analgesia during labor is not a generic procedure, and conclusions regarding the effect of one technique on the progress of labor may not be applicable to other techniques. We do not recommend withholding analgesia until the patient has achieved an arbitrary cervical dilatation during the first stage of labor, and it is equally inappropriate to discontinue analgesia altogether during the second stage.

There remain several unresolved questions with regard to optimal management of epidural anesthesia during labor. *First,* does continuous infusion of local anesthetic affect labor differently than intermittent epidural bolus injection? Purported advantages of continuous epidural infusion during labor include (1) a more stable level of analgesia, (2) reduced risk of hypotension, (3) reduced risk of systemic toxicity, (4) reduced risk of total spinal block, and (5) convenience for the anesthesiologist.[187] An infusion pump delivers a dilute solution of local anesthetic by continuous positive pressure. A potential disadvantage of continuous epidural infusion is that it tends to discourage individualization of the dose of local anesthetic in an individual patient. Thus there is a tendency to give more local anesthetic than one would give if one were using the intermittent epidural bolus injection technique. For example, there have been at least five controlled comparisons of the continuous epidural infusion of bupivacaine versus intermittent epidural bolus injection of bupivacaine.[188–192] In each study, patients in the continuous infusion group received more bupivacaine than did patients in the intermittent bolus group. It is unclear whether the increased dose of bupivacaine is clinically significant and represents a disadvantage. Furthermore, it is unclear whether the continuous epidural infusion technique has more or less effect on the progress of labor and method of delivery than does the intermittent epidural bolus injection technique.

Second, is it advantageous to add opioid to the solution of local anesthetic and thereby reduce the total dose of local anesthetic and the extent of maternal motor block? Chestnut and colleagues[193] observed that the continuous epidural infusion of 0.0625 percent bupivacaine with 0.0002 percent fentanyl produced first-stage analgesia similar to that provided by the infusion of 0.125 percent bupivacaine alone. Women who received bupivacaine and fentanyl experienced less intense motor block, but they did *not* have a shorter second stage or a lower incidence of instrumental delivery than did women who received bupivacaine alone. A legitimate criticism of that study is that the epidural infusion was discontinued at full cervical dilatation in both groups. Had the infusion been continued until delivery, it is possible that there would have been a difference

between groups in the method of delivery. This question deserves further investigation.

Third, should there be more frequent use of oxytocin during the second stage of labor? Goodfellow and colleagues[194] noted a significant increase in maternal blood concentrations of oxytocin between the onset of full cervical dilatation and crowning of the fetal head in patients without epidural anesthesia, but they did not observe a similar increase in patients with epidural anesthesia. Similarly, Bates and colleagues[195] observed significantly less uterine activity during the second stage in patients with epidural anesthesia compared with patients without epidural anesthesia. Both groups of investigators recommended increased utilization of oxytocin during the second stage in order to increase the chance of spontaneous vaginal delivery.

Fourth, is there a role for delayed pushing during the second stage? Maresh and colleagues[155] reported a study of 76 nulliparous patients with epidural anesthesia who were randomly assigned to early pushing or late pushing in the second stage. There was a significant increase in the duration of the second stage but a nonsignificant decrease in the frequency of instrumental delivery in the late-pushing group. The increased second-stage duration was not associated with an increase in fetal heart rate abnormalities or a decrease in Apgar scores or umbilical cord blood pH. It is possible that patients become exhausted when asked to push too early during the second stage. Indeed, it may be preferable to allow the force of uterine contractions to deliver the vertex to a station at which maternal pushing might be effective.

Paracervical Block

Paracervical block analgesia, a simple, effective procedure when performed properly, is used most commonly by obstetricians. Usually, 5 to 6 ml of a dilute solution of local anesthetic without epinephrine (e.g., 1 percent lidocaine or 1 or 2 percent 2-chloroprocaine) is injected into the mucosa of the cervix at either 4 and 8 or 3 and 9 o'clock; an Iowa trumpet prevents deep penetration of the needle (Fig. 15-13). The duration of analgesia depends on the local anesthetic used. Several manufacturers of bupivacaine have stated that bupivacaine, the longest acting local anesthetic, is contraindicated for obstetric paracervical block. In the past, paracervical block enjoyed considerable favor, particularly when anesthesiologist were not available to provide major regional analgesia techniques. Disadvantages of the technique are that the block can only be applied during the first stage of labor and that it must be reapplied frequently during the course of a long labor. Furthermore, it has the widely recognized, major disadvantage of fetal bradycardia, which occurs in 2 to 70 percent of

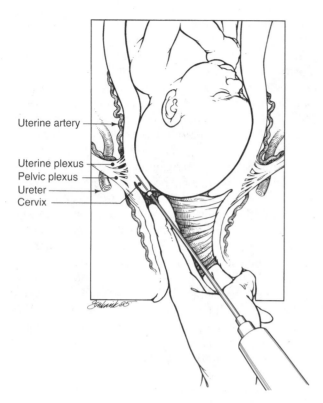

Fig. 15-13 Technique of paracervical block. Schematic coronal section (enlarged) of lower portion of cervix and upper portion of vagina shows relation of needle to paracervical region. (Modified from Bonica,[34] with permission.)

in the fetus, (2) uterine artery vasoconstriction, and (3) postparacervical block increase in uterine activity. A high blood concentration is feasible, because the local anesthetic is injected close to the uterine artery. The anesthetic would traverse the wall of the uterine artery, pass directly to the fetus, and thus result in a high blood concentration and subsequent bradycardia.[196] Clinical support for this theory is that infants who suffer bradycardia frequently have higher anesthetic blood concentrations than do their mothers.[196] Alternatively, the bradycardia may result from uterine artery vasoconstriction secondary to a direct effect of the local anesthetic on the uterine artery.[199,200] This effect has been demonstrated in vitro on human uterine arteries[199] (Fig. 15-14) and is supported by uterine blood flow studies in animals.[200] The fetal electrocardiogram (ECG) pattern during one of these episodes after paracervical block suggests hypoxia, a finding that supports the uterine artery vasoconstriction theory.[201] Although high concentrations of local anesthetic are required to produce vasoconstriction during the administration of a paracervical block, high concentrations are deposited close to the uterine artery (Fig. 15-13). It is unlikely that such levels are obtained with other forms of regional anesthesia. The third theory is based on the possibility that local anesthetic injected directly into the uterine musculature increases uterine tone.

Some have suggested that manipulation of the fetal head, the uterus, or the uterine vasculature during institution of the block might produce reflex bradycardia. It is possible that no one theory is adequate to explain all cases of postparacervical block bradycardia. Regardless of etiology, the severity and duration of the bradycardia correlate with the incidence of fetal acidosis and subsequent neonatal depression. Freeman and colleagues[201] reported a significant fall in pH and a rise

applications. It occurs within 2 to 10 minutes and lasts from 3 to 30 minutes. Although usually benign, it can be associated with fetal acidosis and occasionally with fetal death.[196–198]

There is no consensus regarding the mechanism of postparacervical block bradycardia. The theories include (1) high blood concentrations of local anesthetic

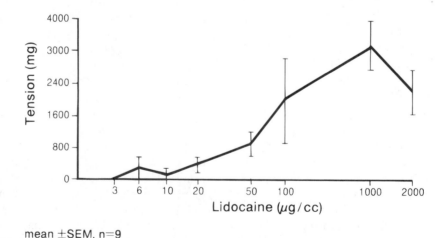

mean ±SEM, n=9

Fig. 15-14 Dose-response curve of the pregnant human uterine artery to lidocaine hydrochloride (mean ± SEM; N = 9). (From Gibbs and Noel,[199] with permission.)

Table 15-4 Anesthetic Procedures Used for Labor in 1992 According to Delivery Service

Delivery Service (births/year)	No Anesthesia (%)	Narcotics Barbiturates Tranquilizers (%)	Paracervical Block (%)	Spinal or Epidural Block (%)
<500	38	46	5	17
500–1,499	15	63	3	32
>1,500	12	49	2	56
All hospitals	22	53	3	34

(From Hawkins et al,[202] with permission)

Table 15-5 Lidocaine Concentrations at Delivery in Maternal Plasma and Umbilical Cord Vein After Perineal Infiltration

Sample (N = 15)	Concentration (ng/ml)	
	Mean ± SD	Range
Maternal plasma		
Peak concentration	648 ± 666	60–2,400
At delivery	548 ± 468	33–1,474
Umbilical cord vein	420 ± 406	45–1,380
Fetal:maternal ratio[a]	1.32 ± 1.46	0.05–4.66

[a] Ratio of level in cord vein to level in maternal vein at delivery (man of individual ratios, not ratio of means).
(From Philipson et al,[203] with permission.)

in base deficit only in those fetuses with bradycardia persisting more than 10 minutes. Paracervical block should be used cautiously at all times and should not be used at all in mothers with fetuses in either acute or chronic distress.

Table 15-4 shows the frequency with which the various forms of analgesia are used during labor. The data are from a joint American Society of Anesthesiologists ACOG survey of 2,265 hospitals in the United States.[202]

Anesthesia for Vaginal Delivery

Pain relief for vaginal delivery can be achieved in a number of ways. Some patients will require no anesthesia. For those who do, the goal is to match the patient's wishes with the requirements of the delivery without subjecting either mother or fetus to unnecessary risk.

Local Anesthesia

In the form of perineal infiltration, local anesthesia is widely used and very safe. Spontaneous vaginal deliveries, episiotomies, and perhaps use of outlet forceps can be accomplished with this simple technique. Local anesthetic toxicity may occur if large amounts of local anesthetic are used or in the unlikely event that an intravascular injection occurs. Usually, 5 to 15 ml of 1 percent lidocaine suffices. Philipson and colleagues[203] demonstrated the rapid and significant transfer of lidocaine to the fetus after perineal infiltration. In 5 of 15 infants, the concentration of lidocaine at delivery was greater in the umbilical vein than in the mother (Table 15-5)[203]

Pudendal Block

Pudendal block is a minor regional block that also is widely used, reasonably effective, and very safe. The obstetrician, using an Iowa trumpet and a 20-gauge needle, injects 5 to 10 ml of local anesthetic just below the ischial spine. Because the hemorrhoidal nerve may be aberrant in 50 percent of patients,[204] some physicians prefer to inject a portion of the local anesthetic

somewhat posterior to the spine (Fig. 15-15). For those inexperienced at identifying the ischial spine, the bony prominence at the inner canthus of one's eye provides a reasonable facsimile of a small and somewhat sharp ischial spine. Although a transperineal approach to the ischial spine is possible, most prefer the transvaginal approach. One percent lidocaine or 2 percent 2-chloroprocaine is used.

The technique is satisfactory for all spontaneous vaginal deliveries and episiotomies and for some outlet or low forceps deliveries, but may not be sufficient for deliveries requiring additional manipulation. For example, a breech delivery or a delivery necessitating more than outlet forceps may require more pain relief, relaxation, and cooperation than pudendal block can ensure. Likewise, a pudendal block may not provide enough anesthesia for the successful and controlled release of shoulder dystocia. In these instances, as in any others that require significant manipulation, more extensive anesthesia will be required. Ideally, such requirements should be anticipated before the event.

More than with perineal infiltration, the potential for local anesthetic toxicity exists with pudendal block because of the proximity of large vessels close to the site of injection (Fig. 15-15). Therefore, aspiration before injection is particularly important. Furthermore, the potential for large amounts of local anesthetic to be used increases when perineal and labial infiltration are required in addition to the pudendal block. In these instances, it is important to monitor closely the amount of local anesthetic given.

Inhalation or Intravenous Analgesia

An anesthesiologist or nurse anesthetist administers inhalation or intravenous analgesia (stage I anesthesia), which provides varying degrees of pain relief and amnesia but maintains protective laryngeal and cough reflexes. Most often the obstetrician will add local infiltration or a pudendal block. The anesthesiologist will

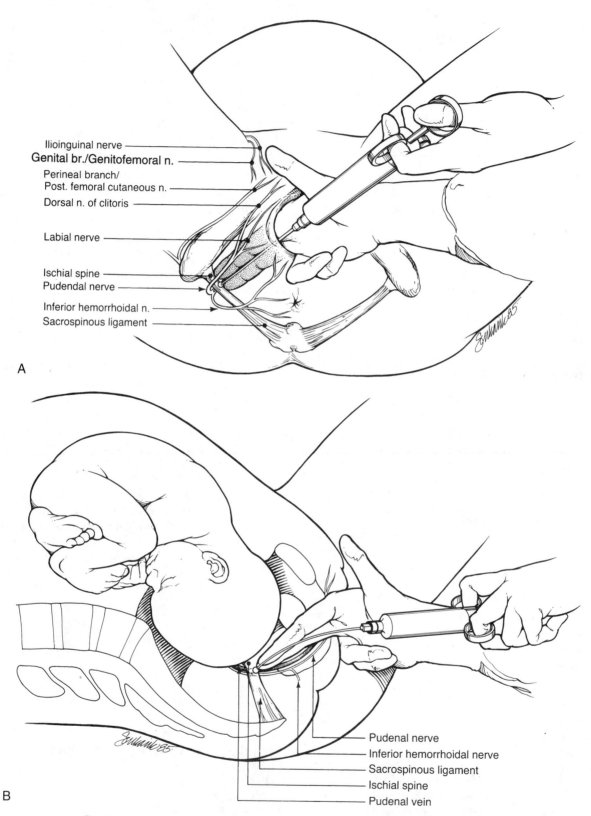

Ilioinguinal nerve

Genital br./Genitofemoral n.

Perineal branch/
Post. femoral cutaneous n.

Dorsal n. of clitoris

Labial nerve

Ischial spine

Pudendal nerve

Inferior hemorrhoidal n.

Sacrospinous ligament

A

Pudenal nerve

Inferior hemorrhoidal nerve

Sacrospinous ligament

Ischial spine

Pudendal vein

B

Fig. 15-15 (A,B) Anatomy of the pudendal nerve and techniques of pudendal block.

frequently question the patient to determine the level of anesthesia and to ensure that deeper planes of anesthesia are avoided. Such precautions are important because, if the patient becomes unconscious and passes beyond stage I, all the hazards associated with general anesthesia are possible, including inadequate airway, hypoxia, and aspiration. Because continual assessment of the patient's state of consciousness is required and is sometimes difficult, only anesthesiologists or nurse anesthetists should administer inhalation analgesia. Furthermore, this technique requires the use of the increasingly complicated anesthesia machine, misuse of which can prove disastrous. Most frequently, the anesthesiologist uses 40 or at most 50 percent nitrous oxide or, for intravenous analgesia, ketamine, 0.25 mg/kg. (This latter agent may be particularly effective for the patient who cannot or will not tolerate an anesthetic face mask.) Less commonly, the anesthesiologist may administer a subanesthetic concentration of a potent halogenated agent (e.g., halothane, enflurane, isoflurane) for a brief period.

Inhalation or intravenous analgesia alone will not be sufficient for performing episiotomies or repairing perineal lacerations. Therefore, these techniques usually require supplemental pudendal block or perineal infiltration. The combined effects of both techniques are additive and satisfactory for spontaneous vaginal deliveries, most outlet forceps deliveries, and even some manipulative deliveries. Inhalation or intravenous analgesia renders some patients amnesic of the event, a characteristic that is often undesirable.

Spinal (Subarachnoid) Block

A saddle block is a spinal block in which the level of anesthesia is limited to little more than the perineum, that is, the saddle area. True saddle blocks are rarely used. Spinal anesthesia is reasonably easy to perform and usually provides total pain relief in the blocked area. Therefore, spontaneous deliveries, forceps deliveries, and episiotomies can be accomplished easily. Likewise, complicated deliveries that require extensive manipulation can be effected in a controlled and pain-free manner. Although the ability to push may be compromised somewhat, the advantage of having a cooperative patient who is receptive to suggestion and able to cooperate because she is pain free may outweigh the disadvantage of moderately diminished strength.

Usually spinal anesthesia is achieved by injecting 4- to 5-mg hyperbaric tetracaine, 25- to 35-mg hyperbaric lidocaine, or 5- to 7.5-mg hyperbaric bupivacaine into the subarachnoid space through a 24- to 27-gauge spinal needle. (It is preferable to use a pencil-point needle of the smallest possible gauge, because these needles produce a minimal risk of spinal headache.)

Because the solution is hyperbaric relative to cerebral spinal fluid, the most important determinant of anesthesia level is gravity. The level is most easily controlled by varying the position of the patient. For example, the sitting position causes the level to fall toward the sacral nerve roots for a perineal block. Other factors may also contribute to the level of anesthesia: amount of drug, volume injected, speed of injection, and height of the patient. Less controllable factors include the Valsalva maneuver, coughing, and straining, any of which will cause the level to rise. If one injects the local anesthetic during a contraction, a higher than expected level of anesthesia may occur. Thus it is best not to inject the local anesthetic during a uterine contraction. Finally, left uterine displacement is maintained by a wedge or by some other effective device placed under the right hip after the local anesthetic has been injected.

Because spinal anesthesia is sometimes administered by persons other than anesthesiologists and is technically easy to perform, the single most important fact to understand is that it is a major regional block; it is not a procedure to be taken lightly. All hazards associated with major blocks are possible, including hypotension and "total spinal." Although these complications can occur, they should not result in disaster if diagnosed early and treated appropriately. The person who administers spinal anesthesia must never leave the patient unattended without ensuring that another competent individual will assume responsibility for monitoring the blood pressure and level of anesthesia. Usually, the level of the spinal block will be complete and fixed within 5 to 10 minutes. However, sometimes the level continues to creep upward for 20 minutes or longer.

Single-Dose Caudal and Lumbar Epidural Anesthesia

Single-dose epidural anesthesia techniques are used much less frequently than in the past. The relative difficulty and the large amounts of local anesthetic required are significant disadvantages for the caudal technique. Usually, when these techniques are used they are instituted during labor as continuous techniques and maintained for the delivery.

General Anesthesia

General anesthesia is rarely indicated for vaginal delivery. Whether given for a brief or a prolonged period of time, general anesthesia engenders considerable risk and should therefore not be used without strong indication. An unanticipated difficult breech, shoulder dystocia, and internal version and extraction of a second twin represent rare indications for general anesthesia. Also, general anesthesia may rarely be indicated for difficult forceps delivery in a patient in whom major

Table 15-6 Anesthetic Procedures Used for Vaginal Delivery in 1992 According to Delivery Service

Delivery Service (births/year)	No Anesthesia (%)	Local or Pudendal Block (%)	Inhalational Analgesia (%)	Preexisting Epidural Block (%)	Spinal Block (%)	General Anesthesia (%)
<500	13	44	1	50	3	1
500–1,499	17	56	1	31	2	1
>1,500	22	65	0	13	3	1
All hospitals	18	55	1	31	3	1

(From Hawkins et al,[202] with permission.)

regional anesthesia is contraindicated. When general anesthesia is indicated, the technique specific for cesarean delivery is used, including administration by experienced and competent personnel, rapid sequence induction, and endotracheal intubation. For breech delivery or delivery of a second twin, one may administer a high concentration of a potent halogenated agent (e.g., halothane, enflurane, isoflurane) to effect uterine and perhaps cervical relaxation. Equipotent doses of any of these three agents will provide equivalent uterine relaxation.[205]

Table 15-6 lists the frequencies with which the various forms of anesthesia are used for vaginal delivery.

Anesthesia for Cesarean Delivery

The patient can be either asleep or awake during cesarean delivery. For those who wish to be awake, either spinal anesthesia or lumbar epidural anesthesia are used most commonly. In the United States, general anesthesia is used for 18 percent of cesarean births, and spinal and epidural anesthesias are used for 41 and 43 percent, respectively (Table 15-7).[202] Local anesthesia for cesarean delivery is possible but only rarely used.[206]

Either general anesthesia or regional anesthesia should be safe for the infant; studies have reported Apgar scores and blood gas values as essentially the same for infants of mothers choosing either technique (Table 15-8).[207–209] In recent years some authors suggested that Apgar scores and acid-base analysis evaluated brain stem activity, but not the activity in higher

brain centers. Therefore, neurobehavioral testing for the newborn was developed.[210] The testing involves eliciting and observing the quality of the infant's responses to certain stimuli in the early postpartum hours. A trained person can accomplish the testing in approximately 15 minutes. Results indicate that infants of mothers who receive regional anesthesia achieve somewhat higher scores than those whose mothers receive general anesthesia, and infants do somewhat better when ketamine is the induction agent for general anesthesia than when thiopental is used.[211] Regarding the choice of local anesthetic for regional anesthesia, infants were originally thought to do better after 2-chloroprocaine and bupivacaine than after lidocaine and mepivacaine.[210,212] Recently, however, lidocaine has been "exonerated" and is associated with neurobehavioral scores equal to those when mothers have received 2-chloroprocaine or bupivacaine.[98] When the Food and Drug Administration (FDA) appointed a committee to study neurobehavioral changes in newborns after anesthesia, the committee concluded that, although anesthetic agents can alter neurobehavioral performance, there was no evidence that they affect later development.[52] Therefore, neurobehavioral con-

Table 15-7 Anesthetic Procedures Used for Cesarean Delivery in 1992 According to Delivery Service

Delivery Service (births/year)	Lumbar Epidural Block (%)	Spinal Block (%)	General Anesthesia (%)
<500	30	49	21
500–1,499	44	38	19
>1,500	54	35	12
All hospitals	43	41	18

(From Hawkins et al,[202] with permission.)

Table 15-8 Elective Cesarean Section—Blood-Gas and Apgar Scores

	General Anesthesia[a] (N = 20)	Epidural Anesthesia[a] (N = 15)	Spinal Anesthesia[b] (N = 15)
Umbilical vein			
pH	7.38	7.359	7.34
P_{O_2} (mmHg)	35	36	37
P_{CO_2} (mmHg)	38	42	48
Apgar <6			
1	1	0	0
5	0	0	0
Umbilical artery			
pH	7.32	7.28	7.28
P_{O_2} (mmHg)	22	18	18
P_{CO_2} (mmHg)	47	55	63
BE (mEq/L)	−1.80	−1.60	−1.40

[a] Data from James et al.[207]
[b] Data from Datta and Brown.[105]

siderations do not weigh heavily in the choice of anesthesia or anesthetic agent; the choice can be based on the preferences of the mother, the obstetrician, and the anesthesiologist as well as on the demands of the particular clinical situation.

General Anesthesia

Although outcomes for the neonate are similar after regional or general anesthesia, failure to intubate and aspiration continue to be major causes of maternal mortality.[213–217] Because these two disadvantages of general anesthesia are of considerable and significant threat to the mother, many anesthesiologists now prefer regional anesthesia over general anesthesia. To understand how these complications arise, the obstetrician should be aware of the sequence of events during general anesthesia. Furthermore, there may be times when the obstetrician must participate in difficult decisions concerning anesthetic management. Those decisions may affect the lives and well-being of both mother and infant.

Premedication

Premedication employing sedative or opioid agents is omitted because these agents cross the placenta and can depress the fetus. Sedation should be unnecessary if the procedure is explained well.

Antacids

Use of a clear antacid is considered routine for all parturients prior to surgery. Additional aspiration prophylaxis using an H_2-receptor blocking agent and/or metoclopramide may be given to parturients with risk factors such as morbid obesity, diabetes, a difficult air-

---

Advantages of General Anesthesia for Cesarean Delivery
   Patient does not have to be awake during a major operation.
   General anesthesia provides total pain relief.
   Operating conditions are optimal.

Disadvantages of General Anesthesia for Cesarean Delivery
   Patient can be awake during childbirth.
   There is a slight risk of fetal depression.
   Intubation causes hypertension and tachycardia, which may be particularly dangerous in severely preeclamptic patients.
   Intubation can be difficult or impossible.
   Aspiration of stomach contents is possible.

---

way, or those who have previously received narcotics. As soon as it is known that the patient requires cesarean delivery, be it with regional or general anesthesia, 30 ml of a clear, nonparticulate antacid, such as 0.3-M sodium citrate,[218] Bicitra,[219] or Alka Seltzer, 2 tablets in 30-ml water,[220] is administered to decrease gastric acidity in order to ameliorate the consequences of aspiration, should it occur. The chalky white particulate antacids are avoided because they can produce lung damage (Fig. 15-16).[221]

Left Uterine Displacement

As during labor, the uterus may compress the inferior vena cava and the aorta during cesarean delivery; aortocaval compression is detrimental to both mother and fetus. The duration of anesthesia makes little difference when left uterine displacement is practiced; however, when patients remain supine, Apgar scores decrease as time of anesthesia increases.[222]

Recent data indicate that the induction-to-delivery time is not the crucial time, rather, it is the uterine incision-to-delivery interval that is predictive of neonatal status.[223] A uterine-incision interval of less than 90 seconds is optimal, whereas an incision-to-delivery interval of 90 to 180 seconds is less satisfactory; after 180 seconds, the incidence of newborn depression is significantly increased. Therefore, it seems that uterine manipulation and difficulty of the delivery are significant factors for the fetus during cesarean delivery.

Preoxygenation

Because patients become unconscious and paralyzed, it is best to wash all nitrogen from the lungs and to replace it with oxygen. This is especially important in pregnant patients, because functional residual capacity is decreased and pregnant patients become hypoxemic more quickly than nonpregnant patients during periods of apnea.[224] Therefore, before starting induction, 100 percent oxygen is administered via face mask for 2 to 3 minutes. In situations of dire emergency, four vital capacity breaths of 100 percent oxygen via a tight circle system will provide similar benefit.[225] Thus, should untoward events occur, the patient can tolerate them for a longer period without becoming hypoxic.

Induction

The anesthesiologist rapidly administers thiopental (a short-acting barbiturate) or ketamine to render the patient unconscious. An appropriate dose of either agent has little effect on the fetus.[226,227]

Muscle Relaxant

Immediately after administration of thiopental or ketamine, the anesthesiologist gives a muscle relaxant to facilitate intubation. Succinylcholine, a rapid-onset,

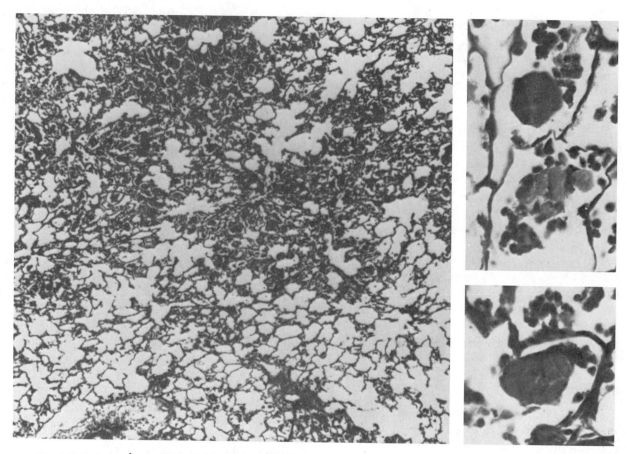

Fig. 15-16 Lung after aspiration of particulate antacid. Compare with normal saline in Figure 15-18. Note marked extensive inflammatory reaction. The alveoli are filled with polymorphonuclear leukocytes and macrophages in approximately equal numbers. Insets at right show large and small intra-alveolar particles surrounded by inflammatory cells (48 hours). Later, the reaction changed to an intra-alveolar cellular collection of clusters of large macrophages with abundant granular cytoplasm, in some of which were small amphophilic particles similar to those seen in the insets. No fibrosis or other inflammatory reaction was seen (28 days). (From Gibbs et al.,[221] with permission.)

short-acting muscle relaxant, remains the agent of choice in most patients.

Cricoid Pressure

In rapid-sequence induction, as the thiopental or ketamine begins to take effect and the patient approaches unconsciousness, an assistant applies pressure to the cricoid cartilage, which is just below the thyroid cartilage, and does not release the pressure until an endotracheal tube is placed, its position verified, and the cuff on the tube inflated.[228,229] Pressure on the cricoid closes off the esophagus and is extremely important in preventing aspiration should regurgitation or vomiting occur. It is a simple, safe, effective maneuver that should not be omitted.

Intubation

Usually intubation proceeds smoothly. However, in approximately 5 percent of patients, it will be difficult or delayed. In some (approximately 0.3 percent of obstet-

ric patients) it will be impossible. The incidence of failed intubation in obstetric patients is about seven times more common than in patients in the general operating room (i.e., 1:280 in the obstetric patient versus 1:2,230 in the surgical patient).[230] When the delay is prolonged or the intubation impossible, the situation becomes a crisis in which the critical factor is to deliver oxygen to the now unconscious and paralyzed patient. Also, because it is during this induction sequence (i.e., before the airway is secured with an endotracheal tube) that the patient is most at risk from aspiration, any delay increases the risk.[214] It is therefore particularly important during a difficult intubation that the person applying cricoid pressure not release that pressure until told to do so by the anesthesiologist.

The patient at risk for a difficult or impossible intubation can often be identified prior to surgery. Examination of the airway is an important part of the anesthetic preoperative evaluation. The most important factors to assess are (1) the ability to visualize oropharyngeal structures (Mallampati classification[231]); (2)

range of motion of the neck; (3) a receding mandible, which indicates the depth of the submandibular space; and (4) whether protruding maxillary incisors are present.[232] When airway abnormalities are recognized by the obstetrician, patients should be referred for an early preoperative evaluation by the anesthesiologist.

Proper Tube Placement

Before the operation begins, the anesthesiologist must ensure that the endotracheal tube is properly positioned within the trachea. End-tidal CO_2 analysis is the preferred method of confirming that the tube is within the trachea.[233] Of course, the anesthesiologist will also confirm that breath sounds are bilateral and equal. If the endotracheal tube is not in the trachea (and therefore is likely in the esophagus), the tube must be removed immediately and the entire situation reassessed. In some instances, the attempt will be repeated. Otherwise, the anesthesiologist will allow the patient to awaken (wherein lies the virtue of the short-acting drugs thiopental and succinylcholine), and another course of action will be chosen. Until the patient completely awakens, ventilation with bag and face mask and continuous application of cricoid pressure may be necessary. Once the patient is awake and breathing spontaneously, the anesthesiologist must choose between awake intubation or regional anesthesia. In most cases, if the endotracheal tube is incorrectly placed, the operation should not proceed until the airway is secure, because the patient cannot be allowed to awaken after the abdomen is opened. If the operation proceeds and ventilation cannot be accomplished, hypoxia, hypercarbia, and cardiac arrest can result; the fetus also will suffer.

When cesarean delivery is not urgent, the decision to delay the operation and to allow the mother to awaken is easy. However, if the operation is being done because of severe fetal distress or maternal hemorrhage, allowing the mother to awaken may further jeopardize the fetus or mother. It is helpful if one continues fetal heart rate monitoring before and even during induction of anesthesia. (In most situations of fetal distress, one can leave the fetal scalp electrode in place until delivery. At that time the circulating nurse can reach under the drapes and disconnect the scalp lead.) Fetal heart rate monitoring may guide anesthetic and obstetric management in situations of failed intubation. Rarely, in situations of dire fetal distress, the anesthesiologist and obstetrician may jointly decide to proceed with cesarean delivery while the anesthesiologist provides oxygenation, ventilation, and anesthesia by face mask ventilation, with an additional person maintaining continuous cricoid pressure. In these emergency situations, it may be necessary to have additional trained personnel to provide assistance. After delivery, the obstetrician should obtain temporary hemostasis and then halt surgery while the anesthesiologist secures the airway by fiberoptic or blind nasal intubation.

The obstetrician and anesthesiologist should address these issues before they become emergent. Such instances should be the subject of combined obstetric/anesthesia conferences during which the concerns of all can be presented and discussed. An algorithm for management of failed intubation in the obstetric patient is shown in Figure 15-17. The anesthesiologist performing a rapid-sequence induction is in a position comparable with the obstetrician confronted with the vaginal delivery of a breech presentation: the anesthesiologist has an unconscious and paralyzed mother whose airway is not yet established, and the obstetrician must deliver the largest part of the baby last. In both instances, one acts before the outcome is certain. In both instances, considerable clinical skill and judgment must be exercised.

Nitrous Oxide and Oxygen

Once the endotracheal tube is in place, a 50:50 mixture of nitrous oxide and oxygen is added to provide analgesia. Such a mixture is safe for both mother and fetus.[234]

Potent Inhalation Agent

Usually, in addition to the nitrous oxide, an analgesic quantity (low concentration) of a potent inhalation agent (e.g., halothane, enflurane, isoflurane, or desflurane) will be added to provide amnesia and additional analgesia. The agents, in low concentrations, are not harmful to mother or fetus. Also, uterine relaxation does not occur, and bleeding is not excessive.[235,236] If one does not add a potent inhalation agent, there will be an unacceptably high incidence of maternal awareness and recall. Even with the use of one of these agents, maternal awareness and recall occasionally occur. Therefore, it is important that all operating room personnel use discretion in conversation and conduct themselves as if the patient were awake.

Postdelivery

Usually the concentration of nitrous oxide can be increased after delivery. In addition, either the potent inhalation agent is continued or an opioid is added to supplement the nitrous oxide and oxygen.

Oxytocin Administration

Ten to 30 units/L are infused intravenously. Bolus injections are avoided, because they can cause hypotension and tachycardia.[237]

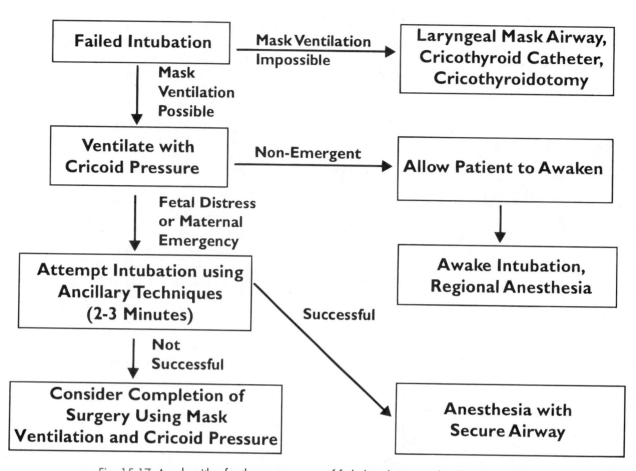

Fig. 15-17 An algorithm for the management of failed intubation in the obstetric patient.

Extubation

Because the patient can aspirate while awakening as well as during induction, extubation is not done until the patient is awake and can respond appropriately to commands. Coughing and bucking do not necessarily indicate that the patient is awake, merely that she is in the second stage, the excitement stage, of anesthesia. It is during this period of anesthesia that laryngospasm is most likely to occur should any foreign body, including the endotracheal tube or bits of stomach contents, stimulate the larynx. The patient must therefore be awake and conscious, not merely active, before extubation.

Recovery

The most important requirement of the recovery room is the presence of personnel trained appropriately and assigned no other duties than those required for the recovery process. The recovery room must contain adequate facilities such as suction, oxygen, and monitoring, and should provide care comparable to that provided patients who have received general or regional anesthesia for other surgical procedures.[3,238–241]

Aspiration

Aspiration is a serious and often fatal complication of general anesthesia and therefore deserves specific attention. In most instances it can be prevented. When it cannot, the consequences depend in part on the volume and nature of the aspirate. The conventional wisdom is that patients are at risk when their stomach contents are greater than 25 ml and when the pH of those contents is less than 2.5.[242] There are several reasons why the pregnant patient is particularly at risk. The enlarged uterus increases intra-abdominal pressure and thus intragastric pressure.[243] The gastroesophageal sphincter is distorted by the enlarged uterus, making it less competent, possibly explaining the high incidence of heartburn that occurs during pregnancy.[244,245] Concentrations of progesterone are increased during pregnancy. Progesterone is a smooth muscle relaxant, and thereby it delays gastric emptying and relaxes the gastroesophageal sphincter. Gastrin, the hormone that increases both acidity and volume of gastric contents, is increased during pregnancy,[246] and motilin, a hormone that speeds gastric emptying, is decreased during pregnancy.[247] Labor itself delays gastric emptying,[248] primarily when patients have received

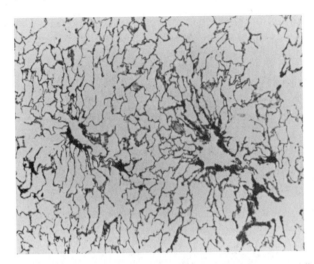

Fig. 15-18 Lung after aspiration of normal saline. Essentially normal lung histology. (From Gibbs and Modell,[273] with permission.)

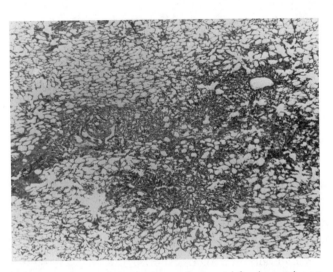

Fig. 15-20 Lung after aspiration of nonacid food particles at pH 5.9. Note inflammatory response around bronchioles and in lung tissues. Edema and hemorrhage exudates are visible. Most of the reaction surrounds the bronchioles. On higher magnification, food particles can be seen as well as polymorphonuclear leukocytes and macrophages. Lung architecture has remained intact. (From Gibbs and Modell,[273] with permission.)

opioids.[249] Many patients undergo cesarean delivery after a prolonged labor, during which they may have received several doses of opioids.[53]

Not all cases of aspiration are the same. The severities of lung damage, morbidity, and mortality vary and depend on the type of material aspirated. Less acid (pH greater than 2.5) liquid significantly decreases PaO_2 physiologically but has very little histologic effect. Liquids with a pH of less than 2.5 decrease PaO_2 further and cause a burn in the lungs that results in hemorrhage, exudate, and edema histologically. The type of aspiration that produces the most severe physiologic and histologic alterations is partially digested food. PaO_2 decreases more than with any other type of aspiration, and lung damage is considerably more destructive[250] (see Table 15-9 and Figs. 15-18 through 15-21).

The variability of the effects is important to the obstetrician and the anesthesiologist. Because the necessity of a cesarean delivery cannot always be predicted, oral intake of anything but small sips of water or ice chips should be prohibited during labor. Eating food during labor is unnecessary and dangerous and should not be encouraged or allowed. Acid liquid can be neutralized safely and effectively with clear antacids or an H_2-receptor antagonist.[218–220,251,252] Partially digested food, however, causes significant hypoxia and lung damage

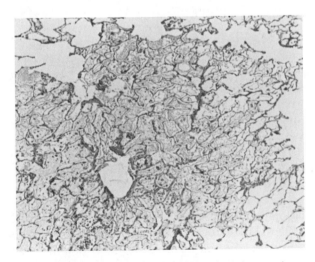

Fig. 15-19 Lung after aspiration of liquid acid. Note hemorrhage (red blood cells) and edema. Lung architecture has remained intact. (From Gibbs and Modell,[273] with permission.)

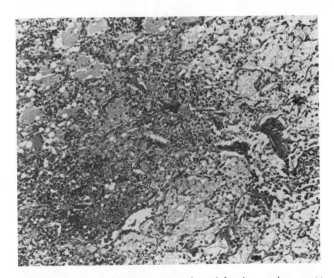

Fig. 15-21 Lung after aspiration of acid food particles at pH 1.8. Hemorrhage exudate and edema are more extensive. Also actual breakdown of alveolar walls and lung architecture has occurred. (From Gibbs and Modell,[273] with permission.)

Table 15-9 Arterial Blood-Gas Tensions and pH of Dogs 30 Minutes After Aspiration of 2 cc/kg of Various Materials

Aspirate		Response		
Composition	pH	PaO_2 (mmHg)	$PaCO_2$ (mmHg)	pH
Saline	5.9	61	34	7.37
HCl	1.8	41	45	7.29
Food particles	5.9	34	51	7.19
Food particles	1.8	23	56	7.13

(From Gibbs and Modell,[273] with permission.)

even at a pH level as high as 5.9.[250] Therefore, the most important and critical preventive measure by the obstetrician is the advice not to eat before coming to the hospital, which should be accompanied by a thorough explanation of the necessity for such advice.

Regional Anesthesia

Hemorrhage is a firm contraindication to regional anesthesia. The blood volume of a hemorrhaging patient is too low for the vascular tree. One compensatory mechanism is vasoconstriction, which reduces the size of the vasculature, making it more commensurate with the blood volume. Major regional anesthesia produces sympathetic blockade, which not only hampers the

---

Advantages of Regional Anesthesia
  The patient is awake and can participate in the birth of her child.
  There is little risk of drug depression or aspiration and no intubation difficulties.
  Newborns generally have good neurobehavioral scores.
  The mother can be given 100 percent oxygen.
  The father is more likely to be allowed in the operating room.

Disadvantages of Regional Anesthesia
  Patients may prefer not to be awake.
  An inadequate block may result.
  Hypotension, perhaps the most common complication of regional anesthesia, occurs during 25 to 75 percent of spinal or epidural procedures.[253–259]
  Total spinal anesthesia may occur.
  Local anesthetic toxicity may occur.
  Although extremely rare, permanent neurologic sequelae may occur.
  There are several contraindications.

---

compensatory mechanism but also dilates the vasculature and makes the discrepancy between volume and vasculature even greater.

Other contraindications to regional anesthesia include infection at the site of needle insertion, coagulopathy, patient refusal, and perhaps some varieties of heart disease. For example, most obstetricians and anesthesiologists have considered epidural anesthesia to be the anesthetic technique of choice for patients with mitral valvular disease, but have considered regional anesthesia to be contraindicated in patients with aortic stenosis, pulmonary hypertension, and/or a right-to-left shunt. The latter group of patients cannot tolerate a decrease in systemic vascular resistance and/or a decrease in venous return of blood to the right side of the heart.[260] Recently there have been several reports of successful administration of epidural anesthesia to patients with aortic stenosis[261] and Eisenmenger syndrome.[262] However, it must be remembered that these reports represent small numbers of cases. Because regional anesthesia results in widespread sympathetic blockade, the pathophysiology of these forms of heart disease would most often dictate that regional anesthesia not be provided. If one chooses to give regional anesthesia to such patients, it is clear that single-dose spinal or epidural anesthesia is inappropriate. Rather, there should be slow, careful induction of epidural anesthesia performed by an anesthesiologist with experience in the use of epidural anesthesia in high-risk obstetric patients. Intrathecal or epidural *opioid* analgesia does not decrease systemic vascular resistance and cause hypotension and has emerged as an attractive choice of analgesia during labor.[263–265]

Fetal distress as a contraindication to regional anesthesia is relative to the type and the degree of fetal distress. If the fetal distress is severe and acute, most often one should not take the additional time necessary to perform a regional technique. Also, if hypotension occurs, the risk to the already compromised fetus is increased. Lesser degrees of fetal distress may well be compatible with regional anesthesia.[266,267] For example, if an epidural catheter has been placed earlier, a partial level of anesthesia already exists, and there is hemodynamic stability, extension of epidural anesthesia may be appropriate for cesarean delivery. The anesthesiologist may give additional local anesthetic while the urethral catheter is inserted and the abdomen is prepared and draped. Often there will be satisfactory anesthesia when the surgeon is ready to make the skin incision. If not, the ongoing fetal heart rate pattern will dictate whether a delay is acceptable. When partial but inadequate epidural anesthesia results, one may consider supplemental local infiltration of local anesthetic. Because the anesthesiologist may have already given a large dose of local anesthetic, the obstetrician should consult with the anesthesiologist to determine the proper choice and concentration of local anesthetic in order to avoid local anesthetic toxicity. (For example, if the anesthesiologist has given lidocaine epidurally, and the patient has an area of inadequate anesthesia, the obstetrician might infiltrate the skin with 1 percent 2-chloroprocaine.)

An improved fetal heart rate tracing may allow one to wait for satisfactory extension of epidural anesthesia, or it may allow the anesthesiologist to perform epidural or spinal anesthesia de novo. Again, this illustrates the usefulness of continuing fetal heart rate monitoring before and during induction of anesthesia. In the absence of satisfactory epidural anesthesia and in the presence of ongoing acute fetal distress, rapid sequence induction of general anesthesia is usually indicated for cesarean delivery. However, one should not indiscriminantly perform rapid sequence induction of general anesthesia. A history and/or suspicion of difficult intubation should prompt performance of either awake intubation or regional anesthesia, despite the presence of fetal distress. One should not endanger the mother in an effort to deliver a distressed fetus. As noted in the ACOG Committee Opinion on Anesthesia for Emergency Deliveries, "the risk of general anesthesia must be weighed against the benefit for those patients who have a greater potential for complications. . . . Cesarean deliveries that are performed for a nonreassuring fetal heart rate pattern do not necessarily preclude the use of regional anesthesia."[268]

Finally, in healthy patients, the choice between epidural and spinal anesthesia will primarily rest with the anesthesiologist. With the recent availability of small-gauge spinal needles with pencil-point tip design, the risk of headache is no different after spinal or epidural anesthesia.[269] Most consider spinal block to be easier and quicker to perform, and most believe that the resulting anesthesia will be more solid and complete. On the other hand, hypotension is more rapid in onset. Perhaps the most significant advantage of spinal anesthesia is that it requires considerably less local anesthetic, and therefore the potential for local anesthetic toxicity is less. Either technique is satisfactory, however, and should provide safe, effective anesthesia for mother, newborn, and obstetrician.

If spinal or epidural anesthesia is used for cesarean delivery, excellent postoperative analgesia can be obtained by addition of narcotics to the local anesthetic solution.[270] In general, the more lipid-soluble narcotics such as fentanyl or sufentanil provide fast onset of analgesia with minimal side effects but have a short duration of 2 to 4 hours. They are often used in a continuous or patient-controlled epidural infusion to extend their duration. In contrast, morphine is quite hydrophilic, which gives it a prolonged duration of up to 24 hours, and it can be given as a single dose at the time of cesarean delivery. Unfortunately its water solubility gives it a long onset time and higher incidence of side effects. The most common side effects of spinal and epidural narcotics are itching and nausea. Respiratory depression is rare in this population.

Several studies have shown that spinal or epidural opioids provide superior pain relief when compared with parenteral (intramuscular or intravenous PCA) narcotics with a trend toward earlier hospital discharge and lower cost.[271,272] Because medications are kept to a minimum with this technique, mothers are rarely sedated and can quickly assume care of the neonate.

Local Anesthesia

The obstetrician can use local anesthesia for a cesarean delivery but must be thoroughly familiar with the recommended maximal dosages of the anesthetic used because large amounts of it may be necessary (Table 15-2). The obstetrician should give a dilute solution of local anesthetic (e.g., 0.5 percent lidocaine or 1.0 percent 2-chloroprocaine) to allow for administration of a sufficiently large volume. (It may be necessary to dilute stock solution of 1 percent lidocaine or 2 percent 2-chloroprocaine to provide the recommended dilute solution.) The patient must be familiar with the procedure and willing to cooperate. When the technique is used successfully, the operation must be done skillfully and with minimal tissue trauma. Such requirements are often difficult to meet during an emergency cesarean delivery, particularly one for severe fetal distress or massive hemorrhage. When a major operation proceeds with local anesthesia, the initial stages of the operation may be accomplished easily, but later the need may arise to progress more rapidly or to use maneuvers that require more tugging and pulling than anticipated. For example, the fetal head may be impacted in the pelvis, or a uterine vein may be lacerated. In these situations the obstetrician must proceed with extreme haste, and a patient under local anesthesia may not be able to tolerate the manipulation. With an anesthesiologist in attendance, general anesthesia can be instituted immediately and the situation resolved. Therefore, the obstetrician must seriously consider all consequences before beginning an emergency cesarean delivery without an anesthesiologist in attendance.

Occasionally local anesthesia is elected in the patient for whom a regional block is technically impossible or contraindicated (e.g., after back injury or surgery) so that the patient can be awake for the delivery of the infant. In these cases, after delivery of the infant general anesthesia is initiated for completion of the operation.

Summary

Obstetric anesthesia has much to offer the obstetric patient. However, as in many other areas of medicine, anesthesia can be dangerous when used inappropriately. To make best use of the available techniques, cooperation and continued communication must exist between all parties: obstetrician, anesthesiologist, and patient.

Key Points

- Analgesia during labor can reduce or prevent adverse hormonal and metabolic stress responses to the pain of labor.

- Use of parenteral opioids for labor analgesia can produce respiratory depression in the mother and newborn and delayed gastric emptying in the mother. However, when used appropriately, opioids are safe and effective.

- Placental transfer of a drug between mother and fetus is governed by the characteristics of the drug (including its size, lipid solubility, and ionization), maternal blood levels and uterine blood flow, placental circulation, and the fetal circulation.

- Regional analgesia is the most effective form of intrapartum pain relief currently available and has the flexibility to provide additional anesthesia for spontaneous or instrumental delivery, cesarean delivery, and postoperative pain control.

- Spinal opioids provide excellent analgesia during much of the first stage of labor while decreasing or avoiding the risks of local anesthetic toxicity, high spinal anesthesia, and motor block. Patients can often ambulate, although most will need additional analgesia later in labor and during the second stage.

- Side effects and complications of regional anesthesia include hypotension, local anesthetic toxicity, total spinal anesthesia, neurologic injury, and spinal headache. Personnel providing anesthesia must be available and competent to treat these problems.

- Epidural analgesia during labor is associated with an increased risk of prolonged labor and operative delivery, but whether there is a cause and effect relationship is controversial. Epidural analgesia is not a generic procedure, and use of a dilute solution of local anesthetic is less likely to result in prolonged labor and malposition of the fetal vertex.

- General anesthesia is utilized for 18 percent of cesarean sections. Although safe for the newborn, general anesthesia can be associated with failed intubation and aspiration, the leading causes of anesthesia-related maternal mortality.

- Aspiration of gastric contents causes the worst physiologic consequences when there are food particles present and/or pH is less than 2.5; therefore, patients should *not* be encouraged to eat during labor.

- Regional anesthesia may be an appropriate choice for cesarean delivery for fetal distress, especially if there is a suspicion of a difficult maternal airway.

References

1. Orkin FW: The Geographical Distribution of Anesthesia Care Providers in the United States. Committee on Manpower, American Society of Anesthesiologists, Park Ridge, IL, 1983

2. Orkin FK: The geographic distribution of anesthesiologists during rapid growth in their supply, abstracted. Anesthesiology 81:A1295, 1994

3. Joint Statement on the Optimal Goals for Anesthesia Care in Obstetrics. American Society of Anesthesiologists/American College of Obstetricians and Gynecologists, Washington, DC, 1988

4. Melzack R, Taenzer P, Feldman P, Kinch RA: Labour is still painful after prepared childbirth training. Can Assoc Med J 125:357, 1981

5. Burns JK: Relation between blood levels of cortisol and duration of human labour. J Physiol (Lond) 254:12P, 1976

6. Tuimala RJ, Kauppila JI, Haapalahti J: Response of pituitary-adrenal axis on partial stress. Obstet Gynecol 46:275, 1975

7. Lederman RP, McCann DS, Work B Jr: Endogenous plasma epinephrine and norepinephrine in last-trimester pregnancy and labor. Am J Obstet Gynecol 129:5, 1977

8. Falconer AD, Powles AB: Plasma noradrenaline levels during labour: influence of elective lumbar epidural blockade. Anaesthesia 37:416, 1982

9. Goland RS, Wardlaw SI, Stark RI, Frantz AG: Human plasma beta-endorphin during pregnancy, labor, and delivery. J Clin Endocrinol Metab 52:74, 1981

10. Fletcher JE, Thomas TA, Hill RG: Beta-endorphin and parturition. Lancet 1:310, 1980

11. Rossier J, French ED, Rivier C et al: Foot-shock induced β-endorphin levels in blood but not brain. Nature 270:618, 1977

12. Dubois M, Pickar D, Cohen MR et al: Surgical stress in humans is accompanied by an increase in plasma beta-endorphin immunoreactivity. Life Sci 29:1249, 1981

13. Wardlaw SL, Stark RI, Bazi L, Frantz AG: Plasma beta-endorphin and beta-lipotropin in human fetus at delivery: correlation with arterial pH and PO_2. J Clin Endocrinol Metab 49:888, 1979

14. Yanagida H, Corssen G: Respiratory distress and beta-endorphin-like immunoreactivity in humans. Anesthesiology 55:515, 1981

15. Lederman RP, Lederman E, Work BA Jr, McCann DS: The relationship of maternal anxiety, plasma catecholamines, and plasma cortisol to progress in labor. Am J Obstet Gynecol 132:495, 1978

16. Adamsons K, Mueller-Heubach E, Myers RE: Production of fetal asphyxia in the rhesus monkey by administration of catecholamines to the mother. Am J Obstet Gynecol 109:248, 1971

17. Rosenfeld CR, Barton MD, Meschia G: Effects of epinephrine on distribution of blood flow in the pregnant ewe. Am J Obstet Gynecol 124:156, 1976

18. Roman-Ponce H, Thatcher WW, Caton D et al: Effects of thermal stress and epinephrine on uterine blood flow in ewes. J Anim Sci 46:167, 1978

19. Myers RE: Maternal psychological stress and fetal asphyxia: a study in the monkey. Am J Obstet Gynecol 122:47, 1975

20. Morishima HO, Yeh M-N, James LS: Reduced uterine blood flow and fetal hypoxemia with acute maternal stress: experimental observation in the pregnant baboon. Am J Obstet Gynecol 134:270, 1979

21. Morishima HO, Pedersen H, Finster M: The influence of maternal psychological stress on the fetus. Am J Obstet Gynecol 131:286, 1978

22. Copher DE, Huber CP: Heart rate response of the human fetus to induced maternal hypoxia. Am J Obstet Gynecol 98:320, 1967

23. Eidelman AI, Hoffmann NW, Kaitz M: Cognitive deficits in women after childbirth. Obstet Gynecol 81:764, 1993

24. Maltau JM, Eielsen OV, Stokke KT: Effect on the stress during labor on the concentration of cortisol and estriol in maternal plasma. Am J Obstet Gynecol 134:681, 1979

25. Buchan PC, Milne MK, Browning MCK: The effect of continuous epidural blockade on plasma 11-hydroxycorticosteroid concentrations in labour. J Obstet Gynaecol Br Commonw 80:974, 1973

26. Thornton CA, Carrie LES, Sayers I et al: A comparison of the effect of extradural and parenteral analgesia on maternal plasma cortisol concentrations during labour and the puerperium. Br J Obstet Gynaecol 83:631, 1976

27. Abboud TK, Sarkis F, Hung TT et al: Effects of epidural anesthesia during labor on maternal plasma beta-endorphin levels. Anesthesiology 59:1, 1983

28. Abboud TK, Artal R, Henriksen EH et al: Effects of spinal anesthesia on maternal circulating catecholamines. Am J Obstet Gynecol 142:252, 1982

29. Myers R, Myers SE: Use of sedative, analgesic, and anesthetic drugs during labor and delivery: bane or boon? Am J Obstet Gynecol 133:83, 1979

30. Pearson JF, Davies P: The effect of continuous lumbar epidural analgesia upon fetal acid-base status during the first stage of labour. J Obstet Gynaecol Br Commonw 81:971, 1974

31. Pearson JF, Davies P: The effect of continuous lumbar epidural analgesia upon fetal acid-base status during the second stage of labour. J Obstet Gynaecol Br Commonw 81:975, 1974

32. Beazley JM, Leaver EP, Morewood JHM, Bircumshaw J: Relief of pain in labour. Lancet 1:1033, 1967

33. Jaffe JH, Martin WR: Narcotic analgesics and antagonists. p. 245. In Goodman LS, Gilman A (eds): The Pharmacological Basis of Therapeutics. 5th Ed. Macmillan, New York, 1975

34. Bonica JJ: Principles and Practice of Obstetric Analgesia and Anesthesia. p. 234. FA Davis, Philadelphia, 1967

35. Shute E, Davis ME: The effect on the infant of morphine administered in labor. Surg Gynecol Obstet 57:727, 1933

36. Kuhnert BR, Kuhnert PM, Tu AL, Lin DCK: Meperidine and normeperidine levels following meperidine

administration during labor. II. Fetus and neonate. Am J Obstet Gynecol 133:909, 1979

37. Pittman KA, Smyth RD, Losada M et al: Human perinatal distribution of butorphanol. Am J Obstet Gynecol 138:797, 1980

38. Shnider S, Moya F: Effects of meperidine on the newborn infant. Am J Obstet Gynecol 89:1009, 1964

39. Way WL, Costley EC, Way EL: Respiratory sensitivity of the newborn infant to meperidine and morphine. Clin Pharmacol Ther 6:454, 1965

40. Gillam JS, Hunter GW, Darner CB, Thompson GR: Meperidine hydrochloride and alphaprodine hydrochloride as obstetric analgesic agents. Am J Obstet Gynecol 75:1105, 1958

41. Gordon DWS, Pinker GD: Increased pethidine dosage in obstetrics associated with the use of nalorphine. J Obstet Gynaecol Br Commonw 65:606, 1958

42. Walker PA: Drugs used in labour: an obstetrician's view. Br J Anaesth 45(suppl):787, 1973

43. Hodgkinson R, Huff RW, Hayashi RH, Husain FJ: Double-blind comparison of maternal analgesia and neonatal neurobehavior following intravenous butorphanol and meperidine. J Int Med Res 7:224, 1979

44. Quilligan EJ, Keegan KA, Donahue MJ: Double-blind comparison of intravenously injected butorphanol and meperidine in parturients. Int J Gynaecol Obstet 18:363, 1980

45. Miller FC, Meuller E, McCart D: Maternal and fetal response to alphaprodine during labor: a preliminary study. J Reprod Med 27:439, 1982

46. Rayburn WF, Smith CV, Parriott JE, Woods RE: Randomized comparison of meperidine and fentanyl during labor. Obstet Gynecol 74:604, 1989

47. Emergency Cardiac Care Committee and Subcommittees, American Heart Association: Neonatal resuscitation. JAMA 268:2276, 1992

48. Committee on Obstetrics: Maternal and Fetal Medicine: Naloxone Use in Newborns. American College of Obstetricians and Gynecologists, Washington, DC, 1989

49. Brackbill Y, Kane J, Manniello RL, Abramson D: Obstetric premedication and infant outcome. Am J Obstet Gynecol 118:377, 1974

50. Stechler G: Newborn attention as affected by medication during labor. Science 144:315, 1964

51. Corke BC: Neurobehavioural responses of the newborn: the effect of different forms of maternal analgesia. Anaesthesia 32:539, 1977

52. Kolata GB: Scientists attack report that obstetrical medications endanger children. Science 204:391, 1979

53. Nimmo WA, Wilson J, Prescott LF: Narcotic analgesics and delayed gastric emptying during labour. Lancet 1:890, 1975

54. Wright PMC, Allen RW, Moore J, et al: Gastric emptying during lumbar extradural analgesia in labour: effect of fentanyl supplementation. Br J Anaesth 68:248, 1992

55. O'Sullivan GM, Sutton AJ, Thompson SA et al: Noninvasive measurement of gastric emptying in obstetric patients. Anesth Analg 66:505, 1987

56. Kuhnert BR, Kuhnert PM, Tu AL et al: Meperidine and normeperidine levels following meperidine administration during labor. I. Mother. Am J Obstet Gynecol 133:904, 1979

57. Kuhnert BR, Philipson EH, Kuhnert PM, Syracuse CD: Disposition of meperidine and normeperidine following multiple doses during labor. I. Mother. Am J Obstet Gynecol 151:406, 1985

58. Kuhnert BR, Kuhnert PM, Philipson EH, Syracuse CD: Disposition of meperidine and normeperidine following multiple doses during labor. II. Fetus and neonate. Am J Obstet Gynecol 151:410, 1985

59. Lazebnik N, Kuhnert BR, Carr PC et al: Intravenous, deltoid, or gluteus administration of meperidine during labor? Am J Obstet Gynecol 160:1184, 1989

60. Rayburn WF, Smith CV, Parriott JE et al: Randomized comparison of meperidine and fentanyl during labor. Obstet Gynecol 74:604, 1989

61. Kleinman SJ, Wiesel S, Tessler MJ: Patient-controlled analgesia (PCA) using fentanyl in a parturient with a platelet function abnormality. Can J Anaesth 38:489, 1991

62. Rosaeg OP, Kitts JB, Koren G et al: Maternal and fetal effects of intravenous patient-controlled fentanyl analgesia during labour in a thrombocytopenic parturient. Can J Anaesth 39:277, 1992

63. Maduska AL, Hajghassemali M: A double-blind comparison of butorphanol and meperidine in labour: maternal pain relief and effect on the newborn. Can Anaesth Soc J 25:398, 1978

64. Nagashima H, Karamanian A, Malovany R et al: Respiratory and circulatory effects of intravenous butorphanol and morphine. Clin Pharmacol Ther 19:738, 1976

65. Kallos T, Caruso FS: Respiratory effects of butorphanol and pethidine. Anaesthesia 34:633, 1979

66. Romagnoli A, Keats AS: Ceiling effect for respiratory depression by nalbuphine. Clin Pharmacol Ther 27:478, 1980

67. Wilson CM, McClean E, Moore J, Dundee JW: A double-blind comparison of intramuscular pethidine and nalbuphine in labour. Anaesthesia 41:1207, 1986

68. Robinson JO, Rosen M, Evans JM et al: Self-administered intravenous and intramuscular pethidine. Anesthesia 35:763, 1980

69. Podlas J, Breland BD: Patient-controlled analgesia with nalbuphine during labor. Obstet Gynecol 70:202, 1987

70. Rayburn W, Leuschen MP, Earl R et al: Intravenous meperidine during labor: a randomized comparison between nursing- and patient-controlled administration. Obstet Gynecol 74:702, 1989

71. Clutton-Brach JC: Some pain threshold studies with particular reference to thiopentone. Anaesthesia 15:71, 1960

72. Dundee JW: Alterations in response to somatic pain associated with anaesthesia. II. The effect of thiopentone and pentobarbitone. Br J Anaesth 32:407, 1960

73. Irving FC: Advantages and disadvantages of the barbiturates in obstetrics. RI Med J 28:493, 1945

74. Powe CE, Kiem IM, Fromhagen C, Cavanagh D: Propiomazine hydrochloride in obstetrical analgesia: a controlled study of 520 patients. JAMA 181:290, 1962

75. Benson C, Benson RC: Hydroxyzine-meperidine anal-

gesia and neonatal response. Am J Obstet Gynecol 84: 37, 1962

76. Zsigmond EK, Patterson RL: Double-blind evaluation of hydroxyzine hydrochloride in obstetric anesthesia. Anesth Analg 46:275, 1967

77. Owen JR, Irani SF, Blair AW: Effect of diazepam administered to mothers during labour on temperature regulation of neonate. Arch Dis Child 47:107, 1972

78. Cree JE, Meyer J, Hailey DM: Diazepam in labour: its metabolism and effect on the clinical condition and thermogenesis of the newborn. BMJ 4:251, 1973

79. Hahn E: An Atlas of Fetal Heart Rate Patterns. Hardy Press, New Haven, CT, 1968

80. Yeh SY, Paul RH, Cordero L, Hon EH: A study of diazepam during labor. Obstet Gynecol 43:363, 1974

81. Schiff D, Chan G, Stern L: Fixed drug combinations and the displacement of bilirubin from albumin. Pediatrics 48:139, 1971

82. Wilson CM, Dundee JW, Moore J et al: A comparison of the early pharmacokinetics of midazolam in pregnant and nonpregnant women. Anaesthesia 42:1057, 1987

83. Ravlo O, Carl P, Crawford ME et al: A randomized comparison between midazolam and thiopental for elective cesarean section anesthesia. II. Neonates. Anesth Analg 68:234, 1989

84. Bland BAR, Lawes EG, Duncan PW et al: Comparison of midazolam and thiopental for rapid sequence anesthetic induction for elective cesarean section. Anesth Analg 66:1165, 1987

85. Camann W, Cohen MB, Ostheimer GW: Is midazolam desireable for sedation in parturients? Anesthesiology 65:441, 1986

86. Gross JB, Weller RS, Conard P: Flumazenil antagonism of midazolam-induced ventilatory depression. Anesthesiology 75:179, 1991

87. Moya F, Thorndike V: Passage of drugs across the placenta. Am J Obstet Gynecol 84:1778, 1962

88. Dilts PV: Placental transfer. Clin Obstet Gynecol 24: 555, 1981

89. Ralston DH: Perinatal pharmacology. p. 50. In Shnider SM, Levinson G (eds): Anesthesia for Obstetrics. 2nd Ed. Williams & Wilkins, Baltimore, 1987

90. Alper MH: What drugs cross the placenta and what happens to them in the fetus? p. I. In Henry SG (ed): Refresher Courses in Anesthesiology. Vol. 4. American Society of Anesthesiologists, Park Ridge, IL, 1976

91. Makowski EL, Meschia G, Droegemueller W, Battaglia FC: Distribution of uterine blood flow in the pregnant sheep. Am J Obstet Gynecol 101:409, 1968

92. Biehl D, Shnider SM, Levinson G, Callender K: Placental transfer of lidocaine: effects of fetal acidosis. Anesthesiology 48:409, 1978

93. Sinclair JC, Fox HA, Lentz JF et al: Intoxication of the fetus by a local anesthetic. N Engl J Med 273:1173, 1965

94. Collis RE, Baxandall ML, Srikantharajah ID et al: Combined spinal epidural (CSE) analgesia: technique, management, and outcome of 300 mothers. Int J Obstet Anesth 3:75, 1994

95. Honet JE, Arkoosh VA, Norris MC et al: Comparison among intrathecal fentanyl, meperidine, and sufentanil for labor analgesia. Anesth Analg 75:734, 1992

96. Norris MC, Grieco WM, Borkowski M et al: Complications of labor analgesia: epidural versus combined spinal epidural techniques. Anesth Analg 79:529, 1994

97. Crawford JS: The second thousand epidural blocks in an obstetric hospital practice. Br J Anaesth 44:1277, 1972

98. Abboud TK, Khoo SS, Miller F et al: Maternal, fetal, and neonatal responses after epidural anesthesia with bupivacaine, 2-chloroprocaine, or lidocaine. Anesth Analg 61:638, 1982

99. Jouppila R, Jouppila P, Karinen JM, Hollmen A: Segmental epidural analgesia in labour: related to the progress of labour, fetal malposition and instrumental delivery. Acta Obstet Gynaecol Scand 58:135, 1979

100. Kandel PF, Spoerel WE, Kinch RAH: Continuous epidural analgesia for labour and delivery: review of 1000 cases. Can Med Assoc J 95:947, 1966

101. Matadial L, Cibils LA: The effect of epidural anesthesia on uterine activity and blood pressure. Am J Obstet Gynecol 125:846, 1976

102. Datta S, Kitzmiller JL, Naulty JS et al: Acid-base status of diabetic mothers and their infants following spinal anesthesia for cesarean section. Anesth Analg 61:662, 1982

103. James FM, Greiss FC Jr, Kemp RA: An evaluation of vasopressor therapy for maternal hypotension during spinal anesthesia. Anesthesiology 33:25, 1970

104. Brizgys RV, Dailey PA, Shnider SM et al: The incidence and neonatal effects of maternal hypotension during epidural anesthesia for cesarean section. Anesthesiology 67:782, 1987

105. Datta S, Brown WU: Acid-base status in diabetic mothers and their infants following general or spinal anesthesia for cesarean section. Anesthesiology 47:272, 1977

106. Kenepp NB, Sheley WC, Kumar S et al: Effects on newborn of hydration with glucose in patients undergoing caesarean section with regional anesthesia. Lancet 1: 645, 1980

107. Ralston DH, Shnider SM, deLorimier AA: Effects of equipotent ephedrine, metaraminol, mephentermine, and methoxamine on uterine blood flow in the pregnant ewe. Anesthesiology 40:354, 1974

108. Moran DH, Perillo M, LaPorta RF et al: Phenylephrine in the prevention of hypotension following spinal anesthesia for cesarean delivery. J Clin Anesth 3:301, 1991

109. Ralston DH, Shnider SM: The fetal and neonatal effects of regional anesthesia in obstetrics. Anesthesiology 48: 34, 1978

110. Chadwick HS, Posner K, Caplan RA et al: A comparison of obstetric and nonobstetric anesthesia malpractice claims. Anesthesiology 74:242, 1991

111. Albright GA: Cardiac arrest following regional anesthesia with etidocaine or bupivacaine. Anesthesiology 51: 285, 1979

112. deJong RH, Gamble CA, Bonin JD: Bupivacaine-induced cardiac arrhythmias and plasma cation concen-

trations in normokalemic cats. Regional Anesth 8:104, 1983

113. Clarkson CW, Hondeghem LM: Mechanism for bupivacaine depression of cardiac conduction: fast block of sodium channels during the action potential with slow recovery from block during diastole. Anesthesiology 62: 396, 1985

114. Morishima HO, Pedersen H, Finster M et al: Bupivacaine toxicity in pregnant and nonpregnant ewes. Anesthesiology 63:134, 1985

115. Abbott Laboratories: Letter to Doctors: Urgent New Recommendations About Bupivacaine. Astra Pharmaceutical Products, Inc., Breon Laboratories, Westboro, MA 1984

116. Writer WDR, Davies JM, Strunin L: Trial by media: the bupivacaine story. Can Anaesth Soc J 31:1, 1984

117. Moore DC, Batra MS: The components of an effective test dose prior to epidural block. Anesthesiology 55: 693, 1981

118. Abraham RA, Harris AP, Maxwell LG, Kaplow S: The efficacy of 1.5 percent lidocaine with 7.5 percent dextrose and epinephrine as an epidural test dose for obstetrics. Anesthesiology 64:116, 1986

119. Leighton BL, Norris MC, Sosis M et al: Limitations of epinephrine as a marker of intravascular injection in laboring women. Anesthesiology 66:688, 1987

120. Moore DC, Crawford RD, Scurlock JE: Severe hypoxia and acidosis following local anesthetic-induced convulsions. Anesthesiology 53:259, 1980

121. Dripps RD, Eckenhoff JE, Vandam LD: Long-term follow-up of patients who received 10,098 spinal anesthetics: failure to discover major neurological sequelae. JAMA 156:1486, 1954

122. Ravindran RS, Bond VK, Tasch MD et al: Prolonged neural blockade following regional analgesia with 2-chloroprocaine. Anesth Analg 59:447, 1980

123. Reisner LS, Hochman BN, Plumer MH: Persistent neurologic deficit and adhesive arachnoiditis following intrathecal 2-chloroprocaine injection. Anesth Analg 59: 452, 1980

124. Moore DC, Spierdijk J, Van Kleef JD et al: Chloroprocaine neurotoxicity: four additional cases. Anesth Analg 61:155, 1982

125. Gissen AJ, Datta S, Lambert D: The chloroprocaine controversy, II. Is chloroprocaine neurotoxic? Regional Anesth 9:135, 1984

126. Fibuch EE, Opper SE: Back pain following epidurally administered Nesacaine-MPF. Anesth Analg 69:113, 1989

127. Levy L, Randel GI, Pandit SK: Does chloroprocaine (Nesacaine MPF) for epidural anesthesia increase the incidence of backache? Anesthesiology 71:476, 1989

128. Cole JT: Maternal obstetric paralysis. Am J Obstet Gynecol 52:374, 1946

129. Goldstein PJ: The lithotomy position. p. 142. In Martin JT (ed): Positioning in Anesthesia and Surgery. WB Saunders, Philadelphia, 1978

130. Deppe G, Hercule J, Gleicher N: Sciatic nerve injury complicating surgical removal of retroperitoneal tumor. Acta Obstet Gynaecol Scand 63:369, 1984

131. Ong BY, Cohen MM, Esmail A et al: Paresthesias and motor dysfunction after labor and delivery. Anesth Analg 66:18, 1987

132. Breen TW, Ransil BJ, Groves PA et al: Factors associated with back pain after childbirth. Anesthesiology 81:29, 1994

133. Groves PA, Breen TW, Ransil BJ et al: Natural history of postpartum back pain and its relationship with epidural anesthesia, abstracted. Anesthesiology 81:A1167, 1994

134. Stride PC, Cooper GM: Dural taps revisited. Anaesthesia 48:247, 1993

135. Carbaat PAT, van Crevel H: Lumbar puncture headache: controlled study on the preventive effect of 24 hours' bed rest. Lancet 2:1133, 1981

136. Craft JB, Epstein BS, Coakley CS: Prophylaxis of dural-puncture headache with epidural saline. Anesth Analg 52:228, 1973

137. Camann WR, Murray RS, Mushlin PS et al: Effects of oral caffeine on postdural puncture headache. Anesth Analg 70:181, 1990

138. Szeinfeld M, Ihmeldan IH, Moser MM et al: Epidural blood patch: evaluation of the volume and spread of blood injected into the epidural space. Anesthesiology 64:820, 1986

139. Ravindran RS: Epidural autologous blood patch on an outpatient basis. Anesth Analg 63:962, 1984

140. DiGiovanni AJ, Galbert MW, Wahle WM: Epidural injection of autologous blood for postlumbar-puncture headache. II. Additional clinical experiences and laboratory investigation. Anesth Analg 51:226, 1972

141. Abouleish E, de la Vega S, Blendinger I, Tio TO: Long-term follow-up of epidural blood patch. Anesth Analg 54:459, 1975

142. Abouleish E, Wadhwa RK, de la Vega S et al: Regional analgesia following epidural blood patch. Anesth Analg 54:634, 1975

143. Loeser EA, Hill GE, Bennett GM, Sederberg JH: Time vs. success rate for epidural blood patch. Anesthesiology 49:147, 1978

144. Quaynor H, Corbey M: Extradural blood patch—why delay? Br J Anaesth 57:538, 1985

145. Berrettini WH, Simmons-Alling S, Nurnberger JI: Epidural blood patch does not prevent headache after lumbar puncture. Lancet 1:856, 1987

146. Cheek TG, Banner R, Sauter J, Gutsche BB: Prophylactic extradural blood patch is effective. Br J Anaesth 61: 340, 1988

147. Chelmow D, Kilpatrick SJ, Laros RK: Maternal and neonatal outcomes after prolonged latent phase. Obstet Gynecol 81:486, 1993

148. Kong AS, Bates SJ, Rizk B: Rupture of membranes before the onset of spontaneous labour increases the likelihood of instrumental delivery. Br J Anaesth 68:252, 1992

149. Naulty JS, Smith R, Ross R: The effect of changes in labor analgesic practice on labor outcome, abstracted. Anesthesiology 69:A660, 1988

150. Friedman EA: Effects of drugs on uterine contractility. Anesthesiology 26:409, 1965

151. Committee on Obstetrics: Maternal and Fetal Medicine:

Dystocia: Etiology, Diagnosis, and Management Guidelines. American College of Obstetricians and Gynecologists, Washington, DC, 1983

152. Peisner DB, Rosen MG: Transition from latent to active labor. Obstet Gynecol 68:448, 1986

153. Chestnut DH, Vandewalker GE, Owen CL et al: The influence of continuous epidural bupivacaine analgesia on the second stage of labor and method of delivery in nulliparous women. Anesthesiology 66:774, 1987

154. Kilpatrick SJ, Laros RK: Characteristics of normal labor. Obstet Gynecol 74:85, 1989

155. Maresh M, Choong KH, Beard RW: Delayed pushing with lumbar epidural analgesia in labour. Br J Obstet Gynaecol 90:623, 1983

156. Cohen WR: Influence of the duration of second stage labor on perinatal outcome and puerperal morbidity. Obstet Gynecol 49:266, 1977

157. Pearson JF: The effect of continuous lumbar epidural analgesia on maternal acid-base balance and arterial lactate concentration during the second state of labour. J Obstet Gynaecol Br Commonw 80:225, 1973

158. Committee on Obstetrics: Maternal and Fetal Medicine: Obstetric Forceps. American College of Obstetricians and Gynecologists, Washington, DC, 1988

159. Robinson JO, Rosen M, Evans JM et al: Maternal opinion about analgesia for labor. Anaesthesia 35:1173, 1980

160. Philipsen T, Jensen NH: Epidural block or parenteral pethidine as analgesic in labour: a randomized study concerning progress in labour and instrumental deliveries. Eur J Obstet Gynecol Reprod Biol 30:27, 1989

161. Phillips KC, Thomas TA: Second stage of labour with or without extradural analgesia. Anaesthesia 38:972, 1983

162. Chestnut DH, Bates JN, Choi WW: Continuous infusion epidural analgesia with lidocaine: efficacy and influence during the second stage of labor. Obstet Gynecol 69:323, 1987

163. Johnsrud ML, Dale PO, Loveland B: Benefits of continuous infusion epidural analgesia throughout vaginal delivery. Acta Obstet Gynecol Scand 67:355, 1988

164. Gribble RK, Meier PR: Effect of epidural analgesia on the primary cesarean rate. Obstet Gynecol 78:231, 1991

165. Larson DD: The effect of initiating an obstetric anesthesiology service on rate of cesarean section and rate of forceps delivery. Soc Obstet Anesth Perinatol 13:1992

166. Iglesias S, Burn R, Saunders LD: Reducing the cesarean section rate in a rural community hospital. Can Med Assoc J 145:1459, 1991

167. Socol ML, Garcia PM, Peaceman AM: Reducing cesarean births at a primarily private university hospital. Am J Obstet Gynecol 168:1748, 1993

168. Robson M, Boylan P, McParland P et al: Epidural analgesia need not influence the spontaneous vaginal delivery rate, abstracted. Am J Obstet Gynecol 168:364, 1993

169. Farabow WS, Roberson VO, Maxey J et al: A twenty-year retrospective analysis of the efficacy of epidural analgesia-anesthesia when administered and/or managed by obstetricians. Am J Obstet Gynecol 169:270, 1993

170. Neuhoff D, Burke S, Porreco RP: Cesarean birth for failed progress in labor. Obstet Gynecol 73:915, 1989

171. Thorp JA, Parisi VM, Boylan PC et al: The effect of continuous epidural analgesia on cesarean section for dystocia in nulliparous women. Am J Obstet Gynecol 161:670, 1989

172. Thorp JA, Eckert LO, Ang MS et al: Epidural analgesia and cesarean section for dystocia: risk factors in nulliparas. Am J Perinatol 8:402, 1991

173. Thorp JA, Hu DH, Albin RM et al: The effect of intrapartum epidural analgesia on nulliparous labor: a randomized, controlled, prospective trial. Am J Obstet Gynecol 169:851, 1993

174. Chestnut DH, Vincent RD, McGrath JM: Does early administration of epidural analgesia affect obstetric outcome in nulliparous women who are receiving intravenous oxytocin? Anesthesiology 80:1193, 1994

175. Chestnut DH, McGrath JM, Vincent RD: Does early administration of epidural analgesia affect obstetric outcome in nulliparous women who are in spontaneous labor? Anesthesiology 80:1201, 1994

176. Dewan DM, Cohen SE: Epidural analgesia and the incidence of cesarean section. Time for a closer look. Anesthesiology 80:1189, 1994

177. American Society of Anesthesiologists and American College of Obstetricians and Gynecologists: Pain relief during labor. Joint Statement on Pain Relief during Labor. Washington, DC, 1992

178. Lowensohn RI, Paul RH, Fales S et al: Intrapartum epidural anesthesia: an evaluation of effects on uterine activity. Obstet Gynecol 44:388, 1974

179. Cheek TG, Samuels P, Tobin M et al: Rapid intravenous saline infusion decreases uterine activity in labor. Epidural analgesia does not, abstracted. Anesthesiology 71:A884, 1989

180. Maltau JM, Andersen HT: Epidural anaesthesia as an alternative to caesarean section in the treatment of prolonged, exhaustive labour. Acta Anaesthesiol Scand 19:349, 1975

181. Craft JB, Epstein BS, Coakley CS: Effect of lidocaine with epinephrine versus lidocaine (plain) on induced labor. Anesth Analg 51:243, 1972

182. Abboud TK, David S, Nagappala S et al: Maternal, fetal, and neonatal effects of lidocaine with and without epinephrine anesthesia in obstetrics. Anesth Analg 63:973, 1984

183. Abboud TK, Sheik-ol-Eslam A, Yanagi T et al: Safety and efficacy of epinephrine added to bupivacaine for lumbar epidural analgesia in obstetrics. Anesth Analg 64:585, 1985

184. Abboud TK, DerSarkissian L, Terrasi J et al: Comparative maternal, fetal, and neonatal effects of chloroprocaine with and without epinephrine for epidural anesthesia in obstetrics. Anesth Analg 66:71, 1987

185. Eisenach JC, Grice SC, Dewan DM: Epinephrine enhances analgesia produced by epidural bupivacaine during labor. Anesth Analg 66:447, 1987

186. Johnson WL, Winter WW, Eng M et al: Effect of pudendal, spinal, and peridural block anesthesia on the second stage of labor. Am J Obstet Gynecol 113:166, 1972

187. Morrison DH, Smedstad KG: Continuous infusion epidurals for obstetric analgesia. Can Anaesth Soc J 32:101, 1985

188. Nadeau S, Elliott RD: Continuous bupivacaine infusion during labour: effects on analgesia and delivery, abstracted. Can Anaesth Soc J 32:S70, 1985

189. Bogod DG, Rosen M, Rees GAD: Extradural infusion of 0.125 percent bupivacaine at 10 ml h^{-1} to women during labour. Br J Anaesth 59:325, 1987

190. Gaylard DG, Wilson IH, Balmer HGR: An epidural infusion technique for labor. Anaesthesia 42:1098, 1987

191. Hicks JA, Jenkins JG, Newton MC et al: Continuous epidural infusion of 0.075 percent bupivacaine for pain relief in labour: a comparison with intermittent top-ups of 0.5 percent bupivacaine. Anaesthesia 43:289, 1988

192. Smedstad KG, Morrison DH: A comparative study of continuous and intermittent epidural analgesia for labour and delivery. Can J Anaesth 35:234, 1988

193. Chestnut DH, Owen CL, Bates JN et al: Continuous infusion epidural analgesia during labor: a randomized, double-blind comparison of 0.0625 percent bupivacaine/0.0002 percent fentanyl versus 0.125 percent bupivacaine. Anesthesiology 68:754, 1988

194. Goodfellow CF, Hull MGR, Swaab DF et al: Oxytocin deficiency at delivery with epidural analgesia. Br J Obstet Gynaecol 90:214, 1983

195. Bates RG, Helm CW, Duncan A, Edmonds DK: Uterine activity in the second stage of labour and the effect of epidural analgesia. Br J Obstet Gynaecol 92:1246, 1985

196. Shnider SM, Asling JH, Holl JW, Margolis AJ: Paracervical block anesthesia in obstetrics. I. Fetal complications and neonatal morbidity. Am J Obstet Gynecol 107:619, 1970

197. Tafeen CH, Freedman HL, Harris H: Combination continuous paracervical and continued pudendal nerve block anesthesia in labor. Am J Obstet Gynecol 100:55, 1968

198. Teramo K, Widholm O: Studies of the effects of anesthetics on foetus. I. The effect of paracervical block with mepivacaine upon fetal-base values. Acta Obstet Gynaecol Scand 46(suppl 2):1, 1967

199. Gibbs CP, Noel SC: Response of arterial segments from gravid human uterus to multiple concentrations of lignocaine. Br J Anaesth 45:409, 1977

200. Greiss FC Jr, Still JG, Anderson SG: Effects of local anesthetic agents on the uterine vasculatures and myometrium. Am J Obstet Gynecol 124:889, 1976

201. Freeman RK, Gutierrez NA, Ray ML et al: Fetal cardiac response to paracervical block anesthesia. Part I. Am J Obstet Gynecol 113:583, 1972

202. Hawkins JL, Gibbs CP, Orleans M et al: Obstetric anesthesia workforce survey—1992 versus 1981, abstracted. Anesthesiology 81:A1128, 1994

203. Philipson EH, Kuhnert BR, Syracuse CD: Maternal, fetal, and neonatal lidocaine levels following local perineal infiltration. Am J Obstet Gynecol 149:403, 1984

204. Klink EW: Perineal nerve block: an anatomic and clinical study in the female. Obstet Gynecol 1:137, 1953

205. Munson ES, Embro WJ: Enflurane, isoflurane and halothane and isolated human uterine muscle. Anesthesiology 46:11, 1977

206. Ranney B, Stanage WF: Advantages of local anesthesia for cesarean section. Obstet Gynecol 45:163, 1975

207. James FM III, Crawford JS, Hopkinson R et al: A comparison of general anesthesia and lumbar epidural analgesia for elective cesarean section. Anesth Analg 56:228, 1977

208. Magno R, Kjellmer I, Karlson K: Anaesthesia for cesarean section. III. Effects of epidural analgesia on the respiratory adaptation of the newborn in elective caesarean section. Acta Anaesthesiol Stand 20:73, 1976

209. Datta S, Alper MH: Anesthesia for cesarean section. Anesthesiology 53:142, 1980

210. Scanlon JW, Brown WU Jr, Weiss JB, Alper MH: Neurobehavioral responses of newborn infants after maternal epidural anesthesia. Anesthesiology 40:121, 1974

211. Hodgkinson R, Bhatt M, Kim SS et al: Neonatal neurobehavioral tests following cesarean section under general and spinal anesthesia. Am J Obstet Gynecol 132:670, 1978

212. McGuinness GA, Merkow AJ, Kennedy RL, Erenberg A: Epidural anesthesia with bupivacaine for cesarean section: neonatal blood levels and neurobehavioral responses. Anesthesiology 49:270, 1978

213. Marx GF, Finster M: Difficulty in endotracheal intubation associated with obstetric anesthesia. Anesthesiology 51:364, 1979

214. Gibbs CP, Rolbin SH, Norman P: Cause and prevention of maternal aspiration. Anesthesiology 61:111, 1984

215. Turnbull AC, Tindall VR, Robson G et al: Report on Confidential Enquiries Into Maternal Deaths in England and Wales 1979–1981. Her Majesty's Stationery Office, London, 1986

216. Morgan M: Anaesthetic contribution to maternal mortality. Br J Anaesth 59:842, 1987

217. Hawkins JL, Koonin L, Palmer SK et al: Anesthesia-related maternal deaths in the United States: a twelve year review 1979–1990, abstracted. Anesthesiology 79:A982, 1993

218. Gibbs CP, Spohr L, Schmidt D: The effectiveness of sodium citrate as an antacid. Anesthesiology 57:44, 1982

219. Gibbs CP, Banner TC: Effectiveness of Bicitra as a preoperative antacid. Anesthesiology 61:97, 1984

220. Chen CT, Toung TJ, Cameron JL: Alka-Seltzer® for prophylactic use in prevention of acid aspiration pneumonia. Anesthesiology 57:A103, 1982

221. Gibbs CP, Schwartz DJ, Wynne JW et al: Antacid pulmonary aspiration in the dog. Anesthesiology 51:380, 1979

222. Crawford JA, Burton M, Davies P: Time and lateral tilt at caesarean section. Br J Anaesth 44:477, 1972

223. Datta S, Ostheimer GW, Weiss JB et al: Neonatal effect of prolonged anesthetic induction for cesarean section. Obstet Gynecol 58:331, 1981

224. Archer GW, Marx GF: Arterial oxygen tension during apnoea in parturient women. Br J Anaesth 46:358, 1974

225. Norris MC, Dewan DM: Preoxygenation for cesarean section: a comparison of two techniques. Anesthesiology 62:827, 1985

226. Kosaka Y, Takahashi T, Mark LC: Intravenous thiobarbiturate anesthesia for cesarean section. Anesthesiology 31:489, 1969

227. Peltz B, Sinclair DM: Induction agents for cesarean sec-

tion: a comparison of thiopental and ketamine. Anaesthesia 28:37, 1973

228. Sellick BA: Cricoid pressure to control regurgitation of stomach contents during induction of anesthesia. Lancet 2:404, 1961

229. Sellick BA: Rupture of the oesophagus following cricoid pressure? Anaesthesia 37:213, 1982

230. Samsoon GLT, Young JRB: Difficult tracheal intubation: a retrospective study. Anaesthesia 42:487, 1987

231. Mallampati SR, Gatt SP, Gugino LD et al: A clinical sign to predict difficult tracheal intubation: a prospective study. Can Anaesth Soc J 32:429, 1985

232. Rocke DA, Murray WB, Rout CC et al: Relative risk analysis of factors associated with difficult intubation in obstetric anesthesia. Anesthesiology 77:67, 1992

233. American Society of Anesthesiologists: Standards for Basic Intra-Operative Monitoring. American Society of Anesthesiologists, Park Ridge, IL, 1995

234. Marx GF, Joshi CW, Orkin LR: Placental transmission of nitrous oxide. Anesthesiology 32:429, 1970

235. Moir DD: Anaesthesia for caesarean section: an evaluation of a method using low concentrations of halothane and 50 percent of oxygen. Br J Anaesth 42:136, 1970

236. Warren TM, Datta S, Ostheimer GW et al: Comparison of the maternal and neonatal effects of halothane, enflurane, and isoflurane for cesarean delivery. Anesth Analg 62:516, 1983

237. Andersen TW, DePadua CB, Stenger V, Prystowsky H: Cardiovascular effects of rapid intravenous injection of synthetic oxytocin during elective cesarean section. Clin Pharmacol Ther 6:345, 1965

238. Orkin LR, Shapiro G: Admission assessment and general monitoring. Int Anesthesiol Clin 21:3, 1983

239. Aldrete JA, Kroulik D: A postanesthetic recovery score. Anesth Analg 49:924, 1970

240. Fisher TL: Responsibility for care in recovery rooms. Can Med Assoc J 102:78, 1970

241. Clark RB, Miller FC: Recovery room and postoperative complications of cesarean section. Anesthesiol Clin North Am 8:173, 1990

242. Roberts RB, Shirley MA: Reducing the risk of acid aspiration during cesarean section. Anesth Analg 53:859, 1974

243. Spence AA, Moir DD, Finlay WEI: Observations on intragastric pressure. Anaesthesia 22:249, 1967

244. Greenan J: The cardio-oesophageal junction. Br J Anaesth 33:432, 1961

245. Williams MH: Variable significance of heartburn. Am J Obstet Gynecol 42:814, 1941

246. Attia RR, Ebeid AM, Fisher JE, Goudsouzian NG: Maternal fetal and placental gastrin concentrations. Anaesthesia 37:18, 1982

247. Christofides ND, Ghatei MA, Bloom SR et al: Decreased plasma motilin concentrations in pregnancy. BMJ 285:1453, 1982

248. Davison JS, Davison MC, Hay DM: Gastric emptying time in late pregnancy and labour. J Obstet Gynaecol Br Commonw 77:37, 1970

249. O'Sullivan GM, Bullingham RE: Noninvasive assessment by radiotelemetry of antacid effect during labor. Anesth Analg 64:95, 1985

250. Schwartz DJ, Wynne JW, Gibbs CP et al: The pulmonary consequences of aspiration of gastric contents at pH values greater than 2.5. Am Rev Respir Dis 121:119, 1980

251. Eyler SW, Cullen BF, Murphy ME, Welch WD: Antacid aspiration in rabbits: a comparison of Mylanta and Bicitra. Anesth Analg 61:288, 1982

252. Hodgkinson R, Glassenberg R, Joyce TH et al: Comparison of cimetidine (Tagamet®) with antacid for safety and effectiveness in reducing gastric acidity before elective cesarean section. Anesthesiology 59:86, 1983

253. James FM III, Dewan DM, Floyd HM et al: Chloroprocaine vs. bupivacaine for lumbar epidural analgesia for elective cesarean section. Anesthesiology 52:488, 1980

254. Caritis SN, Abouleish E, Edelstone DI, Mueller-Heubach E: Fetal acid-base state following spinal or epidural anesthesia for cesarean section. Obstet Gynecol 56:610, 1980

255. Belfrage P, Irestedt L, Raabe N, Arner S: General anaesthesia or lumbar epidural block for caesarean section? Effects on the foetal heart rate. Acta Anaesthesiol Scand 21:67, 1977

256. Corke BC, Datta S, Ostheimer GW et al: Spinal anaesthesia for caesarean section: the influence of hypotension on neonatal outcome. Anaesthesia 37:658, 1982

257. Downing JW, Houlton PC, Barclay A: Extradural analgesia for caesarean section: a comparison with general anaesthesia. Br J Anaesth 51:367, 1979

258. Fox GS, Smith JB, Namba Y, Johnson RC: Anesthesia for cesarean section: further studies. Am J Obstet Gynecol 133:15, 1979

259. Gibbs CP, Werba JV, Banner TE et al: Epidural anesthesia: leg-wrapping prevents hypotension. Anesthesiology 59:A405, 1983

260. Mangano DT: Anesthesia for the pregnant cardiac patient. p. 345. In Shnider SM, Levinson G (eds): Anesthesia for Obstetrics. 2nd Ed. Williams and Wilkins, Baltimore, 1987

261. Easterling TR, Chadwick HS, Otto CM, Benedetti TJ: Aortic stenosis in pregnancy. Obstet Gynecol 72:113, 1988

262. Spinnato JA, Kraynack BJ, Cooper MW: Eisenmenger's syndrome in pregnancy: epidural anesthesia for elective cesarean section. N Engl J Med 304:1215, 1981

263. Ahmad S, Hawes D, Dooley S et al: Intrathecal morphine in a parturient with a single ventricle. Anesthesiology 54:515, 1981

264. Abboud TK, Raya J, Noveihed R, Daniel J: Intrathecal morphine for relief of labor pain in a parturient with severe pulmonary hypertension. Anesthesiology 59:477, 1983

265. Pollack KL, Chest DH, Wenstrom KD: Anesthetic management of a parturient with Eisenmenger's syndrome. Anesth Analg 70:212, 1990

266. Marx GF, Luykx WM, Cohen S: Fetal-neonatal status following caesarean section for fetal distress. Br J Anaesth 56:1009, 1984

267. Chestnut DH: Fetal distress. p. 385. In James FM,

Dewan DM, Wheeler AS (eds): Obstetric Anesthesia: The Complicated Patient. 2nd Ed. FA Davis, Philadelphia, 1988

268. Committee on Obstetrics: Maternal and Fetal Medicine: Anesthesia for emergency deliveries. American College of Obstetricians and Gynecologists, Washington, DC, 1992

269. Hurley RJ, Lambert D, Hertwig L et al: Post dural puncture headache in the obstetric patient: spinal vs epidural anesthesia, abstracted. Anesthesiology 77:A1018, 1992

270. Abouleish E, Rawal N, Rashad MN: The addition of 0.2 mg subarachnoid morphine to hyperbaric bupivacaine for cesarean delivery: a prospective study of 856 cases. Regional Anesth 16:137,1991

271. Cohen SE, Subak LL, Brose WG, Halpern J: Analgesia after cesarean delivery: patient evaluations and costs of five opioid techniques. Regional Anesth 16:141, 1991

272. Baysinger CL, Harkins TL, Horger EO, Chana CH: Intrathecal morphine sulfate versus intravenous patient controlled analgesia following cesarean section: a comparison of hospital costs and duration of stay, abstracted. Anesth Analg 78:S22, 1994

273. Gibbs CP, Modell JH: Management of aspiration pneumonitis. p. 1293. In Miller RD (ed): Anesthesia. 3rd Ed. Vol. 2. Churchill Livingstone, New York, 1990

274. Shnider SM, Wright RG, Levinson G et al: Uterine blood flow and plasma norepinephrine changes during maternal stress in the pregnant ewe. Anesthesiology 50:526, 1979

275. Bonica JJ: Obstetric Analgesia and Anesthesia. World Federation of Societies of Anesthesiologists, Amsterdam, 1980

276. Haymaker L, Woodhall B: Peripheral Nerve Injuries. WB Saunders, Philadelphia, 1945

277. Thomas J, Climmie CR, Long G, Nighjoy LE: The influence of adrenaline on the maternal plasma levels and placental transfer of lignocaine following lumbar epidural administration. Br J Anaesth 41:1031, 1969

Chapter 16

Malpresentations

John W. Seeds and Margaret Walsh

Near term or during labor, the fetus normally assumes a vertical orientation or lie and a cephalic presentation with the fetal vertex flexed on the neck (Fig. 16-1). In about 5 percent of cases, however, deviation occurs from this normal lie, presentation, and flexion attitude, and such deviation constitutes a fetal malpresentation. The word *malpresentation* suggests adverse consequences and is typically associated with increased risk to both the mother and the fetus. Malpresentation once led to a variety of maneuvers intended to facilitate vaginal delivery, and early in this century such interventions included destructive operations leading predictably to fetal death. Later, manual or instrumental attempts to convert the malpresenting fetus to a more favorable orientation were devised. Internal podalic version followed by a complete breech extraction was once advocated as a solution to many malpresentation situations. However, internal podalic version along with most manipulative efforts to achieve vaginal delivery were associated with a high fetal or maternal morbidity or mortality rate and have been largely abandoned. In contemporary practice, cesarean delivery has become the recommended alternative to manipulative vaginal techniques when normal progress toward vaginal delivery is not observed.

This chapter examines malpresentations, possible etiologies, and the mechanics of labor and vaginal delivery unique to each situation.

Clinical Circumstances Associated With Malpresentation

Generally, factors associated with malpresentation include (1) diminished vertical polarity of the uterine cavity, (2) increased or decreased fetal mobility, or (3) obstructed pelvic inlet. The association of great parity with malpresentation is presumably related to laxity of maternal abdominal muscular support and therefore loss of the normal vertical orientation of the uterine cavity. Placentation either high in the fundus or low in the pelvis (Fig. 16-2) is another factor that diminishes the likelihood of a fetus comfortably assuming a longitudinal axis. Uterine myomata, intrauterine synechiae, and müllerian duct abnormalities such as septate uterus or uterus didelph are also associated with a higher than expected rate of malpresentation. Both prematurity and hydramnios permit increased fetal mobility; thus 5 there is an increased probability of a noncephalic presentation if labor or rupture of membranes occurs. In contrast, such conditions as autosomal trisomies, myotonic dystrophy, and fetal neurologic dysfunction that result in decreased fetal muscle tone, strength, or activity are also associated with an increased incidence of malpresentation. Furthermore, preterm birth involves a fetus that is small relative to the maternal pelvis and results in increased fetal mobility. In these cases, pelvic engagement and descent with labor or rupture of membranes can occur despite malpresentation. Finally, the cephalopelvic disproportion associated with severe fetal hydrocephalus or with a frankly contracted pelvis is frequently implicated as an etiology of malpresentation because normal engagement of the fetal head is prevented.

Abnormal Axial Lie

The fetal "lie" indicates the orientation of the fetal spine relative to that of the mother. The normal fetal lie is longitudinal and by itself does not indicate whether the presentation is cephalic or breech. If the

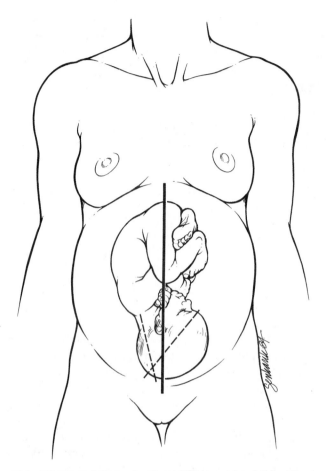

Fig. 16-1 Frontal view of a fetus in a longitudinal lie with fetal vertex flexed on the neck.

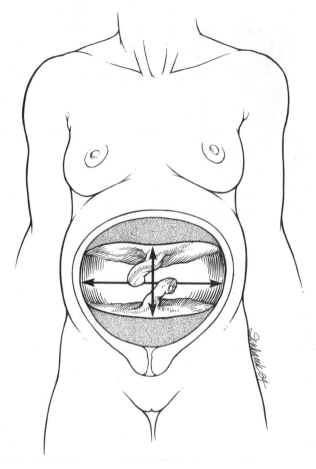

Fig. 16-2 Either the high fundal or low implantation of the placenta illustrated here would normally be in the vertical orientation of the intrauterine cavity and increase the probability of a malpresentation.

Etiologic Factors in Malpresentation

Maternal
  Great parity
  Pelvic tumors
  Pelvic contracture
  Uterine malformation
Fetal
  Prematurity
  Multiple gestation
  Hydramnios
  Macrosomia
  Hydrocephaly
  Trisomies
  Anencephaly
  Myotonic dystrophy
  Placenta previa

fetal spine or long axis crosses that of the mother, the fetus may be said to occupy a transverse or oblique lie (Fig. 16-3), resulting in a shoulder or arm presentation (Fig. 16-4). The presentation is termed unstable if the fetal membranes are intact and there is great fetal mobility.[1]

Abnormal fetal lie is diagnosed on average in approximately 1 in 300 cases, or 0.33 percent.[2-8] Prematurity is often a factor, with abnormal lie reported to occur in about 2 percent of pregnancies at 32 weeks, or six times the rate found at term.[9] Persistence of a transverse, oblique, or unstable lie beyond 37 weeks requires a systematic clinical assessment and plan for management, since rupture of membranes without a fetal part filling the inlet of the pelvis imposes a high risk of cord prolapse, fetal compromise, and maternal morbidity if neglected.

Great parity, prematurity, pelvic contracture, and abnormal placentation are the most commonly reported clinical factors associated with abnormal lie,[2,5-9] although Cockburn and Drake[3] found many cases that manifested none of these. Any condition that alters the normal vertical polarity of the intrauterine cavity will predispose to abnormal lie.

Diagnosis may be by palpation or vaginal examination. Routine use of Leopold's maneuvers may assist detection, but Thorp et al.[10] found the sensitivity of Leopold's maneuvers for the detection of malpresentation to be only 28 percent and the positive predictive value only 24 percent compared with immediate ultrasound verification. Others have observed prenatal detection in as few as 41 percent of cases before labor.[3] A fetal loss rate of 9.2 percent[3] with early diagnosis compares with a mortality of 27.5 percent when the diagnosis was delayed, indicating that early diagnosis improves fetal outcome.

Reported perinatal mortality for unstable or transverse lie (corrected for lethal malformations or extreme prematurity) varies from 3.9 percent[11] to 24 percent,[1] with maternal mortality as high as 10 percent. Maternal deaths are usually related to infection after premature rupture of membranes, hemorrhage secondary to abnormal placentation, complications of operative intervention for cephalopelvic disproportion, or traumatic delivery.[7,9] Fetal loss of the normally developed infant of a viable gestational age is primarily associated with neglect, prolapsed cord, or traumatic delivery.[9] Cord prolapse occurs 20 times as often with abnormal axial lie as it does with a cephalic presentation.

Management

There is a consensus that the normally grown infant at term cannot undergo a safe vaginal delivery from an axial malpresentation.[4,7] Furthermore, a careful search for a potentially dangerous or compromising etiology is indicated. A transverse/oblique or unstable lie late in the third trimester necessitates ultrasound examination to exclude major fetal malformation and abnormal placentation. Elective hospitalization may permit observation and early recognition of cord prolapse.[6,11] Phelan et al.[12] reported a series of 29 patients with transverse lie diagnosed at or beyond 37 weeks' gestation managed expectantly. Eighty three percent (24 of 29) spontaneously converted to breech (9 of 24) or vertex (15 of 24) before labor; however, the overall cesarean delivery rate was 45 percent, and there were two cases of cord prolapse, one uterine rupture, and one neonatal death. Such outcomes suggest that active intervention at or beyond 37 weeks or after confirmation of fetal lung maturity may be of benefit. External cephalic version with subsequent induction of labor if successful might diminish the risk of adverse outcome.

The risk of fetal death varies with the type of obstetric intervention. Fetal mortality of 0 to 10 percent has been reported for cesarean birth compared with 25 to 90

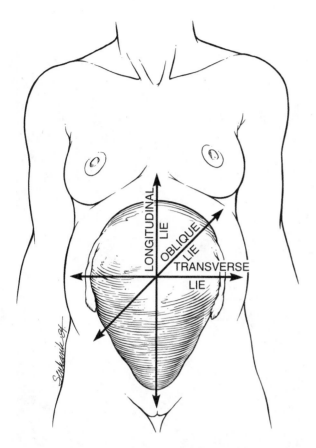

Fig. 16-3 A fetus may occupy a longitudinal, oblique, or transverse axis, as illustrated by these vectors. The lie does not indicate whether the vertex or the breech is closest to the cervix.

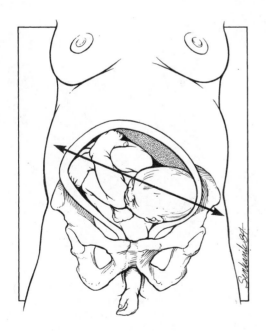

Fig. 16-4 This fetus lies in an oblique axis with an arm prolapsing.

percent when internal podalic version and breech extraction are performed.[3,4,7–9,13] A mortality rate only 6 percent was reported for successful external version and vertex vaginal delivery.[8,9]

External cephalic version followed by induction of labor after 37 weeks in the case of abnormal lie is a reasonable alternative to both expectant management and elective cesarean delivery. Although disputed by some,[3,14] external cephalic version has been found to be safe, with close monitoring, and effective in the majority of cases.[15] Using such a protocol, Edwards and Nicholson[6] reported 86 of 96 cases delivered vaginally, with fetal compromise detected in only four and no fetal losses.

If external version is unsuccessful or unavailable, if spontaneous rupture of membranes occurs, or if active labor has begun with an abnormal lie, cesarean delivery is the treatment of choice for the potentially viable infant.[1,3,14] There is no place for internal podalic version and breech extraction in the management of transverse or oblique lie or unstable presentation in singleton pregnancies because of the unacceptably high rate of fetal and maternal complications.[2]

A persistent abnormal axial lie, particularly if accompanied by ruptured membranes, also alters the choice of uterine incision at cesarean delivery. Although a low transverse cervical incision has many surgical advantages, up to 25 percent of transverse incisions require vertical extension for delivery of an infant from an abnormal lie to allow access to and atraumatic delivery of the vertex entrapped in the muscular fundus.[3,14] Furthermore, the lower uterine segment is often poorly developed. It makes no sense to perform a cesarean to minimize birth trauma, then choose a transverse uterine incision if that incision makes delivery more difficult. Therefore, in cases of transverse or oblique lie with ruptured membranes or a poorly developed lower segment, a vertical incision is more prudent. Intraoperative cephalic version may allow the use of a low transverse incision, as reported by Pelosi et al.,[14] but ruptured membranes with oligohydramnios makes this unlikely.

Deflection Attitudes

The normal "attitude" of the fetal vertex during labor is one of full flexion on the neck, with the fetal chin against the upper chest. Deflection attitudes include various degrees of deflection or even extension of the fetal head on the neck (Fig. 16-5). Spontaneous conversion to a more normal flexed attitude or further extension of an intermediate deflection to a fully extended position will commonly occur as labor progresses. Although safe vaginal delivery is possible in most cases, experience indicates that cesarean delivery is the only

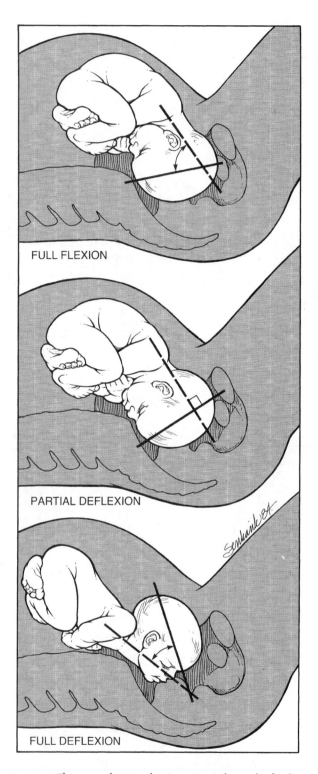

Fig. 16-5 The normal "attitude" (top view) shows the fetal vertex flexed on the neck. Partial deflexion (middle view) shows the fetal vertex intermediate between flexion and extension. Full deflexion (lower view) shows the fetal vertex completely extended, with the face presenting.

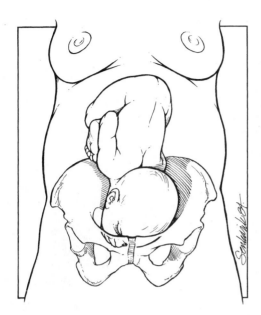

Fig. 16-6 This fetus with the vertex completely extended on the neck enters the maternal pelvis in a face presentation. The cephalic prominence would be palpable on the same side of the maternal abdomen as the fetal spine.

appropriate alternative when arrest of progress is observed.

Face Presentation

A face presentation is characterized by a longitudinal lie and full extension of the fetal head on the neck, with the occiput against the upper back (Fig. 16-6). The fetal chin is chosen as the point of designation at vaginal examination. For example, a fetus presenting by the face whose chin is in the right posterior quadrant of the maternal pelvis would be called a *right mentum posterior* (RMP) (Fig. 16-7). The reported incidence of face presentation ranges from 0.14 to 0.54 percent,[8,16–21] averaging about 0.2 percent, or 1 in 500 live births overall. Reported perinatal mortality, corrected for nonviable malformations and extreme prematurity, varies from 0.6 percent[22] to 5 percent,[23] averaging about 2 to 3 percent.

All clinical factors known to increase the general rate of malpresentation (see box) have been implicated in face presentation, but Browne and Carney[24] emphasized that as many as 60 percent of infants with a face presentation were malformed. Anencephaly, for instance, is found in about one-third of cases of face presentation.[5,25,26] Frequently observed maternal factors include a contracted pelvis or cephalopelvic disproportion in 10 to 40 percent of cases.[17,20,23] In a review of face presentation, Duff[18] found that one of these etiologic factors was found in up to 90 percent of cases.

Early recognition is important, and diagnosis can be suspected anytime abdominal palpation finds the fetal cephalic prominence on the same side of the maternal abdomen as the fetal back (Fig. 16-8); however, face presentation is more often discovered by vaginal examination and confirmed by radiography or ultrasound. In practice, fewer than 1 in 20 infants with face presentation is diagnosed abdominally.[22] In fact, only half of these infants are found to be face presentation by any means prior to the second stage of labor,[20,22,26,27] and half of the remaining cases are undiagnosed until delivery.[20,23] Perinatal mortality may be higher, however, with late diagnosis.[17]

Mechanism of Labor

Knowledge of the early mechanism of labor for the face presentation is incomplete. Many infants with a face presentation probably begin labor in the less extended brow position. With descent into the pelvis, the forces

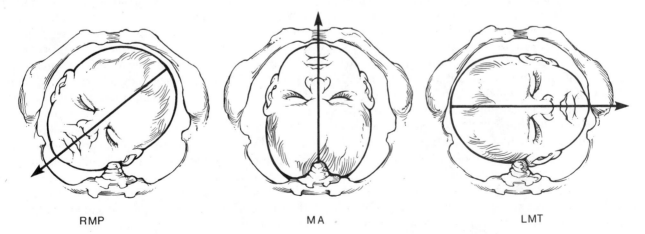

RMP   MA   LMT

Fig. 16-7 The point of designation from digital examination in the case of a face presentation is the fetal chin relative to the maternal pelvis. (A) Right mentum posterior (RMP). (B) Mentum anterior (MA). (C) Left mentum transverse (LMP).

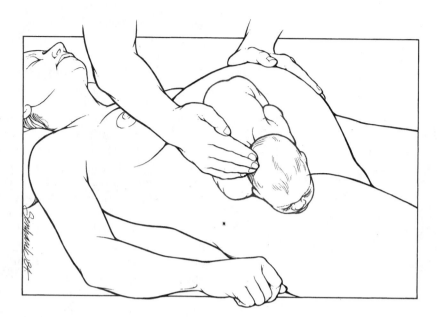

Fig. 16-8 Palpation of the maternal abdomen in the case of a face presentation should find the fetal cephalic prominence on the side away from the fetal small parts instead of on the same side as in the case of a normally flexed fetal head.

of labor press the fetus against maternal tissues, and either flexion or full extension of the head on the spine occurs. The labor of a face presentation must include engagement, descent, internal rotation generally to a mentum anterior position, and delivery by flexion under the symphysis (Fig. 16-9). However, flexion of the occiput may not always occur. Borrell and Fernstrom[28] have proposed that delivery in the full extended attitude may be common.

The prognosis for labor with a face presentation depends on the orientation of the fetal chin. At diagnosis, 60 to 80 percent of infants with a face presentation are mentum anterior,[5,20,22,29] 10 to 12 percent are mentum transverse,[5,22,29] and 20 to 25 percent are mentum posterior.[5,20,22,29] Almost all average-sized infants presenting mentum anterior with adequate pelvic dimensions will achieve spontaneous or easily assisted vaginal delivery.[5,22,30,31] Furthermore, most mentum transverse infants will rotate to the mentum anterior position and deliver vaginally, and even 25 to 33 percent of mentum posterior infants will rotate and deliver vaginally in the mentum anterior position.[5,16,20] In a review of 51 cases of persistent face presentation, Schwartz et al.[29] found that the mean birth weight of those infants in mentum posterior who did rotate and deliver vaginally was 3,425 g, compared with 3,792 g for those infants who did not rotate and deliver vaginally. Persistence of mentum posterior with an infant of normal size, however, makes safe vaginal delivery less likely. Overall, 70 to 80 percent[5,20,22,23] of infants with face presentation can be delivered vaginally, either spontaneously or by low for-

ceps, while 12 to 30 percent require cesarean delivery. Manual attempts to convert the face to a flexed attitude or to rotate a posterior position to a more favorable mentum anterior are rarely successful and increase both maternal and fetal risks.[16,22,26,32] Internal podalic version and breech extraction as a remedy for face presentation is contraindicated. Campbell[22] reported fetal losses of up to 60 percent with this maneuver. Maternal deaths from uterine rupture and trauma after version with extraction have also been documented. Spontaneous delivery or cesarean delivery are therefore the preferred routes for maternal safety as well.[16,22,26]

Prolonged labor is a common feature of face presentation[5,8] and has been associated with an increased number of intrapartum deaths.[17] Therefore, prompt attention to an arrested labor pattern is recommended. The choice between augmentation of a dysfunctional labor or primary cesarean delivery rests on an assessment of uterine activity, pelvic adequacy, and fetal condition. In the case of an average or small fetus, adequate pelvis, and hypotonic labor, oxytocin may be considered. Fetal compromise is common. Salzmann et al.[26] observed a 10-fold increase in fetal compromise with face presentation. Several other observers have also found that abnormal fetal heart rate patterns occur more often with face presentation.[16,18] Continuous intrapartum electronic fetal heart rate monitoring of a fetus with face presentation is considered mandatory, but extreme care must be exercised in the placement of an electrode, as ocular and cosmetic damage might result from this device. If external Doppler heart rate

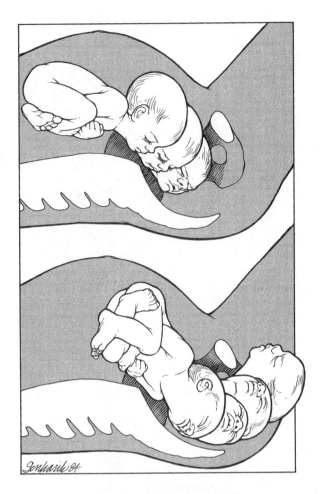

Fig. 16-9 Engagement, descent, and internal rotation remain cardinal elements of vaginal delivery in the case of a face presentation, but successful vaginal delivery of a term size fetus presenting a face generally requires delivery by flexion under the symphysis from a mentum anterior position as illustrated here.

monitoring is inadequate and an internal electrode is considered necessary, placement of the electrode on the fetal chin is often recommended.

Laryngeal and tracheal edema resulting from pressures of the birth process might require immediate nasotracheal intubation.[33] Nuchal teratomas or simple goiter, fetal anomalies that might have caused the malpresentation, require expert neonatal management.

No absolute contraindication to oxytocin augmentation of hypotonic labor in the case of a face presentation exists, but an arrest of progress despite adequate labor or nonreassuring fetal heart rate pattern should call for cesarean delivery.[8] Although cesarean delivery has been reported in up to 60 percent of cases of face presentation,[18,27] safe vaginal delivery may be accomplished in many, and a trial of labor with careful monitoring of fetal condition and progress is not contraindicated unless macrosomia or a small pelvis is identified.

Brow Presentation

An infant in a brow presentation occupies a longitudinal axis, with a partially deflexed cephalic attitude, midway between full flexion and full extension (Fig. 16-10).[24] The frontal bones are the point of designation. If the anterior fontanel is on the mother's left side, with the sagittal suture in the transverse pelvic axis, the fetus would be in a left frontum transverse position (LFT) (Fig. 16-11). The reported incidence of brow presentation varies widely from 1 in 670[34] to 1 in 3,433,[35] averaging about 1 in 1,500 deliveries. Brow presentation will be detected more often in early labor before flexion occurs to a normal attitude. Less frequently, further extension results in a face presentation.

Perinatal mortality corrected for lethal anomalies and very low birth weight varies from 1.28 to 8 percent.[36] In an examination of 88,988 deliveries, Ingolfsson[37] found that corrected perinatal mortality rates for fetuses presenting by the brow depended on the mode of delivery. The highest loss rate, 16 percent, was associated with manipulative vaginal birth.[37]

In general, factors that delay engagement are associated with persistent brow presentation. Cephalopelvic disproportion, prematurity, and great parity are often found and have been implicated in more than 60 percent of cases of persistent brow presentation.[5,35,38,39]

Detection of a brow presentation by abdominal palpation is unusual in practice. More often, a brow is detected on vaginal examination. As in the case of a face presentation, late diagnosis is more likely. Fewer than 50 percent of brow presentations are detected before the second stage of labor, with most of the remainder undiagnosed until delivery.[34,37–39] Frontum anterior is reportedly the most common position at diagnosis, oc-

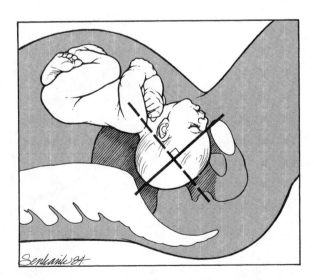

Fig. 16-10 This fetus is a brow presentation in a frontum anterior position. The head is in an intermediate deflexion attitude.

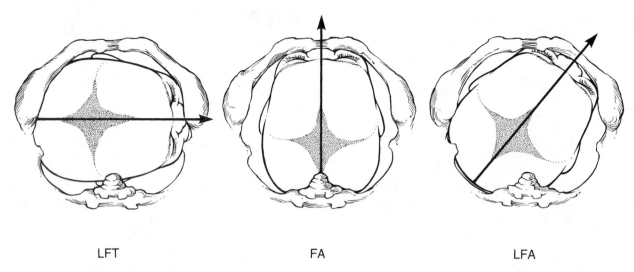

LFT   FA   LFA

Fig. 16-11 In the case of a brow presentation, the anterior fontanel (frontum) relative to the maternal pelvis is the point of designation. (A) Fetus in left frontum transverse (LFT). (B) Frontum anterior (FA). (C) Left frontum anterior (LFA).

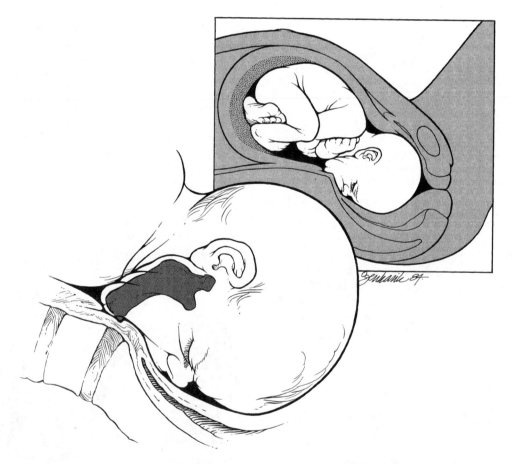

Fig. 16-12 The open fetal mouth against the vaginal sidewall may brace the head in the intermediate deflexion attitude as shown here.

curring about twice as often as either transverse or posterior positions. Although the initial position at diagnosis may be of limited prognostic value, Skalley and Kramer[39] reported the cesarean delivery rate to be higher with frontum transverse or frontum posterior than with frontum anterior.

A persistent brow presentation requires engagement and descent of the largest (mento-occipital) diameter or profile of the fetal head.[40] This process is possible only with a large pelvis or a small infant or both. However, brow presentations convert spontaneously by flexion or further extension to either a vertex or a face presentation and are then managed accordingly.[34,35] The earlier the diagnosis is made, the more likely conversion is to occur spontaneously. Fewer than half of infants with persistent brow presentations undergo spontaneous vaginal delivery, but in most cases a trial of labor is not contraindicated.[5,36]

Prolonged labors have been observed in 33 to 50 percent of brow presentations,[5,20,35,38,39] and secondary arrest is not uncommon.[34] Forced conversion of the brow to a more favorable position with forceps is contraindicated,[34,35,38] as are attempts at manual conversion. One unexpected cause of persistent brow presentation may be an open fetal mouth pressed against the vaginal wall, splinting the head and preventing either flexion or extension[28,35] (Fig. 16-12).

In most cases of brow presentation, as with face presentation, minimal manipulation yields the best results[35,41] if the fetal heart rate pattern remains reassuring. Ingolfsson[37] concluded, however, that expectancy is justified only with a large pelvis, a small infant, and adequate progress. If a brow presentation persists with a large baby, successful vaginal delivery is unlikely, and cesarean delivery may be most prudent.[20]

Although radiographic or computerized tomographic pelvimetry might be helpful, Cruikshank and White[5] reported that while 91 percent of those cases with adequate pelvic dimensions converted to a vertex or a face and delivered vaginally, only 20 percent of those with some form of pelvic contracture did also. Therefore, regardless of pelvic dimensions, consideration of a trial of labor with careful monitoring of maternal and fetal condition may be appropriate. As in the case of a face presentation, oxytocin may be used cautiously to correct hypotonia, but prompt resumption of progress toward delivery should follow.

Compound Presentation

Whenever an extremity is found prolapsed beside a major presenting fetal pole, the situation is referred to as a compound presentation[42] (Fig. 16-13). The reported incidence ranges from 1 in 377 to 1 in 1,213

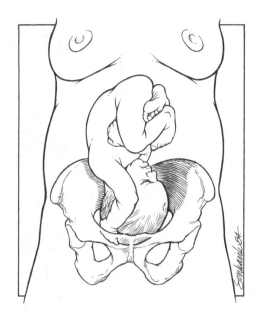

Fig. 16-13 The compound presentation of an upper extremity and the vertex illustrated here most often spontaneously resolves with further labor and descent.

deliveries.[5,42–45] The combination of an upper extremity and the vertex is the most common.

This diagnosis should be suspected with any arrest of labor in the active phase or failure to engage during active labor.[44] The diagnosis is made by vaginal examination that discovers an irregular mobile tissue mass adjacent to the larger presenting part. Diagnosis late in labor is common, and as many as 50 percent of persisting compound presentations are not diagnosed until the second stage.[42] Delay in diagnosis may not be detrimental because it is likely that only the persistent cases require significant intervention.

Although maternal age, race, parity, and pelvic size have all been associated with compound presentation,[43,44] prematurity is the most consistent clinical finding.[5,42] It is primarily the very small fetus that is at great risk of persistent compound presentation. In late pregnancy, external cephalic version of a fetus in breech position may increase the risk of a compound presentation.[46]

Perinatal mortality with compound presentation is typically elevated, with an overall rate of 93 per 1,000 reported by Cruikshank and White.[5] Higher losses of 17 and 19 percent have been reported when the foot prolapses.[43] As with other malpresentations, fetal risk can be directly related to the method of management. A fetal mortality rate of 4.8 percent has been noted if no intervention is required compared with 14.4 percent with intervention other than cesarean delivery. A 30 percent fetal mortality rate has been observed with internal podalic version and breech extraction.[43] There is probably some selection bias in these figures, since it is likely that more difficult cases were chosen for manipulative intervention. When intervention is necessary, cesarean delivery appears to be the only safe choice.

Fetal risk in the case of compound presentation is specifically associated with birth trauma and cord prolapse. Cord prolapse occurs in 11 to 20 percent of cases[5,43,44] and is the most frequent single complication of this malpresentation. It probably occurs because the prolapsed extremity splints the presenting part and results in an irregular fetal aggregate that incompletely fills the pelvic inlet. In addition to the hypoxic risk of cord prolapse, common fetal morbidity includes neurologic and musculoskeletal damage to the involved extremity.

Despite these dangers, labor is not necessarily contraindicated with a compound presentation, but the prolapsed extremity should not be manipulated.[42–44,47] As the major presenting part descends, the accompanying extremity usually retracts. Cruikshank and White[5] found that 75 percent of vertex/upper extremity combinations deliver spontaneously. Occult or undetected cord prolapse is possible, and therefore continuous electronic fetal heart rate monitoring is recommended.

The primary indications for surgical intervention are cord prolapse, nonreassuring fetal heart rate patterns, and failure to progress.[5] Cesarean delivery is the only appropriate clinical intervention,[42] since both version extraction and attempts to reposition the prolapsed extremity are associated with high fetal and maternal morbidity and mortality and are to be avoided.[43,44] Breen and Wiesmeien[42] found that 2 percent of patients with compound presentation required abdominal delivery, whereas Weissberg and O'Leary[44] reported cesarean delivery to be necessary in 25 percent of cases. Protraction of the second stage of labor has been noted to occur more frequently with persistent compound presentation, and dysfunctional labor patterns are said to be common.[42] Again, as in other malpresentations, spontaneous resolution occurs more often and surgical intervention is less frequently necessary in those cases diagnosed early in labor. Persistent compound presentation is more likely with a small infant, as is the prognosis for successful vaginal delivery. Persistent compound presentation with a term-sized infant has a poor prognosis for safe vaginal delivery, and cesarean delivery is usually necessary.

Breech Presentation

The infant presenting as a breech occupies a longitudinal axis with the cephalic pole in the uterine fundus. This presentation occurs in 3 to 4 percent of labors overall, although it is found in 7 percent of pregnancies

Table 16-1   Breech Categories

Type	Overall % of Breeches	Risk (%)	
		Prolapse	Premature
Frank Breech	48–73[31,46,48,50,66]	0.5[64]	38[48]
Complete	4.6–11.5[31,48,50,66]	4–6[64]	12[48]
Footling	12–38[31,48,50]	15–18[64]	50[48]

at 32 weeks and in 25 percent of pregnancies of less than 28 weeks duration.[48] The three types of breech are noted in Table 16-1. The infant in the frank breech position is flexed at the hips with extended knees. The complete breech is flexed at both joints, and the footling breech has one or both hips extended (Fig. 16-14).

The diagnosis of breech presentation may be made by abdominal palpation or vaginal examination and confirmed by ultrasound. Prematurity, fetal malformation, and polar placentation are commonly observed causative factors. High rates of breech presentation are noted in certain fetal genetic disorders, including trisomies 13, 18, and 21, Potter syndrome, and myotonic dystrophy.[49] Thus, conditions that alter fetal muscular tone and mobility also increase the frequency of breech presentation.

Mechanism and Conduct of Labor and Vaginal Delivery

The two most important elements for the safe conduct of vaginal breech delivery are continuous electronic fetal heart rate monitoring and noninterference until spontaneous delivery of the breech to the umbilicus has occurred. Early in labor, the capability for immediate cesarean delivery should be established. Anesthesia should be available, the operating room readied, and appropriate informed consent obtained. Two obstetricians should be in attendance as well as a pediatric team. Appropriate training and experience with vaginal breech delivery are fundamental to success. The instrument table should be prepared in the customary manner, with the addition of Piper forceps and extra towels. There is no contraindication to epidural analgesia once labor is well established, and many view epidural anesthesia as an asset in the control of the second stage.

The infant presenting in the frank breech position usually enters the pelvic inlet in one of the diagonal pelvic diameters (Fig. 16-15). Engagement has occurred when the bitrochanteric diameter of the fetus has passed the plane of the inlet, although by vaginal examination the presenting part may only be palpated at minus two to minus four station (out of five) relative to the ischial spines. As the breech descends and encounters the levator ani muscle sling, internal rotation

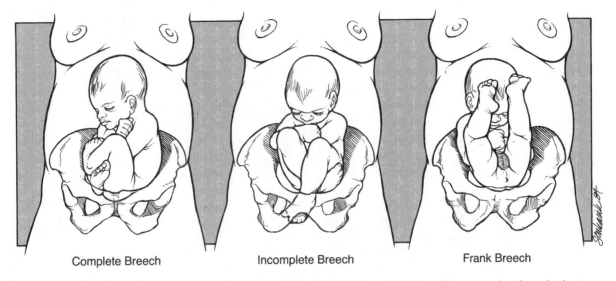

Complete Breech   Incomplete Breech   Frank Breech

Fig. 16-14 The complete breech is flexed at the hips and flexed at the knees. The incomplete breech shows incomplete deflexion of one or both knees or hips. The frank breech is flexed at the hips and extended at the knees.

usually occurs to bring the bitrochanteric diameter into the anteroposterior (AP) axis of the pelvis. The point of designation in a breech labor is the fetal sacrum, and, therefore, when the bitrochanteric diameter is in the AP axis of the pelvis, the fetal sacrum will lie in the transverse pelvic diameter (Fig. 16-16).

If normal descent occurs, the breech will present at the outlet and begin to emerge, first as a sacrum transverse, then rotate to a sacrum anterior. Crowning occurs when the bitrochanteric diameter passes under the pubic symphysis. An episiotomy in the midline to but not through the anal sphincter will facilitate delivery but should be delayed until crowning begins. Some

argue that a mediolateral episiotomy offers more room and less risk of extension through the anal sphincter, but considerable skill and experience are required to repair a mediolateral episiotomy properly, and this incision is associated with greater blood loss and pain. Premature episiotomy will contribute to unnecessary blood loss and to the level of anxiety and perhaps a tendency to rush the delivery. As the infant emerges, rotation begins, usually toward a sacrum anterior position. This direction of rotation may reflect the greater capacity of the hollow of the posterior pelvis to accept the fetal chest and small parts. It is important to emphasize that operator intervention is not yet needed or

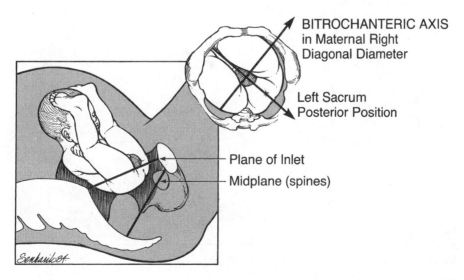

BITROCHANTERIC AXIS
in Maternal Right
Diagonal Diameter

Left Sacrum
Posterior Position

Plane of Inlet
Midplane (spines)

Fig. 16-15 The breech typically enters the inlet with the bitrochanteric diameter aligned with one of the diagonal diameters, with the sacrum as the point of designation in the other diagonal diameter. This is a case of left sacrum posterior (LSP).

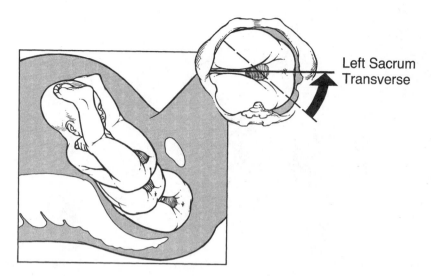

Left Sacrum Transverse

Fig. 16-16 With labor and descent, as illustrated here, the bitrochanteric diameter generally rotates toward the anteroposterior axis and the sacrum toward the transverse.

helpful other than to cut the episiotomy and encourage maternal expulsive efforts.

Premature or aggressive assistance may adversely affect the breech birth in at least two ways. First, cervical dilatation must be maximized and complete dilatation sustained for sufficient duration to retard retraction of the cervix and entrapment of the aftercoming fetal head. Rushing the delivery of the trunk may significantly diminish the effectiveness of this process. Second, the safe descent and delivery of the breech infant must be the result of expulsive forces from above to maintain flexion of the fetal vertex. Any traction from below in an effort to speed delivery would encourage

deflexion of the vertex and result in the presentation of the larger occipitofrontal fetal cranial profile to the pelvic inlet (Fig. 16-17). Such an event could be catastrophic. Rushed delivery also increases the risk of a nuchal arm, with one or both arms trapped behind the head above the pelvic inlet. Entrapment of a nuchal arm makes safe vaginal delivery much more difficult as it dramatically increases the size of the aggregate object that must pass through the birth canal. The safe breech delivery of an average-sized infant, therefore, depends predominantly on maternal expulsive forces, not on traction from below.

As the frank breech emerges further, the fetal thighs

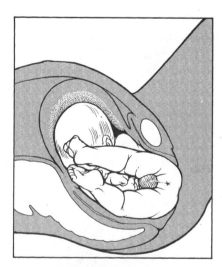

SPONTANEOUS EXPULSION

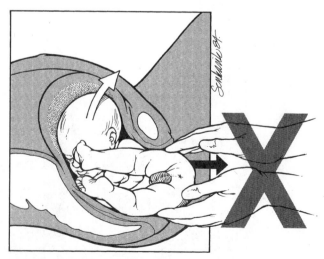

UNDESIRED DEFLEXION

Fig. 16-17 The fetus emerges spontaneously (A), while uterine contractions maintain cephalic flexion. Premature aggressive traction (B) encourages deflexion of the fetal vertex and increases the risk of head entrapment or nuchal arm entrapment.

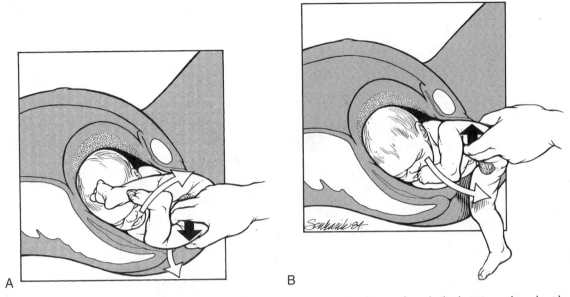

Fig. 16-18 After spontaneous expulsion to the umbilicus, external rotation of each thigh (A) combined with opposite rotation of the fetal pelvis results in flexion of the knee and delivery of each leg (B).

are typically pressed firmly against the fetal abdomen, often splinting and protecting the umbilicus and cord. As the umbilicus appears over the maternal perineum, the operator may align his or her fingers medial to one thigh, then the other, pressing laterally as the fetal pelvis is rotated away from that side (Fig. 16-18). This results in external rotation of the thigh at the hip, flexion of the knee, and delivery of one and then the other leg. The dual movement of counterclockwise rotation of the fetal pelvis as the operator externally rotates the right thigh and clockwise rotation of the fetal pelvis as the operator externally rotates the fetal left thigh is most effective in facilitating delivery. The fetal trunk is then wrapped with a towel to provide secure support of the body while further descent results from expulsive forces from the mother. The operator primarily facilitates the delivery of the fetus. The operator is not applying outward traction on the fetus that might result in deflexion of the fetal head or nuchal arm.

When the scapulae appear at the outlet, the operator may slip a hand over the fetal shoulder from the back (Fig. 16-19), follow the humerus, and, with a lateral movement, sweep first one and then the other arm across the chest and out over the perineum. Gentle rotation of the fetal trunk counterclockwise to assist delivery of the right arm, and clockwise to assist delivery of the left arm, may be applied in a similar manner to that used for delivery of the legs (Fig. 16-20). Once both arms have been delivered, if the vertex has remained flexed on the neck, the chin and face will appear at the outlet, and the airway may be cleared and suctioned (Fig. 16-21).

With further maternal expulsive forces alone, sponta-

neous controlled delivery of the fetal head will often occur. If not, delivery may be accomplished with a simple manual effort to maximize flexion of the vertex using pressure on the fetal maxilla (not mandible) along with suprapubic pressure and gentle downward traction (Fig. 16-22). Although maxillary pressure will maximize cephalic flexion, the main force effecting delivery remains the mother.

Alternatively, the operator may apply Piper forceps to the aftercoming head to facilitate delivery. The application requires slight elevation of the fetal trunk by the assistant, while the operator kneels and applies the Piper forceps directly to the fetal head in the pelvis (Fig. 16-23). Hyperextension of the fetal neck from excessive elevation of the fetal trunk should be avoided.

Examination of the Piper forceps will show that the pelvic curvature characteristic of most forceps has been eliminated. This modification allows direct application to the fetal head and avoids conflict with the fetal body that would occur with the application of standard instruments from below. The forceps are inserted into the vagina from beneath the fetus. The right blade is inserted with the operator's right hand along the right maternal sidewall and placed against the left fetal parietal bone. The left blade is then inserted by the left hand along the left maternal sidewall and placed against the right fetal parietal bone. Forceps application controls the fetal head and prevents extension of the head on the neck. Gentle downward traction on the forceps with the fetal trunk supported on or near the forceps shanks results in controlled delivery of the vertex (Fig. 16-24). Routine use of Piper forceps to the aftercoming head may be advisable both to ensure con-

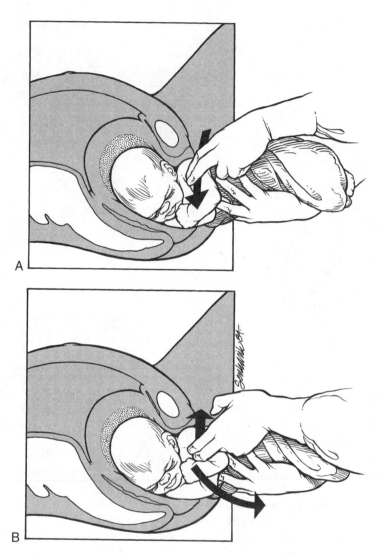

Fig. 16-19 When the scapulae appear under the symphisis, the operator reaches over the left shoulder, sweeps the arm across the chest (A), and delivers the arm (B).

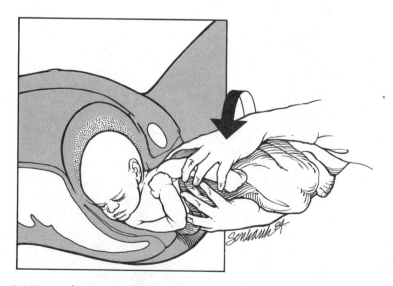

Fig. 16-20 Gentle rotation of the shoulder girdle facilitates delivery of the right arm.

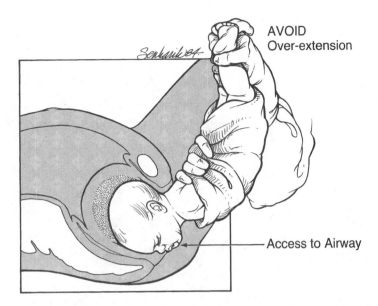

AVOID
Over-extension

Access to Airway

Fig. 16-21 Following delivery of the arms, the fetus is wrapped in a towel for control and slightly elevated. The fetal face and airway may be visible over the perineum. Excessive elevation of the trunk is avoided.

trol of the delivery and to maintain optimal operator proficiency in anticipation of deliveries that may require their use.

Any arrest of spontaneous progress in labor necessitates consideration of cesarean delivery. Any evidence of fetal compromise or sustained cord compression based on continuous electronic fetal monitoring also requires consideration of cesarean delivery. Vaginal interventions directed at facilitating delivery of the breech complicated by an arrest of spontaneous progress are discouraged, because fetal and maternal morbidity and mortality are both greatly increased.

The mechanisms of descent and delivery of the footling and the complete breech are not unlike those of the frank breech described above, except one or both legs might already be extended and thus not require attention. The risk of cord prolapse or entanglement is greater, hence the increased possibility of emergency cesarean delivery. Furthermore, the footling and complete breech are not as effective a dilator of the cervix as either the vertex or the larger aggregate profile of the thighs and buttocks of the frank breech, which might increase the risk of entrapment of the aftercoming head, and, as a result, primary cesarean

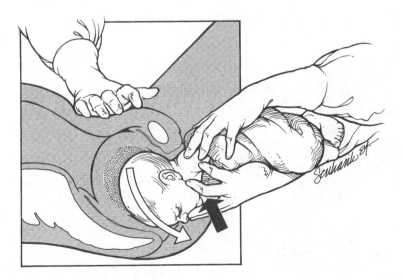

Fig. 16-22 Cephalic flexion is maintained by pressure (heavy arrow) on the fetal maxilla (not mandible!). Often delivery of the head is easily accomplished with continued expulsive forces from above and gentle downward traction.

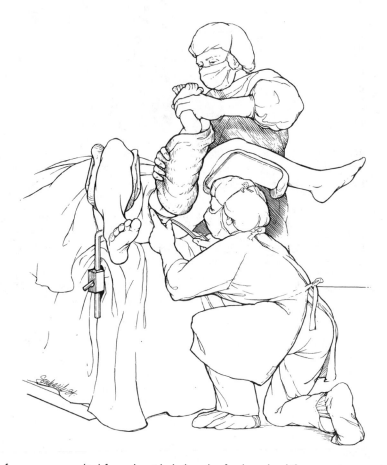

Fig. 16-23 Piper forceps are applied from the side below the fetal trunk while an assistant supports the fetus as illustrated here.

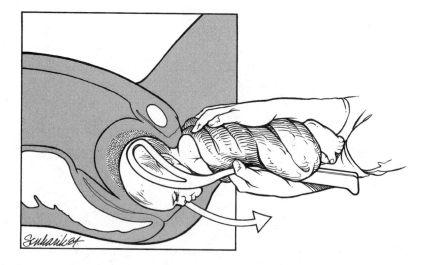

Fig. 16-24 The fetus may be laid on the forceps and delivered with gentle downward traction as illustrated here.

delivery is often advocated for nonfrank breech presentations.

Management of the Term Breech

The reported perinatal mortality associated with breech presentation has varied from 9 to 25 percent,[50,51] which is three to five times that of the nonbreech infant at term.[52–54] The excess deaths associated with breech presentation are largely due to lethal anomalies and complications of prematurity, both of which are found more frequently among breech infants. Excluding anomalies and extreme prematurity, the corrected perinatal mortality reported by some investigators approaches zero regardless of the method of delivery, while others find that, even with exclusion of these factors, the term breech infant is at higher risk for birth trauma and asphyxia.[55–57] The major dangers facing the breech infant are summarized in Table 16-2.

At least a portion of the striking increase in the rate of cesarean deliveries over the past two decades is a response to the risk of morbidity and mortality associated with the breech presentation.[58–61] In 1980, Collea[48] observed that 29 percent of primary cesarean operations performed at his institution during a 12-month period were performed at least in part because of breech presentation. The National Institutes of Health Consensus Report in 1981 found that 12 percent of cesarean deliveries in 1978 were performed for breech presentation and that this indication contributed 10 to 15 percent to the overall rise in the rate of cesarean births. The overall rate of cesarean birth for breech in some institutions is as high as 94 percent, while in the United States generally, the cesarean delivery rate for breech presentation increased from 11.6 percent to 79.1 percent between 1970 and 1985.[61,62] However, even though greater risks appear to face the breech infant,[63] the method of delivery alone has not been conclusively shown to contribute to those risks.[64,65] There remain those who believe that complete abandonment of vaginal delivery for the breech is not yet justified.[66,67]

In some series, improved perinatal survival has been reported for breeches born by cesarean delivery,[51,54,63,68,69] and there is evidence, though inconsistent, that the method of delivery may also impact on the quality of survival. In 1979, Westgren et al.[70] found functional neurologic defects by 2 years of age in 24 percent of breech infants born vaginally, but only in 2.5 percent of those breech infants of similar weights and gestational ages born by cesarean delivery. However, in comparing 175 breech infants having a 94 percent cesarean delivery rate with 595 historical controls having a 22 percent rate of abdominal delivery, Green et al.[61] found no significant differences in outcome. Faber-Nijholt et al.[71] reviewed neurologic outcomes in 348 infants born in breech position. Examinations were performed on 239 children from 3 to 10 years of age. No statistically significant differences were noted between breech infants delivered vaginally and matched vertex controls. These authors concluded that breech outcome relates to degree of prematurity, impact of pregnancy complications, and presence of malformations as well as birth trauma or asphyxia. The benefit of arbitrary cesarean delivery in the case of breech presentation therefore remains uncertain.

Clinical Circumstances and Risks

The various categories of breech presentation clearly demonstrate dissimilar risks, and management plans might vary among these situations.[72,73] The premature breech, the breech with a hyperextended head, and the footling breech are categories that have high rates of fetal morbidity or mortality. Complications associated with incomplete dilatation and cephalic entrapment may be more frequent. In general, for these three breech situations, cesarean delivery appears to optimize fetal outcome and is therefore recommended.

Low birth weight (less than 2,500 g) is a confounding factor in about one-third of all breech presentations.[50,56,59,65,74,75] While the benefit of cesarean delivery to the perinatal mortality rate of the 1,500- to 2,500-g breech infant remains controversial,[11,35,51,74,76–81] improved survival with abdominal delivery has often been found in the 1,000- to 1,500-g weight group.[56,78] Traumatic morbidity is reportedly decreased in both weight groups by the use of cesarean delivery, including a lower rate of both intra- and periventricular hemorrhage.[81] Although some advocate a trial of labor in the frank breech infant weighing over 1,500 g, others recommend labor only when the infant exceeds 2,000 g.[35,59,65,82] There are proportionately fewer frank breech presentations in the low-birth-weight

Table 16-2 Incidence of Complications Seen with Breech Presentation

Complication	Incidence
Intrapartum fetal death	Increased 16-fold[61,63]
Intrapartum asphyxia	Increased 3.8-fold[61,63]
Cord prolapse	Increased 5- to 20-fold[48,51,64]
Birth trauma	Increased 13-fold[48]
Arrest of aftercoming head	8.8%[48]
Spinal cord injuries with extended head	21%[30,89]
Major anomalies	6–18%[51,61,63]
Prematurity	16–33%[31,50,56,59,65,74,75]
Hyperextension of head	5%[88]

group.[31,56] In fact, most infants weighing less than 1,500 g and presenting as a breech are footling.[82] Although most deaths in the very-low-birth-weight breech group are due to prematurity or lethal anomalies,[74,77,82,83] cesarean delivery has been shown by some to decrease corrected perinatal mortality in this weight group compared with that in similar-sized vertex presentations.[56,84] Other authors suggest that improved survival in these studies relates to improved neonatal care of the premature infant when compared with the outcomes of historical controls.[85] When vaginal delivery of the preterm breech is chosen or is unavoidable, however, conduction anesthesia and the use of forceps for the delivery of the aftercoming head appear to decrease fetal morbidity and mortality.[74,86,87]

Hyperextension of the fetal head has been consistently associated with a high (21 percent) risk of spinal cord injury if the breech is delivered vaginally.[30,88,89] In such cases, it is important to differentiate simple deflexion of the head from clear hyperextension, since Ballas et al.[90] have shown that simple deflexion carries no excess risk. The issue of simple deflexion of the fetal vertex as opposed to hyperextension is similar to the relationships between the occipitofrontal cranial plane and the axis of the fetal cervical spine illustrated in Figure 16-5. Often, as labor progresses, spontaneous flexion will occur in response to fundal forces.

Finally, the footling breech carries a prohibitively high (16 to 19 percent) risk of cord prolapse during labor. In many cases, cord prolapse is manifest only late in labor, after commitment to vaginal delivery has been made.[56,77] Cord prolapse necessitates prompt cesarean delivery. Furthermore, the footling breech is a poor cervical dilator, and cephalic entrapment becomes more likely.

Near-Term Frank or Complete Breech

Controversy continues surrounding the method of delivery for the frank or complete breech, as the cesarean delivery rate for breech presentation generally increases to over 90 percent without a continued or proportionate drop in perinatal mortality.[58–60] Maternal mortality is clearly higher with cesarean delivery, ranging from 0.2 to 0.43 percent.[64,72] Maternal morbidity is also higher with abdominal delivery. Some institutions report a 50 percent incidence of postoperative maternal morbidity compared with as little as 5 percent with vaginal delivery.[64] In an attempt to balance both maternal and fetal risks, plans have been proposed to select appropriate candidates for a trial of labor.

Cheng and Hannah[91] examined some of the English language literature regarding breech term deliveries between 1966 and 1992. They reviewed 82 reports, rejecting 58 due to study design inconsistencies or flaws.

The remaining 24 presented outcomes according to intended mode of delivery (vaginal or abdominal). Among the studies reviewed, perinatal mortality was higher for the planned vaginal delivery groups, with an odds ratio of 3.86 (95 percent CI = 2.22 to 6.69). Neonatal short-term morbidity due to trauma was higher in the planned vaginal delivery group, with an odds ratio of 3.96 (95 percent CI = 2.76 to 5.67). Likewise, long-term infant morbidity was more frequent in the planned vaginal delivery group (odds ratio 2.88, with a 95 percent CI = 1.04 to 7.97), but this finding barely achieved significance and resulted from only four foreign studies. Unfortunately, the majority of the 24 reports that were the basis for this review were retrospective, and many presented data gathered without the use of continuous fetal monitoring. One of the most influential reports with a relatively high rate of adverse outcome with vaginal delivery was from West Africa, and continuous fetal monitoring was not used. The meaning of statistical summaries that include data from such widely disparate practice patterns is unclear. The authors acknowledged that differences in outcomes might be due to factors other than the planned method of delivery because of selection bias in most of the studies.[91]

In 1965, Zatuchni and Andros[75] retrospectively analyzed 182 breech births. Of those reviewed, 25 infants had poor outcomes. These investigators concluded that scoring six clinical variables at the time of admission (Table 16-3) identified those patients destined to manifest serious problems in labor and allowed prompt and appropriate intervention. While the parturient herself could increase the score by presenting later in labor, at least three subsequent prospective studies applied the Zatuchni-Andros system and found it to be both sensitive and accurate in selecting candidates for successful vaginal delivery.[92–94] A Zatuchni-Andros score of less than 4 in these studies accurately predicted poor outcomes in patients with infants presenting as a breech. Furthermore, in applying the scoring system, only 21 to 27 percent of patients failed to qualify for a trial of labor.[92,93]

Because most reports dealing with the risks of breech

Table 16-3   Zatuchni-Andros System

Factor	0	1	2
Parity	Nullipara	Multipara	Multipara
Gestational age	39	38	37
Estimated fetal weight	8 lb	7–8 lb	7 lb
Previous breech	No	One	Two
Dilatation	2	3	4 or more
Station	−3 or >	−2	−1 or less

(From Zatuchni and Andros,[75] with permission.)

presentation and method of delivery have been retrospective, serious doubts arise about the validity of recommendations. Much of the data were gathered before electronic fetal heart rate monitoring became commonplace. There has only been one randomized trial that examined term frank breech and method of delivery.[64,95] Singleton term frank breech infants with an estimated fetal weight of between 2,500 and 3,800 g of mothers with adequate radiographic pelvimetry were prospectively randomized into two groups. One hundred fifteen patients were randomized to a vaginal delivery compared with 93 randomized to elective cesarean delivery. One hundred twelve of the 115 women had time for x-ray pelvimetry. Three delivered vaginally before pelvimetry was possible. Fifty-two of the 112 women in the planned vaginal delivery group were not allowed to labor due to inadequate dimensions on pelvimetry, leaving 60 for a planned vaginal delivery. Intrapartum monitoring was used in all patients. Eighty-three percent of those patients allowed to labor delivered vaginally without a perinatal loss.[95] There were no maternal deaths, although 36 percent of patients experienced some postpartum morbidity.[64] The authors found no significant difference in perinatal outcome and concluded that a trial of labor is a safe option with the frank breech of average size, flexed head, adequate pelvis, reassuring heart rate monitoring, and normal progress in labor. The small numbers of patients studied, however, make their acceptance of the null hypothesis inconclusive.

In a similar study, O'Leary[96] allowed those frank breeches estimated to be between 2,500 and 3,500 g in women with a large pelvis to labor vaginally. He used radiographic pelvimetry, ultrasound, and the Zatuchni-Andros score and paid close attention to the labor curve in selecting candidates for cesarean delivery. The results were similar to those of Collea et al.[95] Neither group of investigators found that oxytocin induction of labor was contraindicated if all other criteria were satisfied[95,96]; however, both groups concluded that augmentation of secondary arrest was not appropriate. Neither nulliparity nor multiparity was found to be an accurate prognostic indicator.[31,97] In a similar study, Gimovsky et al.[98] randomized 105 nonfrank term breech infants to cesarean or trial of labor and found that 44 percent of those undergoing trial of labor achieved safe vaginal delivery. There were no differences in neonatal outcomes. Most cesarean deliveries were performed for arrested progress.

Flanagan et al.[99] reported a nonrandomized, retrospective study in which 244 women with breech infants at term (the majority were frank, with some complete, and footling breeches) underwent a trial of labor. Of these, 72 percent delivered vaginally. Of those cesarean deliveries ultimately required, 44 were for abnormal labor (64 percent of those delivered by cesarean), 14 for fetal distress (20 percent), and 11 for cord prolapse (16 percent). The authors noted no increased incidence of significant trauma related to vaginal delivery. However, one child had a facial nerve paralysis with facial asymmetry. The authors stated that this injury was thought to be due to in utero damage from compression, not from trauma at the time of the vaginal delivery. This explanation may or may not be valid. The authors estimate that with the application of external version to a known breech population and a trial of labor for selected frank breech infants, the cesarean rate for these pregnancies could be cut in half.[99]

In conclusion, there does seem to be a place for a trial of labor and attempted vaginal delivery of the uncomplicated term or near term frank breech of average size through a normal pelvis if there is normal progress in labor and fetal heart rate monitoring remains reassuring. The apparent safety of a trial of labor in selected cases, however, is not without dispute.[91,100]

The clinician must possess the necessary training and experience to offer a patient with a persistent breech presentation a trial of labor. Furthermore, the relationship between the patient and the clinician should be well established and the discussions of risk and benefit open and frank. If the training, experience, and relationship are lacking, cesarean delivery becomes the safer choice. However, even if a clinician has made the choice never prospectively to offer a patient with breech presentation a trial of labor, the burden of responsibility to know and understand the mechanism and management of a breech delivery is not relieved. No one active in obstetrics will avoid the occasional emergency breech delivery. Regular review of principles, and practice with simulations using a doll and model pelvis with an experienced colleague, can increase the skills and improve the performance of anyone facing such an emergency.

Those factors that impact on the decision to deliver a breech vaginally or by cesarean section are listed below. The obvious implication of the dramatically decreased experience in training programs with vaginal breech delivery is that inexperience itself will consistute an indication for cesarean delivery. Certainly, in no case should a woman with an infant presenting as a breech be allowed to labor unless (1) anesthesia coverage is immediately available, (2) cesarean delivery can be undertaken promptly, (3) continuous fetal heart rate monitoring is used, and (4) the delivery is attended by a pediatrician and two obstetricians of whom at least one is experienced with vaginal breech birth.

Breech Second Twin

Approximately one-third of all twin gestations present as vertex/breech (i.e., first twin is a vertex, and the second is a breech).[101] The management alternatives in

Management of the Breech

Trial of labor may be considered if
    Estimated fetal weight (EFW) = 2,000 to 3,800 g
    Frank breech
    Adequate pelvis
    Flexed fetal head
    Fetal monitoring
    Zatuchni-Andros score ⩾4
    Rapid cesarean possible
    Good progress maintained in labor
    Experience and training available
    Informed consent possible
Cesarean delivery may be prudent if
    EFW less than 1,500 or over 4,000 g
    Footling presentation
    Small pelvis
    Hyperextended fetal head
    Zatuchni-Andros score under 4
    Absence of expertise
    Nonreassuring fetal heart rate pattern
    Arrest of progress

the case of the vertex/breech twin pregnancy in labor include cesarean delivery, vaginal delivery of the first twin and attempted external cephalic version of the second twin, or internal podalic version and extraction of the second twin. Gocke et al.[102] examined the outcomes of management of 136 pairs of vertex/nonvertex twins weighing over 1,500 g and concluded that breech extraction of the second twin appeared to be a safe alternative to cesarean delivery.[102] Blickstein et al.[101] compared the obstetric outcomes of 39 cases of vertex/breech twins to the outcomes of 48 vertex/vertex twins. Although the breech second twin had a higher incidence of low birth weight and a longer hospital stay, the authors found no basis for elective cesarean in this clinical circumstance. Laros and Dattel[103] studied 206 twin pairs and likewise found no clear advantage to arbitrary cesarean delivery because of a specific presentation. Fishman et al.[104] examined outcomes in 390 vaginally delivered second twins, 207 delivered as a vertex and 183 delivered breech. Ninety-five percent of the breech deliveries were total breech extractions. They found no significant differences between the vertex and breech infants even when stratified by birth weight. Any clinician uncomfortable with the prospective delivery of a singleton breech, however, would be unwise to consider a breech extraction of a second twin.

Vaginal delivery followed by external version may also be a viable alternative. Ultrasound in the delivery room with direct visualization of the fetus during the attempt will facilitate the procedure. Often there is a transient decrease in uterine activity after the delivery of the first infant that can be used to advantage in the performance of a cephalic version. Tchabo and Tomai[105] described an experience with 30 malpositioned second twins (12 transverse and 18 breech). Version after birth of the first twin was successful in 11 of the 12 transverse infants and in 16 of the 18 breech infants. These were all over 35 weeks' gestation, had intact membranes of the second twin after delivery of the first, no evidence of anomalies, and normal amniotic fluid volume.

Internal podalic version/extraction of the second twin can be facilitated by ultrasonic guidance. The goal of the operator is to insert his or her hand into the uterus, identify and grasp both fetal feet with membranes intact, and apply traction to bring the feet into the pelvis and out the introitus, leaving membranes intact until both feet are at the introitus.[106] Maternal expulsive efforts should remain the major force in effecting descent of the fetus. Membranes are ruptured, and the delivery is managed as with any footling breech delivery at that point. The operator can often have difficulty with the identification of the fetal feet; ultrasound may be helpful in the delivery room.

In the case of a breech extraction, and perhaps more often with a breech extraction in the case of the smaller baby, the fetal head can become caught in the cervix. It can be useful in such a case to insert the operator's entire hand into the uterus to cradle the fetal head in it and then withdraw the hand, protecting the fetal head.[107] This splinting technique has also been used for the safe extraction of the breech head at the time of cesarean delivery.

No randomized prospective trials involving preterm twins with vertex/nonvertex presentation have been performed. A small, prospective trial in the near-term gestation (over 35 weeks) by Rabinovici et al.[106] found no difference in neonatal morbidity between vaginal delivery and cesarean birth. They did find increased maternal morbidity with cesarean delivery.

Time Delay Between Delivery of Twins

There are no clearly established time limits for the safe delivery of the second twin after delivery of the first. If frequent or continuous fetal heart rate monitoring is reassuring, there is no specific interval that demands cesarean intervention. There are case reports of intervals of weeks or months between deliveries of the first and second twins. In the very premature gestation, it may be feasible to ligate the umbilical cord, manage the remaining twin expectantly, and monitor growth and well-being with good outcome. Risks such as abruption and/or infection that may be seen with delayed delivery are most acceptable in the case of the very premature gestation, which inherently has a poor prognosis for the second twin if delivered.

External Cephalic Version

External cephalic version is a third alternative to vaginal delivery or cesarean delivery for the breech infant.[15,50,52,108–111] Many have found that external cephalic version significantly reduces the incidence of breech presentation in labor and is associated with few complications such as cord compression or placental abruption.[15,111] Reported success with external version varies from 60 to 75 percent, with a similar percentage of these remaining vertex to labor.[15,112–115] Ylikorkala and Hartikainen-Sorri[111] found that while many infants in breech presentation before 34 weeks will convert

spontaneously to a cephalic presentation, few will do so afterward. Repetitive external version applied weekly after 34 weeks was successful in converting over two thirds of cases and reducing their breech presentation rate by 50 percent.[111] In a randomized trial of external cephalic version in low-risk pregnancies between 37 and 39 weeks, Van Dorsten and colleagues[108] were successful in 68 percent of 25 cases in the version group where only 4 of the 23 controls converted to a vertex spontaneously before labor. All those in whom external version was successful presented in labor as a vertex.[108] van Veelan et al.[117] reported a prospective, controlled study of external cephalic version performed weekly between 33 weeks and term, and 48 percent of the study group were vertex in labor compared with only 26 percent of controls. Hanss[118] reported experience with 112 patients seen for external version, with a success rate

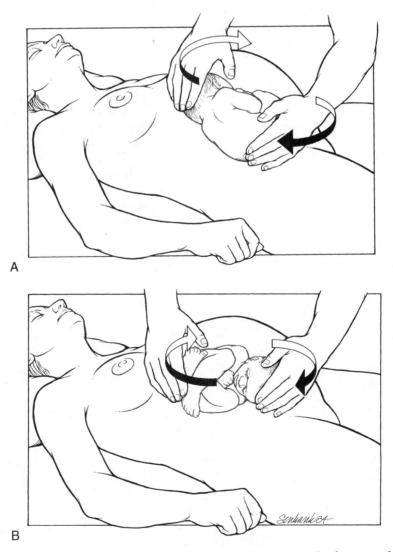

A

B

Fig. 16-25 External cephalic version is accomplished by gently "squeezing" the fetus out of one area of the uterus and into another. Here, the "forward roll," often the most popular, is illustrated.

of 49 percent, with a cesarean rate of 17 percent among those with successful version compared with 78 percent among those patients with unsuccessful version attempt.

Zhang et al.[15] recently reviewed English language reports between 1980 and 1991 that reported the outcomes of pregnancies after external cephalic version and concluded that it was a safe and effective intervention. The overall success rate among investigators in the United States was 65 percent, with an average cesarean delivery rate of 37 percent among those undergoing an attempted version compared with 83 percent among controls. Successful version was reported more often in parous than nulliparous women and more often between 37 and 39 weeks than after 40 weeks.[15]

Gentle constant pressure applied in a relaxed patient with frequent fetal heart rate assessments are elements of the method stressed by all investigators.[50,52,108] Methodology varies, although the "forward roll" is more widely supported than the "back flip" (Fig. 16-25).[108] The mechanical goal is to squeeze the fetal vertex gently out of the fundal area to the transverse and finally into the lower segment of the uterus.

Tocolysis and ultrasound during the procedure may also be helpful, but benefit from tocolysis remains unproven. Most studies of the use of tocolysis are not randomized trials.[115] Robertson et al.,[113] in a randomized trial including 58 patients at 37 to 41 weeks' gestation with breech presentation, found no benefit from β-mimetic tocolysis. The success rate was 66.7 percent with tocolysis and 67.8 percent without tocolysis.[113] Factors associated with failure of version included obesity, deep pelvic engagement of the breech, oligohydramnios, and posterior positioning of the fetal back.[114] Fetomaternal transfusion has been reported to occur in up to 6 percent of patients undergoing external version,[119] and thus Rh-negative unsensitized women should receive Rh-immune globulin.

Shoulder Dystocia

Shoulder dystocia is diagnosed when, after delivery of the fetal head, further expulsion of the infant is prevented by impaction of the fetal shoulders within the maternal pelvis. Specific efforts are necessary to facilitate delivery (Fig. 16-26).

Although a difficult shoulder dystocia occurs infrequently, the clinician does not soon forget the experience. Often, but not always, at the end of a difficult labor, the fetal head may be delivered spontaneously or by forceps, but the neck then retracts. Often, the fetal head appears to be drawn back with the chin against the maternal thigh. It may be difficult to suction the infant's mouth because of its close approximation to the perineum. As maternal expulsive efforts are encouraged,

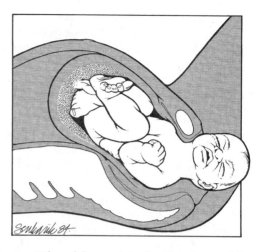

Fig. 16-26 When delivery of the fetal head is not followed by delivery of the shoulders, the anterior shoulder has often become caught behind the symphysis as illustrated here. The head may retract toward the perineum. Desperate traction on the fetal head is not likely to facilitate delivery and may lead to trauma.

the fetal head becomes plethoric, and the danger to the infant is apparent if delivery cannot be promptly accomplished.

Shoulder dystocia has been reported in 0.15 to 1.7 percent of all vaginal deliveries.[120–121] All investigators have documented increased perinatal morbidity and mortality with shoulder dystocia.[120–121] Mortality varies from 21 to 290 in 1,000 when shoulder girdle impaction occurs, and neonatal morbidity has been reported to be immediately obvious in 20 percent of infants.[120] In reviewing 131 macrosomic infants, Boyd et al.[122] found that only half of all cases of brachial palsy occurring in macrosomic infants also carried a diagnosis of shoulder dystocia. Obviously, brachial palsy was noted in the other half of these cases without a clinical diagnosis of shoulder dystocia. Severe asphyxia was observed in 143 of 1,000 births with shoulder dystocia compared with 14 of 1,000 overall.[122] Fetal morbidity is not always immediately apparent. McCall[123] found 28 percent of infants born with shoulder dystocia to demonstrate some neuropsychiatric dysfunction at 5- to 10-year follow up. Fewer than one half of these children had immediate morbidity.

Although shoulder dystocia has traditionally been strongly associated with macrosomia, up to one half of cases of shoulder dystocia occur in neonates under 4,000 g.[124,125] However, Acker et al.[125] found that the relative probability of shoulder dystocia in the 7 percent of infants over 4,000 g was 11 times greater than the average, and in the 2 percent of infants over 4,500 g it was 22 times greater. With macrosomia or continued fetal growth beyond term, the trunk and particularly the chest grow larger relative to the head. The chest circumference exceeds the head circumference in

80 percent of cases.[124] The arms also contribute to the greater dimensions of the upper body. Within a barely adequate pelvis, such bulk might easily block fetal rotation from a disadvantageous AP to the more desirable oblique outlet diameter. Macrosomia shows the strongest correlation with shoulder dystocia of any clinical factor and occurs more often with gestational diabetes and twice as often in postdate pregnancies. Postdate pregnancy also correlates with decreased amniotic fluid volume and perhaps decreased lubricating properties. Other clinical factors associated with shoulder dystocia appear to be related to macrosomia as well and include maternal obesity,[122,126] previous birth of an infant weighing over 4,000 g,[122,124,126] diabetes mellitus[126,127] prolonged second stage of labor[126] prolonged deceleration phase (8 to 10 cm),[118] and instrumental midpelvic delivery.[127] Increased maternal age and excess maternal weight gain have been found by some but not all investigators[122,126,127] to increase the risk of macrosomia and shoulder dystocia.

Macrosomia has been variously defined as a birth weight over either 4,000 g or 4,500 g.[120,122,128–130] A male predominance is routinely observed, and the condition is associated with the clinical features described above. The two most common complications seen with macrosomia are postpartum hemorrhage and shoulder dystocia.[156] Golditch and Kirkman[129] observed shoulder dystocia in 3 percent of deliveries of infants weighing between 4,100 and 4,500 g and in 8.2 percent of those over 4,500 g. Benedetti and Gabbe[120] reported that fetal injury occurred in 47 percent of infants weighing over 4,000 g who were delivered from the midpelvis and had shoulder dystocia.

Clinical efforts to detect macrosomia prenatally could be helpful in anticipating problems with delivery of the shoulders. Such efforts, however, have had imperfect results. Parks and Ziel[126] found that, of 110 macrosomic infants, the diagnosis was made prenatally in only 20 percent. The clinical estimate of birth weight was more than 3 lb in error in 6 percent of cases.

Ultrasonic techniques promoted for the detection of macrosomia include the estimation of fetal weight using a variety of fetal dimensions and the comparison of chest to head circumference. There is a growing trend to consider cesarean delivery of any infant with an estimated weight over 4,500 g or of any infant of a diabetic mother with an estimated weight over 4,000 g.[125,127] Any consideration of elective abdominal delivery based on estimated fetal weight alone, however, must consider the technical error of the method. If 90 percent confidence is desired that the actual fetal weight is at least 4,000 g, the sonographic estimate by most current methods must exceed 4,600 g. This is a result of the expected methodologic error of ± 10 percent (± 1 standard deviation). Furthermore, the fetal vertex is

often too deeply engaged in the pelvis to allow accurate measurement of head circumference. Estimated fetal weight should be only one of several factors considered in the management of the laboring patient. In the case of a diabetic, obese patient with an estimated fetal weight over 4,500 g and making poor progress in labor, cesarean delivery may be the most prudent course of action. However, in most other cases, the risks of cesarean to the mother, the accuracy of prediction of macrosomia, and the alternative of a carefully monitored trial of labor should be discussed. Gross et al.[131] carefully reviewed the clinical characteristics of 394 mothers delivering infants over 4,000 g and concluded that, although birth weight, prolonged deceleration phase, and length of second stage were all individually predictive, no prospective model adequately discriminated the infant destined to sustain trauma from shoulder dystocia from the infant not so destined.[131]

The most effective preventive measure is to be familiar with the normal mechanism of labor and to be constantly prepared to deal with shoulder dystocia. Normally, after the delivery of the head, external rotation (restitution) occurs, returning the head to its natural perpendicular relationship to the shoulder girdle. The fetal sagittal suture is usually oblique to the AP diameter of the outlet, and the shoulders occupy the opposite oblique diameter of the inlet (Fig. 16-27). As the shoulders descend in response to maternal pushing, the anterior shoulder emerges from its oblique axis under one of the pubic rami. If, however, the anterior shoulder descends in the AP diameter of the outlet and the fetus is relatively large for the outlet, impaction behind the symphysis can occur, and further descent is blocked.[121] Shoulder dystocia also occurs with an extremely rapid delivery of the head, as can occur with vacuum extraction or forceps.

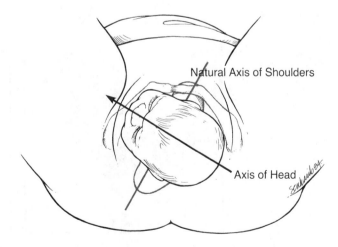

Fig. 16-27 After delivery of the head, "restitution" results in the long axis of the head reassuming its normal orientation to the shoulders as seen here.

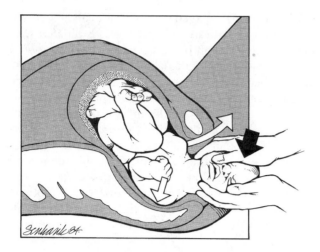

Fig. 16-28 Gentle, symmetric pressure on the head will move the posterior shoulder into the hollow of the sacrum and encourage delivery of the anterior shoulder. Care should be taken not to "pry" the anterior shoulder out asymmetrically, as this might lead to trauma to the anterior brachial plexus.

Successful treatment follows anticipation and preparation. Anticipation involves the prenatal suspicion of macrosomia by clinical and/or sonographic means. One must be aware of the clinical features that have been cited and consider a pregnancy at high risk for macrosomia and therefore for shoulder dystocia.

Such deliveries are best managed in a delivery room. Deliveries in bed increase the difficulty of reducing a shoulder dystocia because the bedding precludes fullest use of the posterior pelvis and outlet. Strong consideration for cesarean delivery is recommended when a prolonged second stage occurs in association with macrosomia.

Once a vaginal delivery has begun, the obstetrician must resist the temptation to rotate the head forcibly to a transverse axis. Maternal expulsive efforts should be used rather than traction. Gentle manual pressure on the fetal head inferiorly and posteriorly will push the posterior shoulder into the hollow of the sacrum, increasing the room for the anterior shoulder to pass under the pubis (Fig. 16-28). This pressure is not out-

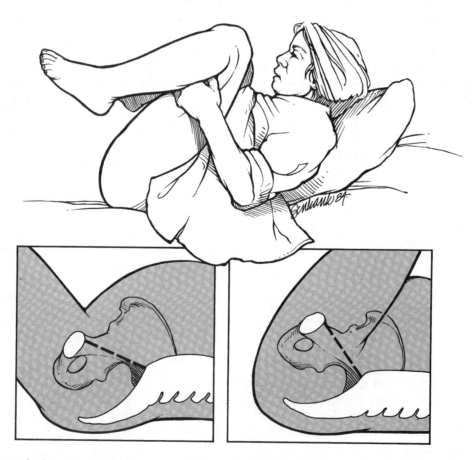

Fig. 16-29 The least invasive maneuver to disimpact the shoulders is the McRoberts maneuver. Sharp ventral flexion of the maternal hips results in ventral rotation of the maternal pelvis and an increase in the useful size of the outlet.

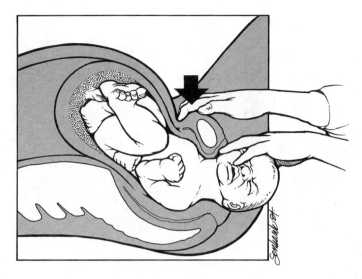

Fig. 16-30 Moderate suprapubic pressure will often disimpact the anterior shoulder.

ward traction and must be symmetric. If the head is pressed asymmetrically, as if to "pry" the anterior shoulder out, brachial injury is more likely.

If delivery is not accomplished, a deliberate, planned sequence of efforts should then be initiated. One must not pull desperately on the fetal head. Fundal expulsive efforts, including maternal pushing and any fundal pressure, should be temporarily stopped. Aggressive fundal pressure prior to disimpaction or rotation of the shoulders will not facilitate delivery and may work against rotation and disimpaction. The McRoberts maneuver[132] a simple, logical, and usually successful measure to promote delivery of the shoulders. The McRoberts maneuver involves hyperflexion of maternal legs on the maternal abdomen that results in flattening of the lumbar spine and ventral rotation of the maternal pelvis and symphasis (Fig. 16-29). This maneuver may increase the useful size of the posterior outlet, resulting in easier disimpaction of the anterior shoulder. Gonik et al.[133] showed that the McRoberts maneuver significantly reduces shoulder extraction forces, brachial plexus stretching, and the likelihood of clavicular fracture.

If the shoulders remain undelivered, often only moderate suprapubic pressure is required to disimpact the anterior shoulder and allow delivery (Fig. 16-30). If this is not effective, the operator's hand may be passed behind the occiput into the vagina, and the anterior shoulder may be pushed forward to the oblique, after which, with maternal efforts and gentle posterior pressure, delivery should occur (Fig. 16-31).[119] Alternatively, the posterior shoulder may be rotated forward, through a 180 degree arc, and passed under the pubic ramus as in turning a screw (Wood's screw maneuver). As the posterior shoulder rotates anteriorly, delivery will often occur.[134]

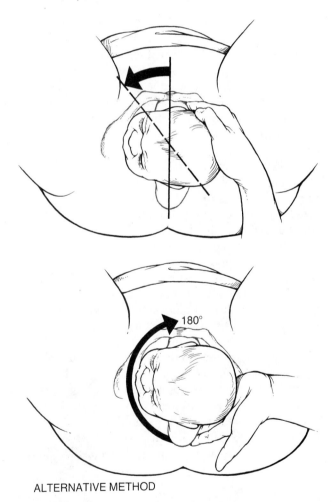

ALTERNATIVE METHOD

Fig. 16-31 Rotation of the anterior shoulder forward through a small arc or the posterior shoulder forward through a larger one will often lead to descent and delivery of the shoulders. Forward rotation is preferred as it tends to compress and diminish the size of the shoulder girdle, while backward rotation would open the shoulder girdle and increase the size.

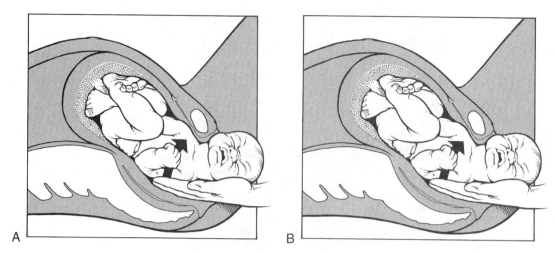

Fig. 16-32 The operator here inserts a hand and sweeps the posterior arm across the chest and over the perineum. Care should be taken to distribute the pressure evenly across the humerus to avoid unnecessary fracture.

Many authorities have advocated delivery of the posterior arm and shoulder should the above methods fail. The operator's hand is passed into the vagina, following the posterior arm of the fetus to the elbow. The arm is flexed and swept out over the chest and the perineum (Fig. 16-32). In some cases, delivery will now occur without further manipulation. In others, rotation of the trunk, bringing the freed posterior arm anteriorly, is required.[119,124]

Deliberate fracture of the clavicle is possible and will facilitate delivery by diminishing the rigidity and size of the shoulder girdle. It is best if the pressure is exerted in a direction away from the lung to avoid puncture. Sharp instrumental transsection of the clavicle is not recommended, since lung puncture is common with such a method, and infection of the bone through the open wound is a serious possible complication.

Two techniques rarely used in the United States for the management of shoulder dystocia include vaginal replacement of the fetal head with cesarean delivery (Zavanelli maneuver) and subcutaneous symphysiotomy. Sanberg[135] reviewed the Zavanelli maneuver and reported that seven of eight infants managed with this technique and delivered by cesarean after replacement of the fetal head for intractable shoulder dystocia had a good outcome. One infant was stillborn.[135] O'Leary and Cuva[136] described 35 cases, 31 of which were considered successful and one of which needed a hysterot-

omy incision to allow manual disimpaction of the fetal shoulders and facilitate vaginal delivery when the fetal head could not be replaced into the vagina from below. Subcutaneous symphysiotomy has been practiced in remote areas of the world for many years as an expedient alternative to cesarean delivery with very good results.[137] However, neither of these techniques has been widely or often used in obstetric practice in the United States. The attempted implementation of either method by the inexperienced practitioner before the trial of more conventional remedies may increase risk to the child, the mother, and the clinician.

In summary, shoulder dystocia is not precisely predictable, but may be anticipated in the case of a variety of predisposing clinical conditions or features such as a history of prior shoulder dystocia, suspected macrosomia, maternal gestational diabetes, maternal obesity, excessive maternal weight gain, prolonged deceleration phase of labor, delayed descent, and postdates. Shoulder dystocia will, in most cases, respond to any or all of several prudent interventions. The specific method used to disimpact the shoulder is probably not as critical as the practice of a careful, methodical approach to the problem and the avoidance of desperate, potentially traumatic or asymmetric traction. There may not be any complication of labor and delivery where forethought is more important to a successful outcome than shoulder dystocia.

Key Points

- The "fetal lie" indicates the orientation of the fetal spine relative to that of the mother. Normal fetal lie is longitudinal and by itself does not indicate whether the presentation is cephalic or breech.

- Cord prolapse occurs 20 times as often with an abnormal axial lie as it does with a cephalic presentation.

- Fetal malformations are observed in more than half of infants with a face presentation.

- Fetal malpresentation requires timely diagnostic exclusion of major fetal malformation and/or abnormal placentation.

- With few exceptions, a closely monitored labor and vaginal delivery is a safe possibility with most malpresentations.

- With few exceptions, cesarean delivery is the only acceptable alternative if normal progress toward spontaneous vaginal delivery is not observed.

- External cephalic version of the infant in breech presentation near term is a safe and often successful management option.

- Appropriate training and experience is a prerequisite to the safe vaginal delivery of selected infants in breech presentation.

- Shoulder dystocia cannot be precisely predicted or prevented but is often associated with macrosomia, maternal obesity, gestational diabetes, and postdates.

- The clinician must be prepared to deal with shoulder dystocia at every vaginal delivery with a deliberate, controlled sequence of interventions.

References

1. Yates MJ: Transverse foetal lie in labour. J Obstet Gynaecol Br Commonw 71:237, 1964

2. MacGregor WG: Aetiology and treatment of the oblique, transverse and unstable lie of the foetus with particular reference to antenatal care. J Obstet Gynaecol Br Commonw 71:237, 1964

3. Cockburn KG, Drake RF: Trasnverse and oblique lie of the foetus. Aust NZ J Obstet Gynaecol 8:211, 1968

4. Sandhu SK: Transverse lie. J Indian Med Assoc 68:205, 1977

5. Cruikshank DP, White CA: Obstetric malpresentations—twenty years' experience. Am J Obstet Gynecol 116:1097, 1973

6. Edwards RI, Nicholson HO: The management of the unstable lie in late pregnancy. J Obstet Gynaecol Br Commonw 76:713, 1969

7. Flowers CE: Shoulder presentation. Am J Obstet Gynecol 96:145, 1966

8. Johnson CE: Abnormal fetal presentations. Lancet 84: 317, 1964

9. Johnson CE: Transverse presentation of the fetus. JAMA 187:642, 1964

10. Thorp JM, Jenkins TJ, Watson W: Utility of Leopold maneuvers in screening for malpresentation. Obstet Gynecol 78:394, 1991

11. Hourihane MJ: Etiology and management of oblique lie. Obstet Gynecol 32:512, 1968

12. Phelan JP, Boucher M, Mueller E et al: The nonlaboring transverse lie. J Reprod Med 31:184, 1986

13. Cackins LA, Pearce EWJ: Transverse presentation. Obstet Gynecol 9:123, 1957

14. Pelosi MA, Apuzzio J, Fricchione D et al: The intraabdominal version technique for delivery of transverse lie by low segment cesarean section. Am J Obstet Gynecol 136:1009, 1979

15. Zhang J, Bowes WA, Fortney JA: Efficacy of external cephalic version: a review. Obstet Gynecol 82:306, 1993

16. Benedetti TJ, Lowensohn RI, Trluscott AM: Face presentation at term. Obstet Gynecol 55:199, 1980

17. Copeland GN, Nicks FI, Christakos AC: Face and brow presentations. NC Med J 29:507, 1968

18. Duff P: Diagnosis and management of face presentation. Obstet Gynecol 57:105, 1981

19. Groenig DC: Face presentation. Obstet Gynecol 2:495, 1953

20. Magid R, Gillespie CF: Face and brow presentation. Obstet Gynecol 9:450, 1957

21. Prevedourakis CN: Face presentation. Am J Obstet Gynecol 94:1092, 1966

22. Campbell JM: Face presentation. Aust NZ Obstet Gynaecol 5:231, 1965

23. Dede JA, Friedman EA: Face presentation. Am J Obstet Gynecol 87:515, 1963

24. Browne ADH, Carney D: Management of malpresentations in obstetrics. BMJ 5393:1295, 1964

25. Gomez HE, Dennen EH: Face presentation. Obstet Gynecol 8:103, 1956

26. Salzmann B, Soled M, Gilmour T: Face presentation. Obstet Gynecol 16:106, 1960

27. Cucco UP: Face presentation. Am J Obstet Gynecol 94: 1085, 1966

28. Borrell U, Fernstrom: Face I: the mechanism of labor. Radiol Clin North Am 5:73, 1966

29. Schwartz A, Dgani R, Lancet M et al: Face presentation. Aust NZ Obstet Gynaecol 26:172, 1986

30. Abroms IF, Bresnan MJ, Zuckerman JE et al: Cervical cord injuries secondary to hyperextension of the head in breech presentations. Obstet Gynecol 41:369, 1973

31. Adams CM: Review of breech presentation. SD J Med 32:15, 1979

32. Gold S: The conduct and management of face presentations. J Int Coll Surg 43:253, 1965

33. Lansford A, Arias D, Smith BE: Respiratory obstruction associated with face presentation. Am J Dis Child 116: 318, 1968

34. Meltzer RM, Sachtleban MR, Friedman EA: Brow presentation. Am J Obstet Gynecol 100:255, 1968

35. Kovacs SG: Brow presentation. Med J Aust 2:820, 1970

36. Levy DL: Persistent brow presentation—a new approach to management. South Med J 69:191, 1976

37. Ingolfsson A: Brow presentations. Acta Obstet Gynecol Scand 48:486, 1969

38. Bednoff SL, Thomas BE: Brow presentation. NY J Med 67:803, 1967

39. Skalley TW, Kramer TF: Brow presentation. Obstet Gynecol 15:616, 1960

40. Moore EJT, Dennen EH: Management of persistent brow presentation. Obstet Gynecol 6:186, 1955

41. Jennings PN: Brow presentation with vaginal delivery. Aust NZ J Obstet Gynaecol 8:219, 1968

42. Breen JL, Wiesmeien E: Compound presentation—a survey of 131 patients. Obstet Gynecol 32:419, 1968

43. Goplerud J, Eastman NJ: Compound presentation. Obstet Gynecol 1:59, 1953

44. Weissberg SM, O'Leary JA: Compound presentation of the fetus. Obstet Gynecol 41:60, 1973

45. Dignam WJ: Difficulties in delivery, including shoulder dystocia and malpresentations of the fetus. Clin Obstet Gynecol 19:577, 1976

46. Ang LT: Compound presentation following external version. Aust NZ J Obstet Gynaecol 19:213, 1978

47. Douglas HGK, Savage PE: An unusual case of compound presentation. J Obstet Gynaecol Br Commonw 77:1036, 1970

48. Collea JV: Current management of breech presentation. Clin Obstet Gynecol 23:525, 1980

49. Braun FHT, Jones KL, Smith DW: Breech presentation as an indicator of fetal abnormality. J Pediatr 86:419, 1975

50. Fall O, Nilsson BA: External cephalic version in breech presentation under tocolysis. Obstet Gynecol 53:712, 1979

51. Kubli F: Risk of vaginal breech delivery. Contrib Gynecol Obstet 3:80, 1977

52. Hibbard LT, Schumann WR: Prophylactic external cephalic version in an obstetric practice. Am J Obstet Gynecol 116:511, 1973

53. Kauppila O, Gronroos M, Aro P et al: Management of low birth weight breech delivery—should cesarean section be routine? Obstet Gynecol 57:289, 1981

54. Rovinsky JJ, Miller JA, Kaplan S: Management of breech presentation at term. Am J Obstet Gynecol 115:497, 1973

55. de la Fuente P, Escalante JM, Hernandez-Garcia JM: Perinatal mortality in breech presentations. Contrib Gynecol Obstet 3:108, 1977

56. Goldenberg RL, Nelson KG: The premature breech. Am J Obstet Gynecol 127:240, 1977

57. NIH consensus development statement on cesarean childbirth. Obstet Gynecol 57:537, 1981

58. Mansani FE, Cerutti M: The risk in breech delivery. Contrib Gynecol Obstet 3:86, 1977

59. Seitchik J: Discussion of "breech delivery—evaluation of the method of delivery on perinatal results and maternal morbidity" by Bowes et al. Am J Obstet Gynecol 135:970, 1979

60. Wolter DF: Patterns of management with breech presentation. Am J Obstet Gynecol 125:733, 1976

61. Green JE, McLean F, Smitt LP et al: Has an increased cesarean section rate for term breech delivery reduced the incidence of birth asphyxia, trauma, and death? Am J Obstet Gynecol 142:643, 1982

62. Croughan-Minihane MS, Petitt DB, Gordis L, Golditch I: Morbidity among breech infants according to method of delivery. Obstet Gynecol 75:821, 1990

63. Brenner WE, Bruce RD, Hendricks CH: The characteristics and perils of breech presentation. Am J Obstet Gynecol 118:700, 1974

64. Collea JV, Rabin SC, Weghorst GR et al: The randomized management of term frank breech presentation—vaginal delivery versus cesarean section. Am J Obstet Gynecol 131:186, 1978

65. De Crespigny LJC, Pepperell RJ: Perinatal mortality and morbidity in breech presentation. Obstet Gynecol 53:141, 1979

66. Graves WK: Breech delivery in twenty years of practice. Am J Obstet Gynecol 137:229, 1980

67. Niswander KR: Discussion of "the randomized management of term frank breech presentation—vaginal delivery versus cesarean section" by Collea et al. Am J Obstet Gynecol 131:193, 1978

68. Lyons ER, Papsin FR: Cesarean section in the management of breech presentation. Am J Obstet Gynecol 130:558, 1978

69. Spanio P, Elia F, DeBonis F et al: Fetal-neonatal mortality and morbidity in cesarean deliveries. Contrib Gynecol Obstet 3:130, 1977

70. Westgren M, Ingemarsson I, Svenningsen NW: Long-term follow up of preterm infants in breech presentation delivered by cesarean section. Dan Med Bull 26:141, 1979

71. Faber-Nijholt R, Huisjes JH, Touwen CL et al: Neurological follow up of 281 children born in breech presentation—a controlled study. BMJ 286, 1983

72. Bowes WA, Taylor ES, O'Brien M et al: Breech delivery—evaluation of the method of delivery on perinatal results and maternal morbidity. Am J Obstet Gynecol 135:965, 1979

73. Lewis BV, Sene Viratne HR: Vaginal breech delivery or cesarean section. Am J Obstet Gynecol 134:615, 1979

74. Cruikshank DP, Pitkin RM: Delivery of the premature breech. Obstet Gynecol 50:367, 1977

75. Zatuchni GI, Andros GJ: Prognostic index for vaginal delivery in breech presentation at term. Am J Obstet Gynecol 93:237, 1965

76. Cruikshank DP: Premature breech (letter to the editor). Am J Obstet Gynecol 130:500, 1978

77. Woods JR: Effects of low birth weight breech delivery on neonatal mortality. Obstet Gynecol 53:735, 1979

78. Ulstein M: Breech delivery. Ann Chir Gynaecol Fenn 69:70, 1980

79. Weissman A, Blazer S, Zimmer EZ et al: Low birthweight breech infant: short term and long term outcome by method of delivery. Am J Perinatol 5:289, 1988

80. Anderson G, Strong C: The premature breech: caesarean section or trial of labour? J Med Ethics 14:18, 1988

81. Tejani N, Verma U, Shiffman R et al: Effect of route of delivery on periventricular/intraventricular hemor-

rhage in the low birthweight fetus with a breech presentation. J Reprod Med 32:911, 1987

82. Karp LE, Doney JR, McCarthy T et al: The premature breech—trial of labor or cesarean section? Obstet Gynecol 53:88, 1979

83. Mann LI, Gallant JM: Modern management of the breech delivery. Am J Obstet Gynecol 134:611, 1979

84. Duenhoelter JH, Wells CE, Reisch JS et al: A paired controlled study of vaginal and abdominal delivery of the low birth weight breech fetus. Obstet Gynecol 54:310, 1979

85. Cox C, Kendall AC, Hommers M: Changed prognosis of breech-presenting low birthweight infants. Br J Obstet Gynaecol 89:881, 1982

86. Milner RDG: Neonatal mortality of breech deliveries with and without forceps to the aftercoming head. Br J Obstet Gynaecol 82:783, 1975

87. Milner RDG: Neonatal mortality of breech deliveries with and without forceps to the aftercoming head. Contrib Gynecol Obstet 3:113, 1977

88. Caterini H, Langer A, Sama JC et al: Fetal risk in hyperextension of the fetal head in breech presentation. Am J Obstet Gynecol 123:632, 1975

89. Daw E: Hyperextension of the head in breech presentation. Am J Obstet Gynecol 119:564, 1974

90. Ballas S, Toaff R, Jaffa AJ: Deflexion of the fetal head in breech presentation. Obstet Gynecol 52:653, 1978

91. Cheng M, Hannah M: Breech delivery at term: a critical review of the literature. Obstet Gynecol 82:605, 1993

92. Bird CC, McElin TW: A six year prospective study of term breech deliveries utilizing the Zatuchni-Andros prognostic scoring index. Am J Obstet Gynecol 121:551, 1975

93. Mark C, Roberts PHR: Breech scoring index. Am J Obstet Gynecol 101:572, 1968

94. Zatuchni GI, Andros GJ: Prognostic index for vaginal delivery in breech presentation at term. Am J Obstet Gynecol 98:854, 1967

95. Collea JV, Chein C, Quilligan EJ: The randomized management of term frank breech presentation—a study of 208 cases. Am J Obstet Gynecol 137:235, 1980

96. O'Leary JA: Vaginal delivery of the term frank breech. Obstet Gynecol 53:341, 1979

97. Selvaggi L, Chieppa M, Loizzi P et al: Intrapartum mortality among breech deliveries. Contrib Gynecol Obstet 3:99, 1977

98. Gimovsky ML, Wallace RL, Schifrin BS et al: Randomized management of the non-frank breech presentation at term—a preliminary report. Am J Obstet Gynecol 146:34, 1983

99. Flanagan TA, Mulchahey KM, Korenbrot CC et al: Management of term breech presentation. Am J Obstet Gynecol 156:1492, 1987

100. Bingham P, Lilford RJ: Management of the selected term breech presentation: assessment of the risks of selected vaginal delivery versus cesarean section for all cases. Obstet Gynecol 69:965, 1987

101. Blickstein I, Schwartz-Shoham Z, Lancet M: Vaginal delivery of the second twin in breech presentation. Obstet Gynecol 69:774, 1987

102. Gocke SE, Nageotte MP, Garite T et al: Management of the nonvertex second twin: primary cesarean section, external version, or primary breech extraction. Am J Obstet Gynecol 161:111, 1989

103. Laros RK, Dattel BJ: Management of twin pregnancy: the vaginal route is still safe. Am J Obstet Gynecol 158:1330, 1988

104. Fishman A, Grubb DK, Kovacs BW: Vaginal delivery of the nonvertex second twin. Am J Obstet Gynecol 168:861, 1993

105. Tchabo JG, Tomai T: Selected intrapartum external cephalic version of the second twin. Obstet Gynecol 79:421, 1992

106. Rabinovici J, Reichman B, Serr DM et al: Internal podalic version with unruptured membranes for the second twin in transverse lie. Obstet Gynecol 71:428, 1988

107. Druzin ML: Atraumatic delivery in cases of malpresentation of the very low birthweight fetus at cesarean section: the splint technique. Am J Obstet Gynecol 154:941, 1986

108. Van Dorsten JP, Schifrin BS, Wallace RL: Randomized control trial of external cephalic version with tocolysis in late pregnancy. Am J Obstet Gynecol 141:417, 1981

109. Hanley BJ: Editorial—fallacy of external version. Obstet Gynecol 4:124, 1954

110. Thornhill PE: Changes in fetal polarity near term spontaneous and external version. Am J Obstet Gynecol 93:306, 1965

111. Ylikorkala O, Hartikainen-Sorri A: Value of external version in fetal malpresentation in combination with use of ultrasound. Acta Obstet Gynecol Scand 56:63, 1977

112. Stine LE, Phalen JP, Wallace R et al: Update on external cephalic version performed at term. Obset Gynecol 65:642, 1985

113. Robertson AW, Kopelman JN, Read JA et al: External cephalic version at term: is a tocolytic necessary? Obstet Gynecol 70:896, 1987

114. Fortunato SJ, Mercer LJ, Guzick DS: External cephalic version with tocolysis: factors associated with success. Obstet Gynecol 72:59, 1988

115. Marchick R: Antepartum external cephalic version with tocolysis: a study of term singleton breech presentations. Am J Obstet Gynecol 158:1339, 1988

116. Scaling ST: External cephalic version without tocolysis. Am J Obstet Gynecol 158:1424, 1988

117. van Veelen AJ, van Cappellen AW, Flu PK et al: Effect of external cephalic version in late pregnancy on presentation at delivery: a randomized control trial. Br J Obstet Gynaecol 96:916, 1989

118. Hanss JW: The efficacy of external cephalic version and its impact on the breech experience. Am J Obstet Gynecol 162:1459, 1990

119. Marcus RG, Crewe-Brown H, Krawitz S et al: Fetomaternal haemorrhage following successful and unsuccessful attempts at external cephalic version. Br J Obstet Gynaecol 82:578, 1975

120. Benedetti TJ, Gabbe SG: Shoulder dystocia—a complication of fetal macrosomia and prolonged second stage of labor with midpelvic delivery. Obstet Gynecol 52:526, 1978

121. Swartz DP: Shoulder girdle dystocia in vertex delivery—clinical study and review. Obstet Gynecol 15:194, 1960

122. Boyd ME, Usher RH, McLean FH: Fetal macrosomia—prediction, risks, and proposed management. Obstet Gynecol 61:715, 1983

123. McCall JO: Shoulder dystocia—a study of after effects. Am J Obstet Gynecol 83:1486, 1962

124. Seigworth GR: Shoulder dystocia—review of 5 years' experience. Obstet Gynecol 28:764, 1966

125. Acker DB, Sachs BP, Friedman EA: Risk factors for Erb-Duchene palsy. Obstet Gynecol 66:764, 1985

126. Parks DG, Ziel HK: Macrosomia—a proposed indication for primary cesarean section. Obstet Gynecol 52:407, 1978

127. Acker DB, Gregory KD, Sachs BP et al: Risk factors for Erb-Duchene palsy. Obstet Gynecol 71:389, 1988

128. Modanlou HD, Dorchester WL, Thorosian A et al: Macrosomia-maternal, fetal, and neonatal implications. Obstet Gynecol 55:420, 1980

129. Golditch IM, Kirkman K: The large fetus—management and outcome. Obstet Gynecol 52:26, 1978

130. Modanlou HD, Komatsu G, Dorchester W et al: Large for gestational age neonates: anthropometric reasons for shoulder dystocia. Obstet Gynecol 60:417, 1982

131. Gross TL, Sokol RJ, Williams T et al: Shoulder dystocia: a fetal-physician risk. Am J Obstet Gynecol 156:1408, 1987

132. Gonik B, Stringer CA, Held B: An alternate maneuver for management of shoulder dystocia. Am J Obstet Gynecol 145:882, 1983

133. Gonik B, Allen R, Sorab J: Objective evaluation of the shoulder dystocia phenomenon: effect of maternal pelvic orientation on force reduction. Obstet Gynecol 74:44, 1989

134. Gross SJ, Shime J, Farine D: Shoulder dystocia: predictors and outcome. Am J Obstet Gynecol 156:334, 1987

135. Sandberg EC: The Zavanelli maneuver extended: progression of a revolutionary concept. Am J Obstet Gynecol 158:1347, 1988

136. O'Leary JA, Cuva A: Abdominal rescue after failed cephalic replacement. Obstet Gynecol 80:514, 1992

137. Hartfield VJ: Symphysiotomy for shoulder dystocia (letter). Am J Obstet Gynecol 155:228, 1986

Chapter 7

Obstetric Hemorrhage

Thomas J. Benedetti

It is critical that the obstetrician be able to estimate rapidly the blood volume deficit in the pregnant patient. Although some have proposed that the pregnant woman fails to show the usual signs and symptoms of blood loss, there is little scientific evidence to support this hypothesis. This confusion may have arisen from an incomplete understanding of the physiologic responses to volume loss and lack of appreciation of normal volume expansion of pregnancy. The normal pregnant patient frequently loses 500 ml of blood at the time of vaginal delivery and 1,000 ml at the time of cesarean delivery. Appreciably more blood can be lost without clinical evidence of a volume deficit as a result of the 40 percent expansion in blood volume that occurs by the 30th week of pregnancy.

To understand why the pregnant patient does not exhibit early signs of volume loss, it is important to understand the normal physiologic responses to hemorrhage (Fig. 17-1). When 1,000 ml is rapidly removed from the circulatory blood volume, vasoconstriction occurs in both the arterial and venous compartments in order to preserve essential body organ flow. As illustrated in Figure 17-1, when intravascular volume is lost, blood pressure is initially maintained by increases in systemic vascular resistance. As volume loss exceeds 20 percent, the fall in cardiac output accelerates and blood pressure can no longer be maintained by increases in resistance. Blood pressure and cardiac output fall in parallel after this point. In addition, if the volume loss has occurred more than 4 hours earlier, significant fluid shifts from the interstitial space into the intravascular space will partially correct the volume deficit. This movement of fluid, termed *transcapillary refill,* can replace as much as 30 percent of lost volume. In more chronic bleeding states, the final blood volume deficit

may amount to as little as 70 percent of the actual blood lost.

Classification Of Hemorrhage

A standard classification for volume loss secondary to hemorrhage is illustrated in Table 17-1. Hemorrhage can be classified as one of four groups, depending on the volume lost. The determination of the class of hemorrhage reflects the volume deficit, which may not be the same as the volume loss. The average 60-kg pregnant woman has a blood volume of 6,000 ml at 30 weeks, and an unreplaced volume loss of less than 900 ml falls into class 1. Such patients rarely exhibit signs or symptoms of volume deficit.

A blood loss of 1,200 to 1,500 ml is characterized as a class 2 hemorrhage. These individuals will begin to show expected physical signs, the first being a rise in pulse rate and/or a rise in respiratory rate. Tachypnea is a nonspecific response to volume loss and, although a relatively early sign of mild volume deficit, is frequently overlooked. A doubling of the respiratory rate may be observed in this circumstance. If the patient appears to be breathing rapidly, the minute ventilation is usually twice its normal value. This finding should not be interpreted as an encouraging sign, but rather one of impending problems.

Patients with class 2 hemorrhage will frequently have orthostatic blood pressure changes and may have decreased perfusion of the extremities. However, this amount of blood loss will not usually result in the classic cold, clammy extremities. Rather, a more subtle test is needed to document this phenomenon. One can simply squeeze the hypothenar area of the hand for 1 to 2 seconds and then release the pressure. A patient with

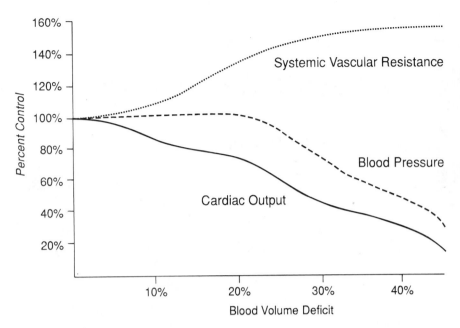

Fig. 17-1 Relationships among systemic vascular pressure, cardiac output, and blood pressure in the face of progressive blood volume deficit.

normal volume status will have an initial blanching of the skin, followed within 1 to 2 seconds by a return to the normal pink coloration. A patient who has a volume deficit of 15 to 25 percent will have delayed refilling of the blanched area of the hand.

Narrowing of the pulse pressure is another sign of class 2 hemorrhage. A thorough understanding of blood pressure readings is necessary in order to interpret subtle volume changes in the pregnant patient. The blood pressure can be viewed as having three components: diastolic pressure, pulse pressure, and systolic pressure. The diastolic pressure reflects the amount of systemic vasoconstriction present, the pulse pressure indicates stroke volume, and the systolic pressure denotes the interrelationship between the level of vasoconstriction and the stroke volume. While pulse pattern is a good clinical approach to the assessment of stroke

volume in a given patient, it is not a reliable method of monitoring stroke volume in larger groups of patients because of individual variations in the many factors that may alter stroke volume (age, aortic stiffness). However, monitoring this parameter in a given patient will provide earlier signs of hypovolemia and reduced blood flow than either systolic or diastolic pressure used individually.

When a patient loses blood, compensatory mechanisms are activated that help ensure perfusion to vital body organs (brain, heart). The initial response, vasoconstriction, diverts blood away from nonvital body organs, (skin, muscle, kidney). Blood loss results in sympathoadrenal stimulation, which causes a rise in diastolic pressure. Since the systolic pressure is usually maintained with small volume deficits (15 to 25 percent), the first blood pressure response seen with volume loss is narrowing of the pulse pressure (120/70 to 120/90 mmHg). That is, pulse pressure changes from 50 to 30 mmHg. When pulse pressure drops to 30 mmHg or less, the patient should be carefully evaluated for other signs of volume loss.

Class 3 hemorrhage is defined as blood loss sufficient to cause overt hypotension. In the pregnant patient, this usually requires a blood loss of 1,800 to 2,100 ml. These patients exhibit marked tachycardia (120 to 60 bpm) and may have cold, clammy skin and tachypnea (respiratory rate of 30 to 50 per minute).

In class 4 patients, the volume deficit exceeds 40 percent. These patients are in profound shock and frequently have no discernible blood pressure. They may have absent pulses in their extremities and are oliguric

Table 17-1 Classification of Hemorrhage in the Pregnant Patient[a]

Hemorrhage Class	Acute Blood Loss[b]	Percentage Lost
1	900	15
2	1,200–1,500	20–25
3	1,800–2,100	30–35
4	2,400	40

[a] Total blood volume = 6,000 ml.

[b] In the usual clinical setting, very few episodes of volume loss occur without some infusion of intravenous fluids, usually crystalloid-containing solutions such as Ringer's lactated solution, or normal saline. Therefore, the amount of blood loss preceding physical signs and symptoms will usually exceed the values listed.

(Adapted from Baker,[90] with permission).

or anuric. If volume therapy is not quickly begun, circulatory collapse and cardiac arrest will soon result.

The hematocrit is another clinical method frequently used to estimate blood loss. After acute blood loss, the hematocrit will not change significantly for at least 4 hours, and complete compensation requires 48 hours. Infusion of intravenous fluids can alter this relationship, resulting in earlier lowering of measured hematocrit. When significant hemorrhage is thought to have occurred, a hematocrit should always be obtained. If this result shows a significant fall from a previous baseline value, a large amount of blood has been lost. Measures should immediately be taken to evaluate the source of the loss and whether the hemorrhage is ongoing but unrecognized.

Cesarean delivery is a frequent cause of excessive blood loss. It must be remembered that narcotics, which are frequently used for pain relief in the immediate postoperative period, can significantly reduce the ability of the sympathetic nervous system to effect vasoconstriction of the arterial and venous compartments. If these medications are given to a hypovolemic patient, serious hypotension can result. Signs and symptoms of hypovolemia should always be sought before the postoperative patient is given narcotic analgesics on the first postpartum day.

Urine Output—"The Window of Body Perfusion"

In hypovolemic patients, urine output must be carefully monitored. In many cases, the urine output will fall before other signs of impaired perfusion are manifest. In contrast, adequate urine volume in patients who have not received diuretics strongly suggests perfusion to vital body organs is adequate.

There is reasonable correlation between renal blood flow and urine output. If the urine output is low, renal blood flow is often low as well. When there is a rapid decrease in renal blood flow, there is usually a reduction in urine output. In such cases, renal blood flow tends to shift from the outer renal cortex to the juxtamedullary portion of the renal cortex. Glomerular filtration rate is further reduced, but absorption of water and sodium is increased because there are fewer glomeruli and longer loops of Henle in this region. Urine will become more concentrated and will have a lower concentration of sodium and a higher osmolarity. With a gradual fall in renal blood flow, the urine sodium and osmolarity will often be affected before any significant fall in urine output. A urine sodium concentration of less than 10 to 20 mEq/L or a urine/serum osmolar ratio of greater than 2 usually indicates reduced renal perfusion.

Blood Loss in Severe Preeclampsia

Major blood loss in a patient with severe preeclampsia may present a confusing picture. One must be aware of the altered hemodynamic status of these patients to appreciate the extent of the volume loss and to ensure appropriate fluid replacement. In severe preeclampsia, the blood volume has frequently failed to expand and is similar to that in a nonpregnant person. These patients will not have the protective effect of the usual volume expansion of pregnancy and will show signs of blood loss earlier. In these cases, however, blood pressure can be a misleading indicator of volume. A blood pressure appropriate for a previously normotensive patient could indicate serious volume depletion in the preeclamptic woman. It is especially important to record serial pressures. If the blood pressure shows a significant drop during the immediate postoperative or postpartum period, a volume deficit should be suspected because hypertension usually persists for days to weeks in patients with severe preeclampsia.

When significant hemorrhage occurs in the woman with hypertension, it may be important to supplement the crystalloid fluid resuscitation with colloidal fluids pending the availability of the best colloid, whole blood. Albumin (5 percent) may be given in the ratio of 500 ml of albumin for every 4 L of crystalloid. This form of therapy will help compensate for the low albumin and total protein concentrations present in the patient with severe preeclampsia. It is not uncommon for these women to have total protein levels less than 5.0 g/dl with an albumin concentration below 2.5 g/dl. If crystalloid fluids are given alone, massive fluid accumulation in the already overexpanded extravascular space can occur and may result in cerebral as well as pulmonary edema.[1]

Treatment

Patients showing signs of class 2 or greater volume loss should receive crystalloid intravenous fluids pending the arrival of blood and blood products. The infusion rate should be rapid, between 1,000 and 2,000 ml in 30 to 45 minutes, or faster if the patient is obviously hypotensive. This infusion may serve as a therapeutic trial to help determine the amount of blood loss. If the physical signs and symptoms return to normal and remain stable after this challenge, no further therapy may be needed. If blood loss has been severe and the patient continues to bleed, however, this favorable response may be only transient. In this situation, typed and cross-matched blood should be given. The initial administration of a balanced salt solution will reduce the amount of whole blood needed to restore an adequate blood volume.[2]

Blood and Blood Products

The use of whole blood has been discouraged by blood banking centers around the United States. In obstetrics, the main indication for whole blood rather than component therapy is massive blood loss requiring more than a 4,000-ml replacement (see Table 17-2).

An anticoagulant (cpda-1) is used to preserve whole blood. This compound contains c, a calcium chelating agent; p, phosphate, to maintain adenosine triphosphate (ATP) levels; d dextrose, food for red blood cells (RBCs) and for preservation of 2,3-diphosphoglyceric acid (DPG) levels; and a, adenine, to preserve ATP levels. Maintenance of ATP is essential to preserve the RBC sodium pump and cell shape, both of which affect cell survival. A byproduct of the normal glycolytic pathway in the RBC, 2,3-DPG, causes a shift to the right of the oxyhemoglobin dissociation curve. This shift permits more oxygen to be dissociated from the hemoglobin molecule and released into the tissues. Despite these alterations, the useful life of a unit of whole blood is only 21 days.

The storage of whole blood has significant effects on its cellular elements as well as coagulation factors. After 24 hours, white blood cells (WBCs) and platelets are either absent or nonfunctional. After 7 days, levels of Factors V and VIII have fallen 50 percent or more. There remains a large amount of plasma protein in stored blood, however, and for which reason it remains the agent of choice for transfusion in the face of major hemorrhage.

Massive Blood Transfusion

Massive transfusion is an ill-defined term but can generally be thought of as the need to replace a patient's entire blood volume in 24 hours.[3] In a pregnant patient, this is usually 10 or more units of blood. Massive transfusion is a medical emergency that often requires the ultimate in surgical and medical skills. Administrative skills are also essential because usually a number of physicians from various medical specialties are involved in the care of such a patient. Events may be occurring rapidly and clinical circumstances changing from minute to minute. Clear lines of communication between the various health care providers must be maintained. During an acute hemorrhage requiring prolonged surgical management, such as a placenta accreta with bladder involvement, it is optimal to have one member of the obstetric team whose job is to coordinate blood replacement and to monitor laboratory results, which are the basis for choosing which components to replace. Communication between the surgeon and the anesthesiologist regarding volume and coagulation status is essential and may be compromised if all physicians are heavily involved in their own work.

The essentials of management of the patient requiring massive transfusion are maintenance of circulation, blood volume, oxygen-carrying capacity, hemostasis, colloid osmotic pressure, and biochemical balance. As soon as it is apparent that more than two units of blood will be required, preparations should be made to have a significant quantity of blood products available. After four units of packed red cells are given, whole blood

Table 17-2   Blood Replacement

Product	Cost/Unit	Contents	Volume (cc)	Effect
Whole blood (WB)	$97	Red blood cells (2,3-DPG) White blood cells (not functional after 24 hours) Coagulation factors (50%—V, VIII after 7 days) Plasma proteins	500	Increase volume (ml/ml) Increase hematocrit 3%/unit
Packed red cells	$97	Red blood cells—same as whole blood White blood cells—less than whole blood Plasma proteins—few	240	Same red blood cells as whole blood Less risk febrile, or WBC transfusion reaction Increase hematocrit 3%/unit
Platelets	$47	55×10^6 platelets/unit, few white blood cells	50	Increase platelet count 5,000–10,000 µl/unit Give 6 packs minimum
Fresh frozen plasma	$50	Clotting Factors V and VIII, fibrinogen	250	Only source of Factors V, XI, XII Increase fibrinogen 10 mg%/unit
Cryoprecipitate	$30	Factor VIII 25% Fibrinogen von Willebrand's factor	40	Increase fibrinogen 10 mg%/unit
Albumin 5%	$54	Albumin	500	
Albumin 25%	$54	Albumin	50	

will provide both the coagulation factors and proteins needed to maintain hemostasis and colloid osmotic pressure. If whole blood is not available, earlier laboratory testing for coagulation deficiencies should be performed because more component therapy will probably be required. As soon as it becomes apparent that massive transfusion therapy is required, baseline coagulation tests should be ordered and the laboratory notified that more tests will be coming on a periodic basis. These tests should include complete blood count (CBC), platelet count, fibrinogen, prothrombin time (PT), and partial thromboplastin time (PTT). The laboratory must be alerted regarding the life-threatening nature of the problem and top priority. A turnaround time of 15 minutes should be the goal.

Previous algorithms for massive transfusion advised transfusion with platelets and fresh frozen plasma after a certain number of units of blood have been used. However, with modern laboratory testing, the overuse of these products can be limited. In general, microvascular oozing will be apparent at platelet counts below 50,000. This drop usually requires the replacement of one and a half blood volumes. However, counts may drop to this level or below in the face of the consumptive process of disseminated intravascular coagulation (DIC) prior to the loss of 15 units of blood. In addition, platelet function itself may be impaired in patients undergoing massive transfusion. If there is continued surgical evidence of microvascular bleeding in the face of laboratory tests near the critical levels, more replacement should be given.

If whole blood is available, there will often be no need for the transfusion of fresh frozen plasma because many of the coagulation factors are present in stored blood. However, if packed cells are used, frequent monitoring of the PT should be performed. When the PT is prolonged by greater than 5 seconds, fresh frozen plasma should be used. In the face of DIC there will also be prolongation of the PTT and fall in fibrinogen. In this case, cryoprecipitate should also be used as a source of Factor VIII and fibrinogen.

Metabolic derangements are frequently mentioned when massive transfusion is discussed. However, traditional formulas for using alkylating agents or calcium supplements are probably unnecessary. Hypocalcemia is a theoretic problem, but clinical syndromes from this problem are infrequently described and the possible complications of prophylactic calcium infusion may be more harmful than hypocalcemia. The one time hypocalcemia can be clinically important is when it is combined with hyperkalemia and hypothermia, a triad that can lead to cardiac arrhythmias. Hypothermia can be a problem if the recently refrigerated blood is administered at a rate of one unit every 5 to 10 minutes. If this rate of administration is required, attempts should be made to warm the blood above 4°C before transfusion. Close attention should be paid to the electrocardiogram. If arrhythmias are noted, supplemental calcium should be considered.

Acid-base problems may arise in the event of massive transfusion. However, citrate toxicity is rarely a problem because the healthy liver can metabolize citrate in a unit of blood in 5 minutes. Unless transfusion rates exceed one unit per 5 minutes or the liver is previously diseased, citrate toxicity should not be a problem. Although stored blood has an acid pH, acidosis is uncommon because the metabolism of citrate produces alkalosis. Prolonged acidosis is more often the result of hypoperfusion and shock rather than blood replacement. Blood gas measurement should guide the therapy with bicarbonate in this instance.

Packed Red Blood Cells

Packed red blood cells (PRBCs) are the most effective and efficient way to provide increased oxygen-carrying capacity to the anemic patient. Unless a patient has suffered massive blood loss, PRBCs and crystalloid will satisfy most clinical needs. Oxygen-carrying capacity may become impaired in the euvolemic patient when the hemoglobin level drops below 7 g/dl. If adequate volume replacement has not been accomplished patients may exhibit orthostatic blood pressure changes or other signs of impaired oxygen-carrying capacity at hemoglobin levels above 7 g/dl. Because this product has small amounts of WBCs and isohemagglutinins (anti-A and anti-B), its use reduces the incidence of nonhemolytic transfusion reactions compared with that of one unit of whole blood. However, care should be taken to administer PRBCs with normal saline rather than Ringer's lactated or dextrose solutions. These solutions can cause the blood to clot or the red cells to lyse.

Platelets

A unit of platelets is derived from a single unit of whole blood and has a shelf life of 72 hours. Transfusion of a single unit of platelets can be expected to raise the platelet count between 5,000 and 10,000/μl. A single unit of platelets should never be given: the smallest single dose of clinical value is four to six units. Platelets should be administered rapidly, over 10 minutes, with repeat laboratory evaluation performed 2 hours after infusion. For the obstetric patient, it is important that the platelets be ABO and Rh specific, since the platelet concentrate usually contains some RBCs that can potentially sensitize an Rh-negative woman. Sensitization can be prevented by concomitant administration of Rh-immune globulin. One 300-μg dose will prevent sensitization for 30 platelet packs. It must also be remembered that six packs of platelets have a volume effect if multiple doses are used. Each unit of platelets carries the transfusion risk of a single unit of blood.

Platelet administration is frequently considered for patients with DIC, massive hemorrhage, severe preeclampsia, and idiopathic thrombocytopenia (ITP). In each of these conditions, the absolute levels at which a platelet transfusion is indicated may vary depending on the time course of the thrombocytopenia (more chronic forms will result in less hemostatic defects than acute loss), the need to perform a surgical procedure, the etiology of the inciting event producing thrombocytopenia, and the level of blood pressure elevation and the bleeding time. In general, platelet counts below 50,000/μl will require transfusion prior to or during surgery. However, when the need for a cesarean delivery arises in patients with platelet counts ranging from 20,000 to 50,000 platelets, transfusion may be avoided or the amount reduced if the transfusion is delayed until the need becomes apparent. This is usually evident from bleeding from skin edges, as hemostasis in the uterus is primarily a function of uterine muscle contraction, not platelet function.

Cryoprecipitate

Prepared by warming fresh frozen plasma and collecting the precipitate, cryoprecipitate contains significant amounts of Factor VIII fibrinogen and von Willebrand factor. Cryoprecipitate is used primarily in patients with von Willebrand disease and in patients with a normal blood volume who require factor replacement. Except for Factor VIII, the same coagulation factors are available in this product as in fresh frozen plasma but in only 15 percent of the volume. As with platelets, cryoprecipitate should be ABO and Rh specific. One unit of cryoprecipitate will raise the serum fibrinogen level 10 mg/dl. This preparation should be used when significant hypofibrinogenemia must be treated.

Fresh Frozen Plasma

Fresh frozen plasma contains all the coagulation factors present in cryoprecipitate, including appreciably higher levels of Factor VIII. Fresh frozen plasma should be administered when both volume replacement and coagulation factors are needed. The main clinical indication for this therapy is the massively hemorrhaging patient. If bleeding continues after the transfusion of four to five units of blood, a coagulation screen should be checked to see whether the replacement of clotting factors and platelets is indicated. If the coagulation parameters and PTT are abnormal, two units of fresh frozen plasma should be administered. Subsequent therapy should be determined by clinical response and follow-up laboratory testing.

Table 17-3 Risks of Blood Transfusion

Complication	Incidence of Complication	Incidence of Death
Human immunodeficiency virus	1/270,000	1/270,000
Hepatitis B	1/100,000	1/2,000,000
Hepatitis C	1/5,000	Less than 1/500,000
Hemolytic transfusion reaction	1/6,000	1/100,000
Nonhemolytic transfusion reaction	1/100	1/10,000,000

Transfusion Risks

PRBCs, fresh frozen plasma, cryoprecipitate, and platelets have the same risk of transmitting infectious diseases as a unit of whole blood. Table 17-3 lists the common risks of blood transfusion when blood is procured from volunteer donors. Significant progress has been made in historical and laboratory screening for common infectious diseases. The risks of serious complications from blood transfusion have fallen to very low rates. Blood obtained from paid sources can be expected to have higher rates of many of the complications listed in the table.

Autologous Transfusion

Primarily as the result of fear of acquiring the acquired immune deficiency syndrome (AIDS) virus from blood transfusion, interest in autologous blood transfusion for pregnant patients has been heightened in recent years. Autologous transfusion can be accomplished in two ways. In the most common approach, blood is collected and stored during the weeks before delivery. This presents some logistic problems for the pregnant patient since 3 weeks is the longest time that the blood can be stored. Most patients are unable to maintain a hematocrit above 33 percent with a donation frequency of less than 2 to 3 weeks. Although predelivery autologous blood donation is generally safe for both mother and fetus, the low incidence of blood transfusion in patients at the time of childbirth and the safety of allogeneic transfusion has limited enthusiasm on the part of health care professionals. Recent studies have questioned the cost effectiveness of autologous transfusion in general.[4] Since the incidence of transfusion in pregnant patients was significantly lower that the incidence of transfusion in the operative patients in that study, predelivery autologous blood donation in pregnant patients is probably not cost effective based on those results.

A second type of autologous donation, intraoperative blood salvage, can occur at the time of excessive blood loss. Intraoperative autotransfusion has been reported in obstetric patients at the time of ruptured ectopic pregnancy and recently after delayed cesarean hysterectomy. This technique has some limitations in the obstetric setting. Heavy bacterial contamination is a contraindication, and the use during cesarean delivery should also be avoided because of the possibility of amniotic fluid, fetal debris, and bacterial contamination. However, in the case of cesarean hysterectomy with massive bleeding or delayed re-operation because of continued bleeding this technique can be considered.[5]

The chance of acquiring the human immune deficiency virus (HIV) from a unit of donated and screened blood is on the order of 1 in 250,000. Furthermore, when blood transfusion is clinically indicated, there is usually the need for more blood than the patient is able to donate unless the blood is frozen which dramatically increases the cost of the procedure. Antepartum patients inquiring about this practice should be carefully counseled that the chance of needing a blood transfusion is about 1/80 overall. It exceeds 1 percent when emergency cesarean delivery becomes necessary or if placenta previa exists.[6,7] These data, coupled with the low risk of acquiring the HIV virus from a donated unit of blood, makes the a priori risk of needing a blood transfusion and subsequently acquiring HIV greater than 1 in 20 million.

Antepartum Hemorrhage

Abruptio Placenta

The premature separation of the normally implanted placenta from its attachment to the uterus is called *abruptio placenta* or *placental abruption*. This event occurs with a frequency of approximately 1 in 120 births but accounts for nearly 15 percent of perinatal mortality. Diagnosis of placental abruption is certain when inspection of the placenta shows an adherent retroplacental clot with depression or disruption of the underlying placental tissue; however, this frequently is not found if the abruption is of recent onset. Clinical findings indicating placental abruption include the triad of external or occult uterine bleeding, uterine hypertonus and/or hyperactivity, and fetal distress and/or fetal death. Placental abruption can be broadly classified into three grades that correlate with clinical and laboratory findings.

Grade 1: Slight vaginal bleeding and some uterine irritability are usually present. Maternal blood pressure is unaffected, and the maternal fibrinogen level is normal. The fetal heart rate pattern is normal.

Grade 2: External uterine bleeding is mild to moderate. The uterus is irritable, and tetanic contractions may be present. Maternal blood pressure is maintained, but the pulse rate may be elevated and postural blood volume deficits may be present. The fibrinogen level is usually reduced to 150 to 250 mg percent. The fetal heart rate often shows signs of fetal distress.

Grade 3: Bleeding is moderate to severe but may be concealed. The uterus is tetanic and painful. Maternal hypotension is frequently present and fetal death has occurred. Fibrinogen levels are often reduced to less than 150 mg percent; other coagulation abnormalities (thrombocytopenia, factor depletion) are present.

Incidence

The reported incidence of placental abruption varies from 1 in 86 to 1 in 206 births.[8–10] This variability reflects differing criteria for diagnosis as well as the increased recognition in recent years of milder forms of the disorder. Grade 1 placental abruption is found in about 40 percent, grade 2 in about 45 percent, and grade 3 in 15 percent of clinically recognized cases of placental abruption.[8,11] Eighty percent of all cases will occur before the onset of labor.[9]

Etiology

The primary etiology of placental abruption is unknown, but several reports have identified statistically significant correlations with common obstetric complications. Studies have suggested an increased incidence of abruption in patients with advanced parity or age, maternal smoking, poor nutrition, cocaine use, and chorioamnionitis.[12–15] However, some of these data may have been subject to selection bias, as only populations of low socioeconomic status were evaluated. The U.S. Perinatal Collaborative project performed during the years 1959 to 1966 and a recent population-based study in Washington state failed to show a relationship between placental abruption and either maternal age or parity.[10,16]

Maternal hypertension (>140/90 mmHg) seems to be the most consistently identified factor predisposing to placental abruption.[17] This relationship is true for all grades of placental abruption but is most strongly associated with grade 3 abruption, in which 40 to 50 percent of cases are found to have hypertensive disease of pregnancy.[16,17] Intrapartum hypertension significantly increases the risk of abruption, but one study failed to show a relationship between the antenatal detection of hypertension and placental abruption.

Blunt external maternal trauma is an increasingly

important cause of placental abruption. Two conditions account for the majority of blunt abdominal trauma leading to placental abruption: motor vehicle collision and maternal battering. Historically 1 to 2 percent of grade 3 abruptions have been attributed to maternal trauma.[17,18] However, recent epidemiologic studies show an alarmingly high incidence of maternal battering in some populations.[19] These data make it incumbent on the obstetrician to consider placental abruption when a history of trauma is elicited and vice versa. Unfortunately, the physical evidence of trauma may be minimal and still be associated with placental abruption that can progress from grade 1 to 3 within 24 hours. Figure 17-2 illustrates fetal heart rate tracings 8 hours apart in a patient who was involved in an automobile accident.

Rapid decompression of the overdistended uterus is an uncommon cause of placental abruption. The two clinical situations in which this may occur are patients with multiple gestations and those with polyhydramnios. The true incidence of placental abruption in twins and other multiple gestations is difficult to ascertain. Abruption usually occurs after the delivery of the first fetus. Delivery of the second twin usually follows soon after, before a retroplacental clot has time to form. Rapid decompression of the uterus should be avoided in a patient with polyhydramnios. Amniotic fluid should be slowly released by amniocentesis before the induction of labor or once spontaneous labor has been established.

In the past, folic acid deficiency, a short umbilical cord, and the supine hypotensive syndrome had been suggested as etiologies for placental abruption. Further evidence has shown, however, that these factors are unlikely causes of placenta abruption.

The pathologic changes in the placental bed in patients with placental abruption show a high incidence of vascular abnormalities. Failure of transformation of uteroplacental arteries is the most common finding (60 percent). Anomalies in the vessels deep in the myometrium, including vessel occlusion with surrounding myometrial hemorrhage, were observed in 33 percent.[20] At the placental level hemorrhage into the decidua basalis causes it to split, leaving a layer adherent to the myometrium. This decidual hematoma may then progress to cause further separation and compression of the adjacent placenta.

There is a significant recurrence rate for placental abruption. This figure has been reported to vary from 5 to 17 percent.[9,13,17] If a patient has suffered an abruption in two pregnancies, the chance for recurrence is 25 percent. Unfortunately, no published data are available to document a prospective plan of management that will reduce this unacceptably high risk. The following case illustrates one plan for managing such a patient.

Illustrative Case

A 32-year-old g5p4 presented at 6 weeks' gestation with the following history: She had suffered grade 3 placental abruption in her third pregnancy at 35 weeks' gestation and had undergone cesarean delivery for severe maternal coagulopathy with a dead fetus. She required 8 units of blood and blood products because of a significant intraoperative hemorrhage and contracted hepatitis C. In her next pregnancy she had an uncomplicated antenatal course and was last seen for a clinic visit at 33 weeks. She was a one pack a day smoker, but all efforts to eliminate smoking from her life had been unsuccessful. At 35 weeks' gestation she presented with syncope followed by severe abdominal pain with a dead fetus. This was the same clinical presentation and gestation as the previous pregnancy. She underwent induction of labor and had a successful vaginal delivery but required 12 units of blood and blood products. In the fifth pregnancy the following management plan was developed: enrollment in a smoking cessation program: clinic visits every 2 weeks: antenatal testing beginning at 28 weeks; amniocentesis at 34 weeks' gestation and delivery by repeat cesarean section with tubal ligation if pulmonary maturity was documented, and, if pulmonary maturity was not present, maternal administration of glucocorticoids with continuous fetal monitoring for 48 hours, followed by caesarean delivery. The patient was unable to comply with the smoking cessation program but maintained her clinic visits. At 34 weeks amniocentesis demonstrated pulmonary maturity, and cesarean section and tubal ligation were accomplished without complication. A 2,500 male had an uncomplicated neonatal course. While this case resulted in a favorable outcome for both mother and fetus, it has been shown that grade 3 placental abruption and fetal death can follow normal antepartum testing by as few as 4 hours.[21]

Diagnosis and Management

Vaginal bleeding in the third trimester of pregnancy is the hallmark of placental abruption and should always prompt an investigation to determine its etiology. After appropriate physical and laboratory examination of the mother and fetus, ultrasound evaluation of the uterus, placenta, and fetus has become the standard of care (Fig. 17-3). The other common and potentially life-threatening cause of third-trimester bleeding, placenta previa, should be recognized in nearly all cases in which it is present. If ultrasound examination fails to show a placenta previa and if other local causes of vaginal bleeding (including cervical or vaginal trauma, labor,

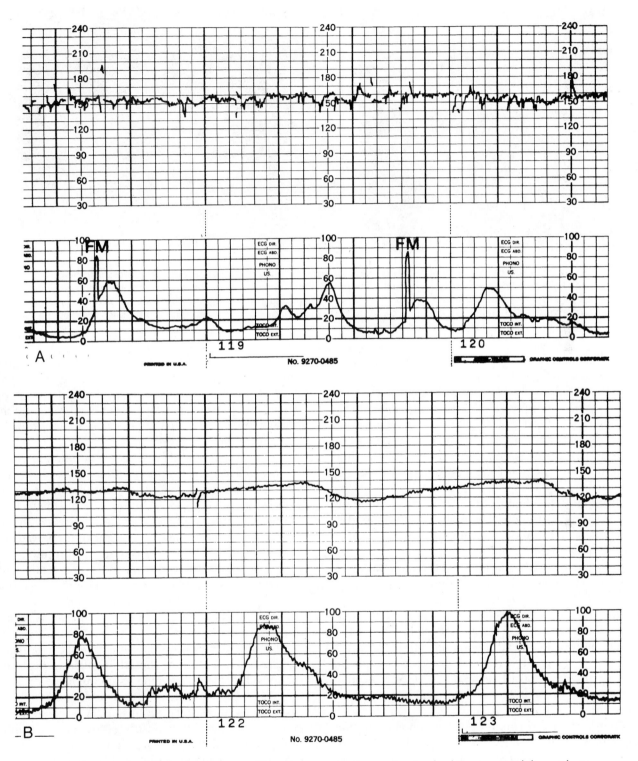

Fig. 17-2 (A) A fetal heart rate tracing at 37 weeks' gestation in a patient involved in an automobile accident in which the maternal abdomen struck the steering wheel. Fetal movements were present, and no periodic changes were observed. Uterine contractions were occurring every 2 to 3 minutes. (B) Eight hours later, repetitive late decelerations are now present. An asphyxiated fetus was delivered, and evidence of grade 3 placental abruption was found at the time of delivery.

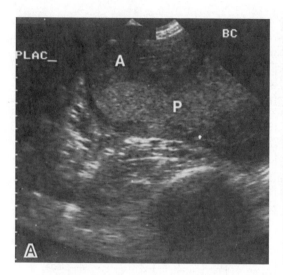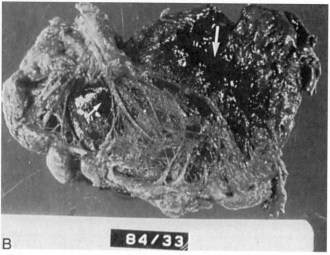

Fig. 17-3 (A) Ultrasound study at 18 weeks' gestation demonstrating a hypoechoic area (A) representing retroplacental bleeding and an enlarged placenta (P). This patient had chronic hypertension. She presented with intermittent dark red vaginal bleeding and abdominal pain, a picture consistent with a chronic abruption. (B) At delivery, the placenta revealed a large clot (small arrow) and fresh hemorrhage (large arrow). The fibrous bands bridging the clot are also consistent with chronic abruption.

or malignancy) have been ruled out, placental abruption becomes a more likely diagnosis.

In the initial studies evaluating ultrasound, less than 2 percent of cases were definitively identifiable with ultrasound. Recent advances in ultrasound imaging and interpretation have improved this rate so that more than 50 percent of patients with confirmed placental abruption will demonstrate ultrasound evidence of hemorrhage.

Ultrasound can identify three predominant locations for placental abruption. These are subchorionic (between the placenta and the membranes), retroplacental (between the placenta and the myometrium), and preplacental (between the placenta and the amniotic fluid). Hematomas identified by ultrasound during the early phases of vaginal bleeding and pain are most likely to be hyperechoic or isoechoic compared with the placenta. As the hematoma resolves, it will become hypoechoic within a week and sonolucent within 2 weeks.[22] Because of the changing character of the hematoma, misinterpretation of a hematoma as uterine myoma, succenturiate placental lobe, chorioangioma, or molar pregnancy has been reported.

The location and extent of the placental abruption identified on ultrasound has definite clinical significance. Retroplacental hematomas carry a worse prognosis for fetal survival than subchorionic hemorrhages. The size of the hemorrhage is also predictive of fetal survival. Large retroplacental hemorrhages (>60 ml/ >50 percent) are associated with a 50 percent or greater fetal mortality, whereas similar-sized subchorionic hemorrhages are associated with a 10 percent mortality.[23]

Gestational age at the time of presentation is an important prognostic factor. Patients present at less than 20 weeks: 82 percent can be expected to have a term delivery despite evidence of placental separation. If the presentation occurs after 20 weeks gestation, only 27 percent will deliver at term.

Nearly 80 percent of patients who eventually prove to have a placental abruption will present with vaginal bleeding. The remaining 20 percent of patients fail to exhibit external signs of bleeding. These patients have a concealed abruption and are commonly given the diagnosis of premature labor. Such cases must be watched very carefully. On some occasions, the abruption may progress despite successful tocolysis, and fetal death may result. Other classic signs of placental abruption include increased uterine tenderness and tone. These findings are uncommon (17 percent) unless the abruption is grade 2 or 3.[9]

Once the diagnosis of placental abruption has been entertained, precautions should be taken to deal with the possible life-threatening consequences for both mother and fetus. At least 4 units of blood should be available for maternal transfusions. A large-bore (16-guage) intravenous line must be secured and the infusion of a crystalloid solution begun. Blood should be drawn for hemoglobin and hematocrit determinations and coagulation studies (fibrinogen, platelet count, fibrin degradation products, PT, PTT). A red-topped tube should also be obtained and used to perform a clot test. This test, a "poor man's" fibrinogen assay, will often give critical information before the laboratory can document a coagulation defect. If a clot does not form within 6 minutes or forms and lyses within 30 minutes, a coagulation defect is probably present and the fibrinogen level is less than 150 mg percent. Because fetal distress will develop in as many as 60 percent of patients who present with a live fetus, continuous fetal monitoring should be used to record fetal heart rate and document uterine activity.

In the patient with a term fetus in whom the diagnosis of grade 1 abruption is made, close observation for signs of fetal or maternal compromise is essential. If the fetus is known to be mature, controlled delivery should be accomplished by induction of labor while the mother and fetus are in stable condition.

The occurrence of a grade 1 placental abruption with a preterm fetus presents greater challenge. Often, a vicious circle is established in which a small placental abruption stimulates uterine irritability, further separating the placenta until fetal compromise becomes evident. In carefully selected cases, it may be possible to inhibit uterine contractions as long as there are no signs of acute fetal distress and no ultrasonographic evidence of intrauterine growth retardation.

Magnesium sulfate has less adverse cardiovascular side effects than β-sympathomimetic agents and has been used in this circumstance. In three separate reports totalling 92 patients, no adverse maternal complications were reported and significant prolongation of gestation (greater than 1 week) was accomplished in over 50 percent of patients.[24–26] No adverse fetal complications were reported, with mortality being attributable only to extreme prematurity. A comparison of other tocolytic agents or a comparison with observation alone has never been evaluated by a clinical trial. Any attempt to arrest preterm labor in known or suspected abruption should be weighed against the likelihood for survival, morbidity if the infant were delivered, and the severity of the abruption.

In many cases of placental abruption, delivery will be the treatment of choice. During labor, careful attention must be paid to several maternal and fetal parameters. Because 60 percent of fetuses may exhibit signs of intrapartum fetal distress, continuous fetal heart rate monitoring is essential. In a similar manner, continuous monitoring of maternal volume status is important. An indwelling Foley catheter will permit accurate assessment of maternal urine output. Serial maternal hematocrit determinations should be made regularly at intervals of 2 to 3 hours. The goal of therapy should be to maintain a maternal urine output of 1 ml/min and a hematocrit of at least 30 percent. An updated flow sheet at the bedside permits the clinician to follow maternal vital signs, urine output, laboratory values, and critical clotting parameters.

Placental abruption frequently stimulates the clotting cascade, resulting in DIC. Intravascular fibrinogen is converted to fibrin by activation of the extrinsic clotting cascade. In the usual clinical setting, platelets and clotting Factors V and VIII are also depleted. Serial measurements of plasma fibrinogen provide valuable information regarding the coagulation status of the patient and will help estimate the volume of blood loss that has occurred.

The normal maternal fibrinogen concentration in the third trimester is 450 mg percent. In grade I abruptions, there is often no alteration in this value and no evidence of DIC. However, when the fibrinogen value drops below 300 mg percent, significant coagulation abnormalities are usually present. Most women with significant falls in fibrinogen will require blood transfusion to maintain a normal circulating volume. If the presenting fibrinogen level is less than 150 mg percent, most patients will have already lost 2,000 ml of blood. The signs and symptoms of such blood loss may not be obvious because, as noted earlier, the normal hypervolemia of pregnancy protects the mother from a volume loss that a nonpregnant individual could not tolerate. In the case of grade 3 placental abruption, the mean blood loss is 2,500 ml or more.[27] In patients with grade 2 and grade 3 abruption, rapid crystalloid infusion of at least 1,000 ml pending the availability of whole blood should be done. Two to 3 ml of crystalloid should be given for each 1 ml of blood lost to maintain euvolemia.

If urine output fails to reach 30 ml/hr despite adequate volume replacement, then consideration should be given to inserting a central venous pressure (CVP) catheter to determine the adequacy of intravascular volume. This catheter is best inserted through a site in the arm rather than the neck or subclavian area because of the severe coagulopathy that is often present. The absolute level of CVP is less important than the response of the CVP to volume infusion, as long as the CVP is less than 7 cm H_2O in response to the preceding 250-ml aliquot. If this response has been achieved but the urine output is still inadequate, consideration should be given to replacing the CVP catheter with a pulmonary artery catheter. This circumstance is uncommon unless there is intrinsic heart disease or severe preeclampsia or the patient has already suffered critical renal ischemia and is in acute renal failure.

Considerable controversy remains regarding the appropriate method of delivery in patients with placental abruption. Concern exists for the fetal outcome in such cases. A number of patients present with a live fetus, only to have that fetus die undelivered while awaiting vaginal delivery.[8,11] Retrospective reviews show a trend for increased fetal survival in patients who have undergone cesarean delivery once the maternal condition has been stabilized. However, none of these reports surveyed a period in which intrapartum fetal monitoring was routine. Currently the use of continuous electronic fetal monitoring in this situation is associated with excellent fetal survival and cesarean delivery can be reserved for cases with fetal distress or other traditional obstetric indications.[9]

The management of mothers with severe coagulopathy and/or fetal demise is also controversial. Restoration of a normal blood volume and coagulation status is the sine qua non of treatment in these patients. Once adequate volume status has been achieved and appropriate coagulation factors administered, attention can be given to effecting delivery. Some clinicians believe that if placental abruption has progressed to fetal death and severe coagulopathy, cesarean delivery will result in the quickest resolution of maternal problems. However, this is usually an unwise choice because operating on such a patient in the presence of a coagulopathy can result in prolonged operative times secondary to surgically uncontrollable bleeding. Fibrinogen levels lower than 125 mg percent lead to generalized bleeding from all surgical incisions. Even in the face of a severe coagulopathy, induction to delivery times exceeding 18 hours may result in equal or better maternal outcome as long as maternal volume status and coagulation status can be maintained.[10]

Contrary to popular belief, the uterus does not need to be evacuated before coagulation status can be restored. Administering blood and blood products and delaying attempts at vaginal delivery for a few hours until hematologic status has improved is associated with good maternal outcome. There are now two reported cases of severe placental abruption with maternal coagulopathy in the second trimester in which blood and blood product administration completely reversed the syndrome and live fetuses were subsequently delivered.[28,29]

When cesarean delivery is necessary, extravasation of blood into the uterine muscle to produce red to purple discoloration of the serosal surface will be found in 8 percent of patients. This finding, known as a Couvelaire uterus, has been feared to result in a high incidence of uterine hemorrhage secondary to atony. However, atony is the exception rather than the rule, and most patients with a Couvelaire uterus demonstrate an appropriate response to the infusion of oxytocin. Hysterectomy should be reserved for cases of atony and hemorrhage unresponsive to conventional uterotonics.

Neonatal Outcome

High perinatal mortality has been uniformly associated with placental abruption with some reports as high as 25 to 30 percent combined fetal and neonatal deaths.[30,31] Recent studies have shown a greater risk for adverse long-term neurobehavioral outcome in infants delivered after placental abruption.[32] In a case-control study of low-birth-weight infants, 40 infants born after placental abruption were compared with 80 infants matched for gestational age at delivery. There was a significant association between abruption and abnormal neonatal outcome (death or cerebral palsy). The chance of a completely normal neonatal outcome tended to decrease in relationship to the severity of the abruption, but small numbers of patients in each group limited the statistical significance of this finding. The most significant obstetric finding in this group was the high incidence of abnormal fetal heart rate (45 percent) and emergency cesarean delivery (53 percent) compared with the control group and (10 and 10 percent, respectively).

Placenta Previa

Placenta previa is defined as the implantation of the placenta over the cervical os. There are three recognized variations of placenta previa: total, partial, and marginal (Fig. 17-4). In total placenta previa, the cervical os is completely covered by the placenta. This type presents the most serious maternal risk, as it is associated with greater blood loss than either marginal or partial placenta previa. The frequency of total placenta previa has been reported to be as low as 20 percent[33] and as high as 43 percent.[34] Partial placenta previa is defined as the partial occlusion of the cervical os by the placenta and occurs in 31 percent of diagnosed cases. A marginal placenta previa is characterized by the encroachment of the placenta to the margin of the cervical os. It does not cover the os. The differentiation of the latter two degrees of placenta previa is dependent on the dilatation of the cervix and the method of diagnosis (ultrasound or direct examination).

A leading cause of third trimester hemorrhage, placenta previa, presents classically as painless bleeding. Bleeding is thought to occur in association with the development of the lower uterine segment in the third trimester. Placental attachment is disrupted as this area gradually thins in preparation for the onset of labor. When this occurs, bleeding occurs at the implantation site, as the uterus is unable to contract adequately and stop the flow of blood from the open vessels.

The incidence of placenta previa is stated to be 1 in 200 live births.[35,34] Significant epidemiologic risk factors are maternal age above 35 years (rate ratio 4.7) and black or other minority races (rate ratio 1.3). Whether the increased risk for older mothers is related to parity or to an independent risk factor is still uncertain. The most important obstetric risk factor in the development of placenta previa is previous cesarean delivery. The risk for placenta previa occurring in the pregnancy following a cesarean delivery has been reported to be between 1 and 4 percent.[33,36–39] There is a linear increase in placenta previa risk with the num-

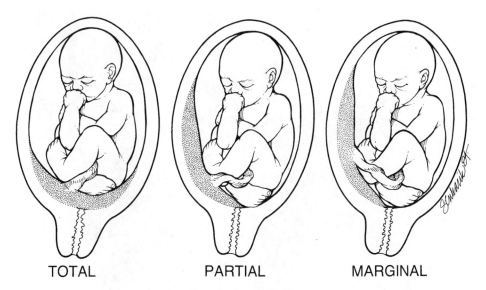

TOTAL   PARTIAL   MARGINAL

Fig. 17-4 Three variations of placenta previa.

ber of prior cesarean deliveries. In patients with four or more cesarean deliveries, the risk of placenta previa approaches 10 percent.[36]

Placenta previa should be suspected in all patients presenting with bleeding after 24 weeks' gestation. Seventy percent of patients who are eventually shown to have placenta previa will present with painless vaginal bleeding. Twenty percent will have evidence of uterine activity accompanying vaginal bleeding; the remaining patients will have the diagnosis made incidentally at the time of cesarean delivery or at ultrasound examination performed for another indication.

Patients with third trimester bleeding should be treated in a manner similar to that outlined in the section on abruptio placenta (e.g., maternal stabilization, blood studies, fetal monitoring). Once fetal and maternal status have been stabilized, ultrasound evaluation should be performed to establish the diagnosis (Fig. 17-5). Gestational age at the time of the ultrasound examination greatly influences the incidence of placenta previa. At 17 weeks' gestation, evidence of placental tissue covering the cervical os will be found in 5 to 15 percent of all patients.[34] However, more than 90 percent of these will resolve by term.[40] This phenomenon has been termed *placental migration*. It is unlikely that the placenta actually separates and reattaches throughout the second and third trimesters. The changes in architecture secondary to differential growth of the lower uterine segment during the second and third trimesters probably account for this observation. Location of the placenta with reference to the cervix will influence the likelihood of resolution of placenta previa with advancing gestation. Total placenta previa diagnosed in the second trimester will persist into the third trimester in 26 percent of cases, while marginal or partial placenta previa will persist in only 2.5 percent of cases.[41]

Once the diagnosis of placenta previa is made, management decisions depend on the gestational age, amount of bleeding, fetal condition, and presentation. In the patient who is unequivocally at 37 weeks gestation' with evidence of uterine activity or with persistent bleeding, delivery is the treatment of choice. In previous years a double setup examination was the initial step in this process. With the advent of rapid and reliable ultrasound availability and interpretation, including transvaginal sonography, this technique is necessary much less often. In the patient in whom there is unequivocal evidence of placenta previa cesarean delivery is the method of choice.

In some patients vaginal delivery may still be considered. Patients with marginal or partial placenta previa who present in labor with minimal bleeding are ideal candidates. It can also be considered for patients with previable gestations or intrauterine fetal demise. Appropriately conducted labor in these selected instances can be safe for both mother and fetus.[42]

When double setup examination is elected, it should be done in an operating room with full preparation made to perform emergency cesarean delivery should excessive vaginal bleeding follow the examination. In performing a double setup examination, the patient should be prepped and draped for cesarean delivery. The anesthesiologist should be present and the operating room team ready. The patient should first undergo a careful speculum examination, which may reveal placental tissue in the cervical os. If the diagnosis of placenta previa cannot be made with a speculum examination, the obstetrician should next examine the vaginal fornices. Fullness in the fornices suggests the presence

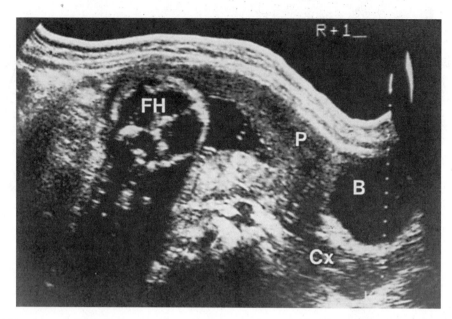

Fig. 17-5 This ultrasound examination at 34 weeks gestation in a patient with painless vaginal bleeding revealed a placenta previa (P) covering the cervical os (Cx). The maternal bladder (B) and fetal head (FH) are also shown.

of the placenta extending down toward the cervix. Finally, examining fingers should be carefully introduced into the cervical os to detect the placenta.

For the patient who is remote from term (24 to 36 weeks' gestation), expectant management is the treatment of choice. The essence of this approach is maintenance of the fetus in a healthy intrauterine environment without jeopardizing maternal condition. Maternal blood loss should be replaced in order to maintain the maternal hematocrit between 30 and 35 percent. This RBC volume will provide a margin of safety in the event of a large hemorrhage. Even an initial blood loss in excess of 500 ml can be expectantly managed with adequate volume replacement.

Although obstetricians are most concerned about maternal hemorrhage, they must remember that fetal blood can also be lost during the process of placental separation. Rh-immune globulin should be given to all at-risk patients with third trimester bleeding who are Rh negative and unsensitized. A Kleihauer-Betke preparation of maternal blood should also be performed in all Rh-negative women. This test will detect the occasional patient with a fetomaternal hemorrhage of greater than 30 ml. Thirty-five percent of infants whose mothers require antepartum transfusion will themselves be anemic and require transfusion when delivered.[34]

Twenty percent of patients with placenta previa will show evidence of uterine contractions. Because a vaginal examination to document cervical dilatation is absolutely contraindicated, it is difficult to make a firm diagnosis of preterm labor. Although no controlled studies are available to show the efficacy of tocolytic therapy in such cases, some studies document that it can be safely attempted.[34,43] The choice of agents in this situation is controversial. If β-mimetics are used in the presence of maternal hypovolemia, serious maternal hypotension can result (Fig. 17-6). In addition, the use of β-mimetics will produce maternal tachycardia, making the evaluation of maternal volume status more difficult. Nonetheless some authors have reported the use of these agents for tocolysis in patients with placenta previa without excessive complications.[44–46]

Because of the reduced risk of cardiovascular complications, magnesium sulfate has become the agent of choice for the treatment of patients in preterm labor with placenta previa at many institutions. Infusion of a 6-g loading dose followed by 3 g/hr or more are often necessary to control uterine irritability because of the increased maternal glomerular filtration rate. Once the patient has been stabilized on magnesium sulfate, the use of oral β-mimetics therapy is an appropriate choice provided that euvolemia has been achieved. Patients may occasionally require more than 1 week of continuous intravenous tocolytic therapy. Such treatment is considered justified since, before 33 weeks' gestation, each day that the fetus remains in utero reduces its stay in the neonatal intensive care nursery by 2 days.[47] The use of antenatal corticosteroids to accelerate fetal pulmonary maturity is effective in reducing the incidence of neonatal respiratory distress syndrome, intracranial hemorrhage, and neonatal death.[48,49] Given a high incidence of respiratory distress syndrome in the infants of mothers requiring delivery after failed expectant

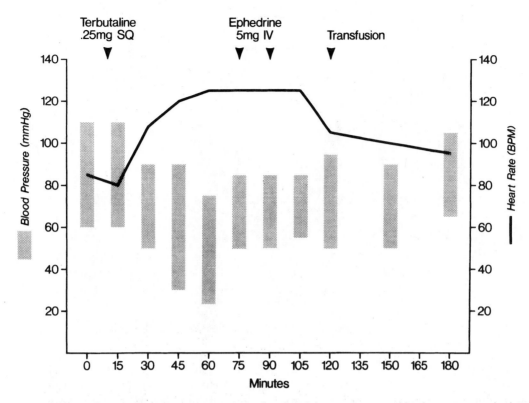

Fig. 17-6 Blood pressure and heart rate response to terbutaline administration in a bleeding patient with placenta previa. Hypotension, which developed acutely, is somewhat resistant to ephedrine and crystalloid administration.

management (24 to 41 percent),[34,50] antenatal steroids should be given in patients presenting between 25 to 33 weeks. However, there are no data on safety or efficacy of repeated weekly doses of steroids administered during a prolonged maternal hospital course. Such therapy should be considered on a case by case basis.

If the mother responds to conservative management, she should be treated with bedrest, preferably in the hospital setting. Blood should always be available for maternal transfusion in the event of sudden hemorrhage. The length of maternal hospitalization in this instance is presently undergoing reevaluation. An initial study suggested that continued hospitalization until delivery was more cost effective than rest at home when total expenses for both mother and baby are calculated.[50] An additional reason for continued hospitalization was the observation that one-half of all patients requiring early delivery because of failed expectant management do so because of excessive bleeding with or without uterine contractions. Two recent studies have challenged this management plan.[51,52] In those retrospective studies no significant advantage in either cost or morbidity was found with conservative hospital management until delivery. Unfortunately no prospective data exist to help in this situation. When this group of patients was reviewed at the University of Washington, we found that a variety of social, demographic, and geographic factors heavily influenced the decisions regarding continued hospitalization. We concluded that so few patients could be safely considered for home management that continued hospitalization with few exceptions was the safest and most cost-effective management plan for our patient population.

Approximately 25 to 30 percent of patients can be expected to complete 36 weeks' gestation without labor or repetitive bleeding forcing earlier delivery. In these patients, amniocentesis should be performed and, if the analysis of amniotic fluid documents pulmonary maturity, cesarean delivery planned.

When encountering a patient with placenta previa, the possibility of a placenta accreta or one of its variations, placenta percreta or placenta increta, should be considered (Fig. 17-7).[53] In this condition, the placenta forms an abnormally firm attachment to the uterine wall. There is absence of the decidua basalis and incomplete development of the fibrinoid layer. The placenta can be attached directly to the myometrium (accreta), invade the myometrium (increta), or penetrate the myometrium (percreta). Antenatal diagnosis with ultrasound has been demonstrated by some authors.[54,55] However, in the largest reported series a false-positive diagnosis was reported in 20 percent of patients. Ultrasound findings most predictive of placenta accreta are

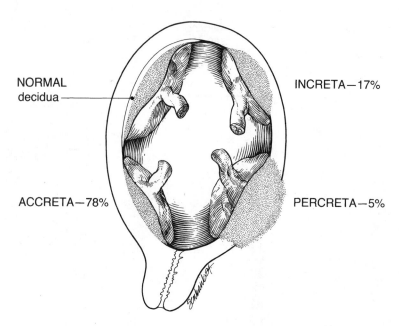

NORMAL
decidua

INCRETA—17%

ACCRETA—78%

PERCRETA—5%

Fig. 17-7 Uteroplacental relationships found in abnormal placentation.

thinning and distortion of the uterine serosa-bladder interface.

Prior cesarean delivery and other uterine surgery are the factors most often associated with placenta accreta. In patients without prior uterine surgery who have placenta previa, the incidence of placenta accreta will be 4 percent. In patients with previous cesarean delivery who have placenta previa, the incidence of placenta accreta is approximately 10 to 35 percent.[36,39] In patients with multiple cesarean deliveries and placenta previa the risk of accreta is 60 to 65 percent. At least two thirds of the patients with placenta previa/placenta accreta will require cesarean hysterectomy.[34,56,57] However, in cases where uterine preservation is highly desired and no bladder invasion has occurred, bleeding after placental removal has been successfully controlled with a variety of surgical techniques. Packing of the lower uterine segment with subsequent removal of the pack through the vagina within 24 hours[57] has been successful. Interrupted circular suture of the lower uterine segment on the serosal surface of the uterus has also been reported to be successful.[58] Predelivery placement of catheters for angiographic embolization of pelvic vessels is another technique recently described.[59,60]

Complete placenta accreta suspected or confirmed before attempted placental removal may permit other treatment options. Bleeding may be minimal unless the placenta has partially separated. If no cleavage plane is identified and a placenta accreta is suspected, one should first make preparations for the possibility of major postpartum blood loss. At least 4 units of blood should be on hand and an anesthesiologist present in the delivery room. If vaginal delivery has occurred, the patient should be in a suite in which a laparotomy can be performed, and surgical instruments for hysterectomy should be sterilized and ready. Whenever possible, the obstetrician should discuss the likely diagnosis with the patient and review possible treatment options.

Five therapeutic plans may be considered. If uterine preservation is not important, or if maternal blood loss is excessive, hysterectomy offers the best chance for survival and will minimize morbidity.[61] If uterine preservation is important, four treatment options are available: (1) placental removal and oversewing the uterine defects: After removing as much of the placenta as possible, the bleeding defects are oversewed and the patient treated with oxytocics and antibiotics (this option is probably most useful when there is significant bleeding from a partially separated placenta with only a focal accreta); (2) localized resection and uterine repair; (3) curettage of the uterine cavity; and leaving the placenta in situ. For the patient who wishes to maximize her chances for uterine preservation and who is not actively bleeding, the placenta may be left in situ. The umbilical cord should be ligated and cut as close to its base as possible. The patient should then be treated with antibiotics. This approach has been successful when bleeding has not necessitated more aggressive surgical procedures.[62] Some authors have advocated treatment with methotrexate in this instance, but there is presently no consensus on whether this therapy is any more effective than observation.

In rare cases placenta accreta invades the maternal bladder. In this instance, it is probably best to treat in a manner similar to abdominal pregnancy and avoid placental removal. However, this may not obviate the need for eventual hysterectomy and cystectomy.[63,64]

Third Trimester Fetal Bleeding

A rare but important cause of third trimester bleeding is that associated with rupture of a fetal vessel. This event is often the result of a velamentous insertion of the umbilical cord and occurs in 0.1 to 1.8 percent of pregnancies. In this instance, the cord inserts at a distance from the placenta, and its vessels must traverse between the chorion and amnion without the protection of Wharton's jelly. When the fetal vessel ruptures, often acute vaginal bleeding is associated with an abrupt change in the fetal heart rate. The fetal heart rate pattern often shows an initial fetal tachycardia fol-

lowed by bradycardia with intermittent accelerations. Short-term variability is frequently maintained.

One must have a high index of suspicion to make the correct diagnosis. In most instances, one must make the diagnosis rapidly and institute definitive therapy and delivery to optimize fetal outcome. The fetal mortality in this condition has been reported to be greater than 50 percent.[65,66] Figure 17-8 illustrates the fetal heart rate tracing of a successfully treated case of spontaneous rupture of a velamentous insertion of the fetal vessel.

On occasion, an examination of the blood passed vaginally, with the Apt test, will reveal its fetal origin. The Apt test is performed by first mixing one part of bloody vaginal fluid with 5 to 10 parts tap water. This

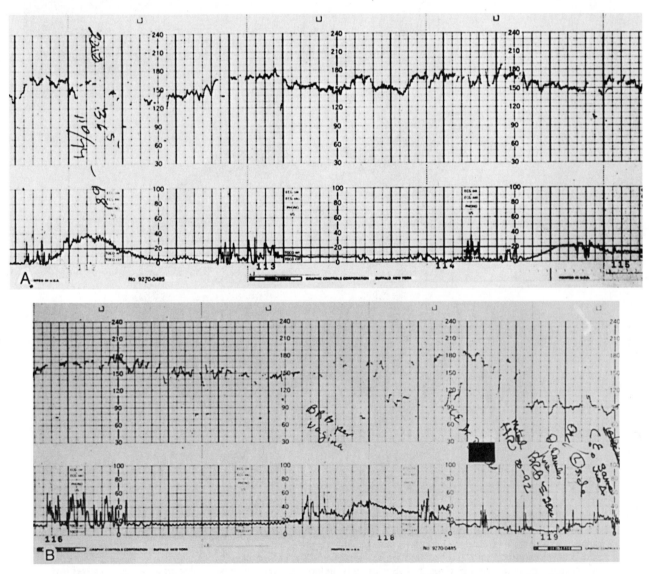

Fig. 17-8 Fetal heart rate tracing after rupture of a velamentous insertion of the cord. (A) Normal fetal heart rate tracing in early labor at term showing accelerations but no other changes. (B) Just before panel 118, bright red vaginal bleeding is noted. Shortly thereafter, the fetal heart rate is noted to be 80 to 90 bpm. (*Figure continues.*)

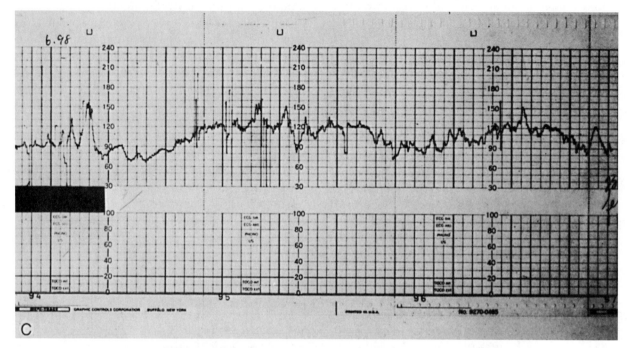

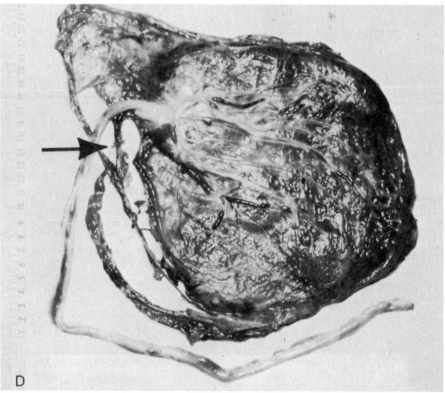

Fig. 17-8 (*Continued*) (C) In the delivery room, the fetal heart rate tracing shows the characteristic bradycardia–tachycardia heart rate response as the fetus attempts to compensate for acute blood loss. An emergency cesarean delivery was performed, and the infant was anemic. After rapid volume infusion and resuscitation, the infant survived and is developing normally. (D) Examination of the placenta showed a velamentous insertion of the umbilical cord and a lacerated fetal vessel as a result of spontaneous rupture of the membranes. In this case, the unprotected fetal vessels passed over the cervical os, a vasa previa.

mixture is then centrifuged for 2 minutes. The supernatant must be pink to proceed with the test. One then takes 5 parts of the supernatant and mixes it with 1 part of 1 percent (0.25 N) sodium hydroxide. This mixture is again centrifuged for 2 minutes. A pink color indicates the presence of fetal blood, and a yellow-brown color indicates maternal blood. Adult oxyhemoglobin is less resistant to alkali than fetal oxyhemoglobin. During the reaction with sodium hydroxide, adult oxyhemoglobin is converted to alkaline globin hematin.[56]

Postpartum Hemorrhage

Acute blood loss is the most common cause of hypotension in obstetrics. Hemorrhage usually occurs immediately preceding or after delivery of the placenta. Excessive blood loss most commonly results when the uterus fails to contract after the delivery of its contents. Effective hemostasis after separation of the placenta is dependent on contraction of the myometrium to compress severed vessels. Failure of the uterus to contract can usually be attributed to myometrial dysfunction and retained placental fragments. Factors predisposing to myometrial dysfunction include overdistension of the uterus as in multiple pregnancy, fetal macrosomia, hydramnios, oxytocin-stimulated labor, uterine relaxants (magnesium, β-mimetics), and amnionitis. At term, approximately 600 ml/min of blood flows through the placental site. However, blood loss from severe uterine atony can easily exceed this rate because blood is lost from the entire intrauterine surface when the uterus fails to contract.

Prevention

The need to deal with excessive blood loss after vaginal birth or cesarean delivery can be limited by recognizing high-risk factors for postpartum hemorrhage (Table 17-4) and by applying proven methods to limit blood loss after delivery. Some techniques with demonstrated effectiveness have still not found their way into general use by many obstetric practitioners, including active management of the third stage of labor and spontaneous delivery of the placenta at time of cesarean delivery. Dilute solutions of oxytocin in addition to gentle cord traction reduces cesarean delivery associated blood loss by 31 percent compared with manual removal of the placenta.[67] Similarly, umbilical cord clamping within 30 seconds of delivery and gentle cord traction followed by administration of intramuscular or dilute solutions of intravenous oxytocin before delivery of the placenta reduce postpartum blood loss and postpartum transfusion requirements.[68] Administration of oxytocin before delivery of the placenta is associated with a reduction in the length of the third stage of labor (mean 5 minutes) and a low incidence of manual removal of the placenta (2 percent) compared with physiologic management of the third stage of labor (15 minutes and 2.5 percent, respectively).[68] When the placenta is retained for 30 minutes or longer randomized studies have shown that injection of the umbilical cord with either saline or oxytocin has no significant benefit in effecting spontaneous delivery of the placenta. In the absence of significant maternal hemorrhage, an additional 30 minutes of expectant management can be allowed because half of the retained placentas will deliver spontaneously during this time, avoiding the need for manual removal, anesthesia, and excessive blood loss.

Upon encountering postpartum hemorrhage, manual digital exploration of the uterus should be quickly accomplished to rule out the possibility of retained placental fragments (Fig. 17-9). If retained tissue is not detected, manual massage of the uterus should be started (Fig. 17-10). Simultaneously, pharmacologic methods should be employed to control uterine bleeding. Initial therapy includes the administration of a dilute solution of oxytocin, usually 10 to 20 units of oxytocin in 1,000 ml of physiologic saline solution. The solution can be administered in rates as high as 500 ml in 10 minutes without cardiovascular complications. However, an intravenous bolus injection of as little as 5 units of oxytocin may be associated with maternal hypotension, further stressing an already compromised maternal cardiovascular system.

When oxytocin fails to produce adequate uterine contraction most clinicians now administer synthetic 15-methyl-$F_{2\alpha}$-prostaglandin (Prostin, Upjohn). Although ergovine (0.2-mg IM) has been a standard second-line drug for many years, the efficacy and safety of prostaglandin medications in this instance have obviated the need to use ergonovine in most instances. Initial studies with prostaglandin medications for postpartum hemorrhage were performed with the naturally occurring $F_{2\alpha}$

Table 17-4 Risk Factors for Obstetric Hemorrhage of Greater Than 1,000 cc

Factor	Risk Increase
Placental abruption	12.6
Placenta previa	13.1
Multiple pregnancy	4.5
Obesity	1.6
Retained placenta	5.2
Induced labor	2.2
Episiotomy	2.1
Birth weight >4 kg	1.9

(From Stones et al.,[91] with permission.)

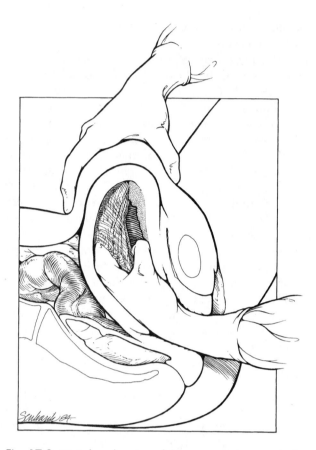

Fig. 17-9 Digital exploration of the uterus and removal of retained membranes. A sponge has been wrapped around the examiner's fingers.

prostaglandin compound, which required direct intrauterine injection. The total dose used was 1 to 2 mg diluted in 10 to 20 ml of saline.[69] Subsequently, clinical trials of the synthetic 15-methyl-$F_{2\alpha}$-prostaglandin produced promising results.[70] This compound should be given in 0.25-mg doses in the deltoid muscle every 1 to 2 hours. As many as five doses may be administered without adverse effect. Experience at the University of Washington would support these observations, as the routine availability of this agent in the delivery unit has arrested a number of otherwise uncontrollable hemorrhages.

When pharmacologic methods fail to control hemorrhage from atony, surgical measures should be undertaken to arrest the bleeding before it becomes life threatening. However, before a laparotomy, a careful inspection of the vagina and cervix should be made to confirm that the uterus is the source of the bleeding.

If the uterus is found to be contracted appropriately and no placental fragments are retained within the uterus, a laceration of maternal soft tissues is the likely cause of continued vaginal bleeding. Careful inspection of the cervix and vagina will often indicate the source of the bleeding. Figures 17-11 through 17-14 illustrate

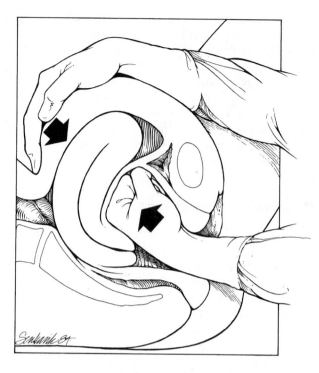

Fig. 17-10 Manual compression and massage of the uterus to control bleeding from uterine atony.

second-, third-, and fourth-degree lacerations of the perineum and techniques for their repair. Adequate exposure for the repair of such lacerations is critical and, if needed, assistance should be summoned to aid in retraction.

In cervical laceration, it is important to secure the base of the laceration, which is often a major source of bleeding. However, this area is frequently the most

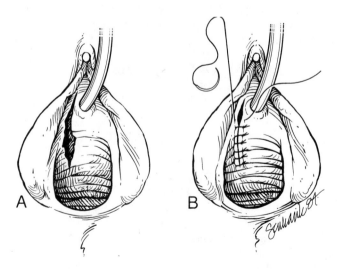

Fig. 17-11 Repair of an anterior periurethral laceration. Either running or interrupted sutures con be used. An indwelling catheter is placed before the repair is made.

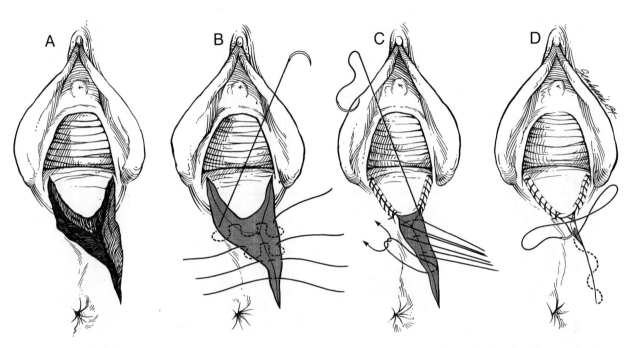

Fig. 17-12 Repair of a second-degree laceration. A first-degree laceration involves the fourchet, the perineal skin, and the vaginal mucous membrane. A second-degree laceration also includes the muscles of the perineal body. The rectal sphincter remains intact.

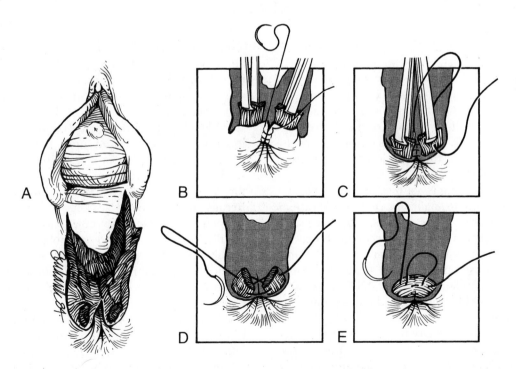

Fig. 17-13 Repair of the sphincter after a third-degree laceration. A third-degree laceration extends not only through the skin, mucous membrane, and perineal body, but includes the anal sphincter. Interrupted figure of eight sutures should be placed in the capsule of the sphincter muscle.

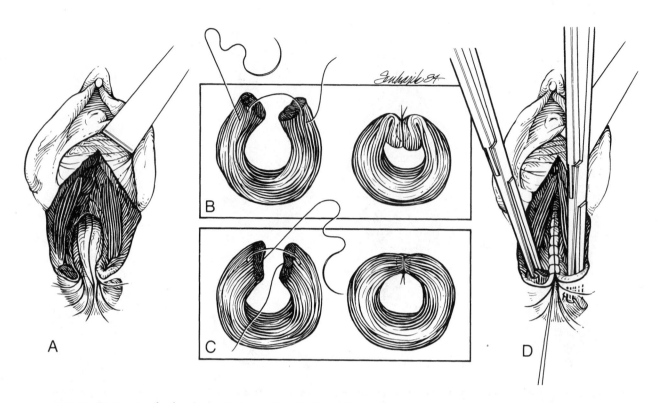

Fig. 17-14 Repair of a fourth-degree laceration. This laceration extends through the rectal mucosa. (A) The extent of this laceration is shown, with a segment of the rectum exposed. (B) Approximation of the rectal submucosa. This is the most commonly recommended method for repair. (C) Alternative method of approximating the rectal mucosa in which the knots are actually buried inside the rectal lumen. (D) After closure of the rectal submucosa, an additional layer of running sutures may be placed. The rectal sphincter is then repaired.

difficult to suture. Valuable time can be lost trying to expose the angle of such a laceration. A helpful technique to use in these cases, especially when help is limited or slow in responding, is to start to suture the laceration at its proximal end, using the suture for traction to expose the more distal portion of the cervix until the apex is in view (Fig. 17-15). This technique has the added advantage of arresting significant bleeding from the edges of laceration.

When uterine bleeding is not responsive to pharmacologic methods and no vaginal or cervical lacerations are present, surgical exploration may be necessary. Laceration of uterine vessels during the birth process will occasionally be found, most commonly after forceps delivery. Substantial episodic hemorrhage followed by periods of relatively little blood flow is often a sign of uterine vessel laceration. In this case, unilateral ligation and repair will stop the blood loss.

If hemorrhage is secondary to atony, vascular ligation will often be necessary to control bleeding. Hypogastric artery ligation, a technique recommended for many decades to control postpartum hemorrhage, has fallen out of favor because of the prolonged operating time, technical difficulties associated with its performance, and an inconsistent clinical response. Instead,

a stepwise progression of uterine vessel ligation should be rapidly accomplished. Ligation of the ascending branch of the uterine arteries should be attempted as a first step if hemorrhage is unresponsive to oxytocin or prostaglandin[71,72] (Fig. 17-16A,B). The uterine artery should be located at the border between the upper and lower uterine segment and suture ligated with 0 or No. 1 chromic suture. The suture should be placed 2 cm medial to the uterine artery and the needle driven from the anterior surface of the uterus posteriorly and tied. Because the suture is placed high in the lower uterine segment, the ureter is not in jeopardy and the bladder usually does not need to be mobilized. In approximately 10 to 15 percent of cases of atony, unilateral ligation of the uterine artery is sufficient to control hemorrhage. Bilateral ligation will control an additional 75 percent.[72]

If bleeding continues, attention should next be paid to interrupting the blood flow to the uterus from the infundibulopelvic ligament (Fig. 17-16C). There are a number of techniques to accomplish this. The easiest involves ligation of the anastomosis of the ovarian and uterine artery, high on the fundus, just below the uterovarian ligament. A large suture on an atraumatic needle can be passed from the uterus, around the ves-

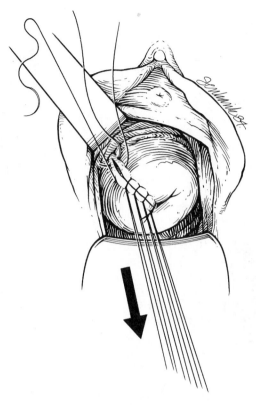

Fig. 17-15 Repair of a cervical laceration, which begins at the proximal part of the laceration, using traction on the previous sutures to aid in exposing the distal portion of the defect.

sel, and tied. If bilateral uterovarian vessel ligation does not stop the bleeding, temporary occlusion of the infundibulopelvic ligament vessels may be attempted. This can be accomplished with digital pressure or with rubber-sleeved clamps. It may be an especially useful technique if the patient is of low parity and future childbearing is of great importance. If this appears to control hemorrhage, ligation of the infundibulopelvic ligament can be performed by passing an absorbable suture from anterior to posterior through the avascular area inferior to and including the ovarian vessels. Although the ovarian blood supply may be decreased, successful pregnancy has been reported after all major pelvic vessels were ligated to arrest postpartum hemorrhage.[73,72]

Pelvic Hematoma

Blood loss leading to cardiovascular instability is not always visible. In some instances traumatic laceration of blood vessels may lead to the formation of a pelvic hematoma. Pelvic hematomas may be divided into three main types: vulvar, vaginal, or retroperitoneal.

Vulvar Hematoma

This type of hematoma results from laceration of vessels in the superficial fascia of either the anterior or posterior pelvic triangle. The usual physical signs are subacute volume loss and vulvar pain. The blood loss in this case is limited by Colle's fascia and the urogenital diaphragm. In the posterior area, the limitations are the anal fascia. Because of these fascial boundaries, the mass will extend to the skin and a visible hematoma will result (Figs. 17-17 and 17-18).

Treatment in these cases requires the volume support outlined previously. Surgical management calls for wide linear incision of the mass through the skin and evacuation of blood and clots. As this condition is often the result of bleeding from small vessels, the lacerated vessel will not usually be identified. Once the clot has been evacuated, the dead space can be closed with sutures. The area should then be compressed by a large sterile dressing and pressure applied. Efforts to pack the cavity are usually futile and only serve to create further bleeding. An indwelling catheter should be placed in the bladder at the start of the surgical evacuation and left in place for 24 to 36 hours. Compression can be removed after 12 hours.

Vaginal Hematoma

Vaginal hematomas may result from trauma to maternal soft tissues during delivery. These hematomas are frequently associated with a forceps delivery but may occur spontaneously. They are less common than vulvar hematomas. In this instance, blood accumulates in the plane above the level of the pelvic diaphragm (Fig. 17-19). It is unusual for large amounts of blood to collect in this space. The most frequent complaint in such cases is severe rectal pressure. Examination will reveal a large mass protruding into the vagina.

Vaginal hematomas should be treated by incision of the vagina and evacuation. As with vulvar hematomas, it is uncommon to find a single bleeding vessel as the source of bleeding. The incision need not be closed, as the edges of the vagina will fall back together after the clot has been removed. A vaginal pack should be inserted to tamponade the raw edges. The pack is then removed in 12 to 18 hours.

Retroperitoneal Hematoma

Retroperitoneal hematomas are the least common of the pelvic hematomas but are the most dangerous to the mother. Symptoms from a retroperitoneal hematoma may not be impressive until the sudden onset of hypotension or shock. A retroperitoneal hematoma occurs after laceration of one of the vessels originating from the hypogastric artery (Fig. 17-20). Such lacerations may result from inadequate hemostasis of the uterine arteries at the time of cesarean delivery or after rupture of a low transverse cesarean delivery scar during a trial of labor. In these patients, blood may dissect up to the renal vasculature.

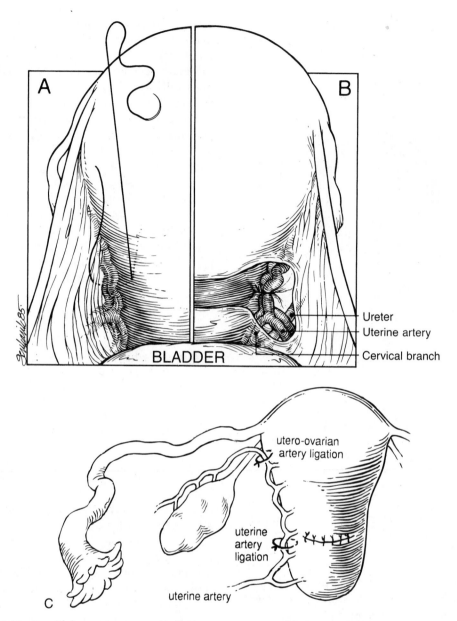

Fig. 17-16 Ligation of the uterine artery. (A,B) This anterior view of the uterus demonstrates the placement of a suture around the ascending branch of the uterine artery and vein as described by O'Leary and O'Leary. Note that 2 to 3 cm of myometrium medial to the vessels has been included in the ligature. The vessels are not divided. (C) View of sutured uterus: ligated uterine artery, and ligated utero-ovarian artery.

Treatment of this life-threatening condition involves surgical exploration and ligation of the hypogastric vessels on both the lacerated side and on the contralateral side if unilateral ligation does not arrest the bleeding. On occasion, it may be possible to open the hematomas and identify the bleeding vessel.

Umbrella Pack

The use of an umbrella pack to control bleeding after hysterectomy is a valuable technique in desperate situations (Fig. 17-21). This technique may be needed after cesarean hysterectomy complicated by persistent bleeding from the vaginal cuff. Such hemorrhage may be encountered after massive blood loss secondary to the washout of platelets or as a result of DIC. In either instance, it may be impossible to control the generalized oozing from the vaginal cuff except with pressure. The umbrella pack will often permit one to tamponade the bleeding surfaces until coagulation factors and platelets can be given and, in addition, enables the surgeon to close the abdomen without the fear of continued blood loss.

The pack itself should be a bag or sack of nonadhesive

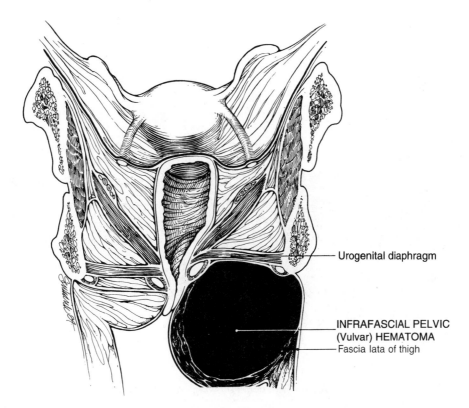

— Urogenital diaphragm

INFRAFASCIAL PELVIC
(Vulvar) HEMATOMA
- Fascia lata of thigh

Fig. 17-17 Vulvar hematoma, showing anatomic landmarks.

material. A small plastic bag serves the purpose very well. The bag can be inserted through the vagina or at laparotomy. When abdominal placement is possible, the bag should be filled with 2-in gauze packing through the vagina to ensure an orderly packing that will facilitate removal at a future time. The bag should be filled with enough gauze to occlude the open vaginal cuff completely and present enough resistance to prevent expulsion when a weight is attached to the end of the pack.

Once the pack is in true pelvis and the gauze has been inserted, a 1,000-ml intravenous bag should be tied to the umbrella pack and traction applied. Traction should be maintained for 24 hours. After 24 hours, the traction may be relieved, but the bag should be left in place for an additional 12 hours. After 36 hours, the gauze packing should be removed by pulling on the tail that has been left protruding through the vagina. After the gauze has been evacuated, the bag should be removed.

Two major complications of this procedure include infection and urinary obstruction. The latter can be obviated by the use of an indwelling Foley catheter. The danger of infection is an ever-present one but is usually of secondary importance in the acute events surrounding such massive bleeding. Prophylactic antibiotics should be used in these cases. Since the publication of this technique in the first edition of this textbook, three cases of successful use of the umbrella pack in obstetric patients have been published.[74,75]

Inversion of the Uterus

Occasionally the third stage of labor is complicated by partial delivery of the placenta followed by rapid onset of shock in the mother. These events characterize uter-

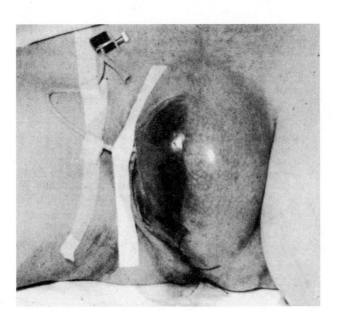

Fig. 17-18 Photograph of vulvar hematoma before evacuation.

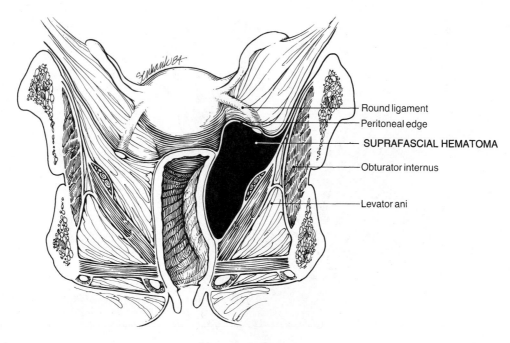

Fig. 17-19 Vaginal hematoma showing anatomic landmarks.

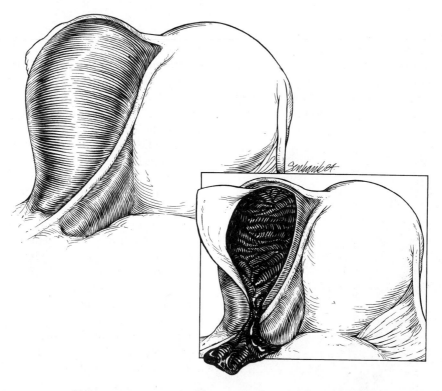

Fig. 17-20 Retroperitoneal hematoma as a result of laceration of one of the branches of the hypogastric artery. Evacuation of the hematoma is illustrated in the accompanying panel.

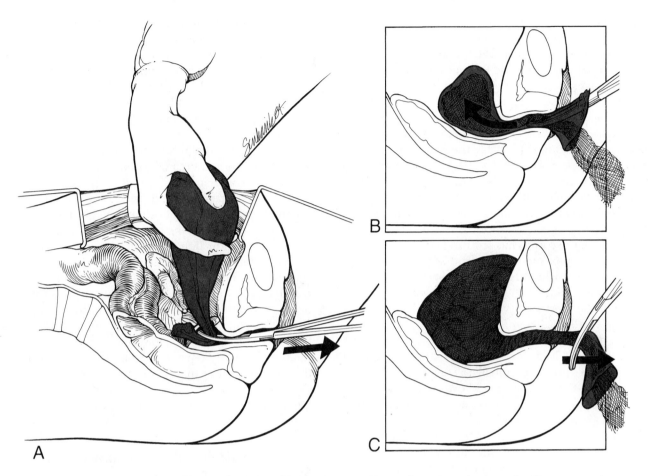

Fig. 17-21 Abdominal placement of an umbrella pack to control hemorrhage from the vaginal cuff. (A) Vaginal route for insertion of gauge packing. The pack is pulled downward over the vaginal cuff (B) and is secured (C).

ine inversion. Hypotension usually results before significant blood loss has occurred. The inexperienced obstetrician may mistake an inversion of the uterus for a partially separated placenta or aborted myoma.

Uterine inversion is an uncommon but life-threatening event. Since 1970, the reported incidence has been 1 in 2,000 deliveries.[76] Inversion of the uterus is termed incomplete if the corpus does not pass through the cervix, complete if the corpus passes through the cervix, and prolapsed if the corpus extends through the vaginal introitus. Uterine inversion usually occurs in association with a fundally inserted placenta. Although previous studies have implicated the use of excessive cord traction and the Crede maneuver as causes of uterine inversion, recent studies have failed to document this association.[76]

Treatment of uterine inversion should include fluid therapy for the mother and restoration of the uterus to its normal position. This latter is best accomplished using the technique illustrated in Figure 17-22 and should be attempted immediately upon recognition of the inversion. Separation of the placenta before re-

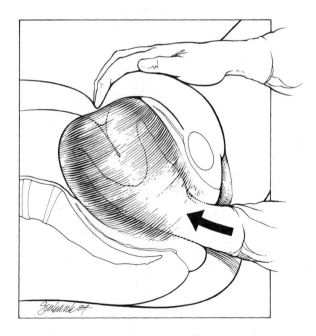

Fig. 17-22 Manual replacement of an inverted uterus.

placement of the uterus will only increase maternal blood loss.[77] If possible, the uterus should be replaced without removing the placenta. Initial efforts to replace the uterus should be made without the use of uterine relaxing agents. If initial efforts fail, the use of either β-mimetic agents or magnesium sulfate should be tried. The choice of these agents depends on the maternal vital signs. In the case of severe maternal hypotension, magnesium sulfate is probably the best choice. These agents have been reported to be safe and associated with an 85 to 90 percent success rate in patients failing initial replacement without pharmacologic therapy. In 10 to 15 percent of remaining cases, general anesthesia should be employed.[78] Subacute inversion of the uterus occurs when the corpus has protruded through the cervix and the cervix and lower uterine segment have subsequently contracted, thereby trapping the corpus. In this instance, general anesthesia is necessary for restoration of the uterus to its proper anatomic position.

Occasionally, it is impossible to reposition the subacutely inverted uterus vaginally and laparotomy is necessary. Figure 17-23 shows the surgical technique used to correct this problem. Initially, a combination of vaginal pressure and traction from above on the round ligaments should be attempted. However, this maneuver may not always be successful, and one may have to resort to a vertical incision on the posterior aspect of the lower uterine segment in order to replace the uterus.

Once the uterine inversion has been corrected, the anesthetic agents used for uterine relaxation should be discontinued and oxytocic agents given to produce uterine contraction. If oxytocin fails to contract the uterus, prostaglandin $F_{2\alpha}$ should be used. The same dosage and intervals used to arrest postpartum hemorrhage with uterine atony are appropriate in this circumstance.

Coagulation Disorders

Continued bleeding in the third stage of labor that is unresponsive to usual treatment should cause the clinician to consider uncommon but serious maternal coagulation disorders.

von Willebrand's Disease

von Willebrand's disease (VWD) is a hemorrhagic disorder that affects both men and women. This coagulopathy is inherited in an autosomal dominant pattern and is characterized by the following laboratory abnormalities: prolonged bleeding time, decreased Factor VIII activity, decreased Factor VIII–related antigen, and decreased von Willebrand factor. The latter is a plasma factor that is essential for proper platelet function and aggregation.

VWD is quite variable in its clinical course, severity,

and laboratory abnormalities, even in the same patient. It is therefore possible for a patient with this disorder to go undetected throughout pregnancy until bleeding problems develop postpartum. The usual increase in Factor VIII coagulant activity associated with pregnancy may also mask VWD. Only those patients with very low levels (<5 percent) before gestation fail to exhibit this rise.

When VWD is diagnosed before parturition, Factor VIII activity should be monitored serially and transfusion with cryoprecipitate given to keep the Factor VIII activity near term at 40 percent. If Factor VIII levels are inadequate, the patient should be given one bag of cryoprecipitate per 10-kg body weight 24 hours before the planned induction of labor or cesarean delivery. This infusion will immediately restore the Factor VIII activity level, but it will take 24 hours for the associated platelet defect to be corrected. If one suspects this disorder in a patient with unexplained postpartum hemorrhage, coagulation studies should be ordered and a hematologist consulted. However, since time is often limited, it would be prudent to notify the blood bank that cryoprecipitate may be needed emergently. In this situation, at least 6 units of cryoprecipitate are required, to be given every 12 hours for the next 3 to 5 days.[79]

Amniotic Fluid Embolism/Anaphylactoid Syndrome of Pregnancy

Amniotic fluid embolism (AFE) is a rare but frequently fatal obstetric emergency clinically recognized in approximately 1 of 8,000 to 1 of 80,000 births. The mortality rate for mothers suffering from AFE is 50 to 60 percent,[80–82] but an additional 30 percent (75 percent of survivors) can be expected to have long-term neurologic deficits.[82] The definitive diagnosis of AFE has traditionally been thought to require demonstration of fetal squames and lanugo in the pulmonary vascular space. However, in the most comprehensive study of this syndrome to date, only 73 percent of patients dying from this syndrome had this finding.[82] Based on mounting clinical and experimental evidence, Clark et al.[83] have suggested renaming this clinical syndrome the *Anaphylactoid syndrome of pregnancy* to emphasize that the clinical findings are secondary to biochemical mediators rather than pulmonary embolic phenomenon.

The classic clinical presentation of the syndrome has been described by five signs that often occur in the following sequence: (1) respiratory distress, (2) cyanosis, (3) cardiovascular collapse, (4) hemorrhage, and (5) coma. In the previously mentioned paper, Clark et al.[83] described a more heterogenous clinical presentation. The most important new findings are the certainty

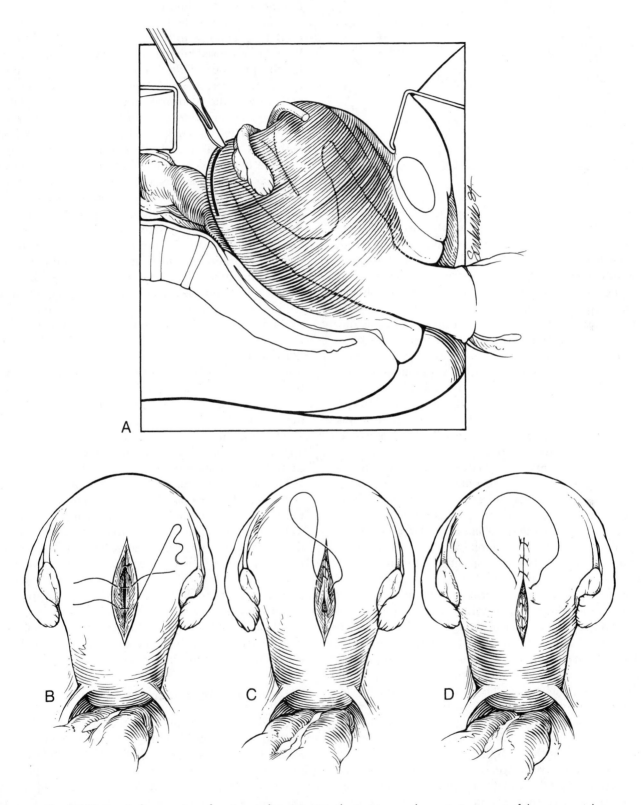

Fig. 17-23 Surgical restoration of an inverted uterus. Note the incision on the posterior aspect of the uterus and subsequent repair.

Table 17-5   Incidence: Signs and Symptoms Occurring in >50% of Patients with AFE[87]

Sign or Symptom	No. of Patients	Percentage
Hypotension	43	100
Fetal distress	30	100
Pulmonary edema/ARDS	28	93
Cardiac arrest	40	87
Cyanosis	38	83
Coagulopathy	38	83
Dyspnea	22	49
Seizure	22	48

(From Clark et al.,[83] with permission.)

of fetal distress accompanying this syndrome and the high incidence of maternal coagulopathy. In many cases, fetal distress is the initial presenting symptom, rapidly followed by maternal distress (see Table 17-5).

The cardiorespiratory effects of acute intravascular injection of amniotic fluid have been studied in pregnant ewes.[84] The initial response to the intravascular injection of amniotic fluid was hypotension. A 40 percent decrease in mean arterial pressure was followed by a 100 percent increase in mean pulmonary artery pressure. Little change occurred in the left atrial pressure or the pulmonary artery wedge pressure. A 40 percent fall in cardiac output was associated with the rapid rise in pulmonary artery pressure. These changes resulted in a two- to threefold increase in pulmonary vascular resistance and a two- to threefold decrease in systemic vascular resistance. In contrast to these findings in sheep, intravascular injection of amniotic fluid in rhesus monkeys failed to produce cardiovascular changes similar to the syndrome observed in humans.[81]

Classic teachings have emphasized the role of uterine hyperstimulation as a predisposing factor in this syndrome. More recent data[82] have shown this to be an erroneous conclusion. Uterine hyperstimulation was found in less than 10 percent of patients prior to the occurrence of AFE. Uterine tetany did occur in 50 percent of patients concomitant with respiratory distress. This most likely represents the uterine response to maternal hypoxemia rather than the event precipitating the AFE. Equally incorrect is the hypothesis that oxytocin administration is a risk factor for the development of the syndrome. There is no higher frequency of oxytocin use in patients suffering AFE than in laboring patients without this complication.

Only scanty information is available on which to base the treatment of the initial syndrome. Early airway control usually necessitating endotracheal intubation has been stressed in the few patients surviving the full-blown syndrome.[85,86] Once maximal ventilation and oxygenation have been achieved, attention should be paid to restoration of cardiovascular equilibrium. Central monitoring of fluid therapy with a pulmonary artery catheter is very helpful if the patient can be stabilized long enough to allow time for its placement. Pulmonary arterial blood may be aspirated and stained for the presence of fetal squames, lanugo hair, and mucin. However, these are found in only 50 percent of patients with the syndrome and there are known false positives. The treatment of shock in the early phase of the syndrome unaccompanied by massive blood loss has not been well studied. Recent data would suggest that the hypotension results from myocardial failure and that efforts should be used to provide myocardial support.[83] These would include inotropic agents such as dopamine, as well as volume therapy.[87] Other investigators have observed reduced systemic vascular resistance and have used vasopressor therapy such as ephedrine or levarterenol with success.[86] If the patient survives the initial cardiorespiratory collapse, there is a high likelihood that coagulopathy will develop if it has not been previously clinically apparent. DIC results in the depletion of fibrinogen, platelets, and coagulation factors, especially Factors V, VIII, and XIII. The fibrinolytic system is activated as well.[88] Most patients will have profound hypofibrinogenemia with values less than 200 mg/dl being the rule. PT and PTT will also be abnormal in nearly all patients. Platelet counts are more variable, with 60 percent having values less than 100,000/ml. Supportive coagulation and volume therapy (blood, fresh frozen plasma, or cryoprecipitate) should be administered as soon as they are available.

The neonatal outcome in patients suffering this catastrophe is better than the maternal outcome. If the fetus is alive at the time of the event, nearly 80 percent will survive the delivery. Unfortunately, 50 percent of the survivors will incur neurologic damage.[82] The two main factors influencing neonatal outcome are the presence or absence of maternal cardiac arrest and the time from arrest to delivery in the later group. In general, fetal outcome is improved when maternal cardiac arrest does not occur. The shortest arrest to delivery time is associated with the best neonatal outcomes in the presence of maternal cardiac arrest.

Disseminated Intravascular Coagulation

DIC results from the loss of local control of the body's clotting mechanisms. Normally, there are four essential elements in the maintenance of local control of the hemostatic system: vascular integrity, platelet function, the coagulation system, and clot lysis.[89] The body must maintain vascular integrity for the survival of the organism. To minimize blood loss, any break in this system initiates the entire hemostatic cascade.

Platelets play an essential role in initiating and localizing clot formation. Platelets circulate until they encounter a break in vascular integrity. They then adhere to the damaged endothelium and release ADP, recruiting additional platelets to form an adhesive mass of platelets. Once the platelet plug extends past the site of damaged endothelium, platelets interact with the normal vessel wall and produce prostacyclin. This substance inhibits further platelet aggregation and localizes the platelet plug to the site of injury.

Platelets also localize the formation of fibrin by the coagulation cascade. Coagulation factors circulate in an inactive form. Aggregated platelets and injured tissue provide a phospholipid surface on which the coagulation factors can act. Once the factors are activated, fibrin is produced. The action of the coagulation cascade is limited to a localized area by a decrease in the amount of activated factors. These factors are reduced by (1) the reticuloendothelial system, (2) dilution by rapid blood flow, and (3) neutralization by a circulating protein (antithrombin 3).[89]

Once a clot has formed, the re-establishment of normal circulation depends on the orderly removal of the clot. Clot lysis is usually a localized process that must proceed in a timely fashion since rapid lysis would lead to rebleeding. Clot lysis is limited in two ways. Since the coagulation cascade and lytic processes both depend on Factor XII, they are triggered simultaneously. Second, activated plasminogen or plasmin is inactivated by antiplasmin, which circulates in concentrations 10 times that of plasminogen. The orderly progression of clot lysis is facilitated by the incorporation of plasminogen directly into the clot, protecting it from rapid neutralization by antiplasmin. Activation of plasminogen within the clot can then proceed at a local level.

During DIC, the body is forming and lysing fibrin clots throughout the circulation rather than in the ubiquitous localized physiologic process. Therefore, the loss of localization of the clotting process is the main defect in DIC. The lytic process may be activated as well but occurs only in response to the activation of the clotting system.

In obstetrics, DIC causing hemorrhage may involve any of the four mechanisms involved in the localization process. However, it is uncommon for DIC to be initiated by a failure of vascular integrity. Similarly, a platelet abnormality leading to diffuse platelet aggregation is an unlikely cause of hemorrhage in obstetrics. However, activation of the coagulation cascade by the presence of large amounts of tissue phospholipid is a common stimulus for DIC in obstetrics. Such conditions include abruptio placenta, retained dead fetus, and amniotic fluid embolism. These tissue phospholipids contribute to the utilization of large amounts of clotting factors and lead to a consumption coagulopathy. Once this widespread coagulation has taken place, the lytic process is called into action. The degradation of large amounts of fibrin produces fibrin split products, or fibrin degradation products (FDP). These factors have their own physiologic activity and, when present in large amounts, contribute to bleeding by inhibiting fibrin cross-linking and producing platelet dysfunction.

The platelet count and fibrinogen level are the most clinically useful tests in evaluating the patient with DIC. They may be repeated on an hourly to every 2-hour basis to provide an accurate reflection of the activity of the coagulation process. PT and PIT are usually abnormal during DIC but are less helpful in evaluating the ongoing severity of the disorder. Because platelets and fibrinogen have a half-life of 4 to 5 days, they are not immediately replaced by the body's own mechanisms and will give an accurate reflection of ongoing consumption as well as the effectiveness of factor replacement.

The sine qua non of successful management of DIC is treatment of the initiating event. Once the cause has been located and treated, the process should resolve. However, depleted factors must be restored to permit orderly repair of injured tissues. Successful therapy involves the replacement of essential factors faster than the body is consuming them. These factors are platelets, coagulation factors derived from fresh frozen plasma or cryoprecipitate, and fibrinogen supplied by cryoprecipitate of fresh frozen plasma. Monitoring replacement therapy should be initiated 20 minutes after the intravenous administration of these products. The obstetrician should attempt to achieve a platelet count of more than $100,000/\mu$l and a fibrinogen level of less than 150 mg percent. In obstetric conditions complicated by hemorrhage, heparin has no use and will only cause the bleeding to worsen.

Key Points

- The rapid assessment of volume loss is dependent on basic vital signs and physical findings.

- Blood product use should be based on objectively determined needs rather than predetermined formulas.

- An action plan should be developed for situations in which massive blood transfusion is anticipated or arises unexpectedly.

- In patients with abruptio placenta, cesarean delivery usually should be performed for obstetric or fetal indications, not maternal coagulopathy.

- Expectant management of patients with abruptio placenta or placenta previa can be safely accomplished in many patients.

- In patients with postpartum hemorrhage secondary to uterine atony, dilute solutions of oxytocin (IV) and 15-methyl-$F_{2\alpha}$-prostaglandin (IM) should be the first two drugs administered.

- The maternal risks from heterologous blood transfusion have decreased significantly in the last 5 years.

- The clinical presentation of amniotic fluid embolism is more hoterogenous than previously described.

- When uterine inversion is encountered, the uterus should be replaced and reinverted before placental removal is attempted.

- Oxytocin should be given before placental expulsion and separation to minimize postpartum blood loss.

References

1. Benedetti T, Quilligan E: Cerebral edema in severe pregnancy induced hypertension. Am J Obstet Gynecol 137: 860, 1979

2. Shires G: Management of hypovolemic shock. Bull NY Acad Med 55:139, 1979

3. Hewitt PE, Machin SJ: Massive blood transfusion. Br Med J 300:107, 1990

4. Etchason J, Petz L, Keeler E et al: The cost effectiveness of preoperative autologous blood donations. N Engl J Med 332:719, 1995

5. Grimes DA: A simplified device for intraoperative autotransfusion. Obstet Gynecol 72:947, 1988

6. Chestnut DH, Dewan DM, Redick LF et al: Anesthetic management for obstetric hysterectomy: a multi-institutional study. Anesthesiology 70:607, 1989

7. Celayeta MA: Comment: Tocolysis in placenta previa. Drug Intell Clin Pharmacol 22:828, 1988

8. Knab D: Abruptio placentae. Obstet Gynecol 52:625, 1978

9. Pritchard J: Obstetric hemorrhage. p. 485. In Pritchard J, MacDonald P (eds): Williams Obstetrics. Appleton-Century-Crofts, New York, 1980

10. Krohn M, Voight L, McKnight B et al: Correlates of placental abruption in birth certificate data. Br J Obstet Gynaecol 94:333, 1987

11. Hurd W, Miodovnik M, Hertzberg V, Lavin J: Selective management of abruptio placentae: a prospective study. Obstet Gynecol 61:467, 1983

12. Paterson M: The aetiology and outcome of abruptio placentae. Acta Obstet Gynecol Scand 58:31, 1979

13. Hibbard B, Jeffcoate T: Abruptio placentae. Obstet Gynecol 27:155, 1966

14. Townsend RR, Laing FC, Jeffrey RB: Placental abruption associated with cocaine abuse. Am J Roentgen 150:1339, 1988

15. Darby MJ, Caritis SN, Shen-Schwarz S: Placental abruption in the preterm gestation: an association with chorioamnionitis. Obstet Gynecol 74:88, 1989

16. Naeye R, Harkness W, Utts J: Abruptio placentae and perinatal death: a prospective study. Am J Obstet Gynecol 128:740, 1977

17. Pritchard J: The genesis of severe placental abruption. Am J Obstet Gynecol 208:22, 1970

18. Douglas R, Stromme W: Operative Obstetrics. Appleton-Century-Crofts, New York, 1976

19. Helton AS, McFarlane J, Anderson ET: Battered and pregnant: a prevalence study. Am J Pub Health 77:1337, 1987

20. Dommisse J, Tiltman A: Placental bed biopsies in placental abruption. Br J Obstet Gynaecol 99:651, 1992

21. Seski JC, Compton AA: Abruptio placenta following a negative oxytocin challenge test. Am J Obstet Gynecol et al. 125:276, 1976

22. Nyberg DA, Cyr DR, Mack LA et al: Sonographic spectrum of placental abruption. A J Roentgen 148:161, 1987

23. Nyberg DA, Mack LA, Benedetti TJ et al: Placental abruption and placental homorrhage: correlation of sonographic findings with fetal outcome. Radiology 358: 357, 1987

24. Bond A, Edersheim T, Curry L et al: Expectant management of abruptio placentae before 35 weeks gestation. Am J Perinatol 6:121, 1989

25. Combs C, Nyberg D, Mack L et al: Expectant management after sonographic diagnosis of placental abruption. Am J Perinatol 9:170, 1992

26. Saller DJ: Tocolysis in the management of third trimester bleeding. J Perinatol 10:125, 1990

27. Pritchard J, Brekken A: Clinical and laboratory studies on severe abruptio placentae. Am J Obstet Gynecol 97: 681, 1967

28. Olah D, Gee H, Deedham P: The management of severe disseminated intravascular coagulopathy complicating placental abruption in the sencond trimester. Br J Obstet Gynaecol 95:419, 1988

29. Montaeiro AA, Onocencio AC, Jorge CS: Placental abruption with disseminated intravascular coagulopathy in the second trimester of pregnancy with fetal survival. Br J Obstet Gynaecol 94:811, 1987

30. Lowe TW, Cunningham FG: Placental abruption. Clin Obstet Gynecol 33:406, 1990

31. Saftlas A, Olson D, Atrash H et al: National trends in the

incidence of abruptio placenta. Obstet Gynecol 78:1081, 1991

32. Spinillo A, Fazzi E, Stronati E et al: Severity of abruptio placenta and neurodevelopmental outcome in low birth weight infants. Early Hum Dev 35:44, 1993

33. Brenner W, Edelman D, Hendricks C: Characteristics of patients with placenta previa and results of "expectant management." Am J Obstet Gynecol 132:180, 1978

34. Cotton D, Ead J, Paul R, Quilligan E: The conservative aggressive management of placenta previa. Am J Obstet Gynecol 17:687, 1980

35. Iyasu S, Saftlas A, Rowley D et al: The epidemiology of placenta previa in the United States, 1979. Am J Obstet Gynecol 168:1424, 1987

36. Clark S, Koonings P, Phelan J: Placenta previa/accreta and prior cesarean section. Obstet Gynecol 66:89, 1985

37. Nielsen TF, Hagberg H, Ljungblad U: Placenta previa and antepartum hemorrhage after previous cesarean section. Gynecol Obstet Invest 27:88, 1989

38. Singh P, Rodrigues C, Gupta PA: Placenta previa and previous cesarean section. Acta Obstet Gynecol Scand 60:367, 1981

39. Chattopadhyay S, Kharif H, Sherbeeni J: Placenta previa and accreta after previous cesarean section. Eur J Obstet Gynecol Reprod Biol 52:151, 1993

40. Rizos N, Doran T, Miskin M et al: Natural history of placenta previa ascertained by diagnostic ultrasound. Am J Obstet Gynecol 133:287, 1979

41. Zelop C, Bromley B, Frigoletto FJ, Benacerraf B: Second trimester sonographically diagnosed placenta previa: prediction of persistent previa at birth. Int J Gynaecol Obstet 44:207, 1994

42. Chervenak F, Lee Y, Hendler M et al: Role of attempted vaginal delivery in the management of placenta previa. Obstet Gynecol 64:798, 1984

43. Watson P, Cefalo R: Magnesium sulfate tocolysis in selected patients with symptomatic placenta previa. Am J Perinatol 7:251, 1990

44. Sampson M, Lastres O, Tomasi A et al: Tocolysis with terbutaline sulfate in patients with placenta previa complicated by premature labor. J Reprod Med 29:248, 1984

45. McShane P, Heyl P, Epstein M: Maternal and perinatal morbidity resulting from placenta previa. Obstet Gynecol 65:176, 1985

46. Tomich P: Prolonged use of tocolytic agent in expectant management of placenta previa. J Reprod Med 30:745, 1985

47. Perkins R: Discussion of paper. Am J Obstet Gynecol 149:323, 1984

48. Liggins G, Howie R: A controlled trial of antepartum glucocorticoid treatment of RDS. Pediatrics 50:515, 1972

49. Ballard R, Ballard P, Goanberg P, Sinderman S: Prenatal administration of betamethasone for prevention of respiratory distress syndrome. J Pediatr 94:97, 1979

50. d'Angelo L, Irwin L: Conservative management of placenta previa: a cost benefit analysis. Am J Obstet Gynecol 149:320, 1984

51. Droste S, Keil K: Expectant management of placenta previa: cost benefit analysis of outpatient treatment. Am J Obstet Gynecol 170:1254, 1994

52. Mouer J: Placenta previa: antepartum conservative management inpatient vs. outpatient. Am J Obstet Gynecol 170:1685, 1994

53. Breen J, Neubecker R, Gregori C, Franklin J: Placenta accreta, increta and percreta. Obstet Gynecol 49:51, 1977

54. Hoffman-Tretin J, Koenigsberg M, Rabin A, Anyaebunam A: Placenta accreta. Additional sonographic observations. J Ultrasound Med 11:326, 1992

55. Finberg H, Williams J: Placenta accreta: prospective sonographic diagnosis in patients with placenta previa and prior cesarean section. J Ultrasound Med 11:333, 1992

56. Read J, Cotton D, Miller F: Placenta accreta: changing clinical aspects and outcome. Obstet Gynecol 56:31, 1980

57. Druzin ML: Packing of lower uterine segment for control of postcesarean bleeding in instances of placenta previa. Surg Gynecol Obstet 169:543, 1980

58. Cho J, Kim S, Cha K et al: Interrupted circular suture: bleeding control during cesarean delivery in placenta previa accreta. Obstet Gynecol 78:876, 1991

59. Alvarez M, Lockwood C, Ghidini A et al: Prophylactic and emergent arterial catheterization for selective embolization in obstetric hemorrhage. Am J Perinatol 9:441, 1992

60. Mitty H, Sterling K, Alvarez M, Gendler R: Obstetric hemorrhage: prophylactic and emergency arterial catheterization and embolotherapy. Radiology 188:183, 1993

61. Fox H: Placenta accreta. Obstet Gynecol Surv 27:475, 1972

62. Gemmell A: Unusual case of adherent placenta treated in unorthodox manner. J Obstet Gynecol 49:43, 1947

63. Jaffe R, DuBeshter B, Sherer D et al: Failure of methotrexate treatment for term placenta percreta. Am J Obstet Gynecol 171:558, 1994

64. Bakrai L: Placenta percreta with bladder invasion: report of three cases. Am J Perinatol 10:468, 1993

65. Torrey E: Vasa previa. Am J Obstet Gynecol 63:146, 1952

66. Sirivongs B: Vasa previa report of 3 cases. J Med Assoc Thai 57:261, 1974

67. McCurdy C, Magann E, McCurdy C, Saltazman A: The effect of placental management at cesarean delivery on operative blood loss. Am J Obstet Gynecol 167:1363, 1992

68. Prendiville W, Harding J, Elburne D, Stirrat G: The Briston third stage trial: active vs. physiological management of the third stage of labor. J Obstet Gynecol 95:3, 1988

69. Takagi S, Yuoshida T, Togo Y et al: The effects of intramyometrial injection of prostaglandin $F_{2\alpha}$ on severe postpartum hemorrhage. Prostaglandins 12:565, 1980

70. Hayashi R, Castillo M, Noah M: Management of severe postpartum hemorrhage due to uterine atony usng an analog of prostaglandin $F_{2\alpha}$. Obstet Gynecol 58:426, 1981

71. O'Leary J, O'Leary J: Uterine artery ligation in control of intractable postpartum hemorrhage. Am J Obstet Gynecol 94:920, 1966

72. Adrabbo F, Salah J: Stepwise uterine devascularization: a novel technique for management of uncontrollable postpartum hemorrhage with preservation of the uterus. Am J Obstet Gynecol 171:694, 1984

73. Mengert W, Burchell R, Blumstein R, Daskal J: Pregnancy after bilateral ligation of internal iliac and ovarian arteries. Obstet Gynecol 34:664, 1969

74. Cassels JJ, Greenberg H, Otterson W: Pelvic tamponade in puerperal hemorrhage. J Reprod Med 30:689, 1985

75. Robie G, Morgan M, Payne G, Wasemiller-Smith L: Logothetopulos pack for the management of uncontrollable postpartum hemorrhage. Am J Perinatol 7:327, 1990

76. Watson P, Desch N, Bowes W: Management of acute and subacute puerperal inversion of the uterus. Obstet Gynecol 55:12, 1980

77. Kichin J, MMBS T, May H, Thornton W: Puerperal inversion of the uterus. Am J Obstet Gynecol 123:51, 1975

78. Brar H, Greenspoon J, Platt L, RH P: Acute puerperal uterine inversion: new approaches to management. J Reprod Med 34:173, 1989

79. Walker E, Dormandy K: The management of pregnancy in von Willebrand's disease. J Obstet Gynaecol Br Commonw 74:459, 1968

80. Courtney L: Amniotic fluid embolism. Obstet Gynecol Surv 29:169, 1974

81. Stolte L, vanKessel H, Seelen H et al: Failure to produce the syndrome of amniotic fluid embolism by infusion of amniotic fluid and meconium into monkeys. Am J Obstet Gynecol 83:694, 1967

82. Clark S, Hankins G, Dudley D et al: Amniotic fluid embolism: analysis of the national registry. Am J Obstet Gynecol 172:1158, 1995

83. Clark S, Montz F, Phelan J: Hemodynamic alterations associated with amniotic fluid embolism: a reappraisal. Am J Obstet Gynecol 151:617, 1985

84. Reis R, Pierce W, Behrendt D: Hemodynamic effects of amniotic fluid embolism. Surg Gynecol Obstet 129:45, 1969

85. Clark S, Morgan M: Amiotic fluid embolism. Anesthesia 34:20, 1979

86. Resnik R, Swartz W, Plummer M et al: Amniotic fluid embolism with survival. Obstet Gynecol 47:295, 1976

87. Schaef R, Campo T, Civetta J: Hemodynamic alterations and rapid diagnosis in a case of amniotic fluid. Anesthesiology 45:155, 1977

88. Ratnoff O, Vosburgh G: Observations on the dotting defect in amniotic fluid embolism. N Engl J Med 247:970, 1952

89. Fishbach D, Fogdall R: Coagulation: The Essentials. Williams and Wilkins, Baltimore, 1981

90. Baker R: Hemorrhage in obstetrics. Obstet Gynecol Annu 6:295, 1977

91. Stones RW, Paterson CM, Saunders NJ: Risk factors for major obstetric hemorrhage. Eur J Obstet Gynecol Reprod Biol 48:15, 1993

Chapter 18

Critical Care Obstetrics

William C. Mabie

In the past decade several large obstetric services in the United States have established intensive care units (ICUs). Although only about 1 percent of obstetric patients require intensive care, these units offer several benefits: (1) intensive observation and organization allows for prevention or early recognition and treatment of complications, (2) familiarity with invasive hemodynamic monitoring permits personnel to exert prompt rational treatment of hemodynamically unstable patients, (3) continuity of care is improved before and after delivery, and (4) residents and fellows learn a great deal about intensive care and the management of rare medical complications of pregnancy.[1]

This chapter is divided into two sections: basic principles and clinical management. In the former, I consider indications, insertion technique, and physiologic principles involved in using the Swan-Ganz catheter in obstetrics. In the latter, I discuss pregnancy-specific diseases and medical complications of pregnancy that often require intensive care.

Basic Principles of Critical Care

Indications for Invasive Hemodynamic Monitoring

The mainstay of intensive obstetric care is pulmonary artery catheterization, common indications for which are listed below. Invasive monitoring is not necessary in every patient with one of these conditions, nor is this an all-inclusive list. Swan-Ganz monitoring should be considered for any critically ill patient whose volume status must be known. The standards and criteria for invasive monitoring should be the same for pregnant as for nonpregnant patients.[2]

The Swan-Ganz catheter is useful in differentiating cardiogenic from noncardiogenic forms of pulmonary edema. It may also be used to guide diuretic therapy and manipulations of cardiac output such as preload and afterload reduction or inotropic therapy. In patients with oliguria, the catheter may be used to assess volume status. In preeclampsia it has been shown that central venous pressure is not adequate for assessing volume status.[3,4] The change in wedge pressure and cardiac output in response to a fluid challenge is the most important guide to intravascular volume. While invasive hemodynamic monitoring is not necessary for acute resuscitation from hemorrhagic shock, it is useful in the subsequent 24 to 72 hours to guide fluid therapy in complex cases in which it is not clear if internal bleeding is continuing or if oliguria, pulmonary edema, liver dysfunction, or severe coagulopathy are present.

Indications for Pulmonary Artery Catheterization in Obstetrics

Refractory or unexplained pulmonary edema

Refractory or unexplained oliguria

Massive hemorrhage

Septic shock

Adult respiratory distress syndrome

Class 3 and 4 cardiac disease

Intraoperative or intrapartum cardiovascular decompensation

Respiratory distress of unknown cause

Definitions of Hemodynamic Terms

Wedge pressure—a measure of left ventricular preload. The pulmonary artery wedge pressure is obtained with a balloon-tipped catheter advanced into a branch of a pulmonary artery until the vessel is occluded, forming a free communication through the pulmonary capillaries and veins to the left atrium. A true wedge position is in a lung zone where both pulmonary artery and pulmonary venous pressures exceed alveolar pressure

Preload—initial stretch of the myocardial fiber at end-diastole. Clinically, the right and left ventricular end-diastolic pressures are assessed by the central venous pressure and wedge pressure, respectively

Afterload—wall tension of the ventricle during ejection. Best reflected by systolic blood pressure

Contractility—the force of myocardial contraction when preload and afterload are held constant

In septic shock, invasive monitoring allows manipulation of cardiovascular parameters with fluid and inotropic therapy as well as assessment of response to therapy through such parameters as oxygen delivery and consumption. In the adult respiratory distress syndrome, the catheter is used to exclude cardiogenic pulmonary edema and to guide supportive therapy with mechanical ventilation, positive end-expiratory pressure, intravenous fluids, diuretics, and inotropic agents. New York Heart Association class 3 and 4 cardiac patients require invasive monitoring to guide fluid and drug therapy, as well as for anesthesia management during labor and delivery. The cause of sudden intraoperative or intrapartum cardiovascular decompensation may be clarified by obtaining wedge pressure and cardiac output. The final indication includes patients in whom the contribution of cardiac or pulmonary disease to respiratory distress is unclear by clinical examination. The pulmonary artery catheter can help to differentiate heart failure from pneumonia, pulmonary emboli, adult respiratory distress syndrome, or chronic pulmonary disorders.

Risks Versus Benefits in Catheter Insertion

Complications associated with invasive hemodynamic monitoring include pneumothorax, ventricular arrhythmias, air embolism, pulmonary infarction, pulmonary artery rupture, sepsis, local vascular thrombo-

sis, intracardiac knotting, and valvular damage.[5] The Swan-Ganz catheter was introduced into clinical practice in 1970.[6] Complications have decreased over the years at least partially due to better physician and nurse awareness. The incidence of pneumothorax has decreased from 1 to 6 percent in the early literature to less than 0.1 percent. Recent studies report that pulmonary infarction has been reduced from 7.2 percent in 1974 to 0 to 1.3 percent. Pulmonary artery rupture has fallen from 0.1 percent to 0.2 percent to almost zero. Local vascular thrombosis has decreased with use of heparin-bonded catheters, and septicemia has fallen from 2 to 0.5 percent. Still complications have not been eliminated.[7]

Interpretive error may also be considered a complication and may result from improper calibration, air or blood in the lines, use of a digital readout instead of hard paper printout, and failure to measure wedge pressure at end expiration when pleural pressure is zero.[7]

The continuous generation of data can be mesmerizing. The obstetrician may spend excessive time calibrating, debugging, and collecting data, yet ignoring such equally important aspects as the fetal heart rate tracing or the progress of labor.

The main benefit of pulmonary artery catheterization is its ability to provide information that clinical examination alone cannot supply.[7] The technique is more accurate than clinical assessment in determining the cause of shock or for assessing the etiology of pulmonary edema. Two studies have shown that prediction of cardiac output and wedge pressure based on history, physical examination, and chest x-ray are about 75 percent accurate in coronary care unit patients[8,9]; however, three studies have shown that wedge pressure and cardiac output may be accurately predicted by clinical criteria only about half of the time in a more heterogeneous group of general ICU patients. Furthermore, information from invasive monitoring made a difference in treatment with fluids, diuretics, vasopressors, or vasodilators about 50 percent of the time.[10–12]

Does use of the Swan-Ganz catheter improve outcome? This question has not been answered rigorously for obstetric patients. There is some evidence for improved outcome in patients with acute myocardial infarction and low cardiac output.[13] There is also evidence of improved outcome in critically ill postoperative patients managed with invasive monitoring targeted to specific hemodynamic endpoints (e.g., wedge pressure, cardiac index, and oxygen delivery).[14] It is important to recognize that the Swan-Ganz catheter is only a monitoring device that can improve patient care and outcome only if the data generated are accurately interpreted and if treatment exists for the condition present.[7]

Inserting the Swan-Ganz Catheter

Technique for Cannulating the Internal Jugular Vein

A pulmonary artery catheter may be inserted at several sites—internal jugular, external jugular, subclavian, basilic, and femoral veins. The right internal jugular is most commonly used because it provides a straight path to the right side of the heart and it has the lowest complication rate (Fig. 18-1). The internal jugular vein emerges from the base of the skull to enter the carotid sheath, which also contains the carotid artery and vagus nerve. Initially the internal jugular vein is posterior and lateral to the carotid artery. However, in the lower portion of the neck it lies lateral and slightly anterior to the carotid artery. The lower portion of the internal jugular vein lies within the triangle formed by the sternal and clavicular heads of the sternocleidomastoid muscle and the clavicle. It is within this triangle that the internal jugular vein is best cannulated (Fig. 18-2).

If the patient is obese or muscular with a short neck, place a small pillow or rolled towel under the shoulders to extend the neck. Have the patient turn her head 60 degrees to the contralateral side. The right internal jugular vein is usually easier to cannulate, and one avoids the risk of injuring the thoracic duct on the left. The patient is asked to raise her head so that the sternal

and clavicular heads of the sternocleidomastoid muscle can be palpated. The carotid artery is palpated; the vein lies lateral to it. The patient is then placed in the Trendelenberg position to distend the veins and to prevent air embolism. Several commercial trays containing the necessary equipment are available for central venous cannulation using the Seldinger technique (i.e., over a guidewire) (Fig. 18-3). The procedure is performed under continuous electrocardiographic (ECG) monitoring.

After the skin is prepared and a sterile drape is applied to the area, the junction of the two heads of the sternocleidomastoid muscle at the apex of the triangle is infiltrated with 1 percent lidocaine. A 1.5 in, 22-gauge needle with a 10-cc syringe may be used to locate the internal jugular vein. When the vein is found and the needle is withdrawn, the tract must be kept in the mind's eye. A large-bore (18-gauge) needle can next be used to follow this path for cannulation of the internal jugular vein. I prefer a slightly different technique in which the vein is cannulated directly using a Teflon catheter over a steel needle, which is used for routine intravenous therapy (18-gauge Cathlon). The needle enters at the apex of the triangle at about 30 degrees from the horizontal plane and is pointed along the medial border of the clavicular head of the sternocleidomastoid muscle toward the ipsilateral nipple. The

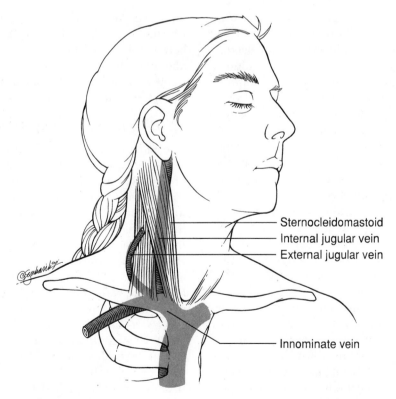

Fig. 18-1 Anatomic relationship of the internal jugular vein and the sternocleidomastoid muscle. The carotid artery lies just medial to the internal jugular vein.

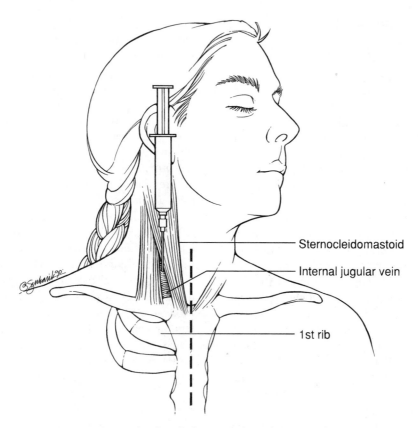

Fig. 18-2 Anatomic landmarks for internal jugular vein catheterization.

Sternocleidomastoid

Internal jugular vein

1st rib

needle is advanced with constant suction until a return of blood is obtained. Occasionally both sides of the vein will be traversed; however, withdrawing the needle slowly and maintaining suction will result in a return of blood. The flexible cannula is then advanced off the needle and is left in place in the vein. The most common problems are failing to locate the vein or puncturing the carotid artery. Usually the latter will be recognizable by pulsatile blood flow. However, occasionally, pressure monitoring is required to determine if the catheter is in the carotid artery. If the carotid has been inadvertently cannulated, the needle can be removed and direct pressure applied for 5 minutes. Another attempt may be made on the right or it may be necessary to go to the left side to insert the catheter.

The J wire (guide wire) is then inserted through the Teflon plastic catheter. This is an important step. If the J wire is introduced easily and moves back and forth freely, one feels confident in placing the vessel dilator and introducer over the J wire. If, on the other hand, one encounters resistance and the patient complains of pain, it is necessary to remove the J wire and aspirate from the catheter to make sure that its position still lies within the vein. Once the J wire is in place, a scalpel blade (No. 11) is used to enlarge the incision. The vessel dilator and introducer are then slipped as one over the

guide wire using firm pressure and a twisting motion, which is particularly important as the catheter passes between the ribs and into the chest. The vessel dilator and guidewire are then withdrawn. Blood should flow freely into the introducer sidearm. Air is removed from the system, and an intravenous infusion is started.

Inserting the Pulmonary Artery Catheter

The catheter is then removed from its sterile packaging. The balloon is checked by inflating with 1.5 ml of air and then deflated passively. The distal port is connected to the transducer that will be used for pulmonary artery pressure monitoring and flushed with heparinized saline. The same is repeated for the proximal infusion port and the central venous pressure port. If disposable transducers are used, it is important to check their calibration and to make sure that all transducers are zeroed to the midchest level. The integrity of the thermostatic wire is then checked by connecting the Swan-Ganz catheter to the cardiac output computer. The computer should register room temperature. The sterility sheath is then placed over the catheter. The tip of the catheter is moved up and down and the oscilloscope checked for pressure variation. The catheter is placed into the introducer with the curvature of the catheter directed to the patient's left side. After

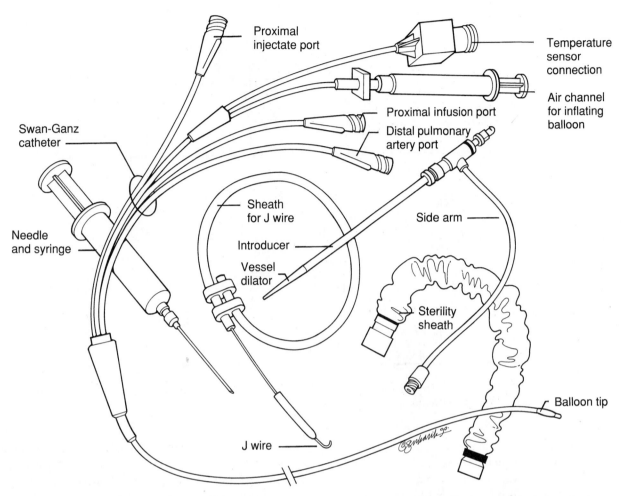

Fig. 18-3 Equipment needed for inserting Swan-Ganz catheter. The use of each piece of equipment is described in detail in the text.

the catheter has been advanced about 15 cm, the balloon is inflated with 1.5 ml of air. The ECG and pressure tracing are observed continuously as the catheter is advanced into the right ventricle. The right ventricle is recognized by its low diastolic pressure (0 to 5 mmHg). Once in the right ventricle, the catheter is moved quickly into the pulmonary artery. The pulmonary artery is recognized because its diastolic pressure is higher than that of the ventricle. The catheter is then passed out to the wedge position, which is usually at approximately the 40-cm mark on the catheter. The wedge tracing is a damped tracing that has a, c, and v waves similar to the right atrium (see below). The wedge pressure is usually slightly lower than the pulmonary artery diastolic pressure. When the balloon is emptied passively, the pulmonary artery tracing should reappear. The introducer is then sewn into place. Antibiotic ointment and an occlusive dressing are applied.

If frequent premature ventricular contractions or ventricular tachycardia develop when the Swan-Ganz catheter passes into the right ventricle, the balloon should be deflated and the catheter withdrawn immediately. If the pulmonary artery is not encountered after 30 cm of catheter has been inserted, the catheter is probably coiling in the ventricle. A chest x-ray should be obtained after the procedure to confirm proper placement of the catheter and to rule out pneumothorax. The strip chart recording of the passage through the heart is then examined and the right atrial, right ventricular, pulmonary artery, and wedge pressures are obtained at end expiration.

Hemodynamic Waveforms

The right atrial pressure tracing (Fig. 18-4A) consists of three distinct waves: a, c, and v. The a wave is a small wave due to atrial systole. The declining pressure that immediately follows the a wave is called the x descent. The c wave may or may not appear as a distinct wave. It reflects the increase in right atrial pressure produced by closure of the tricuspid valve. The negative wave following the c wave is called the x^1 descent. The v wave

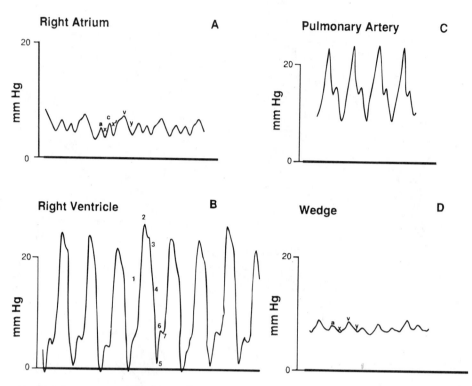

Fig. 18-4 (A–D) Pulmonary artery catheter placement. Waveforms and normal pressures. (Adapted from Daily and Schroeder,[130] with permission.)

is caused by right atrial filling and concomitant right ventricular systole, which causes the leaflets of the closed tricuspid valve to bulge back into the right atrium. The y descent immediately follows the v wave. The pressure changes produced by the a, c, and v waves are usually within 3 to 4 mmHg of each other so that the mean pressure is taken. The normal resting mean right atrial pressure is 2 to 6 mmHg. Elevated right atrial pressures may occur in the following conditions: right ventricular failure, tricuspid stenosis and regurgitation, cardiac tamponade, constrictive pericarditis, pulmonary hypertension, chronic left ventricular failure, and volume overload.

The phases of systole and diastole in the right ventricular pressure tracing can be divided into seven events. Systolic events include (1) isovolumetric contraction, (2) rapid ejection, and (3) reduced ejection. Diastolic events include (4) isovolumetric relaxation, (5) early diastole, (6) atrial systole, and (7) end diastole (Fig. 18-4B).

The pulmonary artery pressure tracing is shown in Figure 18-4C. There is a sharp rise in pressure followed by a decline in pressure as the volume decreases. When the right ventricular pressure falls below the level of the pulmonary artery pressure, the pulmonary valve snaps shut. This sudden closure of the valve leaflets causes the dicrotic notch in the pulmonary artery pressure tracing. Normal pulmonary artery systolic pres-

sure is 20 to 30 mmHg. Normal end-diastolic pressure is 8 to 12 mmHg. Elevated pulmonary artery pressures are seen in pulmonary disease, primary pulmonary hypertension, mitral stenosis or regurgitation, left ventricular failure, and intracardiac left-to-right shunts. Hypoxia increases pulmonary vascular resistance and pulmonary artery pressure.

When a small branch of the pulmonary artery is occluded by inflation of the balloon on the Swan-Ganz catheter, the pressure tracing reflects left atrial pressure. The waveform looks similar to the right atrial pressure tracing described above (Fig. 18-4A). The a wave of the wedge pressure is produced by left atrial contraction followed by the x descent (Fig. 18-4D). The c wave is produced by closure of the mitral valve, but is usually not seen. The v wave is produced by filling of the left atrium and bulging back of the mitral valve during ventricular systole. The decline following the v wave is called the y descent. The normal resting mean wedge pressure is 6 to 12 mmHg. Elevated wedge pressure is seen in left ventricular failure, mitral stenosis or regurgitation, cardiac tamponade, constrictive pericarditis, and volume overload.[15]

Determining the Hemodynamic Profile

Cardiac output is measured by the thermodilution cardiac output computer using five (10 cc) injections of iced saline. Highest and lowest values are discarded,

Table 18-1 Derived Hemodynamic Parameters

Parameter	Symbol	Formula	Units
Pulse pressure	PP	$BP_{syst} - BP_{diast}$	mmHg
Mean arterial pressure	MAP	$BP_{diast} + \frac{1}{3} PP$	mmHg
Cardiac index	CI	$\dfrac{CO}{BSA}$	$L \cdot min^{-1} \cdot m^2$
Stroke volume	SV	$\dfrac{CO \times 1.000}{HR}$	ml
Stroke index	SI	$\dfrac{SV}{BSA}$	$ml \cdot beat \cdot m^2$
Systemic vascular resistance	SVR	$\dfrac{MAP - CVP}{CO} \times 80$	$dynes \cdot sec \cdot cm^{-5}$
Systemic vascular resistance index	SVRI	$SVR \times BSA$	$dynes \cdot sec \cdot cm^{-5} \cdot m^2$
Pulmonary vascular resistance	PVR	$\dfrac{\overline{PAP} - PCWP}{CO} \times 80$	$dynes \cdot sec \cdot cm^{-5}$
Pulmonary vascular resistance index	PVRI	$PVR \times BSA$	$dynes \cdot sec \cdot cm^{-5} \cdot m^2$
Left ventricular stroke work	LVSW	$SV \times MAP \times 0.136$	$gm \cdot m$
Left ventricular stroke work index	LVSWI	$\dfrac{LVSW}{BSA}$	$gm \cdot m \cdot m^2$
Right ventricular stroke work	RVSW	$SV \times \overline{PAP} \times 0.136$	$gm \cdot m$
Right ventricular stroke work index	RVSWI	$\dfrac{RVSW}{BSA}$	$gm \cdot m \cdot m^2$

Abbreviations: BP$_{syst}$, systolic blood pressure; BP$_{diast}$, diastolic blood pressure; CO, cardiac output; HR, heart rate; BSA, body surface area; $\overline{PAP}$, mean pulmonary artery pressure; PCWP, pulmonary capillary wedge pressure.

with the mean of the three remaining values recorded. The following measured hemodynamic variables are then used to calculate the rest of the hemodynamic profile: heart rate, blood pressure, pulmonary artery pressure, pulmonary capillary wedge pressure, central venous pressure, cardiac output, and patient height and weight. The derived variables include cardiac index, stroke volume and index, systemic vascular resistance and index, pulmonary vascular resistance and index, and left and right ventricular stroke work and indices (Table 18-1 provides the formulas).[16]

Oxygen Transport

Arterial oxygen content is the sum of the oxygen bound to hemoglobin and that dissolved in plasma as described by the equation

$$CaO_2 = (Hgb \times 1.36 \times SaO_2) + (PaO_2 \times 0.003)$$

where 1.36 is the milliliters of oxygen bound to 1 g of hemoglobin (Hgb), SaO_2 is the arterial oxygen saturation, and 0.003 is the solubility coefficient of oxygen in human plasma. If $SaO_2 = 1.0$ or 100 percent saturated, Hgb = 15 g/dl, and $PaO_2 = 100$ mmHg. Then:

$$CaO_2 = (15 \times 1.36 \times 1.0) + (100 \times 0.003)$$
$$= 20 + 0.3$$
$$= 20 \text{ ml/dl}$$

The amount of oxygen dissolved in the plasma usually does not make a significant contribution to CaO_2.

Mixed venous blood gives an estimate of the balance between oxygen supply and demand. For example, in low cardiac output states with a high rate of peripheral oxygen extraction, mixed venous oxygen tension ($P\bar{v}O_2$) will be low. Normal $P\bar{v}O_2$ ranges from 35 to 45 mmHg, and mixed venous oxygen saturation ($S\bar{v}O_2$) ranges from 0.68 to 0.76 mmHg. Mixed venous oxygen content is measured on blood drawn from the pulmonary artery rather than from the superior vena cava or the right atrium. This is necessary because inferior vena cava blood has a higher oxygen saturation than superior vena cava blood and because drainage of coronary sinus blood into the right atrium contaminates the chamber with markedly desaturated blood due to the high myocardial oxygen extraction rate. After blood from the three sources passes through the right ventricle, it is thoroughly mixed.[16] A true mixed venous sample can thus be obtained. Mixed venous oxygen content is calculated as follows:

$$C\bar{v}O_2 = (Hgb \times 1.36 \times S\bar{v}O_2) + (P\bar{v}O_2 \times 0.003)$$

If Hgb = 15 g, $S\bar{v}O_2 = 0.75$, and $P\bar{v}O_2 = 40$ mmHg. Then:

$$C\bar{v}O_2 = (15 \times 1.36 \times 0.75) + (40 \times 0.003)$$
$$= 15 + 0.12$$
$$= 15 \text{ ml/dl}$$

The arterovenous (A-V) oxygen content difference is described by the equation:

$$A\text{-}\bar{V}O_2 = CaO_2 - C\bar{v}O_2$$

Substituting the above calculations,

$$A\text{-}\bar{V}O_2 = 20-15 = 5 \text{ ml } O_2/dl$$

The normal range of the arteriovenous oxygen content difference is 3.5 to 5.0 ml/dl.

Oxygen delivery ($\dot{D}O_2$) is the product of CaO_2 and cardiac output (CO) as expressed by the equation:

$$\dot{D}O_2 = CO \times CaO_2 \times 10$$

If cardiac output equals 5 L/min, then

$$\dot{D}O_2 = 5 \times 20 \times 10 = 1{,}000 \text{ ml/min}$$

Oxygen delivery is normally about 1,000 ml/min. Oxygen consumption ($\dot{V}O_2$) is the amount of oxygen that diffuses into the tissues and is expressed by the equation:

$$\dot{V}O_2 = CO \times (CaO_2 - C\bar{v}O_2) \times 10$$
$$= 5 \times 5 \times 10 = 250 \text{ ml/min}$$

Oxygen consumption is normally about 250 ml/min.[17]

Cardiopulmonary Profile

In aggregate, the hemodynamic and oxygen transport parameters described above provide invaluable information for the management of clinical problems. The data shown in Table 18-2 were derived from a single patient with severe preeclampsia near term. Among the measured variables, one notes borderline tachycardia, elevated blood pressure, normal pulmonary artery pressure, wedge pressure, central venous pressure, and cardiac output. Arterial and mixed venous blood gases are also normal, as are all of the derived variables. Because blood pressure = cardiac output × systemic vascular resistance, the hypertension seems to result from a systemic vascular resistance that is inappropriately high for the level of cardiac output.

Oxyhemoglobin Dissociation Curve

Some familiarity with the oxyhemoglobin dissociation curve is necessary to understand oxygen transport and the influence of shifts in the curve. Acidosis, increased red cell 2,3-diphosphoglycerate (DPG), and fever shift the curve to the right, thus reducing the hemoglobin affinity for oxygen and increasing oxygen unloading in the tissues. Alkalosis, reduced red cell 2,3-DPG, and hypothermia cause the curve to shift to the left with the opposite effects on tissue oxygenation. As shown in Figure 18-5, hemoglobin is 50 percent saturated (P_{50}) at a PaO_2 of 27 mmHg. A PaO_2 of 60 mmHg correlates with an oxygen saturation of about 90 percent. Therefore, little is gained in oxygen saturation by increasing PaO_2 much higher than 60 mmHg. On the other hand, below PaO_2 of 60 mmHg, small changes in PaO_2 result in large changes in oxygen saturation. A PaO_2 less than 20 mmHg is incompatible with life.[17]

Hemodynamic Support

Cardiac output is determined by four factors: preload, afterload, rate, and contractility. According to the Frank-Starling principle, the force of striated muscle contraction varies directly with the initial muscle length. The relationship between myocardial fiber length and fiber shortening can be graphically described by the curve in Figure 18-6. Fiber length can best be equated with preload or filling volume of the ventricle. To allow clinical estimation of preload the pressure correlate of the filling volume is used (i.e., right or left ventricular end-diastolic pressure). Varying compliance will alter the pressure-volume relationship. For example, a poorly compliant left ventricle resulting from myocardial hypertrophy or ischemia requires higher intracavitary pressure to achieve a specific end-diastolic volume or fiber stretch.[18]

Afterload is defined as the wall tension of the ventricle during ejection. This is best reflected by the systolic blood pressure. In the absence of aortic or pulmonary stenosis, vascular resistance in the appropriate bed—systemic or pulmonary—will determine the afterload for that side of the heart. The effect of afterload on ventricular output is shown in Figure 18-7.[18]

Heart rate has a marked effect on cardiac output (i.e., cardiac output = heart rate × stroke volume). Increases in head rate are accomplished at the expense of diastolic filling time, systolic emptying time being rate independent. Marked increases in heart rate may lead to circulatory depression when they cause myocardial ischemia or when reduced diastolic filling or loss of atrial "kick" prevents adequate ventricular preload. As a general rule, heart rates exceeding 220-age/min reduce cardiac output and myocardial perfusion.[19]

Contractility is defined as the force of ventricular contraction when preload and afterload are held constant. An increase in contractility is associated with an increase in stroke volume despite no change in preload. Factors that affect contractility include sympathetic impulses, catecholamines, acid-base and electrolyte disturbances, ischemia, loss of myocardium, hypoxia, and drugs or toxins. A third heart sound, distant heart

Table 18-2 Cardiopulmonary Profile in Severe Preeclampsia

Measured Variable	Patient Value	Normal Values for Pregnancy
Heart rate (HR)	93	60–100 beats/min
Blood pressure (BP)	180/105 (130)	70–100 mmHg
Pulmonary artery pressure (PAP)	23/9 (14)	10–20 mmHg
Pulmonary capillary wedge pressure (PCWP)	7	6–12 mmHg
Central venous pressure (CVP)	3	1–7 mmHg
Cardiac output (CO)	7.29	5.0–7.5 L/min
Height	149	NA cm
Weight	67.3	NA kg
Inhaled oxygen fraction (FiO_2)	0.21	0.21
Hemoglobin	10.6	11.0–13.5 gm/dl
Arterial pH (pHa)	7.35	7.36–7.45
Arterial partial pressure of oxygen (PaO_2)	94	80–100 mmHg
Arterial partial pressure of carbon dioxide ($PaCO_2$)	31	28–32 mmHg
Arterial oxygen saturation (SaO_2)	0.97	0.95
Mixed venous oxygen tension ($P\bar{v}O_2$)	44	35–45 mmHg
Mixed venous oxygen saturation ($S\bar{v}O_2$)	0.74	0.68–0.76
Body surface area (BSA)	1.71	NA m^2
Cardiac index (CI)	4.26	3.0–4.6 L/min/m^2
Stroke volume (SV)	78.4	60–90 ml/beat
Stroke index (SI)	45.8	35–53 ml/beat/m^2
Systemic vascular resistance (SVR)	1,393	800–1,500 dynes·sec·cm^{-5}
Systemic vascular resistance index (SVRI)	2,382	1,360–2,550 dynes·sec·cm^{-5}·m^2
Pulmonary vascular resistance (PVR)	77	50–150 dynes·sec·cm^{-5}
Pulmonary vascular resistance index (PVRI)	132	85–255 dynes·sec·cm^{-5}·m^2
Left ventricular stroke work index (LVSWI)	81.1	42–54 gm/m/m^2
Arterial oxygen content (CaO_2)	14.3	20 ml/dl
Mixed venous oxygen content ($C\bar{v}O_2$)	10.8	15 ml/dl
A-V oxygen content difference ($C[a\text{-}\bar{v}]O_2$)	3.46	3.5–5.0 ml/dl
Oxygen delivery ($\dot{D}O_2$)	1040	1,000 ml/dl
Oxygen consumption ($\dot{V}O_2$)	252	250 ml/dl

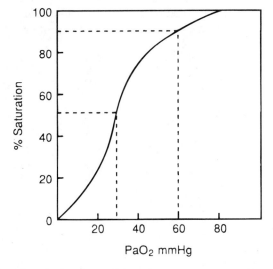

Fig. 18-5 The oxyhemoglobin dissociation curve of normal blood. Hemoglobin is 50 percent saturated at a PaO_2 of 27 mmHg. A PaO_2 of 60 mmHg correlates with an oxygen saturation of about 90 percent.

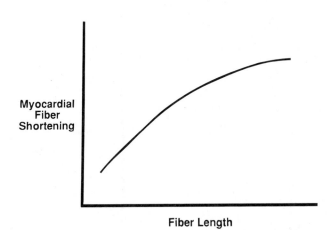

Fig. 18-6 Starling curve relating myocardial fiber length to fiber shortening. (From Rosenthal,[18] with permission.)

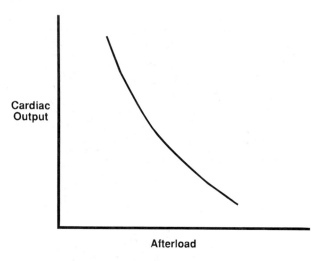

Fig. 18-7 Relationship of afterload to cardiac output at a constant preload. (From Rosenthal,[18] with permission.)

Table 18-3   Hemodynamic Therapy

Decreased preload	Decreased afterload	Contractility
Crystalloid	Volume	Dopamine
Colloid	Inotropic support	Dobutamine
Blood	Vasopressors	Epinephrine
	Norepinephrine	Calcium[a]
	Phenylephrine	Digitalis[b]
	Metaraminol	
Increased preload	Increased afterload	
Diuretics	Arterial dilators	
Furosemide	Hydralazine	
Ethacrynic	Diazoxide	
acid	Mixed arterial-	
Mannitol	venous dilators	
Venodilators	Nitroprusside	
Furosemide	Trimethaphan	
Nitroglycerin	Venous dilators	
Morphine	Nitroglycerin	

[a] May produce marked increase in systemic vascular resistance.
[b] Of questionable value and safety for acute management.
(Adapted from Rosenthal,[18] with permission.)

sounds, and a narrow pulse pressure suggest impaired contractility. Radionuclide ventriculograms and two-dimensional echocardiography allow determination of ventricular size and contractile state. Effects of altered myocardial contractility on cardiac output at a given preload are shown in Figure 18-8.[18,19]

Figure 18-9 uses the Starling curves to summarize the effects of increases and decreases of preload, afterload, and contractility on ventricular function. The agents used to treat hemodynamic instability are grouped in Table 18-3. The therapeutic rationale for supporting the cardiovascular system based on the Frank-Starling relationship is illustrated in Figure 18-10.

The primary adjustment to improve low cardiac output is to optimize preload using volume administration. Because of the lack of correlation between measurements on the right and left sides of the heart in patients with significant cardiopulmonary disease, pulmonary

capillary wedge pressure is monitored to optimize left ventricular preload and to avoid pulmonary edema. If blood pressure and cardiac output do not respond to fluids (e.g., pulmonary capillary wedge pressure of approximately 15 mmHg), then a positive inotropic agent may be needed to increase myocardial contractility. Dopamine is the drug of choice in most situations. It is utilized because its activity is modified at different doses. At 2 to 3 μg/kg/min, renal and splanchnic vasodilatation occur. Positive inotropy occurs up to 10 μg/kg/min. Vasoconstriction predominates over 10 μg/kg/min. These dose ranges reflect a predominance of action only. There is a great deal of overlap and individuality of response. The usual therapeutic range for dopamine in clinical practice is 1 to 10 μg/kg/min. When the requirement exceeds this, a more potent vasopres-

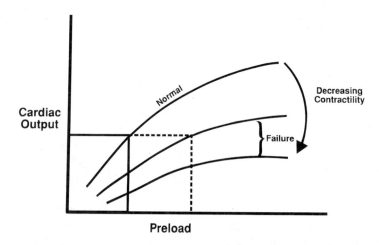

Fig. 18-8 Cardiac function curves demonstrating downward displacement secondary to decreased contractility and failure. Dotted line represents increased preload demands in failure. (From Rosenthal,[18] with permission.)

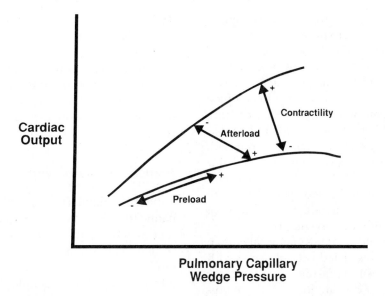

Fig. 18-9 Alteration in Starling curve of ventricular function caused by increases and decreases in preload, afterload, and contractility. (From Rosenthal,[18] with permission.)

sor such as norepinephrine is added; and the dopamine is decreased to renotonic doses in the hope that renal blood flow will be preserved.

Afterload may be manipulated with vasodilators in cardiac failure or in low cardiac output states secondary to severe hypertension. Vasodilators have varying effects on arterial and venous resistances. Nitroglycerin, which is predominantly a venodilator, may cause a greater reduction in preload than in afterload. Nitroprusside, an equal arterial and venular vasodilatator, may be preferred; however, marked decreases in systemic vascular resistance result in hypotension, poor perfusion, and myocardial ischemia. The use of a vaso-

dilator requires careful observation of the adequacy of intravascular volume and the net effect on cardiac output.[18]

Clinical Management

Preeclampsia

The etiology, pathophysiology, and management of preeclampsia are discussed in Chapter 28. Although the indications for invasive hemodynamic monitoring in preeclampsia have not been firmly established, Swan-Ganz monitoring has been recommended for the management of pulmonary edema, oliguria, refractory

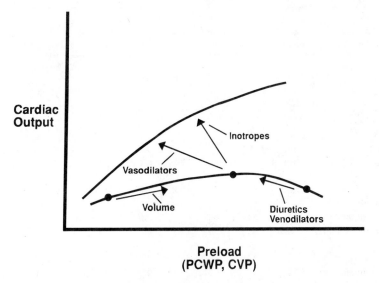

Fig. 18-10 Treatment approaches for altered hemodynamic states based on Starling's law of the heart. PCWP, pulmonary capillary wedge pressure; CVP, central venous pressure. (From Rosenthal[18] with permission.)

hypertension, and epidural anesthesia and as a guide to volume expansion in efforts to prolong pregnancy in early onset severe preeclampsia.[20,21] These indications are rather broad. The great majority of preeclamptic women can be managed with clinical acumen. Invasive hemodynamic monitoring is needed most in complex cases with multiple organ dysfunction or pre-existing cardiac disease or in obese patients with pulmonary edema in whom clinical examination is compromised. Thus, the main value of invasive monitoring in preeclampsia is as a research tool to study the pathophysiology of the disease, to define hemodynamic subsets of patients, and to evaluate the hemodynamic effects of drugs, anesthesia, and other interventions.

The cardiovascular hemodynamics of normal human pregnancy have been investigated over the years with many techniques for measuring cardiac output, including the Fick principle,[22-25] dye dilution,[26-28] thermodilution,[21,29-31] radioiodinated human serum albumin,[32] echocardiography (M-mode, two-dimensional, and Doppler),[33-38] and transthoracic electrical impedance.[39-41] While there is now some consensus on the hemodynamics of normal pregnancy, the data are conflicting.[42] Nearly every author reports different results. There is even more disagreement when one examines serial longitudinal studies of cardiac output in pregnancy and postpartum and the effects of position change, exercise, labor, delivery, and anesthesia. The same lack of agreement is found in studies of preeclampsia. In addition to the above sources of variability, the lack of agreement among hemodynamic studies in preeclamptic patients has been attributed to differences in the definition of preeclampsia, variable severity and duration of disease, underlying cardiac or renal disease, small numbers of patients in each series, the technique for measuring cardiac output, and therapeutic interventions before study entry. In addition, the dynamic, minute-to-minute fluctuation of the cardiovascular system makes it difficult to standardize conditions under which observations are made and limits the value of a single point on a continuum.

Hemodynamics of Normal Pregnancy

Table 18-4 summarizes several of the invasive hemodynamic studies in normal pregnancy. These data represent patients in the third trimester lying in the lateral recumbent position. As previously noted, the mean values for each parameter are quite variable, and there is a broad range. For example, Ueland et al.[27] found a mean cardiac output of 6.7 L/min, ranging from 3.7 to 8.4 L/min. Three of the more important recent studies done with the Swan-Ganz catheter are those by Groenendijk et al.,[30] Wallenburg,[21] and Clark et al.[31] Groenendijk et al. and Wallenburg reported cardiac index, while Clark et al. reported cardiac output. Using 1.7 m^2 for the mean body surface area to convert cardiac index to cardiac output results in a mean output of 7.6 and 6.8 L/min, respectively, for the two Dutch studies compared with 6.2 ± 1.0 L/min in the study by Clark et al. Corresponding systemic vascular resistances are slightly lower in the Dutch studies, although wedge pressures and central venous pressures agree among the three investigations. After synthesizing the hemodynamic data reported in Table 18-4, the author pro-

Table 18-4   Invasive Hemodynamic Findings During the Third Trimester

Author (Year)	Method of Determination	No. of Patients	MAP (mmHg)	HR (beats/ min)	SV (ml)	CO (L/min)	SVR (dynes·sec· cm^{-5})	CI (L·min^{-1}· m^2)	SVRI (dynes·sec· cm^{-5}·m^2)	PCWP (mmHg)	CVP (mmHg)
Hamilton[22] (1948)	Fick					4.6					
Werko[23] (1954)	Fick	11	99	83	71	6.5					
Bader et al[24] (1955)	Fick	11	90	96	58	5.5	1,244	3.4		5	
Walters et al[26] (1966)	Dye Dilution	15		78	79	6.2					
Kerr[25] (1968)	Fick	5	86	84	76	6.3	1,119				
Smith[32] (1970)	RIHSA	10	79			4.5					
Ueland et al[27] (1972)	Dye Dilution	13		86	79	6.7	1,056				
Lim and Walters[28] (1979)	Dye Dilution	23	86	80	93	7.8	1,540				
Lees[29] (1979)	Thermodilution	14	85	84		5.9	1,145				
Groenendijk et al[30] (1984)	Thermodilution	4	95	84			886	4.5		9	
Wallenburg[21] (1988)	Thermodilution	7	83	80				4.0	1,629	6	4
Clark et al[31] (1989)	Thermodilution	10	90	83		6.2	1,210			8	4

Abbreviations: MAP, mean arterial pressure; HR, heart rate; SV, stroke volume; CO, cardiac output; SVR, systemic vascular resistance; CI, cardiac index; SVRI, systemic vascular resistance index; PCWP, pulmonary capillary wedge pressure; CVP, central venous pressure.

Table 18-5   Normal Hemodynamic Values for the Third Trimester of Pregnancy

Parameter	Value
Heart rate	60–100 beats/min
Mean arterial pressure	70–100 mmHg
Pulmonary capillary wedge pressure	6–12 mmHg
Central venous pressure	1–7 mmHg
Cardiac output	5.0–7.5 L/min
Cardiac index	3.0–4.6 L/min^{-1}/m^{-2}
Stroke volume	60–90 ml
Systemic vascular resistance	800–1,500 dynes·sec·cm^{-5}
Systemic vascular resistance index	1,360–2,550 dynes·sec·cm^{-5}·m^2
Pulmonary vascular resistance	50–150 dynes·sec·cm^{-5}
Pulmonary vascular resistance index	85–255 dynes·sec·cm^{-5}·m^2

poses a normal range for hemodynamic parameters in the third trimester of pregnancy (Table 18-5).

Hemodynamics of Preeclampsia

The cardiovascular hemodynamics of preeclampsia are uncertain, having been reported to range from a low output–high resistance state to a high output–low resistance state. In an insightful analysis, Hankins et al.[43] categorized studies by therapy prior to insertion of the Swan-Ganz catheter. They felt that much of the variation in reported data was related to prior treatment (e.g., intravenous fluids, magnesium sulfate, and hydralazine). This categorization of studies has been expanded in Table 18-6.

Actually, prior treatment is only one factor in determining hemodynamics. Before therapy, Cotton et al.[44] found wedge pressure, cardiac output, and systemic vascular resistance to be within the normal range. The findings of Nisell et al.[45] on cardiac output and systemic vascular resistance agreed with those of Cotton et al.[44] On the other hand, Groenendijk et al.,[30] Wallenburg,[21] and Belfort et al.[46,47] found low wedge pressure, normal to low cardiac index, and elevated systemic vascular resistance. In the fluid restriction group,[48–53] all but Hankins et al.[49] found a normal wedge pressure, and all authors found a normal to slightly elevated cardiac output and systemic vascular resistance. Using volume expansion, wedge pressure was normal to high in studies by Rafferty and Berkowitz[54] and Phelan and Yurth[55] but low in the study by Rolbin et al.[56] Cardiac output was elevated in all three studies, and systemic vascular resistance was normal. In the final group in which prior fluid administration and drug therapy were unclear, results were similar to the fluid restriction group with

normal wedge pressure and normal to slightly elevated cardiac output and systemic vascular resistance.[29,57–60]

Phelan and Yurth[55] were the first to propose that a spectrum of hemodynamic changes characterized preeclampsia. The two extremes of the spectrum are represented by the data of Wallenburg[21] and Mabie et al.[51]

Wallenburg's data support the traditional view of preeclampsia—that it is a volume-contracted, vasospastic state. He found a low wedge pressure, low cardiac output, and high systemic vascular resistance in 44 untreated nulliparous preeclamptic patients. In 22 patients who had received various therapies and had been referred to his center, a wide range of hemodynamics was found. He concluded that the untreated patient was significantly volume depleted and that the wide spectrum of hemodynamic findings present in the treated group resulted from prior therapy and the presence of other variables such as labor, multiparity, and pre-existing hypertension. Thus, the disparity in cardiac outputs, peripheral resistances, and wedge pressures among various studies was not due to the hemodynamic variability of preeclampsia but rather to differences in patient selection and therapeutic intervention prior to invasive monitoring.

Mabie et al.[51] studied the hemodynamics of 49 subjects with severe preeclampsia at a large referral center. Despite a heterogeneous population of referred and nonreferred patients, pretreated and nonpretreated individuals, a generally consistent profile emerged. Preeclampsia was in general a high cardiac output state associated with an inappropriately high peripheral resistance. Although the systemic vascular resistance was within the normal range, it was still inappropriately high for the elevated cardiac output. The failure of the circulation to dilate in the setting of increasing cardiac output appeared to be a characteristic feature of preeclampsia. The normal wedge pressure and central venous pressures found in their study suggested central redistribution of intravascular volume if the generally accepted reports of decreased plasma volume in preeclampsia are correct. They postulated splanchnic venoconstriction as the mechanism for this volume shift. Mabie et al.[51] also noted that, while the hemodynamic profile is variable in preeclampsia, it is variable in virtually every other type of experimental and naturally occurring hypertension. They pointed out that Wallenburg had minimized the variable hemodynamic presentation of his untreated group in that 15 percent or more had wedge pressures greater than 8 mmHg, indicating normal central blood volume.

Although there is a wide range of hemodynamic findings, comparing the mean cardiac output and systemic vascular resistance from the studies listed in Table 18-4 to those in Table 18-5 may be instructive. Mean cardiac

Table 18-6 Invasive Hemodynamic Findings in Severe Preeclampsia and Eclampsia

Author	No. of Patients	PCWP (mmHg)	CVP (mmHg)	CO (L/min)	CI (L/min^{-1}/m^2)	SVR (dynes·sec·cm^{-5})	SVRI (dynes·sec·cm^{-5}·m^2)
No therapy[a]							
Cotton et al[44]	5	12.0	6.0	7.6	4.8	1,350	2,256
Nisell et al[45]	21			7.6		1,160	
Groenendijk et al[30]	10	3.3		5.3	2.8	1,943	
Wallenburg[21]	44	4.0	1.0		3.0		2,970
Belfort et al[46]	10	5.0	2.0		3.0	2,392	
Belfort et al[47]	6	6.0	6.0		3.2	1,965	
Magnesium, hydralazine, fluid restriction							
Benedetti et al[48]	10	6.0	3.0	7.4	4.7	1,322	
Hankins et al[49]	8	3.9	1.0	6.7	4.3	1,357	
Cotton et al[50]	45	10.0	4.0	7.5	4.1	1,496	2,726
Mabie et al[51]	41	8.3	4.8	8.4	4.4	1,226	2,293
Wasserstrum et al[52]	8	7.9	3.4		3.7		3,066
Wasserstrum et al[53]	7	11.0	4.0		4.2		
Magnesium, hydralazine, volume expansion							
Rafferty and Berkowitz[54]	3	7.0		11.0	6.2	917	
Phelan and Yurth[55]	10	16.4	9.7	9.3	5.4	1,042	
Rolbin et al[56]	4	5.2		9.7	5.2	1,040	
Unclear about previous treatment							
Graham and Goldstein[57]	10			8.8			
Newsome et al[58]	11				5.0	1,078	
Lees[29]	14			5.8		1,590	
Cotton et al[59]	6	9.0	2.0		3.5		3,330
Clark et al[60]	9	9.2	4.1	8.5	4.2	1,388	

Abbreviations: PWCP, pulmonary capillary wedge pressure; CVP, central venous pressure; CO, cardiac output; CI, cardiac index; SVR, systemic vascular resistance; SVRI, systemic vascular resistance index.

[a] All studies were performed using the Swan-Ganz thermodilution technique except the study by Nisell et al,[45] which used dye dilution.

output is 6.0 L/min, and mean systemic vascular resistance is 1,171 dynes·sec·cm^{-5} in the normotensive, third trimester patients. In severe preeclampsia, mean cardiac output is 8.0 L/min and mean systemic vascular resistance is 1,418 dynes·sec·cm^{-5}. Thus, cardiac output and systemic vascular resistance both tend to be higher in studies of preeclampsia.

In summary, it is too early to draw firm conclusions about the central hemodynamics of preeclampsia. However, there are several points that most authors agree on: (1) preeclampsia includes a spectrum of hemodynamic findings with variable wedge pressures, cardiac outputs, and systemic vascular resistances; (2) pulmonary vascular resistance is unaffected; and (3) systemic vascular resistance is elevated. If not above the normal range for pregnancy, systemic vascular resistance is at least inappropriately high for the level of cardiac output.

Effects of Volume Expansion in Preeclampsia

Because many studies have shown either contracted plasma volume in preeclampsia[61,62] or low wedge pressures,[21,30,46,47] volume expansion has been advocated in the treatment of severe preeclampsia. A few studies of malignant hypertension in the nonpregnant patient have also advocated volume expansion to prevent circulatory collapse precipitated by vasodilator therapy.[63] Advocates of volume expansion have shown that it causes no rise or a fall in blood pressure, yet an increase in cardiac output and a fall in systemic vascular resistance. They suggest that volume expansion prevents precipitous falls in blood pressure during vasodilator therapy; thus, uteroplacental circulation is not compromised.[64–67]

Kirshon et al.[68] managed 15 primigravid patients

with severe preeclampsia using the following protocol: *Step 1:* Colloid osmotic pressure was optimized to 17 mmHg with infusions of 25 percent albumin. *Step 2:* Pulmonary capillary wedge pressure was optimized to 10–15 mmHg with 5 percent albumin infusion. *Step 3:* Mean arterial pressure was reduced by 20 percent or to a mean of 106 mmHg with intravenous nitroglycerin, nitroprusside, or hydralazine.

The results were compared with a control group undergoing Swan-Ganz catheterization but not having volume expansion. The only benefit derived from volume expansion was an absence of acute fetal distress after initiation of antihypertensive therapy. Six of 15 patients (40 percent) still developed fetal distress in labor, suggesting that volume expansion does not affect the overall incidence of fetal distress. No pulmonary edema occurred, but nearly all patients required furosemide postpartum to control wedge pressures.

There are other arguments against volume expansion. The effects of volume loading are transient. If colloid is used, it may "leak" into the alveoli, while crystalloid decreases oncotic pressure, which is already depressed in preeclampsia. In 8 of 10 preeclamptic patients described by Benedetti et al.,[69] colloid had been given prior to the onset of pulmonary edema. Postpartum mobilization of extravascular fluid further predisposes the preeclamptic patient to pulmonary edema.[49] While volume overload may be avoided with central hemodynamic monitoring, such monitoring is not without risk.[5] Moreover, numerous studies indicate that monitoring central venous pressure alone is not adequate in severe preeclampsia.[3,4] Furthermore, volume expansion seems to be counterproductive in that it makes patients more refractory to vasodilators, necessitating higher doses. On the contrary, in the treatment of hypertensive emergencies in the nonpregnant patient, a loop diuretic is advised for its synergistic effect with other antihypertensive agents.[70] Finally, part of the hemodynamic instability characteristic of severe preeclampsia is caused by baroreflex dysfunction. Wasserstrum et al.[53] looked at Δ heart rate/Δ blood pressure and Δ cardiac index/Δ blood pressure in response to hydralazine-induced falls in blood pressure. A high baseline blood pressure was associated with a dramatic reduction in baroreflex sensitivity and control of blood pressure. Baroreflex dysfunction has been described in many other forms of hypertension as well. In summary, it is not yet clear whether or in what circumstances volume expansion is indicated in preeclampsia.[71]

Pulmonary Edema in Preeclampsia

Pulmonary edema in preeclampsia may be divided into cardiogenic (wedge pressure >18 mmHg) and noncardiogenic (wedge pressure <18 mmHg) forms as sum-

Causes of Pulmonary Edema in Preeclampsia

Cardiogenic
  Systolic dysfunction
  Diastolic dysfunction
  Combined

Noncardiogenic
  Increased capillary permeability

Narrowed COP-wedge gradient
  Decreased COP
  Delayed mobilization of extravascular fluid
  Iatrogenic fluid overload

marized below. Cardiogenic pulmonary edema may result from systolic dysfunction or impaired myocardial contractility (e.g., peripartum cardiomyopathy). It may also result from diastolic dysfunction or impaired myocardial relaxation. Patients with left ventricular hypertrophy due to chronic hypertension develop diastolic dysfunction, which precedes the development of systolic dysfunction by several years. These patients, who have thick walls and stiff ventricles, require high filling pressures and are thus predisposed to develop hydrostatic pulmonary edema if they retain excess sodium and water during late pregnancy or receive an iatrogenic fluid overload. Combined systolic and diastolic dysfunction usually occurs in elderly multiparas with long-standing, severe hypertension.[72,73] Echocardiography is a readily available, noninvasive method for assessing ventricular dimensions, mass, and function, as well as valvular morphology and function. It may be used to define subgroups and to tailor therapy according to cardiac structure and function.[74]

Noncardiogenic pulmonary edema results either from a pulmonary capillary leak or from narrowing of the colloid osmotic pressure (COP)–wedge pressure gradient. Plasma proteins such as albumin, globulins, and fibrinogen exert osmotic pressure to hold water in the vasculature, counteracting hydrostatic pressure that pushes water out of the vasculature. Interstitial COP and interstitial hydrostatic pressure have similar antagonistic effects on the other side of the membrane.

Normal intravascular COP in the nonpregnant state is 25.4 ± 2.3 mmHg, whereas normal wedge pressure (a measure of pulmonary vascular hydrostatic pressure) is 6 to 12 mmHg.[75] Therefore, the normal COP–wedge gradient is about 12 mmHg. A COP–wedge gradient of 4 or less has been associated with an increased risk of pulmonary edema.[76] The normal COP in pregnancy at term is 22.4 ± 0.5 mmHg. With delivery accompanied by blood loss and crystalloid replacement, COP decreases to 15.4 ± 2.1 mmHg.[77,78] With preeclampsia, COP has been reported to fall from 17.9 ± 0.7 to 13.7 ± 0.5 mmHg postpartum.[79] This narrowing of the COP–wedge gradient reflects predisposition to pulmonary edema.

Pulmonary edema associated with preeclampsia eclampsia usually occurs postpartum.[69,80] Serum albumin decreases due to renal losses, impaired liver synthesis, and blood loss with crystalloid replacement. Wedge pressure increases due to delayed mobilization of extravascular fluid. Beginning 24 to 72 hours postpartum, edema fluid is mobilized and returned to the intravascular space faster than the diseased kidneys can excrete it. Iatrogenic fluid overload may also contribute to raising the wedge pressure; however, elevations in filling pressure may not be significant enough to account for pulmonary edema without simultaneous lowering of the intravascular COP.

Oliguria in Preeclampsia

Oliguria has been variously defined as, for example, urine output less than 30 ml/h × 3 hr;[60] less than 30 ml/h × 2 hr;[81] less than 0.5 ml/kg/h × 2 hr;[82] and less than 500 ml/24 hr.[83] The pathogenesis of oliguria in severe preeclampsia is not well defined, and appropriate management remains unsettled.

Clark et al.[60] studied nine patients with severe preeclampsia and oliguria (<30 ml/h × 3 hr) using the Swan-Ganz catheter. Eight patients were in labor and one was postpartum. Three hemodynamic subsets were defined. In category 1, five patients had low wedge pressures, normal cardiac indices, and elevated systemic vascular resistances. Their oliguria improved with volume expansion. In category 2, three patients had normal to high wedge pressures and cardiac indices and normal systemic vascular resistances. These patients responded to fluid and/or afterload reduction with hydralazine. They were thought to have renal arterial spasm as the cause of their oliguria. A single patient, in category 3, had high wedge pressure, low cardiac index, and high systemic vascular resistance. She responded to hydralazine and volume restriction. Clark et al.[60] advocated placement of a pulmonary artery catheter to guide management of oliguric patients with severe preeclampsia.

Lee et al.[81] compared urinary diagnostic indices to wedge pressure in seven oliguric, preeclamptic patients. Although urine sodium was high in six patients, indicating intrinsic renal disease, most of the other parameters indicated prerenal disease (e.g., urine osmolality, urine/plasma urea nitrogen, urine/plasma creatinine, renal failure index, and fractional excretion of sodium). Swan-Ganz readings showed predominantly normal wedge pressures (mean 8.7 mmHg, range 4 to 14), indicating euvolemia. Lee et al.[81] concluded that oliguria is a poor index of volume status in preeclamptic women and that urinary diagnostic indices may be misleading if used to guide fluid management in these patients.

Kirshon et al.[82] studied the hemodynamic and renal function effects of low-dose dopamine (1 to 5 µg/kg/min) in six antepartum, oliguric patients with severe preeclampsia. Cardiac output increased from 6.8 ± 1.8 to 8.0 ± 2.3 L/min. Blood pressure, central venous pressure, and wedge pressure did not change significantly from baseline. Urine output increased from a mean of 21 ± 10 to 43 ± 23 ml/hr. The fractional excretion of sodium, negative free water clearance, and osmolal clearance increased during dopamine therapy. The best response in urine flow was seen in patients with the highest wedge pressures. No adverse maternal or fetal effects were noted.

Barton et al.[83] randomized 31 patients into nifedipine (10 mg) or placebo groups, treated every 4 hours beginning immediately after delivery and continuing for 48 hours. Nifedipine did not have a marked effect on blood pressure, since the patients were not very hypertensive; however, the authors observed almost a doubling of urine output (3,934 vs. 2,057 ml) during the first 24 hours after delivery in the nifedipine-treated group. The mechanism of the beneficial effect on urine flow is unknown, but it may have been related to increased renal blood flow or to a natriuretic effect of nifedipine on the proximal convoluted tubule.

One of the first considerations in the oliguric patient is simply to be certain that the Foley catheter is not displaced from the urethra or malfunctioning. It may be helpful to irrigate the catheter with sterile saline and to note whether full return of the irrigant is obtained. Further evaluation of the oliguric patient requires many factors to be considered: antepartum versus postpartum oliguria, history, physical examination, postural changes in blood pressure, blood loss, intake and output, medications, hematocrit, blood urea nitrogen, creatinine, and electrolytes. Urinary diagnostic indices are noninvasive and inexpensive tests, but they must be interpreted with caution in preeclampsia. Prerenal findings suggesting the need for volume expansion include urine sodium less than 20 mEq/L, urine osmolality more than 500 mOsm/kg, urine/plasma urea nitrogen more than 8, urine/plasma creatinine more than 40, renal failure index less than 1, and fractional excretion of sodium below 1.

In treating the oliguric patient, a fluid challenge may be given. For example, 500 ml of normal saline may be administered intravenously over 30 minutes on two occasions. At least 1 hour should be allowed to observe a response in urine output. A trial of furosemide may be given if the patient is thought to be euvolemic or volume overloaded. Dopamine or nifedipine may be tried. Finally, a Swan-Ganz catheter may be placed in order to categorize the central hemodynamics and to guide therapy.

Cardiac Disease

A more complete discussion of cardiac disease is found elsewhere in this volume (Ch. 29). However, the role of invasive monitoring in certain cardiac lesions is considered here. Most New York Heart Association class 3 and 4 patients should have invasive hemodynamic monitoring during labor and delivery. In some patients with complex congenital heart disease, placement of a pulmonary artery catheter is not recommended because the anatomic defect makes it difficult to determine where the catheter is located.

Mitral Stenosis

In the pregnant patient, mitral stenosis is the principal lesion resulting from rheumatic heart disease. Patients with mitral stenosis may have a reasonable cardiac output, albeit relatively fixed. They cannot increase their cardiac output in response to a greater oxygen demand. Normal pregnancy results in increased blood volume, heart rate, and stroke volume. Thus, the pregnant patient with mitral stenosis has a shorter time to get a larger amount of blood across a stenotic valve, resulting in increased left atrial pressure. Because there are no valves in the pulmonary circuit, increased right-sided pressures and eventually right ventricular failure occur. The patient with mitral stenosis is, thus, closer to being in pulmonary edema when she is pregnant than when she is not pregnant.

Clark et al.[84] used invasive hemodynamic monitoring to study 10 pregnant patients with mitral stenosis. A major finding was that postpartum autotransfusion of blood from the contracting uterus resulted in a 10 ± 6 mmHg increase in wedge pressure. This increase in blood volume was thought to explain the occurrence of pulmonary edema in the early postpartum period in patients with mitral stenosis. Clark et al.[84] suggested the following protocol for management using a pulmonary artery catheter: (1) keep the heart rate less than 90 beats/min with a β-blocker (e.g., propranolol or esmolol) to allow sufficient diastolic filling time; (2) maintain wedge pressure during labor at 12 to 14 mmHg with furosemide or fluid restriction in anticipation of a postpartum increase in wedge pressure of 10 mmHg; and (3) use epidural anesthesia to relieve pain and anxiety, thus reducing oxygen demand.

Hypertrophic Obstructive Cardiomyopathy

Resulting from asymmetric hypertrophy of the interventricular septum, this lesion may be of varying severity. These patients have four cardiac problems: (1) dia-

stolic dysfunction, (2) sudden death due to ventricular arrhythmias, (3) obstruction to left ventricular outflow produced by systolic anterior motion of the mitral valve, and (4) mitral regurgitation. During labor, patients should be kept "wet" and "slow." Sufficient fluid should be given so that there is no obstruction to left ventricular outflow, and heart rate should be controlled with a β-blocker if necessary to allow sufficient diastolic filling time.[85]

Eisenmenger Syndrome

Eisenmenger syndrome usually results from an unrecognized ventricular septal defect or a patent ductus arteriosus. Because of their long-standing left-to-right shunt, these patients develop medial hypertrophy of the pulmonary vasculature and pulmonary hypertension. After many years, pulmonary artery pressures equal or exceed systemic pressures; thus, shunt reversal occurs. Ideally, these women should not undertake a pregnancy, because the maternal mortality rate is 25 to 50 percent.[86] During pregnancy, systemic vascular resistance falls due to the vasodilating effects of estrogen, progesterone, prolactin, prostaglandins, and the arteriovenous shunt in the placenta. Pulmonary vascular resistance remains high and fixed. As pregnancy progresses, these patients will shunt more and more blood right to left, thus bypassing their lungs. In labor, they require adequate preload and must be well hydrated before epidural anesthesia is given.[87] A Swan-Ganz catheter is useful to guide management during labor and delivery; however, it is technically difficult to insert a pulmonary artery catheter in patients with severe pulmonary hypertension and to maintain it in position, since it often migrates back into the right ventricle. A distressing feature of Eisenmenger syndrome is sudden death approximately 5 days postpartum. The cause is unknown, but is possibly related to pulmonary embolism or arrhythmia. Hypoxia creates a vicious cycle of pulmonary vasoconstriction resulting in increased right-to-left-shunting, which in turn results in more hypoxia.

Dilated Cardiomyopathy

Patients with poor systolic function are at risk for congestive heart failure in the peripartum period. These patients are usually diagnosed by history, physical examination, chest x-ray, and echocardiography. Invasive hemodynamic monitoring guides fluid management, inotropic therapy, and afterload reduction and prepares patients for the vicissitudes of labor (e.g., hemorrhage, epidural hypotension, or cesarean delivery). Other problems include thromboemboli and both atrial and ventricular arrhythmias.[88,89]

Tocolytic-Induced Pulmonary Edema

Some patients given tocolytics for preterm labor develop pulmonary edema. Early reports suggested the incidence to be as high as 5 percent.[90] With widespread knowledge of this complication, the incidence is now less than 1 percent. Pulmonary edema has occurred with ritodrine, terbutaline, isoxsuprine, and other β-agonists as well as with magnesium sulfate. It has occurred both antepartum and postpartum. The mechanism of tocolytic-induced pulmonary edema is unknown. One of the problems in evaluating the cause is that patients often have a complex clinical course with many interrelating occurrences such as multiple drug administration, blood loss, blood transfusion, anesthesia, vaginal delivery, or cesarean delivery.[91] Perhaps the best explanation for pulmonary edema in this setting is that β-mimetics increase antidiuretic hormone release.[92] Urine output falls, and the hematocrit is diluted down.[93] Indeed, in many of the early cases abruptio placenta or occult bleeding was suspected when, during the evaluation of dyspnea, these patients were found to have had a 5 to 10 point fall in hematocrit. Iatrogenic fluid overload may also have contributed.[94] Nevertheless, invasive hemodynamic monitoring has usually revealed normal wedge pressure, suggesting noncardiogenic pulmonary edema. A significant percentage of patients with tocolytic-induced pulmonary edema do not have a fall in hematocrit. Corticosteroids given to accelerate fetal lung maturity have been blamed, but the mineralocorticoid effect is probably minimal, thus playing no significant role in the development of pulmonary edema. Other proposed mechanisms include myocardial ischemia, endotoxin released from occult chorioamnionitis, high-output cardiac failure, idiosyncratic drug reaction, unrecognized heart disease, reduced intravascular colloid osmotic pressure, and hypokalemia. Pulmonary edema rarely occurs before 24 hours of parenteral therapy and is rare with oral therapy. Predisposing factors include multiple gestation, anemia, low maternal weight, and aggressive fluid-loading. A strategy for prevention includes (1) attention to contraindications to tocolytic therapy; (2) careful intake and output, with total fluid administration limited to 2,500 ml/day; (3) recognition of predisposing factors; and (4) limitation of parenteral therapy to 24 hours.

Patients with tocolytic-induced pulmonary edema usually respond to discontinuation of the drug and administration of oxygen, morphine, and furosemide. Acute respiratory failure requiring mechanical ventilation may still be seen, however. The duration of pulmonary edema is quite variable, ranging from a few hours to 3 to 4 days.[91]

Septic Shock

The American College of Chest Physicians and the Society of Critical Care Medicine held a Consensus Conference in 1991 to standardize definitions for sepsis and organ failure.[95,96] They proposed the phrase *systemic inflammatory response syndrome* (SIRS) to describe the inflammatory process that can be generated by infection or by noninfectious causes such as pancreatitis, burns, and trauma. The response is manifested by two or more of the following conditions: (1) temperature above 38°C or below 36°C; (2) heart rate more than 90 beats per minute; (3) respiratory rate more than 20 breaths per minute or $PaCO_2$ below 32 mmHg; and (4) white blood cell count more than 12,000/mm^3 or less than 4,000/mm^3 or >10 percent band forms. *Sepsis* is SIRS due to infection. *Severe sepsis* is sepsis associated with organ dysfunction, hypoperfusion, or hypotension. Perfusion abnormalities may include, but are not limited to, lactic acidosis, oliguria, or an acute alteration in mental status. *Septic shock* is defined as sepsis-induced hypotension despite adequate fluid resuscitation along with the presence of perfusion abnormalities that may include, but are not limited to, lactic acidosis, oliguria, or an acute alteration in mental status. Patients who are receiving inotropic or vasopressor agents may not be hypotensive at the time that perfusion abnormalities are measured. Hypotension is defined as a systolic blood pressure below 90 mmHg or a reduction of 40 mmHg or more from baseline. The previously used terms "multiple systems organ failure" and "progressive" or "sequential organ failure" were discarded in favor of the term "multiple organ dysfunction syndrome" (MODS). MODS is the presence of altered organ function in an acutely ill patient such that homeostasis cannot be maintained without intervention.

Figure 18-11 shows the pathogenesis of septic shock.[97] Organisms proliferate at the nidus of infection, invade the bloodstream, and release various substances into the blood. These exotoxins and microbial structural components interact with neutrophils, monocytes, macrophages, and endothelial cells, causing release of a myriad of mediators (e.g., cytokines, platelet activating factor, endorphins, endothelium-derived relaxing factor, complement, kinins, coagulation factors, myocardial depressant factor, prostaglandins, and leukotrienes). These mediators cause most of the clinical manifestations of SIRS, including fever, vasodilation, tachycardia, and hypotension. About 50 percent of patients with septic shock survive; the other 50 percent die of refractory hypotension or multiple organ system failure.[97]

During the 1960s and 1970s, gram-negative bacteria were the most common cause of septic shock. Now, the gram-positive microbes, in particular *Staphylococcus au-*

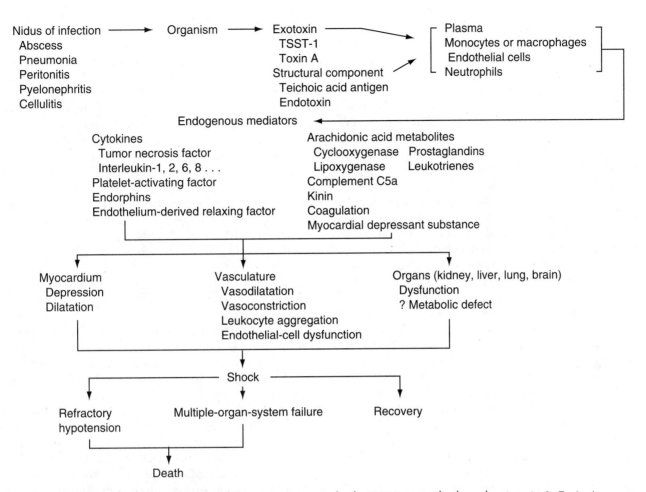

Fig. 18-11 Pathogenetic sequence of the events in septic shock. TSST-1, toxic shock syndrome toxin 1. Toxin A is *Pseudomonas aeruginosa* toxin A. (From Parillo,[97] with permission.)

reus and enterococci, account for 40 to 50 percent of nosocomial infection. Gram-negative microbes are still important, particularly in obstetric and gynecologic infections. Yeast infections (both *Candida albicans* and non-*albicans* species) are also becoming more common. Other fungi, mycobacteria, and viruses (herpes and adenovirus groups) may cause septic shock. The major causes of septic shock in obstetric patients are septic abortion, chorioamnionitis, postpartum endometritis, ruptured appendix, necrotizing fasciitis, pyelonephritis, urinary tract instrumentation, and toxic shock syndrome.

Less than half of patients with septic shock have positive blood cultures.[97] Reliable assays for circulating endotoxin or other microbial toxins have not been developed for purposes other than research.

Management of septic shock consists of resuscitation (hemodynamic monitoring, fluids, vasopressors, antibiotics); source control; and modifying the mediator cascade.[97–100] If possible the patient should be placed in an intensive care unit so that invasive hemodynamic monitoring (Swan-Ganz catheter, arterial line) can be performed to assess intravascular volume and to guide therapy with fluids and vasopressors. Other monitoring consists of urine output, sensorium, skin temperature, electrocardiogram, pulse oximetry, arterial blood gases, lactic acid level, and oxygen delivery and consumption. Supplemental oxygen or mechanical ventilation may be required.

Hypotension should be corrected to a mean arterial pressure of at least 60 mmHg. This can be accomplished with fluids to increase wedge pressure to 12 to 16 mmHg. The superiority of colloid over crystalloid therapy has not been established, and cost concerns favor the latter. Hemoglobin should be maintained above 10 g/dl with packed red blood cells.[101] If hypotension persists despite volume expansion, dopamine is added (3 to 20 μg/kg/min). If high-dose dopamine is unsuccessful, norepinephrine (0.1 to 1 μg/kg/min) should be added and dopamine titrated back to a nephrotonic dose (3 μg/kg/min). Cardiac index should then be optimized to at least 4 L/min/m². Oxygen consumption depends on oxygen delivery in sepsis. Two studies have attempted to treat patients using supranormal levels of oxygen delivery with favorable effects on outcome.[102,103] However, a more recent study has shown no benefit from supranormal oxygen delivery and the idea is highly controversial.[104]

Cultures should be obtained and antibiotics started. Antibiotic choice is based on the suspected source of infection, the anticipated pathogens, and the patterns of resistance. For most obstetric infections, coverage for enterococci, gram-negative microbes, and anaerobic organisms is required. The most commonly used regimen is ampicillin, gentamicin, and clindamycin. An interesting study conducted in dogs with gram-negative sepsis found that antibiotics and cardiovascular support had synergistic beneficial effects. With antibiotics alone, survival was 10 percent; with cardiovascular support alone, survival was 10 percent; however, with antibiotics and cardiovascular support, survival was 40 percent.[105]

Every effort should be made to identify the infection giving rise to sepsis (i.e., source control). In obstetric infections such as septic abortion, pelvic abscess, and necrotizing fasciitis the timing and adequacy of surgical drainage or debridement may be crucial to survival.

The inflammatory response may protect the host from infection, but it may also cause multiple organ dysfunction and death. In the past decade there have been many clinical and animal studies using various blockers of the inflammatory cascade. The results have been disappointing.[106] The experience with antiendotoxin antibody is illustrative. In 1982, Ziegler et al.[107] found that J5 antiserum to endotoxin core antigen reduced mortality in patients with gram-negative bacteremia. The source of this antibody was human volunteers. With the rise of the AIDS epidemic and concerns about transmission of cytomegalovirus, administration of human J5 antitoxin was impractical. Monoclonal antibodies were developed to produce more specific antiendotoxin therapy with less risk for transmission of infection. HA-IA was produced from a human myeloma cell line and E5 from a murine source. In 1991, the first HA-IA study showed benefit in a subgroup of patients with gram-negative bacteremia.[108] However, because many patients had gram-positive sepsis, when the study was analyzed by intention-to-treat, HA-IA did not show a significant effect on survival. In addition, the cost of one dose was over $3,000. A second HA-IA trial was abandoned in 1993 after an interval monitoring of data revealed a higher mortality in patients randomized to receive HA-IA.[109] In the two E5 multicenter trials, no major benefit was found in patients with gram-negative infection.[106,110]

Many other trials have been performed in the past decade with anticytokine antibodies (e.g., antitumor necrosis factor,[111] interleukin-1 receptor antagonist,[112] and antiplatelet-activating factor). We have gained con-siderable knowledge from these studies, in particular knowledge about study design.[101] Many studies used 14-day or 28-day mortality, which is insensitive and requires a large sample size. Reversal of organ dysfunction may be a valid and less stringent endpoint. Severity of illness plays a large role in identifying study subjects who will benefit from immunotherapy. For example, subjects with less than a 25 percent predicted risk of mortality will be unlikely to benefit from immunotherapy and are thus nondiscriminatory. At the other end of the spectrum, patients with greater than a 75 percent predicted risk of mortality are also unlikely to benefit from immunotherapy and are nondiscriminatory. Another problem is that we cannot rapidly identify patients with gram-negative infection at the bedside, yet these are the only patients who would benefit from antiendotoxin therapy. Our greatest problem may be that our level of understanding of septic shock does not permit us to develop successful treatment.[106] Targeting a single microbial toxin or cytokine may not represent a viable strategy for treating a complex inflammatory response. Immune cells and cytokines play both pathogenic and protective roles. In a canine model of human septic shock, when these compensatory molecules were removed by plasmapheresis, mortality was increased.[113]

Two large prospective randomized trials have shown no benefit from corticosteroids in septic shock.[114,115] Naloxone, indomethacin, prostaglandins, granulocyte colony-stimulating factor, and nitric oxide synthase inhibitors have improved survival in animal models of endotoxic shock; however, studies in humans either have not been performed or are inadequately designed to allow accurate interpretation.

In summary, no new therapy for sepsis has shown clinical efficacy. Standard treatment includes hemodynamic support, antibiotics, and surgery.

Adult Respiratory Distress Syndrome

The definition of ARDS includes three components: PaO_2 FIO_2 ratio of 200 or less regardless of the level of positive end-expiratory pressure (PEEP), diffuse bilateral radiographic infiltrates, and either a pulmonary artery wedge pressure of 18 mmHg or less or no clinical or radiographic evidence of increased left atrial pressure.[116] The lung can respond in only a limited number of ways to injury. Therefore, the causes of ARDS are many. In pregnancy the causes include aspiration, pyelonephritis, tocolytics, preeclampsia/eclampsia, chorioamnionitis, endometritis, septic abortion, thromboembolism, amniotic fluid embolism, bacterial or viral pneumonia, and drug overdose. The clinical course is variable, ranging from rapid reversal in a few days (e.g., fat embolism, drug reaction) to delayed reversal requiring weeks of mechanical ventilation (e.g., sepsis with multiple organ failure). Pathologic changes progress from an exudative phase characterized by type I cell destruction, atelectasis, or neutrophil infiltration (days 0 to 4) to a proliferative phase with type II cell proliferation, hyaline membranes, capillary loss, and mononuclear cell infiltration (days 3 to 10) to a late phase with capillary loss and fibrosis (days 7 to 14).[117] Overall mortality from ARDS is 50 to 70 percent with most deaths resulting from the underlying predisposing illness, sepsis, or multiorgan dysfunction.[118,119] In pregnancy the mortality is similar, being reported at 44 and 43 percent in two series.[117,120] In survivors with previously normal lung function, the long-term prognosis is remarkably good. Pulmonary function tests and arterial blood gases return to normal 4 to 6 months after respiratory failure. In some patients, severe fibrotic residua make complete resolution unlikely.

Management of ARDS involves treating the underlying cause, maintaining oxygenation with mechanical ventilation and PEEP, normalizing acid-base derangements, and limiting the accumulation of extravascular lung water.[117] For many years tidal volumes of 12 to 15 ml/kg were recommended for patients receiving mechanical ventilation. This may be inappropriate in patients with ARDS because the lung volume that can be aerated is small. High tidal volumes result in increased barotrauma. Improved hemodynamic performance and fewer pulmonary complications are seen with tidal volumes of 6 to 10 ml/kg. The goal is to maintain peak inspiratory pressure below 45 cm of water.[116]

PEEP reduces shunting and improves matching of ventilation and perfusion, which may allow the use of lower inhaled oxygen fractions. PEEP may be applied in small increments of 3 to 5 cm of water up to a maximum of 15 cm of water. The least PEEP that will provide an acceptable arterial oxygen saturation ($\geq$90 percent) with a nontoxic inhaled oxygen fraction ($\leq$0.6) is chosen.[116]

Normal lungs can be appropriately ventilated at rates of 8 to 14 breaths per minute. Because of the increased physiologic dead space and smaller lung volumes in ARDS, ventilatory rates of 20 to 25 breaths per minute are often required. These ventilatory rates are usually well tolerated unless the patient develops excessive intrathoracic gas trapping ("auto-PEEP"). In these circumstances controlled hypoventilation or permissive hypercapnea may be used. Gradual increases in the partial pressure of arterial carbon dioxide ($\leq$100 mmHg) are usually well tolerated. Intravenous sodium bicarbonate may be required for marked acidosis (pH <7.25)[116]

In ARDS pulmonary edema is due to increased vascular permeability; however, intravascular hydrostatic pressure may still be a contributing factor. Diuretics and fluid restriction may be used to maintain the wedge pressure as low as is compatible with satisfactory oxygen delivery and urine output.[117]

Anecdotal reports suggest that corticosteroids may be useful during the fibroproliferative phase of ARDS, where they appear to decrease collagen deposition and improve lung compliance.[121] In many centers current practice is to begin a 1- to 2-week trial of corticosteroids (2 to 4 mg of prednisone per kilogram per day, or the equivalent) 7 to 14 days after the onset of ARDS in patients with severe disease and no signs of improvement. Before treating with corticosteroids one should rule out or adequately treat pneumonia or other infections.[116]

Inhaled nitric oxide can act as a selective pulmonary vasodilator producing consistent (but limited) decreases in pulmonary artery pressure and intrapulmonary shunting.[122] Further controlled studies are required before its use can be recommended. Unlike infants with neonatal respiratory distress syndrome, patients with ARDS have normal amounts of surfactant, but it is often dysfunctional. Exogenous surfactant has been tried in ARDS with no significant benefit. Other pharmacologic therapies that have been tried and are either ineffective or require more investigation include acetylcysteine (an oxygen-free radical scavenger), ketoconazole (an inhibitor of thromboxane and leukotriene synthesis), pentoxifylline (a phosphodiesterase inhibitor), alprostadil (prostaglandin E_1), nonsteroidal antiinflammatory drugs, and antiendotoxin and anticytokine antibodies.[116]

In two recently published series of ARDS in pregnancy, the incidence was approximately 1 in 3,000 deliveries.[117,120] The major causes of ARDS were hemorrhage, infection, and preeclampsia/eclampsia. Perinatal mortality was 20 percent in the one series in which it was reported.[117] Multiorgan failure developed in many patients. Complications of mechanical ventilation were common, especially barotrauma, right mainstem bronchus intubation, self extubation, and sinusitis. Other complications of ICU supportive care included line sepsis, endocarditis, and deep venous thrombosis. Hypoxic encephalopathy occurred in three patients. Whether delivery would be of net benefit in the course of ARDS is unresolved. Most patients deliver before or soon after admission to the hospital. Management must be individualized. If the patient has an infectious cause that may respond to antimicrobial or antiviral therapy and there is no evidence of fetal compromise, I would not recommend delivery. If delivery is indicated, I would attempt vaginal delivery, reserving cesarean delivery for obstetric indications.

Diabetic Ketoacidosis

Diabetic ketoacidosis (DKA) is due to a relative or absolute insulin deficiency and an excess of insulin counterregulatory hormones. Although the type I insulin-dependent diabetic is more likely to develop DKA, type II noninsulin-dependent diabetics may also develop DKA with sufficient provocation. Investigation of the cause reveals medical illness, usually infection, in 50 percent of the patients. The omission of insulin accounts for an additional 20 percent, and in 30 percent of cases no precipitating cause can be identified.

Symptoms include polyuria, polydipsia, vomiting, vague abdominal pain, hyperventilation, stupor, and coma. Laboratory diagnosis is based on hyperglycemia, ketonemia, and a serum pH below 7.35. In practice, a urinalysis showing 4+ glucose and large ketones is all that is required for the diagnosis of DKA. Other laboratory features may include an anion gap ($Na - [Cl + HCO_3] > 12$ mEq/L), hyponatremia, hyperkalemia, elevated serum urea nitrogen and creatinine, and elevated serum amylase unrelated to pancreatitis.

Some aspects about DKA are different in pregnancy. Patients may have significant DKA with only a modest degree of hyperglycemia. An example of this would be a patient with pH 7.01, PCO_2 7 mmHg, PO_2 132 mmHg, and blood sugar 180 mg/dl. The cause of DKA with modest hyperglycemia is not well understood but may result from the fetus constantly removing glucose, from the expanded blood volume of pregnancy or from rapid clearance of glucose in the urine due to increased glomerular filtration rate. In some cases, glucose administration will be required as substrate for the insulin needed to clear ketonemia. Sodium bicarbonate therapy is normally withheld in the nonpregnant patient until the pH is less than 7.10 or 7.00 because of concern about rapid alkalinization shifting the oxyhemoglobin dissociation curve to the left and metabolic alkalosis occurring as ketones are metabolized to bicarbonate. In pregnancy, bicarbonate should be given for a pH below 7.20 because of the risk of intrauterine fetal demise. Decreased fetal heart rate variability and late decelerations may occur during DKA. This will usually resolve with correction of the maternal metabolic disturbance. Cesarean delivery for fetal distress will usually not be required.[123,124] β-Mimetic drugs and steroids given for preterm labor may worsen glucose control in the diabetic. Magnesium sulfate or nifedipine may be a better tocolytic agent in the diabetic. Treatment of DKA is otherwise the same as for nonpregnant adults.

During the history and physical examination, special attention should be paid to patency of the airway; mental status; cardiovascular, pulmonary, and renal status; source of infection; and state of hydration. Immediate biochemical evaluation should include blood and urine glucose and ketones by chemstrip and ketostix, respectively. Plasma glucose, blood gases and pH, electrolytes, blood urea nitrogen, chest x-ray, ECG, and cultures may be obtained. A liter of normal saline may be given in the first hour followed by 0.5 N saline at a rate depending on the state of hydration. Usually 3 to 5 L of crystalloid will be needed in the first 24 hours. Seven units of regular insulin may be given intravenously and 7 units intramuscularly followed by a constant infusion of 7 to 10 units per hour. Plasma glucose should be determined hourly and electrolytes and blood gases every 4 hours as needed. All laboratory data, intake and output, and medications should be recorded in an organized fashion. If glucose does not fall 10 percent in the first hour, the rate of insulin infusion may be doubled. The biologic effect of insulin is only 10 to 20 percent of normal during DKA. When plasma glucose reaches 250 mg/dl, 5 percent dextrose in water should be added to the regimen. Intravenous glucose and insulin are continued until the urine is cleared of ketones. Unless the serum potassium is more than 5.5 mEq/L or renal insufficiency is present, potassium replacement (20 to 40 mEq/L) should begin with the initial insulin therapy. Sodium bicarbonate (44 or 88 mEq in 1 L of 0.5 N saline) may be given until the arterial pH is above 7.20. Phosphate supplementation is unnecessary. As soon as the patient can eat, she may be restarted on subcutaneous NPH insulin twice daily with regular insulin before each meal based on a sliding scale. Making the transition from intravenous to subcutaneous insulin is often the trickiest part of managing DKA.[125,126]

Thyroid Storm

The diagnosis of thyroid storm is based on three clinical criteria: (1) exaggerated manifestations of hyperthyroidism, (2) rectal temperature greater than 102°F, and (3) central nervous system changes. Alterations in mental state vary from confusion to psychosis to coma. Other common findings include tachycardia out of proportion to fever, arrhythmias, cardiac failure, diarrhea, abdominal pain, vomiting, jaundice, and dehydration.[127]

Interestingly, serum thyroxine (T_4) and triiodothyronine (T_3) levels may be no higher during thyroid storm than they were weeks earlier. Thyroid storm seems to involve loss of refractoriness to the effects of thyroid hormone. There have been reports of thyroid storm with normal serum T_3 levels, presumably illness interfering with normal peripheral conversion of T_4 to T_3.[128] Thyrotoxic crisis associated with pregnancy usually occurs in the early postpartum period. Other precipitating causes include infection, trauma, surgery, myocardial infarction, diabetic ketoacidosis, and cessation of antithyroid drugs.

Treatment of thyroid storm involves the following general measures: (1) replace fluids, glucose, and electrolytes; (2) lower temperature with acetaminophen or a cooling blanket; (3) treat precipitating factors (e.g., infection or trauma); and (4) treat cardiac failure with oxygen and diuretics. Treatment of cardiac failure may involve β-blocker therapy in which case invasive monitoring may be indicated to balance the reduction in heart rate against the negative inotropic effect. Heart failure due to thyrotoxicosis in pregnancy is normally seen in patients with long-standing hyperthyroidism and poor control. Left ventricular ejection fraction is increased at rest in the hyperthyroid state, but there is a significant decrease in ejection fraction during exercise. This cardiomyopathy is reversible with treatment of the underlying thyrotoxicosis.

Specific measures for treating thyroid storm include antithyroid drugs, glucocorticoids, iodides, and propranolol. Propylthiouracil 600 to 1,000 mg administered orally or via nasogastric tube followed by 300 to 600 mg/day prevents further hormone production and blocks peripheral conversion of T_4 to T_3. Methimazole 60 to 100 mg orally followed by 30 to 60 mg daily may be substituted for propylthiouracil, although the former has caused scalp defects in the fetus and does not block peripheral conversion of T_4 to T_3. Iodides given at least 1 hour after the initial dose of propylthiouracil block thyroid hormone release. The 1 hour delay is to allow propylthiouracil to block hormone synthesis and to avoid build up of thyroid hormone stores in the gland. Iodides may be given as Lugol's solution 30 drops PO daily in divided doses, sodium iodide 500 mg IV every 8 to 12 hours, or as radiographic contrast drugs ipodate or iopanoic acid 1 g orally daily. Dexamethasone 2 mg intravenously every 6 hours or equivalent amounts of prednisone or hydrocortisone may be administered to cover the patient for relative adrenal insufficiency and to inhibit peripheral conversion of T_4 to T_3. Propranolol decreases the peripheral effects of thyroid hormone and also blocks the peripheral conversion of T_4 to T_3. It may be given orally 40 to 80 mg every 4 to 6 hours or intravenously 1 mg every 10 minutes up to five doses.

After initial clinical improvement, iododides and glucocorticoids may be discontinued and antithyroid drugs can be continued until the patient becomes euthyroid. Ablative therapy with radioactive iodine or surgery is indicated in nearly all patients after an episode of thyroid storm. In pregnancy, ablative therapy should be postponed until after delivery.[129]

Key Points

- The mainstay of intensive obstetric care is pulmonary artery catheterization
- Supportive care guided by invasive monitoring includes determining the hemodynamic profile and manipulating preload, afterload, heart rate, and myocardial contractility
- The cardiovascular hemodynamics of preeclampsia are uncertain, having been reported to range from a low output–high resistance state to a high output–low resistance state
- Management of complications of preeclampsia such as pulmonary edema or oliguria may be aided by determining hemodynamic subsets
- Management of high-risk cardiac lesions in pregnancy such as mitral stenosis, hypertrophic obstructive cardiomyopathy, Eisenmenger syndrome, and dilated cardiomyopathy must be tailored to the unique pathophysiology of each lesion
- The mechanism of tocolytic-induced pulmonary edema is probably multifactorial and has not been clearly elucidated
- Despite many recent clinical trials using various blockers of inflammation, the therapy of septic shock remains fluids, antibiotics, and surgery
- The management of adult respiratory distress syndrome primarily involves supporting the patient with mechanical ventilation in the intensive care unit until the lung injury heals
- Diabetic ketoacidosis is becoming an uncommon complication in pregnancy, but there are several pitfalls in its management
- Drug therapy of a thyroid storm includes antithyroid medication, β-blockers, iodine, and corticosteroids

References

1. Mabie WC, Sibai BM: Treatment in an obstetric intensive care unit. Am J Obstet Gynecol 162:1, 1990
2. ACOG: Invasive hemodynamic monitoring in obstetrics and gynecology. ACOG Tech Bull No. 175. American College of Obstetricians and Gynecologists, Washington, DC, December 1992
3. Benedetti TJ, Cotton DB, Read JC, Miller FC: Hemodynamic observations in severe preeclampsia with a flow-directed pulmonary artery catheter. Am J Obstet Gynecol 136:467, 1980
4. Cotton DB, Gonik B, Dorman KF, Harrist R: Cardiovascular alterations in severe pregnancy-induced hypertension: relationship of central venous pressure to pulmonary capillary wedge pressure. Am J Obstet Gynecol 151:762, 1985

5. Robin ED: The cult of the Swan-Ganz catheter. Ann Intern Med 103:445, 1985

6. Swan HJ, Ganz W, Forrester J et al: Catheterization of the heart in man with the use of a flow-directed balloon-tipped catheter. N Engl J Med 283:447, 1970

7. Matthay MA, Chatterjee K: Bedside catheterization of the pulmonary artery: risks compared with benefits. Ann Intern Med 109:826, 1988

8. Forrester JC, Diamond G, Swan HJ: Correlative classification of clinical and hemodynamic function after acute myocardial infarction. Am J Cardiol 39:137, 1977

9. Bayliss J, Norell M, Ryan A et al: Bedside hemodynamic monitoring: experience in a general hospital. BMJ 287:187, 1983

10. Connors AF Jr, McCaffree DR, Gray BA: Evaluation of right heart catheterization in the critically ill patient without acute myocardial infarction. N Engl J Med 308:263, 1983

11. Eisenberg PR, Jaffe AS, Schuster DP: Clinical evaluation compared to pulmonary artery catheterization in the hemodynamic assessment of critically ill patients. Crit Care Med 12:549, 1984

12. Fein AM, Goldberg SK, Wahlenstein MD et al: Is pulmonary artery catheterization necessary for the diagnosis of pulmonary edema? Am Rev Respir Dis 129:1006, 1984

13. Gore JM, Goldberg RJ, Spodick DH et al: A community-wide assessment of the use of pulmonary artery catheters in patients with acute myocardial infarction. Chest 92:721, 1987

14. Shoemaker WC, Appel PL, Bland R et al: Clinical trial of an algorithm prediction in acute circulatory failure. Crit Care Med 10:390, 1982

15. Daily EK, Schroeder JS: Techniques in Bedside Hemodynamic Monitoring. CV Mosby, St. Louis, 1989

16. Sprung CL, Rackow EC, Civetta JM: Direct measurements derived calculations using the pulmonary artery catheter. p. 105. In Sprung CL (ed): The Pulmonary Artery Catheter. University Park Press, Baltimore, 1983

17. Snyder JV: Oxygen transport: The model and reality. p. 3. In Snyder JV, Pinsky MR (eds): Oxygen Transport in the Critically Ill. Year Book Medical Chicago, 1987

18. Rosenthal MH: Intrapartum intensive care management of the cardiac patient. Clin Obstet Gynecol 24:789, 1981

19. Marini JJ, Wheeler AP: Critical Care Medicine—The Essentials. Williams & Wilkins, Baltimore, 1989

20. Clark SL, Cotton DB: Clinical indications for pulmonary artery catheterization in the patient with severe preeclampsia. Am J Obstet Gynecol 158:453, 1988

21. Wallenburg HCS: Hemodynamics in hypertensive pregnancy. p. 73. In Rubin PC (ed): Hypertension in Pregnancy. 1st Ed. Elsevier, Amsterdam, 1988

22. Hamilton HFH: The cardiac output in normal pregnancy as determined by the Cournand right heart catheterization technique. J Obstet Gynaecol Br Emp 56:548, 1949

23. Werko L: Pregnancy and heart disease. Acta Obstet Gynecol Scand 33:162, 1954

24. Bader RA, Bader ME, Rose DJ, Braunwald E: Hemodynamics of rest and exercise in normal pregnancy as studied by cardiac catheterization. J Clin Invest 34:1524, 1955

25. Kerr MG: Cardiovascular dynamics in pregnancy and labor. Br Med Bull 24:19, 1968

26. Walters WAW, MacGregor WG, Hills M: Cardiac output at rest during pregnancy and the puerperium. Clin Sci 30:1, 1966

27. Ueland K, Akamatsu TJ, Eng M et al: Maternal cardiovascular dynamics VI. Cesarean section under epidural anesthesia without epinephrine. Am J Obstet Gynecol 114:775, 1972

28. Lim YL, Walters WAW: Hemodynamics of mild hypertension in pregnancy. Brit J Obstet Gynaecol 86:198, 1979

29. Lees MM: Central circulatory responses in normotensive and hypertensive pregnancy. Postgrad Med J 55:311, 1979

30. Groenendijk R, Trimbos JBMJ, Wallenburg HCS: Hemodynamic measurements in preeclampsia: preliminary observations. Am J Obstet Gynecol 150:232, 1984

31. Clark SL, Cotton DB, Lee W et al: Central hemodynamic assessment of normal term pregnancy. Am J Obstet Gynecol 161:1439, 1989

32. Smith RW: Cardiovascular alterations in toxemia. Am J Obstet Gynecol 107:979, 1970

33. Easterling TR, Watts DH, Schmucker BC, Benedetti TJ: Measurement of cardiac output during pregnancy: validation of doppler technique and clinical observations in preeclampsia. Obstet Gynecol 69:845, 1987

34. Katz R, Karliner JS, Resnik R: Effect of a natural volume overload state (pregnancy) on left ventricular performance in normal human subjects. Circulation 58:434, 1978

35. Lee W, Rokey R, Cotton DB: Noninvasive maternal stroke volume and cardiac output determinations by pulsed Doppler echocardiography. Am J Obstet Gynecol 158:505, 1988

36. Mashini IS, Albazzaz SJ, Fadel HE et al: Serial noninvasive evaluation of cardiovascular hemodynamics during pregnancy. Am J Obstet Gynecol 156:1208, 1987

37. Robson SC, Hunter S, Moore M, Dunlop W: Hemodynamic changes during the puerperium: a Doppler and M-mode echocardiographic study. Brit J Obstet Gynaecol 94:1028, 1987

38. Rubler S, Damani P, Pinto ER: Cardiac size and performance during pregnancy estimated by echocardiography. Am J Cardiol 40:534, 1977

39. Masaki DI, Greenspoon JS, Ouzounian JG: Measurement of cardiac output in pregnancy by thoracic electrical bioimpedance and thermodilution. Am J Obstet Gynecol 161:680, 1989

40. Milsom I, Forssman L, Sivertsson R, Dottori O: Measurement of cardiac stroke volume by impedance cardiography in the last trimester of pregnancy. Acta Obstet Gynecol Scand 62:473, 1983

41. Easterling TR, Benedetti TJ, Carlson KL, Watts DH: Measurement of cardiac output in pregnancy by thermodilution and impedance techniques. Brit J Obstet Gynaecol 96:67, 1989

42. Elkayam U, Gleicher N: Hemodynamics and cardiac function during normal pregnancy and the puerperium. p. 5. In Elkayam N, Gleicher N (eds): Cardiac Problems in Pregnancy. 2nd Ed. Alan R. Liss, New York, 1990

43. Hankins GDV, Cunningham FG, Pritchard JA: Cardiopulmonary consequences of hypertension during pregnancy and puerperium. p. 1. In Pritchard, MacDonald, Gant (eds): Williams Obstetrics. 17th Ed. Appleton-Century-Crofts Publishers, New York, 1986

44. Cotton DB, Gonik B, Dorman K: Cardiovascular alterations in severe pregnancy-induced hypertension: acute effects of magnesium sulfate. Am J Obstet Gynecol 148: 162, 1984

45. Nisell H, Lunell NO, Linde B: Maternal hemodynamics and impaired fetal growth in pregnancy-induced hypertension. Obstet Gynecol 71:163, 1988

46. Belfort MA, Uys P, Dommisse J, Davey DA: Hemodynamic changes in gestational proteinuric hypertension: the effects of rapid volume expansion and vasodilator therapy. Br J Obstet Gynaecol 96:634, 1989

47. Belfort MA, Anthony J, Buccimazza A, Davey DA: Hemodynamic changes associated with intravenous infusion of the calcium antagonist verapamil in the treatment of severe gestational proteinuric hypertension. Obstet Gynecol 75:970, 1990

48. Benedetti TJ, Cotton DB, Read JC, Miller FC: Hemodynamic observations in severe preeclampsia with a flow-directed pulmonary artery catheter. Am J Obstet Gynecol 1980;136:465, 1980

49. Hankins GDV, Wendel GD, Cunningham FG, Leveno KJ: Longitudinal evaluation of hemodynamic changes in eclampsia. Am J Obstet Gynecol 150:506, 1984

50. Cotton DB, Lee W, Huhta JC, Dorman KF: Hemodynamic profile of severe pregnancy-induced hypertension. Am J Obstet Gynecol 158:523, 1988

51. Mabie WC, Ratts TE, Sibai BM: The central hemodynamics of severe preeclampsia. Am J Obstet Gynecol 161:1443, 1989

52. Wasserstrum N, Kirshon B, Willis R et al: Quantitative hemodynamic effects of acute volume expansion in severe preeclampsia. Obstet Gynecol 73:546, 1989

53. Wasserstrum N, Kirshon B, Rossavik IK et al: Implications of sino-aortic baroreceptor reflex dysfunction in severe preeclampsia. Obstet Gynecol 74:34, 1989

54. Rafferty TD, Berkowitz RL: Hemodynamics in patients with severe toxemia during labor and delivery. Am J Obstet Gynecol 138:263, 1980

55. Phelan JP, Yurth DA: Severe preeclampsia. 1. Peripartum hemodynamic observations. Am J Obstet Gynecol 144:17, 1982

56. Rolbin SH, Cole AFD, Hew EM: Hemodynamic monitoring in the management of severe preeclampsia and eclampsia. Can Anesth Soc J 28:363, 1981

57. Graham C, Goldstein A: Epidural anesthesia and cardiac output in severe preeclamptics. Anaesthesia 35: 709, 1980

58. Newsome LR, Bramwell RS, Curling PE: Severe preeclampsia: hemodynamic effects of epidural anesthesia. Anesth Analg 65:31, 1986

59. Cotton DB, Longmire S, Jones MM et al: Cardiovascular alterations in severe pregnancy-induced hypertension: effects of intravenous nitroglycerin coupled with blood volume expansion. Am J Obstet Gynecol 154: 1053, 1986

60. Clark SL, Greenspoon JS, Adahl D, Phelan JP: Severe preeclampsia with persistent oliguria: management of hemodynamic subsets. Am J Obstet Gynecol 154:490, 1986

61. Chesley LC: Hypertensive Disorders in Pregnancy. 1st Ed. p. 203. Appleton, Century-Crofts, East Norwalk, CT 1978

62. Hays PM, Cruikshank DP, Dunn LJ: Plasma volume determination in normal and preeclamptic pregnancies. Am J Obstet Gynecol 151:958, 1985

63. Cohn JD: Paroxysmal hypertension and hypovolemia. N Engl J Med 275:643, 1966

64. Goodlin RC, Cotton DB, Haesslein H: Severe edema-proteinuria-hypertension gestosis. Am J Obstet Gynecol 132:595, 1978

65. Gallery EDM, Delprado W, Gyory AZ: Antihypertensive effect of plasma volume expansion in pregnancy-associated hypertension. Aust NZ J Med 11:20, 1981

66. Sehgal NN, Hitt JR: Plasma volume expansion in the treatment of preeclampsia. Am J Obstet Gynecol 138: 165, 1980

67. Wasserstrum N, Cotton DB: Hemodynamic monitoring in severe pregnancy-induced hypertension. Clin Perinatol 13:781, 1986

68. Kirshon B, Moise KJ, Cotton DB et al: Role of volume expansion in severe preeclampsia. Surg Gynecol Obstet 167:367, 1988

69. Benedetti TJ, Kates R, Williams V: Hemodynamic observations in severe preeclampsia complicated by pulmonary edema. Am J Obstet Gynecol 152:330, 1985

70. Ferguson RK, Vlasses PA: Hypertensive emergencies and urgencies. JAMA 255:1607, 1986

71. Duncan SLB: Does volume expansion in preeclampsia help or hinder? Br J Obstet Gynaecol 96:631, 1989

72. Harizi RC, Bianco JA, Alpert JS: Diastolic function of the heart in clinical cardiology. Arch Intern Med 148: 99, 1988

73. Mabie WC, Ratts TE, Ramanathan KB, Sibai BM: Circulatory congestion in obese hypertensive women: a subset of pulmonary edema in pregnancy. Obstet Gynecol 72: 553, 1988

74. Mabie WC, Hackmann BB, Sibai BM: Pulmonary edema associated with pregnancy: echocardiographic insights and implications for treatment. Obstet Gynecol 81:227, 1993

75. Moise KJ, Cotton DB: The use of colloid osmotic pressure in pregnancy. Clin Perinatol 13:827, 1986

76. Rackow EC, Fein IA, Leppo J: Colloid osmotic pressure as a prognostic indication of pulmonary edema and mortality in the critically ill. Chest 72:709, 1977

77. Gonik B, Cotton DB, Spillman T et al: Peripartum colloid osmotic pressure changes: effects of controlled fluid management. Am J Obstet Gynecol 151:812, 1985

78. Cotton DB, Gonik B, Spillman T, Dorman KF: Intrapar-

tum to postpartum changes in colloid osmotic pressure. Am J Obstet Gynecol 149:174, 1984

79. Benedetti TJ, Carlson RW: Studies of colloid osmotic pressure in pregnancy-induced hypertension. Am J Obstet Gynecol 135:308, 1979

80. Sibai BM, Mabie BC, Harvey CJ, Gonzalez AP: Pulmonary edema in severe preeclampsia-eclampsia: analysis of thirty-seven consecutive cases. Am J Obstet Gynecol 156:1174, 1987

81. Lee W, Gonik B, Cotton DB: Urinary diagnostic indices in preeclampsia-associated oliguria: correlation with invasive hemodynamic monitoring. Am J Obstet Gynecol 156:100, 1987

82. Kirshon B, Lee W, Mauer MB, Cotton DB: Effects of low-dose dopamine therapy in the oliguric patient with preeclampsia. Am J Obstet Gynecol 159:604, 1988

83. Barton JR, Hiett AK, Conover WB: The use of nifedipine during the postpartum period in patients with severe preeclampsia. Am J Obstet Gynecol 162:788, 1990

84. Clark SL, Phelan JP, Greenspoon J et al: Labor and delivery in the presence of mitral stenosis: central hemodynamic observations. Am J Obstet Gynecol 152:984, 1985

85. Oakley GDG, McGarry K, Limb DG et al: Management of pregnancy in patients with hypertrophic cardiomyopathy. BMJ 1:1749, 1979

86. Gleicher D, Midwall J, Hockberger D et al: Eisenmenger's syndrome in pregnancy. Obstet Gynecol Surv 34:721, 1979

87. Spinnato JA, Kraynack BJ, Cooper MW: Eisenmenger's syndrome in pregnancy: epidural anesthesia for elective cesarean section. N Engl J Med 304:1215, 1981

88. O'Connell JB, Costanzo-Nordin MR, Subramanian R et al: Peripartum cardiomyopathy: clinical, hemodynamic, histologic, and prognostic characteristics. J Am Coll Cardiol 8:52, 1986

89. Dec GW, Fuster V: Idiopathic dilated cardiomyopathy. N Engl J Med 331:1564, 1994

90. Katz M, Robertson PA, Creasy RK: Caridovascular complications associated with terbutaline treatment for perterm labor. Am J Obstet Gynecol 139:605, 1981

91. Mabie WC, Pernoll ML, Witty JB et al: Pulmonary edema induced by betamimetic drugs. S Med J 76:1354, 1983

92. Schrier RW, Lieberman R, Ufferman RC et al: Mechanism of antidiuretic effect of beta adrenergic stimulation. J Clin Invest 51:97, 1972

93. Kleinman G, Nuwayhid B, Rudelstorfer R et al: Circulatory and renal effects of β-adrenergic receptor stimulation in pregnant sheep. Am J Obstet Gynecol 149:865, 1984

94. Pisani RJ, Rosenow EC: Pulmonary edema associated with tocolytic therapy. Ann Intern Med 110:714, 1989

95. Bone RC, Balk RA, Cerra FB et al: Definitions for sepsis and organ failure and guidelines for the use of innovative therapies in sepsis. Chest 101:1544, 1992

96. Bone RC: Toward an epidemiology and natural history of SIRS (systemic inflammatory response syndrome). JAMA 268:3452, 1992

97. Parillo JE: Pathogenetic mechanisms of septic shock. N Engl J Med 328:1471, 1993

98. Fein AM, Duvivier R: Sepsis in pregnancy. Clin Chest Med 13:709, 1992

99. Lee W, Clark SL, Cotton DB et al: Septic shock during pregnancy. Am J Obstet Gynecol 159:410, 1988

100. Pearlman M, Faro S: Obstetric septic shock: a pathophysiologic basis for management. Clin Obstet Gynecol 33:482, 1990

101. Sibbald WJ, Vincent JL: Roundtable conference on clinical trials for the treatment of sepsis: Brussels, March 12–14, 1994. Chest 107:522, 1995

102. Tuchschmidt J, Fried J, Astiz M, Rackow E: Elevation of cardiac output and oxygen delivery improves outcome in septic shock. Chest 102:216, 1992

103. Shoemaker WC, Appel PL, Kram HB: Role of oxygen debt in the development of organ failure, sepsis, and death in high-risk surgical patients. Chest 102:208, 1992

104. Haynes MA, Timmins AC, Yau EHS et al: Elevation of systemic oxygen delivery in the treatment of critically ill patients. N Engl J Med 330:1717, 1994

105. Natanson C, Danner RL, Reilly JM et al: Antibiotics versus cardiovascular support in a canine model of human septic shock. Am J Physiol 259:H1440, 1990

106. Natanson O, Hoffman WD, Suffredini AF et al: Selected treatment strategies for septic shock based on proposed mechanisms of pathogenesis. Ann Intern Med 120:771, 1994

107. Ziegler EJ, McCutchan JA, Fierer J et al: Treatment of gram-negative bacteremia and shock with human antiserum to a mutant *Escherichia coli*. N Engl J Med 307:1225, 1982

108. Zeigler EJ, Fisher CJ, Sprung C et al: Treatment of gram-negative bacteremia and septic shock with HA-IA human monoclonal antibody against endotoxin. N Engl J Med 324:429, 1991

109. McCloskey RV, Straube RC, Sanders C et al: Treatment of septic shock with human monoclonal antibody HA-IA. A randomized, double-blind, placebo-controlled trial. Ann Intern Med 121:1, 1994

110. Greenman RL, Schein RMH, Martin MA et al: A controlled clinical trial of E5 murine monoclonal IgM antibody to endotoxin in the treatment of gram-negative sepsis. JAMA 266:1097, 1991

111. Tracey KJ, Fong Y, Hesse DG et al: Anti-cachectin/TNF monoclonal antibodies prevent septic shock during lethal bacteremia. Nature 330:662, 1989

112. Ohlsson K, Björk P, Bergenfeldt M et al: Interleukin-1 receptor antagonist reduces mortality from endotoxin shock. Nature 348:550, 1990

113. Natanson C, Hoffman WD, Danner RL et al: A controlled trial of plasmapheresis fails to improve outcome in an antibiotic treated canine model of human septic shock. Transfusion 33:243, 1993

114. Bone RC, Fisher CJ Jr, Clemmer TP et al: A controlled clinical trial of high-dose methylprednisolone in the treatment of severe sepsis and septic shock. N Engl J Med 317:653, 1987

115. Hinshaw L, Peduzzi P, Young E et al: Effects of high-

dose glucocorticoid therapy in patients with clinical signs of systemic sepsis. The Veterans Administration Systemic Sepsis Cooperative Study Group. N Engl J Med 317:659, 1987

116. Kollef MH, Schuster DP: The acute respiratory distress syndrome. N Engl J Med 332:27, 1995

117. Mabie WC, Barton JR, Sibai BM: Adult respiratory distress syndrome in pregnancy. Am J Obstet Gynecol 167:950, 1992

118. Raffin TA: ARDS: mechanisms and management. Hosp Pract 22:65, 1987

119. Montgomery AB, Stager MA, Carrico CJ et al: Causes of mortality in patients with the adult respiratory distress syndrome. 132:485, 1985

120. Smith JL, Thomas F, Orme JF, Clemmer TP: Adult respiratory distress syndrome during pregnancy and immediately postpartum. West J Med 153:508, 1990

121. Meduri GU, Balenchia JM, Estes RJ et al: Fibroproliferative phase of ARDS: clinical findings and effects of corticosteroids. Chest 100:943, 1991

122. Rossaint R, Gerlach H, Schmidt-Ruhnke H et al: Efficacy of inhaled nitric oxide in patients with severe ARDS. Chest 107:1107, 1995

123. Hagay ZJ, Weissman A, Lurie S, Insler V: Reversal of fetal distress following intensive treatment of maternal diabetic ketoacidosis. Am J Perinatol 11:430, 1994

124. Montoro MN, Myers VP, Mestman JH et al: Outcome of pregnancy in DKA. Am J Perinatol 10:17, 1993

125. Kitabchi AE: Low-dose insulin therapy in diabetic ketoacidosis: fact or fiction? Diabetes Metab Rev 5:337, 1989

126. Hagay ZJ: Diabetic ketoacidosis in pregnancy: etiology, pathophysiology, and management. Clin Obstet Gynecol 37:39, 1994

127. Singer PA, Mestman JH: Thyroid storm need not be lethal. Contemp OB/GYN 22:135, 1983

128. Ahmad N, Cohen MP: Thyroid storm with normal serum triiodothyronine level during diabetic ketoacidosis. JAMA 245:2516, 1981

129. Mestman JH: Severe hyperthyroidism in pregnancy. p. 262. In Clark SL, Phelan JB, Cotton DB (eds): Critical Care Obstetrics. Medical Economics Books, Oradell, NJ, 1987

130. Daily EK, Schroeder JP: Hemodynamic Waveforms: Exercises in Identification and Analysis. CV Mosby, St. Louis, 1983

Cesarean Delivery

Richard Depp

The terms *cesarean section, cesarean delivery, and cesarean birth* may be used to describe the delivery of a fetus through a surgical incision of the anterior uterine wall. This definition does not include nonsurgical expulsion on the embryo/fetus from the uterine cavity or tubes following uterine rupture or ectopic pregnancy. *Cesarean section* is a tautology; both words connote incision. Therefore, *cesarean birth* and *cesarean delivery* are preferable terms.

Cesarean birth has become the most common hospital-based operative procedure in the United States, accounting for more than 23.5 percent of all live births in 1993.[1,2] The increase has been attributed to the liberalization of indications for "fetal distress," cephalopelvic disproportion/failure to progress, breech presentations, as well as elective repeat cesarean delivery.[3] In many medical centers the present overall rate would be significantly higher were it not for a recent change in attitude facilitating acceptance of vaginal birth after cesarean birth.[4]

The cesarean delivery-associated maternal mortality rate is approximately 20 per 100,000 births in the United States.[5] Taken as an isolated end point, it is an infrequent complication. Cesarean delivery has many possible immediate untoward consequences: an increased risk for postpartum infectious morbidity despite antibiotic prophylaxis; an increased risk of significant blood loss and need for transfusion with potential problems associated with blood and blood product replacement; and an increased risk of anesthetic complications. There are no reliable data regarding the cumulative long-term maternal morbidity associated with cesarean birth.

Despite a dramatic impact on society, little attention has been focused on the cumulative consequences of this major surgical procedure with its implications not only for the current pregnancy but also for future reproduction. The increase in cesarean birth rates noted in the 1980s has had a dramatic impact on the reproductive future of women. As the percentage of laboring patients presenting with a prior cesarean birth has increased, there has been an associated increase in more difficult repeat cesarean deliveries and complications, including a higher incidence of placenta previa, placenta accreta, symptomatic uterine rupture, hemorrhage, requirement for transfusion, and need for unplanned hysterectomy.

This chapter presents indications for cesarean delivery and peripartum hysterectomy, surgical techniques and procedural complications, and issues surrounding candidacy for and management of a trial of labor (TOL) after a prior cesarean birth (VBAC).

History of Cesarean Delivery

Terms

The origin of the term *cesarean section* is likely the product of two separate reports in 1581 and 1598, the former making reference to *Cesarean* and the second to *Sections*. The origin of the term *cesarean* is somewhat uncertain. The hypothesis that Julius Caesar was the product of a cesarean birth is unlikely to be true in view of the probability of fatality associated with the procedure in ancient times and the observation that his mother, Aurelia, corresponded with him during his campaigns in Europe many years later. The term may have as its origin the Latin verb *cadere*, to cut; the children of such births were referred to as *caesones*. It is also possible that the term stems from the Roman law known as Lex Regis, which mandated postmortem operative delivery so that the mother and child could be buried separately; the specific law is referred to historically as Lex Cesare.[6]

Mythology

According to Greek mythology, Asclepius, the founder of the cult of religious medicine, was removed from the abdomen of his mother, Coronis, by his father, Apollo. Furthermore, there are numerous references to cesarean births in Egyptian, Greek, Hindu, Roman, and other European folklore.

Historical Advances

According to Sewell,[7] cesarean delivery with the expectation of possible survival of the mother and fetus was proposed in the late 1700s and first performed in the early 1800s. However, the procedure was not popularized until the late 1920s. Although surgeons possessed the anatomic knowledge necessary to perform a cesarean delivery in the 1800s, they were limited by their inability to provide anesthesia and control infection. The introduction of diethylether as an anesthetic agent in 1846 at Massachusetts General Hospital increased the feasibility of major abdominal surgery. The credibility of cesarean childbirth as an acceptable option was significantly enhanced when the head of the Church of England, Queen Victoria, had chloroform administered for the birth of her two children, Leopold in 1853 and Beatrice in 1857, thereby popularizing the concept of cesarean birth among the upper classes. Unfortunately, although anesthesia created the potential, mortality rates for cesarean birth remained high secondary to infectious morbidity. Prior to the establishment of the germ theory and the concept of bacteriology in the latter half of the nineteenth century, surgeons were known to wear their street clothes during surgery and to wash their hands only infrequently while passing between patients. In the mid-1860s, British surgeon Joseph Lister introduced carbolic acid as an antiseptic, which, although corrosive, served as the basis for the concept of antisepsis and asepsis.

Surgical techniques were also a limiting factor. Surgeons were hesitant to reapproximate the uterine incision for fear permanent sutures would increase the likelihood of infection and cause uterine rupture in subsequent pregnancies. Not surprisingly women continued to die from blood loss and infection. As a consequence, early physicians employed a number of techniques in an attempt to modify that risk. In 1876, Eduardo Porro, an Italian Professor, recommended hysterectomy combined with cesarean birth to control uterine hemorrhage and prevent systemic infection.[8,9] The Porro procedure combined subtotal cesarean hysterectomy (see discussion of peripartum hysterectomy,

below) with marsupialization of the cervical stump.[8] Fortunately, the need for such an extreme procedure was soon minimized by the proposal to close the uterine incision with sutures. The introduction of suture material, which enabled the surgeon to control bleeding, was of monumental importance in the evolution of the procedure. In 1882, Max Sänger from Leipzig published a monograph based largely on experience from surgeons in the United States who had used internal sutures, explaining the principles and technique of cesarean delivery, including aseptic preparation, with special emphasis on a two-step uterine closure using silver wire and silk and careful attention to hemostasis.[10,11] The use of silver wire stitches were developed by nineteenth century gynecologist J. Marion Sims, who invented his sutures to repair vaginal tears (fistulas) that had resulted from traumatic childbirth. Sänger thought that this approach would obviate the growing tendency for cesarean hysterectomy caused by fear of hemorrhage and infection. It is interesting to note that Sänger attributed much of the early development of suture material to American frontier surgeons, including Frank Polin of Springfield, Kentucky, who in 1852 had reported the use of silver wire sutures in surviving patients who had undergone cesarean delivery.[12]

As the number of procedures increased, clinicians began to focus attention on other details, most notably the type of uterine incision to employ. The low transverse incision was experimented with between 1880 and 1925 and was noted to reduce the risk of infection, as well as uterine rupture, in subsequent pregnancies.[7]

Death from peritonitis remained a major threat. Approximately 30 years later, extraperitoneal cesarean delivery was first described by Frank[13] (1907) and subsequently modified by Latzko[14] (1909) as a technique to reduce the risk of peritonitis in high-risk patients. Subsequently, Krönig[15] (1912) realized that extraperitoneal cesarean birth not only minimized the effects of peritonitis but also allowed access to the lower uterine segment through a vertical midline incision, which could then be covered with peritoneum, an approach that led to the modern-day low vertical procedure. Later, Beck[16] (1919) and DeLee and Cornell[17] (1922) modified the Krönig approach and popularized it in the United States. Finally, Kerr[18] (1926) developed the low transverse incision, which is most commonly employed throughout the world today. The need for an extraperitoneal procedure was essentially eliminated by the development of modern antibiotics. Penicillin was discovered by Alexander Fleming in 1928, and its use became widespread after it was purified as a drug in 1940.

As the risk versus benefit considerations changed, obstetricians became more confident in its use and began to argue against delaying surgery. Surgeons such as

Robert Harris of the United States, Thomas Radford of England, and Franz von Winckel of Germany recommended cesarean delivery as an early solution to labor disorders to improve outcome. In turn, maternal and perinatal mortality rates were reduced as cesarean birth became viewed as one of several approaches to improve perinatal outcome.[7]

Cesarean Birth Rates

The Changing Rate of Cesarean Birth

The early onset of a change in the overall cesarean delivery rate is dramatically demonstrated by data from the Chicago Lying-In Hospital, which had a fivefold increase in the cesarean rate from 0.6 percent in 1910 to 3 percent in 1928.[19] In the ensuing years the reported rate of cesarean delivery (Table 19-1) in the United States increased in dramatic fashion from 4.5 percent in 1965, to 16.5 percent in 1980, finally peaking at 24.7 percent in 1988.[20] Cesarean delivery rates have also increased worldwide during the past 20 years.[21,22] However, the increase in international rates does not approach the high rates seen in the United States. Comparative values are available in 1985 for the United States (22.7 percent), Canada (19 percent), England (10 percent), Denmark (13 percent), Italy (15.8 percent), Sweden (12 percent), Norway (12.5 percent), New Zealand (10 percent), Japan (7 percent).[21,22]

NICHD Task Force on Cesarean Childbirth

Cesarean births increase health-care costs, pose considerable additional risk for maternal mortality and morbidity, and, with few exceptions, provide only marginal proven fetal benefits. In 1979, the National Institutes of Health (NIH) established a Task Force on Cesarean Childbirth and in 1980 sponsored a Consensus Development Conference to consider the issue of cesarean delivery in the United States.[24] The task force recommended that efforts be made to diminish the impact of elective repeat cesarean delivery and the diagnosis of "dystocia" because these indications were the two major causes of the increase in cesarean birth rates that were likely to be susceptible to reduction.

Although an immediate slowing of the rate of increase of cesarean births was not readily apparent, the widespread dissemination of the consensus document did provide the medical community with reassurance that an attempt to reduce the escalating cesarean rate was a reasonable goal. The cesarean rate ultimately peaked at 24.7 percent in 1988.[1] Both the total cesarean rate and the primary rate apparently decreased since then to approximately 23.5 and 17.1 percent, respectively, by 1991.[1] Unfortunately, cesarean rates in some institutions continue to excede 30 percent.

Is There an "Ideal" Cesarean Rate?

It is probably not possible to define an "ideal" cesarean rate. The desired rate will vary from institution to institution on the basis of multiple factors. Quilligan[25] has suggested that it may be better to define a range of values for each indication: failure to progress/cephalopelvic disproportion (2 to 4 percent); repeat cesarean delivery (2 to 6 percent); breech and abnormal lie (1.3 to 3.5 percent); nonreassuring fetal heart rate (FHR) (1.5 to 3 percent); and third trimester bleeding (1 percent).[25] Tertiary centers with associated higher rates of preterm birth and placenta previa can

Table 19-1   Cesarean Birth Rates and Outcomes of Patients with Prior Cesarean Delivery for Selected Years (1965–1991)[1]

| Year | Total Births ×1000 | Cesarean Rate (%) | | Prior Cesarean | |
		Total	Primary	Repeat Cesarean[a] (%)	VBAC[b] (%)
1965	3,760	**4.5**	NA	NA	NA
1970	3,731	5.5	4.2	**25.2**	2.2
1975	3,144	10.4	7.8	27.1	2.0
1980	3,612	**16.5**	12.1	29.9	3.4
1985	3,761	**22.7**	16.3	34.6	6.6
1986	3,757	24.1	17.4	34.3	8.5
1987	3,809	24.4	17.4	35.3	9.8
1988	3,910	**24.7**	**17.5**	**36.3**	12.6
1989	4,041	23.8	17.1	35.6	18.5
1990	4,158	23.5	16.8	35.9	20.4
1991	4,111	23.5	17.1	35.0	24.2

[a]Proportion of *all* cesareans that are repeat cesareans.
[b]Women with vaginal birth per 100 deliveries in women with prior cesareans.

Table 19-2   Goal 14.8: Reduce the Cesarean Delivery Rate to no more than 15 per 100 deliveries[a]

| | | Cesarean Type Specific Targets | |
| | | 1987 Baseline | 2000 Target |
Goal	Delivery		
14.8a	Primary (first time) cesarean delivery	17.4	12
14.8b	Repeat cesarean deliveries	91.2[b]	65[b]

[a]Baseline: 24.4 per 100 deliveries in 1987.
[b]Among women who had a previous cesarean delivery.
(Data from MMWR[1] and U.S. Department of Health and Human Services.[26])

Table 19-4   Total Cesarean Birth Rates (%) by Age of Mother

Age (years)	1980[a]	1989[a]	1991[b]
<20	14.5	18.1	18.2
20–24	15.8	21.1	21.0
25–29	16.7	24.8	24.3
30–34	18.0	26.6	26.7
≥35	20.6	30.3	28.4
Total	16.5	23.8	23.5

[a]Data from Taffel et al.[23]
[b]Data from MMWR.[1]

be expected to have higher cesarean rates. Recently the U.S. Department of Health and Human Services, as part of its Healthy People 2000 program, identified a number of health-related objectives. One goal related to cesarean rates is noted in Table 19-2.[1,26]

Causes of Increased Cesarean Birth Rate

At least 90 percent of the increase between 1980 and 1985 was attributable to three factors: repeat cesarean deliveries (48 percent), dystocia (29 percent), and "fetal distress" (16 percent). There are many complex and interrelated reasons (Table 19-3) for the increase in the cesarean birth rate.[21]

Table 19-3   Causes of Increased Cesarean Rate

Medical advances diminishing maternal risks
Labor- and delivery-related factors
  Repeat cesarean birth[a]
  Continuous electronic fetal monitoring[a]
  Dystocia diagnosis liberalized[a]
  Epidural analgesia/anesthesia
  Macrosomia (> 4,000 vs. > 4,500 g)
  Decreased use of forceps/vacuum[27]
Maternal factors
  More older childbearing women/delay in childbirth[20]
  More nulliparous women with attendant risk
  Increasing maternal risk
Fetal factors
  Fetus as a patient
  Breech presentation[20]
  VLBW fetus
  Active genital herpes
  Post-term pregnancy
  Multiple gestation (especially with nonvertex)
  Failed induction for fetal indication
Physician Factors
  Fear of malpractice litigation
  Physician compensation (possible)
  Physician convenience (possible)

[a](Data from Taffel et al,[20] Notzon et al,[21] and Placek et al,[27] with permission.)

Medical Advances

Early liberalization of the indications for cesarean delivery rose out of the increased availability of effective antibiotics, safer blood banking, and a greater tendency for obstetrics to be practiced in facilities delivering large numbers of patients. Even socioeconomic factors have played a role.

Delay in Childbirth

The widespread availability of contraceptive and sterilization techniques has resulted in women giving birth at an older age.[20]

More Older and Often Nulliparous Patients

Older and often nulliparous patients constitute an increasing proportion of laboring women. In the United States between 1980 and 1985, the number of births in patients at least 30 years of age increased from 20 to 25 percent of all deliveries.[20] It is well known that the cesarean delivery rate increases with advancing age (Table 19-4) as a result of increased likelihood of dystocia and medical complications such as preeclampsia and gestational diabetes.

Dystocia Diagnosis Liberalized

The diagnostic criteria for dystocia accepted by some have been liberalized, and forcep deliveries have fallen into relative disfavor in some medical centers. For the interval 1972 to 1980, Placek et al[27] reported a decline in forceps delivery from 37 to 18 percent, which parallels the increase in the cesarean delivery rate from 7 to 17 percent.[27]

Fetus as a Patient

Historically, cesarean delivery had been performed primarily to reduce the likelihood of maternal morbidity and mortality. In the mid-1970s, the eventual health status of the fetus-neonate began to play a larger role in the decision process. Widespread employment of techniques such as continuous electronic fetal monitoring, ultrasound evaluation of the fetus, and fetal karyotype determinations by amniocentesis or chorionic villus sampling resulted in a change in emphasis to "quality of survival" for newborns, not simply survival. The fetus became viewed more as a person and eventually a patient.

Nonreassuring FHR Indications

Despite dramatic advances in perinatal medicine, the widespread employment of electronic fetal monitoring, and a significant increase in the cesarean birth rate in the last two decades, there has been no reported reduction in the rate of cerebral palsy. There is general consensus that continuous electronic fetal monitoring (EFM) does not reduce the risk of metabolic acidosis-related newborn morbidity or cerebral palsy better than intermittent auscultation.[28-31] Since cesarean delivery for this indication commonly follows the observation of subtle EFM changes in FHR variability or late decelerations, both of which are not detectable by auscultation, the association of subtle findings with later developmental problems may indicate a preexisting fetal abnormality, not likely to benefit from a cesarean delivery.[28-30] The previous "normal" fetus, except in extreme conditions (i.e., severe prolonged decelerations arising from cord prolapse or placental abruption) is likely to have sufficient physiologic adaptability to adjust to the stress responsible for the relatively subtle fetal heart rate patterns that are not detectable by intermittent auscultation. Support for this notion is provided by the obvious contrast between the relatively high frequency of significant FHR alterations but infrequent occurrence of cerebral palsy. The fetus with prior developmental abnormality is more likely to demonstrate nonreassuring FHR patterns during labor than is its neurologically normal peer.

Breech as an Indication

Vaginal breech deliveries have been abandoned by many clinicians in favor of cesarean delivery. Most breech presentations are now delivered by cesarean birth, with rates in some medical centers as high as 79[20] and 92[32] percent, but without notable benefit.[32] Selective vaginal breech delivery can be accomplished safely with good outcome. At this time there is no consensus that will allow the predetermination of the best route of delivery in all cases of breech presentation. Furthermore, cesarean extraction of a breech at cesarean delivery requires skills very similar to those used in a vaginal birth, including avoidance of hyperextension of the fetal head.[33]

Fear of Litigation

Unfortunately, obstetric practice in the United States is adversely influenced by the high rate of malpractice litigation. Medicolegal pressures have forced a liberalization of indications. Concern regarding potential malpractice action for failure to intervene at an alleged "standard" time increased dramatically in the 1980s, particularly among physicians in traditional private practice. Statistics to support this concept indicate that private nulliparous patients are more likely than clinic patients to undergo cesarean delivery if dystocia or malpresentation or so-called fetal distress is diagnosed.[34]

The practice of obstetrics has become more defensive. Many American obstetricians have concluded that one of the best ways to reduce malpractice vulnerability is to "liberalize" indications for cesarean delivery. Obstetricians harbor a fear that they may be criticized in hindsight for failure to perform an earlier cesarean delivery that "may have" resulted in a better outcome. The result is a more defensive approach to practice, including a lower threshold for resorting to cesarean delivery.[35] Unfortunately there are few data to support a benefit to this strategy.

The magnitude of "fear of litigation" as a contributing factor to the current cesarean rates can be inferred from a survey of British and American obstetricians, designed to determine the perceived reason for the rise in cesarean rates. Litigation was the leading reason given by 84 percent of American obstetricians but only 42 percent of British obstetricians.[36] Some physicians have employed cesarean delivery as an answer to all potential problems; an extreme was reached in 1985, when the following was asked: "If an informed patient opts for prophylactic cesarean section at term, can it be denied?"[37] Tort reform is the only likely solution to this particular problem.

Prior Cesarean Birth

As the indications were expanded, it is not surprising that "prior cesarean delivery" became an ever-increasing indication for cesarean birth. Approximately 25 percent (Table 19-1) of all cesarean deliveries were for the indication of prior cesarean birth in 1970.[1] The percentage of all cesarean procedures attributable to this indication peaked at 36.3 percent in 1988.

Determinants of Rate Variation

Physician Factors

The etiology of differences in cesarean birth rates reported by different centers is as yet unresolved. For instance, Blumenthal et al[38] noted a significant difference between the incidence of dystocia in public versus private patients and concluded that the difference was probably the result of differences in indications employed by physicians in the two groups. While it has been suggested that physician convenience or economic gain may be operative in the decision to perform a cesarean delivery in private patients, Phillips et al[39] were unable to demonstrate the predictable distribution of nonscheduled cesarean births that would support this hypothesis. Furthermore, this author's experience with a large number of private physicians in many centers suggests that this is not a major contributor. Rather, it is the fear of not performing a cesarean that is often the main culprit. Furthermore, the difference in compensation for cesarean and vaginal deliveries is small, in most cases well deserved, often following long or difficult labors.

Regional Differences

There are surprisingly dramatic regional difference in total cesarean rates in all hospitals as well as in teaching hospitals.[1,40,41] In 1991, the cesarean rate (Table 19-5) in the South was 27.6 percent, significantly ($p < 0.05$) higher than rates in the West, Midwest, and North-Northeast.[1] Regional variations also exist among teaching hospitals; however in the analysis the rate in the Northeast (23.4 percent) is significantly higher than those in the other three regions ($p = 0.002$).[40]

Teaching Vs. Nonteaching Hospitals

Women delivering in a teaching hospital are less likely to have a cesarean delivery than are those delivering in hospitals without resident programs. In 1990, the estimated rate in all hospitals with resident programs was 20.3 percent compared with an overall national rate of 23.5 percent; the estimated rate for nonteaching hospitals was 24.7 percent (odds ratio, 0.77; 95 percent CI, 0.77–0.78; $p = 0.0001$). Of all cesarean deliveries conducted in teaching hospitals, 64.8 percent were primary and 35.2 percent were repeat.[40] Significantly lower rates were also observed in Illinois teaching hospitals despite the fact that they had more deliveries of

patients 35 years old and older, patients less than 20 years old, patients with medical complications, and patients with labor complications.[41] The hypothesized basis for the lower rate in teaching hospitals include routine consultation prior to performing nonelective cesareans, routine review conferences, and around the clock availability of physicians to manage labor, minimizing any tendency for physician time pressures to influence the decision process.

Obstacles to Rate Reduction

There is an ongoing need to continue to reduce the current cesarean birth rates. Despite an awareness that there is a potential problem, we may have entered a cycle that will make major rate reduction difficult. Respected clinicians vary greatly in their acceptance of procedures such as midforceps or vaginal delivery of the breech, whether it be a singleton or one of a multiple gestation. This author continues to believe that labor can be managed more scientifically, that at least 50 percent of breeches can selectively and safely be delivered vaginally, even the very-low-birth-weight (VLBW) fetus (weighing less than 1,500 g). Many physicians recently trained in obstetrics have had insufficient exposure to operative vaginal procedures to develop a "comfort" level and consequently often opt for a procedure with which they are familiar, cesarean delivery. Furthermore, our specialty is increasingly dominated by the emergence of the subspecialty of maternal-fetal medicine. The traditional obstetrician "teacher" with many years of clinical hands-on experience has been replaced by the young subspecialist who may have greater in-depth scientific knowledge, particularly related to high-risk obstetric problems and invasive procedures, but who often lacks experience or interest in operative vaginal procedures. The questions now are who can and how do we conduct the necessary clinical trial of vaginal delivery versus cesarean delivery, and, if operative vaginal delivery were proven to be safe, who will train future physicians to perform these procedures?

Benefits and Risks of Cesarean Birth

Maternal Mortality

Maternal mortality as a result of cesarean delivery fortunately is an infrequent occurrence, but the overall rate is estimated to be severalfold higher than that following vaginal delivery. Approximately 300 maternal deaths occur annually in the United States out of slightly more than 4 million deliveries of all types per year, an overall rate less than 10 per 100,000 live births. Not surprisingly, the reported incidence of maternal

Table 19-5   Regional Variation in Cesarean Rates (%)

Region	Hospitals	
	All[a]	Teaching[b]
Northeast	22.6	23.4
South	27.6	21.2
Midwest	21.8	20.5
West	19.8	18.7

[a]$p = < 0.05$.
[b]$p = 0.002$.
(Data from MMWR[1] and Sanchez-Ramos et al,[40] with permission.)

mortality following cesarean delivery can vary greatly from series to series, particularly in single institution reports. Maternal mortality following cesarean birth has been assessed in two publications[5,42] with a sufficient number of cesarean deliveries (400,000, 121,000) to provide meaningful estimates. On the basis of these two reports, mortality can be estimated to range from 6.1[5] to 22 per 100,000 live births. Approximately one-third[42] to one-half[5] of maternal deaths of cesarean patients can be attributed directly to the cesarean procedure itself.[5,42]

Perinatal Morbidity and Mortality

The hypothesis that cesarean birth offers a major opportunity to improve perinatal outcome has, with few exceptions, not been proven. It is more likely that the improvement in perinatal mortality is the product of widespread changes in perinatal care. There are no well-documented prospective trials demonstrating benefit to the fetus or to the mother that would justify the extent of the increase in the primary cesarean delivery rate over the past two decades. There was hope that birth-related newborn morbidity, including cerebral palsy, could be dramatically reduced by liberalizing the indications for cesarean delivery. Unfortunately, there are no data to suggest a decline in the incidence of cerebral palsy despite the major perinatal advances put into place since the mid-1970s. Perinatal mortality and morbidity for the most part remain predominantly a function of gestational age, intrauterine growth restriction, and congenital anomalies, as well as the indication for delivery. Nonetheless, any concerted strategy to reduce the cesarean rate can be accepted only if there is evidence to suggest that lowering current rates will not have an adverse effect on perinatal mortality and long-term development. The implied justification for many cesarean births is the protection of the fetus from death and by implication from cerebral palsy. Although national perinatal mortality rates have decreased as cesarean birth rates have increased, the crucial question is, is this simply an association, or does a causal relationship exist?

There has been a heated international debate regarding the role of cesarean birth in reducing perinatal mortality. O'Driscoll and Foley[43] do not attribute improvements in perinatal outcome to liberalization of cesarean indications.[43] Cesarean delivery rates have remained stable at the National Maternity Hospital in Dublin, Ireland, at less than 5 percent between 1965 to 1980, whereas rates in the United States have increased from slightly less than 5 percent in 1965 to more than 15 percent in 1980. Because the perinatal mortality rate at the National Maternity Hospital has progressively fallen from 42.1 to 16.8 per 1,000 births despite a low

cesarean delivery rate, one is forced to consider that, although liberalization of cesarean delivery indicators may contribute to better perinatal outcome, it is likely to be less important than the overall improvement in obstetric and neonatal care.

Leveno et al[44] subsequently countered that the data of O'Driscoll and Foley[43] are limited by their emphasis on mortality rather than morbidity. They suggested that their more liberal use of cesarean delivery (18 percent in 1983) was "associated with" decreased intrapartum deaths and neonatal seizures when compared with the National Maternity Hospital in Dublin, Ireland, where reported cesarean rates are in the 4 to 6 percent range.[44,45]

O'Driscoll and Foley (of the Dublin group) in their response to the critique by Leveno et al, indicated that in order to compare uncommon events, a larger number of births would be required. They compared data from more than 24,000 births (5.1 percent cesarean rate) at The National Maternity Hospital with those from more than 22,000 (17.8 percent cesarean rate) at Parkland Hospital. Despite the dramatic difference in cesarean rates they could detect no difference in perinatal mortality.[46] During the study years (1982–1984) the incidence of neonatal seizures was similar in the two institutions. Caution was also raised regarding the precision of the diagnosis and etiology of seizures between the two institutions.

It is most likely that the decline in perinatal mortality is attributable to major advances in prenatal care (ultrasound, antepartum testing, amniotic fluid surfactant determinations, and so forth), as well as dramatic improvements in neonatal intensive care including the availability of surfactant implemented in the same time frame. Porreco[47] provided data to suggest little, if any, impact arising from cesarean birth. They divided unselected patients into two groups, one with management minimizing the use of cesarean delivery and the other with routine management. The cesarean rate in the first group (5.7 percent) was considerably less than that of the routine group (17.6 percent). Despite the dramatic difference in cesarean rates, the perinatal mortality and morbidity rates were not significantly different between the two groups.[47]

Cesarean Delivery as a Strategy To Reduce Cerebral Palsy

Scheller and Nelson[48] from the NICHD, in a review of the literature of the past 25 years, concluded that there is no evidence to support the hypothesis that the increased cesarean delivery rate has had a favorable impact on the rate of neurologic disorders or on cerebral palsy. When comparing the occurrence rates of cerebral palsy in nations with a broad range of cesarean rates

(7 to 22 percent), the reported cerebral palsy rates in all countries were within a very narrow range of 1.1 to 1.3 per 1,000 in neonatal survivors with birth weights more than 2,500 g.[48] Furthermore, there is no evidence that continuous electronic fetal monitoring provides an advantage over periodic auscultation.[28–30]

It is important that the clinician as well as public health policy leaders consider the balance between the likelihood of salvaging a small number of cases in which the fetus is thought to be threatened by death or later developmental disabilities as a result of intrapartum metabolic acidosis (on the basis of continuous FHR findings) against the significant possibility of maternal morbidity (intraoperative, including serious hemorrhage and postoperative complications of cesarean delivery reported elsewhere in this chapter) arising from cesarean delivery in a larger number of mothers. Most newborns delivered by cesarean birth following the detection of nonreassuring FHR patterns (of a degree to result in physician decision to perform cesarean delivery) during labor do not benefit from the current high rate of surgical intervention, much of which is defensive in nature. Nelson et al[49] assessed (in a population-based case-control study of 155,636 term fetuses) the benefits of continuous electronic fetal monitoring as a means to reduce later cerebral palsy, controlling for the confounding effects of other known major risk factors for cerebral palsy. The authors estimated the false-positive rate of the continuous FHR predictors (multiple late decelerations and/or decreased beat-to-beat variability) that resulted in nonbeneficial cesarean delivery to be 99.9 percent in cases with no risk factors and 99.6 percent in the high-risk (vaginal bleeding, breech presentation, meconium-stained amniotic fluid, gestational age under 37 weeks at delivery, and maternal infection, i.e., sepsis, chorioamnionitis, temperature during labor of 38°C or higher).[49]

For the data to be more easily appreciated, the authors estimated the impact of current cesarean intervention practices on a population of 100,000 singleton term newborns. Summed up, there would be 516 to 2,324 mother-newborn pairs exposed to nonbeneficial cesarean intervention for each newborn in whom cerebral palsy would be prevented under the assumptions of the two models presented below. This range ($\frac{1}{516}$ to $\frac{1}{2,324}$) should be of considerable value in the rational determination of public health policy ordinarily based on risk (maternal intra- and postoperative complications) versus benefit analysis. It also provides a major insight into the present impact of defensive obstetric practice arising in the current medicolegal environment.

In both models the authors predicted that continuous FHR would demonstrate multiple late decelerations or decreased beat-to-beat variability in approxi-

mately 9,300 cases (9.3 percent); of that subset, only 18 children (0.19 percent of 9,300) would be expected to have cerebral palsy. In the authors' first model they assumed a worst case (the literature indicates that 3 to 20 percent of cerebral palsy cases arising in infants born at term are the result of intrapartum metabolic acidosis) scenario, that is, the highest reported estimate (20 percent) of the association. If an obstetric detection and intervention system could be developed that would reliably allow intervention to prevent 100 percent of such cases (in the 20 percent of patients with cerebral palsy that the model attributes to metabolic acidosis) then only 4 (18 × 20 percent = 3.6) of the 100,000 full-term newborns could possibly benefit from continuous fetal monitoring. Unfortunately, the intervention (i.e., cesarean delivery on the basis of a continuous FHR indicator for metabolic acidosis) would occur in 9,296 (9300 − 4) additional deliveries, or 2,324 (9296 ÷ 4) nonbeneficial interventions for each child in which cerebral palsy is prevented.

In the second model the authors further assumed that all cases of cerebral palsy demonstrating the above nonreassuring FHR observations are due to intrapartum metabolic acidosis and that there would be an intervention that is 100 percent effective in the prevention of cerebral palsy (neither assumption is currently correct). Under this ideal scenario the number of interventions resulting in no benefit would be 516 ([9,300 − 18] ÷ 18) for each child in whom cerebral palsy was prevented. Unfortunately neither assumption is correct; nonreassuring FHR observations arise as a result of preexisting central nervous system dysfunction, and there are few diagnosis and intervention systems that are 100 percent effective.

Indications for Cesarean Delivery

Overview of Indications

In general, cesarean delivery is employed when labor is contraindicated or vaginal delivery is unlikely to be accomplished safely or within a time frame necessary to prevent the development of fetal and/or maternal morbidity in excess of that expected following vaginal delivery.

Indications for cesarean delivery can be categorized (Table 19-6) in several ways. Some indications strictly benefit the fetus, whereas others are largely done for maternal benefit to avoid maternal hemorrhage, reduce the potential spread of malignancy, avoid the repeated need for additional procedures such as abdominal cerclage in future pregnancies, and prevent uterine rupture. Some indications will benefit *both* mother and fetus. Some indications are well accepted even though selectively applied on a subjective basis. Placenta previa

Table 19-6 Commonly Reported Indications for Cesarean Delivery

Indications	Selective	Subjective	Controversial[a]	Universally Accepted[b]
Fetal				
Nonreassuring FHR[c]	✓	✓		✓
Breech, frank	✓		✓	
Breech, nonfrank	✓		✓	
Breech, preterm	✓		✓	
Very low birth weight (< 1,500 g)	✓		✓	
Herpes simplex virus	✓			
Immune thrombocytopenic purpura	✓			
Congenital anomalies, major	✓		✓	
Maternal-fetal				
Cephalopelvic disproportion (relative)	✓	✓		✓
Cephalopelvic disproportion (absolute)		✓		✓
Failure to progress	✓	✓		✓
Placental abruption	✓	✓		✓
Placenta previa				✓
Maternal				
Obstructive benign and malignant tumors	✓	✓		✓
Large vulvar condyloma	✓	✓		
Cervical cerclage (abdominal)	✓			
Prior vaginal colporrhaphy	✓			
Conjoined twins				✓

[a]Controversy regarding need for universal application.
[b]Universally accepted if selective/subjective criteria present.
[c]Of a critical degree commonly associated with change in FHR variability.

or conjoined twins are universally accepted as indications for cesarean birth. On the other hand, several indications such as a breech presentation or a VLBW fetus are controversial. It is not feasible to discuss all indications for cesarean delivery in this chapter; however, comparison of cesarean delivery rates associated with specific labor and maternal fetal indications for 1980 and 1989 is noted later in Table 19-12.

Fetal Indications

Fetal indications for cesarean birth are in large part designed to minimize neonatal morbidity and possibly long-term consequences of profound intrapartum metabolic or mixed metabolic acidemia and/or delivery-related trauma (including significant fetal thrombocytopenia) or transmission of infection.[50,51] Accepted indications, often employed selectively, include the following: "significant" nonremediable and nonreassuring FHR patterns, especially when associated with progressive loss of variability; various categories of breech presentation at risk for head entrapment and/or cord prolapse; the VLBW fetus; and active genital herpes. The decision to employ cesarean delivery may be selective, based on the results of ultrasound or cordocentesis studies (i.e., major fetal congenital anom-

alies such as hydrocephalus, gastroschisis, or omphalocele). In such cases a planned, controlled delivery with predictable access to pediatric surgical support may be desirable. The case issue is far from clear, particularly with gastroschisis, for which there is no proven benefit to cesarean birth.

"Significant" Nonreassuring FHR Observations

Approximately 1 to 3 percent of all laboring patients undergo cesarean delivery for a nonremediable and nonreassuring FHR pattern (see Ch. 14). Some clinicians unfortunately continue to designate this indication as "fetal distress," a term not recommended by the American College of Obstetricians and Gynecologists (ACOG).[51] The cesarean delivery rate and the precise criteria for "fetal distress" vary considerably from hospital to hospital and among individual practitioners. In large part, that variation reflects the subjective nature of the interpretation of continuous FHR. In 1978, Haddad and Lundy[52] estimated that approximately 50 percent of cesarean births performed for such nonreassuring FHR patterns in their hospital were not justified on independent peer review.

Infection as a Risk

The impact of vaginal delivery as a risk factor for transmission of infection is organism/problem specific.

Herpes Simplex

Despite the fact that most newborns (70 percent) infected with herpes simplex virus (HSV) are delivered of women who have neither active genital herpes nor a history of these lesions, patients who deliver vaginally with an active genital HSV lesion have a 50 percent risk of transmitting the infection to the neonate if the disease is primary and 0 to 8 percent risk if it is recurrent. Consequently it is generally recommended that patients with a history of genital herpes have a careful perineal examination at the time delivery is contemplated. If an active genital lesion is present, a cesarean delivery should be performed. However, patients with nongenital lesions may deliver vaginally if the lesion can be covered and draped away from the perineum.[53]

Human Immunodeficiency Virus Infection

The human immunodeficiency virus (HIV) provides a contrasting clinical solution, based largely on the observation that the risk of congenital (intrauterine, presumably transplacental) or intrapartum transmission of HIV from an infected woman to her fetus or newborn depends on multiple factors; the best estimates of vertical transmission of HIV from an infected woman ranges from 12.9 to 39 percent. Consequently, cesarean delivery does not appear to protect the neonate from HIV infection.[54]

Maternal-Fetal Indications

Placental abnormalities such as placenta previa or placental abruption in which hemorrhage poses a significant risk to both mother and fetus, as well as labor "dystocia," are indications for which cesarean delivery offers a potential benefit to both mother and fetus. When extreme, each can pose one or more maternal risks, including hemorrhage, uterine rupture and infection, and fetal metabolic acidosis.

Dystocia is a term used to describe indications for cesarean birth arising from one or more of the three "Ps": relatively large fetus (passenger), relatively small "passage" (pelvis), or relatively insufficient or inefficient uterine contractions (power). Some add a fourth "P," the fearful physician. Included in "dystocia" are "failure to progress" (FTP), relative "cephalopelvic disproportion" (CPD), and absolute CPD on the rare occasion when the latter can be diagnosed. Some include "failed inductions" under this designation. CPD is almost always a relative term; the CPD diagnosis is made only after application of a number of diagnostic and thera-

peutic measures including oxytocin. In most instances it involves a normal-sized fetus.[55]

Maternal Indications

There are only a few indications for cesarean delivery that are solely maternal. They include mechanical obstructions of the vagina from large vulvovaginal condylomata, advanced lower genital tract malignancy, and placement of a permanent abdominal cerclage with a desire for future pregnancies.

Hospital Requirements for Cesarean Delivery

The requirements for hospitals offering cesarean delivery appear in several publications.[56–58]

Facility and Personnel Requirements

Any hospital that provides labor and delivery services should be equipped to perform an "emergency" cesarean delivery. A hospital offering obstetric services should provide the professional and institutional resources to respond to "acute obstetric emergencies" (i.e., a cesarean delivery) within 30 minutes, when indicated (see below), from the time a decision is made until the procedure is begun.[58] The nursing, anesthesia, neonatal resuscitation, and obstetric personnel required must be either in the hospital or readily available. Should VBAC-trial of labor be considered a physician who is capable of evaluating the labor and performing the cesarean should be "readily" available.[59] The Canadian Consensus Conference panel has also suggested guidelines similar to those recommended by the ACOG.[57]

Selective Application of Minimum Interval

It is noteworthy that the above recommendation is intended to define the resources necessary for a facility to conduct obstetric services. It is not intended to determine a time frame in which all cesarean deliveries should be initiated. Not all indications for cesarean delivery will require a 30-minute response time. As of this date, there is no consensus standard that defines an acceptable time interval for performance of a cesarean delivery within 30 minutes except in the presence of certain subjective, judgement-dependent, "clinically significant" nonreassuring FHR patterns (see indications above) that fulfill criteria and pose significant risk of profound fetal metabolic acidemia requiring rapid intervention; prolapse of the cord; symptomatic uterine rupture; and certain cases of obvious and symptomatic placental abruption and persistent hemorrhage secondary to placenta previa. Under most circumstances (i.e., protraction and arrest disorders of labor) cesarean delivery is not necessary within a 30-minute time frame. Indeed in certain large units triage may be necessary to determine priority of access to the operating room, anesthesiologists, and other resources.

Feasibility of Recommended Decision to Incision Interval

There was initially some concern regarding the necessity or likelihood of compliance with the recommendation for a 30-minute interval. Porreco and Meier[60] evaluated the likelihood of need for an urgent cesarean birth that would activate the 30-minute recommendation in patients with and without a prior cesarean birth. The indication for the repeat procedure was not urgent in most patients; most patients failed to progress in the first or second stage. The need for a delivery within 30 minutes was similar in patients with no prior cesarean delivery (1.9 percent [two cases]) and in those with a previous low transverse incision (1.4 percent). The two patients with a prior low transverse incision who required an urgent cesarean birth were found to have an intact scar at the time of surgery.[60] The Canadian Consensus Conference on Cesarean Childbirth (four prospective studies) made similar observations, noting the probability of urgent cesarean delivery to be only 2.7 percent among 11,819 births.[57] Symptomatic uterine dehiscence occurred in only 0.22 percent of births.

Surgical Principles and Operative Procedure

Skin Preparation

An abdominal incision interrupts the body's first line of defense against infection. The primary objective of skin preparation for cesarean delivery is to reduce the risk of wound infection by decreasing the bacterial flora of the patient's abdominal wall along the anticipated incision site. It is impossible to sterilize skin. The preparation of the patient's intended incision site in the operating room ordinarily includes mechanical removal of obvious foreign material, application of soap or detergent scrub to remove surface dirt and oil, plus application of a topical antimicrobial agent to reduce the bacteria to a minimal level at the site and adjacent skinfolds and/or umbilicus.[61] In noncesarean patients the duration and choice of the surgical scrub have not been demonstrated to reduce the rate of wound infection significantly in either clean or clean-contaminated (cesarean delivery) wounds.[62–64] There is great variation in the duration of the clinical skin scrub among both physicians and hospitals. Some apply a surgical scrub for up to 5 minutes, whereas others simply scrub the

intended site for approximately 30 seconds and apply a bactericidal solution. Overall, the rate of wound infection is approximately 6 to 8 percent whether the skin preparation is sprayed or mechanically scrubbed. It is likely that simple application by painting or spraying is as effective, if not more effective, than the traditional approach of long-term mechanical scrubbing.[65,66] There are also data that suggest that a rapid alcohol preparation followed by application of iodine-impregnated sterile drapes may safely reduce skin preparation time to 1 to 2 minutes.[67]

Despite years of clinical research, there are few prospective randomized studies to demonstrate benefit of any one of the various skin-cleansing preparations, or even hand washing agents, over another. In general, much of what the physician does is based on long-standing surgical tradition. Some overview of this aspect of surgical practice was provided by Masterson,[68] who indicated that "a surgeon probably would have a lower wound infection rate if he/she did not wash the patient's skin before surgery, than if he/she shaved the patient's operative site the night before surgery. The same author has also indicated that "preoperative skin preparation, whether it is the patient's or the surgeon's, should be a brief event. Successful wound healing is determined more by what is done in the wound than what is done on the wound."

Bacteria such as *Staphylococcus aureus*, which may be normal inhabitants of the hair follicle, may be reduced in the process, but are not totally eliminated. Fortunately "transient" flora are easier to remove from the skin than are the "resident" flora that are attached to the skin by adhesion or adsorption and require friction for removal. Under ordinary circumstances, the number of flora in any one area is relatively stable. The relative risk of infection with skin incisions varies, to some extent, according to the site of the incision; the availability of moisture, which promotes bacterial colonization; and the presence of lipid secretion by sebaceous glands. The indigenous "resident" flora of the skin are mainly diphtheroids and gram-positive rods, including aerobic *Corynebacterium* and anaerobic *Propionibacterium*. Gram-negative organisms can proliferate in moist areas such as under a panniculus or air-tight dressing.[69] The aerobic corynebacteria diphtheroids are the most common organisms in areas of moist skin. The diphtheroids seldom cause clinical infection and are actually important in the ecology of skin by suppressing *Staphylococcus epidermidis* and *S. aureus*.

In contrast to the normal resident skin flora whose numbers are normally stable, "transient" flora are deposited on the skin and in the incision/wound from the environment and, as a consequence, vary greatly in type and number. Other factors that determine whether a wound infection will occur include host resistance, virulence of the organisms deposited on the skin/incisional wound, presence and amount of tissue destruction, size and reactivity of the suture material, vascularity of the incision site, and length of the procedure. In the case of cesarean delivery, leakage of cervical and vaginal secretions into the pelvis and transmittal to the skin incision site are also contributing factors.

Preparation of the vagina prior to cesarean delivery is seldom an issue with the possible exception of cases in which a cesarean hysterectomy is planned. Preparation of the vagina is intended to reduce postoperative infection. However, if the clinician decides to use prophylactic antibiotics, it is doubtful that there is any additional benefit to be gained from preoperative preparation of the vagina with an antiseptic preparation. Should a cesarean hysterectomy be planned, simple irrigation of the vagina with a saline solution will dilute the concentration of bacteria in the vagina and may provide additional benefit.

Hair Removal

In general, the only reason to remove hair from the intended operative site is to eliminate hair that will mechanically interfere with the surgeon's approximation of the wound edges and with adhesion and removal of postoperative dressings.[70] Hair is sterile.[71] Removal of hair with a razor may increase wound infection rates by creating breaks in the skin for bacterial entry. Should shaving be required, it is best done in the operating room. Alexander et al[2] have shown that clipping the hair the morning of surgery results in a significantly lower infection rate than does clipping the hair the evening prior to surgery or shaving at any time.

Suture Selection

Sutures may be synthetic or nonsynthetic in origin. The latter are derived from gut, cotton, or silk. Sutures can be further divided into absorbable and nonabsorbable types (Table 19-7). The *United States Pharmacopeia* categorizes suture materials as nonabsorbable if tensile strength is maintained for more than 60 days. In turn, synthetic suture types are braided or monofilament.

The braided absorbable sutures are either coated (Vicryl or Dexon Plus) or noncoated (Dexon S).

Synthetic sutures offer the benefits of decreased tissue reactivity, prolonged and predictable strength, and low coefficients of friction. Monofilament synthetic sutures elicit somewhat less tissue reaction than their braided counterparts; both are less reactive than their nonsynthetic absorbable and nonabsorbable counterparts. The larger the gauge of the suture, the greater the likelihood of adhesion formation.[73] Knot security is maintained for several weeks longer with synthetic absorbable sutures than with chromic cat gut.

The ideal suture ties easily and offers knot security, minimal tissue inflammatory reaction, and tensile strength compatible with the inherent healing properties of the tissue to be reapproximated. It is also desirable that the suture be flexible, pliable, and easy to handle, resistant to infection, and reabsorbed at a predictable rate. The selection of the suture material to be used should also be based on how rapidly the particular tissue heals. For instance, chromic cat gut, a suture material that maintains tensile strength for a relatively short time, is often appropriate for visceral organs like the bladder, peritoneum, and vagina, surfaces that generally heal quickly, particularly in pregnancy.[74] In contrast, skin and fascia heal more slowly; thus the suture selected should provide more long-term tensile strength. For example, fascia regains only 25 percent of its original strength after 20 days of healing, and the fascial layer is subject to dehiscence if not closed properly. Nonabsorbable synthetic sutures such as polypropylene (Prolene) and polybutester (Novafil) are strong and dependable and are frequently used to repair fascia and for mass closure. Monofilament nylons, braided absorable (Vicryl) Maxon, and PDS are also useful.[75]

Each suture type has definite advantages and disadvantages. When using the synthetic sutures, it is recommended that the clinician add two more knots with longer tails to ensure knot security because these sutures may slip when knots are not properly tied. Manufacturers have introduced coated synthetic sutures (Dexon Plus, coated Vicryl) that have less memory and lie more easily. Should the clinician desire to maintain

Table 19-7   Categories of Suture Material Potentially Available for Cesarean Delivery and/or Peripartum Hysterectomy

	Absorbable	Nonabsorbable
Nonsynthetic	Plain gut Chromic gut	Silk Cotton
Synthetic	Polyglycolic accid (Dexon) Polyglactin (Vicryl) 910 Polydioxanone (PDS) Polyglyconate (Maxon) Monocryl	Polypropylene monofilament (Surgilene, Prolene) Braided (Dacron, Mersilene) Gore-Tex (Polytetraflouroethylene) Nylon (Ethibond)

tensile strength in fascial and subcuticular tissue over longer intervals (e.g., patients who have diabetes, are infected, or on corticosteroid therapy), the newer synthetic monofilament absorbable sutures such as polyglyconate (Maxon) and polydioxanone (PDS) may be preferable because they support the tissues in the wound adequately for more than 6 weeks.

Nonabsorbable monofilament sutures such as Prolene and Novafil may be the suture of choice for closing the patient at risk of infection because they do not allow bacteria to invade and colonize the interstices of the braided polyfilament sutures. This feature is particularly important for infected abdominal wall fascia, where tensile strength is crucial and chronic inflammation least desirable.

Abdominal Incisions

Selection of Incision Type

The surgeon may choose either a vertical or a transverse skin incision (Fig. 19-1) when performing a cesarean delivery. The ultimate choice hinges on factors such as the urgency of the procedure, the presence of prior abdominal scars, and associated nonobstetric pathology, if any. To some degree the decision will be based on the surgeon's past experience and on consumer pressures favoring a low transverse incision.[76,77] The midline vertical, transverse Maylard, and trans-

verse Pfannenstiel incisions are the three most commonly employed types. Transverse Cherney and paramedian vertical incisions are seldom used.

There has been a significant increase recently in the use of transverse incisions as opposed to the traditional low vertical incision. The obstetrician, comfortable with several types of incision, is prepared to make a selective decision for each patient's need. The choice should be based on the relative simplicity and speed of the various incisions, the desired exposure, the estimated fetal weight, the anticipated cosmetic results, and the risk factors for infection or dehiscence. In general, vertical incisions allow more rapid access to the lower uterine segment, have less blood loss, provide greater feasibility for incisional extension around the umbilicus, and allow easier examination of the upper abdomen. In pregnancy, speed of entry through a midline vertical incision is facilitated by the common occurrence of diastasis of the rectus muscles.

Transverse incisions are somewhat more time consuming; the difference in time of entry between the two incision types is approximately 30 to 60 seconds in the hands of an experienced clinician. Transverse incisions are preferred cosmetically, are generally less painful, have been associated with a lower risk of subsequent herniation, and yet provide equal, if not better, visualization of the pelvis. Some argue that there is a lower incidence of postoperative pulmonary complications when a transverse incision is used, particularly in patients with preexisting pulmonary problems such as obstructive lung disease.[78] Whether a transverse incision is less subject to dehiscence and herniation remains controversial.[79,80]

A number of surgical principles are relevant regardless of the incision selected. The surgeon and surgical assistant should apply traction at right angles to the intended incision site in a symmetric manner so that the incision is developed in a uniform vertical plane through its length and depth. The "Allis" test may be used to determine if the abdominal incision will be large enough; if a 15-cm-long Allis clamp fits easily between retractors placed at the ends of the incision, little difficulty will be encountered in delivering the fetus.[81] There is no reason to disturb the fat from the adjacent fascia unless there is difficulty in exposing the fascial edges. Such efforts will simply increase the risk of postoperative seromas and develop unnecessary dead space.

The Pfannenstiel and Maylard incisions are the most commonly employed transverse incisions for cesarean delivery. The Maylard incision is quicker, provides better lateral pelvic and midabdominal visualization, requires less dissection and retraction of the anterior abdominal wall during the procedure, and makes a repeat procedure somewhat easier than the Pfannenstiel.

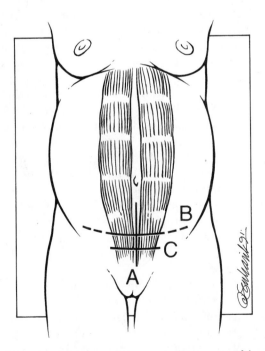

Fig. 19-1 The obstetrician most commonly uses one of three abdominal incisions: (A) midline, (B) Maylard, and (C) Pfannenstiel. Hatched lines indicate possible extension. (Modified from Baker and Shingleton,[313] with permission.)

The Maylard incision (Fig. 19-1) differs from the Pfannenstiel incision in that it involves transverse incision of the anterior rectus sheath and the rectus muscles bilaterally.[82] In the nonobese patient, the skin incision is ordinarily at least 3 to 4 cm above the symphysis. Should there be a large panniculus, the incision may be made considerably higher to avoid placement of the incision on the under surface of the panniculus. The superficial inferior epigastric vessels, generally located in the lateral one-third of the incision, may be individually ligated if necessary. Incision of the rectus muscles is accomplished by placing two fingers or clamps beneath each rectus muscle and lifting the muscles in such a way as to allow surgical incision with either a knife or cutting cautery between the fingers or clamps. In most cesarean procedures, pelvic exposure is sufficient if only the medial two-thirds of the rectus muscles are incised. This avoids the necessity to ligate the deep inferior epigastric vessels, as may be necessary in more extensive gynecologic cases. Nonetheless, the surgeon should palpate for these vessels. Should extension of the incision be necessary, these vessels should be isolated and ligated to avoid hematoma formation. Those favoring a Cherney modification believe it is preferable to partial transsection of the rectus muscles, a technique required with the Maylard incision.[83] After separation of the rectus muscles from the pubic symphysis, the transversalis fascia and peritoneum are then incised transversely, as opposed to the Pfannenstiel incision in which they are incised vertically.

The Pfannenstiel incision (Fig. 19-1) is a curvilinear incision that is best suited for the nonobese patient. The incision is generally made approximately 3 cm above the symphysis pubis within the pubic hair line at its midpoint. The determination of its lateral extension should, to some extent, be a function of the estimated fetal size. Symmetry of the incision can be facilitated by traction of the skin in a cephalad direction during incision that, when released, will result in a curvilinear incision. The incision is generally extended to the lateral border of the rectus muscles at a point 2 to 3 cm inferior and medial to the anterior superior iliac crests. The inferior and superior margin of the fascial incision is elevated to facilitate blunt dissection of the fascial sheath from the underlying rectus muscles. Individual perforating blood vessels between muscle and fascia will require ligation or coagulation to achieve adequate hemostasis. Sharp separation of the muscles from the median raphe, which is facilitated by upward traction on the anterior rectus sheath, is extended superiorly to the level of the umbilicus. Once the rectus muscles are adequately exposed, they are retracted laterally to reveal the underlying transversalis fascia and peritoneum, which is entered via a midline vertical incision

in a manner similar to that of a low vertical abdominal incision.

Abdominal Entry

Surgeons vary in their choice of technique for incising the fascia. Some prefer initial entry by scalpel with subsequent extension with scissors. Others use the scalpel for the entirety of the incision because it is theoretically less traumatic. Once the surgeon becomes familiar with this technique, it allows somewhat faster entry than do scissors. Nonetheless, either technique is appropriate. The site of initial peritoneal entry chosen should be approximately half-way between the umbilicus and symphysis so as to avoid bladder injury, particularly in patients undergoing a repeat cesarean procedure; the peritoneum should be "tented" between two hemostats or pickups and palpated to ascertain that there is no adherent bowel omentum, or even bladder. The peritoneal cavity may be entered using a scalpel or scissors. Should the planned peritoneal incision be in a vertical direction, the peritoneal incision is first extended superiorly for greater exposure and then inferiorly to a point just above the superior pole of the bladder.

Special Considerations

Skin Incision in the Obese Patient

The obese patient is at significant additional risk for wound complications. Reported wound complication rates are 4 and 29 percent in nonobese and obese patients, respectively.[84] Should the patient be massively obese, it may be better to use an incision that does not involve the underside of the panniculus, an area that is more heavily colonized with bacteria and is difficult to prepare surgically, to keep dry, and to inspect in the postoperative period. The objective is to enter the abdomen directly over the lower uterine segment. The surgeon may choose either a vertical midline incision, which is developed peri-umbilically both above and below the umbilicus, or, alternatively, a transverse incision closer to the umbilicus. The actual selection of the site of incision, whether it be vertical or transverse, can be made by retracting the panniculus in a caudad direction so as to place the incision directly overlying the uterine segment.

In closing the fascia of an obese patient, placement of the sutures in the fascia should be at least 1.5 to 2 cm lateral to the cut margin of the fascia, with successive bites approximately 1.5 cm apart along the longitudinal axis of the incision. Should there be major risk factors other than obesity, the clinician may consider use of (1) Smead-Jones monofilament polypropylene internal retention sutures or (2) interrupted or figure-of-eight sutures using either polyglycolic acid or other delayed absorption sutures like monofilament polyglyconate or polydioxanone.

It is also acceptable to use a running continuous large-gauge monofilament polypropylene suture on a large needle in closing the fascial incision. This technique offers the theoretical advantages of distributing tension equally over the continuity of the incision line and increasing the speed of wound closure, thus minimizing the risk of foreign material within the wound. Sutures should not be locked, a technique that reduces vascularization and potentially slows wound healing. Shepherd et al[85] encountered no wound dehiscences employing a mass closure technique in over 200 high-risk gynecology patients. Some advocate placement of a clip on the short end of the suture to avoid knot disruption. If the wound is not entirely dry, closed drainage (anterior to the fascia) exited through a separate stab wound may be employed for 24 to 72 hours until wound drainage is less than 20 cc in 24 hours. Subcutaneous sutures may be used and the skin closed with suture staples, left in place for 10 to 14 days. Some surgeons employ prophylactic postoperative nasal-gastric suction, placed during surgery, for the first 24 hours to avoid distention.

Placenta Previa and Accreta

Although the incidence of placenta accreta has been reported to be approximately 1 in 2,500 deliveries, the incidence increases to approximately 4 percent in patients with a placenta previa.[86] This association is particularly marked in the patient with a previous cesarean birth. Under such circumstances the incidence of placenta accreta may approach 25 percent.[87] For this reason the physician contemplating a cesarean delivery for placenta previa, particularly a repeat procedure, should consider the possibility of hysterectomy.

Selection of Lower Uterine Incision

The most commonly employed uterine incisions (Table 19-8) (Fig. 19-2) are the low transverse incision originally advocated by Kerr[18] and the low vertical incision originally proposed by Krönig.[15] A low transverse (Kerr) incision is employed in more than 90 percent of all cesarean births. The low transverse incision has the following advantages over a vertical incision: less risk of entry into the upper uterine segment, greater ease of entry, less bladder dissection, less operative blood loss, less repair, easier reperitonealization, and less likelihood of adhesion formation to bowel or omentum should it not be possible to apply the bladder flap above the top of the incision line. Importantly, in subsequent pregnancies the obstetrician can feel more comfortable

Table 19-8 Surgical Considerations in Selection of Uterine Incision for Cesarean Delivery

Low Segment Incisions	Transverse	Vertical
Technical ease of		
Extension of incision	−	+
Bladder dissection	+	−
Uterine closure	+	−
Reperitonealization	+	−
Anticipate hysterectomy	−	+
Benefits vs. risks		
Uterine rupture (subsequent)	+	−
Lateral extension into uterine vessels	−	+
Extension inferiorly	+	−
Intraoperative bleeding	+	−
Subsequent adhesions	+	−

+, Advantage to uterine incision type; −, Disadvantage

offering a VBAC trial because there is less likelihood of uterine rupture.[88]

In contrast, a vertical incision (classic or low vertical) may be advantageous if the patient has not been in labor and the lower uterus is narrow and poorly developed or if the fetus is not in a cephalic presentation, particularly a back-down transverse lie or preterm breech. Should a transverse incision be performed under such circumstances, there is a greater likelihood of lateral extension of the incision into the vessels of the broad ligament. However, individualization is reasonable. For instance, the author generally prefers a vertical incision for a transverse lie. However, a low transverse incision is certainly feasible if the lower uterine segment is well developed, as may be the case when the patient presents in active labor with advanced cervical dilatation. Other possible indications for a vertical incision include leiomyomata obstructing exposure to the lower segment and structural uterine anomalies.

The classic uterine incision involves the upper active uterine segment. Its primary advantage is the rapidity of entry into the uterus. Furthermore, some physicians believe that the incision is useful in the presence of an anterior placenta previa, reducing the potential for maternal and fetal hemorrhage.[89] Despite these advantages, this incision is seldom employed except when it is not possible to expose the lower uterine segment or when a hysterectomy is planned. More commonly encountered complications associated with classic incisions include subsequent adhesion formation and greater risk of uterine rupture with later pregnancies.[90] Patients who have had a prior classic incision should consider an appropriately timed elective repeat cesarean birth because of the risk of uterine rupture even before labor has started.

The theoretical advantages of the low vertical (Krönig) incision over the classic incision are similar to those of the low transverse incision. However, unlike

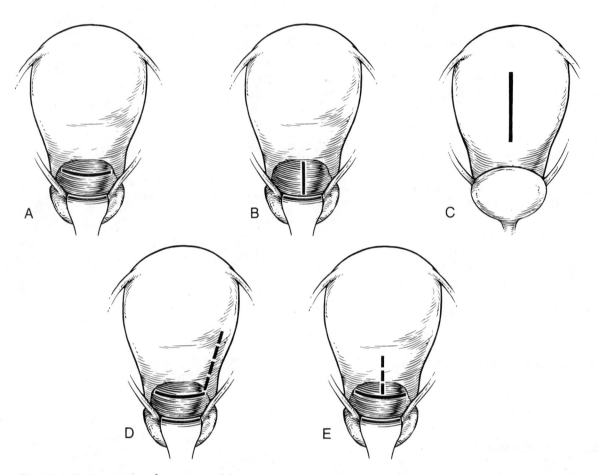

Fig. 19-2 Uterine incisions for cesarean delivery. (A) Low transverse incision. The bladder is retracted downward, and the incision is made in the lower uterine segment, curving gently upward. If the lower segment is poorly developed, the incision can also curve sharply upward at each end to avoid extending into the ascending branches of the uterine arteries. (B) Low vertical incision. The incision is made vertically in the lower uterine segment after reflecting the bladder, avoiding extension into the bladder below. If more room is needed, the incision can be extended upward into the upper uterine segment. (C) Classic incision. The incision is entirely within the upper uterine segment and can be at the level shown or in the fundus. (D) J incision. If more room is needed when an initial transverse incision has been made, either end of the incision can be extended upward into the upper uterine segment and parallel to the ascending branch of the uterine artery. (E) T incision. More room can be obtained in a transverse incision by an upward mid-line extension into the upper uterine segment.

the classic incision, there may occasionally be a caudad (inferior) extension of the incision into the cervix and vagina or even into the bladder. Although the low vertical (Krönig) incision is theoretically limited to the lower uterine segment, it often involves the upper segment.

Performing the Cesarean Delivery

Development of Bladder Flap

After placement of a bladder catheter and entry into the peritoneal cavity, the obstetrician should palpate the uterus to determine the degree and direction of uterine rotation. In most instances the uterus is dextrorotated such that the left round ligament may be visualized more anteriorly and closer to the midline

than is the right. Some obstetricians insert moistened laparotomy pads into each lateral peritoneal gutter prior to making the uterine incision to absorb amniotic fluid and blood escaping from the incision, particularly when there is a strong suspicion of amnionitis. The uterovesical peritoneum (serosa) is grasped in the midline and undermined with Metzenbaum scissors inserted between the peritoneum and underlying myometrium to develop bluntly a retroperitoneal space bilaterally to the lateral margins of the lower uterine segment. The peritoneal reflection is then incised bilaterally in an upward direction and the vesicouterine fold is grasped with forceps and the bladder lifted anteriorly, allowing blunt separation of the bladder from the underlying lower uterine segment. Should adherent adhesions be noted in a repeat procedure, sharp dissection may be necessary to free-up the posterior aspect of the bladder. Once the dissection is complete in the midline, the fingers may be carefully swept laterally in each direction to free the bladder more completely. After the bladder flap is adequately developed, a universal retractor or bladder blade is used to retract the bladder anteriorly and inferiorly to facilitate exposure of the intended incision site. Use of a Richardson retractor to retract the superior margin of a transverse abdominal incision may help to facilitate exposure.

Low Transverse Cesarean Incision

The lower uterine segment incision (Fig. 19-2A) is begun 1 to 2 cm above the site of the original upper margin of the bladder. A small midline incision is first made with a scalpel through the lower uterine segment to the fetal membranes. Continuous suction should be available to facilitate visualization of the operative field and to evacuate amniotic fluid should the incision perforate through the fetal membranes. Care should be taken to avoid laceration of the fetus, which is an occasional complication, especially when the lower uterine segment is thin or when expeditious delivery of the fetus is required.

After suctioning, the incision may be extended laterally and slightly upward (cephalad) to the lateral margin of the lower uterine segment so as to maximize incisional length and avoid extension into the uterine vessels. Extension of the incision may be accomplished

by either of two methods: (1) sharp dissection, taking care to avoid fetal fingers and toes; or (2) blunt dissection by spreading the incision with each index finger. Blunt splitting of the uterine incision, particularly if the lower uterine segment is thin, will result in more rapid entry; however, there is potential for unpredictable extension with this method, particularly if the lower segment is not fully effaced. The choice is largely a function of training and theoretical concerns regarding unintended extension. The relative merits of the two approaches were recently addressed in a prospective randomized study that could detect no difference in the incidence of unintended extension, estimated blood loss, or length of surgery between the two approaches. Rather, the frequency of unintended extensions correlated with the stage of labor (1.4, 15.5, and 35.0 percent for no labor, first stage of labor, and second stage, respectively).[91]

Low Vertical Incision

Should the fetus present as a breech or transverse lie, particularly back down, there is often advantage to a low vertical (Figs. 19-2B, 19-3) uterine incision, particularly if the lower uterine segment is not well developed. The bladder is displaced downward to expose the lower uterine segment more inferiorly so that the low vertical incision will be less likely to extend into the upper segment. Once the anticipated site is exposed, an incision is made at the inferior margin of the lower segment

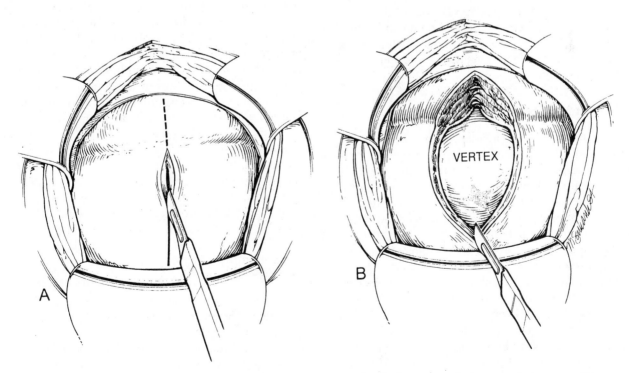

Fig. 19-3 Low vertical incision. (A) Ideally, a vertical incision is contained entirely in the lower uterine segment. (B) Extension into the upper uterine segment, either inadvertently or by choice, is common.

and extended cephalad with either bandage scissors or knife. Should it be necessary to extend the incision into the upper active uterine segment, it should be noted in the operative report.

Although vertical cesarean incisions are traditionally categorized into low vertical and classic types, the performance of a true low vertical incision that does not enter the upper contractile portion of the uterus is actually uncommon. The clinical implication is that the low vertical incision poses considerably less risk in a subsequent VBAC trial than would be the case with a classic incision, the risk of rupture is nonetheless probably somewhat greater than that of a low transverse incision.

Classic Cesarean Incision

The initial incision (Fig. 19-2C) is made with a scalpel 1 to 2 cm above the bladder reflection. Once the fetus or membranes are visualized the incision is extended cephalad with bandage scissors, the size of the incision varying with the estimated size of the fetus. The patient should also be advised of this occurrence and its importance to future pregnancies should a VBAC trial be considered.

Management of the Anterior Placenta

Should the placenta be located in the anterior lower uterine segment, entry can be accomplished by one of three methods. First, the clinician can simply dissect through the placenta; this carries the risk of short-term fetal hemorrhage. Second, the placenta can be separated from the lower uterine segment, facilitating lateral exposure of the fetus. Finally, a classic uterine incision can be employed.

Delivery of the Fetus

Upon completion of the incision, the retractors are removed and a hand is inserted into the uterine cavity to elevate and flex the fetal head through the uterine incision. Initial efforts to deliver the presenting part through the uterine incision will indicate the adequacy of the uterine incision. Should the head be deeply wedged within the pelvis, it can be dislodged by an assistant applying upward pressure vaginally. Once the occiput presents into the incision, moderate fundal pressure may facilitate expulsion. On occasion the head may be delivered with shorthandled Simpson forceps or vacuum. Once delivery of the fetal head is completed, the nose and oropharynx are suctioned with a bulb syringe. If meconium is present, suction can be accomplished with continuous wall suction. When suctioning is complete, expulsion of the remainder of the newborn is facilitated by moderate uterine fundal pres-

sure. The cord is then doubly clamped and cut, and the infant is transferred to the resuscitation team.

Umbilical cord blood gas data may be collected routinely or selectively in high-risk circumstances, such as fetal growth retardation, preterm birth, breech presentations, amnionitis, the presence of thick meconium, cesarean delivery for nonreassuring FHR findings, or unanticipated Apgar scores. To facilitate collection of an adequate arterial sample the umbilical cord is first clamped close to the placenta so as to maintain filling of the umbilical arteries and vein and then clamped close to the newborn. It is then doubly clamped in each location so as to isolate a 10- to 15-cm segment of cord for umbilical arterial and/or venous blood sampling.

Operative Techniques for the Preterm Fetus

The uterine incision to be used for the delivery of the preterm fetus is best selected after entry into the maternal abdomen. At least 50 percent of cases will require a low vertical or classic incision for indications such as malpresentation or a poorly developed lower uterine segment. Among 174 VLBW cesarean births at Los Angeles County Women's Hospital, a low transverse incision was performed in 31 percent of cases, a low vertical incision in 47 percent, and a classic uterine incision in 22 percent.[92] Using ultrasound, Morrison[93] prospectively evaluated the width of the lower uterine segment in the absence of labor and found its transverse dimension to be 0.5, 1.0, and 4.0 cm at 20, 28, and 34 weeks, respectively. Thus without significant labor, the lower uterine segment will probably not be sufficiently developed to provide an adequate transverse dimension for removal of the fetus. The complications of performing a low transverse incision in the absence of adequate development of the lower uterine segment include difficult removal of the fetus, lateral extension of the incision into the broad ligament and uterine vessels, and downward extension of the incision into the cervix and the vagina. It is noteworthy that intraoperative complications including injury to the bladder, broad ligament laceration, and uterine artery laceration are more common in preterm than in term cesarean births. The complication rate is independent of incision type.[94]

Cesarean Delivery of the Breech Presentation

Should an elective cesarean section be planned, it is desirable, prior to performing the procedure, to confirm that the breech has not converted spontaneously to a vertex or to a more unfavorable transverse lie. The lie of the fetus can be verified by palpation prior to making the uterine incision. In the case of a transverse lie, the vertex or the buttocks of the breech can often be guided into a position underlying the planned site of the uterine incision. Should the lower uterine segment be well developed, a transverse or vertical uterine incision can be used. However, a vertical incision is often preferable should the cervix be long and closed, the lower uterine segment poorly developed, or the breech converted to a back-down transverse lie.

The head of a preterm breech infant may be trapped if the incision is not made large enough.[92] Although cesarean delivery is often elected in an attempt to minimize fetal trauma, the actual delivery mechanism via the cesarean incision is essentially identical to that of the vaginal route. Should the fetus present as a non-frank breech or back-up transverse lie, the first step is to identify and grasp a foot and extract the leg through the incision until the second foot can be identified. The surgeon should conduct the delivery process in such a way as to minimize hyperextension of the fetal neck and compression of fetal organs. The mechanism for delivery of the breech is discussed elsewhere (see Ch. 16). However, should there be evidence of head entrapment, the first action should be to extend the abdominal incision and to enlarge the uterine incision. Occasionally it may be necessary to incise perpendicular to a transverse incision (inverted T-shaped incision) or to extend the transverse incision upward parallel to the uterine artery (J incision) (Fig. 19-2D, E). Both the inverted T and J incisions are more subject to uterine rupture with subsequent pregnancies.

Manual Vs. "Spontaneous" Placental Expulsion

Following delivery of the fetus, 20 to 40 units of oxytocin can be administered in an isotonic crystaloid solution. Subsequent removal of the placenta is commonly done manually. McCurdy et al[95] recently compared the manual option to the alternative technique in a prospective randomized trial (N = 62), wherein the placenta is allowed to deliver spontaneously with gentle traction on the umbilical cord, and demonstrated a significantly higher measured blood loss (967 vs. 666 ml) and a surprisingly higher incidence of endometritis (23 vs. 3 percent) in the manual group. Additional data suggesting a benefit for awaiting "spontaneous expulsion" is provided in a 1964 report from Queenan and Nakamoto[96] that demonstrated a reduction in Rh sensitization in the "spontaneous" group. Following its removal, the placenta should be inspected for possible missing cotyledons.

Repair of the Uterine Incision

Closure of the uterine incision may be aided by manual delivery of the uterine fundus through the abdominal incision.[97]

Delivery of the uterine fundus through the abdominal incision facilitates uterine massage and observation of uterine tone, as well as routine examination of the adnexa and tubal ligation. The fundus may be covered with a moistened laparotomy pad and the uterine incision inspected for obvious bleeding points, which are controlled with either Ring forceps or Allis clamps until suture closure can be accomplished. The uterine cavity may then be inspected and wiped clean with a dry laparotomy sponge to remove fetal membranes and placental fragments. If the patient has not been in labor, it may be advantageous to dilate the cervix gently to facilitate later lochial drainage. The dilating instrument should then be discarded from the operating field.

The primary disadvantages of uterine exteriorization are possible peritoneal discomfort and nausea and/or vomiting in patients under inadequate regional anesthesia. Some have hypothesized that exteriorization may temporarily kink and occlude the uterine blood supply, resulting in a delayed onset of bleeding at the incision site. If possible, such a complication must be quite unusual. A recent prospective randomized study by Magann et al[98] addressed the cumulative impact of placenta management and uterine exteriorization and confirmed that blood loss associated with "spontaneous" placental separation was significantly less than that associated with manual removal. When blood loss (uterus exteriorized vs. in situ) was compared, no difference was detectable between the spontaneous separation/expulsion and manual removal groups.[98]

Midline placement of a ring forceps or Allis clamp may be used to elevate the lower portion of the low transverse uterine incision, facilitating visualization of the field and approximation of the incision. Although Allis clamps can be routinely placed at the angles of the incision to control bleeding and to identify the end of the incision, routine placement of more than the one midline clamp in the absence of bleeding simply clutters the field. The perimeter of the uterine incision is then inspected to locate bleeding vessels and to localize the true margins of the uterine incision. Control of uterine bleeding is facilitated by oxytocin administration and massaging the uterus. Oxytocin administration is particularly important following classic cesarean birth. If bleeding is encountered along the margins of the incision, a ring forcep or Allis clamp should be placed at the site of bleeding. If the incisional margin is not carefully identified, on occasion the posterior wall of the lower uterine segment may balloon anteriorly and be confused with the lower margin of the transverse incision, potentially resulting in complete closure of the uterine cavity (i.e., superior edge of the inferior incision margin to the posterior uterine wall).

Reapproximation of the lower uterine incision may be performed in either one or two layers (Fig. 19-4)

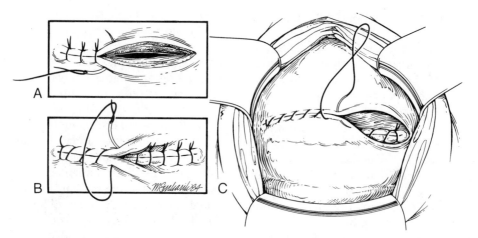

Fig. 19-4 Closure of low transverse incision. (A) The first layer can be either interrupted or continuous. A continuous locking suture is less desirable, despite its reputed hemostatic abilities, because it may interfere with incision vasculature and, hence, with healing and scar formation. (B) A second inverted layer created by using a continuous Lembert's or Cushing's stitch is customary but is really needed only when apposition is unsatisfactory after application of the first layer. Inclusion of too much tissue produces a bulky mass that may delay involution and interfere with healing. (C) The bladder peritoneum is reattached to the uterine peritoneum with fine suture.

using zero or double zero chromic suture or similar absorbable synthetic suture such as Vicryl, the second layer inverting the first. The initial suture should be placed lateral to the angle of a transverse incision or inferior to the lower margin of a vertical incision. Subsequent stitches may be run in a continuous or continuous-locking manner to the opposite end of the incision. The sutures may be placed through the entire myometrium. Some have stressed the importance of avoiding incorporation of decidua in the suture for concern of later development of endometriosis in the scar; however, this is a remote possibility.[99] Although many routinely use a continuous-locking suture, there is questionable advantage to routine suture locking along the entire margin, except at sites of obvious oozing. Locking sutures potentially increase the likelihood of tissue ischemia and potentially may limit wound healing. It has been traditional to place a second continuous layer (Lembert or Cushing) of chromic or similar suture to invert the first layer, with either vertically or horizontally stitches, the latter requiring more frequent placement of the needle upon the needle holder. If the low transverse uterine segment is well effaced and hemostasis adequate, it is reasonable to reapproximate the uterine margins with a single suture layer. Hauth et al[100] have, on the basis of a prospective (N = 906) randomized trial comparing traditional two-layer with single-layer closure, reported that the single-layer closure significantly decreased operating time (39.2 vs. 44.8 minutes), had no increase in postoperative complications, and, surprisingly, required less extra hemostatic sutures (beyond that expected in one or two layers) per patient. Follow-up data regarding subsequent risk of uterine rupture is of interest.

Closure of a classic cesarean incision (Fig. 19-5) involving the more thickened upper segment most often will require a two-layer closure. Should the uterine wall be unusually thick, it may be necessary to use a third layer. Repair of the incision can be done in several ways. A common method is to employ continuous 0 or 1 chromic cat gut suture in layers, the first layer approximating the inner one-half of the uterine wall thickness in a continuous or continuous-locking manner. A second and occasionally a third layer is then used to approximate the uterine musculature. It may be desirable to bury the knot (at the superior end of the incision) of the outer suture line. This can be done by initiating suture entry within the incision, exiting laterally, then reentering from the lateral margin of the opposing side and exiting medially, followed by knot placement. The operative record should state the type of uterine incision, and the patient should be informed about the incision and its impact on care in subsequent pregnancies, including the advisability against a future attempt at a VBAC.[90]

Reapproximation of the Visceral (Bladder Flap) and Parietal Peritoneum

The visceral (vesicouterine) and parietal peritoneum may be reapproximated with a running double or triple zero chromic or similar reabsorbable suture. Alternatively there is increasing acceptance of a practice in which the visceral (bladder flap) and parietal peritoneum are not surgically reapproximated, a principle long accepted in the surgical literature. Unrepaired mesothelial surfaces spontaneously reapproximate within 48 hours and demonstrate healing with no scar formation at 5 days. Clinically this approach is associ-

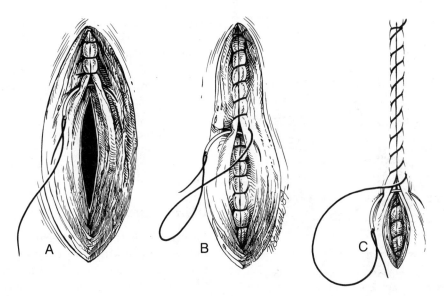

Fig. 19-5 Repair of a classic incision. Three-layer closure of a classic incision, including inversion of the serosal layer to discourage adhesion formation. The knot at the superior end of the incision of the second layer can be buried by medial to lateral placement of the suture from within the depth of the incision and subsequent lateral to medial reentry on the opposing side with resultant knot placement within the incision.

ated with a reduced need for postoperative analgesia and quicker return of bowel function.[101,102] Furthermore, this approach does not promote adhesion formation.[103–106]

Abdominal Closure

Once the uterine incisional reapproximation is completed, the incision should once again be inspected for bleeding points, which can be individually ligated, coagulated, or controlled with figure-of-eight sutures. Before closing the abdomen, the uterus, fallopian tubes, and ovaries should be examined for unsuspected pathology. Some routinely examine the appendix. When surgical sterilization or ovarian cystectomy is required, it is accomplished before replacing the uterus into the abdominal cavity. If used, laparotomy pads are removed and the abdominal contents, lateral gutters, and cul-de-sac are inspected and, where indicated, suctioned. The pelvis and lower abdomen may be irrigated especially if there is coexistent chorioamnionitis or if there has been heavy spillage of meconium outside the operative field. The operating team should confirm that the needle and sponge counts are correct.

There is no need to reapproximate the parietal peritoneum or rectus muscles. The rectus fascia may be closed with either interrupted or continuous (nonlocking) sutures. Suture choice is important in fascial healing. If the suture is absorbed too rapidly, tensile strength may be reduced, thus increasing the likelihood of wound breakdown. Chromic suture should be avoided when possible. Selection of a suture for its duration of strength

is particularly important for patients at risk for wound dehiscence. Unlike their chromic counterparts, synthetic braided sutures maintain tensile strength throughout fascial healing. They are predictably broken down by hydrolysis. In contrast, gut suture has less tensile strength and is degraded less predictably. Local infection may also result in more rapid loss of strength. If the surgeon is dealing with a patient at risk for wound breakdown (from chronic corticosteroid therapy), delayed absorbable material such as PDS or polyglyconate (Maxon) or permanent material such as nylon or polypropylene (Prolene) may have merit.

Once an appropriate suture is chosen, care should be taken in selecting the site of suture placement for fascial closure. In most instances of wound dehiscence, the suture remains intact but has cut through the tissue in which it has been placed. One study indicates that this problem is responsible for up to 88 percent of disrupted wounds.[107]

Large bites using larger gauge suture material are less likely to transect tissue than are small bites with narrow-gauge suture material. Suture entry and exit sites should be well beyond the 1-cm inner zone of collagenolysis at the margin of the wound. Should sutures be placed within this inner zone, there is greater tendency for them to pull through, leading to dehiscence and possible evisceration. Sutures should be placed at approximately 1-cm intervals approximately 1.5 cm from the incision line.

It is acceptable to use a running suture in closing the fascia in patients with a clean incision. Fagniez et al[108] were not able to demonstrate a difference in dehiscence

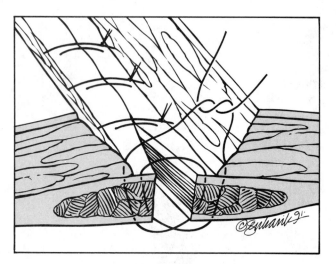

Fig. 19-6 Modification of far-near, near-far Smead-Jones suture. Suture passes deeply through lateral side of anterior rectus fascia and adjacent fat, crosses the midline of the incision to pick up the medial edge of the rectus fascia, then catches the near side of the opposite rectus sheath, and, finally, returns to the far margin of the opposite rectus sheath and subcutaneous fat. (Modified from ACOG,[314] with permission.)

rates in a randomized prospective trial of 3,135 patients employing a running versus interrupted polyglycolic acid suture in midline incisions. Approximation of fascia should allow maintenance of adequate blood flow; unnecessarily tight sutures will cause hypoxia and potentially interfere with predictable wound healing.[109,110] Should a patient be at high risk for wound dehiscence, it is preferable that the fascia not be closed with continuous suturing, particularly on a vertical incision. If the patient is at high risk for abdominal distention and wound breakdown, a mass or Smead-Jones (Fig. 19-6) closure is preferable. This closure is mechanically more sound and allows for a 30 percent increase in abdominal girth.

It is generally not necessary to reapproximate the subcutaneous tissue unless the patient is markedly obese, in which case subcutaneous closure may facilitate skin closure, or, as noted above, to close the peritoneum. No difference in rates of dehiscence was noted between patients who underwent peritoneal closure and those who did not in one large randomized trial.[105] Skin may be closed with staples or a subcuticular stitch. Steristrip adhesive tape (3M Surgical Products, St. Paul, MN) can be used to reduce tension on subcuticular sutures. If staples are used, they may be replaced with Steristrips 3 or 4 days after surgery, depending on regional practice, to decrease scarring.

Intraoperative Complications

The patient undergoing cesarean delivery is at risk for many of the same intra- and postoperative complications as is the patient having a vaginal delivery. Man-

agement problems more commonly associated with cesarean delivery, as well as conditions such as uterine atony and placenta accreta, which are also discussed in Chapter 17, are briefly reviewed in this section.

Although injury to bladder, bowel, or ureters is uncommon, many competent obstetricians, despite careful surgical technique, will encounter complications. When they occur, the primary responsibility is to identify the injury and its extent, to repair the injury, and to obtain consultation should injuries be extensive or unusually complex.

Uterine Lacerations

Lacerations of the lower uterine incision are more common when a low transverse incision is used in the presence of a macrosomic fetus or a noncephalic presentation. Fortunately, these lacerations are usually easily sutured as long as they only extend laterally to the margin of the myometrium or inferiorly into the vagina. Care must be taken to avoid ligation of the ureters. In most circumstances, the lateral apex of the extension can be identified and the suture placed just lateral to that point. Should there be extension into the broad ligament in proximity to the ureters, on occasion it may be necessary to open the broad ligament and identify the ureters before suture placement. Rarely, there may be an advantage to retrograde placement of a No. 8 French ureteral catheter into the ureters. This can be accomplished transurethrally or by performing a vertical incision in the dome of the bladder to visualize the ureteral orifices. The bladder can then be repaired with an initial continuous 2-0 chromic suture followed by a second imbricating layer of 2-0 suture.

Bladder Injuries

Injury to the bladder is an infrequent, but recognized complication of cesarean delivery. More widespread use of the transverse abdominal incision has increased the likelihood of bladder dome injury upon entering the abdomen. Although the risk of bladder injury can be minimized by preoperative catheterization of the bladder and careful entry into the peritoneal cavity, it is not always possible to avoid injury during a repeat procedure. When the bladder is more adherent than usual, sharp dissection of the "webbing" between the bladder base and the lower uterine segment and vagina, as opposed to blunt dissection with a sponge stick or gauze-covered finger, will reduce, but not eliminate, the incidence of unplanned cystotomy.

Bladder injury may also occur at the time of uterine rupture, particularly in patients with a prior cesarean delivery. While rates as high as 10 to 14 percent have been reported, the incidence has decreased somewhat in women attempting VBAC.[111–113] Should hysterectomy be required, cystotomy as a complication of cesarean hysterectomy has been noted to occur in as many as 4 to 5 percent of procedures.[114,115] In most cases the injury occurs at the bladder base. To some extent, if hysterectomy is anticipated, mobilizing the bladder from the lower uterine segment and upper vagina prior to making the uterine incision will diminish this risk.

Should a bladder laceration be encountered, the bladder may be repaired with a two-layer closure with 2-0 or 3-0 chromic. Surgeons may differ significantly in their surgical approach to repair. Controversies focus on the use of continuous versus interrupted sutures, on whether it is important to avoid including the mucosa in the suture line, and on the duration of catheter drainage. The issues are probably of little significance when the cystotomy is in the dome of the bladder. However, a cystotomy in the bladder base is more likely to present problems, because the bladder base is thinner and receives less blood flow. There is also a possibility of laceration into the trigone and injury to the ureteral orifices. Should the trigone be lacerated, there may be an advantage to inserting a ureteral catheter under direct visualization. After the bladder has been repaired, a catheter can be left in place for 7 to 10 days.[113,116]

Ureteral Injury

Although one does not frequently think of ureteral injury during cesarean delivery, this complication has been reported in up to 1 in 1,000 cesarean deliveries.[113] Ureteral injury is also increased with cesarean hysterectomy, with rates of 0.2 to 0.5 percent being documented.[114,115] In most instances, injury occurs during efforts to control bleeding arising from lateral extension of the uterine incision; unfortunately, the injury often goes unrecognized intraoperatively. Should lateral extension of an incision occur in the anatomic region of the ureter, opening the anterior leaf of the broad ligament while controlling blood loss with direct pressure will often facilitate more accurate suture placement, which will diminish the potential for ureteral injury.

Gastrointestinal Tract Injury

Injuries to the bowel are also rare, but nonetheless are reported to occur once in approximately 1,300 cesarean sections.[92] Prior abdominal surgery and pelvic/abdominal infection leading to adhesion formation are common risk factors. Sharp scalpel incision limited to a site of transparent peritoneum will reduce inadvertent bowel or bladder injury.

Should adhesions require lysis to gain access to the lower uterine segment, they should be sharply dissected with scissors tips pointed away from the bowel. Small defects in bowel serosa can be closed simply with interrupted silk sutures on an atraumatic needle. If these defects are very small, no closure may be necessary. Full thickness lacerations should be repaired in a double-layer closure, employing a transverse closure of a longitudinal laceration, to minimize the possibility of narrowing the bowel lumen. The mucosa can be closed with running or interrupted 3-0 absorbable sutures such as chromic or polyglactin. The muscular and serosal layers are then closed with a similar-sized interrupted silk suture. In the event that there are multiple full-thickness small bowel injuries or the colon or sigmoid is entered, consultation with a gynecologic oncologist or general surgeon is appropriate. The small bowel may require resection and reanastomosis. Primary closure of a small laceration (less than 1 cm) of the colon is indicated using a double layer closure as described above. More extensive injury associated with fecal contamination should be treated with copious lavage and may require a temporary colostomy. In either case, gram-negative aerobic and anaerobic coverage should be provided. This is commonly provided by combination therapy with an aminoglycoside and either clindamycin or metronidazole (i.e., clindamycin/gentamicin) and/or cephalosporin with metronidazole. Some have recommended broad-spectrum monotherapy, which has the advantages of lower toxocity, lower drug costs, and lower cost of administration, including eliminating the need for monitoring of aminoglycoside blood levels). Ampicillin/sulbactam (3.0 g IV every 6 hours) is a reasonable first-line choice, with combination therapy reserved for patients with documented penicillin allergy.[119]

Uterine Atony

Initial efforts to control uterine atony include uterine massage and medical therapy with (1) intravenous oxytocin, 20 to 40 units/L; (2) methergotamine, 0.2 mg, or ergonovine administered intramuscularly; or (3) 15 methylprostaglandin $F_{2\alpha}$ (Hemabate), which can be administered either intramuscularly or directly into the myometrium. Should the initial dose of prostaglandin be insufficient, successive dosages of 250 µg, up to a total dose of 1.0 to 1.5 mg, can be used. Should medical treatment fail, the surgeon must decide between ligation of the uterine arteries (see Fig. 17-16), hypogastric artery ligation, and hysterectomy. Uterine or hypogastric artery ligation may be the desirable approach should the patient be stable cardiovascularly and desirous of future pregnancy. Hypogastric artery ligation can be accomplished by ligation of the ascending branch, which can usually be found at the inferior and lateral extreme of the low transverse incision ascending retroperitoneally within the broad ligament (Fig. 19-

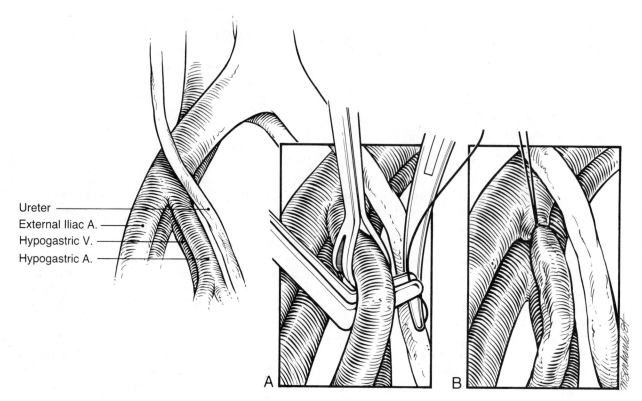

Ureter
External Iliac A.
Hypogastric V.
Hypogastric A.

A   B

Fig. 19-7 Hypogastric artery ligation. Approach to the hypogastric artery via the peritoneum, parallel and just lateral to the ovarian vessels, exposing the interior surface of the posterior layer of the broad ligament. The ureter will be found attached to the medial leaf of the broad ligament. The bifurcation of the common iliac artery into its external and internal (hypogastric) branches is exposed by blunt dissection of the loose overlying areolar tissues. Identification of these structures is essential. (A,B) To avoid traumatizing the underlying hypogastric vein, the hypogastric artery is elevated by means of a Babcock clamp before passing an angled clamp to catch a free tie. (Adapted from Breen et al,[315] with permission.)

7). Unfortunately, even hypogastric artery ligation is actually successful in less than one-half of the cases[20] Should uterine or hypogastric artery ligation also fail to control the hemorrhage it may be necessary to proceed to hysterectomy.

Placenta Accreta

Placenta accreta is now the most common indication for postcesarean hysterectomy. Approximately 25 percent of patients having a cesarean delivery for placenta previa in the presence of a prior uterine incision subsequently require cesarean hysterectomy for placenta accreta. The risk of placenta accreta appears to increase with the number of prior incisions. This obstetric complication may be increasing in frequency because of the increasing incidence of previous cesarean sections.[121,122]

If the accreta is focal and the patient desires future pregnancies, it may be possible to excise the site of trophoblastic invasion, over-sewing bleeding areas with several figure-of-eight sutures. If that is not possible, hysterectomy should be initiated. A complete hysterec-

tomy will usually be required because a placenta accreta commonly involves the lower uterine segment, and, in such cases, a supracervical hysterectomy will not be effective in controlling the bleeding.

Drainage of the Abdominal Incision

The purpose of a drain is to remove the bacterial growth media that can act as a site of infection and reduce potential spaces within the wound. There are few indications for prophylactic drainage, because cesarean delivery is a relatively "short" procedure and operative time and tissue devitalization are ordinarily not an issue. Prophylactic drainage is most commonly employed in situations in which there is an expectation of fluid accumulation in association with likely contamination of the wound, particularly in obese patients.[123] Therapeutic drainage is seldom, if ever, indicated with cesarean delivery or cesarean hysterectomy unless there is a coincidental abscess. Should an abscess be encountered, a continuous suction drain should be inserted via a separate stab wound at a site away from the incision.[124] In some instances in which there is a

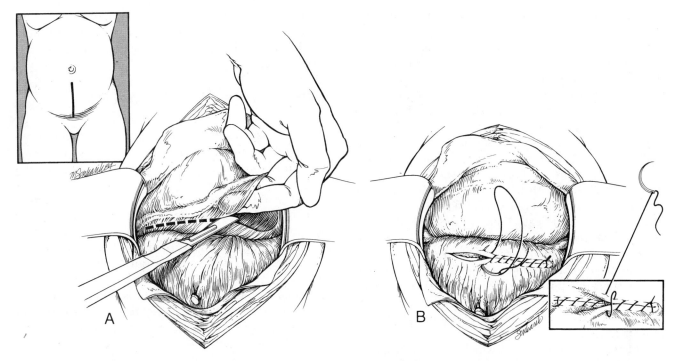

Fig. 19-8 Waters extraperitoneal section. (A) One step in the Waters operation is illustrated. The transversalis fascia has been opened and the vesical peritoneum separated from the muscularis of the bladder dome by sharp dissection. At this point, the uterovesical fold of bladder peritoneum is isolated and is being cut free to expose the lower uterine segment. (B) A successful dissection has left the lower uterine segment widely exposed without having entered the peritoneal cavity. The remainder of the operation is similar to a low transverse cesarean section, except that it will not be necessary to close either a bladder flap or the peritoneum.

suspicion of heavy contamination, particularly in morbidly obese patients, it may be better to plan secondary wound closure as opposed to drainage.

Extraperitoneal Cesarean Delivery

Extraperitoneal cesarean delivery (Fig. 19-8) is mentioned largely for historical purposes. Prior to use of antibiotics, extraperitoneal cesarean delivery was an alternative to cesarean hysterectomy as a means to reduce the risk of infection in patients with chorioamnionitis; Frank[13] and Latzko[14] were prominent early proponents. The operation differs from the more commonly employed modern procedures in that an effort is made to avoid penetrating the peritoneum. The uterus is approached through the space of Retzius, exposing one lateral aspect of the lower uterus and bladder. The bladder is then dissected from its lateral approximation to the anterior surface of the lower uterus and retracted so as to expose the lower uterine segment. Although this procedure is seldom done today, there remain advocates for its use.[125] One prospective study comparing three groups (extraperitoneal cesarean delivery without antibiotic prophylaxis versus extraperitoneal cesarean delivery with antibiotic prophylaxis versus transperitoneal cesarean section with antibiotic prophylaxis)

found that extraperitoneal cesarean delivery was not as effective as systemic prophylactic antibiotics in the prevention of postoperative endomyometritis.[126]

Postmortem Cesarean Delivery

Postmortem cesarean delivery originated with the Catholic Church, which mandated its performance to accomplish baptism. In 1747, the King of Sicily condemned a physician to death for not performing a postmortem cesarean delivery.[127] Obstetric texts continue to discuss the possibility of postmortem cesarean delivery, despite rather dismal success and considerable debate among noted clinicians. The current recommendation is that, if clinically possible, a postmortem cesarean delivery should be begun within 4 to 5 minutes after initiation of cardiopulmonary resuscitation for cardiac arrest. Delivery provides the added benefit of increasing the effectiveness of cardiopulmonary resuscitation by diminishing uterine compression of the inferior vena cava in the supine position.

If a postmortem cesarean delivery is contemplated, successful perinatal outcome will depend on knowledge of preexisting fetal status and realization that death can be reliably anticipated in the near future. There are a number of determinants that favorably affect outcome:

(1) a gestational age compatible with fetal survival, (2) delivery within 10 minutes of cessation of maternal circulation, (3) prompt availability of appropriately trained staff and equipment, and (4) access to personnel capable of neonatal resuscitation.

Unfortunately, in many instances it is not possible to provide one or more of the above, and for this reason outcome is most often poor. Katz et al[128] described 269 cases of postmortem cesarean births between 1879 and 1986 in the English literature. Only 188 newborns survived. In recent history, normal survival following postmortem cesarean birth has been primarily limited to instances in which the baby was delivered within 5 minutes after maternal death. The likelihood of a normal outcome decreases to approximately 10 to 15 percent in the 6- to 15-minute interval and to less than 15 percent at 16 or more minutes after death. The current consensus is that postmortem cesarean delivery may be performed at any time that a viable fetus or the potential for one exists, even without the consent of a family member.[128]

There are limited data with which to assess the ability of modern life-support equipment to maintain the mother for an extended period. A 1988 case report described a mother supported for 10 weeks to gain time for fetal maturation.[129]

Preoperative and Intraoperative Fluid Guidelines

Extracellular (interstitial and intravascular) water constitutes approximately one-third of total body water and 20 percent of total body weight. Ordinary daily physiologic fluid needs approximately 2,000 to 2,500 ml. In the pregnant patient, daily physiologic fluid losses are estimated to be 1,000 ml in excess of urinary output and include urinary output (800 to 1,500 ml), insensible loss (800 ml) from both skin and lungs, and stool loss (200 ml). Insensible loss in the laboring patient can be considerably greater.

Because insensible fluid loss increases significantly in the laboring patient, the woman about to undergo a cesarean delivery for CPD may be quite dehydrated. She may have had insufficient fluid intake since the onset of labor and have increased fluid loss due to the physical exertion and rapid breathing movements associated with labor. The bleeding patient or the patient about to receive epidural anesthesia is particularly sensitive to the effects of dehydration.

There will be little problem with dehydration if intravenous fluid intake has been maintained at 100 to 125 ml per hour. Should this not be the case, fluid losses can be estimated based on the average hourly need (100 to 125 ml) times the cumulative number of hours since the time of last fluid intake. Adjustments, which may

vary from center to center, should be made for ice chips and other fluid intake. An additional intravenous fluid load is required prior to the administration of epidural anesthesia.

Intravenous Fluids Commonly Used

1. Sodium chloride (0.9 percent isotonic saline) is an isotonic solution commonly used to expand plasma volume as well as to correct mild degrees of hyponatremia.
2. Lactated Ringer's solution is also an isotonic solution containing multiple electrolytes in a concentration similar to that found in human plasma. This solution is also used to expand plasma volume and may be preferable to isotonic saline during the first 24 postoperative hours.
3. Sodium chloride 0.45 percent is a hypotonic (half-normal) solution that is useful in the provision of postoperative fluid needs after the first 24 hours when volume expansion is no longer needed.

Fluid and Electrolyte Replacement

Should the patient be only mildly hypovolemic in the first 24 hours, normal isotonic saline or Ringer's lactate solution in 5 percent dextrose is preferable to more hypotonic solutions because there is greater retention of fluids in the intravascular space providing volume expansion. In contrast, infusion of a 5 percent dextrose in water solution will result in distribution of fluid evenly throughout all water spaces, two-thirds being in the intracellular space. Should hypovolemia be more significant, particularly in association with low intravascular colloid osmotic pressure, administration of an albumin-containing solution may minimize the effects of loss of fluids into the interstitial space. Under such circumstances, it may on occasion be advisable to employ a central venous pressure line or a Swan-Ganz catheter.

Special Considerations for Preoperative Fluids

Some patients such as those with vomiting, diarrhea, or fever may require additional fluids. The presence of a fever may increase the need for intravenous fluid replacement, generally on the order of 15 percent above basal levels for every degree centigrade above normal body temperature.[130]

Intraoperative Fluids

Fluid needs during surgery are generally determined by the anesthesiologist or nurse anesthetist and are largely directed to the replacement of estimated blood loss, insensible losses, and urinary output. In general, isotonic solutions are used to maintain adequate circulating blood volume. Actual blood or plasma replacement is rarely needed during cesarean delivery.

Intraoperative fluid requirements, apart from blood replacement, range from 500 to 1,000 ml per hour, up to a maximum of 3 L in a 4-hour interval under ordinary surgical conditions. Such replacement is associated with a low incidence of renal failure and pulmonary edema in instances in which there has been obstetric hemorrhage.[131,132]

Postoperative Complications

Maternal Morbidity and Mortality

The previously noted increase in risk for maternal morbidity and mortality in part is a result of the complications leading to the cesarean delivery and in part is a result of the risk associated with any surgical procedure. Nonetheless, even when morbidity and mortality arising from the indication leading to cesarean delivery have been excluded, maternal morbidity and mortality remain severalfold higher for cesarean delivery than for vaginal delivery.[5,42,132]

In a review of approximately 400,000 cesarean births performed between 1965 and 1978, maternal death occurred in 1 in 1,635 (mortality rate was 6.1/100,000) procedures; approximately one-half of the deaths were attributable to the procedure.[5,42] In another series, Sachs et al[42] reviewed 121,000 cesarean births performed in Massachusetts from 1976 to 1984; 7 (5.8 per 100,000) of 27 total deaths (22 per 100,000) arose as a result of the procedure itself. Lower rates have been described, the most remarkable being from a relatively small sample size (when estimating an infrequent outcome such as maternal mortality), in a study from the Boston Hospital for Women that reported no maternal mortality in 10,231 cesarean deliveries.[133]

Major sources of morbidity and associated mortality relate to complications of maternal sepsis, anesthesia, and thromboembolic disease and its complications. Each has been discussed in Chapters 15 and 38. Much has been done in recent years to reduce the impact of anesthesia-related mortality largely through increased availability of qualified anesthesia personnel and the implementation of rigid protocols, including routine use of antacids prior to cesarean delivery, as well as routine protocols for intubation. Other common causes of morbidity arising from cesarean delivery include hemorrhage and injury to the urinary tract.[134,135] It is important to remember that data describing morbidity for a primary cesarean delivery do not include the consideration of long-term consequences such as the possible need for repeat cesarean births, increased likelihood of placenta accreta, and need for unplanned hysterectomy.

Endomyometritis

Postpartum infection (see also Ch. 38 on perinatal infections) is the most frequent complication arising from cesarean delivery, and indeed primary cesarean delivery is the greatest risk factor with rates up to 20-fold that associated with vaginal delivery. Should prophylactic antibiotics not be used, the incidence of postcesarean endomyometritis varies from as low as 5 to 10 percent to as high as 70 to 85 percent, with a mean of 35 to 40 percent in most series.[136,137] The rate is largely dependent on socioeconomic status and on whether the cesarean delivery is a primary procedure. The lowest incidence occurs in middle- and upper-income women undergoing a scheduled cesarean delivery; the highest occurs in the young indigent patient undergoing primary cesarean delivery after an extended labor and prolonged membrane rupture. Age and socioeconomic status may influence the incidence of infection because they reflect general health and host immunocompetence. The other major risk factors include length of labor, duration of membrane rupture, and number of vaginal examinations and presence of prior chorioamnionitis. These factors exert their effects by influencing the size of the bacterial inoculum. Other weaker risk factors include length of surgery, preoperative hematocrit, intraoperative blood loss, duration of internal fetal monitoring, experience of the surgeon, and type of anesthesia.

Prior to the advent of modern broad-spectrum antibiotics with activity against both anaerobic and aerobic gram-negative bacilli, the incidence of severe complications arising from endomyometritis was as high as 4 to 5 percent.[138,139] When blood cultures were obtained, the frequency of associated bacteremia was approximately 10 percent.[136] Prophylactic antibiotics at the time of cesarean delivery reduce the postoperative infection rate to approximately 5 percent.[138] With the advent of modern antibiotics the incidence of life-threatening complications, including pelvic abscess, septic shock, and septic pelvic thrombophlebitis, is now less than 2 percent.

The microbiology, clinical diagnosis, laboratory aids, treatment, and approaches to reduce the rate of endometritis are detailed in Chapter 38.

Wound Complications

Risk Factors for Poor Wound Healing and Wound Infection

Identifiable medical risk factors that increase the likelihood of poor wound healing include diabetes mellitus and malnutrition. Surgical risk factors to be considered are the duration of surgery, the use of drains, the suture material chosen, and the closure technique employed. Postoperative factors include asthma, pulmonary complications and associated coughing, and vomiting.[140,141] In rare cases, other risk factors such as ascites, long-term corticosteroid therapy, anemia, and even prior irradiation may exist.

Wound infection rates following cesarean delivery vary, according to the patient population evaluated, from 2.5 to as high as 16.1 percent.[140] Determinants include local wound conditions and patient host resistance. Infection rates will vary according to whether the cesarean delivery is performed as an elective repeat (clean procedure) procedure with intact membranes or follows labor, particularly with ruptured membranes (clean contaminated procedure). Risk factors for wound infection interact in a complex manner, making it difficult to determine the independent contribution of any one factor. Clean procedures are generally associated with a wound infection rate of approximately 2 percent, while the corresponding rate for a clean contaminated case is on the order of 5 to 10 percent. Should chorioamnionitis (contaminated procedure) be present, the wound infection rate will approximate 20 percent.

Many studies demonstrate a substantial increase in wound infections with increasing duration of membrane rupture, long labors, and more frequent vaginal examinations.[142–145] Amnionitis and possibly meconium passage are additional risk factors. Up to 75 percent of amniotic fluid cultures done at the time of primary cesarean delivery are positive, with an average of 3.5 organisms, 44 percent being highly virulent bacteria.[146] Flora isolated from amniotic fluid and wound infections exist in a synergistic system of aerobes and anaerobes similar to the situation with endometritis. *S. aureus, Escherichia coli, Proteus mirabilis, Bacteroides* species, and group B streptococci are common isolates; clostridial species are infrequent.[147] Even in the absence of ruptured membranes, patients in preterm labor with unrecognized chorioamnionitis may have pathogens consistent with bowel flora.[148]

Methods To Reduce Wound Infection

Some determinants of wound infection (diabetes mellitus, amnionitis, obesity, and alcoholism) are to a large degree beyond the control of the obstetrician. However, the obstetrician who knows the potential risk factors does have the option to employ a number of measures selectively in an attempt to reduce the risk of wound infection and wound breakdown. These measures include (1) hair removal at the incision site (as opposed to shaving pubic and abdominal hair) if the abdomen is prepared the night prior to surgery; (2) preoperative skin preparation, including careful cleansing of the umbilicus and abdomen prior to surgery;

(3) sterile technique; (4) wound hemostasis; (5) selective use of prophylactic antibiotics; (6) avoidance of reactive (plain gut) or unnecessary suture material, particularly in the patient at risk for a wound infection or breakdown; (7) closed-system drainage if the patient is obese or the wound is "wet" in the absence of an obvious bleeder as opposed to open Penrose drains; (8) skin closure with suture rather than a skin stapler; and (9) delayed wound closure if the wound is grossly contaminated by bowel contents.

Although it is difficult to determine the magnitude of preventable wound infections, Emmons et al[149] suggest that the approximately 25 percent of wound infections that are associated with *S. aureus* represent a potentially preventable condition that presumably arises from exogenous sources. Sixty consecutive wound infections (5.4 percent) were studied among 1,104 women undergoing cesarean delivery. Wound infections caused by cervical-vaginal flora were associated with prolonged labor, particularly with greater duration of continuous electronic FHR monitoring; with more frequent vaginal examinations; and with organisms isolated from the endometrium at cesarean section. In contrast, women with wound infections caused by *S. aureus* had neither prolonged labor nor *S. aureus* isolated at cesarean delivery.[149]

When closing the wound, a balance must be maintained between adequate hemostasis and significant tissue devitalization. Excessive use of electrocautery may result in unnecessary tissue damage and reduced host resistance. Seroma or hematoma formation reduces tissue oxygen tension and phagocyte penetration. Tissues should be carefully reapproximated without major tension. Unnecessarily tight placement of sutures may interfere with adequate tissue oxygenation, which is essential to bacterial phagocytosis.[150]

Morbid obesity is a risk factor for wound infection, regardless of the degree of contamination and length of procedure.[151] Adipose tissue is relatively fragile and tends to heal relatively poorly. As a result, careful handling of the subcutaneous tissue is important. However, there is uncertainty as to the best surgical approach. Gallup[80] recommends a midline incision, a superficial closed suction drain, a nonabsorbable monofilament fascial closure with a Smead-Jones technique, and avoidance of subcutaneous suture. Others favor a transverse incision.[52] The recommendation to avoid subcutaneous suture is based on the theoretical consideration that the suture material acts as an additional foreign body.

Diagnosis and Management of Wound Infection

The diagnosis of a wound infection is generally the result of daily inspection of the wound. Suspicion may be heightened should the patient, previously treated for endometritis, be unresponsive to antibiotic therapy. If fever develops, careful inspection of the wound will often lead to early diagnosis and treatment. Diagnosis of a wound infection is relatively obvious in the febrile patient if the wound is unusually tender, inflamed, and indurated or if drainage of purulent material is observed on palpation. The bacteriology and laboratory approach to diagnosis are discussed in Chapter 38.

Should an infection be found, the involved wound must be opened to allow drainage and debrided to clean the wound margins. A culture for anaerobic and aerobic organisms may be obtained and systemic antibiotics employed to cover the anticipated organisms within the wound. Culturing tissue debris from the wound improves the likelihood of anaerobic organisms. Once the wound is opened, drained, irrigated, and possibly debrided to remove adherent purulent material, the wound can be packed with wet-to-dry dressing three times daily until there is a healthy margin of red granulation tissue. When the infection is controlled, the patient and surgeon must then decide between the inconvenience for the patient associated with healing by secondary intention versus the risk of recurrent infection should primary closure be elected.[153]

Fascial Dehiscence

Dehiscence of a wound through the fascia is infrequent, occurring in approximately 5 percent of wound infections.[145] Dehiscence is suggested by the presence of a large amount of discharge from the wound. If loops of small bowel protrude through the incision, the small bowel should be immediately covered with wet sterile dressings. The wound should be opened and inspected and emergency closure performed in the operating room under sterile conditions. If a dehiscence is confirmed, the wound should be cleansed, debrided, and closed with either Smead-Jones or retention sutures (Fig. 19-6).

Radiologic Imaging as Potential Diagnostic Aid

Resistance to antibiotic therapy, as evidenced by a persistent spiking febrile response, may be an indication for sonography or other imaging techniques (Figs. 19-9 to 19-11) to rule out retained uterine products, seromas, hematomas, or abscesses in the abdominal wall, pelvis, or occasionally the uterine incision. While sonography offers immediate evaluation of the pelvis in the patient resistant to therapy, computed tomography

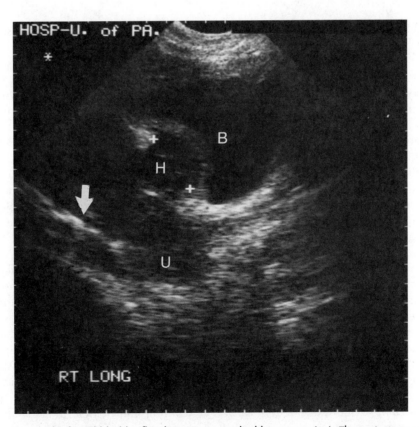

Fig. 19-9 Ultrasound of infected bladder flap hematoma marked by cursors (+). The patient presented approximately 1 week after cesarean delivery with fever. She responded to antibiotics. Note that the full bladder (B) enhances visualization of the hematoma (H). The arrow designates the endometrial cavity of the uterus (U).

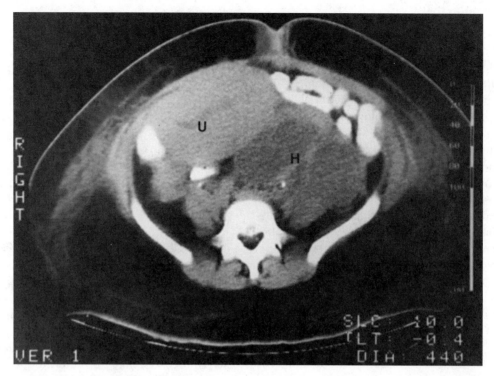

Fig. 19-10 CT scan of pelvis 6 days after a cesarean section showing left-sided broad ligament hematoma (H). The uterus (U) is displaced to the right. The patient responded to antibiotics. (Courtesy of Dr. Michael Blumenfeld, Department of Obstetrics and Gynecology, Ohio State University, Columbus, OH.)

(CT) may be preferable in some cases because it allows complete assessment of the entire peritoneal cavity and may identify fresh hemorrhage within a fluid collection as well as ovarian vein thrombosis. Sonography with a 5- or 7-mHz short-focus transducer also allows detailed examination of the abdominal wall for seromas, hematomas, and abscesses. The sonogram may be normal in the presence of a wound infection. Abscesses commonly present as complex, predominantly cystic masses, occasionally containing fluid levels. A complete examination of the abdomen including the subphrenic space may on occasion reveal a subphrenic abscess; however, these are often difficult to visualize, particularly if there are multiple small abscesses. Scanning the patient in different positions may facilitate more adequate visualization of the subphrenic space. Care should be taken not to mistake the accumulation of subdiaphragmatic fluid for a pleural effusion in the patient with severe preeclampsia. On occasion, a subcapsular liver hematoma may be observed. Sonography may occasionally be difficult in the presence of bowel distention, particularly with the usual placement of the abdominal incision. However, sonography permits the evaluation of peristalsis at the site of a fluid-filled structure (bowel) and, where indicated, may facilitate sonographically guided percutaneous aspiration of a suspected abscess.[154]

By the first postpartum day, the uterus will be at or below the level of the umbilicus. On ultrasound, the uterine wall thickness will vary from 3 to 6.5 cm, being slightly thicker in multiparous patients than in primiparas.[21] The uterine wall ordinarily appears homogenous with an occasional subtle irregularity.[155] The endometrial cavity often presents as a slit whose anteroposterior diameter varies from 0.5 to 1.3 cm.[156] The uterine incision may present a variable sonographic appearance following cesarean section.[157] Strong echoes may arise from the suture material. It is not unusual to see small seromas and hematomas of the uterine incision under the bladder flap. Should a significant fluid collection be observed around the uterine incision in a febrile patient, an abscess should be considered (Fig. 19-9).

When a postpartum abdominal ultrasound examination is performed, the patient should have a full bladder. This will facilitate displacement of the normal anteflexed puerperal uterus posteriorly, positioning the endometrial cavity at right angles to the sound waves and improving visualization.[158] In addition, bladder filling will frequently push any gas-filled loops of bowel out of the pelvis, thus facilitating visualization of the cul-de-sac, adnexa, and uterus. Transvaginal scanning may be helpful if the abdomen is distended, the incision site interferes with adequate abdominal imaging, or the patient is unable to tolerate the pressure of abdominal scanning.

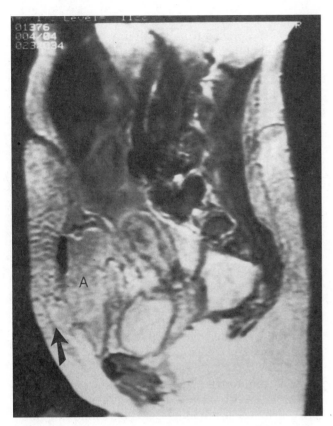

Fig. 19-11 MRI scan of abdominal wall abscess. This patient presented 1 week after a cesarean delivery with fever and an abdominal mass. The differential diagnosis included an intraperitoneal infection with extension or a wound abscess. This MRI shows a wound abscess (A) above fascia that extended to the abdominal wall (arrow). The abscess responded to drainage and antibiotics.

Sonographic findings suggesting endometritis may include a dilated fluid- or gas-filled uterine cavity and fluid in the cul-de-sac. Sonographic evidence of an empty uterus will eliminate the possibility of retained products. However, an abnormal scan may represent either the normal retention of blood or retained products of conception.[159] Abscesses may present with characteristic fluid and gas collections, shaggy walls, and internal echoes in association with cul-de-sac fluid accumulations indicating peritonitis. If gas is detected on sonogram, gas-forming organisms such as *E. coli* or *Clostridium perfringens* may be present. CT may be used to diagnose ovarian vein thrombophlebitis.[160]

Urinary Complications

Urinary tract infections are second to endomyometritis as a cause of postcesarean febrile morbidity. The reported incidence varies from as low as 2 percent to as high as 16 percent.[161] In one study, approximately 7 percent of postoperative clean-catch urine specimens had at least 10^5 bacteria per milliliter in culture. One percent of patients had both bacteriuria and endomyometritis.[162] Urethral catheterization contributes to 80 percent of nosocomial urinary tract infections in hospitalized patients, particularly when indwelling catheters are used. The incidence is increased with longer duration of catheter use, in diabetic patients, and in patients who are critically ill.[160] Attention to detail in terms of proper preparation and insertion of the catheter and the use of a closed drainage system have decreased this risk.

Gastrointestinal Complications

Most patients undergoing cesarean delivery have little if any gastrointestinal problems postoperatively. However, anesthesia and narcotics employed to treat postoperative pain may contribute to bowel dysfunction. As a result, an occasional patient may have postoperative nausea or mild transient abdominal distention in the first 24 hours.

Ileus should be suspected if prolonged nausea or vomiting together with signs such as abdominal distention, absence of bowel sounds, and failure to pass flatus are persistent. Distended loops of bowel with or without air fluid levels on x-ray will provide confirmatory evidence. In most instances simply withholding oral intake, providing adequate fluid replacement, and being observant are sufficient. If the ileus is persistent, nasogastric suction may be required.

Actual mechanical bowel obstruction may initially present as an ileus, but is commonly associated with peristaltic rushes and high-pitched bowel sounds in conjunction with symptoms of nausea, vomiting, and abdominal distension. Once again, some patients will respond to conservative management, including restriction of oral intake and placement of a nasogastric tube or possibly even a long tube. The key to success is maintenance not only of fluids and electrolytes but also of hematocrit and serum protein. Should conservative therapy fail, surgical consultation and possible exploration may be required.

Thromboembolic Disorders

The risk of thrombosis increases during pregnancy because of both higher levels of coagulation factors and diminished fibrinolysis. These changes peak near term and immediately after delivery. Deep venous thrombophlebitis (DVT) of the lower extremities occurs in approximately 0.24 percent of all deliveries.[163,164] The risk of DVT after cesarean delivery is approximately three to five times greater than after vaginal delivery.[165] Compounding risk factors include obesity, inability to ambulate, advanced maternal age, and higher parity. Should the DVT go untreated, approximately 15 to 25 percent of patients will develop pulmonary emboli, and

15 percent will sustain a fatal pulmonary embolus (PE). However, if recognized early and treated appropriately, the risks of PE and death are reduced to 4.5 and 0.7 percent, respectively.[164,166]

Classic symptoms for DVT include unilateral leg pain, tenderness, and swelling. A 2-cm difference in leg circumference between the affected and normal limb is generally required for diagnosis. Other clinical signs include edema, a palpable cord, and a change in limb color. A positive Homan's sign (calf pain on passive dorsiflexion of the foot) or a positive Lowenberg test (pain distal to the site of rapid inflation of a blood pressure cuff to 100 mmHg) suggests DVT.

Unfortunately, the first sign of DVT may be the occurrence of a PE, which can present with symptoms of tachypnea (90 percent), dyspnea (80 percent), pleuritic chest pain with or without splinting (more than 70 percent), apprehension (approximately 60 percent), tachycardia (40 percent), and cough (more than 50 percent).[167,168] Other findings include atelectatic rales, a friction rub, accentuated second heart sound, and a gallop. Patient evaluation is complicated in the postcesarean delivery patient, since splinting from incisional pain and tachypnea are not unusual findings. Doppler studies have a sensitivity of 90 percent for popliteal, femoral, or iliac thromboses, but only 50 percent for calf involvement because of abundant collateral vessels. Impedance plethysmography (IPG) is sensitive in approximately 95 percent of proximal thromboses, but is not as effective as Doppler for pelvic vessel thrombosis and will generally identify most cases, especially above the calves. Should Doppler and IPG be inconclusive, ascending venography, the most accurate of the three tests, should be performed. IPG can be used as a first-line test postpartum in the nonlactating mother. Should PE be suspected, a baseline arterial blood gas, chest x-ray, and electrocardiogram, as well as prothrombin time and partial thromboplastin time, should be obtained. Oxygen therapy should also be administered. Once the diagnosis has been established, heparin therapy should be started (see Ch. 29).

Septic Pelvic Thrombophlebitis

Approximately 0.5 to 2 percent of patients with endomyometritis or wound infection will develop septic pelvic thrombophlebitis, a more common complication of cesarean birth than of vaginal delivery. In large part, this is a result of the higher rate of endomyometritis in patients undergoing cesarean delivery.[169] Largely a diagnosis of exclusion, septic pelvic thrombophlebitis occurs most commonly on the right side and may be suspected should there be fever and unilateral pain. Although tenderness about the incision site may make detection difficult, occasionally one will be able to palpate a tender, rope-like abdominal mass extending laterally and cephalad from the uterus. Sonographic examination of the lower abdomen and pelvis or CT may be of assistance in the diagnosis (see Fig. 38-4).

Postoperative Management

Postoperative Analgesia

Analgesia should be provided in a dose and at a frequency that will neither obtund nor cause respiratory depression and yet allow the patient (1) to avoid the consequences of extremes in analgesic blood levels resulting in unnecessary pain and (2) to cooperate with normal postoperative management. The patient receiving inadequate analgesia may, in an effort to protect her wound, maintain a shallow breathing pattern without deep breaths and, hence, develop atelectasis.[170]

Commonly employed analgesics include meperidone (50 to 75 mg) or morphine (10 mg, depending on maternal size), administered intravenously or intramuscularly every 3 to 4 hours. Intrathecal or epidural narcotic administration employed with agents such as morphine can also be used for postoperative anesthesia, which may last as long as 30 hours following delivery, providing an advantage to a patient who has undergone a regional block.[171]

Ambulation

Early ambulation is important in reinstitution of inflation of the most dependent alveoli and the prevention of pulmonary complications, particularly in the patient who has had general anesthesia. Early ambulation also promotes the return of normal urinary and bowel activity. Under most circumstances, the uncomplicated patient can be allowed to sit up within 8 to 12 hours following the procedure, even after epidural anesthesia. The patient generally can ambulate within the first day after surgery and by the second day can shower without fear of injury to the incision.

Oral Intake

Active bowel sounds are commonly not observed until the second postoperative day. Nonetheless, in most instances the patient will easily tolerate oral fluids the day after surgery. Only rarely, when the patient has been septic or there has been extensive intra-abdominal manipulation, will there be a need to withhold oral fluids, even though the patient may have diminished bowel sounds and not pass gas. Most clinicians feel comfortable in providing clear liquids and ice chips with only a small amount of liquid as soon as nausea subsides to relieve complaints of a dry mouth. The progression of the diet also varies according to clinician. Some advance the patient rapidly to a regular diet, whereas others institute a progression to a full liquid diet by 48 hours, awaiting the return of normal bowel sounds and passage of flatus to indicate return of colonic function. Few wait beyond the third postoperative day to institute a regular diet.

Bladder Management

The urinary catheter is ordinarily removed within 12 to 24 hours following surgery unless there have been intraoperative complications.

Postoperative Wound Care

The incision is generally covered for the first day with a light dressing, until the wound is sealed. The dressing is removed after the first postoperative day.

Laboratory Studies

Blood loss arising from an uncomplicated cesarean delivery is approximately 1,000 ml.[172] As a consequence of blood loss as well as intra- and postoperative hydration, the postoperative hematocrit may be expected to drop by approximately 2 to 3 percentage points during the initial 2 days following surgery, independent of hydration status.

Postoperative Fluids

The normal postpartum period is generally characterized by mobilization of the physiologic accumulation of fluid during pregnancy. As a consequence, large volumes of intravenous fluids are seldom required after cesarean delivery. In the low-risk patient, fluid replacement needs during a 24-hour interval are generally only 1,000 ml above urinary output. Three liters of a salt-containing solution will thus generally suffice during the first 24 hours unless urinary output falls below 30 ml per hour. Under certain circumstances there may be increased requirements for fluids: following prolonged labor, febrile illness, vomiting and diarrhea or even prior use of diuretics or salt restriction. More complex patients may have additional needs. Potassium is ordinarily not required during the first 24 hours by uncomplicated patients because of intracellular potassium release from cell destruction. After the first 24 hours, intravenous fluid replacement with 5 percent dextrose in 0.45 percent sodium chloride is commonly employed, unless volume expansion is an issue. If it is anticipated that the patient will require prolonged intravenous fluids, potassium may be administered as 60 to 80 mEq/day. Should the patient be oliguric, potassium is generally not given until the patient has normal urinary output.

Table 19-9 Average Length of Hospital Stay for Births According to Delivery Route in the United States

	Length of Stay (Days)		
	1980[a]	1989[a]	1991[b]
Primary cesarean	6.7	4.8	4.5
Repeat cesarean	6.1	4.2	4.2
Vaginal delivery	3.2	2.4	2.3
VBAC delivery	—	—	2.2
All deliveries	3.8	2.9	2.8

[a]Data from Taffel et al[23]
[b]Data from MMWR.[1]

Average Length of Stay

Depending on postoperative morbidity/complications and availability of care at home, hospital discharge may occur as early as the second to fifth postoperative day. (Table 19-9)

Discharge Management

Reduction in the length of stay, from over 6 to 7 days to fewer than 4, has had a dramatic impact on many patient-related programs. Table 19-10 provides an example of a typical management guideline that may be used by third party payors as they extend their efforts to "manage care."[173] Elective cesarean patients are no

Table 19-10 Typical Managed Care Goals for Cesarean Delivery (S-350)

Protocol:	(CPT-4:58611, 59510, 59514, 59515, 59525) (ICD-9:74.0, 74.1, 74.4, 74.9) (ICD-9:054.11, 641, 642.5, 642.6, 652.2–652.6, 652.9, 653, 654, 654.2, 654.7, 654.8, 658.2, 658.3, 660, 662.2, 663)
Day 1:	Preadmission patient education and home care assessment. Operating room for cesarean delivery, parenteral fluids and medications, possible PCA or epidural analgesics
Day 2:	Clear liquids to advanced diet as tolerated. Discontinue passive cutaneous analgesics (PCA) or epidural analgesics. Discontinue IV and Foley if not done previously. Parenteral or oral medications. Ambulatory. Flatus present. Possible discharge
Day 3:	Afebrile, ambulatory, oral medications, regular diet. Discharge
Note:	Although most patients recover and may require no more than 36 hours as inpatients postoperatively, the variability in the hour of surgical delivery makes it uncertain how many patients may be able to go home on the first postpartum day. Some who deliver early in the day of delivery may do so

(Data from Milliman & Robertson,[173] with permission.)

longer admitted the night before the intended procedure. It is noteworthy that their goal for length of stay for a cesarean birth is 2 days. One would hope that the managed care payors will divert some of the savings from profit to patient support and medical supervision of mother and newborn at home.

The mother's activities at home for the first week should be limited to personal care and to care of the newborn. By the third to fourth week, the patient can generally resume most activities at home. The length of hospitalization associated with cesarean birth, like those associated with vaginal delivery, has declined dramatically.[1,23]

Reducing the Current Cesarean Birth Rate

Possible Strategies To Reduce the Rate

National Strategies

A number of national strategies have been proposed to reduce the current cesarean birth rate: (1) equalize the reimbursement for vaginal and cesarean deliveries; (2) publish physician-specific cesarean rates; (3) publish hospital-specific cesarean rates; and (4) address physician malpractice concerns through legislation. The ACOG has indicated, with regard to the first strategy, that there is little or no evidence that the decision to perform a cesarean delivery or to offer a trial of labor is in any way motivated by a differential in payment. They recommend that financial incentives should not be used by payors to influence physician or patient decisions relative to the mode of delivery; rather, the decision should be based on standard obstetric indications and maternal fetal safety.[174]

Hospital Administrative Strategies

Bottoms et al[175] concluded that cesarean delivery for dystocia and repeat cesarean deliveries should be points of primary review. If primary indications can be more tightly controlled, the number of candidates for repeat cesarean section will be reduced accordingly. Each hospital review committee should examine its institutional and individual physician cesarean rates. It is important that the review target each indication since variation in total rate among physicians may not be associated with the same indication. Peer review conference screening should support the concept that, with the exception of a failed induction, cesarean delivery conducted on patients while still in the latent phase of labor should be an infrequent indication for cesarean birth. The validity of such a program is evident in a trial conducted in one hospital that evaluated the effects of selected clinical criteria and review mechanisms. Second opinions were required; VBAC-TOL was the pre-

Table 19-11   Potential Approaches To Reduce Cesarean Births

Vaginal birth after cesarean trial of labor (VBAC-TOL)
Dystocia/CPD/FTP
   Disciplined approach to labor management
   Active management of labor
Breech presentation/transverse lie
   External version
   Selective vaginal delivery of breech
Fetal hypoxia/acidosis
   Develop more predictive markers for acidosis
   Fetal capillary blood gases for reassurance
   Fetal stimulation for reassurance

(Data from Taffel et al,[23] with permission.)

ferred clinical approach; and peer review was implemented. After implementation of the program the cesarean rate decreased from 17.5 percent in 1985 to 11.5 percent in 1987, a time when cesarean rates were rising.[176]

Clinical Strategies

Table 19-11 summarizes potential clinical strategies to reduce the current cesarean rate. The strategy most likely to have a significant impact is one that which strongly encourages VBAC trial of labor.

Indications Susceptible to Reduction

In 1991, the last reported year, 996,000 (23.5 percent) of approximately 4.1 million births were by cesarean delivery. Of all cesarean deliveries, approximately 338,000 (35 percent) were associated with a prior cesarean birth and 628,000 (65 percent) were primary cesarean births (30.4 percent with "dystocia," 11.7 percent with breech presentation, 9.2 percent with "fetal distress," and 13.7 percent with all other specified complications.) A comparison of cesarean delivery rates associated with specific labor and fetal maternal indications for 1980 and 1989 is given in Table 19-12. Labor-related indications are largely responsible for the increase in cesarean rates. Although the percentage of women presenting with fetopelvic disproportion remained relatively stable (4.1 and 4.2 percent), the percentage of women with this designation who underwent cesarean delivery increased from 95.7 to 98.5 percent. More dramatic change was observed in the prevalence of other labor-related designations (ICD-9-CM codes 660 and 661). Cesarean delivery as a medicolegal strategy for managing term breech presentation has also played a role. Not only has the prevalence of breech presentation increased (from 3.2 to 4.0 percent), but the percentage of breech fetuses who underwent cesarean birth increased from 67.2 to 83.9 percent. The sub-

Table 19-12 Cesarean Rates per 100 Total Deliveries by Indication

ICD-9-CM Category[a]	Indication	Percent of Women with Diagnosis		Cesarean Rate (%) in Category	
		1980	1989	1980	1989
	Labor related				
653.4	Fetopelvic disprop.	4.1	4.2	95.7	98.5
660.	Obstructed labor	1.1	4.3	25.9	66.3
661.	Abn. labor/inertia	3.0	7.4	53.7	42.7
652.2	Breech presentation	3.2	4.0	67.2	82.9
654.2	Prior cesarean	5.1	10.4	96.6	81.5
656.3	"Fetal distress"	1.7	8.8	66.9	46.0
664.	Early/threat labor	4.1	4.9	25.2	30.2
642.	Hypertens./eclampsia	4.0	5.6	38.3	45.0
645	Prolonged pregnancy	1.3	3.4	34.0	29.5

[a]Categories are not mutually exclusive.
(Data from Taffel et al,[23] with permission.)

jective diagnosis of a "fetal distress" increased even more dramatically, from 1.7 to 8.8 percent; however, the percentage with that designation who required cesarean delivery decreased from 66.9 to 46.0 percent, possibly reflecting a lowering of threshold for this diagnosis.

Reduction in the overall rate will occur only if a strategy is developed for each indication category. For example, O'Driscoll et al[177] attributed much of their success in maintaining a low cesarean rate to a lower rate of dystocia secondary to aggressive utilization of oxytocin; greater use of VBAC-TOL, and liberal criteria for vaginal breech deliveries. Brief mention will be made regarding the above clinical problems associated with cesarean birth with increased emphasis on VBAC-TOL and active management of labor as strategies to reduce current cesarean rates.

Dystocia (Failure to Progress)/ Cephalopelvic Disproportion

There is likely to be significant room for improvement in the current cesarean delivery rate for the clinical entity referred to as "dystocia," the most common indication for primary cesarean birth in the United States. The term includes a broad range of problems, including relative CPD and FTP encountered in the latent and active phases of labor. There is also some basis for a special designation for "failed induction" since a diagnosis of CPD/FTP is more common following labor induction.[178,179]

Determination of the cause of failure to achieve more vaginal deliveries is complex; as a result, any single strategy to reduce the impact of dystocia for cesarean delivery is unlikely to meet with major success.[20,23] Although failure to make sufficient progress in the active phase of the first stage (cervical dilatation) or the sec-

ond stage (descent) has been attributed to deficiencies in uterine "power"/activity, "excess size" of the "passenger," or "relative-small size" of the "pelvic-passage," FTP, may also potentially be the result of different "physician" approaches to the management of the latent and active phases of labor (see discussion of active labor management as a strategy, below)

Prior Cesarean Birth

A reduction in the cesarean birth rate can be achieved only by employing VBAC-TOL as an approach to address and lower the self-perpetuating contribution of the indication of previous cesarean birth.[180–183] Few changes within the specialty of obstetrics and gynecology offer greater potential impact to more women than that of VBAC-TOL, since elective repeat cesarean delivery is estimated to be largely responsible for the increase in cesarean deliveries. The cesarean birth rate rose 44 percent between 1978 and 1984, and 47 percent of the rise was due to the performance of elective repeat cesarean deliveries.[1,3] The total cesarean rate (Table 19-1) in the United States peaked in 1988 at 24.7 percent; of these, 36.3 percent (351,000) were repeat cesarean deliveries. In the 1989–91 interval, the cesarean rate appeared to reduce or plateau. Changing VBAC-TOL rates appear to be largely responsible, increasing 47 percent from 1988 (12.6 percent) to 1989 (18.5 percent), which followed a 29 percent rise in the 1987–88 interval.

Breech Presentation

There is some potential for improvement in the current rate of cesarean births attributable to the breech presentation. The management of both term and preterm breech presentations remains controversial.[184] Nonetheless, the combination of fear of litigation and ever-decreasing opportunities to train residents in the proper approach to the management and technique for vaginal delivery has resulted in a continuing drift in practice toward cesarean births; the cesarean rate for breech presentations increased from 67.2 percent in 1980 to 80.4 percent in 1985 in the United States.[22] Although vaginal delivery can be justified in up to 50 percent of term breech presentations, cesarean births for breech constitute only 10 to 15 percent of all cesarean deliveries, and thus a 50 percent reduction is not likely to have a major impact on the overall cesarean section rate.

Nonreassuring FHR and the Medicolegal Environment

Under better circumstances physicians could reduce the impact of FHR-based indication for cesarean delivery. Some of the blame for the current increase in cesarean delivery is attributed to continuous electronic fetal monitoring and inappropriate overinterpretation of FHR data. However, it is likely that the root cause is physician fear of malpractice litigation. Most FHR alterations, including some rather dramatic (in a visual sense) variable decelerations are likely to reflect only a temporary decrease in fetal oxygenation, as opposed to so-called fetal distress, a diagnosis lacking a consensus for diagnostic criteria. It is well-known that such a diagnosis is associated with a high false-positive rate. There is fairly widespread fear of the medicolegal consequences of not performing a cesarean in the presence of a nonreassuring FHR strip, despite the presence of indicators that ordinarily should provide reassurance. In a less litigious environment, the physician in doubt could gain reassurance that labor can be allowed to continue by a favorable response to fetal scalp or fetal acoustic stimulation or alternatively from a reassuring fetal capillary pH value. The goal is avoidance of rather severe fetal metabolic (cord arterial pH less than 7.00) or mixed acidosis as a means to reduce newborn morbidity and mortality.[185,186] Temporary fetal hypoxemia, without significant associated metabolic or mixed metabolic acidosis poses little risk for major newborn morbidity. Defensive medicine will continue to impact upon this indication. Although cesarean delivery for this indication is not a major contributor to the overall cesarean delivery rate, it is nonetheless likely that the impact of this indication can be reduced if tort reform can be enacted.

Active Management of Labor as a Reduction Strategy

Although the original intent of the active approach to the management of labor was to decrease the incidence of prolonged labor, its application is associated with a significant reduction in the cesarean rate for dystocia.[177,187–189] The active management of labor relies on utilization of strict criteria for the diagnosis of the active phase of labor and on a protocol employing relatively high doses of oxytocin should there be diminished cervical dilatation in the first stage or inadequate descent in the second stage of labor. The benefits of the program are likely to accrue from avoidance of the clinical trap of overly aggressive management of the latent phase of labor as well as early intervention with oxytocin in patients with either protraction or arrest disorders. Patient education and one-on-one supervision by a personal nurse is also important.[177,187]

The medical components of this approach include the early diagnosis of labor (and exclusion of the latent phase of labor), early rupture of intact membranes, and infusion of oxytocin under strict guidelines primarily to term singleton vertex presentations with no fetal indication for delivery. Membranes are artificially ruptured in the approximately 70 percent of women who have not had spontaneous rupture of membranes prior to admission. There are two purposes (1) to ensure efficient uterine activity and (2) to observe volume and color of amniotic fluid.

The efficiency of uterine activity as a "process" of the active phase of the first stage of labor is expressed solely by evaluating the "product" of uterine activity, the rapidity of cervical dilatation; there is no reference to descent of the head during the first stage of labor. Inefficient uterine activity is diagnosed by failure to achieve cervical dilatation at a rate of 1 cm per hour. The patient is first examined upon admission; a second examination is conducted 2 hours thereafter, and in most cases a third is conducted at or near the time of complete dilatation of the cervix. In the second stage, inefficiency of uterine activity is diagnosed when there is insufficient progress in the "product," descent of the vertex. Failure of descent of the head within 1 hour following the diagnosis of complete dilatation is also treated by oxytocin infusion if not already initiated.

Correction of "inefficient uterine activity" is always attempted by employing oxytocin after membrane rupture. Oxytocin infusion rates are relatively high when compared with "traditional" protocols. Oxytocin is initiated at 4 mU per minute; the rate is subsequently increased every 15 minutes in 4-mU increments to a maximum of 32 mU per minute. Oxytocin is not given if there is oligohydramnios or thick meconium (which suggests preexisting oligohydramnios). Either may be suggestive of uteroplacental insufficiency. Employing this protocol, approximately 50 percent of nulliparous patients require oxytocin to accelerate labor in the first stage.

Safety of Active Labor Management as a Strategy

The active management approach has only recently gained increased acceptance in the United States even though it has been employed as early as 1969 in Ireland. Although some had concern regarding the safety of employing a relatively high dose (by the prior practice of some) of oxytocin administered when using this protocol, there is no evidence to suggest a secondary increase in metabolic acidosis.[190–192]

Vaginal Birth After Cesarean Birth

Repeat Cesarean Delivery as a Problem

Despite early reports in the 1960s that VBAC-TOL was both feasible and safe, the American obstetrician was initially reluctant to accept a significant modification in obstetric practice.[193] As late as 1987, more than 90 percent of women (Table 19-1) with a prior cesarean delivery had a repeat procedure.[3] The proportion of all cesarean deliveries that are repeat cesareans peaked in 1988 at 36.3 percent, but subsequently decreased to 35 percent in 1991 in parallel with a 1.2 percent decrease in the total cesarean rate for the same time frame.

Benefits and Risks of VBAC-TOL

VBAC-TOL is successful in 60 to 80 percent of acceptable candidates.[194–197] If applied to all patients presenting with a prior cesarean procedure (8.2 to 8.5 percent), there is a potential to increase the rate of overall vaginal delivery by approximately 5 percent. Furthermore, there is evidence (Evid. Qual. II-2) from a large multicenter trial that VBAC-TOL reduces the incidence of postpartum infection, the need for postpartum transfusion, and maternal length of stay; as a result, there is significant cost savings.[197,198] Adding further impetus is the observation that the associated perinatal mortality rate (7 per 1,000 live births) of the VBAC-TOL study group is not higher than that of the overall rate (10.1 per 1,000 live births).[197]

The potential financial savings arising from a successful national VBAC program was estimated at approximately one-half billion dollars in 1985, assuming a repeat cesarean birth rate of only 6 percent and 3.4 million births.[199] Although the actual costs are not generally available, a recent survey by a national insurance company determined the average total charges in 1993 to be approximately $11,000 and $6,430 for a cesarean procedure and a normal vaginal delivery, respectively.[198]

Evolution of VBAC-TOL Acceptance

Cesarean rates appear to have decreased (Table 19-1) or at the least to have plateaued by 1991. One of the most important contributing factors has been a progressive decrease in clinical acceptance of the historical dictum of "once a cesarean section, always a cesarean section," which had been in practice since the early 1900s. It is logical that such an approach would eventually disappear. First, the clinical environment has changed dramatically since the early 1990s, when the "once a cesarean, always a cesarean" rule was advocated. At that time only 2 percent of births resulted in a cesarean delivery; most often the procedure was performed following a diagnosis of cephalopelvic disproportion; and the procedure commonly employed was a classic uterine incision. The advent of the low cervical segment incision together with better control of postcesarean infections has decreased the risk of uterine incision dehiscence during subsequent pregnancies. Second, there was a need to control rapidly rising national health care costs. Third, elective repeat cesarean delivery was the indication most responsible for the recent increase in cesarean births.

Although western European countries have had a long history of not considering a prior low transverse uterine incision as a contraindication to a subsequent TOL, the concept did not begin to gain momentum in the United States until after 1981, when the NICHD Conference on Child Birth concluded that vaginal delivery after cesarean birth is an appropriate option.[24]

Initial reports indicated that successful VBAC could be achieved in 50 to 80 percent of patients with a prior low transverse uterine incision and in as many as 70 percent of women for whom the indication for the prior cesarean delivery was "failure to progress in labor."[4,200–206] Although uterine rupture was an infrequent possibility, it was noted to be rarely "catastrophic." Maternal and perinatal mortality rates for VBAC-TOL were no higher than those for elective repeat cesarean births.[4,200–206] Acceptance has become more widespread as numerous positive reports, documenting the efficacy and safety of VBAC under a wide variety of clinical settings, have been published.[4,195,207–212] Later reports documented no increase in maternal or fetal risk for candidates who had more than one prior cesarean.[209,210,213]

In 1988, the ACOG published *Guidelines for Vaginal Delivery After a Previous Cesarean Birth*, recommending VBAC-TOL as an option that should be selected based on available evidence available at that time.[57] They further recommended that "each hospital develop its own protocol for management of VBAC-TOL patients; and a woman with one prior cesarean delivery with a low transverse incision should be counseled and encouraged to attempt labor in the absence of a contraindication, such as a prior classical uterine incision." At the time there were insufficient data to provide a complete cost-benefit analysis for patients presenting with a prior low vertical incision, more than one fetus, a breech presentation, or estimated fetal weight greater than 4,000 g. The 1988 Committee Opinion indicated that the use of oxytocin to augment labor does not confer greater risk in a VBAC-TOL in a patient with a prior low transverse incision than would be the case in a general obstetric population; however, it did acknowledge that some physicians would not choose to use oxytocin in VBAC-TOL.[57] Epidural anesthesia was considered appropriate. Suggested 1988 guidelines include the following:

1. Repeat cesarean birth should be by specific indication.
2. Women with two or more prior cesarean deliveries should not be discouraged from attempting a VBAC-TOL.
3. Normal patient activity should be encouraged during the latent phase of labor. There is no need for restriction prior to the onset of the active phase of labor.
4. Professional and institutional resources should be available to respond to "intrapartum obstetric emergencies" such as performing a cesarean delivery within 30 minutes from the time the decision is made until the "surgical procedure is begun."
5. A physician capable of evaluating labor and performing a cesarean delivery should be "readily available."

The most recent ACOG publication has further liberalized the approach as usage has become more widespread[214] (see Tables 19-17 and 19-18, below).

VBAC Trends

VBAC-TOL Rates

Acceptance of the VBAC-TOL concept has not been uniform. Approximately 40 to 50 percent of eligible women who are offered a VBAC-TOL choose the alternative, to have a repeat cesarean delivery.[215–217] A meta-analysis of 29 studies involving 8,770 VBAC-TOLs reflects wide variation in approach as evidenced by "remarkable variation in the percentage of patients accepted for trial of labor, ranging from 16–81%." Of interest, regression analysis indicated that the acceptance and success rates were not significantly associated.[218] Table 19-13 summarizes the dramatic change in acceptance of the validity of the VBAC-TOL concept at a large western university hospital in the 10-year interval from 1983 to 1992. Although the percentage of all patients with a prior cesarean delivery increased,

Table 19-13 Trial of Labor in Women with Prior Cesarean Births (C/S): Trends in Employment and Success

	1983 (%)	1992 (%)
Percent Total deliveries	8.1	14.1
With 1 prior C/S	6.1	11.3
With 2 prior C/S	1.6	2.2
With at least 3 prior C/S	0.4	0.6
Trial of Labor Employed	68	79
With 1 prior C/S	81	85
With 2 prior C/S	31	65
With ≥ 3 prior C/S	12	33
Trial of labor success	82	87
All prior C/S → vaginal delivery	56	69
Repeat C/S as percent of total deliveries	3.5	4.4

(Data from Miller et al,[211] with permission.)

the effect was neutralized by an increase in employment of TOL (68 to 79 percent). The increase was especially evident in patients with two or more prior cesareans.[211]

VBAC Success Rate

Overall VBAC success rates have increased significantly as clinicians have become more confident with the approach. However, even initial attempts were commonly successful. Vaginal delivery was achieved in approximately two out of three attempts between 1950 and 1980.[193,199,200] In view of the current high primary cesarean rate, with the possible exception of prior labor dystocia, it is not surprising that women who are offered a VBAC trial following a prior cesarean delivery appear to be no more likely to require a cesarean delivery than a population of women with no prior cesarean deliveries. A recent report compared VBAC success rates in 1983 with those in 1992 (Table 19-13). TOL success rates remain high (82 and 87 percent) in centers with considerable experience even after the indications have been extended. As a result, the percentage of all prior cesarean delivery patients achieving vaginal delivery increased from 56 to 69 percent.[211]

Vaginal Deliveries in all Prior Cesarean Patients

The impact of increasing national acceptance of the concept and increasing confidence in its clinical application is reflected by an almost threefold change (Table 19-1) in the percentage of women who presented with a prior cesarean who delivered vaginally from 1986 (8.5 percent) to 1991 (24.2 percent).[1,219]

Evaluating the VBAC-TOL Data

Since the publication in 1981 of the NICHD Cesarean Birth Task Force, numerous authors have reported their institution's success rates and morbidity and mortality rates associated with a VBAC-TOL.[24] Unfortunately, it is often difficult for the clinician to integrate VBAC-TOL data from multiple studies since risk factors may vary from study to study; most studies are relatively small; and maternal complications (maternal mortality, uterine dehiscence or rupture) and perinatal complications (death and morbidity) are relatively infrequent. To facilitate interpretation of such data, brief mention is presented regarding two methodologies to evaluate and integrate available data.

U.S. Preventive Task Force Scoring System

Typically under such an approach a Medline database search is conducted for reports of studies published in a predetermined time interval in one or more languages. The selected studies are evaluated, and the quality of the evidence obtained is then assessed on the basis of a scoring system (Table 19-14) scale. In the case of the recently published ACOG Practice Patterns, the first in a series, the literature search only included relevant articles containing at least 50 subjects published between 1985 and 1994.[214] The ACOG subsequently provided recommendations (based on the highest quality level of evidence available). The evidence was graded (Table 19-14) according to the three categories of (A) "good" evidence, (B) fair evidence, and (C) insufficient evidence; but the recommendation can be made on other grounds.

Meta-Analysis as a Tool To Evaluate Infrequent Endpoints

Meta-analysis is a statistical tool that provides access to pooled data from multiple similar selected nonrandomized studies deemed appropriate by the reporting

Table 19-14   U.S. Preventive Services Task Force Scoring System for Evidence Quality

Score	Required Evidence
I	At least one properly designed randomly controlled trial
II-1	Well-designed controlled trial without randomization
II-2	Well-designed cohort or case-control analytic studies, preferably from more than one medical center or research group
II-3	Multiple time series with or without the intervention. Dramatic results in uncontrolled experiments
III	Opinion of respected authorities, based on clinical experience, descriptive studies, or reports of expert committees

(Adapted from ACOG,[214] with permission.)

investigators. This approach provides the most readily available means with which to accumulate sufficient data to evaluate the impact of selected uncommon risk factors or endpoints. Odds ratios (OR) for each of the outcomes of interest can be calculated for each individual study, as well as for the pooled data. In the case of VBAC-TOL data, an OR that is far from 1.0 (i.e., 0.5 or 2.5) indicates a strong relationship between the TOL group and the outcome analyzed. In contrast, an OR that is close to 1 indicates a weak relationship. Similarly a narrow confidence interval (CI) indicates that the summary OR is a precise estimate of the effect, while a wide CI or one that includes the null hypothesis value (1.0) indicates that the observed OR is not a precise effect estimator, which is most often observed when the outcome is a rare event. When outcome measures are rare, the OR for any one particular outcome may appear to reveal a substantial difference between the various birth routes (TOL vs. VBAC vs. elective repeat cesarean delivery); however, when such outcomes are rare, the risk difference between the birth routes will be small. The primary limitation of meta-analysis is that both physician and patient choice are involved in each study and likely to be inconsistent from study to study.

Relevant VBAC-TOL Comparison Groups

To best determine the most appropriate prospective clinical management for patients presenting with a prior cesarean birth, the elective repeat cesarean group is the appropriate reference group with which to evaluate the safety of VBAC-TOL. In prospect, the outcome of the elective group should be compared with the outcome of all patients undergoing TOL. In hindsight, after completion of the TOL, the TOL group may be subdivided into (1) successful TOL (VBAC) and (2) failed trial of labor.

Preexisting Conditions as Predictors of VBAC-TOL Success

One of the first questions to be raised by a patient when considering a VBAC-TOL is, what is the likelihood for a successful vaginal birth according to the indication for the prior cesarean birth? The overall VBAC success rate for all candidates is 60 to 80 percent (Evid. Qual. II-2 and II-3).[194–197] Obstetric history regarding preexisting conditions is helpful in the prediction of VBAC success. Women who have previously given birth vaginally or women whose prior cesarean delivery was for nonrecurring conditions are more likely to succeed (Evid. Qual. II-3).[196,218,220] Despite providing some assistance, there is no system to predict the specific patient who will achieve a VBAC success; even x-ray pelvimetry cannot predict success (Evid. Qual. II-1 and II-3).[221,222] Furthermore, success rates vary because of

Table 19-15 Meta-Analysis of 29 studies (range, 6–24 for Each Indicator) Involving 8,770 VBAC-TOL

Preexisting Indicator in Prior Pregnancy	No. of Studies	Average Success Rate (%)	Odds Ratio[a]	95% CI	Studies Analyzed (Cases)
Previous breech	17	85	2.1	1.8–2.3	17 (1,720)
Prior vaginal delivery	12	84	2.1	1.7–2.5	12 (834)
>1 Prior cesarean	6	75	0.7	0.5–0.9	6 (1,015)
Dystocia[b]	24	67	0.5	0.5–0.6	24 (3,582)
Oxytocin used[a]	10	63	0.3	0.3–0.4	10 (2,289)

[a]Cephalopelvic disproportion, failure to progress.
[b]Odds ratio for a successful trial of labor after cesarean with various preexisting indications.
[c]Used in current pregnancy.
(Data from Rosen and Dickinson,[218] with permission.)

nonclinical variables and patient self-selection, which influences (Evid. Qual. Level II-2 and II-3) VBAC-TOL attempt rates.[215,223,224]

Recurring Vs. Nonrecurring Indications

The likely success of a VBAC trial will depend to some degree on whether the indication for the prior cesarean is a recurring or nonrecurring one. Patients with a nonrecurring indication (breech presentation, so-called fetal distress–nonreassuring FHR pattern, and conditions such as placenta previa, abruption, or maternal hemorrhage) are more likely (82 to 86 percent) to achieve success than is the patient who has undergone a prior cesarean for a potentially recurring condition (70 percent) such as dystocia (failure to progress and/or CPD), approximating the success rate for the so-called low-risk nulliparous patient.[208,218,225]

Rosen employed meta-analysis of 29 individual studies reported between 1982 and 1989 (Table 19-15) to evaluate the association between preexisting conditions and achievement of vaginal delivery (successful VBAC) for the entire subset; the effect of not attempting a VBAC-TOL is included.[218] VBAC-TOL success rates are similar (63 to 85 percent) among the subsets. However, when each subset is considered as a whole, apparently a trial was offered less often or when offered was refused more frequently when the prior indication was dystocia (OR = 0.5) and when oxytocin was used (OR = 0.3), the ORs of achieving vaginal delivery (when one condition is compared to all other preexisting conditions) are listed in Table 19-15 in decreasing order.

Prior Breech

Sixteen of 17 studies selected for meta-analysis indicate that the highest success rate (OR, 2.1; 95 percent CI, 1.8 to 2.3) with the current trial of labor is achieved when the prior indication for cesarean is breech presentation, indicating that the chance of achieving vaginal delivery was more than twice as great for a woman who

had had a prior cesarean for a breech than if she had had a cesarean for all other reasons.[218] Only one study found no association.[201]

Prior Vaginal Delivery

Although all patients have a relatively high rate of successful VBAC attempt, the success rate is increased to over 80 percent for women who have had a prior vaginal birth.[120,226,227] An early report was unable to demonstrate a significant impact of prior vaginal birth on an already high overall success rate (over 80 percent).[208] It may be that the impact of a prior vaginal birth exerts its effect only in patient populations in which VBAC trial management was less aggressive. Eleven of 12 available studies selected for meta-analysis indicate that a prior vaginal delivery improves the likelihood (OR, 2.1; 95 percent CI, 1.7 to 2.5) of a successful trial of labor.[218] Only one selected study indicated that a prior vaginal delivery did not improve the likelihood.[228] Two studies have examined the issue in greater detail, controlling for the order of these deliveries, and determined that vaginal delivery following the prior cesarean is a stronger predictor of success than vaginal delivery before the prior cesarean.[111,208]

More Than One Prior Cesarean (Multiple Prior Cesarean Births)

In 1988, the ACOG Guidelines for vaginal delivery after a previous cesarean birth specified that "A woman with two or more previous cesarean deliveries with low transverse incisions who wishes to attempt birth should not be discouraged from doing so in the absence of contraindications." Recent ACOG guidelines do not specify a maximum number of prior cesarean births as a criterion for VBAC.[58,214] The safety of VBAC-TOL in women having had two or more cesareans is now well established; they can be managed in a manner similar to that for patients with only one prior incision, with few complications.[4,193,201,208–211,213,214,220,229] Meta-

Table 19-16   Use and Success Rates of a VBAC-TOL According to the Number of Prior Cesarean Births

| | No. of Prior Cesareans | | | |
	One	Two	Three	Total
No. of prior cesareans	13,594	2,936	792	17,332
Percent total population	8.2	1.8	0.5	10.5
Trial of labor (TOL) (%)	80	54	30	73
Success (VBAC) (%)	83	75[a]	79[a]	82
Percent potential reduction in total cesarean rate	5.5	0.8	0.1	6.4

[a]Success rate with ≥ 2 prior cesareans was 75.3%, significantly lower than with 1 prior cesarean (OR, 0.612; 95% CI, 0.54–0.69; p < 0.001).
(Data from Miller et al,[211] with permission.)

analysis of six studies, providing data (Table 19-15) on 1,015 women who had more than one prior cesarean before a trial of labor indicate that such patients have historically been 30 percent less likely (OR, 0.7; 95 percent CI, 0.5 to 0.9) to be successful than all other trials of labor.[218] A recent report by Miller et al[211] (Table 19-16) emphasizes the importance of inclusion of patients with two or three prior cesareans if reduction of the total cesarean rate is to be considered a serious goal. They constitute approximately 1.8 and 0.5 percent of the entire obstetric patient population, respectively, and are highly likely (75 and 79 percent, respectively) to achieve vaginal delivery. Although uterine rupture is more likely in this group (OR, 3.06), there is no appreciable increase in perinatal mortality.[211]

Currently available data on the outcome of TOL with three or more prior cesareans are limited; however, VBAC success rate was 79 percent in one study.[211] Until more data are available, there may be some advantage in informing women with more than two prior procedures that they may possibly be at greater risk for uterine rupture if they choose TOL. However, they should not be discouraged from attempting a VBAC-TOL despite the lack of extensive risk versus benefit data. As many as 33 percent of such patients will accept the VBAC-TOL option, and approximately 80 percent of those who do so will be successful.[211]

Prior Dystocia (CPD/FTP)

Absolute cephalopelvic disproportion is virtually never present. Inherent clinical biases would suggest that patients with a previous cesarean delivery for dystocia (FTP or CPD and failed induction) would not only be less likely to achieve a VBAC-TOL, but also would not attempt a trial as often. Meta-analysis of 24 studies involving 3,582 trials in women with a prior cesarean for dystocia (Table 19-16) indicates that if such women attempt a trial, they achieve a 67% VBAC-TOL success rate. However, when the entire group with prior dystocia is considered, they have the lowest success rate for vaginal delivery (Odds Ratio = 0.5–50% of the rate of success [11–16 fewer vaginal deliveries per 100

cases]) achieved by all other women presenting with a history of prior cesarean for other indications (95% CI 0.5–0.6).[218] A more recent (1994) multicenter study (Evid. Qual. II-2) indicates that the patients with prior dystocia (CPD, FTP) who attempted a trial were successful in approximately two of three trials.[197] One study in which 58 patients received oxytocin therapy prior to cesarean delivery for "failure to progress" in the first term pregnancy labors is particularly instructive.[23] Despite the seeming importance of a well-managed initial pregnancy labor trial, 40 (69 percent) of the 58 women achieved vaginal delivery in their subsequent VBAC trial.

Impact of Dystocia-Related Factors

The likelihood of VBAC success is increased in the absence of a prior dystocia diagnosis. Similarly, success is increased by the presence of factors predicting the absence of dystocia, such as absolute fetal weight less than 4,000 g, smaller relative fetal weight than the index pregnancy, and response to oxytocin stimulation within 2 hours.[227] Should oxytocin be required, the absence of a prior CPD diagnosis increases the likelihood of VBAC success.[226] Furthermore, if the issue is indirectly assessed by evaluating other factors possibly related to dystocia, such as the length of the labor prior to the primary cesarean, the fetal birth weight and the extent of dilatation at the time of the prior cesarean, there is no improvement in predictability.[231]

Length of Labor Preceding Prior Cesarean

Two studies reported a tendency for a shorter labor immediately prior to the primary cesarean in women who are successful in a subsequent VBAC-TOL.[231,232]

Fetal Birth Weight

One might hypothesize a linkage between fetal birth rate and VBAC success. Jarrell et al[228] reported a lower trial success rate in women with prior CPD delivering a newborn weighing more than 3,900 g.[228] In contrast, Phelan et al[204] in a report involving 140 trials of labor with "macrosomic" (over 4,000-g) infants, reported that 67 percent of the women delivered vaginally. A statistically significant association between a higher average birth weight and a higher failure rate could not be identified in a subsequent meta-analysis of 10 selected studies providing sufficient data to determine average birth weights (average birth weight ranged from 3,123 to 3,642 g) of VBAC-TOL candidates.[218]

Cervical Dilatation upon Admission for Current Pregnancy

Cervical dilatation greater than 4 cm upon admission has been reported to increase the likelihood of a successful trial of labor significantly in one study but not in the other.[231,232]

Extent of Cervical Dilatation during Prior Primary Cesarean

Should the history indicate that the prior cesarean was for "failure to progress" following a failed induction or in a patient who did not enter the active phase of labor, one might anticipate the success rate to be similar to that of the general VBAC-TOL population. In contrast, should the history indicate that the patient entered the second stage and despite adequate contractile activity and pushing was unable to deliver, one could reasonably hypothesize such a patient to be less likely to achieve success. Despite the possible rationality of the thought process, the data are not supportive. Two studies found no association between the extent of dilatation at the time of the primary cesarean and subsequent success in the present trial of labor.[231,233]

Considerations in Management of VBAC-TOL

Management of the patient undergoing a VBAC-TOL is similar to that of patients attempting to achieve a vaginal delivery.[234] As a consequence, it is appropriate to use oxytocin and epidural anesthesia as one would in other labors. Potential problems such as suspected fetal macrosomia will be encountered and management will be no different from that in normal labor. The major difference will arise from some heightening of concern for uterine dehiscence and/or rupture. Even that concern need not be extreme; the risk is low, and, should dehiscence or rupture occur, in most cases the outcome is favorable for both the mother and fetus.

Prior Uterine Incision

Prior Lower Uterine Segment Incision

The presence of a preexisting incision confined to the lower uterine segment engenders minimal risk of uterine rupture, and the risk does not appear to be modified by the route of delivery.[211,212] Only in hindsight (i.e., should there have been a failed TOL) does the 95 percent confidence interval (1.4 to 5.4) exceed and not overlap the reference value of 1.0, indicating increased risk.

Prior Low Vertical Incision

A prior low vertical uterine incision, limited to the lower, more passive, noncontractile portion of the uterine segment, is not a contraindication for a VBAC-TOL.[58,212] Candidacy for a TOL in a patient with a prior low vertical scar is somewhat controversial. Low vertical incisions are not necessary as often, and most investigators have excluded women with low vertical scars from their reported series of patients. As a consequence, the available data are limited, and the data reported are possibly biased since they are not the product of prospective studies. Some clinicians believe that it is not possible to confine a vertical incision to the lower uterine segment. Some consider any uterine incision that extends into the upper, more contractile portion of the myometrium to be a contraindication to subsequent labor.[235] The theoretical concern does not appear to be warranted. Rosen et al,[212] in a meta-analysis of 170 VBAC patients with a prior low vertical incision, reported that the combined risk of dehiscence and rupture (two cases) was not different from that of VBAC patients with a prior low transverse incision.

Prior Classic Incision

It is likely that we will continue on occasion to be confronted with patients who have had a prior classic incision. A TOL should be strongly discouraged in such cases.[58] Fortunately, classic cesarean incisions are uncommon, and as a result the need to conduct a repeat cesarean in this population subset will make only a small contribution to the overall repeat cesarean rate. Patients with prior classic incision have an associated 12 percent (SE 6 percent) risk (3 cases in 26 women who underwent unplanned TOL) of symptomatic uterine rupture during labor.[212,236] Since approximately one-third of ruptures occur prior to labor, it is currently recommended that women who have a prior classic cesarean delivery be delivered by repeat cesarean procedure upon achieving fetal pulmonary maturity prior to the onset of labor. Such patients should be warned of the hazards of an unintended labor and the signs of possible uterine rupture.[237]

Known Vs. Unknown Incision Type

In an era when prior medical records are not always readily available, it is reassuring that the overall risk of dehiscence or rupture is low even among women undergoing a TOL with an unknown prior cesarean incision type. In large part this is a function of observation that 90 to 95 percent of women with unknown scars will have had a low transverse incision.[202] Some believe, should the extent of an incision be unknown or poorly documented, that a TOL is probably not a reasonable approach.[235] However, this is not a very practical and probably is an unnecessary approach. Meta-analysis reveals no statistically significant difference in rates ($p = 0.95$) between those with versus those without known incision types.[212]

Oxytocin Usage in VBAC Trial

Use of oxytocin is contraindicated only if the patient has a prior classic incision; the indications for use of oxytocin are the same as those for patients without a history of one or more prior cesarean births.[212,238] Oxytocin use should be in general accordance with the guidelines stated in ACOG Technical Bulletin No. 157.[239] Its use during a VBAC-TOL for augmentation does not increase risk and is not associated with an increase in perinatal mortality.[58,240] Some discussion of theoretical questions relating to benefits and risks justifying this conclusion is worthwhile.

Does the Use of Oxytocin Provide Clinical Benefit?

If oxytocin is not used selectively, a significant number of VBAC-TOLs will end up as repeat cesarean procedures. However, when VBAC-TOL patients receiving oxytocin are compared with those not receiving oxytocin, failure is significantly higher in the oxytocin group. Unfortunately, it is not possible to predict prospectively which patient will derive benefit. If there is an early response to oxytocin, one can expect a greater probability of success. In contrast, if a patient fails to progress within approximately 2 hours, cesarean delivery becomes considerably more likely.[227]

Benefit accrues from its use when employed for either induction or augmentation; vaginal delivery can be accomplished in 60 and 68 percent, respectively.[241] Meta-analysis of 10 selected studies indicates that the success rate among TOL patients requiring oxytocin is approximately one-third the rate of success in patients not receiving oxytocin (OR, 0.3; 95 percent CI, 0.3 to 0.4).[218] Only 1 of the 10 studies suggested a higher, but not significantly higher, success rate following the administration of oxytocin.[201] Although the data are not available, selection bias may explain the discrepancy; oxytocin augmentation is seldom employed unless there is recognition of delayed progress in either cervical dilatation in the first stage or descent in the second stage, and induction may be indicated in patients with an unfavorable cervix. The impact of the oxytocin use in VBAC-TOL should be studied further, controlling for multiple variables.

Are There Contraindications to Oxytocin Usage?

With the exception of a prior classic uterine incision, currently there are no absolute contraindications to the use of oxytocin in an appropriate VBAC-TOL candidate. Each case must be considered on the basis of the clinical presentation and a judgment made regarding the relative benefits and risks of its use under the circumstances of the case.

Spontaneous Vs. Induced Uterine Contractions as Risk Factors

Uterine contraction patterns, whether spontaneous or oxytocin induced, may demonstrate hypercontractility (tachysystole or tetany); on occasion there may be associated FHR decelerations. Hypercontractility, if persistent, may potentially increase fetal risk, a risk that is independent of the presence of a prior uterine scar.

Does Oxytocin "Significantly" Increase the Risk of Uterine Rupture and Perinatal Mortality in a VBAC-TOL?

Initial concern that oxytocin usage would significantly increase the risk of uterine rupture/dehiscence has not been confirmed. First the risk is quite low. Its use is not associated with an increase in perinatal mortality.[58] However, a case-control study found that "excessive (overuse of)" oxytocin infusion rates increased the risk for rupture or dehiscence.[242] (Note: No oxytocin dosage data were provided, and the authors seemed to be referring to a poorly documented need for oxytocin, especially in the latent phase of labor.) Although it is known that use of oxytocin is "associated" with an increase in risk of uterine rupture, this risk must be interpreted in an overall clinical context that may include other factors also associated with rupture. Use and duration of administration do not significantly increase the risk above that expected in the absence of oxytocin.[4,87,199,212,241] Meta-analysis of selected studies indicates that the use of oxytocin during a VBAC-TOL does not appear to influence the risk of a dehiscence or rupture ($p = 0.7$), nor does it increase perinatal mortality rates.[212]

Is There an Oxytocin Dose Limitation?

Despite a low risk for dehiscence/rupture, some believe there is strategic advantage to limiting total oxytocin dosage to a maximum of 20 or 30 mU per minute. However, there appears to be no objective medical basis for such a recommendation, and there is no medical consensus that establishes an appropriate dose schedule for oxytocin.[243] Some reassurance is gained by rather widespread employment of oxytocin protocols (associated with active management of labor) that employ 40 mU per minute or more in non-VBAC-TOL patients.[177,243]

Hindsight Analysis of Uterine Rupture

Prior oxytocin usage in a VBAC-TOL complicated by uterine rupture does not provide sufficient basis to conclude that the rupture is the probable product of oxytocin use since rupture or dehiscence can occur in the absence of prior oxytocin use. Oxytocin usage is likely to be relatively common in VBAC candidates. As a result, it is also likely to be common in patients who develop dehiscence or rupture. In a recent large series, Miller et al[211] report that oxytocin was used in only 68 percent of 118 cases of uterine rupture (74 percent of 69 ruptures in women with one prior cesarean and 67 percent of 39 ruptures in women with two prior cesarean deliveries).

Prostaglandin Gel Usage

Although the use of prostaglandin E_2 gel for cervical ripening is extensive and is likely to have been employed in many prior VBAC candidates, reported data are limited. Three authors have reported experience with prostaglandin E_2 gel for cervical ripening.[244–246] Unfortunately, available reports involve insufficient numbers to draw a definite conclusion. At this point its use appears justified. It is likely that this is an area that will be reported on as additional experience with the use of prostaglandin E_2 gel in this group of patients is gained. A randomized trial addressing the efficacy and safety of its use is highly desirable.

Possible Fetal Macrosomia

Prospective management of potential fetal macrosomia presents a significant clinical dilemma in any labor. A fetus whose estimated fetal weight (EFW) is more than 4,000 g is not a contraindication to a TOL.[58,212] Although clinicians might strategically reduce exposure to litigation by routine repeat cesarean delivery when the EFW is greater than 4,000 g, the strategy is flawed. It incorrectly assumes that fetal weight can be predicted reliably and ignores data that indicate that vaginal delivery can be accomplished safely in a large proportion of patients.[204] The decision to perform a cesarean in all patients with an EFW of more than 4,000 g would result in many cesarean deliveries for actual weight less than 4,000 g and with little or no improvement in outcome. The 1988 ACOG VBAC guidelines indicate that "the effects of labor on the patient with an estimated fetal weight of more than 4,000 grams have not been substantiated."[57]

The only way to address the question conclusively is to review retrospectively the outcomes of VBAC-TOLs in which the birth weight is known to be in excess of 4,000 g. Flamm and Goings[247] reviewed the outcomes of 1,776 patients who attempted a TOL in eight California hospitals; 301 newborns weighed at least 4,000 g. Fifty-eight percent of newborns weighing 4,000 to 4,500 g and 43 percent of those with birth weights of at least 4,500 g delivered vaginally. Of interest, when the outcomes of the 301 "macrosomic" TOLs were compared with the outcomes of the 1,475 TOLs with birth weights less than 4,000 g, there was no significant difference in maternal or perinatal morbidity or mortality. This clinical issue should be explored further, particularly for estimated birth weights in excess of 4,500 g.

Possible Fetal Macrosomia and Oxytocin

An EFW above 4,000 g increases the likelihood of labor dystocia, particularly when oxytocin is used and when the EFW exceeds 4,500 g.[204] Although vaginal delivery is less likely, there is no contraindication to a VBAC-TOL or oxytocin use should macrosomia be suspected. Each case will be managed selectively.

Fetal Monitoring

In most cases a significant alteration in FHR pattern is the presenting sign; on occasion, an alteration (increased frequency and/or intensity) in uterine contraction pattern (if monitored externally) or a loss of intrauterine pressure (if monitored with an internal pressure catheter) is the presenting sign.[199] The clinical detection and management of a possible uterine rupture will involve interpretation and reaction to a nonreassuring FHR observation (i.e., a sudden prolonged deceleration or repetitive "significant" variable deceleration of a degree requiring intervention under the circumstances of the case). Although repetitive "significant" variable decelerations or a prolonged deceleration occur all too frequently in non-VBAC-TOL, detection of these findings during a VBAC-TOL strategically may justify a heightened response. The question is not whether a fetal scalp blood sample will confirm fetal metabolic acidosis or if an ultrasound will detect a fetal part outside of the uterine cavity. It may be prudent to proceed more rapidly to cesarean delivery under such circumstances than would be the case in the absence of a prior uterine incision. Undoubtedly such a recommendation will result in some cesarean deliveries in which there is no rupture. However, the occurrence of a significantly nonreassuring FHR observation in a VBAC candidate is so infrequent as to have little impact on the overall cesarean rate of only one institution.

Intrauterine Pressure Catheters

One of the primary justifications for early recommendations by some that intrauterine pressure catheters be employed was the potential to detect intrauterine pressure changes (abrupt change in intrauterine activity or pressure) associated with uterine rupture. Unfortunately, use of intrauterine pressure catheters does reliably assist in the diagnosis of rupture.[248]

Epidural Anesthesia

On the basis of available information, there appears to be little reason to withhold epidural anesthesia in a VBAC-TOL.[4,195,206–208,220] The experience to date suggests that the employment of epidural anesthesia does not delay the diagnosis of uterine rupture and does not decrease the likelihood of a successful VBAC-TOL.[58,206] Although there was natural concern that the use of epidural anesthesia in the first and second stages of labor may obscure symptomatology (pain, tenderness) of an otherwise painful uterine rupture and delay its diagnosis, the safety of epidural anesthesia in patients with a prior low transverse cesarean incision is now well established. Regional anesthesia does not appear to obscure the symptoms associated with uterine rupture.[199,250–252] Furthermore, only a minority of patients experience pain and bleeding.[195,206] Even in the unanesthetized patient, uterine or scar tenderness, a sign of uterine rupture, occurs in only 25 percent of cases.[253]

The signs historically associated with uterine rupture (loss of fetal station, abrupt change in FHR or uterine activity, vaginal bleeding, or signs of intra-abdominal bleeding can be detected despite the activation of epidural anesthesia.[194,240] In balance, any theoretical risk is small compared with the benefits of use, which include pain relief and quick access to safe anesthesia should cesarean delivery be required. Uterine dehiscence/rupture is usually followed by a good outcome for both mother and fetus, especially if fetal monitoring is employed.[199,254] In fact, it may be the reassurance of adequate pain relief during labor that encourages the patient to consider a VBAC-TOL.

A more controversial concern is that epidural anesthesia, particularly when used with epinephrine, may increase the need for cesarean delivery or midforceps delivery by reducing uterine activity.[255,256] This could reduce the incentive for effective maternal pushing in the second stage of labor and limit spontaneous rotation of the fetal head normally anticipated with descent of the vertex into the maternal pelvis.[257,258] However, if this occurs, oxytocin may be administered or the epidural can be discontinued during the second stage of labor until there is satisfactory progress in descent.

Multiple Gestation and Abnormal Fetal Lie

The suitability of a VBAC-TOL in patients with a multiple gestation or breech presentation is not yet resolved.[58] Multiple gestation theoretically increases the risk for uterine rupture/dehiscence because it is associated with increased distension of the uterus. While there are no data demonstrating an increased risk for either problem in this setting, more information regarding VBAC in multiple gestation is required before this can be universally recommended. There are no data to contraindicate a VBAC trial in a frank breech presentation if the obstetrician is comfortable with selective vaginal breech delivery.

Known Vs. Unknown Prior Uterine Incision

A reasonable attempt should be made to document the type of the prior incision. Should the prior operative record be unavailable, the clinician is forced to make a judgment regarding the advisability of a TOL.[58] The patient can be reassured that approximately 99 percent of cesareans performed involve a low transverse incision. Only one percent of "unknown" cases will involve a vertical or classic incision. This seeming dilemma can also be minimized by further examination of the clinical history. If the cesarean was performed for a transverse lie, a placenta previa, or an extremely preterm fetus (either before or in early labor), concern for a low vertical or classic incision may be heightened; classic incisions continue to be used in certain geographic areas under such circumstances. In the absence of such a history, a low segment incision can generally be inferred, particularly if the prior cesarean was for failure to progress or nonreassuring FHR pattern of a degree to require cesarean delivery.

Prior Single-Layer Uterine Incision Closure

There is theoretical reason to suggest that a single-layer closure may actually result in a more functional closure of the lower uterine segment; a second layer of continuous sutures may decrease vascularization, possibly interfering with healing. Clinical experience with a single-layer closure is limited, and unfortunately most operative reports do not distinguish between a single- and a double-layer closure. Two small series have been reported. In the first, Pruett et al[210] reported on 57 TOLs involving a single-layer closure and found no complete uterine ruptures. Tucker et al[259] compared the outcomes of 149 women with a single-layer closure with 143 women with two-layer closure and found no complete uterine ruptures in any of the 292 trials of labor. Partial scar separation was detected in approximately 2 percent of patients in each group.

Routine Uterine Exploration

The relative merits of routine uterine exploration of the lower uterine segment following a successful VBAC is a subject of some controversy, an area where reasonable people may disagree reasonably. Advocates of routine exploration argue that failure to identify a defect does not allow for rational consideration of risk and benefits should a subsequent VBAC trial be considered. It is their belief that should routine exploration detect a "significant defect" that is connected with the peritoneal cavity, laparotomy should be performed either to repair the defect or to perform a hysterectomy. The logic supporting an approach not involving routine exploration is based on two observations. It is not clear how such information would modify future pregnancy management. If active bleeding is suspected, a laparotomy must be performed regardless of pelvic findings. Most agree it is not necessary to repair a small defect dehiscence unless there is significant bleeding or the patient develops significant symptomatology. If a small defect is detected and there are no supporting signs or symptoms, the patient can be followed expectantly with careful observation of vital signs and serial hematocrit determinations.[59,214] Second, should routine exploration occur in a patient with a "uterine window" (the lower uterine segment is intact, but very thin), there is the possibility that the exploration could disrupt an intact but thin lower segment. Although disruption of such a window would be unlikely to result in a significant problem, should abdominal exploration not be performed, one can easily predict an unnecessary sense of anxiety and anticipation by the patient in the ensuing hours until the clinician is confident that the patient will not develop signs or symptoms that would require abdominal exploration.

The ACOG VBAC Practice Pattern

Recently, the ACOG published its first of a series entitled *Practice Patterns* on management of VBAC-TOL candidates. The VBAC Practice Pattern is intended to serve as an acceptable clinical guideline to assist practitioners and patients in making decisions regarding appropriate care.[214] It does not offer an exclusive course of management; it does, however, provide a detailed analysis, including meta-analysis, of factors that should help to determine a reasonable course of action to be chosen after taking into consideration available resources, patient risk factors, and desires of the patient. The relative merits of available data were evaluated employing the U.S. Preventative Task Force Scoring System (Table 19-17) and the evidence (based on the highest level of data available) was graded (Table 19-18) according to the following categories: (A) "good" evidence; (B) fair evidence; and (C) insufficient evidence, but the recommendation can be made on other grounds.

Candidacy for VBAC-TOL

Most patients with a prior cesarean birth are candidates (Table 19-17, Evid. Qual. II-2 and II-3).[59,194,195,197] The only established contraindication is a prior classic

Table 19-17 Candidacy for VBAC-TOL: Clinical Conditions for Which There Are Insufficient Data To Make a Conclusive Recommendation

Condition	Evidence Quality
Prior vertical cesarean (low segment)	II-3
Multiple gestation	II-3
Breech	II-3
EFW >4,000 g (nondiabetic)	II-2
External version	II-2
Prior myomectomy	No data

(Adapted from ACOG,[214] with permission.)

incision (Evid. Qual. III).[214,241] Patients with more than one prior cesarean may be selectively offered a VBAC-TOL (Evid. Qual. II-2 and II-3).[194,220,260–262] Clinical conditions for which there are insufficient data to make a conclusive recommendation are noted in Table 19-17. Limited data (Evid. Qual. II-3) support a VBAC-TOL for patients with a prior low vertical incision, but are insufficient to justify a specific recommendation.[205,263] These statements are likely to be further clarified as additional experience is gained with these conditions.

Oxytocin Usage

Although oxytocin usage is reasonable, the indications for its use and its impact on VBAC success are unresolved.[194,196,264,265] Overall, the success rate associated with its use is decreased (Evid. Qual. II-2); however, the associated decrease in success rate may be a function of oxytocin usage for induction (58 percent) (Evid. Qual. II-2 and II-3); if use for augmentation is assessed separately, success (88 percent) appears to be increased.[265] Some believe that there is no difference in success rates between induction and augmentation (Evid. Qual. II-2 and II-3).[194]

Possible Components of a VBAC-TOL Management Plan

Table 19-19 summarizes the propriety of a number of possible interventions that may be considered in management of a VBAC candidate.[214] It is noteworthy that the issue of routine exploration of the uterus was not addressed.

Uterine Dehiscence and Uterine Rupture

Unfortunately, many studies do not define or differentiate between uterine rupture and dehiscence, and as a result most available data do not reliably specify the risks of rupture vs. dehiscence. Dehiscence has a distinctly different clinical connotation from "uterine rup-

Table 19-18 The ACOG VBAC Practice Pattern Summary

Clinical Issue	Conclusion from Trial	Evidence Level:Quality
Success rate	60%–80%	A:II-2
Benefits of VBAC-TOL	Outweigh risks	A:II-2
Candidates		
Prior LT C/S	Encourage trial	A:II-2
≥ 2 LT C/S	Do not discourage	B:II-2
Contraindications	Prior classic incision	C-III
Clinical problems		
Suspect macrosomia (in nondiabetic)	Not disqualified from VBAC trial	B:II-2
Multiple gestation	Insufficient data	C:II-2; II-3
Breech presentation	Insufficient data	C:II-2; II-3
Nonsubspecialty Hospital	Appropriate site	A:II-3

Abbreviation: LT C/S, low transverse uterine incision with no contraindications.
(Data from ACOG,[214] with permission.)

ture," which historically has been associated with prolonged oxytocin use in multiparous patients or following obstetric manipulations such as internal version or extraction.[266,267] Despite this limitation, the combined threat of uterine dehiscence and rupture during a TOL is not sufficiently high (when compared with the elective repeat cesarean group) to deny women the well-accepted advantages of vaginal delivery.

Definitions (Dehiscence Vs. Rupture)

Uterine incisional dehiscence is commonly used to describe the occult or asymptomatic scar separation or thinning that is occasionally observed at surgery in patients with a prior low transverse incision. A useful operational definition of *dehiscence* is a uterine scar separation that does not penetrate the uterine serosa, does not produce hemorrhage, and does not cause a major clinical problems.[4] Dehiscence is most often detected among women who have experienced a failed TOL. Some patients may develop dehiscence during labor that on occasion may lead to the need for repeat cesarean. The first indication may be observation of a scar defect, a separation, or only a near-transparent uterine "window" at the time of a cesarean procedure. Incomplete ascertainment of uterine dehiscence is likely in women having a successful VBAC-TOL.

Uterine rupture, on the other hand, is symptomatic and may have presenting signs that require acute intervention. Since dehiscence is uncommon (2 percent or less) and rupture is relatively rare (less than 1 percent), most reported studies provide limited statistical power to detect small changes in the risk of dehiscence or rupture among relevant prior cesarean birth compari-

Table 19-19 The ACOG VBAC Practice Pattern: Possible Components of Management Plan

	Indication	Evidence Level: Quality[a]
Latent/early active phase		
Activity: no restriction	Routine	—
Oxytocin induction	As needed	B:II-3
Prostaglandins	As needed (insufficient data)	C:II-2
Active phase of labor		
FHR every 15 minutes	Routine	NA:III
Epidural anesthesia	As needed (not contraindicated)	A:II-2
Oxytocin augmentation	As needed	B:II-3
Second stage of labor		
FHR every 5 minutes	Routine	NA:III
Epidural anesthesia	As needed	A:II-2
Third stage of labor		
Manual exploration for rupture/dehiscence	Not addressed	NA

[a]NA, not available.
(Data from ACOG,[214] with permission.)

son groups.[218] It is, however, unlikely that there is a major increased risk, since dehiscence or rupture is infrequent in all groups.

Combined Risk for Uterine Dehiscence and Rupture

Patients with a prior cesarean delivery who attempt a VBAC-TOL are at no higher risk, antepartum or early intrapartum, for uterine scar disruption (dehiscence and rupture) than are those having an elective repeat cesarean delivery.[4,212,248,268,269] A recent meta-analysis that assessed the relative impact of VBAC-TOL on the combined (did not differentiate) risk of true rupture and asymptomatic dehiscence detected no difference ($p = 0.5$) in the combined risk between patients undergoing a VBAC-TOL (1.8 percent of 2,771) and those undergoing an elective repeat cesarean procedure (1.9 percent of 3,611).[212] However, in hindsight the risk of dehiscence or rupture in the subset that had a failed TOL was 2.8 times that following an elective repeat cesarean ($p < 0.01$). The use of oxytocin did not ($p > 0.1$) influence the risk.

Risk for Dehiscence

Asymptomatic dehiscence is found incidentally in up to 2 percent of prior cesarean patients.[218] The rate is similar in patients with a prior low transverse and low vertical incision.[210] In a series of more than 2,600 patients, dehiscence was noted in only 1.5 percent of 1,465 patients having a successful VBAC-TOL versus 5.1 percent of 331 patients undergoing cesarean delivery for a failed VBAC-TOL. The difference may be partially a function of incomplete ascertainment in the VBAC success group. Nonetheless, these rates were not significantly different from the dehiscence rates in control patients who did not plan a TOL.[4] A recent study (Table 19-20) involving more than 17,000 patients presenting with a prior cesarean, 12,000 of whom under-

went a TOL, may give a more accurate assessment of the true prevalence of dehiscence; the status of the scar was routinely assessed visually or manually, and scar defects were categorized as either dehiscence or rupture. Among 17,332 women, there were 193 (1.1 percent) uterine dehiscences and 117 (0.7 percent) ruptures, for a combined risk in all women of 1.8 percent. The trial-related risk of uterine rupture was 0.5 percent with one prior cesarean, 1.3 percent with two prior cesareans, and 1.1 percent with three or more prior cesareans.[211]

Risk for Uterine Rupture

Two recent series, one involving more than 11,000 and one more than 17,000 women with prior cesarean births, provide data specific for risk of rupture.[195,197,211] In one series, the overall risk (Table 19-20) of rupture (117 cases) was 0.7 percent (0.5 percent for those not undergoing a trial and 0.7 percent for those attempting a trial) in all women presenting with a prior cesarean.[211] In the two other reports summarizing experience from Kaiser-Permanente Hospitals in California, the overall incidence of rupture during the past decade was 0.5 percent ([10 of 5733] in the interval between 1984 and 1988 and 0.8 percent [39 of 5,022] during the 1990–1992 interval).[195,197]

Prospective Risk Scoring for Uterine Dehiscence or Rupture

Unfortunately there are insufficient data for factors other than prior uterine incision type to provide a basis for prospectively identifying the specific patient who is likely to develop uterine rupture. Despite this limitation in prospective clinical care, VBAC-TOL continues to be viewed in a positive manner, largely because of the likelihood of VBAC success, the associated reduction in cesarean deliveries, and reduction in morbidity arising from cesarean delivery.

Table 19-20 Uterine Rupture Vs. Dehiscence among 17,332 Women with One or More Prior Cesarean Births

| | Trial of Labor | | | | Total | |
| | No | | Yes | | | |
	No.	Percent	No.	Percent	No	Percent
Total prior cesarean cases	4,615		12,707		17,322	
Uterine dehiscence	NA[a]		NA[a]		193	1.1
Uterine rupture	22	0.5[b]	95	0.7[c]	117	0.7
Combined risk	NA[a]	NA[a]	NA[a]	NA[a]	**310**	**1.8**

[a]Data not available.

[b]Thirteen non-TOL cases diagnosed at emergency cesarean for FHR indications immediately after admission; 9 discovered at nonemergent cesarean.

[c]One prior cesarean = 0.56%; two prior cesareans = 1.3%; three prior cesareans = 1.1%.

(Data from Leung et al.,[242] with permission.)

Table 19-21   Risk for Uterine Dehiscence (D) or Rupture (R)[a]

Potential Risk Factors	R or D Cases	Odds Ratio	Freq./1,000 Births	95% CI	Studies: (Trials) Comments:
Elective cesarean	69	**1.0**[c]	19	—	11: (N = 3,611)
All trials	50	0.8	18	0.6–1.2	11: (N = 2,771)
VBAC-TOL success[b]	19	0.7	12	0.4–1.2	11: (N = 1,613); $p = 0.3$
VBAC-TOL failure	19	**2.8**	33	**1.4–5.4**	11: (N = 584); $p < .01$
Oxytocin use	23	1.2	23	0.7–2.1	5: (N = 995); $p = 0.7$
Oxytocin not used	32	—	15	—	5: (N = 2,130)
Indications, recurrent	3	0.4	7	0.1–1.1	4: (N = 443)
Indications, nonrecurrent	16	—	26	—	4: (N = 607)
Uterine scar known	25	0.8	11	0.4–1.8	7: (N = 2,315)
Uterine scar unknown	26	—	22	—	7: (N = 1,181)
Low vertical scar	2	—	20	—	5: (N = 170)
Classic cesarean scar	3	—	120[(2)]	—	2: (N = 26)

[a]Meta-analysis of 11 VBAC studies with more than 6,000 VBAC-TOL (1982–1989).
[b]Relative risk versus elective repeat cesarean delivery.
[c]Standard error is 6% or 60 per 1,000 births.
(Data from Rosen et al.[212])

Certain risk factors, including exposure to "excessive amounts" (dose not defined) of oxytocin, dysfunctional labor, and a history of two or more prior cesarean procedures (Evid. Qual. II-2), have been "associated" with uterine rupture.[242] It is noteworthy that in one case-control study of 70 patients with prior cesarean delivery, the term *excessive amounts* of oxytocin was, in the authors' judgment, injudicious initiation (overutilization) of oxytocin during the latent phase of labor without delay following failure of uterine contractions to respond to hydration; the majority of such patients received oxytocin before they had confirmed dysfunctional labor (at 1 to 4 cm dilatation).[242] The frequency and relative impact of a number of possible clinical risk factors, using elective repeat cesarean delivery as a reference, is summarized from a meta-analysis of more than 6,000 VBAC-TOL in Table 19-21.

Maternal Morbidity and Mortality

Maternal Mortality

Because maternal mortality is a rare complication, estimation of relative risk between prior cesarean comparison groups is difficult. In one review of American studies involving 5,400 patients published prior to 1980, there were no maternal deaths arising from uterine rupture, even those involving classic uterine scars.[270] A 1985 summary report of 6,258 women undergoing a TOL over a span of more than 30 years (1950 to 1984) indicated that 5,356 (86 percent) were successful with no maternal mortality, comparing favorably with an expected mortality rate of approximately 1 death per 1,000 cesarean deliveries.[199] Even the increased use of

oxytocin during VBAC has not increased the risk of morbidity or mortality.[2,4,212,226] Other more recent studies support the prior observations of no significant increase in maternal mortality or morbidity.[195,212,261,271] A recent meta-analysis (Table 19-22), summarizing maternal morbidity (dehiscence, rupture, fever) and mortality data from 11,417 VBAC-TOL and 6,147 elective repeat cesareans reported in 31 VBAC studies between 1982 and 1989, confirms low maternal mortality and morbidity rates for both the elective repeat cesarean and TOL groups.[212] There were only two deaths among all TOLs and elective repeat cesarean deliveries. As one would expect, the observed maternal deaths derived from 10 studies were associated with postoperative surgical complications such as pulmonary embolus or following an obstetric complication such as placenta accreta.

Uterine Dehiscence and Rupture

Uterine rupture is the most significant potential risk. However, the risk (Evid. Qual. II-2 and II-3) is less than 1 percent.[194] In a meta-analysis of more than 6,000 deliveries in 11 studies (Table 19-22) there was little difference in the combined rates of dehiscence and rupture between the TOL and elective repeat groups ($p = 0.5$). Although there is the possibility of incomplete ascertainment of dehiscence in the VBAC success group, the authors indicated that an increase of 20 percent in the risk of dehiscence was extremely unlikely. Furthermore, the use of oxytocin did not influence the combined risk of dehiscence and rupture ($p = 0.7$); there was no difference between groups with known vs. unknown scars ($p = 0.95$) or recurrent vs. nonrecurrent

Table 19-22   Maternal Morbidity and Mortality: Meta-Analysis of 31 VBAC Studies Involving 11,417 VBAC-TOL and 6,147 Elective Repeat (ER) Cesarean Deliveries (1982–1989)

	ER Cesarean	All TOL	Failed TOL	Successful TOL	Studies: (Trials)
Prior cesarean cases	3,831	4,617	1,206	3,411	31: (11,417)
Febrile morbidity/1,000[a]	173	96	271	34	17: (N/A)
Odds ratio	**1.0**	0.5	2.0	0.2	
95% CI	—	0.5–0.6	1.7–2.5	0.2–0.2	
Dehiscence/rupture (%)[b]		2.0			11: (> 6,000)
No./1,000 births	19	18	33	12	
Odds ratio	**1.0**	0.8	**2.8**	0.7	
95% CI	—	0.6–1.2	**1.4–5.4**	.4–1.2	
p value		0.5	**<0.01**	0.3	
Maternal mortality/10,000	2.4[c]	2.8[d]			10: (7,830)

[a]Febrile morbidity: amniotic infection, urinary tract infection, endometritis, wound infection/1,000 births.
[b]Combined risk (i.e., data not subdivided).
[c]One death from placenta accreta after ER cesarean.
[d]One death from pulmonary embolus after failed TOL.
(Data from Rosen et al.[212])

indications ($p = 0.1$). Three ruptures (12 percent; SE = 6 percent) occurred among 26 women with a prior classic incision who underwent unplanned TOLs. Two dehiscences (2 percent) occurred in two patients with prior low vertical incisions, a rate similar to that among women with prior low transverse incision.

Maternal Febrile Morbidity

Mothers with successful TOLs (Table 19-22) have the lowest febrile morbidity, while those with a failed TOL (labor plus cesarean) have the highest ($p < .001$).[212] Because such a large percentage of women undergoing a trial of labor following a prior cesarean have a subsequent vaginal delivery, most women undergoing a VBAC-TOL will have less febrile morbidity and are thus likely to require a shorter hospital stay and fewer days lost from employment and family care responsibilities.

Perinatal Mortality and Morbidity Associated with VBAC Trials

Limitations of Available Data

The available perinatal data associated with VBAC-TOL particularly that accumulated prior to 1980, is often flawed. Early reports summarized trials in which monitoring was not consistent with current practice patterns. Some include fetal deaths unrelated to labor or rupture/dehiscence, including antenatal stillbirths, VLBW newborns, and congenital anomalies. Some, like the meta-analysis of Rosen et al,[212] specifically excluded antenatal deaths, newborns weighing less than 750 g, and those with congenital anomalies. Many reports addressing mortality risk associated with uterine

rupture do not provide the number of TOLs giving rise to these ruptures.

Perinatal Morbidity and Mortality

The perinatal risk for patients considering VBAC is no higher than that for patients delivering by elective repeat cesarean birth.[195,197,208,212,260,271] The overall uncorrected perinatal death rate arising from more than 5,500 women presenting with a prior cesarean birth (Table 19-23) was 1.4 percent (14 per 1,000) in a meta-analysis of 10 studies.[212] The uncorrected total perinatal death rate for the subset of women undergoing a TOL was 2.1 times that of women who underwent an elective repeat cesarean ($p < 0.001$); however, when unrelated causes, such as antepartum fetal death (prior to labor), very low birth weight (less than 750 g), and congenital anomalies incompatible with life, were excluded, this difference in perinatal mortality disappeared. The corrected perinatal mortality rate following a TOL was 3 per 1,000 following a trial and 4 per 1,000 following elective repeat cesarean (OR, 0.8; $p = 0.9$). When the perinatal outcome of "true" uterine ruptures was compared (only antepartum deaths excluded) with the outcome with no ruptures, there were 3 (13.6 percent) deaths after 22 ruptures and 28 (0.5 percent) after no rupture in 5,463 trials. Oxytocin use during a TOL did not influence perinatal mortality rate (OR, 1.5; 95 percent CI, 0.5-4.4).

Perinatal Morbidity and Mortality Arising from Dehiscence or Rupture

Intrapartum fetal deaths arising in the subset of patients who experience dehiscence of a low transverse uterine incision are uncommon. Although uterine rup-

Table 19-23 Composite Perinatal Morbidity (5-Minute Apgar Score ≤6) and Mortality Rates[a]

	Elective Repeat Cesarean (N = 2,929)	All TOL (N = 2,549)	Failed TOL (N = NA)	Successful TOL (N = NA)
Perinatal deaths				
No./1,000 births	4	3	—	—
Odds ratio	**1.0**[b]	0.8[c]	—	—
95% CI	—	0.3–2.1	—	—
5-Min Apgar score ≤6				
No./1,000 births	16	24	38	17
Odds ratio	**1.0**[b]	**2.1**[d]	**2.6**[d]	1.8[d]
95% CI	—	1.2–3.6	1.2–5.6	0.8–4.6
p value			0.03	0.2

[a]Ten studies involving more than 5,000 births for perinatal endpoint.
[b]Reference group.
[c]Excludes antenatal death, <750 g, congenital anomalies.
[d]Includes <750 g, congenital anomalies.
(Data from Rosen et al,[212] with permission.)

ture does occur infrequently, it is rarely catastrophic because of the availability of modern fetal monitoring, anesthesia, and obstetric support services.[272] Fetal death data associated with rupture of a vertical (includes classic) fundal incision are less reassuring. No maternal deaths were reported in an early review of published American VBAC studies involving 5,400 patients prior to 1980; fetal deaths were observed in 17 (56.7 percent) cases in which there was dehiscence or rupture of a fundal incision.[270] In contrast, lower uterine segment dehiscence occurred in 25 instances (0.46 percent), with no maternal deaths and only 3 (12 percent) fetal losses; the overall fetal mortality risk was 0.37 percent. Most fetal deaths arising from uterine dehiscence occurred either prior to admission or prior to the advent of widespread employment of continuous electronic FHR monitoring. More recent data suggest that maternal and perinatal outcomes are generally good following uterine rupture. However, uterine rupture under certain circumstances can have serious sequellae. Two reports have summarized the outcomes of 20 uterine ruptures. There were no maternal deaths in either reports, but only 14 of 20 (70 percent) had

good perinatal outcomes. There were four perinatal deaths and four cases with newborn neurologic sequellae. Unfortunately, three of the four perinatal deaths involved women who were laboring at home without fetal monitoring.[248,269] Table 19-24 summarizes the risks of uterine rupture and related perinatal deaths from a series of more than 17,000 women according to the number of prior cesarean births.

Oxytocin as a Risk Factor

Although the number of perinatal deaths reported in the three studies appropriate for meta-analysis is small, it appears that oxytocin use during a VBAC-TOL is unrelated to perinatal mortality rates (OR, 1.5; 95 percent CI; 0.5 to 4.4; $p = 0.2$)[212]

Newborn Depression as Morbidity Endpoint

The uncorrected (for less than 750 g, anomalies) OR for a 5-minute Apgar Score of 6 or less following a VBAC-TOL was 2.1 ($p < 0.001$) versus the elective repeat group. However, the absolute risk for the same

Table 19-24 VBAC-TOL: Risk of a Uterine Rupture and Related Perinatal Deaths per 1,000 Trials According to Number of Prior Cesarean Births

	No. of Prior Cesarean Births							
	One		Two		Three		Total	
	No.	Percent	No.	Percent	No.	Percent	No.	Percent
Uterine rupture:[a]	63	0.6	29	1.8[b]	3	1.2[b]	95	0.7
Related perinatal death (per 1,000 trials)	2	0.2	1	0.6	0	—	3	0.2

[a]In women undergoing a trial of labor.
[b]Incidence of uterine rupture with two or more prior cesarean births was 1.7%, significantly greater than with one prior cesarean (OR, 3.06; 95% CI, 1.95–4.79; p <0.001).
(Data from Miller et al,[211] with permission.)

score is low in both groups (2 percent in VBAC-TOL vs. 1.6 percent in the elective repeat group). This score was also observed 2.1 times more often in newborns born alive after all TOLs than in newborns born following an elective repeat cesarean ($p < 0.001$); unfortunately, these outcome data are flawed since they include newborns weighing less than 750 grams and those with serious congenital anomalies.[212]

In retrospect, should there be a failed TOL, the risk for a low Apgar score is 2.6 times that following an elective repeat cesarean ($p = 0.03$). However, should the TOL succeed, there is no greater risk than after a repeat cesarean ($p = 0.2$). Use of oxytocin does not increase risk (OR, 1.6; 95 percent CI, 0.8 to 3.2; $p = 0.2$).

Interpretation of these Apgar score data as a measure of morbidity is complicated by the tendency of clinicians to deliver infants unlikely to survive via the vaginal route. Inclusion of such cases may unfavorably bias outcome measures for the vaginal route (i.e., if such cases are excluded from analysis, the outcomes would likely be more similar). Supporting this view is the observation of Meyers and Gleicher,[176] who found no difference in Apgar scores as the VBAC rate at their hospital increased from 45 to 86 percent.

Documenting the Medical Record

Unknown Uterine Incision

Although it is highly likely that a prior uterine incision of unknown type involved the lower uterine segment, the best strategy is to make a reasonable effort to document the nature of the prior incision.[58] The Medical Records Office of the prior hospital in many cases can provide the necessary information. In those instances when the clinician is unable to determine the nature of the prior incision, the inability per se should not serve as a contraindication to a TOL.

The Operative Report

A description of the extent of a vertical uterine incision (low vertical vs. classic) in the cesarean operative report can be important in deliberations regarding the decision to pursue a VBAC-TOL in future pregnancies.

Timing of Elective Repeat Cesarean Delivery

Should the patient refuse a VBAC-TOL or have a recurring indication for cesarean delivery, the clinician has four possible options to determine when elective cesarean delivery should occur. According to the ACOG, fetal maturity may be assumed and amniocentesis need not be performed if the criteria of one of the four op-

Table 19-25 Fetal Maturity Assessment Prior to Elective Repeat Cesarean Delivery

Option 1 (FHR)		One or more of the following is present for the stated duration: For 20 weeks: FHR by nonelectronic fetoscope For 30 weeks: FHR by Doppler
Option 2 (HCG)		For 36 weeks: positive serum or urine pregnancy test
Option 3[a] (Ultrasound)		At 6–12 week's gestation: Ultrasound crown–rump length supports gestational age of ≥39 weeks
Option 4[a] (Ultrasound)		At 12–20 weeks multiple ultrasound measures confirm gestational age of ≥39 weeks as determined by clinical history and physical examination
Option 5		Await spontaneous onset of labor
Option 6		Fetal pulmonary maturity documented by amniotic fluid surfactant assessment

Adapted from: ACOG Committee Opinion, Number 98, September 1991[273]
[a]Does not preclude use of menstrual age with agreement within 7 days (option 3) or 10 days (option 4).
(Data from ACOG,[273] with permission.)

tions in Table 19-25 are met.[237,273] The criteria do not preclude use of menstrual dating, particularly if one of the four confirm menstrual dates in a patient with normal menstrual cycles and no immediately recent use of oral contraceptives. Ultrasound is considered confirmatory if there is agreement between menstrual–gestational age and crown–rump age at 6 to 12 weeks or by the average gestational age determined by multiple measurements at 12 to 20 weeks within 1 week and within 10 days, respectively.

Desire for Permanent Sterilization as an Indication for Repeat Cesarean

Approximately 42 percent of patients refuse the VBAC option.[217] The relatively high refusal rate may decline as physicians and patients become more comfortable with the concept. The decision to attempt a VBAC-TOL is often clouded by other clinical factors such as the need for a postpartum tubal ligation. Some would argue that a patient's desire for a permanent sterilization is not an appropriate indication for a repeat cesarean procedure. In most cases such a view is appropriate; the morbidity of vaginal delivery and subsequent postpartum tubal ligation is less than that of a repeat cesarean. In one study, 13 percent of successful VBAC patients had a postpartum tubal ligation with only minor prolongation of their hospital stay.[274]

Many patients, however, will find such an argument unattractive, particularly if the prior cesarean for dystocia was performed after a long labor including ex-

Table 19-26 Most Common Indications for Repeat Cesarean Delivery Without Labor in 17,322 Women with Prior Cesareans

Indication	Occurrence (%)
Elective repeat	47[a]
Malpresentation	20
FHR indication	14
Macrosomia	5
Placenta previa	3
Multiple gestation	2

[a]Twenty-one percent in women with 1 prior cesarean delivery; 56 percent in women with two prior cesarean deliveries; 68 percent in women with ≥3 prior cesarean deliveries. (Data from Miller et al,[211] with permission.)

tended pushing. Unfortunately ligation may not be feasible immediately postpartum following a successful VBAC. Other reasons for refusal are fear of "another long labor" resulting in a cesarean; concern about the likely need for one anesthesia for the cesarean/vaginal delivery and another for the tubal ligation; a preference not to reinitiate contraception; and concern that they cannot easily take time away from family or professional activities, even for an outpatient tubal ligation. More predictable access to tubal ligation immediately following a successful VBAC could potentially blunt the influence of many of the above. This access will vary according to hospital resources, particularly at night and on weekends.

Indication for Repeat Cesarean Delivery

Nearly two-thirds of all repeat cesarean procedures are performed without a trial of labor. The most common indications are listed in Table 19-26.[211]

Informed Consent

Informed Consent Is a Process

Informed consent should be considered a process that includes sharing of information and discussion of the choices reflected in the informed consent document.[275] Ordinarily, effective informed consent requires active participation by both the physician and the patient. It is the physician's responsibility to make sure that the patient is well informed; has under ordinary circumstances reasonable time to contemplate the information provided; and is encouraged to ask questions when necessary. It is the patient's responsibility to provide accurate and complete information and if matters are unclear to pose questions.[276]

The patient and her partner should participate in the decision-making process leading to cesarean delivery. There is considerable variation in both the style and substance of obtaining informed consent for cesarean birth. Although there is certainly merit to nondirected counseling, it should be somewhat obvious that it is difficult to transmit a minimum of 8 years of training and a number of years of clinical experience into a 5- to 10-minute discussion for informed consent, particularly when stress and emotions are high. The provision of informed consent involves walking a fine line; it is part of the so-called "art" of medicine. Much of the information provided will depend on whether the procedure is scheduled or unplanned. A key feature in the process is physician–patient rapport and associated patient trust of the managing physician. Current practice patterns often dictate that the patient receive care from several members of a large group practice, in which case rapport is not always optimal. Some patients want a detailed explanation, while others desire whatever the doctor advises. Sadly, much of what is discussed is often not understood or forgotten when stress is high. Provision of too much information may overwhelm the patient. On the other hand, provision of inadequate or unbalanced information may result in a decision that the patient later regrets.

Content Disclosure Guidelines

There may be variation from state to state regarding the degree of disclosure required for a valid surgical consent (i.e., what is adequate information?). Most states use the "professional" or "reasonable physician standard," while others employ the "materiality" or "patient viewpoint standard."

"Professional" Approach

The "professional" approach to consent is determined by what is customary practice in the medical community. Less information is provided, that is, extremely remote risk even with serious consequences may not necessarily be disclosed. In the case of an anticipated cesarean delivery when time is not an issue, the patient would be informed about the commonly encountered risks of any operative procedure, namely, infection and hemorrhage, as well as major complications associated with anesthesia. Injury to nearby organs, including bladder and ureters, at the time of cesarean delivery is a rare complication that is not ordinarily discussed. Should vaginal delivery be an acceptable alternative, the patient may benefit from knowledge regarding the relative risks and benefits of that approach.

Should primary cesarean delivery be considered for conditions such as a frank breech presentation, much of the focus of the discussion commonly may relate to the potential and theoretical fetal advantages, if any, of cesarean birth. Some mention of the severalfold increase in maternal morbidity and mortality associated with a cesarean delivery and its complications is also appropriate.

The patient should not be asked, "Do you want to do everything possible for your baby?" There are as yet few data to suggest that a cesarean birth, except in the presence of selective indications, has a beneficial effect with regard to survival and long-term outcome. Should cesarean delivery be considered for a VLBW fetus, it may be advantageous to review the anticipated weight and gestational age specific rate of intact survival by either route. If the procedure would not follow labor, discussion of the potentially higher risk of respiratory distress with an elective cesarean birth may be appropriate.

Contingencies can also be important. Should the physician anticipate a repeat cesarean procedure in a patient with a current diagnosis of anterior placenta previa, informed consent may include some discussion regarding the potential need for hysterectomy for placenta accreta, as well as the potential need for transfusion and its associated risks (see Ch. 17). When an elective cesarean delivery likely to require blood replacement is anticipated, the option of autologous transfusion is a possible topic for discussion.

Patient Viewpoint Approach

There may be an evolution to a new conceptual framework, the "materiality" or "patient viewpoint standard." Under the "materiality" or "patient viewpoint standard," even if the risk of a procedure is extremely remote, but has serious consequences, the risk would be disclosed (i.e., the amount of information provided should be based on what a "reasonable person in the patient's position" would "want to know in similar circumstances." This approach would then be based on what a patient would "need to know" to make a decision rather than on professional perception of what a patient "should know." The problem with such an approach is that the "needs" and "the reasonable patient" have not been objectively defined; clearly there are many patients who, in foresight, are happy to rely on the physician's advice, but, in hindsight, would want to know virtually everything. Clearly there are degrees of ability of the physician to communicate and of the patient to comprehend and remember. Such an approach would require physicians to discard their experience regarding what patients are capable of comprehending under similar circumstances or even what the experienced physician, who has an on-going relation with the patient, believes the patient or most patients would like to know or understand.

Possible Components of Consent

Under either approach, the physician should not guarantee or even suggest a guarantee of outcome. To obtain fully informed consent the physician should explain the following:

1. The diagnosis and nature of the condition calling for the intervention
2. The nature and the purpose of the treatment/procedure recommended
3. The material risks and potential complications associated with the recommended treatment/procedure
4. Feasible alternative treatments/procedure, including the option of taking no action
5. Description of material risks and potential complications associated with the alternatives
6. A relative probability of success for the treatment of procedure in understandable terms

Patient Refusal of Treatment/Procedure

On occasion, a patient may refuse a cesarean delivery that is perceived by the physician to be necessary to save either her life or that of the fetus; in most cases there are either religious or ethical considerations. Although there is no "correct" way to manage such a circumstance, the record should reflect the fact that the patient was informed of the benefits anticipated and that the patient refused the procedure. The ACOG Committee on Ethics has released a Committee Opinion that addresses such a situation: "Every reasonable effort should be made to protect the fetus, but the pregnant woman's autonomy should be respected. . . . The role of the obstetrician should be one of an informed educator and counselor, weighing the risks and benefits to both patients, as well as realizing that tests, judgements, and decisions are fallible. Consultation with others, including an Institutional Ethics Committee, should be sought when appropriate, to aid the patient and obstetrician in making decisions. The use of the courts to resolve these conflicts is almost never warranted."[277]

Is Informed Consent a Prerequisite for VBAC-TOL?

The need for specific consent from a patient attempting VBAC seems somewhat superfluous if one acknowledges that the inherent risks of a VBAC are less than or equal to those of an attempted vaginal delivery in other patients. Because likelihood of a successful VBAC is only minimally dependent on the indication for the prior cesarean delivery, the physician should present the chances of success in a positive manner. Obviously written consent can be obtained; however, an equally reasonable approach would be to indicate in the patient's prenatal record that the patient has been informed that labor following a prior cesarean delivery is an acceptable alternative to routine repeat cesarean delivery with only minor attendant risks that are not significantly greater than those of a repeat cesarean procedure.

Patient Refusal of VBAC-TOL

Despite increasingly widespread acknowledgement that VBAC-TOL is safe and has a high successful rate, only 40 to 50 percent of eligible candidates are reported to request an elective repeat procedure.[215,216] A desire to avoid labor-related pain and the convenience of a scheduled elective repeat cesarean are the most common reasons.[278] A woman should not be coerced to undergo a VBAC-TOL. Certain social, geographic, and past obstetric complications may justify the patient's electing to have a repeat cesarean birth.[272] The ACOG has recently stated that "Actions or policies that coerce patients to undergo either a (VBACV) trial of labor or a repeat cesarean procedure interfere with patient autonomy and the physician–patient relationship and undermine informed consent. The mode of delivery ultimately should be based on the clinical circumstances and on the patient's choice after appropriate counseling.[59]

Patient Factors in Consent Process

Factors that influence patient decision-making, including emotional issues, are not generally subject to statistical analysis. Nonetheless, it is apparent that a woman's view of her prior pregnancy is likely to influence future decisions. The decision to accept a VBAC-TOL may be more difficult for the mother who delivers by cesarean than for the one who delivers vaginally.[279] Some limited data on this issue are provided by Nielsen et al,[280] who compared indications for cesarean delivery in Sweden for 1983 (91,000 deliveries) and 1989 (115,000 deliveries). Psychological indications and poor "obstetric history," for which no direct medical or obstetric intervention existed, was employed as a distinct indication; this indication increased significantly from 0.57 percent in 1983 to 1.45 percent ($p < 0.001$) of all deliveries in 1989. Repeat cesarean deliveries (often at the request of a woman after problems with a prior extended or difficult labor) were included in this group since previous cesarean delivery is not considered to be an indication for cesarean delivery in Sweden. Of interest, the total cesarean rate decreased from 12.3 percent (1983) to 11.6 percent (1990) and yet perinatal mortality was halved from 14.2 to 6.3 per 1,000 births and 1-minute Apgar scores less than 4 or 5-minute scores less than 7 decreased from 20 to 14 per 1,000 live births.

Peripartum Hysterectomy

Introduction

Peripartum or obstetric hysterectomy is the surgical removal of the uterus at the time of a planned or unplanned cesarean delivery or in the immediate postpartum period. Peripartum hysterectomies can be classified as total, subtotal, or, occasionally, as radical (with or without node dissection and/or adnexectomy) or alternatively as "unplanned" (emergency), "planned" (scheduled), or "elective" (sterilization being the only indication). Such distinctions are critical when comparing the relative benefits and operative risks of hysterectomy with alternative management options.

Historically, the first cesarean hysterectomy was performed by H.R. Storer, in Boston, in a patient who expired the third postpartum day[281] Eduardo Porro (1876) performed the first procedure on a patient who survived it.[8] In that case, subtotal hysterectomy (amputation of the uterine fundus following hysterotomy with subsequent marsupilization of the stump to the anterior abdominal wall) was performed to increase the chance of survival following cesarean delivery[282] Twenty-five percent of cesarean deliveries were performed as Porro cesarean hysterectomies as late as 1922.[283]

Incidence

Two reports from the same institution over a 10-year span summarize a possible trend of increasing incidence of hysterectomy following cesarean delivery. The rate following cesarean delivery increased from 7.0 (1989) to 8.3 (1993) per 1,000 and continues to be dramatically higher than the rate following vaginal delivery (0.2/1,000 births in 1984 and 0.09/1,000 in 1993)[120,284] The increased rate following cesarean births may reflect the change in prevalence of prior cesarean deliveries. In the early series, only 44 percent of patients requiring hysterectomy had a prior cesarean delivery, whereas 67 percent had a prior cesarean in the more recent cases from 1985 to 1990.

Unplanned Emergency Indications

Most peripartum hysterectomies are unplanned (Table 19-27) and follow cesarean delivery.[120] Most are performed after more conservatives efforts to control bleeding have been unsuccessful. Although hysterectomy may be the ultimate remedy for control of obstetric hemorrhage, conservative measures remain the primary approach; hysterectomy is reserved for circumstances in which conservative measures either fail or are not applicable as would often be the case with abnormal placentation.[284]

Risk Factors for Emergency Hysterectomy

Sixty percent of emergency hysterectomies performed at Harvard were performed in women with a history of a prior cesarean delivery.[285] Prior cesarean delivery increases the risk for subsequent placenta previa, pla-

Table 19-27 Indications for Unplanned Peripartum Hysterectomy

Indication	Clark et al[121] (1978–82)		Stanco et al[284] (1985–90)		Zelop et al[285] (1983–91)	
	No.	Percent	No.	Percent	No.	Percent
Placenta accreta	21	30	55	45	75	64[a]
Placenta percreta	—		6	5	—	
Uterine atony	30	43	25	20	25	21
Bleeding	—		19	16	—	
Uterine rupture	9	13	14	11	10	9
Fibroids with bleeding	3	4	3	2	2	2
Uterine infection	—		1	1	3	3
Scar extension/other	7	10	—		2	2
Total	70	100	123	100[b]	117	101

[a]"Abnormal placentation."

[b]82 (67%) had at least one prior cesarean.

centa accreta, and symptomatic uterine rupture, each of which increases the likelihood of need for an emergency hysterectomy.[284,242,285] The adverse impact of placenta previa as a risk factor for unplanned hysterectomy in patients with a prior cesarean is established.[86,286]

The importance of both previa and prior cesarean delivery as risk factors is supported by several reports from the same institution. In the first of three reports from Southern California, a strong association (25 to 30 percent) between placenta accreta and a preexisting cervical uterine scar was reported.[85] The linkage was even greater in the subset who required hysterectomy. In the second of the series, 52 percent of hysterectomies performed for placenta accreta were associated with a previous cesarean scar.[120] In the third report, 69 percent of 58 patients with placenta previa had one or more prior cesarean births. In that series peripartum hysterectomy followed cesarean delivery in 94 percent of cases; 67 percent had a prior cesarean delivery, 47 percent had a placenta previa, and 50 percent had an accreta or percreta.[284] In another series from Massachusetts, the risk of peripartum hysterectomy in association with placenta previa increases from 7 per 1,000 deliveries in nulliparous women to 1 in 4 deliveries in women with a history of 4 or more prior births ($p < 0.001$).[285]

Placenta Accreta/Percreta

Placenta accreta/percreta with or without previa is now the most common indication for peripartum hysterectomy.[242,284,285]

Until recently, the most common indication for peripartum hysterectomy had been uterine atony. The introduction of prostaglandin $F_{2\alpha}$ as a therapeutic intervention has reduced the relative impact of uterine atony as an indication for hysterectomy. Furthermore,

hysterectomy is seldom performed solely for a Couvelarie uterus in the absence of other more pressing complications or for asymptomatic cesarean scar dehiscence. The shift to abnormal placentation as the most common indication for hysterectomy also reflects the dramatic increase in cesarean deliveries, including repeat cesarean procedures.[85] The shift in relative importance is illustrated (Table 19-27) by two reports from Southern California.[121,284] In the first report, uterine atony was the most common indication; however, in the more recent series from the same institution, Stanco et al[284] reported that abnormal implantation of the placenta had assumed greater relative importance as the most common indication. In a recent series from Harvard, 64 percent of 117 cases were based on this indication; uterine atony was the operative indication in only 21 percent of cases.[285]

Uterine Dehiscence and Rupture

Uterine rupture requiring hysterectomy is reported to occur in 0.2 percent (1 in 555) to 0.8 percent (1 in 122) of VBAC-TOL.[242,284]

In one series, 14 (11 percent) of 123 peripartum hysterectomies (Table 19-27) were performed for uterine rupture in patients undergoing a VBAC TOL, the institutional incidence in such patients being 0.18 percent.[284] These data complement a report from the same institution in which uterine rupture occurred in 0.8 percent of 7,598 patients with a prior cesarean delivery undergoing a TOL.[207]

In early years, hysterectomy for asymptomatic uterine dehiscence was accepted practice. However, this is no longer the case. Even should symptomatic rupture occur, hysterectomy is not always necessary, particularly if the patient has a desire for future fertility and the rupture site is in a favorable location where repair is feasible. The clinician may simply repair the defect, or, should dehiscence be discovered at routine exploration following vaginal delivery, it may be followed by expectant observation as detailed above.

Extension of Uterine Incision

Extension of a uterine incision into the uterine vessels is an uncommon indication for hysterectomy. However, such extensions can pose a therapeutic dilemma. Should hemorrhage be significant, consideration should be given to the alternative of hypogastric or uterine artery ligation (as opposed to hysterectomy), depending on the patient's parity and desire for future pregnancy. Ligation of the anterior division of one or both hypogastric or internal iliac arteries may decrease the arterial pulse pressure up to 85 percent distal to the point of the ligation, thus allowing clot formation.[287] Alternatively, it is possible to ligate the uterine arteries.[288] In some cases it may be advisable to attempt to identify the ureter, which may be in close proximity, by either palpatation or direct visualization before ligating the uterine vessels.[111]

Elective Procedures

Permanent sterilization combined with elimination of potential long-term risks for later uterine pathology were in the 1950s and 1960s, an era of religious prohibitions when women did not have a wide range of contraceptive options, to be an acceptable indication for cesarean hysterectomy. Elective procedures were commonly based on a need for sterilization.[113,114] Justification for hysterectomy was based on an observed need for hysterectomy in 20 percent of patients within a mean interval of 6.3 years from the most recent cesarean delivery.[289] Several reports supported the safety of the planned/elective hysterectomy subset based on a low morbidity rate (Table 19-28).[290,291] Despite the relative safety of this subset, the incidence of elective cesarean hysterectomy has fallen dramatically in recent years. As other contraceptive options became available, authors such as Brenner et al[292] suggested that if hysterectomy is performed primarily for sterilization, the morbidity of a scheduled procedure will outweigh its benefits.[292]

Planned/Nonemergency Cesarean Hysterectomy

Some have included "elective" procedures in this category; however, it is not appropriate to consider planned procedures as "elective"—a term that would imply that there is no indication. In most cases, a planned hysterectomy is performed when a woman requiring cesarean delivery also has a gynecologic problem that is appropriately managed by hysterectomy. Large or symptomatic uterine leiomyomas and cervical intraepithelial neoplasia are the most common indications. Other common indications are benign gynecologic conditions, occasional pelvic malignancy, and prior uterine scars.[293] Several investigators have reported their experience with a scheduled procedure for women referred for surgical cancer and early cervical neoplasia complicating pregnancy.[294,295] Because invasive disease can be excluded by colposcopy during pregnancy, some prefer vaginal delivery after carcinoma in situ of the cervix is confirmed as the most serious lesion. However, in some cases the patient may prefer a single procedure or be noncompliant, in which case cesarean hysterectomy is a reasonable option. An occasional cesarean

Table 19-28. Planned Hysterectomy Morbidity

	Ward and Smith[289] (1953–64)		McNulty[293] (1972–82)		Yancey et al[299] (1979–90)	
	No.	Percent	No.	Percent	No.	Percent
No. of cases	254		80		43	
Operative time	90–120[a]		—		123 ± 36[b]	
Patients transfused	195	77[c]	15	19	17	40[d]
Pelvic hematoma	6	2	4	5	2	5
Febrile morbidity	—		5	6	—	
Pelvic cellulitis	9	4			4	9
Pyelitis	2	1	—		—	
Cystotomy	8	3	4	5	1	2
Ureteral injury	0		0		0	

[a]Minutes skin to skin.
[b]Mean ± standard deviation.
[c]126/195 received 1 unit; indication = Hct <35%.
[d]7/17 received 1 unit transfusions.

hysterectomy may be performed for microinvasive disease. Rarely, invasive cancer of the cervix may be treated with a primary cesarean delivery followed by radical hysterectomy with pelvic lymphadnectomy.[296,297]

Total Vs. Subtotal Hysterectomy

The relative merits of subtotal versus total peripartum hysterectomy will vary according to whether the procedure is a planned or unplanned one. Should the procedure be planned, total hysterectomy is most commonly performed; contrarily if the procedure is unplanned a larger fraction will be subtotal. Some have viewed subtotal hysterectomy as a quicker procedure, one to be employed particularly when the patient is unstable, based on a hypothesis that subtotal hysterectomy has less blood loss and requires less operative time. A recent publication does not support this hypothesis; the authors were unable to detect a significant difference between total and subtotal procedures with respect to blood loss, operating time, or length of hospital stay.[121] Clark et al[121] did suggest the absence of a difference may reflect a selection bias, reflecting the indication and its management prior to the decision to procede to hysterectomy. This possible bias is most evident should the indication be uterine atony or placenta accreta.

Uterine Atony

In one series a subtotal procedure was performed in 77 percent of 30 cases associated with uterine atony.[121] Uterine atony of a degree of severity to require hysterectomy is commonly associated with amnionitis, oxytocin augmentation, preoperative magnesium sulfate infusion, increased fetal weight, and cesarean delivery for labor arrest; however, 23 percent of patients undergoing a hysterectomy for atony have no identifiable risk factors.[121] Not surprisingly, both blood loss and operating time may be increased in patients undergoing hysterectomy for uterine atony.[121] The surgeon, when faced with uterine atony, commonly follows a predetermined series of pharmacologic interventions (oxytocin, methergine, and prostaglandin $F_{2\alpha}$ [Hemabate, Upjohn Co., Kalamazoo, MI]), as well as other maneuvers including currettage and hypogastric artery ligation in an effort to control bleeding and maintain fertility. Such procedures may be effective in controlling hemorrhage; however, if control is not achieved, blood loss experienced prior to the time the procedure is initiated would tend to be greater and the time spent on conservative measures is reflected in a longer operative time, both commonly attributed to the unplanned hysterectomy.

Placenta Accreta/Percreta

In contrast to atony as an indicator, only 23 percent of 21 hysterectomies performed for placenta accreta were of the subtotal variety.[121] Since placenta is less often amenable to conservative management, the transition to a decision for hysterectomy may be somewhat more rapid. Only rarely can accreta be managed by curetting or oversewing the placenta bed. The plantation site involvement is usually too extensive to respond to treatment other than hysterectomy, particularly when it is associated with previa. Subtotal hysterectomy is also less likely to be effective should placentation be in the lower uterine segment, presumably because blood flow via the cervical branch of the uterine artery remains uncontrolled.

Maternal Morbidity and Mortality

It is important to distinguish those procedures performed primarily for gynecologic indications plus or minus sterilization from those performed for obstetric problems requiring emergency intervention, most commonly hemorrhage. Maternal morbidity (Table 19-28) and mortality (Table 19-29) associated with peripartum hysterectomy is not simply the product of the procedure itself. Maternal mortality and morbidity will in large part depend on whether (1) the procedure is a planned/scheduled or an unplanned/emergency procedure, (2) the patient was previously in labor and had significant risk factors for infection, or (3) the patient had coincidental pregnancy-related complications. Unplanned hysterectomies have a greater risk for maternal mortality than planned procedures, since they are commonly performed in response to life-threatening hemorrhage with independent morbidity and mortality consequences. Nonetheless, the risk is very low for both types, and as a result single institution reports seldom report mortality. Only one death (Table 19-28) was reported in three studies (series of 123 and 70 emergency cases from California[121,284] and 117 emergency procedures from Massachusetts[285] the combined mortality rate for the three series is 3.2 per 100,000 (1 in 310).

Unfortunately, population-based mortality data specific for indication/procedure type are not available. However, Wingo et al[298] assessed data collected by the Commission on Professional and Hospital Activities (1979 and 1980) to determine risk factors for 477 deaths among more than 317,000 women having abdominal hysterectomies. Not surprisingly, mortality rates for hysterectomy, when standardized for age and race, were higher when the procedure was associated with pregnancy or cancer than if not associated with these conditions. Although only 8 percent of all hysterectomies performed are associated with pregnancy or cancer, they account for approximately 61 percent of

Table 19-29 Unplanned Hysterectomy Morbidity and Mortality

	Clark et al[121] (1978–82)		Stanco et al[284] (1985–90)		Zelop et al[285] (1983–91)	
	No.	Percent	No.	Percent	No.	Percent
Procedures	70		123		117	
Subtotal	38	54	65	53	25	21
Operative time (Mean)	3.1 hr		NA		3.0[a]	
Blood loss (Mean)	3,575 ml		3,000 ml		3,000 cc[a]	
Hemorrhagic					102	87
Transfused patients	67	96	102	83	102	87
Reexplored	—				3	1
Infect Morbidity					58	50
Febrile	35	50	NA		39	33
UTI			NA		7	6
Wound	8	12	11	9	4	6
Urologic injury	3	4	4	3	10	9
Cystotomy		0	12[b]		9	8
Ureteral	3	4	—		3	3
Maternal death	1[d]	1[c]	0		0	

[a]Median value.

[b]50% ≥3,000 cc and 50% <3,000 cc.

[c]Intentional cystotomies for ureteral stent passage.

[d]Cardiac arrest secondary to amniotic fluid embolus.

(Data from Clark et al,[121] Stanco et al,[284] and Zelop et al.[285])

all deaths. The authors estimated the minimum and maximum standardized mortality rates for pregnancy-related abdominal hysterectomy to be 22.8 and 32.0 per 10,000 procedures, respectively.[298] Although not strictly applicable, the minimum and maximum rate estimates should provide some insight into rates to be associated with planned and unplanned procedures, respectively.

Operative Technique

Should the procedure be an emergency one in which there has been preexisting and ongoing rapid blood loss, it may be necessary to compress the aorta manually until the operative field can be suctioned sufficiently to allow identification and clamping of bleeding points. In some cases bilateral internal iliac, anterior hypogastric, or uterine artery ligation may be required to reduce arterial bleeding from the uterine, vesicle, and pudendal arteries. The operative technique for peripartum hysterectomy employs the general principles applicable to abdominal hysterectomy in the nongravid state. In initiating the surgical procedure, the surgeon should direct attention to (1) early adequate displacement of the bladder from the lower uterine segment and cervix, (2) use of overlapping sutures for successive vascular pedicles, (3) selective as opposed to mass placement of clamps and sutures to control bleeders, (4) periodic inspection of the bladder for an inadvertent cystotomy, (5) possible localization of the ureter should a lateral extension/laceration of the incision be the indication for the procedure, and (6) avoidance of excessive removal of vaginal length, particularly when the cervix is completely effaced.

There is considerable variation in operative technique. Variation involves the use of two versus three clamps for pedicles above the cardinal ligament, use of single versus double ligation of vascular pedicles, the relative desirability for skeletonization of vessels in the broad ligament, and the relative need for an additional step to separate and individually ligate the uterosacral ligaments.

Although the uterine vessels are considerably larger in the pregnant than in the nonpregnant state, tissue planes are more easily developed. Blood loss from a peripartum procedure is greater than (500 to 1,000 cc) that associated with hysterectomy in the nongravid patient, particularly if it is an unplanned one. The altered hemodynamics of normal pregnancy as well as associated obstetric problems are largely responsible. The uterus is enlarged and highly vascular. The associated collateral circulation results in prominence of vessels that would be of little concern in the nonpregnant state. It is for this reason that some surgeons employ a three-clamp rather than a two-clamp technique for pedicle development above the cardinal ligaments. In the case of the three-clamp technique the incision is made between a single medial clamp (to reduce the likelihood of retrograde blood loss from the medial pedicle) and two lateral clamps (to prevent clamp slippage from the lateral pedicle).

Planned Hysterectomy Considerations

Should the hysterectomy be a planned one, the cesarean procedure is performed in the usual manner except that the initial peritoneal/vesicle uterine fold incision may be extended more laterally to the round ligaments. There is also advantage to early mobilization and separation of the bladder from the underlying lower segment in the midline with gentle blunt dissection to a point approximately 1 to 2 cm below the cervical vaginal junction and to some extent laterally. On occasion the bladder may be adherent, requiring sharp dissection with down-turned scissors. This will result in displacement of the bladder and ureters caudad or inferiorly. There is also some advantage in employment of a low vertical incision, particularly if the lower segment is not completely developed, to reduce the possibility of extension into the broad ligament and provide a site for placement of the surgeon's finger in the apex of the incision to facilitate later traction and manipulation of the uterus.

Procedure

Upon completion of the cesarean delivery, the placenta may be delivered and the lower uterine incision quickly reapproximated, or alternatively the surgeon may simply proceed rapidly to gain control of the vascular supply of the uterus while the placenta spontaneously separates. Polyglycolic acid or chromic catgut suture (0 or 1 gauge) may be used throughout the procedure.

Placement of an O'Conner-O'Sullivan retractor or perhaps a large Balfour retractor in the abdominal wall may be helpful, particularly should the patient be obese or exposure difficult. The uterine fundus is then delivered through the incision, and constant traction is maintained on the uterus to maximize pedicle exposure, facilitate development of tissue planes, and stretch the uterine veins, thereby narrowing their lumen and reducing venous blood loss. If a vertical uterine incision has been made, it is often convenient for the assistant to hook an index finger in the upper extreme of the uterine incision to manipulate the fundus and to expose the operative site. If the placenta is still in place, it can be removed. If bleeding of the uterine incision is excessive, further bleeding can be controlled by a variety of techniques, including use of oxytocin, ligation of individual bleeders, or even closure of the uterine incision. In many instances, however, it is possible to complete the isolation of the uterine pedi-

cles in a time period that approximates that required to close the uterine incision.

If the bladder has not been previously mobilized, this can be done with blunt and sharp dissection. Once the bladder separation is completed, the round ligaments (Fig. 19-12) are then clamped with Haney or Kocher clamps, cut, and ligated with transfixing sutures. If not done earlier, the previously made vesicouterine peritoneum incision is extended laterally and cephalad across the anterior leaf of the broad ligament through the point of the previously incised round ligaments.

The ovaries should be inspected; it is seldom necessary to remove them. If the ovaries are normal, placement of the utero-ovarian clamps and a free tie at the intended site is facilitated by perforation of the avascular portion of the posterior leaf of the broad ligament adjacent to the uterus just inferior to the fallopian tube, utero-ovarian ligaments, and ovarian vessels with a curved Kelly clamp. The intent is to provide enough room to insert two or three clamps, either atraumatic (e.g., Masterston) or crushing (e.g., Haney), across the utero-ovarian ligament and fallopian tube between the previously placed utero-ovarian free tie and the uterus. The utero-ovarian ligament and tube may then be ligated with clamps or free tie. An attempt should be made to avoid placement of the clamps or ligature across ovarian tissue, which may result in immediate or delayed bleeding. If the intent is to place three Kocher/Ochsner or Heaney/Masterson clamps on the utero-ovarian ligament and fallopian tube, sequential placement of clamps should move in the direction of the dorsum of the surgeon's dominant hand so as to avoid placement of the surgeon's hand between clamps. If the three-clamp technique is used, the pedicle is incised between the single medial clamp and the two lateral clamps.

If a lateral free tie is employed, the utero-ovarian/adnexal pedicle is then doubly clamped medial to the free tie. The pedicle is incised between the clamps and the lateral pedicle and ligated with a transfixing suture (Fig. 19-12B). Some surgeons also ligate the opposing medial pedicle so as to remove the most medial clamp from the operative field, while avoiding back-bleeding.

Some surgeons then incise the avascular portion of the broad ligaments and skeletonize the large uterine veins. This is more difficult in a cesarean hysterectomy than in a simple abdominal hysterectomy. The ascending uterine vessels adjacent to the uterus near their origin are then identified near the junction of the cervix and uterus and doubly or triply clamped with Haney or Masterson clamps, incised, and ligated, either singularly or doubly. The surgeon should attempt to place the clamp tip snuggly against the uterine margin at a right angle to the ascending uterine vessels to reduce

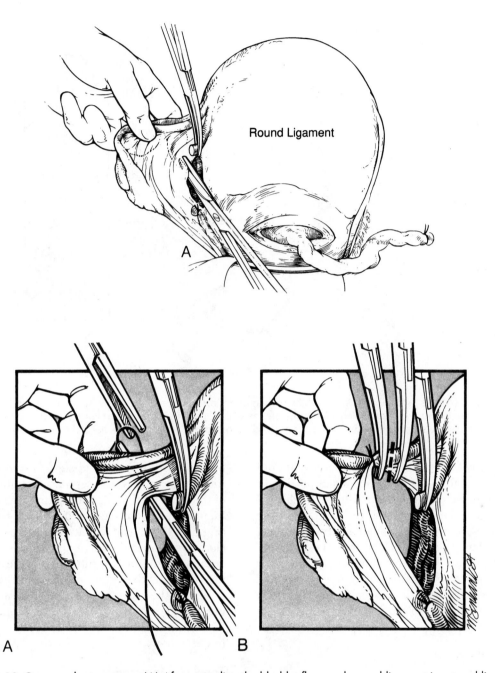

Round Ligament

A

A   B

Fig. 19-12 Cesarean hysterectomy. (A) After extending the bladder flap, each round ligament is cut and ligated. The posterior leaf of the broad ligament can be opened for a short distance, taking care to incise only the surface layer. The avascular space beneath the utero-ovarian ligament may be opened by blunt finger dissection to isolate the adnexal pedicle. (B) (a) A free tie is passed through the avascular space and firmly tied. The advantage of this tie is to secure the vessels within the pedicle before it is cut. (b) The adnexal pedicle is doubly clamped and cut. In addition, a transfixing suture will then be placed around the pedicle.

the likelihood of back-bleeding. Placement of the clamp tip on this vascular pedicle against the lower segment is easy should the cervix be long and uneffaced. However, if the lower segment is well developed, soft, and without distinct margins, palpation of the lateral margin of the lower uterine segment (between thumb and forefinger straddling the intended broad ligament

pedicle) may be required to facilitate closer approximation of the clamp tip to the uterine margin. Prior to placement of the clamps on the uterine vessel, it is often useful to confirm that the bladder is displaced inferiorly, and, should ureteral location be an issue, the ureter can occasionally be palpated between the forefinger and thumb.

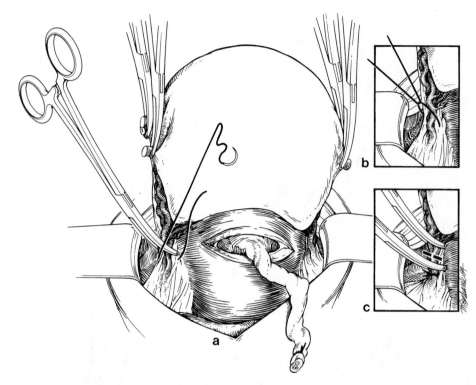

Fig. 19-13 (A) The ascending branches of the uterine artery are clamped, cut, and a suture is placed just below the tip of the clamp and immediately next to the uterine wall. (B) After removing the clamp, the suture is tied, thus securing the vessels before they are cut. (C) The pedicle is regrasped just above the tie and then doubly ligated.

The incision of the uterine vessel pedicle should occur in such a manner as to leave a small portion of tissue medial to the clamp to diminish the likelihood of clamp or later suture slippage. Before incising the uterine pedicle there may be advantage to placement of a medial Haney or Kocher/Ochsner clamp to the uterine vessels above the intended site of incision of the vascular pedicle. Others prefer isolation of the uterine vessels bilaterally prior to incising either pedicle as a technique to avoid back-bleeding. A variation of the two-clamp technique is presented in Figure 19-13.

Subtotal Hysterectomy

Supracervical/subtotal hysterectomy may be a consideration at this point either as a transitional step to remove the fundus and provide better visualization of the lower pelvis or as a permanent strategy (i.e., should the patient be unstable or dissection unusually difficult). The obstetrician should usually plan to perform a total hysterectomy. However, should the patient be unstable or the procedure unusually difficult, a subtotal hysterectomy may occasionally be desirable because it is simpler, particularly should the pathology be confined to the upper uterine segment and the surgeon judge that prolongation of the procedure associated with removal of the cervix will adversely affect the patient.

Once the ascending uterine artery and vein are dou-

bly clamped and the pedicles cut and ligated as in a total hysterectomy, the cervix is amputated at the level of the pedicles. In amputating the cervix it may be useful to cone the amputation downward toward the canal (Fig. 19-14A). The resultant cervical stump can be closed with several interrupted figure-of-eight sutures. Some surgeons doubly suture ligate the ascending uterine vessels by the angles of the cervix (Fig. 19-14B) to minimize the risk of angle bleeding. Additional bleeding points are ligated and reperitonealization performed in a fashion similar to that required for total hysterectomy.

Total Hysterectomy

Should the patient be stable after removal of the fundus, two or more Ochsner/Kocher clamps may be placed on the remaining cervical stump to control bleeding and provide traction for later manipulation while completing the hysterectomy. After the ascending uterine vessels have been ligated, the cervix is separated from the supporting cardinal and uterosacral ligaments and vagina. Pedicles containing descending branches of the uterine vessels and the cardinal and uterosacral ligaments are clamped (doubly or singularly) with either Haney-type curved clamps or Ochsner/Kocher-type straight clamps, attempting to place the clamps as close to the cervix as possible. Ap-

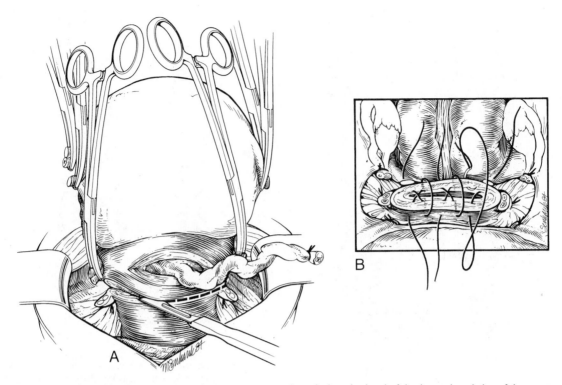

Fig. 19-14 Subtotal hysterectomy. (A) The cervix is incised just below the level of the ligated pedicles of the uterine arteries, amputating the uterine corpus from its cervical stump. (B) The cervical stump may be closed with several interrupted figure-of-eight sutures; reperitonealization is then accomplished as in a total hysterectomy.

proximately 1.0 to 1.5 cm of cardinal pedicle tissue should be encompassed within the instrument with each "bite." Placement of the Haney or Kocher straight clamps should be done in such a manner that the progressively closing jaws of the clamp slide off the firm body of the cervix to decrease the likelihood of inclusion of the adjacent ureters. Should the lower segment be well developed and thinned out, delineation of the margin can be accomplished by palpating the tissues between forefinger and thumb. The resultant wedge-shaped pedicle is then incised and sutured. Inclusion of a portion of the adjacent more superior uterine pedicle in the tie may reduce bleeding between the two pedicles.

Should the lower uterine segment be well developed, it is often necessary to develop more than one pedicle for each cardinal ligament. Successive clamps are placed medial to the preceding clamp, with care to avoid the possibility of unsecured tissue between successive bites. After reconfirming that the bladder reflection is retracted away from the site of intended clamp placement, successive more inferior pedicles are clamped, incised, and suture ligated until the surgeon is confident that the supporting cardinal and uterosacral ligaments have been separated and the level of the lateral vaginal fornix is reached (Fig. 19-15). Although some surgeons attempt to identify and ligate the uterosacral ligaments individually, the uterosacral ligaments

are generally not as distinct at this time as would be the case in the nonpregnant state. In most cases they are included in the cardinal ligament pedicles.

The vagina may be entered anteriorly (or posteriorly) in the midline with the scapel or alternatively following placement of a curved Haney clamp just below the inferior margin of the cervix at the lateral angle. Separation of the cervix from its vaginal attachments can be quite difficult should the lower uterine segment be thinned out and long as a result of effacement. One should avoid both incomplete removal of the cervix and excessive removal of the upper vagina. In some instances it is possible to palpate and milk superiorly the lower margin of the cervix by palpating the approximate site with thumb and forefinger placed anteriorly and posteriorly about the cervicovaginal junction. Should identification of the cervicovaginal junction not be possible by external palpation, there are several alternatives. The surgeon may insert an index finger through a vertical incision in the anterior lower uterine segment/cervical canal into the upper vagina to locate the cervical vaginal margin (Fig. 19-16). Should the index-finger method to locate the lower margin of the cervix be employed, the circulating nurse may re-glove the surgeon. After the vagina is entered, the vagina and cervix are circumferentially separated under direct visualization with large curved Mayo scissors, attempting to maintain the full length of the vagina. Once the cervix is freed

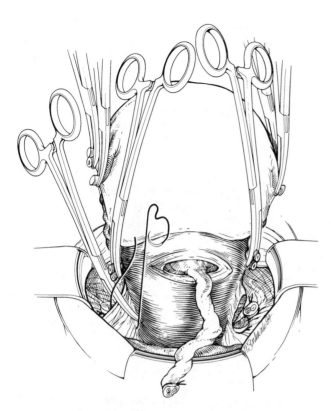

Fig. 19-15 The cardinal ligaments are clamped at their point of insertion, cut, and singly ligated. Because these structures are hypertrophied, several bites may be necessary. Some physicians clamp, cut, and ligate the uterosacral ligaments separately.

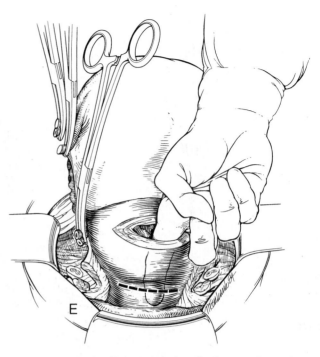

Fig. 19-16 Because the cervix is elongated, it may be useful to insert an index finger through the cervical canal to demarcate the vaginal incision and to ensure complete removal of the cervix and avoid unnecessary removal of vaginal length.

from the vagina, the specimen is then inspected to ensure that the cervix has been completely excised. The two angles of the resultant vaginal cuff are identified and clamped with Kocher/Haney clamps (Fig. 19-17). The vaginal angle containing the vaginal artery can then be secured by a variety of techniques.

The apex of the vaginal cuff is then supported by approximating the vaginal angles to the cardinal ligament pedicle and the uterosacral ligament if previously incised separately. Some incorporate the vaginal angle to the cardinal and uterosacral ligaments via a lock loop suture (Fig. 19-18). The vaginal cuff may be left open or closed. The decision to leave the vaginal cuff open in most instances will depend on the presence of adequate hemostasis and absence of obvious infection. The open cuff will allow excess blood or serous material to drain from the lower pelvis. The vaginal cuff may be closed in either one or two layers, particularly if the pelvis is dry and there are no major additional risks for cuff infection, using either interrupted figure-of-eight sutures or a continuous closure (Fig. 19-19). Alternatively, the cuff can be left open by running a locking circumferential suture about the cuff margins to minimize vaginal cuff bleeding and facilitate drainage; some prefer figure-of-eight sutures.

The cul-de-sac and peritoneal gutters are suctioned of blood and accumulated debris and all previous pedicles examined for bleeding points. Bleeding sites should be individually controlled by picking up as little tissue as possible to avoid ligation or kinking of the ureters. Once the surgeon is assured that hemostasis is adequate and that there have been no lacerations of the bladder, the pelvis may be irrigated.

Should the surgeon decide to reperitonealize the pelvic floor (Fig. 19-20), this can be accomplished in several ways using a continuous suture. The end result is inversion of the pedicle of the ligated fallopian tube and ovarian ligament and round ligament retroperitoneally, avoiding fixation of the ovary to the cuff in the cul-de-sac. A continuous suture reapproximates the medial and lateral leaves of the broad ligament, burying the round ligament stump and approximating the anterior vesicouterine peritoneum over the vaginal vault to the cul-de-sac peritoneum on the posterior margin of the vagina. The procedure is then conducted in reverse order on the opposing side. Some accomplish the dual goals of reperitonealization and support of the apex of the vaginal vault by successive placement of the suture on the anterior vaginal wall to the cardinal ligament to the round ligament pedicle and back to the uterosacral ligaments/posterior vaginal wall, which is then drawn down to the cuff. Many surgeons have discontinued the process of reperitonealizing the pelvic floor and simply

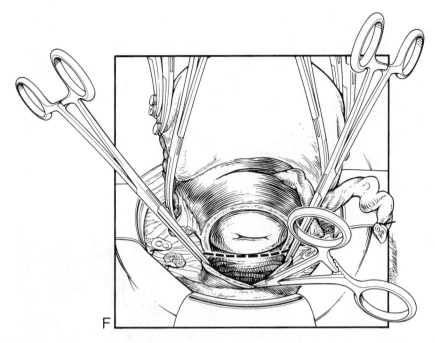

Fig. 19-17 The vagina is circumferentially incised at its cervical attachment and grasped with four clamps.

allow the sigmoid and bladder to fall into place over the vaginal cuff, an approach that may also minimize the admittedly small chance of suturing the ureter during reperitonealization. The surgeon may avoid attachment of the ovarian pedicles to the angle of the vagina by suturing the ovarian pedicle to the ipsilateral round ligament.

Intraoperative Complications

Intraoperative complications associated with peripartum hysterectomy, although similar to those following nonobstetric total abdominal hysterectomy, occur with greater frequency, especially in unplanned procedures. Total hysterectomy may add 30 to 60 minutes to cesarean operating and anesthesia times (Tables 19-28 and 19-29), depending on (1) the surgeon's experience, (2) whether the procedure is emergent or elective, (3) the degree of development of the lower uterine segment, (4) coincidental pelvic pathology such as leiomyomata or obesity, and (5) the presence of ureteral or bladder laceration.

Increased blood loss and occasional injury to either bladder or ureters are the two most commonly encoun-

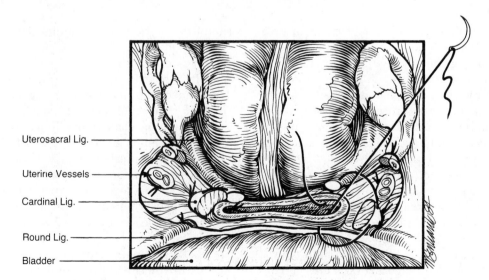

Uterosacral Lig.
Uterine Vessels
Cardinal Lig.
Round Lig.
Bladder

Fig. 19-18 The angles of the vaginal cuff are closed with sutures to include the cardinal and uterosacral ligaments, thus providing fascial support to the vaginal vault. A simple loop suture is commonly used at this location to reduce the likelihood of breakage during the stage of postoperative edema.

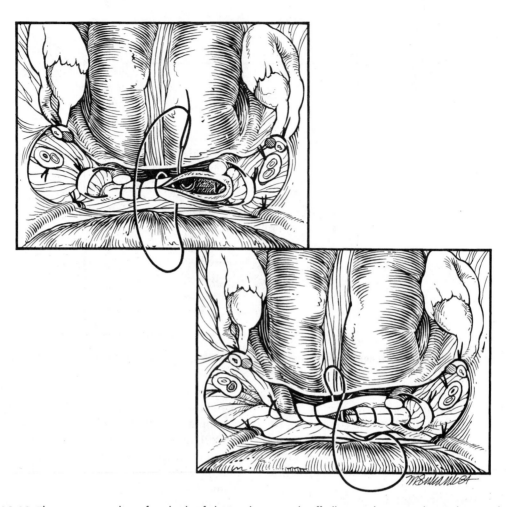

Fig. 19-19 There are a number of methods of closing the vaginal cuff. Illustrated is a two-layer closure. The first layer closes the vagina, and the second layer closes the endopelvic fascia. Many operators prefer to leave the cuff "open" by employing one continuous suture that circles the cuff, approximating the cut edge to its surrounding fascia.

tered intraoperative complications.[300] There is an associated additional blood loss of 500 to 1,000 ml, depending on preexisting blood loss and whether the procedure is planned or unplanned. In emergency procedures, a major portion of the blood loss can be attributed to the indication for the procedure. This is particularly true for uterine atony that has been unresponsive to more conservative obstetric interventions, including prostaglandin $F_{2\alpha}$. Intraoperative blood loss may be secondary to slippage of a clamp off a pedicle or bleeding between pedicles and may be a function of the type of clamp and/or suture placement. It may involve the utero-ovarian or the uterine pedicles, or there may be bleeding at the angle of the vagina and cardinal ligament. On occasion the adnexal bleeding is the result of suture placement through an ovarian vessel. This can often be avoided by the placement of a free-tie suture at the site of the most lateral of two or three clamps and subsequent placement of a transfixing suture at the

site of the more medial (middle) clamp of the lateral pedicle. On occasion it may be necessary to perform a salpingo-oophorectomy to control hematoma formation. In a recent series from Harvard, 17 percent of 117 women who underwent emergency hysterectomy required removal of their adnexa.[285]

Injuries to the bladder and ureter are most common during unplanned/emergency procedures. Most bladder injuries are easily recognized and repaired since they most often occur when dissecting the bladder from the lower uterine segment, particularly in patients with multiple prior cesarean births. The bladder is infrequently included in the lateral margin of the vaginal cuff at the time of the separation of the cardinal ligaments. Rarely spontaneous laceration of the bladder may occur coincident with uterine rupture.

Cystotomy as a complication of cesarean hysterectomy occurred in approximately 4 to 5 percent of procedures in early series.[113,114] Bladder injury can be

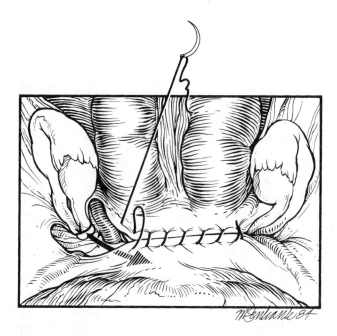

Fig. 19-20 The bladder flap is closed with a continuous suture that inverts the pedicles of the round ligaments and adnexae. Note that these structures have not been attached to the vaginal cuff.

minimized at two points—first by separation and downward displacement of the bladder from the anterior vaginal wall prior to the cesarean delivery while the anterior vaginal wall is still taut and second by rolling the Kocher/Oschner clamps off the cervix when developing the cardinal pedicles.

The incidence of ureteral injury during cesarean delivery is reported to be approximately 1 in 1,000 cesarean deliveries.[112] The risk of ureteral injury is increased even further with cesarean hysterectomy, with rates of 0.2 to 0.5 percent being observed in early series including planned procedures.[113,114] In more recent series typically involving emergency unplanned hysterectomies (Table 19-28), most urinary tract injuries involve the bladder, although on occasion the ureter may be incised or incorporated within a pedicle. Stanco et al,[284] in a 5-year review of 123 (1.3 per 1,000 births) emergency peripartum hysterectomies, found a 3.2 percent incidence of urinary tract injury; in addition, they employed 12 (10 percent) intentional cystotomies to facilitate passage of a ureteral stent.[284] Zelop et al,[285] in an 8-year review of 117 (1.55 per 1,000 births) emergency peripartum hysterectomies, found that 10 (8.5 percent) patients sustained urologic injuries. Of these there were 9 (7.7 percent) cystotomies and 3 (2.5 percent) ureteral injuries that required stenting.

Injury to the ureter is more common in cases where there is a necessity to control a broad ligament bleeding or hematoma formation or to dissect a pelvic tumor. In the case of pelvic tumors careful dissection of the mass, palpation of the lateral cervical margins, and careful placement of the clamps as close to the cervical margin as possible with successive bites more medial to the preceding pedicle will make inclusion of the ureter highly unlikely. Should the surgeon be concerned about the possibility of a ureteral injury, intentional cystotomy in the bladder dome and placement of retrograde ureteral catheters may be employed to assess the patency and integrity of the ureter.

Postoperative Complication

As is the case in any hysterectomy, infection and bleeding are the most common major postoperative complications. The incidence of infectious complications is closely linked to the presence of preexisting risk factors for infection and whether the procedure is planned or unplanned. The incidence of urinary tract infection in the absence of preexisting amnionitis is strongly linked to the duration of indwelling catheter placement. Scheduled procedures performed before labor have an associated incidence of febrile morbidity less than 10 percent; most cases involve the urinary tract, with an occasional wound or vaginal cuff infection. In contrast, febrile morbidity rates approach 30 percent for unplanned procedures.[284,285,299] Postoperative infectious morbidity may be reduced by prophylactic antibiotics to women who have been either in labor or at risk for infection and early removal of indwelling catheters. Prophylactic antibiotics are generally administered intraoperatively, immediately following delivery of the fetus.

The pelvic tissues, if there has been hemorrhage or infection, are frequently quite friable and may tear easily. There may be later ligature slippage as tissue edema resolves. Vaginal bleeding is commonly associated with a bleeder at the lateral angle/junction of the vagina and cardinal ligament; it also may involve the uterine vessels. In some instances bleeding will involve the formation of a broad ligament hematoma arising from the uterine or ovarian vessels. Should the hematoma be small, stable, and asymptomatic, such patients may require no further treatment. The surgeon may evaluate the patient serially using sonography; on occasion it may be necessary to employ computed tomography or magnetic resonance imaging.

Reexploration for bleeding following a peripartum hysterectomy has been reported to be necessary in as many as 2.6 to 4 percent of cases.[284,285] Reexploration may be indicated should the hematoma progressively enlarge. Alternatively, it may be necessary if the patient remains unstable or demonstrates a progressive unanticipated fall in serial hematocrit determinations, after taking into account preoperative and intraoperative blood loss and replacement. Evacuation of the pelvic hematoma and identification and ligation of bleeders are the surgical goals; in some cases it may not be possible to isolate a definite bleeder. On occasion it may be necessary to place cervical drains postoperatively.

Elective Myomectomy and Appendectomy

The propriety of performing an elective myomectomy or appendectomy during a cesarean delivery is a matter of dispute. The majority opinion is that, with the possible exception of a subserosal myoma on a thin pedicle, myomectomy is contraindicated because achieving hemostasis may be difficult. Others assert that hemostasis will be excellent because of the action of the contracting uterus. A better argument for abstention is the knowledge that most myomas will involute to an insignificant size during the puerperium. Although the risk of elective appendectomy is quite low, there are no statistics to prove that the benefits to be gained are greater than the possible surgical complications.

Coincidental Ovarian Neoplasms at Cesarean Delivery

Should an ovarian neoplasm be discovered at the time of cesarean delivery, the surgeon should first rule out the possibility of a theca lutein cyst or the rare luteoma of pregnancy. Other ovarian neoplasms should be excised, sparing the ovary whenever possible.

Postpartum Sterilization

Tubal ligation in the postpartum period offers several major advantages. The patient is often only subjected to one anesthesia (epidural) for the labor and delivery and the ligation process. Should that not be possible, there is still the benefit of only abbreviated hospitalization at a time when maternal responsibilities are less than will be the case just weeks later. Furthermore, additional preoperative work-up is not necessary for a second procedure. Increased tissue vascularity and edema pose a theoretical risk of more difficult hemostasis and possibly contribute to the somewhat higher failure rate compared with interval procedures.

A variety of methods of sterilization are available either at the time of cesarean delivery or during the postpartum period. The tubes can be occluded by banding, clipping, resection, or fulguration. In selecting a method for tubal sterilization, consideration should be given to two factors, should the patient later desire reversal: effectiveness relative to later sterility and reversibility. A rational decision for tubal occlusion may later be proven wrong by different circumstances, particularly should sterilization be performed at a young age.

Patients are also more likely to regret sterilization procedures performed in association with the stress of pregnancy than considered interval procedures.

From the point of view of later reversibility, the use of clips is probably the best method of sterilization, because clips produce the least damage. Occlusion within the tubal isthmus is desirable should later reanastomosis be attempted, because an isthmic-isthmic reapproximation is most likely to succeed. Salpingectomy, cornual resection, extensive fulguration, and fimbriectomy limit the choices for those patients who later seek restoration of fertility. The timing of the operation relative to the time of birth has little impact. In some instances when there is some concern regarding potential newborn outcome, the procedure may be best postponed.

Postoperative complications are infrequent. Hemorrhage is the most commonly encountered problem. Although patient discomfort associated with the procedure may increase the length of hospitalization by 1 day or more, significant discomfort is seldom encountered after 1 or 2 weeks.

Abdominal Incision

In the early puerperium the tubes are easily isolated through a small abdominal incision, since the uterus is enlarged and the abdominal wall is lax. A small, periumbilical incision offers the most cosmetic result and least postpartum discomfort. However, a small 3- to 4-cm midline vertical or transverse incision at the level of the fundus is often used. The only disadvantage to such a small incision is one of limited exposure that may increase the risk of inadvertent ligation of a round ligament rather than a tube. If the operation is delayed, or if the patient has had previous adnexal surgery and adhesions are anticipated, a transverse or midline vertical incision may be desirable.

Techniques

Pomeroy Technique

The Pomeroy technique is the most popular means of postpartum sterilization (Fig. 19-21) because of its simplicity and effectiveness. As originally described, a small knuckle of each tube is picked up approximately 1 inch from its cornual insertion and ligated with a single loop of absorbable suture (plain catgut). A small section of the isolated tubal segment is then resected and submitted to the pathologist to document that the tubal lumina have been interrupted. Presumably the remaining segments of tube will separate when the suture is absorbed, leaving a gap between the proximal and distal ends. A modification wherein the proximal ends of each resected tube are also ligated with a nonabsorbable suture is employed by some in an attempt to reduce the likelihood of recanalization of the proximal

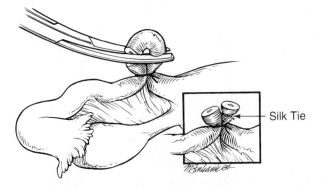

Fig. 19-21 Pomeroy sterilization. A knuckle of tube is ligated with absorbable suture, and a small segment is being excised. Note that the ligation is performed at a site that will favor reanastomosis, should that become desirable. Some surgeons place an extra tie of nonabsorbable suture around the proximal stump as added protection against recanalization.

tubal lumen. The modified operation has a failure rate of approximately 1 in 500.

Uchida Technique

Some clinicians advocate the Uchida technique because of its low failure rate and the theoretically reduced risk of associated disturbance of ovarian blood supply. This technique is more complicated than the Pomeroy technique and requires the surgeon to separate the muscular portion of the tube from its serosal cover, which is then cut and ligated. The proximal segment is then buried in the leaves of the broad ligament, leaving the distal segment exteriorized (Fig. 19-22).

Irving Technique

Although the Irving operation is slightly more complicated than other techniques, it may have the lowest failure rate. After transecting and ligating the cut ends of

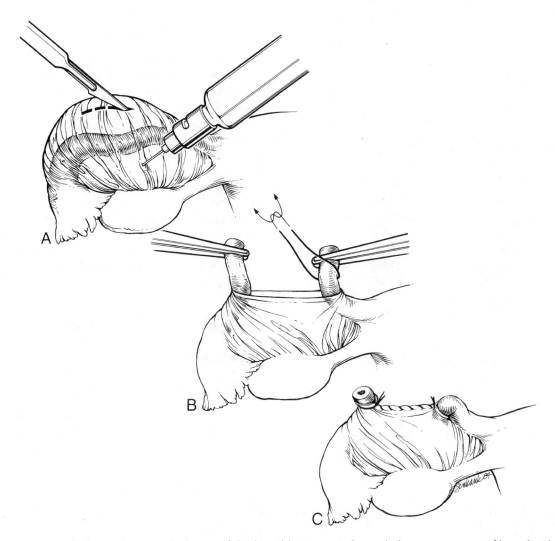

Fig. 19-22 Uchida sterilization. The leaves of the broad ligament and peritubal peritoneum are infiltrated with saline so that the tube can be easily isolated from these structures, divided, and ligated. The broad ligament is then closed, burying the proximal stump between the leaves and including the distal stump in the line of closure.

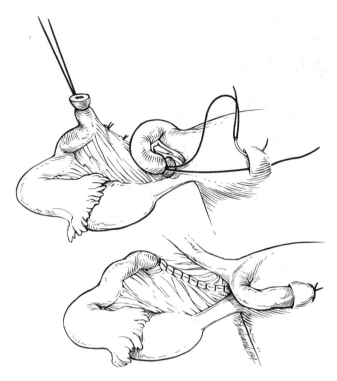

Fig. 19-23 Irving sterilization. The tube is transected 3 to 4 cm from its insertion, and a short tunnel is created by means of a sharp-nosed hemostat in either the anterior or posterior uterine wall. The cut end of the tube can then be buried in the tunnel and, if necessary, further secured by an interrupted suture at the opening of the tunnel. The distal cut end is buried between the leaves of the broad ligament.

the tubes, a tunnel is created by blunt dissection into the adjacent uterine wall at the insertion of the round ligament, a less vascular area. The proximal segment of each tube is carried into the depth of the tunnel by means of a traction suture and transfixed there by an interrupted suture (Fig. 19-23). The cut end of each distal segment is then buried between the leaves of the broad ligament or may be left exposed in the modified Irving procedure.

Kroener Fimbrinectomy

Excision of the distal portion of each tube (Fig. 19-24) and ligation of the cut ends of the tube with nonabsorbable suture (silk) is a highly effective procedure. However, because tubal fimbriae have been excised, reversal of this procedure is not likely.

Other Techniques

Simple ligation of the tubes is not acceptable because of a failure rate approximating 20 percent. The Madliner technique involves ligation of previously crushed tubal loops, and the Aldridge technique results in surgical placement of the free end of each tube in the leaves of

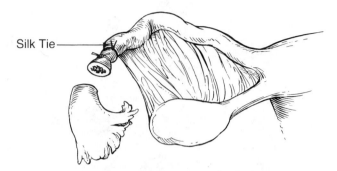

Fig. 19-24 Kroener sterilization. After transecting the distal tube and its fimbria, the proximal tube is religated with a non-absorbable suture to protect against recanalization.

the broad ligament. Both techniques are less effective than the methods described above. On the other hand, no method of tubal sterilization is completely effective.[301]

Counseling for Tubal Ligation

Patient counseling may include a discussion of the risk of failure, alternative methods of contraception including male sterilization, and procedural complications. Some clinicians include a review of the variety of tubal techniques available, as well as the possibility of adverse long-term effects on ovarian function and sexual interest. A sufficient interval should be allowed following the provision of consent to satisfy the legal requirements of various jurisdictions and, of equal importance, to permit the patient and her family to reconsider their decision. Despite attempts to provide detailed information, a number of patients will later desire reversal of the procedure. Because reversal is not always possible, tubal sterilization should only be recommended as a permanent procedure.

Acute Abdomen in Pregnancy

Appendicitis

Appendicitis is the most common acute surgical condition of pregnancy, with an incidence of 1 in 2,000 births. It is encountered with relatively the same frequency in every trimester as well as the puerperium. The diagnosis is reputed to be more difficult and likely to be delayed because the clinical picture tends to be masked by the symptoms and physical changes of pregnancy.[302] Some of the factors confusing the diagnosis are the nausea, vomiting, and abdominal discomfort of early pregnancy, upward displacement of the appendix by the expanding uterus (Fig. 19-25), laxity of the abdominal wall, round ligament spasm, physiologic leukocytosis, and elevated sedimentation rate.

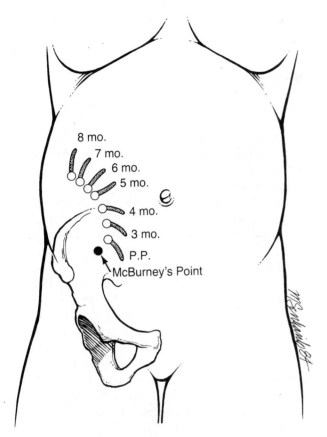

8 mo.
7 mo.
6 mo.
5 mo.
4 mo.
3 mo.
P.P.
McBurney's Point

Fig. 19-25 Locations of the appendix in pregnancy. As modified from Bauer et al,[303] the approximate location of the appendix during succeeding months of pregnancy is diagrammed. In planning an operation, it is better to make the abdominal incision over the point of maximum tenderness unless there is a great disparity between that point and the theoretical location of the appendix. (Modified from Bauer et al,[303] with permission.)

Diagnosis

Despite these confusing factors, the signs and symptoms of appendicitis in pregnancy are similar to those in the nonpregnant patient. The initial visceral pain is typically gradual in onset, often colicky (denoting an element of obstruction), and usually referred to the epigastrium or periumbilical area. During the first trimester, the pain localizes in the right lower quadrant as the overlying parietal peritoneum becomes involved. Past the fourth month, the appendix has been displaced upward and laterally. At 6 months, the point of maximal thickness is above the iliac crest, and at 8 months it rises to the level of the right costal margin.[303] Usually, anorexia accompanied by nausea and vomiting begin 1 to 2 hours after the onset of pain. Right lateral rectal tenderness is commonly found, and about one-half of the patients will have abdominal muscle spasm or guarding. Moving the uterus tends to intensify pain in the appendiceal area. By placing the patient on her left side, the clinician can sometimes differ-entiate pain of uterine origin. If the uterus is the source of the pain, abdominal wall tenderness will diminish as the uterus falls away from the examining fingers.

The patient's temperature can be normal but is usually moderately elevated, up to 101°F. Because of the physiologic leukocytosis of pregnancy, significant alterations of the white blood count depend on finding either a rising count over a period of observation or an increasing left shift. A urinalysis is usually negative unless the inflamed appendix is retroperionteal and lying in close proximity to the right ureter. Roentgenographic studies are rarely helpful. A culdocentesis may demonstrate inflammatory fluid, both before and after rupture.

If the appendix ruptures, either peritonitis follows or the uterus forms the median wall of a localized abscess. In either case, abortion or labor is the usual consequence. As the uterus is emptied, a walled off abscess tends to rupture, producing generalized peritonitis. For these reasons, early diagnosis and operation in all suspicious cases is particularly important. Diagnostic laparoscopy in doubtful cases encountered during early pregnancy may help to avoid an unnecessary laparotomy.

The differential diagnosis includes pyelonephritis, round ligament pain, a placental accident, torsion of an ovarian cyst, degenerating myomata, pancreatitis, and cholecystitis. Appendicitis can also be confused with early labor and postpartum endomyometritis.

Management

A transverse muscle-splitting incision over the point of maximum tenderness is usually adequate and can easily be extended if necessary. If the appendix is unruptured, the incision is closed without drainage. Neither antibiotics nor tocolytic agents are necessary, and abortion and premature labor are unlikely.

When the appendix is ruptured, the patient should receive multiple antibiotic therapy, including an agent effective against anaerobic organisms. Suction drainage through a flank incision will be needed for an abscess or generalized peritonitis. Cul-de-sac drainage is contraindicated, and a cesarean section should be avoided unless a compelling obstetric indication exists. The incision should be separately drained, or the skin should be left open for secondary closure. The value of tocolytic agents to prevent preterm labor in this setting has not been proved.

Acute Cholecystitis

Cholecystitis is more common in pregnancy, presumably because of extrinsic pressure interfering with the circulation and drainage of the gallbladder. The incidence is approximately 1 in 4,000 pregnancies, and attacks are more often associated with increasing age, increasing gravidity, and a history of previous attacks. Preexisting gallstones are rarely a cause of cholecystitis in pregnancy because the ability of the gallbladder to contract is inhibited by high levels of progesterone.

The clinical picture is no different from that in the nonpregnant patient. An attack usually begins with biliary colic, nausea, and vomiting. If the common duct is obstructed by a stone, the pain persists and often radiates to the subscapular area. There is right subcostal tenderness along with fever (i.e., 101°F) and increasing leukocytosis. An ultrasonic study is useful to detect the presence of stones or dilatation of the common duct.[304] If stones are present and Murphy's sign is positive, a diagnosis of cholecystitis is virtually assured.

In most cases, medical therapy suffices. An appropriate antibiotic such as a cephalosporin is combined with intravenous fluids, nasogastric suction, antispasmodics, and anagesics with the expectation of recovery in 48 hours or less. If common duct obstruction or pancreatitis develops, a cholecystectomy or cholecystotomy will be necessary and should not be delayed. Abortion or cesarean section is not indicated. However, there is considerable risk of premature labor following the operative procedure.

Intestinal Obstruction

Mechanical bowel obstruction, a rare complication of pregnancy, usually involves small bowel, is most commonly due to an adhesive band or hernia, and is more likely to be encountered in the second half of pregnancy. Although the clinical picture is variable, typical symptoms include colicky midabdominal pain that increases in severity and may become diffuse and constant as the bowel distends. In the early stages, bouts of pain are accompanied by reflex vomiting. Later, fecal vomiting may occur. There is usually generalized distention without signs of peritoneal irritation. Dehydration and electrolyte imbalance may intervene. If peristaltic rushes are present, a presumptive diagnosis can be made. Repeated roentgenographic studies are indicated despite the theoretical risks of radiation exposure to the fetus. Significant findings include gaseous distention, intraluminal fluid levels, a stepladder arrangement of small bowel loops, and a paucity of large bowel gas. Initial treatment includes an attempt to decompress the small intestine with a long tube plus hydration and correction of any electrolyte imbalance. If after 6 to 8 hours the patient's response is unsatisfactory, an operation should be done before bowel necrosis and perforation are established. The uterus rarely interferes with the operation and should not be disturbed. If labor follows, a well-repaired abdominal incision will

remain intact. The value of postoperative tocolytic agents is speculative.

Trauma

Trauma is the most common nonobstetric cause of maternal death as well as the leading cause of death into the mid-40 age range.[305] Most reported trauma in pregnancy is blunt trauma secondary to automobile accidents, falls, or penetrating injuries. Uterine injury as a result of external trauma is highly unlikely in early pregnancy; however, vulnerability increases as the uterus becomes an abdominal organ in later pregnancy. The fetus is relatively well protected by its amniotic fluid cushion, but placental separation can occur as a result of a direct blow or hypovolemic shock. Uterine rupture is a less likely consequence of a direct blow or seat belt compression. Distortion of the uterus produced by the sudden compression of a waist-type seat belt can produce placental separation (Fig. 19-26). Adverse fetal outcome is closely linked to placental abruption or direct fetal injury. Abruption may occur in up to 50 percent of patients presenting with major injuries.[306] In the absence of uteroplacental insufficiency the reported newborn outcome is not adversely affected.[307]

Clinically, rupture is unlikely unless there is persistent uterine tenderness and a significant FHR alteration. Should there be a penetrating wound from a knife or bullet to the lower abdomen, only 19 percent of injuries involve maternal viscera; however, the fetus is involved in approximately 65 percent of cases.[308]

Should there be evidence of a traumatic injury in a pregnancy with a viable fetus, it is essential to institute supportive care promptly to minimize fetal morbidity. Uterine rupture, some cases of placental separation, and gunshot wounds will require exploration. In the event of a stab wound, an operation can sometimes be avoided if a fistulogram demonstrates that the parietal peritoneum has not been penetrated.

Maternal evaluation may include serial vital signs, radiographic procedures including upright KUB and possibly computed tomography and magnetic resonance imaging. Diagnostic peritoneal lavage may be performed to screen for spillage of bowel contents, meconium, and blood.[309] Fetal assessment with continuous FHR and UC monitoring is employed after maternal stabilization for at least 4 hours. The primary value of fetal monitoring at gestations prior to viability is to detect evolving preterm labor and provide supportive response (O_2, fluids, position) should nonreassuring FHR observations be detected. Frequent contractions may reflect reduced maternal blood volume/uterine blood flow or be a sign of possible abruption. It is note-

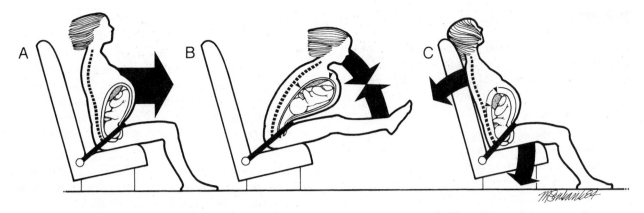

Fig. 19-26 Seat belt injury. The mechanisms by which placental separation might be produced by a waist-type seat belt are illustrated. (A) The force of a collision propels the body forward. (B) Acute flexion of the trunk results in elongation of the uterus, including elongation of the site of placental attachment. (C) As the trunk recoils, the placental site is shortened and the posterior wall of the uterus collides with the vertebral column. (Redrawn from Lees and Singer,[316] with permission.)

worthy that fetal death may occur as late as 48 hours later as a result of abruption.[310]

Management is based on the assumption that fetal survival is closely linked to the degree of maternal injury and mortality, and as a consequence maternal support (airway, respiratory, and circulatory) is paramount. Should there be acute cardiorespiratory arrest that is not successfully corrected by CPR within approximately 4 minutes, cesarean delivery may be indicated.[127] If the patient is not hemodynamically stable, exploratory laparotomy with contingency planning for cesarean birth should be considered.

Consideration should be given to administration of Rh-negative blood until the Rh type is known. If the patient is later determined to be Rh negative, minidose Rh immunoglobulin is appropriate up to 12 to 13 weeks' gestation, whereas 300 μg or more are necessary at more than 13 weeks. Should Kleihauer-Betke test support a large fetal maternal blood, a larger dose may be required based on the estimated volume of the bleed.[311]

Miscellaneous Procedures (Duhrssen's Incisions)

In rare circumstances it may be necessary to incise the cervix as a means to expedite vaginal delivery. Entrapment of the aftercoming head in breech deliveries often following a rapidly progressive labor with expulsion of the fetal body through a partially dilated cervix is probably the most common example. This indication is most likely to involve a preterm breech because of the disproportion between the large fetal head and relatively small body. In such cases, Duhrssen's incisions of the cervix may be attempted.[312] Two or three radial incisions are made in the cervix at the 2, 6, and 10 o'clock

positions (Fig. 19-27). To avoid major hemorrhage, the procedure should seldom if ever be done unless the cervix is at least 7 cm dilated and completely effaced. The incision is facilitated by placement of right angle retractors in the vagina with direct visualization of the remaining cervix, which is then incised with either bandage or Mayo scissors. Following the delivery the cervical incisions are repaired in the same fashion as a cervical laceration (see Fig. 17-15).

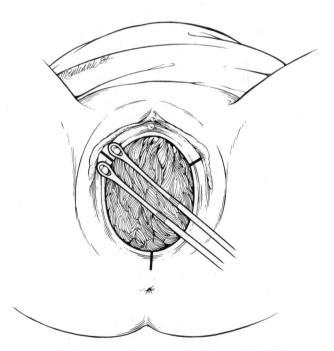

Fig. 19-27 Duhrssen's incision. The location and length of Duhrssen's incisions may be delineated by grasping the cervical rim with two pairs of sponge forceps at the intended point of incision. Either two or three incisions will be sufficient, and repair with interrupted absorbable sutures usually results in satisfactory healing.

Key Points

- Even when morbidity and mortality arising from the indications leading to cesarean delivery are excluded, maternal morbidity and mortality remain many times higher for cesarean delivery than for vaginal delivery.

- As the percentage of laboring patients presenting with prior cesarean births has increased, there have been associated increases in more difficult repeat cesarean deliveries and complications, including a higher incidence of placenta previa, placenta accreta, symptomatic uterine rupture, hemorrhage, requirement for transfusion, and need for unplanned hysterectomy.

- The reported incidence of maternal mortality following cesarean delivery is estimated to range from 6.1 to 22 per 100,000 live births. Approximately one-third to one-half of maternal deaths can be attributed directly to the cesarean procedure itself.

- There are no well-documented prospective trials demonstrating benefit to the fetus or to the mother that would justify the extent of the increase in the primary cesarean delivery rate over the past two decades. Although perinatal mortality rates have decreased as cesarean birth rates have increased, the improvement is largely attributable to major advances in prenatal and intrapartum care, as well as dramatic improvements in neonatal intensive care implemented in the same time frame.

- If the patient is massively obese, it may be better to use an incision directly over the lower uterine segment that does not involve the underside of the panniculus, an area that is more heavily colonized with bacteria and that is difficult to prepare surgically, to keep dry, and to inspect in the postoperative period.

- The physician contemplating a cesarean delivery for placenta previa, particularly a repeat procedure, should consider the possibility of hysterectomy. The reported incidence of placenta accreta (1 in 2,500 deliveries) increases to approximately 4 percent in patients with a placenta previa and may approach 25 percent in patients with a prior cesarean birth.

- Although cesarean delivery is often elected to minimize trauma to the preterm breech fetus, the actual delivery mechanism via the cesarean incision is essentially identical to that of the vaginal route. Should head entrapment be encountered, the first action should be to extend the abdominal incision and to enlarge the uterine incision.

- Elective repeat cesarean delivery is estimated to be responsible for 47 percent of the 44 percent increase in the cesarean birth rate between 1978 and 1984.

VBAC-trial of labor lowers the self-perpetuating contribution of the indication of previous cesarean birth.

- Most patients with a prior cesarean birth are candidates for VBAC. The only established contraindication is a prior classical incision. VBAC reduces the incidence of postpartum infection, the need for postpartum transfusion, maternal length of stay and, as a result, offers the potential to generate significant cost savings.

- VBAC trial candidates are no more likely to require a cesarean delivery than a population of women with no prior cesarean deliveries. VBAC trial of labor is successful in 60–80 percent of acceptable candidates.

References

1. National Center for Health Statistics: Rates of cesarean delivery—United States, 1991. MMWR 42:285, 1993
2. Rutkow I: Obstetric and gynecologic operations in the United States, 1979 to 1984. Obstet Gynecol 67:755, 1986
3. Shiono PA, McNellis D, Rhoads GS: Reasons for the rising cesarean delivery rates 1978–1984. Obstet Gynecol 69:696, 1987
4. Phelan JP, Clark SL, Diaz F et al: Vaginal birth after cesarean. Am J Obstet Gynecol 157:1510, 1987
5. Petitti DB: Maternal mortality and morbidity in cesarean section. Clin Obstet Gynecol 28:763, 1985
6. Horley JMG: Cesarean section. Clin Obstet Gynecol 7:529, 1980
7. Sewell JE: Cesarean Section—A Brief History, The American College of Obstetricians and Gynecologists, Washington, DC, 1993
8. Porro E: Della Amputazione Utero-ovarica, Milan, 1876
9. Harris RP: The results of the first fifty cases of cesarean ovarohysterectomy 1869–1880. Am J Med Sci 80:129, 1880
10. Sänger M: Speaking before the German Gynecology Association 1885. Am J Obstet Dis Women Child 19:883, 1886
11. Sänger M: My work in reference to the cesarean operation. Am J Obstet Dis Women Children 20:593, 1887
12. Eastman NJ: The role of Frontier America in the development of cesarean section. Am J Obstet Gynecol 24:919, 1932
13. Frank F: Suprasymphysial delivery and its relation to other operations in the presence of contracted pelvis. Arch Gynaekol 81:46, 1907
14. Latzko W: Ueber den extraperitonealen Kaiserschnitt, Zentralbl Gynaekol 33:275, 1909
15. Krönig B: Transperitonealer Cervikaler Kaiser-Schnitt, p. 879. In Doderlein A, Kronig B (eds): Operative Gynakologie, F. Enke, Stuttgart, 1912
16. Beck AC: Observations on a series of cesarean sections done at the Long Island College Hospital during the past six years. Am J Obstet Gynecol 79:197, 1919

17. DeLee JB, Cornell EL: Low cervical cesarean section laparotracheotomy. JAMA 79:109, 1922

18. Kerr JMM: The technique of cesarean section with special reference to the lower uterine segment incision. Am J Obstet Gynecol 12:729, 1926

19. DeLee JB: Principles and Practice of Obstetrics, 6th Ed. WB Saunders, Philadelphia, 1933

20. Taffel SM, Placek PJ, Liss T: Trends in the United States cesarean section rate for the 1980–1985 rise. Am J Public Health 77:955, 1987

21. Notzon FC, Placek PJ, Taffel SM: Comparisons of national cesarean-section rates. N Engl J Med 316:386, 1987

22. Notzon FC: International differences in the use of obstetric interventions. JAMA 264:3286, 1990

23. Taffel SM, Placek PJ, Moien M, Kosary CL: 1989 US cesarean section rate steadies—VBAC rises to nearly one in five. Birth 18:73, 1991

24. Cesarean Childbirth: Report of a Consensus Development Conference Sponsored by the National Institute of Child Health and Human Development. DHHS Pub. No. 82–2067. Government Printing Office, Washington, DC, October 1981

25. Quilligan EJ: Making inroads against the C-section rate. Contemp Obstet Gynecol Jan:221, 1983

26. U.S. Department of Health and Human Services: Healthy Children 2000, DHHS Pub. No. HRSA-M-CH 91–2

27. Placek PJ, Taffel SM, Keppel KG: Maternal and infant characteristics associated with cesarean section delivery. Department of Health and Human Services, Pub. No. PHS 84–1232, National Center for Health Statistics, Hyattsville, MD, December 1983

28. Freeman JM, Nelson KB: Intrapartum asphyxia and cerebral palsy. Pediatrics 82:240, 1988

29. Freeman R: Intrapartum fetal monitoring—a disappointing story. N Engl J Med 322:624, 1990

30. Shy KK, Luthy DA, Bennett FC et al: Effects of electronic fetal heart rate monitoring, as compared with periodic auscultation, on the neurologic development of premature infants. N Engl J Med 322:588, 1990

31. American College of Obstetricians and Gynecologists, Committee on Obstetrics: Fetal and neonatal neurologic injury. Technical Bulletin No. 163, January 1992, Washington, DC

32. Green JE, McLean F, Smith LP et al: Has an increased cesarean section rate for term breech delivery reduce the incidence of birth asphyxia, trauma and death? Am J Obstet Gynecol 142:643, 1982

33. American College of Obstetricians and Gynecologists; Technical Bulletin No. 95, August 1986, American College of Obstetrics and Gynecology, Washington, DC

34. Haynes de Regt RH, Minkoff HL, Feldman J, Schwarz RH: Relation of private or clinic care to the cesarean birth rate. N Engl J Med 315:619, 1986

35. NIH Consensus Development Statement on Cesarean Childbirth. Obstet Gynecol 57:537, 1981

36. Savage W, Francome C: British CS rates: have we reached a plateau? Br J Obstet Gynaecol 100:493, 1993

37. Feldman GB, Freiman JA: Prophylactic cesarean section at term? N Engl J Med 312:1264, 1985

38. Blumenthal NJ, Harris RS, O'Connor MC et al: Changing caesarean section rates experience at a Sydney obstetric teaching hospital. Aust NZ J Obstet Gynaecol 24:246, 1984

39. Phillips RN, Thornton J, Gleicher N: Physician bias in cesarean sections. JAMA 248:1082, 1982

40. Sanchez-Ramos L, Moorhead RI, Kaunitz AM: Cesarean section rates in teaching hospitals: a national survey. Birth 21:194, 1994

41. Oleske DM, Glandon GL, Giacomelli GJ, Hohmann SF: The cesarean birth rate: influence of hospital teaching status. Health Serv Res 26:325, 1991

42. Sachs BP, Yeh J, Acker D et al: Cesarean section-related maternal mortality in Massachusetts, 1954–1985. Obstet Gynecol 71:385, 1988

43. O'Driscoll K, Foley M: Correlation of decrease in perinatal mortality and increase in cesarean section rate. Obstet Gynecol 61:1, 1983

44. Leveno KJ, Cunningham FG, Pritchard JA: Cesarean section: an answer to the House of Horne. Am J Obstet Gynecol 153:838, 1985

45. Leveno KJ, Cunningham FG, Prithchard JA: Cesarean section: the House of Horne revisited. Am J Obstet Gynecol 160:78, 1989

46. O'Driscoll K, Foley M, MacDonald D, Stronge J: Cesarean section and perinatal outcome: response from the House of Horne. Am J Obstet Gynecol 158:449, 1988

47. Porreco RP: High cesarean section rate: a new perspective. Obstet Gynecol 65:307, 1985

48. Scheller J, Nelson K: Does cesarean delivery prevent cerebral palsy or other neurologic problems of childhood? Obstet Gynecol 83:624, 1994

49. Nelson KB, Dambrosia JM, Ting TY, Grether JK: Uncertain value of electronic fetal monitoring in predicting cerebral palsy. N Engl J Med 334:613, 1996

50. American College of Obstetricians and Gynecologists; Utility of Umbilical Cord Blood Acid-Base Assessment Committee Opinion No. 91, February 1991

51. American College of Obstetricians and Gynecologists: Fetal Distress and Birth Asphyxia. Committee Opinion No. 137, April 1994

52. Haddad H, Lundy LE: Changing indications for cesarean section: a 38 year experience at a community hospital. Obstet Gynecol 51:133, 1978

53. American Academy of Pediatrics, American College of Obstetricians and Gynecologists; p. 121. Guidelines for Perinatal Care, 3rd Ed. 1992

54. American Academy of Pediatrics, American College of Obstetricians and Gynecologists; p. 124. Guidelines for Perinatal Care. 3rd Ed. 1992

55. NIH Consensus Development Task Force: Statement on Cesarean Childbirth. Am J Obstet Gynecol 139:902, 1981

56. American Academy of Pediatrics, American College of Obstetricians and Gynecologists; p. 80. Guidelines for Perinatal Care, 3rd Ed. 1992

57. Hannah W: Final statement of the panel from the National Consensus Conference on Aspects of Cesarean Birth, Hamilton, Ontario, Canada, 1986

58. American College of Obstetricians and Gynecologists:

Guidelines for Vaginal Delivery After a Previous Cesarean Birth. Committee Opinion No. 64. October 1988

59. American College of Obstetricians and Gynecologists: Vaginal Delivery After a Previous Cesarean Birth, Committee Opinion No. 143 [replaces No. 64, October 1988. October 1994

60. Porreco RP, Meier RP: Repeat cesarean—most unnecessary. Contemp Obstet Gynecol 21:55, 1984

61. Goodenough RD, Molnar JA, Burke JF: Surgical infections. p. 123. In Hardy JD (ed): Hardy's Textbook of Surgery. Philadelphia: JP Lippincott, 1983

62. Cruse PJE, Foord R: The epidemiology of wound infection. Surg Clin North Am 60:27, 1980

63. Dineen P: An evaluation of the duration of the surgical scrub. Surg Gynecol Obstet 129:118, 1969

64. Mead PB, Pories SE, Hall P et al: Decreasing the incidence of surgical wound infections. Arch Surg 121:458, 1986

65. Ritter MS, French MLV, Eitzen HE, Gioe TJ: The antimicrobial effectiveness of operative-site preparative agents. J Bone Joint Surg 62:826, 1980

66. Brown TR, Ehrlich CE, Stehman FB et al: A clinical evaluation of chlorhexidine gluconate spray as compared with iodophor scrub for preoperative skin preparation. Surg Gynecol Obstet 158:363, 1984

67. Alexander JW, Aerni S, Plettner JP: Development of a safe and effective one-minute preoperative skin preparation. Arch Surg 120:1357, 1985

68. Masterson BJ: Skin preparation. Clin Obstet Gynecol 31:736, 1988

69. Larson E: Handwashing and skin physiologic and bacteriologic aspects. Infect Control 6:14, 1985

70. Garner JS: CDC guidelines for the prevention and control of nosocomial infections: guideline for prevention of surgical wound infections, 1985. Am J Infect Control 14:71, 1986

71. Price PB: The bacteriology of normal skin; a new quantitative test applied to a study of the bacterial flora and the disinfectant action of mechanical cleansing. J Infect Dis 63:301, 1938

72. Alexander JW, Fischer JE, Boyajian M et al: The influence of hair-removal methods on wound infections. Arch Surg 118:347, 1983

73. Holtz C: Adhesion induction by suture of varying tissue reactivity and caliber. Int J Fertil 27:134, 1982

74. Kenady DE: Management of abdominal wounds. Surg Clin Orth Am 64:803, 1984

75. Bucknall TE: Abdominal wound closure: choice of suture. JR Soc Med 74:580, 1981

76. Ellis H, Coleridge-Smith PD, Joyce AD: Abdominal incisions—vertical or transverse? Postgrad Med J 60:407, 1984

77. Greenall MJ, Evans M, Pollack AV: Mid-line or transverse laparotomy? A random controlled clinical trial. Br J Surg 67:188, 1980

78. Becquemin J-P, Piquet J, Becquemin M-H et al: Pulmonary function after transverse or midline incision in patients with obstructive pulmonary disease. Int Care Med 11:247, 1985

79. Mowat J, Bonnar J: Abdominal wound dehiscence after cesarean section. BMJ 2:256, 1971

80. Gallup DG: Modification of celiotomy techniques to decrease morbidity in the obese gynecologic patient. Am J Obstet Gynecol 150:171, 1984

81. Finan MA, Mastrogiannis DS, Spellacy WN: The "Allis" test for easy cesarean delivery. Am J Obstet Gynecol 164:772, 1991

82. Maylard AE: Direction of abdominal incisions. BMJ 2: 895, 1907

83. Cherney LS: A modified transverse incision for low abdominal operations. Surg Gynecol Obstet 72:92, 1941

84. Pitkin RM: Abdominal hysterectomy in obese women. Surg Gynecol Obstet 142:532, 1976

85. Shepherd JH, Cavanagh D, Riggs D et al: Abdominal wound closures using a nonabsorbable single layer technique. Obstet Gynecol 61:248, 1983

86. Read JA, Cotton DB, Miller FC: Placenta accreta: changing clinical aspects and outcome. Obstet Gynecol 56:31, 1980

87. Clark SL, Koonings PP, Phelan JP: Placenta previa-accreta and previous cesarean section. Obstet Gynecol 66: 89, 1985

88. Tahilramaney MP, Boucher M, Eglinton GS et al: Previous cesarean section and trial of labor. Factors related to uterine dehiscence. J Reprod Med 29:17, 1984

89. Pritchard JA, McDonald PC, Gant NF (eds): Williams Obstetrics, 17th Ed. Appleton-Century-Crofts, Norwalk, CT 1985

90. Pedowitz P, Schwartz RM: The true incidence of silent rupture of cesarean section scars: a prospective analysis of 403 cases. Am J Obstet Gynecol 74:1701, 1957

91. Rodriguez AI, Porter KB, O'Brien WF: Blunt versus sharp expansion of the uterine incision in low-segment transverse cesarean section. Am J Obstet Gynecol 171: 1022, 1994

92. Janovic R: Incision of the pregnant uterus and delivery of low birthweight infants. Am J Obstet Gynecol 152: 971, 1985

93. Morrison J: The development of the lower uterine segment. Aust NZ J Med 12:182, 1972

94. Nielson TF, Hokegard KH: Cesarean section and intraoperative surgical complications. Acta Obstet Gynaecol Scand 63:103, 1984

95. McCurdy CM Jr, Magann EF, McCurdy CJ, Saltzman AK: The effect of placental management at cesarean delivery on operative blood loss. Am J Obstet Gynecol 167:1363, 1992

96. Queenan JT, Nakamoto M: Postpartum immunization: the hypothetical hazard of manual removal of the placenta. Obstet Gynecol 23:392, 1964

97. Hershey DW, Quilligan EJ: Extraabdominal uterine exteriorization at cesarean section. Obstet Gynecol 52: 189, 1978

98. Magann EF, Dodson MK, Allbert JR et al: Blood loss at time of cesarean section by method of placental removal and exteriorization versus in situ repair of the uterine incision. Surg Gynecol Obstet 177:389, 1993

99. Chatterjee SK: Scar endometriosis: a clinicopathologic study of 17 cases. Obstet Gynecol 56:81, 1980

100. Hauth JC, Owen J, Davis RO: Transverse uterine incision closure: one versus two layers. Am J Obstet Gynecol 167:1108, 1992

101. Hull DB, Varner MW: A randomized study of closure of the peritoneum at cesarean delivery. Obstet Gynecol 77:818, 1991

102. Pietrantoni M, Parsons MT, O'Brien WF et al: Peritoneal closure or non-closure at cesarean. Obstet Gynecol 77:293, 1991

103. Ellis H: The aetiology of post operative abdominal adhesions, an experimental study. Br J Surg 50:10, 1962

104. Ellis H, Heddle R: Does the peritoneum need to be closed at laparotomy? Br J Surg 64:733, 1977

105. Elkins TE, Stovall TG, Warren J: Histological evaluation of peritoneal injury and repair: implications for adhesion formation. Obstet Gynecol 70:225, 1987

106. Tulandi T, Hum HS, Gelfand MM: Closure of laparotomy incisions with or without peritoneal suturing and second-look laparoscopy. Am J Obstet Gynecol 158:536, 1988

107. Sanz LE: Choosing the right wound closure technique. Contemp Ob/Gyn 21:142, 1983

108. Fagniez PL, Hay JM, Lacaine F et al: Abdominal midline incision closure. Arch Surg 120:1351, 1985

109. Sanders RJ, Diclementi, D, Ireland K: Principles of abdominal wound closure. II. Prevention of wound dehiscence. Arch Surg 112:1184, 1977

110. Stone IK, vonFraunhofer JA, Masterson BJ: The biomechanical effects of tight suture closure upon fascia. Surg Gynecol Obstet 163:448, 1986

111. Raghaviah NV, Devi AI: Bladder injury associated with rupture of the uterus. Obstet Gynecol 46:573, 1975

112. Eglinton GS, Phelan JP, Yeh S-Y et al: Outcome of a trial of labor after prior cesarean delivery. J Reprod Med 29:3, 1984

113. Eisenkop SM, Richman R, Platt LD et al: Urinary tract injury during cesarean section. Obstet Gynecol 60:591, 1982

114. Mickal A, Begneaud WP, Hawes TP Jr: Pitfalls and complications of cesarean section hysterectomy. Clin Obstet Gynecol 12:660, 1969

115. Barclay DL: Cesarean hysterectomy. A thirty year experience. Obstet Gynecol 35:120, 1970

116. Everett HS, Mattingly RF: Urinary tract injuries resulting from pelvic surgery. Am J Obstet Gynecol 71:502, 1956

117. Shires GT: Trauma, in Schwartz SI (ed) Principles of Surgery. McGraw-Hill, New York, 1984

118. Carey LC, Catalano PW: The intestinal tract in relation to gynecology. p. 385. In Mattingly RF (ed): TeLinde's Operative Gynecology. JB Lippincott, Philadelphia, 1977

119. Levin S: Selected overview of nongynecologic surgical intraabdominal infections: prophylaxis and therapy. Am J Med, Suppl 79:146, 1985

120. Clark SL, Phelan JP, Yeh SY et al: Hypogastric artery ligation for the control of obstetric hemorrhage. Obstet Gynecol 66:353, 1985

121. Clark SL, Yeh S-Y, Phelan JP et al: Emergency hysterectomy for obstetric hemorrhage. Obstet Gynecol 64:376, 1984

122. Hayashi RH, Castillo MS, Noah ML: Management of severe postpartum hemorrhage due to uterine atony using an analogue of prostaglandin F_2. Obstet Gynecol 58:426, 1981

123. Shaffer D, Benotti PN, Bothe A Jr et al: Subcutaneous drainage in gastric bypass surgery. Infect Surg 5:716, 1986

124. Cruse PJE, Foord R: A five-year prospective study of 23,649 surgical wounds. Arch Surg 107:206, 1973

125. Perkins RP: Extraperitoneal section: a viable alternative. Contemp Obstet Gynecol 9:55, 1977

126. Wallace RL, Eglinton GS, Yonekura ML et al: Extraperitoneal cesarean section: a surgical form of infection prophylaxis? Am J Obstet Gynecol 148:172, 1984

127. Duer EL: Postmortem delivery. Am J Obstet Gynecol 12:1, 1879

128. Katz VL, Dotters DJ, Droegemueller W: Perimortem cesarean delivery. Obstet Gynecol 68:571, 1986

129. Field DR, Gates EA, Creasy R et al: Maternal brain death during pregnancy: medical and ethical issues. JAMA 260:816, 1988

130. Metheny NM: Fluid Balance. 1st Ed. Lippincott, Philadelphia, JB 1984

131. Shires GT, Canizaro PC: Fluid and electrolyte management of the surgical patient. p. 45. In Schwartz S (ed): Principles of Surgery. McGraw-Hill, New York, 1984

132. Rubin GL, Peterson HB, Rochat RW et al: Maternal death after cesarean section in Georgia. Am J Obstet Gynecol 139:681, 1981

133. Frigoletto FD, Phillipe M et al: Avoiding iatrogenic prematurity with elective repeat cesarean section without the use of routine amniocentesis. Am J Obstet Gynecol 137:521, 1980

134. Baskett TF, McMillen RM: Cesarean section: trends and morbidity. Can Med Assoc J 125:723, 1981

135. Danforth DN: Cesarean section. JAMA 253:811, 1985

136. Duff P: Pathophysiology and management of postcesarean endomyometritis. Obstet Gynecol 67:269, 1986

137. Vorherr H: Puerperal genitourinary infection, p. 1. In Sciarra J (ed): Gynecology and Obstetrics, Vol. 2. Harper & Row, Philadelphia, 1982

138. Schwartz WH, Grolle K: The use of prophylactic antibiotics in cesarean section. A review of the literature. J Reprod Med 26:595, 1981

139. Cartwright PS, Pittaway DE, Jones HE et al: The use of prophylactic antibiotics in obstetrics and gynecology: a review. Obstet Gynecol Surv 39:537, 1984

140. Mead PB: Managing infected abdominal wounds. Contemp Obstet/Gynecol 14:69, 1979

141. Wallace D, Hernandez W, Schlaerth JB et al: Prevention of abdominal wound disruption utilizing the Smead-Jones closure technique. Obstet Gynecol 56:26, 1980

142. Green SL, Sarubbi FA: Risk factors associated with postcesarean section febrile morbidity. Obstet Gynecol 49:686, 1977

143. Hawrylyshyn PA, Bernstein P, Papsin FR: Risk factors associated with infection following cesarean section. Am J Obstet Gynecol 139:294, 1981

144. Nielson TF, Hokegard KH: Postoperative cesarean section morbidity: a prospective study. Am J Obstet Gynecol 146:911, 1983

145. Gibbs RS, Blanco JD, St Clair PJ: A case-control study of wound abscess after cesarean delivery. Obstet Gynecol 62:498, 1983

146. Gall SA Jr, Gall SA: Diagnosis and management of post-cesarean wound infections. p. 388. In Phelan JP, Clark SL (eds): Cesarean Delivery. Elsevier Publishers, New York, 1985

147. Sweet RL, Yonekura ML, Hill G et al: Appropriate use of antibiotics in serious obstetric and gynecologic infections. Am J Obstet Gynecol 136:719, 1983

148. Gall SA: Infections in the female genital tract. Comp Ther 9:34, 1983

149. Emmons SL, Krohn M, Jackson M, Eschenbach DA: Development of wound infections among women undergoing cesarean section. Obstet Gynecol 72:559, 1988

150. Kuhn HH, Ullman U, Kuhn FW: New aspects on the pathophysiology of wound infection and wound healing—the problem of lowered oxygen pressure in the tissue. Infection 13:52, 1985

151. Polk HC: Operating room acquired infection: a review of pathogenesis. Am Surg 45:349, 1979

152. Krebs HB, Helmkamp BF: Transverse periumbilical incision in the massively obese patient. Obstet Gynecol 63:241, 1984

153. Dodson MK, Magann EF, Meeks GR: A randomized comparison of secondary closure and secondary intention in patients with superficial wound dehiscence. Obstet Gynecol 80:321, 1992

154. Gerzof SG, Robbins AH, Johnson WC et al: Percutaneous catheter drainage of abdominal abscesses. A five year experience. N Engl J Med 305:653, 1981

155. Gross BH, Callen PW: Ultrasound of the uterus, p. 227. In Callen PW (ed): Ultrasonography in Obstetrics and Gynecology. Philadelphia, WB Saunders, Co, 1982

156. Lee CY, Madrazo BL, Drukker GH: Ultrasonic evaluation of the postpartum uterus in the management of postpartum bleeding. Obstet Gynecol 58:227, 1981

157. Burger NF, Dararas B, Boes EGM: An echographic evaluation during the early puerperium of the uterine wound after cesarean section. J Clin Ultrasound 10:271, 1982

158. Lavery J, Gadwood KA: Postpartum sonography. p. 509. In Sanders RC, Jones E (eds): Ultrasonography in Obstetrics and Gynecology. 4th Ed. Appleton-Century-Crofts Medical, Norwalk, CT, 1991

159. Malvern J, Campbell S, May P: Ultrasonic scanning of the puerperal uterus following secondary postpartum haemorrhage. Br J Obstet Gynaecol 80:320, 1973

160. Shaffer PB, Johnson JC, Bryan D et al: Diagnosis of ovarian vein thrombophlebitis by computed tomography. J Comp Assist Tomogr 5:436, 1981

161. Farrell SJ, Andersen HF, Work BA Jr: Cesarean section: indications and postoperative morbidity. Obstet Gynecol 56:696, 1980

162. Rehu M, Nilsson CG: Risk factors for febrile morbidity associated with cesarean section. Obstet Gynecol 56:269, 1980

163. Bonnar J: Venous thromboembolism and pregnancy. Clin Obstet Gynecol 8:455, 1981

164. Villasanta U: Thromboembolic disease in pregnancy. Am J Obstet Gynecol 93:142, 1965

165. Stead RB: Regulation of hemostasis. p. 27. In Goldhaber AZ (ed): Pulmonary Embolism and Deep Venous Thrombosis. WB Saunders, Philadelphia, 1985

166. Hirsh J, Cade JF, Gallus AS: Anticoagulants in pregnancy: a review of indications and complications. Am Heart J 83:301, 1972

167. Laros RK, Alger LS: Thromboembolism and pregnancy. Clin Obstet Gynecol 22:871, 1979

168. Rosenow ED III, Osmundson PJ, Brown ML: Pulmonary embolism. Mayo Clin Proc 56:161, 1981

169. Duff P, Gibbs RS: Pelvic vein thrombophlebitis: diagnostic dilemma and therapeutic challenge. Obstet Gynecol Surv 38:365, 1983

170. Bartlette RH, Brennan ML, Gazzaniga AB et al: Studies on the pathogenesis and prevention of postoperative pulmonary complications. Surg Gynecol Obstet 137:925, 1973

171. Rosen MA, Hughes SC, Shnider SM: Epidural morphine for the relief of postoperative pain after cesarean delivery. Anesth Analg 62:666, 1983

172. Metcalfe J, Ueland K: Maternal cardiovascular adjustments to pregnancy. Prog Cardiovasc Dis 16:363, 1974

173. Milliman & Robertson: Healthcare Management Guidelines, Vol. 1, Inpatient and Surgical Care. 1995

174. American College of Obstetricians and Gynecologists; Financial Influences on Mode of Delivery. Committee Opinion No. 149. December 1994

175. Bottoms SF, Rosen MG Sokol RJ: The increase in the cesarean birth. N Engl J Med 302:559, 1980

176. Myers SA, Gleicher N: A successful program to lower cesarean-section rates. N Engl J Med 319:1511, 1988

177. O'Driscoll K, Foley M, MacDonald D: Active management of labor as an alternative to cesarean section for dystocia. Obstet Gynecol 63:485, 1984

178. Bergsjo P, Bakketeig LS, Eikhom SN: Case-control analysis of post-term induction of labour. Acta Obstet Gynaecol Scand 61:317, 1982

179. Gibb DMF, Cardozo LD, Studd JWW, Cooper DJ: Prolonged pregnancy: is induction of labour indicated? A prospective study. Br J Obstet Gynaecol 89:292, 1982

180. Hage ML, Helms MJ, Hammond WE, Hammond CB: Changing rates of cesarean delivery: the Duke experience, 1978–1986. Obstet Gynecol 72:98, 1988

181. Porreco RP: Meeting the challenge of the rising cesarean birth rate. Obstet Gynecol 75:133, 1990

182. Sanchez-Ramos L, Kaunitz AM, Peterson HB et al: Reducing cesarean sections at a teching hospital. Am J Obstet Gynecol 163:1081, 1990

183. Pridijian G, Hibbard JU Moawad AH: Cesarean: changing the trends. Obstet Gynecol 77:195, 1991

184. Thorpe-Beeston JG, Banfield PJ, St. G Saunders NJ: Outcome of breech delivery at term. BMJ 305:746, 1992

185. Low JA, Panagiotopoulos C, Derrick EJ: Newborn complications after intrapartum asphyxia with metabolic acidosis in the term fetus. Am J Obstet Gynecol 170:1081, 1994

186. Low JA, Panagiotopoulos C, Derrick EJ: Newborn complications after intrapartum asphyxia with metabolic acidosis in the preterm fetus. Am J Obstet Gynecol 172: 805, 1995

187. Boylan PC, Frankowski R, Rountree R et al: Effective active management of labor on the incidence of cesarean section for dystocia in nulliparous. Am J Perinatol 8:373, 1991

188. Socol ML, Garcia PM, Peaceman AM, Dooley SL: Reducing cesarean births at a primarily private university hospital. Am J Obstet Gynecol 168:1748, 1993

189. Satin AJ, Leveno KJ, Sherman ML et al: High-versus low-dose oxytocin for labor stimulation. Obstet Gynecol 80:111, 1992

190. Cahill DJ, O'Herlihy C, Boylan P: Does oxytocin augmentation increase perinatal risk in primagravid labor? Am J Obstet Gynecol 166:847, 1992

191. Thorpe J, Boylan P, Parisi VM: The influence of high dose oxytocin augmentation on umbilical acid base balance. Am J Obstet Gynecol 159:670, 1988

192. Boylan P: Active management of labor. p. 943. In Flamm BL, Quilligan EJ (eds): Cesarean Section Springer-Verlag, New York, 1995

193. Riva H, Teich J: Vaginal delivery after cesarean section. Am J Obstet Gynecol 81:501, 1961

194. Cowan RK, Kinch RAH, Ellis B, Anderson R: Trial of labor following cesarean delivery. Obstet Gynecol 83: 933, 1994

195. Flamm BL, Newman LA, Thomas SJ et al: Vaginal birth after cesarean delivery: results of a 5-year multicenter collaborative study. Obstet Gynecol 76:750, 1990

196. Nguyen TV, Dinh TV, Suresh MS et al: Vaginal birth after cesarean section at the University of Texas. J Reprod Med 37:880, 1992

197. Flamm B, Goings J, Yunbao L, Wolde-Tsadik G: Elective repeat cesarean delivery versus trial of labor: a prospective multicenter study. Obstet Gynecol 83:927, 1994

198. Average charges for uncomplicated cesarean and vaginal deliveries, United States, 1993. Stat Bull Metrop Insur Co 75:27, 1994

199. Flamm BL: Vaginal birth after cesarean section: controversies old and new. Clin Obstet Gynecol 28:735, 1985

200. Lavin JP, Stephens RJ, Miodovnik M et al: Vaginal delivery in patients with a prior cesarean section. Obstet Gynecol 59:135, 1982

201. Martin JN Jr, Harris BA Jr, Huddleston JF et al: Vaginal delivery following previous cesarean birth. Am J Obstet Gynecol 146:255, 1983

202. Beall M, Eglinton GS, Clark SL et al: Vaginal delivery after cesarean section in women with unknown types of uterine scar. J Reprod Med 29:31, 1984

203. Boucher M, Tahilramaney MP, Eglinton GS et al: Maternal morbidity as related to trial of labor after previous cesarean delivery: a quantitative analysis. J Reprod Med 29:12, 1984

204. Phelan JP, Eglinton GS, Horenstein JM et al: Previous cesarean birth: trial of labor in women with macrosomic infants. J Reprod Med 29:36, 1984

205. Stovall TG, Shaver DC, Solomon SK, Anderson GD: Trial of labor in previous cesarean section patients, excluding classical cesarean sections. Obstet Gynecol 70: 713, 1987

206. Flamm BL, Lim OW, Jones C et al: Vaginal birth after cesarean section: results of a multicenter study. Am J Obstet Gynecol 158:1079, 1988

207. Farmer RM, Kirschbaum T, Potter D et al: Uterine rupture during a trial of labor after previous cesarean section. Am J Obstet Gynecol 165:996, 1991

208. Paul RH, Phelan JP, Yeh S: Trial of labor in the patient with a prior cesarean birth. Am J Obstet Gynecol 151: 297, 1985

209. Farmakides G, Duvivier R, Schulman H et al: Vaginal birth after two or more previous cesarean sections. Am J Obstet Gynecol 154:565, 1987

210. Pruett K, Kirshon B, Cotton D: Unknown uterine scar in trial of labor. Am J Obstet Gynecol 159:807, 1988

211. Miller DA, Diaz FG, Paul RH: Vaginal birth after cesarean: a 10-year experience. Obstet Gynecol 84:255, 1994

212. Rosen MG, Dickinson JC, Westhoff CL: Vaginal birth after cesarean: a meta-analysis of morbidity and mortality. Obstet Gynecol 77:465, 1991

213. Porreco RP, Meier PR: Trial of labor in patients with multiple previous cesarean sections. J Reprod Med 28: 770, 1983

214. American College of Obstetricians and Gynecologists; Vaginal Delivery After Previous Cesarean Birth. Practice Patterns, No. 1. August 1995

215. Hueston WJ, Rudy M: Factors predicting elective repeat cesarean delivery. Obstet Gynecol 83:741, 1994

216. Joseph GF Jr, Stedman CM, Robichaux AG: Vaginal birth after cesarean section: the impact of patient resistance to a trial of labor. Am J Obstet Gynecol 164:1441, 1991

217. American College of Obstetricians and Gynecologists: Vaginal Birth After Cesarean section: Report of 1990 Survey of ACOG's membership, ACOG, Washington, DC, 1990

218. Rosen MG, Dickinson JC: Vaginal birth after cesarean: a meta-analysis of indicators for success. Obstet Gynecol 76:865, 1990

219. Shiono PH, Fielden JR, McNellis D et al: Recent trends in cesarean birth and trial of labor rates in the United States. JAMA 257:494, 1987

220. Phelan JP, Ahn MO, Diaz F et al: Twice a cesarean always a cesarean? Obstet Gynecol 73:161, 1989

221. Thubisi M, Ebrahim A, Moodley J, Shweni PM: Vaginal delivery after previous caesarean section: is X-ray pelvimetry necessary? Br J Obstet Gynaecol 100:421, 1993

222. Krishnamurthy S, Fairlie F, Cameron AD et al: The role of postnatal x-ray pelvimetry after caesarean section in the management of subsequent delivery. Br J Obstet Gynaecol 98:716, 1991

223. Goldman G, Pineault R, Pitvin L et al: Factors influencing the practice of vaginal birth after cesarean section. Am J Public Health 83:1104, 1993

224. Stafford RS: The impact of nonclinical factors on repeat cesarean section. JAMA 265:59, 1991

225. Eglinton GS: Effect of previous indications for cesarean

on subsequent outcome. In Phelan JP, Clark SL (eds): Cesarean Delivery. Elsevier, New York, 1988

226. Horenstein JP, Phelan JP: Previous cesarean section: the risks and benefits of oxytocin usage in a trial of labor. Am J Obstet Gynecol 151:564, 1985

227. Silver RK, Gibbs RS: Prediction of vaginal delivery in patients with a previous cesarean section who require oxytocin. Am J Obstet Gynecol 156:57, 1987

228. Jarrell MA, Ashmead GG, Mann LI: Vaginal delivery after cesarean section: a five year study. Obstet Gynecol 65:628, 1985

229. Saldana LR, Schulman H, Reuss L: Management of pregnancy after cesarean section. Am J Obstet Gynecol 135:555, 1979

230. Miller M, Leader LR: Vaginal delivery after caesarean section. Aust NZJ Obstet Gynaecol 32:213, 1992

231. Seitchik J, Rao VRR: Cesarean delivery in nulliparous women for failed oxytocin-augmented labor: route of delivery in subsequent pregnancy. Am J Obstet Gynecol 143:393, 1982

232. Whiteside DC, Mahan CS, Cook JC: Factors associated with successful vaginal delivery after cesarean delivery after cesarean section. J Reprod Med 28:785, 1983

233. Ollendorff DA, Goldberg JM, Minoque JP, Socol ML: Vaginal birth after cesarean section for arrest of labor: is success determined by maximum cervical dilatation during the prior labor? Am J Obstet Gynecol 159:636, 1988

234. American College of Obstetricians and Gynecologists; Practice perspective: Guidelines for vaginal delivery after previous cesarean birth. Newsletter, February 1985

235. Hankins GDV, Clark SL, Cunningham FG, Gilstrap III LC (eds): Operative Obstetrics, Appleton & Lange, Norwalk, CT, 1995

236. Halperin ME, Moore DC, Hannah WJ: Classical vs. low-segment transverse incision for preterm cesarean section: maternal complications and outcome of subsequent pregnancies. Br J Obstet Gynaecol 95:990, 1988

237. American College of Obstetricians and Gynecologists, Committee on Obstetrics: Maternal and Fetal Medicine: Assessment of Fetal Maturity Prior to Repeat Cesarean Delivery or Elective Induction of Labor. No. 77, January 1990

238. Flamm BL, Goings JR, Fuelberth NJ et al: Oxytocin during labor after previous cesarean section: results of a multicenter study. Obstet Gynecol 70:709, 1987

239. American College of Obstetricians and Gynecologists; Indication and Augmentation of Labor. ACOG Technical Bulletin 157. ACOG, Washington, DC, 1991

240. Arulkumaran S, Chua S, Ratnam SS: Symptoms and signs with scar rupture—value of uterine activity measurements. Aust NZJ Obstet Gynaecol 32:208, 1992

241. Horenstein J, Phelan JP: Vaginal birth after cesarean: the role of oxytocin. In Phelan JP, Clark SL (eds): Cesarean Delivery. Elsevier, New York, 1988

242. Leung AS, Farmer RM, Leung EK et al: Risk factors associated with uterine rupture during trial of labor after cesarean delivery: a case controlled study. Am J Obstet Gynecol 168:1358, 1993

243. Baker ER, D'Alton ME: Management of labor in the nullipara. Clin Consult Obstet Gynecol 4:218, 1992

244. Mackenzie IZ, Bradley S, Embrey MP: Vaginal prostaglandins and labor induction for patients previously delivered by cesarean section. Br J Obstet Gynaecol 91:7, 1984

245. Norman M, Ekman G: Preinductive cervical ripening with prostaglandin E2 in women with one previous cesarean section. Acta Obstet Gynecol Scand 71:351, 1992

246. Blanco JD, Collins M, Willis D, Prien S: Prostaglandin E2 gel induction of patients with a prior low transverse cesarean section. Am J Perinatol 9:80, 1992

247. Flamm BL, Goings JR: Vaginal birth after cesarean section: is suspected fetal macrosomia a contraindication? Obstet Gynecol 74:694, 1989

248. Jones R, Nagashima A, Hartnett-Goodman M, Goodlin R: Rupture of low transverse cesarean scars during trial of labor. Obstet Gynecol 77:815, 1991

249. Rodriguez M, Masaki D, Phelan J, Diaz F: Uterine rupture: are intrauterine pressure catheters useful in the diagnosis? Am J Obstet Gynecol 161:666, 1989

250. Crawford JS: The epidural sieve and and MBC minimal blocking concentration: a hypothesis. Anaesthesia 31:1278, 1976

251. Carlson C, Lybell-Lindahl G, Ingemarsson I: Extradural block in patients who have previously undergone cesarean section. Br J Anaesth 52:827, 1980

252. Uppington J: Epidural analgesia and previous caesarean section. Anaesthesia 38:336, 1983

253. Golan A, Sandbank O, Rubin A: Rupture of the pregnant uterus. Obstet Gynecol 56:349, 1980

254. Flamm BL, Dunnett C, Fischermann E et al: Vaginal delivery following cesarean section: use of oxytocin augmentation and epidural anesthesia with internal tocodynamic and internal fetal monitoring. Am J Obstet Gynecol 148:759, 1984

255. Lowensohn RI, Paul RH, Faless et al: Intrapartum epidural anesthesia: an evaluations of effects on uterine activity. Obstet Gynecol 44:388, 1974

256. Akamatsu TJ, Bonica JJ: Spinal and extradural analgesia-anesthesia for parturition. Clin Obstet Gynecol 17:183, 1974

257. Kaminski HM, Stafl A, Aiman J: The effect of epidural analgesia on the frequency of instrumental obstetric delivery. Obstet Gynecol 69:770, 1987

258. Chestnut DH, Owen CL, Bates JN et al: Continuous infusion epidural analgesia during labor: a randomized, double-blind comparison of 0.625% bupivacaine/0.0002% fentanyl vs 0.125% bupivacaine. Anesthesiology 68:754, 1988

259. Tucker M, Hauth J, Hodgkins P et al: Trial of labor after a one-layer or two-layer closure of a low transverse uterine incision. Obstet Gynecol 168:545, 1993

260. Hansell RS, McMurray KB, Huey GR: Vaginal birth after two or more cesarean sections: a five-year experience. Birth 17:146, 1990

261. Chattopadhyay SK, Sherbeeni MM, Anokute CC: Planned vaginal delivery after two previous caesarean sections. Br J Obstet Gynaecol 101:498, 1994

262. Granovsky-Grisaru S, Shaya M, Diamant YZ: The man-

agement of labor in women with more than one uterine scar: is a repeat cesarean section really the only "safe" option? J Perinat Med 22:13, 1994

263. Pickhardt MG, Martin JN Jr, Meydrech EF et al: Vaginal birth after cesarean delivery: are there useful and valid predictor of success or failure? Am J Obstet Gynecol 166:1811, 1992

264. Chelmow D, Laros RK Jr: Maternal and neonatal outcomes after oxytocin augmentation in patients undergoing a trial of labor after prior cesarean delivery. Obstet Gynecol 80:966, 1992

265. Sakala EP, Kaye S, Murray RD, Munson LJ: Oxytocin use after previous cesarean: why a higher rate of failed labor trial? Obstet Gynecol 356, 1990

266. Plauché WC, Von Almen W, Mueller R: Catastrophic uterine rupture. Obstet Gynecol 64:792, 1984

267. Eden RD, Parker RT, Gall SA: Rupture of the pregnant uterus: a 53 year review. Obstet Gynecol 68:671, 1986

268. Pitkin RM: Once a cesarean? Obstet Gynecol 77:939, 1991

269. Scott J: Mandatory trial of labor after cesarean delivery: an alternative viewpoint. Obstet Gynecol 77:811, 1991

270. Brundenell M, Chakravarti S: Uterine rupture in labour. BMJ 2:122, 1975

271. Eriksen NL, Buttino L Jr: Vaginal birth after cesarean: a comparison of maternal and neonatal morbidity to elective repeat cesarean section. Am J Perinatol 6:375, 1989

272. American Academy of Pediatrics, American College of Obstetricians and Gynecologists; Guidelines for Perinatal Care, 3rd Ed. 1992

273. American College of Obstetricians and Gynecologists, Committee Opinion: Fetal Maturity Assessment Prior to Elective Repeat Cesarean Delivery. No. 98. September 1991.

274. Meier P, Porreco R: Trial of labor following cesarean section: a two year experience. Am J Obstet Gynecol 144:671, 1982

275. American College of Obstetricians and Gynecologists: Ethical Dimensions of Informed Consent. Committee Opinion, No. 108. May 1992

276. Department of Professional Liability, The American College of Obstetricians and Gynecologists; Informed Consent: The Assistant. 1234/89/1 35 40, October, 1987

277. American College of Obstetricians and Gynecologists; Patient Choice: Maternal-Fetal Conflict. Committee Opinion, No. 55. October 1987

278. Abitol MM, Castillo I, Taylor UB et al: Vaginal birth after cesarean section: the patient's point of view. Am Fam Physician 47:129, 1993

279. Lipson JG: Repeat cesarean births: social and psychological issues. JOGN Nurs 13:157, 1984

280. Nielsen TF, Olausson PO, Ingemarsson I: The cesarean section rate in Sweden: the end of the rise. Birth 21:34, 1994

281. Bixby GH: Extirpation of the puerperal uterus by abdominal section. J Gynaecol Soc (Boston) 1:223, 1986

282. Speert H: Eduardo Poor and cesarean hysterectomy. Surg Gynecol Obstet 106:245, 1958

283. Harris JW: A study of the results obtained in sixty-four cesarean sections terminated by supravaginal hysterectomy. Bull Johns Hopkins Hosp 33:318, 1922

284. Stanco LM, Schrimmer DB, Paul RH, Mishell DR Jr: Emergency peripartum hysterectomy and associated risk factors. Am J Obstet Gynecol 168:879, 1993

285. Zelop CM, Harlow BL, Frigoletto FD Jr. et al: Emergency peripartum hysterectomy. Am J Obstet Gynecol 168:1443, 1993

286. Fox H: Placenta accreta, 1945–1969. Obstet Gynecol Surv 17:475, 1972

287. Burchell DR: Physiology of internal iliac artery ligation. J Obstet Gynaecol Br Commonw 75:642, 1968

288. Clark SL, Phelan JP: Surgical control of obstetric hemorrhage. Contemp Obstet Gynecol 24:70, 1984

289. Weed JC: The fate of post cesarean uterus. Obstet Gynecol 14:780, 1959

290. Ward SV, Smith H: Cesarean total hysterectomy: combined section and sterilization. Obstet Gynecol 26:858, 1965

291. Schneider GT, Tyrone CH: Cesarean total hysterectomy: experience of 160 cases. South Med J 59:927, 1968

292. Brenner P, Sall S, Sonnenblick D: Evaluation of cesarean section hysterectomy as a sterilization procedure. Am J Obstet Gynecol 108:335, 1970

293. McNulty JV: Elective cesarean hysterectomy—revisited. Am J Obstet Gynecol 149:29, 1984

294. Park RC, Duff WP: Role of cesarean hysterectomy in modern obstetric practice. Clin Obstet Gynecol 23:601, 1980

295. Hoffman NS, Roberts WS, Fiorica JV et al: Elective cesarean hysterectomy for treatment of cervical neoplasia: an update. J Reprod Med 38:186, 1993

296. Sall S, Rini S, Pineda A: Surgical management of invasive carcinoma of the cervix in pregnancy. Obstet Gynecol 118:1, 1974

297. Thompson JD, Caputo TA, Franklin EW III et al: The surgical management of invasive cancer of the cervix in pregnancy. Am J Obstet Gynecol 121:853, 1975

298. Wingo PA, Huezo CM, Rubin GL et al: The mortality risk associated with hysterectomy. Am J Obstet Gynecol 152:803, 1985

299. Yancey MK, Harlass FE, Benson W, Brady K: The perioperative morbidity of scheduled cesarean hysterectomy. Obstet Gynecol 81:206, 1993

300. Plauché WC, Gruich FG, Bourgeois MO: Hysterectomy at the time of cesarean section: analysis of 108 cases. Obstet Gynecol 58:459, 1981

301. Shepard MK: Female contraceptive sterilization. Obstet Gynecol Surv 29:739, 1974

302. Gomez A, Wood M: Acute appendicitis in pregnancy. Am J Surg 137:180, 1979

303. Bauer JL, Reis RA, Arens RA: Appendicitis in pregnancy with changes in position and areas of normal appendix in pregnancy. JAMA 98:1359, 1932

304. Stauffer RA, Adams A, Wygal J et al: Gallbladder disease in pregnancy. Am J Obstet Gynecol 144:661, 1982

305. Varner MW: Maternal mortality in Iowa from 1952 to 1986. Surg Obstet Gynecol 168:555, 1989

306. Pearlman MD, Tintinalli JE, Lorenz RP: Blunt trauma during pregnancy. N Engl J Med 323:1609, 1990

307. Williams JK, McClain L, Rosemurgy AS, Colorado NM: Evaluation of blunt abdominal trauma in the third trimester of pregnancy: maternal and fetal considerations. Obstet Gynecol 75:33, 1990

308. American College of Obstetricians and Gynecologists: Trauma During Pregnancy. Technical Bulletin 1991

309. Esposito TJ, Gens DR, Gerber-Smith L, Scorpio R: Evaluation of blunt abdominal trauma occurring during pregnancy. J Trauma 29:1628, 1989

310. Higgins SD, Garite TJ: Late abruptio placentae in trauma patients: implications for monitoring. Obstet Gynecol 63:10S, 1984

311. Goodwin TM, Breen MT: Pregnancy outcome and feto-maternal hemorrhage after noncatastrophic trauma. Am J Obstet Gynecol 162:655, 1990

312. Duhrssen A: On the value of deep cervical incisions and episiotomy in obstetrics. Arch Gynaekol 37:27, 1890

313. Baker C, Shingleton HM: Clin Obstet Gynecol 31:701, 1988

314. Prolog. p. 187. In Gynecologic Oncology and Surgery. ACOG, Washington, DC, 1991

315. Breen J, Cregori CA, Kindzierski JA: Hemorrhage in gynecologic surgery. p. 438. Harper Row, Hagerstown, MD, 1981

316. Lees DH, Singer A: Gynecologic Surgery. Vol. 6. Wolfe, 1983

SECTION 4
Postpartum Care

Chapter 20

The Neonate

Adam A. Rosenberg

The first 4 weeks of an infant's life, the neonatal period, are marked by the highest mortality rate in all of childhood. The greatest risk occurs during the first several days after birth. Critical to survival during this period is the infant's ability to adapt successfully to extrauterine life. During the early hours after birth, the newborn must assume responsibility for thermoregulation, metabolic homeostasis, and respiratory gas exchange, as well as undergo the conversion from fetal to postnatal circulatory pathways. This chapter reviews the physiology of a successful transition as well as the implications of circumstances that disrupt this process. Implicit in these considerations is the understanding that the newborn reflects the sum total of its genetic and environmental past as well as any minor or major insults to which it was subjected during gestation and parturition. The period of neonatal adaptation is then most meaningfully viewed as continuum with fetal life.

Cardiopulmonary Transition

Pulmonary Development

Lung development and maturation require a carefully regulated interaction of anatomic, physiologic, and biochemical processes. The outcome of these events provides an organ with adequate surface area, sufficient vascularization, and the metabolic capability to sustain oxygenation and ventilation during the neonatal period. Five stages of morphologic lung development have been identified in the human fetus[1]:

1. Embryonic period—conception to 7 weeks
2. Pseudoglandular period—8th to 16th weeks
3. Canalicular period—17th to 27th weeks
4. Saccular period—28th to 35th weeks
5. Alveolar period—at or after 36 weeks

The lung arises as a ventral diverticulum from the foregut during the fourth week of gestation. During the ensuing weeks, branching of the diverticulum occurs, leading to a tree of narrow tubes with thick epithelial walls composed of columnar-type cells. By 16 weeks, the conducting portion of the tracheobronchial tree up to and including terminal bronchioles has been established. The vasculature derived from the pulmonary circulation develops concurrently with the conducting airways, and by 16 weeks preacinar blood vessels are formed. The canalicular stage is characterized by differentiation of the airways, with widening of the airways and thinning of epithelium. In addition, primitive respiratory bronchioles begin to form, marking the start of the gas-exchanging portion of the lung. Vascular proliferation continues, along with a relative decrease in mesenchyme, bringing the vessels closer to the airway epithelium. The saccular stage is marked by the development of the gas-exchanging portion of the tracheobronchial tree (acinus) composed of respiratory bronchioles, alveolar ducts, terminal saccules, and finally alveoli. During this stage, the pulmonary vessels continue to proliferate with the airways and surround the developing air sacs. The final phase of prenatal lung development (alveolar) is marked by the formation of thin secondary alveolar septae and the remodeling of the capillary bed. Several million alveoli will form before birth, which emphasizes the importance of this last few weeks of pregnancy to pulmonary adaptation. Postnatal lung growth is characterized by generation of alveoli. At birth, there are approximately 20 million airspaces and by 8 years of age, 300 million.[2]

In early gestation, respiratory epithelial cells are simple and columnar in type. A slow transition from columnar epithelium to the lining of a fully developed alveolus starts during the fifth month.[3] By the time of birth, the epithelial lining of the gas-exchanging surface is thin and continuous with two alveolar cell types (types I and II). Type I cells contain few subcellular organelles, while type II cells contain abundant mitochondria, endoplasmic reticulum, Golgi apparatus, and osmiophilic lamellar bodies known to contain surfactant. A scheme for the synthesis of surfactant is presented in Figure 20-1. The kinetics of movement of surfactant from synthesis to lamellar body storage and secretion is slow. Surfactant is secreted as lamellar bodies that unravel into tubular myelin. Tubular myelin is a loose lattice of phospholipids and surfactant-specific proteins. The surface active component of surfactant then adsorbs at the alveolar interface between air and water in a monolayer.[4] With repetitive expansion and compression of the surface monolayer, material is extruded that is either cleared by alveolar macrophages via endocytic pathways or taken up by the type II cell for recycling back into lamellar bodies.[5]

Because of the development of high surface forces along the respiratory epithelium when breathing begins, the availability of surfactants in terminal airspaces is critical to postnatal lung function. Just as surface tension acts to reduce the size of a bubble in water, so too it acts to reduce lung inflation, promoting atelectasis. This is described by the LaPlace relationship, which

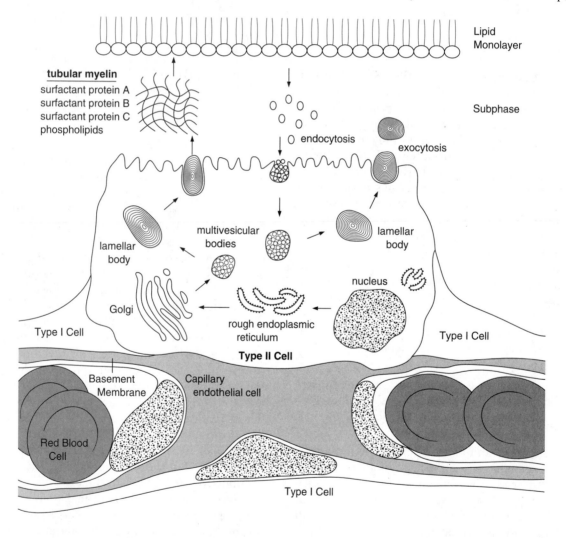

Fig. 20-1 Metabolism of surfactant. Surfactant phospholipids are synthesized in the endoplasmic reticulum, transported through Golgi apparatus to multivesicular bodies, and finally packaged in lamellar bodies. After lamellar body exocytosis, phospholipids are organized into tubular myelin before aligning in a monolayer at the air–fluid interface in the alveolus. Surfactant phospholipids and proteins are taken up by type II cells and either catabolized or reutilized. Surfactant proteins are synthesized in polyribosomes, modified in endoplasmic reticulum, Golgi apparatus, and multivesicular bodies. (Adapted from Whitsett et al.,[154] with permission.)

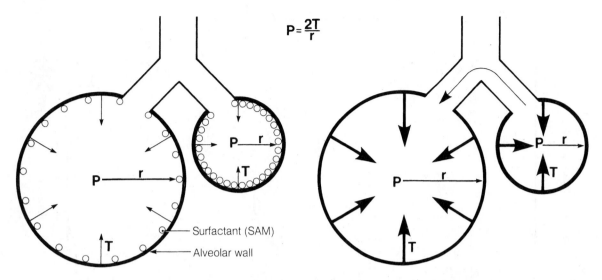

$$P = \frac{2T}{r}$$

Surfactant (SAM)

Alveolar wall

Fig. 20-2 LaPlace's law. The pressure, P, within a sphere is directly proportional to surface tension, T, and inversely proportional to the radius of curvature, r. In the normal lung, as alveolar size decreases, surface tension is reduced because of the presence of surfactant. This serves to decrease the collapsing pressure that needs to be opposed and maintains equal pressures in the small and large interconnected alveoli. (Adapted from Netter,[282] with permission.)

states that the pressure, P, within a sphere is directly proportional to surface tension T and inversely proportional to the radius of curvature r (Fig. 20-2). Surfactant has the physical property of variable surface tension dependent on the degree of surface area compression. In other words, as the radius of the alveolus decreases, surfactant serves to reduce surface tension, preventing collapse of the alveolus. If this property is extrapolated to the lung, smaller alveoli will remain stable due to lower surface tension than other larger alveoli. This feature is emphasized in Figure 20-3, which compares pressure-volume curves from surfactant-deficient and

surfactant-treated preterm rabbits. Surfactant deficiency is characterized by high opening pressure, low maximal lung volume, and lack of deflation stability at low pressures.[6]

Saturated phosphatidylcholine (the surface tension reducing component of surfactant) is found in lung tissue of the human fetus earlier in gestation than in other species (Fig. 20-4).[7] Tissue stores of surfactant are considerable at term. Surfactant is released from storage pools into fetal lung fluid at a basal rate during late gestation. Secretion is stimulated by labor and the initiation of air breathing.[8]

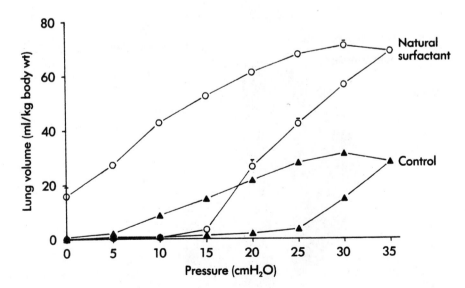

Fig. 20-3 Pressure-volume relationships for the inflation and deflation of surfactant-deficient and surfactant-treated preterm rabbit lungs. (Adapted from Jobe,[6] with permission.)

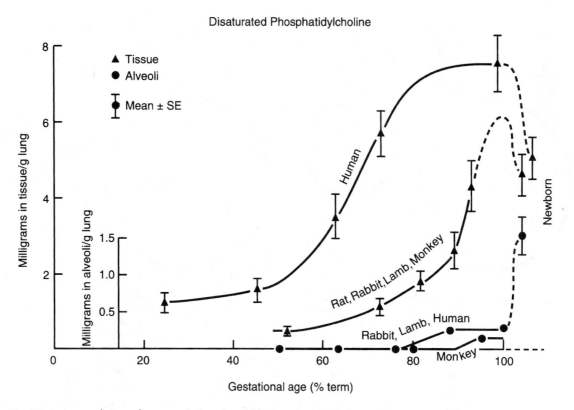

Fig. 20-4 Accumulation of saturated phosphatidylcholine during gestation. Gestational age is plotted as percent age of term. (Adapted from Clements and Tooley,[7] with permission.)

Natural surfactant contains 80 percent phospholipids, 10 percent neutral lipids, and 10 percent protein (Fig. 20-5).[9,10] Approximately half of the protein is specific for surfactant. The principal classes of phospholipids are saturated phosphatidylcholine compounds, 45 percent (more than 80 percent of which are dipalmitoylphosphatidylcholine [DPPC]), 25 percent unsaturated phosphatidylcholine compounds, and 10 percent phosphatidylglycerol, phosphatidylinositol, and phosphatidylethanolamine. Four unique surfactant-associated proteins have been identified.[11–13] All are synthesized and secreted by type II alveolar cells. DPPC is

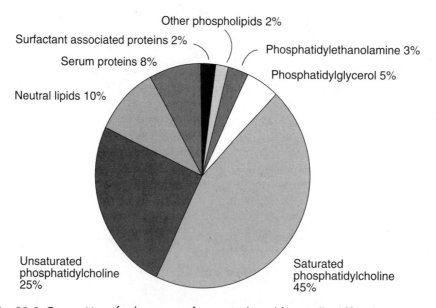

Fig. 20-5 Composition of pulmonary surfactant. (Adapted from Ballard,[10] with permission.)

the molecule critical to the surface tension lowering property of surfactant at the air–liquid interface in the alveolus. Surfactant protein (SP)-A functions cooperatively with the other surfactant proteins and lipids to improve surface properties and regulate secretory and reuptake pathways.[14] SP-B and SP-C are lipophilic proteins that facilitate the adsorption and spreading of lipid to form the surfactant monolayer.[14] SP-D is the least well-described surfactant-associated protein, but appears to function in pulmonary host defense mechanisms.[15]

Several hormones contribute to the regulation of pulmonary phospholipid metabolism: glucocorticords, thyroid hormones, cyclic adenosine mono phosphate (cAMP), and transforming growth factor-β (TGF-β.) The importance of glucocorticoids has been demonstrated in a number of species, and only glucocorticords increase synthesis of each of the known lipid and protein components.[10,16]

Pregnant women with anticipated preterm delivery have received corticosteroid treatment since 1972.[17] Numerous controlled trials have since been done and have been cumulatively evaluated using meta-analysis.[18] Meta-analysis uses quantitative methods to summarize results from a systematic review of randomized controlled trials (Ch. 23). Based on such analysis, a significant reduction of about 50 percent in the incidence of respiratory distress syndrome (RDS) is seen in infants born to mothers who received antenatal corticosteroids. In secondary analysis, a 70 percent reduction in RDS was seen among babies born between 24 hours and 7 days after corticosteroid administration. In addition, evidence suggests a reduction in mortality and RDS even with treatment started less than 24 hours before delivery. Although most babies in the trials were between 30 and 34 weeks' gestation, clear reduction in RDS was evident when the population of babies less than 31 weeks was examined. Gender and race do not influence the protective effect of corticosteroids. In the population of patients with preterm premature rupture of the membranes, antenatal corticosteroids also reduce the frequency of RDS, although the magnitude of reduction was not so great as with intact membranes.

Corticosteroids also accelerate maturation of other organs in the developing fetus, including cardiovascular, gastrointestinal, and central nervous system. Corticosteroid therapy reduces the chances of both periventricular-intraventricular hemorrhage and necrotizing enterocolitis.[18,19] The significant reductions in serious neonatal morbidity are also reflected in a reduction in the risk of early neonatal mortality. The short-term beneficial effects of antenatal corticosteroids are enhanced by reassuring reports about long-term outcome. The children of mothers treated with antenatal corticosteroids show no lag in intellectual or motor development, no increase in learning disabilities or behavioral disturbances, and no effect on growth compared with untreated infants.[20,21]

Since the advent of antenatal steroids for the prevention of RDS, other maternal and neonatal therapies have been introduced that decrease mortality and morbidity. Surfactant replacement therapy to treat specifically the surfactant deficiency that is the cause of RDS has been shown to decrease mortality and the severity of RDS.[9,22–24] The effects of antenatal corticosteroids and postnatal surfactant appear to be additive in terms of decreasing the severity of and mortality due to RDS.[25] Finally, in recent years thyroid-releasing hormone (TRH) has been introduced as an agent to accelerate lung maturation. TRH efficiently crosses the placenta and elicits a striking fetal TSH response.[26] Animal studies have demonstrated improvement in fetal pulmonary maturation after maternal administration of TRH.[27] In addition, thyroid hormone has an additive effect with glucocorticoid on choline incorporation into phosphatidylcholine[28] and is synergistic with cortisol and prolactin in increasing lung compliance and surfactant production.[29] In the largest clinical trial done thus far, betamethesone plus TRH did not affect the total incidence of RDS when compared with betamethasone alone (controls). However, chronic lung disease developed in significantly fewer TRH-treated infants than controls.[30] A review of all available information on antenatal TRH plus glucocorticoids show a decrease in the incidence of RDS, mortality, and chronic lung disease.[16]

The First Breaths

A critical step in the transition from intrauterine to extrauterine life is the conversion of the lung from a dormant fluid-filled organ to one capable of gas exchange. This requires aeration of the lungs, establishment of an adequate pulmonary circulation, ventilation of the aerated parenchyma, and diffusion of oxygen and carbon dioxide through the alveolar-capillary membranes. This process has its roots in utero as fetal breathing.

Fetal Breathing

Fetal breathing has been demonstrated in a large number of mammalian species.[31] Fetal breathing has been most extensively studied in fetal sheep and to a lesser degree in humans. Fetal breathing in third trimester fetal sheep occurs primarily during periods of low voltage electrocortical activity (REM sleep).[32,33] The predominant respiratory pattern is one of rapid, irregular movements varying in amplitude at a rate of 60 to 120/ min. Isolated deep inspiratory efforts can occur at one to three times per minute unassociated with any particular stage of sleep. During high voltage electrocortical activity (quiet sleep), only occasional breaths occur after tonic muscular discharges associated with body movements. During non-REM sleep, the breathing movements are inhibited by a mechanism situated in the midbrain and pons.[34,35] Developmental studies on the ontogeny of fetal breathing have been conducted primarily in the fetal lamb and to a lesser extent the human fetus. The onset of breathing in the fetal sheep has been noted as early as 40 days of gestation. By days 90 through 115, breathing is almost continuous, with rare apneic pauses of less than 2 minutes duration. From day 115 to term, breathing is episodic as described above. Human fetal breathing is quite similar to that observed in fetal sheep.[36] Respiratory activity is initially detectable at 11 weeks. The most prevalent pattern is rapid, small-amplitude movements (60 to 90 per minute) present 60 to 80 percent of the time. Less commonly, irregular low-amplitude movements interspersed with slower larger amplitude movements are seen.

Initially, fetal breathing was thought to depend on behavioral influences. However, subsequent work has shown responses to chemical stimuli and other agents. Acute hypercapnea stimulates breathing in both human and sheep fetuses.[37,38] Hypoxia abolishes fetal breathing,[38] while an increase in oxygen tension to levels above 200 mmHg induces continuous fetal breathing.[39] Hyperglycemia after bolus injections of glucose to the mother or after ingestion of a meal increases fetal breathing in humans.[40,41] Of the pulmonary reflexes, the inflation reflex (decreasing frequency of breathing) is active in fetal life.[42] Peripheral and central chemoreflexes as well as vagal afferent reflexes can be demonstrated in the fetus, but their role in spontaneous fetal breathing appears minimal.[43]

Breathing is intermittent in the fetus and becomes continuous after birth. The mechanism responsible for this transition is unknown. In the fetal lamb, the REM sleep dependence of breathing can be overcome in a number of ways. The most profound continuous intrauterine breathing is caused by prolonged infusion of large doses of prostaglandin synthesis inhibitors,[44] suggesting that prostaglandins may be involved in the transition to continuous postnatal respiration. Other factors surrounding birth, including blood gas changes and various sensory stimuli, are also postulated to be involved.[43,45] Another factor possibly involved is the "release" from a placental inhibitory factor that is removed after cord occlusion.[39,43]

The role of fetal breathing in the continuum from fetal to neonatal life is still not completely understood. Fetal respiratory activity is probably essential to the development of chest wall muscles (including diaphragm) and serves as a regulator of lung fluid volume and thus lung growth.[43]

Mechanics of the First Breath

With its first breaths, the neonate must overcome several forces resisting lung expansion: (1) viscosity of fetal lung fluid, (2) resistance provided by lung tissue itself, and (3) the forces of surface tension at the air–liquid interface.[46] Viscosity of fetal lung fluid is a major factor as the neonate attempts to displace fluid present in the large airways. As the passage of air moves toward small airways and alveoli, surface tension becomes more important. Resistance to expansion by the lung tissue itself is less significant. The process begins as the infant passes through the birth canal. The intrathoracic pressure caused by vaginal squeeze is up to 200 cmH$_2$O.[47,48] With delivery of the head, approximately 5 to 28 ml of tracheal fluid is expressed. Subsequent delivery of the thorax causes an elastic recoil of the chest. With this recoil, a small passive inspiration (no more than 2 ml) occurs.[47] This is accompanied by glossopharyngeal forcing of some air into the proximal airways (frog breathing)[49] and the introduction of some blood into pulmonary capillaries.[50,51] This pulmonary vascular pressure may have a role in producing initial continuous surfaces throughout the small airways of the lung into which surfactant can deploy.[51]

The initial breath is characteristically a short inspiration followed by a more prolonged expiration (Fig. 20-6).[47,52,53] The initial breath begins with no air volume and no transpulmonary pressure gradient. Considerable negative intrathoracic pressure during inspiration is provided by diaphragmatic contraction and chest wall expansion. An opening pressure of about 25 cm H$_2$O usually is necessary to overcome surface tension in the smaller airways and alveoli before air begins to enter. The volume of this first breath varies between

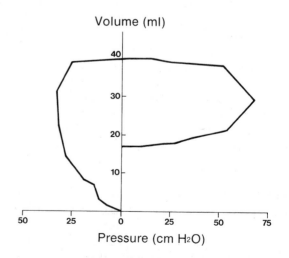

Fig. 20-6 Pressure volume loop of the first breath. Air enters the lung as soon as intrathoracic pressure falls and expiratory pressure greatly exceeds inspiratory pressure. (Modified from Milner and Vyas,[47] with permission.)

30 and 67 ml and correlates with intrathoracic pressure. The expiratory phase is quite prolonged as the infant's expiration is opposed by intermittent closure at the pharyngolaryngeal level[49] with the generation of large positive intrathoracic pressure. This pressure serves to aid both in maintenance of a functional residual capacity (FRC) and with fluid removal from the air sacs. The residual volume after this first breath ranges between 4 and 30 ml, averaging 16 to 20 ml. There are really no major systematic differences among the first three breaths, demonstrating similar pressure patterns of decreasing magnitude. The FRC rapidly increases with the first several breaths and then more gradually. By 30 minutes of age, most infants attain a normal FRC with uniform lung expansion.[54] The presence of functional surfactant is instrumental in the accumulation of an FRC.[7,8]

In utero, alveoli are open and stable at nearly neonatal lung volume because they are filled with fetal lung liquid, probably produced by ultrafiltration of pulmonary capillary blood as well as by secretion by alveolar cells.[55] Thus, normal expansion and aeration of the neonatal lung is also dependent on removal of fetal lung liquid. This process begins before a normal term birth because of either decreased fluid secretion or to increased absorption.[56] Factors involved in this process postnatally are (1) the thoracic squeeze during delivery, (2) a marked increase in pulmonary lymph flow, and (3) removal via the pulmonary circulation.[56,57] The role of the thoracic squeeze in fluid removal is thought to be minimal during a normal birth.[56] With the onset of breathing, residual liquid from the lung lumen moves into the interstitium. Puddling of fluid in connective tissue spaces away from sites of gas exchange allows time for the pulmonary microcirculation and lymphatics to remove the fluid.[58,59] In normal circumstances, the process is complete within six hours of birth. Cesarean-delivered infants without benefit of labor and premature infants have delayed lung fluid clearance. In both groups, the prenatal decrease in lung water does not occur.[56,60] In addition, in the premature, fluid clearance is diminished by increased alveolar surface tension, increased left atrial pressure, and hypoproteinemia.[56,61] Overall, lymphatic pathways remove about 10 percent of lung liquid, with most fluid taken up by the pulmonary circulation.[59]

Circulatory Transition

The circulation in the fetus (Fig. 20-7) has been studied in a variety of species using several techniques (see Ch. 3). These studies have been the subject of a number of excellent reviews.[62–65]

Umbilical venous blood, returning from the placenta, has a P_{O_2} of about 30 to 35 mmHg. Due to the left shift of the oxyhemoglobin disassociation curve due to fetal hemoglobin, this corresponds to a saturation of 80 to 90 percent. About 50 percent of this blood passes through the liver (mainly to the middle and left lobes). This blood will ultimately enter the inferior vena cava (IVC) through the hepatic veins. The remainder bypasses the hepatic circulation via the ductus venosus, which empties directly into the IVC. As it enters the heart, most of the IVC blood is deflected by the crista dividers through the foramen ovale to the left atrium. The remainder of left atrial blood is the small amount of venous return from the pulmonary circulation. Almost all the return from the superior vena cava (SVC) and the coronary sinus passes through the tricuspid valve to the right ventricle, with only 2 to 3 percent crossing the foramen ovale. In the near-term fetus, the combined ventricular output is about 450 ml/kg/min. Two-thirds of the cardiac output is from the right ventricle, and one-third is from the left ventricle. The blood in the left ventricle has a P_{O_2} of 25 to 28 mmHg (saturation of 60 percent) and is distributed to the coronary circulation, brain, head, and upper extremities, with the remainder (10 percent of combined output) passing into the descending aorta. The major portion of the right ventricular output (60 percent of combined output) is carried by the ductus arteriosus to the descending aorta, with only 7 percent of combined output going to the lungs. Thus 70 percent of combined output passes through the descending aorta, with a P_{O_2} of 20 to 23 mmHg (saturation of 55 percent) to supply the abdominal viscera and lower extremities. Fifty percent of combined output will go through the umbilical arteries to the placenta. This arrangement provides blood of a higher P_{O_2} to the critical coronary and cerebral circulations and serves to divert venous blood to where oxygenation occurs.

The diversion of right ventricular output away from the lungs through the ductus arteriosus is due to the very high pulmonary vascular resistance (PVR) in the fetus. This high pulmonary pressure results from chronic exposure to a low P_{O_2} causing vasoconstriction and an increase in the medial muscle layer in pulmonary arteries.[63,66] In addition, compression of capillaries by fetal lung liquid may contribute to pulmonary vascular resistance.[67] With advancing gestational age, an increase in the number of small pulmonary vessels occurs that increases the cross-sectional area of the pulmonary vasculature. This contributes to the gradual decline in PVR that begins during later gestation (Fig. 20-8). With delivery, a variety of factors interact to decrease PVR acutely. Mechanical expansion of the lungs with a hypoxic gas mixture causes a decrease in PVR and a fourfold increase in pulmonary blood flow.[68] When oxygen was used to ventilate in this study, a further increase in pulmonary blood flow was seen due to an

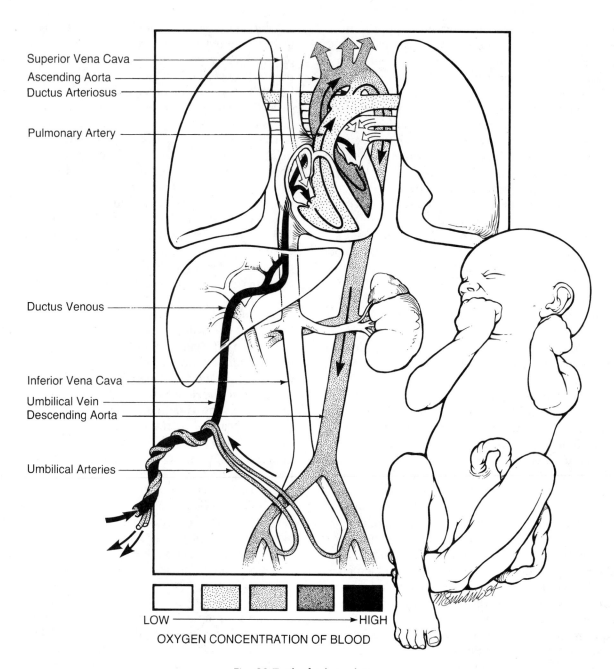

Superior Vena Cava

Ascending Aorta

Ductus Arteriosus

Pulmonary Artery

Ductus Venous

Inferior Vena Cava

Umbilical Vein

Descending Aorta

Umbilical Arteries

LOW ⟶ HIGH

OXYGEN CONCENTRATION OF BLOOD

Fig. 20-7 The fetal circulation.

increase in oxygen tension of the blood. Finally, various hormones and vascular mediators may be involved in the decrease in PVR after birth. Increased production of endothelium-derived relaxing factor or nitric oxide may play an important role in this regard.[69,70]

With the increase in pulmonary flow, left atrial return increases with a rise in left atrial pressure (Table 20-1) In addition, with the removal of the placenta, inferior vena cava return to the right atrium is diminished. The foramen ovale is a flap valve, and, when left atrial pressure increases over that on the right side, the opening is functionally closed. It is still possible to demonstrate

patency with insignificant right to left shunts in the first 12 hours of life in a human neonate, but in a 7- to 12-day newborn such a shunt is rarely seen, although anatomic closure is not complete for a longer time.

With occlusion of the umbilical cord, the large run-off of blood to the placenta is interrupted, causing an increase in systemic pressure. This, coupled with the decrease in right-sided pressures, serves to reverse the shunt through the ductus arteriosus to a predominantly left to right shunt. By 15 hours of age, shunting in either direction is physiologically insignificant.[71] Although functionally closed by 4 days of age,[72] the duc-

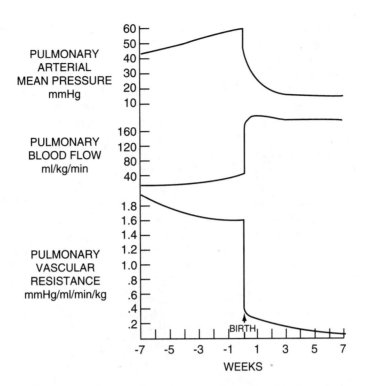

Fig. 20-8 Representative changes in pulmonary hemodynamics during transition from the late-term fetal circulation to the neonatal circulation. (Adapted from Rudolph,[63] with permission.)

tus is not irreversibly and anatomically occluded for 1 month. The role of an increased oxygen environment in ductal closure is well established.[73] Prostaglandin metabolism has also been shown to play an important role in ductal patency in utero and in closure after birth.[74] Ductal closure appears to occur in two phases: constriction and destruction. Initially, the muscular wall constricts followed by permanent closure achieved by endothelial destruction, subintimal proliferation, and connective tissue formation.[75] The ductus venosus is functionally occluded shortly after the umbilical circulation is interrupted.[62]

Shortly after birth in the neonatal lamb, resting cardiac output is about 350 ml/kg/min.[63] This represents an increase in left ventricular output from about 150 (fetal) to 350 (postnatal) ml/kg/min, while right ventricular output increases from 300 (fetal) to 350 (postnatal)

ml/kg/min. The most dramatic increase in individual organ blood flow is that to the lungs (30 to 350 ml/kg/min). Myocardial, renal, and gastrointestinal blood flows also increase, while adrenal, cerebral, and carcass flows decrease.[76]

Abnormalities of Cardiopulmonary Transition

Birth Asphyxia

Even normal infants may experience some asphyxia during the birth process. A variety of circumstances can exaggerate the degree of asphyxia, resulting in a depressed infant, including (1) acute interruption of umbilical blood flow, as occurs during cord compression; (2) premature placental separation; (3) maternal hypotension or hypoxia; (4) any of the above superimposed on chronic uteroplacental insufficiency; and (5) failure to execute a proper resuscitation.[77] Other contributing factors include anesthetics and analgesics used in the mother, mode and difficulty of delivery, maternal health, and prematurity.

Fortunately, some characteristics of the newborn provide protection from these insults. The fetus and neonate are more resistant to asphyxia than are adults.[78] In response to asphyxia, the mature fetus redistributes blood flow to the critical cardiac, cerebral, and adrenal circulations.[79] Unlike adults, who develop

Table 20-1   Pressures in the Perinatal Circulation

	Fetal (mmHg)	Neonatal (mmHg)
Right atrium	4	5
Right ventricle	65/10	40/5
Pulmonary artery	65/40	40/25
Left atrium	3	7
Left ventricle	60/7	70/10
Aorta	60/40	70/45

(Modified from Nelson,[283] with permission.)

tachycardia in response to hypoxia, the fetus responds initially with a reflex bradycardia.[80] As the fetus becomes more hypoxic, it becomes dependent on anaerobic glycolysis to meet energy requirements. During asphyxia, glucose can be released from glycogen stores into the circulation to increase substrate availability.[81,82] In addition, in response to hypoxia, there is a reduction in body movements, a cessation of fetal breathing, and diminished energy utilization by the brain.[83,84] Cumulatively, these features may serve to protect vital organ function.

The neonatal response to asphyxia follows a predictable pattern demonstrable in a number of species. Dawes[85] investigated the responses of the newborn rhesus monkey (Fig. 20-9). After delivery, the umbilical cord was tied and the monkey's head was placed in a plastic bag. Within about 30 seconds, a short series of respiratory efforts began. These were interrupted by a convulsion or a series of clonic movements accompanied by an abrupt fall in heart rate. The animal then lay inert with no muscle tone. Skin color became progressively cyanotic and then blotchy because of vasoconstriction in an effort to maintain systemic blood pressure. This initial period of apnea lasted about 30 to 60 seconds. The monkey then began to gasp at a rate of three to six per minute. The gasping lasted for

about 8 minutes, becoming weaker terminally. The time from onset of asphyxia to last gasp could be related to postnatal age and maturity at birth; the more immature the animal, the longer the time. Secondary or terminal apnea followed and, if resuscitation was not quickly initiated, death ensued. As the animal progressed through the phase of gasping and then on to terminal apnea, heart rate and blood pressure continued to fall, indicating hypoxic depression of myocardial function. As the heart failed, blood flow to critical organs decreased, resulting in organ injury.

The response to resuscitation has also been described in great detail and is qualitatively similar in all species, including humans.[86,87] During the first period of apnea, almost any physical or chemical stimulus will cause the animal to breathe. If gasping has already ceased, the first sign of recovery with initiation of positive pressure ventilation is an increase in heart rate. The blood pressure then rises, rapidly if the last gasp has only just passed, but more slowly if the duration of asphyxia has been longer. The skin then becomes pink, and gasping ensues. Rhythmic spontaneous respiratory efforts become established after a further interval. For each 1 minute past the last gasp, two minutes of positive-pressure breathing is required before gasping begins and 4 minutes to reach rhythmic breathing. Not until some time later do the spinal and corneal reflexes return. Muscle tone gradually improves over the course of several hours.

Delivery Room Management of the Newborn

A number of situations during pregnancy, labor, and delivery place the infant at increased risk for asphyxia. (1) maternal diseases, such as diabetes and hypertension, third trimester bleeding, and prolonged rupture of membranes; (2) fetal conditions, such as prematurity, multiple births, growth retardation, fetal anomalies, and rhesus isoimmunization; and (3) conditions related to labor and delivery, including fetal distress, meconium staining, breech presentation, and administration of anesthetics and analgesics.

When an asphyxiated infant is expected, a resuscitation team should be in the delivery room. The team should have at least two persons, one to manage the airway and one to monitor heart rate and provide whatever assistance is needed. The necessary equipment for an adequate resuscitation is listed in Table 20-2. The equipment should be checked regularly and should be in a continuous state of readiness.

Steps in the resuscitation process[88] are as follows (Fig. 20-10):

1. Dry the infant well and place under the radiant heat source.

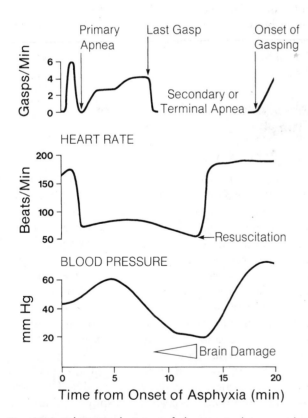

Fig. 20-9 Schematic depiction of changes in rhesus monkeys during asphyxia and on resuscitation by positive pressure ventilation. (Adapted from Dawes,[85] with permission.)

Table 20-2   Equipment for Neonatal Resuscitation

Clinical Needs	Equipment
Thermoregulation	Radiant heat source with platform, mattress covered with warm sterile blankets, servo control heating, temperature probe
Airway management	*Suction:* bulb suction, DeLee suction apparatus, wall vacuum suction with sterile catheters *Ventilation:* manual infant resuscitation bag connected to pressure manometer capable of delivering 100% oxygen, appropriate masks for term and preterm infants *Intubation:* neonatal laryngoscope with #0 and #1 blades; endotracheal tubes 2.5, 3.0, and 3.5 mm OD with stylet
Gastric decompression	Nasogastric tubes 5.0 and 8.0 Fr
Administration of drugs/volume	Sterile umbilical catheterization tray, umbilical catheters (3.5 and 5.0 Fr), volume expanders (Ringer's lactate, 5% albumin), drug box with appropriate neonatal vials and dilutions (Table 20-5), sterile syringes, and needles
Transport	Warmed transport isolette with oxygen source

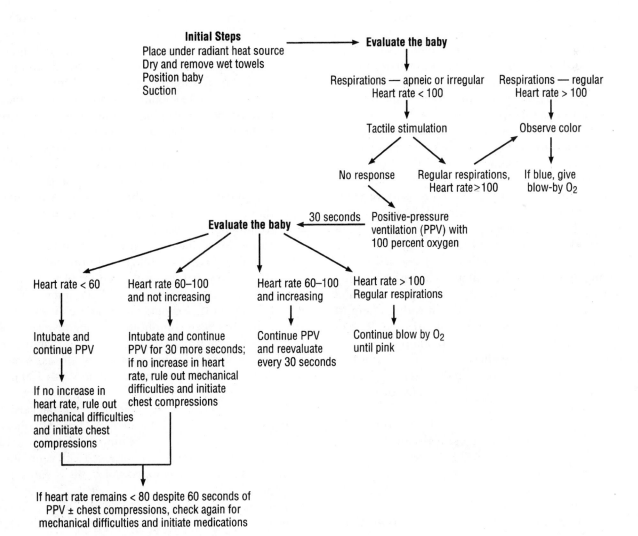

Fig. 20-10 Delivery room management of the newborn. HR, heart rate; PPV, positive-pressure ventilation.

Table 20-3   The Apgar Scoring System

Sign	0	1	2
Heart rate	Absent	<100/min	>100/min
Respiratory effort	Apneic	Weak, irregular, gasping	Regular
Reflex irritability[a]	No response	Some response	Facial grimace, sneeze, cough
Muscle tone	Flaccid	Some flexion	Good flexion of arms and legs
Color	Blue, pale	Body pink, hands and feet blue	Pink

[a] Elicited by suctioning the oropharynx and nose.
(Modified from Apgar,[89] with permission.)

2. Gently suction the oropharynx and nose.

3. Assess the infant's condition (Table 20-3). The best criteria to assess are the infant's respiratory effort (apneic, gasping, regular) and heart rate (more or less than 100). A depressed heart rate indicative of hypoxic myocardial depression is the single most reliable indicator of the need for resuscitation.[87,89]

4. Generally, infants with heart rates over 100 bpm will require no further intervention. Infants with heart rates less than 100 bpm with apnea or irregular respiratory efforts should be vigorously stimulated by rubbing the baby's back with a towel while blowing oxygen over the face.

5. If the baby fails to respond rapidly to tactile stimulation, proceed to bag and face mask ventilation, using a soft mask that seals well around the mouth and nose. For the initial inflations, pressures of 30 to 40 cmH_2O may be necessary to overcome surface active forces in the lungs. A 1- to 2-second inspiratory time may be helpful as well.[90] In the premature infant even higher pressures (40 to 60 cmH_2O) may be needed. Adequacy of ventilation is assessed by observing expansion of the infant's chest with bagging and a gradual improvement in color, perfusion, and heart rate. After the first few breaths, attempts should be made to lower the peak pressure. Rate of bagging should not exceed 40 to 60 bpm.

6. Most neonates can be effectively resuscitated with a bag and face mask. However, if there is not favorable response in 30 to 40 seconds, one must proceed to intubation:

   a. The head should be stable, with the nose in the sniffing position (pointing straight upward).
   b. Insert the laryngoscope blade, and sweep the tongue to the left.
   c. Advance the blade to the base of the tongue, and identify the epiglottis.
   d. Pick up the endotracheal tube with the right hand.
   e. Slide the laryngoscope anterior to the epiglottis, and gently lift along the angle of the handle of the laryngoscope.
   f. Identify the vocal cords.
   g. Insert the tube in the right side of the mouth, and visualize the tube passing through the vocal cords.
   h. Ventilate as described above.
   i. Failure to respond to intubation and ventilation can result from (i) mechanical difficulties (Table 20-4), (ii) profound asphyxia with myocardial depression, and (iii) inadequate circulating blood volume.
   j. The mechanical causes listed in Table 20-4 should be quickly ruled out. Check to be sure the endotracheal tube passes through the vocal cords. Occlusion of the tube should be suspected when there is resistance to bagging and no chest wall movement. If the endotracheal tube is in place, not occluded, and equipment functioning, a trial of bagging with higher pressures is indicated. The other causes listed in Table 20-4 are rare compared with equipment failure or tube problems. A pneumothorax is characterized by asymmetric breath sounds not corrected by repositioning the tube above the carina. Pleural effusions usually occur with fetal hydrops, while a diaphragmatic hernia should be ruled out in the setting of asymmetric breath sounds and a scaphoid abdomen. Pulmonary hypoplasia should be considered if the pregnancy has been complicated by oligohydramnios. It is very unusual for a neonatal resuscitation to require either cardiac massage or drugs. Almost all newborns respond to ventilation with 100 percent oxygen.

7. If mechanical causes are ruled out, external cardiac massage should be performed for persistent heart rate at less than 100 bpm. Compression of 1 to 1.5 cm should be performed, interposed with ventilation at a 3:1 ratio (90 compressions: 30 breaths per minute).

8. If drugs are needed (Table 20-5), the drug of choice is 0.1 to 0.3 ml/kg of 1:10,000 epinephrine through the endotracheal tube or preferably an umbilical venous line. Sodium bicarbonate 1 to 2 mEq/kg of the neonatal dilution can be used for a *documented*. metabolic acidosis. If volume loss is suspected (e.g., docu-

Table 20-4   Mechanical Causes of Failed Resuscitation

Category	Examples
Equipment failure	Malfunctioning bag, oxygen not connected or running
Endotracheal tube malposition	Esophagus, right mainstem bronchus
Occluded endotracheal tube	
Insufficient inflation pressure to expand lungs	
Space-occupying lesions in the thorax	Pneumothorax, pleural effusions, diaphragmatic hernia
Pulmonary hypoplasia	Extreme prematurity, oligohydramnios

mented blood loss with clinical evidence of hypovolemia), 10 ml/kg of a volume expander (5 percent albumin, Ringer's lactate) should be administered through an umbilical venous line. The appropriateness of continued resuscitative efforts should always be reevaluated in an infant who fails to respond to all of the above effort. Today resuscitative efforts are made even in "apparent stillbirths," that is, infants whose 1-minute Apgars scores are 0 to 1. However, efforts should not be sustained in the face of little or no improvement over a reasonable period of time (i.e., 10 to 15 minutes).[91]

A few special circumstances merit discussion at this point. Infants in whom respiratory depression secondary to narcotic administration is suspected may be given naloxone (Narcan). However, this should not be done until the airway has been managed and the infant resuscitated in the usual fashion. A second special group are preterm infants. Minimizing heat loss improves survival so prewarmed towels should be available, and the environmental temperature of the delivery suite should be raised. In the extremely low birth weight infant (less than 1,000 g), proceed quickly to intubation. Volume expanders and sodium bicarbonate should be infused slowly to avoid rapid swings in blood pressure.

Finally, there is the issue of meconium-stained amniotic fluid. Meconium aspiration syndrome (MAS) in a form of aspiration pneumonia that occurs most often in term or post-term infants who have passed meconium in utero (7 to 22 percent of all deliveries[92]). Death rates as high as 40 percent have been reported (although most surveys report 10 to 20 percent[92]) with conventional medical management. Delivery room management of meconium in the amniotic fluid has been based on the notion that aspiration takes place with the initiation of extrauterine respiration and that the pathologic condition is related to the aspirated contents. This resulted in the practice of oropharyngeal suction on the perineum after delivery of the head followed by airway visualization and suction by the resuscitator after delivery.[93] Both of these assumptions are now being questioned. Meconium is found below the vocal cords in 35 percent of births from meconium-stained fluid.[92] In utero aspiration has been induced in animal models[92,94] and confirmed in autopsies of human stillbirths.[92,95] In addition, the combined suction approach to prevention of MAS has not been uniformly successful in decreasing the incidence of MAS.[92,96,97] Further concern has been raised by the experience that routine suctioning of the neonatal airway has been associated itself with respiratory morbidity.[98,99] Of note as well is the finding that infants with meconium-stained fluid in whom only pharyngeal suctioning is performed suffer no increase in the incidence of MAS.[98,99] In terms of the role of meconium in the genesis of MAS, 35 percent of infants born with meconium in the amniotic fluid will have meconium in the lungs. Up to 55 percent will have abnormal chest X-

Table 20-5   Neonatal Drug Doses

Drug	Dose	Route	How Supplied
Epinephrine	0.1–0.3 mL/kg	IV or ET	1:10,000 dilution
Sodium bicarbonate[a]	1–2 mEq/kg	IV	0.5 mEq/ml (4.2% solution)
Volume[b]	10 ml/kg	IV	Whole blood, 5 percent albumin, Ringer's lactate, Normal saline
Naloxone (Narcan)[c]	0.1 mg/kg	IV, ET, IM or SQ	0.4 mg/ml or 1 mg/ml

Abbreviations: IV, intravenous; ET, endotracheal; IM, intramuscular; SQ, subcutaneous.

[a] For correction of metabolic acidosis only after adequate ventilation has been achieved; give slowly over several minutes.

[b] Infuse slowly over several minutes.

[c] After proceeding with proper airway management and other resuscitative techniques.

(Modified from American Heart Association and American Academy of Pediatrics.[88])

rays, yet respiratory distress develops in only 5 to 10 percent of these infants.[92] Severe MAS is associated with persistent pulmonary hypertension of the newborn and is likely the result of a long-standing intra-uterine process with meconium only a marker of intra-uterine hypoxia.[100,101]

Current clinical and experimental data support that MAS is the result of intrauterine asphyxia. The best method of prevention is to identify the fetus at risk (post-term, oligohydramnios). Intrapartum management should emphasize treatments that enhance utero-placental perfusion. Aminoinfusion in cases with oligo-hydramnios may reduce cord compression, gasping, and intrapartum aspiration.[102,103] The management of the infant's airway remains controversial, although postnatal prevention of MAS will often not be possible. A reasonable approach is as follows:

1. The obstetrician carefully suctions the oro- and naso-pharynx after delivery of the head with a DeLee suction apparatus, hooked to wall suction.
2. The delivery is then completed and the baby given to the resuscitator.
3. If the baby is active and breathing and requires no resuscitation, the airway need not be inspected, thus avoiding the risk of inducing vagal bradycardia.
4. Any infant in need of resuscitation should have the airway inspected and suctioned before instituting positive-pressure ventilation.

Sequelae of Birth Asphyxia

The incidence of birth asphyxia varies between 1 and 5 percent, depending on criteria utilized in making the diagnosis.[104,105] As would be expected, the incidence increases in infants of lower gestational age. In a study involving more than 38,000 deliveries, MacDonald et al.[104] reported an incidence of 0.4 percent in infants more than 38 weeks and 62.3 percent in those less than 27 weeks. The acute sequelae that need to be managed in the neonatal period are listed in Table 20-6. It is evident that widespread organ injury occurs. If the infant survives, the major long-term concern is permanent central nervous system (CNS) damage. The challenge is identifying criteria that can provide information about the risk of future problems for a given infant. A variety of markers have been examined to identify birth asphyxia and risk for adverse neurologic outcome.[92,106–111] Meconium in the amniotic fluid considered in isolation does not increase the risk of unfavorable outcome.[92] Marked fetal bradycardia is associated with some increase in risk, but use of electronic fetal monitoring and cesarean delivery have not altered the incidence of cerebral palsy over the last several decades.[106–108] Low Apgar scores at 1 and 5 min-

Table 20-6 The Acute Sequelae of Asphyxia

System	Manifestations
Central nervous system	Cerebral edema, seizures, and hemorrhage
Cardiac	Papillary muscle necrosis–transient tricuspid insufficiency, cardiogenic shock
Pulmonary	Aspiration syndromes (meconium, clear fluid), acquired surfactant deficiency, persistent pulmonary hypertension
Renal	Acute tubular necrosis
Adrenal	Hemorrhage with adrenal insufficiency
Hepatic	Enzyme elevations, liver failure
Gastrointestinal	Necrotizing enterocolitis
Metabolic	Hypoglycemia, hypocalcemia
Hematologic	Clotting disturbances

utes are not very predictive of outcome, but infants with low scores that persist at 15 and 20 minutes after birth have a 50 percent chance of manifesting cerebral palsy if they survive.[109] Cord pH is predictive of adverse outcome only after the pH is less than 7.00.[110] The best predictor of outcome is the severity of the neonatal neurologic syndrome.[111] Infants with mild encephalopathy all survive and are normal on follow-up examination. Moderate encephalpathy carries a 5 percent mortality risk and a 15 percent chance of late disability, while the severe syndrome carries a 100 percent risk of death or disability. Diagnostic aids including electroencephalograms, CT scans, and Doppler flow studies can also aid in predicting outcome.[112] It is also important to keep in mind that the circulatory response to hypoxia is to redistribute blood flow to provide adequate oxygen delivery to critical organs (e.g., brain, heart) at the expense of other organs. Thus, it is hard to imagine an insult severe enough to damage the brain without evidence of other organ dysfunction. In particular, renal dysfunction correlates with neurologic outcome.[113]

The long-term neurologic sequelae of intrapartum asphyxia are cerebral palsy with or without associated cognitive deficits and epilepsy.[106,114,115] Although cerebral palsy can be related to intrapartum events, the large majority of cases are of unknown cause.[115,116] Furthermore, cognitive deficits and epilepsy, unless associated with cerebral palsy, cannot be related to asphyxia or to other intrapartum events.[114,115] To attribute cerebral palsy to peripartum asphyxia, there must be an absence of other demonstrable causes, substantial or prolonged intrapartum asphyxia (fetal heart rate abnormalities, fetal acidosis), and clinical evidence during the first days of life of neurologic dysfunction in the infant.[111,114]

Neonatal Neurology

Intraventricular Hemorrhage

Although related most closely to degree of prematurity, periventricular hemorrhage (PVH) and intraventricular hemorrhage (IVH) should also be considered within the context of sequelae of asphyxia. The incidence of this complication is 20 to 30 percent in infants weighing less than 2,000 g or at 34 weeks' gestation.[117,118] In those infants under 28 weeks' gestation, the incidence is higher.

Bleeding originates in the subependymal germinal matrix located ventrolateral to the lateral ventricles in the caudothalamic groove. The germinal matrix is made up of a rete of thin-walled vessels in the process of remodeling into a capillary network and a mass of undifferentiated cells that are destined to become cortical neurons, astrocytes, and oligodendroglia. Rupture of a germinal matrix hemorrhage into the ventricular system leads to intraventricular hemorrhage. A proposed pathogenesis derived from a review of available information is presented in Figure 20-11. The critical predisposing event is likely an ischemia-reperfusion injury to the capillaries in the germinal matrix. Physiologic data from beagle puppies have shown that the germinal matrix is a low blood flow region prone to ischemia.[119] Furthermore, IVH is most reliably produced in these puppies by a sequence of hemorrhagic hypotension followed by hypertension.[120] The amount of bleeding is then influenced by a variety of factors that affect the pressure gradient across the injured capillary

Table 20-7 Classification of Intraventricular Hemorrhage

Grade	Definition
I	Subependymal hemorrhage
II	Intraventricular hemorrhage without ventricular dilatation
III	Intraventricular hemorrhage with ventricular dilatation
IV	Intraventricular hemorrhage with associated parenchymal hemorrhage

(From Papile et al,[124] with permission.)

wall. Other extrinsic factors, including thrombocytopenia[121] and coagulation abnormalities[122] have been implicated as well. This pathogenic scheme also applies to intraparenchymal bleeding (venous infarction in a region rendered ischemic) and periventricular leukomalacia (PVL; ischemia in a watershed region of arterial supply).[117] Periventricular hemorrhagic infarction is most often an asymmetric lesion, with the more affected areas occurring on the same side as the larger amount of intraventricular blood. PVL can develop independent of IVH and is usually bilateral and symmetric. Up to 50 percent of bleeds occur at less than 24 hours of age, and virtually all occur by day 4 of life.[123] Bleeds are graded according to severity as indicated in Table 20-7.[124]

The neurodevelopmental outcome of infants with IVH is determined by the severity of the original bleed, development of posthemorrhagic hydrocephalus, and the degree of associated parenchymal injury. Infants

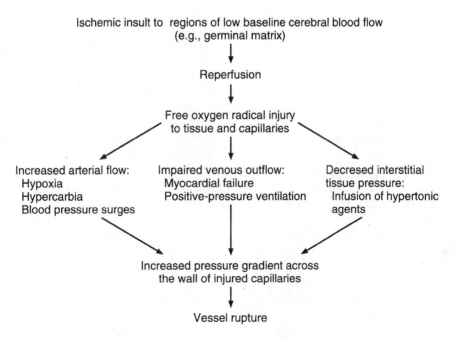

Fig. 20-11 Pathogenesis of periventricular/intraventricular hemorrhage in the preterm infant.

with grade I or II IVH have neurodevelopmental outcomes similar to preterm infants without IVH, although recent reports of outcome in school-aged children do show that survivors of mild IVH display a variety of subtle neurologic and cognitive abnormalities, including motor incoordination, hyperactivity, attention and learning deficits, and visual motor difficulties.[125,126] On the other hand, infants with progressive ventricular dilatation (grade III) or periventricular hemorrhagic infarction (grade IV) are at high risk for major neurodevelopmental handicap as well as less severe neurologic and cognitive disabilities.[127,128] In addition, the presence of severe PVL carries an ominous prognosis.[129]

In recent years, emphasis has been on the prevention of this major neurologic consequence of prematurity. Both antenatal and postnatal approaches have been developed. Overall, incidence of IVH has declined due to improvements in both obstetric and neonatal care.[118] Postnatal pharmacologic strategies have for the most part not had a major effect in decreasing the incidence and severity of IVH, although vitamin E (by ameliorating oxygen free radical damage) and the prostaglandin synthesis inhibitors indomethacin and ethamsylate have shown some promise.[130] Since IVH and PVL are likely perinatal events, antenatal prevention holds the most promise. Both vitamin K and phenobarbital have been administered in this way.[130] Antenatal phenobarbital has resulted in a decrease in both frequency and severity of IVH. The proposed mechanism of action is thought to be scavenging of oxygen-free radicals, although phenobarbital does decrease both brain blood flow and cerebral metabolic rate. Antenatal corticosteroids, although not used specifically to decrease the incidence of IVH, have been shown to decrease the frequency of this complication as well.[18,19]

Seizures

Newborns rarely have well-organized tonic-clonic seizures caused by incomplete cortical organization and a preponderance of inhibitory synapses. Volpe[131] has classified newborn seizures into four essential types. The first is the subtle seizure characterized by ocular phenomena, oral-buccal-lingual movements, peculiar limb movements (e.g., bicycling movements), autonomic alterations, and apnea. Clonic seizures are characterized by rhythmic (one to three jerks per second) movements that can be focal or multifocal. The third seizure type is focal or generalized tonic seizures marked by extensor posturing. The fourth seizure type is myoclonic activity that is distinguished from clonic seizures by the more rapid speed of the myoclonic jerk and the predilection for flexor muscle groups. The differential diagnosis of neonatal seizures is presented in Table 20-8. The most frequent cause of neonatal seizures is hypoxic ischemic encephalopathy, with the second leading cause being intracranial hemorrhage. The prognosis for neonatal seizures depends on the cause. Difficult to control seizure activity caused by hypoxic ischemic encephalopathy and hypoglycemic seizures in particular have a high incidence of long-term sequelae.

Interventions for the Prevention of Periventricular/Intraventricular Hemorrhage

Antenatal interventions
  Pharmacologic
    Phenobarbital
    Vitamin K
    Corticosteroids
  Obstetric
    Prevention of prematurity
    Optimal management of preterm labor and delivery
Postnatal interventions
  Pharmacologic
    Indomethacin
    Vitamin E
    Ethamsylate
  Optimal NICU care
    Aggressive resuscitation
    Careful ventilation to avoid airleaks
    Blood pressure management avoiding hypotension and sudden changes
    Correction of coagulation abnormalities

Birth Injuries

Birth injuries are defined as those sustained during labor and delivery. Although significant birth injury accounts for fewer than 2 percent of neonatal deaths and stillborns, the frequency is six to eight injuries per 1,000 live births (excluding cephalohematomas).[132] Many are avoidable with improved obstetric care, as indicated by a decrease in their incidence as a cause for perinatal mortality from 1953[133] to 1970.[134] However, birth injuries remain the eighth most common cause of neonatal death.[134] Factors predisposing to birth injury include macrosomia, cephalopelvic disproportion, shoulder dystocia, prolonged or difficult labor, precipitous delivery, abnormal presentations (including breech), and use of forceps (especially midforceps). Injuries range from minor (requiring no therapy) to life threatening (Table 20-9).

Soft tissue injuries are most common. Most are related to dystocia and to the use of forceps. Accidental

Table 20-8   Differential Diagnosis of Neonatal Seizures

Diagnosis	Comments
Hypoxic-ischemic encephalopathy	Most common etiology (60%), onset first 24 hours
Intracranial hemorrhage	≤15% of cases; PVH/IVH, subdural or subarachnoid bleeds
Infection	12% of cases
Hypoglycemia	SGA, IDM
Hypocalcemia, hypomagnesemia	Low-birth-weight infant, IDM
Hyponatremia	Rare, seen with syndrome of inappropriate secretion of antidiuretic hormone (SIADH)
Disorders of amino and organic, acid metabolism, hyperammonemia	Associated acidosis, altered level of consciousness
Pyridoxine dependency	Seizures refractory to routine therapy; cessation of seizures after administration of pyridoxine
Developmental defects	Other anomalies, chromosomal syndromes
Drug withdrawal	10% of cases

Abbreviations: PVH/IVH, periventricular/intraventricular hemorrhage; SGA, small for gestational age; IDM, infant of diabetic mother.

lacerations of the scalp, buttocks, and thighs may be inflicted with the scalpel during cesarean delivery. Cumulatively, these injuries are of a minor nature and respond well to therapy. Hyperbilirubinemia, particularly in the premature, is the major neonatal complication related to soft tissue damage.

A cephalhematoma occurs in 0.2 to 2.5 percent of live births.[135] Caused by rupture of blood vessels that traverse from the skull to the periosteum, the bleeding is subperiosteal and therefore limited by suture lines, with the most common site of bleeding being over the

Table 20-9   Birth Injuries

Classification	Example
Soft tissue injuries[a]	Lacerations, abrasions, bruising, fat necrosis
Skull injuries	Cephalhematoma,[a] fractures
Intracranial hemorrhage	Subdural, subarachnoid
Nerve injuries	Facial n.,[a] brachial plexus,[a] phrenic n., recurrent laryngeal n. (vocal cord paralysis), Horner syndrome
Fractures	Clavicle,[a] facial bones, humerus, femur
Dislocations	
Eye injuries	Subconjunctiva[a] and retinal hemorrhages
Torticollis[b]	
Spinal cord injuries	
Visceral rupture	Liver, spleen
Scalp laceration[a]	Fetal scalp electrode, pH
Scalp abscess[a]	Fetal scalp electrode, pH

[a] More common occurrences.
[b] Secondary to hemorrhage into the sternocleidomastoid muscle.

parietal bones. Associations include prolonged or difficult labor and mechanical trauma from forceps. Linear skull fractures beneath the hematoma have been reported in 5.4 percent of cases,[135] but are of no major consequence except in the unlikely event that a leptomeningeal cyst develops. Most cephalhematomas are reabsorbed in 2 weeks to 3 months. Depressed skull fractures are also seen in neonates, but most do not require surgical elevations.

Intracranial hemorrhages related to trauma include subdural and subarachnoid bleeds.[136] With improvements in obstetric care, subdural hemorrhages fortunately are now rare. Three major varieties of subdural bleeds have been described: (1) tentorial laceration with rupture of the straight sinus, vein of Galen, or lateral sinus; (2) falx laceration, with rupture of the inferior sagittal sinus; and (3) rupture of the superficial cerebral veins. The clinical symptomatology is related to the location of bleeding. With tentorial laceration, bleeding is infratentorial, causing brain stem signs and a rapid progression to death. Falx tears will cause bilateral cerebral signs until blood extends infratentorially to the brain stem. Subdural hemorrhage over the cerebral convexities can cause several clinical states, ranging from an asymptomatic newborn to one with seizures and focal neurologic findings. Infants with lacerations of the tentorium and falx have a poor outlook. In contrast, the prognosis for rupture of the superficial cerebral veins is much better, with more than one-half the survivors being normal. Primary subarachnoid hemorrhage is the most common variety of neonatal intracranial hemorrhage.[136] Clinically, these infants are often asymptomatic, although they may present with a characteristic seizure pattern. The seizures begin on day 2 of life, and the infants are "well" between convulsions. In general, the prognosis for subarachnoid bleeds is good.

Trauma to peripheral nerves produces another major group of birth injuries. Brachial plexus injuries are caused by stretching of the cervical roots during delivery, usually when shoulder dystocia is present. Upper arm palsy (Erb-Duchenne), the most common brachial plexus injury, is caused by injury to the fifth and sixth cervical nerves; lower arm paralysis (Klumpke) results from damage to the eighth cervical and first thoracic nerves. Damage to all four nerve roots produces paralysis of the entire arm. Outcome for these injuries is variable, with about 15 percent of infants left with significant residual.[137] Horner syndrome may accompany Klumpke's palsy, and approximately 5 percent of patients with Erb's palsy have an associated phrenic nerve paresis.[132] Facial palsy is another fairly common injury caused either by pressure from the sacral promontory as the infant passes through the birth canal or by forceps. Most of these palsies resolve, although in some infants paralysis is persistent.

The majority of bone fractures resulting from birth trauma involve the clavicle and result from shoulder dystocia or breech extractions that require vigorous manipulations. Clinically many of these fractures are asymptomatic, and symptoms when present are mild. Prognosis for clavicular as well as limb fractures is uniformly good. The most commonly fractured long bone is the humerus.

Spinal cord injuries are a relatively infrequent but often severe form of birth injury. Accurate incidence is difficult to assess, because symptomatology mimics other neonatal diseases and autopsies often do not include a careful examination of the spine. Depressed tone and hyporeflexia are clues to this diagnosis. The type of lesion varies from localized hemorrhage in the anterior cornua to complete destruction of the cord at one or more levels.[138] Excessive longitudinal traction is thought to be the most important cause of neonatal spinal injury, with hyperextension of the head in a footling breech particularly dangerous. Outcomes include death or stillbirth caused by high cervical or brain stem lesions, long-term survival of infants with paralysis from birth, and minimal neurologic symptoms or spasticity.[139]

Respiratory Distress

The establishment of respiratory function at birth is dependent on expansion and maintenance of air sacs, clearance of lung fluid, and provision of adequate pulmonary perfusion. In many premature and other high-risk infants, developmental deficiencies or unfavorable perinatal events hamper a smooth respiratory transition. Furthermore, a neonate has a limited number of ways to respond symptomatically to a variety of pathophysiologic insults. The presentation of respiratory distress is among the most common symptom complexes seen in the newborn and may be secondary to both noncardiopulmonary and cardiopulmonary etiologies (Table 20-10). The symptom complex includes an elevation of the respiratory rate to greater than 60 bpm with or without cyanosis, nasal flaring, intercostal and sternal retractions, and expiratory grunting. The retractions are the result of the neonate's efforts to expand a lung with poor compliance utilizing a very compliant chest wall. The expiratory grunt is caused by closure of the glottis during expiration in an effort to increase expiratory pressure to help maintain functional residual capacity. The evaluation of such an infant requires utilization of history, physical examination, and laboratory data to arrive at a diagnosis. It is important to consider causes other than those related to the heart and lungs, because one's natural tendency is to focus immediately on the more common cardiopulmonary etiologies.

Cardiovascular causes of respiratory distress in the neonatal period can be divided into two major groups—those with structural heart disease and those with persistent right to left shunting through fetal pathways and structurally normal heart. A cardiac defect, some of which may resolve without intervention, is present in approximately 1 percent of live births.[140] Infants presenting in the first week of life with symptoms include those with cyanosis and those with signs of congestive heart failure. Examples of cyanotic heart disease include transposition of the great vessels, tricuspid atresia, certain types of truncus arteriosus, total anomalous pulmonary venous return, and right-sided outflow obstruction, including tetralogy of Fallot and pulmonary stenosis or atresia. Although cyanosis is the central feature in these disorders, tachypnea will develop in many infants because of increased pulmonary blood flow or secondary to metabolic acidosis from hypoxia. Infants with congestive heart failure generally have some form of left-sided outflow obstruction. Left to right shunt lesions such as ventricular septal defect do not present with increased pulmonary blood flow and congestive heart failure until pulmonary vascular resistance is low enough to permit a significant shunt (usually 3 to 4 weeks of age at sea level). Infants with left-sided outflow obstruction generally do well the first day or so until the source of systemic flow, the ductus arteriosus, closes. With ductal narrowing, dyspnea, tachypnea, and tachycardia develop, followed by rapid progression to congestive heart failure and metabolic acidosis. On examination, these infants all have pulse abnormalities. With hypoplastic left heart syndrome and critical aortic stenosis, pulses are profoundly diminished in all extremities, while infants with coarctation of the aorta and interrupted aortic arch will have

Table 20-10   Respiratory Distress in the Newborn

Noncardiopulmonary	Cardiovascular	Pulmonary
Hypo- or hyperthermia	Left-sided outflow obstruction	Upper airway obstruction
Hypoglycemia	Hypoplastic left heart	Choanal atresia
Metabolic acidosis	Aortic stenosis	Vocal cord paralysis
Drug intoxications; withdrawal	Coarctation of the aorta	Meconium aspiration
Central nervous system insult	Cyanotic lesions	Clear fluid aspiration
Asphyxia	Transposition of the great vessels	Transient tachypnea
Hemorrhage	Total anomalous pulmonary	Pneumonia
Neuromuscular disease	venous return	Pulmonary hypoplasia
Werdnig-Hoffman disease	Tricuspid atresia	Primary
Myopathies	Right-sided outflow obstruction	Secondary
Phrenic nerve injury		Hyaline membrane disease
Skeletal abnormalities		Pneumothorax
Asphyxiating thoracic dystrophy		Pleural effusions
		Mass lesions
		Lobar emphysema
		Cystic adenomatoid malformation

differential pulses when the arms and legs are compared.

The syndrome of persistent pulmonary hypertension of the newborn (PPHN) occurs when the normal postnatal decrease in pulmonary vascular resistance does not occur. High pulmonary artery pressures, typical of in utero existence, persist, maintaining right to left shunting across the patent ductus arteriosus and foramen ovale. Most infants with PPHN are full term or postmature and have experienced perinatal asphyxia. Other clinical associations include hypothermia, MAS, hyaline membrane disease, polycythemia, neonatal sepsis, chronic intrauterine hypoxia, pulmonary hypoplasia, and premature closure of the ductus arteriosus in utero.[141–143]

On the basis of developmental considerations, these infants can be separated into three groups[142]: (1) acute vasoconstriction caused by perinatal hypoxia, (2) prenatal increase in pulmonary vascular smooth muscle development, and (3) decreased cross-sectional area of the pulmonary vascular bed caused by inadequate vessel number. In the first group, an acute perinatal event leads to hypoxia and failure of pulmonary vascular resistance to drop. In the second, abnormal muscularization of the pulmonary resistance vessels results in PPHN after birth. The third circumstance includes infants with pulmonary hypoplasia (e.g., diaphragmatic hernia). Clinically, the syndrome is characterized by cyanosis, often unresponsive to increases in F_{IO_2}, respiratory distress, an onset at less than 24 hours, evidence of right ventricular overload, systemic hypotension, acidosis, and no evidence of structural heart disease.

Infants with PPHN make up the majority of patients who are treated in some centers with extracorporeal membrane oxygenation (ECMO).[144] When conventional medical therapy (ventilator, systemic pressors, respiratory alkalosis) fails, infants are placed on bypass with blood exiting the baby from the right atrium and returning to the aortic arch after passing through a membrane oxygenator. Over several days, pulmonary hypertension resolves, and the infants are weaned from ECMO back to conventional ventilator therapy. This treatment can save infants who otherwise would have died with conventional therapy, but it has major side effects that must be considered prior to utilization. In recent years, new modes of treatment have been introduced that are decreasing the need for ECMO. Systemically infused vasodilators (e.g., tolazoline and isuprel) have been used to treat PPHN with variable and often disappointing results. These agents lacked specificity for the pulmonary vascular bed. Recent trials using the inhaled gas nitric oxide (NO), which is very similar to endothelium derived relaxing factor, have shown it to be a very promising and specific pulmonary vasodilator.[145,146] Multicenter clinical trials are currently in progress evaluating this new therapy. In addition, use of high-frequency oscillatory ventilation has proven effective in many of these infants, in particular those with severe associated lung disease.[147]

Of the causes of respiratory distress related to the airways and pulmonary parenchyma listed in Table 20-10, the differential diagnosis in a term infant includes transient tachypnea, aspiration syndromes, and congenital pneumonia. The syndrome of transient tachypnea (wet lung or type II RDS) presents as respiratory distress in nonasphyxiated term infants or slightly preterm infants. The clinical features include various combinations of cyanosis, grunting, nasal flaring, retracting, and tachypnea during the first hours after birth. The chest x-ray is the key to the diagnosis, with prominent perihilar streaking and fluid in the interlobar fissures. The symptoms generally subside in 12 to 24 hours, although they can persist longer. The preferred explanation for the clinical features is delayed reabsorption of fetal lung fluid.[148] Transient tachypnea is seen more commonly in infants delivered by elective cesarean section or in the slightly preterm infant (see Mechanics of the First Breath).

At delivery, the neonate may aspirate clear amniotic fluid or fluid mixed with blood. Whether infants can aspirate a sufficient volume of clear fluid to cause symptoms is controversial. However, there are a group of infants whose clinical course is more prolonged (4 to 7 days) and severe than that of infants with transient tachypnea. These infants have a radiologic picture similar to transient tachypnea often associated with more marked hyperexpansion. Occasionally, the infiltrates are quite impressive, with evidence of far more fluid than is seen with transient tachypnea.

MAS occurs in full-term or postmature infants. The perinatal course is often marked by fetal distress and low Apgar scores. These infants exhibit tachypnea, retractions, cyanosis, overdistended and barrel-shaped chest, and coarse breath sounds. Chest x-ray reveals coarse, irregular pulmonary densities with areas of diminished aeration or consolidation. There is a high incidence of air leaks, and many of the infants exhibit persistent pulmonary hypertension.[92,100]

The lungs represent the most common primary site of infection in the neonate. Both bacterial and viral infections can be acquired before, during, or after birth. The most common route of infection, particularly for bacteria, is ascending from the genital tract before or during labor. Thus prolonged rupture of the membranes in excess of 12 to 18 hours is a major predisposing factor.[149] Major pathogens include group B β-hemolytic *Streptococcus*, gram-negative enterics, and *Listeria monocytogenes*.[150,151] Infants with congenital pneumonia present with symptomatology from very early in life, including tachypnea, retractions, grunting, nasal flaring, and cyanosis. The chest x-ray pattern is often indistinguishable from other causes of respiratory distress, particularly hyaline membrane disease (HMD).[152]

Despite improved understanding and recent advances, HMD remains the most common etiology for respiratory distress in the neonatal period. HMD affects approximately 20,000 infants per year in the United States, developing in 50 percent of infants 26 to 28 weeks of gestation and in 30 percent of those 30 to 31 weeks. It was the initial reports of Avery and Mead[153] demonstrating a high surface tension in extracts of lungs from infants dying of RDS that led to the present understanding of the role of surfactant in the pathogenesis of HMD. The deficiency of surfactant in the premature infant increases alveolar surface tension and, according to LaPlace's law (Fig. 20-2) increases the pressure necessary to maintain patent alveoli. The end result is poor lung compliance, progressive atelectasis, loss of FRC, alterations in ventilation-perfusion match, and uneven distribution of ventilation.[154] HMD is further complicated by the weak respiratory muscles and compliant chest wall of the premature. Hypoxemia and respiratory and metabolic acidemia contribute to increased pulmonary vascular resistance, right to left ductal shunting, and worsening ventilation-perfusion mismatch that exacerbate hypoxemia. Hypoxemia and hypoperfusion result in alveolar epithelial damage, with increased capillary permeability and leakage of plasma into alveolar spaces. Leakage of protein into airspaces serves to inhibit surfactant function, exacerbating the disease process.[155] The materials in plasma and cellular debris combine to form the characteristic hyaline membrane seen pathologically. The recovery phase is characterized by regeneration of alveolar cells, including type II cells, with an increase in surfactant activity.

Clinically, neonates with HMD demonstrate tachypnea, nasal flaring, subcostal and intercostal retractions, cyanosis, and expiratory grunting. As the infant begins to tire with progressive disease, apneic episodes occur. If some intervention is not undertaken at this point, death ensues. The radiologic appearance of the lungs is what would be expected in an extensive atelectatic process. The infiltrate is diffuse, with a ground-glass appearance. Major airways are air filled and contrast with the atelectatic alveoli, creating the appearance of air bronchograms while the diaphragms are elevated because of profound hypoexpansion. Acute complications of HMD include infection, air leaks, and persistent patency of the ductus arteriosus.

Of more concern than acute complications are the long-term sequelae suffered by infants with HMD. The major long-term consequences are chronic lung disease requiring prolonged ventilator and oxygen therapy and significant neurologic impairment. In 1967, Northway et al.[156] first described the syndrome of bronchopulmonary dysplasia in infants surviving severe HMD requiring mechanical ventilation. Today, many infants who develop chronic lung disease are extremely low-birth-weight infants who require prolonged ventilation for apnea and poor respiratory effort. The incidence is now estimated at about 30 percent in preterm infants requiring mechanical ventilation, with the highest rates in babies of the lowest birth weight (>70 percent among survivors <1,000 g).[157] The severity is variable, ranging from very mild pulmonary dysfunction to severe disease with prolonged mechanical ventilation, frequent readmissions for respiratory exacerbations after nursery discharge, and a higher incidence of neurodevelopmental sequelae compared with very-low-

Table 20-11   Cumulative Results of Placebo-Controlled Surfactant Trials[a]

	Modified Natural[b] (%)		Synthetic[c] (%)	
	Surfactant	Control	Surfactant	Control
Mortality	15	24	11	18
Patent ductus arteriosus	46	43	44	48
Severe ICH	19	19	7	8
Chronic lung disease	37	37	11	11

[a] Higher incidences of intracranial hemorrhage (ICH) and chronic lung disease in modified natural surfactant studies reflects the lower gestational age on average in both groups in these studies compared to the artificial surfactant studies.

[b] Studies with Survanta, Curosurf, and Infasurf; 2,000 patients.

[c] Studies with Exosurf; 4,400 patients.

birth-weight controls.[158,159] Although pulmonary function improves over time and most children do quite well, long-term pulmonary sequelae are evident.[160,161] Factors involved in the etiology of chronic lung disease are gestational age, elevated inspired oxygen concentration, positive-pressure ventilation, severity of underlying disease, inflammation, and infection.[162]

One of the exciting areas in neonatology is the development of surfactant replacement therapy for the management of hyaline membrane disease. Modified natural surfactant, which is extracted by alveolar lavage or from lung tissue (usually bovine) and then modified by selective addition and/or removal of components, and true artificial surfactant, which is a mixture of synthetic compounds that may or may not be components of natural surfactant, have been extensively studied.[9,22,–24] In most studies, these agents (administered intratracheally) have shown efficacy in decreasing the severity of acute HMD and the frequency of air leak complications. Efficacy has been demonstrated when used in the delivery room to "prevent" or when used as a rescue treatment for established HMD. Although surfactant replacement therapy has decreased mortality and acute pulmonary morbidity, this therapy has not affected the frequency of other complications of prematurity (Table 20-11). Of note is that, despite resulting in lower ventilator settings and fraction of inspired oxygen concentration over the first several days of life, the incidence of chronic lung disease has not been changed. However, the severity of long-term pulmonary complications is less. Long-term neurodevelopment follow-ups show rates of handicap similar to placebo-treated infants.[163]

Neonatal Thermal Regulation

Physiology

The human newborn is a homeotherm possessing the ability to maintain a stable core body temperature over a range of environmental temperatures.[164] The range of environmental temperatures over which the neonate can operate is narrower than that of an adult due to the infant's inability to dissipate heat effectively in warm environments and, more critically, to maintain temperature in response to cold.

Heat Production

The heat production within the body is a by-product of metabolic processes and must equal heat losses through the skin and lungs. In the adult, heat production in response to cold can come from voluntary muscle activity, involuntary muscle activity (shivering), and nonshivering chemical thermogenesis. While some increases in activity and shivering have been observed, nonshivering thermogenesis is the most important means of increased heat production in the cold-stressed newborn.[165,166] Nonshivering thermogenesis can be defined as an increase in total heat production without detectable (visible or electrical) muscle activity. From both animal[167] and human[168] observations, it has been inferred that the site of this increased heat production is brown fat. More abundant in newborns than adults, brown fat accounts for 2 to 6 percent of total body weight.[164] This fat is located between the scapulae; around the muscles and blood vessels of the neck, axillae, and mediastinum; between the esophagus and trachea; and around the kidneys and adrenal glands. Brown fat differs both morphologically and metabolically from white fat. Brown fat cells contain more mitochondria and fat vacuoles and have a richer blood and sympathetic nerve supply. Brown fat metabolism is stimulated by norepinephrine released through sympathetic innervation causing triglyceride hydrolysis.[167,169] The initiation of nonshivering thermogenesis at birth depends on cooling, separation from the placenta, and a euthyroid state. Sympathetic nervous system stimulation by cold increases local catecholamine turnover within brown fat resulting in a marked increase in oxygen consumption.[170]

Heat Loss

Heat loss to the environment is dependent on both an internal temperature gradient (from within the body to the surface) and an external gradient (from the surface to the environment). The infant can change the internal gradient by altering vasomotor tone and, to a lesser extent, by postural changes that decrease the amount of exposed surface area. The external gradient is dependent on purely physical variables. Heat transfer from the surface to the environment involves four routes: (1) radiation, (2) convection, (3) conduction, and (4) evaporation. Radiant heat loss, heat transfer from a warmer to a cooler object that is not in contact, depends on the temperature gradient between the ob-

Table 20-12   Neonatal Response to Thermal Stress

Stressor	Response	Term	Preterm
Cold	Vasoconstriction	+ +	+ +
	↓ Exposed surface area (posture change)	+/−	+/−
	↑ Oxygen consumption	+ +	+
	↑ Motor activity; shivering	+	−
Heat	Vasodilation	+ +	+ +
	Sweating	+	−

+ +, Maximum response; +, intermediate; +/−, may have a role; −, no response.

jects. Heat loss by convection to the surrounding gaseous environment depends on air speed and temperature. Conduction or heat loss to a contacting cooler object is minimal in most circumstances. Heat loss by evaporation is cooling secondary to water loss at the rate of 0.6 cal/g water evaporated and is affected by relative humidity, air speed, exposed surface area, and skin permeability. In infants in excessively warm environments, under overhead radiant heat sources, or in very immature infants with thin, permeable skin, evaporative losses increase considerably. In the average 2-kg infant under basal conditions, 40 percent of heat loss occurs by radiation, 33 percent by convection, 24 percent by evaporation, and 3 percent by conduction.[171]

Compared with an adult, the newborn is compromised in the ability to conserve as well as dissipate heat. Conservation of heat is impaired because of a large surface area to body weight ratio and less tissue insulation because of less subcutaneous fat.[172] With a cold stress, heat is conserved chiefly by vasoconstriction in both mature and immature neonates. When the environment is too warm, heat loss is augmented by vasodilation of skin vessels and an increase in evaporative heat loss by sweating. Sweating is present in term infants when rectal temperatures rise above 37.2°C.[165,173] With sweating, evaporative heat losses can increase twofold to fourfold in term babies, but this is not enough to prevent a rise in core temperature. Table 20-12 summarizes the neonate's efforts to maintain a stable core temperature in the face of cold or heat stress.

Neutral Thermal Environment

Although most available information confirms that the human neonate is a homeotherm, the range of temperatures over which core body temperature remains stable is narrower than in an adult and decreases with decreasing gestational age. It is therefore advantageous to maintain an infant in a neutral thermal environment (Fig. 20-12). A neutral thermal environment makes minimal demands on the neonate's energy reserves, core body temperature being regulated by changes in skin blood flow and posture. Body temperature remains normal, while oxygen consumption and heat production are minimal and match heat loss.[174] With a drop in environmental temperature out of the thermoneutral range, the infant will increase oxygen consumption and thus heat production to keep up with heat losses and maintain a stable core temperature. Core temperature will be maintained until heat loss exceeds the infant's ability to increase heat production further. When the infant is placed in an environment warmer than neutral thermal zone, hyperthermia rapidly occurs because of the neonate's inability to dissipate heat and an increase in oxygen consumption that ensues as the infant's body temperature rises. The neutral thermal environment for a given infant depends on size, gestational age, and postnatal age.[175] The optimal thermal environment for naked babies and cot nursed (dressed and bundled) babies has been defined (Fig. 20-13).[174,176] It is important to note that the environmental temperatures shown in Figure 20-13 are operative temperatures for an infant in an incubator. The operative temperature can differ from the measured environmental temperature because of changes in relative humidity and temperature of the incubator walls. Incubator wall temperature will vary as a function of room temperature. In general, maintaining the abdominal skin temperature at 36.5°C minimizes oxygen consumption.[177]

Clinical Applications

Delivery Room

In utero, fetal thermoregulation is the responsibility of the placenta and is dependent on maternal core temperature, with fetal temperature 0.5°C higher than maternal temperature.[178] At birth, the infant's core temperature drops rapidly from 37.8°C because of evaporation from its wet body and radiant and convective losses to the cold air and walls of the room. Heat loss can occur at a rate of 0.2 cal/kg/min in the term infant and at a greater rate in premature and sick or unstable infants.[178] Even with an increase in oxygen consumption to the maximum capability of the newborn (15 ml/kg/min), the infant can produce only 0.075 cal/kg/min and will rapidly lose heat. Measures taken to reduce heat loss after birth depend on the clinical situation. For the well term infant, drying the skin and wrapping the baby with warm blankets is sufficient. When it is necessary to leave an infant exposed for close observation or resuscitation, the infant should be dried and placed under a radiant heat source. Room temperature can be elevated as an added precaution for the low-birth-weight infant.

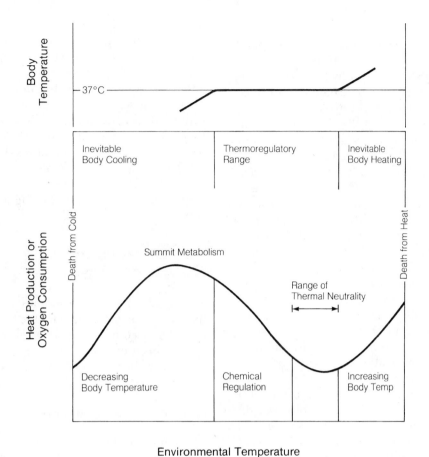

Fig. 20-12 Effect of environmental temperature on oxygen consumption and body temperature. (Adapted from Klaus et al.,[164] with permission.)

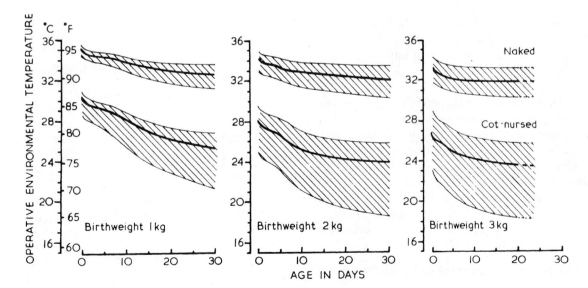

Fig. 20-13 Range of environmental temperatures to maintain naked or cot-nursed 1-kg, 2-kg, and 3-kg infants in a neutral thermal environment. (From Hey,[171] with permission.)

Nursery

Babies are cared for in the newborn nursery wrapped in blankets in bassinets (cot nursed), in isolettes, or under a radiant heat source. Healthy full-term infants (weighing >2.5 kg) need only be clothed and placed in a bassinet under a blanket. A nursery temperature of 25°C should be adequate (Fig. 20-13). Infants weighing 2 to 2.5 kg who are either slightly premature or growth retarded should be allowed 12 to 24 hours to stabilize in an isolette and then advanced to a bassinet. Lower-birth-weight babies (<2 kg) will require care in either isolettes or under radiant heat sources. Adequate thermal protection of the low-birth-weight infant is essential. Several groups have demonstrated decreased mortality in low-birth-weight infants kept in warmer environments.[179-181] This is especially important for the very-low-birth-weight infant (<1.5 kg), who often does not behave like a mature homeotherm. These neonates can react to a small change in environmental temperature with a change in body temperature rather than a change in oxygen consumption. In addition, warmer environments have also been shown to hasten growth of the premature.[182]

The isolette, which heats by convection, is the most commonly used heating device for the low-birth-weight nude infant. The major source of heat loss while in a neutral thermal environment is radiant to the walls of the isolette. The magnitude of this loss is predictable if room temperature is known. These losses can be minimized using double-walled isolettes in which the inner wall temperature is very close to the air temperature within the isolette. An isolette permits adequate observation of the infant and is suitable for caring for the most sick low-birth-weight or full-sized infants. Once clinical status has been stabilized the child can be dressed, which will afford increased thermal stability.

Radiant warmers can also be used to ensure thermal stability of both low-birth-weight and full-sized infants. Radiant warmers are used most effectively for short-term warming during initial resuscitation and stabilization as well as for performing procedures. They provide easy access to the infant while assuring thermal stability. The main heat losses are convection, which can be quite significant because of variable air speed in a room, and evaporation. Evaporative heat loss resulting in significant fluid losses is a major concern for the very-low-birth-weight premature cared for under a radiant warmer. Placing a plastic shield over the infant or covering the skin with a semipermeable membrane can minimize these fluid losses.[183]

Hypothermia and Neonatal Cold Injury

Hypothermia is seen in low-birth-weight infants, particularly following delivery room resuscitation. Hypothermia may also be a sign of infection or intracranial pathology. Neonatal cold injury is a consequence of excessive cold exposure most commonly seen in both term and preterm infants born unexpectedly outside the hospital. Clinical features include poor feeding, lethargy, coolness of skin, bright red color, edema, and occasionally sclerema (hardening of the skin associated with reddening and edema), slow and shallow respiratory effort, and bradycardia.[184] Metabolic derangements include metabolic acidosis, hypoglycemia, hyperkalemia, and elevated blood urea nitrogen. The infant should be warmed slowly in an isolette set at an operative temperature of 2°C higher than the infant's core body temperature.

Neonatal Nutrition and Gastroenterology

At birth, the newborn infant must assume various functions performed during fetal life by the placenta. Cardiopulmonary transition and thermoregulation have already been discussed. The final critical task for the newborn is the assimilation of calories, water, and electrolytes.

Nutritional Requirements

The required caloric, water, and electrolyte intake of the newborn depends on body stores and normal rate of energy expenditure. Body composition varies considerably with gestational age (Fig. 20-14).[185,186] The average 1-kg neonate consists of 85 percent water, 10 percent protein, and 3 percent fat as compared with 74 percent water, 12 percent protein, and 11 percent fat at term. Carbohydrate stores in the term infant are

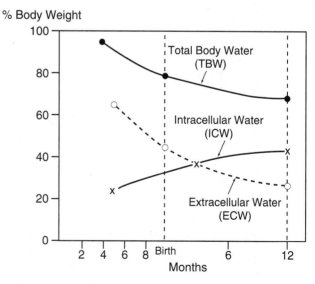

Fig. 20-14 Changes in body water during gestation and infancy. (Adapted from Friis-Hansen,[186] with permission.)

eight times higher. Rates of energy expenditure differ as well. Although basal metabolic rate is lower in premature than in term infants, the premature infant frequently has increased metabolic demand secondary to cold stress and work of breathing. The small-for-gestational-age (SGA) infant provides another special consideration, possessing a higher basal metabolic rate per kilogram than a normally grown infant.[187]

Water and Electrolyte

Maintenance water requirements are dependent on oxygen consumption and rate of generation of renal solute. Other pertinent factors, especially for the premature infant, include variation in insensible water losses and diminished ability to concentrate urine.[188] individual infant's water requirement can be determined by measuring urine and stool losses and estimating insensible losses through skin and mucosa. It is normal during the first 3 to 4 postnatal days for an infant to experience a weight loss of up to 10 percent as the physiologic contraction of extracellular body fluid takes place. Maintenance electrolyte requirements are 2 to 3 mEq/kg/day for sodium, chloride, and bicarbonate and 1 to 2 mEq/kg/day for potassium. During periods of rapid growth, requirements will be higher.

Calories

Caloric needs are primarily dependent on oxygen consumption. The character of the feeding also affects caloric needs by altering specific dynamic action and fecal losses. The average caloric requirement for a normal full-term infant is estimated to be about 100 to 110 kcal/kg/day. The needs of the low-birth-weight infant are more variable, but usually 120 kcal/kg/day is adequate.[189] Standard infant formulas and breast milk provide approximately 20 kcal/ounce. Therefore, volumes of 150 to 180 ml/kg/day will provide the necessary caloric intake of 100 to 120 kcal/kg/day for the average term or preterm infant beyond 32 to 34 weeks gestation. However, infants less than 1,500 g should be fed with either formulas designed specifically for the premature (20 to 24 kcal/ounce) or fortified breast milk.

Protein

Both the quantity and quality of protein intake are important for adequate growth, particularly for the premature infant.[190] Suggested intakes range from 2.0 to 4.0 g/kg/day (3.5 g/kg/day for the premature).[189] The "gold standard" for amino acid content is that which provides a plasma amniogram as close as possible to that seen with human milk.[191] Infants who receive inappropriately high protein intakes or an unbalanced amino acid intake are at risk of developing hyperam-monemia, azotemia, metabolic acidosis acutely, and a lower IQ long term.[192,193] Inadequate protein intake results in growth failure.

Fat and Carbohydrate

Normal full-term infants fail to absorb 10 to 15 percent of ingested fat, while the low-birth-weight infant malabsorbs considerably more.[189,194] Important factors relating to fat absorption are the nature of the fat ingested as well as pancreatic lipase levels and the bile salt pool. Because of the relatively poor digestion of long-chain triglycerides, a theoretically attractive alternative is medium-chain triglycerides with 8 to 12 carbon chain length. Unlike long-chain triglycerides, medium-chain triglycerides do not require bile for emulsification. Medium-chain triglycerides are generally well tolerated by both term and premature infants. Fat should provide 30 to 54 percent total calories, with 3 percent of total calories in the form of linoleic acid.[189]

Intestinal disaccharidases develop early in fetal life, with lactase reaching mature levels at term.[195] Both term and preterm infants can digest lactose, the major sugar in human milk and standard infant formulas, although there is some evidence that digestion may not be fully efficient the first several days of life.[189] Carbohydrate represents 40 to 50 percent of total calories in most formulas as well as human milk. These levels are more than adequate to maintain normal blood glucose levels and prevent ketosis.

Vitamins and Minerals

Published requirements are available for all major minerals and vitamins for term and preterm infants.[189,196,197] Information on trace minerals[189,196,197] available as well.

Infant Feeding

For the well term or slightly preterm infant, institution of oral feeds within the first 2 to 4 hours of life is reasonable practice. For infants who are SGA or large for gestational age (LGA), feeds within the first hour or two of life may be indicated to avoid hypoglycemia. Premature infants (<34 weeks gestation) who are unable to nipple feed present a more complex set of circumstances. In addition to an inability to suck and swallow efficiently, such infants face a number of problems: (1) relatively high caloric demand; (2) small stomach capacity; (3) incompetent esophageal-cardiac sphincter, leading to gastroesophageal reflux; (4) poor gag reflex, creating a tendency for aspiration; and (5) decreased digestive capability (especially for fat). These infants can initially be supported adequately with parenteral nutrition followed by institution of nasogastric tube feedings when their cardiopulmonary status is stable.

Although a wide range of infant formulas satisfy the nutritional needs of most neonates, breast milk remains the standard on which formulas are based. The distribution of calories in human milk is 7 percent protein, 55 percent fat, and 38 percent carbohydrate. The whey: casein ratio is 60:40, allowing ease of protein digestion, while fat digestion is augmented by the presence of a breast milk lipase. In addition to easy digestibility, the amino acid makeup is well suited for the newborn. Despite the low levels of several vitamins and minerals, bioavailability is high. Besides the nutritional features, breast milk's immunochemical and cellular components provide protection against infection.[189]

The major area of controversy regarding breast milk has been its use for the small premature infant. The growth demands of the low-birth-weight infant exceed the contents of human milk for protein, calcium, phosphorus, sodium, zinc, copper, and possibly other nutrients.[198] These shortcomings can be addressed through the addition of human milk fortifiers to mother's preterm breast milk.[199] Advantages of breast milk for the premature include its anti-infective properties, possible protection against necrotizing enterocolitis, and its role in enhancing neurodevelopmental outcome.[199–202]

Under certain circumstances, breast-feeding might be deleterious. For example, phenylketonuria (PKU), a condition requiring special nutritional products, precludes breast-feeding. The presence of environmental pollutants has been documented in breast milk, but to date no serious side effects have been reported. Most drugs do not contraindicate breast-feeding, but there are a few exceptions (see Ch. 10). Transmission of some viral infections via breast milk is a concern as well. Mothers who are hepatitis surface antigen B or HIV positive should not breast-feed. Finally, there is the insufficient milk syndrome and breast-feeding failure. Monographs that deal with this as well as other minor breast-feeding problems are available for mother and physician.[203] The obstetrician and pediatrician should serve as a source of knowledge and, most importantly, support.

Neonatal Hypoglycemia

Glucose is a major fetal fuel transported by facilitated diffusion across the placenta. After birth, before an appropriate supply of exogenous calories is provided, the newborn must maintain blood glucose through endogenous sources. This homeostasis depends on an adequate supply of gluconeogenic substrates (amino acids, lactate, glycerol), functionally intact hepatic glycogenolytic and gluconeogenic enzyme systems, and a normal endocrine counter-regulatory hormone system (gluca-

gon, catacholamines, growth hormone, cortisol) integrating and modulating these processes. Hepatic glycogen stores are almost entirely depleted within the first several hours before birth. Fat and protein stores are then used for energy, while glucose levels are maintained by hepatic gluconeogenesis.

In utero, fetal blood glucose concentration is 20 to 30 percent lower than maternal levels. In the healthy unstressed neonate, glucose falls over the first 1 to 2 hours after birth, stabilizes at a minimum of about 40 mg/dl, and then rises to 45 to 60 mg/dl.[204] Hypoglycemia can be defined as blood glucose levels less than 40 mg/dl.[205] Infants at risk for hypoglycemia and in whom glucose should be monitored include (1) preterm infants, (2) SGA infants, (3) hyperinsulinemic (LGA) infants, and (4) infants with perinatal asphyxia. As in term babies, blood sugar drops after birth in preterm babies, but the latter are less able to mount a counter-regulatory response.[206] In addition, the presence of respiratory distress, hypothermia, and other factors can increase glucose demand, exacerbating hypoglycemia. SGA infants are at risk for hypoglycemia due to decreased glycogen stores as well as impaired gluconeogenesis and ketogenesis.[207] Onset of hypoglycemia in SGA and preterm infants usually occurs at 2 to 6 hours of life. Hyperinsulinemia occurs in the poorly controlled infant of a diabetic mother as well as other rare conditions, including Beckwith-Weidemann syndrome and islet cell dysregulation syndrome (nesidioblastosis).[208] In the case of perinatal asphyxia, hypoglycemia is the result of excessive glucose demand.[205]

Symptoms of hypoglycemia include jitteriness, seizures, cyanosis, respiratory distress, apathy, hypotonia, and eye rolling.[208] However, many infants, particularly prematures, are asymptomatic. Because of the risk of subsequent brain injury,[209,210] hypoglycemia, when present, should be aggressively treated. However, the single best treatment is prevention by identifying infants at risk, including prematures, SGA, LGA, and any stressed infant. These newborns should have blood glucose screened with glucose oxidase impregnated strips. All values less than or equal to 40 mg/dl should be confirmed with a laboratory or rapid glucose analyzer measurement of whole blood glucose.[211] Treatment is provided by early institution of feeds or an intravenous glucose infusion at a rate of 6 mg/kg/min.

Congenital Gastrointestinal Surgical Conditions

Several congenital surgical conditions of the gastrointestinal tract interfere with a normal transition. Many of these conditions can be diagnosed with antenatal ultrasound, allowing transfer of the mother to a perinatal center for delivery.

Gastrointestinal Tract Obstruction

Tracheoesophageal fistula and esophageal atresia are characterized by a blind esophageal pouch and a fistulous connection between either the proximal or distal esophagus and the airway.[212] Eighty-five percent of infants with these conditions have the fistula between the distal esophagus and the airway. Polyhydramnios is common because of the high level of gastrointestinal obstruction. Infants present in the first hours of life with copious secretions, choking, cyanosis, and respiratory distress. Diagnosis can be confirmed with chest x-ray after careful placement of a nasogastric tube to the point where resistance is met. The tube will be seen in the blind pouch. If a tracheoesophageal fistula is present to the distal esophagus, gas will be present in the abdomen.

Infants with high intestinal obstruction present early in life with either bilious or nonbilious vomiting. In duodenal atresia, vomitus may or may not contain bile, whereas malrotation with midgut volvulus and high jejunal atresia are characterized by bilious vomiting. Malrotation and midgut volvulus involve torsion of the intestine around the superior mesenteric artery, causing occlusion of the vascular supply to most of the small intestine. If not treated promptly, the infant can lose most of the small bowel because of ischemic injury. Therefore, bilious vomiting in the neonate demands immediate attention and evaluation. Diagnosis of high intestinal obstruction can be confirmed with x-rays. Duodenal atresia is characterized by a "double bubble sign" (stomach and dilated duodenum). Diagnosis of midgut volvulus can be confirmed with a contrast enema, looking for malposition of the cecum and/or an upper gastrointestinal tract series, looking for contrast not to pass the ligament of Treitz.

Low intestinal obstruction presents with increasing intolerance of feeds (spitting progressing to vomiting), abdominal distention, and decreased or absent stool. Differential diagnosis of lower intestinal obstruction includes imperforate anus, Hirschsprung disease, meconium plug syndrome, small left colon, colonic and ileal atresia, and meconium ileus. Plain x-ray film of the abdomen will show gaseous distension, with air through a considerable portion of the bowel and air-fluid levels. Diagnosis of meconium ileus, meconium plug, and small left colon syndrome can be made by appearance on contrast enema. Rectal biopsy searching for absence of ganglion cells will confirm the diagnosis of Hirschsprung disease.

Abdominal Wall Defects

Omphaloceles[213] are formed by incomplete closure of the anterior abdominal wall after return of the midgut to the abdominal cavity. The size of the defect is variable, but usually the omphalocele sac contains some intestine, stomach, liver, and spleen. The abdominal cavity is small and underdeveloped. The umbilical cord can be seen to insert onto the center of the omphalocele sac. There is a high incidence of associated anomalies, including cardiac, other gastrointestinal anomalies, and chromosal syndromes (trisomy 13). Delivery room treatment involves covering the defect with sterile warm saline to prevent fluid loss and nasogastric tube decompression.

Gastroschisis[213] is a defect in the anterior abdominal wall lateral to the umbilicus with no covering sac, with the herniated viscera usually limited to intestine. Furthermore, the intestine has been exposed to amniotic fluid and has a thickened, beefy red appearance. The herniation is thought to occur as a rupture through an ischemic portion of the abdominal wall. Other than intestinal atresia, associated anomalies are uncommon. Acute therapy is as described for omphalocele.

Diaphragmatic Hernia

In diaphragmatic hernia, herniation of abdominal organs into the hemithorax (usually left) occurs because of a posterolateral defect in the diaphragm. Infants usually present in the delivery room with respiratory distress, cyanosis, decreased breath sounds on the side of the hernia, and shift of the mediastinum to the side opposite the hernia. The infants are often difficult to resuscitate and require early intubation. The rapidity and severity of presentation with respiratory distress is dependent on the degree of associated pulmonary hypoplasia. The ipsilateral and to some extent contralateral lung are compressed in utero because of the hernia. Delivery room treatment is to intubate, to ventilate, and to decompress the gastrointestinal tract with a nasogastric tube. A chest x-ray will confirm the diagnosis.

Necrotizing Enterocolitis

Necrotizing enterocolitis (NEC) is the most common acquired gastrointestinal emergency in the neonatal intensive care unit. This disorder predominantly affects premature infants, with higher incidences present with decreasing gestational age, although it is seen in term infants with polycythemia, congenital heart disease, and birth asphyxia.[214,215] The pathogenesis is multifactorial with intestinal ischemia, infection, provision of enteral feedings, and gut maturity playing roles to varying degrees in individual patients.[214,216] Tocolysis with indomethacin presumably related to changes in intestinal circulation has been associated with an increased incidence of NEC, while antenatal betamethasone may decrease the incidence.[18,217,218]

Clinically there is a varied spectrum of disease from a mild gastrointestinal disturbance to a rapid fulminant course characterized by intestinal gangrene, perforation, sepsis, and shock. The hallmark symptoms are abdominal distention, ileus, delayed gastric emptying, and bloody stools. The radiographic findings are bowel wall edema, pneumatosis intestinalis, biliary free air, and free peritoneal air. Associated symptoms include apnea, bradycardia, hypotension, and temperature instability.

Neonatal Jaundice

The most common "problem" encountered in a term nursery population is jaundice. Neonatal hyperbilirubinemia occurs when the normal pathways of bilirubin metabolism and excretion are altered. Figure 20-15

demonstrates the metabolism of bilirubin.[219] The normal destruction of circulating red cells accounts for about 75 percent of the newborn's daily bilirubin production. The remaining sources include ineffective erythropoiesis and tissue heme proteins. Heme is converted to bilirubin in the reticuloendothelial system. Unconjugated bilirubin is lipid soluble and transported in the plasma reversibly bound to albumin. Bilirubin enters the liver cells by dissociation from albumin in the hepatic sinusoids. Once in the hepatocyte bilirubin is conjugated with glucuronic acid in a reaction catalyzed by glucuronyltransferase. The water-soluble conjugated bilirubin is secreted into the biliary tree for excretion via the gastrointestinal tract. The enzyme β-glucuronidase is present in small bowel and hydrolyzes some of the conjugated bilirubin. This unconjugated

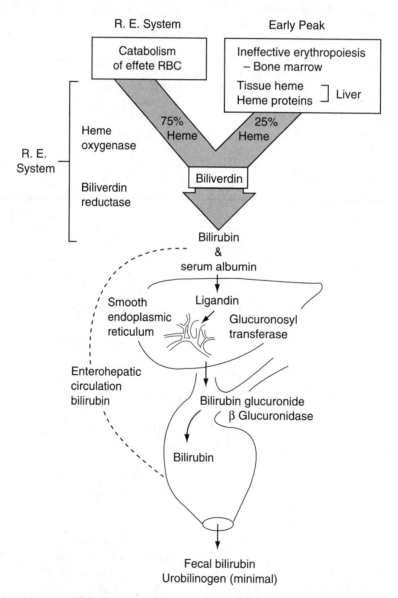

Fig. 20-15 Neonatal bile pigment metabolism. (Adapted from Maisels,[219] with permission.)

bilirubin can be reabsorbed into the circulation, adding to the total unconjugated bilirubin load (enterohepatic circulation).

Almost every newborn will develop a serum unconjugated bilirubin concentration of greater than 2 mg/dl during the first week of life. Approximately 50 percent of all infants above 2,500 g will have levels higher than 5 mg/dl and 6 percent will have 13.0 mg/dl or more.[220] This transient hyperbilirubinemia has been called *physiologic jaundice*. Major predisposing factors of jaundice are (1) increased bilirubin load because of increased red cell volume with decreased cell survival, increased ineffective erythropoiesis, and the enterohepatic circulation; and (2) defective bilirubin conjugation. Impaired hepatic uptake of bilirubin from the plasma and impaired bilirubin excretion contribute to a lesser extent to physiologic jaundice.

Pathologic jaundice during the early neonatal period is indirect hyperbilirubinemia usually caused by overproduction of bilirubin. The leading cause in this group of patients is hemolytic disease, of which fetomaternal blood group incompatibilities (Rh and ABO) are the most common (see Ch. 27). Other causes of hemolysis include genetic disorders such as hereditary spherocytosis and nonspherocytic hemolytic anomies. Other etiologies of bilirubin overproduction include extravasated blood (bruising, hemorrhage), polycythemia, and exaggerated enterohepatic circulation of bilirubin because of mechanical gastrointestinal obstruction or re-

duced peristalsis from inadequate oral intake. Disease states involving decreased bilirubin clearance must be considered in the patients in whom no cause of overproduction can be identified. Causes of indirect hyperbilirubinemia in this category include (1) familial deficiency of glucuronyltransferase (Crigler-Najjar syndrome), (2) Gilbert syndrome, (3) breast milk jaundice, and (4) hypothyroidism. Mixed or direct hyperbilirubinemia are rare during the first week of life.

A strong association exists between breast-feeding and neonatal hyperbilirubinemia. The syndrome of breast milk jaundice is characterized by full-term infants who have jaundice that persists into the second and third weeks of life with maximal bilirubin levels of 10 to 30 mg/dl. If breast-feeding is continued, the levels persist for 4 to 10 days and then decline to normal by 3 to 12 weeks. Interruption of breast-feeding is associated with a prompt decline in 48 hours.[221] In addition to this syndrome, breast-fed infants as a whole have higher bilirubin levels over the first 3 to 5 days of life than their formula-fed counterparts (Fig. 20-16).[220] Rather than interrupting breast-feeding, this early jaundice is responsive to increased frequency of breast-feeding. Suggested mechanisms for breast-feeding associated jaundice include decreased early caloric intake, inhibitors of bilirubin conjugation in breast milk, and increased intestinal reabsorption of bilirubin.[220,222]

The overriding concern with neonatal hyperbilirubinemia is the development of bilirubin toxicity causing

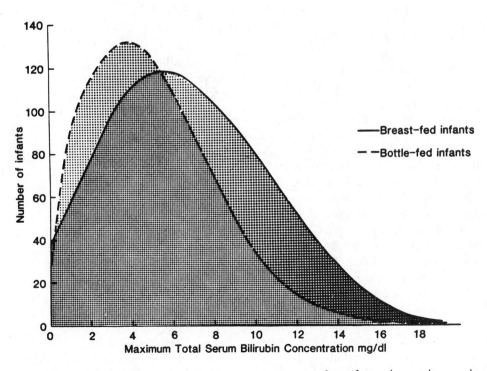

Fig. 20-16 Distribution of maximum serum bilirubin concentrations in white infants who weigh more than 2,500 g. (Adapted from Maisels and Gifford,[220] with permission.)

the pathologic entity of kernicterus, the staining of certain areas of the brain (basal ganglia, hippocampus, geniculate bodies, various brainstem nuclei, and cerebellum) by bilirubin. The clinical syndrome in term infants is marked by refusal to feed, high-pitched cry, hypertonicity, and opisthotonos. Survivors usually suffer sequelae, including athetoid cerebral palsy, high-frequency hearing loss, paralysis of upward gaze, and dental dysplasia.[223] The risk of kernicterus in a given infant is not well defined. The only group that one can speak of with any certainty is those infants with Rh isoimmunization in whom a level of 20 mg/dl has been associated with an increased risk of kernicterus.[224] This observation has been extended to the management of other neonates with hemolytic disease, although no definitive data exist regarding these infants. The risk is probably small for term infants without hemolytic disease even at levels higher than 20 mg/dl.[225–227] The true risk for nonhemolytic hyperbilirubinemia to produce brain damage in the preterm in the current era of liberal use of phototherapy that prevents marked elevation of severe bilirubin in these infants is unknown. However, most currently available data would suggest this risk is low.[228]

Neonatal Hematology

Anemia

Early hematopoietic cells originate in the yolk sac. By 8 weeks gestation, erythropoiesis is taking place in the liver, which remains the primary site of erythroid production through the early fetal period. By 6 months of gestation, the bone marrow becomes the principal site of red cell development. Normal hemoglobin levels at term range from 13.7 to 20.1 g/dl.[229] In the very preterm infant, values as low as 12 g/dl are acceptable.[230] Anemia at birth or appearing in the first few weeks of life is the result of blood loss, hemolysis, or underproduction of erythrocytes.[231] Blood loss resulting in anemia can occur prenatally, at the time of delivery, or postnatally. In utero blood loss can be the result of feto-maternal bleeding or from one fetus to another in a multiple pregnancy. The diagnosis of fetomaternal hemorrhage large enough to cause anemia can be made using the Kleihauer technique of acid elution to identify fetal cells in the maternal circulation. Blood loss at delivery can be due to umbilical cord rupture, incision of the placenta during cesarean delivery, placenta previa, or abruptio placenta. Internal hemorrhage can occur in the newborn, often related to a difficult delivery. Sites include intracranial, into giant cephalhematomas, subgaleal, retroperitoneal, liver capsule, and ruptured spleen. When blood loss has been chronic (e.g., fetomaternal), infants will be pale at birth but well compensated and without signs of volume loss. The initial hematocrit will be low. Acute bleeding will present with signs of hypovolemia (tachycardia, poor perfusion, hypotension). The initial hematocrit can be normal or decreased, but after several hours of equilibration it will be decreased. Anemia due to hemolysis from blood group incompatibilities is common in the newborn period. Less common causes of hemolysis include erythrocyte membrane abnormalities, enzyme deficiencies, and disorders of hemoglobin synthesis. Impaired erythrocyte production is an unusual cause of neonatal anemia.

Polycythemia

Elevated hematocrits occur in 1.5 to 4 percent of live births.[232–234] Although 50 percent of polycythemic infants are appropriate for gestational age (AGA), the proportion of polycythemic infants is greater in the SGA and LGA populations.[232] Causes of polycythemia include (1) twin to twin transfusion, (2) maternal to fetal transfusion, (3) intrapartum transfusion from the placenta associated with fetal distress, (4) chronic intrauterine hypoxia (SGA infants, LGA infants of diabetic mothers), and (5) delayed cord clamping.[235] The consequence of polycythemia is hyperviscosity, resulting in impaired perfusion of capillary beds. Therefore, clinical symptoms can be related to any organ system. As viscosity measurements are not routinely performed at most institutions, hyperviscosity is inferred from hematocrit because the major factor influencing viscosity in the newborn is red cell mass. Cord blood hematocrit greater than or equal to 57 percent[236] and capillary hematocrit of at least 70 percent are indicative of polycythemia. Confirmation of the diagnosis is a peripheral venous hematocrit of at least 64 percent.[236] Reduction of venous hematocrit to less than 60 percent may improve acute symptoms, but it has not been shown to improve long-term neurologic outcome.[237–239]

Thrombocytopenia

Neonatal thrombocytopenia can be isolated or occur associated with deficiency of clotting factors. A differential diagnosis is presented in Table 20-13. The immune thrombocytopenias have important implications for perinatal care. In idiopathic thrombocytopenia purpura (ITP), maternal antiplatelet antibodies that cross the placenta lead to destruction of fetal platelets. Correlation between the degree of thrombocytopenia in mother and fetus is not good[240,241]; thus the severity of thrombocytopenia in an individual fetus cannot be predicted with certainty. In some cases, antenatal administration of prednisone to the mother has improved the fetal platelet count, although this approach has not been uniformly successful.[242,243] There is a small but finite risk of intracranial hemorrhage with a traumatic delivery; thus, fetal platelet count should be determined by percutaneous umbilical blood sampling

Organ-Related Symptoms of Hyperviscosity

Central nervous system	Irritability, jitteriness, seizures, lethargy
Cardiopulmonary	Respiratory distress caused by congestive heart failure or persistent pulmonary hypertension
Gastrointestinal	Vomiting, heme-positive stools, abdominal distention, necrotizing enterocolitis
Renal	Decreased urine output, renal vein thrombosis
Metabolic	Hypoglycemia
Hematologic	Hyperbilirubinemia, thrombocytopenia

(PUBS). In some centers, fetal PC is ascertained by PUBS with cesarean delivery is indicated for fetal platelet count less than 50,000/µl. First-line postnatal therapy is intravenous immunoglobulin.[244] In alloimmune thrombocytopenia, maternal antibody to paternal platelet antigen on fetal platelets crosses the placenta and causes destruction of fetal platelets. In the largest series of cases of suspected alloimmune thrombocytopenic, the majority were due to P1[A1] alloantibodies.[245] As the maternal platelet count is normal, the diagnosis is suspected based on a history of a previously affected pregnancy. Intracranial hemorrhage is more common with this condition than in maternal ITP (10 to 30 percent) and can occur in the antenatal or intrapartum periods.[246] Recurrence risk is 75 percent. PUBS at 18 to 20 weeks can be done to measure platelet count. If severe thrombocytopenia is present, intravenous immunoglobulin should be given weekly to the mother.[246,247] Route of delivery is determined by fetal platelet count on a PUBS sample. Cesarean delivery is done for counts less than 50,000/µl.

Vitamin K Deficiency

Vitamin K_1 oxide (1 mg) should be given intramuscularly to all newborns to prevent hemorrhagic disease caused by a deficiency in vitamin K-dependent clotting factors.[248] Babies born to mothers who are on anticonvulsant medication are particularly at risk of having vitamin K deficiency. Oral vitamin K has been shown to be effective in raising vitamin K levels, but is not as effective in preventing late hemorrhagic disease of the newborn (presenting at 4 to 6 weeks of age). Late hemorrhagic disease of the newborn most commonly occurs in breast-fed infants whose courses have been complicated by diarrhea.

Perinatal Infection

See Chapter 38.

Classification of Newborns by Growth and Gestational Age

In assessing the risk for mortality or morbidity in a given neonate, evaluation of birth weight and gestational age together provide the clearest picture. This requires an accurate assessment of the infant's gestational age. When large populations are considered, maternal dates remain the single best determinant of gestational age. Early obstetric ultrasound is also a very useful adjunct in determining pregnancy dating. However, in the individual neonate, especially when dates are uncertain, a reliable postnatal assessment of gestational age is necessary. A scoring system appraising ges-

Table 20-13 Differential Diagnosis of Neonatal Thrombocytopenia

Diagnosis	Comments
Immune	Passively acquired antibody (e.g., idiopathic thrombocytopenic purpura, systemic lupus erythematosus, drug induced)
	Alloimmune sensitization to PL[A1] antigen
Infections	Bacterial; congenital viral infections (e.g., cytomegalovirus, rubella)
Syndromes	Absent radii; Fanconi's anemia
Giant hemangioma	
Thrombosis	
High-risk infant with respiratory distress syndrome, pulmonary hypertension, and so forth	Disseminated intravascular coagulation
	Isolated thrombocytopenia

Neuromuscular Maturity

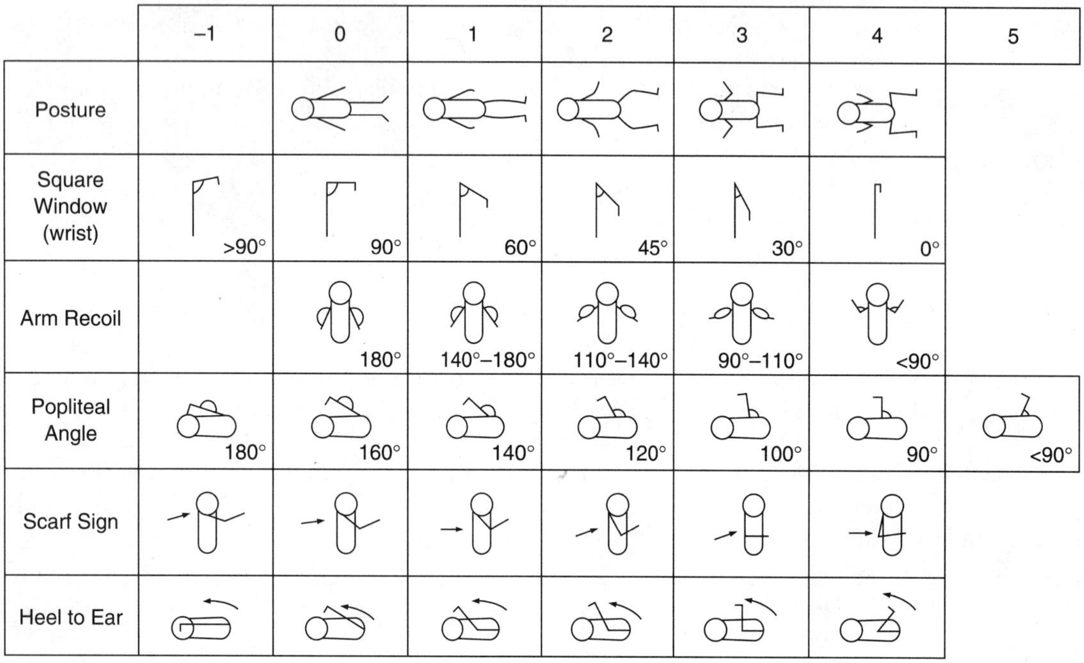

	-1	0	1	2	3	4	5
Posture							
Square Window (wrist)	>90°	90°	60°	45°	30°	0°	
Arm Recoil		180°	140°–180°	110°–140°	90°–110°	<90°	
Popliteal Angle	180°	160°	140°	120°	100°	90°	<90°
Scarf Sign							
Heel to Ear							

Physical Maturity

								Maturity Rating	
Skin	sticky friable transparent	gelatinous red, translucent	smooth pink, visible veins	superficial peeling &/or rash, few veins	cracking pale areas rare veins	parchment deep cracking no vessels	leathery cracked wrinkled	score	weeks
Lanugo	none	sparse	abundant	thinning	bald areas	mostly bald		-10	20
								-5	22
Plantar Surface	heel-toe 40–50 mm: -1 < 40 mm: -2	> 50 mm no crease	faint red marks	anterior transverse crease only	creases ant. 2/3	creases over entire sole		0	24
								5	26
								10	28
Breast	imperceptible	barely perceptible	flat areola no bud	stippled areola 1–2 mm bud	raised areola 3–4 mm bud	full areola 5–10 mm bud		15	30
								20	32
Eye/Ear	lids fused loosely: -1 tightly: -2	lids open pinna flat stays folded	sl. curved pinna; soft; slow recoil	well-curved pinna; soft but ready recoil	formed & firm instant recoil	thick cartilage ear stiff		25	34
								30	36
Genitals male	scrotum flat, smooth	scrotum empty faint rugae	testes in upper canal rare rugae	testes descending few rugae	testes down good rugae	testes pendulous deep rugae		35	38
								40	40
Genitals female	clitoris prominent labia flat	prominent clitoris small labia minora	prominent clitoris enlarging minora	majora & minora equally prominent	majora large minora small	majora cover clitoris & minora		45	42
								50	44

Fig. 20-17 Assessment of gestational age. (From Ballard et al.,[251] with permission.)

tational age on the basis of physical and neurologic criteria was developed by Dubowitz et al.[249] and later simplified and updated by Ballard et al.[250,251] (Fig. 20-17). Infants can then be classified, using growth parameters and gestational age, by means of intrauterine growth curves such as those developed by Lubchenco et al.[252] (Fig. 20-18). Infants born between 38 and 42 weeks are classified as term; less than 38 weeks, as preterm; and greater than 42 weeks, post-term. In each grouping, infants are then identified according to growth as AGA if birth weight falls between the 10th to 90th percentile, SGA if birth weight is below the 10th percentile, and LGA if birth weight is above the 90th percentile. On the basis of a given infant's classification,

the risk of mortality[253] (Fig. 20-19) can be assessed. Not only does mortality risk vary, but specific clinical problems can also be anticipated by an infant's birth weight/gestational age distribution.

There are numerous causes of growth retardation (see Ch. 25). Those operative early in pregnancy such as chromosomal aberrations, congenital viral infections, and some drug exposures induce symmetric retardation of weight, length, and head circumference. In most cases, the phenomenon occurs later in gestation and leads to more selective retardation of birth weight alone. Such factors include hypertension or other maternal vascular disease and multiple gestation.[254] Neonatal problems besides chromosomal ab-

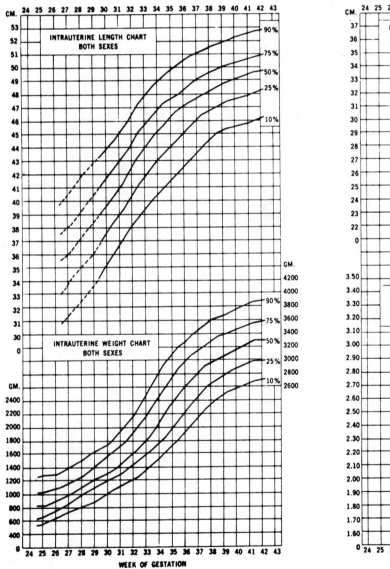

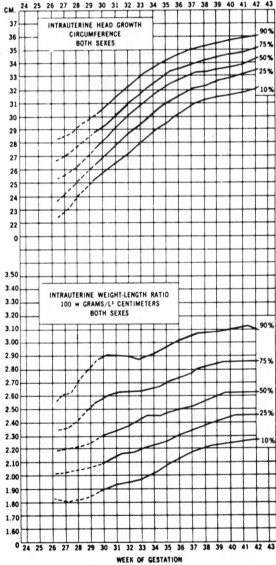

Fig. 20-18 Intrauterine growth curves for weight, length, and head circumference for singleton births in Colorado. (From Lubchenco et al.,[252] with permission.)

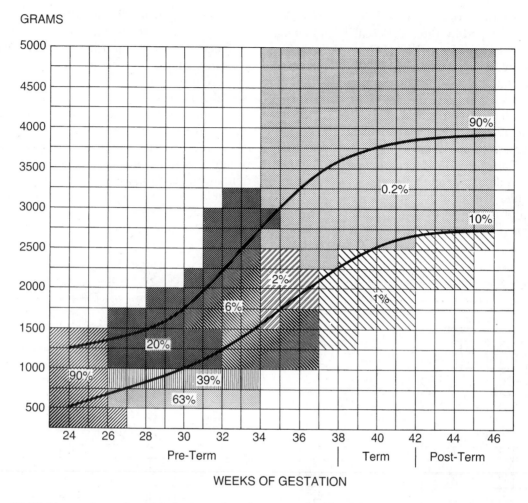

Fig. 20-19 Neonatal mortality risk by birth weight and gestational age based on 14,413 live births at the University of Colorado Health Sciences Center, 1974–1980. (From Koops et al.,[253] with permission.)

normalities and congenital viral infections common in SGA infants include birth asphyxia, hypoglycemia, polycythemia, and hypothermia. In addition, congenital malformations are seen more frequently among undergrown infants.[255]

The most common identifiable conditions leading to excessive infant birth weight are maternal diabetes and maternal obesity.[254] Other conditions associated with macrosomia are erythroblastosis fetalis, other causes of fetal hydrops, and Beckwith-Weidemann syndrome. LGA infants are at particular risk for hypoglycemia and birth trauma.

Nursery Care

Nurseries are classified based on level of care provided. Level I nurseries care for infants presumed healthy, with an emphasis on screening and surveillance. Level II nurseries can care for infants more than 30 weeks gestation, who weigh at least 1,200 g, and who require

special attention short of the need for circulatory or ventilator support and major surgical procedures. Level III nurseries care for all newborn infants who are critically ill regardless of the level of support required. A perinatal center encompasses both high-risk obstetric services and level III nursery services.

Care of the normal newborn involves observation of transition from intra- to extrauterine life, establishing breast or bottle feeds, noting normal patterns of stooling and urination, and surveillance for neonatal problems. Signs suggestive of illness include temperature instability, change in activity, refusal to feed, pallor, cyanosis, jaundice, tachypnea and respiratory distress, delayed (beyond 24 hours) passage of first stool or void, and bilious vomiting. In addition, the following laboratory screens should be performed: (1) blood type and direct and indirect Coombs test on infants born to mothers with type O or Rh-negative blood, (2) glucose screen in infants at risk for hypoglycemia, (3) hematocrit in infants with signs and symptoms of anemia or polycythemia, (4) serologic test for syphilis, and (5)

Infant Criteria for Early Discharge

1. Delivery is vertex, single, sterile, and vaginal.
2. Apgar scores at 1 and 5 minutes are ≥7.
3. The infant is term (38–42 weeks) and weighs 2,700–4,000 g.
4. Minimum length of stay is 20 hours. A transition to normal thermoregulation in an open crib, completion of two successful feedings, evidence of stool and void, completion of neonatal screening for metabolic disease, and blood type and Coomb's test (Rh− and O mothers) prior to discharge.
5. Vital signs within normal ranges at discharge; axillary temperature, 36.1° to 37.2°C; heart rate, 110–150/min; respiratory rate, 40–60/min.
6. The infant has a normal neonatal hospital course and presents no signs or symptoms that require continuous observation:
   Blood dextrose maintained, >40 mg/dl
   ABO-incompatible infants usually held 48 hours and released only if not requiring therapy for jaundice. These infants may leave at 24 hours with good follow-up examination if no jaundice is present.
7. Infants born to Group B streptococcus-positive mothers are observed for 48 hours.
8. Physical examination is completed by physician or trained physician's assistant.
9. Mother demonstrates understanding and ability to provide adequate care for her newborn; infant care education is provided on a one-to-one or classroom basis by the nursing staff before discharge.
10. Signed documentation by the mother that states her obligation to participate in follow-up care.

mandated screening for inborn errors of metabolism, such as PKU, maple syrup urine disease, homocystinuria, galactosemia, sickle cell disease, hypothyroidism, and cystic fibrosis. Finally, babies routinely receive 1 mg intramuscular of vitamin K to prevent vitamin K-deficient hemorrhagic disease of the newborn and either 1 percent silver nitrate or erythromycin ointment to prevent gonococcal ophthalmia neonatorum.

It is now fairly routine on most services for mothers and babies to be discharged within 24 hours of delivery. Criteria for early discharge at the University of Colorado are presented in the box above.[256] These criteria have been adapted from those of the American Academy of Pediatrics.[257]

Care of the Parents

Interest in maternal–infant bonding has grown in the last 20 years in part because of the observation of an excessive incidence of child abuse and nonorganic failure to thrive in infants who experienced a prolonged postdelivery separation from parents.[258] This circumstance had its roots in the historical approach to neonatal care, which emphasized infant isolation for prevention of infection. On the basis of this human experience as well as on studies of maternal–infant bonding in other species,[259] pendulum has now shifted to permit liberal nursery-visiting policies.

Klaus and Kennell[260] outline these steps in maternal–infant attachment: (1) planning the pregnancy, (2) confirming the pregnancy, (3) accepting the pregnancy, (4) noting fetal movement, (5) accepting the fetus as an individual, (6) going through labor, (7) giving birth, (8) hearing and seeing the baby, (9) touching, smelling, and holding the baby, (10) caretaking, and (11) accepting the infant as a separate individual. Numerous influences can affect this process. A mother's and father's actions and responses are derived from their own genetic endowment, their own interfamily relationships, cultural practices, past experiences with this or previous pregnancies, and, most importantly, how they were raised by their parents.[260] Also critical is the in-hospital experience surrounding the birth—how doctors and nurses act, separation from the baby, and hospital practices.

The 60- to 90-minute period after delivery is a very important time. The infant is alert, active, and able to follow with his or her eyes,[261] allowing meaningful interaction to transpire between infant and parents. The infant's array of sensory and motor abilities evokes responses from the mother and initiates communication that may be helpful for attachment and induction of reciprocal actions. Whether a critical time period for these initial interactions exists is not clear, but improved mothering behavior does seem to occur with increased contact over the first 3 postpartum days.[262] The practical implications of this information are that labor and delivery should pose as little anxiety as possible for the mother, and parents and baby should have time together immediately after delivery if the baby's medical condition permits. Eye prophylaxis for gonococcal ophthalmitis should ideally be withheld until after the initial bonding has taken place. It can be performed safely within 1 hour of birth.

Mothers with high-risk pregnancies are at increased risk for subsequent parenting problems. It is important for both obstetrician and pediatrician alike to be involved prenatally, allowing time to prepare the family for anticipated aspects of the baby's care as well as providing reassurance that the odds are heavily in favor of a live baby who will ultimately be healthy. If before birth one can anticipate a need for neonatal intensive care (known congenital anomaly, refractory premature labor), maternal transport to a center with a unit that can care for the baby should be planned. In this way, a mother can be with her baby during its most critical care. Before delivery it is also very helpful to allow the parents to tour the unit their baby will occupy. This practice greatly reduces anxiety after the baby is born.

The single basic principle in dealing with parents of a sick infant is to provide essential information clearly and accurately to both parents, preferably when they are together. With improved survival rates, especially in prematures, most babies, despite early problems, will do well. It is therefore reasonable in most circumstances to be positive about the outcome. There is also no reason to emphasize problems that might occur in the future or to deal with individual worries of the physician. Questions, if asked, need to be answered honestly, but the list of parents' worries does not need to be voluntarily increased.

Before the parents' initial visit to the unit, a physician or nurse should describe what the baby and the equipment look like. When they arrive in the nursery, this can again be reviewed in detail. If a baby must be moved to another hospital, the mother should be given time to see and to touch her infant prior to transfer. The father should be encouraged to meet the baby at the receiving hospital so he can become comfortable with the intensive care unit. He can serve as a link between baby and mother with information and photographs.

As a baby's course proceeds, the nursery staff can help the parents to become comfortable with their infant. This can include participation in caretaking as well as skin-to-skin contact with the infant (Kangaroo care).[263] Individualized developmentally based care has also shown some benefit for high-risk infants.[264] It is also important for the staff to discuss among themselves any problems that parents may be having as well as to keep a record of visits and phone calls. This approach will allow early intervention to deal with potential problems.

The birth of an infant with a congenital malformation provides another situation in which staff support is essential. Parents' reactions to the birth of a malformed infant follow a predictable course. For most, there is initial shock and denial, a period of sadness and anger, gradual adaptation, and finally an increased satisfaction with and the ability to care for the baby. The parents must be allowed to pass through these stages and, in effect, to mourn the loss of the anticipated normal child.[265] Again, information needs to be provided clearly and accurately to both parents, including the prognosis for the particular problem.

The death of an infant or a stillborn is a highly stressful family event. This fact has been emphasized by Cullberg[266] who found that psychiatric disorders developed in 19 of 56 mothers studied 1 to 2 years after the deaths of their neonates. One of the major predispositions was a breakdown of communication between parents. The health care staff needs to encourage the parents to talk with each other, discuss their feelings, and display emotion. The staff should talk with the parents at the time of death and then several months later to review the findings of the autopsy, answer questions, and see how the family is doing.

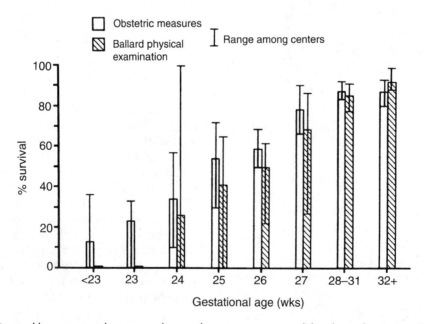

Fig. 20-20 Survival by gestational age according to obstetric measures and the physical component of the Ballard physical examination. (From Hack et al.,[267] with permission.)

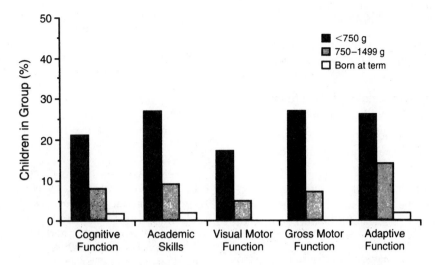

Fig. 20-21 Percentage of children at different birth weights with subnormal functioning. (From Hack et al.,[274] with permission.)

Outcome of Neonatal Intensive Care

More sophisticated neonatal care has resulted in improved survival of very-low-birth-weight ($\leq$1,500 g) infants, in particular those less than 1,000 g (Fig. 20-20). This is very evident if one compares the data in Figures 20-19 and 20-20. Current survival rates are 90 percent or greater for infants 1,000 to 1,500 g, 66 percent for infants 750 to 1,000 g, and 34 percent for infants less than 750 g.[267,268] It is important to note that survival in terms of best obstetric estimate is greater at very low gestational ages than survival in terms of postnatal assessment of gestational age. The numbers in terms of best obstetric estimate should be referred to for antenatal counseling. This improved survival comes with a price, as a variety of morbidities are seen in these infants. However, concern that improved survival would be associated with an increased rate of neurologic sequelae has been largely unfounded. Major neurologic morbidities seen in very-low-birth-weight infants include cerebral palsy (spastic diplegia, quadriplegia, hemiplegia, or paresis), cognitive delay, and hydrocephalus. Lesser disabilities include learning and behavior difficulties that can cause problems when school age is attained. The rate of significant neurologic disability is fairly constant at 10 to 25 percent of all very-low-birth-weight (<1,500 g) survivors. The number trends toward the higher side in infants of extremely low birth weight (<1,000 g).[269–272] In addition to a slight increase in severe disability, extremely low-birth-weight infants have an increased rate of lesser disabili-

ties, including subnormal mental performance and the need for special education in school (Fig. 20-21).[273,274] Risk factors for neurologic morbidity include seizures, major intracranial hemorrhage or periventricular leukomalacia, severe intrauterine growth retardation, need for mechanical ventilation, poor early head growth, and low socioeconomic class.[274–278]

There are other morbidities that need to be considered as well. As the number of less than 1,000-g survivors has increased, a reemergence of retinopathy of prematurity has been seen. This disorder, caused by retinal vascular proliferation leading to hemorrhage, scarring, retinal detachment, and blindness, originally was thought to be due solely to inappropriate exposure to high concentrations of oxygen. It is now thought that the origin is multifactorial, with extreme prematurity a critical factor.[279] Incidence of acute proliferative retinopathy by birth weight is less than 10 percent in infants weighing more than 1,250 g, 15 percent in those 1,000 to 1,250 g, 40 percent in those 750 to 1,000 g, and 50 percent in those less than 750 g.[280] Severe retinopathy is evident in 5 percent of the infants 1,000 to 1,250 g, in 15 percent of the 750 to 1,000 g population, and 25 percent of the less than 750 g infants. Of the infants with severe retinopathy, 10 percent (4 percent of the total population) will go on to have severe visual problems. The other major neurosensory morbidity is hearing loss, which occurs in 2 percent of neonatal intensive care unit survivors.[281] Other sequelae of neonatal intensive care include chronic lung disease, growth failure, short gut, and need for postdischarge rehospitalization.

10 Key Points

- Surfactant maintains lung expansion on expiration by lowering surface tension at the air–liquid interface in the alveolus.

- Respiratory distress syndrome in premature infants is in part due to a deficiency of surfactant.

- A number of hormones including corticosteroids and thyroid hormone contribute to the regulation of pulmonary surfactant production.

- Transition from intra- to extrauterine life requires removal of fluid from the lungs, switching from a fetal to neonatal circulation, and establishment of a normal neonatal lung volume.

- The most important step in neonatal resuscitation is to achieve adequate expansion of the lungs.

- Meconium aspiration syndrome likely is the result of intrauterine asphyxia.

- The best predictor of neurologic sequelae of birth asphyxia is the presence of hypoxic ischemic encephalopathy in the neonatal period. The neurologic sequelae of birth asphyxia is cerebral palsy.

- The major neurologic complication seen in the premature infant is periventricular/intraventricular hemorrhage.

- Hypoglycemia is a predictable and preventable complication in the newborn.

- Survival, in particular for infants less than 1,000 g, has increased with improved methods of neonatal intensive care, including provision of exogenous surfactant.

References

1. Hodson WA: Normal and abnormal structural development of the lung. p. 771. In Polin RA, Fox WW (eds): Fetal and Neonatal Physiology. WB Saunders, Philadelphia, 1992

2. Thurlbeck WM: Postnatal growth and development of the lung. Am Rev Respir Dis 111:803, 1975

3. Campiche MA, Gautier A, Hernandez EI, Reymond A: An electron microscope study of the fetal development of human lung. Pediatrics 32:976, 1963

4. Wright JR, Clements JA: Metabolism and turnover of lung surfactant. Am Rev Respir Dis 136:426, 1987

5. Rider ED, Ikegami M, Jobe AH: Localization of alveolar surfactant clearance in rabbit lung cells. Am J Physiol 283:L201, 1992

6. Jobe AH: The developmental biology of the lung. p. 783. In Fanaroff AA, Martin RI (eds). Neonatal-Perinatal Medicine: Diseases of the Fetus and Infant. 5th Ed. CV Mosby, St. Louis, 1992

7. Clements JA, Tooley WH: Kinetics of surface-active material in the fetal lung. p. 349. In Hodson WA (ed): Development of the Lung. Marcel Dekker, New York, 1977

8. Jobe AH: The role of surfactant in neonatal adaptation. Semin Perinatol 12:113, 1988

9. Jobe AH: Pulmonary surfactant therapy. N Engl J Med 328:861, 1993

10. Ballard PL: Hormonal regulation of pulmonary surfactant. Endocrine Rev 10:165, 1989

11. Weaver TE, Whitsett JA: Function and regulation of expression of pulmonary surfactant-associated proteins. Biochem J 273:249, 1991

12. Hawgood S, Clements JA: Pulmonary surfactant and its apoproteins. J Clin Invest 86:1, 1990

13. Mendelson CR, Alcorn JL, Gao E: The pulmonary surfactant protein genes and their regulation in fetal lung. Semin Perinatol 17:223, 1993

14. Possmayer F: The role of surfactant-associated proteins. Am Rev Respir Dis 142:749, 1990

15. Kuan S, Rust K, Crouch E: Interaction of surfactant protein D with bacterial lipopolysaccharides. J Clin Invest 90:97, 1992

16. Moya FR, Gross I: Combined hormonal therapy for the prevention of respiratory distress syndrome and its consequences. Semin Perinatol 17:267, 1993

17. Liggins GC, Howie RN: A controlled trial of antepartum glucocorticoid treatment for prevention of the respiratory distress syndrome in premature infants. Pediatrics 50:515, 1972

18. Crowley P, Chalmers I, Keirse MJNC: The effects of corticosteroid administration before preterm delivery: an overview of the evidence from controlled trials. Br J Obstet Gynaecol 97:11, 1990

19. Leviton A, Kuban KC, Pagano M et al: Antenatal corticosteroids appear to reduce the risk of postnatal germinal matrix hemorrhage in intubated low birth weight newborns. Pediatrics 91:1083, 1993

20. Schmand B, Neuvel J, Smolders-de-Haas H et al: Psychological development of children who were treated antenatally with corticosteroids to prevent respiratory distress syndrome. Pediatrics 86:58, 1990

21. Smolders-de-Haas H, Neuvel J, Schmand B et al: Physical development and medical history of children who were treated antenatally with corticosteroids to prevent respiratory distress syndrome: a 10- to 12-year follow-up. Pediatrics 86:65, 1990

22. Long W (ed): Surfactant replacement therapy. Clin Perinatol 20:4, 1993

23. Pramanik AK, Holtzman RB, Merritt TA: Surfactant replacement therapy for pulmonary diseases. Pediatr Clin North Am 40:913, 1993

24. Merritt TA, Soll RF, Hallman M: Overview of exogenous surfactant replacement therapy. J Intensive Care Med 8:205, 1993

25. Jobe AH, Mitchell BR, Gunkel JH: Beneficial effects of the combined use of prenatal corticosteroids and postnatal surfactant on preterm infants. Am J Obstet Gynecol 168:508, 1993

26. Thorpe-Beeston JG, Nicolaides KH, Snijders RJM et al: Fetal thyroid stimulating hormone response to mater-

nal administration of thyrotropin-releasing hormone. Am J Obstet Gynecol 164:1244, 1991

27. Rooney SA, Marino PA, Gobran LJ et al: Thyrotropin-releasing hormone increases the amount of surfactant in lung lavage from fetal rabbits. Pediatr Res 13:623, 1979

28. Gross I, Dynia DW, Wilson CW et al: Glucocorticoid-thyroid hormone interaction in the fetal rat lung. Pediatr Res 18:191, 1984

29. Schellenberg J, Liggins GC, Manzai M et al: Synergistic hormonal effects on lung maturation in fetal sheep. J Appl Physiol 65:94, 1988

30. Ballard RA, Ballard PL, Creasy RK et al: Respiratory disease in very-low-birth weight infants after prenatal thyrotropin-releasing hormone and glucocorticoid. Lancet 339:510, 1992

31. Jansen AH, Chernick V: Development of respiratory control. Physiol Rev 63:437, 1983

32. Dawes GS, Fox HE, Leduc BM et al: Respiratory movements and rapid eye movement sleep in the foetal lamb. J Physiol (Lond) 220:119, 1972

33. Rigatto H, Moore M, Cates D et al: Fetal breathing and behavior measured through a double-wall Plexiglas window in sheep. J Appl Physiol 61:160, 1986

34. Dawes GS, Gardner WN, Johnston BM, Walker DW: Breathing in fetal lambs: the effect of brainstem section. J Physiol (Lond) 335:535, 1983

35. Hanson MA, Moore PJ, Nijhuis JG, Parkes MJ: Effects of pilocarpine on breathing movements in normal, chemodenervated and brainstem-transected fetal sheep. J Physiol (Lond) 400:415, 1988

36. Kaplan M: Fetal breathing movements, an update for the pediatrician. Am J Dis Child 137:177, 1983

37. Connors G, Hunse C, Carmichael L et al: The role of carbon dioxide in the generation of human fetal breathing movements. Am J Obstet Gynecol 158:322, 1988

38. Boddy K, Dawes GS, Fisher R et al: Foetal respiratory movements, electrocortical and cardiovascular responses to hypoxaemia and hypercapnia in sheep. J Physiol (Lond) 243:599, 1974

39. Baier RJ, Hasan SU, Cates DB et al: Effects of various concentrations of O_2 and umbilical cord occlusion on fetal breathing and behavior. J Appl Physiol 68:1597, 1990

40. Goodman JDS: The effect of intravenous glucose on human fetal breathing measured by Doppler ultrasound. Br J Obstet Gynecol 87:1080, 1980

41. Patrick J, Campbell K, Carmichael L et al: Patterns of human fetal breathing during the last 10 weeks of pregnancy. Obstet Gynecol 56:24, 1980

42. Maloney JE, Adamson TM, Brodecky V et al: Modification of respiratory center output in the unanesthetized fetal sheep "in utero." J Appl Physiol 39:552, 1975

43. Jansen AH, Chernick V: Fetal breathing and development of control of breathing. J Appl Physiol 70:1431, 1991

44. Kitterman JA, Liggins GC, Clements JA, Tooley WH: Stimulation of breathing movements in fetal sheep by inhibitors of prostaglandin synthesis. J Dev Physiol 1:453, 1979

45. James LS, Weisbrot IM, Prince CE et al: The acid-base status of human infants in relation to birth asphyxia and the onset of respiration. J Pediatr 52:379, 1958

46. Agostoni E, Taglietti A, Agostoni AF, Setnikar I: Mechanical aspects of the first breath. J Appl Physiol 13:344, 1958

47. Milner AD, Vyas H: Lung expansion at birth. J Pediatr 101:879, 1982

48. Karlberg P, Adams FH, Geubelle F, Wallgren G: Alteration of the infant's thorax during vaginal delivery. Acta Obstet Gynaecol Scand 41:223, 1962

49. Bosma J, Lind J: Upper respiratory mechanisms of newborn infants. Acta Paediatr Scand 51(Suppl 135):132, 1962

50. Jäykkä S: Capillary erection and lung expansion. Acta Paediatr Scand 46(Suppl 112), 1957

51. Talbert DG: Role of pulmonary vascular pressure in the first breath: engineering reassessment of Jaykka's experimental findings. Acta Paediatr Scand 81:737, 1992

52. Karlberg P, Cherry RB, Escardó FE, Koch G: Respiratory studies in newborn infants. II. Pulmonary ventilation and mechanics of breathing in the first minutes of life, including the onset of respiration. Acta Paediatr Scand 51:121, 1962

53. Karlberg P: The adaptive changes in the immediate postnatal period, with particular reference to respiration. J Pediatr 56:585, 1960

54. Klaus M, Tooley WH, Weaver KH, Clements JA: Lung volume in the newborn infant. Pediatrics 30:111, 1962

55. Olver RE, Strang LB: Ion fluxes across the pulmonary epithelium and the secretion of lung liquid in the foetal lamb. J Physiol (Lond) 241:327, 1974

56. Bland RD: Formation of fetal lung liquid and its removal near birth. p. 782. In Polin RA, Fox WW (eds): Fetal and Neonatal Physiology. WB Saunders, Philadelphia, 1992

57. Bland RD: Lung liquid clearance before and after birth. Semin Perinatol 12:124, 1988

58. Bland RD, Hansen TN, Haberkern CM et al: Lung fluid balance in lambs before and after birth. J Appl Physiol 53:992, 1982

59. Raj JU, Bland RD: Lung luminal liquid clearance in newborn lambs. Effect of pulmonary microvascular pressure elevation. Am Rev Respir Dis 134:305, 1986

60. Bland RD, Bressack MA, McMillan DD: Labor decreases the lung water content of newborn rabbits. Am J Obstet Gynecol 135:364, 1979

61. Bland RD, Carlton DP, Scheerer RG et al: Lung fluid balance in lambs before and after premature birth. J Clin Invest 84:568, 1989

62. Peltonen T, Hirvonen L: Experimental studies on fetal and neonatal circulation. Acta Paediatr Scand (Suppl 161), 1965

63. Rudolph AM: Fetal circulation and cardiovascular adjustments after birth. p. 1309. In Rudolph AM, Hoffman JIE, Rudolph CD (eds): Rudolph's Pediatrics. 19th Ed. Appleton & Lange, East Norwalk, CT, 1991

64. Teitel DF: Circulatory adjustments to postnatal life. Semin Perinatol 12:96, 1988

65. Friedman AH, Fahey JT: The transition from fetal to neonatal circulation: normal responses and implications for infants with heart disease. Semin Perinatol 17: 106, 1993

66. Naeye RL: Arterial changes during the perinatal period. Arch Pathol Lab Med 71:121, 1961

67. Walker AM, Ritchie BC, Adamson TM, Maloney JE: Effect of changing lung liquid volume on the pulmonary circulation of fetal lambs. J Appl Physiol 64:61, 1988

68. Teitel DF, Iwamato HS, Rudolph AM: Changes in the pulmonary circulation during birth-related events. Pediatr Res 27:372, 1990

69. Kinsella JP, McQueston JA, Rosenberg AA, Abman SH: Hemodynamic effects of exogenous nitric oxide in ovine transitional pulmonary circulation. Am J Physiol 263:H875, 1992

70. Abman SH, Chatfield BA, Hall SL, McMurtry IF: Role of endothelium-derived relaxing factor during transitional pulmonary circulation at birth. Am J Physiol 259: H1921, 1990

71. Moss AJ, Emmanoulides G, Duffie ER Jr: Closure of the ductus arteriosus in the newborn infant. Pediatrics 32: 25, 1963

72. Gentile R, Stevenson G, Dooley T et al: Pulse Doppler echocardiographic determination of time of ductal closure in normal newborn infants. J Pediatr 98:443, 1981

73. Heymann MA, Rudolph AM: Control of the ductus arteriosus. Physiol Rev 55:62, 1975

74. Clyman RI: Ontogeny of the ductus arteriosus response to prostaglandins and inhibitors of their synthesis. Semin Perinatol 4:115, 1980

75. Clyman RI: Ductus arteriosus: current theories of prenatal and postnatal regulation. Semin Perinatol 11:64, 1987

76. Behrman RE, Lees MH: Organ blood flows of the fetal, newborn and adult rhesus monkey. Biol Neonate 18: 330, 1971

77. Phibbs RH: Delivery room management. p. 248. In Avery GB, Fletcher MA, MacDonald MG (eds): Neonatology: Pathophysiology and Management of the Newborn. 4th Ed. JB Lippincott, Philadelphia, 1994

78. Duffy TE, Kohle SJ, Vannucci RC: Carbohydrate and energy metabolism in perinatal rat brain: relation to survival in anoxia. J Neurochem 24:271, 1975

79. Reid DL, Parer JT, Williams K et al: Effects of severe reduction in maternal placental blood flow on blood flow distribution in the sheep fetus. J Dev Physiol 15: 183, 1991

80. Itskovitz J, Goetzman BW, Rudolph AM: The mechanism of late deceleration of the heart rate and its relationship to oxygenation in normoxemic and chronically hypoxemic fetal lambs. Am J Obstet Gynecol 142:66, 1982

81. Gunn AJ, Parer JT, Mallard EC et al: Cerebral histological and electrocorticographic changes after asphyxia in fetal sheep. Pediatr Res 31:486, 1992

82. Jones CT: The development of some metabolic responses to hypoxia in the foetal sheep. J Physiol (Lond) 265:743, 1977

83. Vintzileos AM, Fleming AD, Scorza WE et al: Relation-ship between fetal biophysical activities and umbilical cord blood gas values. Am J Obstet Gynecol 165:707, 1991

84. Holowach-Thurston J, McDougal DB Jr: Effect of ischemia on metabolism of the brain of the newborn mouse. Am J Physiol 216:348, 1969

85. Dawes GS: Foetal and Neonatal Physiology. Year Book, Chicago, 1968

86. Cross KW: Resuscitation of the asphyxiated infant. Br Med Bull 22:73, 1966

87. Gupta JM, Tizard JPM: The sequence of events in neonatal apnea. Lancet 2:55, 1967

88. American Heart Association and American Academy of Pediatrics: Textbook of Neonatal Resuscitation. American Heart Association, Washington DC, 1994

89. Apgar V: A proposal for a new method of evaluation of the newborn infant. Anesth Analg 32:260, 1953

90. Hull D: Lung expansion and ventilation during resuscitation of asphyxiated newborn infants. J Pediatr 75:47, 1969

91. Jain L, Ferre C, Vidyasagar D: Cardiopulmonary resuscitation of apparently stillborn infants: survival and longterm outcome. J Pediatr 118:778, 1991

92. Katz VL, Bowes WA: Meconium aspiration syndrome: reflections on a murky subject. Am J Obstet Gynecol 166:171, 1992

93. Carson BS, Losey RW, Bowes WA, Simmons MA: Combined obstetric and pediatric approach to prevent meconium aspiration syndrome. Am J Obstet Gynecol 126: 712, 1976

94. Block MF, Kallenberger DA, Kern JD, Nepveux RD: In utero meconium aspiration by the baboon fetus. Obstet Gynecol 57:37, 1981

95. Brown BL, Gleicher N: Intrauterine meconium aspiration. Obstet Gynecol 57:26, 1981

96. Falciglia HS: Failure to prevent meconium aspiration syndrome. Obstet Gynecol 71:349, 1988

97. Falciglia HS, Henderschott C, Potter P, Helmchen R: Does DeLee suction at the perineum prevent meconium aspiration syndrome? Am J Obstet Gynecol 167:1243, 1992

98. Linder N, Aranda JV, Tsur M et al: Need for endotracheal intubation and suction in meconium-stained neonates. J Pediatr 112:613, 1988

99. Yoder BA: Meconium-stained amniotic fluid and respiratory complications: impact of selective tracheal suction. Obstet Gynecol 83:77, 1994

100. Murphy JD, Vawter GF, Reid LM: Pulmonary vascular disease in fatal meconium aspiration. J Pediatr 104:758, 1984

101. Jovanovic R, Nguyen HT: Experimental meconium aspiration in guinea pigs. Obstet Gynecol 73:652, 1989

102. Sadovsky Y, Amon E, Bade ME, Petrie RH: Prophylactic amnioinfusion during labor complicated by meconium: a preliminary report. Am J Obstet Gynecol 161:613, 1989

103. Wenstrom KD, Parsons MT: The prevention of meconium aspiration in labor using amnioinfusion. Obstet Gynecol 73:647, 1989

104. MacDonald HM, Mulligan JC, Allen AC, Taylor PM:

Neonatal asphyxia. I. Relationship of obstetric and neonatal complicatons to neonatal mortality in 38,405 consecutive deliveries. J Pediatr 96:898, 1980

105. Brown JK, Purvis RJ, Forfar JO, Cockburn F: Neurologic aspects of perinatal asphyxia. Dev Med Child Neurol 16:567, 1974

106. Nelson KB, Emery ES III: Birth asphyxia and the neonatal brain: what do we know and when do we know it? Clin Perinatol 20:327, 1993

107. Scheller JM, Nelson KB: Does cesarean delivery prevent cerebral palsy or other neurologic problems of childhood? Obstet Gynecol 83:624, 1994

108. Grant A, Joy M-T, O'Brien N et al: Cerebral palsy among children born during the Dublin randomised trial of intrapartum monitoring. Lancet 2:1233, 1989

109. Nelson KB, Ellenberg JH: Obstetric complications as risk factors for cerebral palsy or seizure disorders. JAMA 251:1843, 1984

110. Goldaber KB, Gilstrap LC, Leveno KJ et al: Pathologic fetal acidemia. Obstet Gynecol 78:1103, 1991

111. Finer NN, Robertson CMT: Long-term follow-up of term neonates with perinatal asphyxia. Clin Perinatol 20:483, 1993

112. Gray PH, Tudehope DI, Masel JP et al: Perinatal hypoxic-ischaemic brain injury: prediction of outcome. Dev Med Child Neurol 35:965, 1993

113. Perlman JM, Tack ED: Renal injury in the asphyxiated newborn infant: relationship to neurologic outcome. J Pediatr 113:875, 1988

114. Freeman JM, Nelson KB: Intrapartum asphyxia and cerebral palsy. Pediatrics 82:240, 1988

115. Freeman JM (ed): Prenatal and Perinatal Factors Associated with Brain Disorders. Publication No. 85-1149, NIH, Bethesda, MD, 1985

116. Nelson KB, Ellenberg JH: Antecedents of cerebral palsy: multivariate analysis of risk. N Engl J Med 315:81, 1986

117. Volpe JJ: Intraventricular hemorrhage and brain injury in the premature infant: neuropathology and pathogenesis. Clin Perinatol 16:361, 1989

118. Philip AGS, Allan WC, Tito AM, Wheeler LR: Intraventricular hemorrhage in preterm infants: declining incidence in the 1980s. Pediatrics 84:797, 1989

119. Pasternak JF, Groothuis DR, Fischer JM, Fischer DP: Regional cerebral blood flow in the newborn beagle pup: the germinal matrix is a "low-flow" structure. Pediatr Res 16:499, 1982

120. Goddard J, Lewis RM, Armstrong DL, Zeller RS: Moderate, rapidly induced hypertension as a cause of intraventricular hemorrhage in the newborn beagle model. J Pediatr 96:1057, 1980

121. Andrew M, Castle V, Saigal S et al: Clinical impact of neonatal thrombocytopenia. J Pediatr 110:457, 1987

122. McDonald MM, Johnson ML, Rumack CM et al: Role of coagulopathy in newborn intracranial hemorrhage. Pediatrics 74:26, 1984

123. Partridge JC, Babock DS, Steichen JJ, Han BK: Optimal timing for diagnostic cranial ultrasound in low-birth-weight infants: detection of intracranial hemorrhage and ventricular dilation. J Pediatr 102:281, 1983

124. Papile L-A, Burstein J, Burstein R, Koffler H: Incidence and evolution of subependymal and intraventricular hemorrhage: a study of infants with birth weights less than 1500 gm. J Pediatr 92:529, 1978

125. Ford LM, Steichen J, Steichen Asch PA et al: Neurologic status and intracranial hemorrhage in very-low-birth-weight preterm infants: outcome at 1 and 5 years. Am J Dis Child 143:1186, 1989

126. Lowe J, Papille LA: Neurodevelopmental performance of very-low-birth-weight infants with mild periventricular, intraventricular hemorrhage. Outcome at 5 to 6 years of age. Am J Dis Child 144:1242, 1990

127. Guzzetta F, Shackelford GD, Volpe S et al: Periventricular echodensities in the premature newborn: critical determinant of neurologic outcome. Pediatrics 78:995, 1986

128. Shankaran S, Koepke T, Woldt E et al: Outcome after posthemorrhagic ventriculomegaly in comparison with mild hemorrhage without ventriculomegaly. J Pediatr 114:109, 1989

129. Szymonowicz W, Yu VYH, Bajuk B, Astbury J: Neurodevelopmental outcome of periventricular hemorrhage and leukomalacia in infants 1250g or less at birth. Early Hum Dev 14:1, 1986

130. Abdel-Rahman AM, Rosenberg AA: Preventon of intraventricular hemorrhage in the premature infant. Clin Perinatol 21:505, 1994

131. Volpe JJ: Neonatal seizures: current concepts and revised classificaton. Pediatrics 84:422, 1989

132. Schullinger JN: Birth trauma. Pediatr Clin North Am 40:1351, 1993

133. Arey JB, Dent J: Causes of fetal and neonatal death with special reference to pulmonary and inflammatory lesions. J Pediatr 42:205, 1953

134. Valdes-Dapena MR, Arey JB: The causes of neonatal mortality: an analysis of 501 autopsies on newborn infants. J Pediatr 77:366, 1970.

135. Zelson C, Lee SJ, Pearl M: The incidence of skull fractures underlying cephalohematomas in newborn infants. J Pediatr 85:371, 1974

136. Volpe JJ: Neonatal intracranial hemorrhage: pathophysiology, neuropathology, and clinical features. Clin Perinatol 4:77, 1977

137. Eng GD: Brachial plexus palsy in newborn infants. Pediatrics 48:18, 1971

138. Brans YW, Cassidy G: Neonatal spinal cord injuries. Am J Obstet Gynecol 123:918, 1975

139. Gresham EL: Birth trauma. Pediatr Clin North Am 22:317, 1975

140. Mitchell SC, Korones SB, Berendes HW: Congenital heart disease in 56,109 births: incidence and natural history. Circulation 43:323, 1971

141. Fox WW, Duara S: Persistent pulmonary hypertenson in the neonate: diagnosis and management. J Pediatr 103:505, 1983

142. Rudolph AM: High pulmonary vascular resistance after birth. 1. Pathophysiologic considerations and etiologic classification. Clin Pediatr 19:585, 1980

143. Walsh-Sukys MC: Persistent pulmonary hypertension of

the newborn: the black box revisited. Clin Perinatol 20: 127, 1993

144. Kanto WP: A decade of experience with neonatal extracorporeal membrane oxygenation. J Pediatr 124:335, 1994

145. Kinsella JP, Neish SR, Ivy D et al: Clinical responses to prolonged treatment of persistent pulmonary hypertension of the newborn with low doses of inhaled nitric oxide. J Pediatr 123:103, 1993

146. Roberts JD, Lang P, Polaner DM, Zapol WM: Inhaled nitric oxide in persistent pulmonary hypertension of the newborn. Lancet 340:818, 1992

147. Clark RH: High frequency ventilation. J Pediatr 124: 661, 1994

148. Avery ME, Gatewood OB, Brumley G: Transient tachypnea of the newborn. Am J Dis Child 111:380, 1966

149. St. Geme JW Jr, Murray DL, Carter J et al: Perinatal bacterial infection after prolonged rupture of amniotic membranes: an analysis of risk and management. J Pediatr 104:608, 1984

150. Weisman LE, Stoll BJ, Cruess DF et al: Early onset group B streptococcal sepsis: a current assessment. J Pediatr 121:428, 1992

151. Siegel JD, McCracken GH Jr: Sepsis neonatorum. N Engl J Med 304:642, 1981

152. Ablow RC, Driscoll SG, Effman EL et al: A comparison of early-onset group B streptococcal neonatal infection and the respiratory-distress syndrome of the newborn. N Engl J Med 294:65, 1976

153. Avery ME, Mead J: Surface properties in relation to atelectasis and hyaline membrane disease. Am J Dis Child 97:517, 1959

154. Whitsett JA, Pryhuber GS, Rice WR et al: Acute respiratory disorders. p. 429. In Avery GB, Fletcher MA, MacDonald MG (eds): Neonatology: Pathophysiology and Management of the Newborn. 4th Ed. JB Lippincott, Philadelphia, 1994

155. Jobe AH: Pathophysiology of respiratory distress syndrome. p. 995. In Polin RA, Fox WW (eds): Fetal and Neonatal Physiology. WB Saunders, Philadelphia, 1992

156. Northway WH Jr, Rosan RC, Porter DY: Pulmonary disease following respiratory therapy of hyaline membrane disease. N Engl J Med 276:357, 1967

157. Northway WH Jr: An introduction to bronchopulmonary dysplasia. Clin Perinatol 19:489, 1992

158. Sauve RS, Singhai N: Long term morbidity of infants with bronchopulmonary dysplasia. Pediatrics 76:725, 1985

159. Bregman J, Farrell EE: Neurodevelopmental outcome in infants with bronchopulmonary dysplasia. Clin Perinatol 19:673, 1992

160. Bhutani VK, Abbasi S: Long-term pulmonary consequences in survivors with bronchpulmonary dysplasia. Clin Perinatol 19:649, 1992

161. Northway WH Jr, Moss RB, Carlisle KB et al: Late pulmonary sequelae of bronchopulmonary dysplasia. N Engl J Med 323:1793, 1990

162. Frank L: Pathophysiology of lung injury and repair: special features of the immature lung. p. 914. In Polin RA, Fox WW (eds). Fetal and Neonatal Physiology. WB Saunders, Philadelphia, 1992

163. Survant A: Multidose Study Group: Two-year follow-up of infants treated for neonatal respiratory distress syndrome with bovine surfactant. J Pediatr 124:962, 1994

164. Klaus MH, Martin RJ, Fanaroff AA: The physical environment. p. 114. In Klaus MH, Fanaroff AA (eds): Care of the High-Risk Neonate. 4th Ed. WB Saunders, Philadelphia, 1993

165. Brück K: Temperature regulation in the newborn infant. Biol Neonate 3:65, 1961

166. Adamsons K Jr, Gandy GM, James LS: The influence of thermal factors upon oxygen consumption of the newborn human infant. J Pediatr 66:495, 1965

167. Dawkins MJR, Hull D: Brown adipose tissue and the response of new-born rabbits to cold. J Physiol (Lond) 172:216, 1964

168. Aherne W, Hull D: The site of heat production in the newborn infant. Proc R Soc Med 57:1172, 1962

169. Karlberg P, Moore RE, Oliver TK Jr: The thermogenic response of the newborn infant to noradrenaline. Acta Paediatr Scand 51:284, 1962

170. Gunn TR, Ball KT, Power GG, Gluckman PD: Factors influencing the initiation of nonshivering thermogenesis. Am J Obstet Gynecol 164:210, 1991

171. Hey E: The care of babies in incubators. p. 171. In Gairdner D, Hull D (eds): Recent Advances in Paediatrics. 4th ed. Churchill Livingstone, London, 1971

172. Hey EN, Katz G, O'Connell B: The total thermal insulation of the new-born baby. J Physiol (Lond) 207:683, 1970

173. Hey EN, Katz G: Evaporative water loss in the newborn baby. J Physiol (Lond) 200:605, 1969

174. Hey EN, Katz G: The optimum thermal environment for naked babies. Arch Dis Child 45:328, 1970

175. Scopes JW: Metabolic rate and temperature control in the human body. Br Med Bull 22:88, 1966

176. Hey EN, O'Connell B: Oxygen consumption and heat balance in the cot-nursed baby. Arch Dis Child 45:335, 1970

177. Silverman WA, Sinclair JC, Agate FJ Jr: The oxygen cost of minor changes in heat balance of small newborn infants. Acta Paediatr Scand 55:294, 1966

178. Adamsons K Jr, Towell ME: Thermal homeostasis in the fetus and newborn. Anesthesiology 26:531, 1965

179. Silverman WA, Fertig JW, Berger AP: The influence of the thermal environment upon the survival of newly born premature infants. Pediatrics 22:876, 1958

180. Buetow KC, Klein SW: Effect of maintenance of "normal" skin temperature on survival of infants of low birth weight. Pediatrics 34:163, 1964

181. Day RL, Caliguiri L, Kamenski C, Ehrlich F: Body temperature and survival of premature infants. Pediatrics 34:171, 1964

182. Glass L, Silverman WA, Sinclair JC: Effect of the thermal environment on cold resistance and growth of small infants after the first week of life. Pediatrics 41:1033, 1968

183. Mancini AJ, Sookdeo-Drost S, Madison KC et al: Semi-

permeable dressings improve epidermal barrier function in premature infants. Pediatr Res 36:306, 1994

184. Mann TP, Elliott RIK: Neonatal cold injury due to accidental exposure to cold. Lancet 1:229, 1957

185. Ziegler EE, O'Donnell AM, Nelson SE, Fomon SJ: Body composition of the reference fetus. Growth 40:329, 1976

186. Friis-Hansen B: Water distribution in the foetus and newborn infant. Acta Paediatr Scand Suppl 305:7, 1983

187. Sinclair JC, Silverman WA: Intrauterine growth in active tissue mass of the human fetus, with particular reference to the undergrown baby. Pediatrics 38:48, 1966

188. Bell EF, Oh W: Fluid and electrolyte management. p. 312. In Avery GB, Fletcher MA, MacDonald MG (eds): Neonatology: Pathophysiology and Management of the Newborn. 4th Ed. JB Lippincott, Philadelphia, 1994

189. Committee on Nutrition, American Academy of Pediatrics: Nutritional needs of preterm infants. p. 64. In Barness L (ed). Pediatric Nutrition Handbook. American Academy of Pediatrics, Elk Grove Village, 1993

190. Räihä NCR, Heinonen K, Rassin DK, Gaull GE: Milk protein quantity and quality in low-birth-weight infants. 1. Metabolic responses and effects on growth. Pediatrics 57:659, 1976

191. Hanning RM, Zlotkin SH: Amino acid and protein needs of the neonate: effects of excess and deficiency. Semin Perinatol 13:131, 1989

192. Goldman HI, Freudenthal R, Holland B, Karelitz S: Clinical effects of two different levels of protein intake on low-birth-weight infants. J Pediatr 74:881, 1969

193. Goldman HI, Goldman JS, Kaufman I, Liebman OB: Late effects of early dietary protein intake on low-birth-weight infants. J Pediatr 85:764, 1974

194. Fomon S (Ed): Infant Nutrition. 2nd Ed. WB Saunders, Philadelphia, 1974

195. Auricchio S, Rubino A, Murset G: Intestinal glycosidase activities in the human embryo, fetus, and newborn. Pediatrics 35:944, 1965

196. Ehrenkranz RA: Mineral needs of the very low birth weight infant. Semin Perinatol 13:142, 1989

197. Greene HL, Hambidge KM, Schanler R, Tsang RC: Guidelines for the use of vitamins, trace elements, calcium, magnesium and phosphorus in infants and children receiving total parenteral nutrition. Am J Clin Nutr 48:1324, 1989

198. Schanler RJ: Human milk for preterm infants: nutritional and immune factors. Semin Perinatol 13:69, 1989

199. Gross SJ, Slagle TA: Feeding the low birth weight infant. Clin Perinatol 20:193, 1993

200. Lucas A, Cole TJ: Breast milk and necrotizing enterocolitis. Lancet 336:1519, 1990

201. Lucas A, Morley R, Cole TJ et al: Breast milk and subsequent intelligence quotient in children born preterm. Lancet 339:261, 1992

202. Lucas A, Morley R, Cole TJ, Gore SM: A randomised multicenter study of human milk versus formula and later development in preterm infants. Arch Dis Child 70:F141, 1994

203. Lawrence RA: Breast-Feeding: A Guide for the Medical Profession. 3rd Ed. CV Mosby, St Louis, 1989

204. Cornblath M, Reisner SH: Blood glucose in the neonate and its clinical significance. N Engl J Med 273:378, 1965

205. Hawdon JM, Ward Platt MP, Aynsley-Green A: Prevention and management of neonatal hypoglycemia. Arch Dis Child 70:F60, 1994

206. Hawdon JM, Ward Platt MP, Aynsley-Green A: Patterns of metabolic adaptation for preterm and term infants in the first neonatal week. Arch Dis Child 67:357, 1992

207. Hawdon JM, Ward Platt MP: Metabolic adaptation in small for gestational age infants. Arch Dis Child 68:262, 1993

208. Ogata ES: Carbohydrate homeostasis. p. 568. In Avery GB, Fletcher MA, MacDonald MG (eds): Neonatology. Pathophysiology and Management of the Newborn. 4th Ed. JB Lippincott, Philadelphia, 1994

209. Lucas A, Morley R, Cole TJ: Adverse neurodevelopmental outcome of moderate neonatal hypoglycemia. BMJ 297:1304, 1988

210. Anonymous: Brain damage by neonatal hypoglycemia. Lancet 1:882, 1989

211. Conrad PD, Sparks JW, Osberg I et al: Clinical application of a new glucose analyzer in the neonatal intensive care unit: comparison with other methods. J Pediatr 114:281, 1989

212. Reyes HM, Meller JL, Loeff D: Management of esophageal atresia and tracheoesophageal fistula. Clin Perinatol 16:79, 1989

213. Meller JL, Reyes HN, Loeff DS: Gastroschisis and omphalocoele. Clin Perinatol 16:113, 1989

214. Stoll BJ: Epidemiology of necrotizing enterocolitis. Clin Perinatol 21:205, 1994

215. Wiswell TE, Robertson CF, Jones TA, Tuttle DJ: Necrotizing enterocolitis in full-term infants. A case control study. Am J Dis Child 142:532, 1988

216. Kliegman RM, Walker WA, Yolken RH: Necrotizing enterocolitis. Research agenda for a disease of unknown etiology and pathogenesis. Clin Perinatol 21:437, 1994

217. Norton ME, Merrill J, Cooper BAB et al: Neonatal complications after the administration of indomethacin for preterm labor. N Engl J Med 329:1602, 1993

218. Major CA, Lewis DF, Harding JA et al: Tocolysis with indomethacin increases the incidence of necrotizing enterocolitis in the low-birth-weight neonate. Am J Obstet Gynecol 170:102, 1994

219. Maisels MJ: Jaundice. p. 630. In Avery GB, Fletcher MA, MacDonald MG (eds): Neonatology: Pathophysiology and Management of the Newborn. 4th Ed. JB Lippincott, Philadelphia, 1994

220. Maisels MJ, Gifford KL: Normal serum bilirubin levels in the newborn and the effect of breast-feeding. Pediatrics 78:837, 1986

221. Auerbach KG, Gartner LM: Breast feeding and human milk: their association with jaundice in the neonate. Clin Perinatol 14:89, 1987

222. Gourley GR: Pathophysiiology of breast-milk jaundice. p. 1173. In Polin RA, Fox WW (eds): Fetal and Neonatal Physiology. WB Saunders, Philadelphia, 1992

223. Perlstein MA: The late clinical syndrome of posticteric encephalopathy. Pediatr Clin North Am 7:665, 1960

224. Hsia DY, Allen FH Jr, Gellis SS, Diamond LK: Erythroblastosis fetalis. VIII. Studies of serum bilirubin in relation to kernicterus. N Engl J Med 247:668, 1952

225. Newman TB, Maisels MJ: Does hyperbilirubinemia damage the brain of healthy full-term infants? Clin Perinatol 17:331, 1990

226. Seidman DS, Paz I, Stevenson DK et al: Neonatal hyperbilirubinemia and physical and cognitive performance at 17 years of age. Pediatrics 88:828, 1991

227. Newman TB, Maisels MJ: Evaluation and treatment of jaundice in the term newborn: a kinder, gentler approach. Pediatrics 89:809, 1992

228. Watchko JF, Oski FA: Kernicterus in preterm newborns: past, present, and future. Pediatrics 90:707, 1992

229. Oski FA, Naiman JL: Normal blood values in the newborn period. p. 1. In Oski FA, Naiman JL (eds): Hematologic Problems in the Newborn. 3rd Ed. WB Saunders, Philadelphia, 1982

230. Forestier F, Daffos F, Catherine N et al: Developmental hematopoesis in normal human fetal blood. Blood 77:2360, 1991

231. Pearson HA: Anemia in the newborn: a diagnostic approach and challenge. Semin Perinatol 15(suppl 2):2, 1991

232. Wirth FH, Goldberg KE, Lubchenco LO: Neonatal hyperviscosity. I. Incidence. Pediatrics 63:833, 1979

233. Stevens K, Wirth FH: Incidence of neonatal hyperviscosity at sea level. J Pediatr 97:118, 1980

234. Wiswell TE, Cornish JD, Northam RS: Neonatal polycythemia: frequency of clinical manifestations and other associated findings. Pediatrics 78:26, 1986

235. Black VD, Lubchenco LO: Neonatal polycythemia and hyperviscosity. Pediatr Clin North Am 29:1137, 1982

236. Ramamurthy RS, Berlanga M: Postnatal alteration in hematocrit and viscosity in normal and polycythemic infants. J Pediatr 110:929, 1987

237. Black VD, Camp BW, Lubchenco LO et al: Neonatal hyperviscosity association with lower achievement and IQ scores at school age. Pediatrics 83:662, 1989

238. Black VD, Lubchenco LO, Koops BL et al: Neonatal hyperviscosity: randomized study of effect of partial plasma exchange on long term outcome. Pediatrics 75:1048, 1985

239. Van der Elst CW, Molteno CD, Malan AF, de V Heese H: The management of polycythemia in the newborn infant. Early Hum Dev 4:393, 1980

240. Cines DB, Dusak B, Tomaski A et al: Immune thrombocytopenic purpura and pregnancy. N Engl J Med 306:826, 1982

241. Kelton JG: Management of the pregnant patient with idiopathic thrombocytopenic purpura. Ann Intern Med 99:796, 1983

242. Karpatkin M, Porges RF, Karpatkin S: Platelet counts in infants of women with autoimmune thrombocytopenia: effect of steroid administration to the mother. N Engl J Med 305:936, 1981

243. Christiaens GCML, Nieuwenhuis HK, von dem Borne AEGK et al: Idiopathic thrombocytopenic purpura in pregnancy: a randomized trial on the effect of antenatal low dose corticosteroids on neonatal platelet count. Br J Obstet Gynaecol 97:893, 1990

244. Ballin A, Andrew M, Ling E et al: High-dose intravenous gammaglobulin therapy for neonatal autoimmune thrombocytopenia. J Pediatr 112:789, 1988

245. Mueller-Eckhardt C, Kiefel V, Grubert A et al: 348 cases of suspected neonatal alloimmune thrombocytopenia. Lancet 1:363, 1989

246. Bussel JB, Berkowitz RL, McFarland JG et al: Antenatal treatment of neonatal alloimmune thrombocytopenia. N Engl J Med 319:1374, 1988

247. Bussel J, Kaplan C, McFarland J, and the Working party on Neonatal Immune Thrombocytopenia of the Neonatal Hemostasis Subcommittee of the Scientific and Standardization Committee of the ISTH: Recommendations for the evaluation and treatment of neonatal autoimmune and alloimmune thrombocytopenia. Thromb Haemost 65:631, 1991

248. Lane PA, Hathaway WE: Vitamin K in infancy. J Pediatr 106:351, 1985

249. Dubowitz LMS, Dubowitz V, Goldberg C: Clinical assessment of gestational age in the newborn infant. J Pediatr 77:1, 1970

250. Ballard JL, Kazmaier K, Driver M: A simplified assessment of gestational age. Pediatr Res 11:374, 1977

251. Ballard JL, Khoury JC, Wedig K et al: New Ballard Score, expanded to include extremely premature infants. J Pediatr 119:417, 1991

252. Lubchenco LO, Hansman C, Boyd E: Intrauterine growth in length and head circumference as estimated from live births at gestational ages from 26 to 42 weeks. Pediatrics 37:403, 1966

253. Koops BL, Morgan LJ, Battaglia FC: Neonatal mortality risk in relation to birth weight and gestational age: update. J Pediatr 101:969, 1982.

254. Pittard WB III: Classification of the low-birth-weight infant. p. 86. In Klaus MH, Fanaroff AA (eds): Care of the High-Risk Neonate. 4th Ed. WB Saunders, Philadelphia, 1993

255. Khoury MJ, Erickson JD, Cordero JF, McCarthy BJ: Congenital malformations and intrauterine growth retardation: a population study. Pediatrics 82:83, 1988

256. Conrad PD, Wilkening RB, Rosenberg AA: Safety of newborn discharge in less than 36 hours in an indigent population. Am J Dis Child 143:98, 1989

257. American Academy of Pediatrics, American College of Obstetricians and Gynecologists: Guidelines for Perinatal Care. 3rd Ed. Elk Grove Village, IL, 1992

258. Klein M, Stern L: Low birth weight and the battered child syndrome. Am J Dis Child 122:15, 1971

259. Klaus MH, Kennel JH: Mothers separated from their newborn infants. Pediatr Clin North Am 17:1015, 1970

260. Klaus MH, Kennel JH: Care of the parents. p. 189. In Klaus MH, Fanaroff AA (eds): Care of the High-Risk Neonate. 4th Ed. WB Saunders, Philadelphia, 1993

261. Brazelton TB, Scholl ML, Robey JS: Visual responses in the newborn. Pediatrics 37:284, 1966

262. Klaus MH, Jerauld R, Kreger NC: Maternal attachment: importance of the first post-partum days. N Engl J Med 286:460, 1972

263. Whitelaw A: Kangeroo baby care: just a nice experience or an important advance for preterm infants? Pediatrics 85:604, 1990

264. Als H, Lawhon G, Duffy FH: Individual developmental care for the very low-birth-weight preterm infant. Medical and neurofunctional effects. JAMA 272:853, 1994

265. Solnit AJ, Stark MH: Mourning and the birth of a defective child. Psychoanal Study Child 16:523, 1961

266. Cullberg J: Mental reactions of women to perinatal death. p. 326. In Morris N (ed): Psychosomatic Medicine in Obstetrics and Gynecology. S Karger, New York, 1972

267. Hack M, Horbar JD, Malloy MH et al: Very low birth weight outcomes of the National Institute of Child Health and Human Development National Network. Pediatrics 87:587, 1991

268. Phelps DL, Brown DR, Tung B et al: 28-Day survival rates of 6676 neonates with birth weights of 1250 grams or less. Pediatrics 87:7, 1991

269. Aylward GP, Pfeiffer SI, Wright A, Verhulst SJ: Outcome studies of low birth weight infants published in the last decade: a metaanalysis. J Pediatr 115:515, 1989

270. Escobar GJ, Littenberg B, Petitti DB: Outcome among surviving very low birthweight infants. Arch Dis Child 66:204, 1991

271. Bregman J, Kimberlin LVS: Developmental outcome in extremely premature infants. Impact of surfactant. Pediatr Clin North Am 40:937, 1993

272. Victorian Infant Collaborative Study Group: Improvement of outcome for infants of birthweight under 1000g. Arch Dis Child 66:765, 1991

273. Halsey CL, Collin MF, Anderson CL: Extremely low birth weight children and their peers: a comparison of preschool performance. Pediatrics 91:807, 1993

274. Hack M, Taylor G, Klein N et al: School-age outcomes in children with birth weights under 750g. N Engl J Med 331:753, 1994

275. Bozynski MEA, Nelson MN, Matalon TAS et al: Prolonged mechanical ventilation and intracranial hemorrhage: impact on developmental progress through 18 months in infants weighing 1,200 grams or less at birth. Pediatrics 79:670, 1987

276. Roth SC, Baudin J, McCormick DC et al: Relation between ultrasound appearance of the brain of very preterm infants and neurodeveloopmental impairment at 8 years. Dev Med Child Neurol 35:755, 1993

277. Hack M, Breslau N, Weissman B et al: Effect of very low birth weight and subnormal head size on cognitive abilities at school age. N Engl J Med 325:231, 1991

278. Ornstein M, Ohlsson A, Edmonds J, Asztalos E: Neonatal follow-up of very low birthweight/extremely low birthweight infants to school age: a critical overview. Acta Paediatr Scand 80:741, 1991

279. Lucey JF, Dangman B: A reexamination of the role of oxygen in retrolental fibroplasia. Pediatrics 73:82, 1984

280. Valentine PH, Jackson JC, Kalina RE, Woodrum DE: Increased survival of low birth weight infants: impact on the incidence of retinopathy of prematurity. Pediatrics 84:442, 1989

281. Kramer SJ, Vertes DR, Condom M: Auditory brainstem responses and clinical followup of high risk infants. Pediatrics 83:385, 1989

282. Netter FH: The Ciba Collection of Medical Illustrations. The Respiratory System. Vol. 7. Ciba-Geigy, Summit, NJ, 1979

283. Nelson NM: Respiration and circulation after birth. p. 117. In Smith CA, Nelson NM (eds): The Physiology of the Newborn Infant. 4th Ed. Charles C Thomas, Springfield, II, 1976

Chapter 21

Postpartum Care

Watson A. Bowes, Jr.

Postpartum Involution

The Uterus

The crude weight of the pregnant uterus at term (excluding the fetus, placenta, membranes, and amniotic fluid) is approximately 1,000 g.[1] The weight of the nonpregnant uterus is between 50 and 100 g. It is not known how rapidly this 10-fold involution in organ weight occurs, but within 2 weeks after birth the uterus has usually returned to the pelvis, and by 6 weeks it is usually normal sized, as estimated by palpation.

The involution of the uterus after childbirth has been studied for more than 100 years. The gross anatomic and histologic characteristics of the involutional process are based on the study of autopsy, hysterectomy, and endometrial biopsy specimens. Williams[2] studied 18 hysterectomy specimens from sterilization operations performed from postpartum days 7 through 20. Sharman[3] investigated 10 postmortem uteri (days 1 through 12) and 626 endometrial biopsy specimens obtained from 285 women (day 5 through the ninth month). Anderson and Davis[4] reported findings from 32 uteri, 2 postmortem and 30 hysterectomy specimens (day of delivery through 20 weeks' postpartum).

Immediately after delivery, the decrease in endometrial surface contributes to the shearing off of the placenta at the decidual layer. The average diameter of the placenta is 18 cm; in the immediate postpartum uterus the average diameter of the site of placental attachment measures 9 cm. The placental site in the first 3 days after delivery is infiltrated with granulocytes and mononuclear cells, a reaction that extends into the endometrium and superficial myometrium. By the seventh day, there is evidence of the regeneration of endometrial glands, often appearing atypical, with irregular

chromatin patterns, mishapen and enlarged nuclei, pleomorphism, and increased cytoplasm. By the end of the first week, there is also evidence of the regeneration of endometrial stroma, with mitotic figures noted in gland epithelium; by postpartum day 16, the endometrium is fully restored.

Decidual necrosis begins on the first day, and, by the seventh day, a well-demarcated zone can be seen between necrotic and viable tissue. An area of viable decidua remains between the necrotic slough and the deeper endomyometrium. Sharman[3] described the non-necrotic decidual cells as participating in the reconstruction of the endometrium, a likely role since they were originally endometrial connective tissue cells to which they ultimately revert in the involutional process. By the sixth week, it is rare to find decidual cells.

The immediate inflammatory cell infiltrate of polymorphonuclear leukocytes and lymphocytes persists for about 10 days, presumably serving as an antibacterial barrier. The leukocyte response diminishes rapidly after the tenth day, and plasma cells are seen for the first time. The plasma cell and lymphocyte response may last as long as several months. In fact, endometrial stromal infiltrates of plasma cells and lymphocytes are the sign (and may be the only sign) of a recent pregnancy.

Hemostasis immediately after birth is accomplished by arterial smooth muscle contraction and compression of vessels by the involuting uterine muscle. Vessels in the placental site are characterized during the first 8 days by thrombosis, hyalinization, and endophlebitis in the veins and by hyalinization and obliterative fibrinoid endarteritis in the arteries. The mechanism for hyalinization of arterial walls, which is not completely understood, may be related to the previous trophoblastic infiltration of arterial walls that occurs early in pregnancy. Many of the thrombosed and hyalinized veins are extruded with the slough of the necrotic placental site, but hyalinized arteries remain for extended periods as stigmata of the placental site.

Restoration of the endometrium in areas other than the placental site occurs rapidly, with the process being completed by day 16 after delivery. The gland epithelium does not undergo the reactivity or the pseudoneoplastic appearance noted in placental site glands.[4]

The postpartum uterine discharge or lochia begins as a flow of blood lasting several hours, rapidly diminishing to a reddish-brown discharge through the third or fourth day postpartum. This is followed by a transition to a mucopurulent, somewhat malodorous discharge, lochia serosa, requiring the change of several perineal pads per day. The median duration of lochia serosa is 22 days.[5] However, 15 percent of women will have lochia serosa at the time of the 6-week postpartum examination. In the majority of patients the lochia serosa is followed by a yellow-white discharge, lochia alba. Breast-feeding or the use of oral contraceptive agents does not affect the duration of lochia. Not infrequently there is a sudden but transient increase in uterine bleeding between 7 and 14 days postpartum. This corresponds to the slough of the eschar over the site of placental attachment. Although it can be profuse, this bleeding episode is usually self-limited, requiring nothing more than reassurance of the patient. If it does not subside within 1 or 2 hours, the patient should be evaluated for possible retained placental tissue.

Ultrasound is useful in the management of abnormal postpartum bleeding. The empty uterus with a clear midline echo is quite easy to distinguish from the uterine cavity expanded by clot (sonolucent) or retained tissue (echodense). Serial ultrasound examinations of postpartum patients showed that in 20 to 30 percent there was some retained blood or tissue within 24 hours after delivery. By the fourth postpartum day, only about 8 percent of patients showed endometrial cavity separation, a portion of which eventually had abnormal postpartum bleeding because of retained placental tissue.[6] In cases of abnormal postpartum bleeding, ultrasound examination efficiently detects patients who have retained tissue and who will therefore benefit from uterine evacuation and curettage. Those who have an empty uterine cavity will respond to therapy with oxytocin or methylergonovine.[7]

The Cervix

During pregnancy, the cervical epithelium increases in thickness, and the cervical glands show both hyperplasia and hypertrophy. Within the stroma, a distinct decidual reaction occurs. These changes are accompanied by a substantial increase in the vascularity of the cervix.[8] Colposcopic examination performed after delivery has demonstrated ulceration, laceration, and echymosis of the cervix.[9] Regression of the cervical epithelium begins within the first 4 days after delivery, and by the end of the first week edema and hemorrhage within the cervix are minimal. Vascular hypertrophy and hyperplasia persist throughout the first week postpartum. By 6 weeks' postpartum, most of the antepartum changes have resolved, although round cell infiltration and some edema may persist for several months.[10]

The Fallopian Tube

The epithelium of the fallopian tube during pregnancy is characterized by a predominance of nonciliated cells, a phenomenon that is maintained by the balance between the high levels of progesterone and estrogen.[11] After delivery, in the absence of progesterone and estrogen, there is further extrusion of nuclei from nonciliated cells and diminution in height of both ciliated and nonciliated cells. Andrews[11] demonstrated that the number and height of ciliated cells can be increased in the puerperium by treatment with estrogen.

Fallopian tubes removed between postpartum days 5 and 15 demonstrate inflammatory changes of acute salpingitis in 38 percent of cases, but no bacteria are found. The specific cause of the inflammatory change is unknown.[11] In patients treated with diethylstilbestrol (DES) for lactation suppression, no inflammatory changes in the fallopian tubes were found, suggesting that the number and activity of the ciliated cells are important factors in preventing inflammation. Furthermore, there were no correlations between the presence of histologic inflammation in the fallopian tubes and puerperal fever or other clinical signs of salpingitis.

Ovarian Function

It has long been recognized that women who breast-feed their infants will be amenorrheic for long periods of time, often until the infant is weaned. Several studies, using a variety of methods to indicate ovulation, have demonstrated that ovulation occurs as early as 27 days after delivery, with the mean time being approximately 70 to 75 days in nonlactating women.[12–14] Among those women who are breast-feeding their infants, the mean time to ovulation is about 190 days.

Menstruation resumes by 12 weeks' postpartum in 70 percent of women who are not lactating, and the mean time to the first menstruation is 7 to 9 weeks. In one study of lactating women, it was 36 months before 70 percent began to menstruate. The duration of anovulation depends on the frequency of breast-feeding, the duration of each feed, and the proportion of supplementary feeds.[15] The risk of ovulation within the first 6 months' postpartum in a woman exclusively breast-feeding is 1 to 5 percent.

The hormonal basis for puerperal ovulation suppression in lactating women appears to be the persistence of elevated serum prolactin levels.[16] Prolactin levels fall to the normal range by the third week postpartum in nonlactating women, but remain elevated into the sixth week postpartum in lactating patients. Estrogen levels fall immediately after delivery in both lactating and nonlactating women and remain depressed in lactating patients. In those who are not lactating, estrogen levels begin to rise 2 weeks after delivery and are significantly higher than in lactating women by postpartum day 17. Follicle-stimulating hormone (FSH) levels are identical in breast-feeding and nonbreast-feeding women. It is therefore assumed that the ovary does not respond to FSH stimulation in the presence of increased prolactin levels.

Weight Loss

One of the most welcomed changes for the majority of women who have recently given birth is the loss of the weight that was accumulated during pregnancy. The immediate loss of 10 to 13 lbs is attributed to the delivery of the infant, placenta, and amniotic fluid and to blood loss.[17] By six weeks postpartum 28 percent of women will have returned to their prepregnant weight. The remainder of the weight loss occurs from 6 weeks' postpartum until 6 months after delivery. Women with excess weight gain in pregnancy (>35 lb) are likely to have a net gain of 11 lb. Breast-feeding has relatively little effect on postpartum weight loss.[18]

Thyroid Function

Thyroid size and function throughout pregnancy and the puerperium have been quantitated with ultrasonography and thyroid hormone levels.[19] Thyroid volume increases approximately 30 percent during pregnancy and regresses to normal size gradually over a 12-week period. Thyroxine and triiodothyronine, which are both elevated throughout pregnancy, and triiodothyronine resin uptake, which is decreased during pregnancy, return to normal within 4 weeks' postpartum. It is now recognized that the postpartum period is a time when women are at increased risk of developing autoimmune thryoiditis followed by hypothyroidism.[20]

Cardiovascular System and Coagulation

Blood volume increases throughout pregnancy to levels in the third trimester about 35 percent above nonpregnant values.[21] The greatest proportion of this increase consists of an increase in plasma volume that begins in the first trimester and amounts to an additional 1,200 ml of plasma, representing a 50 percent increase by the third trimester. Red blood cell volume increases by about 250 ml.

Immediately after delivery, plasma volume is diminished by approximately 1,000 ml because of blood loss. By the third postpartum day, plasma volume has increased by 900 to 1,200 ml because of a shift of extracellular fluid into the vascular space.[22] The total blood volume by the third postpartum day, however, declines to 16 percent of the predelivery value.[23] Ueland[23] found that blood volume changes in the puerperium were the same regardless of the method of delivery, but patients who delivered vaginally had a 5 percent increase in hematocrit, whereas those who had a cesarean delivery had a 6 percent decrease in hematocrit. The rate at which red blood cell volume returns to prepregnancy levels is unknown, but when measured at 8 weeks' postpartum it is found to be within the normal range.[24]

Pulse rate increases throughout pregnancy, as does stroke volume and cardiac output. Immediately after delivery, these remain elevated or rise even higher for 30 to 60 minutes. Data are lacking about the rate at which cardiac hemodynamics return to normal levels, but normal values of cardiac output are found when measurements are made 8 to 10 weeks' postpartum.[25] Following delivery there is a transient rise of approximately 5 percent in both diastolic and systolic blood pressures throughout the first 4 days' postpartum.[26] In 12 percent of otherwise normotensive patients, the diastolic blood pressure will exceed 100 mgHg. Monheit et al.[27] viewed data about the cardiovascular changes of the puerperium and stated that the rate of return to the normal physiologic status is hyperbolic, with most of the regression occurring early.

Ygge[28] studied blood coagulation and fibrinolysis in 10 normal pregnant women during the 4 weeks before delivery, during labor and delivery, and 2 weeks' postpartum. Compared with antepartum values, there was a rapid decrease in platelets in some patients and no change or an increase in others. However, 2 weeks after delivery all patients demonstrated an increase in platelet count.

Fibrinolytic activity increased in the first 1 to 4 days after delivery and returned to normal in 1 week. Fibrinogen concentration gradually diminished over the 2-week postpartum period studied. The changes in the coagulation system together with vessel trauma and immobility account for the increased risk of thromboembolism noted in the puerperium, especially when operative delivery has occurred.

The Urinary Tract and Renal Function

It is generally accepted that the urinary tract becomes dilated during pregnancy, especially the renal pelvis and the ureters above the pelvic brim. These findings, demonstrated 50 years ago by Baird,[29] affect the collecting system of the right kidney more than that of the left. It has now been shown that these changes are due predominantly to compression of the ureters by adjacent vasculature and, to a lesser extent, by compression from the enlarged uterus. Ureteral tone above the pelvic brim, which in pregnancy is higher than normal, diminishes in the lateral recumbent position and returns to nonpregnant levels immediately after cesarean delivery.[30]

The intravenous urography studies performed by Dure-Smith[31] demonstrated the ureteral and calyceal dilatation that occurs in pregnancy, presumably because of pressure from the iliac artery. His studies also suggest that subtle anatomic changes take place in the ureters that persist long after the pregnancy has ended. Ultrasound studies of the urinary tract also document the enlargement of the collecting system throughout pregnancy.[32] A study of serial ultrasound examinations of the urinary tract in 20 women throughout pregnancy included a single postpartum examination 6 weeks after delivery.[33] The overall trend was that of dilatation of the collecting system throughout pregnancy, estimated by measurements of the separation of the pelvis–calyceal echo complex, from a mean of 5.0 mm (first trimester) to 10 mm (third trimester) in the right kidney and from 3.0 to 4.0 mm in the left collecting system. Measurements in all but two patients had returned to 0 at the time of the 6-week postpartum examination. Cietak and Newton[34] performed serial nephrosonography on 34 patients throughout pregnancy and the puerperium. Twenty-four patients were followed for 12 weeks' postpartum. However, more than 50 percent of patients at 12 weeks' postpartum demonstrated persistence of urinary stasis, described as a slight separation of the renal pelvis. I interpret this finding as evidence of hyperdistensibility and suggest that pregnancy has a permanent effect on the size of the upper renal tract.

Studies in which water cystometry and uroflowmetry were performed within 48 hours of delivery and again 4 weeks' postpartum demonstrated a slight but significant decrease in bladder capacity (from 395.5 to 331 ml) and volume at first void (from 277 to 224 ml) in the study interval. Nevertheless, all the urodynamic values studied were within normal limits on both occasions. The results were not affected by the weight of the infant or by an episiotomy. However, prolonged labor and the use of epidural anesthesia appeared to diminish postpartum bladder function transiently.[35]

The most detailed study of renal function in normal pregnancy is that of Sims and Krantz,[36] who studied 12 patients with serial renal function tests throughout pregnancy and for up to 1 year after delivery. Glomerular filtration, which increased by 50 percent early in pregnancy and remained elevated until delivery, returned to normal nonpregnant levels by postpartum week 8. Endogenous creatinine clearance, similarly elevated throughout pregnancy, also returned to normal by the eighth postpartum week. Renal plasma flow increased by 25 percent early in pregnancy, gradually diminished in the third trimester (even when measured in the lateral recumbent position), and continued to decrease to below-normal values in the postpartum period for up to 24 weeks. Normal values were finally established by 50 to 60 weeks after delivery. The reason for the prolonged postpartum depression of the renal plasma flow is not clear.

The rate at which changes in renal function return to normal is not known, because studies within the first 6 weeks' postpartum are rare. Renal plasma flow decreases by postpartum day 5, while other measures of renal function continue to be elevated at this time.[37]

Management of the Puerperium

The immediate puerperium for most parturients is spent in the hospital or birthing center. The ideal duration of hospitalization for patients with uncomplicated vaginal births has been controversial, with most authorities recommending a 2-day stay for first time mothers. For patients with an uncomplicated postoperative course following cesarean delivery the postpartum stay is 3 or 4 days.

In a recent study, 1,249 randomly selected patients were questioned 8 weeks following delivery about health problems that occurred during the puerperium.[38] Eighty-five percent reported at least one problem during their hospitalization, and 76 percent reported at least one problem that persisted for 8 weeks. A wide range of problems were reported by the patients, including painful perineum, breast-feeding problems, urinary infections, urinary and fecal incontinence, and headache. Three percent of the patients had been rehospitalized, most commonly for abnormal bleeding or infection. This study draws attention to a substantial amount of symptomatic morbidity that occurs during the puerperium.

If a patient has adequate support at home (i.e., help with housekeeping and meal preparation), there is little value in an extended hospital stay, provided the mother is adequately educated about infant care and feeding, family planning, and identification of danger signs in either the infant or herself. For mothers who do not have adequate support at home and who are insecure about infant care and feeding, extending the hospital stay will provide time for mothers to gain adequate education and some measure of self-confidence. Video presentations are an efficient means of patient education. Also, home nursing visits can be very helpful in providing support, education, and advice to mothers.

In addition to the video presentation, patients should be given ample opportunity to discuss specific questions or concerns with a nurse or physician. It is also important to provide a new mother time and a sympathetic listener so that she can express her feelings and ask questions about her labor and delivery experience.

The time from delivery until complete physiologic involution and psychological adjustment has been called "the fourth trimester."[39] Patients should understand that the lochia will persist for 3 to 8 weeks and that on days 7 to 14 there is likely to be an episode of heavy vaginal bleeding, which occurs when the placental eschar sloughs. Tampons are permissible if they are comfortable upon insertion and are changed frequently and if there are no perineal, vaginal, or cervical lacerations, which preclude insertion of a tampon until healing has occurred.

Physical activity, including walking up and down stairs, lifting heavy objects, riding in or driving a car, and performing muscle-toning exercises, can be resumed without delay if the delivery has been uncomplicated. The most troublesome complaint is lethargy and fatigue. Consequently, every task or activity should be a brief one in the first few days of the puerperium. Mothers whose lethargy persists beyond several weeks must be evaluated, especially as regards thyroid dysfunction. Transient postpartum thyrotoxicosis may occur followed by hypothyroidism. These episodes are characterized by goiter formation, the presence of antithyroid antibodies, and eventual resolution.[40,41]

Sexual activity may be resumed when the perineum is comfortable and when bleeding has diminished. The desire and willingness to resume sexual activity in the puerperium varies greatly among women, depending on the site and state of healing of perineal or vaginal incisions and lacerations, the amount of vaginal atrophy secondary to breast-feeding, and the return of libido.[42] In a study of 50 parturients, Ryding[43] found that 20 percent had little desire for sexual activity 3 months after delivery, and an additional 21 percent had complete loss of desire or aversion to sexual activity. This variation in attitude, desire, and willingness must be acknowledged when counseling women about the resumption of sexual activity.

Many patients will be returning to work situations outside the home after their pregnancies. Frequently the physician must complete insurance or employer forms to establish maternity leave for patients. Six weeks is regarded as the normal period of "disability" following delivery,[44] although some mothers return to work sooner than 6 weeks.

A follow-up examination is frequently scheduled for 6 weeks' postpartum. For many patients, an appointment sooner than this (approximately 2 weeks' postpartum) or a home visit by a visiting nurse or nurse-midwife will be more productive in detecting problems and providing support for a mother. Late puerperal infections, postpartum depression, and problems with infant care and feeding occur long before the 6-week postpartum visit.

Perineal Care

Many women who give birth have an episiotomy or spontaneous lacerations of the perineum or vagina. In the United States, episiotomies are more often performed as midline than as mediolateral incisions. Provided that the incision or the laceration does not extend beyond the transverse perineal muscle, that there is no hematoma or extensive ecchymosis, and that a satisfactory repair has been accomplished, there is little need for perineal care beyond routine cleansing with a bath or shower. Analgesia can be accomplished in most patients with nonsteroidal anti-inflammatory drugs such as ibuprofen. These drugs have been shown to be superior to acetaminophen or propoxyphene for episiotomy pain and uterine cramping.[45] Furthermore, because of a low milk to maternal plasma drug concentration ratio, a short half-life, and transformation into glucuronide metabolites, ibuprofen is safe for nursing mothers.

A patient who has had a mediolateral episiotomy or who has a third- or fourth-degree extension of a midline episiotomy and extensive spontaneous second-degree laceration or extensive perineal bruising may experience considerable perineal pain. Occasionally, the pain and periurethral swelling will prevent the patient from voiding, making urethral catheterization necessary. When a patient complains of inordinate perineal pain, the first and most important step is to re-examine the perineum, vagina, and rectum to detect and drain a hematoma or to identify a perineal infection. Perineal pain may be the first symptom of the very rare but potentially fatal complications of angioedema, necrotizing fasciitis, or perineal cellulitis.[46–48]

In cases of immoderate perineal pain, sitz baths will provide additional pain relief. Although hot sitz baths have long been customary therapy for perineal pain, Droegemueller[49] outlined the rationale for using cold or "iced" sitz baths. This therapy is similar to that for the treatment of athletic injuries, for which considerable success has been achieved with cold therapy. Cold provides immediate pain relief as a result of decreased excitability of free nerve endings and decreased nerve conduction. Further pain relief comes from local vasoconstriction, which reduces edema, inhibits hematoma formation, and decreases muscle irritability and spasm.

Patients who have alternated using hot and cold sitz baths usually prefer the cold.

The technique for administering a cold sitz bath is first to have the patient sit in a tub of water at room temperature to which ice cubes are then added. This avoids the sensation of sudden immersion in ice water. The patient remains in the ice water for 20 to 30 minutes.

Frequently what appears to be severe perineal pain is, in fact, the pain of prolapsed hemorrhoids. Witch hazel compresses, suppositories containing corticosteroids, or local anesthetic sprays or emollients may be helpful. Occasionally a thrombus will occur in a prolapsed hemorrhoid. It is a simple task to remove the thrombus through a small scalpel incision using local anesthesia. Dramatic relief of pain usually follows this procedure.

Patients with perineal incisions or lacerations should be advised to postpone sexual intercourse for 3 weeks or until there is no perineal discomfort. Tampons may be inserted whenever the patient is comfortable doing so. However, to avoid any risk of toxic shock syndrome, the use of tampons should be confined to the daytime to prevent leaving a tampon in the vagina for prolonged periods.

Delayed Postpartum Hemorrhage

Postpartum uterine bleeding of sufficient quantity to require medical attention occurs in 1 to 2 percent of patients. The bleeding occurs most frequently between days 8 and 14 of the puerperium.[50] Often the bleeding is self-limited and of short duration. The cause of most of these cases is presumed to be sloughing of the placental escar. However, when the bleeding is of greater amount requiring curettage, retained gestational products will be found in about 40 percent of cases. In the management of patients with heavy delayed bleeding, ultrasound examination will usually determine if there is retained material, although it is sometimes difficult to distinquish between blood clot and retained placental fragments. Suction evacuation of the uterus is successful in arresting the bleeding in almost all cases whether or not there is histologic confirmation of retained gestational products. If curettage is required at this time in the puerperium, especially if a sharp curette is used, a course of antibiotics is advisable for its possible benefit in reducing the formation of uterine synechiae.

Postpartum Infection

The standard definition of postpartum febrile morbidity is a temperature of 38.0°C (100.4°F) or higher on any 2 of the first 10 days' postpartum, exclusive of the first 24 hours. However, most clinicians do not wait 2 full days to begin evaluation and treatment of patients who develop a fever in the puerperium.[51] The most common cause of postpartum fever is endometritis, which occurs after vaginal delivery in approximately 2 percent of patients and after cesarean delivery in about 10 to 15 percent. The differential diagnosis includes urinary tract infection, lower genital tract infection, wound infections, pulmonary infections, thrombophlebitis, and mastitis.

Endometritis is an ascending infection from pathogens in the lower genital tract, including a variety of aerobic and anaerobic organism.[52] Endometritis that presents within 1 or 2 days after delivery is often Group A *Streptococcus*. When the symptoms begin on the third or fourth day postpartum, the organism is likely to be an enteric pathogen, most commonly *Escherichia coli* or anaerobic organisms. Late onset endometritis (after 7 days) is frequently caused by *Chlamydia trachomatis*. Patients predisposed to puerperal endometritis are those with prolonged rupture of membranes, long labors, multiple vaginal examinations during labor, cesarean delivery especially following a long labor, and anemia.

The symptoms of puerperal endometritis, in addition to fever and chills, are lower abdominal pain, anorexia, malaise, and malodorous vaginal discharge. The signs of endometritis are elevated temperature, abdominal tenderness, mucopurulent vaginal discharge, and uterine and parametrial tenderness on bimanual pelvic examination. Lower abdominal rebound tenderness may be present in some cases because of the associated pelvic cellulitis and peritonitis that occur in many of these infections.

Laboratory studies include a complete blood count, urine culture, and anaerobic and aerobic blood cultures in some instances. Transvaginal endometrial cultures are of limited value, because it is difficult to avoid contamination from vaginal flora.

Treatment of suspected puerperal endometritis is prompt, adequate intravenous antibiotic therapy. The most commonly employed regimen is the combination of clindamycin-gentamicin, which provides coverage of most aerobic and anaerobic organisms involved in these infections. Treatment may also be accomplished with single drug therapy using either a cephalosporin such as cefotetan or cefoxitin, an extended-spectrum penicillin such as piperacillin or mezlocillin, or ampicillin combined with a β lactaminase inhibitor. Single drug regimens are simple, cost effective, and successful in most patients. Metronidazole, which is quite effective against anaerobic infections can be used in combination with clindamycin. When the symptoms and signs of endometritis, including fever, have resolved for 48 hours, parenteral antibiotic therapy can be discontinued. Oral antibiotic therapy thereafter is unnecessary.

If signs and symptoms of infection have not subsided within 48 to 72 hours of intravenous antibiotic therapy, other sources of infection and complications of the original infection must be considered along with the possibility that the offending organism(s) are not adequately covered with the primary antibiotic therapy. Other diagnoses include pelvic abcess, wound infection or dehiscence of the uterine incision in the case of post-cesarean infection, septic pelvic thrombophlebitis, urinary tract infection, and mastitis. Occasionally the cause will be a community-acquired viral infection or other disorder such as systemic lupus erythematosus, appendicitis, or cholecystitis. Pelvic imaging studies including ultrasound, computerized tomography scanning, and magnetic resonance imaging will often be helpful in detecting retained placental tissue, pelvic abcesses, or ovarian vein thrombosis in patients with persistent puerperal febrile morbidity. In patients with persistent fever in whom these studies have failed to detect other sources of infection, a course of intravenous heparin therapy is often recommended. A response to such therapy within 72 hours suggests the diagnosis of septic thrombophlebitis for which there is no definitive clinical, laboratory, or imaging test.

Maternal–Infant Attachment

The reaction of parents to a newborn infant is generally that of joy and exclamation and enlivens the atmosphere in even the most sterile and clinical of circumstances. The total concentration of the parents, especially the mother, on the infant and its welfare and the complete disregard for the surrounding environment and events is evident to even the most untrained observer of this scene. Klaus et al.[53] were among the first investigators to study and quantitate this phenomenon and to bring attention to the importance of the first few hours of maternal–infant association. Their studies as well as those of others have contributed substantially to major changes in hospital policies dealing with patients in labor and delivery and during the postpartum confinement. It is now recognized that there should be opportunities for parents to be with their newborns even from the first few moments after birth and as frequently as possible during the first days thereafter. These associations are usually characterized by fondling, kissing, cuddling, and gazing at the infant, which are manifestations of maternal commitment and protectiveness toward her infant. Separation of mother and infant in the first hours after birth has been shown to diminish or delay the development of these characteristic mothering behaviors,[54] a problem that is intensified when medical, obstetric, or newborn complications require intensive care for either the mother or her newborn infant.

Robson and Powell[55] summarized the literature on early maternal attachment and emphasized how diffi-

cult it is to accomplish good research studies about this phenomenon. While it is generally agreed that early association of the mother and infant is beneficial and should not be interfered with unnecessarily, there are still doubts about the long-term implications, if any, of a lack of early maternal–infant association. In their monograph summarizing their investigations about parent–infant attachment, Klaus and Kennel[56] warn against drawing far-reaching conclusions. Although favoring the theory of a "sensitive period" soon after birth, during which close parent–infant interaction facilitates subsequent attachment and beneficial parenting behavior, these investigators concur that humans are highly adaptable and state that "there are many fail-safe routes to attachment." This appears to be the prevailing view among experts at this time.

The modern hospital maternity ward should enhance and encourage parent–infant attachment by such policies as flexible visiting hours for the father, encouragement of the infant rooming with the mother, and supportive attitudes about breast-feeding. These policies also allow the nursing staff to observe parenting behavior and to identify inept, inexperienced, or even malicious behavior toward the infant. Some situations may call for more intensive follow-up by visiting nurses, home-health visitors, or social workers to provide further support for the family during the posthospital convalescence.

The role of postpartum home visits for enhancing parenting behavior is controversial. Gray et al.[57] found this approach quite beneficial. Siegel et al.[58] studied the effect of early and prolonged in hospital mother–infant contact and a postpartum visitation program on attachment and parenting behavior. They found that early and prolonged maternal–infant contact in the hospital had a significant effect on enhancing subsequent parenting behavior, but the postpartum home visitations had no impact.

The development of the qualities associated with good parenting depends on many things. Certainly it does not depend solely on what transpires in the few hours surrounding the birth experience. There is evidence that specific identification of an infant with its mother's voice begins in utero during the third trimester.[59] Furthermore, the parents' own experiences as children, as well as their intellectual and emotional attitudes about children, must play a large role in their own parenting behavior. Areskog et al.[60] showed that women who expressed fear of childbirth during the antenatal period had more complications and more pain in labor and also had more difficulties in attachment to their infants. Consequently, the peripartum period provides opportunities to enhance parenting behavior and to identify families for which follow-up after birth may be necessary to ensure the most favorable child development.

In summary, the postpartum ward should be an environment that provides parents ample opportunity to interact with their newborn infants. Personnel, including nurses, nurses' aides, and physicians, caring for mothers and infants should be alert to signs of abnormal parenting (e.g., refusal of the mother to care for the infant, the use of negative or abusive names in describing or referring to the infant, inordinate delay in naming the infant, or obsessive and unrealistic concerns about the infant's health). These or other signs that maternal–infant attachment is delayed or endangered are as deserving of frequent follow-up during the postpartum period as are any of the traditional medical or obstetric complications.

Lactation and Breast-Feeding

One of the important objectives of the puerperium is to enhance the maternal–infant interaction as regards nutrition of the infant. After several decades during which interest in breast-feeding languished in Western cultures, there has been renewed interest and enthusiasm for what is clearly the most reasonable means of feeding most newborn infants.[61] Between 1971 and 1981, the number of mothers breast-feeding their infants at the time of discharge from the hospital doubled. Furthermore, the duration of breast-feeding, measured at age 6 months, increased at a faster rate than did the incidence of breast-feeding in the hospital. Although the increase in breast-feeding is seen in all demographic groups, it is greatest in the upper-income and more highly educated groups. The increase in the popularity of breast-feeding is due in part to an increasing awareness of the advantages. The litany of benefits includes improved infant nutrition, increased resistance to infection, decreased expense, and increased convenience.[62]

Successful breast-feeding depends to a great extent on the motivation of the mother and on the support she receives from family, friends, and health-care providers. Undoubtedly the mother's experiences as a child contribute to her attitudes about childbearing and infant feeding. Nevertheless, additional knowledge about breast-feeding may be gained during prenatal care from well-informed, enthusiastic, and supportive physicians and nurses, by reading from one of several lay books on breast-feeding, and by participating in classes on prepared childbirth. A variety of hospital practices, including the use of audiovisual aids, telephone hotlines, and in-service training for personnel, have been shown to increase the incidence of successful breast-feeding.[63]

The prenatal physical examination may identify problems that will affect breast-feeding. These include inverted nipples, which can be corrected in part by wearing breast shields, or *Monilia* vaginal infections, which should be treated to avoid thrush in the infant, and painful *Monilia* infection of the nipples.

The Term Infant

Hospital routines should not interfere with reasonable breast-feeding practices. Allowing the infant to nurse in its wakeful period immediately after birth when the mouthing movements and rooting reflex are active will give the mother confidence and promote milk production and letdown. Furthermore, early suckling not only provides the infant with the important immunologic and anti-infective properties of colostrum, but also has been shown to enhance successful breast-feeding.

Rooming-in allows the parents to become accustomed to demand feeding and provides the mother with opportunities to seek help from the nursing staff while she enhances her breast-feeding skills. Although the rooting and suckling reflexes are intact in a healthy newborn, successful breast-feeding is a learned talent for mother and infant. Neifert and Seacat[64] recommend that the infant be allowed to suckle for 5 minutes per breast per feeding the first day, 10 minutes the second day, and 15 minutes or more per breast per feeding thereafter. If suckling is interrupted before initiation of the letdown reflex, breast engorgement is encouraged and nipple soreness will increase.

The initial breast engorgement that occurs on the second to fourth postpartum days is due to lymphatic and vascular congestion, interstitial edema, and increased tension in the milk ducts. It is best managed with 24-hour demand feedings and, in stubborn cases, the use of oxytocin nasal spray to promote milk letdown. Hot compresses before nursing will facilitate letdown, and cold compresses between feedings may provide additional relief.

A common problem is nipple confusion, in which an infant accepts an artificial nipple but refuses the mother's nipple. This can be avoided by not offering supplemental fluids and by informing the mother of methods to make her nipple more protractile. Breast engorgement enhances this problem, but with patience it usually resolves within 24 to 48 hours.

Nipple soreness, another common complaint during the immediate puerperium, can be relieved by rotating breasts and the infant's position every 5 minutes while nursing; using frequent, shorter feedings rather than prolonged feeding times; avoiding irritating soaps, wet nursing pads, or other applications; and exposing the nipples for air drying followed by the application of hydrous lanolin. In cases of persistent nipple soreness or of sudden appearance of nipple soreness after lactation has been established, *Monilia* infection of the nipple must be considered.[64] The infection, which often occurs in association with thrush or *Monilia* diaper rash, can be documented by culture; it responds promptly to applications of nystatin cream.

An empathetic and knowledgeable nursing staff is essential to successful breast-feeding by the mother who is attempting it for the first time. In the hospital, education and patient confidence can be facilitated with a brief videotape presentation about breast-feeding, which describes some of the problems that might be encountered and offers helpful solutions. Professional lactation counselors are often available to provide education and support in prenatal classes, during the immediate puerperium, and in the home following discharge from the hospital or birthing center. In many areas, the local chapter of the La Leche League will offer valuable advice to women who encounter problems with breast-feeding.

Maternal Nutrition During Lactation

The impact of lactation on the nutritional status of the mother is well reviewed by Casey and Hambidge[65] and in the publication by the Institute of Medicine entitled *Nutrition During Lactation*.[66] A healthy mother breast-feeding a healthy infant will produce approximately 600 to 900 ml breast milk per day and will provide her infant with approximately 520 kcal/day. This requires about 600 kcal/day (including the energy required to produce the milk), which must be made up from the mother's diet or her body stores. For this purpose, the well-nourished woman stores about 5 kg fat throughout pregnancy, which can be called on during lactation to make up any nutritional deficit.

The daily allowances of nutrients recommended for the mother during the first 6 months of lactation by the U.S. National Research Council[67] are listed in Table 21-1.

With the exception of iron and calcium, almost all of the other nutrients are provided in a well-balanced American diet. Even in situations in which there is obvious nutritional deprivation, the quantity and quality of breast milk seem to suffer very little. The composition of breast milk, however, can be influenced to some extent by the mother's diet. The protein content of breast milk is altered very little by the mother's diet, but the fat content is quite susceptible to dietary manipulation. Women who have diets in which the fat is largely of animal origin produce milk with high stearic acid content and low linoleic acid levels, whereas women with diets high in polyunsaturated fatty acids produce milk with high levels of linoleate. The importance of these differences on the subsequent health of breast-fed infants is unknown.

Table 21-1 Daily Allowances of Nutrients Recommended for the Mother During the First 6 Months of Lactation[a]

Nutrients	Recommended Amount
Calories	2,500
Protein	65 g
Vitamin A	1,300 μg (retinol equiv.)
Vitamin D	10 μg (400 IU)
Vitamin E	12 mg (α-tocopherol equiv.)
Thiamine	1.6 mg
Riboflavin	1.8 mg
Niacin	20 mg (niacin equiv.)
Folacin	280 μg
Vitamin B_6	2.1 mg
Vitamin B_{12}	2.6 μg
Ascorbic acid	95 mg
Calcium	1,200 mg
Phosphorus	1,200 mg
Magnesium	355 mg
Iron	15 mg
Zinc	19 mg
Iodine	200 μg

[a] U.S. National Research Council recommendations.

Levels of some but not all vitamins in breast milk can be influenced by maternal intake, but there is little evidence that breast milk in the otherwise well-nourished mother is vitamin deficient. Consequently, the need for vitamin supplementation for the lactating woman on a normal diet is not well established. Some vegetarians may have diets deficient in vitamin B_{12}, and vitamin B_{12} deficiency has been documented in a breast-fed infant of a vegetarian mother.[68] Also, infants of dark-skinned mothers who have had inadequate exposure to sunlight may become vitamin D deficient. This can be avoided by brief daily exposure to sunlight.[69]

Frequently, women inquire about the advisability of dieting and weight loss during lactation. Because of the increased metabolic rate and the increased energy requirements of lactating women, the appetite increases, leading to an increase in caloric intake. However, a persistent weight loss can be achieved through very modest diet restrictions without an untoward effect on the health of either the mother or the infant. Whichelow[70] found that lactating mothers who were losing weight had an average daily intake of 2,509 kcal, whereas women who were not losing weight consumed 2,946 kcal.

Contraindications to Breast-Feeding

There are very few contraindications to breast-feeding. Reduction mammoplasty with autotransplantation of the nipple simply makes breast-feeding impossible.

Puerperal infections including acute mastitis can be managed quite successfully while the mother continues to breast-feed. There is the possibility of transmitting in the breast milk certain viral infections, including cytomegalovirus, herpes simplex, hepatitis B virus (HBV), and human immunodeficiency virus (HIV). The morbidity of cytomegalovirus infection contracted by a healthy term neonate is sufficiently low that potentially infected mothers should not be discouraged from breast-feeding. Although one possible case of viral transmission in the breast milk occurred,[71] the source of neonatal herpes infection is surface contact with the virus; consequently, instruction of the mother in proper handwashing and care of possibly contaminated articles of clothing is sufficient to protect the infant and to permit continued breast-feeding. As regards HBV infection, McGregor and Neifert[72] recommend that breast-feeding not be encouraged in women with acute hepatitis, hepatitis B/e antigenemia (HB_eAg), or other markers of heightened infectivity such as titers of HB_eAg over 1:1,000. However, breast-feeding is permissible in women without active HBV disease and certainly in the uncommon circumstance of an HB_eAg-positive newborn. Thus most mothers with HBV infection before or during pregnancy can be supported in their decision to breast-feed. HIV is present in breast milk, and the risk of vertical transmission is doubled if an infant breast-feeds.[73] Consequently, in developed countries where there is not a high risk of newborn infectious disease associated with bottle feeding, breast-feeding is contraindicated for mothers with HIV infection.

Most medications taken by the mother will enter the breast milk to a small degree (see Ch. 10). Because of the short duration for which most medications are prescribed, however, and the minimal amounts of drug that reach the breast milk (usually in concentrations similar to or less than in maternal plasma), it is usually safe to recommend that the infant continue nursing. The pharmacokinetics of most drugs ingested by breast-feeding women are such that administration of the drug at the time of or immediately after the infant nurses will result in the lowest amount of drug in the milk at the subsequent feeding. If there is any doubt about the effect of a specific drug taken by a mother and whether she should continue breast-feeding, one should consult a recent reference about the effects of drugs in the nursing infant (Ch. 10).[74,75]

Breast Milk for the Premature Infant

There are substantial data confirming the psychological, nutritional, and immunologic advantages to using a mother's breast milk to feed her premature infant.

Very small preterm infants fed their mothers' milk will gain weight at the same rate as when they are fed formula.[76] Metabolic disturbances (azotemia, hyperaminoacidemia, and metabolic acidosis) are more frequent in infants receiving higher intakes of protein from formulas compared with human milk. Furthermore, the immunologically active constituents of breast milk (lactoferrin, lysozyme, lactoperoxidase, complement, leukocytes, and specific immunoglobulins) undoubtedly account for the lower incidence of infectious complications found in premature infants fed breast milk (see Ch. 6).[77]

In addition to the nutritional and immunologic advantages of breast milk for the premature infant, there are the important psychological benefits for the mother. Women who give birth to preterm infants often have a sense of guilt and failure. By providing breast milk, the mother takes an active part in the infant's daily care, which gives her a renewed sense of worth and importance.

In situations in which breast milk will be used for a premature infant, the mother must be instructed in the various methods of milk expression, collection, preservation, and transport. Most intensive care nurseries and many postpartum wards provide written instructions about milk expression and collection techniques.[78] A pump is more efficient and less time-consuming than hand expression. Electric pumps, which simulate the physiologic suckling action of the infant, are available in many nurseries and can be leased from surgical supply companies or rental outlets. Often the local chapter of the La Leche League will provide information on the availability of electric pumps. Hand pumps can also be used.

Occasionally it is difficult to maintain an adequate milk supply using artificial expression. Hopkins et al.[79] have demonstrated that in mothers who have delivered prematurely milk volume is inversely related to the delay in initiation of milk expression. Optimal milk production is associated with five or more milk expressions per day and pumping durations that exceed 100 min/day. Also, nasal oxytocin (Syntocinon) can be helpful in augmenting milk letdown. Breast milk can be refrigerated for 24 hours at 1° to 5°C or frozen at −18° to −23°C for up to 3 months.

Complications of Breast-Feeding

The most common complication of breast-feeding is puerperal mastitis. This condition, which is characterized by fever, myalgias, and an area of pain and redness in either breast, usually has its onset before the end of the second postpartum week, but there is also an increase in its incidence in the fifth and sixth weeks postpartum. Niebyl et al.[80] reported 20 women in whom sporadic (nonepidemic) puerperal mastitis developed. The women were treated with penicillin V, ampicillin, or dicloxacillin and allowed to continue breast-feeding their infants. No abscesss developed. This experience is similar to that of others[81] who have found that in sporadic puerperal mastitis breast-feeding need not be discontinued. In fact, the combination of a penicillinase-resistant penicillin and continued breast-feeding will promptly result in resolution of the infection in 96 percent of cases.

From time to time, a patient will report problems with adequate milk production, sometimes called *lactation failure*. This problem is usually due to infrequent suckling, which can be corrected by decreasing the interval between feedings and by enhancing milk letdown with oxytocin nasal spray. If the milk supply is inadequate in spite of these measures, endogenous suppression of prolactin may be the problem, as in the unusual situation of retained placental fragments inhibiting lactogenesis as described by Neifert et al.[82] Removal of the retained placental tissue by curettage will result in prompt resumption of milk production. In the absence of any obvious source of prolactin inhibition (e.g., ergot preparation, pyridoxine, or diuretics), pharmacologic enhancement of lactation should be considered. Metoclopramide[83] and sulpiride[84] have both been shown to enhance milk production, presumably by blocking dopamine receptors and stimulating prolactin secretion. Metoclopramide is commercially available (Reglan); given in doses of 10 mg three or four times a day, it may be helpful in stubborn cases of lactation failure.

Lactation Suppression

For those patients who for personal or medical reasons will not breast-feed, breast support, ice packs, and analgesic medications are helpful in ameliorating the symptoms of breast engorgement. The new mother should avoid suckling or other means of milk expression, and the natural inhibition of prolactin secretion will result in breast involution. In 30 to 50 percent of patients, this will be associated with 24 to 48 hours of breast engorgement and pain.[85,86]

Bromocriptine is no longer approved by The Food and Drug Administration for lactation suppression. This ergot derivative is a dopamine receptor agonist with prolonged action that inhibits the release of prolactin. Twenty-three percent of patients have side effects, including symptomatic hypotension, nausea, and vomiting, and 18 to 40 percent have rebound breast secretion, congestion, or engorgement following the termination of therapy.[87] Furthermore, there have been reports of puerperal stroke, seizures, and myocar-

dial infarctions in association with the use of bromocriptine prescribed for lactation suppression.[88–91] While these events are rare and a causal relationship with bromocriptine has not been established, the manufacturers' prescription prevention recommendations include instructions to avoid the use of this medication in patients with hypertensive complications of pregnancy and to monitor blood pressure periodically during the time the patient is using the drug. Consequently, it can be questioned whether it is prudent to use a medication for 2 weeks that has this incidence of side effects, possibly life-threatening complications, and the requirement for blood pressure monitoring during the therapy. Puerperal breast engorgement, although painful, is never fatal and in most instances resolves within 72 hours.

Pregnancy Prevention and Birth Control

The immediate postpartum period is a convenient time in which to discuss family planning with patients. Ideally, these conversations begin during the prenatal visits, but once delivery has occurred most patients are disposed to serious considerations about future pregnancies. The period of anovulation infertility lasts from 5 weeks in nonlactating women to 8 weeks or more in women who breast-feed their infants without supplementation.[13] Robson et al.[92] found that most women have resumed intercourse by 3 months, and for many resumption of an active sexual life begins much earlier. Consequently, it is important that a decision be made about pregnancy prevention before the patient leaves the hospital.

A patient should be apprised of the various options of pregnancy prevention and birth control in terms that she and her partner can understand. This may be done by individual instruction from nurses, physicians, or physician assistants or by a variety of films or videotapes. The decision about family planning methods will depend on the patient's motivation, number of children, state of health, whether she is breast-feeding and on the religious background of the couple. It cannot be assumed because a woman has used a method of contraception effectively before the current pregnancy that she will need no counseling thereafter. Debrovner and Winikoff[93] found that more than one-half of patients change contraceptive techniques between pregnancies.

Natural Methods

The natural family planning methods, which depend on predicting the time of ovulation by use of basal body temperature or assessment of cervical mucus, cannot be used until regular menstrual cycles have resumed.[94] In the first weeks or months following birth, provided there is little or no supplemental feeding for the infant, breast-feeding will provide 98 percent contraceptive protection for up to 6 months. At 6 months, or if menses return, or if breast-feeding ceases to be full or nearly full before the sixth month, the risk of pregnancy increases.[95]

Barrier Methods

Barrier methods of contraception and vaginal spermicides were long used in Europe and England before they were manufactured in this country beginning in the 1920s.[96] The failure rate for the diaphragm varies from 2.4 to 19.6 per 100 women-years. Because this method of contraception requires substantial motivation, instruction, and experience, it is more effective in older women who are familiar with the technique. Vessey and Wiggins[97] found a failure rate of 2.4 per 100 women-years among diaphragm users who were over 25 years old and who had a minimum of 5 months' experience using it. This pregnancy rate is comparable to that reported for intrauterine device users.

The proper size of the diaphragm should be determined at the 6-week postpartum visit, even in patients who previously used this form of contraception. In women who are breast-feeding, anovulation leads to vaginal dryness and tightness, which may make the proper fitting of a diaphragm more difficult than in women who are not lactating. The diaphragm should be used with one of the spermicidal lubricants, all of which contain nonoxynol-9.

The use of condoms alone or in combination with spermicides is often advised for women who wish to postpone a decision about sterilization or oral contraceptive therapy until the postpartum visit. Pregnancy rates for the condom are reported to be from 1.6 to 21 per 100 women-years, depending on the age and motivation of the population studied.[98]

Steroid Contraceptive Medications

The combined estrogen-progestin preparations have proved to be the most effective method of contraception, with pregnancy rates reported as less than 0.5 per 100 women-years. Most compounds include 35 μg or less of estrogen and varying amounts of progestins. Compounds containing the progestational components desogestrel, gestodene, or norgestimate appear to be less androgenic and have less impact on carbohydrate and lipid metabolism than compounds containing levonorgestrel or norethindrone.[99] Cardiovascular complications, including hypertension, venous thrombosis, stroke, and myocardial infarction, have been substantially reduced with the reduction in estrogen content. The cardiovascular complications are found predominantly in women who smoke.[100] In nonsmoking women the risk-benefit ratio is clearly in favor of using oral contraceptive agents. This is particularly true when the additional benefits of these agents are considered, which include lowered risks of benign breast disease, ovarian and endometrial cancer, iron-deficiency anemia, toxic shock syndrome, pelvic inflammatory disease, and ectopic pregnancy.[101]

In patients who are not breast-feeding, oral contraceptive agents can be taken as early as 2 to 3 weeks after delivery. The effect of oral contraceptive agents on lactation is controversial. Controlled studies of the combined-type oral contraceptive agents with doses of ethinyl estradiol or mestranol of 50 μg or more demonstrated a suppressive effect on lactation. Progestin-only medications (e.g., norethindrone 0.35 mg q day) do not diminish lactation performance.[102] Combined-type contraceptive agents also decrease the protein, fat, lactose, calcium, and phosphorous concentrations of breast milk, but not to the degree to impair the growth of breast-fed infants.

Diaz et al.[103] studied the effect on lactation and infant growth of a low-dose combination oral contraceptive containing 0.03-mg ethinyl estradiol and 0.15-mg levonorgestrel. The medication was begun after all women were fully nursing 1 month after delivery. Among those women taking the oral contraceptive medications, there was a small but significant decrease in lactation performance and in the weight gain of their infants compared with controls. In women whose motivation to breast-feed is marginal, the slight inhibition of lactation induced by oral contraceptive agents may be sufficient to discourage them from continuing to nurse their infants, and so progestin-only preparations should be offered to these women.

An increasingly popular form of contraception is the use of depot medroxyprogesterone acetate (DMPA), 150 mg IM every 3 months, which has a contraceptive efficacy exceeding 99 percent.[104] DMPA, which had been widely used in other countries, was approved for use in the United States by the FDA in 1992. The most annoying side effect is unpredictable spotting and bleeding. Long-term DMPA use has been associated with reversible reduction in bone density and unfavorable changes in lipid metabolism. The major advantages of this form of contraception is the ease of administration and patient convenience.

Levonorgestrel subdermal implants were approved by the FDA for contraceptive use in the United States in 1990. Each implant consists of six Silastic capsules that contain 36 mg of crystalline levonorgestrel. Pregnancy rates in women using the implants are lower than with any other reversible contraception.[105] Implants inserted 4 weeks after delivery have no effect on lactation or growth of an infant who is nursing even though small amounts of levonorgestrel are excreted in the milk. Although the usual time of insertion is 4 to 6 weeks following delivery, the implants can be inserted in the immediate puerperium. Irregular uterine bleeding, expense, and the occasional difficulty in removing the implants are the major drawbacks to the use of this form of contraception.

Intrauterine Devices

The copper-containing T-shaped device (ParaGard) and the progesterone-releasing device (Progestasert) are highly effective in preventing pregnancy (two to three pregnancies per 100 women-years).[106–108] The advantage of the copper-containing IUD is that it is effective for 10 years; its disadvantage is an increase in irregular uterine bleeding. The device that releases progesterone reduces uterine bleeding, but it must replaced annually.

The biologic action of IUDs is a matter of concern to those who might object to the method if the principal action is to prevent implantation of the blastocyst. The investigations of Alvarez et al.[109] convincingly support the concept that the principal mode of action of IUDs is by a method other than destruction of live embryos. These authors, using techniques to recover ova from the genital tracts of women using no contraception and of women using IUDs, found fertilized eggs in one-half of women using no contraception but none in women using IUDs even though all patients had intercourse within the fertile period.

The pregnancy rate with an IUD is reported to be between 1 and 6 per 100 women-years, with expulsion rates being 4 to 18 and removal for medical reasons being 12 to 16 per 100 women during the first year of use.[110] Addition of bioactive materials such as copper or progesterone to the IUD has not significantly reduced pregnancy rates but has reduced the risk of expulsion or abnormal bleeding.

The major side effects and complications are syncope, uterine perforation, abnormal uterine bleeding, uterine and pelvic infection, and ectopic pregnancy.[107] Syncope is a result of the vagal response that occurs in some women at the time of IUD insertion. Patients with a history of syncope or severe menstrual pain may be at greater risk from a complication, and the use of sedatives, analgesics, or atropine should be considered. These reactions are less common when the IUD is inserted in the puerperium, because functionally the cervix is slightly dilated.

Uterine perforation occurs in 0 to 8 per 1,000 insertions and is highest when the insertion is performed from 1 to 8 weeks after delivery. This is an important consideration when the insertion of the device is planned for the 6-week postpartum visit. If there is any doubt about adequate involution of the uterus, IUD insertion should be postponed for 2 to 3 additional weeks. However, Mishell and Roy[111] demonstrated no increase in perforation with the use of the copper-T inserted 4 to 8 weeks' postpartum, A withdrawal type of insertion appears to reduce the risk of this complication.

Bleeding and uterine cramping occur in 8 to 10 percent of women using an IUD and account for 4 to 15 removals of the device per 100 women in the first year of use. The causes of these symptoms are unknown, although they may be due to the local production of proteolytic enzymes and prostaglandins within the endometrium adjacent to the IUD. A variety of methods have been used to treat this complication, including the use of hormones, vitamins, and prostaglandin synthetase inhibitors, but there are no data establishing the effectiveness of any of these measures.

The relative risk of pelvic infection in IUD users ranges from 1.7 to 9.3. A variety of microorganisms have been implicated, including actinomyces in some cases. Prompt removal of the device and antibiotic therapy are recommended when there is any evidence of salpingitis. However, in parous women who have used the IUD, the risk of infertility caused by pelvic infection is no greater than in patients who have never used an IUD.[112]

Although the overall risk of ectopic pregnancy is lower in women using the IUD when compared with women using no contraception, the chances that a pregnancy will be ectopic is 7 to 10 times higher in the IUD user.

There has been some enthusiasm for insertion of the IUD during the immediate postpartum period. Surprisingly, this practice is associated with fewer perforations than are insertions between 1 and 8 weeks. Not surprising, however, is the finding that much higher expulsion rates are noted (10 to 21 percent).[113]

The IUD has been found to be a satisfactory method of birth control in women who are breast-feeding. Cole et al.[114] reported a multicenter study showing that breast-feeding did not increase the risk of expulsion or other complications regardless of the time of insertion of the device.

Sterilization

Sterilization is the most frequently used method of fertility regulation in the world.[115] The puerperium is a convenient time for tubal ligation procedures to be performed in women who desire sterilization. The procedure can be performed at the time of a cesarean delivery or within the first 24 to 48 hours after delivery. In some hospitals the operation is performed immediately after delivery in uncomplicated patients, especially when epidural anesthesia was given for labor analgesia. With the use of small paraumbilical incision, the procedure seldom prolongs the patient's hospitalization.

The failure rate of postpartum sterilization procedures varies somewhat with the type of tubal ligation performed, but overall it is in the range of 0.5 to 1.0 percent. In the United States, the Pomeroy or Parkland procedures are those most commonly performed, as these are as effective as the more complicated procedures. In either case, a portion of fallopian tube from its middle third is removed, leaving the cut ends ligated together in a single structure, as in the Pomeroy procedure, or separately, as in the Parkland operation.[116] The somewhat more complicated Uchida procedure involves opening the serosa, which has been infiltrated with saline, removing a segment of the muscularis, and burying the proximal-stump fallopian tube beneath the serosa. Uchida[117] also described removing the distal portion of the tube, including the fimbria, although this is not always done. Using this procedure, Uchida reported an extraordinarily low failure rate (0 in 20,000), but there have been reports by others of pregnancies occurring after a Uchida tubal ligation.[118] At the time of a cesarean delivery, an Irving procedure can be performed, which involves removing a segment from the middle third of the tube and then burying the proximal stump in a small tunnel created in the anterior surface of the uterus.[119] This procedure requires a slightly larger incision if done after vaginal delivery.

There are also reports of immediate postpartum sterilization with the laparoscope,[120] but this method lacks widespread enthusiasm. The relaxed abdominal wall and the easy accessibility of the fallopian tubes endows the minilaparotomy with the advantages of convenience and speed without the possible risks of visceral injury that might occur with the trocar of the laparoscope.

Perhaps more important than the type of procedure is the decision about the timing of the procedure or whether it should be performed at all. Puerperal sterilization compared with interval sterilization is associated with increased incidence of guilt and regret.[121,122] With increasing frequency, couples are postponing tubal ligation procedures until 6 to 8 weeks after delivery.[115] This provides time to ensure that the infant is healthy and to review all the implications of the decision. In most patients, laparoscopic tubal ligation can be accomplished as an outpatient procedure with a minimum of morbidity or disruption of family routines.

The risks of tubal ligation procedures, whether performed in the puerperium or as an interval procedure, include the short-term problems of anesthetic accidents, hemorrhage, injury of the viscera, and infection. These complications are infrequent, and deaths from the procedure occur in 2 to 12 per 100,000 procedures. Long-term complications are less well defined and more controversial. About 10 to 15 percent of patients will have irregular menses and increased menstrual pain after tubal sterilization. This so-called post-tubal syndrome is sufficiently severe in some cases to require hysterectomy. Well-controlled prospective studies, however, have failed to provide convincing evidence that these symptoms occur more commonly after tubal sterilization than in control patients of the same age and previous menstrual history.[123,124]

There has also been concern about poststerilization depression.[125] Because depression is common in women of childbearing age and is even more common in the puerperium, it is difficult to know whether sterilization procedures are independent risk factors for depression. It is obvious, however, that the loss of fertility associated with a sterilization procedure will have important conscious and subconscious implications for many women. It is therefore not surprising that some patients manifest transient grief reactions in response to tubal ligation. The loss of libido that may occur in such situations may be frightening to some women and equally disturbing to their partners. Reassurance that such reactions are temporary and are not necessarily symptoms of a seriously disturbed psyche is an important means of support during this crisis. Husbands must be aware of the dynamics of this situation to avoid a sense of estrangement.

Obstetricians must remember that vasectomy is often a more advisable and desirable alternative for a couple considering sterilization.[126] It can be performed as an outpatient procedure under local anesthesia with insignificant loss of time from work. Furthermore, almost all the failures (about 3 to 4 per 1,000 procedures) can be detected by a postoperative semen analysis. This is a decided advantage over the tubal ligation, in which failures are discovered only when a pregnancy occurs. Furthermore, vasectomy is less expensive and overall is associated with fewer complications. In a review of the long-term health effects of vasectomy, Peterson et al.[127] found no evidence that the procedure increases the risk of subsequent myocardial infarction or autoimmune disorders.

Tubal ligation can be reversed, but a patient should not undergo sterilization if she is contemplating reversal. Success as measured by the occurrence of pregnancy following tubal reanastamosis varies from 40 to 85 percent, depending on the type of tubal ligation performed and on the length of functioning tube that remains.[115] Success rates for vas reanastamosis vary from 37 to 90 percent, with higher success rates being associated with shorter intervals from the time of vas ligation.[115]

Hysterectomy has been advocated as a means of sterilization that has the advantage of protecting the patient from future uterine or cervical cancer. However, the morbidity of cesarean or puerperal hysterectomy operations is sufficiently great to preclude their consideration for elective sterilization.[128]

Postpartum Psychological Reactions

The psychological reactions experienced by women following childbirth include the common, relatively mild, and transient "maternity blues" (50 to 70 percent incidence), more prolonged affective disorders regarded as true postpartum depression (PPD; 10 to 15 percent incidence), and frank puerperal psychosis (0.14 to 0.26 percent incidence). Although the specific etiology of these psychological disorders is unknown, they are not necessarily a continuum or progressively severe manifestations of a single underlying disorder.

Maternity Blues

The most common of the psychological manifestations of the puerperium is the transient state of tearfulness, anxiety, irritation, and restlessness, variously described as "maternity blues" or "postpartum blues." As it occurs in up to 70 percent of parturients,[129] it might well be considered a normal involutional phenomenon. The symptoms may appear on any day within the first week after delivery and usually have resolved by postpartum day 10. Occasional patients will note transient recurrence of the symptoms, especially weeping, for several weeks after delivery.[130]

There appear to be no obstetric, social, economic, or personality correlates for maternity blues. While it is tempting to ascribe the symptoms of this syndrome to the changes in steroid hormone levels that occur immediately following delivery, no such correlation has been found.[131] However, lower than expected tryptophan levels have been documented in association with the depressive symptoms in the immediate postpartum period, suggesting a role for neurotransmitters in the elaboration of puerperal mood changes.[132] Hyperactivity of the hypothalamic-pituitary-adrenal axis, blunted responsiveness of the hypothalamic-pituitary-thyroid axis, and altered central neurotransmitter function characterize PPD as well as nonpuerperal major depression.[133]

Patients suffering from maternity blues manifest a wide range of symptoms, including weeping, depression, restlessness, elation, mood lability, headache, confusion, forgetfulness, irritability, depersonalization, insomnia, and negative feelings toward their infants. Not every patient experiences all these symptoms. Investigators who have studied the syndrome have differed in their criteria and definitions of the disorder, to some extent accounting for the varying incidence of maternity blues reported.

Because the syndrome is transient and of short duration, no therapy is indicated. Some of the symptoms may be from sleep deprivation, and increased rest may be helpful. Anticipatory explanation and a sympathetic and understanding attitude on the part of family members and those caring for the patient are all that are required for this troublesome and common complaint.

Postpartum Depression

The incidence of postpartum major depression varies from 8 to 15 percent.[134,135] Pitt[136] was one of the first to document the incidence of neurotic depression in the puerperium. He found that 11 percent of the patients studied at 28 weeks' gestation and at 6 weeks' postpartum developed new cases of depression during the postpartum period.

In a study of 128 women randomly selected and interviewed on several occasions during their pregnancies and for 1 year after birth, Watson et al.[137] used a standardized psychiatric interview. Eight patients (6 percent) were found to have psychiatric disorders when first interviewed before 24 weeks' gestation. Twenty patients (16 percent) had psychiatric disorders identified at 6 weeks' postpartum, 15 of which were classified as affective (depressive) disorders. All but three of the cases of postpartum depression occurred either in women who experienced life situations other than the pregnancy that accounted for the depression or in women who had a previous history of significant depressive reactions. In other words, in the experience of these investigators, it was unusual to find postpartum depression occurring in a patient with an otherwise psychologically uncomplicated pregnancy and past history. They also confirmed a lack of association between postnatal depression and social class, marital status, or parity.

Kumar and Robson[138] obtained repeated psychiatric interviews from 119 primipara throughout and after pregnancy. At 12 weeks' postpartum, these investigators found that 16 patients demonstrated psychiatric disorders, 113 of which were new episodes of depression. Unlike Watson et al.,[137] these observers found little overlap between antenatal and postnatal psychiatric disorders.

The signs and symptoms of postpartum depression are not different from those in the nonpregnant patients, but they may be difficult to differentiate from normal involutional phenomena (e.g., weight loss, sleeplessness) or from the transient "maternity blues."[138] However, in addition to the more common symptoms of depression, the postpartum patient may manifest a sense of incapability of loving her family and manifest ambivalence toward her infant.

There is a high risk of recurrence (50 to 100 percent) of PPD in subsequent pregnancies and a 20 to 30 percent risk of PPD in women who have had a previous depressive reaction not associated with pregnancy. Consequently, it is important to inquire about psychiatric illness when taking the prenatal history.

There are a number of questionnaires or interview techniques to identify the antepartum patient who is at high risk of developing postpartum major depression.[139] Although no specific series of questions for the prediction of PPD has been rigorously validated or widely used in obstetric practice, the work of Posner et al.[140] suggests that one or more of the following 12 characteristics should alert the caretakers that a patient is at increased risk for postpartum major depression:

1. Is under 20 years of age
2. Is unmarried
3. Is medically indigent
4. Comes from a family of six or more children
5. Was separated from one or both parents in childhood or adolescence
6. Received poor parental support and attention in childhood
7. Had limited parental support in adulthood
8. Has poor relationship with husband or boyfriend
9. Has economic problem with housing or income
10. Is dissatisfied with amount of education
11. Shows evidence of emotional problem, past or present
12. Has low self-esteem

It is appropriate that questions addressing some of these risk factors as well as the simple inquiry "are you happy?" be incorporated into the antenatal history.

Puerperal hypothyroidism often presents with symptoms including mild dysphoria; consequently thyroid function studies may be useful in patients presenting with suspected PPD.

Early recognition of the signs and symptoms and supportive care and reassurance from family and health-care professionals are the first line of treatment for PPD. The tricyclic antidepressants (nortriptyline or desipramine) have been helpful, but recent studies suggest that serotonin uptake inhibitors (fluoxetine, paroxetine, or sertraline) are equally effective and have fewer side effects.[133] If there is not prompt response to general supportive measures and initial use of medication, psychiatric consultation is advisable. The prognosis for PPD is good, although symptoms may persist for up to a year.

Vandenberg[141] emphasizes the importance of the family in the therapy of PPD. Being physically and emotionally drained from the stresses of pregnancy and childbirth and further burdened by the incessant demands of her infant, the postpartum patient may be unable to meet the demands of her husband and the other children. This will compound her feeling of self-worthlessness. Helping the husband and other family members to understand the nature of the patient's illness and mobilizing resources to provide the patient with help with her home chores and the care of the other children will help to prevent her sense of entrapment and isolation. If a patient is at high risk of developing PPD or if suspicious signs or symptoms develop during the immediate postpartum period, it is mandatory that the postpartum visits be scheduled sooner than the traditional 6 weeks. The moderately depressed mother will often experience such guilt and embarrassment secondary to her sense of failure in her mothering role that she will be unable to call her physician or admit the symptoms of her depression.[141] Consequently, ample time must be set aside to explore in depth even the slightest symptoms or sign of depression. Home visits in this situation may be appropriate to assess the patient's parenting skills and to determine how she is coping with the increased responsibilities of her new situation.

Postpartum Psychosis

Schizophrenia and manic-depressive reactions are seen with increased frequency in the puerperium, suggesting that there is a psychosis specific to the postpartum condition. In a study of all patients giving birth in 1966 and 1967 in Southampton, England, Nott[142] documented a significant increase in psychiatric referrals for specific psychoses in the 16 weeks after delivery. This confirmed the observation by Kendall et al.,[143] who found a significant increase in admission to psychiatric hospitals during the puerperium compared with the antepartum or the nonpregnant state.

There is considerable debate as to whether the psychotic reactions that occur in the puerperium represent a unique psychiatric entity.[144] The signs and symptoms in general do not differ from those of acute, nonpuerperal psychosis, but the frequency of symptoms differs substantially. Most patients with puerperal psychosis are manic-depressive, with confusion and disorientation prominent features of the clinical presentation. Furthermore, the psychotic reactions occurring in the puerperium appear to have a more favorable prognosis than the nonpuerperal psychosis. The duration of the illness is frequently only 2 or 3 months.

During the immediate postpartum period, the early signs of depression may be difficult to distinguish from "maternity blues," but if suicidal thoughts or attempts occur, or if frankly delusional thoughts are expressed, the diagnosis of postpartum psychosis can be made.[141]

Clearly, all patients with puerperal psychosis require hospitalization for at least initial evaluation and institution of therapy. However, specific therapeutic management of puerperal psychotic disorders is a matter of controversy due to the lack of properly conducted treatment trials in these disorders.[144] Although electroconvulsive therapy, tricyclic antidepressants, neuroleptics, and lithium carbonate have all been recommended for specific subgroups of puerperal psychosis, none has been proven to enhance recovery. Whatever therapy for these conditions is instituted, it should be conducted or supervised by a psychiatrist.

Managing Perinatal Grieving

For the most part, perinatal events are happy ones and are occasions for rejoicing. When a patient and her family experience a loss associated with a pregnancy, special attention must be given to the grieving patient and her family.

The most obvious cases of perinatal loss are those in which a fetal or neonatal death has occurred. Other more subtle losses can be associated with a significant amount of grieving, such as the birth of a critically ill or malformed infant, an unexpected hysterectomy performed for intractable postpartum hemorrhage, or even a planned postpartum sterilization procedure. Grief will occur with any significant loss whether it is the actual death of an infant[145] or the loss of an idealized child in the case of the birth of a handicapped infant.[146]

Mourning is as old as the human race, but the clinical signs and symptoms of grief and their psychological ramifications as they relate to loss suffered by women during their pregnancies have been given special consideration in recent years. In studying the relatives of servicemen who died in World War II, Lindemann[147] recognized five manifestations of normal grieving. These include somatic symptoms of sleeplessness, fatigue, digestive symptoms, and sighing respirations; preoccupation with the image of the deceased; feelings of guilt; feelings of hostility and anger toward others; and disruption of the normal pattern of daily life. He also described the characteristics of what is now recognized as pathologic grief, which may occur if acute mourning is suppressed or interrupted. Some of the manifestations of this so-called morbid grief reaction are overactivity without a sense of loss, appearance or exacerbations of psychosomatic illness, alterations in relationships with friends and relatives, furious hostility toward specific persons, lasting loss of patterns of social interaction, activities detrimental to personal, social, and economic existence, and agitated depression.

Kennel et al.[148] studied the reaction of 20 mothers to the loss of their newborn infants. Characteristic signs and symptoms of mourning occurred in all the patients, even in situations in which the infant was nonviable. Similar grief reactions occurred in most of the parents of 101 critically ill infants who survived after referral to a regional neonatal intensive care unit,[149] showing that separation from a seriously ill newborn is sufficient to provoke typical grief reaction.

It is important that the characteristics of the grieving patient be recognized and understood by health professionals caring for such patients; otherwise, substantial misunderstanding and mismanagement of the patient will occur. For example, if the patient's reaction of anger and hostility is not anticipated, a nurse or physician may take personally statements or actions by the patient or her family and avoid the patient at the very time she needs the most consolation and support. Because of their own discomfort with the implications of death, physicians, nurses, and others on the postpartum unit often find it uncomfortable to deal with patients whose fetus or infant has died. As a consequence, there is a reluctance to discuss the death with the patient and a tendency to rely on the use of sedatives or tranquilizers to deal with the patient's symptoms of grief.[150–152] What is actually beneficial at such a time is a sympathetic listener and an opportunity to express and discuss feelings of guilt, anger, and hopelessness and the other symptoms of mourning.

It is not surprising that PPD is more common and more severe in families that have suffered a perinatal loss. Rowe et al.[153] found that 6 of 26 mothers who experienced a perinatal loss had morbid grief reactions. Interestingly, the prolonged grief response occurred more commonly in those women who became pregnant within 5 months of the death of the infant. This finding suggests that in counseling women after the loss of an infant, one should avoid the traditional advice of encouraging the family to embark soon on another pregnancy as a "replacement" for the infant who died. Just how long the normal grief reaction lasts is not known, and surely it varies with different families. Lockwood and Lewis[154] studied 26 patients who had suffered a stillbirth; they followed several patients for as long as 2 years. Their data suggest that grief in this situation is usually resolved within 18 months, invariably with a resurgency of symptoms at the first anniversary of the loss.

Somatic symptoms of grief, such as anorexia, weakness, and fatigue, are now well recognized; other psychological manifestations are also reported. Spontaneous abortion and infertility increase among couples who attempt to conceive after the loss of an infant.[155] Schleifer et al.[156] found significant suppression of lymphocyte stimulation in the spouses of women with advanced breast carcinoma. Although the most intense suppression was noted within the month after bereavement, a modified response was noted for as long as 14 months. These investigators suggest that this may account for the increase in morbidity and mortality associated with bereavement.

The regionalization of perinatal health care has resulted in a large proportion of the perinatal deaths occurring in tertiary centers. In some of these centers teams of physicians, nurses, social workers, and pastoral counselors have evolved to aid specifically in the management of families suffering a perinatal loss.[157–160] While this approach ensures an enlightened, understanding, and consistent approach to bereaved families, it suggests that the support of a grieving patient is a highly complex endeavor, to be accomplished only by a few specially trained individuals who care for postpartum patients. Kowalski[160] has listed the following guidelines for managing perinatal loss:

1. Keep the mother informed; be honest and forthright
2. Recognize and facilitate anticipatory grieving
3. Encourage the mother's major support person to remain with her throughout labor and delivery
4. Support the couple in seeing or touching the infant
5. Describe the infant in detail, particularly for couples who choose not to see
6. Encourage the mother to make as many choices about her care as possible
7. Teach couple about the grieving process
8. Show infants during postpartum hospitalization on request
9. Allow photographs of the infant
10. Prepare the couple for hospital paperwork, such as autopsy requests
11. Discuss funeral or memorial services
12. Help the couple to think about informing siblings
13. Assist the couple in deciding how to tell friends of the death and in packing away the baby's things
14. Discuss subsequent pregnancy
15. Use public health nurse referral or schedule additional office visits

Clearly, management of grief is not solely a postpartum responsibility. This is particularly true when a prenatal diagnosis is made of fetal death or fetal abnormality. A continuum of support is essential as the patient moves from the prenatal setting, to labor and delivery, to the postpartum ward, and finally to her home. Relaxation of many of the traditional hospital routines may be necessary to provide the type of support these families need. For example, allowing a loved one to remain past visiting hours, providing a couple a private setting to be with their deceased infant, or allowing unusually early discharge with provisions for frequent phone calls and follow-up visits will often facilitate the resolution of grief.

It is also important to realize that the fathers of infants who die have somewhat different grief responses than do the mothers. In a study of 28 fathers who had lost infants, Mandell et al.[161] found their grief characterized by the necessity to keep busy with increased work, feelings of diminished self-worth, self-blame, and limited ability to ask for help. Stoic responses are typical of men and may obstruct the normal resolution of grief.

Key Points

- By six weeks' postpartum 28 percent of women will have returned to their prepregnant weight.

- Approximately 50 percent of parturients experience diminished sexual desire during the three months following delivery.

- Postpartum uterine bleeding of sufficient quantity to require medical attention occurs in 1 to 2 percent of parturients. In patients requiring curettage, 40 percent will be found to have retained placental tissue.

- Late onset endometritis (after 7 days) is frequently caused by *Chlamydia trachomatis*.

- *Monilia* infection is a common cause of persistent nipple soreness in women who are breast-feeding.

- Most women with puerperal mastitis can be adequately prepared with penicillin V, ampicillin, or dicloxacillin while they continue to breast-feed their infants.

- Breast feeding will result in 98 percent contraceptive protection for up to 6 months following delivery provided there is little or no supplemental feeding of the infant.

- Progestin only contraceptive medication (norethindrone 0.35 mg daily) does not diminish lactation performance.

- Postpartum, major depression occurs in 8 to 15 percent of parturients.

- Puerperal hypothyroidism often presents with symptoms that include mild dysphoria; consequently, thyroid function studies are suggested in the evaluation of patients with suspected postpartum depression.

References

1. Hytten FE, Cheyne GA: The size and composition of the human pregnant uterus. J Obstet Gynaecol Br Commonw 76:400, 1969
2. Williams JS: Regeneration of the uterine mucosa after delivery, with special reference to the placental site. Am J Obstet Gynecol 22:664, 1931
3. Sharman A: Postpartum regeneration of the human endometrium. J Anat 87:1, 1953
4. Anderson WR, Davis J: Placental site involution. Am J Obstet Gynecol 102:23, 1968
5. Oppenheimer LS, Sheriff EA, Goodman JDS et al: The duration of lochia. Br J Obstet Gynaecol 93:754, 1986
6. Lipinski JK, Adam AH: Ultrasonic prediction of complications following normal vaginal delivery. J Clin Ultrasound 9:17, 1981
7. Chang YL, Madrozo B, Drukker BH: Ultrasonic evaluation of the postpartum uterus in management of postpartum bleeding. Obstet Gynecol 58:227, 1981
8. Glass M, Rosenthal AH: Cervical changes in pregnancy, labor and puerperium. Am J Obstet Gynecol 60:353, 1950
9. Coppleson M, Reid BL: A colposcopic study of the cervix during pregnancy and the puerperium. J Obstet Gynaecol Br Commonw 73:575, 1966
10. McLaren HC: The involution of the cervix. BMJ 1:347, 1952
11. Andrews MC: Epithelial changes in the puerperal fallopian tube. Am J Obstet Gynecol 62:28, 1951
12. Cronin TJ: Influence of lactation upon ovulation. Lancet 2:422, 1968
13. Perex A, Uela P, Masnick GS et al: First ovulation after childbirth: the effect of breast feeding. Am J Obstet Gynecol 114:1041, 1972
14. Sharman A: Ovulation after pregnancy. Fertil Steril 2:371, 1951
15. Gray RH, Campbell ON, Apelo R et al: Risk of ovulation during lactation. Lancet 335:25, 1990
16. Bonnar J, Franklin M, Nott PN et al: Effect of breast-feeding on pituitary-ovarian function after childbirth. BMJ 4:82, 1975
17. Crowell DT: Weight change in the postpartum period: a review of the literature. J Nurse Midwifery 40:418, 1995
18. Scholl TO, Hediger ML, Schall JI et al: Gestational weight gain, pregnancy outcome, and postpartum weight retention. Obstet Gynecol 1995:86, 423
19. Rasmusen NG, Hornnes PJ, Hegedus L: Ultrasonographically determined thyroid size in pregnancy and postpartum: the goitrogenic effect of pregnancy. Am J Obstet Gynecol 160:1216, 1989
20. Jausson R, Dahlberg PA, Winsa B et al: The postpartum period constitutes an important risk for the development of clinical Graves disease in young women. Acta Endocrinol 116:321, 1987
21. Walters WAW, Limm VL: Blood volume and haemodynamics in pregnancy. Clin Obstet Gynaecol 2:301, 1975
22. Lindesman R, Miller MM: Blood volume changes during the immediate postpartum period. Obstet Gynecol 21:40, 1963
23. Ueland K: Maternal cardiovascular dynamics. VIII. Intrapartum blood volume changes. Am J Obstet Gynecol 126:671, 1976
24. Paintin DB: The size of the total red cell volume in pregnancy. J Obstet Gynaecol Br Commonw 69:719, 1962
25. Walters WAW, MacGregor WG, Hills M: Cardiac output at rest during pregnancy and the puerperium. Clin Sci 30:1, 1966
26. Walters BNJ, Thompson ME, Lea E, DeSwiet M: Blood pressure in the puerperium. Clin Sci 71:589, 1986
27. Monheit AG, Cousins L, Resnik R: The puerperium: anatomic and physiologic readjustments. Clin Obstet Gynecol 23:973, 1980
28. Ygge J: Changes in blood coagulation and fibrinolysis during the puerperium. Am J Obstet Gynecol 104:2, 1969
29. Baird D: The upper urinary tract in pregnancy and pu-

erperium, with special reference to pyelitis of pregnancy. J Obstet Gynaecol Br Emp 42:733, 1935

30. Rubi RA, Sala NC: Ureteral function in pregnant women. III. Effect of different positions and of fetal delivery upon ureteral tonus. Am J Obstet Gynecol 101: 230, 1968

31. Dure-Smith P: Pregnancy dilatation of the urinary tract. Radiology 96:545, 1970

32. Peake SL, Roxburgh HB, Langlois SL: Ultrasonic assessment of hydronephrosis of pregnancy. Radiology 146:167, 1983

33. Fried AM, Woodring JH, Thompson DJ: Hydronephrosis of pregnancy: a prospective sequential study of the course of dilatation. J Ultrasound Med 2:255, 1983

34. Cietak KA, Newton JR: Serial qualitative maternal nephrosonography in pregnancy. Br J Radiol 58:399, 1985

35. Kerr-Wilson RHJ, Thompson SW, Orr JW Jr et al: Effect of labor on the postpartum bladder. Obstet Gynecol 64: 115, 1984

36. Sims EAH, Krantz KE: Serial studies of renal function during pregnancy and the puerperium in normal women. J Clin Invest 37:1764, 1958

37. DeAlvarez RR: Renal glomerulotubular mechanisms during normal pregnancy. Am J Obstet Gynecol 75:931, 1958

38. Glazener CMA, Abdalla M, Stroud P et al: Postnatal maternal morbidity: extent, causes, prevention and treatment. Br J Obstet Gynaecol 102:282, 1995

39. Jennings B, Edmundson M: The postpartum periods: after confinement: the fourth trimester. Clin Obstet Gynecol 23:1093, 1980

40. Fein J, Goldman JM, Weintraub BD: Postpartum lymphocytic thyroiditis in American women: a spectrum of thyroid dysfunction. Am J Obstet Gynecol 138:504, 1980

41. Amino N, Mori H, Iwatani Y et al: High prevalence of transient postpartum thyrotoxicosis and hypothyroidism. N Engl J Med 306:849, 1983

42. Reamy K, White SE: Sexuality in pregnancy and the puerperium: a review. Obstet Gynecol Surv 40:1, 1985

43. Ryding E-L: Sexuality during and after pregnancy. Acta Obstet Gynecol Scand 63:679, 1984

44. American College of Obstetricians and Gynecologists: Pregnancy, Work, and Disability. Technical Bulletin No. 58. ACOG, Washington, DC, 1980

45. Windle ML, Booker LA, Rayburn WF: Postpartum pain after vaginal delivery: a review of comparative analgesic trials. J Reprod Med 34:891, 1989

46. Shy KK, Eschenback DA: Fatal perineal cellulitis from episiotomy site. Obstet Gynecol 54:929, 1979

47. Stiller RJ, Kaplan BM, Andreoli JW Jr: Hereditary angioedema and pregnancy. Obstet Gynecol 64:133, 1984

48. Ewing TL, Smale LE, Eliot FA: Maternal deaths associated with postpartum vulvar edema. Am J Obstet Gynecol 134:173, 1979

49. Droegemueller W: Cold sitz baths for relief of postpartum perineal pain. Clin Obstet Gynecol 23:1039, 1980

50. King PA, Duthie SJ, Dip V et al: Secondary postpartum hemorrhage. Aust NZ J Obstet Gynaecol 29:394: 1989

51. Charles J, Charles D: Postpartum infection. p. 60. In Charles D (ed): Obstetric and Perinatal Infections. Mosby Year Book, St Louis, 1993

52. Duff P: Pathophysicology and management of post-cesarean endomyometritis. Obstet Gynecol 67:26, 1985

53. Klaus MH, Jerauld R, Kreger NC et al: Maternal attachment: importance of the first postpartum days. N Engl J Med 286:460, 1972

54. McClellan MS, Cabianca WC: Effects of early mother–infant contact following cesarean birth. Obstet Gynecol 56:52, 1980

55. Robson KM, Powell E: Early maternal attachment. p.155. In Brickington IF, Kumar R (eds): Motherhood and Mental Illness. Acadmic Press, San Diego, 1982

56. Klaus M, Kennel J: Parent–Infant Bonding. CV Mosby, St Louis, 1982

57. Gray J, Butler C, Dean J et al: Prediction and prevention of child abuse and neglect. Child Abuse Neglect 1:45, 1977

58. Siegel E, Cauman KE, Schaefer ES et al: Hospital and home support during infancy: impact on maternal attachment, child abuse and neglect and health care utilization. Pediatrics 66:183, 1980

59. DeCasper AJ, Fifer W: Of human bonding: newborns prefer their mother's voices. Science 208:1174, 1980

60. Aerskog B, Uddenberg N, Kjessler B: Experience of delivery in women with and without antenatal fear of childbirth. Gynecol Obstet Invest 16:1, 1983

61. Martinex GA, Dodd DA: Milk feeding patterns in the United States: first 12 months of life. Pediatrics 71:166, 1983

62. Jeliffe DB, Jeliffe EFP: "Breast is best": modern meanings. N Engl J Med 297:912, 1977

63. Winikoff B, Myers D, Laukaran VH, Stone R: Overcoming obstacles to breast-feeding in a large municipal hospital: applications of lessons learned. Pediatrics 80:423, 1987

64. Neifert MR, Seacat JM: Medical management of successful breast-feeding. Pediatr Clin North Am 33:743, 1986

65. Casey CE, Hambidge KM: Nutritional aspects of human lactation. p. 199. In Neville MC, Neifert MR (eds): Lactation, Physiology, Nutrition, and Breast-Feeding. Plenum Press, New York, 1983

66. Institute of Medicine (Subcommittee on Nutrition During Lactation): Nutrition During Lactation. National Academy Press, Washington, DC, 1991

67. National Research Council, Food and Nutrition Board: Recommended Dietary Allowances. 10th Ed. National Academy of Sciences, Washington, DC, 1989

68. Higginbottom MC, Sweetman L, Nyhan WL: A syndrome of methylmalonic acidemia, homocystinuria, megaloblastic anemia and neurologic abnormalities in a vitamin B12 deficient breast-fed infant of a strict vegetarian. N Engl J Med 299:317, 1978

69. O'Connor P: Vitamin D deficiency in rickets in two breast-fed infants who were not receiving vitamin D supplementation. Clin Pediatr 16:361, 1977

70. Whichelow MJ: Success and failure of breast-feeding in relation to energy intake. Proc Nutr Soc 35:62A, 1975

71. Dunkle LM, Schmidt RR, O'Connor DP: Neonatal herpes simplex infection possibly acquired via maternal breast milk. Pediatrics 63:250, 1979

72. McGregor JA, Neifert MR: Maternal problems in lactation. p. 333. In Neville MC, Neifert MR (eds): Lactation: Phyiology, Nutrition and Breast-Feeding. Plenum Press, New York, 1983

73. Peckham C, Gibb D: Mother-to-child transmission of the human immunodeficiency virus. N Engl J Med 333:298, 1995

74. Briggs GC, Freeman RK, Yaffe SJ: Drugs in Pregnancy and Lactation: Williams & Wilkins, Baltimore, 1994

75. American Academy of Pediatrics: Committee on Drugs. The transfer of drugs and other chemicals into human milk. Pediatrics 93:137, 1994

76. Atkinson SA, Bryan MH, Anderson GH: Human milk feeding in premature infants: protein, fat, and carbohydrate balances in the first two weeks of life. J Pediatr 99:617, 1981

77. Haywood AR: The immunology of breast milk. p. 249. In Neville MC, Neifert MR (eds): Lactation: Physiology, Nutrition, and Breast-Feeding. Plenum Press, New York, 1983

78. Neifert MR: The infant problems in breast-feeding. p. 273. In Neville MR, Neifert MR (eds): Lactation: Physiology, Nutrition, and Breast Feeding. Plenum Press, New York, 1983

79. Hopkins JM, Schanler RJ, Garza C: Milk production by mothers of premature infants. Pediatrics 81:815, 1988

80. Niebyl JR, Spence MR, Parmley TH: Sporadic (nonepidemic) puerperal mastitis. J Reprod Med 20:97, 1978

81. Thomsen AC, Espersen T, Maigaard S: Course and treatment of milk statis, noninfectious inflammation of the breast, and infectious mastitis in nursing women. Am J Obstet Gynecol 149:492, 1984

82. Neifert MR, McDonough SI, Neville MC: Failure of lactogenesis associated with placental retention. Am J Obstet Gynecol 140:477, 1981

83. Sousa PSR: Metoclopramide and breast feeding. BMJ 1:512, 1975

84. Aono R, Shigi T, Aki T et al: Augmentation of puerperal lactation by oral administration of sulpiride. J Clin Endocrinol Metab 48:478, 1979

85. Morris JA, Creasy RK, Hohe PT: Inhibition of puerperal lactation: double-blind comparison of chlorotrianisene, testosterone enanthate with estradiol valerate and placebo. Obstet Gynecol 36:107, 1970

86. Niebyl JR, Bell Wr, Schaaf ME et al: The effect of chlorotrianisene as postpartum lactation suppression on blood coagulation factors. Am J Obstet Gynecol 134:518, 1979

87. Sandoz Pharmaceuticals: Drug Information Brochure re. Pariodel (Bromocriptine Mesylate). Sandoz Pharmaceuticals, East Hanover, NJ, 1987

88. Willis J (ed): Postpartum hypertension, seizures, and strokes reported with bromocriptine. FDA Drug Bull 14:3, 1984

89. Katz M, Kroll I, Pak I et al: Puerperal hypertension, stroke, and seizures after suppression of lactation with bromocriptine. Obstet Gynecol 66:822, 1985

90. Iffy L, TenHove W, Frisoli G: Acute myocardial infarction in the puerperium in patients receiving bromocriptine. Am J Obstet Gynecol 155:371, 1986

91. Ruch A, Duhring JL: Postpartum myocardial infarction in a patient receiving bromocriptine. Obstet Gynecol 74:448, 1989

92. Robson KM, Brant H, Kumar R: Maternal sexuality during first pregnancy after childbirth. Br J Obstet Gynaecol 88:882, 1981

93. Debrovner CH, Winikoff B: Trends in postpartum contraceptive choice. Obstet Gynecol 63:65, 1984

94. Flynn AM: Natural methods of family planning. Clin Obstet Gynaecol 11:661, 1984

95. Rojnik B, Kosmelj K, Andolsek-Jeras L: Initiation of contraception postpartum. Contraception 51:75, 1995

96. Wortman J: The diaphragm and other intravaginal barriers—a review. Popul Rep H:58, 1979

97. Vessey M, Wiggins P: Use-effectiveness of the diaphragm in a selected family planning clinic population in the United Kingdom. Contraception 9:15, 1974

98. Mills A: Barrier contraception. Clin Obstet Gynaecol 11:641, 1984

99. Speroff L, DeCherney A et al: Evaluation of a new generation of oral contraceptives. Obstet Gynecol 81:1034, 1993

100. Kay CR: The Royal College of General Practitioners' oral contraceptive study: some recent observations. Clin Obstet Gynaecol 11:759, 1984

101. Baird DT, Glasier AF: Hormonal contraception. N Engl J Med 328:1543, 1993

102. Buchanan R: Breastfeeding aid to infant health and fertility control. Popul Rep JO:49, 1975

103. Diaz S, Peralta G, Juez C et al: Fertility regulation in nursing women: III, Short-term influence of low-dose combined contraceptive upon lactation and infant growth. Contraception 27:1, 1983

104. Kaunitz AM: Long-acting injectable contraception with depot medroxyprogesterone acetate. Am J Obstet Gynecol 170:1543, 1994

105. Darney PD: Hormonal implants: contraception for a new century. Am J Obstet Gynecol 170:1536, 1994

106. Mishell DR Jr: Intrauterine devices. Clin Obstet Gynaecol 11:679, 1984

107. Harlap S, Kost K, Forrest JD: Preventing Pregnancy, Protecting Health: A New Look at Birth Control Choices in the United States. The Alan Guttmacher Institute, New York, 1991

108. Willis J (ed): Copper T 380A IUD marketed in U.S. FDA Drug Bull 18:19, 1988

109. Alvarez T, Brache V, Fernandez E et al: New insights on the mode of action of intrauterine contraceptive devices in women. Fertil Steril 49:768, 1988

110. U.S. Department of Health, Education and Welfare: Second Report on Intrauterine Contraceptive Devices, The Medical Device and Drug Advisory Committees on Obstetrics and Gynecology. Food and Drug Administration, Washington, DC, 1978

111. Mishell DR Jr, Roy S: Copper intrauterine contraceptive device event rate rollowing insertion 4 to 8 weeks postpartum. Am J Obstet Gynecol 143:29, 1982

112. Daling JR, Weiss NS, Metch BJ et al: Primary tubal in-

fertility in relation to use of an IUD. N Engl J Med 312: 937, 1985

113. Cole LP, Edelman DA, Potts DM et al: Postpartum insertion of modified intrauterine devices. J Reprod Med 29:677, 1984

114. Cole LP, McCann MF, Higgins JE et al: Effects of breast feeding on IUD performance. Am J Public Health 73: 384, 1983

115. Newton JR: Sterilization. Clin Obstet Gynaecol 11:603, 1984

116. Cunningham FG, MacDonald PC, Leveno KJ et al: Williams Obstetrics. 19th Ed. Appleton & Lange, Norwalk, CT, 1993

117. Uchida H: Uchida tubal sterilization. Am J Obstet Gynecol 121:153, 1975

118. Benedetti TJ, Miller FC: Uchida tubal sterilization failure: a report of four cases. Am J Obstet Gynecol 132: 116, 1978

119. Irving FC: A new method of insuring sterility following cesarean section. Am J Obstet Gynecol 8:335, 1924

120. Aranda C, Prada C, Broutin A et al: Laparoscopic sterilization immediately after term delivery: preliminary report. J Reprod Med 14:171, 1963

121. Sim M, Emens JM, Jordon JA: Psychiatric aspects of female sterilization. BMJ 3:220, 1973

122. Emens JM, Olive JE: Timing of female sterilization. BMJ 2:1126, 1978

123. Vessy M, Huggins G, Lawless M et al: Tubal sterilization: findings in a large prospective study. Br J Obstet Gynaecol 90:203, 1983

124. Bhiwandiwala PP, Mumford SD, Feldblum PJ: Menstrual pattern changes following laparoscopic sterilization with different occlusion techniques: a review of 10,004 cases. Am J Obstet Gynecol 145:684, 1983

125. Bledin KD, Brice B: Psychological conditions in pregnancy and the puerperium and their relevance to postpartum sterilization: a review. Bull WHO 61:533, 1983

126. Peterson HB, Huber DH, Belker Am: Vasectomy: an appraisal for the obstetrician-gynecologist. Obstet Gynecol 76:568, 1990

127. Walker MW, Jick H, Hunter JR: Vasectomy and nonfatal myocardial infarction. Lancet 1:13, 1981

128. Haynes DM, Martin BJ: Cesarean hysterectomy: a twenty-five year review. Am J Obstet Gynecol 46:215, 1975

129. Yalom I, Lunde D, Moos R et al: Postpartum blues syndrome. Arch Gen Psychiatry 18:16, 1968

130. Stein G: The maternity blues. p. 119. In Brockington IF, Kumar R (eds): Motherhood and Mental Illness. Academic Press, London, 1982

131. Nott PN, Franklin M, Armitage C et al: Hormonal changes and mood in the early puerperium. Br J Psychiatry 128:379, 1976

132. Handley SL, Sunn TL, Waldron S et al: Tryptophan, cortisol and puerperal mood. Br J Psychiatry 136:498, 1980

133. Stowe ZN, Nemeroff CB: Women at risk for postpartum-onset major depression. Am J Obstet Gynecol 173: 639, 1995

134. Cox JL, Murray D, Chapman G: A controlled study of the onset, duration and prevalence of postnatal depression. Br J Psychiatry 163:27, 1993

135. Pop VJM, Essed GGM, de Geus CA et al: Prevalence of post partum depression—or is it post-puerperium depression? Acta Obstet Gynaecol Scand 72:354, 1993

136. Pitt B: Atypical depression following childbirth. Br J Psychiatry 114:1325, 1968

137. Watson JP, Elliot SA, Rugg AJ et al: Psychiatric disorders in pregnancy and the first postnatal year. Br J Psychiatry 144:453, 1984

138. Kumar R, Robson K: Neurotic disturbance during pregnancy and the puerperium: preliminary report of a prospective survey of 119 primiparae. p. 40. In Sand M (ed): Mental Illness in Pregnancy and the Puerperium. Oxford University Press, London, 1978

139. Horowitz JA, Damato E, Solon L et al: Postpartum depression: issues in clinical assessment. J Perinatol 15: 268, 1995

140. Posner NA, Unterman RR, Williams KN: Postpartum depression: the obstetrician's concerns. p. 69. In Inwood DG (ed): Recent Advances in Postpartum Psychiatric Disorders. American Psychiatric Press, Inc., Washington, DC, 1985

141. Vandenberg RL: Postpartum depression. Clin Obstet Gynaecol 23:1105, 1980

142. Nott PN: Psychiatric illness following childbirth in Southampton: a case register study. Psychol Med 12: 557, 1982

143. Kendell RE, Rennie D, Clark JA et al: The social and obstetric correlates of psychiatric admission in the puerperium. Psychol Med 11:341, 1981

144. Brockington IF, Winokur G, Dean C: Puerperal psychosis. p. 37. In Brockington IF, Kumar R (eds): Motherhood and Mental Illness. Academic Press, London, 1982

145. Leppert PC, Pahlka BS: Grieving characteristics after spontaneous abortion: a mangement approach. Obstet Gynecol 64:119, 1984

146. Drotar D, Baskiewicz A, Irvin N et al: The adaptation of parents to the birth of an infant with a congenital malformation: a hypothetical model. Pediatrics 56:710, 1975

147. Lindemann E: Symptomatology and management of acute grief. Am J Psychol 101:141, 1944

148. Kennel JH, Slyter H, Claus MKH: The mourning response of parents to the death of a newborn. N Engl J Med 83:344, 1970

149. Benfield DG, Leib SA, Reuter J: Grief response of parents after referral of the critically ill newborn to a regional center. N Engl J Med 294:975, 1976

150. Giles PFH: reactions of women to perinatal death. Aust NZ J Obstet Gynaecol 10:207, 1970

151. Zahourek R, Jensen J: Grieving and the loss of the newborn. Am J Nurs 73:836, 1973

152. Seitz PM, Warrick LH: Perinatal death: the grieving mother. Am J Nurs 74:2028, 1974

153. Rowe J, Clyman R, Green C et al: Follow-up of families who experience perinatal death. Pediatrics 62:166, 1978

154. Lockwood S, Lewis IC: Management of grieving after stillbirth. Med J Aust 2:308, 1980

155. Mandell F, Wolf LC: Sudden infant death syndrome and subsequent pregnancy. Pediatrics 56:774, 1975

156. Schleifer SJ, Keller SE, Camerimo M et al: Supression of lymphocyte stimulation following bereavement. JAMA 250:374, 1983

157. Lake M, Knuppel R, Murphy J et al: The role of a grief support team following stillbirths. Am J Obstet Gynecol 61:497, 1983

158. Furlong R, Hobbins J: Grief in the perinatal period. Obstet Gynecol 61:497, 1983

159. Condon JT: Management of established pathological grief reaction after stillbirth. Am J Psychiatry 143:987, 1986

160. Kowalski K: Managing perinatal loss. Clin Obstet Gynecol 23:1113, 1980

161. Mandell F, McAnulty E, Race RM: Observations of paternal response to sudden unanticipated infant deaths. Pediatrics 65:221, 1980

Complicated Pregnancies

Fetal Wastage

Joe Leigh Simpson

Chapter 22

Not all conceptions result in a liveborn infant. Of clinically recognized pregnancies, 10 to 15 percent are lost. Of married women in the United States, 4 percent have experienced two fetal losses and 3 percent have experienced three or more.[1] It is accepted that a subset of women genuinely manifest repetitive spontaneous abortions as opposed to merely representing random untoward events. This chapter will consider the causes of fetal wastage, the management of couples experiencing repetitive losses, and the topic of ectopic gestations.

Frequency and Timing of Pregnancy Losses

Pregnancy is not generally recognized clinically until 5 to 6 weeks after the last menstrual period, but before this time β-human chorionic gonadotropin (β-hCG) assays can detect preclinical pregnancies. Wilcox et al.[2] performed daily urinary hCG assays beginning around the expected time of implantation (day 20 of gestation). Of pregnancies detected in this fashion, 31 percent (61/198) were lost; the preclinical loss rate was 22 percent (43/198), and the clinically recognized loss rate was 12 percent (19/155). These rates are consistent with data gathered by this author and colleagues[3] in a National Institute of Child Health and Human Development collaborative study in which serum β-hCG assays were performed 28 to 35 days after the previous menses. The total fetal loss rate (preclinical and clinical) for pregnancies detected at 4 to 5 weeks or approximately 10 days later than those ascertained by Wilcox et al.[2] was 16 percent.

Clinically recognized first trimester fetal loss rates of 10 to 12 percent overall are well documented in both retrospective and prospective cohort studies.[4] The higher loss rates reported in some older studies probably reflect unwitting inclusion of surreptitious illicit abortions, a common occurrence during the era in which legal termination was proscribed. Loss rates reflect many factors that will be discussed in this chapter, but two associations are worth emphasizing here. First, maternal age greatly increases risk, a 40-year-old woman carrying twice the risk of a 20-year-old woman. Second, prior pregnancy history is pivotal. Loss rates are lowest (6 percent) among nulliparous women who have never experienced a loss,[5] rising to 25 to 30 percent after three or more losses. Most recurrence risk data were derived from studying women whose losses were usually not recognized until 9 to 12 weeks gestation. However, the same counseling figures are appropriate for couples whose pregnancies are ascertained in the fifth week of gestation.[6]

Studies utilizing ultrasonography have now made it clear that fetal demise occurs before overt clinical signs are manifested. This conclusion is based on cohort studies showing that only 3 percent of viable pregnancies are lost after 8 weeks' gestation.[7] Given an accepted clinical loss rate of 10 to 12 percent, fetal viability must cease weeks before maternal symptoms appear; thus, most fetuses aborting clinically at 9 to 12 weeks must have died weeks previously. Most pregnancy losses after 8 weeks likely occur in the next two gestational months, as loss rates are only 1 percent in women confirmed by ultrasound to have viable pregnancies at 16 weeks. Overall, almost all losses are "missed abortions" (retained in utero for an interval prior to clinical recognition); thus, the term is archaic.

Etiology of Preclinical Losses

Establishing an etiology for preclinical losses is not easy, but the one proven explanation is morphologic and genetic abnormalities in the early embryo. Decades ago Hertig and Rock[8-10] examined the fallopian tubes, uterine cavities, and endometria of women undergoing elective hysterectomy. These women were of proved fertility, with a mean age 33.6 years. Coital times were recorded before hysterectomy. Eight preimplantation embryos (less than 6 days from conception) were recovered. Four of these eight embryos were morphologically abnormal. The four abnormal embryos presumably would not have implanted or, if implanted, would not have survived long thereafter. Nine of 26 implanted embryos (6 to 14 embryonic days) were morphologically abnormal (Fig. 22-1).

Another line of investigation has revealed that chromosomal abnormalities exist in approximately 25 percent of preimplantation embryos that are fertilized in vitro[11,12] and appear morphologically normal. In turn,

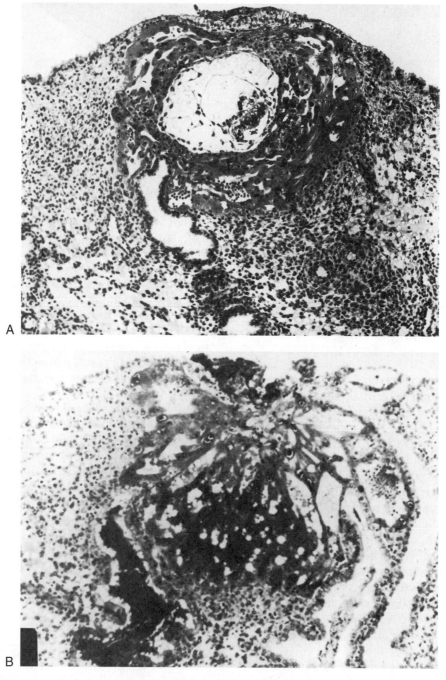

Fig. 22-1 Cross section of endometrium containing an abnormal 14-day-old embryo **(A)** compared with a normal 11-day-old embryo. **(B)** In the abnormal embryo no embryonic disc is present and only syncytiotroblasts are identifiable. (From Hertig and Rock,[166] with permission.)

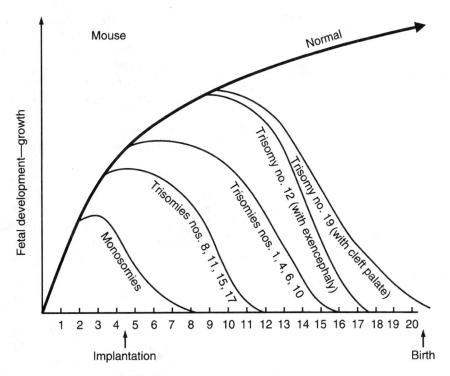

Fig. 22-2 Timing for loss of murine autosomal monosomy and murine autosomal trisomy. (From Gropp,[15] with permission.)

this figure is consistent with chromosomal abnormalities existing in 10 percent of sperm of ostensibly normal males and in perhaps 20 percent of oocytes.[13,14] One can conclude that chromosomal abnormalities are not only frequent in morphologically *normal* embryos but even more frequent in morphologically *abnormal* embryos. That is, cytogenetic abnormalities would be expected to be very frequent in the morphologically abnormal embryos recovered by Hertig and Rock.[8–10]

Consistent with this conclusion are elegant studies in the mouse by Gropp.[15] Mice heterozygous for a variety of Robertsonian translocations were mated to produce various monosomies and trisomies. By selective mating and sacrifice of pregnant animals at varying gestational ages, both survivability and phenotypic characteristics of the aberrant complements could be determined. In mice, as presumably in humans, autosomal monosomy proved inviable. Most monosomes aborted around the time of implantation (4 to 5 days after conception) (Fig. 22-2). Most trisomies survived longer, but only rarely to term. These findings are analogous to those observed in aneuploid human fetuses.

Cytogenetic Etiology in Clinically Recognized Losses

The major cause of clinically recognized pregnancy losses is chromosomal abnormalities. At least 50 percent of clinically recognized pregnancy losses result from a chromosomal abnormality.[16–18] The frequency is probably even higher. If one analyzes chorionic villi after ultrasound diagnosis of fetal demise, rather than relying on later recovery of spontaneously expelled products, the frequency of chromosomal abnormalities proves to be 75 to 90 percent.[19,20]

Among second trimester losses, one also observes chromosomal abnormalities similar to those observed in liveborn infants: trisomies 13, 18, and 21; monosomy X; and sex chromosomal polysomies. Among third trimester losses (stillborn infants) the frequency of chromosomal abnormalities is approximately 5 percent.[21] This frequency is less than that observed in earlier abortuses, but still higher than found among liveborns (0.6 percent).

Autosomal Trisomy

Autosomal trisomies comprise the largest (approximately 50 percent) single class of chromosomal complements in cytogenetically abnormal spontaneous abortions. Frequencies of these trisomies are listed in Table 22-1. Trisomy for every chromosome except No. 1 has been reported, and trisomy for that chromosome has been observed in an eight-cell embryo.[22] The most common trisomy is No. 16. Most trisomies show a maternal age effect, but the effect is variably marked among certain chromosomes. The maternal age effect is especially impressive for double trisomies.

Table 22-1   Chromosomal Complements in Spontaneous Abortions: Recognized Clinically in the First Trimester[a]

Complement	Frequency	(%)
Normal 46, XX or 46, XY		54.1
Triploidy		7.7
69, XXX	2.7	
69, XYX	0.2	
69, XXY	4.0	
Other	0.8	
Tetraploidy		2.6
92, XXX	1.5	
92, XXYY	0.55	
Not Stated	0.55	
Monosomy X		8.6
Structural abnormalities		1.5
Sex chromosomal polysomy		0.2
47, XXX	0.05	
47, XXY	0.15	
Autosomal monosomy (G)		0.1
Autosomal trisomy for chromosomes		22.3
1	0	
2	1.11	
3	0.25	
4	0.64	
5	0.04	
6	0.14	
7	0.89	
8	0.79	
9	0.72	
10	0.36	
11	0.04	
12	0.18	
13	1.07	
14	0.82	
15	1.68	
16	7.27	
17	0.18	
18	1.15	
19	0.01	
20	0.61	
21	2.11	
22	2.26	
Double trisomy		0.7
Mosaic trisomy		1.3
Other abnormalities or not specified		0.9
		100.0

[a] Pooled data from several series, as referenced elsewhere by Simpson and Bombard.[18]

Various attempts have been made to correlate morphologic abnormalities with specific trisomies,[23,24] but relationships are imprecise. Trisomies incompatible with life predictably show slower growth than trisomies compatible with life (trisomies 13, 18, and 21). For example, the mean crown-to-rump length in abortuses shown to be trisomic (13, 18, and 21) is 20.65 mm compared with only 10.66 mm for trisomies that virtually never survive to term (e.g., trisomy 10 or 16).[23] Either the former survive longer or the latter show greater intrauterine growth retardation, or both. Potentially viable trisomies tend to show anomalies consistent with those found in full-term liveborn trisomic infants.[23,24] The malformations present have been said to be more severe than those found in induced abortuses detected after prenatal diagnosis.

Autosomal trisomies are more likely to arise cytologically in maternal meiosis than in paternal meiosis. Most (90 percent) trisomies arise during maternal meiosis, usually maternal meiosis I.[25] Therefore, periconceptional events (exposure to toxins or fertilization involving gametes aged in vivo by delayed fertilization) are less likely to play an etiologic role in most trisomies, since errors in maternal meiosis I originated years before.

Polyploidy

In polyploidy more than two haploid chromosomal complements exist. Triploidy (3n = 69) and tetraploidy (4n = 92) occur often in abortuses. Triploid abortuses are usually 69,XXY or 69,XXX, resulting from dispermy.[26,27] Pathologic findings in triploid placentas include a disproportionately large gestational sac, cystic degeneration of placental villi, intrachorial hemorrhage, and hydropic trophoblasts (pseudomolar degeneration).[23,24] Malformations include neural tube defects and omphaloceles, anomalies reminiscent of those observed in triploid conceptuses progressing to term. Facial dysmorphia and limb abnormalities have also been reported. An association exists between triploidy and hydatidiform mole, a "partial mole" said to exist if molar tissue and fetal parts coexist. The more common "complete" hydatidiform mole is 46,XX, of androgenetic origin.[27]

Tetraploidy is uncommon, rarely progressing beyond 2 to 3 weeks of embryonic life.

Monosomy X

Monosomy X is the single most common chromosomal abnormality among spontaneous abortions, accounting for 15 to 20 percent of abnormal specimens. (Fig. 22-3) Monosomy X embryos usually consist of only an umbilical cord stump. Later in gestation, anomalies characteristic of the Turner syndrome may be seen, specifically cystic hygromas and generalized edema. Although liveborn 45,X individuals usually lack germ cells, 45,X abortuses show germ cells; however, these germ cells rarely develop beyond the primordial germ cell stage. The pathogenesis of 45,X germ cell failure thus involves not so much failure of germ cell development as more rapid attrition in 45,X than in 46,XX embryos.[28,29] Incidentally, this observation makes plausi-

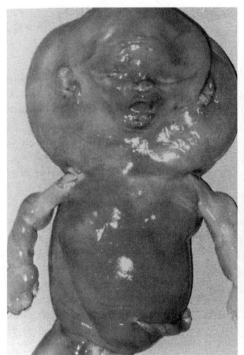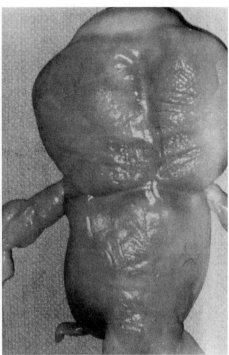

Fig. 22-3 Photograph of a 45,X abortus. (From Simpson and Bombard,[18] with permission.)

ble the rare but well-documented pregnancies occurring in 45,X individuals.[30]

Monosomy X usually (80 percent) occurs as result of paternal sex chromosome loss.[31] This observation is consistent with the lack of a maternal age effect in 45,X or possibly even an inverse effect.

Structural Chromosomal Rearrangement

Structural chromosomal rearrangement account for 1.5 percent of all abortuses (Table 22-1). Rearrangements (e.g., translocation) may either arise de novo during gametogenesis or be inherited from a parent carrying a "balanced" translocation or inversion. Phenotypic consequences depend on the specific duplicated or deficient chromosomal segments. Although not a common cause of sporadic losses, inherited translocations are an important cause of *repeated* fetal wastage.

Sex Chromosomal Polysomy (X or Y)

The complements 47,XXY and 47,XYY each occur in about 1 per 800 liveborn male births; 47,XXX occurs in 1 per 800 female births. X or Y polysomies are only slightly more common in abortuses than in liveborns.

Mendelian and Polygenic/Multifactorial Etiology

The 30 to 50 percent of first trimester abortuses that show no chromosomal abnormalities could still have undergone fetal demise as a result of other genetic etiologies. Neither mendelian nor polygenic/multifactorial disorders show chromosomal abnormalities. Many excellent anatomic studies of abortuses have demonstrated structural abnormalities, but lack of cytogenetic data on the dissected specimens makes it nearly impossible to determine the precise role of noncytogenetic mechanisms in early embryonic maldevelopment. Doubtless pivotal to early development are many mendeliam genes, mutation of which would be expected to result in embryonic death and pregnancy loss.

Novel Cytogenetic Mechanisms

Beyond the scope of this chapter are several novel cytogenetic mechanisms that have been shown to explain certain placental abnormalities and, hence, fetal losses in conceptuses with a diploid number of chromosomes.

One possibility is mosaicism restricted to the placenta, the embryo per se being normal. This phenomenon is termed "confined placental mosaicism." Losses caused by this mechanism may already be reflected in extant data because most studies have involved analysis only of villous material. Not reflected would be a more recently recognized possibility—uniparental disomy. In this phenomenon, both homologues for a given chromosome are derived from a single parent, probably as a result of expulsion of a chromosome from a trisomic zygote. The karyotype would appear normal (46,XX or 46,XY), but genes on the involved chromosome would actually lack contribution of one parent.

For example, uniparental disomy for chromosome 21 has been detected in an embryonic abortus.[32]

Anatomic defects caused by polygenic or multifactorial etiologies would be expected to represent isolated anatomic defects. These could be responsible for losses throughout gestation, but perhaps a relatively greater proportion of later fetal losses. However, lack of concomitant cytogenetic data makes it nearly impossible to delineate precisely the role of noncytogenetic mechanisms in late fetal losses. One problem is that an ostensibly isolated anatomic defect occurring in a late fetal death actually may augur multiple system defects, thus suggesting an underlying cytogenetic abnormality or mutant gene.

Genetic Counseling and Recurrent Risks

The obstetrician faced with a couple experiencing spontaneous abortion has several immediate obligations: (1)inform the couple concerning the frequency of fetal wastage (10 to 12 percent clinically recognized pregnancies) and its likely etiology (at least 50 percent cytogenetic), (2) provide recurrence risk rates, and (3) determine the necessity of a formal clinical evaluation.

Patient Information

The responsibility of informing patients can be fulfilled by summarizing the salient facts cited in this chapter and emphasizing common etiologies responsible for fetal losses. Worth citing explicitly is the positive correlation between loss rates and both advancing maternal age and prior losses (see below). The maternal age effect is not solely the result of increased trisomic abortions, but presumably reflects endometrial factors as well.

Recurrence Risks

Loss rates are definitely increased among women who have experienced previous losses, but not nearly to the extent once thought (Table 22-2). For decades, obste-

tricians fervently believed in the concept of "habitual abortion." After three losses, the risk of subsequent losses was thought to rise sharply. Such beliefs were based on calculations made in 1938 by Malpas,[33] who concluded that following three abortions the likelihood of a subsequent one was 80 to 90 percent. Occurrence of three consecutive spontaneous abortions was thus said for decades to confer upon a women the designation of "habitual aborter." These risk figures not only proved incorrect but also were and unfortunately still seem subconsciously to be used as "controls" for clinical studies evaluating various treatment plans. This practice led to unwarranted acceptance of certain interventions, the most famous of which was diethylstilbestrol (DES) treatment.

In 1964, Warburton and Fraser[34] showed that the likelihood of recurrent abortion rose only to 25 to 30 percent, irrespective of whether a woman had previously experienced one, two, three, or even four spontaneous abortions. This concept has been confirmed in many subsequent studies, although if no previous liveborns have occurred the likelihood of fetal loss is somewhat higher.[35] Lowest risks (5 percent) are observed in nulliparous women with no prior losses.[5] Women who smoke cigarettes or drink alcohol moderately are probably at slightly higher risk.[36] Recurrence risks are higher if the abortus is cytogenetically normal than cytogenetically abnormal.[37]

Taking all the above into account, the prognosis is reasonably good even without therapy, the predicted success rate being 70 percent. Indeed, Vlaanderen and Treffers[38] reported successful pregnancies in each of 21 women having unexplained prior repetitive losses but subjected to no intervention. Other groups reached similar conclusions.[39,40] To be judged efficacious, therapeutic regimens must achieve successes greater than 70 percent.

Necessity of Formal Evaluation

Every couple experiencing a fetal loss should be counseled and provided recurrence risk rates, but not every couple requires formal assessment. Infertile couples who are in their fourth decade may choose to be evaluated after only two losses. After three losses, all couples should be offered formal evaluation. Once a couple enters evaluation, they should undergo all tests standard for a given practitioner. There is no scientific rationale for performing some studies after three losses but deferring others until after four losses. Any couple having a stillborn or anomalous liveborn infant should undergo cytogenetic studies unless the stillborn was known to have a normal chromosome complement. Parental chromosomal rearrangements (i.e., translocations or inversions) should be excluded.

Table 22-2   Approximate Recurrence Risk Figures Useful for Counseling Women with Repeated Spontaneous Abortions[a]

	Prior Abortions	Risk (%)
Women with liveborn infants	0	5–10
	1	20–25
	2	25
	3	30
	4	30
Women without liveborn infants	3	30–40

[a] Recurrence risks are slightly higher for older women and for those who smoke cigarettes or drink alcohol and for those exposed to high levels of selected chemical toxins.
(Based on data from Warbuton and Fraser,[34] Poland et al.[35] and others.)

Etiology and Clinical Evaluation or Repetitive Abortions

Translocations

Structural chromosomal abnormalities are generally accepted as one explanation for repetitive abortions. The most common structural rearrangement encountered is a translocation, found in about 5 percent of couples experiencing repeated losses.[41-43] Individuals with balanced translocations are phenotypically normal, but abortuses or abnormal liveborns may show chromosomal duplications or deficiencies as a result of normal meiotic segregation. About 60 percent of the translocations detected are reciprocal, and 40 percent are Robertsonian. Females are about twice as likely as males to show a balanced translocation.[41]

The clinical significance of translocations is illustrated in Figure 22-4. If a child has Down syndrome as result of such a translocation, the rearrangement will prove to have originated de novo in 50 to 75 percent of cases. That is, a balanced translocation will not exist in either parent. The likelihood of Down syndrome recurring in subsequent offspring is minimal. On the other hand, the risk is significant in the 25 to 50 percent of families in which individuals have Down syndrome as the result of a balanced parental translocation (e.g., parental complement 45,XX, − 14, − 21, + [14q;21q]). The theoretical risk of having a child with Down syndrome is 33 percent, but empirical risks are considerably less. The likelihood is only 2 percent if the father carries the translocation and 10 percent if the mother carries the translocation.[44,45] If Robertsonian (centric-fusion) translocations involve other chromosomes, empiric risks are lower. In t(13q;14q), the risk for liveborn trisomy 13 is 1 percent or less.

Reciprocal translocations are those that do not involve centromeric fusion. Empirical data for specific translocations are usually not available, but useful generalizations can be made on the basis of pooled data derived from many different translocations. Studies of sperm chromosomes[46] theoretically might provide data specific for a given translocation in a specific individual, but this is not readily available. Of interest is that sperm of fathers experiencing repeated losses show no more than the expected 10 percent of cytogenetic abnormalities.[47]

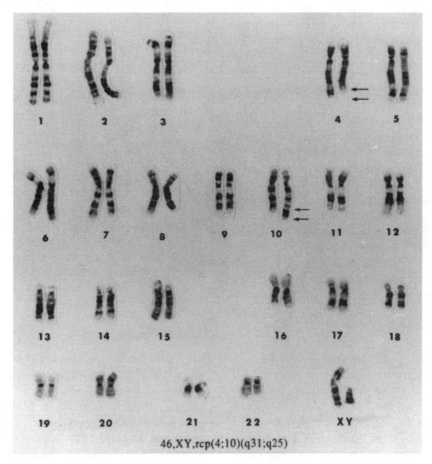

46,XY,rcp(4;10)(q31;q25)

Fig. 22-4 Balanced translocation detected in a woman experiencing multiple abortions. (From Simpson and Tharapel,[163] with permission.)

Irrespective, theoretical risks for abnormal offspring (unbalanced reciprocal translocations) are far greater than empiric risks. Overall, the risk is 12 percent for offspring of either female heterozygotes or male heterozygotes.[44,45] Detecting a parental chromosomal rearrangement thus profoundly affects subsequent pregnancy management. Antenatal cytogenetic studies should be offered in subsequent pregnancies. The frequency of unbalanced fetuses is lower if parental balanced translocations are ascertained through repetitive abortions (3 percent) than through anomalous liveborns (nearly 20 percent).[44]

A few translocations preclude the possibility of normal liveborn infants, namely, translocations involving homologous chromosomes (e.g., t[13q13q] or t[21q21q]). If the father carries such a structural rearrangement, artificial insemination may be appropriate. If the mother carries the rearrangement, donor oocytes or donor embryos (assisted reproductive technologies) should be considered.

Inversions

A less common parental chromosomal rearrangement responsible for repetitive pregnancy losses is an inversion. In inversions the order of genes is reversed. Analogous to translocations, individuals heterozygous for an inversion should be normal if their genes are merely rearranged. However, individuals with inversions suffer abnormal reproductive consequences as a result of normal meiotic phenomena, namely, crossing-over in their gametes, yielding unbalanced gametes. Pericentric inversions (see Ch. 9) are present in perhaps 0.1 percent of females and 0.1 percent of males experiencing repeated spontaneous abortions. Paracentric inversions are even rarer.

Counseling a couple having an inversion is complex. Inversions involving only a small portion of the total chromosomal length paradoxically may be less significant clinically because the large duplications or large deficiencies that follow crossing-over are usually lethal. By contrast, inversions involving only 30 to 60 percent of the total chromosomal length are relatively more likely to be characterized by duplications or deficiencies compatible with survival.[48]

Overall, females with a *pericentric* inversion have a 7 percent risk of abnormal liveborns; males carry a 5 percent risk. Pericentric inversions ascertained through phenotypically normal probands are less likely to result in abnormal liveborns.

Few data are available on recurrence risks for *paracentric* inversions. Theoretically there should be less risk for detecting unbalanced products at chorionic villus sampling (CVS) or amniocentesis than with pericentric inversions because paracentric recombinants are usu-

ally lethal. On the other hand, abortions and abnormal liveborns have been observed within the same kindred, and the risk for unbalanced viable offsprings has been tabulated at 4 percent.[49] Antenatal cytogenetic studies should be offered.

Recurrent Aneuploidy

Already discussed at length as the most common overall cause for sporadic abortions, numerical chromosomal abnormalities (aneuploidy) may be responsible for both recurrent as well as sporadic losses. This reasoning is based on observations that the complements of successive abortuses in a given family are more likely to be either recurrently normal or recurrently abnormal (Table 22-3). If the complement of the first abortus is abnormal, the likelihood is 80 percent that the complement of the second abortus also will be abnormal.[50] The recurrent abnormality usually is trisomy.

These data suggest that certain couples are predisposed toward chromosomally abnormal conceptions. Although it can be argued that corrections for maternal age render the ostensible nonrandom distribution nonsignificant, this author counsels increased risks compared with normal women of comparable age. If couples are predisposed to recurrent aneuploidy, they might logically be at increased risk not only for aneuploid abortuses but also for aneuploid liveborns. The trisomic autosome in a subsequent pregnancy might not always confer lethality, but rather might be compatible with life (e.g., trisomy 21). Indeed, the risk of liveborn trisomy 21 following an aneuploid abortus is about 1 percent.[51]

Information concerning fetal chromosomal status may be lacking for couples having repetitive abortions. Antenatal diagnosis then may or may not be appropriate. Risks for abnormal offspring are probably increased, but the risk of amniocentesis or CVS is especially troublesome to couples who have had difficulty achieving pregnancy. Finally, there is some evidence that abortion rates are *lowest* in couples with prior losses when conception occurred in midcycle.[52] Midcycle fertilization would not involve oocytes or sperm aged in vivo before fertilization.

Luteal Phase Defects

Implantation in an inhospitable endometrium is a plausible explanation for spontaneous abortion. The hormone usually hypothesized to be deficient is progesterone, a deficiency of which might fail to prepare the estrogen-primed endometrium for implantation. Luteal phase defects (LPD) is used to describe the endometrium manifesting an inadequate progesterone effect. Progesterone secreted by the corpus luteum is necessary to support the endometrium until the tro-

Table 22-3 Recurrent Aneuploidy: The Relationship Between Karyotypes of Successive Abortuses

Complement of First Abortus	Complement of Second Abortus					De Novo Rearrangement
	Normal	Trisomy	Monosomy	Triploidy	Tetraploidy	
Normal	142	18	5	7	3	2
Trisomy	31	30	1	4	3	1
Monosomy X	7	5	3	3	0	0
Triploidy	7	4	1	4	0	0
Tetraploidy	3	1	0	2	0	0
De novo rearrangement	1	3	0	0	0	0

(Tabulation by Warburton et al.[50])

phoblast produces sufficient progesterone to maintain pregnancy, an event occurring around 7 gestational (menstrual) weeks or 5 weeks after conception. Plausible pathogenic mechanisms underlying LPD include decreased gonadotropin-releasing hormone (GNRH), decreased follicle-stimulating hormone (FSH), inadequate luteinizing hormone (LH), inadequate ovarian steroidogenesis, or endometrial receptor defects.

Once almost universally accepted as a common cause for fetal wastage, LPD now seems to be considered an uncommon cause. Although plausible clinically, there are no randomized studies verifying efficacy of treatment. Moreover, histology identical to that observed with luteal phase "defects" exists in fertile women. When regularly menstruating fertile women with no history of abortions were biopsied in serial cycles, the frequency of LPD was 51.4 percent in any single cycle and 26.7 percent in sequential cycles.[53]

A major difficulty in determining the frequency as well as validity of LPD is lack of standard diagnostic criteria. LPD was originally defined on the basis of an endometrial biopsy lagging at least 2 days behind the actual postovulation date. This was determined by counting backward from the next menstrual period, assuming 14 days from the date of ovulation to menses. However, the original reports of Noyes et al.[54] showed a mean error of 1.81 days in dating, suggesting that an endometrial biopsy should be designated "out-of-phase" only if it lags 3 or more days behind the actual postovulation date. Not surprisingly, interobserver variation is considerable. Endometrial biopsies (N = 62) read by five different pathologists resulted in differences in interpretation that would have altered management in approximately one-third of patients.[55] Reading coded endometrial biopsy slides a second time, the same pathologist agreed with his or her initial diagnosis in only 25 percent of samples.[56] At a minimum, at least two out of phase biopsies are necessary to make the diagnosis of LPD. Other diagnostic criteria have been proposed, such as integrated serum progesterone (three values) levels.[57] However, most investigators believe hormone levels are no better than endome-

trial biopsy. (Indeed, in patients with two or more spontaneous abortions, a low serum progesterone in the luteal phase is only 71 percent predictive of an LPD as defined on the basis of an abnormal endometrial biopsy.[58]) Perturbations of endometrial receptors have not yet been correlated with pregnancy loss, but, with the gene for the progesterone receptor now cloned, specific molecular studies can be expected.

A study frequently cited as showing efficacy of progesterone therapy is that of Tho et al.[59] Of 100 women with repetitive spontaneous abortions, 23 showed documented LPDs on the basis of out-of-phase endometrial biopsies. All 23 women were treated with progesterone suppositories, with 21 completing their pregnancies. A quasicontrol group consisted of 37 other women who had no ostensible etiology for their losses. Twenty-two (22) of these 37 women were treated empirically with progesterone; 15 were not. Seventy-three percent of the treated women had successful pregnancies compared with 47 percent of untreated women. Daya and Ward[60] found that 26 of 65 women with recurrent abortions (40 percent) had not only two consecutive out-of-phase biopsies but also low serum progesterone. When the 26 were treated with progesterone, only three (19 percent) of 16 subsequent pregnancies aborted. Again, however, the lack of controls makes it unclear whether the 81 percent success rate is greater than the expected 70 percent. Another study suggesting a beneficial effect of treating LPD involved 33 infertile women whose LPD was documented by two out-of-phase biopsies.[61] (Note that this study involved infertile women rather than those with recurrent abortions.) No abortions occurred in the 14 women who conceived after documentation of an in-phase endometrial biopsy produced by progesterone treatment. Of the 16 women whose biopsy was not corrected, there were 4 pregnancies; all ended in spontaneous abortion.

Other recent observations have suggested a relationship between fetal loss and either oligomenorrhea[62] or polycystic ovary disease (PCO),[63] either of which could be related to endometrial dysynchrony. In one study, PCO was diagnosed only by ultrasound,[63] but Regan et al.[64] have also reported elevated serum LH in women experiencing pregnancy loss. Additional data are necessary.

In summary, LPD probably exists, but it is far less common than once believed. The consensus is that LPD is either an arguable entity or cannot be proved to be treated successfully with progesterone therapy. Indeed, a meta-analysis by Karamardian and Grimes[65] showed no beneficial effect (pregnancy rate) of treatment. Treatment should be initiated only if the diagnosis is firmly established and only if couples are apprised of the unfounded claims of progesterone teratogenicity (see Ch. 10). Patients should probably be informed that therapeutic efficacy is unproved. If instituted, treatment usually consists of vaginal progesterone suppositories 25 mg twice daily beginning with the basal body temperature elevation and continuing at least 6 to 8 weeks.

Thyroid Abnormalities

Decreased conception rates and increased fetal losses are associated with overt hypothyroidism or hyperthyroidism. However, subclinical thyroid dysfunction is probably not an explanation for repeated losses.[66] One recent study observed an increased frequency of antithyroid antibodies among couples experiencing repeated losses.[67]

Diabetes Mellitus

Women whose diabetes mellitus is poorly controlled are at increased risk for fetal loss.[3] In one study, women whose glycosylated hemoglobin level was greater than 4 SD above the mean showed higher pregnancy loss rates than women with lower glycosylated hemoglobin levels. This finding was also found in retrospective studies.[68] Poorly controlled diabetes mellitus should be considered one cause for early pregnancy loss, but well-controlled or subclinical diabetes is probably not a cause of early miscarriage.

Intrauterine Adhesions (Synechiae)

Intrauterine adhesions could interfere with implantation or early embryonic development. Adhesions may follow overzealous uterine curettage during the postpartum period, intrauterine surgery (e.g., myomectomy), or endometritis. Curettage is the usual explanation, with adhesions most likely to develop if curettage is performed 3 or 4 weeks postpartum. Individuals with uterine synechiae usually manifest hypomenorrhea or amenorrhea, but 15 to 30 percent show repeated abortions. If adhesions are detected in a woman experiencing repetitive losses, lysis under direct hyperoscopic visualization should be performed. Postoperatively, an intrauterine device or inflated Foley catheter may be inserted in the uterus to discourage reapposition of healing uterine surfaces. Estrogen administration should also be initiated. Approximately 50 percent of patients conceive after surgery, but the frequency of abortions remains high.

Incomplete Müllerian Fusion

Müllerian fusion defects (Fig. 22-5) are an accepted cause of *second* trimester losses and pregnancy complications. Low birth weight, breech presentation, and uterine bleeding are other abnormalities associated with müllerian fusion defects. Ben Rafael et al.[69] confirmed these conclusions after comparison with women with hysterosalpingogram-proven normal uteri; however, most other reports lack controls.[70–76] A few studies claim that the worst outcomes are associated with either septate uteri[72] or T-shaped uteri,[71] but others discern few differences among various anomalies.[75] Some authors[77] believe that minor structural defects may be just as deleterious as overt defects, but this does not seem completely plausible.

The major problem in attributing cause and effect for second trimester complications and uterine anomalies is that the latter are so frequent that adverse outcomes could often be coincidental. For example, Stampe-Sorensen[78] found unsuspected bicornuate uteri in 1.2 percent of 167 women undergoing laparoscopic sterilization; 3.6 percent had a severely septate uterus, and 15.3 percent had fundal anomalies. Simon et al.[79] found müllerian defects in 3.2 percent (22/679) of fertile women; 20 of the 22 defects were septate. Treatment has traditionally involved surgical correction, such as metroplasty. Ludmire et al.[80] wondered if conservative treatment might not be just as efficacious as surgical correction, following 101 women with an uncorrected malformation through a standardized protocol to decrease physical activity. Fetal survival rates in both bicornuate and septate groups (58 and 65 percent, respectively) did not differ significantly from rates in the same patients prior to institution of the protocol (52 and 53 percent, respectively).

First trimester abortions might also be due to müllerian fusion defects. Septate uteri might raise the risk of poor implantation on a poorly vascularized and inhospitable surface. Abortions occurring after ultrasonographic confirmation of a viable pregnancy at 8 or 9 weeks may properly be attributed to uterine fusion defects if the latter is present; however, losses having no confirmation of fetal viability at that time are statistically more likely to represent missed abortions in which fetal demise occurred prior to 8 weeks. Women experiencing second trimester abortions can be assumed to benefit from uterine reconstruction, but reconstructive

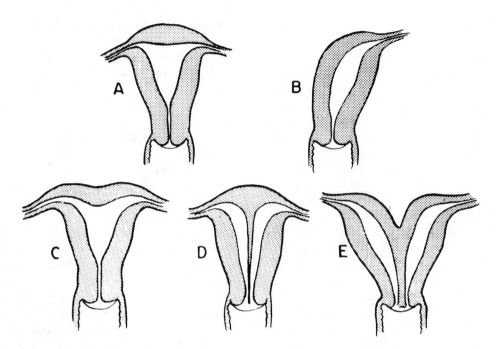

Fig. 22-5 Diagrammatic representation of some müllerian fusion anomalies: **(A)** normal uterus, fallopian tubes, and cervix; **(B)** uterus unicornis (absence of one uterine horn); **(C)** uterus arcuatus (broadening and medial depression of a portion of the uterine septum); **(D)** uterus septus (persistence of a complete uterine septum; and **(E)** uterus bicornis unicollis (two hemiuteri, each leading to same cervix). (From Simpson,[164] with permission.)

surgery is not necessarily advisable if losses are restricted to the first trimester.

Leiomyomas

Although leiomyomas are very frequent, relatively few affected women with leiomyomas develop symptoms requiring medical or surgical therapy. That leiomyomas cause pregnancy wastage per se rather than obstetric complications like prematurity is thus plausible but probably rare. Analogous to uterine anomalies, the coexistence of uterine leiomyomas and reproductive losses need not necessarily imply a causal relationship. Location of leiomyomas is probably more important than size, submucous leiomyomas being most likely to cause abortion. Postulated mechanisms leading to pregnancy loss include (1) thinning of the endometrium over the surface of a submucous leiomyoma, predisposing to implantation in a poorly decidualized site; (2) rapid growth caused by the hormonal milieu of pregnancy, compromising the blood supply of the leiomyoma and resulting in necrosis ("red degeneration") that in turn leads to uterine contractions and eventually fetal expulsion; and (3) encroachment of leiomyomas upon the space required by the developing fetus, leading to premature delivery through mechanisms presumably analogous to those operative in incomplete müllerian fusion. Relative lack of space can also lead to fetal deformations (i.e., positional abnormalities arising in a genetically normal fetus).

In conclusion, surgical procedures to reduce leiomyomata may occasionally be warranted for women experiencing repetitive second trimester abortions. More often leiomyomata will have no etiologic relationship to pregnancy loss. Ideally, surgery should be reserved for women whose abortuses were both phenotypically and karyotypically normal and in which viability until at least 9 to 10 weeks was documented.

Incompetent Internal Cervical Os

A functionally intact cervix and lower uterine cavity are obvious prerequisites for a successful intrauterine pregnancy. Characterized by painless dilation and effacement, cervical incompetence usually occurs during the middle second or early third trimester. This condition frequently follows traumatic events like cervical amputation, cervical lacerations, forceful cervical dilatation, or conization. A relationship to various connective tissue disorders is plausible but yet unproved. The various surgical techniques to correct cervical incompetence are discussed in Chapter 23.

Infections

Infections are accepted causes of late fetal wastage and logically could be responsible for early fetal loss as well. Microorganisms reported to be associated with spontaneous abortion include *Variola, Vaccinia, Salmonella typhi, Vibrio fetus, Malaria, Cytomegalovirus, Brucella,*

Toxoplasmosis, Mycoplasma hominis, Chlamydia trachomatis, and *Ureaplasma urealyticum.* Transplacental infection doubtless occurs with each of these microorganisms, and sporadic losses could logically be caused by any. As an example, Sompolinsky et al.[81] isolated *Ureaplasma, M. hominis,* or both from 32 midtrimester placentas and 24 abortuses. Among 28 *induced* (control) midtrimester abortions, such organisms were recovered from only one placenta and no abortuses. Indirectly supporting an important role for infectious agents are studies in which empiric antibiotic therapy appears to benefit couples experiencing repeated losses. Among repetitive aborters treated for 4 weeks while not pregnant with tetracycline, Toth et al.[82] reported recurrent fetal losses in only 10 percent. By contrast, 38 percent of aborters who chose not to receive tetracycline experienced further fetal loss. However, the two groups were not randomized and therefore were not necessarily comparable. (Recall also that tetracycline is contraindicated in the second trimester; See Ch. 11). Moreover, other studies have found no difference in outcome between women treated and not treated with antibiotics.[83] Unanswered is whether the infectious agents were causative in the fetal losses or merely arose secondarily after demise due to a noninfectious etiology. Confounding variables (e.g., maternal age, prior pregnancy history) are also rarely taken into account. Overall, a purported association between a common microorganism and pregnancy loss could easily reflect chance findings or be explained by other factors.

Of all organisms mentioned, *Ureaplasma* and *Chlamydia* are not only the most commonly implicated in *repetitive* abortion but also fulfill certain prerequisites necessary to assume a causal relationship. Both can exist in an asymptomatic state, and neither necessarily are so severe as to cause infertility. From 46 women with histories of three or more consecutive losses of unknown etiology, Stray-Pedersen et al.[84] recovered *Ureaplasma* significantly more often among women with repetitive abortions (28 percent) than among female controls (7 percent). Of 43 women in the former group, 13 harbored *Ureaplasma* in both cervix and endometrium. In 12 other women, the organism was recovered only in the cervix, a circumstance less likely to cause abortions, given that *Ureaplasma* is ubiquitous in the vagina. All 43 women and their husbands were then treated with doxycycline, with subsequent cultures confirming eradication of *Ureaplasma.* Nineteen of the 43 women became pregnant; of the 19, three experienced another spontaneous abortion and 16 had normal full-term infants. Among 18 women with untreated *Ureaplasma,* only 5 full-term pregnancies occurred. Some other workers have also found an association between pregnancy loss and *Ureaplasma.*[85]

Other ubiquitous organisms have also been the subject of recent interest. Based on the presence of chlamydial antibodies in the sera of women who experienced repeated losses, an association has been claimed on the basis of presence of high titers.[86,87] However, other data show no relationship.[88,89] An immunohistochemical study found no difference in the frequency of cytomegalovirus antigen in karyotypically normal and abnormal abortuses, suggesting no causal association.[90] Toxoplasmosis antibodies have been observed in Mexican and in Egyptian women having repetitive losses,[91,92] but whether frequencies are higher in those general populations is unclear.

What evaluation and management is recommended? Culturing the endometrium for *U. urealyticum* seems reasonable, with culture-positive women having such infections treated. Alternatively, tetracycline therapy can be reasoned to be so innocuous that empiric treatment with doxycycline (100 mg orally twice times a day for 10 days, both husband and nonpregnant wife) could be recommended.

Anti-Fetal Antibodies

Perturbations of the immune system can be responsible for fetal wastage. However, the nature of the immunologic process responsible for maintaining pregnancy has proved to be complex. Several different immunologic processes may play a role.

In one immunologic process, an otherwise normal mother produces antibodies against her fetus on the basis of genetic dissimilarities. Fetal loss is well documented in Rh-negative (D-negative) women having anti-D antibodies. More apropos for early pregnancy loss is the presence of anti-P antibodies. Most individuals are genotype Pp or PP, but one may be homozygous for p (pp). If a woman of genotype pp has a Pp or PP mate, resulting offspring may or must be Pp. If the mother develops anti-P antibodies, Pp fetuses will be rejected (aborted) early in gestation. Plasmapheresis and other modalities may be therapeutically efficacious.[93,94]

Autoimmune Disease

An association between pregnancy loss and certain autoimmune diseases is generally accepted.[95,96] It seems clear that women with autoimmune diseases like lupus erythermatosis have increased pregnancy loss. Less clear is the significance of various antibodies in healthy women having repetitive spontaneous abortion. Claims have been made on the basis of increased antibody titers or low complement levels indicating active antigen–antibody interaction. The types of antibodies sought in women with pregnancy losses are diverse, ranging from nonspecific antinuclear antibodies to antibodies against cellular components like phospholipids, histones, or double- or single-stranded DNA.

Individuals having antiphospholipid antibodies, including lupus anticoagulant (LAC) antibodies and anticardiolipin antibodies (aCL) constitute the group most often associated with fetal wastage. Almost all[97] agree that the frequency of midtrimester fetal death in women who show LAC or aCL is increased, perhaps dramatically so. Other pregnancy complications (e.g., growth retardation, preeclampsia) are also more common. These antibodies have closely related specificities and could be members of the same family of autoantibodies. LAC in particular has been associated with subplacental clotting and fetal losses in all trimesters.[98] The abortifacient mechanism is thus presumably decidual. Incidentally, LAC antibody is actually a misnomer. In vitro LAC is an anticoagulant, but in vivo LAC increases the likelihood of thrombosis. Treatment with heparin and low-dose aspirin is more effective than prednisone therapy.[99]

Although a relationship between aCL and *second/third* trimester losses seems reasonably well established, data are far less clear for *first* trimester pregnancy losses. Initially studies seemed to show increased aCA in aborters, but no control data were provided. For controlled studies, the frequencies of various related antibodies (LAC, ACA, aPL) proved similar in first trimester aborters and controls.[100–103]

Even less consensus exists concerning other antibodies. An illustrative example is antisperm antibodies. Unequivocally important in infertility, antisperm antibodies develop in approximately 50 percent of males after vasectomy. These antibodies adversely affect the ability to conceive if vas reversal is undertaken, the mechanism being sperm immobilization. Women may also manifest antisperm antibodies that predictably interfere with fertilization. Some studies also show an increased frequency of antisperm antibodies among women experiencing repeated abortions,[104–108] but others, including one by the author, show no such relationship.[109,110] If an association does exist, the biologic basis might reflect antibody cross reaction with paternally derived whole body antigens needed for embryonic survival (or cross reaction with aPL antibodies on the placenta). If so, however, why would the manifestation be clinically recognized losses and not simply preclinical losses?

In conclusion, repetitive pregnancy losses in clinically asymptomatic women dictates a search for both LAC (activated thromboplastin time or platelet neutralization tests) and aCL. However, a search for other antibodies is not generally recommended. Treatment with heparin and low-dose aspirin is best restricted to couples with second or third trimester losses.

Alloimmune Disease (Shared Parental Antigens)

Fetal rejection is apparently eschewed because the maternal immune system mitigates against the phenomenon through blocking or suppressive factors that protect the fetus. Although such reasoning has been assumed to be the explanation for pregnant women developing antipaternal antileukocytotoxic antibodies,[111] many women with three or more recurrent abortions fail to show these antibodies. Moreover, these antibodies do not develop until midtrimester and thus probably arise only secondarily. Sargent et al.[112] observed cytotoxic antibodies (T cell and B cell) in only 1 of 16 successful pregnancies (through 17 weeks) compared with 0 of 9 pregnancies ending in abortion.

That parental histo*in*compatibility could be beneficial in pregnancy maintenance continues to be the source of considerable investigation, although any relationship may or may not be related to blocking antibodies. Considerable experimental support for a beneficial effect of fetomaternal incompatibility in animals can be cited: (1) Increased placental size in mice results from matings in which paternal and maternal histocompatibility antigens differ. (2) Higher implantation frequencies occur in histoincompatible murine zygotes.[113] In the mouse, this can be attributed to the H-2 locus (the mouse equivalent to human HLA) because differences in implantation frequencies reflect differences at that locus. Whether increased HLA sharing per se constitutes the mechanism underlying lack of parental differences in humans is less certain. Some couples sharing HLA-DR antigens experience no spontaneous abortions despite 10 or more pregnancies.[114] About half the reported studies[115,116] show differences in HLA sharing between couples experiencing abortions and controls. Ober et al.[117] observed an association between losses and HLA-B sharing in an analysis of the Hutterites, an inbred population on whom rigorous genetic analyses are possible.

An alternative interpretation that could explain how some but not all couples sharing HLA antigens experience deleterious effects would be for the normal pregnancy to require fetomaternal histo*in*compatibility but not at the HLA locus. The locus could be closely linked, specifically to HLA-B. This hypothesis is consistent with HLA-G being the only HLA antigen expressed on trophoblasts.

Another possibility is that the deleterious effect of parental antigen sharing may not be immunologic at all. All observations could be explained entirely on a nonimmunologic basis by postulating existence of a lethal recessive gene closely linked to HLA. Murine embryos homozygous for certain alleles at the T/t locus die at various stages of embryogenesis; a T/t-like complex could exist in humans. If so, deleterious parental HLA sharing between mother and father (and, hence, between mother and fetus) could merely secondarily reflect homozygosity for a linked gene. This is one of several potential mechanisms that would explain kindreds in which multiple family members have repeated losses.[118] However, the necessity of postulating existence of the same mutant gene in heterozygous form in multiple unrelated spouses makes a genetic basis less appealing. Moreover, if only homozygous offspring were lethal, the abortus to liveborn ratio would be 1:3 (25 to 75 percent) if the parents were heterozygous, rather than the ratio of 1:0 (100 to 0 percent) seen with consecutive abortuses.

The above is not simply an academic exercise. If fetal rejection truly occurs as the result of diminished fetomaternal immunologic interaction (alloimmunte factors), it follows that immunotherapy to enhance interaction at the few potentially differing loci is not unreasonable. This rationale followed observations that blood transfusions prior to kidney transplantation decreased allograft rejection.[119] Women lacking blocking antibodies but sharing HLA antigens with their spouse have been immunized with paternal leukocytes, third party leukocytes, or trophoblast membranes.

However, efficacy of immunotherapy remains highly controversial. In the first prospective randomized trial, 209 couples with repeated abortions were studied.[120] Of these, 104 women had no antibody against paternal lymphocytes and no other apparent cause for the losses. A paired sequential trial was conducted, the experimental group receiving purified lymphocytes derived from their husbands. Seventeen of 22 (77 percent) treated women had a successful pregnancy, compared with 10 of 27 (37 percent) controls given their own cells. The ostensibly better outcome in the immunized group is tempered by lower than expected successes in the control group. (Recall that the expected rate is 60 to 70 percent.)

Several other studies later claimed benefit from leukocyte "vaccination." However, the consensus is that benefit remains limited if existent at all. A meta-analysis by Fraser et al.[121] found an odds ratio of 1.3 toward a beneficial effect; the authors thus concluded that immunotherapy with lymphocytes was not efficacious. These conclusions generally apply to leukocyte injections. Data specific to injection of trophoblast membranes, seminal fluid via suppositories, or intravenous immunoglobin therapy are even more limited.

Attempts to clarify the confusion continue. A multicenter effort tabulating results of immunotherapy by injection of paternal leukocytes shows an 11% beneficial effect in treated couples.[122] Data that show a small beneficial effect in selected centers are puzzling, suggesting existence of unwitting confounding variables.

Conversely, advocates of immunotherapy point out that the volume of paternal leukocytes injected is often less than advocated by Mowbray et al.[120] and not necessarily given in timely fashion.

Given the uncertainty concerning the role of immunologic factors in repetitive abortions, the standard of care clearly does not require physicians to direct couples with repetitive abortions either into diagnostic evaluation to detect the presence of alloimmune factors or into immunotherapy. It is reasonable to discuss immunologic factors, particularly if no other explanation exists. However, alloimmune immunologic evaluation should be initiated only by those few centers prepared to pursue a thorough effort and, in the author's opinion, to subject results to the scrutiny of randomized studies. Merely determining HLA status without other studies is certainly not recommended. All except a few obstetricians/gynecologists should refer any couples desiring immunologic evaluation to colleagues having special expertise.

Drugs, Chemicals, and Noxious Agents

Various exogenous agents have been implicated in fetal losses. Indeed, women are exposed frequently to relatively low doses of ubiquitous agents. However, few agents can be implicated with confidence. Rarely are data adequate to determine the true role of these exogenous factors in early pregnancy losses.

Outcomes following exposures to exogenous agents are usually deduced on the basis of case–control studies. In such studies, women who aborted claimed exposure to the agent in question more often than controls. However, case–control studies suffer certain inherent biases, as reviewed in Chapter 8. The primary bias is that controls have less incentive to recall antecedent events than subjects experiencing an abnormal outcome (recall bias). Employers attempt to limit exposure of women in the reproductive age group; thus, exposures to potentially dangerous chemicals are usually unwitting and, hence, poorly documented. Moreover, pregnant women usually are exposed to many agents concurrently, making it nearly impossible to attribute adverse effects to a single agent. Given these caveats, physicians should be cautious about attributing pregnancy loss to exogenous agents. On the other hand, common sense dictates that exposure to potentially noxious agents be minimized.

X-Irradiation

Irradiation and antineoplastic agents in high doses are accepted abortifacients. Of course, therapeutic x-rays or chemotherapeutic drugs are administered during pregnancy only to seriously ill women whose pregnancies often must be terminated for maternal indications.

On the other hand, pelvic x-ray exposure of up to perhaps 10 rads places a woman at little to no increased risk. Exposure doses are usually far less (1 to 2 rads). Still, it is prudent for pregnant hospital workers to avoid handling chemotherapeutic agents and minimize potential exposures during diagnostic x-ray procedures.

Cigarette Smoking

Smoking during pregnancy is accepted as associated with spontaneous abortion. Kline et al.[123] found increased abortion rates in smokers, independent of maternal age and independent of alcohol consumption. A modest dose-response curve led Alberman et al.[124] to conclude that smokers showed a nonsignificantly higher proportion of abortuses with normal karyotypes. This observation suggests that smoking affects the conceptus directly.

Caffeine

The consensus has long been that no deleterious effects of caffeine exist, while most studies were retrospective and case-control in design. Recent data gathered in cohort fashion by Mills et al.[125] are reassuring. The odds ratio for an association between caffeine (coffee and other dietary forms) was only 1.15 (95 percent CI 0.89 to 1.49).[125] Additional data from women exposed to very high levels (>300 mg caffeine daily) would be useful, but general reassurance can be given concerning moderate caffeine exposure and pregnancy loss.

Alcohol

An association between alcohol consumption and fetal loss once seemed generally accepted. In one study,[123] 616 women suffering spontaneous abortions were compared with 632 women delivering at 28 gestational weeks or more. Among women whose pregnancies ended in spontaneous abortion, 17 percent drank at least twice per week; only 8.1 percent of controls drank similar quantities of alcohol. Harlap and Shiono[126] also found a slightly increased risk for abortion in women who drank in the first trimester. More recent studies have not reported a relationship in moderate drinkers. Halmesmäki et al.[127] found that alcohol consumption was nearly identical in women who did and did not experience an abortion; 13 percent of aborters and 11 percent of control women drank on average three to four drinks per week; other investigations have reached a similar conclusion.[128]

Alcohol consumption should be avoided or minimized during pregnancy for many reasons, but abstinence may only minimally if at all decrease pregnancy loss rate. Avoidance has other benefits that can be better substantiated.

Contraceptive Agents

Conception with an intrauterine device in place clearly increases the risk of fetal loss. However, if the device is removed prior to pregnancy, there is no increased risk of spontaneous abortions. Use of oral contraceptives before or during pregnancy is not associated with fetal loss, nor is spermicide exposure either prior to or after conception (see Ch. 10.).

Environmental Chemicals

Limiting exposure to potential toxins in the work place is recognized as prudent for pregnant women. Among the many chemical agents variously claimed to be associated with fetal losses,[130,131] consensus seems to be evolving around a selected few.[132] These include anesthetic gases, arsenic, aniline dyes, benzene, solvents, ethylene oxide, formaldehyde, pesticides, and certain divalent cations (lead, mercury, cadmium). Workers in rubber industries, battery factories, and chemical production plants are among those at potential risk. The difficulty lies in defining the precise effect of lower exposures and attributing a specific risk. False alarms concerning potential toxins are frequent. A study claiming an association between pregnancy loss and video display terminal exposure of greater than 20 hours per week generated enormous media attention,[133] until considerable data became available to the contrary.[134] The same holds true, in the author's opinion, for exposure in moderation to saunas or hot tubs. Data show no increased risk in general for pregnant laboratory workers[135] or pregnant pharmaceutical industry workers.[136]

Trauma

Women commonly attribute pregnancy losses to trauma, such as a fall or blow to the abdomen. However, fetuses are actually well protected from external trauma by intervening maternal structures and amniotic fluid. The temptation to attribute a loss to minor traumatic events should be avoided.

Psychological Factors

That impaired psychological well-being predisposes to early fetal losses has been claimed but never proved. Certainly neurotic or mentally ill women experience losses just like normal women. Whether the frequency of losses is higher in the former is less certain because potential confounding variables have not been taken into account.

Investigations cited as proving a benefit of psychological well-being are those of Stray-Pedersen et al.[138] Pregnant women who previously experienced repetitive abortions received increased attention but no specific medical therapy ("tender loving care"). These women (N = 16) proved more likely (85 percent) to complete their pregnancy than 42 women not offered such close attention (36 percent successful outcome). One potential pitfall was that only women living "close" to the university were eligible to be placed in the increased attention group. Women living farther away served as "controls"; however, these women may have differed from the experimental group in other ways as well. Although other studies can be cited as consistent with a beneficial effect of psychological well-being,[39,40] any ostensible positive effect of psychological well-being is probably either more apparent than real or secondary to other factors. Empathy is always an admirable trait for physicians, and all couples deserve this attention; however, lack thereof does not necessarily lead to fetal loss.

Severe Maternal Illness

Many debilitating maternal diseases have been implicated in early abortion. Pathogenesis is not necessarily independent of mechanisms discussed previously, specifically endocrinologic or immunologic. Symptomatic maternal diseases established as causes of fetal wastage include Wilson disease, maternal phenylketonuria, cyanotic heart disease, hemoglobinopathies, and inflammatory bowel disease. Actually, any life-threatening disease would be expected to be associated with an increased abortion rate. Seriously ill women rarely become pregnant, but the disease process may deteriorate after the onset of pregnancy. Overall, relatively few fetal losses will be the result of severe maternal disease, with the same even more applicable for repetitive losses.

Ectopic Pregnancy

In ectopic pregnancy, implantation occupies at a site other than the endometrium. Ectopic pregnancies are responsible for approximately 10 percent of all maternal mortality.[139] Moreover, the prognosis for future reproduction is poor. Only one-half of women having an ectopic pregnancy are eventually delivered of a liveborn infant. Most of these never become pregnant, and up to 25 percent of those who do suffer a repeat ectopic pregnancy.[140] Various factors contribute to ectopic pregnancies, the most common being infection. Unlike intrauterine spontaneous abortions, genetic factors are not paramount in the etiology of ectopic pregnancy. Ectopic embryos show chromosomal abnormalities no more often than predicted on the basis of embryonic age.[141]

Incidence

The incidence of recorded ectopic gestation is increasing. Some of this increase seems real and some spurious. A true increase can be hypothesized as result of

(1) improved treatment for pelvic inflammatory disease, a condition that in the past would have conferred sterility; (2) an increase in surgical corrections of fallopian tube occlusion; and (3) a greater number of elective sterilizations, some of which are later reversed surgically. However, there is also an artificial increase related to improved diagnostic techniques. Ectopic pregnancies that in the past would have been mislabeled as unexplained abdominal pain or bleeding are readily recognized today because pregnancy tests have become very sensitive.

Most ectopic pregnancies (96 percent) are tubal. The remainder are interstitial uterine ectopic pregnancies and, rarely, cervical, abdominal, or ovarian pregnancies.[142] Most tubal pregnancies are located in the distal (ampullary) two-thirds of the tube. A few ectopic pregnancies are isthmic, located in the proximal portion of the extrauterine part of the tube. On rare occasions both intrauterine and extrauterine gestations occur can coexist (heterotopic pregnancy).

Signs and Symptoms

Abdominal pain and irregular vaginal bleeding are the most common presenting symptoms in ectopic pregnancy.[143,144] In a 1983 report of 328 patients presenting with ectopic pregnancy, 94 percent had pain, 89 percent a missed menstrual period, 80 percent vaginal bleeding, and 20 percent hypotension.[145] An abdominal mass is palpable in only one-half of patients with an ectopic pregnancy. Of course, passage of a decidual cast in association with vaginal bleeding nearly unequivocally indicates ectopic pregnancy, but this is uncommon. The Arias-Stella phenomenon is frequently found in the endometrium in association with ectopic pregnancies; however, this phenomenon is also seen in 70 to 80 percent of therapeutic and spontaneous abortions,[146] so it is not specific for ectopic gestation.

Ectopic pregnancies should be diagnosed before the onset of hypotension, bleeding, pain, and overt rupture. Patients with a history of tubal surgery, pelvic inflammatory disease, tubal disease, or previous ectopic pregnancy are at special risk for ectopic pregnancy and would benefit not only from their physicians' vigilance but also from routine hormone screening of the type discussed below. Fortunately, *early* diagnosis of ectopic gestation is now quite feasible. Ectopic pregnancy can be detected by 6 weeks' gestation, often as early as at 4 1/2 gestational weeks.

Chronic ectopic pregnancy is a distinct entity. Diagnosis may be difficult because normal anatomic landmarks are distorted by the formation of adhesions resulting from chronic inflammatory processes. Chronic ectopic pregnancies present a management quandary because the significance of the associated declining β-hCG levels is difficult to determine. The dilemma is whether resolution will occur spontaneously or require surgical intervention to prevent catastrophic hemorrhage and permanent adhesion formation resulting in tubal damage.

Diagnosis

Direct vision by laparoscopy has been the diagnostic standard for ectopic pregnancy. However, if the pregnancy is early and the gestational sac small, the gestation may not be visualized. Thus, algorithms incorporating a single measurement of serum progesterone, serial measurement of the β-subunit of hCG, pelvic ultrasonography, and uterine curettage are accepted.[146] Figure 22-6 shows a useful approach.

Single Measurement of Serum Progesterone

Serum progesterone reflects production of progesterone (P) by the corpus luteum, which is stimulated by a viable pregnancy. Measurement of P is an inexpensive screening test that can identify patients who need to undergo further testing. Ectopic pregnancy can be excluded and viable intrauterine pregnancy diagnosed with 97.5 percent sensitivity if serum P levels are 25 ng/ml (≥79.5 nmol/L) or higher, obviating the need for further testing. Conversely, serum P can identify nonviable pregnancies with 100 percent sensitivity if P levels are 5 ng/ml (≤15.9 nmol/L) or lower.[147–150] If a single progesterone is 5 ng/ml or lower, diagnostic uterine evacuation can be performed even if ectopic pregnancy cannot otherwise be distinguished from a spontaneous intrauterine abortion. P values above 5 but below 25 ng/ml necessitate establishing viability by ultrasonography.

Serial Serum β-hCG Measurements

β-hCG is produced by trophoblastic cells. In normal pregnancies, β-hCG concentration increases 67 percent over a 2-day interval.[151] Abnormal intrauterine or ectopic pregnancies have impaired β-hCG production and, hence, a prolonged hCG doubling time. Thus, se-

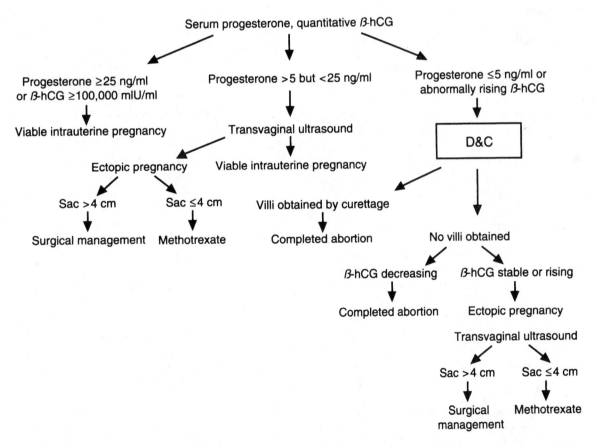

Fig. 22-6 Algorithm for the diagnosis of unruptured ectopic pregnancy without laparoscopy. Progesterone measurements increase the sensitivity of the algorithm by inexpensively screening large numbers of patients during the first trimester of pregnancy. The definitive diagnosis is made by transvaginal ultrasound or uterine curettage and does not depend on the serum progesterone concentrations obtained during screening. (From Carson and Buster,[147] with permission.)

rial β-hCG measurements can be used to assess the viability of pregnancy, signal the optimal time for ultrasonography, and document the effectiveness of diagnostic curettage.

Transvaginal Ultrasound

If β-hCG is greater than 1,500 mIU/ml and the pregnancy is intrauterine, a gestational sac should be visualized by transvaginal ultrasound. By transabdominal ultrasound the gestational sac may not be identified until β-hCG reaches 6,000 mIU/ml. If β-hCG is greater than these levels but the gestational sac cannot be visualized, an ectopic location should be assumed. Conversely, intrauterine pregnancies may also be confirmed by ultrasound, specifically excluding ectopic pregnancy.[147–150]

Widely available in gynecologic offices and emergency rooms, ultrasonography with a 5-mHz transvaginal ultrasound probe can document intrauterine gestation earlier than transabdominal ultrasonography. Transvaginal color Doppler sonography may further enhance early diagnostic sensitivity and specificity through the identification of characteristic uterine and adnexal flow patterns.[152]

Uterine Curettage

Villi float in saline, a characteristic permitting identification of tissue obtained by curettage. If no villi are recognized and a decrease in the β-hCG level of 15 percent or more 8 to 12 hours occurs after curettage, a completed abortion can be assumed to exist. If villi are not visualized and β-hCG titers plateau or rise, trophoblasts can be assumed *not* to have been removed by the uterine curettage; thus, an ectopic pregnancy can be presumed to be present.

Surgical Treatment

Salpingectomy by laparotomy has long offered almost a 100 percent cure. However, current emphasis is not just to prevent death but also to facilitate rapid recovery, preserve fertility, and reduce costs. Laparoscopic salpingostomy and partial salpingectomy are thus rapidly replacing laparotomy. Laparotomy should be performed only when a laparoscopic approach is too difficult, the surgeon is not trained in operative laparoscopy, or the patient is hemodynamically unstable.

Linear salpingostomy is the standard laparoscopic operation when an ectopic mass is unruptured yet more than 4 cm in length by ultrasound.[147,153–157] Over the bulging antimesenteric border of the implantation site, a longitudinal incision is made by electrocautery, scissors, or laser. The products of conception are removed by forceps or suction. After hemostasis is achieved, the incision is allowed to heal by secondary intention. Alternatively, sutures can be placed. Approximately 95 percent of laparoscopic salpingostomies are successful (i.e., no additional procedures are needed).[147] Of the 93 women evaluated in one study, 86 percent were later shown to have patent oviducts; 66 percent of 430 women who were followed subsequently became pregnant, with 23 percent of those pregnancies being ectopic.[158]

Segmental resection is necessary if ectopic pregnancies are located in the isthmus (the midportion of the oviduct). Subsequent laparotomy is then necessary for reanastomosis of the surgically divided oviduct. Laparoscopic salpingectomy is also desirable for patients who do not wish to become pregnant again.

Postoperative bleeding, elevated β-hCG levels indicative of persistent viable trophoblastic tissue, and other symptoms occur in up to 20 percent of cases after conservative laparoscopic surgery. Excision of the involved oviduct or medical therapy may then be necessary.

Medical Treatment

Although operative laparoscopy has substantially fewer complications than laparotomy, there remains irreducible morbidity intrinsic to surgery and anesthesia. Medical treatments can greatly reduce this morbidity. To supplant surgery, however, medical therapies must match the high success rates, low complication rates, and good reproductive potential achieved with laparoscopic operations. This appears to be true.[147,159] The agent used is the folic acid antagonist methotrexate, which inhibits synthesis of purines and pyrimidines and thus interferes with DNA synthesis and cell multiplication. Actively proliferating trophoblasts have long been known to be vulnerable to methotrexate, as illustrated by its successful use in the treatment of gestational trophoblastic disease.

Hemodynamically stable patients with ectopic pregnancies are eligible for treatment with methotrexate if the mass is unruptured and measures 4 cm or less in diameter by ultrasound.[147] Patients with larger ectopic masses, embryonic cardiac activity, or evidence of acute intra-abdominal bleeding (acute abdomen, hypotension, or falling hematocrit) are not eligible for methotrexate therapy.[147] Outcome of treatment with systemic methotrexate (Table 22-4)[147,161] compares favorably with that of laparoscopic salpingostomy; 94 percent of women successfully treated with systemic methotrexate needed no subsequent therapy. Of women tested, 81 percent had patent oviducts; 71 percent subsequently became pregnant, with 11 percent of those being ectopic.

High doses of methotrexate can cause bone marrow suppression, acute and chronic hepatotoxicity, stomati-

Table 22-4 Summary of the Methotrexate Regimens Used

Regimen	Monitor
Multiple dose Methotrexate, 1 mg/k of body weight intramuscularly every other day (days 1, 3, and so on) Leucovorin, 0.1 mg/kg intramuscularly every other day (days 2, 4, and so on) Continue treatment until β-hCG drops ≥15% in 48 hours or 4 doses of methotrexate have been given	Serum β-hCG weekly until undetectable; blood count, platelet count, liver-enzymes levels
Single dose Methotrexate, 50 mg/m² of body surface area intramuscularly No leucovorin	Serum β-hCG level days 4 and 7, then weekly until undetectable; initial blood count, platelet count, liver-enzyme levels

(From Carson and Buster,[147] with permission.)

tis, pulmonary fibrosis, alopecia, and photosensitivity. Fortunately, these side effects are not only infrequent with the shorter treatment schedules used for an ectopic pregnancy but can be mitigated against by the administration of leucovorin (citrovorum factor). Experience with methotrexate in gestational trophoblastic disease provides little reason for concern about the risks of subsequent neoplasia or congenital anomalies in later pregnancies.[162]

Safeguards are necessary to enhance the success and minimize the toxicity of systemic methotrexate. First, the patient should undergo a pelvic examination by only a single examiner and then only once. Self-control concerning this part of management should be similar to that employed with placenta previa. Second, both physician and patient must recognize that transient pain is common, usually occurring 3 to 7 days after initiation of methotrexate therapy. The pain, presumably caused by tubal abortion, normally lasts 4 to 12 hours. Perhaps the most difficult aspect of methotrexate therapy is distinguishing the transient abdominal pain associated with successful therapy from that of rupturing ectopic pregnancy. Surgical intervention becomes necessary only when pain is accompanied by orthostatic tachycardia, hypotension, or a falling hematocrit. If uncertainty exists concerning the patient's hemodynamic stability, physicians may prefer to hospitalize the patient with pain for observation. Because colicky abdominal pain is common during the first 2 or 3 days of methotrexate therapy, patients should also be warned to avoid gas-producing foods such as leeks and cabbage. Patients should also avoid exposure to the sun because of the photosensitivity methotrexate produces.

Intramuscular methotrexate is not the only route of therapy, but less experience exists with other methods. These include the direct injection of methotrexate into the ectopic, methotrexate administered by tubal cannulation, or prostaglandins by direct injection.

Finally, few medical advances evolve without negative consequences. As ectopic pregnancy is detected earlier and more efficiently, some pregnancies that would otherwise have been spontaneously absorbed are now treated, in retrospect, needlessly. Identifying early ectopic pregnancies that are destined for spontaneous remission would thus be useful, although efforts to do so have so far been unsuccessful. "Overtreatment" of ectopic pregnancy will thus be the inevitable corollary of early intervention.

Relative Benefits of Surgical Versus Medical Therapy

Conservative laparoscopic surgery is very efficacious, as is that of systemic methotrexate therapy. Systemic methotrexate therapy is less expensive than operative laparoscopy, and patients lose less time from work. On the other hand, some patients prefer surgical therapy because they wish to avoid the possible side effects of systemic chemotherapy and a more protracted counsel of treatment. However, even after laparoscopic removal of ectopic tissue, residual tissue remains to cause hemorrhage and other complications in 20 percent of cases. With either surgical or medical treatment, weekly blood tests are thus necessary until β-hCH becomes undetectable. Only a small subgroup of patients treated with either medical or surgical therapy have been followed to determine subsequent reproductive capabilities; thus, it is difficult to state conclusively whether the rates of pregnancy, tubal patency, and recurrent ectopic pregnancy differ between medical and surgical treatment. Not until a prospective randomized study is conducted will the optimal choice of the therapy for each patient be known.

In conclusion, removal of the ectopic pregnancy is recommended by salpingostomy when laparoscopy is needed for diagnosis. We recommend systemic methotrexate when laparoscopy is not required for diagnosis. Laparoscopic surgery is also preferable when the ectopic mass is larger than 4.0 cm. A laparotomy is performed only for catastrophic hemorrhage or hemodynamic instability.

Recommended Evaluation for Recurrent Pregnancy Losses

1. Couples experiencing only one first trimester abortion should receive pertinent information, but not necessarily be evaluated formally. Mention the relatively high (10 to 15 percent) pregnancy loss rate in the general population and the beneficial effects of abortion in eliminating abnormal conceptuses. Provide the relevant recurrence risks, usually 20 to 25 percent subsequent loss in the presence of a prior liveborn and somewhat higher in the absence of a prior liveborn. Risks are higher for older women and those who smoke. If a specific medical illness exists, treatment is obviously necessary. Intrauterine adhesions should be lysed. Otherwise, no further evaluation need be undertaken, even if uterine anomalies or leiomyomas are detected. On the other hand, occurrence of an anomalous stillborn or liveborn warrants genetic evaluation irrespective of the number of pregnancy losses.

2. Investigation may or may not be necessary after two spontaneous abortions, depending upon the patient's age and personal desires. After three spontaneous abortions, evaluation is usually indicated. One should then (a) obtain a detailed family history, (b) perform a complete physical examination, (c) discuss recurrence risks, and (d) order the selected tests cited below.

3. Parental chromosomal studies should be performed on all couples having repetitive losses. Antenatal chromosomal studies should be offered if a balanced chromosomal rearrangement is detected in either parent or if autosomal trisomy occurred in any previous abortus.

4. Although it is impractical to karyotype all abortuses, cytogenetic information on abortuses may exist. Detection of a trisomic abortus suggests the phenomenon of recurrent aneuploidy, justifying prenatal cytogenetic studies in future pregnancies. Performing prenatal cytogenetic studies solely on the basis of repeated losses is more arguable, but not unreasonable among women aged 30 to 34 years.

5. The validity of LPD as a discrete entity increasingly seems arguable. To detect LPD, timed endometrial biopsies should be performed late in the luteal phase in two or more cycles. Results should be correlated with the date of ovulation. If histologic dating reveals an endometrium 2 or more days less than expected, the diagnosis can be made. Diagnosis on the basis of progesterone levels is preferred

by some. Progesterone therapy has been proposed, but its efficacy has not been proved.

6. Other endocrine causes for repeated fetal losses seem unlikely except poorly controlled diabetes mellitus (hyperglycemia). It is reasonable to screen for thyroid dysfunction and carbohydrate intolerance, but not exhaustively in the absence of clinical symptoms. These etiologies are very rare causes of pregnancy losses.

7. To determine the role of infectious agents, the endometrium may be cultured for *Ureaplasma urealyticum*. Alternatively, a couple could be treated empirically with doxycycline (100 mg two times per day for 10 days) before pregnancy. Of other infections agents, only *Chlamydia trachomatis* seems genuinely possible.

8. If an abortion occurs after 8 to 10 weeks gestation, a uterine anomaly or submucous leiomyoma should be considered. The uterine cavity should be explored by hysteroscopy or hysterosalpingography. If a müllerian fusion defect (septate or bicornuate uterus) is detected in a woman experiencing one or more second trimester spontaneous abortions, surgical correction may be warranted. A large submucous leiomyoma may also justify myomectomy or reduction. However, the same statements do not necessarily apply following *first* trimester losses. Cervical incompetence should be managed by surgical cerclage during the next pregnancy.

9. To exclude autoimmune disease involving antiphospholipid antibodies, assessment should include LAC and aCA. Women with antibodies who experience midtrimester losses may benefit from treatment with heparin and aspirin, but the same does not necessarily hold when these antibodies are detected in asymptomatic women having first trimester pregnancy losses. Testing for antisperm antibodies or other autoantibodies (e.g., DNA) is not indicated.

10. Controversy persists concerning the propriety of immunologic evaluations and especially the role of immunotherapy for couples sharing HLA antigens or otherwise having blunted maternal response to paternal antigens. Determining parental HLA types in the absence of other immunologic testing is not recommended. Couples desiring evaluation for immunologic causes of fetal wastage should be referred to the few centers undertaking a systematic approach under experimental protocols.

11. One should discourage exposure to cigarettes and alcohol, yet remain cautious in ascribing cause and effect in individual cases. Similar counsel should apply for exposures to other potential toxins.

10 Key Points

- Approximately 22 percent of all pregnancies detected on the basis of urinary hCG assays are lost, usually before clinical recognition.
- The clinical loss rate is 10 to 12 percent. Most of these pregnancies are lost before 8 weeks' gestation. Only 3 percent of pregnancies are lost after an ultrasonographically viable pregnancy at 8 to 9 weeks, and only 1 percent are lost after 16 weeks' gestations.
- Pregnancy losses may be recurrent, 4 percent of U.S. women experiencing two losses and 3 percent three or more losses. Although increasing after one loss, the recurrence risk generally reaches no more than 25 percent after three or four losses. Loss rates for 40-year-old women are approximately twice that of 20-year-old women.
- By far the most common causes of pregnancy losses are chromosomal abnormalities. At least 50 percent of clinically recognized pregnancy losses show a chromosomal abnormality. The types of chromosomal abnormalities differ from those found in liveborns, but autosomal trisomy still accounts for 50 percent of abnormalities. A balanced translocation is present in about 5 percent of couples having repeated spontaneous abortions.
- Many other causes of repetitive abortions have been proposed, but few are proved. These include luteal phase defects and infectious processes (e.g., *Ureaplasma*). It is reasonable to evaluate couples for these conditions, but efficacy of treatment remains uncertain.
- Uterine anomalies are accepted causes of second trimester pregnancies. Couples experiencing such losses may benefit from metroplasty or hysteroscopic resection of a uterine septum. Uterine anomalies are less common causes of first trimester losses.
- Drugs, toxins, and physical agents are associated with spontaneous abortion, but usually not in repetitive pregnancies. Avoiding potential toxins is obviously desirable, but one should not assume that such exposures explain repetitive losses.
- LAC antibodies and aCL are clearly associated with second trimester losses, but their role in first trimester losses is more arguable. Controversy persists concerning the propriety of immunologic evaluations and immunotherapy for couples sharing HLA antigens or otherwise showing blunted maternal response to paternal antigens (alloimmune disease). Determining parental HLA types in the absence of other immunologic evaluations is not recommended. Detailed immunologic evaluation should be restricted to centers performing the gamut of immunologic tests.
- The incidence of ectopic pregnancy is rising, partly through earlier detection by ultrasound and sensitive β-hCG assays. Treatment may be surgical (linear salpingostomy performed through the laparoscope) or medical (methotrexate).
- Management of ectopic pregnancy has undergone significant modification over recent years. The condition is less commonly an acute emergency and more easily diagnosed early in gestation on the basis of maternal serum progesterone, maternal β-hCG, transvaginal ultrasound, and uterine curettage. The earlier detection of an unruptured ectopic pregnancy has greatly modified treatment. Laparotomy is now rarely necessary. Laparoscopic procedures are commonly employed, with an increase in subsequent pregnancy rates and a decrease in repeat ectopic gestations. About one third of women with ectopic pregnancies prove eligible for medical treatment (methotrexate). Patients at high risk for ectopic pregnancy may benefit from a screening serum progesterone determination at the time of initial pregnancy test.

References

1. U.S. Department Health and Human Services: Reproductive impairments among married couples. p. 5. In U.S. Vital and Health Statistics Series 23, No. 11. National Center for Health Statistics, Hyattsville, MD, 1982
2. Wilcox AJ, Weinberg CR, O'Connor JF et al: Incidence of early pregnancy loss. N Engl J Med 319:189, 1988
3. Mills JL, Simpson JL, Driscoll SG et al: NICHD-DIEP Study: incidence of spontaneous abortion among normal women with insulin-dependent diabetic women whose pregnancies were identified within 21 days of conception. N Engl J Med 319:1617, 1988
4. Simpson JL, Carson SA: Genetic and non-genetic causes of spontaneous abortions. In Sciarra JJ (ed): Gynecology and Obstetrics, Vol. 3. JB Lippincott, Philadelphia, 1995.
5. Regan L: A prospective study on spontaneous abortion. p. 22. In Beard RW, Sharp F (eds): Early Pregnancy Loss: Mechanisms and Treatment. The Royal College of Obstetricians and Gynaecologists, London, 1988
6. Simpson JL, Gray RH, Queenan JT et al: Risk of recurrent spontaneous abortion for pregnancies discovered in the fifth week of gestation. Lancet 344:964, 1994
7. Simpson JL, Mills JL, Holmes LB et al: Low fetal loss rates after demonstration of a live fetus in the first trimester. JAMA 258:2555, 1987
8. Hertig AT, Rock J, Adams EC: Description of human ova within the first 17 days of development. Am J Anat 98:435, 1956
9. Hertig AT, Rock J, Adams EC, Menkin MC: Thirty-four fertilized human ova, good, bad and indifferent, recovered from 210 women of known fertility. A study

of biologic wastage in early human pregnancy. Pediatrics 25:202, 1959

10. Hertig AT, Rock J: Searching for early human ova. Gynecol Invest 4:121, 1973

11. Plachot M, Junca AM, Mandelbaum J et al: Chromosome investigations in early life. Human preimplantation embryos. Hum Reprod 2:29, 1987

12. Papadopoulos G, Templeton AA, Fisk N, Randall J: The frequency of chromosome anomalies in human preimplantation embryos after in-vitro fertilization. Hum Reprod 4:91, 1989

13. Plachot M: Genetics of human oocytes. p. 367. In Boutaleb Y, Gzouli A (eds): New Concepts in Reproduction. Vol. 88. Parthenon, Lanes, England, 1992

14. Martin R: Chromosomal analysis of human spermatozoa. p. 91. In Verlinsky Y, Kuliev A (eds): Preimplantation Genetics. Plenum Press, New York, 1991

15. Gropp A: Chromosomal animal model of human disease. Fetal trisomy and development failure. p. 17. In Berry L, Poswillo DE (eds): Teratology. Springer-Verlag, Berlin, 1975

16. Boué J, Boué A, Lazar P: Retrospective and prospective epidemiological studies of 1500 karyotyped spontaneous human abortions. Teratology 12:11, 1975

17. Hassold T: A cytogenetic study of repeated spontaneous abortions. Am J Hum Genet 32:723, 1980

18. Simpson JL, Bombard AT: Chromosomal abnormalities in spontaneous abortion: frequency, pathology and genetic counseling. p. 51. In Edmonds K, Bennett MJ (eds): Spontaneous Abortion. Blackwell, London, 1987

19. Sorokin Y, Johnson MP, Zadoe IE et al: Postmortem chorionic villus sampling: correlation of cytogenetic and ultrasound findings. Am J Med Genet 39:314, 1991

20. Strom C, Ginsberg N, Applebaum M et al: Analyses of 95 first trimester spontaneous abortions by chorionic villus sampling and karyotype. J Assist Reprod Genet 9:458, 1992

21. Kuleshov NP: Chromosome anomalies of infants dying during the perinatal period and premature newborn. Hum Genet 34:151, 1976

22. Watt JL, Templeton AA, Messinis I et al: Trisomy 1 in an eight cell human pre-embryo. J Med Genet 24:60, 1987

23. Warburton D, Byrne J, Canik N: Chromosome Anomalies and Prenatal Development: An Atlas. New York, Oxford University Press, 1991

24. Kalousek DK: Pathology of abortion: chromosomal and genetic correlations. p. 228. In Kraus FT, Damjanov I, Kaufman N (eds): Pathology of Reproductive Failure. Williams & Wilkins, Baltimore, 1991

25. Zaragoza MV, Jacobs PA, James RS: Nondisjunction of human acrocentric chromosomes: studies of 432 trisomic fetuses and liveborns. Hum Genet 94:411, 1994

26. Jacobs PA, Angell RR, Buchanan IM et al: The origin of human triploids. Ann Hum Genet 42:49, 1978

27. Beatty RA: The origin of human triploidy: an integration of qualitative and quantitative evidence. Ann Hum Genet 41:299, 1978

28. Singh RJ, Carr DH: The anatomy and histology of XO embryos and fetuses. Anat Rec 155:369, 1966

29. Jirásek JE: Principles of reproductive embryology. p. 51. In Simpson JL (ed): Disorders of Sex Differentiation: Etiology and Clinical Delineation. Academic Press, San Diego, 1976

30. Simpson JL: Pregnancies in women with chromosmal abnormalities. p. 439. In Shulman JD, Simpson JL (eds): Genetic Diseases in Pregnancy. Academic Press, San Diego, 1981

31. Chandley AC: The origin of chromosome aberrations in man and their potential for survival and reproduction in the adult human populations. Ann Genet 24:5, 1981

32. Henderson DJ, Sherman LS, Loughna SC et al: Early embryonic failure associated with uniparental disomy for human chromosome 21. Hum Mol Genet 3:1373, 1994

33. Malpas P: A study of abortion sequences. J Obstet Gynaecol Br Emp 45:932, 1938

34. Warburton D, Fraser FC: Spontaneous abortion risks in man: data from reproductive histories collected in a medical genetics units. Am J Human Genet 16:1, 1964

35. Poland BJ, Miller JR, Jones DC et al: Reproductive counseling in patients who have had a spontaneous abortion. Am J Obstet Gynecol 127:685, 1977

36. Kline J, Stein ZA, Susser M, Warburton D: Smoking: a risk factor for spontaneous abortion. N Engl J Med 297:793, 1977

37. Boué J, Boué A: Chromosomal analysis of 2 consecutive abortions in each of 43 women. Humangenetik 19:275, 1973

38. Vlaanderen W, Treffers PE: Prognosis of subsequent pregnancies after recurrent spontaneous abortion in first trimester. BMJ 295:92, 1987

39. Liddell HS, Pattison NS, Zanderigo A: Recurrent miscarriage—outcome after supportive care in early pregnancy. Aust NZJ Obstet Gynaecol 31:320, 1991

40. Houwert DE, Jong MH, Termijtelen A et al: The natural course of habitual abortion. Eur J Obstet Gynecol Reprod Biol 33:221, 1989

41. Simpson JL, Elias S, Martin AO: Parental chromosomal rearrangements associated with repetitive spontaneous abortion. Fertil Steril 24:1023, 1981

42. Simpson JL, Meyers CM, Martin AO et al: Translocations are infrequent among couples having repeated spontaneous abortions but no other abnormal pregnancies. Fertil Steril 51:811, 1989

43. De Braekeleer M, Dao TN: Cytogenetic studies in couples experiencing repeated pregnancy losses. Hum Reprod 5:519, 1990

44. Boué A, Gallano P: A collaborative study of the segregation of inherited chromosome structural arrangements in 1356 prenatal diagnoses. Prenat Diagn 4:45, 1973

45. Daniel A, Hook EB, Wulf G: Risks of unbalanced progeny at amniocentesis to carriers of chromosome rearrangements: data from United States and Candian Laboratories. Am J Med Genet 31:14, 1989

46. Martin RH: Segregation analysis of translocations by the study of human sperm chromosome complements. Am J Hum Genet 44:461, 1989

47. Rosenbusch B, Sterzik K, Lauritzen C: Cytogenetic anal-

ysis of sperm chromosomes in couples with habitual abortion. Geburtshilfe Frauenheilkd 51:369, 1991

48. Sutherland GR, Gardiner AJ, Carter RF: Familial pericentric inversion of chromosome 19 inv (19) (p13q13) with a note on genetic counseling of pericentric inversion carries. Clin Genet 10:53, 1976

49. Schwartz S, VanDyke DL, Palmer CG: Paracentric inversions in humans: a review of 446 paracentric inversions with presentation of 120 new cases. Am J Med Genet 55:171, 1995

50. Warburton D, Kline J, Stein Z et al: Does the karyotype of a spontaneous abortion predict the karyotype of a subsequent abortion? Evidence from 273 women with two karyotyped spontaneous abortions. Am J Hum Genet 41:465, 1987

51. Alberman ED: The abortus as a predictor of future trisomy 21. p. 69. In De la Cruz FF, Gerald PS (eds): Trisomy 21 (Down Syndrome). University Park Press, Baltimore, 1981

52. Gray RH, Simpson JL, Kambic RT et al: Timing of conception and the risk of spontaneous abortion among pregnancies occurring during the use of natural family planning. Am J Obstet Gynecol 172:1567, 1995 (in press)

53. Davis OK, Berkley AS, Cholst IN et al: The incidence of luteal phase defect in normal, fertile women, determined by serial endometrial biopsy. Fertil Steril 51:582, 1989

54. Noyes RW, Hertig ATR, Rock J: Dating the endometrial biopsy. Fertil Steril 1:3, 1950

55. Scott RT, Synder RR, Strickland DM et al: The effect of interobserver variation in dating endometrial history on the diagnosis of luteal phase defects. Fertil Steril 50:888, 1988

56. Li TC, Dockery P, Rogers AW, Cooke ID: How precise is histologic dating of endometrium using the standard dating criteria. Fertil Steril 759:51, 1989

57. Jordan J, Craig K, Clifton DK, Soules MR: Luteal phase defect: the sensitivity and specificity of diagnostic methods in common clinical use. Fertil Steril 62:54, 1994

58. Daya S, Ward S, Burrows E: Progesterone profiles in luteal phase defect cycles and outcome of progesterone treatment in patients with recurrent spontaneous abortions. Am J Obstet Gynecol 158:225, 1988

59. Tho PT, Byrd JR, McDonough PC: Etiologies and subsequent reproductive performance of 100 couples with recurrent abortions. Fertil Steril 32:389, 1979

60. Daya S, Ward S: Diagnostic test properties of serum progesterone in the evaluation of luteal phase defects. Fertil Steril 49:168, 1988

61. Daly DC, Walters CA, Soto-Albers CE et al: Endometrial biopsy during treatment of luteal phase defects is predictive of therapeutic outcome. Fertil Steril 40:305, 1983

62. Quenby SM, Farquharson RG: Predicting recurring miscarriage: what is important? Obstet Gynecol 82:132, 1993

63. Sagle M, Bishop K, Ridley N et al: Recurrent early miscarriage and polycystic ovaries. BMJ 297:1027, 1988

64. Regan L, Owen EJ, Jacobs HS: Hypersecretion of lutenising hormone, infertility, and miscarriage. Lancet 336:1141, 1990

65. Karamardian LM, Grimes DA: Luteal phase deficiency: effect of treatment on pregnancy rates. Am J Obstet Gynecol 167:1391, 1992

66. Montero M, Collea JV, Frasier D, Mestman J: Successful outcome of pregnancy in women with hypothyroidism. Ann Intern Med 94:31, 1981

67. Pratt DE, Kaberlein G, Dudkiewicz A: The association of antithyroid antibodies in euthyroid nonpregnant women with recurrent first trimester abortions in the next pregnancy. Fertil Steril 60:1001, 1993

68. Miodovnik M, Mimouni F, Tsang RL et al: Glycemic control and spontaneous abortion in insulin dependent diabetic women. Obstet Gynecol 68:366, 1986

69. Ben Rafael Z, Seidman DS, Recabi K et al: Uterine anomalies. A retrospective, matched control study. J Reprod Med 36:723, 1991

70. Michalas SP: Outcome of pregnancy in women with uterine malformation: evaluation of 62 cases. Int J Gynaecol Obstet 35:215, 1991

71. Makino T, Sakai A, Sugi T et al: Current comprehensive therapy of habitual abortion. Ann NY Acad Sci 626:597, 1991

72. Mouton DM, Damewood MD, Schlaff WD, Rock JA: A comparison of the reproductive outcome between women with a unicornuate uterus and women with a didelphic uterus. Fertil Steril 58:88, 1992

73. Golan A, Langer R, Neuman M et al: Obstetric outcome in women with congenital uterine malformations. J Reprod Med 37:233, 1992

74. Candiani GB, Fedele L, Parazzini F, Zamberletti D: Reproductive prognosis after abdominal metroplasty in bicornuate or septate uterus: a life table analysis. Br J Obstet Gynaecol 97:613, 1990

75. Stein AL, March CM: Pregnancy outcome in women with mullerian duct anomalies. J Reprod Med 35:411, 1990

76. Makino T: Management of uterine congenital malformations: evaluation of outcome. In Hedon B, Springer J, Mores P (eds): Proceedings of the 15th World Congress on Fertility and Sterility, Montpellier, France, 17–22 September, 1995. Parthenon, New York, 1995.

77. Makino T, Umeuchi M, Nakada K et al: Incidence on congenital uterine anomalies in repeated reproductive wastage and prognosis for pregnancy after metroplasty. Int J Fertil 37:167, 1992

78. Stampe-Sorensen S: Estimated prevalence of mullerian anomalies. Acta Obstet Gynecol Scand 67:441, 1988

79. Simon C, Marinex L, Pardo F et al: Müllerian defects in women with normal reproductive outcome. Fertil Steril 56:1192, 1991

80. Ludmire J, Samuels P, Brooks S, Mennuti MT: Pregnancy outcome of patients with uncorrected uterine anomalies managed in a high-risk obstetric setting. Obstet Gynecol 75:906, 1990

81. Sompolinsky D, Solomon F, Elikina L et al: Infections with mycoplasma and bacteria. Individual midtrimester abortion and fetal loss. Am J Obstet Gynecol 121:610, 1975

82. Toth A, Lesser ML, Brooks-Toth CW et al: Outcome of subsequent pregnancies following antibiotic therapy after primary or multiple spontaneous abortions. Surgery Gynecol Obstet 163:243, 1986

83. Van Iddekinge B, Hofmeyr GJ: Recurrent spontaneous abortion—aetiological factors and subsequent reproductive performance in 76 couples. S Afr Med J 80:223, 1991

84. Stray-Pedersen B, Eng J, Reikvan TM: Uterine T-mycoplasma colonization in reproductive failure. Am J Obstet Gynecol 130:307, 1978

85. Troshima OI, Gamove NA, Vulfovich IuV, Rakovskaia IV: *Mycoplasma* and *Ureaplasma* infections in chronic genital inflammatory processes, abortion and infertility. Vestn Akad Med Nauk SSSR 6:23, 1991

86. Quinn PA, Petric M, Barkin M et al: Prevalence of antibody to *Chlamydia trachomatis* in spontaneous abortion and infertility. Am J Obstet Gynecol 156:291, 1987

87. Witkin SS, Ledger WJ: Antibodies to chlamydia trachomatis in sera of women with recurrent spontaneous abortions. Am J Obstet Gynecol 167:135, 1992

88. Rae R, Smith IW, Liston WA, Kilpatrick DC: Chlamydial serologic studies and recurrent spontaneous abortion. Am J Obstet Gynecol 170:782, 1994

89. Olliaro R, Regazzetti A, Gorini G et al: Chlamydia trachomatis infection in "sine causa" recurrent abortion. Boll 1st Sieroter Milan 70:467, 1991

90. van Lijnschoten G, Stals F, Evers JLH et al: The presence of cytomegalovirus antigens in karyotyped abortions. p. 79. In van Lijnschoten G (ed): Morphology and Karyotype in Early Abortion. University Press Maastricht, Amsterdam, 1993

91. Zavala-Vlazquez J, Guzman-Marin E, Barrera-Perez M, Rodriguez-Feliz ME: Toxoplasmosis and abortion in patients at the O'Horan Hospital of Merida, Yucatan. Salud Publica Mex 31:664, 1989

92. el Ridi AM, Nada SM, Aly AS et al: Toxoplasmosis and pregnancy: an analytical study in Zagazig, Egypt. J Egypt Soc Parasitol 21:81, 1991

93. Rock JA, Shirey RS, Braine HG et al: Plasmapheresis for the treatment of repeated early pregnancy wastage associated with anti-P. Obstet Gynecol 66:57S, 1985

94. Strowitzki T, Wiedemann R, Heim MU et al: Pregnancy with an extremely rare P blood group with anti-PP1Pk. Geburtshilfe-Frauenheilkd 51:710, 1991

95. Cowchock S: Autoantibodies and pregnancy wastage. Am J Reprod Immun 26:38–41, 1991

96. Branch DW, Ward K: Autoimmunity and pregnancy loss. Semin Reprod Endocrinol 7:168, 1989

97. Scott JR, Rote NS, Branch DW: Immunologic aspects of recurrent abortions and fetal death. Obstet Gynecol 70:645, 1987

98. Elias S, Eldor A: Thrombombolism in patients with "lupus" type circulating anticoagulant. Arch Intern Med 1244:510, 1984

99. Cowchock FS, Reece AE, Balaban D et al: Repeated fetal losses associated with antiphospholipid antibodies: a collaborative randomized trial comparing prednisone with low-dose heparin treatment. Am J Obstet Gynecol 166, 1318, 1992

100. Petri M, Golbus M, Anderson R et al: Antinuclear antibody, lupus anticoagulant, and anticardiolipin antibody in women with idiopathic habitual abortion. Arth Rheum 30:601, 1987

101. Carp HJ, Menashe Y, Frenkel Y et al: Lupus anticoagulant. Significance in habitual first-trimester abortion. J Reprod Med 38:549, 1993

102. Mishall DR Jr: Recurrent abortion. J Reprod Med 38:250, 1993

103. Eroglu GE, Scopelitis E: Antinuclear and antiphospholipid antibodies in healthy women with recurrent spontaneous abortion. Am J Reprod Immunol 31:1, 1994

104. Witkin SS, Chaudhry A: Association between recurrent spontaneous abortions and circulation IgG antibodies to sperm tails in women. J Reprod Immunol 15:151, 1989

105. Hass GG, Kubota K, Quebbeman JF et al: Circulating antisperm antibodies in recurrent aborting women. Fertil Steril 45:209, 1986

106. Erguven S, Asar G, Gulmezoglu AM, Yergok YZ: Antisperm and anticardiolipin antibodies in recurrent abortions. Mikrobiyol Bul 24:1, 1990

107. Yan JH: Evaluation of circulating antisperm anti bodies and seminal emmunosuppressive material in repeatedly aborting couples. Chung Hua Fu Chan Ko Tsa Chih 25:343, 1990

108. Clarke GN, Baker HW: Lack of association between sperm antibodies and recurrent spontaneous abortion. Fertil Steril 59:463, 1993

109. Zhang XC: Clinical study on circulating antisperm antibodies in women with recurrent abortion. Chung Hua Fu chan Ko Tsa Chih 25:21, 1990

110. Carson SA, Simpson JL, Mills JL et al: Cohort study showing that IgA antisperm antibodies (20% binding) but not IgG or IgM antibodies are associated with pregnancy losses. Society of Gynecologic Investigation 40th Annual Meeting, P313, March 31–April 3, 1993

111. Beard RW, Baude P, Mowbray JF et al: Protective antibodies and spontaneous abortion. Lancet 1:1090, 1983

112. Sargent IL, Wilkins T, Redman CWG: Maternal immune responses to the fetus in early pregnancy and recurrent miscarriage. Lancet 11:1099, 1988

113. Beer AE, Billingham RF: The Immunology of Mammalian Reproduction. Prentice-Hall, Englewood, NJ, 1976

114. Ober CL, Martin AO, Simpson JL et al: Shared HLA antigens and reproductive performance among Hutterites. Am J Hum Genet 35:994, 1983

115. Coulam CB: Immunologic tests in the evaluation of reproductive disorders: a critical review. Am J Obstet Gynecol 167:1844, 1992

116. Laitinen T, Koskimies S, Westman P: Foeto-maternal compatibility in HLA-DR, -DQ, and -DP loci in Finnish couples suffering from recurrent spontaneous abortions. Eur J Immmunogenet 20:249, 1993

117. Ober C, Elias S, Kostyu DD, Hauck WW: Decreased fecundability in Hutterite couples sharing HLA-DR. Am J Hum Genet 50:6, 1992

118. Christiansen OB, Mathiesen O, Lauritsen JG, Grunnet N: Idiopathic recurrent spontaneous abortion: evidence

of a familial predisposition. Acta Obstet Gynecol Scand 69:597, 1990

119. Norman DJ, Barry JM, Fischer S: The beneficial effect of pretransplant third-party blood transfusions on allograft rejection in HLA identical sibling kidney transplants. Transplantation 41:125, 1986

120. Mowbray JF, Gibbings C, Liddell et al: Controlled trial of treatment of recurrent spontaneous abortion by immunization with paternal cells. Lancet 1:941, 1985

121. Fraser EJ, Grimes DA, Schultz KF: Immunization as therapy for recurrent spontaneous abortion: a review and meta-analysis. Obstet Gynecol 82:854, 1993

122. Recurrent Miscarriage Immunotherapy Trialists Group: Worldwide collaborative observational study and meta-analysis on allogenic leukocyte immunotherapy for recurrent spontaneous abortion. Am J Reprod Immunol 32:55, 1994

123. Kline J, Shrout P, Stein ZA et al: Drinking during pregnancy and spontaneous abortion. Lancet 2:176, 1980

124. Alberman ED, Creasy M, Elliott M et al: Maternal effects associated with fetal chromosomal anomalies in spontaneous abortions. Br J Obstet Gynecol 83:621, 1976

125. Mills JL, Holmes L, Aarons JH et al: Moderate caffeine use and the risk of spontaneous abortion and intrauterine growth retardation. JAMA 269:593, 1993

126. Harlap S, Shiono PH: Alcohol, smoking and incidence of spontaneous abortions in the first and second trimester. Lancet 2:173, 1980

127. Halmesmärki E, Valimaki M, Roine R et al: Maternal and paternal alcohol consumption and miscarriage. Br J Obstet Gynaecol 96:188, 1989

128. Parazzini F, Bocciolone L, LaVecchia C et al: Maternal and paternal moderate daily alcohol consumption and unexplained miscarriages. Br J Obstet Gynaecol 97:618, 1990

129. Simpson JL: Relationship between congenital anomalies and contraception. Adv Contracept 1:3, 1985

130. Fija-Talamanca I, Settimi L: Occupational factors and reproductive outcome. p. 61. In Hafez ESE (ed): Spontaneous Abortion. MTP Press, Lancaster, 1984

131. Barlow S, Sullivan FM: Reproductive Hazards of Industrial Chemicals: An Evaluation of Animal and Human Data. Academic Press, San Diego, 1982

132. Savitz DA, Sonnenfeld NL, Olshan AF: Review of epidemiologic studies of paternal occupational exposure and spontaneous abortion. Am J Ind Med 25:361, 1994

133. Goldhaber MK, Polen MR, Hiatt RA: The risk of miscarriage and birth defects among women who use visual display terminals during pregnancy. Am J Indust Med 13:695, 1988

134. Parazzini F, Luchini L, La Vecchia C, Crosignani PG: Video display terminal use during pregnancy and reproductive outcome—a meta analysis. J Epidemiol Comm Health 47:265, 1993

135. Heidam LZ: Spontaneous abortions among laboratory workers: A follow up study. J Epidemiol Comm Health 38:36, 1984

136. Taskinen H, Lindbohm M-L, Hemminki K et al: Spontaneous abortions among women working in the pharmaceutical industry. Br J Indust Med 43:199, 1984

137. Stray-Pedersen B, Stray-Pedersen S: Etiologic factors and subsequent reproductive performance in 195 couples with a prior history of habitual abortion. Am J Obstet Gynecol 148:140, 1984

138. Stray-Pedersen B, Stray-Pedersen S: Recurrent abortion: the role of psychotherapy. p. 433. In Beard RW, Sharp F (eds): Early Pregnancy Loss: Mechanism and Treatment. Royal College of Obstetricians and Gynaecologists, London, 1988

139. Dorfman SF: Deaths from ectopic pregnancy, United States, 1979 to 1980. Obstet Gynecol 62:334, 1983

140. Thorburn J, Philipson M, Lindblom B: Fertility after ectopic pregnancy in relation to background factors and surgical treatment. Fertil Steril 49:595, 1988

141. Elias S, LeBeau M, Simpson JL, Martin AO: Chromosome analysis of ectopic human conceptuses. Am Jm Obstet Gynecol 141:698, 1981

142. Breen JL: A 21 year study of 654 ectopic pregnancies. J Obstet Gynecol 106:1004, 1970

143. Brenner PF, Roy S, Mishell DR Jr: Ectopic pregnancy: a study of 300 consecutive surgically treated cases. JAMA 243:673, 1980

144. DeCherney AH, Maheux R: Modern management of tubal pregnancy. p. 61. In Leventhal JM et al: Current Problems in Obstetrics and Gynecology. Year Book, Chicago, 1983

145. Thornburn JEK, Janson PO, Lindstedt G: Early diagnosis of ectopic pregnancy. Acta Obstet Gynecol Scand 62:543, 1983

146. Silverberg SG: Arias-Stella phenomenon in spontaneous and therapeutic abortion. Am J Obstet Gynecol 112:777, 1972

147. Carson SA, Buster JE: The ectopic pregnancy: new advances in diagnosis and treatment. N Engl J Med 329:1174, 1993

148. Stovall TG, Ling FW, Carson SA, Buster JE: Nonsurgical diagnosis and treatment of tubal pregnancy. Fertil Steril 54:537, 1990

149. Stoval TG, Ling FW, Gray LA et al: Methotrexate treatment of unruptured ectopic pregnancy: a report of 100 cases. Obstet Gynecol 77:749, 1991

150. Stovall TG, Ling FW, Carson SA, Buster JE: Serum progesterone and uterine curettage in differential diagnosis of ectopic pregnancy. Fertil Steril 57:456, 1992

151. Lenton EA, Neal LM, Sulaiman R: Plasma concentrations of human chorionic gonacotropin from the time of implantation until the second week of pregnancy. Fertil Steril 37:773, 1982

152. Emerson DS, Carier MS, Altieri LA et al: Diagnostic efficacy of endovaginal color Doppler flow imaging in an ectopic pregnancy screening program. Radiology. 183:413, 1992

153. DeCherney AH, Diamond MP: Laparoscopic salpingostomy for ectopic pregnancy. Obstet Gynecol 70:948, 1987

154. Lindblom B: Ectopic pregnancy: laparoscopic and medical treatment. Curr Opin Obstet Gynecol 4:400, 1992

155. Chapron C, Querleu D, Crepin G: Laparoscopic tratment of ectopic pregnancies: a one hundred cases study. Eur J Obstet Gynecol Reprod Biol 41:187, 1991

156. Vermesh M, Silva PD, Rosen GF et al: Mangement of unruptured ectopic gestation by lineal salpingostomy: a prospective, randomized clinical trial of laparoscopy versus laparotomy. Obstet Gynecol 73:400, 1989

157. Brumsted J, Kessler C, Gibson C et al: A comparison of laparoscopy and laparotomy foe the tratment of ectopic pregnancy. Obstet Gynecol 71:889, 1988

158. Seifer DB, Gutmann JN, Doyle MB et al: Persistent ectopic pregnancy following laparoscopic linear salpingostomy. Obstet Gynecol 76:1121, 1990

159. Stovall TG, Ling FW, Gray LA: Single-dose methotrexate for tratment of ectopic pregnancy. Obstet Gynecol 77:754, 1991

160. Tanaka T, Hayashi H, Kutsuzawa T et al: Treatment of ectopic pregnancy with methotrexate: report of a successful case. Fertil Steril 37:851, 1982

161. Ory SJ, Villanueva AL, Sand PK, Tamura RK: Conservative treatment of ectopic pregnancy with methotrexate. Am J Obstet Gynecol 154:1299, 1986

162. Ross GT: Congenital anomalies among children born of mothers receiving chemotheralpy for gestational trophoblatic neoplasms. Cancer, Suppl. 37:1043, 1976

163. Simpson JL, Tharapel AT: Principles of cytogenetics. p. 27. In Philip E, Barnes J (eds): Scientific Foundations of Obstetrics and Gynaecology. 4th Ed. Heinemann Medical Books, London, 1991

164. Simpson JL: Disorders of Sexual Differentiation, Etiology and Clinical Delineation. Academic Press, San Diego, 1976

165. Hook EB, Cross PK, Schreinemachers DM et al: Chromosomal abnormality rates at amniocentesis and liveborn infants. JAMA 249:2043, 1983

166. Hertig A, Rock J: A series of potentially abortive ova recovered from fertile women prior to the first missed menstrual period. Am J Obstet Gynecol: 58:968, 1949

167. Hertig AT, Rock J: On the development of the early human ovum with special reference to the trophoblast of the previllous stage: a description of seven normal and five pathologic ova. Am J Obstet Gynecol 47:149, 1944

Chapter 23

Preterm Birth

Jay D. Iams

Premature birth is the single largest cause of perinatal mortality and morbidity in nonanomalous infants in developed nations. In the United States, complications of prematurity account for more than 70 percent of fetal and neonatal deaths annually in babies without anomalies.[1] Long-term sequelae of prematurity disproportionately contribute to developmental delay, visual and hearing impairment, chronic lung disease, and cerebral palsy.[2] For example, an infant born weighing less than 1,500 g is approximately 200 times more likely to die in infancy and, if a survivor, 10 times more likely to be neurologically impaired than a peer born weighing more than 2,500 g. Even in seemingly intact preterm survivors, poor school performance and family disruption are more common. Advances in neonatal care during the last 30 years have led to increased survival and reduced short- and long-term morbidity for infants born before 37 weeks of pregnancy, but the rate of preterm birth has actually increased since 1970. The incidence of delivery before 37 completed weeks' gestation was 93 per 1,000 live births in 1970, 101 per 1,000 live births in 1987, and 109 in 1993.[3] Significant improvements in infant, child, and family health are clearly dependent on prevention of preterm birth.

Efforts to identify and treat the conditions leading to prematurity have intensified over the past 15 to 20 years, but have been largely disappointing, fulfilling the prophetic words of Nicholson Eastman in 1947: "Only when the factors underlying prematurity are completely understood can any intelligent attempt at prevention be made."[4] In the last decade, significant progress has been made toward understanding the factors that underlie preterm birth. The decade to come may yet see Eastman's hope fulfilled.

This chapter begins with the epidemiology of prematurity as a basis for understanding the difference between *spontaneous* and *indicated* preterm births. A pathophysiologic model of prevention and treatment for spontaneous preterm births and the concepts of primary, secondary, and tertiary care for spontaneous prematurity are introduced. Remaining sections of the chapter consider tertiary care of clinical presentations of spontaneous preterm birth and techniques of secondary and primary care.

The Problem of Prematurity

Definitions

Discussions of the problems of premature and low-birth-weight infants are complicated by use of data that incorrectly interchange the definitions of *prematurity*, defined by the duration of pregnancy, and *low birth weight*, defined by the size of the infant at birth. Infants born before 37 weeks' gestation (259 days from the first day of the mother's last menstrual period, or 245 days after conception) are *premature*. *Low-birth-weight* (LBW) infants weigh less than 2,500 g at birth, regardless of gestational age. *Very-low-birth-weight* (VLBW) infants weigh less than 1,500 g at birth. Extremely-low-birth-weight infants weigh less than 1,000 g at birth. Obviously, age does not equal size. The confusion occurred because of difficulty in determining gestational age with confidence prior to the availability of sensitive serologic and ultrasonographic means of pregnancy dating. It is now possible to determine gestational age very accurately by correlation of menstrual history with sensitive pregnancy tests and by measurements of fetal size with ultrasound in the first half of pregnancy. Unfortunately, these methods of pregnancy dating are still not available for some pregnancies. Because gestational age and birth weight are directly correlated throughout most of gestation, birth weight has been used as an indirect indicator of gestational age in many studies, especially those in which data are obtained from poorly dated pregnancies. Interchanging the two measures has led to significant misinterpretation of data at every level of analysis, because the problems of LBW infants may be the result of prematurity in some instances, of poor intrauterine growth in others, and of both in still others. Similarly, problems due to prematurity in infants whose birth weight exceeds 2,500 g may go unrecognized because of their apparently "full-term" appearance.

The proportion of LBW infants who are preterm versus term varies widely between developed and underdeveloped nations. In underdeveloped areas, most LBW infants are born after 37 weeks, their low birth weight the result of poor intrauterine nutrition and chronic maternal illness and/or malnutrition. In developed nations, most LBW infants are premature, although there are wide variations within the United States according to race, parity, fetal sex, and environmental factors such as maternal cigarette smoking and altitude. The birth weight data reported by Brenner and associates[5] (Fig. 23-1) are based on a racially mixed population near sea level in North Carolina. Ideally, each region or state should generate a birth weight versus gestational age chart for its own population. In the absence of such data,

a published chart based on a similar population can be used.

The incidences of LBW and VLBW deliveries have changed little since 1975 (Fig. 23-2).[6] There were 288,482 infants born in 1993 who weighed less than 2,500 g, an LBW rate of 72 per 1,000 liveborn infants. The rate of VLBW (less than 1,500 g) was stable at 13 per 1,000 liveborns in 1992 and 1993, increasing slightly from 12 per 1,000 since the last edition of this text. Rates of LBW and VLBW newborn blacks are consistently about twice as high as corresponding rates for nonblacks (Fig. 23-2). Even when corrected for age and educational level, black women continue to deliver more LBW infants than do white women. A slight decline in the incidence of LBW newborns occurred during the 1970s. The major portion of this decrease resulted from a decrease in term LBW infants rather than in preterm LBW infants,[7] a trend observed equally in white and nonwhite populations. There has been no change in these trends despite the availability of drugs to stop preterm labor.

Perinatal Mortality and Morbidity

Analysis of perinatal mortality and morbidity statistics has long been confounded by the various definitions of fetal, perinatal, neonatal, and infant time periods that

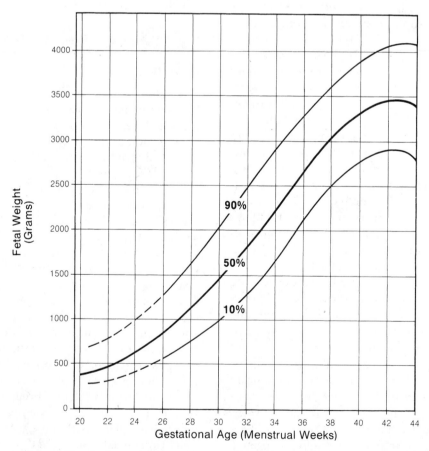

Fig. 23-1. Percentage of low birth weight infants by race: 1975–1992. (From Brenner et al,[5] with permission.)

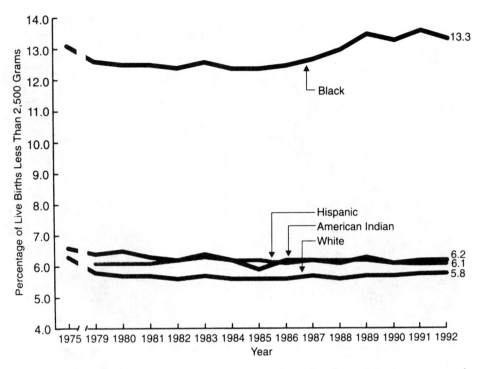

Fig. 23-2. Rate (%) of low birth weight infants in the United States by maternal race: 1975–1995. (From the National Center for Health Statistics,[6] with permission.)

have been used across the United States and around the world.[8] The definitions endorsed by the American College of Obstetricians and Gynecologists are used here (Figs 23-3, 23-4, and 23-5).[9]

Significant improvements in survival rates for extremely preterm infants (26 weeks or younger) weighing less than 1,000 g have been observed in several studies. Data from 1982 to 1986, before the introduction of neonatal artificial surfactant (Fig. 23-6,[10] show survival rates of only 1.8 percent at 23 weeks, 9.9 percent at 24 weeks, 15.5 percent at 25 weeks, and 54.7 percent at 26 weeks gestation. From 1988 to 1991, after the introduction of neonatal surfactant therapy, survival (Fig. 23-7)[11] increased to 15 percent at 23 weeks, 56 percent at 24 weeks, and 80 percent at 25 weeks. Fanaroff et al[9] reported similar survival data from the National Institute of Child Health and Human Development (NICHD) Neonatal Network in a large cohort of infants born in 1991 to 1992 (Fig. 23-8). The survival figures cited include all liveborn infants born at the reporting institutions, even those not successfully transferred from the delivery room to the nursery. Not surprisingly, higher survival rates are reported when only neonatal unit admissions are analyzed. Nevertheless, obstetric reports have shown similar trends of improved survival. Bottoms et al[12] reported data from 799 nonanomalous infants born between 22 and 26 weeks studied in the NICHD Maternal Fetal Network as shown in Table 23-1.

Other variables such as infant sex (more girls survive than boys)[9] and race (black infants weighing less than 3,000 g do better than white infants) also influence survival significantly. Several reviewers have demonstrated significant survival differences not explained by the above-listed demographic factors[13,14] Thus, when available, it is always best to use local statistics when evaluating patients.

Despite the marked improvement in neonatal survival over the past 40 years, the United States still compares relatively unfavorably with other developed countries with respect to neonatal mortality. In the past, this poor international ranking was blamed on an excess of LBW infants at all gestational ages in the United States. However, a study[15] of linked birth and perinatal death records from 105,084 Norwegian and 7,445,914 American births in 1986 to 1987 found that the higher rate of perinatal deaths in the United States is due entirely to a small excess of preterm births in the United States (2.9 percent) versus Norway (2.1 percent) and that a reduction in preterm delivery in the United States to the rate observed in Norway would produce a perinatal mortality rate equivalent to that in Norway. The authors concluded that the prevention of excess perinatal mortality in the United States depends more on prevention of prematurity, especially extreme prematurity, than on prevention of low birth weight.

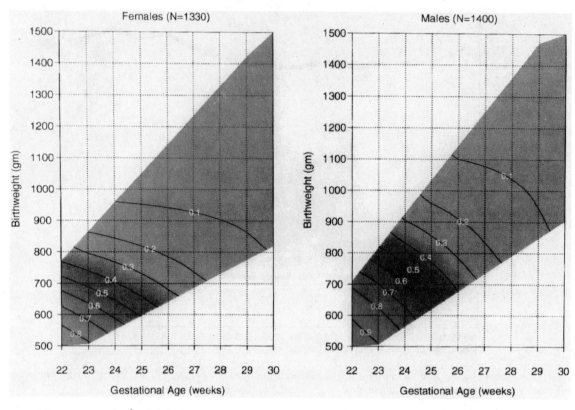

Fig. 23-3. Estimated mortality for preterm infants at 20 to 30 weeks' gestation and 500 to 1,500 g according to gender, birth weight, and gestational age in the National Institute of Child Health and Human Development Neonatal Network in 1991–1992. (From Fanaroff et al,[9] with permission.)

Perinatal Morbidity

Preterm infants are at risk for specific disease relating to the immaturity of various organ systems. Common complications in these very premature infants include respiratory distress syndrome, intraventricular hemorrhage, bronchopulmonary dysplasia, patent ductus arteriosus, necrotizing enterocolitis, sepsis, apnea, and retinopathy of prematurity. Extremely preterm infants are at greatest risk. There is wide interinstitutional variation in the frequencies of these sequelae, which may reflect in part differences in definitions as well as in clinical practices.[13] Robertson et al[16] reported gestational age specific morbidities for 20,662 infants born from well-dated pregnancies; 1,539 of the infants were born at 36 weeks or before. Rates of neonatal morbidities by gestational age for respiratory distress syndrome, intraventicular hemorrhage (grades III and IV), sepsis, necrotizing enterocolitis, patent ductus arteriosus, hyperbilirubinemia, and hypoglycemia and of *no* morbidity are shown in Figure 23-9.

Long-Term Morbidity

During the 1950s, preterm infants were found to be at increased risk for neurodevelopmental handicaps such as severe mental retardation (IQ or DQ [developmental quotient] less than 70), cerebral palsy, seizure disorders, blindness, and deafness. Since then, concern about long-term neurologic sequelae has focused on smaller and smaller infants of increasingly earlier gestational ages. Between 1975 and 1992, the rate of intact survival has steadily increased for VLBW and ELBW infants (see Fig. 23-8). Data comparing rates of death and major disability in 1987 to 1988 compared with 1989 to 1990 reveal two important observations: increased survival rates have not been accompanied by an increase in morbidity, but the prevalence of significant long-term morbidity among survivors remains high (Fig 23-8).

Despite fears to the contrary, the proportion of survivors within each birth weight group who have serious handicaps has not increased since the introduction of neonatal intensive care. For infants born between 1975 and 1985, 26 percent of surviving infants with birth weights below 800 g, 17 percent of survivors with birth weights between 750 and 1,000 g, and 11 percent of survivors with birth weights between 1,000 and 1,500 g have major handicaps at 1 or 2 years of age. More moderate impairment defined as an IQ between 70 and 80 was reported in an additional 41 percent of neonates born at less than 800 g, 31 percent born between 750 and 1,000

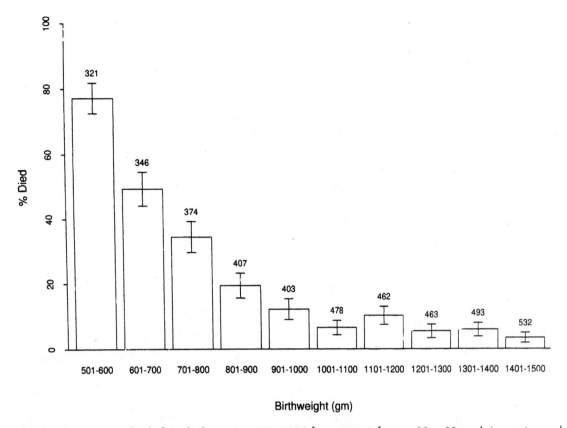

Fig. 23-4. Percent mortality before discharge in 1991–1992 for preterm infants at 20 to 30 weeks' gestation and 500 to 1,500 grams in the National Institute of Child Health and Human Development Neonatal Network in 1991–1992 by 100-g birth weight subgroups with 95% confidence intervals. Number of infants in each birth weight category are shown above each bar. (From Fanaroff et al,[9] with permission.)

g, and 16 percent between 1,000 and 1,500 g birth weight.[14] A 1994 study of school age outcomes found higher rates of cererbral palsy, severe visual impairment, and reduced head size and height for children with birth weights under 750 g when compared with children with birth weights of 750 to 1,449 g and children born at term (Fig. 23-10).[2] Abnormal cognitive, academic, visual motor, gross motor, and adaptive performance were also more frequent among children with birth weights below 750 g (Fig. 23-11). These children were all born before the introduction of surfactant and aggressive use of antenatal corticosteroids.

Preterm infants are also at greater risk of experiencing non-neurologic morbidity, such as chronic pulmonary disease. In addition to prolonged hospitalization at birth, many VLBW infants are rehospitalized during the first year of life.[17] Although much less well studied, there is concern that preterm birth disrupts maternal–infant bonding, which can have a major impact on family function, with increased likelihood of child abuse and family separation. Sudden infant death syndrome has also been reported more frequently among prematurely born infants.

Overview of the Pathogenesis of Prematurity

The Epidemiology of Preterm Birth

It is commonly said that prematurity is a multifactorial problem due to diverse and often unrelated maternal and/or fetal disorders. The list of maternal and fetal diagnoses antecedent to preterm deliveries is indeed long and broad: preterm labor, preterm ruptured membranes, preeclampsia, abruptio placenta, multiple gestation, placenta previa, fetal growth retardation, excessive or inadequate amniotic fluid volume, fetal anomalies, amnionitis, incompetent cervix, and maternal medical problems such as diabetes, asthma, drug abuse, and pyelonephritis may all lead to preterm delivery. Maternal characteristics that have been associated with an increased risk of preterm delivery are also diverse: maternal race (black more than nonblack), low socioeconomic status, poor nutrition and low prepregnancy weight, a history of previous preterm birth, absent or inadequate prenatal care, age less than 18 or more than 40, strenuous work, high personal stress, anemia (hemoglobin level below 10 g/dl), cigarette

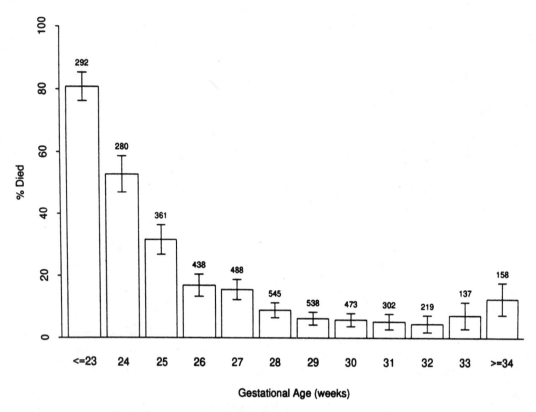

Fig. 23-5. Percent mortality before discharge in 1991–1992 for preterm infants at 20 to 30 weeks' gestation and 500 to 1,500 g in the National Institute of Child Health and Human Development Neonatal Network in 1991–1992 by best obstetric estimate of gestational age with 95% confidence intervals. Number of infants at each week of gestational age is shown above each bar. (From Fanaroff et al,[9] with permission.)

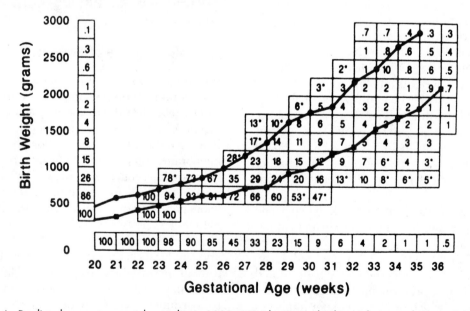

Fig. 23-6. Predicted percent neonatal mortality in 1982–1986 by 250-g birth weight intervals (y axis), by 1-week gestational age intervals (x axis), and by combined 250-g birth weight and weekly gestational intervals (center cells) derived from multiple regression model of data collected from five perinatal centers between 1982 and 1986. Upper line indicates the 90th percentile and lower line the 10th percentile. An asterisk indicates fewer than five infants per cell. (From Copper et al,[10] with permission.)

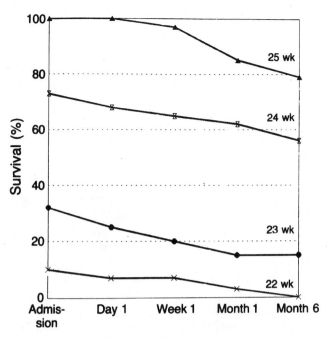

Fig. 23-7. Survival rates between admission and 6 months of age for infants born between 22 and 25 weeks' gestational age (by best obstetric estimate) in 1988 to 1991. (From Allen et al,[11] with permission.)

smoking, bacteriuria, genital colonization or infection (e.g., bacterial vaginosis, *Neisseria gonorrhea*, *Chlamydia trachomatis*, *Mycoplasma*, and *Ureaplasma*), cervical injury or abnormality (e.g., in utero exposure to diethylstilbestrol, a history of cervical conization, or second trimester induced abortion), uterine anomaly or fibroids, excessive uterine contractility, and premature cervical dilation of more than 1 cm or effacement of 80 percent or more.

Spontaneous Vs. Indicated Preterm Delivery

Are the risk factors for preterm birth related in some way, or does each disease or risk factor lead to preterm delivery by a unique pathway? The multitude of clinical disorders and risk factors has been usefully organized into two broad categories called *spontaneous* or *indicated* preterm birth, based on the presumed health of the mother and fetus prior to the clinical presentation that led to premature delivery.[18] Approximately 75 percent of preterm births occur "spontaneously" after preterm labor (PTL), preterm prematurely ruptured membranes (preterm PROM), or related diagnoses. (*PROM* refers to rupture of membranes before the onset of labor at *any* gestational age, hence the apparently re-

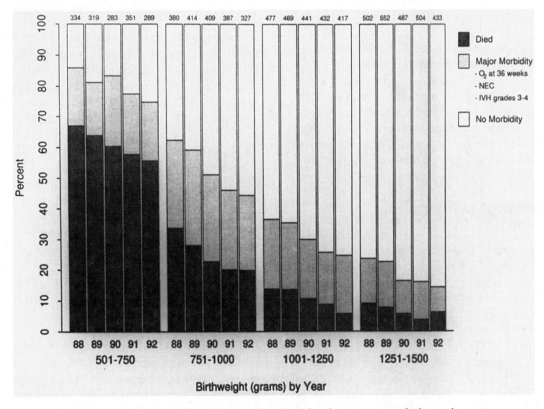

Fig. 23-8. Change in neonatal mortality and survival with and without major morbidity in the NICHD Neonatal Network between 1988 and 1992. NEC, necrotizing enterocolitis; IVH, intraventricular hemorrhage. (From Fanaroff et al,[9] with permission.)

Table 23-1   Morbidity and Survival to 120 Days of Life According to Obstetrical Gestational Age

Weeks	Obstetric Estimate of Gestational Age					
	21	22	23	24	25	26
Number	42	72	97	121	127	110
Intrapartum death (%)	19	14	11	2	1	0
Survived to 120 days (%)	3	18	30	48	70	75
Major Morbidity at 120 days (%)	100	73	62	68	51	48

(From Bottoms et al.[12], with permission.)

dundant *preterm PROM*). The *spontaneous preterm delivery* category also includes deliveries after amnionitis, with or without preterm PROM, and, for reasons that will become clear later in the chapter, patients with "incompetent" cervix. Complications of PTL and preterm PROM may lead to an "indication" for delivery (e.g., intrauterine infection), but these births are nevertheless termed *spontaneous* because they follow spontaneous PTL or preterm PROM. *Indicated preterm births* follow medical or obstetric disorders that place the fetus at risk (e.g., acute or chronic maternal hypertension, diabetes, placenta previa or abruption, and intrauterine growth restriction). Indicated preterm births account for 20 to 30 percent of births before 37 weeks in most series.[18] Prevention of indicated premature deliveries is based on prevention and treatment of the underlying disease to avert the consequent preterm delivery.

The distinction between indicated and spontaneous preterm births can be difficult and seemingly arcane clinically (see later), but the distinction is useful conceptually because it has led to a model of spontaneous preterm birth in which a common conceptual pathway explains and relates several conditions previously thought to be largely unrelated. The remainder of this chapter is focused on spontaneous prematurity, the principal unsolved problem in obstetrics.

The Epidemiology of Spontaneous Preterm Birth

Although the list of risk factors associated with PTL and preterm PROM is extensive, more than one-half of spontaneous preterm births (SPTBs) occur in women who have no *apparent* risk factors. The risk factors commonly associated with SPTB have relatively high prevalences in the population and consequently a low predictive value for SPTB. Efforts to create scoring systems to identify pregnancies with increased risk of SPTB based on epidemiologic risk factors have faltered for this reason. The prematurity prediction scoring system most widely studied[19,20] was able to identify two-thirds of preterm births in a middle-class population in San Francisco, but did not perform as well when employed in indigent populations with higher prevalence rates of factors related to preterm delivery.[21]

Risk factors are similar for PTL and preterm PROM, with just a few exceptions. Women with preterm PROM are more likely to be indigent,[18] more likely to smoke,[22,23] and more likely to have experienced bleeding in the current pregnancy[24] than are women who present with preterm labor (Table 23-2).

Both preterm PROM and PTL are more common among women who are indigent, poorly nourished, black, or have a history of genital infection, in particular bacterial vaginosis. In parous women, the risk of SPTB is increased by a history of prior preterm delivery. The recurrence risk rises as the number of prior preterm births increases and increases still further as the gestational age of the prior preterm birth decreases (Table 23-3).

Although the exact mechanisms of SPTB are not yet fully understood, the ultimate result may be premature initiation of labor, rupture of the amniotic sac, or, less commonly, intra-amniotic infection or a clinical presentation of incompetent cervix. The final clinical presentation as PTL or preterm PROM, and the epidemiologic characteristics of the women who experience SPTB, are clues to understanding how these clinical endpoints occur. Risk factors associated with SPTB in univariate surveys are numerous and diverse, ranging from medical and obstetric factors to socioeconomic status and race. The list can be confusing if each risk factor is considered individually, but when they are evaluated as potential pieces of a larger puzzle, plausible theories of pathogenesis have begun to emerge. Investigation of the potential relation of such clues has led investigators to see many of the clinical presentations of spontaneous prematurity as different faces of the same underlying disease process.

It is helpful to look at risk factors as either unique to the affected pregnancy and therefore nonrecurrent or as potentially operative in successive pregnancies. Risk factors such as placenta previa and abruption, polyhydramnios and oligohydramnios, second-trimester bleeding, and multiple gestation typically are not recurrent. Risk factors that may be expected to influence

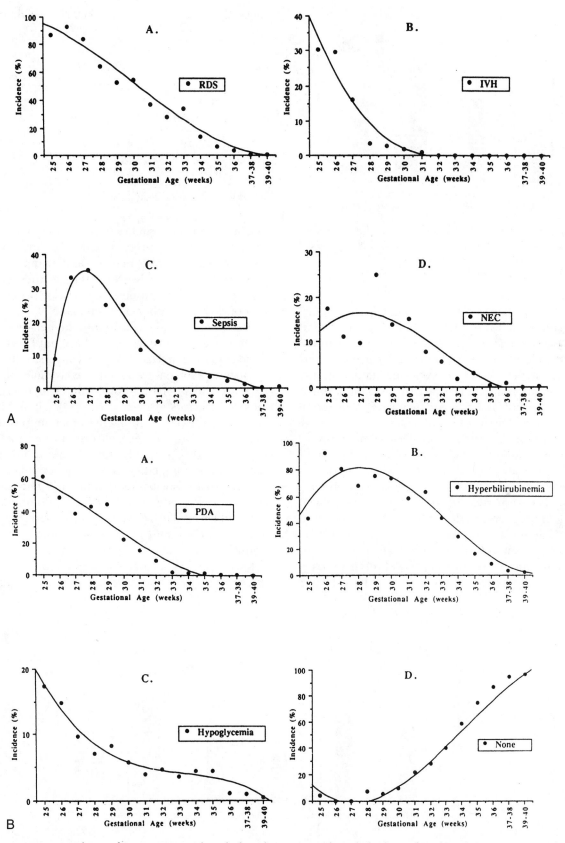

Fig. 23-9. Incidence of various neonatal morbidities by gestational age at birth in infants born between 1982 and 1986 in a five-center prospective trial. (A) Rates of (A) respiratory distress syndrome (RDS; A), intraventricular hemorrhage (IVH; B) sepsis (C), and; necrotizing enterocolitis (NEC; D). (B) Rates of (A) patent ductus arteriosus (PDA; A), hyperbilirubinemia (B), hypoglycemia (C), and of no morbidity (D). (From Robertson et al,[16] with permission.)

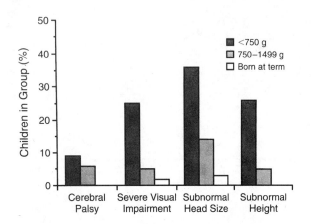

Fig. 23-10. Percentage of children with cerebral palsy, severe visual impairment, subnormal head size, and subnormal height in infants born less than 750 g birth weight, 750 to 1,499 g birth weight, and at term. (From Hack et al,[2] with permission.)

Table 23-2 Risk Factors for Preterm Delivery and Preterm PROM (Relative Risks, with 95% CI)

Preterm	PROM	Preterm Delivery Without PROM
Prior preterm delivery	6.3 (1.9–21)	21.0 (4–105)
Smoking	4.9 (1.5–16.8)	2.9 (0.6–12)
Bleeding		
1st Trimester	0.8 (0.2–2.4)	1.8 (0.2–13)
2nd Trimester	15.1 (2.8–81)	19.7 (2.1–186)
3rd Trimester	4.6 (0.9–17)	1.5 (0.4–5.4)

(From Ekwo et al.,[24] with permission.)

successive pregnancies may be immutable (e.g., a history of preterm delivery, black race) or as recurrent but potentially amenable to intervention (e.g., maternal genital tract infection and/or colonization, reduced cervical competence, low socioeconomic status, uterine malformations, limited prenatal care visits, poor nutritional status and low prepregnancy weight, maternal work, and sexual activity).

Recurrent and immutable risk factors may provide clues to the etiology of SPTB: an obstetric history of preterm birth and black race are the two most frequently noted (Table 23-4). A history of prior preterm birth predicts recurrent SPTB in 15 to 80 percent of subsequent pregnancies, depending on the population studied. The most recent birth is the most predictive. For example, among women pregnant for the third time, those whose first infant was delivered preterm and whose second infant was born at term have a lower

risk in the third pregnancy than do women whose most recent delivery was preterm. The likelihood of recurrent preterm birth also increases as the number of prior preterm births increase. Nevertheless, these data sets also show that most women with a prior preterm birth do not deliver another preterm baby.

Black women have consistently higher rates of preterm delivery, for reasons that have until recently defined explanation. Data from the University of Alabama at Birmingham have opened new avenues of inquiry to address this persistent problem. Goldenberg et al[27] looked at factors associated with LBW in 1,029 black and 462 white parous indigent women in Alabama and found that black women delivered preterm and LBW infants more frequently than white women, even though white indigent women in the population studied had greater sociodemographic risk. The study concluded that sociodemographic factors commonly cited as the likely explanation for the increased incidence of low birth weight and prematurity in blacks are in fact unlikely to be causative.

Recurrent risk factors that are potentially treatable offer information about etiology and also suggest po-

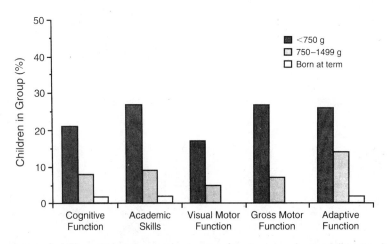

Fig. 23-11. Percentage of children with subnormal cognitive function, academic skills, visual and gross motor function, and adaptive function in infants born less than 750 gram birth weight, 750 to 1,499 g birth weight, and at term. (From Hack et al,[2] with permission.)

Table 23-3   Incidence of SPTB According to Gestational Age of Prior SPTB in Women with a Previous SPTB

Gestational Age at Prior SPTB	Current Pregnancy Outcome: % SPTB and (Relative Risk)			
	SPTB ≤ 28	SPTB ≤ 30	SPTB ≤ 32	SPTB ≤ 35
None	0.2%	0.4%	0.8%	2.6%
23–27 weeks	7.0 (34.5)*	7.0 (17.3)*	14 (17.3)*	26 (9.7)*
28–34 weeks	3.2 (16.0)*	4.0 (10.0)*	5.7 (7.0)*	15.3 (5.8)*
35–36 weeks	1.5 (7.3)	1.5 (3.6)	2.9 (3.6)	13.2 (5.0)*

*$p < 0.001$.
(From Mercer et al.,[25] with permission.)

tential avenues of treatment. A reduction in preterm birth in an interventional trial would suggest that the risk factor being eliminated or reduced had an important causal role. No such trial has been reported. In fact, unifactorial interventional trials have reported almost completely unsuccessful results: programs to reduce or eliminate the risk of uterine contractions, cervical competence, social stress, smoking, access to prenatal care, maternal physical activity and employment, coitus and/or orgasm, nutritional status and weight gain in pregnancy, and maternal genital tract infection and/or colonization have all been targets of unsuccessful interventional trials. Does this mean that these risks are factitious? Perhaps, but the failure of unifactorial interventions to reduce prematurity rates is more likely due to simplistic unifactorial theories of pathogenesis that are being replaced by the understanding of spontaneous prematurity as a syndrome of collaborative and continuous risk factors. Since the last edition of this text, there have been several new themes that link risk factors previously thought to be unrelated.

Decidual Ischemia and Prematurity

The distinction between *spontaneous* and *indicated* preterm births is predicated on the assumption that fetal growth and well-being have been satisfactory before the spontaneous occurrence of uncomplicated preterm labor or preterm PROM. Although most data support this general assumption, there are contrary observations indicating that the prevalence of poor intrauterine growth is increased among prematurely born infants, even in the absence of apparent maternal disease.[28–31] These clinical observations have been supported first by pathologic studies[32–34] and later by Doppler velocimetry evaluation of uterine artery systolic/diastolic (S/D) ratios showing increased impedance in the uterine arteries of women who delivered after PTL.[35] Salafia et al[32] studied placentas from preterm births between 22 and 32 weeks and found decidual vascular abnormalities significantly more often than in controls (odds ratio [OR], 4.1, 95 percent; confidence interval [CI], 2.3 to 7.4). In a case–control study, Arias et al[33] also found that placental vascular lesions were significantly more common in the placentas from noninfected women who delivered after PTL than in controls (OR, 3.8, 95 percent CI, 1.3 to 11.1) Lockwood[36] has postulated that the contribution of fetal stress to the onset of PTL may be mediated and accelerated by uteroplacental corticotropin-releasing hormone (CRH), a peptide produced by the placenta, amniochorion, and decidua and known to enhance prostanoid production in the same cells. These reports provide a convincing and biologically plausible mechanism by which abnormalities of the placenta and uteroplacental blood flow may lead to SPTB, either directly

Table 23-4   Risk of Preterm Birth According to Obstetric History

First Birth	Second Birth	Number	Subsequent/Preterm Birth	
			Percent	Relative Risk
Term	—	25,817	4.4	1.0
Preterm	—	1,860	17.2	3.9
Term	Term	24,689	2.6	0.6
Preterm	Term	1,540	5.7	1.3
Term	Preterm	1,128	11.1	2.5
Preterm	Preterm	320	28.4	6.5

(From Bakketeig and Hoffman,[26] with permission.)

through decidual and/or membrane injury or indirectly by inducing fetal stress.

Infection and Prematurity

There have been numerous reports, some dating back more than four decades, of an association between preterm birth and infection.[37,38] The first lines of evidence were clinical. Positive amniotic fluid cultures have been reported in 20 to 30 percent of women with preterm labor[39–41] and especially in women whose preterm labor was refractory to tocolytic drugs.[42] The incidences of maternal and neonatal infections following preterm birth is higher than for term birth. In fact, the association between both clinical infection and histologic amnionitis increases as the gestational age at delivery decreases, especially before 30 to 32 weeks.[43]

Microbiologic studies have observed an association between preterm birth and maternal vaginal colonization with various microflora, including bacterial vaginosis, group B streptococcus, *C. trachomatis*, and *Trichomonas*. Increasingly, the attention of investigators and clinicians has turned to the persistent association between maternal bacterial vaginosis and increased risk of spontaneous preterm birth.[44–46] Rather than a specific infection caused by a single organism, bacterial vaginosis is now understood as an alteration of the maternal vaginal flora in which the normally predominant lactobacillus is largely replaced by gram-negative anaerobic bacteria such as *Gardnerella vaginalis*, *Bacteroides*, *Prevotella*, *Mobiluncus* species, and *Mycoplasma* species. The association between bacterial vaginosis and prematurity has been noted in microbiologic, histologic, and clinical studies. Gravett et al[47] noted that women who tested positive for bacterial vaginosis in the second and third trimesters had an increased risk of PTL (OR, 2.0; 95 percent CI, 1.1 to 3.5), preterm PROM (OR, 2.0; CI, 1.1 to 3.7), and intra-amniotic infection (OR, 2.7; CI, 1.1 to 6.1). Bacteria isolated from women with bacterial vaginosis may produce proteases and collagenases that are capable of injuring fetal membranes and affecting the likelihood of membrane rupture.[48] Meis et al[49] studied the association of vaginal colonization with bacterial vaginosis and *Trichomonas* and SPTB in 2,929 women. There was no relationship between *Trichomonas* and prematurity, but maternal colonization with bacterial vaginosis at 28 weeks was significantly associated with SPTB (OR, 1.85, 95 percent CI, 1.15 to 2.95; $p < 0.01$).

Infections, Contractions, and the Cervix

Given the high prevalence of maternal lower genital colonization with bacterial vaginosis (10 to 40 percent) and other microorganisms, why does spontaneous prematurity occur in some but not most colonized gravi-

dae? Is the association causal, or is it incidental to some other process? The maternal inflammatory response to genital tract colonization may vary according to the number and invasive properties of the microorganisms and the maternal immunologic function in general. In particular, host defenses that fail to prevent colonization of the *upper* tract may allow microbial growth at the decidual membrane interface and thus trigger a host response at that site that results in production of cytokines and eventually in labor or preterm PROM. But how and when do bacteria in the lower genital tract reach the intrauterine environment? There are two current theories:

1. One theory is that uterine contractions open the cervix, allowing ascent of organisms into the uterus only *after* the process has been initiated by an idiopathic increase in contractions. This theory argues that PTL occurs as the result of the loss of hormonal inhibition of natural uterine contractile activity that leads to cervical ripening and ultimately to cervical dilatation and effacement. Inflammation noted in the membranes of women delivered preterm is seen not as the cause but rather as the result of the increase in contractions.[50]

2. An alternate theory[51] places uterine contractions at the *end* of a process in which cytokines produced by the host response to microorganisms in the decidua act to initiate prostaglandin production, which leads to cervical ripening and uterine contractions. This theory fits well with the multifactorial model of spontaneous prematurity advanced throughout this chapter but does not explain *how* and *when* the microorganisms arrive at the membrane–decidual interface. An ascending route from the vagina through the cervix is consistent with data showing relationships between both cervical dilatation[52–54] and cervical length and the risk of SPTB.[55,56] These studies support a "host defense" role for the cervix and cervical mucus as a barrier to the ascent of bacteria during pregnancy. Another suggested explanation for the presence of microorganisms within the uterus has been based in part on the work of Korn et al[57] who observed a chronic plasma cell endometritis in endometrial biopsy specimens from 10 of 22 women with bacterial vaginosis compared with only 1 of 19 controls (OR, 15, 95 percent CI, 2 to 686). The chronicity of bacterial vaginosis colonization of the endometrium has led Goldenberg et al[58,59] to the intriguing hypothesis of a chronic intrauterine infection of the endometrium with bacterial vaginosis *before conception*, with subsequent proliferation of these low-virulence organisms within the uterus in the altered immune environment of pregnancy. This pathway is supported as well by the observation[60] of increased

levels of amniotic fluid tumor necrosis factor-α, a cytokine released in response to inflammation or ischemia, in samples obtained at *mid-trimester* genetic amniocentesis from women who experienced spontaneous PTL weeks later.

Rather than viewing these theories as competing and mutually exclusive, the model of SPTB advanced in this chapter allows multiple mechanisms to participate to variable degrees in the steps preceding preterm birth. This model has been given additional support by results from a large prospective study of multiple risk factors in a single population, the NICHD Preterm Birth Prediction Study, a prospective observational study of risk factors for SPTB that collected demographic and medical–obstetric information about nearly 3,000 subjects who were representative of the population at 10 participating university centers. Multiple potential risk factors, including serial cervical and vaginal cultures,[49] digital and transvaginal ultrasound examination of the cervix,[56] and an assay for the presence of oncofetal fibronectin (fFN) in cervical and vaginal secretions[61] were obtained at regular intervals between 24 and 34 weeks of pregnancy. Fibronectin is an extracellular matrix protein that is best described as the "glue" that attaches the fetal membranes to the underlying uterine decidua.[62] Fibronectin is normally found in the cervicovaginal secretions before 20 to 22 weeks of pregnancy and again at the end of normal pregnancy as labor approaches. It is not normally present in cervicovaginal secretions between 22 and 37 weeks.

This study has elucidated interrelationships of the epidemiologic and current pregnancy risk factors discussed previously.[61] The study confirmed univariate associations of SPTB with black race, maternal nutritional status (expressed as a body mass index less than $19.8/m^2$),[63] bacterial vaginosis diagnosed by a Gram's stain score[64] of 7 or more, and pH above 4.5, cervical dilatation and effacement expressed as a Bishop score, vaginal bleeding, self-reported frequent uterine contractions, history of prior pelvic infection, and prior SPTB. Characteristics that were *not* associated with SPTB in this study included maternal age less than 18, educational level, obstetric conditions other than bleeding, urinary tract infection, smoking, drug and alcohol use, prior first and second trimester abortions, symptoms of pelvic pressure, and most medical conditions.[58]

Multivariate analysis revealed that the strongest predictors of SPTB were cervicovaginal fFN,[59] transvaginal sonographic cervical length,[56] an obstetric history of previous preterm birth,[25] and presence of bacterial vaginosis,[49] respectively. The presence of fibronectin is a marker of disruption of the decidual–chorionic interface and thus is not itself etiologic. Its presence in cervicovaginal secretions has predictive value for delivery within 14 days of sampling. Interestingly, fFN was strongly correlated with the presence of bacterial vaginosis, almost completely predicting which subjects with bacterial vaginosis were at risk for SPTB. Twenty percent of the NICHD study population had bacterial vaginosis. Of the bacterial vaginosis positive women who delivered prematurely (3 percent of the total population), almost all were fFN positive, suggesting that bacterial vaginosis either causes or is a marker for disruption of the choriodecidual interface in subjects with bacterial vaginosis.[65]

In the NICHD study, sonographic cervical length and obstetric history were also strongly and continuously correlated with each other and with the risk of SPTB in a *continuous* manner.[58] That is, for subjects with a history of prior SPTB, the risk of recurrent SPTB increased as the gestational age at the time of the prior PTB decreased. The length of the cervix as measured by transvaginal sonography was inversely and continuously related to the likelihood of SPTB in the current pregnancy and to a history of SPTB, especially for SPTB before 32 weeks' gestation. This study and others[55,66] indicate that cervical length is a marker for the functional ability of the cervix to resist delivery and that cervical competence operates as a continuum. This view is a major departure from the previous understanding of the cervix as a categorical rather than a continuous variable (i.e., either competent or incompetent) and has changed our understanding of the contribution of the cervix to spontaneous preterm delivery: if the cervix is a structure with degrees of "competence," then cervical incompetence may not be a distinct and uncommon disorder, but instead may be viewed as the end of a spectrum. The impact of these new studies is further discussed in the section on abnormal cervical competence.

The Spontaneous Preterm Birth Syndrome

The information in the preceding paragraphs has been integrated into a basic model for the majority of SPTB. Romero et al[51] have termed this the *preterm labor syndrome*. In this model, the fetal membranes and decidua, in response to an inflammatory insult—usually infectious or ischemic, but occasionally traumatic or even "allergic" in origin (delayed-type hypersensitivity-like immune responses[67]—produce cytokines (tumor necrosis factor-α [TNFα], interleukin-1 [IL-1], and interleukin 6 [IL-6]). These cytokines then elicit the elaboration of uterotonic bioactive lipids (prostaglandin E_2, prostaglandin $F_{2\alpha}$, thromboxane A_2, leukotrienes B_4 and C_4,[68] 5-HETE [hydroperoxyeicosotetraenoic acid], and others) that stimulate myometrial contractions and may ini-

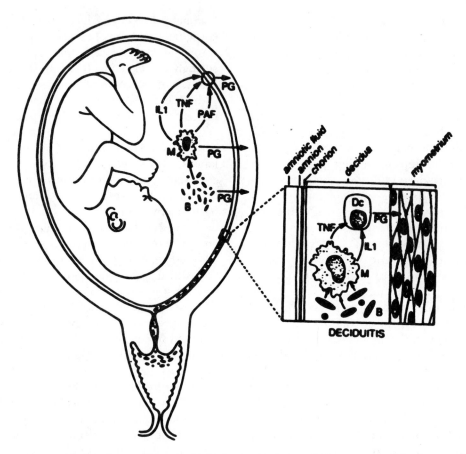

Fig. 23-12. Model of ascending microbial infection leading to SPTB as proposed by Romero.[51]

tiate release of proteases that are capable of injuring the membranes and underlying decidua, finally resulting via prostaglandin stimulation in cervical ripening, dilatation, and/or membrane rupture (Fig. 23-12).

Whether an inflammatory insult actually leads to preterm delivery is influenced by the intensity and dura-

tion of the insult, the gestational age at the time of insult, and the host response to the injury. The gestational age is important, because the responsiveness of the uterus to stimulation increases with gestational age, especially after 30 to 32 weeks. We have found the relationship depicted in Figure 23-13 to be useful to under-

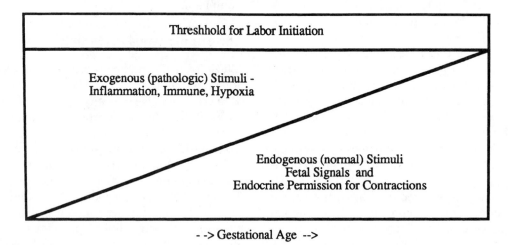

Fig. 23-13. Hypothetical model of combined influence of multiple exogenous and endogenous stimuli leading to SPTB.

standing the various possible interactions that may reach or exceed a hypothetical "threshold" required to establish labor. The exogenous stimulus required to reach this hypothetical threshold decreases as pregnancy progresses closer to term, when endogenous factors presumed to derive from both mother (e.g., maternal uterine contraction frequency, estrogen, and progesterone levels) and fetus (maturity-related signals, e.g., epidermal growth factor) are sufficient to cause normal labor.[69] In some cases, a single risk factor may by itself create sufficient stimulation to reach the threshold required for initiation of labor or rupture of membranes, but such factors are rare: overwhelming maternal sepsis and extreme uterine distention due to higher order multifetal gestation or severe polyhydramnios are two. More commonly, exogenous and endogenous factors combine to create a sufficient stimulus for labor or amniorrhexis.

A Model for the Pathogenesis and Treatment of SPTB

Recurrent SPTB is best understood as a syndrome of multiple interactive risk factors that operate synergistically and repeatedly to produce premature labor, preterm PROM, amnionitis, or cervical incompetence. This syndrome is analagous to atherosclerotic cardiovascular disease. Integrating the findings of the NICHD Preterm Prediction study with previous literature, a model of the pathogenesis of SPTB has been postulated that is analogous to the current understanding of the pathogenesis, treatment, and prevention of atherosclerotic cardiovascular disease (ASCVD).[70] In the case of ASCVD, the clinical endpoint is complete or partial occlusion of a vessel; in the case of SPTB, the clinical endpoint is sufficient "injury" or stimulus to the fetoplacental unit to trigger labor or membrane rupture. That ASCVD is a disease caused by the interaction of multiple contributing continuous variables is no longer controversial, but use of this model in perinatal medicine represents a departure from traditional obstetric assumptions in that risk factors are viewed as continuous and collaborative, not as absolute and independent. For example, in the cardiovascular model, a myocardial infarction is just one of several potential presenting complaints that occur as the result of occlusion of cardiac vessels. Other clinical presentations such as angina without infarction or rhythm disturbances are also the result of a common pathophysiology, one in which multiple continuous and potentially mutable variables, e.g., LDL cholesterol, blood pressure, cigarette smoking, and blood glucose, act together to increase risk of disease in an epidemiologic setting of immutable variables such as family history, age, and gender. In any individual patient, some risk factors play a greater role than others; some are uncommon, but powerful when present; others, like smoking, are relatively weak in an individual but are so common that the attributable risk for the population is great. In the obstetric example of spontaneous prematurity, the continuous variables are uterine volume, uterine contraction frequency, microbial colonization of the lower and upper genital tract, hypoxic or hemorrhagic injury to the fetal–maternal interface, fetal paracrine signals for labor that are gestational age related, and host resistance to labor, including cervical "competence" and resistance to infection.

Preterm labor and PROM are not "idiopathic" events that just "happen." The increased contractions we call preterm labor occur for a reason. The cervix softens and thins for a reason. Membranes rupture for a reason. Successful treatment requires a search for the reason in each patient.

Prevention and Treatment of Preterm Birth

Prevention and treatment strategies for SPTB may also be compared to those employed for atherosclerosis, using the concepts of tertiary, secondary, and primary care.[71–73]

Tertiary care is treatment of an individual patient *after* the diagnosis has been made. Tertiary care has no effect on the incidence of the disease, but rather is aimed at reducing morbidity and mortality after an index illness has occurred. For SPTB, tertiary care includes prompt diagnosis and referral to the appropriate care site, treatment of the primary diagnosis with appropriate medication (e.g., tocolytic drugs for PTL or antibiotics for amnionitis), and ancillary treatments such as corticosteroids to reduce neonatal mortality and morbidity.

Secondary care selects individuals with increased risk for surveillance and/or prophylactic treatment. Key steps in secondary care are identification of the appropriate group of subjects to receive special care and the availability of effective intervention measures to prevent or reduce risk. For SPTB, secondary care efforts have included risk scoring systems, early diagnosis programs (patient education programs, frequent contact with a special nurse, and ambulatory uterine activity monitoring), prophylactic medications (e.g., tocolytic drugs, progesterone supplementation, antibiotics), and reduced activity.

Primary care is the elimination or reduction of risk in an entire population. Effective primary care requires a good understanding of the pathophysiology of the disease and public health educational efforts to modify behaviors and eliminate risk factors. ASCVD has reached this level of care in that the media are active participants

Synthesis of Clinical, Epidemiologic, and Basic Information about SPTB

Resistance to labor
  Endocrine milieu: local progesterone as smooth muscle relaxant versus estrogen as stimulant (endocrine "permission" for contractions increases with gestational age)
  Cervical resistance a continuous variable

Stimuli for labor
  Normal
    Maternal—estrogen increases
    Fetal endogenous signals—also increase with gestational age
  Abnormal
    Inflammatory—infection, immune, hypoxia (stimulation via cytokines of endogenous prostaglandins)

Preterm labor = Synthesis of stimuli versus resistance
  Spontaneous preterm delivery is the result of interplay of multiple *continuous* variables
    Uterine volume
    Uterine contraction frequency in normal pregnancy
    Microbial/ischemic/inflammatory stimuli
    Host resistance—cervical competence as a continuum, both structural and immune

A multifactorial disease with multiple clinical presentations
  Preterm labor
  Preterm PROM
  Premature cervical effacement/dilatation or "competence"

Analogous to atherosclerotic cardiovascular disease

in educating the public about diet and life style choices to reduce risk of cardiovascular disease. For SPTB, the population is clear (women of childbearing age), but effective primary interventions have not been demonstrated. The contents of a public health program to reduce prematurity have not been fully elucidated but will certainly include some or all of the following:

Smoking and STD prevention

Fertility management to avoid higher order multifetal gestation

Planned pregnancy

Policies for women in the workforce that allow individually variable work schedules

Physical and sexual activity advice

A cervical assessment at 20 to 26 weeks

Tertiary Care

Diagnosis and Treatment of Spontaneous Preterm Birth

Clinical Assessment of Spontaneous Vs. Indicated Preterm Delivery

The distinction between indicated and spontaneous prematurity, although helpful in understanding the pathogenesis of prematurity, is often very difficult to apply in practice. The clinical presentation of several serious maternal or fetal disorders may mimic spontaneous PTL or preterm PROM. Therefore, the clinical evaluation of a patient with apparent preterm labor or ruptured membranes begins with a search for the underlying cause of PTL or preterm PROM and an assessment of fetal well-being. For example, PTL labor and preterm PROM accompanied by abnormal amniotic fluid volume and/or bleeding may be especially difficult to categorize as either spontaneous or indicated. In a patient with polyhydramnios, was PTL the result of preexisting polyhydramnios caused by a fetal anomaly or by an intrauterine viral infection? Does the patient with light bleeding and oligohydramnios have spontaneously ruptured membranes, or is the oligohydramnios caused by a fetal renal anomaly? The distinction is important not only for the management of the current pregnancy, but also for the care of future pregnancies. SPTB is an obstetric syndrome with a recurrence risk that increases as the gestational age at the time of presentation decreases.[25] In contrast, the recurrence risk of PTL or preterm PROM due to polyhydramnios is the recurrence risk of the underlying cause of the abnormal fluid volume. Key features of the history that suggest diagnoses other than SPTB include a history of first or second trimester bleeding in the current pregnancy (may indicate a blighted second twin), elevation of the maternal serum α-fetoprotein (may indicate fetal anomaly or, if no anomaly is found, may have been caused by occult intrauterine bleeding), and fetal death at presentation (PTL and preterm PROM with fetal demise are rare; aneuploidy, structural anomalies, and maternal connective tissue or hypertensive disorders should be suspected).

Clinical decision-making for patients with impending preterm delivery is based on a careful assessment of the risks for both mother and infant of continuing the pregnancy versus delivery. Decisions made prior to SPTB typically focus on assessment of risks for the infant, but maternal interests must always be considered.

Premature Birth and Assessment of Fetal Maturity

The principal goal of tertiary care of PTL and preterm PROM is to reduce perinatal morbidity and mortality, most of which is caused by immaturity of the respiratory, gastrointestinal, coagulation, and central nervous systems of the premature infant. Although not the only determinant of neonatal morbidity and mortality, pulmonary immaturity is the most frequent cause of serious newborn illness and death and is the only organ system whose function is directly testable before delivery. Assessment of fetal pulmonary maturity by amniotic fluid studies or other means is consequently an important part of the evaluation of the patient with impending preterm delivery. If the quality of obstetric dating is good and intrauterine fetal well-being is not compromised, the likelihood of neonatal respiratory distress syndrome can often be satisfactorily estimated from the gestational age (Fig. 23-9).

The need to assess fetal pulmonary maturity directly through studies of amniotic fluid is greater in two settings: First, when dates are uncertain (e.g., fetal size larger than expected for dates, suggesting a more advanced gestation or maternal glucose intolerance; or size less than expected, suggesting fetal growth restriction) and, second, when fetal jeopardy is not now present (prompt delivery would be indicated) but may occur during the remaining days or weeks of pregnancy (e.g., when membranes have ruptured, fetal heart rate patterns are nonreassuring, or growth restriction is suspected). Occasionally, amniocentesis may be indicated for studies in addition to fetal lung maturity (e.g., fetal karyotype in cases of PTL complicated by polyhydramnios; culture, glucose, and Gram stain when amnionitis is suspected).

Diagnosis of Preterm Labor

The diagnosis of PTL is traditionally made by the combination of persistent uterine contractions and change in the dilatation and/or effacement of the cervix by digital examination.[74] However, the accuracy of these criteria is poor. Randomized trials of drugs to arrest PTL have found that approximately 40 percent of subjects diagnosed by these criteria and treated with placebo will deliver at term,[75] indicating a large number of false-positive diagnoses. The high rate of false-positive diagnoses has been justified in the past by the need for early detection and treatment because of studies showing that as many as 25 to 50 percent of women with PTL are diagnosed after the membranes have rup-

tured or the cervix has dilated beyond 3 cm, when successful tocolysis is unlikely. The consequence of this approach to diagnosis has been the unnecessary treatment of women with persistent uterine activity who do not actually have PTL. On the other hand, false-negative diagnosis is also a significant problem. One study found an 18 percent rate of preterm birth in women who were sent home without treatment after evaluation for possible PTL.[76]

Difficulty in accurate diagnosis is the product of the high prevalence of the symptoms and signs of early PTL among normal healthy women and the imprecision of the digital examination of the cervix. Symptoms of PTL are nonspecific, and, it is important to note, *are not necessarily those of labor at term*. Women treated for PTL may report symptoms of pelvic pressure, an increase in vaginal discharge, backache, and menstrual-like cramps, all of which may occur in normal pregnancy. Contractions may be painful or painless and may be distinguished from the normal contractions of pregnancy (Braxton-Hicks contractions) only by their persistence. Two prospective studies of the symptoms of PTL[54,77] found that symptoms were poorly predictive because of the common occurrence of the same symptoms in women without PTL (Fig. 23-14).

Contraction frequency can also be misleading. A prospective study[78] of uterine contractions in normal pregnancies in 109 low-risk subjects, who all delivered at term and who were monitored for 24 hours twice weekly from 20 weeks until delivery, found a wide variation in contraction frequency according to gestational age and time of day (Fig. 23-15). A strong clustering of contractions occurred at night and became more pronounced after 24 weeks. The night:day ratio of contractions per hour was 1.8:1 at 21 to 24 weeks, 2.3:1 at 28 to 32 weeks, and 2.0:1 at 38 to 40 weeks ($p < 0.001$) Uterine contraction frequency was decreased following maternal rest and increased after coitus in this study. Prior to 37 weeks' gestation, as many as seven contractions per hour fell within 2 SD above the 95th percentile, depending on the time of day. An occasional patient had more than 15 contractions per hour, yet still delivered at term. Therefore, contraction frequency alone can be seen to be insufficient to establish the diagnosis of PTL. Too often, women who have frequent contractions are treated with oral or even parenteral medication, usually terbutaline, without waiting for overt cervical change or other definitive evidence of labor. This practice reduces contraction frequency but does nothing to establish the diagnosis of PTL and often leads to unnecessary oral "prophylaxis" of recurrent contractions in otherwise normal pregnancies. Recent improvements in diagnostic accuracy for PTL should result in fewer women receiving unnecessary medication.

Although digital assessment of cervical dilation of at

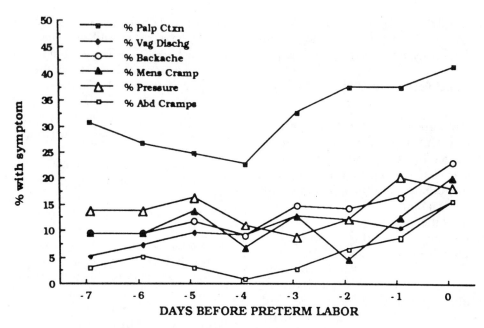

Fig. 23-14. Symptoms reported by 57 women with increased risk of preterm birth who were contacted daily during the 7 days prior to and on the day of the diagnosis of PTL. No individual symptom or combination of symptoms was predictive of impending PTL. Palp Ctxn, % who reported increased or persistent self-palpated contractions; Vag dischg, % who reported a change or increase in vaginal discharge; Backache, % who reported a persistent backache; Mens cramp, % who reported menstrual-like cramps; Pressure, % who reported abdominal or pelvic pressure; Abd Cramps, % who reported abdominal cramps. (From Iams et al,[77] with permission.)

least 3 cm is relatively straightforward, assessment of dilation of less than 3 cm, effacement, and cervical consistency (soft or firm) are highly subjective. Nevertheless, these early subtle changes in the cervix often form the basis of a diagnosis of PTL.[79] Copper et al[54] studied digital examination of high-risk patients and found that softening of the lower segment and effacement were more predictive of impending labor than were other features of the cervical examination, including

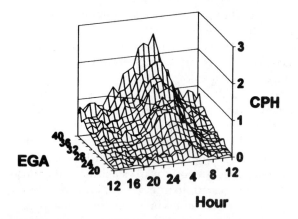

Fig. 23-15. Mean hourly frequency of monitored uterine contractions by gestational age and time of day in 109 normal pregnant women who delivered at term after uncomplicated pregnancies. (From Moore et al,[78] with permission.)

dilatation. Unfortunately, effacement is poorly reproducible among examiners.[80]

A number of studies have reported that failed tocolysis, defined as delivery within 24 to 48 hours despite tocolysis, was associated with cervical dilation above 3 cm at presentation. Thus patients with persistent contractions whose cervix is effaced at least 80 percent and dilated more than 2 cm should be treated without waiting for additional information. But what about women with lesser degrees of dilation? If cervical change detected by digital examination is not very reliable, except at the extremes, is it safe to wait for obvious cervical change before initiating treatment? A retrospective study of 209 patients with PTL[81] suggested that for patients whose initial digital examination was 2 cm or less there was no change in perinatal outcome if treatment was initiated only after obvious change in dilatation. An initial examination showing dilation of 3 or more cm was associated with failed tocolysis.

Patients with possible early PTL whose cervical dilation is less than 3 cm present a diagnostic challenge. Recently, two new methods of improving the accuracy of diagnosis in symptomatic women have been reported: transvaginal sonography to measure cervical length, and the presence of fetal fibronectin in cervicovaginal fluid. As described later in this chapter, both tests are also being evaluated as screening tests for risk of SPTB in asymptomatic women.

Cervical Sonography

Transabdominal sonographic measurement of cervical length is affected variably by maternal body habitus and bladder filling and is not possible in many patients. Transvaginal sonography performed with an empty maternal bladder is unaffected by maternal habitus and provides satisfactory images in more than 95 percent of subjects. The accuracy of PTL diagnosis has been improved with this technique (Fig. 23-16).[82,83] Cervical sonography appears to be useful in excluding preterm labor in some patients and in making a positive diagno-

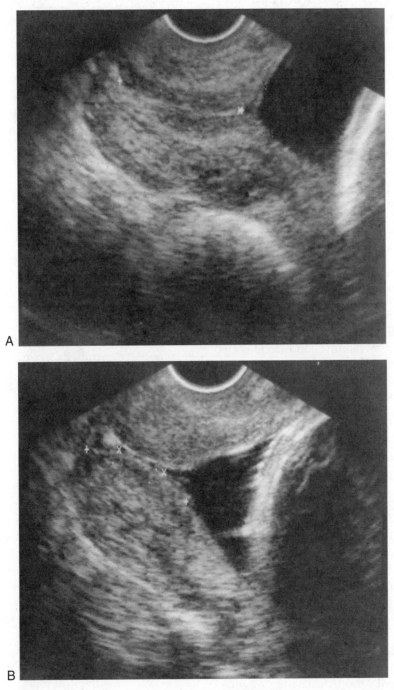

Fig. 23-16. (A) Transvaginal ultrasound image of the cervix at 28 weeks in normal pregnancy. Calipers (+) are placed at the notches marking the internal and external os, where the anterior and posterior walls of the cervical canal touch. (B) Transvaginal ultrasound image of the cervix at 28 weeks in a patient with preterm labor. The (X) calipers mark the length of the cervical canal that is used for clinical evaluation. The (+) calipers are placed at the outer edges of the cervix; this length is *not* useful clinically because of wide variation among patients (see Anderson et al[55] and Iams et al[56,82]).

sis in others. A cervical length of 30 mm or more by transvaginal sonography is good evidence that significant effacement has not occurred (30 mm is approximately the 25th percentile of length). In a study of 60 women with early PTL (dilation less than 3 cm) diagnosed by traditional criteria,[82] all 15 subjects whose sonographic cervical length was 30 mm or more delivered at term, and all 24 subjects who delivered preterm had cervical lengths less than 30 mm. Another study of 59 women with PTL and cervical dilation less than 3 cm employed transvaginal sonography before tocolysis was initiated and found that a sonographic length of 18 mm or less and funneling of the internal os were superior to digital examination in predicting which women would deliver preterm.[83] Cervical sonography is not available in every labor suite at present, but these studies suggest that it will be useful in the management of PTL, especially to allow avoidance or cessation of tocolysis in patients in whom contractions persist without evident cervical change and to evaluate patients whose contractions are accompanied by vaginal bleeding of uncertain origin.

Fibronectin

A clinical assay for fetal fibronectin was approved by the FDA in 1995 as an aid in the diagnosis of preterm labor. fFN is an extracellular matrix protein that is normally found in the fetal membranes and decidua. As the gestational sac implants and attaches to the interior of the uterus in the first half of pregnancy, fFN is normally found in cervicovaginal fluid. The presence of fFN in the cervix or vagina after the 20th week is abnormal and may indicate disruption of the attachment of the membranes to the decidua. Fibronectin reappears in cervicovaginal secretions as labor approaches at term. In contrast to other potential predictors of premature delivery such as obstetric history or frequent uterine contractions, the presence of fFN in cervicovaginal fluid provides direct evidence of current pathologic changes at the interface of fetal and maternal tissues. Lockwood and associates[84] collected cervicovaginal fluid and measured fFN by immunoassay using the monoclonal antibody FDC-6. They observed an association of preterm birth and fFN in 117 women with possible preterm labor, half of whom delivered before 37 weeks' gestation (Table 23-5).

Three subsequent studies[85–87] have found fibronectin to be superior to the traditional methods of diagnosis of PTL in predicting SPTB with 7 days of presentation. As can be seen in Table 23-6, fibronectin had superior sensitivity, specificity, and predictive values compared with contraction frequency, cervical dilation more than 1 cm, and vaginal bleeding.

When fibronectin results were compared in the same

Table 23-5 Fetal Fibronectin and Prediction of Preterm Birth <37 Weeks in Symptomatic Women[a]

Fetal Fibronectin	Delivery	
	<37 Weeks	>37 Weeks
Present	49	10
Absent	11	47
Total	60	57

[a] n = 117 symptomatic women with intact membranes and possible PTL. Sensitivity = 82%; specificity = 83%; Positive predictive value = 83%; Negative predictive value = 81%.

(From Lockwood et al,[84] with permission.)

study to a clinician's decision to use tocolysis, it can be seen (Table 23-7) that when used in women with cervical dilation less than 3 cm, the fibronectin assay improved both sensitivity and specificity.[88] Only 7 of the 14 women who delivered within 7 days received tocolysis; all 7 who did not receive tocolysis were missed by the clinician but were identified by fibronectin. Addition of the fibronectin assay to clinical decision-making in this population would have led to tocolytic treatment for 20 additional women (7 of whom delivered less than 7 days) and might have averted tocolysis in 60 women, only 1 of whom delivered within 7 days[85,88]

Peaceman et al[86] found similar results in a 10-center study of 763 symptomatic women, 129 of whom were diagnosed clinically as having PTL and treated with tocolysis. Of the 86 who were fibronectin negative, 3 (3.5 percent) delivered at 7 days or less (negative predictive value = 96.5 percent in a population of women diagnosed and treated for PTL). There were only 9 women who delivered within 7 days among the 634 symptomatic women who were not diagnosed with preterm labor, and all 9 were fibronectin positive. A companion trial was conducted in 200 symptomatic women at a center in which tocolysis was not employed.[87] The sensitivity, specificity, positive predictive value, and negative predictive value for delivery at 7 days or less in this setting were 62.5, 87.0, 16.7, and 98.2 percent, respectively. Three of 170 fibronectin-negative women (1.8 percent) delivered at 7 days or less at this center. The clinical utility of the fibronectin assay lies primarily in the negative predictive value as a test to avoid overdiagnosis and unnecessary treatment. It may also improve sensitivity by identifying additional women who may benefit from further observation and/or treatment. Based on these data presented to the FDA, the fibronectin assay was approved for use as an aid to the accurate diagnosis of PTL in women who present with symptoms and a cervical dilation less than 3 cm. Fibronectin may have additional clinical utility as a screen for risk of spontaneous prematurity in asymptomatic women.

Table 23-6   Comparison of Fibronectin to Other Predictors of Delivery Within 7 Days[a]

| Predictor | Sensitivity | Specificity | Predictive Value | |
			Positive	Negative
Fibronectin	93	82	29	99
Vaginal bleeding	36	89	21	97
Cervix >1 cm	29	82	11	94
Contractions				
≥4/hr	58	45	7	94
≥8/hr	42	67	9	94

[a]n = 192 women with possible PTL and cervix <3 cm.
(From Iams et al,[85] with permission.)

Experience with combined use of the fibronectin assay and cervical sonography in clinical practice is limited, but suggests that the two tests are complementary. A positive fibronectin assay indicates the presence of an acute process that may lead to SPTB within 7 to 14 days in 15 to 30 percent of symptomatic women, while sonographic cervical length measurement correlates best with risk of SPTB at less than 35 weeks. Fibronectin appears to be the better test for acute risk: the presence of fibronectin indicates that the membrane–decidual interface has been injured and that a pathologic process is currently present. The likelihood that this process will in fact progress to preterm birth may in part be a function of the sonographic cervical length. A positive fibronectin assay is more likely to be associated with delivery in women with a short cervix. Both a long cervix (more than 30 mm by transvaginal ultrasound) and a negative fibronectin assay have excellent negative predictive value for preterm delivery in symptomatic women. A short cervix with a negative fibronectin assay suggests that labor is not currently present, but would be difficult to arrest if it did occur. These impressions have been confirmed by a recent study in Italy.[89]

The suggested protocol for evaluation and treatment of women with possible PTL in the box below incorporates fibronectin into current clinical care patterns and should always be preceded by an evaluation of the etiology of SPTB. Transvaginal sonography can be used as an adjunctive test in patients with persistent contractions and cervical dilation of 2 cm or less. Because of variation introduced by maternal bladder filling, transabdominal sonography is not sufficiently reproducible to be useful.

To summarize, the diagnosis of preterm labor is often uncertain, and, as can be seen in the next section, the treatment is not always benign. To increase the sensitivity of diagnosis without treating unnecessarily, it is best to be *liberal* in looking for PTL but *conservative* in diagnosis and treatment. The goal of first contact with a patient who may have PTL should be sensitivity, while the goal of evaluation in labor and delivery should be specificity. We recommend the following maxims:

1. Invite any patient complaining of possible symptoms of PTL to come in for a period of contraction monitoring and a cervical examination. Severity of symptoms bears little relation to their clinical significance.
2. Wait for a cervical change of at least 1 cm, a dilation of 2 cm, or a positive fibronectin assay before accepting the diagnosis of PTL in a patient with persistent contractions.
3. Use cervical sonography (length 30 mm or longer) as test to support continued observation.
4. Be wary of "incidental" diagnosis of PTL, especially in the afternoon and early evening.

Remember the wide range of contraction frequency in normal pregnancy.

Treatment of Preterm Labor

Goals of Treatment

Once diagnosed, the ultimate goal of therapy for PTL is delivery at term of an infant who suffers none of the sequelae of prematurity. Given the uncertainty of the original diagnosis in the pre-fibronectin era and the consequent inclusion of women without PTL in studies of tocolysis, it has been difficult to demonstrate that

Table 23-7   Number of Women with Symptoms of PTL Delivered Within 7 Days Stratified by Fibronectin Results and Physician's Clinical Diagnosis of PTL[88]

Fibronectin	Clinical Dx of PTL	No Clinical Dx of PTL
Positive	$^6/_{25}$ (24%)	$^7/_{20}$ (35%)
Negative	$^1/_{60}$ (1.7%)	$^0/_{87}$ (0%)

Clinical Evaluation of Patients With Possible Preterm Labor

Patient presents with signs/symptoms suggesting preterm labor
  Persistent contractions (painful or painless)
  Intermittent abdominal cramping, pelvic pressure, or backache
  Increase or change in vaginal discharge
  Vaginal spotting or bleeding

Sterile speculum examination for pH, fern, pooled fluid, cultures for group B *Streptococcus* (outer one-third of vagina and perineum), *Chlamydia* (cervix), and *N. gonorrhoea* (cervix), and fibronectin swab (external cervical os and posterior fornix, avoiding areas with bleeding)

Transabdominal ultrasound examination for placental location, amniotic fluid volume, estimated fetal weight and presentation, and fetal well-being

Digital examination (If preterm PROM ruled out by above)
  Cervix ≥ 3 cm dilation → The diagnosis of PTL confirmed. Candidate for tocolysis
  Cervix 2–3 cm dilation → The diagnosis of PTL likely but not established. Assay fibronectin and monitor contraction frequency. Repeat digital examination 30–60 minutes. Candidate for tocolysis if any cervical change, contractions increase in frequency, or fibronectin is positive
  Cervix < 2 cm dilation → The diagnosis of PTL uncertain. Monitor contraction frequency, assay fibronectin, and repeat digital examination in 1–2 hours. Candidate for tocolysis if there is a 1-cm change in cervical dilatation or if fibronectin is positive

Treatments for symptomatic fibronectin-positive results
  Parenteral tocolysis
  Maternal transfer
  Steroids
  Hospitalize × 3–7 days
  Group B *Streptococcus* prophylaxis

Treatments for symptomatic fibronectin-negative results
  Parenteral tocolysis begun (cx ≥2 cm)
    Risk of delivery ≤7 days = 1.7%–3.5%
    Conclude course of tocolysis
    Reduce hospital stay
  Tocolysis not begun
    Risk of delivery ≤7 days = 0%–1.8%
    Observe in outpatient setting
  Cervical sonography should be considered in these patients to assess risk of SPTB

current treatment of PTL achieves this endpoint. Treatment with tocolytic drugs has not been shown to reduce premature delivery for treated subjects. However, there is good evidence that tocolytics can delay delivery for at least 48 hours, an important interval during which the mother and fetus may be transferred to a tertiary center and treated with steroids. The immediate goals of tocolytic therapy are sufficient delay in delivery to allow antepartum transfer of the mother to the most appropriate hospital, treatment of underlying causes of PTL (e.g., maternal pyelonephritis), and corticosteroid treatment. Because both antepartum maternal transport and steroid therapy have been shown to reduce neonatal morbidity and mortality, aggressive pursuit of these achievable goals may be expected to lead to further improvements in neonatal outcomes.

As noted previously, the initial evaluation of preterm labor is focused on the risks and benefits of continuing the pregnancy for both mother and fetus. The mother's well being is always the primary consideration. Common maternal contraindications to tocolysis include severe hypertension, significant bleeding, and maternal cardiac disease. PTL accompanied by maternal hypertension places both mother and fetus at risk of acute hypertensive crises and may occur in response to fetal stress or distress, uterine ischemia, or occult placental abruption. Although vaginal spotting may occur in women with PTL because of cervical effacement or dilatation, any bleeding beyond light spotting is rarely due to labor alone. Placenta previa and abruption must be considered, because both may be accompanied by uterine contractions. In general, both diagnoses contraindicate tocolytic treatment. However, in rare instances prophylactic use of tocolysis in patients with these dangerous diagnoses may be considered to achieve time for corticosteroids in the setting of extreme prematurity and when the bleeding is believed to occur in response to contractions. Such treatment is fraught with difficulty, because even low doses of some tocolytic agents can be hazardous in a patient with bleeding. β-Mimetic agents and calcium channel blockers may

Contraindications to Tocolysis

Maternal contraindications to tocolysis
   Significant hypertension (eclampsia, severe pre-eclampsia, chronic hypertension)
   Antepartum hemorrhage
   Cardiac disease
   Any medical or obstetric condition that contraindicates prolongation of pregnancy
   Hypersensitivity to a specific tocolytic agent

Fetal contraindications to tocolysis
   Gestational age ≥ 37 weeks
   Advanced dilatation/effacement
   Birth weight ≥ 2,500 g
   Demise or lethal anomaly
   Chorioamnionitis
   In utero fetal compromise
      -Acute: fetal distress
      -Chronic: IUGR or substance abuse

Uterine Muscle Physiology

Actin plus myosin → (myosin light chain kinase [MLCK]) → contraction

MLCK becomes active in presence of free intracellular calcium

Increased free intracellular calcium → increased MLCK → contractions

Decreased free intracellular calcium → decreased contractions

hamper maternal cardiovascular response to hypotension, and prostaglandin inhibitors are known to impair maternal platelet function. Cardiac disease is a contraindication because of the risks of tocolytic drug treatment in these patients.

Potential causes of PTL should be not only sought in the initial evaluation of the patient, but also reassessed during the course of treatment. An underlying cause for labor may be found that is best treated by delivery (e.g., abruptio placenta or chorioamnionitis), that may influence the choice of tocolytic (e.g., a degenerating myoma often responds best to a prostaglandin inhibitor), or that may require adjunctive treatment (e.g., antibiotic for pyelonephritis or a therapeutic amniocentesis for polyhydramnios).

Biochemistry of Myometrial Contractility and Tocolytic Action

A review of myometrial activity and the site(s) of action of the various tocolytic agents is appropriate before individual drugs are described. Figure 23-17 summarizes the current knowledge of the regulatory mechanisms of uterine smooth muscle contractility. The key process in actin–myosin interaction, and thus contraction, is myosin light chain phosphorylation. This reaction is controlled by myosin light chain kinase (MLCK). The activity of tocolytic agents can be explained by their effect on the factors regulating the activity of this enzyme, notably calcium and cAMP (Fig. 23-17A). Cal-

cium is essential for the activation of MLCK and binds to the kinase as a calmodulin–calcium complex. Intracellular calcium levels are regulated by two general mechanisms: (1) influx across the cell membrane and (2) release from intracellular storage sites. Entry of calcium into cells occurs by at least two mechanisms. Depolarization leads to calcium influx through specific calcium channels that are voltage dependent. This is the site of action of the calcium channel blockers. Calcium can also enter through voltage-independent mechanisms, most notably the calcium—magnesium—ATPase system. Magnesium ions may interact here and also may compete with calcium for the voltage-dependent channels. Calcium is stored within cells in the sarcoplasmic reticulum and in mitochondria. Progesterone and cAMP promote calcium storage at these sites, while prostaglandin $F_{2\alpha}$ ($PGF_{2\alpha}$) and oxytocin stimulate its release (Fig. 23-17B). MLCK is also regulated by cAMP. cAMP directly inhibits MLCK function via phosphorylation. Levels of cAMP are increased by the action of adenylate cyclase, which in turn is stimulated by β-adrenergic agents. Therefore, β-mimetic tocolytics act through adenylate cyclase to increase cAMP, which inhibits MLCK activity both by direct phosphorylation and by reducing intracellular free calcium (by inhibiting calcium release from storage vesicles) (Fig. 23-17C). β-Mimetics also interact with surface receptors on the trophoblast, leading to increased cAMP, which in this tissue increases production of progesterone. Hormonal production is a lengthy process, and significant production is not seen for at least 18 hours. For the myometrium to contract in a coordinated and effective manner (i.e., labor, whether term or preterm), individual smooth muscle cells must be functionally interconnected and able to communicate with adjacent cells. The key element of this coordination and hence one of the keys for labor is the gap junction. The formation

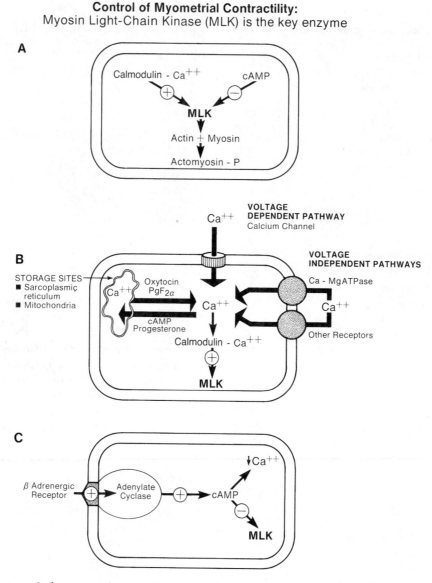

Control of Myometrial Contractility:
Myosin Light-Chain Kinase (MLK) is the key enzyme

Fig. 23-17. Control of myometrial contractility: myosin light-chain kinase (MLK) is the key enzyme. See text for details.

of gap junctions and the concentration of oxytocin receptors is regulated by estrogens and progesterone.[90]

Choosing a Tocolytic Agent

Tocolytic drugs are reasonably safe when used according to published protocols. However, their reported safety is due more to the youth and general good health of the patients treated than to the inherent safety of the drugs. The choice of tocolytic requires careful consideration of the efficacy, risks, and side effects of each of the available agents and on an assessment of the suitability of the agent for each individual patient. The following sections described the parenteral administration of current tocolytic drugs. The use of these agents

in oral form following the acute care of an episode of PTL is controversial because of the absence of evidence of effectiveness in prolonging pregnancy.

The β-Mimetic Tocolytics

The β-mimetic drugs have been the most commonly used tocolytics for more than 30 years. They are structurally related to epinephrine and norepinephrine and include ritodrine (the only agent approved by the FDA for use as a tocolytic), terbutaline (marketed in the United States only as a drug for asthma but widely used as a tocolytic), albuterol, fenoterol, hexoprenaline, isoxuprine, metaproterenol, nylidrin, orciprenaline, and salbutamol. Only the first two are in common use as tocolytics in the United States and will be described here.

Efficacy of β-Mimetics. There is good evidence that β-mimetic agents are successful in prolonging pregnancy for at least 48 hours and perhaps longer. King et al[75] conducted a meta-analysis of the randomized trials of β-sympathomimetic tocolytic drugs and found that treated subjects had better outcomes than placebo for delivery within 24 (OR, 0.29, CI, 0.21 to 0.41) and 48 (OR, 0.59, 0.42 to 0.83) hours of admission. There was a reduction in preterm births less than 37 weeks in treated subjects in 3 of 15 studies (OR, 0.71, CI, 0.53 to 0.96). However, there was no advantage for the treated group compared with placebo controls in the frequency of low birth weight less than 2,500 g (OR, 0.75, CI, 0.55 to 1.02), severe respiratory distress syndrome (OR, 1.07, CI, 0.71 to 1.61), or perinatal death (OR, 0.96, CI, 0.55 to 1.68). The trials analyzed by King et al[75] were conducted prior to the introduction of neonatal surfactant therapy and at a time when antepartum use of corticosteroids was cautious. A large multicenter Canadian prospective randomized trial of ritodrine reported similar results (Table 23-8).[91] A reduction in deliveries within 2 to 7 days of diagnosis was noted, but there was no significant difference in births before 37 weeks. The trend toward fewer deliveries before 32 weeks did not achieve statistical significance.

Critics of the Canadian study have particularly cited two features of design: the inclusion of a large number of subjects with ruptured membranes and the use of a standard but, in the opinion of critics, suboptimal dosage of oral medication. The first objection is easily countered by noting that subjects with PROM were randomly allotted to both treatment arms, and that the King et al[75] meta-analysis found the same result in populations with intact membranes. The concern about the adequacy of the oral ritodrine dosage in the Canadian study is ultimately a question about the efficacy of any dose of any oral tocolytic to suppress recurrent PTL. This unanswered question is addressed later in the section on aftercare of PTL with oral tocolysis. The ability of β-mimetic agents to delay delivery longer than 48 hours remains controversial and unproven at present, but there is a consensus that short-term tocolysis with these agents is effective in delaying delivery long enough to allow maternal transport and to administer steroids and antibiotics for group B streptococcal prophylaxis.

Pharmacology of β-Mimetics. Sympathomimetic or adrenergic drugs act through either α- or β-receptors. Stimulation of α-receptors leads to contraction of smooth muscles, while β-receptor stimulation carries the opposite effect, leading to smooth muscle relaxation at all sites: vascular, gastrointestinal, and uterine. The presence of β-receptors in other tissues (e.g., the heart) accounts for the side effects of beta-mimetics. Beta-receptors are divided into β_1- and β_2-subtypes. The β_1-receptors are largely responsible for the cardiac effects, while β_2-receptors mediate the smooth muscle relaxation as well as hepatic glycogen production and islet cell release of insulin. All β-mimetics are structurally related to epinephrine, with two carbons separating a benzene ring from an amino group. Relative β_2-activity appears to be associated with large alkyl substitutions on the amino group while maintaining hydroxyl groups at the 3 or 5 position on the benzene ring.[92] It should be noted that when drugs are referred to as β_2-selective or β_2-specific, whether they be agonist or blocker, the selectivity is only relative and not absolute. First, β-receptors are not distributed on an "either/or" basis, but rather have variable ratios of β_2- to β_1-receptors. For example, the heart is primarily stimulated by β_1-agonists, but 14 percent of its β-receptors are β_2. Second, not all β_2-specific drugs are perfectly selective and will stimulate β_1-receptors to a certain extent. This is particularly true when serum concentrations are elevated.

Pharmacokinetics of Ritodrine

The therapeutic blood level of ritodrine has not been clearly established but appears to vary according to the degree of uterine activity rather than to cervical dilation or status of the membranes.[93] Ritodrine is conjugated in the liver to inactive glucuronic and sulfuric

Table 23-8   Results of the Canadian Ritodrine Study

	Ritodrine (%) (n = 352)	Placebo (%) (n = 356)	Relative Risk (95% CI)
Entry to delivery			
% <24 hours	7.1	19.7	−12.6 (17.5 to −7.7)
% <48 hours	21.4	35.4	−14.0 (−20.6 to −7.4)
<7 days	38.2	47.2	−9.0 (−14.8 to −3.2)
Delivery <32 weeks	49	58	−9.3 (−18.6 to 0.2)
Delivery <37 weeks	68	69	−0.6 (−7.4 to 6.2)

(Data from Canadian Preterm Labor Investigators Group.[91])

esters. Both unconjugated and conjugated drugs are then excreted in the urine. Actual serum ritodrine levels vary greatly at a given infusion rate; for example, at an infusion rate of 50 µg/min, ritodrine levels may vary from 15 to 35 ng/ml from one patient to another.[93] The variability in serum levels among individuals at the same infusion rates appears to be related to differences in hepatic blood flow or serum concentrations of protein rather than maternal weight.[94] Concentrations of 80 ng/ml or more are commonly required initially to inhibit PTL. Ritodrine crosses the placenta readily, and fetal concentrations average 30 percent of maternal levels after a 2-hour infusion and are equal to those of the mother after longer infusions. In kinetics studies, it appears that serum ritodrine levels reach 75 percent of maximum levels within 20 minutes of a constant intravenous infusion.[94] The manufacturer's recommended protocol for intravenous therapy starts at 0.1 mg (100 µg) per minute and is increased by 0.05 mg (50 µg) every 10 minutes until contractions cease, side effects occur, or the maximum rate (0.35 mg [350 µg]/min) is reached. The infusion is then maintained at the effective level for 12 hours after contractions cease.[95] Caritis et al[93] noted that side effects occur most often when the infusion rate and concentration of ritodrine are increasing. The authors found that the rate of change in the infusion rate or drug concentration was more important than absolute drug level[94] and proposed an alternative protocol with equal efficacy and fewer side effects. The Caritis protocol uses as little drug as necessary, starting at 50 µg/min and increasing by 50 µg/min every 20 minutes only if contractions are more frequent than every 10 minutes. The dose may exceed 350 µg/min in some patients if the maternal pulse remains below 110 bpm, as some of these individuals are exhibiting rapid clearance of the drug. Once labor is stopped, the infusion rate is maintained for 1 hour and then reduced every 20 minutes to the lowest rate that inhibits contractions adequately. This rate is then maintained for 12 hours.

A single intramuscular injection of 5 to 10 mg of ritodrine results in labor-inhibiting concentrations with clinically insignificant cardiovascular effects. After intramuscular injection, ritodrine causes a dose-related increase in heart rate and blood pressure and a dose-related decrease in diastolic blood pressure. After a 10-mg injection, the maximal changes in heart rate, systolic blood pressure, and diastolic blood pressure are 22, 10, and 19 percent, respectively.[96] The intramuscular route is preferable for women who are being transferred to another hospital.

Terbutaline

Pharmacokinetics. Serum levels of terbutaline range from 10 to 14 ng/ml following a 1-hour infusion of 0.010 mg (10 µg)/min. At infusion rates above 5 µg/min, this drug can be accumulated with raised serum levels and increased symptoms,[94] probably reflecting the longer half-life of terbutaline over ritodrine. Drug levels are 30 percent lower in pregnant patients than in nonpregnant volunteers. The onset of action is rapid with both intravenous bolus (1 to 2 minutes) and subcutaneous administration (3 to 5 minutes).

Dosage of Terbutaline. Terbutaline has not been approved by the FDA for tocolysis. Consequently there is no manufacturer's protocol for its use for this indication. Currently published protocols often employ subcutaneous administration, with the usual dose being 0.25 mg (250 µg) every 3 hours.[97] A single subcutaneous dose of terbutaline may be used to arrest contractions during the initial evaluation, pending results of the fibronectin assay (see algorithm). Intravenous administration is also employed in some centers, beginning at 2.5 µg/min and increasing by 2.5 µg/min every 20 minutes in a manner similar to ritodrine until a maximum of 17.5 to 20 µg/min is reached.[98]

Tachyphylaxis with β-Mimetic Drugs

Tachyphylaxis or desensitization of the adrenergic receptor occurs throughout the body after prolonged exposure to β-agonists and affects the clinical use of β-mimetic drugs as tocolytics. Animal studies suggest that contractions resume after only several hours of *continuous* intravenous therapy with high-dose β-mimetic therapy; the myometrium remains quiescent longer with

---

Caritis Intravenous Ritodrine Protocol

Begin infusion at 50 µg/min (0.05 mg/min)

Increase by 50 µg/min every 20 minutes

Maximum dose: 350 µg/min

If contractions are less frequent than every 10 minutes, wait another 20 minutes before increasing dose

Once labor is stopped, maintain infusion rate for 1 hour; then reduce every 20 minutes to the lowest rate that inhibits contractions adequately

Continue this maintenance rate for 12 hours

Potassium replacement is unnecessary on routine basis

pulsatile administration of lower doses of the same tocolytic agent.[99] Caritis et al[100,101] have documented reduced β-receptor sensitivity to continuous versus intermittent administration of ritodrine and have shown that the mechanism of this altered sensitivity occurs via reduced receptor density and adenyl cyclase activity. Interestingly, dexamethasone treatment ameliorated these effects and preserved the tocolytic effect. These observations have led to alternate protocols for ritodrine (see above) and to studies of intermittent administration of β-mimetic agents. Spatling et al[102] reported that a reduced amount and duration of fenoterol was required when the drug was given in a pulsatile compared with a continuous regimen.

Side Effects and Complications of Parenteral β-Mimetic Tocolysis

Maternal side effects of the β-adrenergic agonists are common and diverse, as shown in Table 23-9, taken from a recent comprehensive review. Most are mild and of limited duration, but serious maternal cardiopulmonary and metabolic complications have been reported, including maternal death when β-adrenergic agents were given to mothers with unrecognized or occult car-

diac disease. A thorough history and review of possible cardiac symptoms before initiating treatment and prompt attention to any patient with persistent symptoms during treatment are important in preventing these complications. Some centers obtain routine electrocardiograms before beginning treatment with β-mimetic agents, but a normal electrocardiogram (ECG) does not exclude underlying cardiac disease and is probably not cost-effective in women without a worrisome history or persistent symptoms.

β-Mimetic Complications

β-Mimetic therapy for PTL has been associated with a series of maternal deaths, largely from pulmonary edema, but the drugs appear to have acceptable margins of safety if (1) the interaction between the pharmacology of β-mimetic drugs and the physiology of pregnancy is well understood, (2) there is careful attention to detail in the care of patients receiving these drugs, and (3) the potential for serious complications with these drugs is respected and contraindications are strictly observed. Symptomatic side effects are frequent with high-dose therapy. About 20 to 30 percent of patients experience nausea, and more than 50 percent of

Table 23-9   Side Effects and Complications of β-Mimetic Tocolysis

Maternal	Fetal and Neonatal
Physiologic	Fetal
Apprehension	Tachycardia
Jitteriness	Cardiac arrhythmia
Headache	Myocardial and septal
Nausea and vomiting	hypertrophy
Fever	Myocardial ischemia
Hallucinations	Heart failure
Metabolic	Hyperglycemia
Hyperglycemia	Hyperinsulinemia
Hyperinsulinemia	Death
Hyperlactic acidemia	Neonatal
Hypokalemia	Tachycardia
Hypocalcemia	Hypoglycemia
Antidiuresis, water retention	Hypocalcemia
Altered thyroid function	Hyperbilirubinemia
Elevated transaminases	Tachycardia
Cardiac	Myocardial ischemia
Tachycardia	Hypotension
Pulmonary edema	Intraventricular hemorrhage
Hypotension	Decreased myocardial contractility
Arrhythmias/palpitations	
Heart failure	
Myocardial ischemia, altered ECG and chest pain	
Shortness of breath	
Other	
Skin rash	
Pruritis	
Ileus	
Death (cardiac)	

(Data from Hill[103].)

patients develop tachycardias greater than 120 bpm.[98,104]

Pulmonary Edema. Pulmonary edema is the most serious complication of tocolytic therapy and can often be prevented. A recent review is recommended for a detailed discussion.[105] The reason for its frequent occurrence can be understood by reviewing the physiologic factors predisposing to pulmonary edema in normal pregnancy that add to the stress of β-mimetic therapy, especially in the face of certain medical factors. Pulmonary edema in association with tocolysis was thought to be secondary to volume overload/left heart failure, but evaluation of cardiac function with Swan-Ganz catheters or echocardiography has failed to demonstrate left ventricular failure in all but a few cases of pulmonary edema, most of which were associated with underlying hypertension.[106] Noncardiogenic causes that may be important are decreased colloid oncotic pressure and increased pulmonary vascular permeability, especially when premature labor is associated with amnionitis. In one study, tocolysis for PTL was associated with a higher incidence of pulmonary edema in the presence of maternal infection (21 percent) than when it was absent (1 percent).[107] Of note, nearly all patients with pulmonary edema were receiving either physiologic saline solutions or Ringer's lactated solution, which further decreases colloid oncotic pressure and expands vascular volume.[106] In any case, patients treated with β-mimetics should be considered as having a compromised cardiovascular system and should not receive large amounts of saline or Ringer's lactated solution.

It is uncommon for pulmonary edema to develop in the first 24 hours of β-mimetic therapy unless one of the predisposing factors is present. In fact, more than 90 percent of reported cases of pulmonary edema occur after 24 hours of β-mimetic therapy. Glucocorticoids have often been associated with pulmonary edema in this setting, and many investigators consider them a predisposing factor. However, betamethasone and dexamethasone have essentially no mineralocorticoid activity, and their association with maternal pulmonary edema may be coincidental. There are now many cases of pulmonary edema reported without concomitant use of corticosteroids and with tocolytics other than the β-mimetics. Recommendations to avoid pulmonary edema related to tocolytic treatment are outlined in the box.

Myocardial Ischemia and Cardiac Dysrhythmias. Symptomatic cardiac dysrhythmias and symptomatic myocardial ischemia have occurred during β-agonist tocolytic therapy. Myocardial infarction with resultant maternal death has been reported.[104] Ischemia appears to be localized to the subendocardial region. The subendocardial oxygen supply:demand ratio can be re-

---

Pulmonary Edema and Tocolytic Therapy: Predisposing Factors

Underlying predisposing factors in normal pregnancy
- Increased intravascular volume
- Decreased peripheral vascular resistance
- Decreased blood viscosity
- Increased heart rate
- Decreased plasma colloid oncotic pressure
- Increased pulmonary vascular permeability (?)
- Intrapartum volume shifts

Additive effects of β-mimetic therapy
- Further expansion of intravascular volume
- Further decrease in peripheral vascular resistance
- Further decrease in blood viscosity
- Further increase in heart rate
- Further decrease in plasma colloid oncotic pressure
- Further increase in pulmonary vascular permeability (?)

Extra predisposing medical or treatment factors
- Twins
- Injudicious fluid management
- Heart rate >130 bpm
- Treatment >24 hours
- Unsuspected heart lesions (e.g., mitral stenosis)
- Amnionitis
- Hypertension
- Glucocorticoids (?)

---

duced by two factors that are known to be operative during pregnancy and β-mimetic therapy: the placental arterial-venous fistula that diminishes aortic diastolic blood pressure and the induced tachycardia resulting in a shortened diastole, which is the time for myocardial perfusion. If a patient develops chest pain during therapy, one should discontinue the β-mimetic and administer oxygen. With severe pain, therapy with nitrates may be necessary. Premature ventricular contraction, premature nodal contractions, and atrial fibrillation have been noted in association with β-mimetic therapy.[104] These usually respond well to discontinuation of the drug and oxygen administration. The most important steps to prevent these cardiac complications are (1) excluding patients with prior cardiac disease and (2) limiting infusion rates so that maternal pulse does not exceed 130 bpm. Baseline ECGs

Recommendations To Avoid Tocolytic-Related Pulmonary Edema

Restrict fluid intake to 2.5 liters/day (total IV and PO)

Limit salt content of fluids (avoid saline or Ringer's lactated solution)

Restrict total dose and length of intravenous β-mimetic therapy

Respect contraindications to β-mimetic use

Table 23-10   Increased Rate of Intraventricular Hemorrhage (IVH) in Neonates After In Utero Therapy with β-Mimetic Agents (All intraventricular bleeding)

Tocolytic Rx	% IVH	OR	CI	p Value
β-mimetic	16	2.47	1.3 –4.6	0.004
Mg SO$_4$	4	0.87	0.3 –2.4	0.79
None	4	0.90	0.5 –1.6	0.73
Grades 3 and 4 hemorrhages				
β-Mimetic	5.8	2.50	0.96–6.5	0.06
Mg SO$_4$	1.9	0.91	0.21–3.9	0.90
None	1.2	0.72	0.27–1.9	0.52

(Data from Groome et al.[112])

or routine ECGs during treatment are not helpful. There is a very poor correlation between symptoms of myocardial ischemia and ECG changes in these patients.[108,109] Nonetheless, if a patient does not quickly respond to oxygen and discontinuation of β-mimetic therapy, an ECG is in order.

Hypotension. The β-mimetics in current use produce a mild (5 to 10 mmHg) fall in diastolic blood pressure. However, the extensive peripheral vasodilation makes it difficult for the patient to mount a normal, vasoconstrictive response to hypovolemia. This is one of the reasons β-mimetics are dangerous in the face of antepartum hemorrhage. Another is that the important early signs of excessive blood loss such as maternal and fetal tachycardia are masked by these drugs.[104]

Hyperglycemia and Hypokalemia. β-Mimetic agents compound the problems of patients with overt or gestational diabetes mellitus. Increased glycogenolysis with resultant hyperglycemia, increased lactic acid release from skeletal muscles, and ketone formation from fat stores, as well as a fall in bicarbonate, markedly increase the risk of ketoacidosis.[110] These drugs should in general be avoided in women with diabetes. If it is absolutely necessary to use β-mimetics, a simultaneous intravenous insulin infusion should be employed to avoid ketoacidosis. In the nondiabetic woman, β-mimetics will cause a significant increase in serum glucose level, although rarely over 180 mg/dl.[98] β-Mimetics also lead to potassium flux from plasma into cells, thereby causing a fall in serum measurements without a change in excretion. Hence there is no change in total body potassium. We recommend measurement of glucose and potassium before initiating therapy and on occasion during the first 24 hours of treatment. This will ensure that the unrecognized gestational diabetic and the occasional normal patient in whom significant hyperglyce-

mia (> 180 mg/dl) develops will not be missed. After 24 hours of therapy, both the serum glucose and potassium levels will have begun to return to baseline even without specific therapy.[111] No potassium replacement is needed unless the serum potassium level falls below 2.5 mEq/L.

Neonatal Side Effects of β-Mimetics. β-Mimetic tocolysis has been linked to an increased risk of neonatal intraventricular hemorrhage (Table 23-10).[112] These data have led many centers to reevaluate the use of the β-mimetic drugs as the first line agents for tocolysis. Neonatal hypoglycemia and ileus have also been reported with β-mimetics and can be clinically significant if the maternal infusion is not discontinued more than 2 hours before delivery.[113] Neonatal hypocalcemia may also occur. On a positive note, some reports link β-mimetic drugs with improved neonatal lung function and with a decreased incidence of respiratory distress syndrome. These effects are not uniformly found and are not of the magnitude associated with corticosteroids. With all tocolytic drugs, and particularly β-mimetics and magnesium sulfate, adverse neonatal effects are greatest when the fetus is born close to a period of high-dose parenteral therapy.[114] These drugs must be used with great caution if at all when there is advanced cervical dilatation and delivery appears inevitable. Situations in which the patient is at increased risk for β-mimetic complications (relative contraindications) are listed below. Careful risk/benefit evaluation needs to be performed on an individual basis in these cases.

Summary of β-Mimetic Tocolysis

β-mimetic drugs have been the tocolytics of first choice for almost three decades, but have lost ground recently to other agents with better safety and side-effect profiles. Although terbutaline and ritodrine (still the only FDA-approved tocolytic), are familiar choices, concern about the potential increase in intraventricular hemorrhage associated with β-mimetics has already led many

---

Contraindications to β-mimetic tocolytics

Absolute
  Maternal cardiac disease (structural, ischemia, or dysrhythmia)
  Eclampsia, severe preeclampsia, or other significant hypertensive disease
  Significant antepartum hemorrhage
  Uncontrolled diabetes mellitus
  Maternal hyperthyroidism
Relative
  Diabetes, whether diet or insulin controlled
  Hypertension
  History of severe migraine headaches
  Febrile patient
  Increased risk of pulmonary edema

---

centers to choose other agents as first line therapy. However, as will become obvious in the following paragraphs, there is no clearly superior agent to suppress uterine contractions.

Magnesium Sulfate

Intravenous magnesium sulfate has been used in obstetrics for seizure prophylaxis in preeclampsia for almost 60 years, but was not used specifically for the inhibition of PTL until the 1970s.[115,116] The mechanism of tocolytic activity of magnesium is unclear. In vitro studies of uterine muscle strips show reduced contractility in the presence of magnesium ion. It has been suggested that it acts by competition with calcium either at the motor end plate, reducing excitation, or at the cell membrane, reducing calcium influx into the cell at depolarization.

Efficacy. The efficacy of magnesium as a tocolytic agent has been studied in relatively few trials that enrolled relatively few subjects. A report by Steer and Petrie[115] defined successful treatment as cessation of contractions for 24 hours. Twenty-four of 31 women treated with magnesium sulfate were undelivered 24 hours after beginning therapy compared with 14 of 31 treated with intravenous ethanol. An observational study of magnesium-treated singleton pregnancies with intact membranes and cervical dilation of 3 to 4 cm reported that 64 percent of subjects were undelivered at 48 hours and 56 percent were undelivered at 7 days.[117] Subsequent randomized studies of magnesium compared with β-mimetics[118,119] found no differences in tocolytic effect, but had too little power to conclude

efficacy. A study in which 120 subjects with PTL were randomly assigned to receive either ritodrine or magnesium reported that only 4 and 8 percent of subjects, respectively, were delivered within 48 hours of entry; only 17 and 20 percent of ritodrine- and magnesium-treated subjects had delivered at 7 days.[120] More than 45 percent of subjects in each group remained undelivered at 37 weeks, consistent with findings from the King et al,[75] meta-analysis and suggesting liberal diagnostic criteria for preterm labor at that center. In contrast, Cox et al[121] reported an open randomized trial of 156 women treated between 24 and 34 weeks' gestation with either magnesium or no tocolysis in which there were no differences in duration of pregnancy, birth weight, neonatal morbidity, or perinatal mortality. The rate of delivery within 24 hours of enrollment was about 30 percent in each group. Delivery within 7 days of enrollment occurred in 47 percent of magnesium-treated subjects compared with 37 percent of controls (NS). Interestingly, about 35 percent of subjects in each group delivered more than 28 days after enrollment, again suggesting overdiagnosis of PTL in about a third of subjects diagnosed prior to FDA approval of fibronectin, even within a rigorous study protocol at a center known for therapeutic restraint. Although these studies suggest some delay in delivery associated with magnesium, the agent does not appear to be a highly effective tocolytic.

Dosage. Magnesium sulfate must be administered parenterally in order to elevate serum levels above the normal range. Therapeutic dosage and serum levels have not been formally established but empirically are similar to those used for intravenous treatment of preeclampsia: a 4- to 6-g loading dose given over 20 minutes, followed by an infusion of 2 to 4 g/hr, dropping to 1 to 2 g/hr once contractions cease.[117] Madden et al[122] were unable to show that serum levels correlated with successful tocolytic therapy. In 101 episodes of PTL treated with magnesium sulfate, no difference was found in the proportions of tocolytic success when serum levels were less than 6 mg/dl compared with when levels were more than 6 mg/dl. Mean serum magnesium levels in patients with successful tocolysis were similar to those in patients in whom tocolysis failed. The investigators concluded that serum magnesium levels alone should not serve as the endpoint of therapy and that the drug should be titrated on the basis of clinical efficacy or maternal toxicity. Excess magnesium is rapidly excreted by the kidney, provided there is normal renal function. Should there be any evidence of renal impairment, such as oliguria or a serum creatinine level over 0.9 mg/dl, magnesium therapy should be approached cautiously, the patient followed with serum levels, and doses adjusted accordingly. Magne-

Protocol for Magnesium Sulfate Tocolysis

Administer loading dose of 6 g magnesium sulfate in 10%–20% solution over 15 minutes (60 ml of 10% magnesium sulfate in D5 0.9 normal saline)

Maintenance dose of 2 g/hr (40 g of magnesium sulfate added to 1 liter D5 0.9 normal saline or Ringer's lactate at 50 ml/hour)

Increase magnesium sulfate by 1 g/hr until the patient has no more than one contraction per 10 minutes or maximum dose of 4–5 g/hr is reached

Limit IV fluid to 125 cc/hr. Follow fluid status closely with an indwelling urinary catheter if needed

Maintain magnesium sulfate tocolysis for 12–24 hours once successful

Decrease magnesium sulfate therapy by 1 g/hr every 30 minutes when ending therapy. Stop when 2 g/hr is reached

If contractions reoccur, reevaluate patient to assess need for further tocolytic therapy. Consider an underlying cause of the preterm labor that has not been diagnosed, such as amnionitis or occult abruption. An amniocentesis should be considered. Also, reconsider the accuracy of the original diagnosis of preterm labor

While on magnesium sulfate, check
  Deep tendon reflexes and vital signs hourly
  Intake and output every 2–4 hours
  Magnesium levels only if using doses above 4 g/hr or if clinical concern about toxicity

sium sulfate should not be used in patients with myasthenia gravis. The clinical protocol for magnesium sulfate as a tocolytic at The Ohio State University Medical Center is shown in the box.

Maternal Side Effects. Magnesium has a relatively low rate of symptomatic side effects compared with other tocolytic drugs. Flushing, nausea, vomiting, headache, generalized muscle weakness including especially complaints of diplopia and shortness of breath, and pulmonary edema have all been reported. Beall et al[123] randomized patients to ritodrine, terbutaline, or magnesium sulfate as the initial intravenous tocolytic. Although the rate of failure (defined as changing medication because of persistent contractions or intolerance of side effects) was approximately 30 percent in the

magnesium and β-mimetic groups, the reasons for discontinuing the agents differed. Subjects receiving β-mimetics experience greater side effects but rarely failed because of persistent contractions. Magnesium failed because of persistent contractions, but the agent was tolerated relatively well. It has therefore become the tocolytic agent of choice in a number of major medical centers. There can be, however, major and life-threatening complications with magnesium therapy, including chest pain and pulmonary edema. In the largest clinical experience, 355 patients reported by Elliott,[117] side effects were noted in 7 percent. Four patients (1.1 percent) developed pulmonary edema, a rate similar to that seen with β-mimetics. It should be pointed out that Elliott[117] used higher magnesium sulfate doses than other investigators, and it is not clear whether maternal fluids were restricted. In two other studies comparing ritodrine and magnesium sulfate, the incidence of side effects rose significantly when both drugs were used together.[119,120]

Neonatal Side Effects. Although magnesium crosses the placenta and achieves serum levels comparable to maternal levels, serious neonatal complications are uncommon. Lethargy, hypotonia, and even respiratory depression may occur. Neonatal bony anomalies were reported in 6 of 11 infants who were exposed to magnesium for more than 7 days, but the clinical significance of this phenomenon is unknown.[124]

Antenatal maternal magnesium treatment has also been associated with improved neonatal outcome in several recent studies. Nelson and Grether,[125] in a case–control study from the California Cerebral Palsy Project, found that maternal magnesium treatment for either preeclampsia or PTL was associated with lower rates of cerebral palsy at examinations up to 7 years after birth. Only 7.1 percent of 42 children with cerebral palsy had been exposed to antenatal magnesium compared with 36 percent of 75 controls without cerebral palsy (OR, 0.14 [0.05, 0.51]). Bottoms et al[12] reported improved survival and decreased intraventricular hemorrhage in a study of 808 VLBW infants less than 1,000 g who had been exposed to antepartum magnesium. Hauth et al[126] followed 389 infants whose birth weight was below 1,000 g and who were born between 24 and 28 weeks' gestation, and they assessed the relationship of in utero magnesium exposure to cerebral palsy at 1 year of age. Among infants exposed to magnesium, the rate of cerebral palsy was 7.6 percent compared with 19 percent for infants whose mothers did not receive magnesium.[126] These are preliminary reports, but are consistent with an unpublished meta-analysis of neonatal database outcomes performed by the NICHD.

Summary of Magnesium.

Magnesium sulfate is a safe agent with limited and unproven tocolytic effectiveness. The quality and sample size of published studies do not allow a conclusion about the appropriate role for magnesium as a tocolytic agent at this time. Because of its favorable safety profile, magnesium may be an especially useful choice when the diagnosis of PTL is early and uncertain and in patients for whom other agents are contraindicated (e.g., insulin dependent diabetes). Recent reports of reduced rates of intraventricular hemorrhage and cerebral palsy in infants born to magnesium-treated women may lead to the inclusion of this agent in future protocols of multiple drug therapy for preterm labor.

Indomethacin

Prostaglandins are important mediators of the final pathways of uterine muscle contraction. Labor at term is associated with increased concentrations of arachidonic acid and prostaglandins E_2 and $F_{2\alpha}$ in amniotic fluid. Administration of prostaglandins to pregnant women can ripen the cervix and/or induce labor, depending on the dosage and route of administration. Prostaglandin synthetase inhibitors interfere with these effects and therefore have theoretical appeal as tocolytic agents. Prostaglandins cause an increase in free intracellular calcium levels in myometrial cells, thus increased activation of MLCK and consequent uterine contractions. Myometrial gap junction formation, an important step in synchronized uterine activity, is also enhanced by prostaglandins. Prostaglandin synthesis is stimulated by cytokines, bacterial products including phospholipases and endotoxins, and corticosteroids. Inhibition of cyclooxygenase, the enzyme that converts arachidonic acid to prostaglandin F_2, by nonsteroidal antiinflammatory drugs (NSAIDs) leads to reduced synthesis of prostaglandins. The NSAID agents vary in their activity, potency and side effect profiles. Indomethacin is the most widely used agent in this class, which also includes sulindac, naproxen, aspirin, and fenoprofen.

The potential for clinical use of these agents was observed in studies showing prolonged pregnancy and longer mean duration of labor in women taking therapeutic doses of salicylates.[127] In 1974, indomethacin was reported to delay delivery by more than 7 days in 80 percent of treated subjects.[128]

Efficacy. Indomethacin has been reported to be effective in two small randomized, placebo-controlled trials. Niebyl et al[129] found indomethacin superior to placebo in delaying delivery for 48 hours (80 percent vs. 33 percent). Zuckerman et al[130,131] reported sustained delay in delivery for indomethacin-treated subjects (95

percent at 48 hours and 83 percent at 7 days) compared with placebo (23 percent at 48 hours and 16 percent at 7 days). A randomized comparison of indomethacin to ritodrine[132] found prolongation of pregnancy for 7 days in about two-thirds of subjects in each group; the indomethacin group had significantly fewer maternal side effects. There are numerous other reports that describe indomethacin tocolysis favorably, but many employed other tocolytics simultaneously or sequentially.

Dosage. Indomethacin is well absorbed orally or per rectum. The usual dose is a 50-mg loading dose by mouth or 50 to 100 mg per rectum if the patient cannot tolerate the oral dose. Subsequently, 25 to 50 mg is administered orally every 4 to 6 hours, depending on the response. Therapy is usually limited to 2 to 4 days because of concern about side effects of oligohydramnios and neonatal pulmonary hypertension (see below). The dosage regimen used at our center is shown in the box.

Protocol for Indomethacin Tocolysis

Limit use to PTL before 32 weeks' gestation in subjects with normal amniotic fluid volume

Loading dose of 100 mg rectally or 50 mg orally; repeat in 1 hour if no decrease in contractions

Give 25–50 mg every 4–6 hours for 48 hours

Check amniotic fluid volume prior to initiation and at 48–72 hours. If oligohydramnios is present, the drug should be discontinued or, in desperate cases, decreased in dosage

We do not use the drug for longer than 48 consecutive hours, but occasionally repeat a course of treatment after a 5-day drug-free interval. Use of indomethacin for more than 48 hours requires extraordinary circumstances. Ductal flow and tricuspid regurgitation should be evaluated with Doppler echocardiography. Repeat the evaluation at least weekly and discontinue if constriction found. Amniotic fluid volume should be checked twice weekly

Discontinue therapy promptly if delivery seems imminent

Fetal contraindications to use of indomethacin include growth retardation, renal anomalies, chorioamnionitis, oligohydramnios, ductal dependent cardiac defects, and twin–twin transfusion syndrome

Maternal Side Effects. Prostaglandin inhibition may have multiple and diverse side effects because of the abundance of prostaglandin-mediated physiologic functions. Nevertheless, the principal advantage of this agent is the relative infrequency of serious maternal side effects when the agent is used in a brief course of tocolysis. As with any NSAID, gastrointestinal side effects such as nausea, heartburn, and vomiting are the most common, but are usually mild. More serious complications include gastrointestinal bleeding, alterations in coagulation, thrombocytopenia, and asthma in aspirin-sensitive patients. Lunt et al[133] reported normal prothrombin and activated partial thromboplastin times, but found abnormal prolonged bleeding times in 65 percent of women treated for 48 hours and recommended that a bleeding time be obtained before operative delivery or anesthesia. Prolonged treatment can lead to renal injury, especially when other nephrotoxic drugs such as aminoglycoside antibiotics are employed. Hypertensive women may experience acute increased blood pressure after indomethacin treatment. Drugs of this class are antipyretic agents and may obscure a clinically significant fever. Maternal contraindications to indomethacin tocolysis include renal or hepatic disease, active peptic ulcer disease, poorly controlled hypertension, asthma, and coagulation disorders.

Fetal and Neonatal Side Effects. In contrast to the generally favorable maternal side effect profile, the potential for fetal and neonatal complications of indomethacin tocolysis is worrisome. In actual practice, serious complications have been rare, but the potential for significant injury to the fetus is real if treatment protocols are not followed carefully. There are case reports of neonatal deaths following maternal indomethacin tocolysis in the 1970s and early 1980s, before the pathologic mechanisms of potential fetal injury were recognized. Three principal side effects of indomethacin have been of concern: constriction of the ductus arteriosus, oligohydramnios, and neonatal pulmonary hypertension. The ductal constriction occurs because formation of prostacyclin and prostaglandin E_2, which maintain ductal vasodilatation, is inhibited by indomethacin.[134] Moise et al[135] first reported Doppler evidence of ductal constriction in 7 of 14 women who were treated with indomethacin between 27 and 31 weeks of pregnancy. Tricuspid regurgitation occurred in three fetuses; all ductal abnormalities resolved within 24 hours after the medication was discontinued. The likelihood of ductal constriction increased after 32 weeks of pregnancy.[134] Prior to 32 weeks the incidence of ductal constriction was 5 to 10 percent. At 32 to 35 weeks, the incidence increased to 50 percent after 48 hours of indomethacin exposure. Although potentially serious,

ductal contriction is usually transient and responds to discontinuation of the drug. However, persistent ductal constriction and right heart failure that did not reverse after the drug was stopped have been reported.[136]

Oligohydramnios associated with indomethacin tocolysis is common, dose related, and reversible, but there is a report of neonatal renal insufficiency and death after prolonged administration.[137] The oligohydramnios is a consequence of reduced fetal urine production due in turn to reduction by indomethacin of the normal prostaglandin inhibition of antidiuretic hormone and by direct effects on fetal renal blood flow.

Primary pulmonary hypertension in the neonate is a potentially fatal illness that has also been associated with prolonged (more than 48 hours) indomethacin therapy.[138,139] Primary neonatal pulmonary hypertension has not been reported with 24 to 48 hours of therapy, but the incidence may be as high as 5 to 10 percent with long-term therapy.[132]

Other complications, including necrotizing enterocolitis, small bowel perforation, patent ductus arteriosus, jaundice, and intraventricular hemorrhage, have been observed when indomethacin was used outside of standardized protocols that did not limit the duration of treatment and/or employed the drug after 32 weeks.[140] Niebyl and Witter,[141] Dudley and Hardie,[142] and Gardner et al[143] have performed follow-up studies of children treated in utero with indomethacin and have not found significant long-term effects.

Sulindac is an alternate NSAID that has been favorably compared to indomethacin as a tocolytic. Placental transfer of this drug is less than with indomethacin, but the tocolytic efficacy of sulindac has not been studied in large numbers of subjects.[144] Rasanen and Jouppila[145] found fewer fetal cardiovascular effects detected by Doppler with sulindac than with indomethacin.

Because of the effect on fetal urine production and amniotic fluid volume, indomethacin may be an appropriate tocolytic when PTL is associated with polyhydramnios. Several studies report successful treatment of PTL with indomethacin for patients with polyhydramnios and for polyhydramnios without labor.[146–150] We have found that uterine activity and pain associated with degenerating uterine fibroids in pregnancy also respond well to indomethacin.

Summary

Indomethacin is an effective tocolytic agent that is well tolerated by the mother. Concern about fetal side effects has appropriately limited use of indomethacin to brief courses of therapy for patients experiencing PTL before 32 weeks. In a review of tocolytic efficacy and safety, Higby[151] concluded that indomethacin was the only tocolytic for which there was convincing evidence of effectiveness and that there was "little risk to the fetus" when used before 32 weeks according to published protocols. However, indiscriminate use of prostaglandin inhibitors (e.g., for patients beyond 32 weeks or who have frequent contractions in the absence of a positive fibronectin or cervical dilation of 2 cm or more) may not have a favorable risk/benefit ratio for the fetus. Perhaps with additional experience more favorable fetal safety profiles will be confirmed for other antiprostaglandins such as sulindac.

Calcium Channel Blockers

Inhibitors of intracellular calcium entry have potent effects on the contraction of smooth muscle and thus have potential use as tocolytics. Calcium channel blockers are FDA approved for treatment of cardiovascular diseases, including certain types of hypertension, angina, and arrhythmias, but have been used for several years as tocolytic drugs. The primary pharmacologic effect is believed to occur via inhibition of the voltage-dependent channels of calcium entry into smooth muscle cells, resulting in a direct decrease in intracellular calcium as well as decreased release of calcium from intracellular storage sites. Of several classes of calcium blockers, nifedipine and nicardipine have received the most attention as tocolytic agents because they more selectively inhibit uterine contractions than others such as verapamil. These drugs differ from other tocolytics in that they are rapidly absorbed via oral or sublingual administration. The pharmacokinetics in pregnancy are apparently similar to that seen in nonpregnant individuals, with appearance of nifedipine within plasma within just a few minutes, peak concentrations at 15 to 90 minutes, and a half-life of 81 minutes after sublingual or oral administration.[152] Placental transfer of nifedipine was documented in this study in two patients who delivered 2 to 3 hours after receiving nifedipine. The duration of action of a single dose can be as long as 6 hours.

Efficacy. Nifedipine was reported by Ulmsten et al[153] in a small observational study to be effective in suppressing contractions and well tolerated by mother and fetus. Read and Welby[154] compared nifedipine to ritodrine in 40 patients who were randomly assigned to receive intravenous and then oral ritodrine in standard doses (n = 20) or nifedipine 30 mg PO, followed by 20 mg Q8h; these 40 were also compared with an additional nonrandomly selected group that did not receive a tocolytic agent. Seventy-five percent of the nifedipine group, 45 percent of the ritodrine group, and 29 percent of the untreated subjects remained undelivered after 3 days. Several subsequent reports have compared nifedipine with either ritodrine or terbutaline, with generally favorable results. In each trial, nifedipine was equal or superior to the β-mimetic agents in delaying delivery with fewer side effects.

Side Effects. Maternal cardiovascular side effects of the calcium channel blockers are similar to but milder than those with the β-mimetics. A mild decrease in blood pressure and a rise in pulse have been noted by most authors, with occasional cases of significant hypotension.[155] Unlike the β-mimetics, nifedipine is not associated with a decrease in serum potassium, although modest increases in glucose have been noted. Maternal symptoms are infrequent but include headache (20 percent), flushing (8 percent), dizziness, and nausea (6 percent). A case of hepatotoxicity requiring discontinuation of the drug has been reported. Two reports describe skeletal muscle blockade when used in conjunction with magnesium sulfate,[156,157] so this combination therapy should be avoided. Both reports describe a prompt response to cessation of magnesium and/or treatment with calcium gluconate.

Widespread acceptance of nifedipine as a tocolytic has been restrained by initial animal studies that reported reduction in uteroplacental blood flow, fetal bradycardia, and hypoxic myocardial depression with other calcium channel blockers, including verapamil, nicardipine, and diltiazem.[158,159] However, animal studies of nifedipine have not shown such effects unless supertherapeutic doses were infused. Reports of Doppler assessment of fetal and uteroplacental circulation during nifedipine use in women for treatment of PTL have also been reassuring.[160] No changes in middle cerebral artery, renal artery, ductus arteriosus, umbilical artery, or maternal vessels were noted in one study of 11 women treated with nifedipine for PTL. Murray et al[161] have reported an observational series of 102 mothers and 120 neonates treated with nifedipine. Fetal well-being and neonatal complications such as low Apgar scores and cord pH less than 7.20 were typical of premature infants. Ray et al[162] found no significant differences in Apgar scores or umbilical venous blood gas values in infants exposed to nifedipine compared with infants not exposed to any tocolytic medicines. These human studies have provided sufficient reassurance that many centers have begun to use nifedipine as the tocolytic of first choice.

Summary. Nifedipine is the only calcium channel blocker that should be used at present as a tocolytic. It has become the tocolytic agent of choice at an increasing number of hospitals because of the low incidence of significant maternal side effects and ease of administration. There are few remaining concerns about fetal side effects because animal studies suggesting fetal compromise were performed with agents other than nifedipine and because of an increasing number of reports of safe use in humans. Nifedipine should not be

Nifedipine Tocolysis

Nifedipine is usually given as a 10- to 20-mg dose every 6 hours orally. Patients in active PTL may be given a loading dose of 10 mg sublingually every 20 minutes for up to three doses, followed by oral administration every 6 hours

combined with magnesium. Use should follow published dosage schedules closely until more extensive clinical experience has been reported.

New Tocolytic Agents

Tocolytic agents that are under study at present include the oxytocin antagonist atosiban and the nitric oxide donor glyceryl trinitrate. Preliminary studies of atosiban indicate short-term efficacy in arresting contractions with few maternal or fetal side effects.[163] The nitroglycerin patch has also been reported to be a promising tocolytic,[164] but maternal headache has been a significant side effect in anecdotal reports.

Treatment with Multiple Tocolytics

All tocolytic drugs have significant failure rates, especially in advanced PTL. Therapy with multiple agents has been studied in an effort to improve efficacy. It should be recalled that patients whose contractions persist or recur during intravenous tocolytic treatment have a high incidence of underlying amnionitis and partial abruption. Other patients with persistent contractions without cervical change will stop contracting spontaneously and are not in PTL at all. Therefore, these diagnoses should be considered before considering multidrug therapy. It should also be remembered that the definition of "successful" tocolysis does not necessarily require that *no* contractions occur, only that the frequency be reduced to less than 4 to 6 per hour without further cervical change. Most often, use of a second agent will be considered when there has been no response to treatment with the primary tocolytic drug. The β-mimetics and calcium channel blockers are the most rapidly effective agents, often leading to at least a temporary cessation of contractions in less than 30 minutes; magnesium and indomethacin often require more than 1 to 2 hours to observe an effect. Centers using magnesium as the first line tocolytic agent often add one or two

supplemental doses of subcutaneous terbutaline 0.25 mg for patients with active PTL and advanced cervical effacement. This combination is reasonably effective and is safe if supplemental terbutaline is given only once or twice. Sustained treatment with the combination of magnesium and a β-mimetic has been found to increase the risk of significant side effects and should be avoided. One randomized trial compared ritodrine treatment alone with combination ritodrine-magnesium sulfate therapy and found improved pregnancy prolongation with combination therapy.[165] However, almost one-half of patients in both groups had tachycardia in excess of 140 bpm. Another group compared ritodrine with ritodrine-magnesium sulfate and was forced to halt the study when nearly one-half the 24 patients receiving combination therapy developed cardiovascular symptoms.[166] Both β-mimetics and magnesium sulfate can have similar effects on the cardiovascular system, increased cardiac output and cardiac performance with decreased peripheral vascular resistance, so the increased occurrence of side effects is not surprising. Beall and associates[123] studied sequential treatment with patients randomized to a β-mimetic or to magnesium sulfate therapy. Patients who failed the first agent were switched to the other. Initial success rates were comparable at approximately 70 percent for either ritodrine or magnesium sulfate. Most failures with ritodrine were due to maternal side effects, while most failures with magnesium sulfate were because of persistent contractions. Almost 90 percent of women who failed the initial agent responded favorably to the alternative. As noted previously, the combination of magnesium and calcium channel blockers may lead to skeletal muscle blockade.

Ancillary Treatment for Women with Preterm Labor

The initial goal of treatment of women with PTL is to delay delivery long enough to allow three interventions that have been shown to reduce the neonatal morbidity and mortality caused by prematurity:

1. Transfer of mother and fetus to a hospital equipped to care for a premature infant
2. Administration of glucocorticoids to reduce neonatal respiratory distress syndrome and intraventricular hemorrhage
3. Administration of antibiotic prophylaxis to prevent neonatal group B **Streptococcus** infection

Maternal and Neonatal Transfer

Regionalization of neonatal intensive care and maternal perinatal care has been shown to improve the rates of morbidity and mortality for LBW and especially for

VLBW infants. Transfer of the LBW infant after birth was instituted in the 1970s and led to dramatic improvements in neonatal outcomes. When it was recognized that some VLBW infants died before a regional center's neonatal care team could arrive, transfer of the mother with fetus in utero became the preferred alternative whenever possible. Most states have adopted systems of regionalized perinatal care[167] that recognize the advantages of concentrating care for VLBW infants in special centers. Hospitals and birth centers caring for normal mothers and infants are designated as Level I. Most larger urban hospitals that care for the majority of maternal and infant complications are designated as level II centers; these hospitals have neonatal intensive care units staffed and equipped to care for most infants with birth weights above 1,250 to 1,500 g. Level III centers typically provide care for the sickest and smallest infants and for maternal complications requiring intensive care.

Antenatal Glucocorticoids

In 1972, Liggins and Howie[168] reported a reduction in hyaline membrane disease or respiratory distress syndrome in infants born to women treated with antenatal corticosteroids. Since then, numerous studies have confirmed the beneficial effects of maternal steroid treatment in reducing newborn respiratory distress syndrome and have demonstrated additional benefits, including reduced incidence and severity of intraventricular hemorrhage and necrotizing enterocolitis and, most importantly, decreased perinatal mortality.

Physiologic Effects. Antenatal steroids influence the synthesis of fetal proteins and peptides. In general it may be said that they enhance cell differentiation and maturation rather than cell growth. In the fetal lung, steroids induce several changes that favorably affect neonatal pulmonary performance: production of surfactant is enhanced by the effect of glucocorticoids on the activity of enzymes important in the synthesis of phosphatidylcholine, a major component of surfactant; neonatal lung compliance is increased; production of proteins that enhance surfactant activity (SP-B and SP-C) is increased; and alveolar protein leakage is decreased. Steroids also affect other organ systems, inducing maturation in the fetal brain, skin and gastrointestinal tract. Animal studies have suggested that steroids promote maturation of the germinal matrix and thereby reduce the occurrence of perinatal intraventricular hemorrhage.[169,170]

Dosage. Two essentially identical glucocorticoid regimens have been studied and found equally effective; betamethasone 12 mg IM Q24h for two doses or dexamethasone 6 mg IM Q6h for four doses. Other steroid preparations, such as prednisone, may not be effective because of poor placental transfer and should not be used.

Therapeutic Effects of Antenatal Corticosteroids.
Pulmonary Function. The original study of Liggins and Howie[168] reported a 50 percent reduction in respiratory distress syndrome in steroid-treated neonates, an observation that has been repeatedly confirmed. A recent meta-analysis by Crowley[171] of 15 trials found an OR of 0.51 (95 percent; CI, 0.42 to 0.61) in the cumulative data for the occurrence of respiratory distress syndrome in infants born to mothers treated with antepartum steroids compared with placebo-treated controls (Fig. 23-18). Some questions remain about the efficacy of steroids in reducing respiratory distress syndrome in patients with preterm PROM (see later section), but the magnitude and the consistency of the benefit across multiple trials have eliminated any doubt of efficacy of antenatal steroids in reducing respiratory distress syndrome in patients with intact membranes. Questions raised by earlier trials[172] that the effectiveness of steroids might be limited to certain subgroups (e.g., female and/or black infants or infants only between 28 and 32 weeks' gestation) have been answered by the larger numbers accumulated in the Crowley meta-analysis: the benefit is significant for male and female, and for black and nonblack, infants across a wide range of gestational ages from 24 through 34 weeks. The earlier questions about efficacy in subgroups are now seen to derive entirely from inadequate statistical power due to small sample sizes for subgroup analysis in the initial trials. Readers wishing to learn about the importance of statistical power and β-error in clinical medicine could find no better example than the misunderstood and "under-powered" secondary analyses of steroid efficacy in subgroups of larger trials. At our center, the "Elephant Gun Story" has been useful to illustrate the effect of power and sample size and is offered for readers less comfortable with statistics.

Imagine a gun (steroids) that is guaranteed to shoot elephants (respiratory distress syndrome [RDS]) rendering them harmless (no RDS) or at least less hostile (milder RDS). The most efficient way to demonstrate the efficacy of the gun would be to go to a place where there are many elephants. In India (28 to 32 weeks), where many elephants are found, the efficacy of the gun is easily demonstrated, but in Ohio (after 32 weeks), it would take a long time to find enough elephants to provide a convincing demonstration of the gun. However, if an elephant should be encountered in Ohio (after 32 weeks), there is no reason to believe that the gun would be any less effective when used at 32 to 34 weeks than at 30 weeks. After 34 weeks,

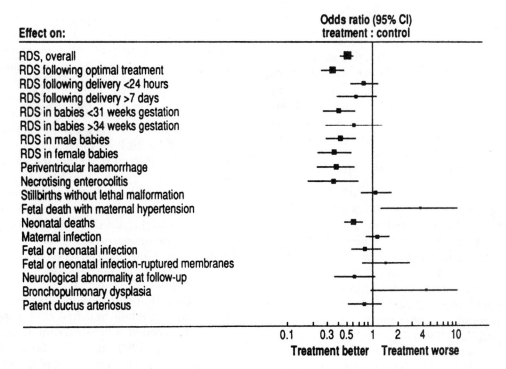

Fig. 23-18. Summary of meta-analysis of 15 trials of the effect of corticosteroid use before preterm delivery on maternal and newborn outcome. RDS, respiratory distress syndrome. (From Crowley[171], with permission.)

RDS is so rare that shooting the steroid gun without first being certain that one has identified a fetus at risk for RDS (via amniotic fluid studies) is not justified. Before 34 weeks, RDS is so common that documentation of fetal immaturity is not necessary.

Maternal steroid treatment is not uniformly effective in eliminating respiratory distress syndrome entirely, but has been shown to ameliorate its severity when it does occur. One trial[173] found no reduction in respiratory distress syndrome in treated patients studied between 24 and 28 weeks, but did observe decreased severity of respiratory distress syndrome in treated infants manifested by reduced ventilator pressure settings and fewer NICU days. Other trials[174,175] have confirmed these results. It is important to emphasize that exogenous surfactant, now shown to be an effective postnatal treatment for respiratory distress syndrome, does not replace the important respiratory benefits of antenatal steroid treatment. The effects of steroids and surfactant have been found to be additive for infants who receive both treatments, including significant reduction in mortality for infants who received both treatments (0 percent) compared with those who received either therapy alone (19 percent).[175–178]

Intraventricular Hemorrhage. Analyses of placebo-controlled trials of antenatal steroids[171,179,180] have confirmed the original observation by Howie and Liggins[181] that antenatal steroid treatment is associated with a significant (50 percent) reduction in the incidence of intraventricular hemorrhage (see Fig. 23-18). The mechanism by which steroids produce this benefit was originally attributed entirely to the reduced frequency and severity of respiratory distress syndrome, but effects independent of respiratory distress syndrome have been postulated based on studies that controlled for respiratory distress syndrome severity[182] and cranial ultrasound studies of neonates performed shortly after birth.[183] A study confined to patients treated between 24 and 28 weeks[173] in which there was no reduction in respiratory distress syndrome in treated patients nevertheless found a reduction in intraventricular hemorrhage from 25 percent in untreated to 3 percent ($p = 0.012$) in treated infants. A reduction in the size of cerebral infarction has been shown in animals treated with dexamethasone prior to but not after an experimental hypoxic brain injury.[169] In contrast to these findings, a recent observational study of infants less than 1,000 g found no relationship between the occurrence of neonatal intraventricular hemorrhage and maternal steroid administration.[184]

Other Effects. Antenatal steroid treatment has been associated with other favorable effects on neonatal outcome, including a 65 percent reduction in the incidence of necrotizing enterocolitis (OR, 0.35, CI, 0.18–0.68).[171] Reductions in the incidence of patent ductus arteriosus and circulatory instability and improved Apgar scores[185] have also been reported.

Perinatal Mortality. The most persuasive evidence of the benefit of antenatal steroids comes from analyses indicating that perinatal mortality is reduced in infants born to treated mothers. In the meta-analysis cited earlier,[171] the OR for neonatal mortality after antenatal steroids was 0.61 (CI, 0.49–0.78). This figure is consistent with the data from the original report[168] showing a 40 percent reduction in early neonatal mortality after steroid treatment.

Risks. The major short-term concern is the risk of reduced resistance to infection for both the mother and infant. Neither of the two largest studies[172,186] noted any increased incidence of neonatal or maternal infections. There may be some excess risk in mothers and infants when steroids are given in the face of preterm rupture of the membranes (see discussion below). Increased fetal jeopardy in pregnancies complicated by proteinuric hypertension was suggested by the original study of Liggins and Howie,[168] but was not confirmed in subsequent series.[187,188] Another short-term result of prenatal glucocorticoid therapy is impairment of maternal glucose tolerance, particularly in a woman with insulin-dependent diabetes. To prevent ketoacidosis, these patients may require management with insulin infusions for several days and should be observed carefully. In most patients without diabetes, the hyperglycemic effect of glucocorticoids is limited to 2 to 3 days following administration, but may be prolonged if other traditional risk factors such as maternal age, obesity, or family history are present. The hyperglycemic effect of steroid treatment is one reason to avoid routine weekly injections of steroids in high-risk pregnancies.

Although antenatal steroids can inhibit adrenal responsiveness in the newborn, the effect is biochemical only and is without apparent clinical significance. The doses given produce levels of corticoids comparable to those endogenously produced by the neonatal adrenal gland in response to the stress of respiratory distress syndrome.

There is some evidence that maternal steroid treatment given chronically as in therapy of connective tissue disease can affect the tensile strength of the amniotic membranes and lead to an increased risk of PROM, but this has not been reported when steroids are given in the dosage regimen recommended for neonatal respiratory distress syndrome prophylaxis.

Long-term risks for the fetus are only theoretical at present, there being no evidence of delayed adverse effects after in utero therapy. Any concern about long-term effects is founded on the general effect of steroids to accelerate fetal cellular and organ maturation at the expense of cell and organ growth.[189] Antenatal steroid therapy given in a rodent model at a gestational age analogous to the early third trimester in humans was associated with reduced brain cell number and decreased brain DNA content.[190] It is reassuring to note that the original cohort of fetuses treated by Liggins and Howie and in the Collaborative Trial[191] have displayed no differences when compared with gestational age-matched controls in physical or mental function, but Slotkin[192] cautions that "therapeutic use of antenatal steroids . . . occupies precisely the timeframe of maximum vulnerability of the central nervous system (CNS) . . . (and) . . . low doses of glucocorticoids that lie at or below the threshold for eliciting changes in lung surfactant production are capable of altering CNS development" and may also affect tissue response to hypoxia in organ systems other than the CNS.

Clinical Use. Despite the impressive evidence of both medical and economic benefits[193,194] maternal steroid treatment preceded only 26 percent of low birth weight deliveries in a 1990 survey.[195] Fewer than half of treated infants in this review had received a full course of treatment. The underutilization apparently occurred for diverse reasons. Some did not receive treatment for unavoidable causes such as presentation in advanced labor or maternal illness requiring immediate delivery (e.g., eclampsia or significant obstetric hemorrhage). Others were not treated because of previously inadequate supportive data or misinterpretations of the literature (e.g., underestimation by obstetricians of neonatal survival rates for ELBW babies,[196] concern about maternal or neonatal risks of infectious morbidity, or questions about the effectiveness of partial treatment or of population subsets such as white male fetuses).

In response to these concerns, the NICHD convened a Consensus Development Conference on Antenatal Steroids in 1994.[197] Their recommendations were reviewed by the Committee on Obstetric Practice Opinion (No. 147) of the American College of Obstetricians and Gynecologists.[198] Both organizations recommended increased use of antenatal steroids for mothers expected to deliver imminently before 32 weeks' gestation to reduce mortality and the incidence of respiratory distress syndrome and intraventricular hemorrhage, regardless of the status of the fetal membranes. At 32 to 34 weeks, both NICHD and ACOG recommended antenatal steroid treatment for mothers with intact membranes who were likely to deliver within 7 days, but noted that the benefit for infants born to women with ruptured membranes after 32 weeks is still controversial. The controversy centers on whether a large trial[199] that found a substantial benefit with steroids should be included in meta-analyses. The results of the trial in question may have been confounded by issues involving concomitant treatments and by a remarkably high rate of respiratory distress syndrome in the control group. When meta-analyses of steroid trials in patients with preterm PROM exclude the data from this trial, the beneficial effect of steroids on the incidence of respiratory distress syndrome is lost, but the effect on intraventricular hemorrhage is retained.

In addition to the preterm PROM issues, questions regarding the need for and risk of repeated weekly courses of steroids remain unanswered. The opportunity for long-term risk would seem to be greater with repeated dosing but is not proved to occur. The risk and consequences of imminent preterm birth, in contrast, are immediate and real and will vary in individual ways as the pregnancy continues. A weekly reassessment of the need for steroids, rather than a policy of routinely administering steroids each week to high-risk patients, is probably the wisest course.

The NICHD Consensus Panel's campaign to increase the use of steroids has also led to new unanswered questions about the indications for steroid treatment of high-risk patients. What risk of "imminent preterm delivery" is sufficient to treat the patient with antenatal corticoids? Is actual PTL or preterm PROM required, or is a history of a previous preterm delivery or a dilated or effaced cervix enough? At our center, we have used admission to the hospital as the criterion for steroid treatment: with rare exception, steroids are not likely to be necessary until the risk of preterm delivery has required hospitalization. In response to many questions from physicians who refer patients to The Ohio State University Medical Center, we have distributed the guidelines shown in the box.

Antibiotics for Women with Preterm Labor

There are two potential uses for antibiotics in women with PTL. The first is prophylaxis of neonatal group B streptococcal infection, an intervention that is clearly effective (as discussed elsewhere in this volume). The second is antibiotic therapy aimed at prolonging gestation in women with PTL by targeting a broad range of microorganisms that have been implicated in the pathogenesis of SPTB. Administration of antibiotics to women being treated for PTL has been studied extensively and has not been particularly successful. Randomized placebo-controlled trials[200–207] are summarized in Table 23-11, and the data from the largest trial[205] is shown in detail in Table 23-12.

Given the extensive and persuasive literature that links genital tract colonization and infection with spontaneous prematurity, what can be the reasons for the failure of supplemental prophylactic antibiotics to enhance tocolysis? The first is the problem that has hampered all studies of PTL, the inaccurate overdiagnosis of PTL in the pre-fibronectin era. The inclusion of women who do not actually have PTL in trials of interventions for PTL confounds interpretation of the results. Antibiotic trials limited to subjects who are fibronectin positive might produce different results. The second reason is that the clinical diagnosis of PTL, even when accurate, may occur so late in the pathologic sequence that it is simply too late for antibiotics to exert any favorable effect. Regardless of the explanation, it is clear from the number and diversity of the studies displayed in Table 23-12 that supplemental antimicrobial therapy for reasons other than treatment of a specific pathogen such as gonorrhea or prophylaxis of group B *Streptococcus* is not justified at present for women with PTL.

Other Adjunctive Antenatal Treatments To Reduce Fetal Morbidity

The persistence of cases of respiratory distress syndrome among infants born to women treated with steroid therapy has led to alternative treatment approaches to further enhance pulmonary maturation. Neonatal treatment with surfactant has become an established adjunctive therapy that adds independently and synergistically to the benefit of corticosteroids in reducing morbidity related to respiratory distress syndrome. Maternal adjunctive treatment with thyroid-releasing hormone has also been studied, but promising initial studies have not been confirmed in subsequent trials.

Studies of other agents given to the mother before delivery to reduce or prevent neonatal morbidity have been reported for phenobarbital and vitamin K, with mixed results. The goal of treatment with both agents was to reduce the incidence of intraventricular hemorrhage. Phenobarbital was investigated after studies in primates suggested that the drug reduced cerebral glucose requirements. Vitamin K supplementation was intended to improve fetal coagulation to limit the extent of cerebral hemorrhage. Initial studies of both agents appeared, promising but a larger trial (n = 372) that compared phenobarbital and vitamin K with placebo found no benefit to treatment with these agents. Rates of grades III and IV intraventricular hemorrhage, of any intraventricular hemorrhage, and of neonatal mortality did not differ between 181 infants born to mothers who received placebo and 191 whose mothers received both vitamin K and phenobarbital.[208]

Recent reports have noted the association of a reduced incidence of intraventricular hemorrhage and cerebral palsy in premature infants with antepartum maternal magnesium sulfate treatment for both PTL tocolysis and seizure prophylaxis.[125,126] Though preliminary, the studies are promising enough to support magnesium sulfate as a reasonable tocolytic choice despite its modest ability to arrest contractions. However,

Current Recommendations for Antenatal Use of Corticosteroids at The Ohio State University

ACOG and the NICHD Panel have issued similar but not identical position statements. Both ACOG and NICHD agree that steroids are highly effective to reduce both respiratory distress (RDS) and intraventricular hemorrhage (IVH) in premature infants and to reduce the perinatal morbidity and mortality due to these problems. Both ACOG and NICHD agree that steroids have been underutilized, and both have encouraged obstetricians to use antenatal steroids more liberally. The questions have come when these general guidelines are translated into our care of individual patients. Here are our recommendations:

1. How do I decide who should get steroids? Any woman whose risk of preterm birth is sufficient to require hospitalization is probably a candidate for steroids. The usual indications are PTL and preterm PROM (see below), but women with preeclampsia, placenta previa or abruption, or IUGR fetuses are also candidates. The key question is "Is this patient likely to deliver within the week?". If the answer is yes with a probability high enough to need hospital care, give steroids. Women with risk (e.g., twins or prior preterm birth) who do not require hospitalization probably do not need to be treated at home except in very rare circumstances. Weekly treatment of outpatients with risk is not recommended.

2. What about ruptured membranes? There is still some doubt about the efficacy of steroids to reduce RDS in women with preterm PROM (ACOG says no, NICHD says maybe yes), but steroids appear to reduce IVH in babies born to women with preterm PROM. Because IVH rarely occurs after 32 and 6/7ths weeks, we now use steroids in preterm PROM patients up through 32 and 6/7ths weeks, provided there is no evidence of infection.

3. Should I treat women before 28 and/or after 32 weeks? The answer is yes. We begin treatment with steroids at 23–24 weeks and will treat without an amniocentesis up through 34 weeks for patients with intact membranes. Women with preterm PROM at ≥33 weeks, and with intact membranes at ≥35 weeks, may be treated if amniotic fluid studies show immature lungs.

4. What about repeated courses of steroids? There is no clear answer to this question. There are theoretical reasons to worry that repeated courses might affect fetal neurological development or immune function, but there is no evidence that this has occurred in humans after 20+ years of use. Both ACOG and NICHD say that more research is needed but take no stand for or against weekly treatment. The best guide is still to treat anyone whose risk of preterm birth is high enough to require hospital care and to reconsider that question each week.

5. What drug and dose should be used? The standard regimen is betamethasone 12 mg IM twice, given 24 hours apart. Some doctors at Ohio State University and elsewhere use 12 mg IM × 2, given 12 hours apart, for women whose risk of preterm delivery within 48 hours is thought to be very high.

6. Can I give steroids along with tocolytics?
For women with intact membranes: Yes. Just be careful to follow intake and output and to listen to the lungs frequently.
For women with ruptured membranes: This is controversial. At present, we recommend using tocolytics in these patients only to allow maternal transfer.

the evidence at present to support adjunctive use of magnesium as an agent intended to protect against neonatal intraventricular hemorrhage is inconclusive.

Problems and Controversies with Tocolytic Therapy

Persistent Contractions Despite Maximum Dose Therapy

Persistent contractions despite aggressive and prolonged tocolysis may occur at the opposite ends of the spectrum of PTL. The most common reason is an inaccurate diagnosis of PTL, in which contractions persist but the cervix does not change. In the past, such patients were often treated with oral or even subcutaneous tocolytics rather than risk the persistence of frequent contractions. The availability of fibronectin and cervical sonography has provided methods to reassure these patients that their contractions do not indicate the presence of PTL. At the opposite extreme, persistent contractions may indicate an underlying stimulus of PTL such as chorioamnionitis or abruption. Women whose contractions persist for more than 12 to 24 hours of aggressive tocolysis should be reevaluated as follows:

Table 23-11 Randomized Placebo-Controlled Trials of Adjunctive Antibiotics in Preterm Labor

Author	No. With PTL	Antibiotic Rx	Effect
McGregor et al[200]	17 (refractory to tocolysis)	Erythromycin 333 mg TID	> Interval to delivery > Deliver at term, >birth weight
Winkler et al[201]	19	Ampicillin 500 QID	> Interval to delivery
Newton et al[202]	103	Ampicillin 2 g IV Q6 and Erythromycin 333 TID	No effect
McGregor et al[203]	117	Clindamycin IV/PO	> Interval to delivery
Newton et al[204]	86	Ampicillin and sulbactam	No effect
Romero et al[205]	277	Ampicillin IV/PO and erythromycin IV/PO	No effect
Norman et al[206]	81	Ampicillin IV/PO and metronidazole PR/PO	> Interval to delivery
Gordon et al[207]	117	Ceftizoxime IV	No effect

Is the cervix changing? Perform a transvaginal cervical ultrasound to measure cervical length and look for funneling or separation of the membranes from the lower segment. Obtain a swab for fibronectin.

Is the patient infected? Review white blood cell counts and consider amniocentesis for glucose, Gram stain, and culture.

Is there fetal compromise? Review fetal heart tracings and do a biophysical assessment.

Is there evidence of abruption? Repeat hemoglobin, hematocrit, and coagulation profiles and abdominal sonography for placental implantation site. Is there a suspicion of abruption or of uterine anomaly with implantation of the placenta on the septum?

If infection, fetal compromise, and abruption are excluded, stop parenteral tocolysis for 24 hours and observe. Most patients will stop contracting spontaneously.

Table 23-12 Supplemental Antibiotic Treatment in Women with Preterm Labor[a]

	Outcome	
	Antibiotic Rx	Placebo
	n = 131	n = 144
Delivery <37 weeks	53%	52%
Entry to delivery (days)	35 days	32 days
Mean Birth Weight	2,535 g	2,883 g
Preterm PROM	19%	15%
Amnionitis	2%	5%

[a]Prospective, randomized trial by NICHD MFMU Network. Ampicillin + erythromycin vs. placebo; 277 subjects with PTL at 24–34 weeks, intact membranes.
(Data from Romero et al[205])

Who Needs an Amniocentesis?

Amniocentesis can be helpful in the management of some women with PTL. Evaluation of amniotic fluid for fetal pulmonary maturity studies is especially helpful when the gestational age is in doubt, when the size of the fetus suggests poor or excessive intrauterine growth, when there is any question of a hostile intrauterine environment (e.g., maternal medical or obstetric illness, decreased amniotic fluid volume, history of substance abuse). Amniotic fluid glucose, Gram stain, and culture may be indicated when infection is suspected because of maternal fever, leukocytosis, or persistent contractions. Amniocentesis should also be considered prior to corticosteroid treatment of patients after 34 weeks. Routine use of amniocentesis to assess pulmonary maturity in all patients with PTL is not practiced in most hospitals, but may be justified in centers that care for populations having poor dates, high rates of maternal substance abuse, or fetal growth restriction.

How Long a Hospital Stay?

The duration of hospitalization for an episode of PTL will vary according to several factors, including the dilatation, effacement, and sonographic length of the cervix, ease of tocolysis, fibronectin status, gestational age, obstetric history, distance from hospital, and availability of home care and family support. As noted previously, a negative fibronectin and/or sonographic cervical length of more than 30 mm provide strong evidence that the short-term risk of preterm delivery is low. In contrast, women with complete cervical effacement at a gestational age at the margins of perinatal viability are particularly likely to benefit from prolonged hospital care. Associated risk factors that may complicate or increase the risk of recurrent PTL, such as a positive genital culture for group B *Streptococcus*, *chlamydia*, or *gonorrhea*, urinary tract infection, and anemia should be controlled before discharge from hospital care. Social issues such as homelessness, the availability of child care, or protection from an abusive partner are often the most important determinants of a patient's ability to comply with medical care and must always be considered before the patient is discharged from the hospital.

What Is the Role of Home Uterine Activity Monitoring After Preterm Labor?

Four studies have described home uterine activity monitoring (HUAM) in posthospitalization management of women with PTL in the current pregnancy.[209–212] An observational study reported fewer preterm births in women who used a home contraction monitor after the diagnosis of PTL compared to nonrandomly selected controls.[209] In contrast, two prospective randomized trials of HUAM after preterm labor found no advantage to monitored contraction data compared with self-palpation and frequent nursing contact.[210,211] A 1995 multicenter randomized trial of HUAM versus (sham) HUAM found no improvement in the rate of preterm birth when HUAM data were used.[212] In these studies, the monitored contraction data were typically used to adjust the dose of oral β-mimetic drugs to suppress contractions. The inability to demonstrate an advantage for patients who used the home monitor in these studies may be explained in part by the ineffectiveness of oral tocolysis as described in the following section.

Oral Tocolytic Treatment: Is There a Role for Oral Tocolytic Medications After Parenteral Therapy?

Although commonly employed, oral tocolytic medication after suppression of an acute episode of PTL is poorly supported by existing literature. Published studies have enrolled only limited numbers of subjects, mak-

ing meta-analysis the most appropriate basis for evaluation. Two meta-analyses[213,214] of randomized controlled trials of oral β-mimetics, the drugs most frequently prescribed, found no reduction in preterm birth, no prolongation of pregnancy, and no reduction in recurrent PTL associated with this treatment (Fig. 23-19). It should be noted that chronic administration of β-mimetic tocolytics can have significant side effects, both fetal and maternal. One case report[215] describes a woman whose fetus developed hypertrophy of the myocardial septum, apparently as a result of prolonged β-mimetic-induced fetal tachycardia. Several studies[111,216] have documented a clear deterioration in glucose tolerance with more than 5 days of oral terbutaline. Women treated with continuous β-mimetic drugs, whether by the oral or subcutaneous route, should be screened (and rescreened if previously tested) for glucose intolerance.

There are several possible reasons for the apparent inability of oral tocolytics to improve outcome. The most obvious reasons relate to the pharmacology of the agents used. First, the dosages of oral β-mimetics and magnesium do not achieve levels in the blood comparable to levels produced by parenteral therapy.[217] Second, treatment with oral β-mimetic agents for more than 2 to 3 weeks is associated with tachyphylaxis, a decreased pharmacologic effect caused by down-regulation of the β-receptor after prolonged use. Neither of these issues has been addressed directly in the literature. The Canadian ritodrine study[91] indicated prolongation of pregnancy for 2 to 5 days while the drug was given parenterally; there was no additional prolongation of pregnancy when the medication was administered orally in a dose insufficient to achieve therapeutic blood levels. The FDA has withdrawn its approval for oral ritodrine based largely on the results of the Cana-

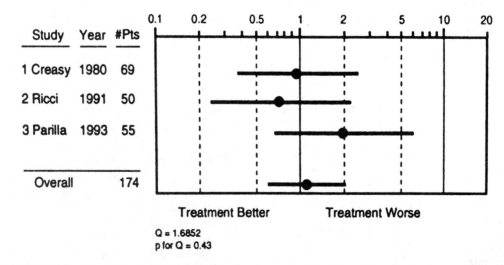

Fig. 23-19. Odds ratios in three trials of the effect of oral β-sympathomimetic drugs on incidence of preterm birth in women previously treated for preterm labor with parenteral tocolysis. (From Macones et al,[213] with permission.)

dian trial. Tachyphylaxis, although a well-known phenomenon, has never been addressed in a study of proper design or size. Administration of terbutaline via a subcutaneous infusion pump has been marketed as a method of reducing the likelihood of tachyphylaxis. Unfortunately, there are no studies of the effect of this expensive intervention on the rates of preterm delivery or recurrent PTL. In the absence of studies showing benefit, and because of the high cost of continuous subcutaneous administration by pump, this method is used in our center only in women who have PTL complicated by maternal diabetes in whom it may reduce the adverse effects of terbutaline on control of blood sugar.

Another more fundamental explanation of the inability of both parenteral and oral tocolytics to delay delivery by more than a few days is that suppression of contractions is a poor strategy for prevention of preterm birth because it is based on an erroneous understanding of PTL as an event that occurs (and may recur) as a result of a spontaneous and accidental coalescence of subclinical uterine activity. According to this view, the underlying cause(s) of PTL are usually infectious or ischemic processes that are not directly affected by tocolytics. This conclusion is consistent with studies showing no decrease in prematurity for women followed with HUAM, another intervention aimed at preventing premature birth by early detection and suppression of contractions (see also later section on HUAM as an aid to detection of PTL). Finally, studies of oral tocolysis have been few in number and small in size, and, like all studies of PTL interventions, have enrolled a high number of subjects with poorly diagnosed PTL. The inability to identify any benefit of oral tocolysis may be due to methodologic problems, to subtherapeutic dosing regimens, and to a wholly erroneous underlying theory of PTL. In summary, the utility of oral tocolytic treatment for women with PTL has not been established.

Abnormal Cervical Competence

Few subjects in obstetrics have been the subject of greater or more prolonged controversy than has cervical incompetence. The diagnosis of incompetent cervix has traditionally been made and is still most confidently established by an obstetric history of passive and painless dilatation of the cervix in the second trimester. The controversy has centered on whether this classic picture is the only true presentation for this disorder or whether there are other clinical presentations that are also the result of poor cervical competence. A history of the amniotic sac found bulging through a well-effaced and partially dilated cervix in the absence of contractions, bleeding, infection, or amniorrhexis is classic but is not common. There are many other women who present for care in the second trimester with uterine cramps, leaking amniotic fluid, chorioamnionitis, or even bleeding, and whose cervical dilation and effacement seem out of proportion to the duration and/or severity of the presenting complaints. Do these women have an incompetent cervix with subsequent development of labor, PPROM, and so forth, or did they simply dismiss or fail to notice the presence of uterine contractions? Arguments about the presentation and incidence of incompetent cervix are ultimately based on two different theories of how and why the cervix dilates and effaces prematurely. According to the traditional view, the cervix operates as a categorical variable in which it is either fully functional (competent) or is nonfunctional (incompetent). PTL, ruptured membranes, bleeding, or intra-amniotic infection in women presenting at 16 to 26 weeks are assumed to be primary etiologic diagnoses in which a competent cervix changes only in response to uterine activity, whether overt or occult. This understanding of cervical competence as either categorically competent or incompetent is based on studies of the cervix in which digital examination was used to assess cervical dilation and length. A 1961 study[218] stated the question clearly: The authors "wondered whether there can be any degrees in the incompetence of the internal os. If an incompetent os can cause abortion, is it possible that a lesser degree of incompetency can lead to premature labour?" They performed digital examination of the cervix in 655 subjects and concluded that "a degree of incompetence of the internal os that would lead to a premature labour does not seem to exist." This conclusion has been dominant in texts for the past three decades, but has occasionally been questioned by clinical studies suggesting that women with a history of second trimester delivery might benefit from treatment with prophylactic cerclage.[219,220] These studies suggested that the traditional clinical presentation of incompetent cervix may be simply fortuitous, i.e., that some women with a passively dilated cervix and bulging amniotic sac might develop contractions, infection, or membrane rupture as the consequence of incompetent cervix. The view that cervical competence was categorical was not questioned, only that the clinical presentation was more diverse.

Recent studies of the cervix using ultrasound have gone further, challenging the idea that cervical competence is categorical and suggesting instead that it has variable function along a continuum of "competence."[55] Studies of transabdominal sonography of the cervix[221,222] noted that cervical incompetence could be detected earlier by ultrasound than by digital examination. However, because of the variable effect of maternal body habitus and bladder filling on transabdominal sonographic measurement of the cervix, this method is not reliable.[223] Iams et al[66] used transvaginal ultrasound to investigate whether cervical competence was catgorical or continuous. Cervical length measurements were obtained during pregnancy from three groups of patients: women with an obstetric history typical of incompetent cervix, women with a history of a prior spontaneous preterm birth, and women who had normal obstetric histories and normal current pregnancies. The authors hypothesized that if cervical function were categorical, cervical length would be short in women with incompetent cervix but would be normal in the women who delivered preterm. Alternately, if cervical function were continuous, cervical length would decrease as the gestational age at delivery in the previous pregnancy decreased. The results were consistent with the latter hypothesis: the earlier the gestational age at delivery in the prior pregnancy, the shorter the cervix in the current pregnancy.[66]

Additional support for the view of cervical competence as a continuum comes from two prospective studies in which transvaginal sonographic measurements of the cervix in the late second and early third trimesters were correlated with risk of preterm delivery in the current pregnancy. In a cross-sectional study of 178 women, Andersen et al[55] noted a striking increase in the risk of preterm delivery as cervical length decreased; the increase in risk was not confined to women with the very shortest cervical length, but rather extended into the normal ranges of length. The NICHD Prediction of Prematurity study cited earlier[56] confirmed and extended the work of Andersen et al in a study of 2,915 pregnant women who received blinded transvaginal sonographic measurement of cervical length at 24 and 28 weeks' gestation. The relative risk of preterm birth increased as cervical length decreased across the range of cervical lengths and was noted at both 24 and 28 weeks (Fig. 23-20). As in the Andersen et al study, an increase in risk of SPTB as the cervix shortened was observed even within the normal range (i.e., the risk of preterm birth was higher for women whose cervical length was at the 50th percentile than for women whose cervical length was at the 75th percentile; (Fig. 23-21). The same cervical changes (shortened cervix, funnelled internal os) that are associated with increased risk of SPTB have also been described in women who present with typical cervical incompetence.[224] The only difference is the duration of pregnancy at the time of examination.

These studies have changed our understanding of the cervix from the traditional categorical concept of cervical "incompetence" versus "competence" to one of *variable* competence, in which cervical function is described by a bell-shaped curve that roughly corresponds to length. The risk of SPTB increases as cervical length decreases. Women with cervical lengths below the 5th or 10th percentile clearly have the greatest risk

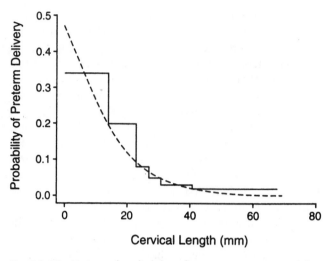

Fig. 23-20. Estimated probability of spontaneous preterm delivery before 35 weeks of gestation from the logistic regression analysis (dashed line) and observed frequency of spontaneous preterm delivery (solid line) according to cervical length measured by transvaginal ultrasonography at 24 weeks. (From Iams et al[56] with permission.)

for SPTB (see Fig. 23-21), but the clinical presentation is not uniform. Some will present with PTL, others with preterm PROM, and still others with the classic picture of incompetent cervix. The importance of reduced cervical "competence" as a contributing factor in the pathogenesis of preterm delivery increases as the gestational age at the time of delivery decreases. It is important here to reemphasize the concept discussed earlier of multiple contributing variables: cervical resis-

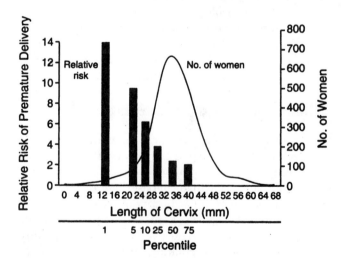

Fig. 23-21. Distribution of subjects by percentile of cervical length measured by transvaginal sonography at 24 weeks (solid line) and relative risk of spontaneous preterm birth before 35 weeks according to percentiles of cervical length (bars). Relative risk of spontaneous preterm delivery for women at the 1st, 5th, 10th, 25th, 50th, and 75th percentiles are compared with the risks among women with cervical lengths above the 75th percentile. (From Iams et al[56] with permission.)

tance to delivery is a continuous variable, but so also are the factors favoring delivery, such as uterine volume and contractile activity, infectious insults, and time spent standing. Competence is therefore relative to the circumstances of a given pregnancy. For example, a cervix at the 10th to 25th percentiles of length may be adequate for a singleton pregnancy in a woman who does not perform manual labor but inadequate to resist delivery in a twin pregnancy in a woman who works 60 hours per week as a house officer. The concepts of a continuum of cervical competence and of multiple interactive variables provide an explanation for some of the controversies about patients said to have an "incompetent cervix": Why do they not always present with the typical classic presentation in every pregnancy? Why do some women with the typical history do well without a cerclage? Why is there so much disagreement about the role of cerclage? What should be the criteria for placing a cerclage? Why does the baby not just "fall out" after a cerclage is removed? Why is cerclage not uniformly effective? The answer in each case is that pregnancy outcome is influenced by more than just a uniformly and totally incompetent cervix.

Length Vs. Competence

If cervical length is normally distributed and correlates with risk of SPTB, is it possible to define reduced cervical competence according to a cervical length below, for example, the 5th percentile? The answer is no: Cervical length alone is not sufficient to determine the function of the cervix in pregnancy. The ratio of muscle to collagen has been shown to be increased in women with a history of incompetent cervix.[225] We have found that women with a history of cervical cone biopsy may have significant cervical shortening without increased risk of preterm birth, perhaps because of the scarring that occurs as the cervix heals. The assumption thus far in this discussion has been that "competence" is a physical property, related to length as a marker of apparent strength. Length may instead simply reflect the host defense function of the cervix, the ability to resist the ascent of vaginal flora into the decidual space. A short but scarred and closed cervix might then be fully competent.

There are still many questions yet unanswered, including the mechanisms by which effacement occurs and the gestational age at which the cervix first begins to efface or shorten. Does the cervix shorten because of intracervical or systemic inflammatory stimuli, because of changes in the hormonal milieu, or because of intrinsic variations in the resistance of cervical collagen to the increase in uterine volume as pregnancy progresses? Are the changes mediated by prostaglandins, or is there subclinical uterine activity that produces a

shortened cervix? Despite the unanswered questions, this much is clear: cervical competence is variable and so is the clinical presentation. The only clearly diagnostic presentation is still a history of painless dilation, but any patient with a history of early preterm birth before 26 weeks may have *reduced cervical competence*, a term that more accurately reflects the data described above.

Etiology

It is clear from the obstetric histories of affected women that reduced cervical competence may be congenital and/or acquired. Some women have typical histories of painless dilation in the first and every subsequent pregnancy, while others experience progressively earlier delivery with each pregnancy until a typical "incompetent" history occurs. Still others have several term births before an obstetric injury in the penultimate pregnancy creates a damaged cervix. The concept of percentiles of competence suggests that women with cervical lengths below the 25th to 50th percentiles may suffer clinically meaningful injury to the cervix as a result of obstetric or gynecologic trauma that would not have clinical consequences had the initial cervical length been longer.

Cervical trauma may occur in the course of either vaginal or cesarean delivery. The cervix may be lacerated and heal poorly or may be stretched beyond tolerance. Our center has seen an increasing number of women whose typical presentation of incompetent cervix followed a prior cesarean delivery performed for disproportion after prolonged pushing in the second stage of labor. Obstetric trauma may accompany dilatation and curettage for completion of spontaneous or induced abortion. The current practice of pretreating nulliparous patients with *Laminaria* and using tapered cervical dilators before dilatation and extraction or dilatation and curettage has greatly reduced cervical trauma. A history of prior first trimester elective abortion carries a risk of injury so small as to be insignificant if it were performed by an experienced operator using local anesthesia only and if *Laminaria* were used in nulliparas.[226] Depending on the amount of tissue removed, cervical cone biopsy may lead to reduced cervical competence, but has less risk than is commonly thought.[227,228] Patients with a higher concentration of smooth muscle relative to collagen fibers in the cervix may be at increased risk for cervical incompetence.[225] Congenital structure changes in the cervix can occur in association with müllerian uterine malformations or after diethylstilbestrol exposure. We have followed women with prior conization, müllerian anomalies, and in utero diethylstibestrol exposure with serial transvaginal sonography and have had success in selecting candidates for cerclage when funneling or shortening below

20 mm occurs, thus limiting cerclage to relatively few patients with these risk factors.

Diagnosis

Reduced cervical competence is a clinical diagnosis marked by gradual, painless dilatation and effacement of the cervix with membranes visible through the cervix. As noted above, this history establishes the diagnosis, but is probably a fortuitous presentation; eventually, women with this cervical status may develop membrane rupture, labor, or even amnionitis with intact membranes. Short labors with the delivery of an immature fetus or loss of the pregnancy at progressively earlier gestational ages in successive pregnancies is characteristic of reduced competence. Until recently, objective criteria in the absence of the typical history have been lacking. The use of dilators or balloons to determine cervical resistance and/or hysterosalpingograms to measure the width of the cervical canal between pregnancies have not been sensitive or specific, and digital examination of the cervix is highly subjective. Sonography has provided a reproducible method of evaluating the cervix. The sonographic characteristics of reduced competence are a short cervix, with a length of less than 20 mm, often but not always accompanied by funneling of the internal os. Funneling may be thought of as "effacement in progress": the process procedes from the inside out, beginning at the internal os and moving caudad. It may be first identified on digital examination by a subtle softening of the lower segment and on ultrasound examination by a narrow funnel or echolucent proximal third of the endocervical canal (Fig. 23-22A). As the process continues, the opening of the internal os becomes broader and the shoulders of the funnel more pronounced (Fig. 23-22B). Eventually, the shoulders disappear, leaving only a short cervical length. Remarkably, the process is dynamic, with the internal os opening and closing in response to fundal or suprapubic pressure or assumption of the standing position. Local or coordinated uterine activity may accompany the funneling of the internal os, but more commonly there is no palpable or measurable uterine contraction. Note that these criteria are essentially identical to those seen in PTL, differing only in the absence of contractions and the earlier gestational age at which the reduced competence phenomenon occurs. Zilianti et al[229] have suggested a useful acronym to describe the process of effacement as seen by transvaginal sonography: TYVU. These letters form, in chronologic sequence, the sonographic appearance of the cervical canal and lower segment as it changes from the uneffaced T to the beginning funnel Y with further shortening to V and finally to a fully developed lower uterine segment, U. Because of the variation in the appearance of the internal or cephalad portion of the cervix, we have concentrated on accurate measurement of the residual lower cervical length, as the most consistent over time, both serially for each woman and for comparison with data from other centers.

A diagnosis of reduced cervical competence may be made prior to pregnancy or in the first trimester, if a typical history of painless dilatation and effacement of the cervix in a prior pregnancy can be documented. Women with a history of a previous second trimester loss in which cervical sonography documented the classic picture of funneling and shortened cervical length are also candidates for prophylactic cerclage sutures. However, when the history is atypical or uncertain, it is more appropriate to follow the patient closely with frequent transvaginal ultrasound examinations beginning at 16 to 18 weeks' gestation, looking for the criteria noted above, and for funneling in response to fundal pressure. Guzman et al[230] have confirmed a report[231] that transfundal pressure may be useful in eliciting cervical funneling as an aid in making or excluding a diagnosis of incompetent cervix. Funneling did not occur in response to fundal pressure in 150 normal pregnancies, but was seen in 14 of 31 women with a history suggestive of abnormal competence.

What then is the significance of funneling in the absence of a worrisome obstetric history? The prognostic significance would appear to increase as the gestational age at which it is noted decreases. In the NICHD study[56] the positive predictive value for preterm birth before 35 weeks was only 17.3 percent when funneling was noted at 24 weeks and just 11.6 percent at 28 weeks. Data from this trial indicate that in marked contrast to measurement of cervical length, funneling is inconsistently observed because of wide interexaminer variation. Funneling is probably the normal mechanism of effacement after 30 to 32 weeks. In the absence of a history of early preterm birth, the appearance of spontaneous or induced funneling after 24 weeks of pregnancy certainly does not establish a diagnosis of cervical incompetence, nor does it require a cerclage. For all these reasons, we place greater significance on the cervical length exclusive of any funneling and believe that the appearance of a "funnel" with a normal residual length has little import.

When reduced cervical competence presents unexpectedly in a patient without a worrisome history, the initial symptoms may include a sense of pelvic pressure, low backache, or premenstrual molimina accompanied by an increase in vaginal discharge that may be light tan or blood streaked. Sonography at this point will usually reveal a large funnel and substantial shortening, with or without dilatation of the external os. Later, overt fluid leakage or contractions may ensue.

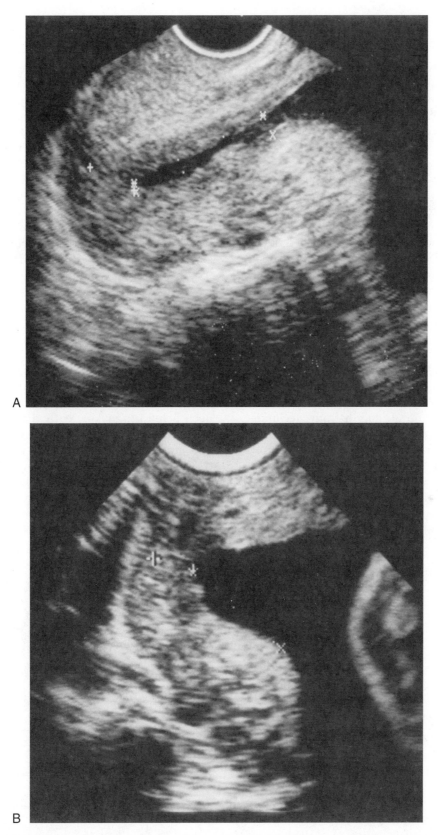

Fig. 23-22. (A) Transvaginal ultrasound image of the cervix in a woman with abnormal cervical competence showing mild separation of the canal, or early evidence of funneling. Cervical length is marked by the (+) caliper; the other calipers define the funnel. (B) Transvaginal ultrasound image of the cervix in a woman with abnormal cervical competence showing a marked funnel. The (+) caliper shows the length of the remaining cervix and the (X) caliper the length of the funnel.

Cerclage Technique

Prophylactic Cerclage

Since the early 1950s, obstetricians have sought an effective surgical technique to strengthen the cervix and thereby prevent premature cervical dilatation. In 1950, Lash and Lash[232] described a repair in the nonpregnant patient that involved partial excision of the cervix, presumably removing the areas of weakness. However, this technique was associated with a high incidence of subsequent infertility. In 1955, Shirodkar[233] reported successful management of cervical incompetence with the use of a submucosal band, first of fascia lata and later of mersilene, placed at the level of the internal os. This procedure, which could be performed during pregnancy, required anterior displacement of the bladder and a fair amount of submucosal dissection. The Shirodkar cerclage was also difficult to remove so that most successful pregnancies were delivered via cesarean section. Several years later, McDonald[234] described the use of a purse-string technique that could easily be performed during pregnancy. This approach involves either four or five "bites" as high on the cervix as possible. A metal catheter may be used to help identify the posterior extent of the bladder. The knot is placed anteriorly to facilitate removal. This operative technique is illustrated in Figure 23-23. The optimal choice for the suture material has not been established, but obviously a permanent suture is required. We use two purse-string stitches with 5 Ethibond, but there are many suitable variations. The McDonald procedure has proved to be as effective as the Shirodkar technique[235] and requires considerably less dissection. Therefore,

we consider it to be the method of choice. Prophylactic cerclage sutures may be placed at 10 to 14 weeks' gestation if the criteria listed above are met. We do not use prophylactic tocolytics at the time of prophylactic cerclage, but do give perioperative penicillin to women with positive vaginal cultures for group B *Streptococcus*. After prophylactic cerclage, intercourse, prolonged standing (more than 90 minutes), and heavy lifting are omitted. We follow these patients with periodic vaginal sonography to assess stitch location and funneling.[236-238] No additional restrictions are recommended as long as the stitches remain within the middle or upper third of the cervix without the development of a funnel, and the length of the cervix is 25 mm or longer. Some shortening of the cervix should be expected after 20 weeks. In fact, if the cervical length remains 35 mm or longer throughout the second trimester, the accuracy of the original diagnosis may be questioned.[239]

Emergency Cerclage

Care of the patient with newly detected reduced cervical competence in the second trimester is both difficult and controversial. The introduction of sonography has been helpful in making early diagnoses and avoiding the complications that accompany advanced dilatation and effacement. When the diagnosis is made before cervical dilatation has occurred and when there is still 10 to 15 mm or more of cervical length, we admit the patient for 12 to 24 hours of treatment with perioperative indomethacin and broad spectrum antibiotics before placing the cerclage sutures and observe the pa-

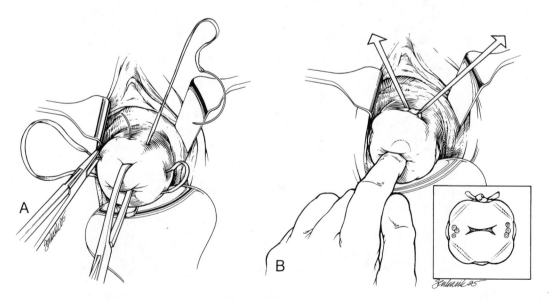

Fig. 23-23. Placement of sutures for McDonald cervical cerclage. (A) We use a double-headed Mersilene band with four "bites" in the cervix, avoiding the vessels. (B) The suture is placed high upon the cervix close to the cervical–vaginal junction, approximately the level of the internal os.

tient for 48 to 96 hours, postoperatively. However, if the cervix has dilated to allow visualization of the membranes, the patient is hospitalized for at least 5 to 7 days and often longer after cerclage placement. The prognosis for these patients is better than generally expected, with many women delivering a "viable" (usually defined as more than 1,000 g) infant (Table 23-13), but aggressive therapy is required to achieve these results. The prognosis is influenced by the gestational age at the time the heroic suture is placed.[240] If the sutures appear tenuous, prolonged hospitalization with Trendelenberg position may be required.

In the setting of advanced dilatation with bulging membranes, several techniques may be helpful. First, careful inspection of the membranes to identify separation or loss of the chorion from the intact amnion should be routine. If only the amnion remains, prolongation of pregnancy beyond a few days is unlikely. Precerclage amniocentesis to remove sufficient fluid to reduce the bulging membranes (and obtain cultures) has been helpful in the most advanced cases. Overfilling the bladder with 1,000 cc os saline may help by elevating the membranes out of the operative field, but may also obstruct the surgeon's view.[241] We often place a Foley catheter balloon inside the cervix and overfill it with 50 cc of saline or more to push the membranes gently out of the lower segment. The cerclage can then be placed and tied as the balloon fluid is evacuated.

For patients who have a very short or amputated cervix or who have failed a vaginal suture, a transabdominal cerclage may be necessary. For a more thorough discussion of this procedure, the reader is referred to an excellent review by Novy.[242] After the cerclage, patients should decrease their physical activity and have periods of bed rest during the day. Sexual activity is usually prohibited. The status of the cervix is followed by weekly or biweekly pelvic examinations. If there is progressive cervical shortening, activity can be further

Table 23-13 Outcome After Emergent Second Trimester Cerclage

Author	No.	Cx Dilation (cm)	Percent Salvaged
Kuhn and Pepperell	42	2–5	60
Peters et al	13	>3	23
Olatubosun and Dyck	12	>4	83
Conradt et al	11	6	45
Harger	10	>3	50
Barth et al	15	4–5	73
Lombardi et al	14	>4	71
MacDougall et al	19	5	68
Others	15	3–4	67
Total	141		65

decreased. Monitoring may indicate contractions that are not recognized by the patient. The cerclage is removed electively at 37 weeks' gestation, a procedure that can usually be accomplished in the office.

Cerclage is uncommonly performed after 26 weeks' gestation. The great risk of inducing PROM or PTL and the ability to prolong gestation with bed rest and suppressive medications argue against surgical intervention in such cases.

Risks of Cerclage

Cervical injury at the time of delivery is the most commonly reported morbidity from a McDonald cerclage. While fibrous scar tissue may form at the site of the stitch, producing an abnormal labor curve, most patients will labor normally after cerclage removal.[243] A fibrous "band" may rupture, leading to a cervical laceration (1 to 13 percent), or never dilate (cervical dystocia, 2 to 5 percent), requiring cesarean birth.[227] Rarely, a laceration may extend to the broad ligament or corpus of the uterus, requiring extensive repair or even hysterectomy.

For elective cerclage at the beginning of the second trimester, the risk of infection is very small, estimated at no more than 1 percent. Later in the pregnancy, displacement of the suture also can occur (3 to 12 percent). A second cerclage has a much lower success rate.[227] Late complications of cerclage include PROM or PTL and chorioamnionitis; the risk varies with the duration of gestation and the presence of cervical dilation. When fluid leakage occurs in a patient with a cerclage, the suture(s) should be removed immediately[244] to reduce the risk of infection. The patient may then be managed according to protocols for preterm PROM (see later).

Efficacy of Cervical Cerclage

The utility of cerclage was established in the era before randomized trials became standard. There has never been a randomized prospective study documenting the benefit of cerclage for women with a "classic" history of cervical incompetence. Success, defined as fetal survival, is impressive. In every study since 1965 of reasonable size (at least 100 patients), 80 to 90 percent of the pregnancies have resulted in viable live births.[227] In the absence of a controlled prospective trial, investigators have compared postcerclage outcome with fetal survival before cerclage, a suboptimal control group. Past obstetric and neonatal practices typically differ substantially from current practice.

Three prospective randomized trials of cerclage[220,245,246] have been conducted in patients with increased risk of preterm birth, *excluding* women with classic indications for cerclage. Two trials[245,246] found no benefit from cervical cerclage in this patient population, and one noted an increase in the need for antepartum hospitalization.[246] The third, a prospective and randomized study[220] limited to women (n = 905) in whom the obstetrician was uncertain about the need for cerclage, found a decrease in the occurrence of preterm births before 33 weeks in women treated with a cerclage compared with controls (13 vs. 18 percent, $p = 0.03$). There were similar statistically significant reductions in birth weight under 1,500 g and in neonatal deaths.

In summary, there has been a substantial increase in our knowledge of the role of the cervix in the pathogenesis of spontaneous prematurity since the previous edition of this text. Understanding the cervix as one of several continuous interactive variables has helped to explain many of the controversies about the "incompetent" cervix. Although it is clear that the cervix is an important contributor to many preterm births before 28 weeks, it is also clear that cerclage is not always the appropriate therapy. Diagnostic criteria incorporating both obstetric history and sonographic results have been proposed but have not been widely tested in practice. Selection of appropriate patients for cerclage with ultrasound and the role of ancillary treatment of cerclage patients with antibiotics and/or tocolytics should be investigated.

Preterm Premature Rupture of The Membranes

PROM is defined as leakage of amniotic fluid beginning at least 1 hour prior to the onset of labor at any gestational age. The following discussion is limited to the diagnosis and management of preterm PROM, defined as PROM that occurs before 37 weeks' gestation. The etiology, complications, and sequelae of preterm PROM overlap those of PROM at term, but differ in one major respect. Infection of the choriodecidual interface often *precedes* preterm PROM and is thought to play a role in causing membrane rupture. In contrast, infection of the chorioamnion more often *follows* membrane rupture at term.

Etiology

The fetal membranes are made up of a thin layer of amnion and a thicker outer layer of chorion that is directly apposed to maternal decidual tissue. Interspersed between the amnion and chorion is a collagen-rich connective tissue zone that serves in part to replenish the amnion. By 26 weeks' gestation, the amnion is composed of a single layer of cuboidal cells. The chorion is four to six cell layers in thickness. The amnion has greater tensile strength than the chorion, although both membrane layers together withstand

greater bursting pressures than they do separately. The amount of physical stress tolerated by the membranes decreases as pregnancy progresses. Membranes supported by a closed cervix require much greater pressures to rupture than do membranes covering an open area of 3 to 4 cm in diameter.[247] As gestational age advances, the relative concentration of collagen decreases as well.[248] All these factors help to maintain membrane integrity throughout pregnancy but facilitate rupture of membranes in labor at term.

Why then do some membranes rupture early? Epidemiologic studies have identified several risk factors associated with a higher risk of preterm PROM. Genital tract infection or colonization with various microorganisms, coitus, low socioeconomic status, poor nutrition, smoking, and bleeding in pregnancy have all been linked to an increased chance of preterm PROM. These risk factors are consistent with a syndrome of spontaneous premature delivery in which preterm PROM is just one of several possible clinical presentations. Although other scenarios certainly occur (see later section on bleeding), most evidence points to a pathway in which various genital microorganisms gain access to the decidual–membrane interface. Organisms may ascend through a short or dilated cervix that poorly defends the intrauterine contents during pregnancy, may reach this space via hematogenous spread, or may even have colonized the endometrium *before* conception.[57] According to this paradigm, it is the inflammatory interaction between host defenses and microorganisms that initiates a process that may ultimately result in several clinical presentations, including both preterm PROM and PTL. The likelihood of clinical illness is a function of the number and kind of organisms involved and of host factors such as the physical and immune function of the cervix, myometrial contractile response, and physical strength of membranes, the last of which may be influenced by maternal nutritional status, direct injury via trauma or bleeding, and smoking. The injury to fetal membranes may occur either directly as the result of proteases and other enzymes produced by microorganisms or indirectly through membrane injury caused by cytokines produced as part of the maternal immune response. This hypothesis is supported by epidemiologic, histologic, microbiologic, and clinical studies.

A study of SPTBs in North Carolina[18] found that preterm PROM was the predominant clinical presentation in indigent patients, while PTL was more common than PROM among women who received private obstetric care. Several studies have linked preterm PROM with cigarette smoking. Meyer and Tonascia[22] reported that smokers were three times more likely than nonsmokers to experience PROM before 34 weeks' gestation. This study observed an apparent dose-dependent effect for smoking: heavier smokers in this study experienced more PROM than lighter smokers. Case–control studies by Harger et al[249] and by Hadley et al[23] demonstrated both smoking and a history of previous preterm PROM to be significant risk factors. Harger et al[249] also found a strong relationship to antepartum bleeding in more than one trimester (OR, 7.4, 95 percent Cl, 2.2–25.6). Ekwo et al[24] confirmed the association of preterm PROM with smoking and found an especially strong relationship of preterm PROM to second trimester bleeding (see Table 23-2). In contrast to these observations, the NICHD Preterm Prediction Study[250] did not identify an association between smoking and preterm PROM, finding instead that a short cervical length (25 mm or less as determined with transvaginal ultrasound) was the best predictor of preterm PROM.

Histologic studies have revealed local defects within the membranes that may predispose to rupture. Bourne[251] stained the fetal membranes through the cervix with Trypan blue dye and demonstrated that the site of rupture is usually immediately above the cervix, an area of membranes that is poorly supported physically and nutritionally. At term, intact membranes excised at the time of cesarean section show localized areas of weakness over the internal os and in the area opposite the placental site.[252] Possible explanations for these areas of weakness include damage to the membranes from bleeding earlier in pregnancy with subsequent scarring, leading to rupture when these areas are stretched by uterine contractions and/or fetal growth. The membranes respond to physical stress in part as an "elastic" substance with full return to prior configuration and in part as a "viscous" substance with persistent deformation and thinning after application and removal of a stress.[253] Thus a scarred area may rupture rather than expand. Changes in collagen content in membranes that rupture prematurely have also been identified, compared with gestational age-matched control membranes.[248,254]

Evidence of the association of infection with preterm PROM is abundant and diverse.[255] Naeye[256] observed an association between preterm deliveries caused by PROM and the combination of coitus within 9 days of delivery and the histologic diagnosis of chorioamnionitis. In the absence of chorioamnionitis, the association with coitus and preterm PROM persisted, but with a much lower relative risk. This relationship has not been consistently observed in other studies. Histologic studies of membranes after preterm PROM often demonstrate significant bacterial contamination diffusely along the choriodecidual interface with minimal involvement of the amnion. This suggests spread of the organisms along the maternal-fetal surfaces before membrane rupture.[257] Sbarra et al[258] have shown reduced bursting pressure when membranes grown in tissue culture were exposed to either group B *Streptococcus* or *Escherichia coli*.[258]

Specific genital tract pathogens have also been correlated with the occurrence of PROM. The organisms include *Bacteroides fragilis* and other anaerobes, *Neisseria gonorrhoeae*, *Chlamydia trachomatis*, *Trichomonas vaginalis*, and group B β-hemolytic streptococci.[257] In most of these cases, the suspected pathogen was isolated twice as often in women with PROM. For example, PROM occurred in 15.3 percent of women colonized with group B streptococci compared with 7 percent of women not colonized, a highly statistically significant association in this report involving 6,706 parturients.[259] The strongest association has been found for bacterial vaginosis and SPTB due to both preterm PROM and preterm labor. The NICHD Preterm Prediction Study[49] found a significant relationship between maternal acquisition of bacterial vaginosis between 24 and 28 weeks of pregnancy and SPTB due to both preterm PROM and PTL (OR, 1.84, 95 percent CI, 1.15–2.95). However, a significant relationship between bacterial vaginosis and SPTB was not observed for women who were colonized with bacterial vaginosis at both 24 and 28 weeks, suggesting that it was the acquisition of bacterial vaginosis during pregnancy that was important in this study.

Additional support for the importance of infectious agents in the etiology of preterm PROM comes from observations concerning maternal, fetal, and neonatal infections. Many of these infections are evident soon after the membranes have ruptured, suggesting that subclinical infection may have preceded fluid leakage. Similar inferences may be drawn from a study of cord blood that found increased levels of immunoglobulins in infants born after preterm PROM compared with other preterm infants.[260] Two peaks in immunoglobulin levels were observed, the first at 12 hours after birth and the second at 72 hours after birth, suggesting that significant fetal exposure to infectious agents occurred before delivery in the first group and at or after delivery in the second.

Diagnosis

The most common presentation is a gush of fluid from the vagina followed by persistent, uncontrolled leakage, but some patients report only small, intermittent leakage or perineal wetness. It is not possible to exclude the diagnosis without examining the patient. Therefore, any history of passing fluid through the vagina should be evaluated by a sterile speculum examination to collect fluid for confirmatory tests. Digital examination of the cervix in women with possible PTL or preterm PROM should be avoided until after ruptured membranes have been excluded. Once preterm PROM

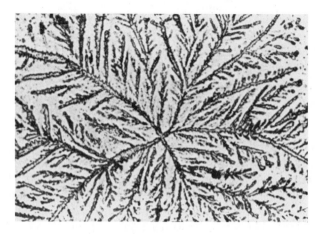

Fig. 23-24. Demonstration of amniotic fluid arborization pattern (From Reece et al,[265] with permission.)

is diagnosed, digital examination should be avoided until delivery is anticipated within 24 hours, because of the risk of introducing bacteria into the endocervix. Even a single digital examination has been found to increase the likelihood of subsequent amnionitis and neonatal infection. A significant increase in neonatal infection and neonatal mortality was observed when a digital examination preceded delivery by more than 24 hours in the presence of PROM.[261] Another study of women with preterm PROM found that the mean interval from rupture to delivery was 2.1 days in 121 women who had a digital examination compared with 11.3 days in 144 women who had only a sterile speculum examination.[262] Often a visual estimate at the time of sterile speculum examination can identify women with advanced dilatation.[263] The sterile speculum examination may also reveal a collection or "pool" of fluid that can be tested for pH with nitrazine paper. Since amniotic fluid is slightly alkaline (the pH is about 7.15), vaginal secretions containing amniotic fluid will usually result in pH changes in the blue-green range, 6.5 to 7.5. Nitrazine testing is accurate in 90 to 98 percent of cases.[264] False-positive values can result from vaginal infections that raise vaginal pH, especially *T. vaginalis*, the presence of blood, or, more rarely, cervical mucus. False-negative reactions are frequent when only a scant amount of fluid is present.

Another helpful test relies on the property of amniotic fluid to "fern." When placed on a clean slide and allowed to air dry, amniotic fluid produces a microscopic crystallization in a "fern" pattern (Fig. 23-24). This phenomenon is due to the interaction of amniotic fluid proteins and salts and accurately confirms PROM in 85 to 98 percent of cases. False-positive tests can result from the collection of cervical mucus, which also "ferns," but usually in a more floral pattern. The fern test is unaffected by meconium, changes in vaginal pH, and blood:amniotic fluid ratios of up to 1:5.[265, 266] The

fern pattern in samples heavily contaminated with blood is atypical and appears more "skeletonized."[266]

An ultrasound evaluation for amniotic fluid volume should be performed in all cases of confirmed preterm PROM to determine fetal presentation and to estimate fetal weight and gestational age. In patients in whom the diagnosis of membrane rupture is equivocal, the volume of amniotic fluid seen on ultrasound may be helpful in evaluating the patient. Although nonspecific, a finding of decreased or absent fluid supports a diagnosis of ruptured membranes. When abundant residual fluid is observed in women after a confirmed diagnosis of PROM, the possibility of polyhydramnios prior to rupture should be considered. Another useful step in equivocal cases is to repeat the sterile speculum examination after the patient has rested in a semiupright position for approximately 1 hour to encourage the pooling of secretions in the posterior vagina. During this time, the woman may be monitored to evaluate fetal well-being and uterine contractions. Particular attention should be paid to the occurrence of variable decelerations that might suggest compression of the umbilical cord secondary to reduced amniotic fluid volume. Fibronectin is present in amniotic fluid, and the fibronectin assay will be strongly positive in the presence of ruptured membranes. It may prove useful when other tests are equivocal in a patient with reduced fluid and a good history. In rare instances, a dilute solution of dye (e.g., indigo carmine) may be injected via amniocentesis to look for subsequent transcervical leakage onto a tampon, thus making an absolute diagnosis. Methylene blue dye has been associated with hemolytic anemia and hyperbilirubinemia in the infant and should not be used. Amniocentesis is seldom indicated, but its use illustrates the importance of making a definite diagnosis of ruptured membranes. A complete evaluation is required whenever the diagnosis is suggested by a report of wetness or leaking at any gestational age. Preterm PROM is not a diagnosis that can be made casually and should never be entirely excluded in any patient with either oligohydramnios or symptoms of persistent leakage.

Natural History

Decisions about care of patients with preterm PROM rest on an understanding of the likely course of pregnancy in the absence of medical intervention. Studies that report aggregate outcomes for all women with preterm PROM between 20 and 34 weeks have observed that the duration of pregnancy after PROM is inversely related to the gestational age at time of membrane rupture. When PROM occurs prior to 26 weeks gestation, 30 to 40 percent of cases will gain at least one additional week before delivery and 20 percent will gain over 4 weeks.[267] In contrast, 70 to 80 percent of patients who experience PROM between 28 to 36 weeks' gestation deliver within the first week after PROM and more than one-half of these within the first 4 days.[268] At term, 80 percent of women go into labor within the first 24 hours after rupture of the membranes. While these data accurately describe the total population of women who experience preterm PROM, it is difficult to predict the clinical course of an individual patient following preterm PROM. It is commonly said that socioeconomic status is related to the likelihood of both delivery and infection after preterm PROM. For example, Cox et al[269] found that 93 percent of 298 indigent women at Parkland Hospital with preterm PROM before 34 weeks (lower limit not stated) were in labor within 48 hours after membrane rupture. The rate of chorioamnionitis in those managed expectantly was 16 percent. However, Nelson et al[270] compared interval from rupture to delivery and the rate of chorioamnionitis in 317 women on the clinic service with 194 women on the private service experiencing preterm PROM and found no difference between them.

Maternal Risks

Whether a cause or a result of PPROM, intrauterine infection is a potentially serious complication to the mother. A clinical diagnosis of chorioamnionitis accompanies preterm PROM in approximately 10 percent of cases (range 3 to 30 percent).[257] Regardless of clinical signs of infection, as many as 25 to 30 percent of women with PPROM (range, 14.6 to 43.3 percent) will have a positive amniotic fluid culture. Although most instances of amnionitis respond well to antibiotic administration and delivery, maternal deaths from sepsis can occur.[271] As would be expected from studies of the pathogenesis and epidemiology of spontaneous preterm birth, amnionitis is more common when PROM occurs before 30 to 32 weeks than later in pregnancy.

Fetal and Neonatal Risks

Infection is a major potential complication for the fetus and neonate as well as for the mother. The same vaginal organisms that lead to maternal infection can result in congenital pneumonia, sepsis, or meningitis. However, the presence of obvious culture-documented amnionitis usually does not result in neonatal infection. In published series, the range of neonatal sepsis in cases of preterm PROM with or without clinical amnionitis has ranged from 2 to 19 percent and the range of neonatal deaths caused by infection from 1 to 7 percent. The frequency of neonatal infection varies considerably with gestational age, race, and maternal antepartum course, as well as the definition used by the investiga-

tors. Studies requiring positive cultures for diagnosis tend to detect lower sepsis rates than those combining clinical course, radiographic findings, and neonatal bacterial colonization for diagnosis.

There are also serious noninfectious fetal complications that may occur after preterm PROM. There is a higher risk of frank or occult cord prolapse, particularly if the fetus is not in a cephalic presentation. Regardless of presentation, the risks of fetal distress in labor leading to cesarean delivery are significantly higher with preterm PROM than with isolated preterm labor (7.9 vs. 1.5 percent).[272] The most common fetal heart rate tracing leading to operative delivery is severe variable decelerations due to cord compression. Amnioinfusion may be used to prevent or reduce cord compression secondary to oligohydramnios.

Placental abruption occurs in 4 to 6 percent of cases of preterm PROM, especially when PROM is accompanied by bleeding.[273, 274] A 15 percent rate of abruption has been observed when patients with prolonged preterm PROM manifest vaginal bleeding in addition to fluid leakage. When abruption occurred after PROM, nearly half of these pregnancies were complicated by acute intrapartum fetal distress.[275]

Pulmonary hypoplasia is a particular concern when fetal membranes are ruptured prior to 26 weeks' gestation. About 25 percent of babies delivered after 26 weeks' gestation following PROM that occurred before 26 weeks' gestation were found to have pulmonary hy-

---

Noninfectious Risks with Preterm PROM

Cord prolapse
   More common in nonvertex presentations
Cesarean delivery more common
   Failed induction: 44% cesarean delivery in one series, all failure to progress
Abruption: three studies associated prolonged PROM and abruption
   5%–6% of premature PROMs; 25% abruption rate if bleeding after PROM
Pulmonary hypoplasia
   Correlates with gestational age at rupture[278]
      19 weeks, 50%
      22 weeks, 25%
      26 weeks, <10% (lower rates in other studies)
Respiratory distress syndrome
   Altered rates of respiratory distress after PPROM? Literature nearly equally divided on this subject

poplasia following birth.[267] The duration and degree of oligohydramnios are associated with the chance of pulmonary hypoplasia. Rotschild et al[276] found that the frequency of pulmonary hypoplasia was correlated with gestational age at rupture. When rupture occurred at 19 weeks or earlier, 50 percent of infants were affected (Fig. 23-25). The rate fell to 25 percent for infants born at 22 weeks and to less than 10 percent at 26 weeks. Carroll et al[277] compared the relative risk of neonatal death due to pulmonary hypoplasia and complications of prematurity in a study of 172 singleton infants liveborn after preterm PROM. Thirty infants died, 18 due to pulmonary hypoplasia and 12 because of prematurity. Both overall survival and the risk of pulmonary hypoplasia were related to the gestational age at the time of amniorrhexis. When rupture occurred after 23 weeks, there were no neonatal deaths due to pulmonary hypoplasia. For infants born at 23 weeks or earlier, the likelihood of pulmonary hypoplasia increased as gestational age at rupture decreased to a maximum of 50 percent before 20 weeks, the same figure reported by Rotschild et al[276] Prediction of pulmonary hypoplasia has been attempted by measuring residual fluid volume, lung length, comparison of the thoracic and abdominal circumferences, assessment of fetal breathing, and Doppler studies of blood flow in the ductus arteriosus and of perinasal amniotic fluid movement, but none of these tests have added significantly to estimates of risk based on the gestational age at the time of rupture.

Skeletal deformities related to compression following oligohydramnios may also occur but often resolve in the first year of life. Twenty-seven percent of fetuses with PROM prior to 26 weeks who experienced prolonged rupture before delivery developed skeletal deformations.[278]

Initial Evaluation and Management

After the diagnosis of preterm PROM has been confirmed, maternal and fetal indications for immediate delivery should be ruled out before considering other management options. The most urgent fetal indications are prolapse of the umbilical cord, a complication that occurs more commonly when the fetus is in the breech presentation, and fetal bradycardia caused by cord compression due to oligohydramnios. The principal maternal indication for delivery is chorioamnionitis. When a firm diagnosis of chorioamnionitis can be made by the presence of maternal fever of 101°F or higher, uterine tenderness, and leukocytosis at least 20,000 mm³, delivery should be undertaken promptly regardless of the gestational age. Unfortunately, many cases of chorioamnionitis do not fulfill these criteria, and most confirmatory tests lack adequate sensitivity and specificity.

Gestational age should be carefully reassessed or established in order to estimate the relative risks for the fetus of delivery versus expectant management (see below). All clinical and ultrasound dating criteria should be reviewed. Because oligohydramnios may flatten the fetal head, biparietal diameter measurements to estimate fetal weight by ultrasound may be inaccurate in women with preterm PROM.[279, 280] Use of formulas based on head circumference, femur length, or cerebellar diameter are more reliable indicators of gestational age and fetal weight in these situations.

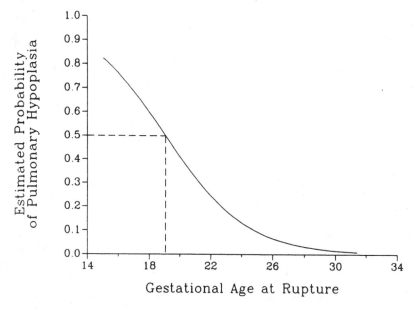

Fig. 23-25.   Curve relating probability of pulmonary hypoplasia to gestational age at time of rupture of membranes. (From Rotschild et al,[276] with permission.)

Before 30 to 32 weeks gestation, the neonatal risks of prematurity will usually outweigh the in utero risks of infection and fetal compromise caused by oligohydramnios, while the reverse is usually the case after 34 to 35 weeks' gestation.[281] Exactly where the relative risk ratio shifts depends on factors unique to each patient. Consideration of these individual risks forms the basis for management for women with preterm PROM and is among the most challenging tasks in obstetrics. The relative risks of prematurity, infection, and fetal well-being must be repeatedly evaluated for women with preterm PROM. As will be evident in the following paragraphs, the methods of risk assessment are not uniformly satisfactory.

Amniocentesis for Women with Preterm PROM

In contrast to women with PTL and intact membranes for whom amniocentesis is occasionally indicated, assessment of amniotic fluid for infection and maturity studies should always be considered in women with preterm PROM. The difference lies in the greater risks that attend continued pregnancy when membranes are ruptured. Continuing the pregnancy, called *expectant management*, is accompanied by ongoing risks of maternal and fetal infection, cord prolapse, and abruption that must be reassessed at least daily by means of tests that are not entirely reliable. Demonstration of either fetal pulmonary maturity or intraamniotic bacteria often leads to a decision for delivery, thus obviating the difficulties of fetal and maternal surveillance. Amniotic fluid may be obtained from either free-flowing vaginal fluid or amniocentesis for studies of fetal maturity, but amniocentesis is required to obtain fluid for culture, Gram stain, and glucose tests for infection. Placing the patient in the Trendelenburg position prior to the amniocentesis may facilitate the procedure by favoring intrauterine retention of fluid. Amniocentesis has been successfully accomplished in 50 percent[268] to 96 percent[286] of reported series of patients with preterm PROM. The success rate is apparently influenced primarily by the aggressiveness of the investigators. Although the amniotic fluid pocket may be small, amniocentesis is reasonably safe when performed with ultrasound guidance. Yeast et al[283] reviewed charts from 138 patients with PROM at 28 to 34 weeks' gestation who were not in labor or clinically infected. Amniocentesis was performed in 91 women compared with 46 women for whom amniocentesis was considered impossible because of the absence of fluid pocket or placenta-free window. There was no difference in time to onset of labor between the two groups. There was no evidence of fetal injury from the amniocentesis needle. One mother had a small hematoma of the superior

broad ligament noted at cesarean delivery. Other reported complications of third-trimester amniocentesis include perforation of maternal epigastric and uterine vessels and intraperitoneal and uterine hematomas. A literature review reported the risk of fetal injury to be between 0.6 and 2.0 percent and that of placenta and cord injury to be 0.3 to 1.1 percent.[284]

If there is free-flowing amniotic fluid in the vaginal vault at the time of sterile speculum examination, it may be used for lung maturity testing with phosphatidylglycerol, the lecithin/shingomyelin (L/S) ratio, but is obviously not reliable for infection studies.[285, 286] Bacterial contaminants in vaginally collected fluid have been reported to produce phosphatidylglycerol, creating a false impression of fetal lung maturity.[287]

Garite and colleagues[268] reported their experience with amniocentesis performed in women with PROM between 28 and 34 weeks of pregnancy. None of the 98 patients who had an amniocentesis demonstrated signs of clinical amnionitis, and none were in labor. A mature L/S ratio of at least 1.8:1 was found in 39 percent of samples. An additional 13 percent had Gram stains of unspun amniotic fluid that demonstrated the presence of bacteria. Thus 52 percent of these asymptomatic women were delivered expeditiously because of amniotic fluid findings. Mercer et al[288] studied the clinical value of amniotic fluid results between 32 and 36 weeks' gestation in a prospective trial of 164 women with preterm PROM. There were 13 (7.9 percent) with immature maturity studies, 12 (7.3 percent) in whom fluid could not be obtained, and 4 (2.4 percent) with chorioamnionitis. There were 93 with mature amniotic fluid studies and reassuring fetal heart rate testing who consented to be randomized to either induction of labor or expectant management. Women in whom labor was induced had a lower rate of chorioamnionitis (10.9 vs 27.7 percent) and shorter hospital stays (2.3 vs. 3.5 days). There was no difference in the cesarean delivery rate. Infants born after expectant management were treated more often for suspected sepsis, but there was no difference in neonatal survival or significant morbidity. These trials support the value of obtaining and acting upon the results of amniotic fluid maturity testing in women with preterm PROM after 32 weeks' gestation.

Tests for Infection in Patients with Preterm PROM

Expectant management of preterm PROM requires initial and continued surveillance for infection. Ultimately, the endpoint for tests of "infection" in this clinical setting should be clinically important maternal or fetal/neonatal infection. Intermediate endpoints, such as amniotic fluid bacteria, white blood cells, glucose, and even culture, while associated with perinatal infection, do not equate uniformly with clinical infectious morbidity or mortality. At the outset of this discussion, it is well to remember that the incidence of clinical amnionitis approximates 10 percent (range 3 to 30 percent) in women with preterm PROM. Of infants born to mothers with clinical amnionitis, only 1 to 15 percent will have positive cultures, confirming a diagnosis of neonatal sepsis. Finally, the rate of perinatal mortality caused by infection has ranged from 0 to 13 percent in studies of infants born after preterm PROM. The principal causes of perinatal morbidity and mortality after preterm PROM are still related more to prematurity (e.g., respiratory distress syndrome, intraventricular hemorrhage) than to infection. Nevertheless, it is important to make an early diagnosis of infection. A two- to fourfold increase in perinatal mortality, intraventricular hemorrhage, and neonatal sepsis has been reported in infants born after amnionitis compared with gestationally matched controls born to noninfected mothers.[289] Most importantly, antepartum treatment of maternal amnionitis clearly decreases the incidence of neonatal sepsis (Table 23-14).[290–292]

Ohlsson and Wang[293] reviewed tests to detect intrauterine infection and concluded that no test was wholly satisfactory. An elevated maternal leukocyte count had a reported sensitivity of 23 to 80 percent, a specificity of 60 to 95 percent, a positive predictive value of 50 to 75 percent, and a negative predictive value of 40 to 90 percent to predict clinical or histologic amnionitis. Increased maternal serum C-reactive protein had a sensitivity of 37 to 100 percent, a specificity of 44 to 100 percent, a positive predictive value of 10 to 100 percent; and a negative predictive value of 50 to 100 percent, again using clinical or histologic amnionitis as the endpoint.

Amniotic fluid obtained by amniocentesis can be used to detect amnionitis, based on demonstration of bacteria on a Gram stain of unspun fluid, amniotic fluid glucose levels, or the presence of interleukin 6. Approximately 10^5 organisms per milliliter is needed before a Gram stain will be positive. Thus, not all culture-positive fluids have positive Gram stains, though virtually all positive Gram stains result from culture-positive fluids. Gram stain for bacteria has a reported sensitivity ranging from 36 to 80 percent, and a specificity of 80 to 97 percent to predict a subsequent positive culture. Amniotic fluid culture has a reported sensitivity of 65 to 85 percent and a specificity of 85 percent to predict clinical chorioamnionitis. The presence of white blood cells (WBCs) in amniotic fluid has not proven helpful in predicting infection, but a low amniotic fluid glucose level (16 to 20 mg% or less) has been found to correlate well with a positive fluid culture, with sensitivity and specificity of approximately 90 percent. The amniotic fluid glucose is simple, rapid, and available around the clock, all big advantages over the other tests. Asrat et al[294] studied 108 women with preterm PROM to identify clinical characteristics that were associated with a positive Gram stain and found associations with earlier gestational age, maternal temperature and white blood cell count, and fetal tachycardia and nonreactive fetal heart rate tracings. Interleukin-6 is a promising test that is not yet available for clinical use.[295]

White blood cell counts from peripheral blood are customary in patients with preterm PROM but are not always predictive of the presence or absence of chorioamnionitis. Maternal serum C-reactive protein, a nonspecific indicator of inflammation, has been employed as a predictor of subclinical or overt infection,[296] but others have reported considerable overlap between C-reactive protein in infected and noninfected pregnancies.[297] Because of its low specificity, most centers do not consider this test clinically useful.

Nonstress testing for patients with preterm PROM is widely and appropriately practiced to look for evidence of cord compression, but may not be a reliable test for incipient or occult infection. Mercer et al[298] studied 133 women with preterm PROM and observed that a nonreactive nonstress test (NST) was associated with a 48 percent rate of amnionitis and/or neonatal sepsis. However, the NST was insufficiently sensitive: 29 percent of patients with a reactive NST also developed amnionitis and/or neonatal sepsis. Another study of 245 NSTs in women with preterm PROM reported that there were two intrauterine fetal deaths due to sepsis within 24 hours of a reactive NST.[272] Thus the NST alone would appear to be inadequate as a primary test for fetal infection. Ultrasound assessment has also been studied as a predictor of subsequent maternal or neonatal infection. Vintzileos et al[299] compared sonographic estimation of qualitative amniotic fluid volume (vertical measurement of largest pocket less than 1 cm) and amniocentesis performed on admission in 54 pregnancies and found each to be similarly efficacious. However, the association of low amniotic fluid index and the chance of later infection has not been confirmed in subsequent studies.[298,300] A more consistent relationship has been reported between a biophysical profile

Table 23-14 Importance of Antepartum Diagnosis and Treatment of Amnionitis

Author	No.	% Neonatal Sepsis	
		If Treated Antepartum	If Treated Postpartum
Sperling et al[290]	257	2.8	19.6
Gilstrap et al[292]	273	1.5	5.7
Gibbs et al[291]	45	0	21.0

score of 6 or less and subsequent maternal or neonatal infection. Goldstein et al[301] studied fetal behavior and intra-amniotic infection defined as positive amniotic fluid cultures. All fetuses demonstrating an episode of fetal activity (breathing and body movements) of more than 30 seconds in a 30-minute period had negative cultures, while the absence of fetal breathing and less than 50 seconds of gross body movements in 30 minutes identified only women with infection. In patients with some fetal breathing lasting less than 30 seconds but body movements of more than 50 seconds, 64 percent of cultures were positive.

Management Strategies

When a thorough assessment reveals no evidence of fetal distress or infection and fetal pulmonary maturity cannot be confirmed, three basic management options remain. The first is conservative or expectant management, in which the patient is hospitalized for intensive surveillance for signs of fetal compromise or infection, at which time labor is allowed or induced if necessary. This approach is associated with a low rate of cesarean delivery, but relies on methods of fetal assessment that must be performed at least daily and, as described previously, are not always accurate. An alternate choice is immediate delivery for pregnancies beyond a certain gestational age (e.g., 32 weeks or more) or estimated fetal weight (e.g., 1,500 to 1,800 g or more). This strategy avoids the need for ongoing surveillance for fetal well-being and infection, but commits to delivery some women who might have continued the pregnancy long enough to allow additional fetal development and reduced neonatal morbidity. This strategy has a high rate of cesarean delivery for failed induction. The third strategy is an attempt to delay delivery in order to influence the relative risks of prematurity and infection, e.g., by reducing the risk of infection with antibiotic treatment, administering steroids to accelerate fetal lung maturation, and/or treatment with tocolytic drugs to allow the steroids and antibiotics to have a therapeutic effect. All three strategies are appropriate choices, depending on the gestational age and individual and population-based assessments of the risk of infection and prematurity. For example, expectant management is often chosen for women who present before 26 to 28 weeks, immediate delivery for women after 32 to 34 weeks, with interventionist strategies employed between 26 and 34 weeks. Adherence to a single strategy for all women with preterm PROM ignores the important individual differences among patients' risks of infection and immaturity.[302]

Use of Corticosteroids

As noted earlier in this chapter, antenatal corticosteroid have an unequivocal benefit on the risk of intraventricular hemorrhage for infants born at 32 weeks or earlier, regardless of the status of the membranes before delivery. Because grades III and IV intraventricular hemorrhages are rare after 32 weeks, the decision to use steroids in women with preterm PROM after 32 weeks depends on analyses of the effects of steroids on respiratory distress syndrome. Randomized trials of the effects of corticosteroids on respiratory distress syndrome in the presence of PROM have revealed conflicting results. A meta-analysis[171] that included the controversial Morales trial found a reduction in respiratory distress syndrome after corticosteroid use in subjects with preterm PROM. A meta-analysis that excluded the Morales trial[303] found no benefit in respiratory distress syndrome. The NICHD summary statement[197] encouraged more study of steroids for reduction of respiratory distress syndrome in preterm PROM after 32 weeks; the ACOG[198] also advocated caution in using steroids for preterm PROM after 32 weeks. At our center, we do not administer steroids to women with preterm PROM after 32 weeks.

Use of Antibiotics

Because the risk of perinatal group B streptococcal infection is associated with both premature birth and duration of membrane rupture before delivery, women with preterm PROM should be cultured for group B streptococcal colonization and treated presumptively with an appropriate antibiotic pending culture results. The importance of prophylactic maternal antibiotics in preterm PROM has been well established and is endorsed by both the ACOG and the American Academy of Pediatrics. Antibiotic prophylaxis has also been studied as a method of prolonging the interval from rupture to delivery by reducing the risk of infection in an effort to reduce perinatal morbidity and mortality due to infection and prematurity. Recent trials of various antibiotics are summarized in Table 23-15.

Mercer et al[304] enrolled 614 women in an NICHD trial that compared combined neonatal morbidity and mortality in 614 women with preterm PROM between 24 and 32 weeks of pregnancy who were managed expectantly and treated with either antibiotics or placebo within 72 hours of amniorrhexis (Table 23-16). The antibiotic group received 48 hours of intravenous ampicillin and erythromycin followed by oral amoxicillin and erythromycin for 5 days or until delivery. Women in both groups who were colonized with group B *Streptococcus* were treated with open-label ampicillin or erythromycin in addition to their assigned study regimen; these 118 subjects were analyzed separately. The primary outcome was combined mortality and morbidity including sepsis within 72 hours of birth, respiratory distress syndrome, grade III-IV intraventricular hemorrhage, and stage 2–3 necrotizing enterocolitis. The

Table 23-15   Prospective Random Trials of Antibiotics in Preterm PROM

Author	Treatment	Protocol Effect
Dunlop	Cephalexin PO	No effect on NN sepsis
Amon	Ampicillin IV, then PO	Prolonged latency, decreased NN sepsis
Johnston	Mezlo IV, then PO Amp	Prolonged latency, decreased NN sepsis
McGregor	Erythromycin PO	Prolonged latency, NN sepsis same
Mercer	Erythromycin PO	Prolonged latency, NN sepsis same
Christmas	Amp/Gent/Clind IV then PO Augmentin	Prolonged latency, decreased NN sepsis
Lockwood	Piperacillin IV	Prolonged latency, NN sepsis same
Owen	Amp or Erythro	Prolonged latency, NN sepsis same
Blanco	Ceftizoxime IV	No effect on latency or NN sepsis
Mercer	Amp + E-mycin IV/PO	Prolonged latency and reduced NN morbidity including sepsis

mortality rate was 5 percent in both groups, but the antibiotic group had significantly less morbidity, as shown in Table 23-16. Latency was prolonged in the antibiotic group. The group B streptococcal carriers, all of whom were treated with antibiotics, did as well as the group receiving antibiotic. Erythromycin was used in addition to ampicillin to treat *Mycoplasma* and *Ureaplasma*. As might be expected in a study from a study that enrolled a largely indigent population, the rate of chorioamnionitis was relatively high in both groups. It is interesting that women treated for group B streptococcal colonization did not benefit further from the prolonged broad-spectrum therapy.

In summary, prophylactic antibiotics should be given to all women with preterm PROM to reduce the risk of neonatal group B streptococcal infection. Recent data indicate that significant reductions in neonatal morbidity can also be achieved with broad-spectrum antibiotic treatment, especially in populations with a high prevalence of chorioamnionitis.

Use of Tocolytics

There is currently little evidence to support the routine use of tocolytic agents in patients with preterm PROM. A report from the National Institutes of Health Collaborative Study on Antenatal Steroids noted an association between tocolytic use in PROM and a higher rate of respiratory distress syndrome.[305] Prospective randomized trials by Garite et al[306] and Weiner et al[307] of prophylactic tocolysis revealed no consistent benefit to adjunctive tocolytics for these patients. However, as reviewed in the preceding paragraphs, the studies indicating benefit for adjunctive antibiotics and steroids have raised anew the question of short-term tocolysis in order to allow a course of steroids and possibly antibiotics. Adjunctive tocolysis is routine in some medical centers, but the majority, including ours, are waiting for more definitive studies before discarding our long-standing concern about suppressing labor in potentially infected patients.

Preterm PROM in Special Circumstances

Preterm PROM before 26 weeks of pregnancy has diverse etiologies that may alter the plans of management described previously. For instance, PROM may occur following amniocentesis. If the amniocentesis was performed for genetic studies or evaluation of rhesus disease, a good outcome should be expected. A brief course of bedrest and expectant management until the leakage stops and does not resume is usually all that is

Table 23-16   Effect of Prophylactic Antibiotics on Perinatal Morbidity in Infants Born to Women with Preterm PROM

	Ampicillin + Erythromycin (%) (n = 239)	Placebo (%) (n = 257)	RR	95% CI
All morbidity	45	55	0.82	0.69–0.98
RDS	41	51	0.80	0.66–0.97
Sepsis	8	15	0.54	0.33–0.88
Pneumonia	3	7	0.42	0.18–0.96
Chronic lung disease	14	21	0.68	0.46–1.00
Amnionitis	24	34	0.70	0.53–0.93

(Data from Mercer et al.[304])

required. However, infection and/or delivery are likely if the amniocentesis was performed to evaluate a patient with advanced cervical dilatation or PTL. It should be noted that PROM should not automatically be attributed to a genetic studies amniocentesis performed more than 10 to 14 days before rupture. Other causes should be considered.

When preterm PROM occurs in a woman who has experienced persistent second trimester bleeding, especially when accompanied as well by a history of pre-rupture oligohydramnios and/or an elevated maternal serum α-fetoprotein level, the prognosis for a surviving infant is very poor. These patients typically have had abnormal placental implantation noted on ultrasound evaluation. Management of these patients should include a thorough history and placental evaluation, looking for evidence of placental trauma or loss of a blighted twin and an attempt to obtain both placental and fetal samples for karyotype. Other possible diagnoses for second trimester losses (e.g., fetal anomaly or aneuploidy, uterine anomalies, diethylstilbestrol, incompetent cervix, and maternal trauma, both exogenous and self-induced) should all be considered.

Women with extremely preterm PROM deserve special attention to the psychosocial as well as the medical aspects of care. Often the transition from an apparently healthy pregnancy to disaster is abrupt. Medical professionals frequently get ahead of the patient in foreseeing a poor outcome in this setting. In the absence of compelling medical indications for delivery, recent literature support the maternal safety of a brief period of observation for these women. A review of 898 women with early preterm PROM[308] found that only six women (0.7 percent) developed sepsis; however, there was a single maternal death. As described previously, fetal outcome varies by the gestational age at rupture (25 or less survival before 24 weeks, and more than 59 percent survival between 24 and 26 weeks). In the review by Ghidini and Romero,[308] 417 of 914 (46 percent) of infants survived. Among 195 who were followed, 119 (61 percent) were neurologically normal. Orthopedic malformations are common at birth, but often resolve with time and physical therapy. Pulmonary hypoplasia was observed in nearly 100 percent of infants when rupture occurred before 20 weeks.

Management of PPROM in Women with Herpes

Major et al[309] reported an observational study of 18 women with preterm PROM complicated by a history of maternal genital herpes simplex infection and estimated that the theoretical maximum risk of neonatal herpes simplex virus was approximately 19 percent. At our center, we administer acyclovir prophylactically to women with this history based on the low reported incidence of adverse effects of acyclovir in neonates.

Management of Preterm PROM in Women with a Cerclage in Place

Ludmir et al[244] studied subjects with a cerclage in situ who later developed preterm PROM and observed that the risk of amnionitis was substantially higher when the stitch was not removed immediately.

Conduct of Labor and Delivery for the Preterm Infant

Gestational Age-Specific Neonatal Mortality and Morbidity

Obstetricians must repeatedly make decisions regarding the management of VLBW preterm fetuses. One of the most important determinants of good neonatal outcome is the obstetrician's assessment of potential viability. Unfortunately, obstetricians often underestimate the potential for intact survival in premature infants.[310] Paul and colleagues[311] have shown that infants misjudged to be previable experience significantly higher mortality rates than do infants of the same weight and gestational age who are correctly estimated to be viable and receive intensive intrapartum care. This study was repeated in 1994 with the same result: an attitude of aggressive attempts to "save" the infant is associated with increased overall survival, increased intact survival, and, unfortunately, increased severe neurologic morbidity as well.[312] Neonatal survival data are often best presented for obstetricians in terms of best obstetric estimation of gestational age, as shown in Table 23-1. Estimates of fetal weight by ultrasound are commonly used and, although accurate within 10 to 20 percent, may lead to inappropriate clinical decisions. Bottoms et al[12] recognized that the least accurate fetal measurement, abdominal circumference, had a substantial influence on weight estimates and therefore reported survival data that allow more accurate survival estimates based on measurement of fetal biparietal (BPD) and femur length. There were no survivors when the femur length was less than 40 mm or the BPD was below 54 mm and only a 10 percent chance of survival to 120 days if the femur was less than 43 mm or the BPD was less than 58 mm.

As neonatal and perinatal care has improved, the lower limit of "viability" has been a progressively earlier gestational age. The use of surfactant has pushed the limits beyond the predictions of the last edition of this text.[9,12] As many as 15 percent of infants born at 23 weeks, 56 percent at 24 weeks, and 80 percent at 25 weeks may now survive to hospital discharge in the postsurfactant era.[11]

Fetal Monitoring

Intensive maternal and fetal monitoring is especially important when the fetus is premature. The preterm fetus may tolerate labor poorly, and the cause of the preterm birth may create additional intrapartum risks. Careful and intensive fetal surveillance of these fetuses has been associated with significantly improved outcome in every major study.[313,314] Luthy et al[315] showed that attentive nursing care (one on one) for preterm fetuses with auscultation every 15 minutes gives perinatal mortality results equal to those with electronic fetal monitoring. However, the same authors subsequently showed that electronic fetal monitoring gives better information about fetal and neonatal well-being.[316] Ominous heart rate tracings have the same associations with fetal acidosis as they do later in gestation. Prompt intervention can minimize their effect on perinatal morbidity and mortality.[316,318]

Fetal Heart Rate

Mean fetal heart rate falls continuously, from 160 bpm at 22 weeks' gestation to 140 bpm at term. This is apparently due to a gradual increase in parasympathetic tone. At no age after 26 to 28 weeks should the normal baseline heart rate be above 170 bpm.

Variability

Changes in fetal heart rate variability in the preterm fetus carry the same significance for risk of acidosis as in term infants. Zanini et al[317] clearly demonstrated that, for any periodic change in premature infants, fetal pH is significantly less if variability is absent.

Resistance to Hypoxia

Some have reported an apparent tolerance in premature infants to prolonged periods of hypoxia both in utero and in the neonatal nursery. This has led to a concept of "plasticity," the ability of the premature brain to absorb insults and "bounce back." While this idea may have some validity, particularly in considering prognosis, it is dangerous to use it when managing patients in labor. Premature infants do sustain hypoxic-ischemic insults and have higher rates of cerebral palsy. Ominous patterns should be viewed with the same or greater level of concern as appropriate in term labor.

Anesthesia and Analgesia

There is no one method of anesthesia or analgesia for labor with a preterm fetus that is superior for all conditions. The goal of intrapartum care is to provide the neonatologist with the least traumatized least depressed, and least acidotic fetus consistent with mater-

nal health. Epidural anesthesia offers the advantage of pelvic floor and outlet muscle relaxation, minimizing an important sourse of resistance to the soft premature fetal head. Hypotension sometimes associated with this method can largely be avoided by adequate preloading with a crystalloid and more gradual onset of the block. Paracervical block is undesirable because of the risk of fetal bradycardia secondary either to transplacental passage of the anesthetic agent causing direct myocardial depression or to local uterine vascular vasospasm with diminished uteroplacental perfusion. The use of parenteral narcotics, even early in labor, is generally minimized because of concern for respiratory depression and because of the uncertain speed of PTL. Analgesia that allows maternal self-control is particularly helpful in the second stage of labor.

Anesthesia for cesarean delivery creates special concerns for each potential method when the fetus is preterm. The epidural technique requires a deeper, more intense block, involving more spinal segments than vaginal delivery. This may increase the chance of hypotension. Preloading the mother with large volumes of dextrose-containing fluid may lead to fetal acidosis.[319] General anesthesia is quicker to administer in an emergency situation and usually involves less changes in uteroplacental perfusion. However, it does entail greater risks to the mother, can lead to fetal depression if the surgery is difficult, and deprives the mother of perhaps her only chance to see and bond with a sick premature infant during its first hours of life.

Labor

The course of labor in preterm gestation is often significantly shorter than that of term pregnancy. Of particular importance are the rapidity of the active phase and the short second stage of labor. These need to be considered as one follows the labor to ensure that the fetus does not have a precipitous delivery without control of the fetal head. Multiparous women can have particularly short active phases, with 30 to 90 minutes not uncommon. Monitoring the course of labor after preterm PROM is always problematic because of the proscription of vaginal examinations until the woman is in active labor. It is often the case that women with preterm PROM are found to be in advanced labor after only minimally apparent uterine activity. This recurrent problem can never be entirely avoided and requires constant vigilance by both nurses and physicians.

Delivery

The two predominant goals for the intrapartum management of the preterm infant are avoidance of asphyxia and birth trauma. The critical role of asphyxia is demonstrated by a study from Michael Reese Hospital.[320] In 136 neonates of less than 32 weeks' gestation, the 1-minute Apgar score was highly correlated with survival. Babies with 1-minute Apgar scores of 4 or more had a 95 percent survival rate, while infants with a score or 3 or less had only a 56 percent survival rate. The implication from this and other studies is that initial condition at birth substantially affects survival. How then can one "optimize" the birth process for the VLBW (less than 1,500-g) infant?

Episiotomy

A generous episiotomy is recommended by many investigators, based on common sense, to minimize the forces of outlet perineal resistance on the small soft head. In fact, these forces are probably much less than those of the cervix and muscles of the vagina through which the fetus has already passed. Data demonstrating improved outcome associated with the use of episiotomy are very difficult to find.[321] When delivering a VLBW infant, we perform an early episiotomy if there is perineal resistance. Few multiparous women will be in this group.

"Prophylactic" Forceps

An analysis of the National Collaborative Perinatal Project data concluded that the premature infants (less than 2,500 g birth weight) who had the best outcome were the ones delivered by low forceps[322] and suggested that "prophylactic" forceps protected the fragile premature infant's head. Subsequent studies have not shown this benefit,[321,323] and one report described traumatic intracranial hemorrhage in preterm infants delivered with outlet forceps.[324] Forceps may be employed for premature infants for the customary indications, but should not be used prophylactically. Careful attention should be paid to the often rapid second stage to avoid the head "bursting" through the perineum.

Cesarean Delivery

Despite anecdotal opinion to the contrary, routine cesarean delivery of all preterm infants is not justified by current literature. For infants in breech presentation, there are intuitive reasons for cesarean birth—to avoid trapping of the aftercoming head, an infrequent but disastrous complication; and other manipulations that could lead to trauma and hypoxia. Most retrospective studies have suggested a benefit from cesarean delivery for the VLBW breech. A study of 216 breeches of 750- to 1,500-g birth weight infants delivered over 4 years revealed a mortality rate in the cesarean group of 29 percent, significantly less than the 58 percent mortality rate for breech infants born vaginally ($p < 0.001$).[325] This advantage remained after correction for hospital setting, birth weight, and presence of growth retardation. However, in this study as in many others, the smallest VLBW breeches were more apt to have been delivered vaginally and their higher mortality rate may have had as much to do with their size as with their method of delivery. Other studies with somewhat smaller numbers of VLBW breeches found trends toward improvement with cesarean birth that did not reach statistical significance or that lost significance when confounding variables were considered.[326–328] Therefore, we remain comfortable with the current American custom of cesarean delivery of all VLBW nonvertex infants, but acknowledge that supporting data are not conclusive.

A critical technical point cannot be overstressed. One does not want to avoid a traumatic vaginal delivery only to struggle and have a difficult cesarean birth because of an undeveloped lower uterine segment or an inadequate incision.[327] Clearly, the operation must be carried out in a way that will fulfill its purpose, atraumatic delivery. While some have recommended routine use of a low vertical or classic incision, the exact uterine incision can depend on the fetal position and on the anatomy of the individual patient. If the lower uterine segment is well developed and the fetus is in the lower one-third of the uterus, a transverse incision is reasonable.

Routine cesarean delivery of VLBW vertex infants can no longer be supported. Several large studies have failed to note improvement in perinatal morbidity or mortality with cesarean birth for indications other than classic obstetric ones.[328–331] The trend favoring cesarean delivery seen in some studies disappears after adjustment for confounding factors.[331,332] Neonatal intracranial hemorrhage appears to occur as often before and after as it does during labor and delivery. One study[333] suggested that cesarean-delivered VLBW infants had a significantly reduced incidence of intracranial hemorrhage but was immediately followed by four studies that did not find such an advantage. Some have suggested that the route of delivery may be less important than the presence of active labor in the development of intracranial hemorrhage,[334] but studies corrected for gestational age, presentation, and labor complications fail to support this finding. In a study[335] that carefully separated out "high-risk" VLBW labor (e.g., preeclampsia, vaginal bleeding, abnormal heart rate tracing) from "low-risk" VLBW (e.g., preterm labor, incompetent cervix), cesarean delivery was of no value in the low-risk group, but was associated with significantly improved survival rates in the high-risk group. Thus there are situations requiring delivery in the face of a long closed cervix that may lead to a decision for cesarean delivery for VLBW fetuses rather than a long and potentially morbid induction of labor. However, studies to date have failed to provide clear evidence that this approach is of great benefit to the infant and mother.

Secondary Care for Preterm Birth

Identification of Women with Increased Risk of Preterm Birth

All secondary health care strategies are based on identification of a population with an increased risk of disease. This population becomes the target of various interventions, e.g., identification and elimination of medical or behavioral risk factors, increased diagnostic surveillance to initiate prompt treatment, and/or prophylactic treatment. For SPTB, secondary care strategies include risk scoring systems to select high-risk pregnancies, early diagnosis programs (patient education programs, frequent contact with a special nurse, and ambulatory uterine activity monitoring), and therapeutic interventions such as prophylactic medications, reduced activity, and even cerclage.

Until recently, treatment of women with disorders leading to SPTB has been entirely tertiary, that is, occurring *after* the patient presented with a clinical problem such as preterm PROM or PTL. Secondary care of "prematurity" as a clinical problem to be solved has in the past been seen either as a pointless exercise ("Only when the factors causing prematurity are clearly understood can any intelligent attempt at prevention be made"[4]) or as a social problem beyond the purview of obstetricians ("I do not think that . . . prematurity can be reduced . . . by better obstetrics. . . . These problems are social, not obstetric"[336]). These sentiments retain some validity today, but have been challenged as unduly nihilistic by the pioneering work of Papiernik et al[337] in France and by Creasy et al[19] in the United States, who argued that premature birth could and should be addressed proactively, even though the pathophysiology was not (and is not) entirely clear and despite the frustrating social correlates that often accompany preterm birth. Although the specific screening and intervention programs proposed by these investi-

gators have not been uniformly effective in reducing preterm birth, their efforts spawned a generation of research that has nearly overcome the therapeutic nihilism of prior decades.[338]

Scoring Systems

Creasy and colleagues[19] and Papiernik et al[339] developed a risk scoring system that assigned points for various medical, obstetric, and demographic risk factors, with a score of 10 or more being "high risk." Risk factors were selected and weighted empirically, based on univariate analyses of epidemiologic data. The system had a sensitivity of 40 to 60 percent in most populations in which it was tested, but the specificity and positive predictive value were poor; many normal subjects were labeled as being at risk (Table 23-17).

Although the Creasy score has been abandoned by most centers, the concept of evaluating all pregnant women for risk of preterm delivery remains attractive. Rather than a complex point system, a simple obstetric history can be helpful, placing emphasis on just a few major risk factors:

1. *A prior preterm delivery* between 16 and 36 weeks carries a two- to threefold increase in risk of recurrent preterm birth (interestingly, the magnitude of risk is related to the outcome of the most recent pregnancy[26] and increases substantially as the gestational age of the previous preterm birth decreases[25])
2. *Multiple gestation,* an increasingly prevalent risk factor with the increased number of pregnancies achieved with assisted reproductive technologies
3. *Vaginal bleeding* after the first trimester (see Table 23-2)
4. *Low pre-pregnancy weight* (less than 19.8 kg/m[258,63]

These major risk factors are easily elicited, but no system has been sufficiently sensitive to identify more than about half of women who will deliver prematurely. Just as screening for preeclampsia is part of every woman's prenatal care, all pregnant women must also receive

Table 23-17 Application of Creasy Scoring System

Author	No.; Location	% Preterm Delivery	% High Risk	Sensitivity	Positive Predictive Value
Creasy	966; New Zealand	6.2	13	64	30
Herron	1150; San Francisco	2.4	15	44	4
Iams	3,049; Columbus, OH	12.0	23	44	24
Main	380; Philadelphia	16.3	35	48	23
Ross	8,240; Los Angeles	6.4	33	56	10
Holbrook	7,329; San Francisco	8.4	14	41	25

care and education aimed at the problem of prematurity. Education about the importance of early prenatal care, the significance of second trimester bleeding, and the need to report often-ignored symptoms of PTL should be a part of routine antenatal care.

Detection of risk factors that arise during pregnancy has been difficult. Research has focused on uterine contractions, cervical examination, the vaginal microflora, serologic markers, and, most recently, on the presence of fetal fibronectin in the cervix and vagina.

Biophysical Assessment of Prematurity Risk

Because labor is ultimately defined by the presence of uterine contractions accompanied by cervical dilatation and effacement, assessment of contraction frequency and/or cervical dilatation and effacement might be expected to predict risk of premature birth. In fact, there are clear associations of the likelihood of preterm birth with both contractions and cervical examination. However, the clinical value of this information has been disappointing.

Uterine Contractions

Studies of uterine activity in human pregnancy performed in women with risk factors for preterm birth have shown a rise in uterine activity as pregnancy progresses and more frequent contractions in women destined to labor or deliver prematurely. Two types of contractile activity have been reported: a high-frequency, low-amplitude contraction pattern and higher amplitude contractions that occur with increasing frequency in late pregnancy. Aubry and Pennington[340] demonstrated an increase in uterine activity in women who delivered preterm that was apparent several weeks before overt PTL occurred. Katz et al[341] monitored uterine activity four times daily for 30 to 60 minutes in the second and third trimesters in 34 ambulatory women with risk factors for preterm birth. Contraction frequency data were not analyzed by time of day or patient activity level, but showed a steady rise until term. There were more contractions per hour in the 21 subjects who delivered preterm than in the 13 who delivered at term, a phenomenon again evident several weeks prior to delivery. Among those who delivered at term, the mean number of contractions per hour was 2 or less up to 28 weeks, 3 or less between 28 and 32 weeks, and 4 or less between 32 and 36 weeks. A study of uterine activity recorded during antenatal fetal heart rate testing in 2,446 women between 30 weeks' gestation and delivery found that uterine activity increased by 4.7 percent per week.[342] Women who delivered preterm had more, and who delivered post-term had fewer, uterine contractions per 10-minute window of observation. In this

study, there was an increase in uterine activity during the 3 days preceding labor, a finding that has not been observed in other studies.[77]

These studies all suggested that frequent assessment of uterine contractions might accurately identify a group of women with increased risk of preterm birth who would be candidates for further diagnostic assessment (e.g., cervical examination) or for prophylactic interventions such as oral tocolytics or reduced activity. In response to data showing a correlation between risk of prematurity and contraction frequency, an entire industry has arisen to provide daily monitoring of uterine contractions for women with risk factors such as multiple gestation or a prior preterm delivery. Monitored contraction data are transmitted over telephone lines and read by specially trained nurses in the expectation that an early diagnosis of preterm labor might lead to prompt and therefore more effective use of tocolysis. Numerous studies of the effects of this strategy have been performed, with conflicting conclusions.[212,343–350] There is consensus that the monitoring technique produces accurate data and that frequent supportive nursing contact and education for high-risk women is associated with a small but significant decline in the incidence of preterm birth. The mechanism of this effect is not understood. The independent value of uterine activity monitoring data as either a screen for risk or an aid to early detection of PTL has not been demonstrated. Meta-analyses of published reports have largely concluded that HUAM as currently employed is ineffective in reducing preterm birth in at-risk women,[351–354] although a recent analysis found benefit.[355] The reasons for this disappointing chapter in the annals of prematurity prevention are explored in the next section.

Uterine Contractility in Normal and High-Risk Pregnancies

If contractions are an integral part of labor, and if HUAM monitors detect contractions accurately, why has frequent assessment of uterine activity not produced an obvious benefit in early detection and treatment of PTL? The principal reason seems to be an incomplete understanding of normal uterine activity in pregnancy that has made detection of abnormal activity difficult. Longitudinal (rather than cross-sectional) studies of uterine activity patterns in normal and high-risk pregnancies are relatively recent. Uterine activity was recorded in 81 black women who delivered at term without complication.[356] Subjects wore a tocodynamometer for three 72-hour sessions during the second and third trimesters of pregnancy. Data were obtained between 22 and 25 weeks, 26 and 29 weeks, and 30 and 33 weeks. There was a steady increase in mean hourly uterine activity with advancing gestation in both primigravid and parous women and an increase in contraction frequency at night.

Moore et al[78] studied 109 women without antepartum complications who delivered after spontaneous labor at term. Subjects recorded uterine activity for 24 hours twice a week for a total of 71,683 hours. No contractions were recorded in 73 percent of hours, and 96 percent of hours had fewer than four contractions per hour (see Fig. 23-15). Contraction frequency was similar in nulliparous and parous subjects. Contractions increased with gestational age but rarely exceeded three contractions per hour before 37 weeks. The 95th percentile of uterine activity was 1.3 ± 0.5 (SD) contractions per hour at 21 to 24 weeks, 2.9 ± 1.0 at 28 to 32 weeks, and 4.9 ± 1.7 at 38 to 40 weeks ($p < 0.0001$). The normal range of contraction frequency varied with time of day, gestational age, and maternal activity. The increased occurrence of contractions at night was pronounced after 24 weeks. The night:day ratio of contractions per hour was 1.8:1 at 21 to 24 weeks, 2.3:1 at 28 to 32 weeks, and 2.0:1 at 38 to 40 weeks ($p < 0.001$). Depending on the time of day, as many as seven contractions per hour could fall within 2 SD above the 95th percentile before 37 weeks. A few women recorded more than 15 contractions per hour, yet still delivered at term without intervention. Physical activity, but not emotional status, had a significant effect on contraction frequency. Contractions were diminished after recumbency and increased after coitus. No changes were associated with self-reported stress. The effect of physical activity on uterine activity has been documented in a Dutch study of 30 women at term.[357] A standard program of exercise was associated with a more than fivefold increase in contractions, which subsided promptly after concluding exercise.

Subjects with a history of preterm birth were enrolled in a small study by Germain et al.[358] Diurnal uterine activity patterns in normal subjects were compared with patterns recorded from women with a history of preterm birth. Uterine activity was measured for 1 hour at 4-hour intervals for 24 hours at 94, 79, 65, 52, 39, 24, and 9 days before delivery. They observed a loss of the daily diurnal pattern of uterine activity in high-risk subjects who delivered preterm, but reported no change in diurnal pattern in high-risk subjects who delivered at term or in normal subjects. The loss of the expected diurnal increase in contractions in the afternoon and evening occurred at least 9 and sometimes as long as 24 days before the onset of PTL. The *pattern* of contractions was predictive of subsequent preterm delivery, but the *number of contractions per hour* was not. The effects of gestational age, time of day, and diurnal patterns of activity were not considered in the clinical studies of HUAM programs cited above.

Another potential explanation for the outcome of the HUAM trials may lie in the theory of prematurity that forms the basis for use of this technology. If premature labor occurs as the result of the loss of hormonal inhibition of natural uterine contractile activity, in which normal contractions coalesce into pathologic contractions that result in cervical dilatation and effacement, then early detection of contractions (e.g., with HUAM) should be an effective means of assessing risk. The inability to demonstrate benefit for HUAM may indicate that this theory is either incorrect or is applicable only to relatively few cases of PTL. The experience with HUAM is a clear instance in which the dictum of Eastman[4] noted previously has proved to be correct.

The HUAM literature should not be interpreted to mean that there is no relationship between uterine contraction frequency and risk of preterm birth, only that the association has not been clinically useful when applied in the HUAM model. The NICHD Preterm Birth Prediction Study recently confirmed that women who noted contractions had a higher relative risk of SPTB.[58,59]

Digital Cervical Examination

Several studies have an observed association between digital examination showing premature cervical dilatation and effacement and risk of subsequent preterm birth (Fig. 23-26).[52–54] As with uterine contractions, however, the observation of an association has not led to a clinical benefit such as reduced incidence of PTL or delivery. In a randomized study, Buekens et al[359] found no difference in rates of preterm birth among 2,803 women who were followed with serial cervical examination as compared with 2,799 women in whom examination was not routinely performed.

Cervical Sonography

Digital examination of the cervix is reasonably accurate in active labor, but is subject to great interexaminer variation when dilatation is less than 3 cm or effacement is less than 80 percent.[80] Measurement of cervical length using transvaginal sonography[56] has been reported to identify women at risk for preterm birth on the basis of a cervical length less than the 10th percentile, or about 25 mm at 24 to 28 weeks of pregnancy. The data from this trial, although useful in redefining the contribution of cervical factors to the pathogenesis of early preterm birth, have not been tested as part of any program of intervention (e.g., prophylactic use of maternal rest, tocolysis, antibiotics, or cerclage). An evaluation of transabdominal cervical sonography compared with digital examination of the cervix[360] in the care of high-risk women found no benefit to sonography, probably because of the unpredictable effect of

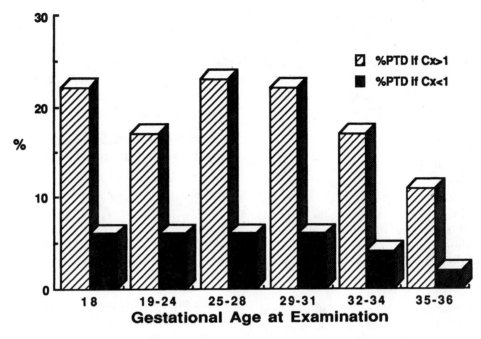

Fig. 23-26. Percent of women who delivered prematurely according to cervical dilation of less than 1 cm vs. 1 cm or more and gestational age at the time of the examination. (Data from Papiernik et al.[53])

bladder volume on transabdominal cervical imaging.[361,362]

Genital Colonization with Microorganisms

The association of maternal colonization with various genital microorganisms and risk of preterm birth has led to investigations of screening tests to identify and treat women at risk. In the Vaginal Infections and Prematurity (VIP) Study,[363,364] parturients who were culture positive for various microorganisms were randomly assigned to receive placebo or antibiotic treatment. No reduction in preterm birth was associated with screening and treatment for *C. trachomatis, Ureaplasma urealyticum,* or group B *Streptococcus,* despite preliminary data suggesting an association of these organisms with increased risk of preterm birth for *Ureaplasma*[363] and for group B *Streptococcus.*[364] Antibiotic treatment was employed after 25 weeks in this trial; the authors speculated that earlier treatment might have been more successful. Interestingly, a randomized trial of screening and treatment for bacterial vaginosis, in which treatment with metronidazole and erythromycin was provided after 26 weeks, reported a significantly reduced rate of SPTB, from 49 percent in the placebo group to 31 percent in the antibiotic group.[365] Unlike the VIP study, in which all colonized subjects were eligible for randomization, the trial of bacterial vaginosis treatment was limited to women with a history of prior preterm birth. The epidemiologic association of bacterial vaginosis with spontaneous preterm delivery in

multiple regression analyses[49] together with the data by Hauth et al[365] has led some to recommend routine screening and treatment, at least for high-risk women. This conclusion may be warranted soon if additional confirmatory reports are forthcoming, but, as of this writing, there are two reasons to withhold judgment. First, there is no accurate and economical method to screen for bacterial vaginosis—the published report used a research laboratory. Second, the effect has been confirmed by only one prospective, blinded and randomized study conducted in a very high-risk population in Alabama. If obstetricians have learned anything from the last 10 years of prematurity intervention trials, it should be that an apparently useful intervention should not be universally embraced on the basis of early reports.

Vaginal pH readings of 5.0 or higher have been associated with an increased risk of SPTB.[366,367] This finding is apparently a result of the association between bacterial vaginosis and spontaneous prematurity. There is no evidence that vaginal pH can be used as a substitute for bacterial vaginosis screening or that treatment of low- or high-risk pregnant women with a vaginal pH of 5.0 or higher will affect the duration of pregnancy.

Biochemical Markers of Risk for SPTB

Biochemical markers have long been sought to identify women who will deliver premature infants. Maternal blood assays for progesterone, prolactin, relaxin, major basic protein, C-reactive protein, interleukins, and collagenase have all been tested in attempts to identify pregnancies with increased risk. Increased levels of estriol in maternal saliva have also been reported to correlate with the risk of preterm birth[368] and appear to be the most promising of the biochemical screens being evaluated.

Fibronectin

The presence of fetal fibronectin in cervicovaginal mucus has been described earlier in the chapter in a discussion of its use (approved by FDA) as an aid to the diagnosis of early PTL in symptomatic subjects. Recent data have suggested that there may be a broader use for the fibronectin assay as a screen for risk of preterm delivery in asymptomatic subjects. Goldenberg et al[61] have reported data from 2,929 women enrolled in the NICHD Preterm Prediction Study indicating that a single positive fibronectin assay performed at 24 to 26 weeks may identify up to 60 percent of women destined to deliver before 28 weeks' gestation. The sensitivity of the 24- to 26-week fibronectin assay for predicting preterm birth declined after 30 weeks. Remarkably, this test has similar predictive value for women who are otherwise categorized as low or high risk by other traditional methods. However, as with every screening test described here, there are as yet no reports describing use of fibronectin as a screening test leading to a successful intervention to reduce prematurity. Based on the reported association of fibronectin and bacterial vaginosis,[65] randomized trials of antibiotic prophylaxis in fibronectin-positive women are ongoing.

Unifactorial Interventions To Prevent Preterm Birth

Attempts to prevent prematurity over the last 15 years have been based on a traditional medical model of identifying and correcting a potential "cause" of preterm birth, with the expectation that the rate of preterm birth would decline. Reported intervention trials have addressed individual risk factors such as early identification of PTL through patient education, pharmacologic suppression of uterine contractions, antimicrobial therapy of vaginal microorganisms, cerclage sutures to bolster the cervix, reduction of maternal stress, improved access to prenatal care, and reduced physical activity. Some trials have enrolled women with the risk factor in question without regard to obstetric history (e.g., the VIP studies[363,364]), while others have been limited to women with a prior preterm delivery (e.g., the European cerclage trials[220,245,246]). In no case has a study that focused on elimination of a single risk factor led to a decrease in preterm birth, but there have

been hopeful if statistically insignificant trends identified in some of them. In virtually every trial, reports of an association between a risk factor and SPTB have been followed by small trials, usually observational in design, that describe promising early results, only to find minimal if any benefit when carried out in other populations.

Education of At-Risk Women About the Signs and Symptoms of Preterm Labor

Initial studies[19,20,337] described substantial reductions in SPTB, but subsequent reports showed inconsistent results.[21,369,370] In a multicenter investigations, the March of Dimes Collaborative Trial[370] found significant benefits in two centers, but no benefits at all in three other participating centers. The authors could not explain the differences in outcome by center.

Antibiotics To Eliminate Various Pathogens from the Genital Tract

The story of antibiotics to prevent preterm birth has been an erratic one. The serendipitous observation[371] of a reduced frequency of preterm birth in women who received tetracycline as prophylaxis for urinary tract infection was followed by reports of success (erythromycin treatment leads to higher birth weight[372]), then of failure for women colonized with *Ureaplasma*[363] and group B *Streptococcus*,[364] and, most recently, by success again for women colonized with bacterial vaginosis[373] (metronidazole and erythromycin for women with bacterial vaginosis and a history of SPTB[365]). Clearly there is a relationship between genital microorganisms and preterm birth, but the results of all these trials just as clearly indicate that infection does not operate independently as a cause of preterm birth. The selection of appropriate candidates for antibiotic prophylaxis is the next challenge.

Social Support and Improved Access to Prenatal Care

Prenatal care has something to do with the rate of SPTB in both black and white women, but the specific contribution of prenatal care to lower rates of SPTB is not clear. Prospective interventions designed to reduce preterm birth through better access to care, reduced stress, and so forth have been unsuccessful,[374,375] another univariate association that is important but whose elimination is not sufficient to reduce prematurity.

Prophylactic Cerclage for Women with a History of Preterm Birth

A historical study[219] described significant improvements in pregnancy outcome for women with a history of early preterm birth but subsequent attempts to reduce the incidence of preterm birth with cerclage have been mixed. Two studies[245,246] observed no benefit at all, while another[220] found a significant reduction in the incidence of early preterm births, but no effect on the overall rate of SPTB.

Prophylactic Medications

Tocolytic agents have been widely used without cervical change (i.e., prophylactically) in this country. However, the large-scale use of ritodrine has not been associated with a reduction in either preterm or LBW deliveries.[376] Some would argue that the entire US experience with HUAM described previously has been in effect a trial of early labor suppression with β-mimetics for women with risk factors for SPTB. If so, it is strong evidence that prophylaxis with these agents in not effective.

Parenteral progesterone (17α-hydroprogesterone caproate) has been used for prophylaxis against PTL after reports[377] suggested a decreased incidence of preterm births in treated women. Another study in an active-duty military population failed to demonstrate any reduction in preterm delivery rates compared with a placebo group.[378]

Bedrest and Activity Modification

There is substantial evidence of a relationship between maternal physical activity and risk of SPTB. Colie[379] reviewed the subject and concluded that there was consistent evidence of a weak relationship between maternal physical activity and risk of SPTB. Luke et al[380] observed strong relationships between hours worked per week, occupational fatigue score, and risk of SPTB. However, a recent scholarly review of bedrest in pregnancy[381] concluded that there was no evidence that bedrest offered any benefit to pregnant women, once again indicating unsuccessful interventions based on a persistent association.

Unifactorial vs. Multifactorial Approaches to Preterm Birth Prevention

The foregoing would appear to indicate that for every factor associated with spontaneous preterm birth there has been an ineffective intervention trial. What other conclusion could be drawn from the investigations described? It has been the thesis of this chapter that SPTBs occur when the sum of the "triggers" or stimuli for labor exceed the ability of the maternal host to resist labor and that the stimulus or trigger represented by each individual "risk factor" is rarely sufficient to reach the threshold necessary to initiate SPTB. If the reports of unifactorial interventions are reviewed with the cardiovascular model of multiple collaborative risk conditions in mind, then the failure of each individual trial to affect the rate of SPTB becomes not only understandable but expected. However, it remains to be seen whether multifactorial interventions will succeed against SPTB. The cardiovascular model would suggest that identification and simultaneous elimination of multiple factors will be necessary to reduce prematurity and that ultimately a national strategy of *primary* prevention will be required. As Bastian said in *The Neverending Story*, "there is still a long way to go."

Conclusion

1. Ultimate prevention of preterm birth will require replacement of the current tertiary treatment approach by aggressive secondary and primary interventions to reduce risk in the population.
2. Tocolytics, glucocorticoids, and antibiotics are effective tertiary therapies in the problem of preterm birth, but can never be wholly effective in eliminating the morbidity and mortality due to prematurity.
3. Inaccurate diagnosis of PTL has been one of the largest impediments to evaluation of treatment strategies for premature labor. New methods hold great promise for improvement in this key step in patient care.

Key Points

- Preterm birth is the single greatest cause of perinatal morbidity and mortality in nonanomalous infants, being responsible for 70 percent of fetal, neonatal, and infant deaths.

- The outcomes for premature and LBW infants are better than most medical professionals believe it to be.

- Spontaneous preterm birth (those that follow PTL, preterm PROM, and abnormal cervical competence) is a syndrome that is analogous to atherosclerosis: multiple continuous risk variables operate collaboratively via injury to the maternal–fetal interface to produce several related clinical disorders.

- The mechanism of injury may be infectious, ischemic, or "allergic," alone or in or combination.

- Major risk factors for preterm birth are a prior history of preterm delivery, multifetal gestation, bleeding after the first trimester of pregnancy, and a low maternal body mass index, but these factors precede no more than 50 percent of preterm births. Every pregnancy is potentially at risk.

- Cervical "competence" is not an absolute or categorical property of the cervix, but rather is a continuum. The risk of SPTB increases as the length of the cervix decreases.

- Accurate early diagnosis of PTL is a major problem. Up to 50 percent of patients diagnosed with PTL do not actually have PTL, yet as many as 20 percent of symptomatic patients diagnosed as not being in labor will deliver prematurely. The addition of fetal fibronectin and cervical sonography to the evaluation should improve the accuracy of diagnosis.

- Tertiary care of the clinical disorders that precede spontaneous preterm birth that can reduce perinatal morbidity and mortality are (1) transfer of the mother and fetus to an appropriate hospital; (2) administration of antibiotics to prevent neonatal group B *Streptococcus* infection; (3) administration of corticosteroids to reduce neonatal respiratory distress syndrome and intraventricular hemorrhage, a treatment that has been underutilized in the past; and (4) administration of labor-arresting (tocolytic) medications to allow the above to occur.

- There is no truly reliable test for fetal well-being or infection in women with preterm PROM.

- Prevention of preterm birth will require prevention of risk in the population.

References

1. Guyer B, Strobino DM, Ventura SJ et al: Annual summary of vital statistics—1994. Pediatrics 96:1029, 1995

2. Hack M, Taylor HG, Klein N et al: School-age outcomes in children with birth weights under 750 g. N Engl J Med 331:756, 1994

3. Monthly Vital Statistics Report, Advance Report of Final Natality Statistics for 1993, National Center for Health Statistics

4. Eastman NT: Prematurity from the viewpoint of the obstetrician. Am Pract 1:343, 1947

5. Brenner WE, Edelman DA, Hendricks CH: A standard of fetal growth for the United States of America. Am J Obstet Gynecol 126:555, 1976

6. National Center for Health Statistics, p. 21. DHHS Publ. No. HSRA-MCH-95–1, July 1995

7. Kessel S, Villar J, Berendes H, Nugent R: The changing pattern of low birth weight in the United States. JAMA 251:1978, 1984

8. Sachs BP, Fretts RC, Gardner R et al: The impact of extreme prematurity and congenital anomalies on the interpretation of international comparisons of infant mortality. Obstet Gynecol 85:941, 1995

9. Fanaroff AA, Wright LL, Stevenson DK et al: Very low-birth-weight outcomes of The National Institute of Child Health and Human Development Neonatal Research Network, May 1991 through December 1992. Am J Obstet Gynecol 173:1423, 1995

10. Copper RL, Goldenberg RL, Creasy RK et al: A multicenter study of preterm birth weight and gestational age-specific neonatal mortality. Am J Obstet Gynecol 168:78, 1993

11. Allen MC, Donohue PK, Dusman AE: The limit of viability—neonatal outcome of infants born at 22 to 25 weeks' gestation. N Engl J Med 329:1597, 1993

12. Bottoms S, Paul R, Iams JD et al: Obstetrical determinants of neonatal survival in extremely low birth weight infants. Am J Obstet Gynecol 170:383, 1994

13. Horbar JD, McAuliffe TL, Adler SM et al: Variability in 28-day outcomes for very low birth weight infants: an analysis of 11 neonatal intensive care units. Pediatrics 82:554, 1988

14. Ehrenhaft PM, Wagner JL, Herdman RC: Changing prognosis for very low birth weight infants. Obstet Gynecol 74:528, 1989

15. Wilcox A, Buekens P, Kiely J: Birth weight and perinatal mortality: a comparison of the United States and Norway. JAMA 273:709, 1995

16. Robertson PA, Sniderman SH, Laros RK et al: Neonatal morbidity according to gestational age and birth weight from five tertiary care centers in the United States, 1983 through 1986. Am J Obstet Gynecol 166:1629, 1992

17. McCormick MC, Shapiro S, Starfield BH: Rehospitalization during the first year of life for high risk survivors. Pediatrics 66:991, 1980

18. Meis PJ, Ernest JM, Moore ML: Causes of low birth-weight births in public and private patients. Am J Obstet Gynecol 156:1165, 1987

19. Creasy R, Gummer B, Liggins G: System for predicting spontaneous preterm birth. Obstet Gynecol 55:692, 1980

20. Herron M, Katz M, Creasy RK: Evaluation of a preterm birth prevention program: preliminary report. Obstet Gynecol 59:452, 1982

21. Main DM, Gabbe SG, Richardson D et al: Can preterm

deliveries be prevented? Am J Obstet Gynecol 151:892, 1985

22. Meyer M, Tonascia J: Maternal smoking, pregnancy complications, and perinatal mortality. Am J Obstet Gynecol 128:494, 1977

23. Hadley CB, Main DM, Gabbe SG: Risk factors for preterm premature rupture of the fetal membranes. Am J Perinatol 7:374, 1990

24. Ekwo EE, Gosselink CA, Moawad A: Unfavorable outcome in penultimate pregnancy and premature rupture of membranes in successive pregnancy. Obstet Gynecol 80:166, 1992

25. Mercer BM, Goldenberg RL, Moawad A et al: Prediction of spontaneous prematurity based on prior obstetric outcome (abstract). Am J Obstet Gynecol 172:404, 1995

26. Bakketeig LS, Hoffman HJ: Epidemiology of preterm birth: results from a longitudinal study of births in Norway. p. 17. In Elder LS, Hendricks CH (eds): Preterm Labor. Butterworths, London/Boston, 1981

27. Goldenberg et al: Low birthweight, preterm birth, and fetal growth retardation in black and white women. Am J Obstet Gynecol, 1996 (in press)

28. Tamura RK, Sabbagha RE, Depp OR et al: Diminished growth in fetuses born preterm after spontaneous labor or rupture of membranes. Am J Obstet Gynecol 148:1105, 1984

29. MacGregor SN, Sabbagha RE, Tamura RK et al: Differing fetal growth patterns in pregnancies complicated by preterm labor. Obstet Gynecol 72:834, 1988

30. Ott WJ: Intrauterine growth retardation and preterm delivery. Am J Obstet Gynecol 168:1710, 1993

31. Hediger ML, Scholl TO, Schall JI, Fischer RL: Fetal growth and the etiology of preterm delivery. Obstet Gynecol 85:175, 1995

32. Salafia CM, Vogel CA, Vintzeleos AM et al: Placental pathologic findings in preterm birth. Am J Obstet Gynecol 165:934, 1991

33. Arias F, Rodriguez L, Rayne SC, Kraus FT: Maternal placental vasculopathy and infection: two distinct subgroups among patients with preterm labor and preterm ruptured membranes. Am J Obstet Gynecol 168:585, 1993

34. Arias F, Victoria A, Cho K et al: There are different histologic groups with distinct clinical characteristics among patients with preterm premature rupture of membranes (abstract). Am J Obstet Gynecol 174:464, 1996

35. Strigini FA, Lencioni G, DeLuca G et al: Uterine artery velocimetry and spontaneous preterm delivery. Obstet Gynecol 85:374, 1995

36. Lockwood CJ: The diagnosis of preterm labor and the prediction of preterm delivery. Clin Obstet Gynecol 38:675, 1995

37. Knox IC, Hoerner JK: The role of infection in premature rupture of the membranes. Am J Obstet Gynecol 59:190, 1950

38. Gibbs RS, Romero R, Hillier SL et al: A review of premature birth and subclinical infection. Am J Obstet Gynecol 166:1515, 1992

39. Bobitt JR, Hayslip CC, Damato JD: Amniotic fluid infection as determined by transabdominal amniocentesis in patients with intact membranes in preterm labor. Am J Obstet Gynecol 140:947, 1981

40. Wahbeh CJ, Hill GB, Eden RD et al: Intraamniotic bacterial colonization in premature labor. Am J Obstet Gynecol 148:739, 1984

41. Romero R, Sirtori M, Oyarzun E et al: Infection and labor V: prevalence, microbiology, and clinical significance of intraamniotic infection in women with preterm labor and intact membranes. Am J Obstet Gynecol 161:817, 1989

42. Duff P, Kopelman JN: Subclinical intra-amniotic infection in asymptomatic patients with refractory preterm labor. Obstet Gynecol 69:756, 1987

43. Russell P: Inflammatory lesions of the human placenta I. Clinical significance of acute chorioamniotis. Am J Diagn Gynecol Obstet 1:127, 1979

44. Hillier SL, Martius J, Krohn M et al: A case control study of chorioamniotic infection and histologic chorioamnionitis in prematurity. N Engl J Med 319:972, 1988

45. Martius J, Krohn M, Hillier SL et al: Relationships of vaginal *Lactobacillus* species, cervical *Chlamydia trachomatis*, and bacterial vaginosis to preterm birth. Obstet Gynecol 71:89, 1988

46. Krohn MA, Hillier SL, Lee ML et al: Vaginal *Bacteroides* are associated with an increased rate of preterm delivery among women in preterm labor. J Infect Dis 164:88, 1991

47. Gravett MG, Nelson HP, DeRouen T et al: Independent associations of bacterial vaginosis and *Chlamydia trachomatis* infection with adverse pregnancy outcome. JAMA 256:1899, 1986

48. Schoonmaker JN, Lawellin DW, Lunt B, McGregor JA: Bacteria and inflammatory cells reduce chorioamniotic membrane integrity and tensile strength. Obstet Gynecol 74:590, 1989

49. Meis PJ, Goldenberg RL, Mercer B et al: The preterm prediction study: significance of vaginal infections. Am J Obstet Gynecol 173:1231, 1995

50. MacDonald PC, Casey ML: The accumulation of prostaglandins (Pgs) in amniotic fluid is an after effect of labor and not indicative of a role for PGE2 or PGF2 alpha in the initiation of human parturition. J Clin Endocrinol Metab 76:1332, 1993

51. Romero R, Mazor M, Munoz H et al: The preterm labor syndrome. Ann NY Acad Sci 734:414, 1994

52. Leveno KJ, Cox K, Roark M: Cervical dilatation and prematurity revisited. Obstet Gynecol 68:434, 1986

53. Papiernik E, Bouyer J, Collin D et al: Precocious cervical ripening and preterm labor. Obstet Gynecol 67:238, 1986

54. Copper R, Goldenberg RL, Davis RO et al: Warning symptoms, uterine contractions and cervical examination findings in women at risk of preterm delivery. Am J Obstet Gynecol 162:748, 1990

55. Andersen HF, Nugent CE, Wanty SD et al: Prediction of risk for preterm delivery by ultrasonographic measurement of cervical length. Am J Obstet Gynecol 163:859, 1990

56. Iams JD, Goldenberg RL, Meis PJ et al: The length of the cervix and the risk of spontaneous premature delivery. N Engl J Med 334:567, 1996

57. Korn AP, Bolan G, Padian N et al: Plasma cell endometritis in women with symptomatic bacterial vaginosis. Obstet Gynecol 85:387, 1995

58. Goldenberg RL, Iams JD, Mercer BM et al: Pathways to prematurity (abstract). Am J Obstet Gynecol 174:308, 1996

59. Goldenberg RL, Thom E, Moawad A et al: The Preterm Prediction Study: Fetal fibronectin, bacterial vaginosis, and peripartum infection. JAMA, 1996 (in press)

60. Ghidini A, Eglinton GS, Spong CY et al: Elevated midtrimester amniotic fluid tumor necrosis alpha levels: A predictor of preterm delivery (abstract). Am J Obstet Gynecol 174:397, 1996

61. Goldenberg RL, Mercer BM, Meis PJ et al: The preterm prediction study: Early fetal fibronectin testing predicts early spontaneous preterm birth. Am J Obstet Gynecol 87:643, 1996

62. Feinberg RF, Kleiman HJ, Lockwood CJ: Is oncofetal fibronectin a trophoblast glue for human implantation? Am J Pathol 138:537, 1991

63. Kramer MS, Coates AL, Michoud MC et al: Maternal anthropometry and idiopathic preterm labor. Obstet Gynecol 86:744, 1995

64. Spiegel CA, Amstel R, Holmes KK: Diagnosis of bacterial vaginosis by direct Gram's stain of vaginal fluid. J Clin Microbiol 18:170, 1983

65. Goldenberg R, Iams J, Mercer B et al: Fetal fibronectin, bacterial vaginosis and peripartum infection (abstract). Am J Obstet Gynecol 174:303, 1996

66. Iams JD, Johnson F, Sonek J et al: Cervical competence as a continuum: a study of sonographic cervical length and obstetrical performance. Am J Obstet Gynecol 172:1097, 1995

67. Mosmann TR: Cytokines, differentiation and functions of subsets of CD4 and CD8 T cells. Behring Inst Mitt 1995; 96:1–6.

68. Feinberg BB, Stellar MA, Walsh SW: Cytokine regulation of trophoblast steroidogenesis (abstract 479) Soc Gynecol Invest 1992

69. Albert TJ, SU HC, Zimmerman PD et al: Interleukin-1-beta regulates the inducible cyclooxygenase in amnion-derived WISH cells. Prostaglandins 48:401, 1994

70. Creasy RK: Preterm birth prevention: where are we? Am J Obstet Gynecol 168:1223, 1993

71. Thompson RS et al: Primary and secondary prevention services in clinical practice. JAMA 273:1130, 1995

72. Manson JE et al: The primary prevention of myocardial infarction. N Engl J Med 326:1406, 1992

73. Frank E: Improved cholesterol-related knowledge and behavior and plasma control levels in adults during the 1980s. JAMA 268:1566, 1992

74. Gonik B, Creasy RK: Preterm labor: its diagnosis and management. Am J Obstet Gynecol 154:3, 1986

75. King JF, Grand A, Keirse MJN et al: Betamimetics in preterm labour: an overview of randomised controlled trials. Br J Obstet Gynaecol 95:211, 1988

76. Pircon RA, Strassner HT, Kirz DS et al: Controlled trial of hydration and bed rest versus rest alone in the evaluation of preterm uterine contractions. Am J Obstet Gynecol 161:775, 1989

77. Iams JD, Johnson FF, Parker M: A prospective evaluation of the signs and symptoms of preterm labor. Obstet Gynecol 84:227, 1994

78. Moore TR, Iams JD, Creasy RK et al: Diurnal and gestational patterns of uterine activity in normal human pregnancy. Obstet Gynecol 83:517, 1994

79. Stubbs TM, Van Dorsten JP, Miller MC: The preterm cervix and preterm labor: relative risks, predictive values, and change over time. Am J Obstet Gynecol 155:829, 1986

80. Holcomb WL, Smeltzer JS: Cervical effacement: variations in belief among clinicians. Obstet Gynecol 78:43, 1991

81. Utter GO, Dooley SL, Tamura RK, Socol ML: Awaiting cervical change for the diagnosis of preterm labor does not compromise the efficacy of ritodrine tocolysis. Am J Obstet Gynecol 163:882, 1990

82. Iams JD, Paraskos J, Landon MG et al: Cervical sonography in preterm labor. Obstet Gynecol 84:40, 1994

83. Gomez R, Galasso M, Romero R et al: Ultrasonographic examination of the uterine cervix is better than cervical digital examinations as a predictor of the likelihood of premature delivery in patients with preterm labor and intact membranes. Am J Obstet Gynecol 171:956, 1994

84. Lockwood CJ, Senyei AE, Dische MR et al: Fetal fibronectin in cervical and vaginal secretions as a predictor of preterm delivery. N Engl J Med 325:669, 1991

85. Iams JD, Casal D, McGregor JA et al: Fetal fibronectin improves the accuracy of diagnosis of preterm labor. Am J Obstet Gynecol 173:141, 1995

86. Peaceman AM, Andrews WW, Thorp JM et al: Fetal fibronectin as a predictor of preterm birth in symptomatic patients—A multicenter trial (abstract). Am J Obstet Gynecol 174:303, 1996

87. Adeza Biomedical: Presentation to the United States Food and Drug Administration. April 6, 1995

88. Iams JD: Reply to a letter from M. Plaut. Am J Obstet Gynecol 174:79, 1996

89. Rizzo G, Capponi A, Arduini D et al: The value of fetal fibronectin in cervical and vaginal secretions and of ultrasonographic examination of the uterine cervix in predicting premature delivery in patients with preterm labor and intact membranes. Am J Obstet Gynecol 1996 (in press)

90. Huszar G, Naftolin F: The myometrium and uterine cervix in normal and preterm labor. N Engl J Med 311:571, 1984

91. Canadian Preterm Labor Investigators Group: Treatment of preterm labor with the beta-agonist ritodrine. N Engl J Med 327:308, 1992

92. Weiner N: Norepinephrine, epinephrine and the sympathomimetic amines. p. 143. In Gilman AG, Goodman LS, Gilman A (eds): The Pharmacological Basis of Therapeutics. 6th Ed. Macmillan, New York, 1980

93. Caritis S, Lin LS, Toig G et al: Pharmacodynamics of ritodrine in pregnant women during preterm labor. Am J Obstet Gynecol 147:752, 1983

94. Caritis SN, Venkataramanan R, Darby MJ et al: Pharmacokinetics of ritodrine administered intravenously: recommendations for changes in the current regimen. Am J Obstet Gynecol 162:429, 1990

95. Barden T, Peter J, Merkatz I: Ritodrine hydrochloride:

a betamimetic agent for use in preterm labor. Obstet Gynecol 56:1, 1980

96. Caritis SN, Venkataramanan R, Cotroneo M et al: Pharmacokinetics and pharmacodynamics of ritodrine after intramuscular administration to pregnant women. Am J Obstet Gynecol 162:1215, 1990

97. Stubblefield P, Heyl P: Treatment of premature labor with subcutaneous terbutaline. Obstet Gynecol 59:457, 1982

98. Caritis S, Toig G, Heddinger L et al: A double-blind study comparing ritodrine and terbutaline in the treatment of preterm labor. Am J Obstet Gynecol 150:7, 1984

99. Casper RF, Lye SJ: Myometrial desensitization to continuous but not to intermittent β-adrenergic agonist infusion in the sheep. Am J Obstet Gynecol 154:301, 1986

100. Caritis SN, Chiao JP, Moore JJ, Ward SM: Myometrial desensitization after ritodrine infusion. Am J Physiol 253:410, 1987

101. Caritis SN, Chiao JP, Kridgen P: Comparison of pulsatile and continuous ritodrine administration: effects on uterine contractility and beta-adrenergic receptor cascade. Am J Obstet Gynecol 164:1005, 1991

102. Spatling L, Fallenstein F, Schneider H et al: Bolus tocolysis: treatment of preterm labor with pulsatile administration of a beta-adrenergic agonist. Am J Obstet Gynecol 160:713, 1989

103. Hill WC: Risks and complications of tocolysis. Clin Obstet Gynecol 38:725, 1995

104. Benedetti T: Maternal complications of parenteral beta-sympathomimetic therapy for premature labor. Am J Obstet Gynecol 145:1, 1983

105. Lamont RF: The contemporary use of beta-agonists. Br J Obstet Gynaecol 100(10):890, 1993

106. Philipsen T, Eriksen PS, Lynggard F: Pulmonary edema following ritodrine-saline infusion in premature labor. Obstet Gynecol 58:304, 1981

107. Hatjis CG, Swain M: Systemic tocolysis for premature labor is associated with an increased incidence of pulmonary edema in the presence of maternal infection. Am J Obstet Gynecol 159:723, 1988

108. Hendricks SK, Keroes J, Katz M: Electrocardiographic changes associated with ritodrine-induced maternal tachycardia and hypokalemia. Am J Obstet Gynecol 154:921, 1986

109. Ying Y-K, Tejani N: Angina pectoris as a complication of ritodrine hydrochloride therapy in premature labor. Obstet Gynecol 60:385, 1982

110. Young D, Toofanian A, Leveno K: Potassium and glucose concentrations without treatment during ritodrine tocolysis. Am J Obstet Gynecol 98:105, 1983

111. Main EK, Main DM, Gabbe SG: Chronic oral terbutaline tocolytic therapy is associated with maternal glucose intolerance. Am J Obstet Gynecol 157:644, 1987

112. Groome LJ, Goldenberg RL, Cliver SP et al: Neonatal periventricular-intraventricular hemorrhage after maternal beta-sympathomimetic tocolysis. The March of Dimes Multicenter Study Group. Am J Obstet Gynecol 167:873, 1992

113. Epstein M, Nicholls E, Stubblefield P: Neonatal hypoglycemia after beta-sympathomimetic tocolytic therapy. Pediatrics 94:449, 1979

114. Lipsitz P: The clinical and biochemical effects of excess magnesium in the newborn. Pediatrics 47:501, 1971

115. Steer C, Petrie R: A comparison of magnesium sulfate and alcohol for the prevention of premature labor. Am J Obstet Gynecol 129:1, 1977

116. Spisso K, Harbert G, Thiagarajah S: The use of magnesium sulfate as the primary tocolytic agent to prevent premature delivery. Am J Obstet Gynecol 142:840, 1982

117. Elliott J: Magnesium sulfate as a tocolytic agent. Am J Obstet Gynecol 147:277, 1983

118. Miller YM, Keane MWD, Horger EO: A comparison of magnesium sulfate and terbutaline for the arrest of preterm labor. J Reprod Med 27:348, 1982

119. Hollander DI, Nagey DA, Pupkin MJ: Magnesium sulphate and ritodrine hydrochloride: a randomized comparison. Am J Obstet Gynecol 156:631, 1987

120. Wilkens IA, Lynch L, Mehaleb KE et al: Efficacy and side effects of magnesium sulphate and ritodrine as tocolytic agents. Am J Obstet Gynecol 159:685, 1988

121. Cox SM, Sherman LM, Leveno KJ: Randomized investigation of magnesium sulfate for prevention of preterm birth. Am J Obstet Gynecol 163:767, 1990

122. Madden C, Owen J, Hauth JC: Magnesium tocolysis: serum levels versus success. Am J Obstet Gynecol 162:1177, 1990

123. Beall MH, Edgar BW, Paril RH et al: A comparison of ritodrine, terbutaline, and magnesium sulfate for the suppression of preterm labor. Am J Obstet Gynecol 153:854, 1985

124. Holcomb WL, Shackelford GD, Petrie RH: Magnesium tocolysis and neonatal bone abnormalities: a controlled study. Obstet Gynecol 78:611, 1991

125. Nelson KB, Grether J: Effect of $MgSO_4$ therapy on cerebral palsy rates in infants < 1500 grams. J Pediatr 95:263, 1995

126. Hauth, JL, Goldenberg RL, Nelson KG et al: Reduction of cerebral palsy rates with maternal $MgSO_4$ treatment in newborns weighing 500–1000 grams (abstract). Am J Obstet Gynecol 172:419, 1995

127. Lewis RB, Schulman JD: Influence of acetylsalicylic acid, an inhibitor of prostaglandin synthesis, on the duration of human gestation and labour. Lancet 2:1159, 1973

128. Zuckerman H, Reiss U, Rubenstein I: Inhibition of human premature labor with indomethacin. Obstet Gynecol 44:787, 1974

129. Niebyl J, Blake D, White R et al: The inhibition of premature labor with indomethacin. Am J Obstet Gynecol 136:1014, 1980

130. Zuckerman H, Shalev E, Gilad G et al: Further study of the inhibition of premature labor by indomethacin. Part I. J Perinat Med 12:19, 1984

131. Zuckerman H, Shalev E, Gilad G et al: Further study of the inhibition of premature labor by indomethacin. Part II. J Perinat Med 12:25, 1984

132. Besinger RE, Niebyl JR, Keyes WG et al: A randomized comparative trial of indomethacin and ritodrine for the

longterm treatment of preterm labor. Am J Obstet Gynecol 164:981, 1991

133. Lunt CC, Satin AJ, Barth WH et al: The effect of indomethacin tocolysis on maternal coagulation status. Obstet Gynecol 84:820, 1994

134. Moise K: Effect of advancing gestational age on the frequency of fetal ductal constriction in association with maternal indomethacin use. Am J Obstet Gynecol 168:1350, 1994

135. Moise KJ, Huhta JC, Sharif DS et al: Indomethacin in the treatment of premature labor: effects on the fetal ductus arteriosus. N Engl J Med 319:327, 1988

136. Mohen D, Newnharn JP, Orsogna LD: Indomethacin for the treatment of polyhydramnios: a case of constriction of the ductus arteriosus. Aust NZ J Obstet Gynecol 32:243, 1992

137. van der Heijden BJ, Carlus C, Nancy F et al: Persistent anuria, neonatal death, and renal microcystic lesions after prenatal exposure to indomethacin. Am J Obstet Gynecol 171:617, 1994

138. Manchester D, Margolis H, Sheldon R: Possible association between maternal indomethacin therapy and primary pulmonary hypertension of the newborn. Am J Obstet Gynecol 126:467, 1976

139. Csaba I, Sulyok E, Ertl T: Relationship of maternal treatment with indomethacin to persistence of fetal circulation syndrome. J Pediatr 92:484, 1978

140. Norton ME, Merrill J, Cooper BAB et al: Neonatal complications after the administration of indomethacin for preterm labor. N Engl J Med 329:1602, 1993

141. Niebyl JR, Witter FR: Neonatal outcome after indomethacin treatment for preterm labor. Am J Obstet Gynecol 155:747, 1986

142. Dudley DKL, Hardie MJ: Fetal and neonatal effects of indomethacin used as a tocolytic agent. Am J Obstet Gynecol 151:181, 1985

143. Gardner M, Skelly S, Owen J et al: Neonatal complications associated with prenatal use of indomethacin (abstract). Am J Obstet Gynecol 172:414, 1995

144. Carlan SJ, O'Brien WF, O'Leary TD, Mastrogiannis D: Randomized comparative trial of indomethacin and sulindac for the treatment of refractory preterm labor. Obstet Gynecol 79:223, 1992

145. Rasanen J, Jouppila P: Fetal cardiac function and ductus arteriosus during indomethacin and sulindac therapy for threatened preterm labor: a randomized study. Am J Obstet Gynecol 173:20, 1995

146. Cabrol D, Landesman R, Muller J et al: Treatment of polyhydramnios with prostaglandin synthetase inhibitor (indomethacin). Am J Obstet Gynecol 157:422, 1987

147. Mamopoulos M, Assimakopoulos E, Reece AE et al: Maternal indomethacin therapy in the treatment of polyhydramnios. Am J Obstet Gynecol 162:1225, 1990

148. Kirshon B, Mari G, Moise KJ: Indomethacin therapy in the treatment of symptomatic polyhydramnios. Obstet Gynecol 75:202, 1990

149. Lange IR, Harman CR, Ash KM et al: Twin with hydramnios: treating premature labor at source. Am J Obstet Gynecol 160:552, 1989

150. Moise KJ: Indomethacin as treatment for symptomatic polyhydramnios. Contemp Obstet Gynecol 40:53, 1995

151. Higby K, Xenakis EM, Paverstein CJ: Do tocolytic agents stop preterm labor? A critical and comprehensive review of safety and efficacy. Am J Obstet Gynecol 168:1247, 1993

152. Ferguson JE, Schutz T, Pershe R et al: Nifedipine pharmocokinetics during preterm labor tocolysis. Am J Obstet Gynecol 161:1485, 1989

153. Ulmsten U, Andersson KE, Wingerup L: Treatment of preterm labor with the calcium antagonist nifedipine. Arch Gynecol 229:1, 1980

154. Read MD, Wellby DE: The use of a calcium antagonist (nifedipine) to suppress preterm labor. Br J Obstet Gynaecol 93:933, 1986

155. Ferguson JE, Dyson DC, Holbrook H et al: Cardiovascular and metabolic effects associated with nifedipine and ritodrine tocolysis. Am J Obstet Gynecol 161:788, 1989

156. Snyder SW, Cardwell MS: Neuromuscular blockade with magnesium sulfate and nifedipine. Am J Obstet Gynecol 161:35, 1989

157. Ben-Ami M, Giladi Y, Shalev E: The combination of magnesium sulphate and nifedipine: a cause of neuromuscular blockade. Br J Obstet Gynaecol 101:262, 1944

158. Parisi VM, Salinas J, Stockmar EJ: Fetal vascular responses to maternal nicardipine administration in the hypertensive ewe. Am J Obstet Gynecol 161:1035, 1989

159. Parisi VM, Salinas J, Stockmar EJ: Placental vascular responses to maternal nicardipine administration in the hypertensive ewe. Am J Obstet Gynecol 161:1039, 1989

160. Mari G, Kirshon B, Moise KJ et al: Doppler assessment of the fetal and uteroplacental circulation during nifedipine therapy for preterm labor. Am J Obstet Gynecol 161:1514, 1989

161. Murray C, Haverkamp AD, Orleans M et al: Nifedipine for the treatment of preterm labor. Am J Obstet Gynecol 167:52, 1992

162. Ray D et al: Am J Obstet Gynecol 170:387, 1994

163. Goodwin TM, Paul R, Silver HM et al: The effect of the oxytocin antagonist atosiban on preterm uterine activity in the human. Am J Obstet Gynecol 170:474, 1994

164. Lees C, Campbells, Jauniaux E et al: Arrest of preterm labour and prolongation of gestation with glyceryl trinatrate, a nitric oxide donor: Lancet 343:1325, 1994

165. Hatjis CG, Swain M, Nelson LH: Efficacy of combined administration of magnesium sulfate and ritodrine in the treatment of premature labor. Obstet Gynecol 69:317, 1987

166. Ferguson JE, Hensleigh PA, Kredenster D: Adjunctive use of magnesium sulfate with ritodrine for preterm labor tocolysis. Am J Obstet Gynecol 148:166, 1984

167. Toward Improving the Outcome of Pregnancy II. March of Dimes, 1994

168. Liggins GC, Howie RN: A controlled trial of antepartum glucocorticoid treatment for prevention of the respiratory distress syndrome in premature infants. Pediatrics 50:515, 1972

169. Barks JDE, Post M, Tuor UI: Dexamethasone prevents hypoxic-ischemic brain damage in the neonatal rat. Pediatr Res 29:558, 1991

170. Volpe JJ: Brain injury in the premature infant: is it preventable? Pediatr Res 27:528, 1990

171. Crowley PA: Antenatal corticosteroid therapy. A meta-

analysis of the randomized trials. Am J Obstet Gynecol 173:322, 1995

172. Collaborative Group on Antenatal Steroid Therapy: Effect of antenatal dexamethasone administration on the prevention of respiratory distress syndrome. Am J Obstet Gynecol 141:276, 1981

173. Garite TJ, Rumney PJ, Briggs GG et al: A randomized, placebo-controlled trial of betamethasone for the prevention of respiratory distress syndrome. Am J Obstet Gynecol 166:646, 1992

174. Eronen M, Kari A, Posonon E: The effect of antenatal dexamethasone administration on the fetal and neonatal ductus arteriosus. A randomized double-blind study. Am J Dis Child 147:187, 1993

175. Kari MA, Hallman M: Prenatal doxamethasone treatment in conjunction with rescue therapy of human surfactantia randomized placebo-controlled multicenter study et al: Pediatrics 93:730, 1994

176. Jobe AH, Mitchell BR, Gunkel JH: Beneficial effects of the combined use of prenatal corticosteroids and postnatal surfactant on preterm infants. Am J Obstet Gynecol 168:508, 1993

177. Andrews EB, Marcucci G, White A et al: Associations between use of antenatal corticosteroids and neonatal outcomes within the Exosurf Neonatal Treatment Investigational New Drug Study Group. Am J Obstet Gynecol 173:290, 1995

178. Farrell EE, Silver RK, Kimberlin LV et al: Impact of antenatal dexamethasone administration on respiratory distress syndrome in surfactant-treated infants. Am J Obstet Gynecol 161:628, 1989

179. Shankaran S, Bauer CR, Bain R et al: Relationship between antenatal steroid administration and grades III and IV intracranial hemorrhage in low birth weight infants. Am J Obstet Gynecol 173:305, 1995

180. Wright L, Verter J, Younes N et al: Antenatal corticosteroid administration and neonatal outcome in very low birth weight infants: The NICHD Neonatal Research Network. Am J Obstet Gynecol 173:269, 1995

181. Howie RN, Liggins GC: Clinical trial of antepartum betamethasone for prevention of respiratory distress in preterm infants. p. 281. In Anderson AB et al (eds): Preterm Labor. Proceedings of the 5th Study Group of the Royal College of Obstetricians and Gynecologists, London, 1977. Royal College of Obstetricians and Gynecologists, London, 1977

182. Leviton A, Kuban KC, Pagano M et al: Antenatal corticosteroids appear to reduce the risk of postnatal germinal matrix hemorrhage in preterm infants. Pediatrics 91:1083, 1993

183. Ment LR, Oh W, Ehrenkrantz RA et al: Antenatal steroids, delivery mode, and intraventricular hemorrhage in preterm infants. Am J Obstet Gynecol 172:795, 1995

184. Chapman S, Hauth JC, Goldenberg RL et al: Lack of apparent corticosteroid benefit in ≤1000 g infants born after preterm amnion rupture (abstract). Am J Obstet Gynecol 174:316, 1996

185. Gardner MO, Goldenberg RL, Gaudier FL et al: Predicting low Apgar scores of infants weighing less than 1000 grams: the effect of corticosteroids. Obstet Gynecol 85:170, 1995

186. Liggins GC: The prevention of RDS by maternal betamethasone administration. p. 97. In Moore TD (ed): Lung Maturation and the Prevention of Hyaline Membrane Disease. Report of the Seventieth Ross Conference on Pediatric Research. Ross Laboratories, Columbus, OH, 1976

187. Nochimson D, Petrie R: Glucocorticoid therapy for the induction of pulmonary maturity in severely hypertensive gravid women. Am J Obstet Gynecol 133:449, 1979

188. Ricke PS, Elliott JP, Freeman R: Use of corticosteroids in pregnancy-induced hypertension. Obstet Gynecol 55:206, 1980

189. Loeb JN: Corticosteroids and growth. N Engl J Med 295:547, 1976

190. Cotterrell M, Balazs R, Johnson AL: Effects of corticosteroids on the biochemical maturation of rat brain. Postnatal cell formation. J Neurochem 19:2151, 1972

191. Collaborative Group on Antenatal Steroid Therapy: Effects of antenatal dexamethasone administration in the infant: long-term follow-up. J Pediatr 104:259, 1984

192. Slotkin TA: Adverse effects of antenatal steroids on nervous system development: animal models. National Institute of Health Consensus Development Conference on Effect of Corticosteroids for Fetal Maturation on Perinatal Outcomes, February 28–March 2, 1994

193. Mugford M, Piercy J, Chalmers I: Cost implications of different approaches to the prevention of respiratory distress syndrome. Arch Dis Child 66:757, 1991

194. Simpson KN, Lynch SR: Cost savings from the use of antenatal steroids to prevent respiratory distress syndrome and related conditions in premature infants. Am J Obstet Gynecol 173:316, 1995

195. Vermont-Oxford Trials Network: Very low birthweight outcomes for 1990. Pediatrics 91:540, 1993

196. Gardner MO, Bronstein JM, Goldenberg RL et al: Physical opinions of preterm infant outcome and their effect on antenatal corticosteroid use. J Perinatol 1995 (in press)

197. Effect of corticosteroids for fetal maturation on perinatal outcomes. National Institutes of Health Consensus Development Conference, February 28–March 2, 1994. Am J Obstet Gynecol 173:246, 1995

198. American College of Obstetricians and Gynecologists Committee on Obstetric Practice. Clinical Opinion 147. Antenatal Corticosteroid Therapy for Fetal Maturation. December 1994

199. Morales WJ, Deibel ND, Lazar AJ, Zadrozny D: The effect of antenatal dexamethasone on the prevention of respiratory distress syndrome in preterm gestation with premature rupture of the membranes. Am J Obstet Gynecol 154:591, 1986

200. McGregor JA, French JI, Reller LB et al: Adjunctive erythromycin treatment for idiopathic preterm labor. Am J Obstet Gynecol 154:498, 1986

201. Winkler M, Baumann L, Ruckhaberle K, Schiller E: Erythromycin therapy for subclinical intrauterine infections on threatened preterm delivery. J Perinat Med 16:253, 1988

202. Newton ER, Dinsmoor MJ, Gibbs RS: A randomized, blinded, placebo-controlled trial of antibiotics in idiopathic term labor. Obstet Gynecol 74:562, 1989

203. McGregor JA, French JI, Seo K: Adjunctive clindamycin therapy for preterm labor: results of a double-blinded, placebo-controlled trial. Am J Obstet Gynecol 165:867, 1991

204. Newton ER, Shields L, Ridgway LE et al: Combination antibiotics and indomethacin in idiopathic preterm labor: a randomized double blind clinical trial. Am J Obstet Gynecol 165:1753, 1991

205. Romero R, Sibai B, Caritis S et al: Antibiotic treatment of preterm labor with intact membranes: a multicenter, randomized, double-blinded, placebo-controlled trial. Am J Obstet Gynecol 169:764, 1993

206. Norman K, Pattinson RC, deSouza J et al: Ampicillin and metronidazole treatment in preterm labour: a multicentre, randomised controlled trial. Br J Obstet Gynaecol 101:404, 1994

207. Gordon M, Samuels P, Shubert P et al: A randomized, prospective study of adjunctive ceftizoxime in preterm labor. Am J Obstet Gynecol 172:1546, 1995

208. Thorp JA, Ferrette-Smith D, Gaston LA et al: Combined antenatal vitamin K and phenobarbital for preventing intracranial hemorrhage in newborns less than 34 weeks gestation. Obstet Gynecol 86:1, 1995

209. Katz M, Gill PJ, Newman RB: Detection of preterm labor by ambulatory monitoring of uterine activity for the management of oral tocolysis. Am J Obstet Gynecol 154:1253, 1986

210. Iams JD, Johnson FF, O'Shaughnessy RW: Ambulatory uterine activity monitoring in the posthospital care of patients with preterm labor. Am J Perinatol 7:170, 1990

211. Nagey DA, Bailey-Jones C, Herman AA: Randomized comparison of home uterine activity monitoring and routine care in patients discharged after treatment for preterm labor. Obstet Gynecol 82:319, 1993

212. The CHUMS Group: A multicenter randomized controlled trial of home uterine activity monitoring. Am J Obstet Gynecol 173:1120, 1995

213. Macones GA, Berlin M, Berlin J: Efficacy of oral beta-agonist maintenance therapy in preterm labor: a meta-analysis. Obstet Gynecol 85:313, 1995

214. Keirse MJNC, Grant A, King JF: p. 694. In Chalmers I, Enkin M, Keirse MJNC (eds): Effective Care in Pregnancy and Childbirth. Oxford University Press, New York, 1989

215. Fletcher SE, Fyfe DA, Case CL et al: Myocardial necrosis after long-term maternal subcutaneous terbutaline infusion for suppression of preterm labor. Am J Obstet Gynecol 165:1401, 1991

216. Foley MR, Landon MB, Gabbe SG et al: Effect of prolonged oral terbutaline therapy on glucose tolerance in pregnancy. Am J Obstet Gynecol 168:100, 1993

217. Caritis SN, Venkataramanan R, Cotroneo M et al: Pharmacokinetics of orally administered ritodrine. Am J Obstet Gynecol 161:32, 1989

218. Parikh MN, Mehta AC: Internal cervical os during the second half of pregnancy. J Obstet Gynaecol Br Commonw 68:818, 1961

219. Crombleholme W, Minkoff H, Delke I et al: Cervical cerclage: an aggressive approach to threatened or recurrent pregnancy wastage. Am J Obstet Gynecol 146:168, 1983

220. MRC/RCOG Working Party on Cervical Cerclage: Final report of the Medical Research Council/Royal College of Obstetricians and Gynaecologists multicentre randomised trial of cervical cerclage. Br J Obstet Gynaecol 100:516, 1993

221. Ayers JW, DeGrood RM, Compton AA et al: Sonographic evaluation of cervical length in pregnancy. Obstet Gynecol 71:939, 1988

222. Michaels WH, Montgomery C, Karo J et al: Ultrasound differentiation of the competent from the incompetent cervix: prevention of preterm delivery. Am J Obstet Gynecol 154:537, 1986

223. Andersen HF: Transvaginal and transabdominal ultrasonography of the uterine cervix during pregnancy. J Clin Ultrasound 19:77, 1991

224. Brook I, Feingold M, Schwartz A et al: Ultrasonography in the diagnosis of cervical incompetence in pregnancy—a new diagnostic approach. Br J Obstet Gynaecol 88:640, 1981

225. Buckingham JC, Buethe RA, Danforth DN: Collagen-muscle ratio in clinically normal and clinically incompetent cervices. Am J Obstet Gynecol 91:231, 1965

226. Schuly KF, Grimes DA, Cates W Jr: Measures to prevent cervical injury during suction curettage abortion. Lancet 1:1182, 1983

227. Harger JH: Cervical cerclage: patient selection, morbidity, and success rates. Clin Perinatol 10:321, 1983

228. Jones JM, Sweetnam P, Hibbard BM: The outcome of pregnancy after cone biopsy of the cervix: a case control study. Br J Obstet Gynaecol 86:913, 1979

229. Zilianti M, Azuaga A, Calderon F et al: Monitoring the effacement of the uterine cervix by transperineal sonography: A new perspective. J Ultrasound Med 14:719, 1995

230. Guzman ER, Rosenberg JC, Houlihan C et al: A new method using ultrasound and transfundal pressure to evaluate the asymptomatic incompetent cervix. Obstet Gynecol 83:248, 1994

231. Sonek J, Blumenfeld M, Foley M et al: Cervical length may change during ultrasonographic examination. Am J Obstet Gynecol 162:1355, 1990

232. Lash AF, Lash SR: Habitual abortion: the competent internal os of the cervix. Am J Obstet Gynecol 59:68, 1950

233. Shirodkar VN: A method of operative treatment for habitual abortions in the second trimester of pregnancy. Antiseptic 52:299, 1955

234. McDonald IA: Suture of the cervix for inevitable abortion. J Obstet Gynaecol Br Emp 64:346, 1957

235. Harger J: Comparison of success and morbidity in cervical cerclage procedures. Obstet Gynecol 56:543, 1980

236. Parelukar SG, Kiwi R: Dynamic incompetent cervix uteri: sonographic observations. J Ultrasound Med 1:223, 1982

237. Rana J, Davis SE, Harrigan JT: Improving the outcome of cervical cerclage: a prospective study. Ultrasound Obstet Gynecol 9:275, 1990

238. Andersen HF, Karimi A, Sakala EP, Kalugdan R: Prediction of cervical cerclage outcome by endovaginal ultrasonography. Am J Obstet Gynecol 171:1102, 1994

239. Quinn MJ: Vaginal ultrasound and cervical cerclage: a

prospective study. Ultrasound Obstet Gynecol 2:410, 1992

240. Aarts JM, Brons JT, Bruinse HW et al: Emergency cerclage: A review. Obstet Gynecol Surv 50:459, 1995

241. Scheerer LJ, Lam F, Bartolucci L et al: A new technique for reduction of prolapsed fetal membranes for emergency cervical cerclage. Obstet Gynecol 74:408, 1989

242. Novy MJ: Transabdominal cervicoisthmic cerclage: a reappraisal 25 years after its introduction. Am J Obstet Gynecol 164:163, 1991

243. Weissman A, Jakobi P, Zahi S, Zimmer EZ: The effect of cervical cerclage on the course of labor. Obstet Gynecol 76:168, 1990

244. Ludmir J, Bader T, Chen L et al: Poor perinatal outcome associated with retained cerclage in patients with premature rupture of membranes. Obstet Gynecol 84:823, 1994

245. Rush RW, Issacs S, McPherson K et al: A randomized controlled trial of cervical cerclage in women at high risk of spontaneous preterm delivery. Br J Obstet Gynaecol 91:724, 1984

246. Lazar P, Gueguen S, Dreyfus J et al: Multicentred controlled trial of cervical cerclage in women at moderate risk of preterm delivery. Br J Obstet Gynaecol 91:731, 1984

247. Kitzmiller J: Preterm premature rupture of the membranes. p. 298. In Fuchs F, Stubblefield PG (eds): Preterm Birth Causes, Prevention and Management. Macmillan, New York, 1984

248. Skinner S, Campos G, Liggins G: Collagen content of human amniotic membranes: effect of gestation length and premature rupture. Obstet Gynecol 57:487, 1981

249. Harger JH, Hsing AW, Tuomala RE et al: Risk factors for preterm premature rupture of fetal membranes: a multicenter case–control study. Am J Obstet Gynecol 163:130, 1990

250. Mercer BM, Goldenberg RL, Iams JD et al: The Preterm Prediction Study: analysis of risk factors for preterm premature rupture of the membranes. J Soc Gynecol Invest 3:350A, 1996

251. Bourne G: The Human Amnion and Chorion. Lloyd-Luke Medical Books, London, 1960

252. Ibrahim M, Bou-Resli M, Al-Zaid N, Bishay L: Intact fetal membranes: morphological predisposal to rupture. Acta Obstet Gynecol Scand 62:481, 1983

253. Lavery J, Miller C: Deformation and creep in the human chorioamniotic sac. Am J Obstet Gynecol 134:366, 1979

254. Al-Zaid NS, Gumaa KA, Bou-Resli MN et al: Premature rupture of fetal membranes: changes in collagen type. Acta Obstet Gynecol Scand 67:291, 1988

255. Lonky NM, Hayashi RH: A proposed mechanism for premature rupture of membranes. Obstet Gynecol Surv 43:1:22, 1988

256. Naeye R: Factors that predispose to premature rupture of the fetal membranes. Obstet Gynecol 60:93, 1982

257. Romero R, Mazor M: Infection and preterm labor. Clin Obstet Gynecol 31:3:553, 1988

258. Sbarra AJ, Thomas GB, Cetrulo CL et al: Effect of bacterial growth on the bursting pressure of fetal membranes in vivo. Obstet Gynecol 70:107, 1987

259. Regan J, Chao S, James LS: Premature rupture of membranes, preterm delivery, and group B streptococcal colonization of mothers. Am J Obstet Gynecol 141:184, 1981

260. Cedarqvist LL, Zerroudakis IA, Ewoll LC, Litwin SD: The relationship between prematurely ruptured membranes and fetal immunoglobulin production. Am J Obstet Gynecol 134:784, 1979

261. Schutte M, Treffers P, Kloosterman G et al: Management of premature rupture of membranes: the risk of vaginal examination to the infant. Am J Obstet Gynecol 146:395, 1983

262. Lewis DF, Major CA, Towers CV et al: Effects of digital vaginal examinations on latency period in preterm premature rupture of membranes. Obstet Gynecol 80:630, 1992

263. Brown CL, Ludwiczak MH, Blanco JD et al: Cervical dilation: accuracy of visual and digital examinations. Obstet Gynecol 81:215, 1993

264. Smith R: A technic for the detection of rupture of the membranes: a review and preliminary report. Obstet Gynecol 48:172, 1976

265. Reece EA, Chervenak F, Moya F et al: Amniotic fluid arborization: effect of blood, meconium, and pH alterations. Obstet Gynecol 64:248, 1984

266. Rosemond RL, Lombardi SJ, Boehm FH: Ferning of amniotic fluid contaminated with blood. Obstet Gynecol 75:338, 1990

267. Taylor J, Garite T: Premature rupture of membranes before fetal viability. Obstet Gynecol 64:615, 1984

268. Garite T, Freeman R, Linzey E et al: Prospective randomized study of corticosteroids in the management of premature rupture of the membranes and the premature gestation. Am J Obstet Gynecol 141:508, 1981

269. Cox SM, Williams ML, Leveno KJ: The natural history of preterm ruptured membranes: what to expect of expectant management. Obstet Gynecol 71:558, 1988

270. Nelson LH, Anderson RL, O'Shea TM, Swain M: Expectant management of preterm premature rupture of the membranes. Am J Obstet Gynecol 171:350, 1994

271. Moretti M, Sibai BM: Maternal and perinatal outcome of expectant management of premature rupture of membranes in the midtrimester. Am J Obstet Gynecol 159:390, 1988

272. Moberg L, Garite T, Freeman R: Fetal heart rate patterns and fetal distress in patients with preterm premature rupture of membranes. Obstet Gynecol 64:60, 1984

273. Nelson DM, Stempel LE, Zuspan FP et al: Association of prolonged preterm premature rupture of the membranes and abruptio placentae. J Reprod Med 31:249, 1986

274. Vintzileos AM, Campbell WA, Nochimson DJ et al: Preterm premature rupture of the membranes: a risk factor for the development of abruptio placentae. Am J Obstet Gynecol 156:1235, 1987

275. Major CA, de Veciana M, Lewis DF, Morgan MA: Preterm premature rupture of the membranes and abruptio placentae: is there an association between these pregnancy complications? Am J Obstet Gynecol 172:672, 1995

276. Rotschild A, Ling EW, Peterman ML, Farquharson D:

Neonatal outcome after prolonged preterm rupture of the membranes. Am J Obstet Gynecol 162:46, 1990

277. Carroll SG, Blott M, Nicolaides KH: Preterm prelabor amniorrhexis: outcome of live births. Obstet Gynecol 86:18, 1995

278. Nimrod C, Varela-Gittings F, Machin G et al: The effect of very prolonged membrane rupture on fetal development. Am J Obstet Gynecol 148:540, 1984

279. O'Keeffe DF, Garite TJ, Elliott JP et al: The accuracy of estimated gestational age based on ultrasound measurement of biparietal diameter in preterm premature rupture of the membranes. Am J Obstet Gynecol 151:309, 1985

280. Bottoms SF, Welch RA, Zador IE et al: Clinical interpretation of ultrasound measurements in preterm pregnancies with premature rupture of the membranes. Obstet Gynecol 69:358, 1987

281. Garite T: Premature rupture of the membranes: the enigma of the obstetrician. Am J Obstet Gynecol 151:1001, 1985

282. Romero R, Quintero R, Oyarzun E et al: Intraamniotic infection and the onset of labor in preterm premature rupture of the membranes. Am J Obstet Gynecol 159:661, 1988

283. Yeast J, Garite T, Dorchester W: The risks of amniocentesis in the management of premature rupture of the membranes. Am J Obstet Gynecol 149:505, 1984

284. Galle P, Meis P: Complications of amniocentesis. J Reprod Med 27:149, 1982

285. Dombroski R, MacKenna J, Brame K: Comparison of amniotic fluid maturity profiles in paired vaginal and amniocentesis specimens. Am J Obstet Gynecol 140:461, 1981

286. Shaver DC, Spinnato JA, Whybrew D et al: Comparison of phospholipids in vaginal and amniocentesis specimens of patients with premature rupture of membranes. Am J Obstet Gynecol 156:454, 1987

287. Schumacher RE, Parisi VM, Steady HM et al: Bacteria causing false positive test for phosphatidylglycerol in amniotic fluid. Am J Obstet Gynecol 151:1067, 1985

288. Mercer BM, Crocker LG, Boe NM et al: Induction versus expectant management in prematurity of the membranes with mature amniotic fluid at 32–36 weeks: A randomized trial. Am J Obstet Gynecol 1679:775, 1993

289. Garite TJ, Freeman RK: Chorioamnionitis in the preterm gestation. Obstet Gynecol 59:539, 1982

290. Sperling RS, Ramamurthy RS, Gibbs RS: A comparison of intrapartum versus immediate postpartum treatment of intraamniotic infection. Obstet Gynecol 70:861, 1987

291. Gibbs RS, Dinsmoor MJ, Newton ER, Ramamurthy RS: A randomized trial of intrapartum versus immediate postpartum treatment of women with intra-amniotic infection. Obstet Gynecol 72:823, 1988

292. Gilstrap LC, Leveno KJ, Cox SM et al: Intrapartum treatment of acute chorioamnionitis: impact on neonatal sepsis. Am J Obstet Gynecol 159:579, 1988

293. Ohlsson A, Wang E: An analysis of antenatal tests to detect infection in preterm premature rupture of the membranes. Am J Obstet Gynecol 162:809, 1990

294. Asrat T, Nageotte MP, Garite SE, Dorchester W: Gram stain results from amniocentesis in patients with pre-term premature rupture of the membranes—comparison of maternal and fetal characteristics. Am J Obstet Gynecol 163:887, 1990

295. Romero R, Yoon BH, Mazor M et al: A comparative study of the diagnostic performance of amniotic fluid glucose, white blood cell count, interleukin-6, and Gram stain in the detection of microbial invasion in patients with preterm premature rupture of membranes. Am J Obstet Gynecol 169:839, 1993

296. Evans M, Hajj S, Devoe L et al: C-reactive protein as a predictor of infectious morbidity with premature rupture of membranes. Am J Obstet Gynecol 138:648, 1980

297. Fisk NM, Fysh J, Child AG et al: Is C-reactive protein really useful in preterm premature rupture of the membranes? Br J Obstet Gynaecol 94:1159, 1987

298. Mercer B, Moretti M, Shaver D et al: Intensive antenatal testing for women with preterm prematurity of the membranes (abstract). Am J Obstet Gynecol 164:362, 1991

299. Vintzileos AM, Campbell WA, Nochimson DJ et al: Qualitative amniotic fluid volume versus amniocentesis in predicting infection in preterm premature rupture of the membranes. Obstet Gynecol 67:579, 1986

300. Miller KM, Kho MS, Brown HL, Gabert HA: Clinical chorioamnionitis is not predicted by an ultrasonic biophysical profile in patients with premature rupture of the membranes. Obstet Gynecol 76:1051, 1990

301. Goldstein I, Romero R, Merrill S et al: Fetal body and breathing movements as predictors of intraamniotic infection in preterm premature rupture of membranes. Am J Obstet Gynecol 159:363, 1988

302. Arias et al: Am J Obstet Gynecol 174:304, 1996

303. Ohlsson A: Treatments of preterm premature rupture of the membranes: a meta-analysis. Am J Obstet Gynecol 160:890, 1989

304. Mercer M, Miodovnik M, Thurnau G et al: A multicenter randomized masked trial of antibiotic vs. placebo therapy after preterm premature rupture of the membranes (abstract). Am J Obstet Gynecol 174:304, 1996

305. Curet L, Rao V, Zachman R et al: Association between ruptured membranes, tocolytic therapy, and respiratory distress syndrome. Am J Obstet Gynecol 148:263, 1984

306. Garite TJ, Keegan KA, Freeman RK et al: A randomized trial of ritodrine tocolysis versus expectant management in patients with premature rupture of membranes at 25 to 30 weeks of gestation. Am J Obstet Gynecol 157:388, 1987

307. Weiner CP, Renk K, Klugman M: The therapeutic efficacy and cost-effectiveness of aggressive tocolysis for premature labor associated with premature rupture of the membranes. Am J Obstet Gynecol 159:216, 1988

308. Ghidini A, Romero R: Premature rupture of the membranes: when it occurs in the second trimester. Contemp Obstet Gynecol 39:66, 1994

309. Major CA, Towers CV, Lewis DF, Asrat T: Expectant management of patients with both preterm premature rupture of the membranes and genital herpes. Am J Obstet Gynecol 164:248, 1991

310. Haywood JL, Goldenberg RL, Bronstein J et al: Comparison of perceived and actual rates of survival and

freedom from handicap in premature infants. Am J Obstet Gynecol 171:432, 1994

311. Paul R, Koh K, Monfared A: Obstetric factors influencing outcome in infants weighing from 1,001 to 1,500 grams. Am J Obstet Gynecol 133:503, 1979

312. Bottoms S, Paul R, Iams J et al: Obstetrician's attitude and neonatal survival of extremely low birth weight infants (abstract). Am J Obstet Gynecol 170:296, 1994

313. Hon E, Zanini D, Quilligan E: The neonatal value of fetal monitoring. Am J Obstet Gynecol 122:508, 1975

314. Neutra RR, Fienberg SE, Greeland S, Friedman EA: Effect of fetal monitoring on neonatal death rates. N Engl J Med 299:324, 1978

315. Luthy DA, Shy KK, van Belle G et al: A randomized trial of electronic fetal monitoring in preterm labor. Obstet Gynecol 69:687, 1987

316. Larson EB, van Belle G, Shy KK et al: Fetal monitoring and predictions by clinicians: observations during a randomized clinical trial in very low birth weight infants. Obstet Gynecol 74:584, 1989

317. Zanini B, Paul R, Huey J: Intrapartum fetal heart rate: correlation with scalp pH in the preterm fetus. Am J Obstet Gynecol 136:43, 1980

318. Bowes W, Gabbe S, Bowes C: Fetal heart rate monitoring in premature infants weighing 1,500 gm or less. Am J Obstet Gynecol 137:791, 1980

319. Kenepp N, Shelley W, Gabbe S et al: Fetal and neonatal hazards of maternal hydration with 5% dextrose before cesarean section. Lancet 1:1150, 1982

320. Myers S, Paton J, Fisher D: Neonatal survival of the tiny infant: the challenge. Presented at the Annual Meeting, Society of Perinatal Obstetricians, 1985

321. Barrett J, Boehm F, Vaughn W: The effect of type of delivery on neonatal outcome in singleton infants of birth weight of 1,000 g or less. JAMA 250:625, 1983

322. Bishop E, Israel S, Briscoe C: Obstetric influences on the premature infant's first year of development: a report from the Collaborative Study of Cerebral Palsy. Obstet Gynecol 26:628, 1965

323. Schwartz D, Miodovnik M, Lavin J: Neonatal outcome among low birth weight infants delivered spontaneously or by low forceps. Obstet Gynecol 62:283, 1983

324. O'Driscoll K, Meagher D, MacDonald D et al: Traumatic intracranial haemorrhage in firstborn infants and delivery with obstetric forceps. Br J Obstet Gynaecol 88:577, 1981

325. Main D, Main E, Maurer M: Cesarean section versus vaginal delivery for the breech fetus weighing less than 1,500 grams. Am J Obstet Gynecol 146:580, 1983

326. Westgren LMR, Songster G, Paul RH: Preterm breech delivery: another retrospective study. Obstet Gynecol 66:481, 1985

327. Haesslein I, Goodlin R: Delivery of the tiny newborn. Am J Obstet Gynecol 134:192, 1979

328. Malloy MH, Rhoads GG, Schramm W, Land G: Increasing cesarean section rates in very-low-birth-weight infants, effect on outcome. JAMA 262:1475, 1989

329. Kitchen W, Ford GW, Doyle LW et al: Cesarean section or vaginal delivery at 24 to 28 weeks gestation: comparison of survival and neonatal and two-year morbidity. Obstet Gynecol 66:149, 1985

330. Malloy MH, Rhoads GG, Schramm W et al: Increasing cesarean section rates in very low birthweight infants: effect on outcome. JAMA 262:1475, 1989

331. Malloy MH, Onstad L, Wright E et al: The effect of cesarean delivery on birth outcome in very low birth weight infants. Obstet Gynecol 77:498, 1991

332. Olshan A, Shy K, Luthy D et al: Cesarean birth and neonatal mortality in very low birth weight infants. Obstet Gynecol 64:267, 1984

333. Kosmetatos N, Dinton C, Williams M et al: Intracranial hemorrhage in the premature: its predictive features and outcome. Am J Dis Child 134:855, 1980

334. Anderson GD, Bada HS, Sibai BM et al: The relationship between labor and route of delivery in the preterm infant. Am J Obstet Gynecol 158:1382, 1988

335. Dietl J, Arnold H, Mentzel H et al: Effect of cesarean section on outcome in high- and low-risk very preterm infants. Arch Gynecol Obstet 246:91, 1989

336. Taylor ES: Discussion of a paper by Main DM, Gabbe SG, Richardson, et al. Am J Obstet Gynecol 151:892, 1985

337. Papiernik E, Bouyer J, Dreyfus J et al: Prevention of premature births: a perinatal study in Haguenau, France. Pediatrics 76:154, 1985

338. Iams JD: Obstetric inertia: an obstacle to the prevention of prematurity. Am J Obstet Gynecol 159:796, 1988

339. Papiernik E, Kaminski M: Multifactorial study of the risk of prematurity at 32 weeks of gestation. J Perinat Med 2:30, 1974

340. Aubry RH, Pennington JC: Identification and evaluation of the high risk pregnancy: the perinatal concept. Clin Obstet Gynecol 16:3, 1973

341. Katz M, Newman RB, Gill PJ: Assessment of uterine activity in ambulatory patients at high risk of preterm labor and delivery. Am J Obstet Gynecol 154:44, 1986

342. Nageotte MP, Dorchester W, Porto M et al: Quantitation of uterine activity preceding preterm, term, and postterm labor. Am J Obstet Gynecol 158:1254, 1988

343. Katz M, Gill PJ, Newman RB: Detection of preterm labor by ambulatory monitoring of uterine activity: a preliminary report. Obstet Gynecol 65:773, 1986

344. Morrison JC, Martin JN Jr, Martin RW et al: Prevention of preterm birth by ambulatory assessment of uterine activity: a randomized study. Am J Obstet Gynecol 156:536, 1987

345. Porto M, Nageotte MP, Hill O et al: The role of home monitoring in the prevention of preterm birth, abstracted. Society of Perinatal Obstetricians February 5–7, 1987

346. Iams JD, Johnson FF, O'Shaughnessy RW: A prospective random trial of home uterine activity monitoring in pregnancies at increased risk of preterm labor II. Am J Obstet Gynecol 159:595, 1988

347. Hill WC, Flemming AD, Martin RW et al: Home uterine activity monitoring is associated with a reduction in preterm birth. Obstet Gynecol 76:13S, 1990

348. Dyson DC, Crites YM, Ray DA, Armstrong MA: Prevention of preterm birth in high risk patients: the role of education and provider contact versus home uterine monitoring. Am J Obstet Gynecol 164:756, 1991

349. Mou SM, Sunderji SG, Gall S et al: Multicenter random-

ized clinical trial of home uterine monitoring for detection of preterm labor. Am J Obstet Gynecol 165:858, 1991

350. Wapner RJ, Cotton DB, Artal R et al: A randomized multicenter trial assessing a home uterine activity monitoring device used in the absence of daily nursing contact. Am J Obstet Gynecol 172:1026, 1991

351. Grimes DA, Schultz KF: Randomized controlled trials of home uterine activity monitoring: a review and critique. Obstet Gynecol 79:137, 1992

352. United States Preventive Services Task Force: Home uterine activity monitoring for preterm labor. JAMA 270:371, 1992

353. Sachs BP, Hellerstein S, Freeman R et al: Home monitoring of uterine activity: does it prevent prematurity? N Engl J Med. 325:1374, 1991

354. Rhoads GG, McNellis DC, Kessel SS: Home monitoring of uterine activity. Am J Obstet Gynecol 165:2, 1991

355. Colton T, Kayne HL, Zhang Y, Heeron T: A metaanalysis of home uterine activity monitoring. Am J Obstet Gynecol 173:1499, 1995

356. Main DM, Grisso JA, Wold T et al: Extended longitudinal study of uterine activity among low-risk women. Am J Obstet Gynecol 165:1317, 1991

357. Spinnewijn WEM, Lotgering FK, Struijk PC et al: Fetal heart rate and uterine contractility during maternal exercise at term. Am J Obstet Gynecol 174:43, 1996

358. Germain AM, Valenzuela GJ, Ivankovic M et al: Relationship of circadian rhythms of uterine activity with term and preterm labor. Am J Obstet Gynecol 168:1271, 1993

359. Buekens P, Alexander S, Boutsen M et al: Randomized controlled trial of routine cervical examinations in pregnancy. Lancet 344:841, 1994

360. Lorenz RP, Comstock CH, Bottoms SF, Marx SR: Randomized prospective trial comparing ultrasonography and pelvic examination for preterm labor surveillance. Am J Obstet Gynecol 162:1603, 1990

361. Zemlyn W: The effect of the urinary bladder in obstetrical sonography. Radiology 169:169, 1978

362. Brown JE, Thiemee GA, Shah DM et al: Transabdominal and transvaginal endosonography: evaluation of the cervix and lower uterine segment in pregnancy. Am J Obstet Gynecol 155:721, 1986

363. Eschenbach DA, Nugent RP, Rao AV et al: Am J Obstet Gynecol 164:734, 1991

364. Klebanoff MA, Regan JA, Rao AV et al: Outcome of the Vaginal Infections and Prematurity Study: results of a clinical trial of erythromycin among pregnant women colonized with group B streptococci. Am J Obstet Gynecol 172:1540, 1995

365. Hauth JC, Goldenberg RL: Reduced incidence of preterm delivery with metronidazole and erythromycin in women with bacterial vaginosis. N Engl J Med 333:1732, 1995

366. Ernest JM, Meis PJ, Moore ML et al: Vaginal pH: a marker of preterm premature rupture of the membranes. Obstet Gynecol 74:734, 1989

367. Gleeson RP, Elder AM, Turner MJ et al: Vaginal pH in pregnancy in women delivered at and before term. Br J Obstet Gynaecol 96:183, 1989

368. McGregor JA, Jackson GM, Lachelin GC et al: Salivary estriol as risk assessment for preterm labor: a prospective trial. Am J Obstet Gynecol 173:1337, 1995

369. Meis PJ, Ernest JM, Moore ML et al: Regional program for prevention of premature birth in northwestern North Carolina. Am J Obstet Gynecol 157:550, 1987

370. Collaborative Group on Preterm Birth Prevention. Multicenter randomized, controlled trial of a preterm birth prevention program. Am J Obstet Gynecol 169:352, 1993

371. Elder HA, Santamaria BAG, Smith S et al: The natural history of asymptomatic bacteriuria during pregnancy: the effect of tetracycline on the clinical course and the outcome of pregnancy. Am J Obstet Gynecol 111:441, 1971

372. McCormack WM, Rosner B, Yhu-Hsung L et al: Effect on birthweight of erythromycin treatment of pregnant women. Obstet Gynecol 69:202, 1987

373. McGregor JA, French JI, Parker R et al: Prevention of premature birth by screening and treatment for common genital tract infections: results of a prospective controlled evaluation. Am J Obstet Gynecol 173:157, 1995

374. Olds DL, Henderson CR, Tatelbaum R, Chamberlain R: Improving the delivery of prenatal care and outcomes of pregnancy: a randomized trial of nurse home visitation. Pediatrics 77:16, 1986

375. Spencer B, Thomas H, Morris J: A randomized controlled trial of the provision of a social support service during pregnancy: the South Manchester Family Worker Project. Br J Obstet Gynaecol 96:281, 1989

376. Leveno KJ, Little BB, Cunningham FG: The national impact of ritodrine hydrochloride for inhibition of preterm labor. Obstet Gynecol 76:12, 1990

377. Johnson J, Lee P, Zachary A et al: High-risk prematurity—progestin treatment and steroid studies. Obstet Gynecol 54:412, 1979

378. Hauth J, Gilstrap L, Brekken A et al: The effect of 17 alpha-hydroxyprogesterone caproate on pregnancy outcome in an active-duty military population. Am J Obstet Gynecol 146:187, 1983

379. Colie CF: Preterm labor and delivery in working women Semin Perinatol 17:37, 1993

380. Luke B, Mamelle N, Keith L et al: The association between occupational factors and preterm birth: a United States nurses' study. Am J Obstet Gynecol 173:849, 1995

381. Goldenberg RL, Cliver SP, Bronstein J et al: Bedrest in pregnancy. Obstet Gynecol 84:131, 1994

Multiple Gestations

Usha Chitkara and Richard L. Berkowitz

The phenomenon of twinning has fascinated mankind throughout its recorded history. Twins have often been regarded as being inherently "different" from singletons, and societal responses to their birth have ranged from awe to fear. Researchers have been interested in exploiting their uniqueness in an attempt to separate the influences of genetic and environmental factors on both fetal and postpartum development.[1] Obstetricians have long been aware that pregnancies complicated by twinning are by their very nature at higher risk than those of most singletons. Finally, parents and future siblings are often overjoyed or overwhelmed when they are told that twins are expected but are virtually never neutral in their response.

Twins are either monozygotic (MZ) or dizygotic (DZ). In the former case a single fertilized ovum splits into two distinct individuals after a variable number of divisions. Such twins are almost always genetically identical and therefore of the same sex. On rare occasions mutations can cause genetic discordance resulting in phenotypic and chromosomal dissimilarities between MZ twins. On the other hand, when two separate ova are fertilized, DZ twins result. These individuals are as genetically distinct as any other children born to the same couple. Sets of DZ twins may have the same or opposite sex. DZ half-siblings have been reported in which two ova were fertilized by different fathers, and it has been hypothesized that monovular dispermic fertilization may occur. These latter situations are very uncommon, however. In most cases, DZ twins are genetically dissimilar true siblings, while MZ twins are genetically identical.

The frequency of MZ twins is fairly constant throughout the world at a rate of approximately 4 per 1,000 births. This rate does not seem to vary with maternal characteristics such as age or parity. DZ twinning, however, is associated with multiple ovulation, and its frequency varies between races and within countries and is affected by several identifiable factors. In general, the frequency of DZ twins is low in Asians, intermediate in whites, and high in blacks. In the United States, the overall incidence of twins is approximately 12 per 1,000 births, and two-thirds are DZ.[1] The Yorubas of Western Nigeria, however, have a frequency of 45 twins per 1,000 births, and about 90 percent are DZ.[2]

The frequency of DZ births is affected by maternal age, increasing from a rate of 3 in 1,000 in women under age 20 to 14 in 1,000 at ages 35 to 40. Above age 40 the rate declines. The frequency of DZ twinning also increases with parity independent of maternal age.[1]

The different rates of DZ twinning may be due to racial or individual variations in pituitary gonadotropin production. Infertility patients treated with menopausal urinary gonadotropins (Pergonal) or clomiphene citrate are well known to have a dose-dependent increase in multiple births when compared with women who conceive without these agents. While DZ twins predominate in these patients, triplets and higher numbers of conceptuses may also occur. The use of in vitro fertilization and embryo transfer has further increased the incidence of multiple pregnancies. Reports of in vitro fertilization pregnancies suggest that the incidence of multiple gestations in these patients may be as high as 22 percent.[3,4]

The cause of MZ twinning is unclear. Benirschke and Kim[5] state that it is probably an uncommon occurrence among other mammals. In two species of armadillo, however, polyembryony regularly follows implantation of a single blastocyst. Oxygen deprivation has been experimentally shown to enhance fission in fish embryos, and some teratogens have been associated with increased MZ twinning rates in laboratory animals, but there is currently no satisfactory explanation for the fact that MZ twins occur in humans with such a constant frequency around the world.

Placentation

Twin placentas are described in terms of their membranes (Fig. 24-1). The sac of a singleton pregnancy consists of an outer chorion and an inner amnion. Each DZ twin develops within a similar sac because both blastocysts generate their own placentas. If implantation of these blastocysts is not proximal to each other, two separate placentas will result, each of which will have a chorion and an amnion. Should they implant

side by side, intimate fusion of the placental discs will occur, but these placentas are always diamniotic and dichorionic, and vascular anastomoses rarely occur. While MZ twins may also have placentas with two amnions and two chorions, this generally is not the case. Monochorionic placentas have a single chorion that usually surrounds two amnions, but occasionally there is only a single amnion. Regardless of whether these monochorial placentas are diamniotic or monoamniotic, they are always a single disc and only occur in MZ twins. Triplets and quadruplets have also been delivered with monochorial placentas and shown to be MZ. Almost all monochorial placentas have blood vessel communications between the fetal circulations.

The type of placenta that develops in an MZ pregnancy is determined by the timing of cleavage of the fertilized ovum. If twinning is accomplished during the

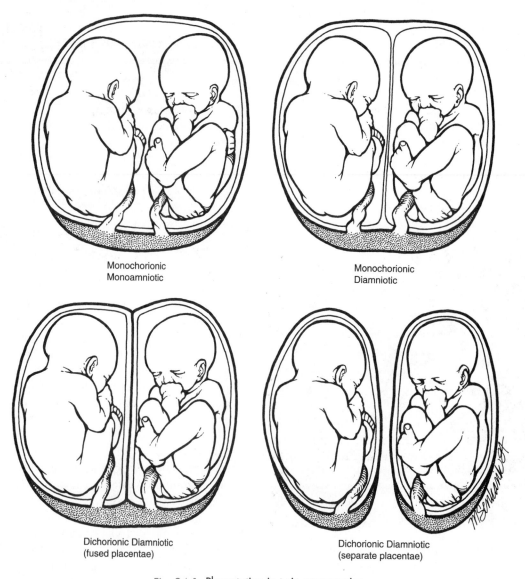

Monochorionic
Monoamniotic

Monochorionic
Diamniotic

Dichorionic Diamniotic
(fused placentae)

Dichorionic Diamniotic
(separate placentae)

Fig. 24-1 Placentation in twin pregnancies.

first 2 to 3 days, it precedes the setting aside of cells that eventually become the chorion. In that case, two chorions and two amnions will be formed. After approximately 3 days, however, twinning cannot split the chorionic cavity, and from that time on a monochorial placenta must result. If the split occurs between the third and eighth days, a diamniotic monochorial placenta will develop. Between the eighth and thirteenth days, the amnion has already formed, and the placenta will therefore be monoamniotic and monochorionic. Embryonic cleavage between the thirteenth and fifteenth days will result in conjoined twins within a single amnion and chorion; beyond that point, the process of twinning cannot occur.

The frequency of placental types within a population is influenced by the rate of DZ twinning. In the United States approximately 80 percent of twin placentas are dichorionic, and 20 percent are monochorionic. In Nigeria, where DZ twinning is much more common, the frequency of dichorionic placentas approaches 95 percent.[5] With triplets, quadruplets, and higher orders of multiple gestation, monochorionic and dichorionic placentations may coexist.

Because monochorial placentas can only occur in MZ pregnancies, study of the membranes will establish zygosity in 20 percent of cases in the United States. In approximately 35 percent of cases the twins will be of opposite sex and therefore necessarily DZ. This leaves only 45 percent of cases (twins of like sex having dichorionic placentas) in which further studies are necessary in order to determine zygosity. Cameron[6] found that this 45 percent breaks down into 8 percent MZ and 37 percent DZ. He states that "the percentage of monozygotic dichorionic pairs is inversely proportional to the completeness of the genotyping." In other words, the more genotypic markers that are studied, the greater the likelihood of demonstrating dizygosity. Cameron used six blood group markers, four red blood cell (RBC) enzymes, and placental alkaline phosphatase in order to determine zygosity. However, at present, the most accurate method for determination of twin zygosity is by analysis of DNA polymorphism.[7,8]

The often cited Weinberg rule states that in a population of twins the estimated number of MZ pairs is almost exactly equal to the total minus twice the number of twins of unlike sex. The assumption underlying this rule is that among DZ pairs the sex of one twin is independent of that of the other, resulting in almost exactly equal numbers of like and unlike sexed pairs. The small difference anticipated from exact equality is due to the fact that the sex ratio is not precisely 0.5. This rule has been questioned by several authorities who present evidence that in DZ populations there seems to be a higher frequency of like-sex than opposite-sex twins at birth.[9] Cameron's data[6] would favor the latter view.

Perinatal Morbidity and Mortality

Numerous reports have documented that perinatal morbidity and mortality are greater in twins than in singletons. A collaborative study has been published regarding 6,503 sets of twins delivered at 32 different hospitals between 1961 and 1972.[10] The overall perinatal mortality in this series was 124 per 1,000 births. When only those twins weighing more than 1,000 g were considered, the perinatal loss was 62 per 1,000 births, which was approximately three times greater than that of comparable singletons at the same institutions.

A high incidence of low-birth-weight infants is the major cause of the increased perinatal mortality in twins. Both preterm delivery and intrauterine growth restriction (IUGR) contribute to this problem. In addition to prematurity and growth restriction, twins have an increased frequency of congenital anomalies, placenta previa, abruptio placenta, preeclampsia, cord accidents, and malpresentations.

Because of advances in both maternal-fetal medicine and neonatal care, a general decline in perinatal mortality has been reported over the past two decades from centers around the world. In general, this overall trend has also been noted for multiple gestations. Desgranges et al.[11] reported a perinatal mortality rate of 95/1,000 in 213 twins delivered between 1969 and 1973 compared with 56/1,000 in 221 twins delivered between 1974 and 1979 at the Hopital Notre-Dame in Montreal. During these periods, there was essentially no change in the fetal death rates (28/1,000 vs. 32/1,000), but the neonatal mortality fell from 68/1,000 to 24/1,000. The frequency of anomalies during the entire period was 23/1,000, and these accounted for 18 percent of all deaths. The average length of pregnancy in both study periods was identical, and the improved neonatal outcome was found to be due to increased survival rates in neonates weighing 1,000 to 1,500 g at birth.

With the routine use of antenatal fetal heart rate testing, Rattan and colleagues[12] noted a marked reduction in fetal mortality after 32 weeks when 153 twins delivered between 1975 and 1979 were compared with 160 twins delivered between 1980 and 1983. The rate of stillbirths fell from 23 per 1,000 in the former period to 0 per 1,000 in the latter.

Despite these encouraging trends, the problems associated with multiple gestations continue to place these infants at higher risk than their singleton counterparts. Hawrylyshyn et al.[13] reported an overall perinatal mortality rate of 91 per 1,000 births in 177 twin pairs delivered between 1975 and 1979 in Toronto. The number of cases in each year was fairly small, but there was no demonstrable decline in perinatal mortality during the study period. In this series, more than

70 percent of the deaths occurred before 30 weeks' gestation. Those deaths either took place in utero or during the neonatal period in association with respiratory distress syndrome, intracerebral hemorrhage, or necrotizing enterocolitis. These workers concluded that if obstetricians are to have a major impact on the perinatal survival of twins, they must concentrate on the period between 25 and 30 weeks' gestation.

In multifetal gestations with three or more fetuses the most important complication again is premature delivery with its concomitant increase in perinatal morbidity and mortality. Accurate knowledge regarding outcome of these pregnancies remains limited because of the relatively small numbers in any reported series, especially for quadruplets and higher order births. Among three fairly large series published before 1983, Holcberg et al.[14] reported a perinatal mortality rate of 312 per 1,000 among 31 triplet pregnancies managed in their institution between 1960 and 1979. Ron-El et al.[15] reported a perinatal mortality of 185 per 1,000 in their series of 29 triplet and 6 quadruplet gestations managed between 1970 and 1978. Loucopoulos and Jewelewicz,[16] in a series of 27 triplets, 7 quadruplets, and 1 quintuplet cared for from 1965 to 1981, noted a perinatal mortality rate of 148 per 1,000.

Major improvements in perinatal and neonatal care over the past two decades have resulted in significantly better survival rates for triplets and perhaps higher order pregnancies. This is reflected in the results of some of the more recent published reports on multiple gestations. Lipitz et al.[17] reported a perinatal mortality of 93/1,000 among 78 triplet gestations managed in their institution between 1975 and 1988. Gonen et al.,[18] presenting their data on 30 multiple gestations (24 triplets, 5 quadruplets, and 1 quintuplet) from 1978 to 1988, reported a perinatal mortality rate of 51.5 per 1,000; and the experience of Newman et al.[19] with 198 triplet pregnancies delivered between 1985 and 1988 was similar. Three recent publications from Britain, Switzerland, and Australia report outcome data on multiple gestations conceived spontaneously or by assisted reproductive technology. The British report[20] contained 143 sets of triplets and 12 sets of quadruplets with perinatal mortality rates of 70 per 1,000 and 104 per 1,000, respectively. The Swiss data[21] included 77 sets of triplets with a perinatal mortality of 89 per 1,000 and 9 quadruplet sets with a perinatal mortality of 147 per 1,000; whereas the Australian series, including 133 sets of triplets and 6 sets of quadruplets, reported perinatal mortality of 108 per 1,000 and 250 per 1,000, respectively.[22]

A review of the subject by Alvarez and Berkowitz[23] in 1990 concluded that although perinatal mortality rates had decreased, the risk of prematurity in multifetal gestations had not changed significantly over the past 20 to 30 years. The average gestational age at delivery for triplets consistently seems to be 33 to 35 weeks. Approximately 75 percent of these patients deliver prior to 37 weeks, and at least 20 percent deliver prior to 32 weeks. The number of reported patients with four or more fetuses remains too small for a meaningful analysis of perinatal morbidity and mortality rates. However, one can assume that at best the outcome in those pregnancies is the same as with triplets, and it probably is worse.

The infant mortality rate for multiple births is also high. Luke and Keith[24] analyzed the National Infant Mortality Surveillance (NIMS) Project based on the 1980 U.S. birth cohort and reported an overall infant mortality rate of 8.6 per 1,000 for singletons, 56.6 per 1,000 for twins, and 166.7 per 1,000 for triplets. This represents a 6.6-fold and 19.4-fold higher mortality in twins and triplets, respectively, compared with singletons. Likewise, among survivors, the incidence of severe handicap was significantly higher among multiple births, being 19.7, 34.0 and 57.5 per 1,000 postneonatal survivors in singletons, twins, and triplets, respectively, and representing a 1.7-fold and 2.9-fold higher rate among twins and triplets compared with singletons. The overall risk for infant mortality and severe handicap was also noted to be substantially higher in black infants than in whites.

Diagnosis

It is obviously impossible to offer specialized antepartum care if multiple gestation remains undiagnosed until the intrapartum period. An often quoted statistic in the older literature is that 50 percent of twins remain undiagnosed until the time of delivery.[25] Because of the current widespread use of diagnostic ultrasound, this is certainly no longer true. The number of twins in the United States diagnosed during the antenatal period is currently unknown, but there must be substantial variations from one institution to another, depending on the degree to which ultrasound is used. In a report from Yale–New Haven Hospital,[26] 91 percent of 385 twin sets delivered between 1977 and 1981 were diagnosed before the onset of labor.

Multiple gestations should be suspected whenever (1) the uterus seems to be larger than dates, (2) hydramnios or unexplained maternal anemia develops, (3) auscultation of more than one fetal heart is suspected, or (4) the pregnancy has occurred following ovulation induction or in vitro fertilization. Multiple gestation may also be diagnosed serendipitously at the time of ultrasound scanning before a genetic amniocentesis or as a result of an elevated serum α-fetoprotein (AFP) level in mass-screening programs.

An argument often used in support of universal ultrasound screening for all pregnant women during the second trimester is that it would result in the early diagnosis of multiple pregnancies with almost 100 percent accuracy.[27] Persson and Kullander[28] reported the results of this type of screening program, which has been in effect at the Malmo General Hospital in Sweden since 1973. Originally the program began with a single scan performed in the thirtieth week, but subsequently all women were offered examinations at both 17 and 33 weeks. Between 1974 and 1982, 98 percent of 254 multiple gestations were detected by ultrasound screening. There were no false-positive diagnoses, but 2 percent of multiple gestations were missed on the first examination. These authors also reported a reduction in perinatal mortality from 107 per 1,000 to 34 per 1,000 when similar numbers of twins delivered between 1970 and 1974 were compared with those delivered from 1975 to 1982. Major morbidity (e.g., cerebral palsy, mental retardation, late motor development, and hearing defects) decreased from 9.6 to 3.6 percent, and the frequency of delivery prior to 38 weeks dropped from 34 to 15.8 percent. The marked improvement in these figures was obviously due to multiple factors, but early diagnosis was among them. Results of the recent Routine Antenatal Diagnostic Imaging with Ultrasound (RADIUS) study from the United States indicate a similar experience.[29] This study compared a group of low-risk pregnant women who underwent routine ultrasound screening in the second and third trimesters of pregnancy with a control group who had an ultrasound examination only when medically indicated. The diagnosis of multiple gestation, when present, was made before 26 weeks' gestation in all women who had the screening ultrasound examination. In contrast, among women in the control group, 37 percent of multiple gestations were not identified until after 26 weeks' gestation, and in 13 percent the diagnosis was not made until the delivery admission.

Separate gestational sacs can be identified ultrasonically as early as 6 weeks from the first day of the last menstrual period. With transabdominal scanning, an embryo within each sac should be visible by 7 weeks, and beating fetal hearts should be seen by 7.5 to 8 weeks.[30] With good equipment the fetal cranial pole is also identifiable during this period, but the intracranial landmarks used for accurate biparietal diameter measurements are usually not seen until 14 to 16 weeks. Increasing sophistication in the development and use of endovaginal scanning has made it possible to visualize these developmental landmarks 1 to 2 weeks earlier than with abdominal scanning techniques so that the embryonic pole and fetal heart can be seen by 6 weeks and the intracranial landmarks are visible by 10 to 12 weeks' gestation.[31] The earliest reported diagnosis of

twins was strongly suspected 10 days after ovulation and confirmed 23 days later.[32]

In general, the ultrasonic diagnosis of multiple gestations within the first trimester is relatively straightforward. It is mandatory, however, to visualize separate fetuses (Fig. 24-2). Retromembranous collections of blood or fluid or a prominent fetal yolk sac should not be confused with a twin gestation. Demonstration of the viability of each fetus at the time of the examination requires visualization of independent cardiac activity. Unfortunately, mistakes can be made regarding the number of fetuses present when scans are hastily interpreted. This is particularly true in the third trimester, but may also occur in the first and second trimesters, especially with four or more fetuses. It must be remembered that an ultrasound image, unlike a flat plate of the abdomen, does not provide a composite overview. The image displayed is only a tomographic slice through the area being studied. It is therefore possible to display two circular structures that may represent different fetal heads or, alternatively, the head and thorax of the same fetus in a tucked position. Misinterpretation in this setting has resulted in the incorrect diagnosis of twins when only one fetus was present. On the other hand, rapid and careless scanning may result in failure to detect a second fetus whose head is deeply engaged in the pelvis or pushed up under the ribs. If a multiple gestation is suspected, the ultrasonologist must be compulsive in examining the entire uterine cavity. A scan should not be completed until the orientation of all the visualized fetal parts is understood.[33]

Early Wastage in Multiple Gestations

As a result of ultrasound studies performed during the first trimester, there is evidence to suggest that the incidence of multiple gestations in humans is higher than is usually appreciated and that a significant amount of early wastage occurs in these pregnancies. This has led to the concept of the "vanishing twin" (Figs. 24-3 and 24-4). Landy et al.[34] reviewed nine series that have addressed this phenomenon. The series vary in regard to the populations studied, timing of the ultrasonography, and number of scans performed. Frequencies of twin "disappearance" in patients scanned before 14 weeks gestational age reportedly range from 13 to 78 percent. The higher rates were found in studies performed before 10 weeks' gestation.

One explanation for the disappearance of a gestational sac is resorption, which has been documented to occur in both human singleton pregnancies and lower animals (Fig. 24-5). This phenomenon has been ultrasonically described in human multiple gestations between 7 to 12 weeks. The true incidence of resorption of

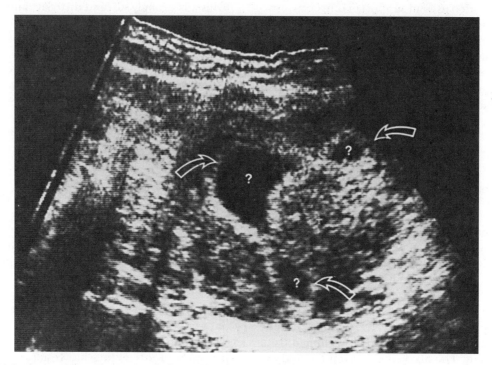

Fig. 24-2 The scanning plane may artifactually transact a sac in such a fashion as to give the impression of multiple sacs. In this case, the three gestational sacs were all part of the single normal larger one. (From Jeanty and Romero,[30] with permission.)

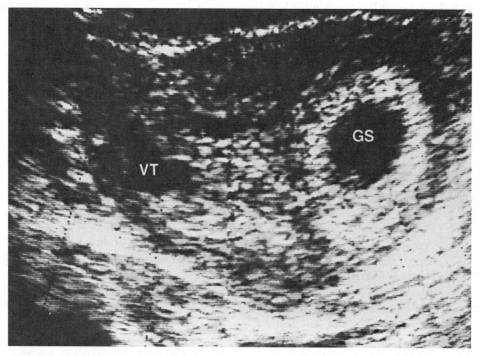

Fig. 24-3 This scan shows an early gestational sac (GS) with a well-formed trophoblastic rim and an adjacent vanishing twin (VT). (From Jeanty and Romero,[30] with permission.)

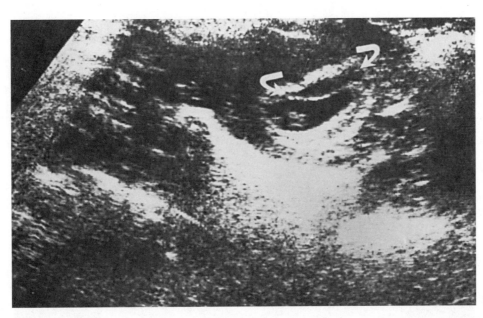

Fig. 24-4 Vanishing twin with an incomplete trophoblastic rim (arrows) (From Jeanty and Romero,[30] with permission.)

one or more gestational sacs is unknown, but it can occur without adverse effects on a coexisting fetus. Another explanation for sac disappearance is the presence of a blighted ovum or anembryonic pregnancy. Robinson and Caines[35] define a blighted ovum as a gestational sac having a volume of 2.5 cc or more in which no fetus can be identified on ultrasound examination. It should be noted that the sac need not be totally anechoic, because disorganized echoes may be present in some cases. Several studies have reported that the only apparent complication of regression of a blighted ovum is slight vaginal bleeding. Regardless of whether vaginal bleeding accompanies regression of a blighted ovum, a coexisting normal pregnancy has a good prognosis for carrying to term. Furthermore, experience with patients undergoing elective first trimester reduction of multifetal pregnancies suggests that the clinical course and outcome of these pregnancies is similar to that observed with the naturally occurring phenomenon of a blighted or "disappearing" co-twin.[36–38]

Landy et al.[34] point out that pathologic evidence to confirm "disappearance" rates as high as 78 percent is lacking. Examination of the placenta and membranes after delivery of a singleton thought to be a surviving twin rarely shows evidence of the one that disappeared. It is also true that examination of the products of an abortion is usually not helpful in verifying the presence of a sac that has "vanished." The difficulty encountered in obtaining positive pathologic confirmation of the diagnosis, however, does not mean that it is incorrect. On the other hand, false diagnoses are certainly possible as a result of poor ultrasound studies. If equipment with inferior resolution is used, or if the types of artifacts

described earlier are misread as being second sacs, the presence of multiple gestations may be overdiagnosed. Particular attention should be paid to the fact that pressure from the scanning transducer can create an hourglass appearance in a normal single sac that may be incorrectly interpreted as demonstrating two separate sacs.

Aside from first trimester bleeding, there are no reported maternal complications associated with the early disappearance of a fetus.[34] The associated overall abortion rates in reported series range from 7 to 37 percent. However, in two studies when a vanished sac was associated with vaginal bleeding during the first trimester, spontaneous abortions occurred in 26 percent[39] and 92 percent[40] of cases. In a retrospective review of the first trimester ultrasound data for 260 twin pregnancies in which one or both fetuses delivered at term, Dickey et al.[41] found that disparities in gestational sac diameter and crown–rump length (CRL) were good predictors of eventual outcome. When disparities of 3 mm or more were observed either between the twin gestational sac diameters (at ≤49 days gestation) or between the twin crown–rump length measurements (at ≤63 days gestation), these were associated with an embryo loss rate of 50 percent or more. The incidence of these disparities was lower in pregnancies resulting from assisted reproductive technologies than spontaneous conceptions and was unrelated to differences in birth weight, length, or gender of the neonate.

Landy et al.[34] conclude that the phenomenon of the vanishing twin seems to truly exist. While on the basis of current information it is impossible to determine the exact prevalence of this occurrence, their data suggest

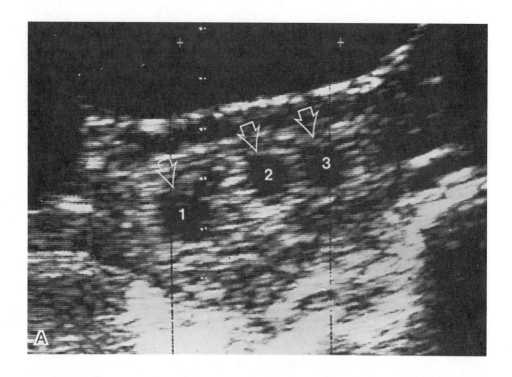

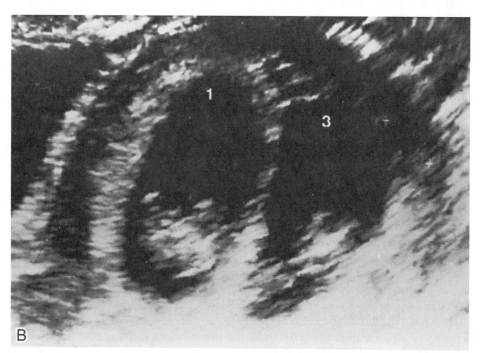

Fig. 24-5 **(A)** Three gestational sacs seen early in the first trimester. **(B)** Two weeks later, the second sac has disappeared, and only the two lateral ones remain. (From Jeanty and Romero,[30] with permission.)

that a reasonable figure for its incidence may be as high as 21 percent.[42] These authors caution, however, that it is necessary to make "an accurate, faultless diagnosis" of multiple gestation in the first trimester before sharing this information with the mother because of its inevitable emotional and social impact.

Growth and Development

Normal individual twins grow at the same rate as singletons up to 30 to 32 weeks' gestation. After that time, they do not gain weight as rapidly as singletons of the same gestational age.[43] Daw and Walker[44] stated that after 32 weeks the combined weight gain of both twins is approximately equivalent to that gained by a singleton for the remaining portion of the pregnancy. The retardation in each twin's somatic growth is thought to be related to "crowding" in utero. The implication of this concept is that at some point in the third trimester the placenta can no longer keep pace with the nutrient requirements of both developing fetuses. This process occurs even earlier than 30 weeks when more than two fetuses are present.

A study of specimens obtained by induced abortion performed between 8.5 and 21 weeks showed the relationship between body weight and length in twins to be the same as that for singletons.[45] This finding supports the concept that twins are not growth retarded during the first half of pregnancy. Fenner et al.[46] have provided some insight into the other end of the gestational age spectrum by studying 146 twins admitted to their neonatal unit with gestational ages at birth ranging from 30 weeks to term. When data from these infants were plotted on Lubchenco's growth charts for singletons, these workers found that the twins' birth weights dropped below the mean for singletons by 32 weeks but remained within the low normal range until the thirty-sixth week, after which time they fell progressively below the tenth percentile. Twin birth lengths and head circumferences, however, remained within the low normal range for singletons throughout the entire pregnancy. The disparity between relatively normal head size and body length in association with somatic deprivation is compatible with the concept of asymmetric growth retardation. The latter is a mechanism whereby growth-retarded fetuses preferentially favor head growth at the expense of increases in body weight.[47] These studies suggest that alterations in twin growth occur primarily in the third trimester, worsen as gestational age progresses, and are usually asymmetric in nature.

In the large collaborative study conducted by Kohl and Casey,[10] birth weights differed between 500 and 999 g in 18 percent of the twin sets and were in excess of 1,000 g in 3 percent. Obviously these discrepancies in birth weight could be due, in part, to constitutional factors. Because DZ twins are genetically distinct individuals, it is not surprising that they should be programmed to have very different weights at birth. There are, however, several pathologic situations in which twins may be born with substantial weight differences. These include the twin-to-twin transfusion syndrome, the combination of an anomalous fetus with a normal co-twin, and growth retardation affecting only one twin because of local placental factors.[33] IUGR, on the other hand, can affect both twins relatively equally, in which case they would both be small, but not discordant in size. Detection of differences in size in utero therefore

suggests that IUGR may be present but is not diagnostic of that condition. Conversely, the demonstration that twin fetuses have similar sizes does not rule out abnormal growth. It therefore is necessary to assess each twin individually if abnormal growth in utero is to be detected.

Assessing Fetal Growth With Ultrasound

Ultrasound is the most accurate method for assessing fetal growth. Regular ultrasonic scanning permits ongoing assessment of individual growth.

Are Singleton Nomograms Applicable to Twins?

The first question to be asked is whether ultrasound nomograms devised for singletons can be used to follow twins. Conflicting data exist in the published literature regarding this issue. Some investigators have found twins to have smaller biparietal diameters (BPDs) than those of singletons at all gestational ages,[48] while others have found mean BPD values corresponding to those of singletons until the third trimester but demonstrate progressive slowing in growth of the twin BPDs thereafter.[49–53] When, however, 18 sets of concordant twins with verified menstrual dates were compared with values from singletons that were appropriate for gestational age (AGA) at birth, Crane et al.[54] found the two groups to have mean BPD values that were essentially identical throughout gestation. These authors conclude that normal twin BPD growth is similar to that of AGA singletons at all stages of gestation, and the conflicting results of earlier studies are due to the inclusion of discordant twins with IUGR in the study group. A similar conclusion was reached by Graham et al.,[55] who studied 104 twins with concordant growth, excellent gestational age assessment, and delivery after 36 weeks; they found almost identical results when BPD and femur length values were compared with those from a selected population of singletons. Other investigators[53,56] also found no significant difference in BPD between uncomplicated singleton and twin pregnancies, suggesting that charts derived from singleton pregnancies may be reliably used to estimate gestational age of twins.

Neonatal anthropometric data obtained from concordant twins suggests that although there is significant reduction of birth weights of twins in late pregnancy, head circumference and body lengths are generally similar to those of normal singletons at corresponding gestational age.[52,54] These findings are consistent with ultrasound observations showing twin femur length growth patterns similar to singletons throughout gestation,[51,55,57] but a reduction in the abdominal circumference growth in twins after 32 weeks.[51,52]

The Significance of Divergent Biparietal Diameters

In 1976, Dorros[58] reported a case in which BPD values in a set of twins were discordant by 7 to 10 mm on three examinations performed between 38 and 41 weeks. At delivery one infant was found to be severely growth retarded, while the other was AGA. The placenta had an infarct covering approximately 20 percent of the total surface area and was located near the origin of the growth-retarded twin's umbilical cord. Several series have subsequently shown that as the difference between twin BPDs increases, the likelihood that the smaller fetus will be growth retarded increases. Leveno et al.[59] reported that a comparison of BPD differences of 4 mm or less with those of 5 mm or greater was associated with an increase from 7 to 22 percent in the number of twin pairs with one growth-retarded infant. Houlton[60] noted an overall increase in small for gestational age (SGA) infants from 40 to 71 percent in a comparison of BPD differentials below 6 mm with those of 6 mm or greater.

Crane et al.[54] defined discordance in utero as an intrapair difference in BPD of 5 mm or more and a fall in BPD below 2 standard deviation (SD) for gestational age on their normal twin curve. Twelve sets of twins met this criterion for discordancy, nine of whom were subsequently shown to have a difference in birth weight of more than 25 percent. They suggested that head circumferences (HC) be measured if BPD intrapair differences exceed 5 mm. Since HC is less likely to be affected by molding in utero, an intrapair HC difference of less than 5 percent suggests that true discrepancy does not exist. Chitkara et al.[61] also found that BPD intrapair differentials of 5 mm or greater correlated with an increased incidence of significant birth weight differences. However, estimated fetal weight and abdominal circumference measurements were found to be better predictors of discordant size. Other investigators have corroborated these observations.[62]

This compilation of confusing and seemingly conflicting data can probably be summarized as follows. Significant differences in twin BPDs may indicate that one twin is growth retarded. However, the finding could be purely artifactual because of flattening of the head in association with malpresentation or in utero crowding. Measurements of several parameters, along with serial examinations, will help distinguish fetal growth abnormalities in most cases. Nevertheless, while major intrapair BPD differences may reflect IUGR in one fetus, it is not the only criterion that should be used to look for abnormal development in utero because it will not be present when both twins are growth retarded.

The Use of Multiple Parameters to Assess for IUGR and Growth Discordance

How then should growth in utero be followed in multiple pregnancies? BPD alone, as an isolated variable, is a poor predictor of IUGR in twins. Neilson[63] retrospectively analyzed 66 twin pregnancies with good dates by plotting BPD values on a singleton nomogram. Only 56 percent of the 43 SGA neonates were found to have abnormal BPD growth, while 49 percent of the fetuses with abnormal BPD curves were found not to be growth retarded at delivery. In a subsequent prospective study of 31 twin pregnancies, Neilson[64] did an initial scan for dating before 20 weeks and a "second stage" examination between 34 and 36 weeks. At the second examination, fetal size was assessed by calculating the product of CRL and trunk area (TA), plotted on a nomogram devised for singletons. In this series, 19 of the 62 neonates were SGA, and all of them fell below the tenth percentile on the CRL and TA nomogram. In addition, 23 percent of the AGA babies were in the abnormal zone. Interestingly, the numbers calculated for each fetus did not prove useful in predicting weight differences within twin pairs at delivery.

Our experience[61] and that of others[52,61,65–67] suggest that a survey of multiple parameters on serial ultrasound examinations provides the most accurate assessment of the size of each individual fetus in twin gestations. The highest accuracy for predicting either appropriate or retarded growth is obtained by estimating the fetal weight. Among individual parameters, abdominal circumference is the single most sensitive measurement in predicting both IUGR and growth discordance.[61,62,66,67] Recent studies suggest that an intrapair difference in abdominal circumference measurement of 2 cm or more can be effectively used as a screening test for discordant fetal growth and IUGR in the smaller twin.[62,66,67] On the other hand, individual measurements of BPD, HC, or femur length are relatively poor predictors for either IUGR or growth discordance.[61,66,67]

Probably the most important conclusions that can be drawn from these various studies are that it is technically feasible to measure multiple ultrasound parameters in twin pregnancies and that a consideration of as many variables as possible will maximize the effectiveness of an ultrasonic assessment of fetal size. The same general principles can be applied to the assessment of growth in triplets and higher order multiple gestations. Another point that should be stressed is that growth is a dynamic process and therefore patients with multiple gestations should be followed with serial scans. Since growth retardation is a process that usually occurs during the third trimester and the predictive accuracy of any fetal measurement in utero is inversely proportional to the scan–delivery interval, we recommend that women with twins be scanned every 3 to 4 weeks after the 26th week and more frequently than that if IUGR or growth discordance is suspected.

Ultrasonographic Prediction of Amnionicity and Chorionicity

The risk for many of the complications occurring in multiple gestation depends on whether the placentation is monochorionic or dichorionic. The incidences of IUGR and fetal death are higher in monochorionic than dichorionic twins, and the twin-to-twin transfusion syndrome (TTS) occurs only in monochorionic twins. Antenatal knowledge of the type of placentation and chorionicity is not only helpful but in some cases is critical for determining optimal management. This is true when deciding whether IUGR in one fetus of a twin gestation is due to TTS or uteroplacental insufficiency, when contemplating the selective termination of one abnormal twin, or performing an elective first-trimester multifetal pregnancy reduction procedure. In these latter situations, if the gestation is monochorionic a shared placental circulation could result in death or damage to a surviving fetus.

The sonographic prediction of chorionicity and amnionicity should be systematically approached by determining the number of placentas visualized and the sex of each fetus and then by assessing the membranes that divide the sacs. The pregnancy is clearly dichorionic if two separate placental discs are seen or if the twins are of different sex. When a single placenta is present and the twins are of the same sex, careful sonographic examination of the dividing membrane will usually result in a correct diagnosis. Evaluation of three features in the intertwin membrane will provide an almost certain diagnosis about the mono- or dichorionicity of a twin pregnancy. These three features are (1) thickness of the intertwin membrane, (2) the number of layers visualized in the membrane, and (3) assessment of the junction of the membrane with the placental site for what has been described as the "twin peak" sign. In dichorionic diamniotic pregnancies the dividing membrane appears "thick"[69–71] and has a measured diameter of ≥2 mm,[72] and either three or four layers can often be identified (Fig. 24-6).[73,74] With a monochorionic diamniotic pregnancy only 2 layers of membranes will be identified, and the membrane appears to be "thin and hairlike"[73] (Fig. 24-7). D'Alton and Dudley[74] caution that a floating monochorionic diamniotic membrane may fold back upon itself and give a false impression of having four layers. These authors suggest that inspection of the membranes near their placental insertion will reduce this artifact. It should be mentioned that signifi-

cant magnification of the image is helpful in counting the number of layers. Determination of membrane thickness allows correct identification of di- or monochorionic gestation in 80 to 90 percent of cases.[68–70] Counting the number of layers adds a few extra minutes to the total scanning time but can increase the predictive accuracy to almost 100 percent.[73,74]

Initially described as the *lambda sign* by Bessis and Papiernik[75] in 1981, the "twin peak" sign was identified by Finberg[76] in 15 twin and 5 triplet pregnancies undergoing ultrasound studies during the second and third trimesters. All twin pregnancies were proven to be dichorionic and all triplet pregnancies were proven to be trichorionic by placental pathology. They described the *twin peak sign* as a triangular projection of tissue with the same echogenicity as the placenta extending beyond the chorionic surface of the placenta. This tissue is insinuated between the layers of the intertwin membrane, wider at the chorionic surface and tapering to a point at some distance inward from that surface (Fig. 24-8). This finding is produced by extension of chorionic villi into the potential interchorionic space of the twin membrane. This space exists only in a dichorionic pregnancy and is produced by reflection of each chorion away from its placenta at the place where it encounters the chorion and placenta of the co-twin (Fig. 24-9A). The *twin peak sign* cannot occur in monochorionic placentation because the single continuous chorion serves as an impenetrable barrier to the growth of the placental villi. These villi are thus excluded from extension into the potential interamniotic space of the monochorionic diamniotic twin membrane (Fig. 24-9B). In assessing the *twin peak sign* with ultrasonography, it is important that the zone of intersection of the membrane with the placenta be carefully scrutinized over as much length as can be detected. It should be mentioned that the absence of the *twin peak sign* alone does not guarantee that the pregnancy is monochorionic. Under these circumstances, evaluation of other features of the membrane previously described (i.e., thickness and number of layers) will give additional diagnostic clues regarding chorionicity and amnionicity. During first trimester transabdominal ultrasound studies on twin pregnancies, Kurtz et al.[77] found the *lambda* or *twin peak sign* to be unreliable for predicting chorionicity and amnionicity. Monteagudo et al.,[78] however, found excellent correlation of this sign with first trimester transvaginal ultrasound examinations, especially at around 9 to 10 weeks' gestation.

In some pregnancies with monochorionic diamniotic placentation, the dividing membranes may not be sonographically visualized because they are very thin. In other cases they may not be seen because severe oligohydramnios causes them to be closely apposed to the

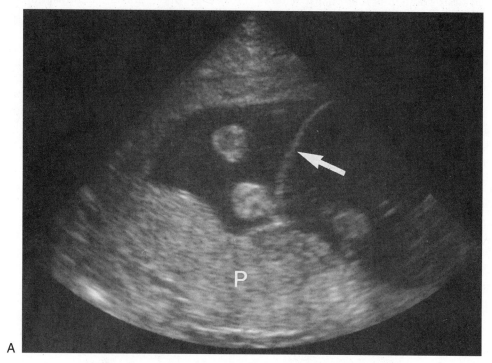

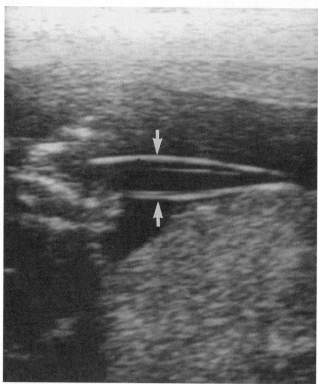

Fig. 24-6 **(A)** The dividing membrane (arrow) is thick, suggestive of a DC/DA placentation. **(B)** Visualization of four layers in the dividing membrane suggests DC/DA placentation.

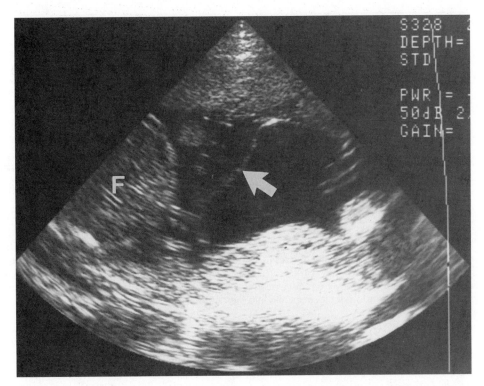

Fig. 24-7 The dividing membrane (arrow) is thin and hair-like, suggestive of MC/DA placentation.

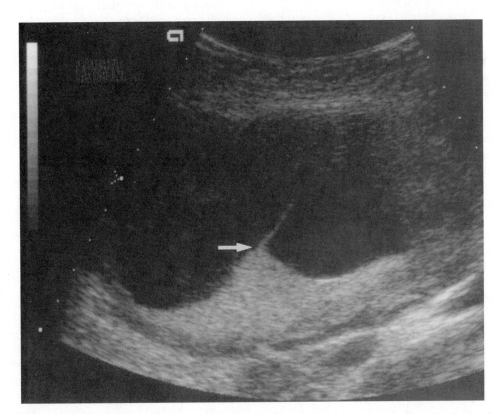

Fig. 24-8 "Twin peak" sign appears as a triangular extension of placental tissue, wide at the placental surface and tapering to a point at its junction with the intertwin membrane (arrow).

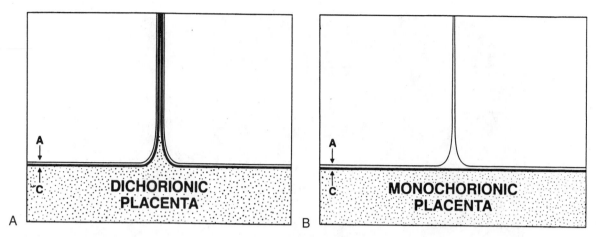

Fig. 24-9 **(A)** In a dichorionic pregnancy with fused placentas, both the amnions (A) and the chorions (C) reflect away from the placental surface at the point of origin of the septum. This creates a potential space in direct continuity with the chorionic villi and into which they can extend. **(B)** In a monochorionic twin pregnancy, the septum is formed by reflection of the two amnions away from the placenta. There is a continuous single chorion, which provides an intact barrier, preventing extension of placental villi into the potential interamniotic space.

fetus in that sac. This results in a "stuck twin" appearance, where the trapped fetus remains firmly held against the uterine wall despite changes in maternal position (Fig. 24-10).[68] Diagnosis of this condition confirms the presence of a diamniotic gestation, which should be distinguished from a monoamniotic gestation where dividing membranes are absent. In the latter situation free movement of both twins, and occasionally entanglement of their umbilical cords, can be demonstrated.[79]

Doppler Studies in Multiple Gestation

Advances in Doppler ultrasound technology within the past decade have made it possible to evaluate fetoplacental hemodynamics in normal and abnormal pregnancies. Several studies in singleton pregnancies have demonstrated that abnormal Doppler velocimetry in the umbilical artery (UA) and other fetal vessels is often associated with fetal IUGR, pregnancy complications, and adverse perinatal outcome.[80-83] Although some investigators favor continuous wave systems, we think that Doppler studies in multiple gestations are best performed using a pulsed Doppler duplex system to be certain that the vessel being studied belongs to a targeted fetus.

In 32 uncomplicated twin pregnancies where both fetuses were AGA, Giles et al.[84] found that the umbilical artery systolic/diastolic (S/D) ratios were similar to those of normal singleton AGA fetuses. Their findings were confirmed by Gerson et al.,[85] who prospectively studied 65 normal twin pregnancies between 20 and 39 weeks' gestation. These authors reported that umbilical artery S/D ratios in normal twins decrease with advancing ges-

tation and that the relationship between S/D ratio and gestational age is the same in singleton and normal AGA twins. These studies, and our own observations, suggest that the umbilical artery S/D ratios in fetuses of a twin gestation can be evaluated as if two singleton fetuses were being assessed.

Fetal growth retardation in singleton pregnancies is often associated with abnormal Doppler studies, which may precede documentation of the IUGR by sonographic biometry or abnormalities in other tests of fetal well-being.[83] These observations are consistent with histologic evidence that abnormal umbilical artery wave forms may reflect vascular lesions in the placenta, which can be presumed to increase resistance to blood flow through the umbilical arteries.[86] Similar alterations in umbilical artery S/D ratios have been documented in some growth-retarded twins. In their study of 76 twin pregnancies, Giles et al.[84] had 33 patients in whom one or both twins were SGA; in 78 percent of these pregnancies at least one fetus had an elevated S/D ratio. Farmakides et al.[87] performed Doppler studies in 43 twin pregnancies and tried to predict growth discordancy by examining S/D ratio differences in each twin pair. They found that a ratio difference of 0.4 or more between the twins was predictive of a weight difference of more than 349 g, with a sensitivity of 73 percent and specificity of 82 percent. Similar observations were reported by Saldana et al.[88] These investigators found that an S/D ratio difference of 0.4 or more was a better predictor than ultrasound for birth weight discordancy in the SGA/AGA twin pairs, but was poor in predicting discordant weight in the SGA/SGA, AGA/AGA, or AGA/LGA twin pairs. They also suggested that in order to obtain maximal information the absolute S/D ratios as well as differences in these ratios must be carefully evaluated in all cases.

Opinions vary regarding the usefullness of routinely performing Doppler studies in all twin pregnancies. Two studies illustrate this controversy. The first, by Giles et al.,[89] described the clinical management and pregnancy outcome in a study group of 112 women with twin gestations in whom results of two or more Doppler studies were made available to the patients' obstetricians. These results were compared with a group of 95 patients in whom Doppler studies were performed, but not reported to the clinicians. In the study group the first test was performed at 28 to 32 weeks' gestation, and this was repeated 4 to 5 weeks

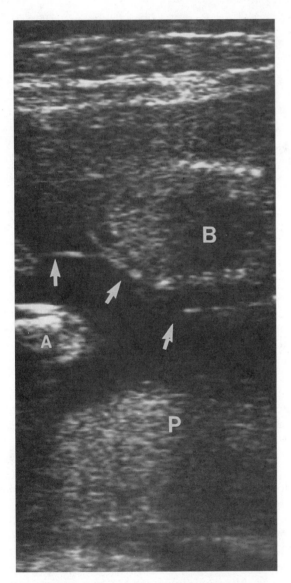

Fig. 24-10 Twin gestation with severe oligohydramnios in sac of twin B. The separating membrane (*arrows*) is closely apposed to this fetus and was visualized with difficulty. Sac of twin A showed severe polyhydramnios. P, placenta.

later if the initial study was normal. If, however, a Doppler evaluation was abnormal, further studies were repeated as often as once a week, along with nonstress tests and sonographic studies. Patients were delivered if their nonstress tests were persistently abnormal or serial sonographic studies showed failure of fetal growth. In this series a significant reduction in perinatal mortality and morbidity was noted in the study group. It is interesting that the improvement in outcome was achieved without any appreciable differences in gestational age at delivery or mode of delivery between the two study groups. The second study[90] was a prospective evaluation of 89 twin pregnancies where an attempt was made to determine the predictive value of umbilical artery Doppler studies in identifying twin fetuses destined to be SGA at birth. Serial Doppler recordings were made from each twin once a month from 22 weeks' gestation until delivery, but the results were not made available to the patients' clinicians. Thirty-two of the 178 infants in this series were SGA at birth, but only 24 of the 82 Doppler studies performed in the growth-retarded fetuses were abnormal, giving an overall sensitivity of 29 percent and a positive predictive value of 34 percent. This study, therefore, did not confirm the relatively high predictive value of Doppler studies for SGA twins reported by other investigators.[84,87]

A few more recent studies have also attempted to evaluate the usefulness of Doppler velocimetry in predicting twin fetuses, that are small for gestational age, those with TTS, and those with discordant growth.[91-94] In a longitudinal prospective study by Degani et al.,[92] serial ultrasound biometry and Doppler studies were performed at monthly intervals in 37 twin pregnancies. While the overall sensitivity of Doppler alone for predicting an SGA fetus was only 58 percent, abnormal Doppler findings preceded sonographic diagnosis of SGA by about 3.7 weeks. A combination of sonographic and Doppler parameters improved the sensitivity to 84 percent, suggesting that Doppler velocimetry complements real-time ultrasonography in the early detection of abnormal growth in twin pregnancies. Gaziano et al.[91] found an increased incidence of SGA infants in patients with abnormal Doppler studies, and the incidence of other adverse pregnancy complications, including stillbirth and major anomalies, was also found to be high in this group.

From our review of the current literature, we are not convinced that Doppler studies need to be routinely performed as part of the antepartum surveillance of women with multiple gestations. However, when IUGR is suspected in one or more fetuses, Doppler velocimetry is a useful adjunct in assessing and following these pregnancies.

Our routine for the surveillance of patients with multiple gestations is as follows:

1. Initial ultrasound evaluation is performed at 18 to 20 weeks' gestation. This includes standard biometry to confirm gestational age and the size of each fetus, assessment of amniotic fluid volume in each sac, and evaluation of each fetus's anatomy to rule out morphologic anomalies. An attempt is made to determine chorionicity by examining fetal gender, the number of placentas, the thickness as well as number of layers in the membrane separating the sacs, and the presence or absence of the *twin peak sign*.

2. If the first study is normal, subsequent scans for fetal growth are performed at 24 to 26 weeks and every 3 to 4 weeks thereafter as long as fetal growth and amniotic fluid volume in each sac remains normal.

3. If there is evidence of IUGR, discordant fetal growth, or discordant fluid volumes, fetal surveillance is intensified and includes frequent nonstress testing along with biophysical profile and Doppler velocimetry studies. Because absent end diastolic or reversed diastolic flow can be a predictor of poor outcome or imminent death in utero, serious consideration is given to delivering patients with these findings if the healthy fetus is mature enough for an elective delivery.

Abnormalities Associated With Multiple Gestation

Twin to Twin Transfusion Syndrome

Benirschke and Kim[5] state that, as a group, MZ monochorial twins have greater disparity in weight than do dichorial twins. A comparison of dichorial MZ and DZ twins with MZ twins having a monochorial placenta shows this effect on birth weight to be due entirely to the type of placentation and not zygosity. This finding is best explained by the twin-to-twin transfusion syndrome (TTS).

To our knowledge, TTS in humans has only been reported in association with monochorionic placentas. On very rare occasions, vascular communications may exist between dichorial placentas, even in the case of DZ twins as evidenced by the occurrence of blood group chimeras,[5] but these anastomoses are the rule rather than the unusual exception among monochorionic twins. The potential for the transfusion syndrome occurs when the arterial circulation of one twin is in communication with the venous circulation of the other through arteriovenous shunts in a "common villous district" (Figs. 24-11 and 24-12).[5] In this situation, one fetus becomes a donor that transfuses its co-twin. The donor becomes anemic and growth retarded. Although occasionally it may become hydropic as a result of high-

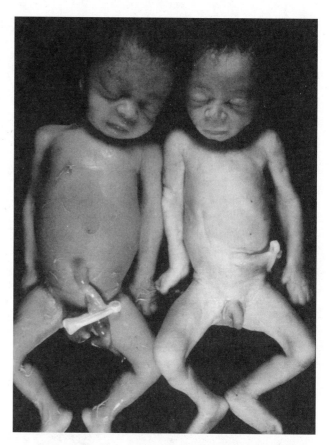

Fig. 24-11 Stillborn male twins at 31 weeks' gestation, secdary to the TTS. The plethoric twin on the left weighed 1,670 g and the anemic growth retarded twin on the right weighed 1,300 g.

output failure, more frequently this twin is significantly smaller than the other. The recipient, on the other hand, becomes polycythemic and can suffer from congestive heart failure as a result of circulatory overload. Thromboses of peripheral vessels may also develop in association with its hypertransfused state.

The perinatal mortality associated with TTS may be as high as 70 percent. Two studies[96,97] suggest that the three antenatal factors that almost invariably predict a fatal outcome in these pregnancies are (1) an early gestational age at diagnosis with delivery before 28 weeks, (2) severe hydramnios requiring therapeutic amniocentesis, and (3) fetal hydrops. If hydramnios develops early, premature labor often occurs before the third trimester.

Furthermore, it appears that if the birth weights of MZ twins differ by less than 20 percent, the difference will usually not persist during later development. If, however, the weights are discrepant by more than 25 percent, differences in height, and in some cases developmental delay, may persist into adult life.[95]

TTS can be ultrasonically detected in utero.[98] When severe, the syndrome usually manifests itself clinically as a result of hydramnios that is almost always found to exist in the sac of the larger twin. Sonographic criteria that provide an almost unequivocal antenatal diagnosis of TTS include (1) the presence of same-sex twins with a single placenta; (2) thin (two-layer) separating membrane between the sacs; (3) significant discordance in fetal growth (although this is not inevitably present); (4) discordant amniotic fluid volume with polyhydramnios in the sac of the larger recipient twin and possibly a "stuck twin" appearance as a result of oligohydramnios in the sac of the donor twin; and (5) signs of hydrops or cardiac failure in either fetus, but this generally occurs more frequently in the larger twin.

When twins of unequal size are discovered on ultrasound examination, it is important to distinguish the transfusion syndrome from a pregnancy in which one fetus is growth retarded but the other is developing normally. In the latter situation the normal twin is usually surrounded by an appropriate quantity of amniotic fluid, and oligohydramnios may or may not be present in the other sac. In TTS, however, hydramnios and ultrasonic evidence of hydrops are often noted in association with the larger twin, while the donor is smaller than it should be and not simply smaller than its larger sibling. This latter point may be useful in ruling out a third uncommon situation, namely, that of a normal fetus and a larger hydropic co-twin that is anomalous or erythroblastotic.

In addition to the usual fetal biometry and amniotic fluid volume assessment by ultrasonography, several investigators have attempted to evaluate the role of Doppler velocimetry studies in making or confirming a diagnosis of TTS. To date, these studies have only provided conflicting data. Farmakides et al.[87] reported two cases in which umbilical artery waveforms of the twins were discordant and concluded that a simultaneous observation of high and low resistance S/D ratios was highly suggestive of this diagnosis. On the other hand, in eight cases where the diagnosis was documented or strongly suspected, Giles et al.[84] found no difference in interpair S/D ratios. Pretorius et al.[99] also reported eight cases of TTS and found no consistent pattern of umbilical artery doppler S/D ratios. Other studies have reported similar observations on umbilical Doppler velocimetry in twin pregnancies with TTS.[91,92,94] The mortality rate in the study by Pretorius et al.[99] was very high, with five of eight pregnancies ending in fetal or neonatal death of both twins. In all five instances of perinatal loss, one or both of the twins had either absent or reversed diastolic flow. The authors concluded that, although evidence of greatly increased placental resistance (i.e., absent or reversed diastolic flow) is not helpful in identifying the donor from the recipient twin, it invariably predicts a poor outcome. In their study of umbilical artery blood flow velocity waveforms, Ishimatsu et al.[100] were also unable to identify any distinctive findings in patients with TTS. However, the presence of cardiomegaly in five recipient twins, with tricuspid regurgitation and a biphasic umbilical vein waveform in three others, led them to suggest that these findings may be more diagnostic than umbilical artery Doppler velocimetry and representative of the hemodynamic changes that occur in TTS.

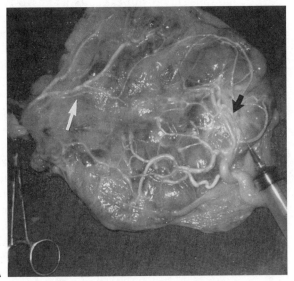

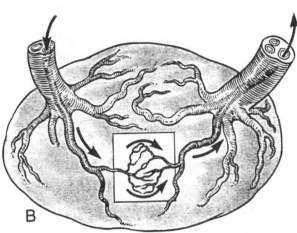

Fig. 24-12 **(A)** The placenta of a pregnancy complicated by the TTS. Milk has been injected into an artery on the "donor" side of the placenta (*black arrow*). It can be seen returning through the venous circulation on that side but is also evident in the venous circulation of the "recipient" (*white arrow*). **(B)** The arteriovenous shunt shown in **(A)**.

Other investigators have utilized much more invasive techniques in an attempt to make a definitive prenatal diagnosis of TTS. Bruner and Rosemund[101] performed cordocentesis on both twins and were unable to demonstrate consistently a hemoglobin difference of 5 g or more between the recipient and donor twins. Tanaka et al.[102] suggested the "pancuronium test," which involves cordocentesis and intravascular injection of pancuronium bromide, a nondepolarizing neuromuscular blocking agent, into one twin. Paralysis of both twins under these circumstances would confirm transplacental vascular communications and a diagnosis of TTS. The role of such invasive methods for the diagnosis of this condition is unclear, and, in our opinion, the potential risks from a cordocentesis probably outweigh the benefits of definitively establishing the diagnosis.

The pathophysiology of polyhydramnios in TTS is poorly understood. Based on their observation of significantly increased concentrations of atrial natriuretic factor (ANF) in the cord blood of recipient twins compared with donor twins in three cases of TTS, Wieacker et al.[103] suggest that chronic overload of circulatory volume in the recipient twin causes increased release of ANF from the fetal heart. This in turn results in increased fetal urine production leading to polyhydramnios. Fries et al.,[104] on the other hand, proposed a more mechanical explanation for the presence of polyhydramnios in TTS. These authors found a high prevalence of velamentous cord insertion associated with this syndrome. They concluded that this might contribute to the development of profound disparity in amniotic fluid volume because the easy compressibility of the membranously inserted cord could result in reduced blood flow to one twin. They also suggested that removal of a large volume of amniotic fluid by amniocentesis may help reduce this compressive force on the cord insertion site, thereby leading to a reversal of the fluid imbalance.

Pregnancy outcome in patients with TTS appears to depend on the number and type of vascular anastomoses between the placentas, the pressures and directions of blood flow, and the timing of the imbalanced transfusion during the pregnancy. Even though the majority of monozygotic twins have monochorial placentas and communicating vessels, only 5 to 17 percent are reported to develop a significant transfusion syndrome.[105–107] It is possible, however, that the actual incidence of TTS may be underestimated either because of the selection bias of studying liveborn twins or because the majority of dead monochorionic twins escape diagnosis at their co-twin's birth.[107] Clinical manifestations of TTS are usually characterized by the onset of acute polyhydramnios with or without associated preterm labor. Mortality rates associated with this presentation can range from 60 to 100 percent, the highest rates occurring in cases where the manifestation of this syndrome appears before 24 weeks gestation.[5,107,110,111]

Various therapeutic maneuvers have been attempted in an effort to improve pregnancy outcome in severe cases of TTS. These approaches include therapeutic amniocentesis,[112–115] laser ablation of vascular anastomoses,[116] selective feticide,[117,118] and maternal treatment with digoxin or indomethacin.[119–121] In a review of the subject in 1990, Blickstein[122] concluded that therapeutic amniocentesis had poor efficacy in these cases. However, three more recent reports consisting of 17, 9, and 27 cases of TTS[112–114] suggest that a much better pregnancy outcome can be achieved with the use of serial therapeutic amniocentesis than has so far been achieved with any other treatment modality. The overall survival in these three series ranged from 74 to 83 percent. The results of a fourth series of 19 patients were less promising, with an overall survival rate of only 37 percent. These latter investigators observed that in pregnancies with poor outcomes the intertwin disparity in fetal size and the mean amniotic fluid volume drained at each amniocentesis were greater than in pregnancies in which one or both twins survived.[115]

Isolated maternal treatment with either digoxin or indomethacin for this syndrome has not proven beneficial in improving fetal outcome.[119–121] Selective feticide of one twin in the presence of the placental vascular communications expected in TTS can have devastating consequences, including death or survival with permanent damage of the co-twin.[123] Fetoscopically directed YAG laser occlusion of placental vascular communications as suggested and reported by De Lia et al.[116] has tremendous appeal, since it aims to address the problem at its source. However, the technical expertise and special equipment required for this procedure limit its use to a very few specialized centers. Furthermore, since the sites of the vascular anastamoses must be visually located, this procedure can only be performed in patients with posterior placentas. Therefore, until such a time that a larger number of successfully treated patients is reported, this technique remains experimental and of limited applicability.

The weight of evidence from clinical reports suggests that repeated therapeutic amniocenteses provide the best option for treatment until delivery is possible.[112–114] The total number and frequency of amniocenteses must be individualized since some patients show improvement following one or two procedures whereas others may require that it be performed far more frequently. Elliott et al.[112] described one patient who underwent 10 amniocenteses between 20 and 30 weeks' gestation for the treatment of this syndrome. The volume of fluid aspirated at any one time should again be individualized, with an aim to removing as much fluid as possible from the polyhydramniotic sac and attaining a relatively "normal" fluid volume or a maximum vertical fluid pocket of about 7 cm at the end of the procedure. The role of prophylactic tocolysis in these cases remains unproven. Our clinical observations suggest that there is no particular benefit to administering routine tocolysis, unless the patient is already taking this type of medication for documented preterm labor before the amniocentesis.

Congenital Anomalies in Multiple Gestations

There is general agreement that anomalies occur more frequently in twins than in singletons, but controversy exists regarding the degree of difference. A large series from Czechoslovakia[124] reported a rate of anomalies of 1.4 percent for singletons, 2.7 percent for twins, and 6.1 percent for triplets. Among cases of twins in which anomalies were detected, both twins were affected in 14.8 percent. There were no cases of triplets in which all three infants were affected. Hendricks[125] found the frequency of anomalies to be more than three times higher in twins than in singletons, while in Kohl and Casey's series[10] the frequency was 1.5 to 2 times higher. Other studies cited by Benirschke and Kim[5] report smaller increases.

The diagnosis of a variety of morphologic abnormalities in multiple gestations has been made in utero with ultrasound. It is possible to detect anomalies of one or both fetuses or conversely to rule out specific disorders in twins who are known to be at increased risk for them. As is true for singletons, however, an ultrasonic diagnosis can only be made when a potentially detectable anatomic abnormality has become manifest at the time the fetus is studied. Neilson et al.[126] describe four cases in which anomalies in one or both twins were heralded by elevated serum AFP values. In all these patients, the abnormalities were detected by ultrasound. They also reported one case in which an elevated serum AFP value was found to be due to an intrauterine death of one twin in association with a healthy co-twin.

Anomalies Related to Twinning

Some anomalies such as acardia and conjoined twins are directly related to the twinning process. *Acardia* is a malformation that occurs in one of MZ twins, triplets, or even quintuplets with a frequency of approximately 1 per 30,000 deliveries.[5] These extremely malformed fetuses either have no heart at all (holoacardia) or only some rudimentary cardiac tissue (pseudoacardia) in association with other multiple developmental abnormal-

ities (Fig. 24-13). Aside from a single case report[127] to the contrary, these patients always have monochorial placentas and vascular anastomoses that sustain the life of the acardiac twin. Because of their isosexual status and monochorial relationship, they are considered to be MZ and therefore represent the ultimate of discordance in the development of genetically identical individuals.

Controversy exists regarding the etiology of this condition. Kaplan and Benirschke[128] believe that reversal of flow through the acardiac twin secondary to at least one artery-to-artery and one vein-to-vein connection in the placenta leads to the anomaly of twin reversed arterial perfusion (TRAP) sequence. Retrograde fetal perfusion has been documented to occur by Doppler studies in two cases.[129,130] Other authors,[95,127] however, believe that acardia is a primary defect in cardiac development, and, while the placental vascular anastomoses are necessary for survival of the affected twin, these are not responsible for the abnormalities.

There is also a high incidence of chromosomal abnormalities in these pregnancies. In 6 out of the 12 acardiac cases reported by Van Allen et al.,[131] an abnormal karyotype was found in the perfused twin, while the karyotype of the pump twin was normal. The remaining six perfused twins were chromosomally normal.

Antenatal diagnosis by ultrasound of an acardiac fetus coexisting with a normal co-twin is fairly straightforward. The anomalous twin may appear to be an amorphous mass or may show a wide range of abnormalities that depend on which organ system has failed to develop. The lower extremities and body are typically more completely developed, while the most severe abnormalities involve the upper body. The heart is frequently absent or rudimentary, and a single umbilical artery is present in approximately half the cases. As mentioned above, a retrograde pattern of fetal perfusion can be demonstrated to occur through the umbilical arteries by Doppler studies.

The pump twin, although structurally normal, is at increased risk for in utero cardiac failure, and mortality rates of 50 percent or higher have been reported.[132] When the size ratio of the acardiac to that of the pump twin is less than 25 percent, the mortality rate is diminished. However, the prognosis worsens when polyhydramnios, preterm labor, or cardiac decompensation of the pump twin are present.[132] Various techniques have been used to interrupt the vascular communication between the twins in an effort to improve outcome of the normal pump twin. These methods have included hysterotomy with physical removal of the acardiac twin,[133–135] ultrasound-guided injection of thrombogenic materials into the umbilical circulation of the acardiac twin,[136–138] and, more recently, ligation of the

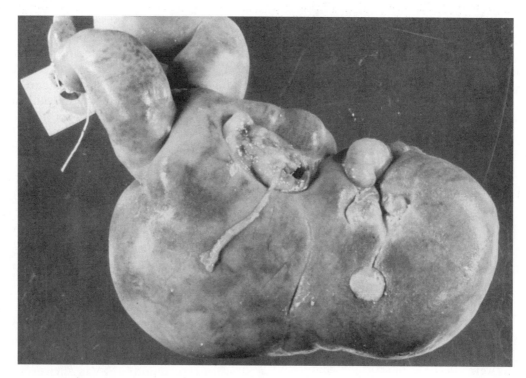

Fig. 24-13 Acardiac twin. (Courtesy of Dr. James Wheeler, Department of Surgical Pathology, Hospital of the University of Pennsylvania, Philadelphia, PA.)

umbilical cord of the acardiac twin under fetoscopic guidance.[140]

Nance[95] presents evidence to suggest that a group of birth defects involving midline structures, including symmelia, extrophy of the cloaca, and midline neural tube defects, may be associated in some way with the twinning process. Symmelia is a rare severe defect that results from fusion of the preaxial halves of the developing hindlimb buds. This produces a single lower extremity with a knee that flexes in the opposite direction from normal. The incidence of this condition is 100 times higher in MZ births than in singletons. MZ twins have also been shown to have a higher frequency of neural tube defects than singletons,[141] and they are often discordant for the abnormality. Nance[95] suggests that the MZ twinning process, with its attendant opportunities for asymmetry, cytoplasmic deficiency, and competition in utero, may favor the discordant expression of midline neurologic defects in these twins. He also cites evidence that 10 percent of all cases of extrophy of the cloaca occur in like-sex twins. In each of these instances, it is unclear whether the occurrence of a malformation somehow initiates the twinning process or whether a common factor predisposes to both events. Discordance is often, but not always, a feature of these midline defects in MZ twins.

Conjoined twins occur with a frequency of about 1 per 50,000 deliveries and in approximately 1 per 600 twin births.[142–144] The most famous conjoined twins were Chang and Eng Bunker, who were born in Siam in 1811. These xiphopagus twins (i.e., joined by a band of tissue extending from the umbilicus to the xiphoid cartilage) lived unseparated for 63 years. P.T. Barnum exhibited them extensively for a number of years. At the age of 31, they married two sisters who bore them a total of 26 children. They died within hours of each other.[142–144]

The precise etiology of conjoined twinning is unknown, but the most widely accepted theory is that incomplete division of an MZ embryo occurs at approximately 13 to 15 days postovulation. Most conjoined twins are female, with the ratio of females to males being reported as 2:1 or 3:1. The majority of these infants are delivered prematurely and are stillborn.[143] They are classified according to their site of union. The most common location is the chest (thoracopagus)(Fig. 24-14), followed by the anterior abdominal wall from the xiphoid to the umbilicus (xiphopagus), the buttocks (pygopagus), the ischium (ischiopagus), and the head (craniopagus).[143] Organs may be shared to varying degrees in different sets of twins. Major congenital anomalies of one or both twins are not uncommon and must be carefully searched for before definitive therapy is attempted. The success of surgical separation depends on the degree of union, the absence of major anomalies, and the presence of separate hearts.

In 1950, Gray et al.[145] proposed a set of radiographic criteria for diagnosing ventrally fused twins. These include the twins facing each other with their heads at the same level and thoracic cages in close proximity, loss of the usual flexion of the fetal spines and occasionally hyperextension of the cervical spines, and no change in position of the twins relative to each other in response to external manipulations or spontaneous fetal movement. Hydramnios is said to be present in almost one-half the reported cases of conjoined twins. Amniography or fetography and even contrast magnetic resonance has been used in establishing the diagnosis radiographically because these procedures outline the fetal body contours and can demonstrate a shared gastrointestinal tract.[146] Ultrasound, however, has become the safest and most reliable way to make this diagnosis in utero. Several reports have been published in which sonographic detection of this condition has been made antenatally.[146–154] In some cases the diagnosis has been made as early as the first trimester of pregnancy by transvaginal ultrasound.[155,156] Since fetal soft tissues are so well visualized with today's sonographic equipment, invasive imaging procedures such as amniography should no longer be necessary.

Once antenatal diagnosis has been established, the

mode of delivery can be planned. Vaughn and Powell[143] point out that dystocia, previously thought to be rare since the union between conjoined twins is usually soft and pliable, may be a frequent and serious complication if vaginal delivery is attempted at term. When dystocia occurs in this setting, intrauterine surgical separation may be required that could result in devastating consequences for the fetuses and significant trauma to the mother. Craniopagus twins will not develop this type of dystocia, since it can be anticipated that they will deliver "in series" rather than "in parallel." It is therefore recommended that most conjoined twins be delivered by cesarean section at term or if they present in premature labor and are potentially salvageable.[143] If they are considered to have a poor chance of surviving and are small enough to pass through the birth canal without damaging the mother, vaginal delivery might be the preferable option. Compton[157] states that with near-term-sized twins, cesarean delivery seems indicated even if the fetuses are dead. This is based on the premise that maternal morbidity from elective cesarean delivery is predictably lower than that associated with failed partial vaginal delivery necessitating an emergency operative delivery.

Chromosomal Anomalies in Twins

Most known chromosomal anomalies have been reported in twins.[158] DZ twins are usually discordant for these anomalies, and, surprisingly, MZ twins may be as well. Such MZ twins are known as heterokaryotypes, and, in these cases it is assumed that a maldistribution of chromosomal material occurred at about the same time as the twinning process itself (postzygotic nondisjunction). Phenotypically dissimilar MZ twins may have similar chromosome mosaicisms in lymphocyte cultures due to the shared fetal circulation in a monochorionic placenta, but show different karyotypes in fibroblast cultures.[159,160] Since most cytogenetic studies are done on lymphocytes, it is likely that some heterokaryotypic twins have gone unrecognized.

The incidence of Down syndrome is no more common in twins than in singletons. Although most pregnancies with one affected fetus are DZ, there have been rare cases of MZ twins discordant for trisomy 21.[161] Concordance for Down syndrome in DZ twins is unusual, but several investigators have reported a somewhat higher concordance rate in DZ pairs than would be expected, even allowing for maternal age.[162,163] This suggests that some women may have a unique predisposition to this chromosomal anomaly.

Death of One Twin in Utero

The death of one twin in utero is not an exceptionally rare event. Hanna and Hill[164] report a frequency of 2.2 percent over an 8-year period at their institution and

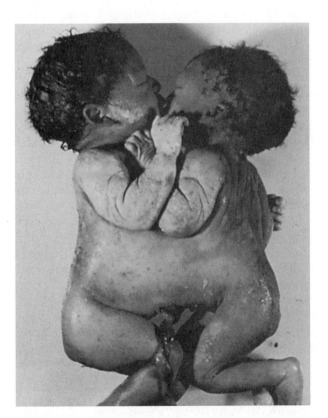

Fig. 24-14 Conjoined twins attached at the chest orthorocopagus, the most common form of conjoined twins. They originate at the primitive streak stage of the embryonic plate (13 to 15 days). (Courtesy of Dr. James Wheeler, Department of Surgical Pathology, Hospital of the University of Pennsylvania, Philadelphia, PA.)

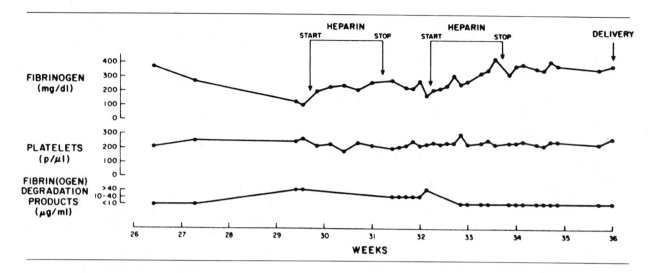

Fig. 24-15 Effect of heparin therapy after 26 weeks' gestation on the platelet count and the plasma concentrations of fibrinogen and fibrin/fibrinogen degradation products in a pregnancy complicated by the death of one twin in utero. (From Romero et al.[167] with permission.)

cite a Swiss study in which the frequency was 6.8 percent over a period of almost 10 years. When only one twin dies in utero, it may become a fetus papyraceous. In that condition, the fluid is resorbed from the dead twin's body, and it is compressed into the adjacent membranes by the growth of the living fetus. Benirschke and Kim[5] observed that this process can occur with any kind of placentation and that it is occasionally seen as a result of TTS.

When a dead twin remains undelivered, a legitimate medical concern is the potential for disseminated intravascular coagulation (DIC) in the mother. DIC is well known to complicate some cases of retained dead fetuses in singleton pregnancies.[165] This is usually a chronic process that develops slowly in response to the release of thromboplastic material from the degenerating fetus into the maternal circulation. Although most cases of this type of DIC have been reported in the setting of a singleton gestation, it can occur after the death of one fetus in a multiple gestation.[166]

Romero and colleagues[167] have reported a case in which death of one twin in utero was detected at 26 weeks' gestation (Fig. 24-15). Three and a half weeks later, the patient's fibrinogen level had fallen from an initial value of 370 to 95 mg/dl. In response to an intravenous infusion of heparin, the hypofibrinogenemia was reversed. After a total of 25 days of therapy, the heparin was stopped and the patient went on to vaginally deliver a 2,040 g infant with Apgar scores of 9 and 9 and a macerated 350-g stillborn at 36 weeks. Successful reversal of maternal antepartum DIC with the use of heparin has been documented in two other patients. In each case, the pregnancy was prolonged by 10 weeks, with a normal outcome of the surviving

twin.[166,168] These cases demonstrate that in selected situations it may be possible to treat the chronic maternal coagulopathy associated with a retained dead twin in order to allow a premature living co-twin to continue to develop in utero. Fortunately, however, this is usually not necessary because the incidence of this complication must be very low. In our experience with 61 cases in which death of an anomalous twin fetus was selectively induced during the second trimester, none of the patients developed evidence of clinical DIC. Similar experiences have been reported by other groups.[123,169–171] Therefore, as Hanna and Hill[164] have suggested, when death in utero of one twin is detected before 34 weeks, conservative management is the wisest course. This should include weekly maternal clotting profiles and serial assessments of fetal growth and well-being. Since no coagulation disorders have been observed after spontaneous or induced first trimester death of one or more fetuses in a multiple gestation, monitoring of coagulation factors may not be necessary when losses occur prior to 13 weeks.

It should be noted that normal maternal fibrinogen levels or successful reversal of a consumption coagulopathy within the maternal circulation does not ensure that the surviving fetus will be unaffected by the process. If vascular anastomoses exist within a monochorial placenta, the shared circulation may permit embolization of thromboplastic material from the dead fetus directly into its living sibling. This phenomenon has been cited as the cause of intrauterine DIC and bilateral cortical necrosis,[172] multicystic encephalomalacia,[173] and other structural abnormalities[174,176] in liveborn MZ twins with stillborn macerated co-twins. Another mechanism that may lead to death or damage of the living twin could be massive loss of blood from the survivor into the circulation of the other twin because of the lowered resistance that results from its death.[178] By contrast, because of the virtual absence of shared circulations, damage to the survivor should occur far less frequently in the case of DZ twins or MZ twins with dichorionic placentas. Carlson and Towers[177] presented a series of 17 multiple gestations in which one fetus had died and also reviewed the literature on this subject. They concluded that there is a 17 percent chance that the "surviving twin" in a monochorionic gestation will either die or suffer major morbidity, whereas these possibilities are unlikely to occur in the surviving twin in a dichorionic gestation. These authors also observed a high incidence of lesser morbidities, including abnormal fetal heart rate tests, cesarean delivery for fetal distress, IUGR, and hyperbilirubinemia in the surviving infant, but the rates of these complications were similar in mono- and dichorionic twin pregnancies.

In a series of 43 twin pregnancies with single fetal death occurring at various times during pregnancy, Prompeler et al.[179] observed that the loss of one of the twins in the first trimester did not impair the development of the surviving twin. If, however, fetal death occurred after 17 weeks' gestation, there was an increased risk of IUGR, preterm labor, and perinatal mortality.

Selective Termination of an Anomalous Fetus

The diagnosis of discordancy for a major genetic disease before the time limit for legal termination of pregnancy in the second trimester places the parents in an extremely difficult position. Traditional choices in this setting are to terminate the pregnancy and sacrifice one normal child or to continue the pregnancy with the certain knowledge that one child will be afflicted with a devastating condition. A third choice is to perform selective termination of the affected fetus, anticipating healthy survival of the normal twin. Technical difficulties associated with this latter procedure in DZ twin gestations have, to a large extent, been resolved since its first description over a decade ago.[180] However, several issues pertaining to technical, medical, ethical, and psychological problems related to this procedure must be carefully considered and discussed with the parents.

Several techniques that have been successfully used to perform selective terminations in the second trimester include cardiac puncture with exsanguination,[180,181] removal of the affected twin at hysterotomy,[182] cardiac puncture with intracardiac injection of calcium gluconate,[170] air embolization through the umbilical vessels with fetoscopic guidance,[169] and intracar-

diac injection of potassium chloride.[183] The latter approach has gained acceptance because of its safety and is currently preferred both for selective termination procedures in the second trimester and for elective reduction of fetal numbers in the first trimester.[36–38,125,171,182]

Immediate problems and complications associated with selective termination procedures include selecting the wrong fetus, technical inability to accomplish the objective of the procedure, premature rupture of the membranes, infection, and loss of the entire pregnancy. Before initiating the procedure, it is critical that the abnormal fetus be correctly identified. When the indication for selective termination is an abnormal karyotype diagnosed by amniocentesis or chorionic villus sampling, a sonographically identifiable marker may or may not be present. If the gender of the twins is different, or the affected fetus has a gross morphologic anomaly such as hydrocephaly or omphalocele, the abnormal twin can be easily identified by sonography. However, in the absence of such visible signs, one must rely on the information provided from the original diagnostic procedure, which frequently has been performed elsewhere and several days or weeks before the patient presents herself to undergo the termination. In those cases where accurate localizing information is lacking, fetal blood sampling and rapid karyotype determination should be performed to re-identify the abnormal fetus before selective termination is attempted. Furthermore, in all cases a sample of fetal tissue must be obtained from the terminated twin to confirm that the correct fetus has been selected.

In a series of 61 patients who underwent this procedure at the Mount Sinai Medical Center, the abnormal fetus was correctly identified in all cases (unpublished data). The first seven cases in this series were performed with a variety of techniques (e.g., exsanguination, pericardial tamponade with normal saline, or intracardiac injection of air), and four of those pregnancies were lost completely as a result of complications of the procedure. The next 56 cases, however, were all performed by injection of potassium chloride into the umbilical vein or a cardiac chamber of the affected fetus. Only three (5.4 percent) of these latter pregnancies were lost completely, and those losses all occurred from 3 to 4 weeks after the procedure had been performed. Fifty of the 56 potassium chloride cases were performed on twins, 5 on triplets, and 1 on quadruplets. Forty-nine of these cases were done between 17 + 5 and 23 + 3 weeks and the other seven between 13 + 5 and 16 + 0 weeks.

In the 50 cases of twins who underwent selective termination to a singleton by injection of potassium chloride, there were two complete pregnancy losses (4.9 percent), and the mean gestational age at delivery was

35.5 ± 4.9 weeks. When the 16 patients whose procedures were performed before 20 weeks were compared with the 34 done after that time, the latter had a statistically increased chance of delivering earlier than 37 weeks, to undergo premature rupture of the membrane or preterm labor, and to have birth weights less than 2,500 g. Furthermore, if the presenting twin was the one that was terminated, there was a trend toward an increased incidence of premature rupture of the membrane and preterm delivery, but only having a birth weight less than 2,500 g was statistically significant.[184]

In considering selective termination of an abnormal twin, particular caution must be exercised to exclude the possibility of a monochorionic gestation. Vascular connections between fetal circulations occur in approximately 70 percent of MZ twins. In this situation, a lethal agent injected into the anomalous twin could enter the circulation of its normal sibling and result in death or permanent damage.[123] To avoid this possibility, it has been suggested that pericardial tamponade with an innocuous agent such as normal saline might be attempted.[185] However, even if this were technically successful it is possible that the living normal twin could exsanguinate into the vasculature of its dead co-twin because of marked decrease in peripheral resistance of the shared circulations.[123] To date most reported attempts at selective termination in monochorionic pregnancies have been followed by death of the second twin within a short time. This has led perinatologists to attempt to occlude completely the circulation of the anomalous monochorionic twin at the time of the procedure by performing cord ligation with surgical removal of the fetus by hysterotomy[123,186,187] or cord ligation by fetoscopy[140] or use of a helical metal coil,[138] biological glue (Dumez, personal communication, 1995), or surgical silk suture soaked in 96 percent ethanol[188] to induce thrombosis.

In summary, the therapeutic option of selective termination requires extensive counseling, the need to establish placental chorionicity prior to the procedure, significant technical competence, and verification of the diagnosis on the fetus that is terminated. When everything has been considered, selective termination may be the best choice for a particular set of parents in this unenviable predicament, but detailed and truly informed consent is mandatory.

First Trimester Multifetal Pregnancy Reduction

The increasingly successful use of ovulatory drugs, in vitro fertilization, and related therapies has resulted in a growing incidence of multifetal pregnancies with three or more fetuses. Because of a high risk of perinatal morbidity and mortality from premature delivery in these pregnancies, first trimester reduction[36–38] of the number of fetuses has been advocated as a method to improve outcome. The original method of transcervical aspiration of gestational sacs described by Dumez and Oury[189] has largely been abandoned. Currently, the method of choice consists of injecting a small dose of potassium chloride into the fetal thorax under real-time sonographic guidance using either a transabdominal[171,190–192] or transvaginal[193,194] approach.

At the Mount Sinai Medical Center 300 consecutive women who underwent transabdominal multifetal pregnancy reduction procedures have completed their pregnancies. Eighty-seven percent of these patients presented with either triplets or quadruplets, but 37 women initially had between five and nine fetuses. Two hundred eighty-two of these pregnancies were reduced to twins, 8 to triplets, and 10 to singletons. The latter were all done for medical indications i.e., the women were thought to be unlikely to successfully complete a twin pregnancy (unpublished data).

Two hundred seventy-four of these patients delivered one or more living fetuses at or beyond 24 weeks, and 26 (8.7 percent) of the pregnancies were lost completely. It should be noted, however, that the spontaneous loss rate prior to 24 weeks in a series of 106 triplets following documentation of cardiac activity was reported to be 20.7 percent.[195] Therefore, the losses in the multifetal pregnancy reduction series cited above almost certainly do not accurately reflect wastage due to the procedure and may, in fact, represent an improvement over natural loss rates in multifetal pregnancies.

In the Mount Sinai series the mean gestational age at delivery was 35.4 weeks for those patients delivering viable fetuses. In these 274 cases, 147 delivered at or after 36 weeks (54 percent), 96 between 32 and 36 weeks (35 percent), 23 between 28 and 32 weeks (8 percent), and 8 between 24 and 28 weeks (3 percent). Neonatal morbidity and mortality were confined to six of the pregnancies where delivery occurred between 24 + 5 and 27 + 6 weeks. Two of these infants died and four developed intracranial hemorrhages of varying degrees of severity. One infant died at 10 months of age from brochopulmonary dysplasia as a consequence of its severe prematurity. To the best of our knowledge, all of the other infants in this series have developed normally.

The experience cited above, as well as that reported in other series,[171,191–193] indicates that first trimester pregnancy reduction is technically feasible and results in the delivery of healthy infants close to term in the majority of cases. While most people would agree that perinatal morbidity and mortality are likely to improve when pregnancies with four or more fetuses are reduced to smaller numbers, the advantages of reducing triplets to twins is far more controversial. In the absence of special circumstances, we do not believe that a first trimester reduction from three to two fetuses can be justified on the basis of improving perinatal mortality. However, since three recently published series containing data on 198, 133, and 106 sets of triplets[19,195,196] indicated that 20, 32, and 24 percent, respectively, delivered at 32 weeks or earlier, a reduction in the morbidity associated with severe prematurity may result from reducing triplets to twins. Until more detailed data are available from triplet pregnancies managed conservatively under modern circumstances, it is not possible to know whether multifetal pregnancy reduction does truly reduce perinatal morbidity in these cases.

Problems Related to Placentation

Benirschke and Kim[5] note that prolapse of the cord and rupture of a vasa previa with fetal exsanguination are more common in twins than in singletons. They attribute the latter to the fact that a velamentous cord insertion occurs in 7 percent of twin placentas as opposed to 1 percent in singletons. Robinson et al.[197] found that 7.1 percent of 72 pregnancies having a velamentous insertion of the cord had associated deformational defects of the neonate. This is defined as an alteration in shape and/or structure of a part of the fetus that has differentiated normally (e.g., clubfoot). These workers speculate that competition for space between the developing fetus and the placenta due to mechanical factors that cause crowding in utero leads to fetal structural defects of a deformational nature and also alters the direction in which the placenta can grow. The latter situation secondarily causes velamentous insertion to occur when the bulk of the placental tissue is forced to grow laterally leaving the umbilical cord, which initially was located centrally, in an area that eventually becomes atrophic chorion laeve. The increased incidence of velamentous cord insertions in twin pregnancies may result from competition for space when two blastocysts happen to implant in close proximity. In support of this theory is the observation that velamentous insertions are more common in the most closely approximated twin placentas.

Monoamniotic twins are rare and have a high risk of fetal mortality. In a study from 1935, the survival rate of both twins was only 16 percent, while more recent series report double survival rates of 40 percent.[198] The high fetal mortality associated with a single amniotic sac is due to prematurity, vascular anastomoses in the placenta, and, most commonly, entanglement of the umbilical cords (Fig. 24-16). The latter is said to occur in as many as 70 percent of monoamniotic twins. Cord entanglement has been detected ultrasonically at 19 weeks in a case of monoamniotic twins discordant for an open neural tube defect.[199] Inability to visualize a membrane separating two sacs in a twin gestation is suggestive of a monoamniotic pregnancy but is not diagnostic because occasionally the membrane can remain undetected even though it is present. Townsend and Filly[200] suggest that the observation of entangled umbilical cords in the absence of a membrane separating twin fetuses provides a reliable sign for the sonographic diagnosis of monoamniotic twin gestation. They point out, though, that it is essential to trace both cords into the entangled mass before making this diagnosis. Another uncommon mishap that can result from this type of placentation is inadvertent clamping of the undelivered twin's cord after delivery of the first twin. McLeod and McCoy[201] present just such a case in which a tight cord around the neck of twin A was clamped and divided and then found to belong to twin B. After abdominal manipulation, the second twin was rapidly delivered by forceps, and both neonates survived. These workers suggest that, whenever possible, division of a cord around the first twin's neck should be avoided. They end their paper with the reminder that if the wrong cord has been severed, "immediate extraction of the second twin is essential."

The optimal management of monoamniotic twin pregnancies with respect to timing and route of delivery remains controversial. Because of an impression of increasing morbidity and mortality rates in monoamniotic twins with advancing gestations, prophylactic preterm delivery by 30 to 32 weeks has been advocated to prevent cord-related deaths late in pregnancy.[202] However, two recent retrospective studies[203,204] reviewing the outcome of 44 monoamniotic twin pregnancies found no fetal deaths after 30 to 32 weeks' gestation. The authors of the latter study[204] suggested that the decreased intrauterine space available in the third trimester may prevent extensive fetal movements and therefore cord entanglement. The investigators of both studies concluded that their data did not support any particular advantage to elective delivery of these pregnancies at 30 to 32 weeks' gestation. We believe that demonstration of fetal pulmonic maturity should be taken into account as an important determinant for timing of delivery and generally target a gestational age of 32 to 34 weeks for delivering monoamniotic twins. There is less controversy regarding the mode of delivery of these patients. Although anecdotal cases of a successful monoamniotic twin vaginal delivery may be mentioned, the potential for a disastrous outcome either from complications of cord entanglement or from fetal interlocking is substantial and makes vaginal delivery in these cases less than ideal. Therefore, cesarean delivery is recommended in all viable monoamniotic twin pregnancies.

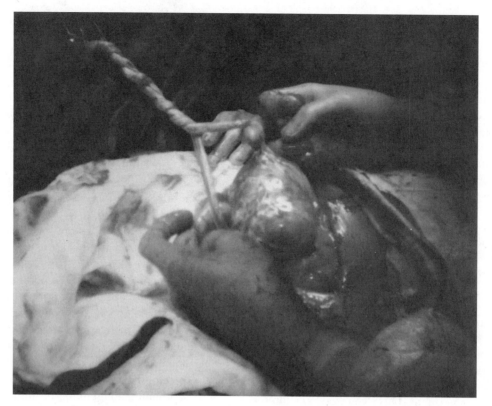

Fig. 24-16 Entangled cords found during cesarean delivery in a case of MC/MA twins.

Amniocentesis in Multiple Gestations

When Should Both Sacs Be Tapped?

In some situations it is obviously necessary to perform amniocentesis on each twin sac. Genetic studies must be performed on fluid surrounding each twin because, if DZ, they are genetically distinct individuals. Twins at risk of erythroblastosis fetalis must also have each sac tapped for optical density determinations, since one twin may be Rh positive and the other Rh negative.[205] It should be noted that twins in Rh-sensitized pregnancies have been successfully transfused in utero.[206]

The issue of pulmonary maturity studies in twins is more complex. Two series have found a close correlation between L/S ratios in amniotic fluid samples from twin sets. Spellacy et al.[207] found no significant difference in fluids obtained from both sacs when L/S ratios were studied in 14 pregnancies. Sims and colleagues[208] also found the L/S ratios of both sacs to be closely related in 20 sets of twins. Obladen and Gluck,[209] however, noted significant discrepancies in postnatal phospholipid profiles of tracheal effluent in eight pairs of twins, six of whom were delivered vaginally.

Wilkinson et al.[216] reported a case of quadruplets cesarean delivered at 30 weeks in which the presenting baby had amniotic fluid and pharyngeal aspirate L/S ratio values that were on the borderline of maturity, while those of the other three infants were clearly immature and almost identical to each other. The firstborn infant had mild respiratory distress, while the other three developed severe hyaline membrane disease. None of the neonates experienced birth asphyxia or postnatal hypothermia, and all the pharyngeal aspirates were collected within 10 minutes of birth. These investigators cite an earlier publication from their group in which the firstborn of triplets and quadruplets had also been found to have higher pharyngeal L/S ratios and less severe respiratory distress than those of their siblings delivered subsequently. This relationship was found regardless of whether the firstborn was delivered vaginally following spontaneous labor or was the presenting fetus in a cesarean delivery.

Norman et al.[211] studied 30 African women with twins, all of whom had both sacs tapped immediately before cesarean delivery. Twenty-four of these patients were not in labor at the time of their delivery, and no significant intrapair differences in L/S ratio were found in this group. Six women who were in labor, however, were found to have a significant increase in the L/S ratio of their presenting twin when compared with its sibling. In addition, both free and unconjugated glucocorticoids were found to be increased in the amniotic fluid of the presenting twin after labor had begun, but no significant difference was noted within twin sets when labor had not commenced. These latter reports suggest that the onset of labor in a multiple pregnancy may be determined by the fetus with the most mature lungs, which apparently is often the one presenting.

It is possible that one twin may be significantly more stressed in utero than the other. The concept of accelerated lung maturation in response to antenatal stress has become widely accepted.[212] It is therefore certainly conceivable that one twin may be pulmonically mature, while the other is not. Leveno et al.[213] presented a series of 42 cesarean-delivered twin pregnancies in whom amniocentesis on each sac was performed immediately before delivery. The cesarean deliveries were done for a variety of indications, and no mention was made of the presence or absence of labor. In this group of patients, there were four instances in which one twin had an L/S ratio less than 2, while the sibling's value was 2 or greater. The pair with the greatest difference had L/S ratios of 0.7 and 3.5. However, only one of these eight neonates developed hyaline membrane disease and that was a twin whose L/S ratio was 1.4 while the sibling's was 2.2. Interestingly, in this series there were seven pairs in whom only one fetus was growth retarded; IUGR was not found to increase the L/S ratio significantly in these cases. Similarly, Norman et al.[211] compared the L/S ratios from each sac before the onset of labor in eight sets of twins with only one growth-retarded fetus and were unable to find significant differences.

It appears that the stress associated with IUGR may not be sufficient to cause a significant difference in lung maturity when only one twin is affected. There has been one case report,[214] however, that raises the possibility that the stress associated with premature rupture of membranes for more than 16 hours in a presenting fetus may give it a pulmonary advantage over its co-twin with intact membranes. It is likely that other stressful processes could affect twins unequally and result in major differences regarding pulmonary surfactant production.

We believe it is reasonable to assume that in most cases of nonlaboring patients with twins, an L/S ratio from one sac will accurately reflect the status of both fetuses. If one twin appears to be abnormal for any reason, however, or if the patient is in premature labor, both sacs should be tapped to assess pulmonary maturity. Should the operator elect to tap only one sac in these situations, it should be that of the twin who appears to be normal in the former case and that of the second twin in the latter. The stressed twin, or the presenting twin in these two instances, can be assumed to have an L/S ratio at least as mature as that of its sibling, and probably more so.

The Technique of Tapping Multiple Sacs

Elias et al.[215] reported that they were successful in obtaining fluid from both amniotic sacs in 19 of 20 pregnancies during the second trimester. These workers used ultrasound to identify the lie of each fetus and then introduced an amniocentesis needle into one sac using a standard insertion technique. After aspirating some fluid they introduced a blue dye, to serve as a marker, and then removed the needle. A different needle was then inserted and the aspiration of untinged fluid indicated that the second sac had been successfully entered.

Several points should be stressed:

1. The usual precautions applying to all cases of amniocentesis must certainly be followed when multiple sacs are to be tapped. A thorough ultrasound examination should precede the amniocentesis, at which time the viability of all fetuses should be verified and their gestational ages and relative sizes assessed. The position of the placenta(s) and dividing membranes should be noted (Figs. 24-17 and 24-18) and a search for gross fetal, uterine, and adnexal pathology performed. It is particularly important to note the position of one fetus relative to the other(s) and to label the aspirated fluids appropriately, as well as placing a drawing in the patient's chart so that at a later date it is possible to correlate a particular fetus with its fluid specimen. This becomes even more critically important in the case of genetic studies if at a later date selective termination of one fetus is to be considered.

2. Direct ultrasonic visualization of the needle tip during its insertion allows for much greater precision in guiding the needle to an optimal sampling site. It also reduces the potential for traumatizing the fetus. Jeanty et al.[216] published a description of how this can easily be accomplished.

3. Use of a marker dye is very helpful in performing amniocentesis on more than one sac, but methylene blue has been associated with fetal hemolysis when injected intra-amniotically.[217] Furthermore, multiple ileal obstructions[218] or jejunal atresia[219,220] have been reported in twins whose sacs have been injected with 1 percent methylene blue at the time of a diagnostic tap in the second trimester. It is therefore recommended that either indigo carmine or Evan's blue be used rather than methylene blue. Whatever dye is used, it should not be red so as to avoid confusion in the event of a bloody tap.

4. When failure to see a separating membrane between the sacs suggests the possibility of a monoamniotic twin gestation, use of a marker dye alone may not definitively rule out this diagnosis since aspiration of colored fluid on a second needle insertion may

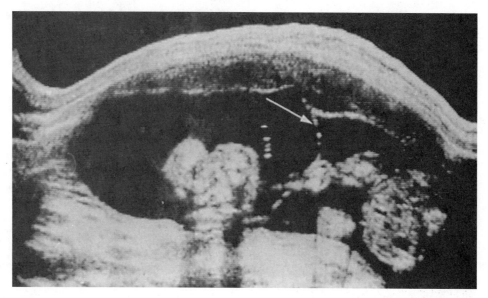

Fig. 24-17 Sagittal scan with a single anterior placenta demonstrating a vertical membrane (arrow) separating the two sacs.

represent re-entry into the first sac. Under these circumstances a technique described by Tabsh[221] may be useful in differentiating a single monoamniotic sac from separate diamniotic sacs where the membrane is simply not being visualized. Leaving the needle in place after an initial sample of fluid is withdrawn, 0.1 ml of air drawn into the syringe through a micropore filter is mixed with 0.5 ml of marker dye and 5 ml of aspirated amniotic fluid. This mixture is then injected back into the sac under firm, gentle pressure in order to create microbubbles within the

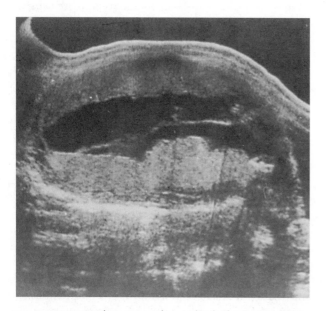

Fig. 24-18 Sagittal scan revealing individual anterior and posterior placentas with the membranes running horizontally between the two sacs.

amniotic fluid The microbubbles serve as ultrasonic contrast agents within the first sac and should demarcate it from a second sac if one is present. A site for needle insertion into the second sac can then be selected. Aspiration of colorless fluid confirms that a second sac has been entered, whereas fluid colored with dye indicates that the original sac has been re-entered. If the microbubbles are seen around both fetuses, a diagnosis of monoamniotic twins can be confirmed.

Although second trimester amniocentesis for genetic indications has become a well-accepted procedure, some studies have suggested a higher postprocedural fetal loss rate in twin pregnancies than in those with singletons.[222–224] Loss rates as high as 4.9 percent[223] to 16.7 percent[222] have been reported. These studies, however, did not address the question of whether the increased fetal wastage following amniocentesis is attributable to the procedure or to the twin gestation itself. In a recent case-controlled study, Ghidini et al.[225] concluded that second trimester amniocentesis in twin pregnancies was not associated with excess pregnancy loss and that the likelihood of fetal loss secondary to this procedure is probably of the same order of magnitude as that in singletons.

Management of Multiple Gestations

The Antepartum Period

Specialized antenatal care cannot be offered to women with multiple gestations unless they are known to be carrying more than one fetus. In areas in which universal ultrasound screening is not performed, the early diagnosis of twins depends on maintaining a high index of suspicion whenever uterine size appears to be larger than dates. Once suspected, twins can be easily diagnosed by performing a thorough ultrasound examination. After confirmation of a multiple gestation, the issue arises as to which, if any, of the various methods used in an attempt to improve perinatal outcome in these patients is worthy of consideration.

The value of bedrest in the hospital for a patient carrying twins is controversial. Marivate and Norman[2] cite five studies that reported a reduction in perinatal mortality and prematurity rates and two others that found no difference in those variables when patients with twins routinely admitted to the hospital were compared with those treated on an outpatient basis. Two prospective randomized trials published in 1984 and 1985 found no benefit from late hospital admission,[226,227] and in the latter study preterm delivery was more common among the hospitalized group.

Hawrylyshyn et al.[13] reported that in their series of 175 consecutive twin deliveries bedrest after 30 weeks had no effect on perinatal mortality. Since 70 percent of the perinatal deaths in their study occurred before the thirtieth week, these workers concluded that elective hospitalization must include the period from 25 to 30 weeks in order to exert any significant impact on both the survival and the quality of survival of twins. In support of this concept, it should be noted that Chervenak et al.[26] found that 81 percent of the perinatal mortality in their series of 385 twin pregnancies occurred before the twenty-ninth week of gestation.

Two other studies evaluated the role of early routine hospital admission for twin gestations and came to similar conclusions. The first was a multicenter randomized study from Australia in which 11 hospitals participated.[228] Of 141 women with twins in the study, 72 were assigned to outpatient care and 69 were hospitalized from 26 to 30 weeks' gestation. No differences between the groups could be demonstrated in the frequencies of major maternal complications, preterm delivery, or mean birth weights at delivery. Surprisingly, in fact, there was a trend toward greater frequency of preterm delivery and admission of neonates to the NICU in the group admitted to the hospital. Leveno et al.[229] similarly observed no differences in pregnancy outcome between 134 patients with twin gestations that were hospitalized from 24 to 32 weeks versus 177 patients who were not routinely hospitalized.

Bedrest in the hospital is expensive and disrupts normal family life. Since there is no evidence to suggest that elective hospitalization is universally beneficial for patients with twins, we feel that these women should only be hospitalized for the same indications that would be used to admit women with singletons.

Prophylactic administration of tocolytic agents to women with twins has been tried with varying degrees of success. Marivate and Norman[2] cite one report in which pregnancy prolongation and increased birth weight was associated with this approach and three other series that found no improvement in these variables when prophylactic tocolysis was administered to patients with twins. Since an increased incidence of maternal cardiovascular complications has been reported in women with multiple gestations who have been treated with β-agonists,[230] it seems prudent to restrict the use of these agents to women who are confirmed to be in preterm labor.

Results of studies using prophylactic cervical cerclage in women with multiple gestations have been disappointing.[2] Since this surgical procedure may be associated with adverse sequelae for both the mother and her fetuses, it is recommended that cerclage placement be limited to women with either a strong suggestive history or with objectively documented cervical incompetence.

In an attempt to predict the onset of labor in a series of women with twins, Houlton et al.[231] evaluated the effectiveness of a cervical assessment score based on the length of the cervical canal in centimeters minus the dilatation of the internal os in centimeters. These workers found a significant relationship between a cervical score of 0, or a decrease in cervical score, and the onset of labor within the subsequent 14 days. Similar effectiveness of this scoring system was reported by Neilson et al.[232] On the other hand, O'Connor et al.[233] found that routine cervical assessment and uterine activity measurements were not helpful in predicting preterm delivery. Nevertheless, Marivate and Norman[2] suggest that the use of the simple scoring system described above permits the selection of a group of patients with twins at increased risk for preterm delivery.

Another concept regarding early detection of preterm labor involves ambulatory home monitoring of uterine contractions with a mobile tocodynamometer. Although the efficacy of this method for detecting preterm labor in multiple gestations has not yet been evaluated with prospective randomized trials, clinical studies suggest that this may be a useful adjunct in the intensified antepartum surveillance of these patients.[19] It has been suggested that these women might benefit maximally from prophylactic bedrest in the hospital and aggressive early tocolysis for documented preterm labor. A randomized prospective study would shed some light on the efficacy of this approach, but to our knowledge this has not yet been performed.

The value of special twin clinics has been described by several investigators.[2,233] In these clinics, where all women known to be carrying twins are seen at regular intervals by the same medical team, several advantages accrue. Patients have the opportunity in this type of clinical setting to develop rapport with a small group of caregivers. This should result in an increased awareness of their special problems and may increase compliance with therapeutic directives. The patients can also talk with other women who are expecting twins and learn that their antenatal experiences are not unique. Furthermore, the medical personnel become more adept at detecting early signs of the special problems associated with twin pregnancies. Finally, and perhaps most importantly, the team of caregivers has the opportunity to develop an antenatal management protocol that is maximally effective for their population of patients.

The value of performing serial ultrasound studies to evaluate the growth and development of each fetus in a multiple gestation has been mentioned earlier in this chapter. It should also be noted that assessment of fetal well-being by simultaneous nonstress heart rate testing in twin pregnancies seems both feasible and efficacious. DeVoe and Azor[234] reported 24 sets of twins who underwent 120 simultaneously recorded nonstress tests in the third trimester. Technical problems in obtaining readable tracings were encountered in only 15 percent of cases. Reactive nostress tests were found to be associated with a good prognosis if delivery occurred within 1 week, while nonreactive nonstress tests were less specific but in some cases reflected significant distress in utero. These authors concluded that nonstress tests in twins, whether reactive or nonreactive, appear to be prognostically comparable to those previously reported in singleton third trimester pregnancies. They point out, however, that contraction stress tests are of more limited applicability in twin gestations. The two major problems encountered when contractions are stimulated in these patients are the technical difficulties associated with obtaining two interpretable external fetal heart rate tracings and the potential for initiating preterm labor.

Before 1983, three relatively large series were published describing the management of pregnancies in which three or more fetuses were involved Ron-El et al.[15] reported their experience with 29 triplet and 6 quadruplet pregnancies in Tel Aviv between 1970 and 1978. Seven of these pregnancies were conceived spontaneously, and the other 19 followed the administration of fertility drugs. Hospitalization was recommended at the beginning of the third trimester or with the onset of complications. Patients were given prophylactic oral tocolysis beginning in the second trimester and intravenous β-agonist therapy if premature contractions occurred. Depot hydroxyprogesterone caproate was administered twice weekly from mid-second trimester until pulmonary maturity was demonstrated. Dexamethasone was administered when premature contractions were documented. Cervical cerclage was per-

formed in women with prepregnancy evidence of cervical incompetence or when signs of painless cervical dilatation were recognized during prenatal examinations. The cesarean delivery rate was 44 percent and the mean birth weight was $1,830 \pm 536$ g. The overall perinatal mortality rate was 185 per 1,000.

In another series from Israel, Holcberg et al.[14] described the outcome of 31 triplet pregnancies managed between 1960 and 1979 at their institution in Beersheba. Twenty-one of these pregnancies were conceived spontaneously, and 10 followed the induction of ovulation. Triplet gestation was diagnosed earlier in the group with induced ovulation, and their period of hospitalization before delivery was longer than the group that conceived spontaneously. The most frequent antenatal complications for the entire group were preterm delivery (97 percent), pregnancy-induced hypertension (46 percent), and anemia (29 percent). Thirteen percent of patients required postpartum blood transfusions for excessive bleeding from an atonic uterus. The overall perinatal mortality rate was 312 per 1,000. The only neonatal death occurring in an infant born after 31 weeks was due to congenital malformations incompatible with life. The incidence of cesarean delivery was 32 percent. In this series, patients in whom ovulation had been induced fared significantly better than those who conceived spontaneously. The birth weights were higher, the duration of pregnancy was longer, and the incidence of pregnancy-induced hypertension and perinatal death was lower. Holcberg et al.[14] attribute these differences in outcome to the earlier diagnosis and longer hospitalizations mentioned above.

Loucopoulos and Jewelewicz[16] reported the outcome of 35 pregnancies involving 27 sets of triplets, 7 sets of quadruplets, and 1 set of quintuplets at the Sloane Hospital for Women in New York between 1965 and 1981. Six patients conceived triplets spontaneously, and the remainder became pregnant after the use of ovulatory agents. Bedrest was advised as soon as the diagnosis of multifetal pregnancy was made and hospitalization was planned at 28 to 30 weeks unless complications occurred earlier. Betamethasone was administered electively at 26 to 28 weeks and repeated weekly thereafter. Oral phenobarbitol administration, at a dose of 30 mg three times a day, was begun at the same time in an attempt to reduce the degree of neonatal hyperbilirubinemia. Tocolytic agents were not routinely used, and cervical cerclage was not performed. The cesarean delivery rate was 42 percent, and the mean birth weight was $1,815 \pm 628$ g. The overall perinatal mortality rate was 148 per 1,000.

Among four studies evaluating various management protocols in multiple gestations involving three or more fetuses, Goldman et al.[235] assessed the efficacy of elective cerclage. Out of 27 multiple pregnancies, 12 with triplets and 3 with quadruplets received elective cerclage, whereas 10 triplet and 2 quadruplet gestations did not. These investigators found that the cerclage group achieved a significantly longer mean gestation, higher birth weights, higher Apgar scores, lower rates of respiratory distress syndrome, and a significantly lower perinatal mortality rate. Lipitz et al.,[17] however, reporting their experience with 78 triplets managed between 1975 and 1988, concluded that there was no benefit of elective cervical cerclage either in prolonging gestation or decreasing fetal loss. Their observations are supported by a recent study also evaluating the role of elective cerclage in triplet pregnancies.[237] In the report of Lipitz et al.,[17] 86 percent of the patients delivered prematurely, with the mean gestational age at delivery being 33.2 weeks. The perinatal and neonatal mortality rates were 93 per 1,000 and 51 per 1,000 livebirths, respectively. A higher proportion of low Apgar scores and respiratory disorders occurred in the third infant in patients delivered vaginally. These authors recommend cesarean delivery for triplet pregnancies.

Gonen et al.[18] reported the outcome and follow-up data of 30 multiple gestations (24 triplets, 5 quadruplets, and 1 quintuplet) managed over a 10-year period from 1978 to 1988. In their study, the early neonatal mortality rate was 31.6 per 1,000, late neonatal mortality was 21 per 1,000, and the perinatal mortality was 51.5 per 1,000 live births. The incidence of respiratory distress syndrome was 43 percent, bronchopulmonary dysplasia 6 percent, retinopathy of prematurity 3 percent, intraventricular hemorrhage 4 percent, and cerebral palsy 2 percent. Follow-up of 84 infants for a period of 1 to 10 years showed 75 percent of them to be free from any neurologic or developmental handicap, 22 percent had mild functional delay, one infant was mildly handicapped, and one was moderately handicapped. Although all patients were not managed with the same protocol, the authors concluded that the most likely determinants of the excellent outcome in this series were early diagnosis, meticulous antenatal care, early hospitalization, frequent evaluation of fetal well-being, cesarean delivery, presence of a trained neonatologist for each neonate at the time of delivery, and the resources of a highly skilled neonatal intensive care unit.

Newman et al.[19] evaluated outpatient antepartum management and pregnancy outcome of 198 women who delivered triplets between 1985 and 1988. The study involved 24 centers, with individual patients managed at the discretion of obstetricians in both private and academic practices. All patients were managed with the assistance of ambulatory perinatal nursing to provide outpatient surveillance. Uterine activity was monitored twice a day with a portable tocodynamometer,

and daily telephone contact along with around the clock availability of the nursing staff provided a liaison between the patient and her physician. Modified bedrest was prescribed for almost all patients, but prophylactic tocolytic agents or betamethasone were used at the discretion of the individual physician. Although patients were hospitalized for either preterm labor or other medical complications, the average stay for antepartum hospitalization was only 15 days in this series. The mean gestational age and birth weight at delivery were 33.6 ± 3 weeks and 1,871 ± 555 g, respectively. The corrected perinatal survival was 95 percent, leading the authors to conclude that routine hospitalization is unnecessary for patients with triplets, and intensive outpatient surveillance is justifiable and is associated with excellent outcomes in these pregnancies.

In a recent report, 10 cases of quadruplet pregnancies managed over a 5-year period were reported by Elliott and Radin[236] with unusually excellent outcomes, including a perinatal mortality rate of zero. Their protocol involved prophylactic use of low-dose aspirin, home contraction monitoring, terbutaline pump tocolysis, and bedrest at home starting at 16 weeks gestation. The superb results obtained by this group of clinicians merit further assessment of their management approach in a larger group of patients with higher order multiple gestations.

Based on a review of the published studies and our own clinical experience, we believe that management of multifetal gestations with three or more fetuses can be achieved on an outpatient basis in most cases, but must include intensified surveillance of the mother and fetuses. Our protocol includes (1) modified bedrest at home initiated at 16 weeks gestation; (2) frequent prenatal visits with cervical assessment for evidence of effacement or dilatation (routine cerclage is not recommended, but is offered to patients with clinical documentation or historical evidence of cervical incompetence); (3) home contraction monitoring for evidence of increased uterine activity or signs of preterm labor beginning at 20 weeks gestation; (4) serial ultrasound studies for evaluation of fetal growth; (5) early initiation of weekly nonstress tests at 26 to 28 weeks' gestation; (6) hospitalization for any evidence of preterm labor or other obstetric/medical complications; (7) tocolytic agents and betamethasone restricted to patients with documented preterm labor; and (8) elective cesarean delivery recommended in all cases either at onset of labor near term or at 36 completed weeks' gestation following documentation of lung maturity.

The Intrapartum Period

A number of factors must be considered when evaluating a laboring patient with twins or reviewing series that present delivery outcomes in women with multiple gestations. These variables include the gestational age and estimated weights of fetuses, their positions relative to each other, the availability of real-time ultrasound on the labor floor and in the delivery room, and the capability of monitoring each twin independently during the entire intrapartum period. Older series may not be applicable to current practice because our ability to monitor both twins closely during labor and delivery has increased considerably in recent years.

All combinations of intrapartum twin presentations can be classified into three groups: twin A vertex, twin B vertex; twin A vertex, twin B nonvertex; and twin A nonvertex, twin B either vertex or nonvertex. In a series of 362 twin deliveries presented by Chervenak et al.,[238] these presentations were found in 42.5, 38.4, and 19.1 percent of cases, respectively. These data were similar to the findings of other investigators.[10,25]

In the series by Chervenak et al.,[238] 81.2 percent of the vertex–vertex twin gestations were delivered vaginally. These investigators, and several others cited in their paper, believe that when both twins are in vertex presentation, a cesarean delivery should only be performed for the same indications applied to singletons. This recommendation implies that both twins can be monitored during labor.

Currently, cesarean delivery seems to be the method of choice when the presenting twin is in a nonvertex position, as there are no studies documenting the safety of vaginal delivery for this group. External cephalic version of the presenting twin would be difficult, if not impossible in these patients. Furthermore, if the second twin is in a vertex presentation and faces its sibling the potential for locking exists. Khunda[239] states that frequency of locking is approximately 1 per 1,000 twin deliveries, with an associated fetal mortality of 31 percent. This condition occurs most commonly in breech–vertex presentations when the fetal chins overlie each other. It is usually not recognized until the body of the presenting twin is out of the vagina and the aftercoming head cannot be delivered. Eventually it becomes clear that entry of the first twin's head into the pelvis is being obstructed by that of the second twin. Sevitz and Merrell[240] published a case in which a vaginal delivery was accomplished and one twin survived after intravenous administration of a β-mimetic agent to a woman whose twins had locked during delivery. The more devastating consequences of this disorder, however, have been aptly described by Nissen.[241] Finally, it is possible that the second twin could complicate the delivery of the first twin in more subtle ways, such as by deflexing its head. It may eventually be shown that in some circumstances fears regarding a vaginal delivery when the leading twin presents in a nonvertex position are unwarranted, but this has not yet been convincingly demonstrated.

The management of that subset of women whose twins are in vertex–breech or vertex–transverse lies is particularly controversial. Chervenak et al.[238] cite 11 references in which depressed Apgar scores and increased perinatal mortality rates associated with vaginal breech delivery of the second twin have led some of the investigators to recommend cesarean delivery whenever twin B is in a nonvertex lie. Conflicting data have been reported, however. Acker et al.[242] found no perinatal deaths when 74 nonvertex first or second twins weighing more than 1,499 g were delivered by cesarean section or when 76 nonvertex second twins with similar birth weights were delivered vaginally. Furthermore, no statistically significant difference was found in low 5-minute Apgar scores when these two groups were compared.

Chervenak and colleagues[243] presented the intrapartum management of 93 vertex–breech and 42 vertex–transverse twin sets. Seventy-eight percent of the vertex–breech group and 53 percent of the vertex–transverse group were delivered vaginally. Seventy-six second twins were delivered vaginally by breech extraction, 16 of whom had birth weights of less than 1,500 g. Within that group there were six neonatal deaths, four intraventricular hemorrhages, and a 67 percent occurrence of depressed 5-minute Apgar scores. It should be noted, however, that there were also seven neonatal deaths and four intraventricular hemorrhages in the firstborn fetuses of the same pregnancies, all of whom were delivered in vertex presentation. At birth weights above 1,500 g, there were no neonatal deaths or documented intraventricular hemorrhages and only three cases (5 percent) of 5-minute Apgar scores of less than 7 in the group of second twins delivered vaginally by breech extraction. Chervenak et al.[243] state that their data do not prove vaginal breech delivery of the low-birth-weight second twin to be more damaging than cesarean delivery. Nevertheless, because of the documented ill effects of vaginal delivery on low-birth-weight singleton breech infants[244,245] and the absence of evidence that being a second twin gives these infants an advantage relative to their singleton counterparts, vaginal breech delivery was not advised for second twins weighing less than 1,500 g. On the other hand, if a second twin weighs between 1,500 and 3,500 g and the criteria for vaginal delivery of a singleton breech are met, this series suggests that vaginal breech delivery is an acceptable option.

The same group has also reported their experience with 25 external cephalic versions performed on 14 transverse and 11 breech malpositioned second twins.[246] Version to vertex presentation was successful in 71 and 73 percent of cases, respectively. Among the 25 attempted cases only two neonates had 5-minute

Apgar scores below 7. However, in a study reported by Gocke et al.[247] the success rate for external cephalic version of the second twin was only 46 percent. Their study analyzed 136 sets of vertex–nonvertex twins with birth weights above 1,500 g in whom delivery of the second twin was managed by primary cesarean delivery, external version, or primary breech extraction. A primary attempt at delivery of the second twin by external version was performed on 41 twins, 55 underwent attempted breech extraction, and 40 patients had a primary cesarean delivery. No differences were noted in the incidence of neonatal mortality or morbidity among the three modes of delivery. External version was associated not only with a higher failure rate than breech extraction, but also a higher rate of fetal distress, cord prolapse, and compound presentation. The authors, therefore, suggest that primary breech extraction of the second nonvertex twin weighing more than 1,500 g is a reasonable alternative to either cesarean delivery or external version.

Analyzing their own extensive experience along with a review of the published literature, Chervenak et al.[238] have made the following recommendations for patients presenting with twins in vertex–nonvertex lies. During the intrapartum period, a sonographic EFW for twin B should be determined. With current methods,[248] there is a 10 percent SD in the sonographic estimation of fetal weight so that 95 percent of the time estimates are accurate to within ± 20 percent. Therefore, using a cutoff for EFW of 2,000 g is unlikely to result in the birth of a neonate weighing less than 1,500 g. On the basis of the arguments cited above, the investigators believe that a birth weight in excess of 1,500 g is sufficient for a vaginal breech delivery, but a lesser weight is not. Regardless of the estimated weight, they suggest that an attempt be made to convert the second twin to a vertex presentation by performing an external version after the first twin has been delivered. If this proves successful, a vaginal delivery can be anticipated. If the attempted version is unsuccessful and the EFW is between 2,000 and 3,500 g, a breech extraction can be performed unless the other criteria for a singleton vaginal breech delivery are not satisfied. Recent reports support these recommendations and have documented the efficacy and safety of either external cephalic version[249] or total breech extraction[250,251] for the delivery of second nonvertex twins weighing more than 1,500 g. However, if the EFW of the second twin is less than 2,000 g, or the criteria for a singleton vaginal breech delivery are not met, a cesarean delivery should be performed following a failed external version. Evrard and Gold[252] discuss the reluctance of some obstetricians to ever consider a combined vaginal–abdominal approach to delivering twins but point out that there are some situations in which it is appropriate. Other workers have made reference to this form of delivery in a small number of patients in their twin series.[238,253]

In commenting on their series of triplets, quadruplets, and quintuplets, Loucopoulos and Jewelewicz[16] state that "the mode of delivery does not seem to play any particular role insofar as outcome is concerned. Continuous fetal surveillance, speed, and atraumatic delivery are the hallmarks of successful intrapartum management. In experienced hands, vaginal delivery should be attempted unless there is a medical indication for cesarean section." They caution, however, that general anesthesia should be used if one is contemplating vaginal delivery, since the absence of adequate uterine relaxation could make an internal version or extraction impossible and thereby increase the risk of neonatal injury. It is fair to point out that great skill with external versions and/or breech deliveries might be required in order to achieve the atraumatic but speedy delivery called for by these authors. In our opinion, only an experienced obstetrician with demonstrated expertise in these maneuvers should even consider attempting the vaginal delivery of a patient who is known to have three or more viable fetuses. We currently feel that elective cesarean delivery is the safest mode for these pregnancies.

Time Interval Between Deliveries

Another variable that many investigators have considered important in the outcome of twin pregnancies is the time interval between their deliveries. After delivery of the first twin, uterine inertia may develop, the second twin's cord can prolapse, and partial separation of its placenta may render the second twin hypoxic. In addition, the cervix can clamp down, making rapid delivery of the second twin extremely difficult if fetal distress develops. Many reports have suggested that the interval between deliveries should ideally be within 15 minutes and certainly not more than 30 minutes.[5,10,25,254,255] Most of the data in support of this view, however, were obtained before the advent of intrapartum fetal monitoring.

There are obviously situations in which expeditious delivery of the second twin is desirable shortly after the birth of the first, but this is not always the case. Several extraordinary examples attest to this fact. Mashiach et al.[256] reported a case of a woman with a triplet pregnancy in a uterus didelphys, with fetuses A and B in the right uterine horn and fetus C in the left horn. A missed abortion of fetus A was noted at 22 weeks. At 27 weeks the right horn began to contract and a macerated fetus A was delivered vaginally, but the passage of fetus B was obstructed by the vertex of fetus C. A cesarean section was then performed on the right uterine horn and a 1,080 g infant was delivered who died in 2 weeks.

Since the left horn was not contracting, it was left intact. At 37 weeks, 72 days after the first two deliveries, an elective cesarean delivery was performed, and a 2,490 g healthy infant was delivered who went home with the mother on the seventh postpartum day. These workers cite several other examples of significant delays in the delivery of twins who were located in separate uterine horns.

Woolfson et al.[257] reported the case of a woman with a single normally shaped uterus who delivered a 570 g first twin vaginally as a breech at 25 weeks. This infant died of respiratory distress in 5 days. The first twin's placenta was retained within the uterus, and the cervical os closed to less than 3 cm after delivery. The cord was cut at the level of the cervix, and prophylactic antibiotics were administered. The patient was followed with serial maternal clotting profiles and ultrasound examinations of the remaining fetus. At 32 weeks, after 53 days in the hospital following delivery of the first twin, labor resumed and spontaneous rupture of the membranes occurred. A cesarean delivery was performed and a 1,600 g infant with Apgar scores of 7 and 9 was delivered. The placentas weighed 310 and 110 g, and the patient's postoperative course was uneventful. These authors cite four other reports in which intervals varying from 14 to 84 days were reported in twin deliveries wherein tocolytics, cervical cerclage, or simple observation were the mainstays of management.

Another such case reported by Feichtinger et al.[258] achieved 12 additional weeks and delivery of a healthy second twin, following delivery and death of the first twin at 21 weeks gestation. This patient presented with preterm labor and ruptured membranes at 21 weeks. A cerclage suture that had been prophylactically placed at 12 weeks gestation was removed to allow delivery of a nonviable twin A. There was no evidence of placental separation, the sac of twin B was intact, and its heart rate monitoring was nornal. A Shirodkar type of cerclage was then placed, and the patient was treated with tocolytics, intravenous antibiotics, and vaginal antiseptic suppositories. Her subsequent antepartum course after discharge from the hospital at 24 weeks was apparently unremarkable, until readmission for preterm labor and uneventful delivery at 33 weeks gestation. The infant weighed 1,750 g and had an uncomplicated neonatal course.

The total number of reported cases in which delayed delivery of a second twin has been attempted are limited. Three recent publications report the authors' experience and a review of the literature on this subject.[259–261] These reports suggest general agreement on a management protocol for these patients, which should include high ligation of the umbilical cord of the delivered twin with an absorbable suture, prophylactic use of tocolytics, bedrest, ongoing monitoring of the patient for evidence of infection and/or coagulation disorders, and serial monitoring for growth and well-being of the viable fetus(es). Three remaining areas of controversy are the routine use of cervical cerclage, prophylactic antibiotics, and corticosteriods for enhancement of fetal lung maturity of the viable fetus(es).

It must be recognized that most of the reported cases represent spectacular successes. This type of management, however, should not be considered "standard of care." If an individual case is considered for such a treatment protocol, the potential risks, which may be considerable, along with the benefits must be discussed in detail and a fully informed consent obtained from the patient and her partner.

Rayburn et al.[253] reported the outcome of 115 second twins delivered vaginally at or beyond 34 weeks gestation after the vertex delivery of their siblings. The second twin was visually monitored ultrasonically on some occasions, and continuous monitoring of the fetal heart was performed in all cases. Oxytocin was used if uterine contractions subsided within 10 minutes after delivery of the first twin. In this series 70 second twins delivered within 15 minutes of the first twin, 28 within 16 and 30 minutes, and 17 more than 30 minutes later. The longest interdelivery interval was 134 minutes. All these infants survived, and none of them had traumatic deliveries. All 17 of the neonates delivering beyond 30 minutes had 5-minute Apgar scores of 8 and 10. In those cases with delivery intervals in excess of 15 minutes, the birth weight differential was not in excess of ±200 g when first and second twins were compared In the series reported by Chervenak et al.,[246] the fetal heart of the second twin was monitored with ultrasound visualization throughout the period between twin deliveries, and no difference in the occurrence of low 5-minute Apgar scores was noted in relationship to the length of the interdelivery interval.

It therefore seems apparent that while some second twins may require rapid delivery, others can be safely followed with fetal heart rate surveillance and remain undelivered for substantial periods of time. This less hurried approach when twin B is not in distress may reduce the incidence of both maternal and fetal trauma associated with difficult deliveries performed to meet arbitrary deadlines.

Ultrasound and the Intrapartum Management of Multiple Gestations

Ultrasound can also be useful during labor and delivery. On admission to the delivery floor, the position of each twin can be quickly and accurately assessed and viability of both fetuses confirmed by direct visualization of their hearts. Knowledge of the presentation of each twin permits the establishment of a management protocol regarding the anticipated route of delivery. If a vaginal delivery is to be attempted, the weights of both twins can be rapidly estimated. This information is particularly important for the second twin because if it is thought to weigh less than 1,500 g or more than 3,500 g, a vaginal breech delivery might not be attempted. It is also possible to rule out extension of the head when a fetus is in breech presentation by using the method described by Berkowitz and Hobbins.[262] Ballas et al.[263] cited an incidence of more than 70 percent for cord transection when 11 breeches with extended heads were delivered vaginally compared with no cord injuries when nine infants with deflexed heads were delivered by cesarean section. Although these data were derived from singleton breeches, there is no reason to believe that they could not apply to twins as well.

Both fetuses must be monitored electronically throughout labor in order to ensure their well-being. When membranes are already ruptured, a scalp electrode can easily be attached to the presenting part of twin A, and the second twin can be monitored with an external Doppler transducer. In practice, however, it is sometimes difficult to find the optimal spot from which to monitor the second twin. By using real-time ultrasound twin B's heart can be precisely located and the Doppler transducer placed accordingly. If movement of the second twin results in loss of a readable tracing, the transducer can be repositioned after real-time ultrasound has revealed the new position of twin B's heart.

When a patient with twins is taken to the delivery room, the real-time scanner should accompany her. After delivery of the first infant, real-time examination immediately and precisely establishes the position of the second twin. Visualization of the fetal heart allows twin B to be monitored for evidence of bradycardia until one fetal pole settles into the pelvis, membranes are ruptured, and a scalp electrode is applied. While visual monitoring of the heart does not provide subtle information such as a loss of baseline variability, it does permit early detection of significant deviations from the normal fetal heart rate range.

In addition to monitoring heart rate, visualization of the second twin permits both external and internal manipulations to be performed in a more controlled fashion. Externally, it is often possible to guide the vertex over the inlet by directing pressure from the ultrasound transducer over the fetal head while pushing the buttocks toward the fundus with the other hand.[262] If this is unsuccessful, an internal version can be made less difficult by visualizing the operator's hand within the uterus and directing it toward the fetal feet. This technique can reduce the confusion often experienced when a small fetal part is blindly caught, and it is unclear whether it belongs to an upper or a lower extremity.

Conclusion

The patient carrying more than one fetus presents a formidable challenge to the obstetrician. The high perinatal morbidity and mortality rates traditionally associated with multiple gestations are due to many factors, some of which can still not be altered. The extraordinary advances in technology during the past 25 years, however, have given us new insights into some problems peculiar to multifetal pregnancies as well as some tools with which to detect those problems. Early diagnosis of multiple gestations and follow-up with serial studies hold the potential for administering specialized regimens to selected patients, and this should have a beneficial impact on the outcome of those pregnancies.

10 Key Points

- Perinatal/neonatal morbidity and mortality are significantly higher in multiple gestations than singleton pregnancies.

- Any patient with a multiple gestation should be clinically managed as a high-risk pregnancy.

- The incidence of congenital structural malformations is two to three times higher in fetuses of multiple gestations when compared with those of singleton gestations.

- Ultrasound evaluation is the single most important diagnostic test in multiple gestations.

- All patients with multiple gestations should have a thorough second trimester ultrasound examination to assess for individual fetal growth, congenital malformations, amnionicity, and chorionicity.

- Twin-to-twin transfusion syndrome is a serious potential complication in monozygotic twins.

- Prophylactic cerclage, tocolytics, or hospitalization for bedrest do not have any proven advantage in the management of multiple gestations.

- In twin pregnancies with discordant growth, fetal lung maturity studies obtained from amniotic fluid of the larger twin will usually also represent similar or greater lung maturity of the smaller twin.

- The presentation of each fetus must be sonographically verified as soon as a patient with twin pregnancy comes in labor.

- As a general rule, mode of delivery should be vaginal when both twins are vertex, individualized for vertex/nonvertex twins, and cesarean section when the first twin is nonvertex. For triplets or more, the safest mode of delivery is by cesarean section.

References

1. Hrubec Z, Robinette CD: The study of human twins in medical research. N Engl J Med 310:435, 1984

2. Marivate M, Norman RJ: Twins. Clin Obstet Gynaecol 9:723, 1982

3. Kurachi K, Aono T, Susuki M et al: Results of HMG (Hurregon)–HCG therapy in 6,096 treatment cycles of 2,166 Japanese women with anovulatory infertility. Eur J Obstet Gynecol Reprod Biol 19:43, 1985

4. Australian In-Vitro Fertilization Collaborative Group: In-vitro fertilization pregnancies in Australia and New Zealand. Med J Aust 148:429, 1988

5. Benirschke K, Kim CK: Multiple pregnancy (first of two parts). N Engl J Med 288:1276, 1973

6. Cameron AH: The Birmingham twin survey. Proc R Soc Med 61:229, 1968

7. Derom C, Bakker E, Vlietnick R et al: Zygosity determi-nation in newborn twins using DNA variants. J Med Genet 22:279, 1985

8. Hill AVS, Jeffreys AJ: Use of minisatellite DNA probes for determination of twin zygosity at birth. Lancet 2:1394, 1985

9. James WH: Is Weinberg's differential rule valid? Acta Genet Med Gemellol 28:69, 1979

10. Kohl SG, Casey G: Twin gestation. Mt Sinai J Med 42:523, 1975

11. Desgranges MF, De Muylder X, Moutquin JM et al: Perinatal profile of twin pregnancies: a retrospective review of 11 years (1969–1979) at Hopital Notre-Dame, Montreal, Canada. Acta Genet Med Gemollol 31:157, 1982

12. Rattan PK, Knuppel RA, O'Brien WF: Intrauterine fetal death in twins after thirty-two weeks of gestation. Abstract 132. Society of Perinatal Obstetricians. Annual Meeting, February 1984

13. Hawrylyshyn PA, Barkin M, Bernstein A, Papsin FR: Twin pregnancies—a continuing perinatal challenge. Obstet Gynecol 59:463, 1982

14. Holcberg G, Biele Y, Jewenthal H, Insler V: Outcome of pregnancy in 31 triplet gestations. Obstet Gynecol 59:472, 1982

15. Ron-El R, Caspi E, Schreyers P et al: Triplet and quad-ruplet pregnancies and management. Obstet Gynecol 57:458, 1981

16. Loucopoulos A, Jewelewicz R: Management of multifetal pregnancies: sixteen years' experience at the Sloane Hospital for Women. Am J Obstet Gynecol 143:902, 1982

17. Lipitz S, Reichman B, Paret G et al: The improving outcome of triplet pregnancies. Am J Obstet Gynecol 161:1279, 1989

18. Gonen R, Heyman E, Asztalos EV et al: The outcome of triplet, quadruplet, and quintuplet pregnancies managed in a perinatal unit: obstetric, neonatal, and follow-up data. Am J Obstet Gynecol 162:454, 1990

19. Newman RB, Hamer C, Clinton Miller M: Outpatient triplet management: a contemporary review. Am J Obstet Gynecol 161:547, 1989

20. Levene MI, Wild J, Steer P: Higher multiple births and the modern management of infertility in Britain. Br J Obstet Gynaecol 99:607, 1992

21. Arlettaz R, Duc G: Triplets and quadruplets in Switzerland, 1985–88. Schweiz Med Wochenschr 122:511, 1992

22. Jones HA, Lumley J: Triplets and quadruplets born in Victoria between 1982 and 1990. The impact of IVF and GIFT on rising birthrates. Med J Aust 158:659, 1993

23. Alvarez M, Berkowitz RL: Multifetal gestation. Clin Obstet Gynecol 33:79, 1990

24. Luke B, Keith LG: The contribution of singletons, twins and triplets to low birth weight, infant mortality and handicap in the United States. J Reprod Med 37:661, 1992

25. Farooqui MO, Grossman JH, Shannon RA: A review of twin pregnancy and perinatal mortality. Obstet Gynecol Surv 28:144, 1973

26. Chervenak FA, Youcha S, Johnson RE et al: Antenatal diagnosis and perinatal outcome in a series of 385 consecutive twin pregnancies. J Reprod Med 29:727, 1984

27. Cetrulo CL, Ingardia CJ, Sbarra AJ: Management of multiple gestation. Clin Obstet Gynecol 23:533, 1980

28. Persson PH, Kullander S: Long-term experience of general ultrasound screening in pregnancy. Am J Obstet Gynecol 146:942, 1983

29. LeFevre ML, Bain RP, Ewigman BG et al: A randomized trial of prenatal ultrasonographic screening: impact on maternal management and outcome. Am J Obstet Gynecol 169:483, 1993

30. Jeanty P, Romero R: What does an early gestation look like? p. 34. In: Obstetrical Ultrasound. McGraw-Hill, New York, 1984

31. Timor-Tritsch IE, Blumenfeld Z et al: Sonoembryology p. 225. In Timor-Tritsch IE, Rottem S (eds): Transvaginal Sonography. Elsevier, New York, 1991

32. Smith DH, Picker RH, Saunders DM: Twin pregnancy suspected before implantation. Obstet Gynecol 56:252, 1980

33. Berkowitz RL: Ultrasound in the antenatal management of multiple gestations. p. 69. In Hobbins JC (ed): Diagnostic Ultrasound in Obstetrics. Vol. 3. Churchill Livingstone, New York, 1979

34. Landy HJ, Keith L, Keith D: The vanishing twin. Acta Genet Med Gemellol 31:179, 1982

35. Robinson HP, Caines JS: Sonar evidence of early pregnancy failure in patients with twin conceptions. Br J Obstet Gynaecol 84:22, 1977

36. Berkowitz RL, Lynch L, Chitkara U et al: Selective reduction of multifetal pregnancies in the first trimester. N Engl J Med 318:1043, 1988

37. Khalil M, Tabsh A: Transabdominal multifetal pregnancy reduction: report of 40 cases. Obstet Gynecol 75:739, 1990

38. Lynch L, Berkowitz RL, Chitkara U, Alvarez M: First-trimester transabdominal multifetal pregnancy reduction: a report of 85 cases. Obstet Gynecol 75:735, 1990

39. Finberg HJ, Birnholz JC: Ultrasound observations in multiple gestation with first trimester bleeding. The blighted twin. Radiology 132:137, 1979

40. Varma TR: Ultrasound evidence of early pregnancy failure in patients with multiple conceptions. Br J Obstet Gynaecol 86:290, 1979

41. Dickey RP, Olar TT, Taylor SN et al: Incidence and significance of unequal gestational sac diameter or embryo crown-rump length in twin pregnancy. Hum Reprod 7:1170, 1992

42. Landy HJ, Weiner S, Corson SL et al: The "vanishing twin": ultrasonographic assessment of fetal disappearance in the first trimester. Am J Obstet Gynecol 155:14, 1986

43. McKeown T, Record RG: Observations on foetal growth in multiple pregnancy in man. J Endocrinol 8:386, 1952

44. Daw E, Walker J: Growth differences in twin pregnancy. Br J Clin Pract 29:150, 1975

45. Iffy L, Lavenhar MA, Jakobovits A, Kaminetzky HA: The rate of early intrauterine growth in twin gestation. Am J Obstet Gynecol 146:970, 1983

46. Fenner A, Malm T, Kusserow U: Intrauterine growth of twins. Eur J Pediatr 133:119, 1980

47. Winick M, Brasel JA, Velasco EG: Effects of prenatal nutrition upon pregnancy risk. Clin Obstet Gynecol 16:184, 1973

48. Leveno KJ, Santos-Ramos R, Duenhoelter JH et al: Sonar cephalometry in twins: a table of biparietal diameters for normal twin fetuses and a comparison with singletons. Am J Obstet Gynecol 135:727, 1979

49. Bleker OP, Kloosterman GJ, Huidekoper BL, Breur W: Intrauterine growth of twins as estimated from birthweight and the fetal biparietal diameter. Eur J Obstet Reprod Biol 7:85, 1977

50. Schneider L, Bessis R, Tabaste JL et al: Echographic survey of twin foetal growth: a plea for specific charts for twins. p. 137. In WE Nance (ed): Twin Research: Clinical Studies. Alan R Liss, New York, 1977

51. Grumbach K, Coleman BG, Arger PH et al: Twin and singleton growth patterns compared using ultrasound. Radiology 158:237, 1986

52. Socol ML, Tamura RK, Sabbagha RE et al: Diminished biparietal diameter and abdominal circumference growth in twins. Obstet Gynecol 64:235, 1984

53. Scheer K: Ultrasound in twin gestations. J Clin Ultrasound 2:197, 1975

54. Crane JP, Tomich PG, Kopta M: Ultrasonic growth patterns in normal and discordant twins. Obstet Gynecol 55:678, 1980

55. Graham D, Shah Y, Moodley S et al: Biparietal diameter femoral length growth in normal twin pregnancies. Abstract 112. Society of Perinatal Obstetricians. Annual Meeting, February 1984

56. Shah YG, Graham D, Stinson SK et al: Biparietal diameter growth in uncomplicated twin gestation. Am J Perinatol 4:229, 1987

57. Haines CJ, Langlois SL, Jones WR: Ultrasonic measurement of fetal femoral length in singleton and twin pregnancies. Am J Obstet Gynecol 155:838, 1986

58. Dorros G: The prenatal diagnosis of intrauterine growth retardation in one fetus of a twin gestation. Obstet Gynecol, suppl. 48:46, 1976

59. Leveno KJ, Santos-Ramos R, Duenhoelter JH et al: Sonar cephalometry in twin pregnancy: discordancy of the biparietal diameter after 28 weeks' gestation. Am J Obstet Gynecol 138:615, 1980

60. Houlton MCC: Divergent biparietal diameter growth rates in twin pregnancies. Obstet Gynecol 49:542, 1977

61. Chitkara U, Berkowitz GS, Levine R et al: Twin pregnancy: routine use of ultrasound examinations in the prenatal diagnosis of IUGR and discordant growth. Am J Perinatol 2:49, 1985

62. Hill LM, Guzick D, Chenevey P et al: The sonographic assessment of twin growth discordancy. Obstet Gynecol 84:501, 1994

63. Neilson JP: Detection of the small-for dates twin fetus by ultrasound. Br J Obstet Gynaecol 88:27, 1981

64. Neilson JP: Detection of the small-for-gestational age twin fetus by a two-stage ultrasound examination schedule. Acta Genet Med Gemellol 31:235, 1982

65. Yarkouni S, Reece EA, Holford T et al: Estimated fetal

weight in the evaluation of growth in twin gestations: a prospective longitudinal study. Obstet Gynecol 69:636, 1987

66. Storlazzi E, Vintzileos AM, Campbell WA et al: Ultrasonic diagnosis of discordant fetal growth in twin gestations. Obstet Gynecol 69:363, 1987

67. Brown CEL, Guzick DS, Leveno KJ et al: Prediction of discordant twins using ultrasound measurement of biparietal diameter and abdominal perimeter. Obstet Gynecol 70:677, 1987

68. Barss VA, Benacerraf BR, Frigoletto FD: Ultrasonographic determination of chorion type in twin gestation. Obstet Gynecol 66:779, 1985

69. Mahony BS, Filly RA, Callen PW: Amnionicity and chorionicity in twin pregnancies: prediction using ultrasound. Radiology 155:205, 1985

70. Hertzberg BS, Kurtz AB, Choi HY et al: Significance of membrane thickness in the sonographic evaluation of twin gestations. AJR 148:151, 1987

71. Townsend RR, Simpson GF, Filly RA: Membrane thickness in ultrasound prediction of chorionicity of twin gestations. J Ultrasound Med 7:327, 1988

72. Winn HN, Gabrielli S, Reece EA et al: Ultrasonographic criteria for the prenatal diagnosis of placental chorionicity in twin gestations. Am J Obstet Gynecol 161:1540, 1989

73. D'Alton ME, Dudley DKL: Ultrasound in the antenatal management of twin gestation. Semin Perinatol 10:30, 1986

74. D'Alton ME, Dudley DK: The ultrasonographic prediction of chorionicity in twin gestation. Am J Obstet Gynecol 160:557, 1989

75. Bessis R, Papiernik E: Echographic imagery of amniotic membranes in twin pregnancies. p. 183. In Twin Research 3: Twin Biology and Multiple Pregnancy. Alan R Liss, New York, 1981

76. Finberg HJ: The "twin peak" sign: reliable evidence of dichorionic twinning. J Ultrasound Med 11:571, 1992

77. Kurtz AB, Wopner RJ, Mata J et al: Twin pregnancies: accuracy of first trimester abdominal US in predicting chorionicity and amnionicity. Radiology 185:759, 1992

78. Monteagudo A, Timor-Tritsch IE, Sharma S: Early and simple determination of chorionic and amniotic type in multifetal gestations in the first fourteen weeks by high-frequency transvaginal ultrasonography. Am J Obstet Gynecol 170:824, 1994

79. Nyberg DA, Filly RA, Golbus MS et al: Entangled umbilical cords: a sign of monoamniotic twins. J Ultrasound Med 3:29, 1984

80. Trudinger BJ, Giles WB, Cook CM: Flow velocity waveforms in the maternal uteroplacental and fetal umbilical placental circulations. Am J Obstet Gynecol 152:155, 1985

81. Campbell S, Pearce JMF, Hackett G et al: Qualitative assessment of uteroplacental blood flow: early screening test for high-risk pregnancies. Obstet Gynecol 68:649, 1986

82. Fleischer A, Schulman H, Farmakides G et al: Uterine artery Doppler velocimetry in pregnant women with hypertension. Am J Obstet Gynecol 154:806, 1986

83. Berkowitz GS, Chitkara U, Rosenberg J et al: Sonographic estimation of fetal weight and Doppler analysis of umbilical artery velocimetry in the prediction of intrauterine growth retardation: a prospective study. Am J Obstet Gynecol 158:1149, 1988

84. Giles WB, Trudinger BJ, Cook CM: Fetal umbilical artery flow velocity-time waveforms in twin pregnancies. Br J Obstet Gynaecol 92:490, 1985

85. Gerson A, Johnson A, Wallace D et al: Umbilical arterial systolic/diastolic values in normal twin gestation. Obstet Gynecol 72:205, 1988

86. Giles WB, Trudinger BJ, Baird PJ: Fetal umbilical artery flow velocity waveforms and placental resistance: pathological correlation. Br J Obstet Gynaecol 92:31, 1985

87. Farmakides G, Schulman H, Saldana LR et al: Surveillance of twin pregnancy with umbilical arterial velocimetry. Am J Obstet Gynecol 153:789, 1985

88. Saldana LR, Eads MC, Schaefer TR: Umbilical blood waveforms in fetal surveillance of twins. Am J Obstet Gynecol 157:712, 1987

89. Giles WB, Trudinger BJ, Cook CM, Connelly A: Umbilical artery flow velocity waveforms and twin pregnancy outcome. Obstet Gynecol 72:894, 1988

90. Hastie SJ, Danskin F, Neilson JP, Whittle MJ: Prediction of the small for gestational age twin fetus by Doppler umbilical artery waveform analysis. Obstet Gynecol 74:730, 1989

91. Gaziano E, Knox E, Bendel R et al: Is pulsed doppler velocimetry useful in the management of multiple gestation pregnancies? Am J Obstet Gynecol 164:1426, 1991

92. Degani S, Gonen R, Shapiro I et al: Dopler flow velocimetry waveforms in fetal surveillance of twins: a prospective longitudinal study. J Ultrasound Med 11:537, 1992

93. Kurmanavicius J, Hebisch G, Huch R et al: Umbilical artery blood flow velocity waveforms in twin pregnancies. J Perinat Med 20:307, 1992

94. Shah Y, Gragg L, Moodley S et al: Doppler velocimetry in concordant and discordant twin gestations. Obstet Gynecol 80:272, 1992

95. Nance WE: Malformations unique to the twinning process. Prog Clin Biol Res 69A:123, 1981

96. Bebbington MW, Wittmann BK: Fetal transfusion syndrome: antenatal factors predicting outcome. Am J Obstet Gynecol 160:913, 1989

97. Gonsoulin W, Moise KJ, Kirshon B et al: Outcome of twin–twin transfusion diagnosed before 28 weeks of gestation. Obstet Gynecol 75:214, 1990

98. Wittman BK, Baldwin VJ, Nichol B: Antenatal diagnosis of twin transfusion syndrome by ultrasound. Obstet Gynecol 58:123, 1981

99. Pretorius DH, Manchester D, Barkin S et al: Doppler ultrasound of twin transfusion syndrome. J Ultrasound Med 7:117, 1988

100. Ishimatsu J, Yoshimura O, Manabe A et al: Ultrasonography and Doppler studies in twin-to-twin transfusion syndrome. Asia Oceania J Obstet Gynecol 18:325, 1992

101. Bruner JP, Rosemund RL: Twin-to-twin transfusion syndrome: a subset of the twin oligohydramnios-polyhy-

dramnios sequence. Am J Obstet Gynecol 169:925, 1993

102. Tanaka M, Natori M, Ishimoto H et al: Intravascular pancuronium bromide infusion for prenatal diagnosis of twin-twin transfusion syndrome. Fetal Diagn Ther 7: 36, 1992

103. Wieacker P, Wilhelm C, Prompeler H et al: Pathophysiology of polyhydramnios in twin transfusion syndrome. Fetal Diagn Ther 7:87, 1992

104. Fries MH, Goldstern RB, Kilpatrick SJ et al: The role of velamentous cord insertion in the etiology of twin–twin transfusion syndrome. Obstet Gynecol 81:569, 1993

105. Robertson EG, Neer KJ: Placental injection studies in twin gestation. Am J Obstet Gynecol 147:170, 1983

106. Naeye RL: Functionally important disorders of the placenta, umbilical cord, and fetal membranes. Hum Pathol 18:680, 1985

107. Rausen AR, Seki M, Strauss L: Twin transfusion syndrome. A review of 19 cases studied at one institution. J Pediatr 66:613, 1965

108. Hoyme HE, Higginbottom MC, Jones KL: Vascular etiology of disruptive structural defects in monozygotic twins. Pediatrics 67:288, 1981

109. Brown DL, Benson DL, Driscoll SG et al: Twin–twin transfusion syndrome: sonographic findings. Radiology 170:761, 1989

110. Chescheir NC, Seeds JW: Polyhydramnios and oligohydramnios in twin gestations. Obstet Gynecol 71:882, 1987

111. Bebbington MW, Wittmann BK: Fetal transfusion syndrome: antenatal factors predicting outcome. Am J Obstet Gynecol 160:913, 1989

112. Elliott JP, Urig MA, Clewell WH: Aggressive therapeutic amniocentesis for treatment of twin–twin transfusion syndrome. Obstet Gynecol 77:537, 1991

113. Pinette MG, Pan Y, Pinette SG et al: Treatment of twin–twin transfusion syndrome. Obstet Gynecol 82: 841, 1993

114. Reisner DP, Mahony BS, Petty CN et al: Stuck twin syndrome: outcome in thirty-seven consecutive cases. Am J Obstet Gynecol 169:991, 1993

115. Saunders NJ, Snijders RJ, Nicolaides KH: Therapeutic amniocentesis in twin–twin transfusion syndrome appearing in the second trimester of pregnancy. Am J Obstet Gynecol 166:820, 1992

116. De Lia JE, Cruikshank DP, Keye WR: Fetoscopic neodymium: YAG laser occlusion of placental vessels in severe twin–twin transfusion syndrome. Obstet Gynecol 75:1046, 1990

117. Wittmann BK, Farquharson DF, Thomas WD et al: The role of fetocide in the management of severe twin transfusion syndrome. Am J Obstet Gynecol 155:1023, 1986

118. Weiner CP: Diagnosis and treatment of twin to twin transfusion in the mid-second trimester of pregnancy. Fetal Ther 2:71, 1987

119. De Lia JR, Emery MG, Sheafor SA et al: Twin transfusion syndrome: successful in utero treatment with digoxin. Int J Gynecol Obstet 23:197, 1985

120. Simpson PC, Trudinger BJ, Walker A et al: The intrauterine treatment of fetal cardiac failure in a twin pregnancy with an acardiac, acephalic monster. Am J Obstet Gynecol 147:842, 1983

121. Jones JM, Sbarra AJ, Dilillo L et al: Indomethacin in severe twin-to-twin transfusion syndrome. Am J Perinatol 10:24, 1993

122. Blickstein I: The twin–twin transfusion syndrome. Obstet Gynecol 76:714, 1990

123. Golbus MS, Cunningham N, Goldberg JD et al: Selective termination of multiple gestations. Am J Med Genet 34:339, 1988

124. Onyskowova A, Dolezal A, Jedlicka V: The frequency and the character of malformations in multiple birth (a preliminary report). Teratology 4:496, 1971

125. Hendricks CH: Twinning in relation to birth weight, mortality, and congenital anomalies. Obstet Gynecol 27:47, 1966

126. Neilson JP, Hood VD, Cupples W: Ultrasonic evaluation of twin pregnancies associated with raised serum alpha-fetoprotein levels. Acta Genet Med Gemellol 31:229, 1982

127. Gewolb IH, Freedman RM, Kleinman CS, Hobbins JC: Prenatal diagnosis of a human pseudoacardiac anomaly. Obstet Gynecol 61:657, 1983

128. Kaplan C, Benirschke K: The acardiac anomaly: new case reports and current status. Acta Genet Med Gemellol 28:51, 1979

129. Pretorius DH, Leopold GR, Moore TR et al: Acardiac twin: report of Doppler sonography. J Ultrasound Med 7:413, 1988

130. Benson CB, Bieber FR, Genest DR, Doubilet PM: Doppler demonstration of reversed umbilical blood flow in an acardiac twin. J Clin Ultrasound 17:291, 1989

131. Van Allen MI, Smith DW, Shepard TH: Twin reversed arterial perfusion (TRAP) sequence: a study of 14 twin pregnancies with acardius. Semin Perinatol 7:285, 1983

132. Moore TR, Gale S, Benirschke K: Perinatal outcome of forty-nine pregnancies complicated by acardiac twinning. Am J Obstet Gynecol 163:907, 1990

133. Robie GF, Payne GG Jr, Morgan MA: Selective delivery of an acardiac, acephalic twin. N Engl J Med 320:512, 1989

134. Fries MH, Goldberg JD, Golbus MS: Treatment of acardiac-acephalus twin gestations by hysterotomy and selective delivery. Obstet Gynecol 79:601, 1992

135. Ginsberg NA, Applebaum M, Rabin SA et al: Term birth after midtrimester hysterotomy and selective delivery of an acardiac twin. Am J Obstet Gynecol 167:33, 1992

136. Hamada H, Okane M, Koresawa M et al: Fetal therapy in utero by blockage of the umbilical blood flow of acardiac monster in twin pregnancy. Nippon Sanka Fujinka Gakkai Zasshi 41:1803, 1989

137. Roberts RM, Shah DM, Jeanty P, Beattie JF: Twin, acardiac, ultrasound-guided embolization. Fetus 1:5, 1991

138. Porreco RP, Barton SM, Haverkamp AD: Occlusion of umbilical artery in acardiac, acephalic twin. Lancet 337: 326, 1991

139. Grab D, Schneider V, Keckstein J, Terinde R: Twin, acardiac, outcome. Fetus 2:11, 1992

140. Quintero RA, Reich H, Puder KS et al: Brief report:

umbilical-cord ligation of an acardiac twin by fetoscopy at 19 weeks of gestation. N Engl J Med 330:469, 1994

141. Windham GC, Bjerkedal T, Sever LE: The association of twinning and neural tube defects: studies in Los Angeles, California, and Norway. Acta Genet Med Gemellol 31:165, 1982

142. Harper RG, Kenigsberg K, Sia CG: Xiphopagus conjoined twins: a 300-year review of the obstetric, morphopathologic, neonatal and surgical parameters. Am J Obstet 137:617, 1980

143. Vaughn TC, Powell C: The obstetrical management of conjoined twins. Obstet Gynecol, suppl. 53:67, 1979

144. Wedberg R, Kaplan C, Leopold G et al: Cephalothoracopagus (Janiceps) twinning. Obstet Gynecol 54:392, 1979

145. Gray CM, Nix HG, Wallace AJ: Thoracopagus twins: prenatal diagnosis. Radiology 54:398, 1950

146. Apuzzio JJ, Ganesh V, Landau I, Pelosi M: Prenatal diagnosis of conjoined twins. Am J Obstet Gynecol 148:343, 1984

147. Zoppini C, Vanzulli A, Kustermann A et al: Prenatal diagnosis of anatomical connections in conjoined twins by use of contrast magnetic resonance imaging. Prenat Diagn 13:995, 1993

148. Austin E, Schifrin BS, Pomerance JJ et al: The antepartum diagnosis of conjoined twins. J Pediatr Surg 15:332, 1980

149. Fagan CJ: Antepartum diagnosis of conjoined twins by ultrasonography. AJR 129:921, 1977

150. Gore RM, Filly RA, Parer JT: Sonographic antepartum diagnosis of conjoined twins. JAMA 247:3351, 1982

151. Morgan CL, Trought WS, Sheldon G et al: B-scan and real time ultrasound in the antepartum diagnosis of conjoined twins and pericardial effusion. AJR 130:578, 1978

152. Schmidt W, Herberling D, Kubli F: Antepartum ultrasonographic diagnosis of conjoined twins in early pregnancy. Am J Obstet Gynecol 139:961, 1981

153. Wilson RL, Shaub MS, Cetrulo CJ: The antepartum findings of conjoined twins. J Clin Ultrasound 5:35, 1977

154. Wood MJ, Thompson HE, Roberson FM: Real-time ultrasound diagnosis of conjoined twins. J Clin Ultrasound 9:195, 1981

155. Fontanarosa M, Bagnoli G, Ciolini P et al: First trimester sonographic diagnosis of diprosus twins with craniorachischisis. J Clin Ultrasound 20:69, 1992

156. Meizner I, Levy A, Katz M et al: Early ultrasonic diagnosis of conjoined twins. Harefuah 124:741, 1993

157. Compton HL: Conjoined twins. Obstet Gynecol 37:27, 1971

158. Benirschke K, Kim CK: Multiple pregnancy (second of two parts). N Engl J Med 288:1329, 1973

159. Uchida IA, deSa DJ, Whelan DT: 45/46XX mosaicism in discordant monozygotic twins. Pediatrics 71:413, 1983

160. Potter AM, Taitz LS: Turner's syndrome in one of monozygotic twins with mosaicism. Acta Pediatr Scand 61:473, 1972

161. Rogers JG, Voullaire L, Gold H: Monozygotic twins discordant for trisomy 21. Am J Med Genet 11:143, 1982

162. Macdonald AD: Mongolism in twins. J Med Genet 1:39, 1964

163. Avni A, Amir J, Wilunsky E et al: Down's syndrome in twins of unlike sex. J Med Genet 20:94, 1983

164. Hanna JH, Hill JM: Single intrauterine fetal demise in multiple gestation. Obstet Gynecol 63:126, 1984

165. Pritchard JA, Ratnoff OD: Studies of fibrinogen and other hemostatic factors in women with intrauterine death and delayed delivery. Surg Obstet Gynecol 101:467, 1955

166. Skelly H, Marivate M, Norman R et al: Consumptive coagulopathy following fetal death in a triplet pregnancy. Am J Obstet Gynecol 142:595, 1982

167. Romero R, Duffy TP, Berkowitz RL et al: Prolongation of a preterm pregnancy complicated by death of a single twin in utero and disseminated intravascular coagulation. N Engl J Med 310:772, 1984

168. Angel JL, O'Brien WF: Management of the dead fetus syndrome with a surviving twin. Clin Decisions Obstet Gynecol 1:6, 1987

169. Rodeck CH, Mibeshan RS, Abramowicz J, Campbell S: Selective fetocide of the affected twin by fetoscopic air embolism. Prenat Diagn 2:189, 1982

170. Antsaklis A, Politis J, Karagiannopoulos C, Kaskarelis D: Selective survival of only the healthy fetus following prenatal diagnosis of thalassaemia major in binovular twin gestation. Prenat Diagn 4:289, 1984

171. Wapner RJ, Davis G, Johnson A et al: Selective reduction of multifetal pregnancies. Lancet 335:90, 1990

172. Moore CM, McAdams AJ, Sutherland J: Intrauterine disseminated intravascular coagulation: a syndrome of multiple pregnancy with a dead twin fetus. J Pediatr 74:523, 1969

173. Yoshioka H, Kadomoto Y, Mino M et al: Multicystic encephalomalacia in liveborn twin with a stillborn macerated co-twin. J Pediatr 95:798, 1979

174. Benirschke K: Twin placenta in perinatal mortality. NY State J Med 61:1499, 1961

175. Hoyme HE, Higginbottom MC, Jones KL: Vascular etiology of disruptive structural defects in monozygotic twins. Pediatrics 67:288, 1981

176. Schinzel AAGL, Smith DW, Miller JR: Monozygotic twinning and structural defects. J Pediatr 95:921, 1979

177. Carlson NJ, Towers CV: Multiple gestation complicated by the death of one fetus. Obstet Gynecol 73:685, 1989

178. Benirschke K: Intrauterine death of a twin: mechanisms, implications for surviving twin, and placental pathology. Semin Diagn Pathol 10:222, 1993

179. Prompeler HJ, Madjar H, Klosa W et al: Twin pregnancies with single fetal death. Acta Obstet Gynecol Scand 73:205, 1994

180. Aberg A, Mitelman F, Cantz M, Gehler J: Cardiac puncture of fetus with Hurler's disease avoiding abortion of unaffected co-twin. Lancet 2:990, 1978

181. Kerenyi TD, Chitkara U: Selective birth in twin pregnancy with discordancy for Down's syndrome. N Engl J Med 304:1525, 1981

182. Beck L, Terinde R, Rohrborn G et al: Twin pregnancy, abortion of one fetus with Down's syndrome by sectioparva, the other delivered mature and healthy. Eur J Obstet Gynaecol Reprod Biol 12:267, 1981

183. Chitkara U, Berkowitz RL, Wilkins IA et al: Selective second-trimester termination of the anomalous fetus in twin pregnancies. Obstet Gynecol 73:690, 1989

184. Lynch L, Berkowitz RL, Stone J et al: Preterm delivery after selective termination in twin pregnancies. Am J Obstet Gynecol 172:262, 1995

185. Wittman BK, Farquharson DF, Thomas WDS: The role of feticide in the management of severe twin transfusion syndrome. Am J Obstet Gynecol 155:1023, 1986

186. Robie GF, Payne GG, Morgan MA: Selective delivery of an acardiac acephalic twin. N Engl J Med 320:512, 1989

187. Urig MA, Simpson GF, Elliott JP, Clewell WH: Twin–twin transfusion syndrome: the surgical removal of one twin as a treatment option. Fetal Ther 3:185, 1988

188. Holzgreve W, Tercanli S, Krings W et al: Letter to the Editor. N Engl J Med 331:56, 1994

189. Dumez Y, Oury JF: Method for first trimester selective abortion in multiple pregnancy. Contrib Gynecol Obstet 15:50, 1986

190. Berkowitz RL, Lynch L, Lapinski R, Bergh P: First-trimester transabdominal multifetal pregnancy reduction: a report of two hundred completed cases. Am J Obstet Gynecol 169:17, 1993

191. Khalil MA, Tabsh A: A report of 131 cases of multifetal pregnancy reduction. Obstet Gynecol 82:57, 1993

192. Evans MI, Dommergues M, Wapner RJ et al: Efficacy of transabdominal multifetal pregnancy reduction: collaborative experience among the world's largest centers. Obstet Gynecol 82:61, 1993

193. Timor-Tritsch IE, Peisner DB, Monteagudo A et al: Multifetal pregnancy reduction by transvaginal puncture: evaluation of the technique used in 134 cases. Am J Obstet Gynecol 168:799, 1993

194. Gonen Y, Blankier J, Casper RF: Transvaginal ultrasound in selective embryo reduction for multiple pregnancy. Obstet Gynecol 75:720, 1990

195. Lipitz S, Reichman BN, Uval J et al: A prospective comparison of the outcome of triplet pregnancies managed expectantly or by multifetal reduction to twins. Am J Obstet Gynecol 170:874, 1994

196. Jonas HA, Lumley J: Triplets and quadruplets born in Victoria between 1982 and 1990: the impact of IVF and GIFT on rising birthrates. Med J Austr 158:659, 1993

197. Robinson LK, Jones KL, Benirschke K: The nature of structural defects associated with velamentous and marginal insertion of the umbilical cord. Am J Obstet Gynecol 146:191, 1983

198. Colburn DW, Pasquale SA: Monoamniotic twin pregnancy. J Reprod Med 27:165, 1982

199. Nyberg DA, Filly RA, Golbus MS, Stephens JD: Entangled umbilical cords: a sign of monoamniotic twins. J Ultrasound Med 3:29, 1984

200. Townsend RR, Filly RA: Sonography of nonconjoined monoamniotic twin pregnancies. J Ultrasound Med 7:665, 1988

201. McLeod FN, McCoy DR: Monoamniotic twins with an unusual cord complication. Br J Obstet Gynaecol 88:774, 1981

202. Rodis JF, Vintzeleos AM, Campbell WA et al: Antenatal diagnosis and management of monoamniotic twins. Am J Obstet Gynecol 157:1255, 1987

203. Carr SR, Aronson MP, Coustan DR: Survival rates of monoamniotic twins do not decrease after 30 weeks' gestation. Am J Obstet Gynecol 163:719, 1990

204. Tessen JA, Zlatnik FJ: Monoamniotic twins: a retrospective controlled study. Obstet Gynecol 77:832, 1991

205. Beischer NA, Pepperell RJ, Barrie JU: Twin pregnancy and erythroblastosis. Obstet Gynecol 34:22, 1969

206. Ellis MI, Coxon A, Noble C: Intrauterine transfusion of twins. BMJ 1:609, 1970

207. Spellacy WN, Cruz AC, Buhi WC, Birk SA: Amniotic fluid L/S ratio in twin gestation. Obstet Gynecol 50:68, 1977

208. Sims CD, Cowan DB, Parkinson CE: The lecithin sphingomyelin (L/S) ratio in twin pregnancies. Br J Obstet Gynaecol 83:447, 1976

209. Obladen M, Gluck L: RDS and tracheal phospholipid composition in twins: independent of gestational age. J Pediatr 90:799, 1977

210. Wilkinson AR, Jenkins PA, Baum JD: Uterine position and fetal lung maturity in triplet and quadruplet pregnancy. Lancet 2:663, 1982

211. Norman RJ, Joubert SM, Marivate M: Amniotic fluid phospholipids and glucocorticoids in multiple pregnancy. Br J Obstet Gynaecol 90:51, 1983

212. Gluck L, Kulovich MV: Maturation of the fetal lung, RDS, and amniotic fluid. In Villee CA, Villee DB, Zuckerman J (eds): Respiratory Distress Syndrome. Academic Press, New York, 1973

213. Leveno KJ, Quirk JG, Whalley PJ et al: Fetal lung maturation in twin gestation. Am J Obstet Gynecol 148:405, 1984

214. Wender DF, Kandall C, Leppert PC, Berkowitz RL: Hyaline membrane disease in twin B following prolonged rupture of membranes for twin A. Conn Med 45:83, 1981

215. Elias S, Gerbie AB, Simpson JL et al: Genetic amniocentesis in twin gestations. Am J Obstet Gynecol 138:169, 1980

216. Jeanty P, Rodesch F, Romero R et al: How to improve your amniocentesis technique. Am J Obstet Gynecol 146:593, 1983

217. McEnerney JK, McEnerney LN: Unfavorable neonatal outcome after intraamniotic injection of methylene blue. Obstet Gynecol, suppl. 61:35, 1983

218. Nicolini U, Monni G: Intestinal obstruction in babies exposed in utero to methylene blue. Lancet 336:1258, 1990

219. Van Der Pol JG, Wolf H, Boer K et al: Jejunal atresia related to the use of methylene blue in genetic amniocentesis in twins. Br J Obstet Gynaecol 99:141, 1992

220. McFadyen I: The dangers of intraamniotic methylene blue. Br J Obstet Gynaecol 99:89, 1992

221. Tabsh K: Genetic amniocentesis in multiple gestation. A new technique to diagnose monoamniotic twins. Obstet Gynecol 75:296, 1990

222. Palle C, Andersen JW, Tabor A et al: Increased risk of abortion after genetic amniocentesis in twin pregnancies. Prenat Diagn 3:83, 1983

223. Pijpers L, Jahoda MGJ, Vosters RPL et al: Genetic amniocentesis in twin pregnancies. Br J Obstet Gynaecol 95:323, 1988

224. Anderson RL, Goldberg JD, Golbus MS: Prenatal diagnosis in multiple gestation: 20 years' experience with amniocentesis. Prenat Diagn 11:263, 1991

225. Ghidini A, Lynch L, Hicks C et al: The risk of second-trimester amniocentesis in twin gestations: a case–control study. Am J Obstet Gynecol 169:1013, 1994

226. Hartikainen-Sorri AL, Jouppila P: Is routine hospitalization needed in antenatal care of twin pregnancy? J Perinat Med 12:31, 1984

227. Saunders MC, Dick JS, Brown IM: The effects of hospital admission for bed rest on the duration of twin pregnancy: a randomized trial. Lancet 2:793, 1985

228. MacLennan AH, Green RC, O'Shea R et al: Routine hospital admission in twin pregnancy between 26 and 30 weeks' gestation. Lancet 335:267, 1990

229. Leveno KJ, Andrews WW, Gilstrap LC et al: Impact of elective hospitalization on outcome of twin pregnancy. Presented at the Tenth Annual Meeting, Society of Perinatal Obstetricians, Houston, Texas, January 1990

230. Katz M, Robertson PA, Creasy RK: Cardiovascular complications associated with terbutaline treatment for preterm labor. Am J Obstet Gynecol 139:605, 1981

231. Houlton MCC, Marivate M, Philpott RH: Factors associated with preterm labour and changes in the cervix before labour in twin pregnancy. Br J Obstet Gynaecol 89:190, 1982

232. Neilson JP, Verkuyl AA, Crowther CA, Bannerman C: Preterm labor in twin pregnancies: prediction by cervical assessment. Obstet Gynecol 72:719, 1988

233. O'Connor MC, Arias E, Royston JP, Dalrymple IJ: The merits of special antenatal care for twin pregnancies. Br J Obstet Gynaecol 88:222, 1981

234. DeVoe LD, Azor H: Simultaneous nonstress fetal heart rate testing in twin pregnancy. Obstet Gynecol 58:450, 1981

235. Goldman GA, Dicker D, Peleg A, Goldman JA: Is elective cerclage justified in the management of triplet and quadruplet pregnancy? Aust NZ J Obstet Gynaecol 29:9, 1989

236. Elliott JP, Radin TG: Quadruplet pregnancy: contemporary management and outcome. Obstet Gynecol 80:421, 1992

237. Mordel N, Zajicek G, Benshushan A et al: Elective suture of uterine cervix in triplets. Am J Perinatol 10:14, 1993

238. Chervenak FA, Johnson RE, Youcha S: Intrapartum management of twin gestation. Obstet Gynecol 65:119, 1985

239. Khunda S: Locked twins. Obstet Gynecol 39:453, 1972

240. Sevitz H, Merrell DA: The use of a beta-sympathomimetic drug in locked twins. Br J Obstet Gynaecol 88:76, 1981

241. Nissen ED: Twins: collision, impaction, compaction, and interlocking. Obstet Gynecol 11:514, 1958

242. Acker D, Lieberman M, Holbrook H et al: Delivery of the second twin. Obstet Gynecol 59:710, 1982

243. Chervenak FA, Johnson RE, Berkowitz RI et al: Is routine cesarean section necessary for vertex-breech and vertex-transverse twin gestations? Am J Obstet Gynecol 148:1, 1984

244. Duenhoelter JH, Wells CE, Reisch JS: A paired controlled study of vaginal and abdominal delivery of the low birth weight breech fetus. Obstet Gynecol 54:310, 1979

245. Goldenberg RL, Nelson KG: The premature breech. Am J Obstet Gynecol 127:240, 1977

246. Chervenak FA, Johnson RE, Berkowitz RL, Hobbins JC: Intrapartum external version of the second twin. Obstet Gynecol 62:160, 1983

247. Gocke SE, Nageotte MP, Garite T et al: Management of the nonvertex second twin: primary cesarean section, external version, or primary breech extraction. Am J Obstet Gynecol 161:111, 1989

248. Shepard MJ, Richards VA, Berkowitz RL et al: An evaluation of the two equations for predicting fetal weight by ultrasound. Am J Obstet Gynecol 142:47, 1982

249. Tchabo JG, Tomai T: Selected intrapartum external cephalic version of the second twin. Obstet Gynecol 79:421, 1992

250. Fishman A, Grubb DK, Kovacs BW: Vaginal delivery of the nonvertex second twin. Am J Obstet Gynecol 168:861, 1993

251. Greig PC, Veille JC, Morgan T et al: The effect of presentation and mode of delivery on neonatal outcome in the second twin. Am J Obstet Gynecol 167:901, 1992

252. Evrard JR, Gold EM: Cesarean section for delivery of the second twin. Obstet Gynecol 57:581, 1981

253. Rayburn WF, Lavin JP, Miodovnik M, Varner MW: Multiple gestation: time interval between delivery of the first and second twins. Obstet Gynecol 63:502, 1984

254. Ferguson WF: Perinatal mortality in multiple gestations. A review of perinatal deaths from 1609 multiple gestations. Obstet Gynecol 23:861, 1964

255. Spurway JH: The fate and management of the second twin. Am J Obstet Gynecol 83:1377, 1962

256. Mashiach S, Ben-Rafael Z, Dor J, Serr DM: Triplet pregnancy in uterus didelphys with delivery interval of 72 days. Obstet Gynecol 58:519, 1981

257. Woolfson J, Fay T, Bates A: Twins with 54 days between deliveries. Case report. Br J Obstet Gynaecol 90:685, 1983

258. Feichtinger W, Breitenecker G, Frohlich H: Prolongation of pregnancy and survival of twin B after loss of twin A at 21 weeks' gestation. Am J Obstet Gynecol 161:891, 1989

259. Wittmann BK, Farquharson D, Wong GP et al: Delayed delivery of second twin: report of four cases and review of the literature. Obstet Gynecol 79:260, 1992

260. Poeschmann PP, Van Oppen CAC, Bruinse HW: Delayed interval delivery in multiple pregnancies: report of three cases and review of the literature. Obstet Gynecol Surv 47:139, 1992

261. Arias F: Delayed delivery of multifetal pregnancies with premature rupture of membranes in the second trimester. Am J Obstet Gynecol 170:1233, 1994

262. Berkowitz RL, Hobbins JC: Delivering twins with the help of ultrasound. Contemp Obstet Gynecol 19:128, 1982

263. Ballas S, Toaff R, Jaffa AJ: Deflexion of the fetal head in breech presentation. Obstet Gynecol 52:653, 1978

Chapter 25

Intrauterine Growth Restriction

Ira Bernstein and Steven G. Gabbe

The identification of pregnancies at risk for preventable perinatal morbidity and mortality is a primary goal of the obstetric care provider. This identification allows for the directed utilization of resources aimed at minimizing perinatal complications. Intrauterine growth restriction (IUGR) is the second leading contributor to the perinatal mortality rate.[1] The perinatal mortality rate for these infants is 6 to 10 times greater than that for a normally grown population, 120 per 1,000 for all cases of growth restriction and 100 per 1,000 if anomalous infants are excluded. Approximately 30 percent of all stillborn infants are growth restricted. The incidence of intrapartum asphyxia in cases complicated by IUGR has been reported to be 50 percent.[2] A portion of these perinatal complications are preventable. If the growth-restricted fetus is appropriately identified and managed, the perinatal mortality can be lowered.[3] This chapter presents the varied etiologies of the growth restriction syndromes, recent advances in the detection and management of this problem, and the available information on the long-term prognosis for infants who have suffered from impaired intrauterine growth.

Nomenclature

A variety of terms have been used to identify the fetus who is small relative to its peers. They include "premature," "low birth weight," "small for gestational age," "fetal growth retarded." "small for dates," and "intrauterine growth restricted." All represent the small fetus and have intentional distinctions based on their origins, found primarily in the pediatric literature.

The evolution of terms used to classify the small newborn is illustrative of the difficulty in identifying the appropriate descriptive term for the growth-restricted fetus. The recognition and identification of the small neonate has its modern origin in 1919. Ylppo[4] suggested that all children with birth weights under 2,500 g be labeled "premature" while recognizing that many small children were the products of normal length gestations. This label persisted until 1961, when the WHO Expert Committee on Maternal and Child Health acknowledged that many babies defined as premature were not born prematurely and reclassified birth weight below 2,500 g as "low birth weight."[5] As early as 1946 McBurney[6] reported cases of "undernourished full-term infants," and this phenomenon was further highlighted in 1963 by Gruenwald,[7] who noted the important differences between the neonate with low birth weight secondary to prematurity, the infant born too soon, and the infant who was small compared with other newborns of the same gestational age. Lubchenco et al.,[8] Usher and McLean,[9] and others[10,11] throughout the 1960s laid the groundwork for the classification of the growth-deficient infant through population studies that established the relationship between gestational age and weight. In 1974, at the WHO Scientific Meeting in Geneva, the concepts of "light" and "heavy" for dates emerged.[12] These concepts correlate most closely with the current classification of the growth-restricted neonate. However, the definition used to define "light for dates" (either by percentile rank or standard deviations [SD]) was not established. A commonly used subclassification has developed that reserves the obstetric label of IUGR for the fetus who suffers morbidity and/or mortality association with the failure to reach growth potential (Fig. 25-1) and the pediatric term "small for gestational age" as the more general term for the small fetus for whom no pathology has yet emerged. For the purposes of this chapter, we have chosen the terms

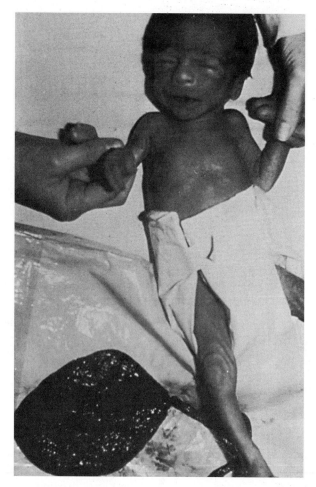

Fig. 25-1 A growth-retarded infant exhibiting subcutaneous wasting.

"fetal" or "intrauterine growth restriction" and apply the label in the prenatal period based on estimates of fetal size alone. We believe that this term appropriately characterizes the syndrome and eliminates the negative cognitive associations of the term "retardation."

Definition

Neonatal growth restriction is recognized as a syndrome encompassing small size as well as specific metabolic abnormalities including hypoglycemia, hypothermia, and polycythemia. In contrast, IUGR is currently characterized as a syndrome in which failure to reach growth potential is both a necessary and sufficient condition. Additional prenatal diagnostic criteria that support the diagnosis of fetal growth restriction exist but are generally not required for the diagnosis to be applied. Small size is therefore the hallmark of the syndrome, and varying criteria have been used to identify the growth-restricted fetus.

While failure to reach growth potential is the abnormality recognized in this disorder, individual growth

capacity is not routinely established, and as a result fetal size is most often compared with appropriate population-based "growth curves." On occasion, individual growth projections may be available, and this allows for a more direct examination of a failure to achieve growth potential.

Ultrasound criteria have emerged as the diagnostic standard employed in the identification of fetal growth restriction. Wilcocks et al.[13] in 1964 first demonstrated the correlation between ultrasound measurement of the fetal head and birth weight. Campbell and Dewhurst[14] published the first sonographic descriptions of fetal growth restriction with their analysis of the changes in biparietal diameter over time. Two patterns of altered head growth were described. In "late flattening," which represents approximately two-thirds of all cases of IUGR, the biparietal diameter (BPD) increases normally until late pregnancy and then lags behind. In the "low-profile" or symmetric type, impaired head growth occurs much earlier in gestation. These abnormal growth patterns were later labeled types 1 (late flattening) and 2 (low profile), and these concepts would become generalized to describe asymmetric and symmetric growth deficiencies, respectively.

As an individual parameter, abdominal circumference AC has demonstrated the greatest sensitivity in the identification of the small child.[15] The use of abdominal circumference, a directly measurable fetal parameter, in combination with head circumference has been adopted for the identification of growth restriction by some laboratories.[3]

The most common assessment of fetal size in the United States is the estimation of fetal weight. This was first described by Campbell and Wilkin[16] employing a combination of BPD and abdominal circumference. Since that report numerous investigators have identified distinct fetal parameters identifiable by ultrasound that are useful in the estimation of fetal size.[17-20] All of the techniques incorporate an index of abdominal size as a variable contributing to the estimation of fetal weight. These techniques generally have 95 percent confidence limits that deviate approximately 15 percent around the actual value. Numerous population-specific formulas have been derived.[21]

An absolute threshold used for the definition of growth restriction can be applied to any of the parameters evaluated (BPD, AC or estimated fetal weight (EFW)). These criteria are statistically defined rather than outcome based and employ either a threshold percentile ranking (non-normative data) or a number of standard deviations below the mean (normative data) for the definition to be fulfilled. Birth weight below the population 10th percentile, corrected for gestational age, has been the most widely used criterion for defining growth restriction at birth, and this has been generalized to imply a sonographically estimated fetal weight below the 10th percentile for appropriate population-based cross-sectional growth charts.

The major aim of identifying this syndrome sonographically should be sensitivity in the identification of a group of infants who have increased morbidity and mortality. Using the birth weight 10th percentile cutoff, approximately 70 percent of the infants thus identified as growth restricted are normally or constitutionally small, so-called light for gestational age or small for gestational age (SGA).[22] These neonates are *not* at increased risk for poor outcome, but represent one end of the spectrum of normal neonatal size. This group, however, does include infants who are truly growth restricted and who are at risk for increased perinatal morbidity and mortality. Usher and McLean[9] have pointed out that, when restricting the cutoff weight for IUGR to 2 SD below the mean, only infants below the 3rd percentile are considered growth restricted. The exact thresholds are a matter of debate. Using the 3rd percentile overlooks an increased number of growth-restricted infants, while the 10th percentile cutoff includes normal infants who will be monitored unnecessarily. Manning and Hohler[3] have suggested a cutoff of the 5th percentile based on the distribution of short-term morbidity in their population.

The biologic significance of any definition of IUGR can only be measured by discovering which parameters most accurately predict infants at risk for both short- and long-term impairment. The prognostic values of the 3rd, 5th, and 10th percentiles still remain to be clinically validated. Until a definition of growth restriction is uniformly applied by perinatologists using appropriate population-specific growth curves, we will be unable to determine how effectively we have detected and treated IUGR.[23,24]

Etiology

When considering the definition and detection of IUGR, one must also review the etiologies of IUGR and their appropriate therapies. Etiologies for fetal growth restriction can be crudely separated into fetoplacental and maternal in origin. The fetoplacental origins of growth restriction include those etiologies that have been traditionally ascribed to the fetus, including the chromosomal abnormalities, the genetic syndromes, and the infectious etiologies, as well as those secondary to placental abnormalities.

Fetoplacental Origins

Intrauterine infection, though long recognized as a cause of growth restriction, accounts for less than 10 percent of all cases. Herpes, cytomegalovirus, rubella, and toxoplasmosis are well documented, and other intrauterine infections are strongly suspected (Ch. 38). The infectious process produces early disruption of

Fetoplacental Etiologies of Fetal Growth Retardation

Chromosomal abnormalities
  Trisomies (13, 18, 21)
  Trisomy 9 mosaicism
  Trisomy 4P
  4P−, 5P−, 11P−, 13Q− syndromes
  Partial trisomy 10Q

Genetic syndromes
  Cretinism (hypothyoidism)
  Russell-Silver
  Bloom
  Lowe
  De Lange
  Progeria
  Leprechaunism

Congenital malformations
Infectious diseases
  Cytomegalovirus
  Toxoplasmosis
  Rubella

Placental pathology
  Previa
  Abruption
  Circumvallate
  Mosaicism
  Infarctions
  Twins

fetal growth during the stage of cell hyperplasia and is, therefore, associated with a poor prognosis for normal development. For the agents associated with IUGR, prevention of the infection is the most important therapy.

Chromosomal abnormalities, congenital malformations, and genetic syndromes have been associated with less than 10 percent of cases of IUGR. Abnormalities in cell replication and reduced cell number produce a pattern of impaired growth that is early in onset and symmetric. Neonatal prognosis in these cases is determined by the specific abnormality identified. Growth restriction has been observed in 53 percent of cases of trisomy 13 and 64 percent of cases of trisomy 18.[25] Congenital anomalies such as renal agenesis represent a related situation.[26]

Placental abnormalities can be a cause of fetal growth restriction. An absolute or relative decrease in placental mass affects the quantity of substrate the fetus receives and has been recognized ultrasonographically to ante-date fetal growth restriction.[27] Thus, a circumvallate placenta, partial placental abruption, placenta accreta, placental infarction, or hemangioma may result in growth restriction. An elevated maternal serum α-feto-protein or human chorionic gonadotropin (hCG) level in the second trimester has been associated with an in-creased risk for IUGR and may result from abnormal placentation.[28-30] Intrinsic placental pathology has been identified in some cases of growth restriction, in-cluding the presence of a single umbilical artery or the presence of placental mosaicism, either of which may act to impair normal fetoplacental exchange mecha-nisms.[31-33] Placental location has also been linked to growth restriction. Placenta previa without bleeding has been suggested as a risk factor, because the low implantation site may not be optimal for nutrient transfer.[34]

Twin gestation represents a relative decrease in pla-cental mass in relation to fetal mass and is, therefore, often associated with IUGR (Ch. 24). In 1966, Gruen-wald[35] observed that the growth curve of twins deviated from that of singletons with a progressive fall of growth after 32 weeks. This finding implies relative placental insufficiency as opposed to intrinsic fetal compromise and suggests that the longer the twin pregnancy contin-ues the greater the delay in intrauterine growth with "catch-up" growth observed after birth. Thus, twins represent a group of fetuses at high risk for IUGR as confirmed by an incidence of 17.5 percent in one study.[36] Although twins have an increased incidence of perinatal mortality that relates primarily to prematur-ity and subsequent respiratory distress syndrome (RDS), growth restriction represents the second most prevalent cause of morbidity for these infants.

Maternal Origins

Decreased uteroplacental blood flow with its associated reduction in transfer of nutrients to the fetus is respon-sible for the majority of clinically recognized cases of IUGR. Maternal vascular disease, whether chronic hy-pertension, preeclampsia, or diabetes with vasculopa-thy, has been associated with impaired fetal growth.[37-39] In preeclampsia, failure of trophoblastic invasion of maternal spiral arterioles by 20 to 22 weeks' gestation and intimal thickening accompanied by fi-brinoid degeneration of the media of these arterioles result in luminal narrowing and, therefore, decreased blood flow through the placental bed.[40] Such cases are generally marked by asymmetric IUGR with mainte-nance of normal fetal head growth and reduction in the size of the fetal liver, heart, thymus, spleen, pan-creas, and adrenal glands. Ward et al.[41] have demon-strated that mutations in the angiotensinogen gene contribute to the development of both preeclampsia and the associated incidence of fetal growth restriction

(personal communication). Thus, a portion of this com-promised maternal vascular expansion may be ex-plained by specific genetic deficiencies. Decreased pla-cental blood flow from postural maternal hypotension and maternal hyperviscosity with sludging has also been reported to cause IUGR. Some patients with hy-pertension have been noted to demonstrate a reduction in the normal expansion of blood volume seen in preg-nancy. This contracted circulating blood volume has been correlated with IUGR. A reduction in maternal oxygenation in women living at high altitude or those with cyanotic heart disease or parenchymal lung dis-ease may be responsible for IUGR. Those hemoglobin-opathies and anemias that impair maternal and fetal oxygenation have also been linked to limited fetal growth.[42]

Poor maternal weight gain has long been recognized as a risk factor for growth restriction. Controversy still exists about the contribution maternal malnutrition can make to IUGR. Studies of the offspring of women preg-nant during the siege of Leningrad in 1942 and the Dutch famine in 1945 indicate little effect on fetal growth by such dietary restriction.[43] In Holland, de-spite a maternal intake of 600 to 900 calories daily for 6 months, the average birth weight fell only 240 g in women with good prepregnancy nutritional status. However, investigation of Guatemalan Indian tribes has indicated that protein malnutrition before 26 weeks can result in symmetric growth restriction.[44] Protein restriction after 26 weeks did not limit fetal growth. The degree of malnourishment observed in Guatemala or during the Dutch famine would not ordinarily be found in the United States. Nevertheless maternal pre-pregnancy weight and weight gain in pregnancy are two of the most important variables contributing to birth weight.[45,46]

Pregnant women may be subject to poor nutrition through limited gastrointestinal absorption imposed by Crohn's disease or ulcerative colitis. These conditions have not been generally associated with increased num-bers of growth-restricted infants. Massively obese women who have undergone ileojejunal bypass are re-ported to have smaller infants than average, but they usually fall above the 10th percentile in birth weight.

Glucose is a critical fetal nutrient, and if its supply is reduced growth restriction may result. Using cord blood sampling, Economides and Nicolaides[47] ob-served significantly lower maternal and fetal glucose levels in cases of growth restriction and speculated that the major cause of fetal hypoglycemia in these cases was reduced glucose supply from the mother due to impaired placental perfusion. Khouzami et al.[48] docu-mented a significant association between maternal hy-poglycemia on a 3-hour oral glucose tolerance test (GTT) and subsequent birth of non-low-birth-weight but growth-restricted babies. Sokol et al.[49] and Langer et al.[50] have confirmed that a flat maternal response to glucose loading is associated with an increased risk for fetal growth restriction. Langer et al.[50] demonstrated that a "flat" GTT was associated with a 20-fold increase in IUGR in normotensive patients. They suggest that the 3-hour GTT may be used as a screening test to identify women at high risk for IUGR.

Maternal drug ingestion may produce IUGR by a direct effect on fetal growth as well as through inadequate dietary intake. Smoking produces a symmetrically smaller fetus through reduced uterine blood flow and impaired fetal oxygenation.[51] The consumption of alcohol and the use of coumarin or hydantoin derivatives are now well known to produce particular dysmorphic features in association with impaired fetal growth. Mills et al.[52] have demonstrated a significant increase in the risk of IUGR with the consumption of one to two drinks daily, in the absence of fetal alcohol syndrome. Maternal use of cocaine has been associated with not only IUGR but also reduced head circumference growth.[53]

In 1971, Lobi et al.[54] reported that advanced maternal age was a factor in the etiology of IUGR. More recently, Berkowitz et al.[55] found no evidence that the first births of women between 30 and 34 years or those over 35 years were at increased risk for growth restriction. Miller and Merritt[56] confirmed that if one controls for underlying medical complications, maternal age is not related to restricted fetal growth.

A history of poor pregnancy outcome is clearly correlated with the subsequent delivery of a growth-restricted infant.[57] Galbraith et al.[58] and Tejani[59] have shown that prior birth of an IUGR infant is the obstetric factor most often associated with the subsequent birth of a growth-restricted infant. The study populations did include women with underlying medical problems. Tejani and Mann[60] in a retrospective study of 83 multigravidas who had delivered IUGR infants noted that the perinatal wastage from their 200 prior pregnancies was 41 percent. This striking figure, which includes spontaneous abortions as well as neonatal and intrauterine deaths, points to the significance of poor obstetric history as a risk factor for IUGR. Women whose first pregnancy results in a growth-restricted infant have a 1 in 4 risk of delivering a second infant below the 10th percentile. After two pregnancies complicated by IUGR, there is a fourfold increase in the risk of a subsequent growth-restricted infant.[57] When all indices of risk have been applied, the one-third of the population considered at highest risk accounts for two-thirds of the infants identified as growth restricted. Two-thirds of pregnancies, although not judged to be "at risk" for IUGR, yield one-third of neonates below the 10th percentile.[58] Most of these babies are constitutionally small.

In summary, a framework does exist for considering the causes of growth restriction. Is the fetus abnormal? The delivery system disrupted? The maternal supply line compromised? These questions categorize the source of the problem without explaining the mechanism by which the growth process is disturbed. Even when one is aware of these clinical associations, the sum of the many factors affecting the growth of an individual fetus is unpredictable.

Diagnosis

Significant improvements have been made in detecting and characterizing the growth-restricted fetus. These improvements have served as the basis for plans designed to reduce the associated perinatal morbidity and mortality. In the past, clinical parameters such as maternal weight gain and measurement of fundal height were used to reflect fetal growth. Belizan et al.[61] observed that curvilinear fundal height measurements in centimeters from the symphysis pubis could be closely correlated with gestational age: a lag of 4 cm or more suggests growth restriction. Persson et al.[62] reported a sensitivity of only 27 percent and a positive predictive value of 18 percent using carefully performed fundal height measurements to detect IUGR. Additional studies have confirmed the lack of sensitivity of fundal height measurements for detecting fetal growth restriction.[63] The presence of risk factors should therefore prompt ultrasound estimation of fetal size independent of maternal weight gain or fundal height growth.

Risk Factors for Fetal Growth Restriction: Indications for Ultrasound

History of fetal growth retardation
Hypertension
Diabetes mellitus
Elevated MSAFP/hCG
Antiphospholipid syndrome
Chronic medical illnesses
Low maternal prepregnancy weight (<90% IBW)
Poor maternal weight gain
Twin gestation
Substance abuse (tobacco, alcohol, drugs)
Preterm labor
Abnormalities of placentation
Vaginal bleeding
Matenal anemia (hgb < 10)
Maternal hypoxia (cyanotic cardiac or pulmonary disease, altitude)
Maternal hemoglobinopathies
Drug ingestion (hydantoin, Coumarin)

Fetal Measurements

The use of estimated fetal weight has been the most common method for characterizing fetal size and thereby growth abnormalities. An accurate ultrasonographic assessment of fetal weight is essential in detecting and following patients suspected of having growth-restricted infants.[64] Using a multifactorial equation and a measurement of abdominal size, a weight can be predicted and related to BPD. Formulas that incorporate the femur length (FL) may increase the accuracy of in utero weight estimation for the fetus with IUGR.[65]

A significant limitation of employing estimated fetal weight to measure fetal size is that it cannot be measured directly, but must be calculated from a combination of directly measured parameters. This results in an increased error in the estimate. In addition, the lack of directly measured normative data creates difficulty in establishing normal growth curves. Commonly, cross-sectional birth weight data have been utilized to characterize ultrasound-estimated fetal weight. These birth weight criteria, however, do not appropriately describe sonographic estimated fetal weights, as there is a significant association of preterm birth with fetal growth restriction.[66,67] Thus, the weights of preterm infants are not normally distributed as they are at term. This association has been highlighted by several investigators who have identified the discrepancy between birth weight defined growth curves and sonographically estimated fetal weight defined growth curves in preterm gestation.[68–70] Ultrasound generated estimated fetal weight growth curves consistently demonstrate higher fetal weights over the range of preterm gestation than do birth weight generated growth curves. This discrepancy results from the fact that ultrasound examinations represent a larger breadth of the entire population at any gestational age. Preterm birth weight reflects only those individuals who have delivered under abnormal circumstances. It is therefore most appropriate to compare estimated fetal weights by ultrasound with ultrasound derived growth curves in order to characterize preterm estimated fetal weight appropriately.

The use of the individualized growth model has been supported by several investigators.[71,72] The obvious advantage is the lack of dependency on population-based normative data and the ability to detect a true personal growth restriction. This can be done even when the estimated fetal weight is greater than the 10th percentile for the population. The disadvantages of these models are that they require baseline ultrasound morphometric data in the second trimester as well as an additional later scan to establish growth potential for an individual morphometric parameter. A third scan is then necessary to identify that a growth abnormality exists. This volume of information is frequently not available, limiting the practical application of these individual growth models. In addition, the diagnostic advantages of the individualized growth modeling has been questioned when compared with the sequential comparison of the percentile ranking of individual or composite growth parameters to population-based growth curves.[73]

Fetal growth as opposed to fetal size is a dynamic process and requires more than a single evaluation for its estimation. The absence of fetal growth over a sustained period is a concern. The routine clinical evaluation of fetal growth is based on fundal height enlargement during the course of pregnancy. In pregnancies at risk or in those in whom fetal size is already estimated to be below the 10th percentile, serial ultrasound estimations of fetal size are performed. The appropriate observation interval for the evaluation of fetal growth has been based on two assumptions: (1) growth is continuous rather than sporadic and (2) the identification of growth is limited by the technical capability of the ultrasound equipment employed to measure the fetus.[3] The most commonly recommended interval between evaluations is 2 weeks.[3,74] Recent data have demonstrated that early childhood growth, up to 21 months of age, is characterized by sporadic growth pulses that punctuate prolonged periods of growth stasis.[75] While the fetal growth rate of the third trimester is greater than the early childhood growth rate, it may be that fetal growth is also saltatory and that the detection of growth is limited by the physiologic interval of growth pulses rather than by the technical limitations of the measuring tool. Preliminary data from Bernstein and Blake[76] suggest that normal fetal growth can be characterized by significant periods of stasis, with 2 week intervals being too short to detect the normal changes in fetal size.

In an attempt to increase detection of the fetus with asymmetric growth restriction, head circumference (HC) to AC ratios can be assessed (Figs. 25-2 and 25-3).[77,78] In the normally growing fetus, the HC/AC ratio exceeds 1.0 before 32 weeks' gestation, is approximately 1.0 at 32 to 34 weeks' gestation, and falls below 1.0 after 34 weeks' gestation. In fetuses affected by asymmetric growth restriction, the HC remains larger than that of the body (Fig. 25-2). The HC/AC ratio is then elevated. In symmetric IUGR, both the HC and the AC are reduced, and the HC/AC ratio remains normal (Fig. 25-3). Using the HC/AC ratio, 85 percent of growth-restricted fetuses are detected, with a reduction in false-negative diagnoses. Thus, a single set of measurements, even when determined in the latter part of pregnancy, can be very helpful in evaluating the status of intrauterine growth.

In some cases, measurement of the HC may be diffi-

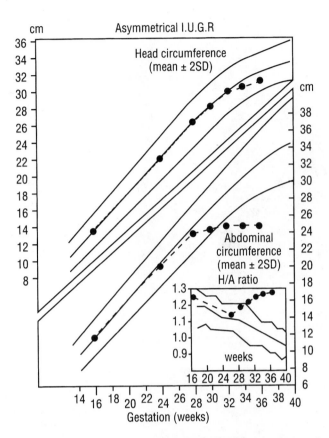

Fig. 25-2 Growth chart in a case of asymmetric IUGR. Although head circumference is preserved, AC growth falls off early in the third trimester. For this reason, the H/A ratio shown in the lower right corner of the graph becomes elevated. IUGR, intrauterine growth retardation. (From Chudleigh and Pearce,[196] with permission.)

cult as a result of fetal position. One can then compare the FL, which is relatively spared in asymmetric IUGR, to the AC.[79] The FL/AC is 22 at all gestational ages from 21 weeks to term and so can be applied without knowledge of the number of weeks gestation. An FL/AC ratio greater than 23.5 suggests IUGR.

Oligohydramnios

Decreased amniotic fluid volume has been associated clinically with IUGR and may be the earliest sign detected on ultrasonography, preceding an elevation in HC/AC ratio and lagging fetal growth (Fig. 25-4). Decreased perfusion of the fetal kidneys and reduced urine production explain this observation.[80] In an early study, Manning et al.[82] reported that a vertical pocket of amniotic fluid measuring 1 cm or more reflected an adequate fluid volume. Of fetuses with fluid pockets less than 1 cm, 96 percent were actually growth restricted. Only 5 of 91 cases with an adequate amount of amniotic fluid exhibited IUGR. The patient with an uncertain gestational age who presents late in preg-

nancy poses a difficult diagnostic dilemma because interpretation of BPD and HC/AC ratios must be related to accurate gestational age. Under these conditions, measuring an amniotic fluid pocket, or an FL/AC ratio, may be helpful, as these do not rely on knowledge of the gestational age. More recently, Manning and his colleagues[82] have broadened their criteria. A 2-cm vertical pocket is considered normal, 1 to 2 cm is marginal, and less than 1 cm is decreased. Using this definition, they observed a 6 percent incidence of IUGR with a pocket 2 cm or larger, 20 percent with a pocket 1 to 2 cm, and 39 percent with a pocket less than 1 cm. One may also use the amniotic fluid index to quantitate amniotic fluid volume (Ch. 11), although this technique requires a knowledge of gestational age. The overall clinical impression of reduced amniotic fluid on ultrasonography may be most important. The volume of amniotic fluid also has prognostic significance for the course of labor. Groome et al.[83] demonstrated that oligohydramnios associated with fetal oliguria is associated with a higher rate of intrapartum complications seemingly associated with reduced placental reserve.

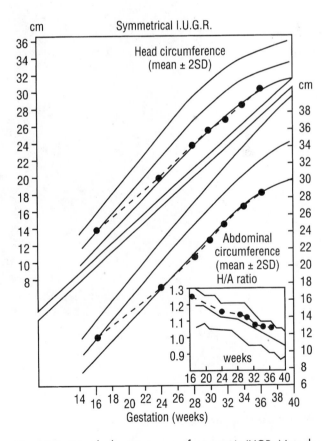

Fig. 25-3 Growth chart in a case of symmetric IUGR. Note the early onset of both HC and AC growth retardation. For this reason, the H/A ratio shown in the lower right corner remains normal. IUGR, intrauterine growth retardation. (From Chudleigh and Pearce,[196] with permission.)

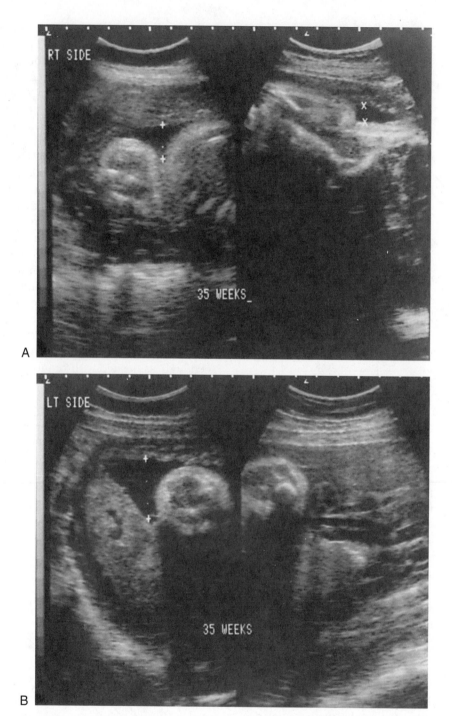

Fig. 25-4 **(A & B)** Amniotic fluid index (AFI) performed at 35 weeks on a patient whose fundal height measured 30 cm. Findings consistent with asymmetric growth retardation were observed, including estimated fetal weight of 1,500 g, HC/AC ratio of 1.15, and AFI of 5.0 cm, as illustrated. At 35 weeks, the 50th percentile for the AFI is 14.0 cm; the 5th percentile is 11.9 cm. Note that one amniotic fluid pocket greater than 2.0 cm was found.

Maternal Doppler Velocimetry

Doppler velocimetry of the maternal uterine artery has been examined to establish its usefulness in the prediction of pregnancies destined to produce a growth-restricted newborn. Schulman[84] found that women with hypertensive disorders who had an elevated uterine artery systolic/diastolic (S/D) ratio (greater than 2.6) and/or diastolic notching were more likely to have pregnancies complicated by IUGR and intrauterine fetal death. He noted that the changes in uterine artery flow patterns might precede those observed in the umbilical artery and antedate fetal growth restriction. Jacobson et al.[85] observed that an elevated uteroplacental artery resistance index (RI) predicted fetal growth restriction with a sensitivity of 70.6 percent and had a positive predictive value of 33.3 percent in women at high risk for either preeclampsia or growth restriction. Additional studies have been performed with low-risk populations. However, in low-risk patients, the examination of second trimester maternal uterine artery waveforms has produced sensitivities and positive predictive values for fetal growth restriction as high as 50 percent and 35 percent, respectively; values only marginally better than routine clinical indicators of fetal growth.[86–89] Valensise and Romanini[90] have demonstrated that the combination of abnormal second trimester maternal uterine artery Doppler velocimetry and maternal glucose tolerance testing demonstrating a "flat" response results in a positive predictive value of 94 percent and a sensitivity of 54 percent for the detection of fetal growth restriction. In summary, the overall value of second trimester maternal uterine artery Doppler waveforms in screening of pregnancies at risk for growth restriction is unclear. At present there are no data suggesting that sensitivity is improved beyond that achieved with standard clinical assessment. The availability of second trimester stratification of risk for fetal growth restriction has not yet demonstrated an impact on perinatal morbidity or mortality.

Fetal Body Composition

The ponderal index was first described by Rohrer[91] in 1921 as an index of corpulence. This index of neonatal size (weight/length[3]) that is normally distributed accurately described the nutritional state of the neonate. When compared with birth weight percentile, the ponderal index demonstrates an improved ability to predict neonatal asphyxia, acidosis, hypoglycemia, and hypothermia.[92] The ponderal index also correlates with direct measures of neonatal fat as estimated by skinfold thickness.[93] Attempts to translate the ponderal index directly to the fetus have been hampered by the difficulty in accurately assessing fetal length. Attempts to modify the ponderal index for fetal sonographic estimation have been made. Yagel et al.[94] demonstrated that the addition of a fetal ponderal index improved the prediction of perinatal morbidity in fetuses already suspected of having IUGR. Alternative methods for the characterization of fetal growth by physiologic compartments have recently been attempted. Several studies have examined fetal subcutaneous fat content employing ultrasound examination. Subcutaneous fat deposition has been examined in the face, abdomen, arm, and thigh.[95–99] Reduction in facial fat stores has been strongly associated with being SGA. This reduc-

tion in fat content is consistent with the reduction observed in the growth-restricted neonate and may prove to be a sensitive indicator of the small fetus at increased risk for perinatal complications.[100] The optimal method of in utero assessment for fetal fat has not yet been determined.

Biochemical Markers

Biochemical markers have been utilized to assist in the identification of the small fetus who is at increased risk for the morbidity and mortality associated with fetal growth restriction. The most widely examined include fetal erythropoietin and amino acid concentrations.

Erythropoietin production in the fetus, as in the adult, is stimulated by the presence of anemia or hypoxia.[101,102] Numerous studies have demonstrated the ability of the fetus to respond to hypoxic conditions with the production of erythropoietin. This increase in erythropoietin may or may not lead to increased red cell production, depending on erythropoietic reserve.[101,103] Erythropoietin, identified in the cord blood of growth-restricted fetuses by cordocentesis, amniotic fluid, or cord blood at delivery, may prove to be of benefit in the identification of the child at risk for long-term morbidity.[103–106] Ruth et al.[107] identified an association between cord blood erythropoietin levels and developmental outcome (including cerebral palsy and death) at 2 years in nonpreeclamptic patients with evidence of acute asphyxia at birth. Neonates from pregnancies complicated by preeclampsia had elevated cord erythropoietin levels regardless of outcome.[107]

Altered amino acid concentrations, particularly the relationship between the branched chain amino acids such as valine and the gluconeogenic amino acids like glycine, have been identified in the growth-restricted fetus and newborn. These changes reflect a specific fetal response that is independent of maternal amino acid levels. The observed increase in the glycine/valine ratio appears to result from a reduction in phophoenolpyruvate carboxykinase activity, a rate-limiting enzyme for gluconeogenesis.[108] Studies have demonstrated that cord blood samples from growth-restricted neonates demonstrate an increased glycine/valine ratio within the first few hours of life.[109–112] This profile of amino acids parallels the aminogram observed in children who suffer from protein calorie malnutrition.[113] In the growth-restricted neonate the glycine/valine ratio of umbilical cord blood has been correlated with specific neonatal risk, including hypoglycemia and death.[114] Amino acid data from umbilical venous plasma obtained by percutaneous umbilical blood sampling and amniotic fluid confirms that the elevation in glycine/valine ratio precedes parturition in the growth-restricted fetus.[115–118] Fetal cord blood glycine/valine ratios have been shown to be inversely proportional to fetal arterial oxygen content.[116] No relationship with short-term or long-term morbidity has been established.

In summary, the ability to determine appropriate fetal growth using fundal height measurements in a normal population is limited. Fundal height measurements lack both sensitivity and specificity in the identification of the small fetus. It is therefore reasonable to employ a better tool (ultrasound) whenever clinical circumstances point to an increased risk for a growth-restricted fetus. A number of clinical conditions that increase the risk for a small child were listed earlier. In the absence of routine clinical indications, ultrasound screening of these high-risk pregnancies should be performed at 16 to 18 weeks for dating (if not otherwise established) and again at 32 to 34 weeks.

Management

In developing a plan for the management of suspected growth restriction, it is important to remember the major etiologic groups. Most infants thought to be growth restricted are constitutionally small and require no intervention. Unfortunately, this diagnosis is usually made retrospectively. Approximately 15 percent exhibit symmetric growth restriction due to an early fetal insult for which there is no effective therapy. Here, an accurate diagnosis is essential. Finally, approximately 15 percent have growth restriction or extrinsic growth failure due to placental disease or reduced uteroplacental blood flow. In such cases, antepartum fetal monitoring and carefully timed delivery may be critical.

Once growth restriction is suspected, a well-organized approach to management should be undertaken. The clinician should evaluate and treat problems that may be contributing to growth restriction. Therapy of growth restriction is often nonspecific but should be directed at the underlying cause of poor fetal growth if one can be determined. When a maternal medical problem such as inflammatory bowel disease is contributing to poor growth, specific therapy should be instituted. Alleviation of hypoxia, therapy of high blood pressure and anemia, and hyperalimentation are three examples.

When placental infarction was implicated as the underlying etiology, Moe[119] reported subcutaneous heparin therapy to have a favorable influence on pregnancy outcome. Certainly, mothers should be counseled to stop smoking and ingesting alcohol. Nonspecific therapies include bedrest in the left lateral decubitus position to increase placental blood flow. While an inadequate diet has not been clearly established as a cause of growth restriction in this country, dietary supplementation may be helpful in those with poor weight gain or low prepregnancy weight.

Testing

Serial evaluations of fetal growth should be instituted as soon as the diagnosis of growth restriction is confirmed or for patients in whom the suspicion for growth restriction is high. In the clinic setting, special effort should be made to have the same examiner see the patient each visit to measure the fundal height and assess fetal weight. Ultrasound examinations should be scheduled every 3 to 4 weeks and should include determinations of the BPD, HC/AC, fetal weight, and amniotic fluid volume (Table 25-1). Arrested head growth is of great concern, especially in light of the most recent data available on ultimate developmental potential for the growth-restricted infant.[120] Clear documentation of arrested head growth over a 4-week period is alarming, and the feasibility and safety of delivery should be reviewed.[121]

Ultrasound should be used not only to document abnormal growth but also to detect lethal congenital malformations such as renal agenesis. In cases of severe symmetric growth restriction, amniocentesis, placental biopsy, or cordocentesis should be considered to rule out a chromosomal abnormality such as trisomy 13, 18, or 21 (Table 25-2).[25] Trisomy 18 may present with growth restriction and polyhydramnios. If the diagnosis of a lethal anomaly can be made with certainty, an unnecessary cesarean delivery for fetal distress may be prevented.

Fetal well-being should also be assessed regularly once the diagnosis of growth restriction is entertained. These infants have an increased incidence of intrauterine demise, presumably from cord compression as well as placental insufficiency. Monitoring these infants decreases the stillbirth rate by detecting the compromised fetus and allowing timely intervention.[3]

Appropriate antepartum testing should be instituted as soon as the diagnosis of growth restriction is suspected. Experience with the nonstress test (NST) in cases of growth restriction has confirmed that a reactive NST correlates highly with a fetus that is not in immediate danger of intrauterine demise. Twice weekly nonstress testing is an appropriate interval.[122] Visser and associates[123] performed antepartum fetal heart rate monitoring immediately before cordocentesis in 58 growth-restricted and 29 appropriately grown fetuses. In the appropriately grown fetuses, blood PO_2 and pH values were within the normal range for gestation in 27 cases demonstrating a reactive heart rate pattern and in 2 in which the tracing was nonreactive. In contrast, abnormal antepartum heart rate patterns were found in 15 of the 19 growth-restricted fetuses with hypoxemia, acidemia, or both. The best heart rate marker for fetal hypoxemia was a pattern characterized by repetitive decelerations. In that group, only two fe-

Table 25-1 Utilization of Ultrasonography in the Diagnosis and Evaluation of IUGR

Parameter	Results	Diagnosis	Plan
BPD	Appropriate for dates (within 2 weeks of dates)	No IUGR	Repeat only if indicated by clinical parameters (e.g., lagging fundal growth)
EFW	Above 10th percentile		
HC/AC ratio	In normal range		
Amniotic fluid volume	Normal		
BPD	Appropriate for dates (within 2 weeks of dates)	Probable asymmetric IUGR	Repeat ultrasound examination every 2–3 weeks if not delivered
EFW	Below 10th percentile		Start antepartum surveillance and continue until delivery
HC/AC ratio	Above 95th percentile		
Amniotic fluid volume	Low		
BPD	2 weeks or more; smaller than expected for menstrual dates	Probable symmetric IUGR	Repeat ultrasound examination every 2–3 weeks if not delivered
EFW	Below 10th percentile		Start antepartum surveillance and continue until delivery
HC/AC ratio	In normal range		
Amniotic fluid volume	Normal or low		If IUGR present before 20 weeks, scan for anomalies and consider fetal karyotype

(Modified from Grannum,[121] with permission.)

tuses demonstrated normal PO_2 and pH values. In none of the cases with a reactive heart rate pattern was the growth-restricted fetus acidemic. However, many growth-restricted fetuses with a normal heart rate pattern were found to have fetal PO_2 values in the lower range of normal. Overall, antepartum fetal heart rate patterns in both normal and growth-restricted fetuses were found to correlate well with fetal oxygenation. The appearance of spontaneous decelerations during the NST may reflect oligohydramnios and cord compression and has been associated with a high perinatal mortality rate.[124] The addition of a measure of amniotic fluid volume to the NST has been called a "modified biophysical profile". When compared with a weekly contraction stress test, the twice weekly modified biophysical profile results in similar perinatal outcome.[125]

Nonreactive NST results are often falsely positive and should be further evaluated before any manage-

ment decision is made. Contraction stress testing (CST) is one option for additional testing. A negative CST result, even when the CST is performed early in the third trimester, is an indication of adequate placental respiratory reserve.[126] Conversely, positive CST results occur in 30 percent of the pregnancies complicated by proven growth restriction. In a study by Lin et al.,[127] 30 percent of growth-restricted infants had nonreactive NST results and 40 percent had positive CST results. Ninety-two percent of IUGR infants with a nonreactive positive pattern exhibited perinatal morbidity. However, a 25 to 50 percent false-positive rate has been associated with the CST by some investigators.[126] Therefore, information from antepartum fetal heart rate testing must always be reviewed in concert with the gestational age of the fetus, as well as other indices of fetal well-being and fetal growth.

The fetal biophysical profile score developed by Manning et al.[128] can provide appropriate follow up to nonreassuring fetal heart rate testing or can be used as an alternative method for primary antenatal surveillance. Several studies have demonstrated good correlation between these test results and the level of fetal acidemia as determined by percutaneous umbilical blood sampling in the growth-restricted fetus without anomalies.[129,130] Vintzileos et al.[131] have demonstrated that the components of the biophysical score are affected at different levels of hypoxemia and acidemia, the earliest manifestations of abnormal fetal biophysi-

Table 25-2 Chromosomal Abnormalities and IUGR

	Ultrasound Findings Present		
IUGR	Anomaly	Hydramnios	Abnormal Karyotype
X			12/180 (7%)
X	X		18/57 (32%)
X		X	6/22 (27%)
X	X	X	7/15 (47%)

(From Eydoux et al.,[25] with permission.)

cal activity being the loss of reactivity in the NST along with the absence of fetal breathing. This is followed by decreased fetal tone and movement in association with more advanced acidemia, hypoxemia, and hypercapnia. As a backup test for nonreassuring fetal heart rate testing the biophysical profile leads to lower rates of intervention when compared with the CST, with no impact on perinatal outcome.[132]

Maternal monitoring of fetal activity has been used extensively in Great Britain, Scandinavia, and Israel for the assessment of pregnancies complicated by IUGR. In a study of 50 cases, Matthews[133] clearly showed the predictive value of fetal activity charting for growth-restricted fetuses subsequently demonstrating distress in labor. The techniques available for monitoring fetal movement are reviewed in Chapter 12.

Doppler flow studies of the fetal vasculature have been applied to assess the condition of the fetus thought to be growth restricted. These studies have also contributed to our understanding of the pathophysiology of IUGR. Wladimiroff et al.[134] observed an increase in the pulsatility index of the umbilical artery associated with a reduced pulsatility index in the internal carotid artery, suggesting "brain sparing" in cases of asymmetric growth restriction. An increase in the pulsatility index in the fetal renal artery was observed by Veille and Kanaan,[80] consistent with decreased renal blood flow. These findings and others have confirmed some of the basic fetal responses to growth restriction.

The major focus of Doppler studies for the assessment of fetal health has been the umbilical-placental circulation. Studies by Giles et al.[135] demonstrated that the small arterial vessel count in the tertiary stem villi of the placenta is significantly lower in patients with high umbilical artery S/D ratios than in those with normal S/D ratios. These observations suggest that the increased resistance to flow as demonstrated by a high S/D ratio is associated with and may be due to obliteration of the small muscular arteries in the tertiary stem villi. Rochelson et al.[136] also confirmed a significant reduction in the small muscular artery count and the small muscular artery/villus ratio in the placentas of trisomic fetuses. Abnormal umbilical artery Doppler waveforms could be closely correlated with reduced small muscular artery counts. This study suggests that growth restriction in the fetus with a chromosomal abnormality may be due to not only poor intrinsic growth potential but also abnormalities in placental morphology and fetoplacental blood flow. Fok et al.[137] demonstrated that the percentage of abnormal arterial vessels in the placentas of 14 growth-restricted fetuses could be correlated with the Doppler resistance index.

Abnormal Doppler flow studies indicate increased likelihood of significant perinatal morbidity and mortality in cases of IUGR. Soothill et al.[138] measured um-

bilical venous PO_2, PCO_2, pH, and plasma lactate levels in 29 growth-restricted fetuses. They found significant negative correlations between the severity of fetal hypoxia, hypercapnia, acidosis, and hyperlacticemia and the mean velocity of flow in the fetal aorta. Hackett et al.[139] reported that fetuses with absent end-diastolic flow in the fetal aorta were significantly more growth restricted and required delivery at an earlier gestational age than those in whom end diastolic flow was observed. These fetuses were also more likely to suffer perinatal death, necrotizing enterocolitis, and hemorrhage.

Randomized prospective trials have been performed to examine the impact of Doppler velocimetry on perinatal outcome. Trudinger et al.[140] demonstrated that the availability of umbilical Doppler information resulted in a reduction in fetal distress in labor and emergency cesarean delivery in a group of women considered at high risk. Infants from the control group spent more time in the intensive care nursery and required longer respiratory support. Eighteen percent of the study group and 11 percent of the control group were growth restricted at delivery.[140] Omtzigt et al.[141] demonstrated that the availability of umbilical Doppler velocimetry resulted in reduced perinatal mortality in a referral population when it was used to influence the frequency of other antepartum testing. Fourteen percent of the infants in this study had birth weights below the 10th percentile.[141] Primary antenatal surveillance using umbilical artery velocimetry was compared to cardiotocography in the growth-restricted fetus by Almstrom et al.[142] IUGR fetuses who had primary surveillance with umbilical Doppler velocimetry had fewer antenatal hospital admissions, inductions of labor, emergency cesarean deliveries for fetal distress, and fewer admissions to the intensive care nursery. In contrast, Newham et al.[143] demonstrated no improvement in perinatal morbidity and only a small beneficial effect on antepartum management when umbilical artery Doppler velocimetry results were available in a high-risk obstetric group. In a nonrandomized trial, umbilical Doppler velocimetry was able to predict neonatal morbidity in the growth-restricted newborn, while fetal heart rate variability and biophysical profile evaluation were not.[144] Chang et al.[145] have demonstrated that of the ultrasound parameters routinely available, fetal growth rate and the ratio of peripheral to central nervous system Doppler indices provided the greatest sensitivity in the prediction of neonatal morbidity for the small newborn, with sensitivities of 54 and 69 percent, respectively.

Absent end-diastolic velocity in the umbilical artery has repeatedly been associated with poor perinatal outcome (Fig. 25-5) In a study of 31 fetuses with absent end-diastolic velocity in the umbilical artery, Brar and

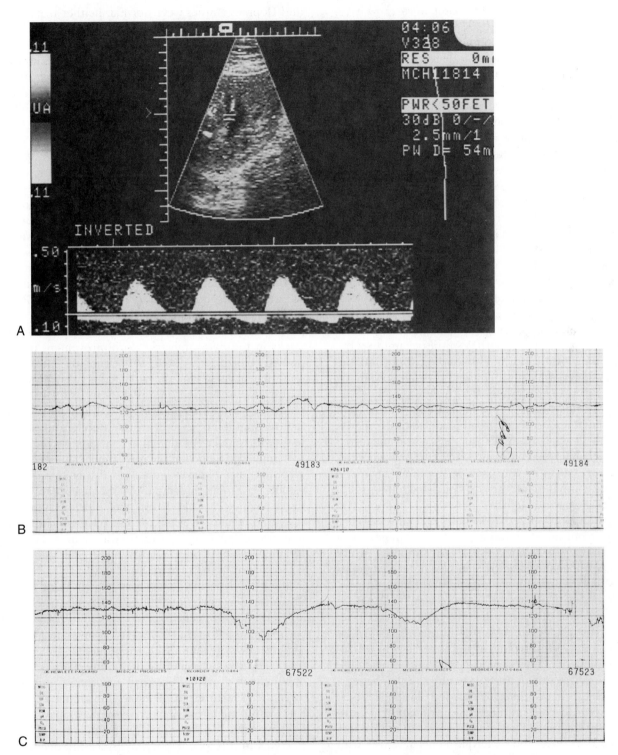

Fig. 25-5 A 30-year-old G1P0 at 28 + 3 weeks gestation who was found to have an estimated fetal weight below the 10th percentile for population-based norms. Doppler flow studies **(A)** demonstrated reversed end-diastolic flow in the umbilical artery. The patient was taken to labor and delivery, where she was placed on face mask oxygen and betamethasone was administered. The fetal heart heart tracing **(B)** was considered reassuring. Within 24 hours the fetal heart rate tracing deteriorated **(C)** and the patient was taken for primary cesarean delivery. A viable male infant weighing 480 g was delivered and received Apgar scores of 3 and 8.

Platt[146] noted that over 80 percent were growth restricted. There were 10 perinatal deaths, for a perinatal mortality rate of 32 percent. Of note, five fetuses showed improvement in umbilical artery waveforms in response to bedrest. Brar and Platt[146] warned that it appeared premature to intervene in a pregnancy solely on the basis of such abnormal waveforms because antepartum improvement could occur. McGowan et al.[147] reported similar findings in a study of 15 singleton preterm pregnancies evaluated on the day of delivery. Absent end-diastolic velocity in the umbilical artery was associated with a high incidence of early delivery, growth restriction, oligohydramnios, pregnancy-induced hypertension, cesarean delivery for fetal distress, and low Apgar scores. These fetuses usually had evidence of acute or chronic hypoxia. Absent end-diastolic umbilical flow signals the need for aggressive antenatal surveillance at a level greater than that usually provided for the small fetus.[148] Reversed end-diastolic flow in the umbilical artery reflects severe fetal compromise and is an ominous finding. Perinatal mortality rates were 50 and 64 percent in two studies examining the prognostic significance of this finding. Both authors recommended that consideration for delivery be made when reversed end-diastolic flow is detected.[149,150]

Doppler velocimetry of the fetal umbilical artery and aorta has demonstrated prognostic relevance in the IUGR fetus when the waveform response to maternal hyperoxygenation is examined.[151,152] Improvement in waveform indices is associated with a more favorable outcome compared with growth-restricted fetuses demonstrating no improvement.

In summary, Doppler velocimetry of fetal vessels has improved our understanding of the pathophysiology of fetal growth restriction. Additionally, umbilical artery Doppler velocimetry identifies the IUGR fetus at greatest risk for neonatal morbidity and mortality. In controlled trials the use of fetal Doppler waveform analysis has been associated with improved perinatal outcome.

As previously noted cordocentesis may be indicated for the rapid karyotyping of the severely growth-restricted fetus. Evaluation of fetal acid-base status in the growth-restricted fetus appears to offer limited benefit. Nicolini et al.[153] examined 58 growth-restricted fetuses, utilizing cordocentesis for acid-base evaluation in addition to karyotyping. They found significant differences in pH, PCO_2, PO_2, and base equivalents in fetuses who had no evidence of end-diastolic flow by umbilical artery Doppler velocimetry. However, they observed no relationship between acid-base determination and perinatal outcome. Pardi et al.[154] examined umbilical blood acid-base status in 56 growth-restricted fetuses and demonstrated an association between acid-base status and the results of cardiotocographic and umbilical artery Doppler waveform analysis. If both fetal heart rate

and Doppler studies were normal, neither hypoxemia nor acidemia was noted. When both tests were abnormal, 64 percent of the growth-restricted fetuses demonstrated abnormal acid-base analysis. Unfortunately the prognostic significance of these abnormalities is uncertain. In summary, there would appear to be no direct fetal benefit from the use of percutaneous umbilical blood sampling in the setting of fetal growth restriction.

Therapy

Several studies have examined the potential benefits of maternal hyperoxygenation in the treatment of the compromised growth-restricted fetus. Nicolaides et al.[155] administered 55 percent oxygen by face mask to mothers whose pregnancies were complicated by severe growth restriction, oligohydramnios, and decreased blood flow in the fetal descending aorta. Ten minutes of maternal hyperoxygenation raised the fetal P_{O_2} to normal or near-normal in five of six cases. Therapy was provided for an average duration of approximately 5 weeks in the five survivors. No improvement in fetal growth velocity was noted. Ribbert et al.[156] provided maternal oxygen therapy (2.5 L/min nasal prong) to four growth-restricted infants at 27 to 28 weeks. Pregnancy was prolonged an average of 9 days beyond the first recognition of fetal heart rate decelerations. Neonates who were exposed to maternal hyperoxygenation had improved blood gas measurements but more hypoglycemia, thrombocytopenia, and disseminated intravascular coagulation compared with concordant gestational age and fetal heart rate matched growth-restricted controls not exposed to oxygen. The ability to improve fetal blood gas values with maternal oxygen therapy has also been confirmed in the growth-restricted fetus by Battaglia et al.[157]

Maternal hyperoxygenation may be of value for the safe, short-term prolongation of pregnancy. Such therapy may be of benefit to allow the administration of corticosteroids to reduce the risk of neonatal respiratory distress syndrome in anticipation of a preterm delivery. In addition, maternal hyperoxygenation may be of benefit in providing for prolongation of pregnancy when the growth-restricted fetus is too immature to survive. While maternal hyperoxygenation may reduce fetal hypoxia, overall neonatal outcome may not be improved with prolonged therapy, since the deleterious effects of continued intrauterine substrate deprivation may extend beyond the benefits of improved fetal oxygen tension.

In 1987, Wallenburg and Rotmans[158] significantly reduced the incidence of fetal growth restriction in women with a history of recurrent IUGR using low-dose aspirin and dipyridamole beginning at 16 weeks gestation. Women receiving therapy had a rate of fetal growth restriction of 13 percent compared with 61 percent in an untreated control group. No treated woman had a child with severe growth restriction (birth weight <2.3 percentile) compared with 27 percent in the untreated group (CH). Trudinger et al.[159] examined aspirin alone (150 mg) versus placebo in the treatment of women with abnormal fetal umbilical Doppler indices in the third trimester and found a significant improvement in both birth weight and head circumference in the treated group. No improvement in Doppler indices was seen in those fetuses with extreme (>99.95 percentile) abnormalities. The EPREDA multicenter trial examined the impact of aspirin (150 mg), aspirin and dipyridamole (225 mg), or placebo in the prevention of IUGR in high-risk pregnancies.[160] Treatment resulted in improved birth weight and lower rates of stillbirth, abruptio placentae, and IUGR. No added benefit of dipyridamole over aspirin alone was noted. In contrast, in the Italian study of aspirin to prevent IUGR, aspirin (50 mg) was compared with placebo in women judged to be at moderate risk.[161] No difference was detected in birth weight or in the rate of IUGR. In summary, there would appear to be some benefit associated with the use of low-dose aspirin in the prevention of IUGR in those patients with significant risk factors. This benefit may well be dose dependent.

Delivery

Proper timing of delivery is often the critical management issue when dealing with the growth-restricted fetus. Frigoletto[162] has emphasized, "The majority of fetal deaths occur after the 36th week of gestation and before labor which leads to the conclusion that many deaths could be prevented by accurate recognition of growth restriction and appropriately timed and conducted intervention." The crux of management is to balance the hazards of prematurity with the threat of intrauterine demise. Careful consideration should be given to the reliability of the information on which the gestational age of the fetus has been established, the fetal growth curve, and the results of antepartum fetal monitoring.

Amniocentesis may be an important adjunct to this decision-making process. The lecithin/sphingomyelin (L/S) ratio may also provide information that allows more accurate dating of the pregnancy. A surprisingly low L/S ratio would suggest an earlier gestational age rather than fetal growth restriction. In cases of symmetric growth restriction, a late amniocentesis may also be employed to obtain amniotic fluid for a fetal karyotype.

To review, if growth restriction is suspected or anticipated, appropriate fetal testing and daily maternal assessment of fetal activity should be instituted. Ultra-

sound examinations to assess fetal growth should be scheduled every 3 to 4 weeks. As long as studies show continued fetal head growth and test results remain reassuring, no intervention is required. If the patient fails a primary surveillance tool such as the NST, follow-up testing must be done. If the CST result is positive or the fetal biophysical profile score is either 6 with oligohydramnios or 4 or less, delivery should be considered. An assessment of fetal lung maturity should be made if possible. In the face of a mature L/S ratio and ominous antepartum test results, delivery should be effected. If the patient has an immature L/S ratio and abnormal test findings, then consideration can be given to steroid administration with continuous heart rate monitoring and oxygen supplementation until delivery or until antepartum test results improve. If amniotic fluid cannot be obtained for an L/S ratio as a result of oligohydramnios and the clinical picture supports the diagnosis of severe IUGR, early delivery should be considered. In these difficult cases, the pediatricians who will care for the baby should be included in the decision-making process.

Because a large proportion of growth-restricted infants suffer intrapartum asphyxia, intrapartum management demands continuous fetal heart rate monitoring. Cord blood sampling has demonstrated that these fetuses may exhibit increased lactic acid levels, polycythemia, hypoglycemia, and acidosis before labor.[167] During labor, a tracing without late decelerations is predictive of a good outcome in cases complicated by IUGR. However, with late decelerations, the incidence of asphyxia in growth-restricted infants is far greater than in normally grown infants. Therefore, earlier intervention may be indicated.[164] As many growth-restricted fetuses require preterm delivery, an unfavorable cervix is not uncommon. The presence of IUGR has been considered a relative contraindication to the use of prostaglandin for cervical preparation by some authors.[165] An unfavorable cervix may also preclude internal fetal heart rate monitoring. In the face of an inadequate external tracing, cesarean delivery may be necessary.

Neonatal Outcome

Neonatal morbidity must be anticipated when the growth-restricted fetus is delivered. These infants suffer more frequently from meconium aspiration than do appropriately grown infants. Gasping in utero in response to asphyxia appears to contribute to this problem. Meconium aspiration is rarely seen before 34 weeks gestation and is, therefore, largely a problem of the mature growth-restricted infant. At delivery, careful suctioning of the nasopharynx and oropharynx with the DeLee

---

Early Neonatal Morbidities in IUGR

Birth asphyxia
Meconium aspiration
Hypoglycemia
Hypocalcemia
Hypothermia
Polycythemia, hyperviscosity, hyperbilirubinemia
Thrombocytopenia
Pulmonary hemorrhage
Malformations
Sepsis

---

catheter decreases the incidence of this complication.[166] Further clearing of the airway can be accomplished at delivery by direct laryngoscopy and aspiration by an experienced pediatrician. Because immediate attention to the many neonatal problems experienced by these infants is essential, appropriate pediatric support should be present in the delivery room when an infant suspected of being growth restricted is to be delivered.

Hypoglycemia is a frequent problem in growth-restricted infants, a result of both inadequate glycogen reserves secondary to intrauterine malnutrition and a gluconeogenic pathway that is less responsive to hypoglycemia than that of the normally grown infant.[167] Hypoglycemia should be anticipated in all growth-restricted infants and frequent blood glucose monitoring instituted. Hypocalcemia, another well-recognized problem in growth-restricted babies, may be due to relative hypoparathyroidism, a result of acidosis associated with intrauterine asphyxia.[168] Hyperphosphatemia secondary to tissue breakdown may also contribute. Frequent calcium monitoring is essential as symptoms are nonspecific and similar to those associated with hypoglycemia.

Polycythemia is observed three to four times more frequently in the growth-restricted infant than in weight-matched controls. Polycythemia results from hypoxia, which leads to increased production of red blood cells, and from transfer of blood volume from the placental circulation to the fetal circulation in the face of intrauterine asphyxia.[167] Thus, these infants produce more red blood cells that are shunted to them if hypoxia occurs during labor. Polycythemia leads to increased red blood cell breakdown, accounting in part for the high incidence of hyperbilirubinemia in these infants. Polycythemia is a criterion for, but does not necessarily lead to, hyperviscosity, which can result in

capillary bed sludging and thrombosis. Multiple organ systems can be affected, leading to pulmonary hypertension, cerebral infarction, and necrotizing enterocolitis.

Hyponatremia resulting from impaired renal function is also frequently reported in growth-restricted infants. The renal complications associated with IUGR may be attributed to asphyxia, which can produce central nervous system injury leading to inappropriate antidiuretic hormone (ADH) secretion.[167]

Hypothermia is another common problem for the growth-restricted infant and results from decreased body fat stores secondary to intrauterine malnourishment.[167] Hypothermia, if unrecognized and untreated, can contribute to the metabolic deterioration of an already unstable growth-restricted infant.

The relationship of RDS and intraventricular hemorrhage (IVH) to gestational age in growth-restricted premature infants compared with normally grown premature infants is unclear. Procianoy and colleagues[169] demonstrated that RDS occurred in 74 percent of appropriately grown infants but was diagnosed in only 5 percent of growth-restricted infants. Similarly, appropriately grown neonates had a 42 percent incidence of IVH hemorrhage, whereas this complication was detected in just 11 percent of growth-restricted infants.[169] In contrast, Piper and Langer[170] found no difference in indices of fetal lung maturity comparing gestational age matched SGA and appropriate for gestational age (AGA) fetuses. Similarly, Thompson et al.[171] found no difference in the frequency of ventilatory support when growth-restricted and AGA infants were matched for gestational age and mode of delivery. Mortality rates were higher in the IUGR group.

The past two decades have seen tremendous advances in the overall management of the low-birthweight infant. Obstetricians are more aware of the syndrome of IUGR, and improved techniques for the detection of impaired intrauterine growth and the assessment of well-being are now available. Technology required for the neonatal care of these infants advances each year. Have improvements in obstetric and pediatric care favorably affected the outcome of the growth-restricted infant? The perinatal mortality rate for those infants who receive optimal intrapartum and neonatal management is decreased when compared with that for age-matched controls who did not have intensive care.[172] The ultimate growth potential for these infants also appears to be good. Although Babson's data[173] in 1970 indicated that only partial "catch-up growth" could be expected in growth-restricted term infants, the degree of catch-up growth observed in several longitudinal studies made since that time suggests that these infants can be expected to have normal growth curves and normal albeit slightly reduced size as adults. In the

8-year follow-up of children weighing less than 1,500 g at birth by Kitchen et al.,[174] 75 percent of growth-restricted infants achieved a height and weight above the 10th percentile. Of infants whose birth weight fell below the 3rd percentile, 60 percent had reached the 25th percentile for weight at 8 years. In Kitchen and associates' study,[174] however, 50 percent of the children with small head circumferences still had head circumferences below the 10th percentile at the 8-year follow-up visit in spite of their growth in height and weight. Similarly, the study of preterm infants with IUGR by Vohr et al.[175] showed a pattern of catch-up to normal levels by 2 years of age. Low et al.[176] studied this same weight group for 1 year and confirmed that the differences between the growth-restricted and appropriately grown groups disappeared at 12 months of age. Kumar et al.[177] noted that in infants whose birth weights were less than 1,250 g, at 1 year 46 percent of the growth-restricted infants remained less than the 3rd percentile for weight and 38 percent remained less than the 3rd percentile for height. In general, those infants suffering growth restriction near the time of delivery do tend to catch up. However, those neonates with earlier onset and more long-standing growth restriction in utero continue to lag behind.

The issue of long-term neurologic sequelae remains unresolved. In 1972, Fitzhardinge and Steven,[178] evaluating a group of 96 growth-restricted infants, noted that between 50 percent of males and 36 percent of females had poor school performance and overall 25 percent had minimal cerebral dysfunction. Major neurologic deficits were much less frequent. Other studies have shown low birth weight and short gestation to be risk factors for cerebral palsy. However, the vast majority of children with cerebral palsy are not growth restricted. Commey and Fitzhardinge[179] studied a group of outborn infants, most but not all of whom weighed less than 1,500 g, and found that 49 percent had developmental handicaps at 2 years. Twenty-one percent had major neurologic sequelae. They attributed this poor neurologic outcome to hypoxic insults sustained in the intrapartum or immediate neonatal period.[179] Their study population was admittedly skewed, since only the sickest infants were transferred to their care. The large number of severe neurologic deficits observed in this group of infants in whom more than 90 percent had no intrapartum fetal monitoring underscores the potential impact that recognition and prevention of intrapartum asphyxia can have on ultimate outcome.

The positive effect of intrapartum surveillance is reflected in the data of Low et al.[176] In a study of 88 growth-restricted infants, they reported no severe neurologic sequelae. They did detect a lag in mental development that was significant in the growth-restricted ba-

bies when compared with appropriately grown controls, especially in the group with birth weights less than 2,300 g. This study correlates well with the data of Lipper et al.[180] on low-birth-weight babies. She observed that growth-restricted infants with a head circumference below the 10th percentile have two to three times the number of serious neurologic sequelae of their normocephalic counterparts. The study by Kumar et al.[177] of infants with a mean birth weight of 1,066 g showed that 30 percent of these very-low-birth-weight growth-restricted premature infants had major neurologic problems. Walther,[181] in an examination of 7 year olds who suffered no perinatal complications despite IUGR and who were matched for social class with a control group, showed an increase in teacher-identified hyperactivity, poor concentration and clumsiness. In a study of school performance in 8 year olds matched for socioeconomic status, Robertson et al.[182] demonstrated a tendency toward hyperactivity in preterm growth-restricted children compared with control groups. Low et al.[183] have shown that in 9 to 11 year olds only fetal growth restriction and the Blishen score (an index of socioeconomic status) contributed independently to the presence of learning deficits. Intrapartum fetal asphyxia, assessed by umbilical artery base deficit, was not associated with learning deficits in this group of children.

The pattern that emerges from evaluation of these data emphasizes that neurologic outcome depends on the degree of growth restriction, its time of onset, and the immaturity of the infant at birth. An early intrauterine insult, between 10 to 17 weeks' gestation, could limit neuronal cellular multiplication and would obviously have a profound effect on neurologic function.[184] In the third trimester, brain development is characterized by glial multiplication, dendritic arborization, establishment of synaptic connections, and myelinization, all of which continue during the first 2 years of life. Recovery after a period of impaired growth in the third trimester is, therefore, more likely to occur. Thus, the preterm appropriately grown infant has more normal neurologic development and fewer severe neurologic deficits than its preterm growth-restricted counterpart. Developmental milestones and neurologic development of mature infants with IUGR and mature infants of normal birth weight are similar. Presumably, this also reflects heightened physician awareness of the growth-restricted infant that allows detection, appropriate antepartum management, intrapartum therapy, and early pediatric intervention.[185–187] The premature growth-restricted infant suffers from increased susceptibility to intrauterine asphyxia and all of the neonatal complications of the premature, as well as those of the infant with IUGR. If growth restriction is associated with lagging head growth before 26 weeks, even mature infants have significant developmental delay at 4 years of age.[188]

Diseases commonly associated with adulthood may have their origins during fetal life. Recent data from two English cohorts have linked IUGR with an increased risk of developing cardiovascular disease, abdominal obesity, noninsulin-dependent diabetes mellitus, and hyperlipidemia.[189–192] These diseases have all been linked to insulin resistance and labeled Syndrome X when they coexist. The risk of developing these abnormalities appears to be inversely proportional to birth weight and independent of gestational age at birth. The mechanism for this association may be a congenital deficiency in pancreatic β-cell endocrine function, which manifests in later life as insulin resistance.[193,194] These data appear to contrast with the World War II Dutch famine experience in which the cohort of children exposed to maternal caloric deficiency in the second half of pregnancy experienced both a reduction in birth weight and a reduction in the incidence of obesity as they entered adulthood when compared with nonfamine-exposed peers.[195]

Overall, increased awareness of the IUGR syndrome and an improved ability to observe intrauterine growth and evaluate fetal well-being in utero have improved along with our understanding of this disease. Continued assessment of the underlying physiology, the efficacy of therapy, and the relationship of fetal status to specific short- and long-term developmental outcome are necessary if overall morbidity and mortality are to be decreased.

Key Points

- Fetal growth restriction is the second leading cause of perinatal morbidity and mortality. Intrauterine growth restriction is currently defined by fetal size alone.

- Characterization of fetal size should be performed using growth curves that are population specific and appropriate.

- The definition of fetal growth restriction has not been based on correlations with short- and long-term morbidity.

- Preterm delivery is associated with an increased incidence of fetal growth restriction.

- Fundal height measurements have low sensitivity in the identification of fetal growth restriction.

- Mortality resulting from fetal growth restriction can be reduced with appropriate antenatal surveillance strategies, which may include early delivery.

- Low-dose aspirin therapy can prevent recurrent IUGR.

- The use of fetal umbilical Doppler flow studies in the management of the growth-restricted fetus reduces perinatal morbidity and mortality.

- Fetal growth restriction is associated with high rates of intrapartum asphyxia.

- Intrauterine growth restriction can result in both short-term and lifelong morbidities.

References

1. Wolfe HM, Gross TL: Increased risk to the growth retarded fetus. p. 111. In Gross TM, Sokol RJ (eds): Intrauterine Growth Retardation. Year Book Medical Publishers, Chicago, 1989

2. Low JA, Boston RW, Pancham SR: Fetal asphyxia during the intrapartum period in intrauterine growth-retarded infants. Am J Obstet Gynecol 113:351, 1972

3. Manning FA, Hohler C: Intrauterine growth retardation: diagnosis, prognostication, and management based on ultrasound methods. p. 331. In Fleischer AC, Romero R, Manning FA et al (eds): The Principles and Practice of Ultrasonography in Obsterics and Gynecology. Appleton and Lange, Norwalk, 1991

4. Ylppo A: Zur Physiologie, Klinik und zum Schicksal der Fruhgeborenen. Ztschr Kinderh 24:1 1920

5. Dunn PM: The search for perinatal definitions and standards. Acta Paediatr Scand 319:7, 1985

6. McBurney RD: The undernourished fullterm infant. West J Surg 55:363, 1946

7. Gruenwald P: Chronic fetal distress and placental insufficiency. Biol Neonate 5:215, 1963

8. Lubchenco LO, Hansman C, Boyd E: Intrauterine growth in length and head circumference as estimated

from live births at gestational ages from 26 to 42 weeks. Pediatrics 37:403, 1966

9. Usher R, McLean F: Intrauterine growth of live-born Caucasian infants at sea level: standards obtained from measurements in 7 dimensions of infants born between 25 and 44 weeks of gestation. J Pediatr 74:901, 1969

10. Battaglia FC, Lubchenco LO: A practical classification of newborn infants by weight and gestational age. J Pediatr 71:159, 1967

11. Babson SG, Behrman RE, Lessel R: Fetal growth: live-born birth weight for gestational age of white middle class infants. Pediatrics 45:937, 1970

12. World Health Organization: Report of a Scientific Group on Health Statistics Methodology Related to Perinatal Events, Document ICD/PE/74.4:1–32, 1974

13. Wilcocks J, Donald J, Duggan TC, Day N: Fetal cephalometry by ultrasound. J Obstet Gynaecol Br Commonw 71:11, 1964

14. Campbell S, Dewhurst CJ: Diagnosis of the small-for-dates fetus by serial ultrasonic cephalometry. Lancet 2: 1002, 1971

15. Chang TC, Robson SC, Boys RJ, Spencer JAD: Prediction of the small for gestational age infant: which ultrasonic measurement is best? Obstet Gynecol 80:1030, 1992

16. Campbell S, Wilkin D: Ultrasonic measurement of fetal abdomen circumference in the estimation of fetal weight. Br J Obstet Gynaecol 82:689, 1975

17. Favre R, Nisand G, Bettahar K et al: Measurement of limb circumferences with three-dimensional ultrasound for fetal weight estimation. Ultrasound Obstet Gynecol 3:176, 1993

18. Hadlock FP, Harrist RB, Sharman RS et al: Estimation of fetal weight with the use of head, body, and femur measurements—a prospective study. Am J Obstet Gynecol 151:333, 1985

19. Vintzileos AM, Campbell WA, Rodis JF et al: Fetal weight estimation formulas with head, abdominal, femur and thigh circumference measurements. Am J Obstet Gynecol 157:410, 1987

20. Combs CA, Jaekle RK, Rosenn B et al: Sonographic estimation of fetal weight based on a model of fetal volume. Obstet Gynecol 82:365, 1993

21. Sabbagha RE, Minogue J, Tamura RK, Hungerford SA: Estimation of birth weight by use of ultrasonographic formulas targeted to large-, appropriate-, and small-for-gestational age fetuses. Am J Obstet Gynecol 160: 854, 1989

22. Ott WJ: The diagnosis of altered fetal growth. Obstet Gynecol Clin North Am 15:237, 1988

23. Seeds JW: Impaired fetal growth: definition and clinical diagnosis. Obstet Gynecol 64:303, 1984

24. Goldenberg RL, Cutter GR, Hoffman HJ et al: Intrauterine growth retardation: standards for diagnosis. Am J Obstet Gynecol 161:271, 1989

25. Eydoux P, Choiset A, LePorrier N et al: Chromosomal prenatal diagnosis: study of 936 cases of intrauterine abnormalities after ultrasound assessment. Prenat Diagn 9:255, 1989

26. Wald NJ, Cuckle HS, Boreham J et al: Birth weight of infants with spina bifida cystica. Br J Obstet Gynaecol 87:578, 1980

27. Hoogland HJ, de Haan J, Martin CB Jr: Placental size during early pregnancy and fetal outcome. a preliminary report of a sequential ultrasonographic study. Am J Obstet Gynecol 138:441, 1980

28. Robinson L, Grau P, Crandall BF: Pregnancy outcomes after increasing maternal serum alpha-fetoprotein levels. Obstet Gynecol 74:17, 1989

29. Wenstrom KD, Owen J, Boots LR, Dubard MB: Elevated second trimester human chorionic gonadotropin levels in association with poor pregnancy outcome. Am J Obstet Gynecol 171:1038, 1994

30. Gonen R, Perez R, David M et al: The association between unexplained second trimester maternal serum hCG elevation and pregnancy complications. Obstet Gynecol 80:83, 1992

31. Cowles T, Tatlor S, Zneimer S, Elder F: Association of confined placental mosaicism with intrauterine growth restriction, abstracted. Am J Obstet Gynecol 170:273, 1994

32. Kalousek DK, Howard-Peebles PN, Olson SB et al: Confirmation of CVS mosaicism in term placentae and high frequency of intrauterine growth retardation association with confined placental mosaicism. Prenat Diagn 11:743, 1991

33. Salafia CM, Vintzileos AM, Silberman L et al: Placental pathology of idiopathic intrauterine growth retardation at term. Am J Perinatol 9:179, 1992

34. Chapman MG, Furness ET, Jones WR et al: Significance of the ultrasound location of placental site in early pregnancy. Br J Obstet Gynaecol 86:846, 1979

35. Gruenwald P: Growth of the human fetus. II: Abnormal growth in twins and infants of mothers with diabetes, hypertension, or isoimmunization. Am J Obstet Gynecol 94:1120, 1966

36. Houlton MCC, Marivate M, Philpott RH: The prediction of fetal growth retardation in twin pregnancy. Br J Obstet Gynaecol 88:264, 1981

37. Long PA, Abell DA, Beischer NA: Fetal growth retardation and preeclampsia. Br J Obstet Gynaecol 87:13, 1980

38. Katz AE, Davison JM, Hayslett JP et al: Pregnancy in women with kidney disease. Kidney Int 18:192, 1980

39. Zulman JI, Alal N, Hoffman GS et al: Problems associated with the management of pregnancies in patients with systemic lupus erythematosus. J Rheumatol 7:327, 1980

40. DeWolf F, Brosens I, Renaer M: Fetal growth retardation and the maternal arterial supply of the human placenta in the absence of sustained hypertension. Br J Obstet Gynaecol 87:678, 1980

41. Ward K, Hata A, Jeunemaitre X et al: A molecular variant of angiotensinogen associated with preeclampsia. Nature Genet 4:59, 1993

42. Pritchard JA, Scott DE, Whalley PJ et al: The effects of maternal sickle cell hemoglobinopathies and sickle cell trait on reproductive performance. Am J Obstet Gynecol 117:662, 1973

43. Smith CA: Effects of maternal undernutrition upon the

newborn infant in Holland (1944–1945). Am J Obstet Gynecol 30:229, 1947

44. Lechtig A, Yarbrough C, Delgado H et al: Effect of moderate maternal malnutrition on the placenta. Am J Obstet Gynecol 123:191, 1975

45. Singer JE, Westphal M, Niswander K: Relationship of maternal weight gain during pregnancy to birth weight and infant growth and development in the first year of life. Obstet Gynecol 31:417, 1968

46. Abrams BF, Laros RK: Prepregnancy weight, weight gain and birth weight Am J Obstet Gynecol 154:503, 1986

47. Economides DL, Nicolaides KH: Blood glucose and oxygen tension levels in small-for-gestational-age fetuses. Am J Obstet Gynecol 160:385, 1989

48. Khouzami VA, Ginsburg DS, Daikoku NH et al: The glucose tolerance test as a means of identifying intrauterine growth retardation. Am J Obstet Gynecol 139:423, 1981

49. Sokol RJ, Kazzi GM, Kalhan SC, Pillay SK: Identifying the pregnancy at risk for intrauterine growth retardation: possible usefulness of the intravenous glucose tolerance test. Am J Obstet Gynecol 143:220, 1983

50. Langer O, Damus K, Maiman M et al: A link between relative hypoglycemia-hypoinsulinemia during oral glucose tolerance tests and intrauterine growth retardation. Am J Obstet Gynecol 155:711, 1986

51. Haworth JC, Ellestad-Sayed JJ, King J et al: Fetal growth retardation in cigarette-smoking mothers is not due to decreased maternal food intake. Am J Obstet Gynecol 137:719, 1980

52. Mills JL, Graubard BI, Harley EE et al: Maternal alcohol consumption and birth weight. how much drinking during pregnancy is safe? JAMA 252:1875, 1984

53. Little BB, Snell LM, Klein VR et al: Cocaine abuse during pregnancy: maternal and fetal implications. Obstet Gynecol 74:157, 1989

54. Lobi M, Welcher DW, Mellits ED: Maternal age and intellectual function of offspring. Johns Hopkins Med J 128:347, 1971

55. Berkowitz GS, Skovron ML, Lapinski RH et al: Delayed childbearing and the outcome of pregnancy. N Engl J Med 322:659, 1990

56. Miller H, Merritt TA: Fetal Growth in Humans. Year Book Medical Publishers, Chicago, 1979

57. Wolfe HM, Gross TL, Sokol RJ: Recurrent small for gestational age birth: perinatal risks and outcomes. Am J Obstet Gynecol 157:288, 1987

58. Galbraith RS, Karchman EJ, Piercy WN et al: The clinical prediction of intrauterine growth retardation. Am J Obstet Gynecol 133:231, 1979

59. Tejani NA: Recurrence of intrauterine growth retardation. Obstet Gynecol 59:329, 1982

60. Tejani N, Mann LI: Diagnosis and management of the small for gestational age fetus. p. 943. In Frigoletto FD (ed): Clinical Obstetrics and Gynecology. Harper & Row, Hagerstown, MD, 1977

61. Belizan JM, Villar J, Nardin JC et al: Diagnosis of intrauterine growth retardation by a simple clinical method:

62. Persson B, Stangenberg M, Lunell NO et al: Prediction of size of infants at birth by measurement of symphysis fundus height. Br J Obstet Gynaecol 93:206, 1986

63. Hepburn M, Rosenburg K: An audit of the detection and management of small-for-gestational age babies. Br J Obstet Gynaecol 93:212, 1986

64. Sabbagha RE, Minogue J, Tamura RK et al: Estimation of birth weight by use of ultrasonographic formulas targeted to large-, appropriate-, and small-for-gestational-age fetuses. Am J Obstet Gynecol 160:854, 1989

65. Guidetti DA, Divon MY, Braverman JJ et al: Sonographic estimates of fetal weight in the intrauterine growth retardation population. Am J Perinatol 6:457, 1989

66. Wilcox AJ: Birth weight, gestation, and the fetal curve. Am J Obstet Gynecol 139:863, 1981

67. Weiner CP, Sabbagha RE, Vaisrub N, Depp R: A hypothetical model suggesting suboptimal intra-uterine growth in infants delivered preterm. Obstet Gynecol 65:323, 6 1985

68. Ott WJ: Intrauteri growth retardation and preterm delivery. Am J Obstet Gynecol 168:1710, 1993

69. Bernstein IM, Meyer MC, Capeless EL: "Fetal growth charts": comparison of cross-sectional ultrasound examinations with birthweight. Maternal-Fetal Med 3:182, 1994

70. Hadlock FP, Harrist RB, Martinez-Poyer J: In utero analysis of fetal growth: a sonographic weight standard. Radiology 181:129, 1991

71. Eik-Nes SH, Grottum P, Persson PH, Marsal K: Prediction of fetal growth by ultrasound biometry. I. Meth Acta Obstet Gynecol 61:53, 1982

72. Rossavik IK, Deter RL: Mathematical modeling of fetal growth. I. Basic principles. J Clin Ultrasound 12:529, 1984

73. Shields LE, Huff RW, Jackson GM et al: Fetal growth: a comparison of growth curves with mathematical modeling. J Ultrasound Med 5:271, 1993

74. Gabbe SG: Intrauterine growth retardation. p. 923. In Gabbe SG, Niebyl JR, Simpson JL (eds): Obstetrics: Normal and Problem pregnancies. 2nd Ed. Churchill Livingston, New York, 1991

75. Lampl M, Veldhuis JD, Johnson ML: Saltation and stasis: a model of human growth. Science 258:801, 1992

76. Bernstein IM, Blake K: Evidence that normal fetal growth is not continuous, abstract ed. Maternal Fetal Med 4:197, 1995

77. Crane JP, Kopta MM: Prediction of intrauterine growth retardation via ultrasonically measured head/abdominalcircumference ratios. Obstet Gynecol 54:597, 1979

78. Seeds JW: Impaired fetal growth: ultrasonic evaluation and clinical management. Obstet Gynecol 64:577, 1984

79. Hadlock FP, Deter RL, Harrist RB et al: A date-independent predictor of intrauterine growth retardation: femur length/abdominal circumference ratio. AJR 141:979, 1983

80. Veille JC, Kanaan C: Duplex Doppler ultrasonographic

evaluation of the fetal renal artery in normal and abnormal fetuses. Am J Obstet Gynecol 161:1502, 1989

81. Manning FA, Hill LM, Platt LD: Qualitative amniotic fluid volume determination by ultrasound: antepartum detection of intrauterine growth retardation. Am J Obstet Gynecol 193:254, 1981

82. Manning FA, Lange IR, Morrison I, Harman CR: Determination of fetal health: Methods for antepartum and intrapartum fetal assessment. Curr Probl Obstet Gynecol 7:1, 1983

83. Groome LJ, Owen J, Neely CL, Hauth JC: Oligohydramics: antepartum fetal urine production and intrapertum fetal distress Am J Obstet Gynecol 165:1077, 1991

84. Schulman H: The clinical implications of Doppler ultrasound analysis of the uterine and umbilical arteries. Am J Obstet Gynecol 157:889, 1987

85. Jacobson S-L, Imhof R, Manning N et al: The value of Doppler assessment of the uteroplacental circulation in predicting preeclampsia or intrauterine growth retardation. Am J Obstet Gynecol 162:110, 1990

86. North RA, Ferrier C, Long D et al: Uterine artery doppler velocity waveforms in the second trimester for the prediction of preeclampsia and fetal growth retardation. Obstet Gynecol 83:378, 1994

87. Bewley S, Cooper D, Campbell S: Doppler investigation of uteroplacental blood flow resistance in the second trimester: a screening study for preeclampsia and intrauterine growth retardation. Br J Obstet Gynaecol 98:871, 1991

88. Steele SA, Pearce JM, Mcparland PM, Chamberlain GVP: Early Doppler ultrasound screening in prediction of hypertensive disorders of pregnancy. Lancet 335:1548, 1990

89. Bower S, Schuchter K, Campbell S: Doppler ultrasound screening as part of routine antenatal scanning: prediction of preeclampsia and intrauterine growth retardation. Br J Obstet Gynaecol 100:989, 1993

90. Valensise H, Romanini C: Second-trimester uterine artery flow velocity waveform and oral glucose tolerance test as a means of predicting intrauterine growth retardation. Ultrasound Obstet Gynecol 3:412, 1993

91. Rohrer VF: Der index der korperfulle als mass des ernahrungszustandes. Munchener Medizinsche Wochenschrift 19:580, 1921

92. Walther FJ, Ramaekers LHJ: The ponderal index as a measure of the nutritional status at birth and its relation to some aspects of neonatal morbidity. J Perinat Med 10:42, 1982

93. Miller HC, Hassanein K: Diagnosis of impaired fetal growth in newborn infants. Pediatrics 48:511, 1971

94. Yagel S, Zacut D, Igelstein S et al: In utero ponderal index as a prognostic factor in the evaluation of intrauterine growth retardation. Am J Obstet Gynecol 157:415, 1987

95. Bernstein IM, Catalano PM: Ultrasonographic estimation of fetal body composition for children of diabetic mothers. Invest Radiol 26:722, 1991

96. Landon MB, Sonek J, Foy P et al: Sonographic measurement of fetal humeral soft tissue thickness in pregnancy complicated by GDM. Diabetes, suppl 2 40:66, 1991

97. Abramowicz JS, Sherer DM, Woods JR: Ultrasonographic measurement of cheek-to-cheek diameter in fetal growth disturbances. Am J Obstet Gynecol 169:405, 1993

98. Hill LM, Guzick D, Boyles D et al: Subcutaneous tissue thickness cannot be used to distinguish abnormalities of fetal growth. Obstet Gynecol 80:268, 1992

99. Winn HN, Holcomb WL: Fetal nonmuscular soft tissue. a prenatal assessment. J Ultrasound Med 4:197, 1993

100. Sparks JW: Human intrauterine growth and nutrient accretion. Semin Perinatol 8:74, 1984

101. Cox WL, Daffos F, Forestier F et al: Physiology and management of intrauterine growth retardation. a biologic approach with fetal blood sampling. Am J Obstet Gynecol 159:36, 1988

102. Fisher JW: Control of erythropoietin production. Proc Soc Exp Biol Med 173:289, 1983

103. Finne PH: Erythropoietin levels in cord blood as an indicator of intrauterine hypoxia. Acta Pediatr Scand 55:478, 1966

104. Maier RF, Bohme K, Dudenhausen JW, Obladen M: Cord blood erythropoietin in relation to different markers of fetal hypoxia. Obstet Gynecol 81:575, 1993

105. Snijders RJM, Abbas A, Melby O et al: Fetal plasma erythropoietin concentration in severe growth retardation. Am J Obstet Gynecol 168:615, 1993

106. Teramo KA, Widness JA, Clemons GK et al: Amniotic fluid eyrthropoietin correlates with umbilical plasma erythropoietin in normal and abnormal pregnancy. Obstet Gynecol 69:710, 1987

107. Ruth V, Autti-Ramo I, Granstrom ML et al: Prediction of perinatal brain damage by cord plasma vasopressin, erythropoietin, and hypoxanthine values. J Pediatr 113:880, 1988

108. Pollack A, Susa JB, Stonestreet BS et al: Phosphoenolpyruvate carboxykinase in experimental intrauterine growth retardation in rats. Pediatr Res 13:175, 1979

109. Gebre-Medhin M, Larsson U, Lindblad BS, Zetterstrom R: Subclinical protein energy malnutrition in under priviledged Ethiopian mothers and their newborn infants. Acta Pediat Scand 67:213, 1978

110. Lindblad BS, Zetterstrom R: The venous free amino acid levels of mother and child during delivery. Acta Pediatr Scand 57:195, 1968

111. Lindblad BS, Rahimtoola RJ, Said M et al: The venous plasma free amino acid levels of mother and child during delivery. III. Acta Pediatr Scand 58:497, 1969

112. Haymond MW, Karl IE, Pagliara AS: Increased gluconeogenic substrates in the small for gestational age infant. N Engl J Med 291:322, 1974

113. Edozien JC, Phillips EJ, Collis WRF: The free aminoacids of plasma and urine in kwashiorkor. Lancet i:615, 1960

114. Mestyan J, Soltesz G, Schultz K, Horvath M: Hyperaminoacidemia due to the accumulation of gluconeogenic amino acid precursors in hypoglycemic small for gestational age infants. J Pediatr 87:409, 1975

115. Cetin I, Corbetta C, Sereni LP et al: Umbilical amino

acid concentrations in normal and growth retarded fetuses sampled in utero by cordocentesis. Am J Obstet Gynecol 162:253, 1990

116. Economides DL, Nicolaides KH, Gahl WA et al: Cordocentesis in the diagnosis of intrauterine starvation. Am J Obstet Gynecol 161:1004, 1989

117. Economides DL, Nicolaides KH, Gahl WA et al: Plasma amino acids in appropriate and small for gestational age fetuses. Am J Obstet Gynecol 161:1219, 1989

118. Bernstein IM, Rhodes S, Stirewalt WS: Amniotic fluid glycine/valine ratio is elevated in fetuses with growth retardation. Maternal Fetal Med 3:251, 1994

119. Moe N. Anticoagulant therapy in the prevention of placental infarction and perinatal death. Obstet Gynecol 58:481, 1981

120. Hobbins JC, Berkowitz RL, Grannum P: Diagnosis and antepartum management of intrauterine growth retardation. J Reprod Med 21:319, 1978

121. Grannum PAT: Ultrasonic measurements for diagnosis. p. 123. In Gross TM, Sokol RJ (eds): Intrauterine Growth Retardation. Year Book Medical Publishers, Chicago, 1989

122. Flynn AM, Kelly J, O'Connor M: Unstressed antepartum cardiotocography in the management of the fetus suspected of growth retardation. Br J Obstet Gynaecol 86:106, 1979

123. Visser GHA, Sadovsky G, Nicolaides KH: Antepartum heart rate patterns in small-for-gestational-age third-trimester fetuses: correlations with blood gas values obtained at cordocentesis. Am J Obstet Gynecol 162:698, 1990

124. Pazos R, Vuolo K, Aladjem S et al: Association of spontaneous fetal heart rate decelerations during antepartum nonstress testing and intrauterine growth retardation. Am J Obstet Gynecol 144:574, 1982

125. Nageotte MP, Towers CV, Asrat T et al: The value of a negative antepartum test: contraction stress test and modified biophysical profile. Obstet Gynecol 84:231, 1994

126. Gabbe SG, Freeman RD, Goebelsmann U: Evaluation of the contraction stress test before 33 weeks' gestation. Obstet Gynecol 52:649, 1978

127. Lin CC, Devoe LD, River P et al: Oxytocin challenge test and intrauterine growth retardation. Am J Obstet Gynecol 140:282, 1981

128. Manning FA, Platt FA, Sipos L: Antepartum fetal evaluation: development of a fetal biophysical profile. Am J Obstet Gynecol 136:787, 1980

129. Manning FA, Snijders R, Harman CR et al: Fetal biophysical prfolie score: VI. Correlation with antepartum umbilical venous fetal pH. Am J Obstet Gynecol 169:755, 1993

130. Ribbert LSM, Snijders RFM, Nicolaides KH, Visser GHA: Relationship of fetal biophysical profile and blood gas values at cordocentesis in severely growth-retarded fetuses. Am J Obstet Gynecol 163:569, 1990

131. Vintzileos AM, Fleming AD, Scorza WE et al: Relationship between fetal biophysical activities and umbilical cord blood gas values. Am J Obstet Gynecol 165:707, 1991

132. Nageotte MP, Towers CV, Asrat A, Freeman RK: Perinatal outcome with the modified biophysical profile. Am J Obstet Gynecol 170:1672, 1994

133. Matthews DD: Maternal assessment of fetal activity in small-for-dates infants. Obstet Gynecol 45:488, 1975

134. Wladimiroff JW, Wijngaard JAGW, Degani S et al: Cerebral and umbilical arterial blood flow velocity waveforms in normal and growth-retarded pregnancies. Obstet Gynecol 69:705, 1987

135. Giles WB, Trudinger BJ, Bard PJ: Fetal umbilical artery flow velocity waveforms and placental resistance: pathological correlation. Br J Obstet Gynaecol 92:31, 1985

136. Rochelson B, Kaplan C, Guzman E et al: A quantitative analysis of placental vasculature in the third-trimester fetus with autosomal trisomy. Obstet Gynecol 75:59, 1990

137. Fok RY, Pavlova Z, Benirschke K et al: The correlation of arterial lesions with umbilical artery Doppler velocimetry in the placentas of small-for-dates pregnancies. Obstet Gynecol 75:578, 1990

138. Soothill PW, Bilardo CM, Nicolaides KH et al: Relation of fetal hypoxia in growth retardation to mean blood velocity in the fetal aorta. Lancet 2:118, 1986

139. Hackett GA, Campbell S, Gamsu H et al: Doppler studies in the growth retarded fetus and prediction of neonatal necrotizing enterocolitis, haemorrhage, and neonatal morbidity. BMJ 294:13, 1987

140. Trudinger BJ, Cook CM, Giles WB et al: Umbilical artery flow velocity wavefroms in high-risk pregnancy: randomized control trial. Lancet 1:188, 1987

141. Omtzigt AMWJ, Reuwer PJHM, Bruinse HW: A randomized controlled trial on the clinical value of umbilical Doppler velocimetry in antenatal care. Am J Obstet Gynecol 170:625, 1994

142. Alstrom H, Axelsson O, Cnattingius S et al: Comparison of umbilical-artery velocimetry and cardiotocography for surveillance of small-for-gestational-age fetuses. Lancet 340:936, 1992

143. Newham JP, O'Dea MRA, Reid KP, Diepeveen DA: Doppler flow velocity wavefrom analysis in high risk pregnancy: a randomized controlled trial. Br J Obstet Gynaecol 98:956, 1991

144. Soothill PW, Ajayi RA, Campbell S, Nicolaides KH: Prediction of morbidity in small and normally grown fetuses by fetal heart rate variability, biophysical profile score and umbilical artery Doppler studies. Br J Obstet Gynaecol 100:742, 1993

145. Chang TC, Robson SC, Spencer JAD, Gallivan S: Prediction of perinatal morbidity at erm in small fetuses: comparison of fetal growth and Doppler ultrasound. Br J Obstet Gynaecol 101:422, 1994

146. Brar HS, Platt LD: Antepartum improvement of abnormal umbilical artery velocimetry: does it occur? Am J Obstet Gynecol 160:36, 1989

147. McGowan LM, Erskine LA, Ritchie K: Umbilical artery Doppler blood flow studies in the preterm, small for gestational age fetus. Am J Obstet Gynecol 156:655, 1987

148. Divon MY, Girz BA, Lieblich R, Langer O: Clinical management of the fetus with markedly diminished umbili-

cal artery end-diastolic flow. Am J Obstet Gynecol 161: 1523, 1989

149. Brar HS, Platt LD: Reverse end-diastolic flow velocity on umbilical artery velocimetry in high-risk pregnancies: an ominous finding with adverse pregnancy outcome. Am J Obstet Gynecol 159:559, 1988

150. Mandruzzato GP, Bogatti P, Fischer L, Gigli C: The clinical significance of absent or reverse end-diastolic flow in the fetal aorta and umbilical artery. Ultrasound Obstet Gynecol 1:192, 1991

151. Bilardo CM, Snijders RM, Campbell S, Nicolaides KH: Doppler study of the fetal circulation during long-term maternal hyperoxygenation for severe early onset intrauterine growth retardation. Ultraound Obstet Gynecol 1:250, 1991

152. de Rochambeau B, Poix D, Mellier G: Maternal hyperoxygenation: a fetal blood flow velocity prognosis test in small-for-gestational-age fetuses? Ultrasound Obstet Gynecol 2:279, 1992

153. Nicolini U, Nicolaidis P, Fisk NM et al: Limited role of fetal blood sampling in prediction of outcome in intrauterine growth retardation. Lancet 336:768, 1990

154. Pardi G, Cetin I, Marconi AM et al: Diagnostic value of blood sampling in fetuses with growth retardation. N Engl J Med 328:692, 1993

155. Nicolaides KH, Bradley RJ, Soothill PW et al: Maternal oxygen therapy for intrauterine growth retardation. Lancet 1:942, 1987

156. Ribbert LSM, van Lingen RA, Visser GHA: Continuous maternal hyperoxygenation in the treatment of early fetal growth retardation. Ultrasound Obstet Gynecol 1: 331, 1991

157. Battaglia C, Artini PG, D'Ambrogio G et al: Maternal hyperoxygenation in the treatment of intrauterine growth retardation. Am J Obstet Gynecol 167:430, 1992

158. Wallenburg HCS, Rotmans N: Prevention of recurrent idiopathic fetal growth retardation by low-dose aspirin and dipyridamole. Am J Obstet Gynecol 157:1230, 1987

159. Trudinger BJ, Cook CM, Thompsom RS et al: Low-dose aspirin therapy improves fetal weight in umbilical placental insufficiency. Am J Obstet Gynecol 159:681, 1988

160. Uzan S, Beaufils M, Breart G et al: Prevention of fetal growth retardation with low-dose aspirin: findings of the EPREDA trial. Lancet 337:1427, 1991

161. Parazzini F, Benedetto C, Frusca T et al: Low dose aspirin in prevention and treatment of inrauterine growth retardation and pregnancy induced hypertension. Italian study of aspirin in pregnancy. Lancet 341:396, 1993

162. Frigoletto FD: Evaluation and management of deferred-fetal growth. p. 922. In Frigoletto FD (ed): Clinical Obstetrics and Gynecology. Harper & Row, Hagerstown, MD, 1977

163. Soothill PW, Nicolaides KH, Campbell S: Prenatal asphyxia, hyperlacticaemia, hypoglycaemia, and erythroblastosis in growth retarded fetuses. BMJ 294:1051, 1987

164. Lin C-C, Moawad AH, Rosenow PJ et al: Acid-base characteristics of fetuses with intrauterine growth retardation during labor and delivery. Am J Obstet Gynecol 137, 1980

165. Sawai SK, Williams MC, O'Brien WF et al: Sequential outpatietn application of intravaginal prostaglandin E₂ gel in the management of postdates pregnancies. Obstet Gynecol 78:19, 1991

166. Carson BS, Losey RW, Bowes WA Jr et al: Combined obstetric and pediatric approach to prevent meconium aspiration syndrome. Am J Obstet Gynecol 126:712, 1976

167. Oh W: Considerations in neonates with intrauterine growth retardation. p. 989. In Frigoletto FD (ed): Clinical Obstetrics and Gynecology. Harper & Row, Hagerstown, MD, 1977

168. Tsang RC, Oh W: Neonatal hypocalcemia in low birthweight infants. Pediatrics 45:773, 1970

169. Procianoy RS, Garcia-Prats FA, Adams JM et al: Hyaline membrane disease and intraventricular haemorrhage in small for gestational age infants. Arch Dis Child 55: 502, 1980

170. Piper JM, Langer O: Is lung maturation related to fetal growth in diabetic or hypertensive pregnancies? Eur J Obstet Gynecol Reprod Biol 51:15, 1993

171. Thompson PJ, Greenough A, Gamsu HR, Nicolaides KH: Ventilatory requirements for repiratory distress syndrome in small-for-gestational-age infants. Eur J Pediatr 151:528, 1992

172. Kitchen WH, Richards A, Ryan MM et al: A longitudinal study of very low-birthweight infants. II: Results of controlled trial of intensive care and incidence of handicaps. Dev Med Child Neurol 21.582, 1979

173. Babson SG: Growth of low-birthweight infants. J Pediatr 77:11, 1970

174. Kitchen WH, McDougass AB, Naylor FD: A longitudinal study of very low-birthweight infants. III: Distance growth at eight years of age. Dev Med Child Neurol 22: 1633, 1980

175. Vohr BR, Oh W, Rosenfield AG et al: The preterm small-for-gestational age infant: a two-year follow-up study. Am J Obstet Gynecol 133:425, 1979

176. Low JA, Galbraith RS, Muir D et al: Intrauterine growth retardation: a preliminary report of long-term morbidity. Am J Obstet Gynecol 130:534, 1978

177. Kumar SP, Anday EK, Sacks LM et al: Follow-up studies of very low birthweight infants. (1,250 grams or less) born and treated within a perinatal center. Pediatrics 66:438, 1980

178. Fitzhardinge PM, Steven EM: The small-for-dates infant. II: Neurological and intellectual sequelae. Pediatrics 50:50, 1972

179. Commey JOO, Fitzhardinge PM: Handicap in the preterm small-for-gestational age infant. J Pediatr 94:779, 1979

180. Lipper E, Lee K-S, Gartner LM et al: Determinants of neurobehavioral outcome in low birthweight infants. Pediatrics 67:502, 1981

181. Walther FJ: Growth and development of term disproportionate small-for-gestational age infants at the age of 7 years. Early Hum Dev 18:1, 1988

182. Robertson CMT, Etches PC, Kyle JM: Eight-year school

performance and growth of preterm, small for gestational age infants: a comparative study with subjects matched for birth weight or for gestational age. J Pediatr 116:19, 1990

183. Low JA, Handley-Derry MH, Burke SO et al: Association of intrauterine fetal growth retardation and learning deficits at age 9 to 11 years. Am J Obstet Gynecol 167:1499, 1992

184. Dobbing J: The later development of the brain and its vulnerability. p. 565. In Davis JA, Dobbing J (eds): Scientific Foundations of Paediatrics. WB Saunders, Philadelphia, 1974

185. Breart G, Poisson-Salomon A-S: Intrauterine growth retardation and mental handicap: epidemiological evidence. Bailliere's Clin Obstet Gynaecol 2:91, 1988

186. Wennergren M, Wennergren G, Vilbergsson G: Obstetric characteristics and neonatal performance in a four-year small for gestational age population. Obstet Gynecol 72:615, 1988

187. Achenbach TM, Phares V, Howell CT et al: Seven year outcome of the Vermont intervention preogram for low birthweight infants. Child Dev 61:1672, 1990

188. Fancourt R, Campbell S, Harvey D et al: Follow-up study of small-for-dates babies. BMJ 1:1435, 1976

189. Law CM, Barker DJP, Osmond C et al: Early growth and abdominal fatness in adult life. J Epidemiol Comm Health 46:184, 1992

190. Phipps K, Barker DJP, Hales CHD et al: Fetal growth and impaired glucose tolerance in men and women Diabetologica 36:225, 1993

191. Barker DJP, Hales CN, Fall CHD et al: Type 2 diabetes mellitus, hypertension and hyperlipidemia (syndrome X): relation to reduced fetal growth. Diabetologia 36: 62, 1993

192. Barker DJP, Gluckman PD, Godfrey KM et al: Fetal nutrition and cardiovascular disease in-adult life. Lancet 341:938, 1993

193. Hubinont C, Nicolini U, Fisk NM et al: Endocrine pancreatic function in growth retared fetuses. Obstet Gynecol 77:541, 1991

194. Van Assche FA, Aerts L, Holemans K: Fetal growth retardation is associated with a reduced function of insulin producing B cells and may explain insulin resistance in later life, abstracted. Am J Obstet Gynecol 170:315, 1994

195. Ravelli GP, Stein ZA, Susser MW: Obesity in young men after famine exposure in utero and early infancy. N Engl J Med 295:349, 1976

196. Chudleigh P, Pearce JM: Obstetric Ultrasound. Churchill Livingstone, Edinburgh, 1986

Chapter 26

Postdate Pregnancy

Roger K. Freeman and David C. Lagrew, Jr

Postdate pregnancy is a common problem in the practice of obstetrics. Previously, the diagnosis of postdate pregnancy was often the result of poor dating. Today, postdate patients are fewer in number due to better dating through the use of first and second trimester ultrasound. Because this group now contains fewer patients with poor dating, these patients as a whole are at higher risk for complications.

Comprehensive management of postdate pregnancy involves both fetal testing and consideration for delivery, with the choice for each individual pregnancy dependent on several clinical factors. If the management choice is fetal testing, there are several methods available. If delivery is chosen, the clinician must determine the timing, route, and method. This chapter will address specific problems related to intrapartum management, examine neonatal issues that pose special problems for the pediatrician, and develop an approach to the management of these challenging and complex clinical dilemmas.

Background

Post-term pregnancy has not always been of universal concern. Until the development of accurate dating techniques there was controversy over whether it was physiologically possible for pregnancy to exceed the 42nd week. Despite a description of postmaturity by Ballantyne[1] as early as the turn of the century, the American medical community viewed the problem with less concern than Europeans. As recently as the early 1960s, American obstetricians were skeptical of McClure-Brown's data[2] showing a twofold increase in fetal mortality when the patient reached 42 weeks gestation. Conversely, American pediatricians sided more with the British position that a post-term pregnancy endan-

gered the fetus. This position was clarified by Clifford's postmaturity classification system[3] in 1952 that helped define the degree of affliction these children suffered. The accumulation of other pediatric data[4] supported Clifford's conclusions, and gradually evidence began to suggest increased risk to both fetus and neonate. By the late 1960s and 1970s, the American obstetrical literature recognized these risks, and with the advent of ultrasound dating, it became clear that gestations could truly exceed 42 weeks.

Controversy has also existed in the management of post-term pregnancy. British authors recommended routine induction of labor between the 42nd and 43rd weeks to prevent poor outcome. They demonstrated beneficial birth results from such aggressive management.[2] Subsequent to this recommendation, investigators attempted, without success, to demonstrate the efficacy of routine inductions. A large study by Lucas et al.,[5] involving more than 60,000 pregnancies, did not show improvement in fetal and neonatal outcomes from routine induction at 42 weeks. Other studies suggested elective induction increased the cesarean delivery.[6] During this time, however, the fetus could not be evaluated before or during labor; therefore, the risks of induction were imposed on many fetuses with adequate uteroplacental reserve. In addition, fetuses with uteroplacental insufficiency and oligohydramnios underwent prolonged inductions without intrapartum monitoring. Some researchers theorized that the better statistics in Great Britain were actually the result of closer intrapartum attention, including frequent auscultation by nurse midwives during labor.

Definition and Incidence

In this chapter, the terms *postdate* and *post-term* will be used interchangeably. Most authors define a postdate pregnancy as that which has reached 42 weeks of amen-

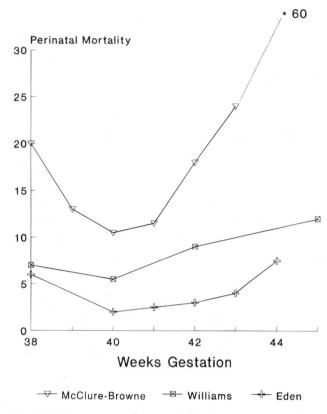

Fig. 26-1 Comparison of perinatal mortality rates versus gestational age through the past three decades. (McClure-Browne[2] data collected in 1958, Williams[68] in 1970–1976, and Eden et al.[9] in 1983–1985.)

orrhea. The incidence of morbidity increases after 40 weeks (Fig. 26-1).[2] At 42 weeks, perinatal mortality doubles, making this an appropriate cut-off point.

Accurate diagnosis of post-term pregnancy depends on proper clinical dating of the pregnancy. Approximately 50 percent of patients deliver by their estimated date of confinement, and about 35 to 40 percent deliver within the following two weeks (Fig. 26-2). Saito et al.[7] estimate that two-thirds of patients thought to be postdate from menstrual history deliver at normal ovulatory ages. Rayburn et al.[8] calculate the incidence of patients reaching the 42nd week as varying from 3 to 12 percent. With accurate gestational age estimation, the lower range is more appropriate.[8] Early prenatal examination and ultrasound clearly improve the accuracy of dating.

Morbidity and Mortality

The rate of maternal, fetal, and neonatal complications increases exponentially with gestational age.[2-4] The primary maternal risk is cesarean delivery, with an associated increased incidence of postpartum infections, hemorrhage from uterine atony, prolonged hospitalization, wound complications, and pulmonary emboli. Eden et al.[9] found the cesarean delivery rate more than doubled when passing the 42nd week compared with term (38 to 40 weeks). They attributed this increase to the incidence of cephalopelvic disproportion resulting from larger infants. Some cesarean deliveries are ac-

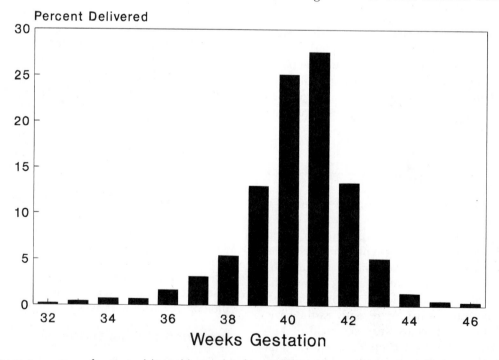

Fig. 26-2 Percentage of patients delivered by weeks of amenorrhea. More recent studies with better gestational age assessment have decreased the percentage of 42 weeks and beyond to less than 10 percent. (Data from Treloar et al.[69])

counted for by attempted induction of patients with unripe cervices. The overall incidence of fetal distress is minimally elevated compared with term populations.[10]

Maternal complications also include trauma from the vaginal delivery of large babies.[11] Vaginal side wall and cervical lacerations and fourth-degree extensions are all more common with instrumented and macrosomic deliveries. These complications carry the potential for urinary retention, fistula formation, hemorrhage, infection, and wound breakdown.

Neonatal complications from postmaturity include placental insufficiency, birth trauma from macrosomia, and meconium aspiration syndrome. Each of these may result in acute and chronic injury to the child. While the incidence of fetal demise has declined with improved perinatal management, perinatal mortality increases past term.[12] Although the attendant risks have been lowered in postdate pregnancy, they have not been eliminated.

Most early work in postdate pregnancy focused on the dysmature infant, the incidence of which reaches 10 percent by the 43rd week.[8] Clifford[3] described these infants as withered, meconium stained, long nailed, fragile, with a small placenta, and at risk for stillbirth. In the neonatal period there is a increased risk of hypoglycemia, heat instability, and meconium aspiration.[3] Growth retardation from postmaturity is the result of uteroplacental insufficiency.[12] First the placenta deprives the fetus of adequate nutrients, and then birth weight diminishes as the fetus uses energy stores in the adipose tissue and liver. Diminished fetal plasma volume leads to oligohydramnios. With further deterioration the placenta loses respiratory function and the fetus faces asphyxial damage and possible stillbirth.[11]

Fortunately, long-term problems appear to arise less with postmaturity than with other forms of growth retardation.[13] Manning[13] reported that these infants regain normal weight quickly and exhibit few long-term neurologic problems. Unlike the deprivation of other forms of fetal dysmaturity, postmaturity has a rapid onset and is of short duration.

While fetal growth can cease with postmaturity, a number of infants will continue growing and exceed 4,000 g, particularly in male gestations (Fig. 26-3).

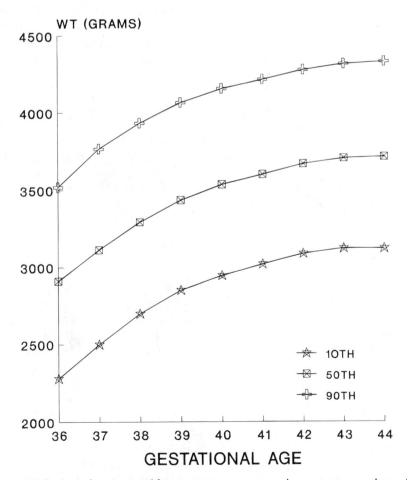

Fig. 26-3 Birth weight for male fetuses in California 1970–1976. Note the increasing numbers of infants greater than 4,000 g after term. (From Williams et al.,[68] with permission.)

Sechen et al.[14] showed that most infants continue interval growth after 40 weeks, leading to macrosomia. About 25 to 30 percent of post-term neonates weigh over 4,000 g, a rate that is three times greater than that of term newborns.[9,15] Large infants frequently undergo prolonged labors and difficult deliveries and have an increased risk of birth trauma. The incidence of shoulder dystocia reaches 1.9 times that of average-sized infants.[9] Macrosomic infants are also subject to asphyxia. Callenbach and Hall[16] found that long-term neurologic damage was as prevalent in larger post-term infants as in poorly grown post-term infants. This differs from data presented by Shime et al.,[17] who suggest that poor neurologic outcome is more likely in small infants. Based on these conflicting data, antenatal surveillance is necessary in *all* post-term pregnancies regardless of growth.

The post-term infant is more likely to have meconium-stained fluid with possible risk for meconium aspiration syndrome. Meconium is found in 25 to 30 percent of post-term pregnancies, double the incidence at term.[9,15] Meconium passage results from increased hypoxic stimulation to the parasympathetic system or is a function of the mere presence of a more mature, active vagal reflex. The diminished amniotic fluid causes the meconium to be thicker and more likely to obstruct airways. Aspiration into the alveoli can cause significant respiratory embarrassment and death.

Management

Recent changes in obstetric care have affected the management recommendations of postdate pregnancy. Postdate pregnancies identified by accurate gestational age assessment will be more likely to have complications. In previous studies, poorly dated patients diluted these risks. Obstetric management must reflect this higher risk and warrants an aggressive delivery and fetal surveillance policy. The increased number of large infants also changes management recommendations. Many authors feel that induction of labor avoids further growth and prevents fetal deprivation.[18] Although older studies of routine induction failed to demonstrate improvement in maternal or neonatal outcome, most were before the development of cervical ripening agents and included many "poor dates" pregnancies.

Diagnosis

The accurate diagnosis of postdate pregnancy can be made only by proper dating. Accurate diagnosis allows concentration of management on the highest risk patients. A major problem of determining gestational age is that all methods of estimating gestational age lose accuracy in the third trimester, when fetal growth diminishes. Therefore, we must determine an accurately estimated date of delivery before the third trimester. Since we cannot predict who will be undelivered by 42 weeks, we must accurately date all prenatal patients (see Ch. 11).

It is important to review clinical parameters in all patients since they are helpful in establishing gestational age at minimal cost. Anderson et al.[19] found that the last menstrual period was the best clinical predictor of gestational age. Seventy-one percent of their patients could recall the exact date of the last period, 25 percent an approximate date, and 4 percent no date. The regularity, date, amount, and length of menses are important clinical factors in gestational age estimation. The use of oral contraceptives may explain delayed ovulation. First trimester pelvic examination can be helpful in confirming menstrual dates. Other clinical parameters include date of first pregnancy test, first fetal heart tones (12 weeks with Doppler, 18 weeks with fetoscope), timing of the fundal height reaching the umbilicus (20 weeks), and quickening.

Ultrasound has become the standard for the determination of gestational age. Routine first or second trimester ultrasound of all pregnant patients decreases the incidence of post-term pregnancy.[20] In patients with regular menses, confirmation by a first trimester pelvic examination, ovulation data, or timed insemination, ultrasound is of less importance. Ultrasound is clearly beneficial in patients without known or reliable clinical data.

Ultrasound is most accurate in early gestation. Measurement of crown–rump length between 6 to 10 weeks can define gestational age within 3 to 5 days.[21] The crown–rump length becomes less accurate after 12 weeks in determining gestational age because the fetus begins to curve. Kopta et al.[22] showed that second trimester biparietal diameter and femur length measurements were as predictive of gestational age as a late crown–rump length. A screening ultrasound at 16 to 20 weeks also allows review of fetal anatomy. During this period, range of error is within plus or minus 1.5 weeks. The most cost-effective period for ultrasound dating, therefore, is between 16 to 20 weeks.

Sonographic accuracy lessens in the third trimester as the rate of bone growth decreases. At this time in gestation, the range of error with ultrasound dating is 3 to 4 weeks; therefore, it is of little help in confirming gestational age unless other dating parameters are poor. A third trimester ultrasound should not be used to disprove a postdate pregnancy. Such late estimation of gestational age may cause inappropriate intervention or inaction leading to poor outcome.

The Choice: Expectant Management Versus Induction of Labor

The first major decision in management is dependent on the certainty of the dates. The accuracy of the gestational age assessment is important when planning intervention. Patients with unsure dates should be managed in a less aggressive fashion when considering delivery if the cervix is not clearly inducible. However, these patients should receive the same program of antenatal surveillance as well-dated pregnancies. There are two basic schemes of management for well-dated postdate patients (Fig. 26-4).

Patients with favorable cervices benefit from induction of labor. Unfortunately, these are the minority of postdate pregnancies. Harris et al.[24] found that only 8.2 percent of pregnancies at 42 weeks had a ripe cervix (Bishop score >7). There are two major reasons for inducing patients with favorable cervices. First, some fetuses will continue growing after term and may develop macrosomia and cephalopelvic disproportion. Second, although antenatal surveillance with appropriate methods is quite reliable, there are occasional mispredictions that result in 0.5 to 1 per thousand unexpected stillbirths in nonanomalous fetuses even with

good patient compliance.[24] Therefore, if the cervix is favorable, delivery provides the safest alternative for mother and baby. Induction is a reasonable option in such patients after the 41st week has passed and spontaneous labor has not ensued.

With confirmed dates and an unfavorable cervix there are two major management methods. The most established method is to initiate antepartum surveillance while awaiting spontaneous labor[25] and/or spontaneous cervical ripening. The other method is to administer prostaglandin gel for cervical ripening and proceed with induction.[26]

There are clinical problems with both management schemes that must be considered. The purpose of expectant management with testing is to await cervical ripening and spontaneous labor, which should decrease the need for cesarean delivery. Previous clinical trials of routine induction at 42 weeks failed to demonstrate benefit[5] or found higher cesarean delivery rates.[6] In contrast, Dyson et al.[26] found that induction at 41 weeks with the utilization of prostaglandin cervical ripening led to a lowered cesarean delivery rate. They attributed these findings to the increasing incidence of larger babies and fetal distress when delaying delivery.

Two large prospective randomized trials[27,28] and a

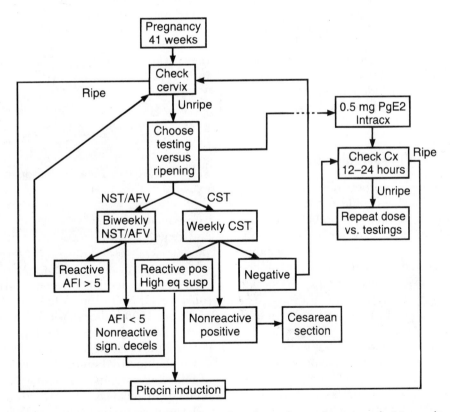

Fig. 26-4 Postdate pregnancy management flow chart. The scheme depicts the various decision-making processes involved in the management of the post-term pregnancy with respect to delivery. The decision whether to use intracervical prostaglandin should be based on clinical data regarding patient safety and ripeness of the cervix. It has been our practice to attempt a trial of induction in well-dated pregnancies at 43 weeks' gestation.

recent meta-analysis[29] have reevaluated the risks and benefits of routine induction versus expectant management. The American trial involved randomizing 440 patients between induction versus expectant management.[27] The induction group was then subdivided into those receiving a single insertion of intracervical prostaglandin gel or placebo. There were no differences in incidences of adverse perinatal outcomes, macrosomia, or cesarean delivery between the groups. It was concluded that either management protocol was acceptable.[27] The Canadian trial randomized 3,407 women at 41 weeks.[28] The induction group received three doses of prostaglandin gel followed by oxytocin induction. These patients had a significantly lower cesarean delivery rate (21.2 vs. 24.5 percent) when compared with women managed expectantly due to a reduced incidence of fetal distress. There was no statistical difference in the rate of stillbirth. Grant[29] performed a meta-analysis of 11 trials and found that routine induction had a lower rate of perinatal mortality, cesarean delivery, and meconium staining.

Prostaglandin ripening, though less studied in postdate pregnancies, appears to have some shortcomings. Dyson et al.[26] found that 50 percent of patients in whom the gel did not ripen the cervix required cesarean delivery. In addition, uterine hyperstimulation can be occasionally seen with prostaglandin gel. Therefore, prostaglandin gel ripening should be used with caution in patients with equivocal antepartum testing. Other factors may also play a role in explaining failure of cervical ripening. Boyd et al.[30] found that uterine dysfunction in primigravid pregnancies, independent of induction of labor and size of the infant, increased the cesarean delivery rate.

Cervical Ripening with Prostaglandin

Previous well-controlled prospectively randomized trials of postdate pregnancies could not demonstrate the benefit of routine induction,[5,6,31] probably because an unripe cervix is found in up to 80 percent of patients reaching the 42nd week of gestation.[23] The availability of prostaglandin gel can improve the likelihood of successful induction. Prostaglandin E_2 gel applied locally to the cervix softens, dilates, and effaces the cervix. The clinical effects are shortened labor, fewer failed inductions, and less need for artificial amniotomy.[26]

The protocol for prostaglandin ripening should be used in patients with an unripe cervix at or beyond 41 weeks gestation when induction is elected. The gel is given on the afternoon or evening before scheduled induction. Before administration, a reassuring fetal heart rate and uterine activity pattern is documented. If the fetus has a nonreassuring fetal heart rate tracing or there is excessive uterine activity, the use of prosta-

glandin gel may not be advisable. After evaluating cervical status, 0.5 mg of prostaglandin E_2 gel is placed intracervically. The patient is observed on the monitor for approximately 2 hours or until uterine activity has subsided. Fifteen percent of patients in the Dyson et al.[26] study went into spontaneous labor and did not require oxytocin induction. When needed, oxytocin induction should be started the next morning after examination has documented ripening of the cervix. If the cervix remains unfavorable, a second dose of prostaglandin gel may be given or expectant management with fetal surveillance initiated while awaiting cervical ripening.

Expectant Management with Antenatal Surveillance

Most expectant management schemes require some form of antenatal surveillance of fetal well-being. There is no uniform agreement about the best method or time to initiate testing. The decision is based on which test has the lowest failure rate, is most cost effective, and has a reasonable intervention rate in your population. Antenatal testing is also recommended for patients undergoing cervical ripening with repeated doses of gel but who remain uninducible.

Previously most schemes have suggested beginning testing at 42 weeks, since this represents the highest risk population and a manageable proportion of patients. The general trend in the United States has been to begin testing during the 41st week of pregnancy. This practice appears to be reasonable in light of the increased incidence of perinatal mortality following 40 weeks. Porto et al.[42] demonstrated an increasing incidence of positive contraction stress tests from 40 to 42 weeks. Since cost effectiveness becomes an issue, fetal movement charting may be reasonable prior to the 41st week (see Ch. 12).

Most antepartum testing in the United States is done with the nonstress test (NST). This test is simple, brief, and requires only inexpensive equipment. The NST yields few equivocal results, and interventions are rarely necessary for an abnormal test result.[33] The major concern using this modality has been falsely reassuring results. Weekly NSTs appear to have a false-negative rate of 6.1 per 1000 (stillbirth within 1 week of a reassuring test).[34] With twice weekly testing, Boehm et al.[34] decreased the false-negative rate from 6.1 to 1.9 per 1,000. Randomized studies have failed to show a benefit of following patients with weekly NST compared with no fetal surveillance.[35,36]

To improve predictability, NSTs are performed twice weekly. Spontaneous decelerations are significant. Phelan et al.[37] demonstrated that the majority of poor perinatal outcomes were confined to patients with decelerations on their NST. Small et al.[38] showed improvement in fetal and neonatal outcomes with induction of labor for significant decelerations on an NST. Unfortunately, this liberal policy increased the intervention rate from 0.97 to 31.8 percent.

Another surveillance choice is the contraction stress test (CST). The major benefit of the CST is that negative results appear to predict fetal well-being for 7 days. Weekly CSTs are effective in preventing stillbirth and have a false-negative rate of only 0.71 per 1,000.[24] The CST is performed with inexpensive equipment and has an acceptable intervention rate for abnormal tests of 10.4 percent.[10] Nipple stimulation techniques have significantly reduced testing time while not sacrificing accuracy.[39] The major problem of the CST is the high rate of equivocal results.[24,33]

The major benefit of the CST for primary surveillance in postdate pregnancy is that, following a reactive negative result, the patient does not require repeat testing for 7 days. By contrast, patients with equivocal tests require repeat testing in 24 hours. This is the major disadvantage of the CST, since up to 35.5 percent of tests will be equivocal in post-term testing.[10] For positive and highly suspicious tests, attempted delivery is indicated. If the CST result is reactive and positive, a trial of labor may be attempted, since up to 66 percent of such patients will deliver vaginally.[24] Should the test result be nonreactive and positive, the patient should have constant electronic fetal monitoring while preparations for cesarean delivery are made. If the fetus remains nonreactive, a cesarean delivery is used.[24] With clinically significant oligohydramnios, cord compression may occur as manifested by variable decelerations. Variable decelerations on the NST should be followed up with an estimate of amniotic fluid volume.

The introduction of real-time ultrasound has opened a new view of fetal biophysical observations for the evaluation of fetal status. Manning et al.[40] have used the combination of fetal movement, fetal tone, amniotic fluid volume, fetal breathing, and heart rate reactivity to assess fetal condition. This biophysical profile (BPR) was initially used on a weekly basis to evaluate post-term pregnancies. Weekly testing yielded results similar to the weekly NST, with false-negative rates of approximately 7 per 1,000.[40] Johnson et al.[41] showed improved efficacy by twice weekly testing and aggressive intervention for diminished fluid volume. They followed 307 patients with such surveillance without a demise. Intervention for abnormal results was an acceptable 10.4 percent of patients followed with the BPP.

Realizing that a reactive fetus will invariably demonstrate fetal tone and movement, another group of investigators have introduced the modified biophysical profile (mBPP). This twice weekly test uses the NST and amniotic fluid volume. Eden et al.[42] introduced this approach in a series of 109 post-term patients without a stillbirth. Clark et al.[43] have confirmed these initial results in a group of 6,000 consecutive patients followed without a fetal demise. In this study, some 40 percent of the pregnancies were post-term.[43] The intervention rate was 23.9 percent in the Eden et al. group and 3 percent in the Clark et al. for all diagnoses group. The incidence of intervention appears to depend on the definition of oligohydramnios and aggressiveness of intervention for significant decelerations. The mBPP has a minimal number of equivocal results.[43] Grubb et al.[44] reported results of 8,038 patients followed with the mBPP in post-term pregnancies. They documented an acceptable fetal mortality rate of 1.12 per 1,000. The intervention rate to achieve this success was not reported.

Assessment of amniotic fluid volume can be performed with varying techniques and intervention thresholds. Subjective estimation by skilled sonographers has been shown to correlate with findings at delivery.[45] This method makes serial observation difficult since observers vary. The utilization of fluid estimates is hampered by the poor understanding of amniotic fluid dynamics as highlighted by the description of Clement et al.[46] of six post-term pregnancies in which the amniotic fluid volume dropped abruptly within 24 hours including one stillbirth. Our own data have demonstrated that, compared with term patients, post-term patients are five times more likely to develop oligohydramnios in 3 to 4 days following a normal amniotic fluid index (AFI).[47] These data suggest the AFI should be repeated *twice weekly* in post-term patients.[47]

Semiquantitative techniques have been proposed by various authors. Initial BPP methods utilized the deepest vertical pocket to assign numeric values to fluid volume. The thresholds for calling the finding abnormal varied from 1 to 3 cm. Chamberlain et al.[48] found that the perinatal mortality in fetuses with 1-cm pockets was 187.5 per 1,000 (109.4 per 1,000 corrected). These data included fetuses of all gestational ages, and those with oligohydramnios made up only 0.85 percent of the total population.[48] Johnson et al.[40] found that only 3.7 percent (11/293) of post-term fetuses develop this degree of oligohydramnios. Six of the 11 fetuses had meconium below the cords, requiring admission to the neonatal intensive care unit.[41] In the 1- to 2-cm group, considered to have marginally decreased fluid, one of nine neonates were admitted to the NICU. The 6.8 percent of patients with fluid less than 2 cm[41] is considerably lower than the 19.4 percent of post-term patients with less than a 3-cm pocket.[49] Eleven percent of the Crouley and O'Herlihy[49] patients with decreased fluid had a cesarean delivery for fetal distress compared with 0.75 percent in the normal fluid group. As noted above, the 3-cm cut-off included nearly 20 percent of patients, leading to a large number of interventions.

We prefer to assess fluid volume with the AFI. This method involves measuring the deepest vertical fluid pocket in centimeters of each uterine quadrant and summing the four together. Phelan et al.[50] found a mean AFI of 14.1 pm 3.5 cm ($\pm$ SD) at 42 weeks' gestation. Less than 5 cm is considered oligohydramnios, 5 to 8 cm borderline, and greater than 8 cm normal.[51] This method is not overly time consuming and can be taught to technicians and nurses who have minimal ultrasound experience.

If the patient remains undelivered by the 43rd week of gestation, it has been our policy to attempt induction of labor. This policy should only apply to well-dated gestations. However, there are no data in the literature, to our knowledge, that have proven that this approach will improve outcome.

Intrapartum Management

Careful intrapartum management is also important to guarantee continued fetal and subsequent neonatal well-being. The major complications in the intrapartum period are meconium staining, macrosomia, and fetal intolerance to labor. The key to proper management is timely recognition, prompt reaction, and skilled actions.

Meconium staining is four times more common in the post-term pregnancy than in term gestations. Before the institution of suctioning techniques, meconium aspiration syndrome was the leading cause of mortality in infants over 2,500 g. Clifford[3] based his staging system to predict clinical outcome of dysmature infants largely on the degree of meconium staining present. There are two primary reasons that meconium is more common in the post-term pregnancy. First, the greater length of time in utero, the more chance for activation of the mature vagal system with excretion of meconium. Second, hypoxia is more likely to occur in the infant who shows the stigmata of dysmaturity and placental insufficiency. The other factor that makes post-term meconium a higher risk for morbidity is the diminished amniotic fluid volume of advanced pregnancy. With oligohydramnios, there is less dilution and meconium is more likely to cause airway obstruction.

When minimal fluid is encountered at the time of membrane rupture, the risk for thick tenacious meconium is increased. Amnioinfusion dilutes meconium, improves 1-minute Apgar scores, and decreases the number of infants with meconium below the cords.[52] Instillation of normal saline through an intrauterine pressure catheter is a relatively benign procedure and may reduce variable decelerations (see Ch. 14).[53]

Meconium aspiration syndrome may be reduced by aggressive suctioning at the time of delivery of the head. Most cases of aspiration appear to occur when the infant takes its first few breaths of life. Carson et al.[54] showed that thorough suctioning of the nasopharynx and oropharynx before delivery of the shoulders could prevent aspiration. This technique should be combined with neonatal tracheal aspiration when meconium is present at or below the vocal cords.[55] While these techniques have been shown to make meconium aspiration syndrome less common, they will not prevent the disease completely. It has become evident that fetal asphyxia in utero before labor may lead to pulmonary injury such that the lungs cannot clear meconium. This problem combined with pulmonary vascular damage followed by persistent fetal circulation after birth can lead to significant neonatal morbidity and mortality.[56] Autopsy data on stillbirth infants have shown the presence of meconium in the bronchial airways.[57]

Another important aspect of management is preventing birth trauma associated with macrosomia. Macrosomia should be suspected in all post-term gestations. Fetal weight should be estimated immediately before or in the early stages of labor of all post-term pregnancies in which vaginal delivery is considered.

Estimation of accurate fetal weight is difficult in post-term pregnancy, but the use of ultrasound has improved accuracy. If clinical estimates of the fetus are large or the maternal pelvis is small, an ultrasound-estimated fetal weight may be helpful. Ultrasonic weight predictions generally fall within 20 percent of the actual birthweight.[58] Chervenak et al.[59] found ultrasonic estimation of fetal weight to have a sensitivity of 60.5 percent and specificity of 90.7 percent for predicting birthweight over 4,000 g.

Another tool in the assessment of suspected macrosomia is the fetal pelvic index (FPI) as described by Morgan and Thurnau.[60-62] This method compares ultrasonic fetal measurements of the abdomen and head with X-ray pelvimetry measurements of maternal pelvic inlet and midpelvis circumferences.[60] The latter are easily obtain by CT scan using the Colcher-Sussman method. The FPI has been shown to predict accurately the need for cesarean delivery[61] and shoulder dystocia[62] in mothers with suspected fetal macrosomia. This technique may aid in choosing which patients are appropriately taken to cesarean delivery without a trial of labor. The theoretical risk of childhood leukemia from in utero X-ray exposure should be discussed with the patient prior to the procedure.[63] Because of these concerns and the cost involved, consideration for use of the FPI should be limited to post-term patients with probable macrosomia by ultrasound, borderline clinical pelvimetry, and/or an unengaged vertex.

There are several steps to take with suspected macrosomia. Midpelvic operative vaginal delivery should be avoided, particularly with a prolonged second stage. Benedetti and Gabbe[64] noted that patients with a prolonged second stage and midpelvic delivery increased their risk of shoulder dystocia from 0.16 to 4.57 percent. The pediatrician and anesthesiologist should be notified so they can prepare for delivery. Someone skilled in the various maneuvers for dealing with shoulder dystocia should be present for the delivery. Lastly, cesarean delivery should be considered for suspected macrosomia in patients with an estimated fetal weight greater than 4,500 g, a marginal pelvis, or previous difficult vaginal delivery with the same or smaller sized infant.

Intrapartum asphyxia is also more common in the post-term pregnancy; therefore, close observation of the fetal heart rate is necessary. Some of the factors that may cause fetal compromise are placental deterioration, long labor and oligohydramnios. The incidence of cesarean delivery for fetal distress increases from 5.4 to 13.1 percent in post-term patients who develop oligohydramnios.[65]

Cord compression is more likely in these gestations since oligohydramnios is combined with a thin, easily compressible umbilical cord.[66] Cord compression can be prevented with normal saline amnioinfusion, which can reduce severe variable decelerations.[53] These patterns alone do not require immediate intervention as long as the fetal heart rate variability and baseline remain within normal limits. Variable decelerations primarily result from cord compression not hypoxia. Variable decelerations should be closely followed for evidence of developing hypoxia. A slow return to baseline, blunting of the shape and of the variable deceleration, and overshoot of the baseline after the variable deceleration of concern.

Late decelerations indicate more direct evidence of fetal hypoxia. If intermittent, late decelerations are managed conservatively with positioning and oxygen. If vaginal delivery is not imminent, cesarean delivery should be considered when late decelerations are frequent and persistent. If persistent late decelerations are associated with decreased variability or an elevated baseline fetal heart rate, delivery is indicated. Decreased heart rate variability may be due to a fetal sleep state. Fetal sleep cycles may be differentiated from true depression by the use of fetal scalp stimulation. Clark et al.[67] showed the virtual absence of acidosis in fetuses whose heart rates rose in response to this technique (see Ch. 14).

Conclusion

While postdate pregnancy increases the risks to the fetus and mother, satisfactory outcome can be expected with appropriate pregnancy dating, fetal surveillance, intervention when necessary, and careful intrapartum and neonatal management.

Key Points

- Postdatism has not always been of universal concern, but with improving gestational age assessment and closer follow up, the problem has become more well defined.

- The primary risk to the mother from postdatism includes an increase in postpartum infections, hemorrhage from uterine atony, prolonged hospitalization, wound complications, and an increased incidence of cesarean delivery.

- Neonatal complications from postmaturity include placental insufficiency, birth trauma from macrosomia, and meconium aspiration syndrome.

- The accuracy of diagnosis of the post-term pregnancy can be made only by proper dating, since all methods of estimating gestational age lose accuracy in the third trimester. It is important to determine an accurate estimated delivery date in early pregnancy.

- Post-date management can be divided into two clear choices, (1) expectant management and (2) induction of labor.

- Patients with favorable cervices benefit from induction of labor.

- When the cervix is uninducible, consideration of cervical ripening is weighed against expectant management with antepartum testing.

- Recent prospective randomized trials have suggested a slightly decreased cesarean delivery rate is associated with induction of labor. Expectant management should be accompanied by antepartum testing.

- Oligohydramnios is an important clinical development in the post-date pregnancy. All pregnancies should be followed closely for this development.

- Intrapartum, management should include careful fetal surveillance, identification of and prevention of trauma from macrosomia, and suctioning of meconium-stained fluid at delivery.

References

1. Ballantyne JW: The problem of the postmature infant. J Obstet Gynaecol Br Emp 11:6
2. McClure-Browne JC: Postmaturity. Am J Obstet Gynecol 85:373, 1963
3. Clifford SH: Postmaturity—with placental dysfunction. J Pediatr 44:1, 1954
4. Zwerdling MA: Factors pertaining to prolonged pregnancy and its outcome. J Pediatr 40:202, 1967
5. Lucas WE, Anctil A, Callagan DA: The problem of post-term pregnancy. Am J Obstet Gynecol 91:241, 1965
6. Gibb DM, Cardozo LD, Studd JW et al: Prolonged preg-

nancy: is induction of labour indicated? A prospective study. Br J Obstet Gynaecol 89:292, 1982

7. Saito M, Yazawa K, Hashiguchi A: Time of ovulation and prolonged pregnancy. Am J Obstet Gynecol 112:31, 1972

8. Rayburn WF, Motley ME, Stempel LE: Antepartum prediction of the postmature infant. Obstet Gynecol 160: 148, 1982

9. Eden RD, Seifert JS, Winegar A: Perinatal characteristics of uncomplicated postdate pregnancies. Obstet Gynecol 69:296, 1987

10. Lagrew DC, Freeman RK, Dorchester W: Antepartum surveillance in postterm pregnancy with the contraction stress test. Society of Perinatal Obstetricians Abstract/ Las Vegas, February 1988

11. Sack RA: The large infant: a study of maternal, obstetrical, fetal, and newborn characteristics including a long-term pediatric follow-up. Am J Obstet Gynecol 104:195, 1969

12. Vorherr H: Placental insufficiency in relation of postterm pregnancy and fetal postmaturity. Am J Obstet Gynecol 123:67, 1975

13. Manning F: Neonatal complications of postterm gestation. J Reprod Med 33:271, 1988

14. Secher NJ, Hansen PK, Lenstrup C et al: Birth weight for gestational age charts based on early ultrasound estimation of gestational age. Br J Obstet Gynaecol 93:128, 1986

15. Freeman RK, Garite TJ, Mondanlou H et al: Postdate pregnancy: utilization of contraction stress testing for primary fetal surveillance. Am J Obstet Gynecol 140:128, 1981

16. Callenbach JC, Hall RT: Morbidity and mortality of advanced gestational age: post-term or postmature. Obstet Gynecol 53:721, 1978

17. Shime J, Librach CL, Gare DJ et al: The influence of prolonged pregnancy on infant development at one and two years of age: a prospective controlled study. Am J Obstet Gynecol 154:341, 1986

18. Dyson DC: Fetal surveillance vs. labor induction at 42 weeks in postterm gestation. J Reprod Med 33:262, 1988

19. Anderson HF, Johnson TRB, Glora JD et al: Gestational age assessment. II. Prediction from combined clinical observations. Am J Obstet Gynecol 140:770, 1981

20. Grennert L, Persson P, Gennser G et al: Benefits of ultrasound screening of a pregnant population. Acta Obstet Gynecol Scand Suppl 78:5, 1978

21. Robinson HP, Fleming JEE: A critical evaluation of sonar "crown–rump" length measurements. Br J Obstet Gynaecol 82:702, 1975

22. Kopta MM, May RR, Crane JP: A comparison of the reliability of the estimated date of confinement predicted by crown–rump length and biparietal diameter. Am J Obstet Gynecol 145:562, 1983

23. Harris BA, Huddleston JF, Sutliff G et al: The unfavorable cervix in prolonged pregnancy. Obstet Gynecol 62: 171, 1983

24. Lagrew DC, Freeman RK: Contraction stress test in assessment and care of the fetus. p. 351, In Eden RD, Boehn FH (eds): Assessment and Care of the Fetus: Phys-

iologic, Clinical and Medicolegal Principles. Appleton & Lange, East Nowalk, CT, 1990

25. Lagrew DC, Freeman RK: Management of postdate pregnancy. Am J Obstet Gynecol 154, 1986

26. Dyson DC, Miller PD, Armstrong MA: Management of prolonged pregnancy: induction of labor versus antepartum fetal testing. Am J Obstet Gynecol 156:928, 1987

27. A clinical trial of induction of labor versus expectant management in postterm prengnacy. The NICHHD Network of Maternal-Fetal Medicine Units. Am J Obstet Gynecol 170:716, 1994

28. Hannah ME, Hannah WJ, Hellman J et al: Induction of labor vs. antenatal monitoring in postterm pregnancy. N Engl J Med 326:1587, 1992

29. Grant JM: Induction of labour confers benefits in prolonged pregnancy. Br J Obstet Gynaecol 101:99, 1994

30. Boyd ME, Usher RH, McClean FH et al: Obstetric consequences of postmaturity. Am J Obstet Gynecol 158:334, 1988

31. Katz Z, Yemini M, Lancet M et al: Non-aggressive management of post-date pregnancies. Eur J Obstet Gynecol Reprod Biol 15:71, 1983

32. Porto M, Merrill PA, Lovett SM et al: When should antepartum testing begin in post-term pregnancy? Society of Perinatal Obstetricians, San Antonio, Texas, January 1986

33. Lagrew DC, Freeman RK: Fetal monitoring in the prolonged pregnancy. p. 123. In Spencer J (ed): Fetal Monitoring. Royal Postgraduate Medical School, University of London, 1989

34. Boehm FH, Salyer S, Shah DM et al: Improved outcome of twice weekly nonstress testing. Obstet Gynecol 67:566, 1986

35. Lumley J, Lester A, Anderson E et al: A randomized trial of weekly cardiotocography in high risk obstetrical patients. Br J Obstet Gynaecol 90:101, 1983

36. Kidd L, Panel N, Smith R: Non-stress antenatal cardiotocography—a prospective randomized clinical trial. Br Obstet Gynaecol 92:115, 1985

37. Phelan JP, Platt PD, Yeh SY et al: Continuing role of the nonstress test in the management of postdates pregnancy. Obstet Gynecol 64:624, 1984

38. Small ML, Phelan JP, Smith CV et al: An active management approach to the postdate fetus with a reactive nonstress test and fetal heart rate decelerations. Obstet Gynecol 70:636, 1987

39. Huddelson JF, Sutliff G, Robinson D: Contraction stress test by intermittent nipple stimulation. Obstet Gynecol 63:669, 1984

40. Manning FA, Platt LK, Sipos L: Antepartum fetal evaluation: development of a fetal biophysical profile. Am J Obstet Gynecol 136:787, 1980

41. Johnson JM, Harman JCR, Lange IR et al: Biophysical profile scoring in the management of the postterm pregnancy: an analysis of 307 patients. Am J Obstet Gynecol 154:269, 1986

42. Eden RD, Gergely RZ, Schifrin BS et al: Comparison of antepartum testing schemes for the management of the postdate pregnancy. Am J Obstet Gynecol 144:683, 1982

43. Clark SL, Sabey P, Jolley K: Nonstress testing with acous-

tic stimulation and amniotic fluid volume assessment: 5973 tests without unexpected fetal death. Am J Obstet Gynecol 160:694, 1989

44. Grubb DK, Rabello YA, Paul RH: Post-term pregnancy: fetal death rate with antepartum surveillance. Obstet Gynecol 79:1024, 1992

45. Goldstein RB, Filly RA: Sonographic estimation of amniotic fluid volume. J Ultrasound Med 7:363, 1988

46. Clement D, Schifrin BS, Kates RB: Acute oligohydramnios in postdate pregnancy. Am J Obstet Gynecol 157:884, 1987

47. Lagrew DC, Pircon RA, Nageotte M et al: How frequently should the amniotic fluid index be repeated. Am J Obstet Gynecol, 167:4, 1992

48. Chamberlain PF, Manning FA, Morrison T et al: Ultrasound evaluation of amniotic fluid volume. Am J Obstet Gynecol 150:245, 1984

49. Crowley P, O'Herlihy C: The value of ultrasound measurement of amniotic fluid volume in the management of prolonged pregnancies. Br J Obstet Gynaecol 91:444, 1984

50. Phelan JP, Ahn MY, Smith CV et al: Amniotic fluid index measurements during pregnancy. J Reprod Med 32:601, 1987

51. Rutherford SE, Phelan JP, Smith CV et al: The four quadrant assessment of amniotic fluid volume: an adjunct to antepartum fetal heart rate testing. Obstet Gynecol 70:353, 1987

52. Wenstrom KD, Parsons MT: The prevention of meconium aspiration in labor using amnioinfusion. Obstet Gynecol 73:647, 1989

53. Miyazaki FS, Taylor NA: Saline amnioinfusion for relief of variable or prolonged decelerations. Am J Obstet Gynecol 146:670, 1983

54. Carson BS, Losey RW, Bowes WA: Combined obstetric and pediatric approach to prevent meconium aspiration syndrome. Am J Obstet Gynecol 126:712, 1976

55. Bloom RD, Copley C: Meconium in amniotic fluid, lesson 2. p. 17. In American Heart Association Textbook of Neonatal Resuscitation.

56. Katz VL, Bowes WA Jr: Meconium aspiration syndrome: reflections on a murky subject. Am J Obstet Gynecol 166:171, 1992

57. Brown BL, Gleicher N: Intrauterine meconium aspiration. Obstet Gynecol 57:26, 1981

58. Shepard MJ, Richards VA, Berkowitz RL: An evaluation of two equations for predicting fetal weight by ultrasound. Am J Obstet Gynecol 142:47, 1982

59. Chervenak JL, Divon MY, Hirsch J et al: Macrosomia in the postdate pregnancy: is routine ultrasonographic screening indicated? Am J Obstet Gynecol 161:753, 1989

60. Morgan MA, Thurnau GR, Fishburne JI Jr: The fetal-pelvic index, an indicator of fetal-pelvic disproportion. A preliminary report. Am J Obstet Gyencol 155:608, 1986

61. Thurnau GR, Morgan MA: Efficacy of the fetal-pelvic index as a predictor of fetal-pelvic disproportion in patients with abnormal labor patterns requiring labor augmentations. Am J Obstet Gynecol 159:1168, 1988

62. Morgan MA, Thurnau GR: Efficacy of fetal-pelvic index for delivery of neonates weighing 4,000 grams or greater: a preliminary report. Am J Obstet Gynecol 158:1133, 1988

63. Morgan MA, Thurnau GR: Detecting fetal-pelvic disproportion. Contemp Obstet Gynecol 38:53, 1993

64. Benedetti TJ, Gabbe SG: Shoulder dystocia: a complication of fetal macrosomia and prolonged second stage of labor with mid-pelvic delivery. Obstet Gynecol 52:526, 1978

65. Leveno KJ, Quirk JG, Cunningham FG et al: Prolonged pregnancy: observations concerning the causes of fetal distress. Am J Obstet Gynecol 150:465, 1984

66. Silver RK, Dooley SL, Ramura RK et al: Umbilical cord size and amniotic fluid volume in prolonged pregnancy. Am J Obstet Gynecol 157:716, 1987

67. Clark SL, Gimovsky ML, Miller FC: Fetal heart rate response to scalp blood sampling. Am J Obstet Gynecol 144:706, 1982

68. Williams RL, Creasy RK, Cunningham CG et al: Fetal growth and perinatal viability in California. Obstet Gynecol 59:624, 1982

69. Treloar AE, Behn BG, Cowan DW: Analysis of gestational interval. Am J Obstet Gynecol 99:34, 1967

Isoimmunization in Pregnancy

Marc Jackson and D. Ware Branch

This chapter reviews the causes and management of isoimmunization in pregnancy. Topics included are Rh isoimmunization, sensitization caused by other erythrocyte antigens, and platelet isoimmunization. Rh isoimmunization is emphasized because it remains a leading cause of fetal or neonatal death from hemolytic disease. Also, to a great extent, the principles of pathophysiology and management discussed under Rh isoimmunization apply to the other causes of isoimmunization. With regard to Rh isoimmunization, the following are discussed: the genetics and biochemistry of the Rh antigen, the causes of Rh isoimmunization, the use of Rh-immune globulin, and the assessment and management of the Rh-isoimmunized pregnancy. Throughout this chapter, the traditional term *sensitization* is used interchangeably with *isoimmunization*.

History of Erythroblastosis Fetalis

In 1932, Diamond et al.[1] observed that erythroblastosis fetalis was associated with fetal edema, neonatal hyperbilirubinemia, and neonatal anemia. Later, Darrow[2] proposed that these related conditions were caused by the passage of maternal antibodies across the placenta and that it was the antibodies that caused the destruction of the fetal erythrocytes. In 1939, Levine and Stetson[3] observed the presence of atypical agglutinins in the serum of a woman who had just delivered a hydropic stillborn infant; these agglutinins were found to be active against her husband's erythrocytes even though he was of the same ABO blood group. Levine and Stetson suggested that an immunizing property in the blood or tissues of the fetus had been inherited from the father and passed into the maternal circulation, causing her to develop the agglutinin. This was the first suggestion that erythroblastosis fetalis was an isoimmune disorder, and within 3 years the role of isoimmunization in the pathogenesis of erythroblastosis was established.[4]

Although many erythrocyte antigens have subsequently been described, only a few are clinically important causes of maternal isoimmunization leading to hemolysis of fetal and neonatal cells. Fortunately, the number of cases of fetal and neonatal hemolytic disease resulting from Rh antigen incompatibility is decreasing due to the widespread use of Rh-immunoglobulin prophylaxis. This has led to an increase in the importance of the "minor antigens" of the erythrocyte membrane as a cause of isoimmunization.

Genetics and Biochemistry of the Rh Antigen

Nomenclature

In 1940, Landsteiner and Wiener[5] announced that they had produced rabbit immune sera to rhesus monkey erythrocytes that, even after adsorption, agglutinated the majority (85 percent) of human erythrocytes; they designated this newly discovered property of serum the *Rh factor*. Agglutinated cells were called *Rh positive*. It is now recognized that the "Rh factor" is an antibody directed against an erythrocyte surface antigen of the rhesus blood group system.

Since its discovery, the development of an adequate nomenclature for the Rh blood group system has been hampered by its high degree of polymorphism. Five major antigens can be identified with known typing sera, and there are many variant antigens. Unfortunately, three different systems of nomenclature have been suggested since the discovery of the Rh antigen. Two of these, the Fisher-Race system and the Wiener system, were established during the 1940s and are the ones most frequently used in the literature. The HLA-like system of Rosenfield and colleagues[6] was proposed in 1962.

In obstetrics, the Fisher-Race nomenclature is best known. Although this system has some limitations in terms of our current understanding of genetics and in its classification of the numerous variant antigens, it is well suited to understanding the inheritance of the Rh antigen and the clinical management of Rh isoimmunization.[7]

The Fisher-Race nomenclature assumes the presence of three genetic loci, each with two major alleles. The antigens produced by these alleles were originally identified by specific antisera and have been lettered C, c, D, E, and e. No antiserum specific for a "d" antigen has been found, and use of the letter "d" indicates the absence of a discernible allelic product. Anti-C, anti-c, anti-D, anti-E, and anti-e designate specific antisera directed against the respective antigens.

An Rh gene complex is described by the three appropriate letters; thus, eight gene complexes could exist (listed in decreasing order of frequency in the white population): CDe, cde, cDE, cDe, Cde, cdE, CDE, and CdE. Genotypes are indicated as pairs of gene complexes, such as CDe/cde. Certain genotypes, and thus certain phenotypes, are more common in the population than others (Table 27-1).[8] The genotypes CDe/cde

and CDe/CDe are the most common, with approximately 55 percent of all whites having the CcDe or CDe phenotype. The genotype CdE has actually never been demonstrated.[7] Although the alleles are always written in the order C(c), D(d), E(e), the actual order of the genes on chromosome 1 is D, C(c), E(e).

According to the Fisher-Race concept, the Rh antigen complex is the final expression of a group of at least five possible antigens (C, D, E, c, e). The vast majority of Rh isoimmunization causing transfusion reactions or serious hemolytic disease of the fetus and newborn are the result of incompatibility with respect to the D antigen. For this reason, common convention holds that *Rh positive* indicates the presence of the D antigen and *Rh negative* indicates the absence of D antigen on erythrocytes.

Working at the same time as Fisher and Race, Wiener[9] developed a system of nomenclature based on the assumption of only one genetic locus. In the Wiener system, the eight genotypes are designated (in decreasing order of frequency in the white population) R^1, r, R^2, R^0 r', r", R^Z, and r^v (Table 27-1).

In the 1970s, Rosenfield and co-workers[6,10] suggested that none of the previously described models could explain the vast quantitative differences observed in the expression of Rh antigens. Furthermore, they pointed out that genetic concepts such as the operon model of gene function with nonlinked regulator genes were poorly accommodated by the simple mendelian model of Fisher and Race. Rosenfield therefore proposed an updated system of nomenclature that numbered the antigens, currently designated Rh1 through Rh48.

Unique Rh antibodies have been used to identify more than 30 antigenic variants in the Rh blood group system. Two of the most common (albeit infrequent in absolute terms) are the C^W antigen and the D^u antigen, which is also known as *weak D*. The latter is a heterogeneous group of clinically important D antigen variants most often found in blacks. The erythrocytes of most D^u-positive individuals appear to have a quantitative decrease in expression of the normal D antigen, although some D^u variants are significantly different, antigenically speaking, from D. Thus, it appears that there are at least two cellular expressions responsible for the D^u phenotype, including a reduction in the number of D antigen sites with all epitopes represented, and expression of only some of the various D antigen epitopes with some epitopes missing. D^u-positive erythrocytes can be shown to bind anti-D typing sera, but in some cases only by sensitive indirect antiglobulin methods. At least some D^u-positive patients are capable of producing anti-D, presumably by sensitization to missing D epitopes. Theoretically, this could

Table 27-1   Frequency of Rh Phenotypes and Genotypes Among Whites

Phenotype	Population Frequency (%)	Frequency Within	
		Genotype	(%)
CcDe	35	CDe/cde (R^1/r)	94
		CDe/cDe (R^1/R^0)	6
		cDe/Cde (R^0/r')	<1
CDe	20	CDe/CDe (R^1/R^1)	95
		CDe/Cde (R^1/r')	5
ce	16	cde/cde (r/r)	100
CcDEe	13	CDe/cDE (R^1/R^2)	89
		CDe/cdE (R^1/r")	7
		cDE/Cde (R^2/r')	2
		CDE/cde (R^z/r)	1
		CDE/cDe (R^z/R^0)	<1
cDEe	10	cDE/cde (R^2/r)	93
		cDE/cDe (R^2/R^0)	6
		cDe/cdE (R^0/r")	1
cDE	3	cDE/cDE (R^2/R^2)	86
		cDE/cdE (R^2/r")	14
cDe	2	cDe/cde (R^0/r)	97
		cDe/cDe (R^0/R^0)	3
Cce	1	Cde/cde (r'/r)	100

result in a D^u-positive mother becoming sensitized to her D-positive fetus.

Genetic Expression

The genetic locus for the Rh antigen is on the short arm of chromosome 1.[11,12] Within the Rh locus are two distinct structural genes adjacent to one another, RhCcEe and RhD. These two genes likely share a single genetic ancestor, as they are identical in more than 95 percent of their coding sequences.[13] The first gene codes for the C/c and E/e antigens, and the second gene codes for the D antigen; patients who are D-negative lack the RhD gene on both their chromosomes. Thus, D-negative patients have a deletion of the D gene on both their chromosomes 1.

The expression of the Rh antigen on the erythrocyte membrane is genetically controlled, not only in terms of the structure of the antigen but also in terms of the number of specific Rh-antigen sites (e.g., D, E, C, c, or e). Several genetic factors have been shown to alter the number of specific Rh-antigen sites; these include the gene dose, the relative position of the alleles, and the presence or absence of regulator genes.

There is a relatively constant amount of Rh antigen sites available on the erythrocyte surface, totaling about 100,000 sites per cell; these sites appear to be approximately evenly divided between C(c), D, and E(e) antigens.[14,15]

Gene dosage has an effect on the number of specific Rh antigen sites that express antigen; individuals homozygous for a particular genotype have up to twice as many antigen sites as individuals who are heterozygous.[16] For example, the erythrocytes of individuals homozygous for the c allele have twice as many c antigen sites expressed as are found on the erythrocytes of heterozygotes. Similar observations have been made with regard to the other alleles (E, e, and C).[16,17]

An effect of allelic interaction on Rh antigen sites has been described: erythrocytes of genotype CDe/cde express less D antigen than do the erythrocytes of genotype cDE/cde.[18] Thus, the presence of the C antigen seems to affect the expression of the D antigen. Similarly, individuals of genotype CDe/cDE express less C antigen than individuals of genotype CDe/cde.[8] In addition, genes other than those coding for the Rh antigen may affect the final antigenic expression; two independently segregating regulator genes have been described.[10]

Biochemistry and Immunology

The Rh antigens on human erythrocytes are polypeptides embedded in the lipid phase of the erythrocyte membrane, distributed throughout the membrane in a nonrandom fashion. D antigen sites are spaced in a lattice-like pattern across the red cell membrane, at a mean distance of 92 nm in Rh(D) heterozygotes and 64 nm in homozygotes.[19,20] The Rh polypeptides are polymorphic, with the molecular weight of the D antigen being approximately 31,900 daltons and the C(c) and E(e) polypeptides having a molecular weight of about 33,100 daltons.[21] The final tertiary structure and antigenic expression of the protein is dependent on its association with lipids in the membrane, and in this context it may be thought of as a protein–lipid complex, or proteolipid.[22,23] It appears that most of the Rh polypeptide lies within the phospholipid bilayer of the erythrocyte membrane, spanning the membrane 13 times, with short segments extending outside the red cell and extruding into the cytoplasm.[24,25]

The D antigen appears very early in embryonic life and has been demonstrated on the red blood cells of a 38-day-old fetus.[26] The antigen is also expressed early in the erythroid cell series; with ^{125}I-labeled anti-D, pronormoblasts have been shown to contain D antigen.[27]

Seven different D antigen epitopes have been identified or deduced using human monoclonal anti-D antibodies, and others may exist.[28] One hypothesis suggests that these different epitopes are part of the same protein–lipid complex, but are more or less expressed according to the depth that the polypeptide portion is embedded in the red cell membrane lipid bilayer.[29] It is possible that some of the immunologic variation in the Rh blood group system (and fetal hemolytic disease) is explained by the variable expression of the D antigen epitopes and the specificity of the antibodies formed against them.

The precise function of the Rh antigens are unknown, although they probably have a role in maintaining red cell membrane integrity. Rh$_{null}$ erythrocytes, which lack all of the Rh antigens, manifest several membrane defects. The Rh antigens may interact with a membrane adenosine triphosphatase,[23] possibly functioning as part of a proton or cation pump that controls volume or electrolyte flux across the erythrocyte membrane. Supporting this hypothesis, Rh$_{null}$ erythrocytes have increased osmotic fragility and abnormal shapes.[30] It has also been proposed that Rh antigens regulate the asymmetric distribution of different phospholipids through the red cell membrane as a component of the enzyme phosphatidyl flippase.[31,32]

Causes of Rh Isoimmunization

For Rh isoimmunization to occur in a pregnancy, at least three circumstances must exist:
1. The fetus must have Rh-positive erythrocytes, and the mother must have Rh-negative erythrocytes.
2. A sufficient number of fetal erythrocytes must gain access to the maternal circulation.
3. The mother must have the immunogenic capacity to produce antibody directed against the D antigen.

Incidence of Rh-Incompatible Pregnancy

About 15 percent of whites of European extraction are Rh negative; only 5 to 8 percent of American blacks and 1 to 2 percent of Asians and Native Americans are Rh negative. In the white population, an Rh-negative woman has about an 85 percent chance of mating with an Rh-positive man. About 60 percent of Rh-positive men are heterozygous and 40 percent are homozygous at the D locus. Given that one-half of conceptions due to heterozygous men will be Rh positive, the overall chance of an Rh-positive man producing an Rh-positive fetus is about 70 percent. Thus, without knowing the father's blood type, an Rh-negative woman has about a 60 percent chance of bearing an Rh-positive fetus (0.85 × 0.70). Among whites, the net result is that about 10 percent of pregnancies are Rh incompatible (0.15 × 0.60). However, because sufficient fetomaternal hemorrhage and a subsequent maternal antibody response do not occur in every case, less than 20 percent of incompatible pregnancies eventuate in maternal sensitization. Thus, in the era before Rh-immune globulin prophylaxis, about 1 percent of pregnant women had anti-D antibody.

Fetomaternal Hemorrhage

Although transplacental passage of fetal erythrocytes was proposed to be the cause of maternal isoimmunization in the 1940s,[4] it was not until the mid-1950s that fetal erythrocytes were first demonstrated in the maternal circulation.[33] Since then, numerous studies have confirmed that fetal red cells gain access to the maternal circulation during pregnancy and the immediate postpartum period. Fetomaternal hemorrhage in a volume sufficient to cause isoimmunization is most common at delivery, occurring in about 15 to 50 percent of births.[33–36] In more than half of these intrapartum fetomaternal bleeds, the amount of fetal blood entering the maternal circulation is 0.1 ml or less.[36,37] However, in 0.2 to 1 percent of cases, the estimated volume of fetomaternal hemorrhage is 30 ml or more.[34,38,39] Clinical factors such as cesarean delivery, multiple gestation, bleeding placenta previa or abruption, manual removal of the placenta, and intrauterine manipulation may increase the chance of substantial hemorrhage. However, the majority of excessive fetomaternal hemorrhages occur in patients without risk factors who have an uncomplicated vaginal delivery.[39,40]

The amount of fetomaternal hemorrhage necessary to cause isoimmunization varies from patient to patient, probably due to the immunogenic capacity of the Rh-positive erythrocytes and the immune responsiveness of the mother. As little as 0.1 ml of Rh-positive red blood cells has been shown to sensitize some Rh-negative volunteers, and about 3 percent of women found to have 0.1 ml of fetal erythrocytes in their circulation after an Rh-incompatible delivery develop anti-D antibodies within 6 to 12 months.[36]

Overall, about 16 percent of Rh-negative women will become isoimmunized by their first Rh-incompatible (ABO-compatible) pregnancy if not treated with Rh-immune globulin.[37] Half of these women respond with the production of sufficient anti-D antibody to be detectable within the first 6 months after delivery; in the remainder, anti-D is not detected until early in the next incompatible pregnancy. In this latter group, sensitization likely occurred during the first pregnancy, but the primary immune response was too slight for detectable antibody levels to develop. Though not all Rh-negative women bearing Rh-positive infants will become sensitized, the risk of sensitization approaches 50 percent after several incompatible pregnancies.

Even without labor or obvious disruption of the choriodecidual junction, antepartum fetomaternal hemorrhage occurs in sufficient volume to result in isoimmunization in a small percentage of cases. In one large series, fetomaternal hemorrhage was detected in the first trimester in 7 percent of patients, in 16 percent of patients during the second trimester, and in 29 percent of the third trimester determinations.[33] The result of this antepartum fetomaternal hemorrhage is an overall rate of Rh sensitization of about 1 to 2 percent before delivery.[41] However, antepartum sensitization rarely occurs before the third trimester.

Fetomaternal hemorrhage leading to isoimmunization has also been described with abortion and tubal pregnancy.[42–45] As mentioned above, fetal Rh antigens are present at least by the 38th day after conception and, assuming that as little as 0.1 ml of fetal blood can cause isoimmunization, a fetomaternal hemorrhage leading to sensitization could occur by the seventh week after the last menses.[46] In one case, a significant number of fetal red blood cells was demonstrated in the maternal circulation after an elective termination of pregnancy at 6 weeks after the last menses.[47]

Estimates of the incidence and the amount of fetomaternal hemorrhage after spontaneous abortion have varied, but review of the literature suggests that between 5 and 25 percent of spontaneous abortions result in detectable fetomaternal hemorrhage.[35] For the unsensitized Rh-negative woman, a spontaneous first trimester abortion carries a 3 to 4 percent risk of isoimmunization.[48] Induced abortions are also likely to produce detectable fetomaternal hemorrhage (in 7 to 27 percent of cases); the overall risk of sensitization is about 5 percent.[45] In the second trimester, pregnancy termination by saline injection and hysterotomy is associated with significant fetomaternal hemorrhage.[44,45]

Threatened abortion in the first trimester also appears to increase the risk of sensitization. Fetomaternal hemorrhage can be demonstrated in 11 to 45 percent of such patients,[49,50] and a case of sensitization following threatened first trimester miscarriage has been reported.[51]

All Rh-negative unsensitized women should receive 50 μg of Rh-immune globulin within 72 hours of induced or spontaneous first trimester abortion. Patients in the midtrimester, 13 weeks or more, are routinely given a full dose, 300 μg.

Ectopic pregnancy can result in isoimmunization in a susceptible woman.[42] The risk of significant fetomaternal hemorrhage may be greater in cases of ruptured tubal pregnancy, presumably because of the absorption of fetal erythrocytes into the maternal circulation across the peritoneum.[52]

Amniocentesis in the second and third trimester is associated with fetomaternal hemorrhage in 15 to 25 percent of cases, even when ultrasound is used to identify placental location.[53,54] Isoimmunization occurring after amniocentesis has been reported.[55]

Maternal Immunologic Response

At least two characteristics affect whether isoimmunization will occur in a susceptible Rh-negative woman. First, as many as 30 percent of Rh-negative individuals appear to be immunologic "nonresponders" who will not become sensitized, even when challenged with large volumes of Rh-positive blood.[56,57] Second, ABO incompatibility exerts a protective effect against the development of Rh sensitization.[58] Levine and Stetson[3] are credited with first recognizing the association between ABO incompatibility and a lower-than-expected incidence of Rh sensitization, and fetomaternal ABO incompatibility is now well accepted as being partially protective.[58,59]

Two mechanisms explaining the protective effect of ABO incompatibility have been proposed. The first suggests that the ABO-incompatible fetal cells are more rapidly cleared from the maternal circulation so that trapping of the antigen in the spleen, where sensitization can be initiated, does not occur. Although the incidence of fetomaternal hemorrhage is no different in ABO-incompatible pregnancies, the number of fetal cells in the maternal circulation is less than in ABO-compatible pregancies, suggesting an increased clearance rate.[34,35] A second mechanism for the protective effect of ABO incompatibility proposes that maternal anti-A or anti-B antibodies damage or alter the fetal Rh antigen so that it is no longer immunogenic.[59]

Whatever the mechanism, ABO incompatibility diminishes the risk of isoimmunization to about 1.5 to 2 percent after the delivery of an Rh-positive fetus.[60] This effect is most pronounced in matings in which the mother is type O and the father is type A, type B, or type AB.[61]

The Use of Rh-Immune Globulin

The principle that a passively administered antibody will prevent active immunization by its specific antigen is termed *antibody-mediated immune suppression* (AMIS) and was well known to immunologists for decades before being applied to the prevention of Rh disease. During the early 1960s, Freda et al.[62] in the United States and Clarke et al.[63] in Great Britain simultaneously undertook to evaluate AMIS in humans. Both groups achieved a high degree of protection from isoimmunization by administering anti-D immune globulin (Rh-immune globulin) to Rh-negative male volunteers who had been infused with Rh-positive red cells.[62,63] In 1963, Pollack et al.[64] established that 300 μg of Rh-immune globulin would reliably prevent isoimmunization in male volunteers who had received 10 ml of Rh-positive cells. By an extrapolation of the data, Pollack et al. showed that 20 μg of Rh-immune globulin per milliliter of fetal erythrocytes or 10 μg/ml of whole fetal blood was required to prevent isoimmunization; thus, the rule was established that 10-μg Rh-immune globulin should be given for every 1 ml of fetal blood in the maternal circulation.

The early trials using AMIS to prevent isoimmunization in Rh-negative women delivering Rh-positive infants were excitingly successful.[65–67] The administration of Rh-immune globulin within 72 hours of delivery reduced isoimmunization to less than 1.5 percent in the Rh-negative women who were followed through a subsequent incompatible pregnancy. This represented a 7- to 10-fold decrease in isoimmunization compared with the controls. Although 300 μg or more of Rh-immune globulin was used, it has subsequently been shown that a dose of 100 μ to 150 μg is probably adequate for routine use.[67,68] Nonetheless, the standard approved dose for Rh prophylaxis in the United States remains 300 μg.

The 72-hour time limit set for the postpartum administration of Rh-immune globulin is an artifact of the design of the early male prisoner volunteer studies. Prison officials would only allow the investigators to visit the volunteers at 3-day intervals[69]; thus, the use of Rh-immune globulin at intervals of more than 3 days after a challenge with Rh-positive cells was never extensively evaluated. However, to be effective, Rh-immune globulin must be given before the primary immune response is established. The time required to mount a primary immune response doubtlessly varies from case to case, and it is prudent to administer Rh-immune globulin to appropriate mothers as soon as possible after delivery. If for some reason the neonatal Rh status is unknown by the third day after delivery, it is preferable to administer Rh-immune globulin to an Rh-negative mother rather than to continue to await the neonatal results. Finally, if an Rh-negative mother who is a candidate for Rh-immune prophylaxis is mistakenly not treated within the recommended 72 hours following delivery, she may be given Rh-immune globulin up to 14 to 28 days after delivery in an effort to avoid sensitization.

Antepartum Prophylaxis

Early trials showed that 1 to 2 percent of susceptible women became sensitized in spite of postpartum Rh-immune prophylaxis. The majority of these "prophylaxis failures" resulted from antepartum fetomaternal hemorrhage. In an effort to address this problem, Bowman and colleagues[70] in Canada conducted an antepartum Rh prophylaxis trial in which 300 µg of Rh-immune globulin was given at 28 and 34 weeks gestation. Antenatal sensitization was reduced from 1.8 to 0.1 percent. Subsequently, it was shown that 300 µg of Rh-immune globulin given only at 28 weeks gestation is nearly as effective.[71] Reviewing several large studies, the 1979 McMaster University Conference on the prevention of Rh disease confirmed that the antepartum administration of Rh-immune globulin could reduce the risk of antepartum isoimmunization by more than one half.[41] In more than 18,000 control cases, the incidence of antepartum sensitization was 1.05 percent, whereas in the 10,000 treated cases it was only 0.17 percent.

Despite these results, antepartum Rh prophylaxis remains controversial. From a safety perspective, there is a risk of infection (although exceedingly small) to the donors who provide plasma for human anti-D immunoglobulin, which is produced by immunization and antibody boosting by injecting incompatible Rh-positive red cells into Rh-negative volunteers. Also, Hensleigh[72] has argued that the safety of Rh-immune globulin prophylaxis to the recipient mother and fetus has not been convincingly demonstrated. However, decades of experience with Rh-immune globulin have not produced any suspicion of detrimental effects, and a systematic evaluation of a large cohort of women receiving Rh-immune globulin failed to detect any untoward side effects.[73]

The cost-effectiveness of antepartum prophylaxis has also been addressed. Setting aside the ethical issues of witholding Rh-immune globulin prophylaxis because of financial concerns, it nonetheless appears that routine antepartum prophylaxis is much less expensive than managing later sensitized pregnancies.[74,75] Baskett and Parsons[76] calculated that the cost per case of

Rh isoimmunization prevented was less than half of the cost per case treated, with 80 percent of treatment costs being accounted for by neonatal intensive care.

More recently, monoclonal antibody techniques have been used to produce human anti-D.[77] This technology has the potential to produce a standardized antibody in essentially unlimited supply. Human donor risk will be eliminated, and production costs are certain to decrease, improving the cost-benefit ratio even further. Initial in vitro testing of monoclonal anti-D has been favorable,[78] and preliminary human trials to determine effectiveness in blocking endogenous anti-D production are underway.[79]

Mechanism

The precise mechanism of AMIS is not clearly understood. There are three theories: (1) antigen deviation, (2) antigen blocking-competitive inhibition, and (3) central inhibition. The hypothesis that AMIS works by deviation of the antigen away from the immunologic apparatus that is responsible for the formation of antibody was first suggested by Race and Sanger.[7] Support for this theory came from the observation of an increased clearance of ^{51}Cr-labeled Rh-positive red cells in Rh-negative volunteers who were treated with Rh-immune globulin. This increase in clearance was presumed to be caused by intravascular hemolysis that resulted in the destruction or alteration of the Rh antigen so that it did not incite the production of anti-D antibody. However, it is now known that IgG anti-D does not cause intravascular hemolysis of Rh-positive cells; instead, the intact, antibody-coated cells are removed from the circulation by the spleen or lymph nodes,[80] the very site of antibody formation.

Antigen deviation could also occur by the phagocytosis of the antibody-coated Rh-positive cells; this could, and presumably does, occur in the spleen and lymph nodes. However, macrophage ingestion and processing of antigen are essential for immunization to occur, and passive immunization that is directed against red cell antigens has been shown to be specific.[81] Also, if antigen deviation through phagocytosis was the primary mechanism of AMIS, it seems likely that all red cell antigens would be destroyed. For these reasons, antigen deviation is probably not the mechanism of AMIS.

Antigen blocking by anti-D antibody is also not the probable mechanism for AMIS: antibody preparations that lack the Fc portion have been shown to bind avidly to antigen, yet they do not suppress the immune response.[82] In addition, with the usual doses of anti-D used to effect immune suppression, less than 20 percent of the Rh antigen is bound.[81]

The most likely mechanism for AMIS is that of central inhibition, as proposed by Gorman and elaborated upon by Pollack.[81] In this hypothesis, fetal erythrocytes coated with exogenously administered anti-D are filtered out of the circulation by the spleen and lymph nodes. The increase in the local concentrations of anti-D bound to the D antigen appears to "suppress" the primary immune response by interrupting the commitment of B cells to IgG-producing plasma cell clones. Exactly how this suppression is effected is poorly understood, but the binding of antibody–antigen complexes (anti-D–D antigen complexes) by immune effector cells results in the release of cytokines that inhibit the proliferation of B cells specific for the antigen. The process appears to be dependent on the presence of Fc receptor on the IgG; Fab' fragments do not inhibit AMIS.

Management of the Unsensitized Rh-Negative Pregant Woman

At the first prenatal visit of each pregnancy, every patient should have her ABO blood group, Rh type, and antibody screen checked (Fig. 27-1). It is essential that these determinations are made in each subsequent pregnancy, as previous maternal antibody screening is not an adequate assessment.

If the patient is Rh negative, D^u negative, and has no demonstrable antibody, she is a candidate for Rh-immune globulin prophylaxis at 28 weeks gestation and again immediately postpartum. Before administration of 300 μg of Rh-immune globulin at the beginning of the third trimester, it is probably unnecessary to obtain a second antibody screen to ensure that the patient is not already sensitized and producing anti-D.[83,84] Similarly, a repeat antepartum antibody screen at 35 to 36 weeks gestation is unwarranted.

When the Rh-negative, unsensitized patient is admitted for delivery, an antibody screen is routinely done. If the antibody screen is negative and the newborn is Rh positive or D^u positive, the patient should again be given Rh-immune globulin.

Because up to 1 percent of deliveries result in a fetomaternal hemorrhage of greater than 30 ml (the largest volume of fetal blood adequately covered by a standard 300-μg dose of Rh-immune globulin), Rh-negative patients with an Rh-positive or D^u-positive newborn should be screened for "excessive" fetomaternal hemorrhage immediately postpartum.[85] An erythrocyte rosette test has been shown to be a simple and sensitive method for detecting excessive fetomaternal bleed-

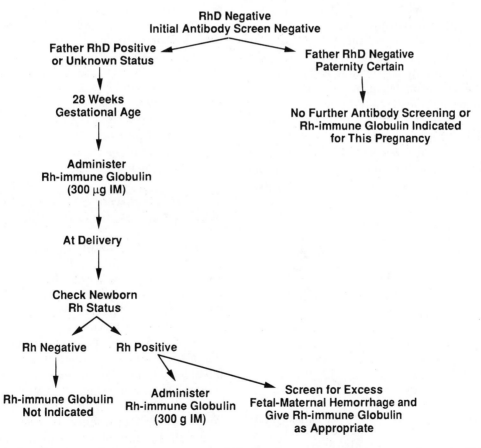

Fig. 27-1 Flow diagram outlining the management of Rh-negative, nonimmunized pregnancies at the University of Utah Medical Center.

ing,[39] and most laboratories use one of the commercially available versions of the erythrocyte rosette test as a screening test. For patients with a positive screen, Kleihauer-Betke testing can be used to quantitate the volume of fetal red cells in the maternal circulation. In this way, the appropriate dose of Rh-immune globulin can be calculated. If the volume of hemorrhage is estimated to be greater than 30 ml whole blood, a dose of Rh-immune globulin calculated at 10 μg/ml of whole fetal blood should be administered.

Management of the D^u-positive patient is sometimes confusing. A D^u-positive mother who delivers an Rh-positive infant is not at significant risk of Rh sensitization, probably because the D^u antigen is actually a weakly expressed D antigen. Thus, D^u-positive mothers may be clinically treated as if they were Rh positive. However, occasionaly a woman previously typed as Rh-negative is unexpectedly found to be D^u-positive during pregnancy or after delivery. In this situation, the clinician should be suspicious that the patient's "new" D^u-positive status is actually due to a large number of fetal cells in the maternal circulation. Appropriate diagnostic studies should be performed, and if fetomaternal hemorrhage is found, the mother should be treated with Rh-immune globulin.

Because of the risk of significant fetomaternal hemorrhage with abortion or ectopic pregnancy, Rh-immune globulin prophylaxis is indicated if the patient is Rh negative and unsensitized. If the pregnancy loss occurs at 12 weeks' gestation or less, a 50-μg dose of Rh-immune globulin is adequate to cover the entire fetal blood volume[86] (Table 27-2). If the gestational age is unknown or beyond 12 weeks, a full 300-μg dose of Rh-immune globulin is indicated.

An Rh-negative, unsensitized patient who has antepartum bleeding or suffers an unexplained second or third trimester fetal death should be evaluated for the possibility of massive fetomaternal hemorrhage. If fetal cells are found in the maternal circulation, Rh-immune globulin is indicated at a dose of 10 μg per estimated milliliter of whole fetal blood (Table 27-2).

Antenatal Rh-immune globulin is indicated at the time of chorionic villus sampling or amniocentesis in an Rh-negative, unsensitized patient. For first trimester procedures, 50 μg of Rh-immune globulin is protective. However, for second or third trimester procedures, a full 300-μg dose is indicated even if the procedure is not associated with detectable hemorrhage (Table 27-2). When amniocentesis is performed within 72 hours of delivery, such as for the determination of fetal pulmonary maturity, Rh-immune globulin may be withheld and administered immediately postpartum if the infant is found to be Rh positive or D^u positive; if delivery is to be delayed for more than 72 hours, Rh-immune globulin should be given.

Since Rh-immune globulin became available in the United States in the late 1960s, the incidence of Rh isoimmunization has been drastically reduced. Antepartum sensitizations have markedly declined with the now-widespread practice of antepartum prophylaxis; however, postpartum prophylaxis failures still represent a significant problem.[87] The routine use of postpartum screening programs to detect "excessive" fetomaternal hemorrhage will likely avoid the majority of these postpartum sensitizations.

Failure to administer Rh-immune globulin when it is indicated also remains a problem.[87] In one study, nearly one-fourth of the cases of new sensitization were due to this inexcusable oversight.[88] It is imperative that the physician be responsible for determining the Rh type in every patient who undergoes abortion, chorionic villus sampling, or amniocentesis, blood transfusion, or pregnancy.

The Rh-Isoimmunized Pregnancy: Assessment of the Fetus

Any patient with an anti-D antibody titer of greater than 1:4 should be considered Rh sensitized and her pregnancies managed accordingly. The eventual goal of management is to minimize fetal and neonatal morbidity and mortality. Patients (fetuses) can be roughly categorized as (1) those who are unlikely to require intrauterine intervention and who can be delivered when they achieve pulmonary maturity and (2) those who will likely have moderate-to-severe hemolytic disease and require intrauterine transfusion and early delivery. An accurate assignment of gestational age using menstrual dates and early ultrasound is crucial in management of the Rh-isoimmunized pregnancy, as the timing of amniocentesis, umbilical cord blood sampling, in utero treatment, and delivery will depend on it.

Table 27-2 Recommended Doses of Rh-Imune Globulin

Indication	Dose (μg) of Rh-Immune Globulin
First trimester spontaneous or induced abortion	50
First trimester chorionic villus sampling	50
Ectopic pregnancy	
Prior to 12 weeks gestation	50
After 12 weeks gestation	300
Amniocentesis or second trimester chorionic villus sampling	300
Fetomaternal hemorrhage	10 per estimated ml of whole fetal blood

(From American College of Obstetrics and Gynecologists,[84] with permission.)

Determination of the Fetal Antigen Status

When first confronted with an Rh-immunized pregnancy, the possibility that the fetus might be Rh negative and therefore not need expensive and potentially hazardous procedures should be considered. If the woman might have become sensitized during a pregnancy fathered by another partner or by a mismatched blood transfusion, determining the paternal Rh-antigen status is reasonable since the father of the current pregnancy might be Rh negative. If he is Rh negative (and it is certain that he is the father of the fetus), further assessment and intervention are unnecessary. If the father is Rh positive, the blood bank laboratory can reliably estimate the probability that he is heterozygous for the D antigen by using Rh antisera to determine his most likely genotype (Table 27-1). Alternatively, DNA analysis can be used to determine his zygosity with a high degree of certainty.[89] Of course, if the man has fathered Rh-negative children, he is a known heterozygote.

If the father is homozygous for the D antigen, all his children will be Rh positive; if he is heterozygous, there is a 50 percent likelihood that each pregnancy will have an Rh-negative fetus who is at no risk of anemia and does not require further assessment or treatment.

In the past, cordocentesis with analysis of fetal red blood cells was required to determine fetal antigen status. Some have advocated routine fetal blood sampling for fetal Rh antigen status at 18 to 20 weeks gestation in all Rh-immunized pregnancies with a heterozygous father.[90] However, this approach never gained widespread acceptance, probably because of the increased risks of fetal loss and fetomaternal hemorrhage associated with cordocentesis.[91]

Recently, advances in molecular genetics have made it possible to determine fetal Rh status without analysis of fetal red blood cells. The Rh locus on chromosome 1p34-p36 has been cloned,[92] and polymerase chain reaction (PCR) now allows determination of fetal Rh status from the uncultured amniocytes in 2 ml of amniotic fluid or as little as 5 mg of chorionic villi.[93,94]

Several PCR techniques using different primers have been reported.[93,95–97] The accuracies of the various methods are still being defined, and the sensitivities and specificities of these PCR assays are not yet well established. Despite the potential limitations, early experience with DNA amplification of the RhD gene is very promising. Dildy et al.[98] recently reported our laboratory's experience, with 100 percent accuracy in determining fetal Rh status in 223 amniotic fluid samples from Rh-negative gravidas.

At the University of Utah, we now routinely include DNA analysis of fetal cells in our Rh assessment protocol. If an Rh-sensitized patient (with a partner who is heterozygous or whose status is unknown) is having a chorionic villus sampling or second trimester amniocentesis for another, unrelated indication, we perform fetal Rh typing at that time. In other cases, fetal Rh typing is performed at the time of the first amniocentesis for amniotic fluid bilirubin analysis. In cases where the PCR results indicate an Rh-negative fetus, we offer patients surveillance with fetal kick counts and serial ultrasounds, after a full discussion and explanation that the sensitivity and specificity of the PCR technique are still uncertain.

Because of the added risk and expense, we do not offer chorionic villus sampling or early amniocentesis solely for Rh typing, except for patients with severe Rh sensitization who would consider termination of an Rh-positive pregnancy. In the near future, it seems likely that fetal Rh status may be routinely available from analysis of fetal cells in the maternal circulation. Favorable early experience with this technology has been reported.[99] Preimplantation genetic diagnosis of RhD type on single blastomeres has also been described.[97]

Antibody Titer

In the first sensitized pregnancy, the level of the anti-D antibody titer determines the need for amniocentesis. Several authors have noted that severe erythroblastosis or perinatal death does not occur when the antibody levels remain below a certain "critical titer".[59,100,101] This titer varies from laboratory to laboratory but is usually 1:16 or 1:32. Freda[101] found no perinatal deaths caused by hemolytic disease when the anti-D titer within 1 week of delivery was 1:16 or less. Queenan[59] reported no intrauterine deaths with a maternal anti-D titer of 1:16 or less and only one fetal death with an anti-D titer of 1:32. However, the reliability and method of antibody titration vary greatly from one laboratory to another. As the number of sensitized pregnancies diminishes, the familiarity of laboratory personnel with titration techniques also decreases. Because of this potential difficulty, an anti-D titer of 1:8 or greater is usually considered at the University of Utah Medical Center an indication for amniocentesis to manage the sensitized pregnancy (Fig. 27-2). If the initial anti-D titer is less than 1:8, and if the patient does not have a history of a previously affected infant, the pregnancy may be followed with anti-D titers every 2 to 4 weeks and serial ultrasound assessment of the fetus.

Except for using the "critical titer" to establish the need for amniocentesis in the first sensitized pregnancy, maternal serum anti-D titers are not particularly useful in the management of most Rh-isoimmunized pregnancies; indeed, titers may remain stable throughout gestation in as many as 80 percent of the severely

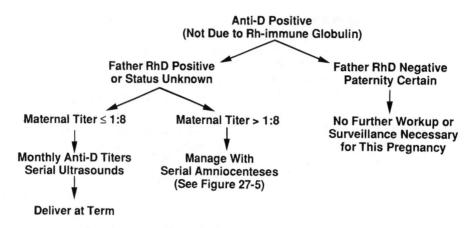

Fig. 27-2 Flow diagram outlining the management of a first Rh-senstized pregnancy.

affected pregnancies.[101] Several possible explanations for this observation are that (1) the binding constant of anti-D varies between individuals; (2) the Rh-antigen expression on the fetal erythrocyte membrane varies between individuals,[29] and (3) the ability of the fetus to replace erythrocytes without compromising liver function varies between individuals.

Obstetric History

A well-documented obstetric history can be an important management guide for the Rh-isoimmunized patient. Fetal hemolytic disease tends to be either as severe, or more severe, in subsequent pregnancies. A history of previous intrauterine or neonatal death from hemolytic disease carries a particularly grave prognosis.[100,102] As a general rule of thumb, if a mother has had a hydropic fetus, the chance that the next Rh-incompatible fetus will become hydropic (if left untreated) is more than 80 percent. Only occasionally will an Rh-incompatible fetus be less severely affected than its previous sibling.

In general, hemolysis and hydrops develop at about the same time or somewhat earlier in subsequent pregnancies; this can be used as a rough guide for timing initial fetal studies and transfusions. However, the history is not particularly helpful if the previous pregnancy was the first sensitized pregnancy, since relatively few fetuses develop hydrops in a first sensitized pregnancy.

Amniotic Fluid Analysis

Assessment of amniotic fluid in Rh immunization is based on the original observations of Bevis[103] that spectrophotometric determinations of amniotic fluid bilirubin correlated with the severity of fetal hemolysis. The bilirubin in amniotic fluid is a by-product of fetal hemolysis that reaches the amniotic fluid primarily by excre-

tion into fetal pulmonary and tracheal secretions and diffusion across the fetal membranes and the umbilical cord. Using a semilogarithmic plot, the curve of optical density of normal amniotic fluid is approximately linear between wavelengths of 525 and 375 nm. Bilirubin causes a shift in the spectrophotometric density with a peak at a wavelength of 450 nm. The amount of shift in optical density from linearity at 450 nm (the ΔOD_{450}) is used to estimate the degree of fetal red cell hemolysis (Fig. 27-3).

Liley[104] provided a framework for the management of Rh-immunized pregnancies based on ΔOD_{450} values in the third trimester. Retrospectively, he correlated amniotic fluid ΔOD_{450} values with newborn outcome by dividing the graph of gestational age versus ΔOD_{450} into three zones. Unaffected fetuses and those with mild anemia had ΔOD_{450} values in zone I (the lowest zone), while severely affected fetuses had ΔOD_{450} values in zone III (the highest zone). Fetuses with zone II values (the middle zone) had disease ranging from mild to severe, indicated primarily by the trend of the amniotic fluid bilirubin determinations. There is a normal tendency for amniotic fluid bilirubin to decrease as pregnancy advances; thus, the boundaries of the zones slope downward as gestational age increases. (Figure 27-4).

Management prior to this time consisted primarily of early induced delivery, but Liley's method identified pregnancies that could be safely allowed to continue without great risk of hydrops and stillbirth. In this way, iatrogenic prematurity was avoided in many cases, with a reduction in perinatal mortality from 22 to 9 percent over a 5-year period.[104]

It became clear with further study that a single measurement of ΔOD_{450} was poorly predictive of fetal condition unless it was very high or very low.[105] Also, because of the wide range of severity of disease in the middle zone, Liley emphasized the need for repeating

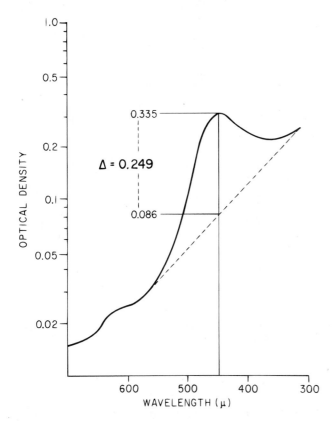

Fig. 27-3 Graph of spectrophotometric analysis of amniotic fluid taken from an Rh-sensitized pregnancy with fetal hydrops. The solid line is the plot of the optical density of the bilirubin-containing fluid across the wavelengths on the x-axis. The interrupted line represents the curve expected from amniotic fluid without increased bilirubin. The difference between the optical density of the solid line and the interrupted line at 450 nm is the ΔOD_{450} value.

the amniotic fluid analyses to establish the ΔOD_{450} trend. Queenan[106] subsequently analyzed serial amniotic fluid ΔOD_{450} values in patients delivering unaffected (Rh negative), mildly affected (cord hemoglobin greater than 14 g/dl), severely affected (cord blood hemoglobin less than 10 g/dl), and stillborn infants. There was a clear downward trend in the ΔOD_{450} values in unaffected and mildly affected infants, and values from the severely affected fetuses showed a mixed pattern of higher values. The amniotic fluid ΔOD_{450} values from infants who died in utero from erythroblastosis showed upward trends except in a single case that was complicated by polyhydramnios. Thus, a horizontal or rising trend is ominous and indicates the need for intervention either by intrauterine transfusion or delivery. Management now includes serial amniocenteses to determine the trend of ΔOD_{450} values over time.[106,107]

The usefulness of the late-second and early-third trimester amniotic fluid ΔOD_{450} determinations for the management of Rh-immunized pregnancies has been confirmed by decades of experience in many centers.

However, several practical caveats deserve emphasis. First, a single ΔOD_{450} value is often insufficient for management purposes; the ΔOD_{450} trend, as established by serial amniocenteses, provides more reliable information about the fetal status. Second, amniotic fluid bilirubin levels are an indirect measure of fetal anemia, and relying solely on the ΔOD_{450} values occasionally leads to the false impression that a mildly or moderately involved fetus is severely anemic or vice versa. Finally, the fairly common practice of extrapolating Liley's original graph for use prior to 26 weeks' gestation is controversial.

Data for ΔOD_{450} analysis were originally obtained from third trimester pregnancies, and several investigators have arbitrarily extrapolated the Liley graph backward and interpreted the results as for third trimester fetuses.[108] Nicolaides and colleagues[109] questioned this approach. They obtained amniotic fluid and umbilical cord blood samples from 59 fetuses with Rh immunization between 18 and 25 weeks' gestation and correlated ΔOD_{450} values with fetal hemoglobin. While the ΔOD_{450} roughly correlated with the degree of fetal anemia, the ΔOD_{450} values were widely scattered and did not accurately predict the hematocrit in an individual fetus. Also, two-thirds of severely affected fetuses (hemoglobin <6 g/dl) had ΔOD_{450} values in the middle or lower zone, incorrectly suggesting only mild to moderate anemia. The authors concluded that second trimester amniotic fluid bilirubin analysis is unreliable and that umbilical cord blood sampling is the only accurate method of assessing fetal anemia.[109] These results were widely accepted, and standard recommendations for second trimester fetal assessment were modified to include fetal blood sampling instead of amniocentesis.[110]

However, some authors disagreed with these conclusions. Spinnato and co-workers[111] suggested that the ΔOD_{450} results of Nicolaides et al.[109] were misleading because no correction for amniotic fluid contamination was utilized. They found that chloroform extraction of amniotic fluid in Rh-immunized pregnancies (to recover bilirubin and remove contaminants such as blood and meconium) resulted in a decrease in ΔOD_{450} values in 90 percent of samples by a mean of 20 percent and allowed accurate clinical categorization of each patient tested. Nicolaides' group also included hydropic fetuses in their analysis, relied more on single ΔOD_{450} values than on trends, and did not address the risk/benefit ratio for routine umbilical cord blood sampling. Spinnato et al.[111] concluded that second trimester chloroform-extracted amniotic fluid bilirubin analysis permits accurate fetal assessment and avoids umbilical cord blood sampling in all but 15 percent of patients.

Others have found amniotic fluid bilirubin analysis before 28 weeks to be valuable as well. Ananth and

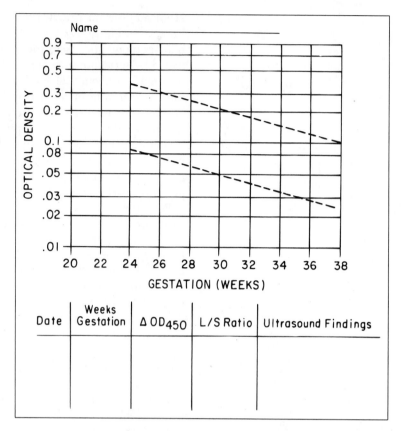

Fig. 27-4 Liley graph used at the University of Utah Medical Center.

Queenan[112] studied ΔOD_{450} values and trends in 32 Rh-immunized pregnancies between 16 and 20 weeks' gestation. They found that ΔOD_{450} values greater than or trending above 0.15 predicted severe isoimmunization, whereas ΔOD_{450} values below 0.09 indicated mild or absent disease. They concluded that umbilical blood sampling is necessary only in pregnancies with ΔOD_{450} values greater than 0.15; fetuses with ΔOD_{450} values below 0.15 can be managed with serial amniocenteses to determine whether the trend indicates severe disease.

In a subsequent analysis of nearly 800 amniotic fluid bilirubin levels obtained between 14 and 40 weeks gestation, Queenan et al.[113] defined the trends in ΔOD_{450} values in unffected and Rh-immunized pregnancies. In unaffected pregnancies, normal amniotic fluid ΔOD_{450} values trend upward between 14 and 22 weeks, level off until 26 weeks, then decline steadily until term. Using the mean and standard deviation of values across the gestational age range, these authors proposed a new graphic framework for assessment of ΔOD_{450} values in Rh-sensitized pregnancies, with four zones: Rh negative, indeterminate, Rh positive (affected), and intrauterine death risk. Although valuable in assessing Rh-sensitized pregnancies prior to 28 weeks, further

work and independent confirmation of this new management scheme will be necessary before it supplants the Liley curve.

Fetal Blood Analysis

Direct fetal vascular access with fetoscopy and ultrasound-guided umbilical vein puncture was developed in the 1980s, thus enabling accurate assessment of the degree of fetal anemia and fetal intravascular transfusion.[114–116] Fetal blood sampling also allows determination of the presence or absence of the offending antigen on the fetal erythrocytes when the antigen status or zygosity of the father is unknown or uncertain.[90,117] As a result, direct fetal blood sampling is now considered by many to be a first step in the analysis of the fetus at risk for severe hemolytic disease.

MacKenzie and colleagues[118] have confirmed the utility of fetal blood sampling in the management of Rh-isoimmunized pregnancies. In 51 consecutive sensitized pregnancies, 11 fetuses were found by blood sampling to be Rh negative and thus required no further evaluation. Of the continuing pregnancies, the fetal hematocrit and the amniotic fluid ΔOD_{450} values were in agreement in 79 percent of instances. However, the amniotic fluid ΔOD_{450} value underestimated the degree of fetal anemia in 11 percent of comparisons and overestimated the degree of fetal anemia in 10 percent.

Adoption of routine umbilical cord blood sampling has not been universal because of concern for potential fetal and maternal morbidity. The procedure is successful in greater than 95 percent of cases, but attributable fetal loss rates between 0.5 and 2 percent per procedure have been reported even by experienced investigators.[117,119,120] In approximately 5 percent of patients, other morbidity occurs; complications such as acute refractory fetal distress, umbilical cord hematoma, amnionitis with maternal adult respiratory distress syndrome, and placental abruption have been described.[121-123]

Additionally, there appears to be a significant risk of fetomaternal bleeding with umbilical cord blood sampling, with the potential for worsened maternal sensitization and fetal involvement.[124-126] Although most studies of this issue have described patients undergoing cordocentesis with intravascular transfusion rather than umbilical blood sampling alone, it appears that significant fetomaternal hemorrhage occurs in 25 to 50 percent of procedures.

Traversing an anterior placenta with the sampling needle is generally thought to increase the likelihood of fetomaternal hemorrhage. In the series of Nicolini et al.[91] 65 percent of patients with an anterior placenta had significant increases in maternal serum α-fetoprotein (used as a marker for fetomaternal bleeding) compared with 17 percent of patients with a posterior placenta. However, Bowman et al.[126] found little effect of placental location on the incidence of fetomaternal hemorrhage. Using Kleihauer-Betke testing for the presence of fetal cells in the maternal circulation, they identified transplacental hemorrhage greater than 0.05 ml in 61 percent of those with an anterior placenta and 48 percent with a posterior placenta. Similarly, they found a significant increase in maternal antibody levels in approximately one-half of the patients, regardless of placental location. Also, they reported that 56 percent of patients having a cordocentesis without transfusion had significant transplacental hemorrhage.

Although concern for worsened maternal sensitization as a consequence of fetal blood sampling has been raised, there are no longitudinal data available with which to determine whether cordocentesis with fetomaternal bleeding and increased antibody titers worsen the prognosis for subsequent pregnancies. Because of the technical difficulty and increased hazard (both immediate and remote) associated with the procedure, umbilical cord blood sampling should be used with caution and performed only by properly trained personnel.

Ultrasound and Doppler Studies

Ultrasonographic examination of the fetus has become an extremely important adjunct in the management of the Rh-sensitized pregnancy, primarily as a guide to amniocenteses and intrauterine transfusions. Ultrasound has also been studied in an effort to identify sonographic findings that might predict the severity of erythroblastosis fetalis so as to avoid the need for invasive assessments. Polyhydramnios, placental thickness greater than 4 cm, pericardial effusion, dilation of the cardiac chambers (especially the right atrium), chronic enlargement of the spleen and liver, visualization of both sides of the fetal bowel wall, and dilation of the umbilical vein have all been proposed as indicators of significant prehydropic fetal anemia.[127-134]

In an effort to determine which, if any, ultrasound parameters are most predictive, Chitkara et al.[131] reviewed the ultrasound findings just prior to umbilical cord blood sampling on 35 occasions between 21 and 33.5 weeks' gestation in 15 severely sensitized pregnancies. The relationship between sonographic findings of polyhydramnios, increased placental thickness, increased umbilical vein diameter, and hydrops to fetal hematocrit was studied. All fetuses with hydrops had a hematocrit less than 15 percent, but two of eight fetuses with a hematocrit below 15 percent had a normal ultrasound and another had only moderate polyhydramnios. Of 19 fetuses with a hematocrit between 16 and 29 percent, more than half had a normal ultrasound, 42 percent had mild to moderate polyhydramnios, and 17 percent had placental thickening. Polyhydramnios was the first and only sonographic sign before fetal anemia (hematocrit less than 26 percent) in 6 of 10 patients studied serially. Although polyhydramnios may be an early indication of significant hemolysis and fetal anemia, the absence of this sonographic finding did not preclude significant anemia; half of fetuses with normal ultrasound examinations had hematocrits less than 30 percent. Although these results indicate that ultrasound is insensitive for detection of fetal anemia, it is important to note that there was no normal control group for comparison, and many of these sonograms were performed when fetuses had already undergone at least one transfusion.

Nicolaides et al.[132] measured fetal head circumference, abdominal circumference, head/abdomen ratio, estimated intraperitoneal volume, placental thickness, and extrahepatic and intrahepatic umbilical vein diameters in 50 patients prior to umbilical cord blood sampling for severe Rh disease. No fetus had been transfused, and the measurements were compared with those from 410 healthy women with normal singleton pregnancies. The presence of hydrops predicted a fetal hemoglobin less than 5 g/dl in all 12 cases so affected.

In the absence of hydropic changes on ultrasound, none of the other ultrasonographic parameters differentiated mild from severe anemia. Half of the fetuses with a hemoglobin <5 g/dl had no sonographic abnormality, and no consistent pattern was apparent in those with abnormal ultrasound findings. Of the fetuses with a hemoglobin level of 5 to 10 g/dl, two-thirds had a normal ultrasound examination. Thus, it appears that at the present time sonographic findings other than hydrops are not reliable in distinguishing mild from severe hemolytic disease even in experienced hands, and the role of ultrasound in the monitoring of fetuses with severe Rh immunization is limited to the establishment of gestational age, monitoring for hydropic changes, and guidance for amniocentesis, umbilical blood sampling, and transfusion.

Doppler flow velocity waveforms have also been extensively investigated as noninvasive predictors of fetal anemia[135–143] and acidosis.[144,145] Fetal cardiac output and blood velocities in the umbilical artery, umbilical vein, fetal descending aorta, fetal ductus venosus, and fetal middle cerebral artery have all been studied in isoimmunized pregnancies. In general, fetal blood flow velocity waveforms have not been predictive of acid-base status in Rh-isoimmunized pregnancies. Similarly, although many studies have found significant differences in blood flow indices between anemic and nonanemic fetuses, the wide range and overlap of values in both groups of patients have limited the utility of Doppler technology.

Nicolaides et al.[137] compared fetal aorta Doppler blood velocities in 68 severely immunized fetuses and 218 normal controls. In nonhydropic fetuses, an aortic mean velocity above the normal range suggested fetal anemia, and a normal mean velocity made significant anemia unlikely. However, the authors concluded that because of the large overlap in values between anemic and nonanemic fetuses Doppler measurements of the aortic blood flow cannot accurately predict the degree of fetal anemia.

In a similar study, Copel et al.[138] retrospectively found that a calculation based on the peak velocity in the descending aorta was predictive of a fetal hematocrit above or below 25 percent with a high degree of sensitivity. However, their formula and its modifications were not useful in predicting the hematocrit after fetal transfusion. Most importantly, this group was unable to predict the degree of fetal anemia in a prospective evaluation of their method.[139]

Legarth and colleagues[142] compared Doppler blood flow velocities to umbilical vein hematocrit during 49 fetal blood sampling or transfusion procedures. Using the S/D ratio, the pulsatility index, and the resistance index, they found no correlation between umbilical artery Doppler indices and fetal hematocrit at the time of blood sampling, and the blood flow velocity indices did not predict fetal hematocrit.

Ultrasound and Doppler ultrasound technology continue to advance rapidly. These noninvasive tools someday may be used to determine accurately and reliably the degree of fetal anemia and, thus, to direct fetal management. However, at present, neither ultrasound nor Doppler blood flow analysis can be recommended in lieu of amniotic fluid ΔOD_{450} determinations or fetal blood sampling for determining the need for intrauterine transfusion or delivery in Rh-immunized pregnancies.

Determining the Need for Intrauterine Transfusion

About one-half of susceptible infants of Rh-immunized pregnancies do not require intrauterine transfusion or extensive extrauterine therapy. Such fetuses are considered to have mild-to-moderate hemolytic disease. In general, mild-to-moderate fetal hemolysis is expected when (1) the involved pregnancy is the first sensitized pregnancy or (2) previously delivered Rh-positive infants have been mildly to moderately affected (mild-to-moderate anemia without hydrops). In such cases, we perform ultrasound examinations of the fetus every 2 to 4 weeks from 18 weeks gestation until delivery. If the fetus shows no evidence of hydrops, we use amniotic fluid ΔOD_{450} determinations for the initial management, performing the first amniocentesis at 24 to 28 weeks gestation. The timing of repeat amniocenteses and determination of the need for intrauterine transfusion or delivery are based on the ΔOD_{450} values and trend (Fig. 27-5). If the values fall within the low zone or the lower half of the middle zone, amniocentesis is repeated every 2 to 4 weeks, depending on the ΔOD_{450} trend. Severe anemia requiring intrauterine transfusion is suspected when the ΔOD_{450} values rise into the upper quarter of the middle zone or into zone III, especially before 30 weeks gestation. Depending on the clinical situation, a single ΔOD_{450} value in zone III also may be taken as an indication of severe anemia. If at any time the fetus has evidence of hydrops by ultrasound, one can assume a fetal hematocrit less than 15 percent,[16,131] and fetal blood sampling and transfusion should be arranged immediately.

The need for cordocentesis in the management of nonhydropic fetuses with ΔOD_{450} values indicative of severe anemia (and requiring intrauterine transfusion) is controversial. As discussed below, there is no proven advantage to cordocentesis and intravascular transfusion in nonhydropic fetuses, and experienced practitioners have described excellent perinatal outcomes using amniotic fluid ΔOD_{450} values with intraperitoneal transfusions.[146–148] However, because of the mor-

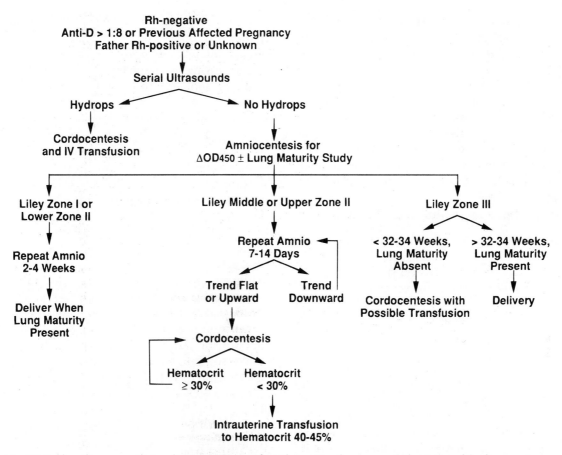

Fig. 27-5 Flow diagram outlining the management of an Rh-sensitized pregnancy. The timing of the first amniocentesis is based on the history, maternal titer, and gestational age. In addition to assessment of amniotic fluid bilirubin or umbilical cord hematocrit, all patients monitor fetal movements on a daily basis after 26 to 28 weeks and have nonstress tests one to two times weekly and ultrasound exams every 1 to 2 weeks.

bidity associated with fetal transfusion regardless of route, it seems appropriate to obtain umbilical cord blood when practical to determine fetal Rh status and to confirm anemia prior to transfusion. The optimum management in any individual case will be determined by the clinical presentation and the experience and expertise of the physicians involved.

When the obstetric history suggests that the fetus is at risk for moderate-to-severe hemolysis and hydrops, we are more likely to begin the search for fetal anemia earlier in the pregnancy. In this situation, we usually follow the trend of ΔOD_{450} values, using a modification of the Liley curve, with the understanding that interpretation of ΔOD_{450} values before 24 weeks is difficult. Between 18 and 24 weeks, we stress ΔOD_{450} trends over single values and typically use Queenan's horizontal zones,[112] with ΔOD_{450} values below 0.09 suggesting an unaffected or mildly affected infant and ΔOD_{450} values above 0.15 suggesting fetal anemia. In some cases, especially those with a history of severe second trimester disease or previous severe disease with misleading ΔOD_{450} values, cordocentesis to determine the fetal

hematocrit and antigen status is a reasonable first step. Again, the optimum management in an individual case will be determined by history, clinical findings, and the experience and expertise of the management team.

At any gestational age, the presence of fetal hydrops should be taken as evidence of severe fetal anemia, and cordocentesis with immediate intravascular transfusion is indicated.

Intrauterine Transfusion in the Rh-Isoimmunized Pregnancy

In 1963, Liley[149] reported the first successful intrauterine transfusion, and a new therapy was created, one that provided obstetricians with a much-needed alternative to preterm delivery in severe erythroblastosis fetalis. The administration of erythrocytes to the involved fetus accomplishes two goals: (1) it corrects fetal anemia and consequently improves fetal oxygenation, and (2) it reduces extramedullary hematopoietic demand, leading to a fall in portal venous pressure and improved hepatic function.

Originally, intrauterine transfusions were done by the intraperitoneal route, and this approach was the mainstay of transfusion therapy until the last decade. In 1981, Rodeck et al.[114] reported the successful intravenous transfusion of two erythroblastotic fetuses using a fetoscopic technique. Although the fetoscopic approach was quite successful,[115] introduction of the transfusion needle by ultrasound guidance (without the fetoscope) has become the most popular technique.[150–158] The umbilical vein is the most commonly used vessel, usually at its insertion into the placenta.

Intrauterine Intraperitoneal Transfusion

Placement of erythrocytes in the fetal peritoneal cavity reverses fetal anemia by gradual uptake of the red cells into the fetal circulatory system via subdiaphragmatic lymphatics. Perinatal survival following intraperitoneal transfusion is related to gestational age at delivery and the severity of fetal disease, particularly with regard to whether hydrops develops. When transfusions were performed with x-ray guidance, overall neonatal survival was approximately 60 percent, survival of nonhydropic infants was near 70 percent, and less than 40 percent of those developing hydrops survived.[159] The routine use of ultrasound for transfusion and monitoring, improvements in transfusion technique, and advances in neonatal care have now resulted in more favorable outcomes (Table 27-3).

Prior to intraperitoneal transfusion, an intravenous line is placed in the mother, and she is sedated with an IV narcotic and short-acting benzodiazapine. Many practitioners also administer an antiemetic and a prophylactic antibiotic. Using real-time ultrasound, fetal position and condition, placental location, and amniotic fluid volume are determined. Intraperitoneal access is best accomplished with the fetus on its side or back. Some workers have suggested external manipulation of the fetus for positioning.[108,160] Peritoneal access is ideally accomplished through the lateral or anterolateral abdominal wall, with the fetal bladder and pelvic bones serving as landmarks. Care should be taken to avoid the umbilical cord and its insertion into the fetal abdomen.

After a site for needle insertion is chosen on the maternal abdomen, the area is prepped and draped in sterile fashion, and a local anesthetic is injected. Using a sterile technique, an 18- or 20-gauge needle is directed under continuous real-time ultrasound guidance into the fetal peritoneum, ideally just cephalad and lateral to the fetal bladder. When it appears that the needle tip has entered the fetal peritoneal cavity, saline or a small air bubble is introduced through the needle to verify its location (Fig. 27-6). Although we usually infuse the blood through the needle, Bowman[107] suggests using an epidural catheter passed through a 16-gauge Tuohy needle for the actual transfusion. When the catheter is clearly seen in the fetal peritoneal cavity, the needle is then withdrawn from the maternal abdomen, leaving the catheter threaded for transfusion.

After confirmation that the needle tip or catheter is in the fetal peritoneal cavity, the transfusion is performed at a rate no faster than 5 to 10 ml per minute. With real-time ultrasound, the flow of red cells into the peritoneum can usually be visualized. Type O-negative, leukocyte-poor, packed erythrocytes cross-matched with the maternal serum are used; the desired hematocrit for the packed cells is 75 to 85 percent. The transfusion is carried out manually with a 20- or 30-ml syringe connected to the transfusion line with a three-way stopcock.

The volume of blood for intraperitoneal transfusion in milliliters is calculated by subtracting 20 from the gestational age in weeks and then multiplying by 10.

Table 27-3 Perinatal Survival Rates with Intrauterine Transfusion

	Nonhydropic	Hydropic	Overall
Intraperitoneal transfusion: neonatal survival			
Bowman and Manning[146]	16/16 (100%)	6/8 (75%)	22/24 (92%)
Scott et al.[147]	12/14 (86%)	4/6 (67%)	16/20 (80%)
Watts et al.[148]	26/26 (100%)	4/9 (44%)	30/35 (86%)
Harman et al.[157]	19/23 (83%)	10/21 (48%)	29/44 (66%)
Total	73/79 (92%)	24/44 (55%)	97/123 (79%)
Intravascular transfusion: neonatal survival			
Grannum et al.[153]	5/6 (83%)	16/20 (80%)	21/26 (81%)
Nicolaides et al.[154]	8/8 (100%)	9/10 (90%)	17/18 (94%)
Berkowitz et al.[155]	13/16 (81%)	0/1 (0%)	13/17 (76%)
Poissonnier et al.[156]	55/60 (92%)	29/47 (62%)	84/107 (79%)
Harman et al.[157]	22/23 (96%)	18/21 (86%)	40/44 (91%)
Weiner et al.[158]	35/35 (100%)	11/13 (85%)	46/48 (92%)
Total	138/148 (93%)	83/112 (74%)	221/260 (85%)

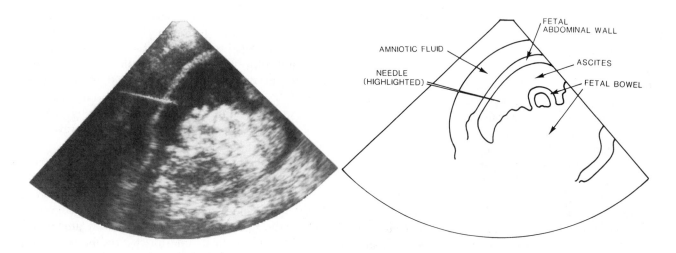

Fig. 27-6 Sonogram showing intrauterine transfusion needle in the fetal peritoneal cavity.

Thus, a 28-week fetus would receive 80 ml of blood. This simple formula is intended to provide a reasonable amount of blood to the fetus without creating undue intraperitoneal pressure. When fetal ascites is present, some of this fluid should be gently aspirated before transfusion. Bowman[37] has suggested that no more than twice the volume of the proposed transfusion should be removed, with a maximum being 150 ml. The rate of absorption of the transfused blood from the peritoneal cavity into the bloodstream is said to be about 12 percent per day in the nonhydropic fetus. In our experience, little or none of the transfused blood is detectable by ultrasonographic examination 3 to 5 days after transfusion in cases in which the fetus was not hydropic. If the fetus is hydropic, red cell uptake is variable and unpredictable; in some cases it is adequate,[37] but in others absorption is quite poor.

It is important that the fetal heart rate be monitored periodically during the transfusion in case fetal bradycardia occurs. Bradycardia early in the procedure presages fetal death.[107] Late in the procedure, a fall in the fetal heart rate may indicate compression of the vena cava by increased intraperitoneal pressure. Measurement of fetal heart rate during the transfusion can easily be done with ultrasound.

Bowman[107] has developed a formula for estimating the residual donor hemoglobin in the fetus following transfusion. His calculation assumes that 55 percent of the transfusion hemoglobin enters the fetal circulation after intraperitoneal transfusion and that the daily red cell loss is about 1/120th of the total. The amount of remaining donor hemoglobin (g/dl) is estimated with the following calculation:

$$\frac{0.55 \times a}{85 \times b} \times \frac{120 - c}{120}$$

where a is donor transfusion hemoglobin (g/dl), b is estimated fetal weight, and c is number of days since transfusion. According to Bowman, the goal is to keep the donor hemoglobin in the fetus above 10 g/dl. This necessarily requires that the first and second transfusions be done about 10 days apart. The timing of subsequent transfusions is calculated according to the above formula, which predicts a repeat intraperitoneal transfusion about every 4 weeks. Thus, the basic intraperitoneal transfusion schedule puts the second transfusion about 10 days after the first and a repeat transfusion every 4 weeks thereafter.

The routine use of ultrasound for needle guidance has dramatically reduced the procedure-related morbidity and mortality associated with intraperitoneal transfusion. Confirmation of appropriate needle placement is usually straightforward, but inadvertent transfusion into the bowel, liver, abdominal wall, and retroperitoneum may occur. Infection, premature rupture of the membranes, refractory preterm labor, and fetal distress necessitating immediate delivery continue to be hazards. Bowman and Manning[146] reported 5 traumatic deaths in 53 transfusions (9.4 percent) during the 2 years prior to instituting ultrasound guidance; there were no deaths in the 64 transfusions immediately afterward. In a similar analysis, Scott et al.[147] observed a reduction in traumatic death rate from 8.0 to 2.3 percent per transfusion. Most recently, Harman et al.[157] have reported a traumatic death rate of 7.6 percent per procedure; nearly three fourths of the fetal and neonatal deaths in this series were due to trauma or complications of prematurity and not to Rh disease. Thus, while intraperitoneal transfusion has evolved into a relatively safe procedure, it is not without risk for fetal loss.

Intrauterine Intravascular Transfusion

First described by Rodeck et al.[114] with fetoscopy, intravascular fetal transfusion has been widely adopted in modified form using ultrasound to guide placement of a needle into the umbilical vein. Direct access to the fetal circulation for transfusion offers a number of advantages over the intraperitoneal approach: (1) fetal hematocrit can be measured, allowing a more precise calculation of the volume of blood required for transfusion; (2) in some cases, the fetus will have a higher hematocrit than expected and transfusion can be delayed; (3) occasionally, the fetus will be found to be Rh negative; and (4) a post-transfusion hematocrit can be used to determine whether the transfusion was adequate and when the next one should be scheduled. Also, transfusion into the fetal vascular system ensures complete uptake of the intended red blood cell mass with a more rapid correction of fetal anemia. This is especially important for hydropic fetuses who often do not adequately absorb intraperitoneally transfused erythrocytes. Potential disadvantages of intravascular fetal transfusion include the rare possibility of volume overload in the compromised fetus, procedure-related complications, and the risk of increasing the severity of maternal sensitization due to fetomaternal hemorrhage.

Despite the recent popularity of intravascular over intraperitoneal transfusion, perinatal survival in pregnancies managed with intravascular transfusion is convincingly improved only for hydropic fetuses. Reported overall survival rates range from 76 to 94 percent (Table 27-3). The perinatal survival of nonhydropic fetuses exceeds 90 percent, and approximately 75 percent of hydropic fetuses survive with intravascular transfusion.

Preparation of the patient is the same as for fetal intraperitoneal transfusion, and the approach to the umbilical cord is determined with real-time ultrasound. A 20- or 22-gauge needle is used, and the progress of the needle tip is guided with continuous ultrasound. When the placenta is anterior, we prefer to use the transplacental approach into the umbilical vein (Fig. 27-7). Otherwise, we attempt to enter the vessel by traversing the amniotic sac and puncturing the cord near its insertion into the placenta. If the fetus is particularly active (in spite of the sedation administered to the mother) or if the needle passes near the fetal extremities, the fetus can be paralyzed immediately upon entry into the vein by injecting pancuronium bromide, 0.1 to 0.3 mg/kg of estimated fetal weight.[161,162] As with intraperitoneal transfusion, O-negative, leukocyte-

ANTERIOR or FUNDAL PLACENTA
Needle (highlighted)

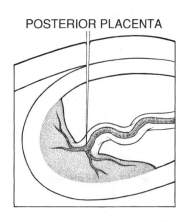

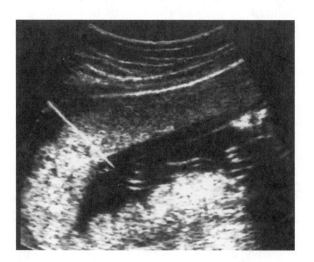

Fig. 27-7 Needle placement for intravascular fetal transfusion.

poor, packed erythrocytes cross-matched with the maternal serum are used.

When vascular access is attained, a small amount of blood is withdrawn into one to three heparinized 1-ml syringes and the initial fetal hematocrit immediately determined. With adequate visualization using ultrasound, there is usually little doubt about the proper placement of the needle tip in the fetal circulation. Comparison of the red cell indices to those of a maternal sample can help confirm that the blood sample is of fetal origin; in addition to the expected difference in hematocrit, fetal red cells have a higher mean corpuscular volume than adult erythrocytes. One sample should be used to determine the fetal antigen status if it is still uncertain.

Several different methods of estimating the volume of blood needed for transfusion have been reported.[163,164] We determine the volume of blood to be transfused according to the method described by Nicolaides et al.,[163] with a post-transfusion hematocrit of 40

to 45 percent as the goal. The initial fetal hematocrit, the hematocrit of the donor blood, and the gestational age are used in conjunction with the graphs shown in Figure 27-8 to determine the amount of blood to be infused. When the infusion is started, streaming or turbulence can be seen within the vessel, confirming that the needle tip is still within the vein. We infuse the blood at a rate of about 10 ml per minute. At the end of the transfusion and before withdrawing the needle, a minute or so of circulation time is allowed; then a post-transfusion sample is drawn for measurement of the final hematocrit.

Following intravascular transfusion, the decline in the donor hematocrit is dependent on the life span of the donor erythrocytes, the rate of fetal growth (and increased vascular volume), and the ratio of fetal to donor erythrocytes (since the fetal erythrocytes are subject to continued hemolysis). The latter is most influential between the first and second intravascular transfusions, during which time the ratio of fetal cells to donor

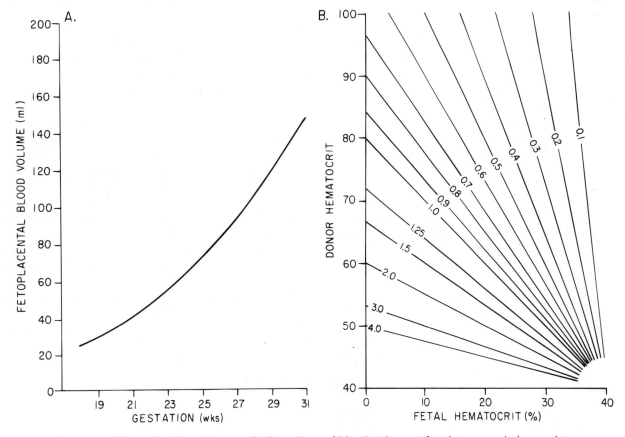

Fig. 27-8 Graphs used to determine rapidly the volume of blood to be transfused intravascularly to achieve a post-transfusion hematocrit of 40 to 45 percent. First, the estimated fetoplacental blood volume (EFBV) is determined using the gestational age and (A). Second, the pretransfusion fetal hematocrit and the donor blood hematocrit are used in conjunction with (B) to derive the multiplying factor. This factor is then multiplied by the EFBV to determine the amount of blood to be transfused. For example, at 26 weeks gestation, the EFBV is found on the abscissa of (A) to be 85 ml. If the pretransfusion hematocrit is 20 percent and the donor blood hematocrit is 80 percent, the multiplying factor derived from (B) is 0.5. Multiplying this number by the EFBV (0.5 × 85 ml) shows that about 42 ml should be transfused. (Adapted from Nicolaides et al.[163] with permission).

cells is greatest. MacGregor and colleagues[165] have used the following equations to predict the fetal hematocrit after transfusion:

Predicted Hct

$$= \frac{(\text{Hct f} - \text{Hct i}) \times (\text{EFW1/EFW2}) \times (120 - \text{days elapsed})}{120}$$

Predicted Hct

$$= \frac{\text{Hct f} \times (\text{EFW1/EFW2}) \times (120 - \text{days elapsed})}{120}$$

where Hct f is the post-transfusion hematocrit, Hct i is the initial (pretransfusion) hematocrit, EFW1 is the estimated fetal weight at the index transfusion, and EFW2 is the estimated fetal weight at the subsequent transfusion. The first equation is used to predict the fetal hematocrit after the first transfusion, and the second equation is used to predict the fetal hematocrit between subsequent transfusions. On average, the decline in the fetal hematocrit following the first transfusion is about 1.5 percent per day; following subsequent transfusions, the decline in fetal hematocrit is about 1.0 to 1.2 percent per day. Using intravascular transfusions for the management of severe fetal hemolysis, repeat transfusions are scheduled to keep the fetal hematocrit above 25 to 30 percent.

Although most authors recommend simple transfusion, some perform intravascular exchange transfusions, feeling that exchange transfusion may allow a longer interval between intravascular transfusions by replacing a greater volume of the fetal cells with donor cells.[153] Also, exchange transfusion is preferred in some centers because of the fear that the increase in blood volume with simple transfusion might compromise fetal cardiac capacity.[153,156] These fears are probably unfounded, as it seems that even a hydropic fetus can tolerate a bolus infusion of red cells without further compromise.[166]

Morbidity and mortality related to the technique of vascular access and transfusion are similar to those with intraperitoneal transfusion.[154,156–158,167] Fetal bradycardia is the most common problem, occurring in 8 to 12 percent of cases, although it is usually transient and only rarely requires immediate delivery. Postprocedure infection and premature rupture of the membranes have also been reported. The reported fetal death rate ranges between 0.6 percent[157] and 4.7 percent[167] per procedure, with hydropic fetuses being at greatest risk. Overall, it appears that intravascular transfusion in experienced hands seems to have a procedure-related complication rate of around 10 to 15 percent and a mortality rate of between 1 and 5 percent.

Using intravascular transfusions alone probably increases the total number of procedures required for each pregnancy because the volume of blood transfused at each procedure is smaller than that given via the intraperitoneal route. Also, up to 80 percent of blood transfused into the peritoneal cavity of nonhydropic fetuses appears in the fetal circulation,[168] a figure considerably higher than previously thought. Finally, as discussed above, concern about the intravascular route has been raised because of the possibility of increasing maternal sensitization due to iatrogenically worsened disease.[91,124–126] It appears that umbilical cord blood sampling and intravascular transfusion can be associated with significant fetomaternal bleeding and a heightened maternal immune response, but actual clinical data from subsequent pregnancies do not yet exist. Additionally, comparative data from intraperitoneal procedures are not available, and it is not certain whether increases in α-fetoprotein and anti-D are worse following intravascular transfusion than following intraperitoneal transfusion.

Intraperitoneal Versus Intravascular Transfusion

For the hydropic fetus, analysis of the collective experience of the last decade definitely shows an improved survival rate using intravascular transfusion when compared with treatment with intraperitoneal transfusion. However, the difference in outcome between the two techniques is much less clear in nonhydropic fetuses. In the absence of hydrops, survival rates of 80 to 100 percent have been documented for both methods, with near-identical rates of survival when the published series are combined (Table 27-3). Unfortunately, a prospective, randomized clinical trial designed to determine the superior technique in the nonhydropic fetus has not been performed.

In an attempt to compare the two methods, Harman et al.[157] analyzed results from patients who underwent intravascular and intraperitoneal transfusions for severe fetal anemia. Forty-four patients undergoing 173 intravascular transfusions were compared retrospectively to 44 fetuses treated with 104 intraperitoneal transfusions in the same institution and matched for severity of disease, placental location, and gestational age. The authors concluded that intravascular transfusion was superior, based on a higher survival rate, a greater gestational age at delivery, and significant reductions in low Apgar scores, cesarean delivery rate, the need for and number of neonatal exchange transfusions, and intensive care nursery admissions and duration of stay. Additionally, the intraperitoneal group had a higher procedure-related mortality (7.7 percent vs. 0.6 percent per transfusion) and a greater overall rate of maternal complication (12.5 percent vs. 3 percent). However, the survival of nonhydropic fetuses was not significantly different between the two treatment groups, and the morbidity data were not analyzed separately for hydropic and nonhydropic fetuses. Acknowledging that the difference in survival for nonhydropic fetuses was statistically unconvincing, the authors nonetheless argued that the lower procedure-related loss rate with intravascular treatment was clinically significant and that intraperitoneal transfusion should be reserved for those situations where intravascular transfusion is impossible due to position of the fetus and cord.

Combined Intravascular Intraperitoneal Transfusion

In an effort to reduce the number of transfusions necessary during treatment of a severely involved pregnancy, Nicolini et al.[169] have combined intravascular and intraperitoneal transfusions. After intravascular transfusion to a fetal hematocrit of approximately 40 percent, enough blood to raise the intravascular hematocrit to 60 percent was then transfused intraperitoneally. The amount of blood transfused intravascularly was calculated as described above, and the amount of blood subsequently transfused intraperitoneally was calculated according to the following equation:

$$V_{IPT} = V_{IVT} \times \frac{(\text{desired Hct} - \text{Hct f})}{(\text{Hct f} - \text{Hct i})}$$

where V_{IPT} is the volume of blood to be transfused intraperitoneally, V_{IVT} is the volume of blood transfused intravascularly, Hct f is the fetal hematocrit after the intravascular transfusion, and Hct i is the initial (pretransfusion) hematocrit. Using the estimated decline in fetal hematocrit and clinical parameters to decide upon the timing of the next transfusion, the authors performed only 3.2 procedures per patient, and the mean fall in hematocrit was slightly less than 1 percent per day. Comparison of 32 patients who had combined procedures to another 17 who received only intravascular transfusions revealed a slightly increased mean interval between transfusions (24.2 vs. 21.6 days) and a higher fetal hematocrit at the time of the subsequent procedure (27.0 vs. 23.2 percent). Although these differences achieved statistical significance, their clinical importance is unclear. While some authors have advocated routinely combining intravascular and intraperitoneal transfusion,[170] it is unknown whether the addition of intraperitoneal erythrocytes can reduce the number of transfusions per pregnancy or improve the outcomes achieved with intravascular transfusion alone. Because the increased morbidity associated with intraperitoneal transfusion likely offsets any benefits of the combined procedure, we do not routinely perform combined intravascular and intraperitoneal transfusions.

Other Therapies

A number of noninvasive alternatives to intrauterine transfusion have been sought for the treatment of fetal hemolysis. Most of these have been aimed at modifying the maternal immune response so as to decrease the severity of erythroblastosis. Two of these, promethazine and oral ingestion of Rh-positive erythrocytes, are of historical interest only and were never proven to be of benefit.[171-174]

Plasmapheresis to reduce the level of maternal anti-D has been used in the treatment of severe Rh isoimmunization. Although the removal of several liters of plasma per week will result in a transient reduction in the anti-D titer during or immediately after treatment, a chronic, significant reduction in antibody titer is difficult, if not impossible, to achieve by this technique.[175-177] Some studies have suggested a benefit to plasmapheresis, but these results are difficult to interpret because of the use of other treatments and the lack of controls.[178,179] Furthermore, all studies of plasmapheresis in which several or more liters of plasma were removed weekly demonstrated an increase in anti-D titers or concentration soon after plasmapheresis was stopped. This "rebound" phenomenon has been attributed to the removal of the negative feedback influence on further anti-D production by high circulating titers of anti-D antibody.[180] Repeated, "small-volume" plasmapheresis may avoid antibody rebound.[180] The potential usefulness of plasmapheresis must be tempered by its potential for serious consequences for the mother and fetus; there are reports in the literature of maternal sepsis in Rh-sensitized patients undergoing plasmapheresis.[176,178] In view of the lack of a clearly documented benefit, plasmapheresis is not currently used at most centers in the treatment of severe Rh sensitization.

Plasmaphersis in combination with immunosuppression to prevent antibody rebound has also been used to treat severe Rh isoimmunization. Odendaal et al.[181] reported their experience with nine patients, seven of whom had a previous pregnancy loss or neonatal death directly or indirectly due to isoimmunization.[181] Using plasmapheresis three to seven times a week and immunosuppression with azathioprine and prednisome, eight patients delivered liveborns between 28 and 33 weeks' gestation, with the single fetal death being associated with a placental abruption. Again, because of the potential for morbidity with plasmapheresis and immunosuppression, and because benefit has not yet been demonstrated in adequate numbers of patients, such therapy is not commonly used.

The successful use of intravenous high-dose immunoglobulin (IgG) in platelet isoimmunization has led to its use in the treatment of severe Rh isoimmunization. The supposed mechanism of action is via either Fc receptor blockade in the fetal reticuloendothelial system (inhibiting the removal and destruction of anti-D-coated erythrocytes in the fetal spleen and liver) or blockade of Fc-mediated antibody placental transport (limiting the transplacental passage of anti-D to the fetus). The success of IgG therapy in ameliorating some cases of severe Rh disease presents exciting possibilities.[182-184] Intravenous IgG has been given to women in doses of 0.4 g/kg each day for 5 days, with the assumption that significant amounts cross the placenta and thereby has a beneficial effect on the fetus. However, placental transport of exogenous IgG may be limited before 32 weeks' gestation.[185] If the effectiveness of intravenous IgG therapy is due to effects on the fetal side, placement of the IgG directly into the fetal circulation via cordocentesis may be the most effective route of administration prior to 32 weeks' gestation. Further study and experience with more patients will be necessary before IgG therapy has a place in the routine management of severe Rh immunization.

Timing of Delivery

During the early 1960s, liberalized use of preterm delivery markedly reduced the incidence of perinatal death in Rh-sensitized pregnancies, primarily by decreasing the incidence of intrauterine death.[102,186] However, severely affected fetuses continued to die in utero or from complications of prematurity. Fortunately, refinements in the technique of intrauterine transfusion have made possible the prolongation of pregnancy until a gestational age compatible with neonatal survival is reached. Also, the analysis of the phospholipid content of amniotic fluid to determine fetal pulmonary maturity has greatly clarified the timing of delivery in relation to neonatal risk. Finally, the tremendous improvements in neonatal care over the past two decades have led to excellent survival rates, with acceptable morbidity rates, for even the very preterm infant.

If the history and antenatal studies indicate only mild fetal hemolysis, we await fetal pulmonary maturity before undertaking delivery by induction of labor, usually at 36 to 37 weeks' gestation. In these cases, fetal pulmonary maturation does not seem to be either delayed or accelerated by disease, and amniotic fluid studies accurately reflect fetal maturity.[187,188] If the cervix is not ripe, we typically use intracervical prostaglandin gel prior to oxytocin induction.

Rather than subject the fetus to the risk of continued intrauterine transfusions, severely sensitized pregnancies are generally delivered at the University of Utah after 32 to 34 weeks' gestation. This policy is based on an overall neonatal survival rate greater than 95 per-

cent after 32 weeks' gestation in our neonatal intensive care unit. If preterm delivery is anticipated, maternal steroids are administered to enhance fetal pulmonary maturity.

Some authors, in the interest of limiting morbidity, recommend the judicious use of intrauterine transfusion after 32 weeks' gestation when pulmonary phospholipid studies at that time indicate that the fetus is immature.[107] Delivery is then accomplished between 34 and 36 weeks' gestation. Regardless of the usual institutional practices, individual case circumstances need to be carefully weighed when making the decision as to when the fetus should be delivered.

Sensitization Caused by Minor Antigens

In addition to the D antigen, hundreds of other distinct antigens exist on the red blood cell surface. Known as "minor," "atypical," or "irregular" antigens, their frequencies vary between different populations. For instance, over 95 percent of whites and 80 percent of blacks are Duffy antigen negative. On the other hand, 80 percent of men are c antigen positive, and nearly half are homozygous.

In the past, minor antigens were an infrequent cause of maternal sensitization or fetal or neonatal hemolytic disease. Because of the reduction in Rh disease brought about by Rh-immune globulin prophylaxis, minor antigen sensitization has become relatively more frequent in pregnancy. In fact, antibodies to minor antigens are much more common in the general population than antibodies to the D antigen.[88]

The large majority of cases of minor antigen sensitization are due to incompatibile blood transfusion, as most blood banks do not routinely assess donor–recipient compatability for antigens other than ABO and RhD. Overall, antibodies to minor antigens occur in about 1.5 to 2.5 percent of obstetric patients.[189,190] Fortunately, some of the most common atypical antibodies, such as anti-Le[a], anti-Le[b], and anti-I, do not cause fetal or neonatal hemolysis. Le[a] and Le[b], the Lewis antigens, are not true erythrocyte antigens, but are secreted by other tissues and then adsorbed onto the red cell surface.[191] Fetal erythrocytes acquire very little antigen in utero and thus react only weakly to anti-Lewis.

However, a number of the minor antigens can result in fetal anemia and hydrops. Of the potentially serious antibodies, anti-E, anti-Kell, anti-c, anti c + E, and anti-Fy[a] (Duffy) are the most common.[88] A complete listing of the irregular antigens and antibodies as compiled by Weinstein[192] is shown in Table 27-4, with the potential severity of fetal involvement and proposed management listed.

In general, management of the pregnant patient with

Table 27-4   Atypical Antibodies and Their Relationship to Fetal Hemolytic Disease

Blood Group System	Antigens Related to Hemolytic Disease	Hemolytic Disease Severity	Proposed Management
Lewis	Not a proven cause of hemolytic disease of the newborn		
I	Not a proven cause of hemolytic disease of the newborn		
Kell	K	Mild to severe with hydrops fetalis	Amniotic fluid bilirubin studies
	k	Mild	Expectant
	Ko	Mild	Expectant
	Kp^a	Mild	Expectant
	Kp^b	Mild	Expectant
	Js^a	Mild	Expectant
	Js^b	Mild	Expectant
Rh (non-D)	E	Mild to severe with hydrops fetalis	Amniotic fluid bilirubin studies
	C	Mild to severe with hydrops fetalis	Amniotic fluid bilirubin studies
	c	Mild to severe with hydrops fetalis	Amniotic fluid bilirubin studies
Duffy	Fy^a	Mild to severe with hydrops fetalis	Amniotic fluid bilirubin studies
	Fy^b	Not a cause of hemolytic disease in the newborn	
	By^3	Mild	Expectant
Kidd	Jk^a	Mild to severe	Amniotic fluid bilirubin studies
	Jk^b	Mild	Expectant
	Jk^3	Mild	Expectant
MNSs	M	Mild to severe	Amniotic fluid bilirubin studies
	N	Mild	Expectant
	S	Mild to severe	Amniotic fluid bilirubin studies
	s	Mild to severe	Ambiotic fluid bilirubin studies
	U	Mild to severe	Amniotic fluid bilirubin studies
	Mi^a	Moderate	Amniotic fluid
MSSs	Mt^a	Moderate	Amniotic fluid bilirubin studies
	Vw	Mild	Expectant
	Mur	Mild	Expectant
	Hil	Mild	Expectant
	Hut	Mild	Expectant
Lutheran	Lu^a	Mild	Expectant
	Lu^b	Mild	Expectant
Diego	D1^a	Mild to severe	Amniotic fluid bilirubin studies
	Di^b	Mild to severe	Amniotic fluid bilirubin studies
Xg	Xg^a	Mild	Expectant
P	PP$_{1pk}$(Tj^a)	Mild to severe	Amniotic fluid bilirubin studies
Public antigens	Yt^a	Moderaqte to severe	Amniotic fluid bilirubin studies
	Yt^b	Mild	Expectant
	Lan	Mild	Expectant
	En^a	Moderate	Amniotic fluid bilirubin studies
	Ge	Mild	Expectant
	Jr^a	Mild	Expectant
	Co^a	Severe	Amniotic fluid bilirubin studies
	Co^{a-b-}	Mild	Expectant
Private antigens	Batty	Mild	Expectant
	Becker	Mild	Expectant
	Berrens	Mild	Expectant
	Biles	Moderate	Amniotic fluic bilirubin studies
	Evans	Mild	Expectant
	Gonzales	Mild	Expectant
	Good	Severe	Amniotic fluid bilirubin studies
	Heibel	Moderate	Amniotic fluid
	Hunt	Mild	Expectant
	Jobbins	Mild	Expectant
	Radin	Moderate	Amniotic fluid bilirubin studies
	Rm	Mild	Expectant
	Ven	Mild	Expectant
	Wright^a	Severe	Amniotic fluid bilirubin studies
	Wright^b	Mild	Expectant
	Zd	Moderate	Amniotic fluid bilirubin studies

(Modified from Weinstein,[192] with permission.)

antibody to one of the significant minor antigens has been much the same as for Rh immunization, using previous history, frequent measurement of maternal antibody titers, serial amniocenteses after a critical titer is reached, and transfusion or delivery based on the ΔOD_{450} values and trends.[107,192] However, few centers have a large number of pregnancies affected by minor antigen sensitization; thus, establishment of a critical maternal titer is difficult, and it is uncertain whether amniotic fluid bilirubin studies are as reliable as with RhD isoimmunization.

Pregnancy with Kell sensitization, which can result in severe fetal anemia, hydrops, and death, deserves special mention. In common usage, "Kell" refers to the K or K1 antigen of the Kell blood group system. Only about 9 percent of whites are positive for the Kell antigen; the gene frequency for kk is 91.1 percent, Kk 8.7 percent, and KK 0.2 percent.[7] About 0.2 percent of pregnant women are positive for anti-Kell, and, as mentioned above, nearly all cases of immunization are the result of Kell-incompatible transfusion.

A number of investigators have suggested that the fetal anemia associated with Kell sensitization is qualitatively different from that of Rh disease and requires a different management protocol.[193–197] Specifically, maternal titers and amniotic fluid ΔOD_{450} values may not be as predictive of the degree of fetal anemia as with Rh disease. For example, Berkowitz et al.[193] reported a case of fetal hydrops and death due to Kell sensitization despite amniotic fluid ΔOD_{450} values trending downward in the lower third of the Liley midzone. Similarly, Copel et al.[195] reported a case of fetal hydrops with a maternal anti-Kell titer of 1:4; in another patient, the anti-Kell titer spontaneously rose from 1:32 to 1:2,048 even though the fetus was Kell negative.

It may be that the mechanism of anemia is different than with RhD disease. Although Kell antibody can activate the complement cascade to attach C3 to red cell membranes,[198] it also appears that suppression of fetal erythropoiesis is important in the development of fetal anemia due to anti-Kell.[199]

Caine and Mueller-Huebach[194] described their experience with 127 Kell-sensitized pregnancies. Thirteen (10 percent) had an affected Kell-positive fetus, and five (38 percent of those affected) had severe disease. Only 3 percent of pregnancies with a maternal titer ≤1:16 had a Kell-positive fetus compared with 29 percent of those with a titer >1:16. No patient with a titer ≤1:16 had a fetal death, and all patients with a poor perinatal outcome had a titer ≥1:128 at delivery. Importantly, no patient with a poor outcome had an amniotic fluid ΔOD_{450} value in the highest Liley zone, suggesting that serious hemolytic disease develops at lower ΔOD_{450} values than with Rh sensitization.

Leggat and co-workers[196] described 194 pregnancies

over 25 years in which anti-Kell was the only antibody identified. Of the 178 unaffected babies, 106 (60 percent) had maternal titers ≥1:16. There were 16 affected infants (9 percent of the total), 10 with mild disease and 6 with moderate or severe anemia. Of the six mothers who delivered affected infants, four had titers ≥1:16 while two had titers ≤1:8. Amniotic fluid analysis was also performed in pregnancies that resulted in 16 unaffected and 5 affected newborns; fetuses with disease of moderate or greater severity had ΔOD_{450} values trending upward or in the upper part of the Liley midzone, but four unaffected fetuses had ΔOD_{450} values associated with moderate-to-severe hemolysis in Rh disease. The authors concluded that neither maternal antibody titer nor amniotic fluid analysis was a satisfactory predictor of fetal status.

Bowman et al.,[200] on the other hand, found that amniotic fluid ΔOD_{450} measurements were accurate in predicting fetal status in 16 of 18 Kell-negative pregnancies. In 10 of 12 Kell-positive fetuses, ΔOD_{450} values appropriately predicted disease severity, although the ΔOD_{450} level of one fetus with a hydropic death was in the lower half of zone II, and those of another fetus with only moderate disease reached the line between zones II and III.

In light of these data, several authors have suggested a management scheme for Kell-sensitized pregnancies that includes umbilical cord blood sampling at 20 weeks gestation when the father is either Kell positive or of uncertain status.[197,201] With this protocol, at least half of the fetuses will be found to be Kell negative, and no further testing will be necessary; rarely, a fetus will be found to be significantly anemic and can be promptly transfused. However, management after 20 weeks' gestation of the approximately 80 percent of Kell-positive fetuses destined to have mild or moderate disease is not addressed by this cord sampling protocol.

Recognizing that amniotic fluid bilirubin studies may be misleading in some pregnancies and that more liberal use of umbilical cord blood sampling is appropriate, we agree with Bowman et al.[200] that serial ΔOD_{450} measurements are still of value. When the father is known to be Kell negative, the fetus will also be Kell negative, and no surveillance or testing is necessary. When the father is Kell positive or of uncertain status and there is no history of severe fetal involvement, we follow maternal anti-Kell titers, track fetal movements, and perform serial ultrasounds as long as the maternal titer remains below 1:8. For patients whose titers rise above 1:8 or who have a history of fetal involvement, we perform serial amniocenteses every 1 to 4 weeks unless the fetus is known to be Kell negative, beginning at 20 to 28 weeks depending on history, maternal titer, and previous ΔOD_{450} value. Additionally, we offer umbilical cord blood sampling at the time of the first amniocentesis if the procedure seems to be technically feasible. As with RhD disease, we use a modified Liley curve extrapolated back to 24 weeks (Fig. 27-4); between 16 and 24 weeks gestation, we typically use Queenan's horizontal boundaries[112] with an emphasis on ΔOD_{450} trends. If ΔOD_{450} levels rise into or above the middle of zone II, we recommend umbilical cord blood sampling for hematocrit and Kell status, with blood ready for transfusion if necessary. Between amniocenteses and/or fetal blood samplings, we perform nonstress tests and frequent ultrasounds looking for developing hydrops.

The gene for the Kell antigen has been identified on the long arm of chromosome 7,[202,203] and prenatal diagnosis of fetal Kell status with PCR on uncultured amniocytes will likely soon be available. This will greatly reduce the need for umbilical blood sampling, as about half of fetuses of sensitized pregnancies will be identified as Kell negative with amniocentesis.

ABO Incompatibility

Twenty to 25 percent of pregnancies are ABO incompatible, meaning that the mother's serum contains anti-A or anti-B, while the erythrocytes of the fetus contain the respective antigen. This results in ABO incompatibility being a common cause of hemolytic disease of the newborn, accounting for over 60 percent of all cases.[204] Fortunately, the disease is nearly always manifested as no worse than moderate neonatal anemia and mild-to-moderate neonatal hyperbilirubinemia, and less than 1 percent of cases require exchange transfusion. ABO incompatibility has never clearly been shown to be a cause of fetal hemolysis and can generally be regarded as a pediatric rather than an obstetric problem.[205]

There are several reasons why ABO incompatibility rarely results in severe hemolytic disease. Individuals with group A or B blood type produce predominantly IgM anti-B or anti-A, both of which cross the placenta poorly. Also, there are fewer A and B antigen sites on the fetal erythrocyte than on the adult erythrocyte; thus, less antibody can bind to fetal red cell membranes. Finally, maternal and fetal tissues other than erythrocytes contain the A and B antigens, and some investigators believe that anti-A or anti-B antibodies are absorbed by these sites so that less of the antibodies are available for erythrocyte binding.[204]

The A and B antigens are "naturally occurring" antigens; that is, they occur widely in nature unassociated with erythrocyte membranes. Therefore, A or B sensitization does not require prior exposure to red cells through pregnancy or by transfusion, and it is not unusual for ABO hemolytic disease to affect the firstborn child. Clinically apparent hemolytic disease of the newborn resulting from ABO incompatibility is mostly confined to the situation wherein the mother is type O and the infant is type A or B, because group O individuals produce anti-A and anti-B that is predominantly of the IgG class and can therefore cross the placenta to bind to the fetal erythrocytes.[204]

In most cases, ABO hemolytic disease manifests itself as mild to moderate hyperbilirubinemia during the first 24 to 48 hours of life. It is rarely associated with significant anemia. High levels of bilirubin can cause kernicterus, with preterm neonates being most susceptible. Phototherapy is the first line of treatment, although exchange transfusion may be indicated according to the degree of hyperbilirubinemia.

Because ABO incompatibility is likely to occur in subsequent pregnancies, the delivery of an affected newborn should be documented in the patient's record. However, since significant fetal hemolysis does not occur, screening for anti-A or anti-B antibodies in the mother's serum and analysis of the amniotic fluid for bilirubin are not required.

Platelet Isoimmunization

Like erythrocytes, platelets contain specific surface antigens, and maternal sensitization to platelet antigens can occur when there is an incompatibility between fetus and mother. In a situation analogous to Rh isoimmunization, alloimmune thrombocytopenia is the result of maternal sensitization to incompatible fetal platelets and transfer of antiplatelet antibody to the fetus with subsequent sequestration of platelets in the reticuloendothelial system.[206] In affected cases, the maternal platelet count is normal, with fetal–neonatal thrombocytopenia ranging from mild to profound.

Five biallelic systems of platelet-specific antigens have been well described: Pl^A1/Pl^A2, Ko^b/Ko^a, Bak^a/Bak^b (Lek^a/Lek^b), Pen^a/Pen^b (Yuk^b/Yuk^a), and Br^b/Br^a. A new and simplified system of nomenclature for the human platelet antigens has been suggested,[207] numbering the antigen families in chronological order of discovery (HPA-1 through HPA-5), but many clinicians continue to use the older system. Platelets also express HLA class I antigens but not those of class II.[208,209]

Sensitization to the Pl^A1 antigen is the etiology in about three-fourths of cases of neonatal alloimmune thrombocytopenia. Approximately 2 percent of whites, 0.4 percent of blacks, and less than 0.1 percent of Asians are negative for Pl^A1. Sensitization to Br^a is the second most common cause of neonatal alloimmune thrombocytopenia, about 10 to 15 percent of cases; less than 1 percent of whites are negative for Br^a.[208,209]

Although HLA antigens are less immunogenic on platelets than on other cells, anti-HLA antibodies may rarely cause neonatal isoimmune thrombocytopenia.[210] Also, maternal HLA class II type appears to influence susceptibility to platelet isoimmunization; HLA-DR3 is associated with Pl[A1] isoimmunization, and HLA-DRw6 is associated with sensitization to Br[a].[211]

Neonatal alloimmune thrombocytopenia occurs in about 1:1,000 to 1:2,000 births and is probably the most common reason for severe thrombocytopenia in the newborn.[206,212–214] The clinical severity of neonatal alloimmune thrombocytopenia varies widely. Approximately 90 percent of affected newborns have diffuse petechiae, and 9 to 12 percent suffer intracranial bleeding, with a neonatal mortality of 5 to 13 percent.[208,212] About 45 percent of cases of central nervous system hemorrhage occur before birth, often resulting in porencephalic cysts.[215] Fetal thrombocytopenia appears to be most common in the third trimester, but has been detected as early as 20 weeks gestation.[216,217]

Unlike Rh isoimmunization, maternal titers of antibody to the platelet antigen are not predictive of clinical outcome, anti-platelet IgG production can occur in the first pregnancy, and firstborn children are often affected. Primiparas account for between 20 and 60 percent of identified cases,[208,218] and mothers at risk are usually identified only after the birth of an affected newborn. There are several reasons why all pregnant women are not screened for the presence of antiplatelet antibodies: (1) at least one-fourth of cases of alloimmune neonatal thrombocytopenia are not due to the Pl[A1] antigen; (2) the maternal immune response seems to be influenced by other factors such as HLA type, and only a minority of infants of mothers negative for the Pl[A1] antigen will develop significant thrombocytopenia; and (3) no relationship exists between the level of antibody to Pl[A1] and the degree of thrombocytopenia. Following delivery of an affected newborn, though, the incidence of recurrent fetal–neonatal thrombocytopenia of equal or greater severity is up to 95 percent in the next pregnancy.[208,209]

The management of patients at risk for neonatal isoimmune thrombocytopenia is directed at preventing hemorrhage in the fetus and neonate. Before the availability of umbilical cord blood sampling, the management strategy for pregnancies at risk for alloimmune thrombocytopenia was to avoid fetal trauma with bedrest during the pregnancy and cesarean delivery before labor.[219,220] However, since approximately half of fetuses who suffer intracranial bleeding do so before labor, avoidance of labor and vaginal delivery only partially reduces the associated morbidity and mortality. As mentioned, maternal platelet counts are normal, and maternal antibody levels are not predictive of fetal platelet count. Umbilical cord blood sampling and direct measurement of fetal platelet count is currently the only method to assess fetal status accurately.

Several strategies have recently been proposed for the management of pregnancies at risk for alloimmune thrombocytopenia. Transfusions of maternal (antigen-negative) platelets into the fetal circulation and maternally administered high-dose immunoglobulin (with and without concurrent administration of corticosteroids) both appear to raise the fetal platelet count in utero, and each therapy has its supporters.

One group has suggested that the diagnosis of fetal thrombocytopenia be made by cordocentesis at 20 to 22 weeks' gestation, and patients with an affected fetus should be advised to rest carefully and avoid abdominal trauma.[221,222] At 37 weeks gestation, umbilical cord blood sampling can be repeated, and if the fetal platelet count is normal, labor can be induced; if the platelet count is less than 50,000 cells/μl, maternal platelets are transfused into the fetal circulation using the following formula, allowing safe induction of labor and vaginal delivery:

$$V = \frac{EFBV \times (\text{desired FPC} - \text{pretransfusion FPC})}{\text{count of platelet concentrate}}$$

where V is volume of platelet concentrate to be transfused, EFBV is estimated fetal blood volume, and FPC is fetal platelet count.[222] This approach, with a single fetal platelet transfusion immediately before delivery, does not address the possibility of spontaneous hemorrhage in utero, but may be the most reasonable management plan for fetuses considered to be at low risk for antepartum bleeding.

In an effort to prevent antepartum intracranial bleeding, Nicolini et al.[223] and Murphy et al.[224] have described the use of serial platelet transfusions throughout the third trimester. Both patients cited had previous infants with Pl[A1] antigen alloimmune thrombocytopenia leading to severe antepartum intracranial hemorrhage with neurologic sequelae. Fetal thrombocytopenia was documented, and weekly platelet transfusions were begun at 26 to 29 weeks. Platelets transfused in utero (even Pl[A1]-negative platelets) have a short lifespan, and counts dropped from post-transfusion levels of over 150,000 cells/μl to less than 50,000 cells/μl at the next weekly transfusion. The pregnancies were carried to 32 and 35 weeks, respectively, and delivered by cesarean section. Neonatal platelet counts were greater than 44,000 cells/μl, and neither infant suffered intracranial bleeding. Further experience and data are needed to confirm the efficacy of this approach because of the potentially high fetal morbidity and mortality associated with frequent cordocentesis in alloimmune thrombocytopenia[225] and the difficulty and risks of repeated maternal platelet pheresis. Also, fetal intracranial hemorrhage is rare before the third trimester, and it has been suggested that the weekly intrauterine platelet transfusion might be limited to the third trimester, with delivery as soon as pulmonary maturity is documented.[226,227]

The most widely used management for fetal thrombocytopenia involves the maternal administration of high-dose immunoglobulin (IgG).[228,229] This treatment is based on the well-established observation that most cases of neonatal alloimmune thrombocytopenia are effectively treated by giving the neonate intravenous IgG.[230–232] The mechanism of action is uncertain but may involve Fc-receptor blockade in the fetal reticuloendothelial system and inhibition of uptake of IgG-coated platelets by reticuloendothelial cells, or Fc-receptor binding in the placenta, inhibiting the transplacental transfer of antiplatelet antibody. Reports of umbilical cord infusion of IgG failing to improve fetal platelet count suggest that any beneficial effect of maternal immunoglobulin infusion is due to maternal or placental factors.[233]

Expanding on an earlier report,[228] Lynch and coworkers[229] administered intravenous (maternal) immunoglobulin and serially measured fetal platelet counts in 18 women who had previously delivered an infant with severe alloimmune thrombocytopenia. After confirming thrombocytopenia at 20 to 22 weeks' gestation or at referral, weekly infusions of intravenous immunoglobulin (1.0 g/kg body weight) were initiated. Umbilical blood sampling was repeated in 4 to 6 weeks to assess the effect of the therapy and then again at term to determine the mode of delivery. Nine of the 18 patients also received corticosteriods. The median platelet count rose from 32,000 cells/μl before treatment to 60,000 cells/μl at birth. Only three infants had a fetal platelet count less than 30,000 cells/μl at term, and there were no cases of intracranial hemorrhage (compared with seven of the previous, untreated siblings). Steroid treatment did not appear to have a beneficial effect on fetal platelet count.

Although these results are encouraging, fetal platelet count is not always increased with maternal high-dose immunoglobulin infusion, even with a documented increase in fetal immunoglobulin levels.[222,234–236] One problem with maternally administered IgG is that it may not cross the placenta effectively prior to 32 weeks gestation.[185] Also, intravenous immunoglobulin is quite expensive (over $1,000 per weekly infusion), and the infectious risk (albeit small) of blood product infu-sion is highlighted by the recent outbreak of acute hepatitis C associated with use of some brands of intravenous immunoglobulin.[237]

In the management of patients at risk for alloimmune thrombocytopenia, we offer weekly infusions of intravenous immunoglobulin beginning at 20 to 24 weeks' gestation after a full discussion of the risks and potential benefits and after cordocentesis to confirm fetal thrombocytopenia. For those whose fetal platelet count is normal, and for those who decline umbilical blood sampling and immunoglobulin treatment, we advocate bedrest with avoidance of abdominal trauma and serial sonograms during the third trimester to detect intracranial bleeding. Regardless of the regimen used, all patients undergo cordocentesis at 36 to 37 weeks gestation to determine the fetal platelet count. If the fetal platelet count is greater than 50,000 cells/μl, labor is induced. If the fetal platelet count is less than 50,000 cells/μl, immediate platelet tranfusion into the umbilical vein, with documentation of an adequate post-transfusion platelet count, is followed by induction of labor.

Patients with a previous severely thrombocytopenic fetus and significant antepartum morbidity are generally offered surveillance at an earlier gestational age, but the risks of repeated umbilical blood sampling and serial platelet transfusions do not seem to be warranted except in extreme cases. If the fetus remains severely thrombocytopenic (<50,000 platelets/μl) in spite of attempts to raise the platelet count, cesarean delivery is preferred.

In all cases of documented fetal-neonatal alloimmune thrombocytopenia, maternal platelets should be available for transfusion after delivery, regardless of the treatment protocol used or the antepartum fetal platelet count.

Determination of platelet antigen genotypes using polymerase chain reaction has been described,[238,239] and reports of diagnosis of fetal platelet antigen status from uncultured amniocytes obtained at amniocentesis should be forthcoming. As with Rh disease, this advance will allow determination of fetal antigen status (and risk of thrombocytopenia) in sensitized pregnancies without umbilical cord blood sampling. Also in the very near future, preimplantation genetic testing will be available, given the ability to determine genotype from a single cell.

Key Points

- To reduce the incidence of Rh sensitization, Rh-immune globulin should be given to Rh-negative unsensitized women at 28 weeks' gestational age and again after delivery if the newborn is Rh positive. Rh-immune globulin is also indicated for these patients in cases of miscarriage, ectopic pregnancy, chorionic villus sampling, amniocentesis, or fetomaternal hemorrhage.

- The gene coding for the D antigen has been cloned, and in the near future prenatal determination of fetal Rh status should be routinely available from uncultured amniocytes obtained at amniocentesis.

- Measurement of amniotic fluid bilirubin remains the standard for assessment of pregnancies at risk for significant fetal anemia. Neither ultrasound alone nor Doppler are adequately sensitive to identify anemic fetuses.

- The timing of the first amniocentesis is based on history, maternal anti-D titers, gestational age, and ultrasound findings. The timing of subsequent amniocenteses is based on the ΔOD_{450} values and trends.

- Analysis of amniotic fluid bilirubin before 26 weeks is controversial. Although most data suggest that ΔOD_{450} values and trends are accurate before the third trimester, more liberal use of cordocentesis may be appropriate.

- Fetal transfusion can be performed using either the intraperitoneal or intravascular route. For hydropic fetuses, intravascular transfusion is clearly superior. For nonhydropic fetuses, perinatal survival rates are similar with either method.

- With the reduction in Rh disease brought about by widespread use of Rh-immune globulin prophylaxis, sensitization to the minor or atypical antigens has become relatively more common. A number of these minor antigens can cause several fetal anemia.

- Management of pregnancies complicated by sensitization to one of the serious minor antigens (such as Kell) is based on the experience with Rh disease. However, amniotic fluid bilirubin analysis may not be as accurate an indicator of fetal anemia with Kell sensitization as with Rh disease.

- Platelets also carry distinct antigens, and, in a process similar to Rh sensitization, platelet sensitization can occur. Unlike Rh disease, firstborn fetuses can be affected, and maternal antibody titers do not predict fetal platelet count.

- The optimal management scheme for pregnancies affected with platelet sensitization is unclear. A protocol involving (1) cordocentesis at 28 weeks for documentation of thrombocytopenia, (2) weekly maternal administration of intravenous immunoglobulin, and (3) cordocentesis at about 37 weeks to determine platelet count before delivery has been suggested and seems to balance risk and potential benefit.

References

1. Diamond LK, Blackfan KD, Baty JM: Erythroblastosis fetalis and its association with universal edema of the fetus, icterus gravis neonatorum and anemia of the newborn. J Pediatr 1:269, 1932
2. Darrow RR: Icterus gravis (erythroblastosis) neonatorum: examination of etiologic considerations. Arch Pathol Lab Med 25:378, 1938
3. Levine P, Stetson RE: An unusual case of intragroup agglutination. JAMA 113:126, 1939
4. Levin P, Burnham L, Katzin EM et al: The role of isoimmunization in the pathogenesis of erythroblastosis fetalis. Am J Obstet Gynecol 42:925, 1941
5. Landsteiner K, Wiener AS: An agglutinable factor in human blood recognized by immune sera for rhesus blood. Proc Soc Exp Biol Med 43:223, 1940
6. Rosenfield RE, Allen FH Jr, Swisher SN, Kochwa S: A review of Rh serology and presentation of a new terminology. Transfusion 2:287, 1962
7. Race RR, Sanger R: Blood Groups in Man. 6th Ed. Blackwell, Oxford, 1975
8. Rote NS: Pathophysiology of Rh isoimmunization. Clin Obstet Gynecol 25:243, 1982
9. Wiener AS: The Rh series of allelic genes. Science 100:595, 1944
10. Rosenfield RE, Allen FH, Rubenstein P: Genetic model for the Rh blood-group system. Proc Natl Acad Sci USA 70:1303, 1973
11. Marsh WL, Chaganti RSK, Mayer K et al: Mapping human autosomes: evidence supporting assignment of rhesus to the short arm of chromosome number 1. Science 183:966, 1974
12. Marsh W, Kimball LF: Mapping assignment of the Rh and Duffy blood group genes to chromosome 1. Mayo Clin Proc 52:145, 1977
13. Colin Y, Cherif-Zahar B, Le Van Kim C et al: Genetic basis of the RhD-positive and RhD-negative blood group polymorphism as determined by Southern analysis. Blood 80:1074, 1991
14. Merry AH, Thomson EE, Anstee DJ et al: The quantification of erythrocyte antigen sites with monoclonal antibodies. Immunology 51:793, 1984
15. Bloy C, Blanchard D, Lambin P et al: Characterization of the C, c, E, and G antigens of the Rh blood group system with human monoclonal antibodies. Mol Immunol 225:925, 1988
16. Hughes-Jones NC, Gardner B, Lincoln PJ: Observations on the number of available c, D, and E antigen sites on red cells. Vox Sang 21:210, 1971
17. Skov F, Hughes-Jones NC: Observations on the number of available C antigen sites on red cells. Vox Sang 33:170, 1977

18. Masouredis SP: Relationship between Rho(D) genotype and quantity of I[131] anti-Rho(D) bound to red cells. J Clin Invest 39:1450, 1960

19. James NT, James V: Nearest neighbor analysis on the distribution of Rh antigens on erythrocyte membranes. Br J Haematol 40:657, 1978

20. Masouredis SP, Sudora EJ, Mahan L, Victoria EJ: Antigen site densities and ultrastructural distribution patterns of red cell Rh antigens. Transfusion 16:94, 1976

21. Moore S, Green C: The identification of specific Rhesus polypeptide blood group ABH active glycoprotein complexes in the human red cell membrane. Biochem J 244:735, 1987

22. Bloy C, Blanchard D, Lambin P et al: Human monoclonal antibody against Rh(D) antigen: partial characterization of the Rh(D) polypeptide from human erythrocytes. Blood 69:1491, 1987

23. Brown PJ, Evans JP, Sinor LT et al: The rhesus antigen. A dicyclohexylcarbodiimide-binding proteolipid. Am J Pathol 110:127, 1983

24. Avent ND, Ridgwell K, Tanner MJA: cDNA cloning of a 30 kDA erythrocyte membrane protein associated with Rh (Rhesus)-blood-group-antigen expression. Biochem J 271:821, 1990

25. Cherif-Zahar B, Bloy C, Le Van Kim et al: Molecular cloning and protein structure of a human blood group Rh polypeptide. Proc Natl Acad Sci USA 87:6243, 1990

26. Bergstrom H, Nilsson LA, Nilsson L et al: Demonstration of Rh antigens in a 38-day-old fetus. Am J Obstet Gynecol 99:130, 1967

27. Reardon A, Masouredis SP: Blood group D antigen content of nucleated red cell precursors. Blood 50:981, 1977

28. Lomas C, Tippett P, Thompson KM et al: Demonstration of seven epitopes on the Rh antigen D using human monoclonal anti-D antibodies and red cells from D categories. Vox Sang 57:261, 1989

29. Gorick BD, Thompson KM, Melamed MD, Hughes-Jones NC: Three epitopes on the human Rh antigen D recognized by ^{125}I-labelled human monoclonal IgG antibodies. Vox Sang 55:165, 1988

30. Lauf PK, Clinton HJ: Increased potassium transport and ouabain binding in human Rh null red blood cells. Blood 48:457, 1976

31. Kuypers F, van Linde-Sibenius-Trip M, Roelofsen B et al: Rh[null] human erythrocytes have an abnormal membrane phospholipid organization. Biochem J 221:931, 1984

32. Issitt PD: The Rh blood groups. p. 111. In Garrity G (ed): Immunobiology of Transfusion Medicine. Marcel Dekker, New York, 1994

33. Cohen F, Zuelzer WW, Gustafson DC et al: Mechanisms of isoimmunization. I. The transplacental passage of fetal erythrocytes in homospecific pregnancies. Blood 23:621, 1964

34. Lloyd LK, Miya F, Hebertson RM et al: Intrapartum fetomaternal bleeding in Rh-negative women. Obstet Gynecol 56:285, 1980

35. Woodrow JC: Transplacental hemorrhage. Ser Haematol 111:15, 1970

36. Zipursky A, Israels LG: The pathogenesis and prevention of Rh immunization. Can Med Assoc J 97:1245, 1967

37. Bowman JM: The management of Rh-isoimmunization. Obstet Gynecol 52:1, 1978

38. Sebring ES, Polesky HF: Detection of fetal maternal hemorrhage in Rh immune globulin candidates: a rosetting technique using enzyme-treated Rh₂Rh₂ indicator erythrocytes. Transfusion 22:486, 1982

39. Stedman CM, Baudin JC, White CA, Cooper ES: Use of the erythrocyte rosette test to screen for excessive fetomaternal hemorrhage in Rh-negative women. Am J Obstet Gynecol 154:1363, 1986

40. Ness PM, Baldwin ML, Niebyl JR: Clinical high-risk designation does not predict excess fetal-maternal hemorrhage. Am J Obstet Gynecol 156:154, 1987

41. Davey MG, Zipursky A: McMaster conference on prevention of Rh immunization. Vox Sang 36:50, 1979

42. Aborjaily AN: Rh sensitization after tubal pregnancy. N Engl J Med 281:1076, 1969

43. Litwak O, Taswell HF, Banner EA et al: Fetal erythrocytes in maternal circulation after spontaneous abortion. JAMA 214:531, 1970

44. Matthews CD, Matthews AEB, Gilbey BE: Antibody development in rhesus-negative patients following abortion. Lancet 2:318, 1969

45. Queenan JT, Shah S, Kubarych SF et al: Role of induced abortion in Rhesus immunization. Lancet 1:815, 1971

46. Ascari WQ: Abortion and maternal Rh immunization. Clin Obstet Gynecol 14:625, 1971

47. Leong M, Duby S, Kinch RA: Fetal-maternal transfusion following early abortion. Obstet Gynecol 54:424, 1979

48. Freda VJ, Gorman JG, Galen RS et al: The threat of Rh immunization from abortion. Lancet 2:147, 1970

49. Litwalk O, Taswell H, Banner E, Keith L: Fetal erythrocytes in maternal circulation after spontaneous abortion. JAMA 215:521, 1970

50. Von Stein GA, Munsick RA, Stiver K, Ryder K: Fetomaternal hemorrhage in threatened abortion. Obstet Gynecol 79:383, 1992

51. Dayton VD, Anderson DS, Crosson FT, Cruikshank SH: A case of Rh isoimmunization: should threatened first-trimester abortion be an indication for Rh immune globulin prophylaxis? Am J Obstet Gynecol 163:63, 1990

52. Katz J, Marcus RG: The risk of Rh isoimmunization in ruptured tubal pregnancy. BMJ 3:667, 1972

53. Harrison R, Campbell S, Craft I: Risks of fetomaternal hemorrhage resulting from amniocentesis with and without ultrasound placental localization. Obstet Gynecol 48:557, 1976

54. Mennuti MT, Brummond W, Crombleholme WR et al: Fetal maternal bleeding associated with genetic amniocentesis. Obstet Gynecol 55:48, 1980

55. Henry G, Wexler P, Robinson A: Rh-immune globulin after amniocentesis for genetic diagnosis. Obstet Gynecol 48:557, 1976

56. Pollack W, Ascari WQ, Crispen JF et al: Studies on Rh prophylaxis after transfusion with Rh-positive blood. Transfusion 11:340, 1971

57. Pollack W, Ascari WQ, Kochesky RJ et al: Studies on Rh prophylaxis. I. Relationship between doses of anti-Rh and size of antigenic stimulus. Transfusion 11:333, 1971

58. Nevanlinna HR, Vainio T: The influence of mother–child ABO incompatibility on Rh immunization. Vox Sang 1:26, 1956

59. Queenan JT: Modern Management of the Rh Problem. 2nd Ed. Harper & Row, Hagerstown, MD, 1977

60. Woodrow JC: Rh Immunization and Its Prevention. Series Hematologica, Vol. 3. Copenhagen, Munksgaard, 1970

61. Ascari WQ, Levin P, Pollack W: Incidence of maternal Rh immunization by ABO compatible and incompatible pregnancies. BMJ 1:399, 1969

62. Freda VJ, Gorman JG, Pollack W: Successful prevention of experimental Rh sensitization in man with anti-Rh gamma 2-globulin antibody preparation. Transfusion 4:26, 1964

63. Clarke CA, Donohoe WTA, Finn R et al: Further extraperitoneal studies on the prevention of Rh haemolytic disease. BMJ 1:979, 1963

64. Pollack W, Gorman JG, Freda VJ: Rh immune suppression: past, present, and future. p. 9. In Frigoletto FD, Jewett JR, Konugres AD (eds): Rh Hemolytic Disease: New Strategy for Eradication. GK Hall, Boston, 1982

65. Hamilton EG: Prevention of Rh isoimmunization by injection of anti-D antibody. Obstet Gynecol 30:812, 1967

66. Pollack W, Singer HO, Gorman JG et al: The prevention of isoimmunization to the Rh factor by passive immunization with Rh D immune globulin. Haematology 2:1, 1968

67. Chown B, Duff Am, James J et al: Prevention of primary Rh immunization: first report of the Western Canadian Trial. Can Med Assoc J 100:1021, 1969

68. Mollison PL, Barron SL, Bowley C et al: Controlled trial of various anti-D dosages in suppression of Rh sensitization following pregnancy. BMJ 2:75, 1974

69. Freda VJ, Gorman JG, Pollack W et al: Prevention of Rh hemolytic disease—ten years clinical experience with Rh immune globulin. N Engl J Med 292:1014, 1975

70. Bowman JM, Chown B, Lewis M, Pollack JM: Rho-isoimmunization during pregnancy. Can Med Assoc J 118:623, 1978

71. Bowman JM, Pollock JM: Antenatal Rh prophylaxis: 28 weeks' gestation service program. Can Med Assoc J 118:627, 1978

72. Hensleigh PA: Preventing Rhesus isoimmunization. Antepartum Rh immune globulin prophylaxis versus a sensitive test for risk identification. Am J Obstet Gynecol 146:749, 1983

73. Thornton JG, Page C, Foote G et al: Efficacy and long term effects of antenatal prophylaxis with anti-D immunoglobulin. BMJ 298:1671, 1989

74. Kochenour NK, Beeson JH: The use of Rh-immune globulin. Clin Obstet Gynecol 25:283, 1982

75. Bowman JM: Controversies in Rh prophylaxis. Who needs Rh immune globulin and when should it be used? Am J Obstet Gynecol 151:289, 1985

76. Baskett TF, Parsons ML: Prevention of Rh(D) alloimmunization: a cost-benefit analysis. Can Med Assoc J 142:337, 1990

77. Kumpel BM, Poole D, Bradley BA: Human monoclonal antibodies. Their production, serology, quantitation, and potential use as blood grouping reagents. Br J Haematol 71:125, 1989

78. Thomson A, Contreras M, Gorick B et al: Clearance of Rh D-positive cells with monoclonal anti-D. Lancet 336:1147, 1990

79. Selinger M: Immunoprophylaxis for rhesus disease—expensive but worth it? Br J Obstet Gynaecol 98:509, 1991

80. Mollison PL: The reticulo-endothelial system and red cell destruction. Proc R Soc Med 55:915, 1962

81. Pollack W: Recent understanding for the mechanism by which passively administered antibody suppresses the immune response to Rh antigen in unimmunized Rh-negative women. Clin Obstet Gynecol 25:255, 1982

82. Chan PL, Sinclair NR: Regulation of the immune response. VI. Inability of F(ab)2 antibody to terminate established immune responses and its ability to interfere with IgG antibody-mediated immunosuppression. Immunology 24:289, 1973

83. Barss VA, Frigoletto FD, Konugres A: The cost of irregular antibody screening. Am J Obstet Gynecol 159:428, 1988

84. American College of Obstetricians and Gynecologists: Prevention of D isoimmunization. ACOG Technical Bulletin 147. American College of Obstetricians and Gynecologists, Washington DC, 1990

85. Standards Committee, American Association of Blood Banks: Standards for Blood Banks and Transfusion Services. 16th Ed. American Association of Blood Banks, Washington DC, 1994

86. Keith LG, Berger GS: The risk of Rh immunization associated with abortion, spontaneous and induced. p. 111. In Frigoletto FD, Jewett JF, Konugres AA (eds): Rh Hemolytic Disease: New Strategy for Eradication. GK Hall, Boston, 1982

87. Baskett TF, Parsons ML, Peddle LJ: The experience and effectiveness of the Nova Scotia Rh Program, 1964–84. Can Med Assoc J 134:1259, 1986

88. Tovey LAD: Haemolytic disease of the newborn—the changing scene. Br J Obstet Gynecol 93:960, 1986

89. Kanter MH: Derivation of new mathematic formulas for determining whether a D-positive father is heterozygous or homozygous for the D antigen. Am J Obstet Gynecol 166:61, 1992

90. Reece EA, Copel JA, Scioscia AL et al: Diagnostic fetal umbilical blood sampling in the management of isoimmunization. Am J Obstet Gynecol 159:1057, 1988

91. Nicolini U, Kochenour NK, Greco P et al: Consequences of fetomaternal hemorrhage after intrauterine transfusion. BMJ 297:1379, 1988

92. Le Van Kim C, Mouro I, Cherif-Zachar B et al: Molecular cloning and primary structure of the human blood group RhD polypeptide. Proc Natl Acad Sci USA 89:10,900, 1992

93. Bennett PR, Warwick R, Vaughan JV et al: Prenatal de-

termination of fetal RhD type by DNA amplification. N Engl J Med 329:607, 1993

94. Fisk NM, Bennett P, Warwick RB et al: Clinical utility of fetal RhD typing in alloimmunized pregnancies by means of polymerase chain reaction on amniocytes or chorionic villi. Am J Obstet Gynecol 171:50, 1994

95. Simsek S, Bleker PMM, von den Borne AEGK: Prenatal determination of fetal Rh type. N Engl J Med 330:795, 1994

96. Rossiter JP, Blakemore KJ, Kickler TS et al: The use of polymerase chain reaction to determine fetal RhD status. Am J Obstet Gynecol 171:1047, 1994

97. Van den Veyver IB, Chong SS et al: Single-cell analysis of the RhD blood type for use in preimplantation diagnosis in the prevention of severe hemolytic disease of the newborn. Am J Obstet Gynecol 172:533, 1995

98. Dildy GA, Jackson GM, Ward K: Determination of fetal RhD status from uncultured amniocytes. Obstet Gynecol [in press].

99. Lo M-YD, Bowell PJ, Selinger M et al: Prenatal determination of fetal RhD status by analysis of peripheral blood of rhesus negative mothers. Lancet 341:1147, 1993

100. Allen H, Diamond LK, Jones AR: Erythroblastosis fetalis. IX. Problems of stillbirth. N Engl J Med 251:453, 1954

101. Freda VJ: The Rh problem in obstetrics and a new concept of its management using amniocenteses and spectrophotometric scanning of amniotic fluid. Am J Obstet Gynecol 92:341, 1965

102. McElin TW, Buckingham JC, Danforth DN: The outcome and treatment of Rh-Sensitized pregnancies. Am J Obstet Gynecol 84:4678, 1962

103. Bevis DCA: Blood pigments in haemolytic disease of the newborn. J Obstet Gynaecol Br Emp 63:65, 1956

104. Liley AW: Liquor amnii analysis in the management of pregnancy complicated by rhesus sensitization. Am J Obstet Gynecol 82:1359, 1961

105. Liley AW: Errors in the assessment of hemolytic disease from amniotic fluid. Am J Obstet Gynecol 86:485, 1963

106. Queenan JT: Current management of the Rh-sensitized patient. Clin Obstet Gynecol 25:293, 1982

107. Bowman JM: Hemolytic disease (erythroblastosis fetalis). p. 711. In Creasy RK, Resnik R (eds): Maternal Fetal Medicine: Principles of Practice. 3rd Ed. WB Saunders, Philadelphia, 1994

108. Berkowitz RL, Hobbins JC: Intrauterine transfusion utilizing ultrasound. Obstet Gynecol 57:33, 1981

109. Nicolaides KH, Rodeck Ch, Mibashan RS, Kemp JR: Have Liley charts outlived their usefulness? Am J Obstet Gynecol 155:90, 1986

110. American College of Obstetricians and Gynecologists: Management of D isoimmunization in pregnancy. ACOG Technical Bulletin 148. American College of Obstetricians and Gynecologists, Washington DC, 1990

111. Spinnato JA, Ralston KK, Greenwell ER et al: Amniotic fluid bilirubin and fetal hemolytic disease. Am J Obstet Gynecol 165:1030, 1991

112. Ananth U, Queenan JT: Does midtrimester ΔOD_{450} of amniotic fluid reflect the severity of Rh disease? Am J Obstet Gynecol 161:47, 1989

113. Queenan JT, Tomai TP, Ural SH, King JC: Deviation in amniotic fluid optical density at a wavelength of 450 nm in Rh-immunized pregnancies from 14 to 40 weeks' gestation: a proposal for clinical management. Am J Obstet Gynecol 168:1370, 1993

114. Rodeck CH, Holman CA, Karnicki J et al: Direct intravascular fetal blood transfusion by fetoscopy in severe rhesus isoimmunization. Lancet 1:625, 1981

115. Rodeck CH, Nicolaides KH, Warsof SL et al: The management of severe rhesus isoimmunization by fetoscopic intravascular transfusion. Am J Obstet Gynecol 150:749, 1984

116. Nicolaides KH, Rodeck CH, Millar DS, Mibashan RS: Fetal haematology in rhesus isoimmunization. BMJ 290:661, 1985

117. Daffos F, Capella-Pavlovsky M, Forestier F: Fetal blood sampling during pregnancy with use of a needle guided by ultrasound: a study of 606 consecutive cases. Am J Obstet Gynecol 153:655, 1985

118. MacKenzie IA, Bowell PF, Castle BM et al: Serial fetal blood sampling for the management of pregnancies complicated by severe rhesus (D) isoimmunization. Br J Obstet Gynecol 95:735, 1988

119. Daffos F, Forestier F, Kaplan C, Cox W: Prenatal diagnosis and management of bleeding disorders with fetal blood sampling. Am J Obstet Gynecol 158:939, 1988

120. Ghidini A, Sepulveda W, Lockwood CJ, Romero R: Complications of fetal blood sampling. Am J Obstet Gynecol 168:1339, 1993

121. Pielet BW, Socol ML, MacGregor SN et al: Cordocentesis: an appraisal of risks. Am J Obstet Gynecol 159:1497, 1988

122. Wilkins I, Mezrow G, Lynch L et al: Amnionitis and life-threatening respiratory distress after percutaneous umbilical blood sampling. Am J Obstet Gynecol 160:427, 1989

123. Feinkind L, Nanda D, Delke I, Minkoff H: Abruptio placentae after percutaneous umbilical cord sampling: a case report. Am J Obstet Gynecol 162:1203, 1990

124. Bowell PJ, Selinger M, Ferguson J et al: Antenatal fetal blood sampling for the management of alloimmunized pregnancies: effect upon maternal anti-D potency levels. Br J Obstet Gynaecol 95:759, 1988

125. MacGregor SN, Silver RK, Sholl JS: Enhanced sensitization after cordocentesis in a rhesus-isoimmunized pregnancy. Am J Obstet Gynecol 165:382, 1991

126. Bowman JM, Pollock LM, Peterson LE et al: Fetomaternal hemorrhage following funipuncture: increase in severity of maternal red-cell alloimmunization. Obstet Gynecol 84:839, 1994

127. Frigoletto FD, Greene MF, Benacerraf BR et al: Ultrasonographic fetal surveillance in the management of the immunized pregnancy. N Engl J Med 315:430, 1986

128. Benacerraf BR, Frigoletto FD: Sonographic sign for the detection of early fetal ascites in the management of severe isoimmune disease without intrauterine transfusion. Am J Obstet Gynecol 152:1039, 1985

129. DeVore GR, Mayden K, Tortora M et al: Dilatation of

the umbilical vein in rhesus hemolytic anemia: a predictor of severe disease. Am J Obstet Gynecol 141:464, 1981

130. Witter FR, Graham D: The utility of ultrasonically measured umbilical vein diameters in isoimmunized pregnancies. Am J Obstet Gynecol 146:225, 1983

131. Chitkara U, Wilkins I, Lynch L et al: The role of sonography in assessing severity of fetal anemia in Rh and Kell-isoimmunized pregnancies. Obstet Gynecol 71: 393, 1988

132. Nicolaides KH, Fontanarosa M, Gabbe SG, Rodeck CH: Failure of ultrasonographic parameters to predict the severity of fetal anemia in rhesus isoimmunization. Am J Obstet Gynecol 158:920, 1988

133. Vintzileos AM, Campbell WA, Storlazzi E et al: Fetal liver ultrasound measurements in isoimmunized pregnancies. Obstet Gynecol 68:162, 1986

134. Roberts AB, Mitchell JM, Pattison NS: Fetal liver length in normal and isoimmunized pregnancies. Am J Obstet Gynecol 161:42, 1989

135. Kirkinen P, Jouppila P: Umbilical vein blood flow in rhesus isoimmunization. Br J Obstet Gynecol 90:640, 1983

136. Rightmire DA, Nicolaides KH, Rodeck CH, Campbell S: Fetal blood velocities in Rh isoimmunization: relationship to gestational age and to fetal hematocrit. Obstet Gynecol 68:233, 1986

137. Nicolaides KH, Bilardo CM, Campbell S: Prediction of fetal anemia by measurement of the mean blood velocity in the fetal aorta. Am J Obstet Gynecol 162:209, 1990

138. Copel JA, Grannum PA, Belanger K et al: Pulsed Doppler flow-velocity waveforms before and after intrauterine intravascular transfusion for severe erythroblastosis fetalis. Am J Obstet Gynecol 158:768, 1988

139. Copel JA, Grannum PA, Green JJ et al: Pulsed Doppler flow-velocity waveforms in the prediction of fetal hematocrit of the severely isoimmunized pregnancy. Am J Obstet Gynecol 161:341, 1989

140. Copel JA, Grannum PA, Green JJ et al: Fetal cardiac output in the isoimmunized pregnancy: a pulsed Doppler-echocardiographic study of patients undergoing intravascular intrauterine transfusion. Am J Obstet Gynecol 161:361, 1989

141. Oepkes D, Vandenbussche FP, Van Bel F, Kanhai HHH: Fetal ductus venosus blood flow velocities before and after transfusion in red-cell alloimmunized pregnancies. Obstet Gynecol 82:237, 1993

142. Legarth J, Lingman G, Stangenberg M, Rahman F: Umbilical artery Doppler flow-velocity waveforms in rhesus-isoimmunized fetuses before and after fetal blood sampling or transfusion. J Clin Ultrasound 22:43, 1994

143. Mari G, Adrignolo A, Abuhamad A et al: Doppler ultrasound in the management of the pregnancy complicated by fetal anemia, abstracted. Am J Obstet Gynecol 168:318, 1993

144. Legarth J, Lingman G, Stangenberg M, Rahman F: Lack of relation between fetal blood gases and fetal blood flow velocity waveform indices found in rhesus isoimmunised pregnancies. Br J Obstet Gynaecol 99: 813, 1992

145. Legarth J, Lingman G, Stangenberg M, Rahman F: Umbilical artery Doppler flow-velocity waveforms and fetal acid-base balance in rhesus-isoimmunized pregnancies. J Clin Ultrasound 22:37, 1994

146. Bowman JM, Manning FA: Intrauterine fetal transfusions: Winnipeg, 1982. Obstet Gynecol 61:201, 1983

147. Scott JR, Kochenour NK, Larkin RM et al: Changes in the management of severely Rh-immunized patients. Am J Obstet Gynecol 149:336, 1984

148. Watts DH, Luthy DA, Benedetti TJ et al: Intraperitoneal fetal transfusion under direct ultrasound guidance. Obstet Gynecol 71:84, 1988

149. Liley AW: Intrauterine transfusion of foetus in haemolytic disease. BMJ 2:1107, 1963

150. Bang J, Bock J, Trolle D: Ultrasound guided fetal intravenous transfusion for severe rhesus haemolytic disease. BMJ 284:373, 1982

151. Berkowitz RL, Chitkara U, Goldberg JD et al: Intrauterine intravascular transfusions for severe red blood cell isoimmunization: ultrasound-guided percutaneous approach. Am J Obstet Gynecol 155:574, 1986

152. Seeds JW, Bowes WA: Ultrasound-guided fetal intravascular transfusion in severe rhesus isoimmunization. Am J Obstet Gynecol 154:1105, 1986

153. Grannum PA, Copel JA, Plaxe SC et al: In utero exchange transfusion by direct intravascular injection in severe erythroblastosis fetalis. N Engl J Med 314:1431, 1986

154. Nicolaides KH, Soothill PW, Rodeck CH et al: Rh disease: intravascular blood transfusion by cordocentesis. Fetal Ther 1:185, 1986

155. Berkowitz RL, Chitkara U, Wilkins IA et al: Intravascular monitoring and management of erythroblastosis fetalis. Am J Obstet Gynecol 158:83, 1988

156. Poissonnier H-M, Brossard Y, Demedeiros N et al: Two hundred intrauterine exchange transfusions in severe blood incompatibilities. Am J Obstet Gynecol 161:709, 1989

157. Harman CR, Bowman JM, Manning FA, Menticoglou SM: Intrauterine transfusion—intraperitoneal versus intravascular approach: a case–control comparison. Am J Obstet Gynecol 162:1053, 1990

158. Weiner CP, Williamson RA, Wenstrom KD et al: Management of fetal hemolytic disease by cordocentesis. II. Outcome of treatment. Am J Obstet Gynecol 165:1302, 1991

159. Bowman JM: The management of Rh isoimmunization. Obstet Gynecol 52:1, 1978

160. Clewell WH, Dunne MG, Johnson ML, Bowes WA: Fetal transfusion with real-time ultrasound guidance. Obstet Gynecol 57:516, 1981

161. Copel JA, Grannum PA, Harrison D, Hobbins J: The use of intravenous pancuronium bromide to produce fetal paralysis during intravascular transfusion. Am J Obstet Gynecol 158:170, 1988

162. Moise KJ, Deter R, Kirshon B et al: Intravenous pancuronium bromide for fetal neuromuscular blockade during intrauterine transfusion for red-cell alloimmunization. Obstet Gynecol 74:905, 1989

163. Nicolaides KH, Clewell WH, Mibashan RS et al: Fetal

haemoglobin measurement in the assessment of red cell isoimmunization. Lancet 1:1073, 1988

164. Christmas JT, Little BB, Johnston WL et al: Nomograms for rapid estimation of intravascular intrauterine exchange transfusion. Obstet Gynecol 75:887, 1990

165. MacGregor SN, Socol ML, Pielet BW et al: Prediction of hematocrit decline after intravascular fetal transfusion. Am J Obstet Gynecol 161:1491, 1989

166. Rodeck CH, Letsky E: How the management of erythroblastosis fetalis has changed. Br J Obstet Gynaecol 96:759, 1989

167. Pielet BW, Socol ML, MacGregor SN et al: Cordocentesis: an appraisal of risks. Am J Obstet Gynecol 159:1497, 1988

168. Pattison N, Roberts A: The management of severe erythroblastosis fetalis by fetal transfusion: survival of transfused adult erythrocytes in the fetus. Obstet Gynecol 74:901, 1989

169. Nicolini U, Kochenour NK, Greco P et al: When to perform the next intrauterine transfusion in patients with Rh allo-immunization: combined intravascular and intraperitoneal transfusion allows longer intervals. Fetal Ther 4:14, 1990

170. Lenke RR, Persutte WH, Nemes JM: Combined intravascular and intraperitoneal transfusions for erythroblastosis fetalis. A report of two cases. J Reprod Med 35:425, 1990

171. Gusdon JP, Moore V, Myrvik QN et al: Promethazine HCl as an immunosuppressant. J Immunol 108:1340, 1972

172. Gusdon JP: The treatment of erythroblastosis with promethazine hydrochloride. J Reprod Med 26:454, 1981

173. Bierme SJ, Blanc M, Abbal M, Fournie A: Oral Rh treatment for severely immunized mothers. Lancet 1:604, 1979

174. Bierme SJ, Blanc M, Fournie A et al: Desensitization by oral antigen. p. 249. In Frigoletto FD, Jewett JF, Konugres AA (eds): Rh Hemolytic Disease: New Strategy for Eradication. GK Hall, Boston, 1982

175. Bowman JM, Peddle LJ, Anderson C: Plasmapheresis in severe Rh isoimmunization. Vox Sang 15:272, 1968

176. Clarke CA, Bradley J, Elson CJ et al: Intensive plasmapheresis as a therapeutic measure in rhesus-immunized women. Lancet 1:793, 1970

177. Powell LC: Intense plasmapheresis in the pregnant Rh-sensitized woman. Am J Obstet Gynecol 101:153, 1968

178. Fraser ID, Bennett MO, Bothamley JE et al: Intensive antenatal plasmapheresis in severe rhesus isoimmunization. Lancet 1:6, 1976

179. Graham-Pole J, Barr W, Willoughby MLN: Continuous-flow plasmapheresis in management of severe rhesus disease. BMJ 1:1185, 1974

180. Rubinstein P: Repeated small volume plasmapheresis in the management of hemolytic disease of the newborn. p. 211. In Frigoletto FD, Jewett JF, Konugres AA (eds): Rh Hemolytic Disease: New Strategy for Eradication. GK Hall, Boston, 1982

181. Odendaal HJ, Tribe R, Kriel CJ et al: Successful treatment of severe Rh isoimmunization with immunosuppression and plasmapheresis. Vox Sang 60:169, 1991

182. Berlin G, Selbing A, Ryden G: Rhesus haemolytic disease treated with high-dose intravenous immunoglobulin. Lancet 1:1153, 1985

183. de la Camara C, Arrieta R, Gonzalez A et al: High-dose intravenous immunoglobulin as the sole prenatal treatment for severe Rh immunization. N Engl J Med 318:519, 1988

184. Scott JR, Branch DW, Kochenour NK, Ward K: Intravenous immunoglobulin treatment of pregnant patients with recurrent pregnancy loss caused by antiphospholipid antibodies and Rh immunization. Am J Obstet Gynecol 159:1055, 1988

185. Sidiropoulos D, Herrmann U, Morell A et al: Transplacental passage of intravenous immunoglobulin in the last trimester of pregnancy. J Pediatr 109:505, 1986

186. Boggs TR: Survival rates in Rh sensitizations. Pediatrics 33:758, 1964

187. Quinlan RW, Buhi WC, Cruz A: Fetal pulmonary maturity in isoimmunized pregnancies. Am J Obstet Gynecol 148:787, 1984

188. Horenstein J, Golde S, Platt LD: Lung profiles in the isoimmunized pregnancy. Am J Obstet Gynecol 153:443, 1985

189. Queenan JT, Smith BD, Haber JM et al: Irregular antibodies in the obstetric patient. Obstet Gynecol 34:767, 1969

190. Polesky HF: Blood group antibodies in prenatal sera. Minn Med 50:601, 1967

191. Giblett ER: Blood group antibodies causing hemolytic disease of the newborn. Obstet Gynecol 7:1044, 1964

192. Weinstein L: Irregular antibodies causing hemolytic disease of the newborn: a continuing problem. Clin Obstet Gynecol 25:321, 1982

193. Berkowitz RL, Beyta Y, Sadovsky E: Death in utero due to Kell sensitization without excessive elevation of the ΔOD_{450} value in amniotic fluid. Obstet Gynecol 60:746, 1982

194. Caine ME, Mueller-Heubach E: Kell sensitization in pregnancy. Am J Obstet Gynecol 154:85, 1986

195. Copel JA, Scioscia A, Grannum PA et al: Percutaneous umbilical blood sampling in the management of Kell isoimmunization. Am J Obstet Gynecol 67:288, 1986

196. Leggat JM, Gibson JM, Barron SL, Reid MM: Anti-Kell in pregnancy. Br J Obstet Gynaecol 98:162, 1991

197. Goh JTW, Kretowicz EM, Weinstein S, Ramsden GH: Anti-Kell in pregnancy and hydrops fetalis. Aust NZ J Obstet Gynaecol 33:210, 1993

198. Marsh WL, Redman CM: The Kell blood group system: a review. Transfusion 30:158, 1990

199. Vaughan JI, Warwick R, Letsky E et al: Erythropoietic suppression in fetal anemia because of Kell alloimmunization. Am J Obstet Gynecol 171:247, 1994

200. Bowman JM, Pollock JT, Manning FA et al: Maternal Kell blood group alloimmunization. Obstet Gynecol 79:239, 1992

201. Constantine G, Fitzgibbon N, Weaver JB: Anti-Kell in pregnancy. Br J Obstet Gynecol 98:943, 1991

202. Murphy MT, Morrison N, Miles JS et al: Regional chromosomal assignment of the Kell blood group locus (KEL) to chromosome 7q33–q35 by fluorescence in situ hybridization: evidence for the polypeptide nature of antigenic variation. Hum Genet 91:585, 1993

203. Lee S, Zambas ED, Marsh WL, Redman CM: The human Kell blood group gene maps to chromosome 7q33 and its expression is restricted to erythroid cells. Blood 81:2804, 1993

204. Cook LN: ABO hemolytic disease. Clin Obstet Gynecol 25:333, 1982

205. Zlatnick FJ: Non-Rh₀(D) hemolytic disease of the newborn: an obstetric viewpoint. Semin Perinatol 1:169, 1977

206. Resnikoff-Etievant MF: Management of alloimmune neonatal and antenatal thrombocytopenia. Vox Sang 55:193, 1988

207. von dem Borne AEGKr, Decary F: Nomenclature of platelet-specific antigens. Transfusion 30:477, 1990

208. Shulman NR, Reid DM: Platelet immunology. p. 414. In Colman RW, Hirsh J, Marder VJ, Salzman EW (eds): Hemostasis and Thrombosis: Basic Principles and Clinical Practice. 3rd Ed. JB Lippincott, Philadelphia, 1994

209. von dem Borne AEGKr, Simsek S, van der Schoot CE, Goldschmeding R: Platelet and neutrophil alloantigens: their nature and role in immune-mediated cytopenias. p. 149. In Garrity G (ed): Immunobiology of Transfusion Medicine. Marcel Dekker, New York, 1994

210. Sternbach MS, Malette M, Nadon F, Guevin RM: Severe alloimmune neonatal thrombocytopenia due to specific HLA antibodies. Curr Stud Hematol Blood Transf 52:97, 1986

211. Mueller-Eckhardt C: Platelet allo- and autoantigens and their clinical implications. p. 63. In Nance SJ (ed): Transfusion Medicine in the 1990's. American Association of Blood Banks, Arlington, VA, 1990

212. Mueller-Eckhardt C, Grubert A, Weisheit M et al: 384 cases of suspected neonatal alloimmune thrombocytopenia. Lancet 1:363, 1989

213. Burrows RF, Kelton JG: Incidentally detected thrombocytopenia in healthy mothers and their infants. N Engl J Med 319:142, 1988

214. Blanchette VS, Chen L, Salomon de Friedberg Z et al: Alloimmunization to the PL^A1 antigen: results of a prospective study. Br J Haematol 74:209, 1990

215. Herman JH, Jumbelic MI, Ancona RJ, Kickler TS: In utero cerebral hemorrhage in alloimmune thrombocytopenia. Am J Pediatr Hematol Oncol 8:312, 1986

216. Daffos F, Forestier F, Kaplan C, Cox W: Prenatal diagnosis and management of bleeding disorders with fetal blood sampling. Am J Obstet Gynecol 158:939, 1988

217. Bussel JB, Berkowitz RL, McFarland JH et al: Antenatal treatment of neonatal alloimmune thrombocytopenia. N Engl J Med 319:1374, 1988

218. Pearson HA, Shulman NR, Marder VJ, Cone TE: Isoimmune neonatal thrombocytopenic purpura: clinical and therapeutic considerations. Blood 23:154, 1964

219. Mennuti M, Schwarz RH, Gill F: Obstetric management of isoimmune thrombocytopenia. Am J Obstet Gynecol 118:565, 1974

220. Sitarz AL, Driscoll Jr JM, Wolff JA: Management of isoimmune neonatal thrombocytopenia. Am J Obstet Gynecol 124:39, 1976

221. Daffos F, Forestier F, Muller JY et al: Prenatal treatment of alloimmune thrombocytopenia. Lancet 2:632, 1984

222. Kaplan C, Daffos F, Forestier F et al: Management of alloimmune thrombocytopenia: antenatal diagnosis and in utero transfusion of maternal platelets. Blood 72:340, 1988

223. Nicolini U, Rodeck CH, Kochenour NK et al: In-utero platelet transfusions for alloimmune thrombocytopenia. Lancet 2:506, 1988

224. Murphy MF, Pullon HWH, Metclfe P et al: Management of fetal alloimmune thrombocytopenia by weekly in utero platelet transfusions. Vox Sang 58:45, 1990

225. Paidas JM, Berkowitz RL, Lynch L et al: Alloimmune thrombocytopenia: fetal and neonatal losses related to cordocentesis. Am J Obstet Gynecol 172:475, 1995

226. Mueller-Eckhardt C, Kiefel V, Jovanovic V et al: Prenatal treatment of fetal alloimmune thrombocytopenia. Lancet 2:910, 1988

227. Management of alloimmune neonatal thrombocytopenia. Editorial. Lancet 1:137, 1989

228. Bussel JB, Berkowitz RL, McFarland JG et al: Antenatal treatment of neonatal alloimmune thrombocytopenia. N Engl J Med 319:1374, 1988

229. Lynch L, Bussel JB, McFarland JG et al: Antenatal treatment of alloimmune thrombocytopenia. Obstet Gynecol 80:67, 1992

230. Derycke M, Drysus M, Ropert JC, Tchernia G: Intravenous immunoglobulin for neonatal isoimmune thrombocytopenia. Arch Dis Child 60:667, 1985

231. Sidiropoulos D, Straume B: Treatment of neonatal isoimmune thrombocytopenia with intravenous immunoglobulin. Blut 48:383, 1984

232. Massey GV, McWilliams NB, Mueller DG et al: Intravenous immunoglobulin in treatment of neonatal isoimmune thrombocytopenia. Pediatrics 111:133, 1987

233. Marzusch K, Wiest E, Pfeiffer K-H et al: Antenatal fetal therapy for neonatal allo-immune thrombocytopenia with high dose immunoglobulin. Br J Obstet Gynaecol 101:1011, 1994

234. Water AH, Ireland R, Mibashan RS et al: Fetal platelet transfusions in the management of alloimmune thrombocytopenia. Thromb Haemost 58:323, 1987

235. Mir N, Samson D, House MJ, Kovar IZ: Failure of antenatal high-dose immunoglobulin to improve fetal platelet count in neonatal alloimmune thrombocytopenia. Vox Sang 55:188, 1988

236. Nicolini U, Tannirandorn Y, Gonzalez P et al: Continuing controversy in alloimmune thrombocytopenia: fetal hyperimmunoglobulinemia fails to prevent thrombocytopenia. Am J Obstet Gynecol 163:1144, 1990

237. Morbidity and Mortality Weekly Report: Outbreak of hepatitis C associated with intravenous immunoglobulin administration—United States, October 1993–June 1994. MMWR 43:505, 1994

238. Skogen B, Bellissimo DB, Hessner MJ et al: Rapid determination of platelet alloantigen genotypes by polymerase chain reaction using allele-specific primers. Transfusion 34:955, 1994

239. Bray PF, Jin Y, Kickler T. Rapid genotyping of the five major platelet alloantigens by reverse dot-blot hybridization. Blood 84:4361, 1994

Pregnancy and Coexisting Disease

Chapter 28

Hypertension in Pregnancy

Baha M. Sibai

Hypertensive disorders are the most common medical complications of pregnancy, with a reported incidence ranging between 5 and 10 percent.[1] The incidence varies among different hospitals, regions, and countries. In addition, these disorders are a major cause of maternal and perinatal mortality and morbidity worldwide.[2] The term *hypertension in pregnancy* is usually used to describe a wide spectrum of patients who may have only mild elevations in blood pressure or severe hypertension with various organ dysfunctions. The manifestations in these patients may be clinically similar (e.g., hypertension, proteinuria); however, they may result from different underlying causes such as chronic hypertension, renal disease, or pure preeclampsia. The three most common forms of hypertension are acute pregnancy-induced hypertension, preeclampsia, and chronic essential hypertension.

The terminology used to classify the hypertensive disorders of pregnancy has been confusing and inconsistent, making comparison of studies difficult and often impossible. For many years, the hypertensive disorders of gestation were labeled *toxemia of pregnancy*. This term was used because it was felt that this wide variety of disorders had as a common etiologic agent a circulating toxin. We now know this to be untrue.

Definitions

The Committee on Terminology of the American College of Obstetricians and Gynecologists has classified the hypertensive disorders of pregnancy as follows.[3]

Preeclampsia and Eclampsia

The so-called classic triad of preeclampsia includes hypertension, proteinuria, and edema. The diagnosis of preeclampsia is based on blood pressure criteria, as well as proteinuria or edema or both. Blood pressure must increase by at least 30 mmHg systolic or 15 mmHg diastolic. Readings of 140/90 mmHg after 20 weeks' gestation, if prior blood pressure is unknown, are considered sufficiently elevated for the diagnosis of preeclampsia. The elevation must be present on two measurements taken 6 hours apart. The Committee defines either an increase in mean arterial pressure of 20 mmHg or, if the prior blood pressure is unknown, a mean arterial pressure of 105 mmHg as indications of hypertension. Mean arterial pressure is one-third the pulse pressure plus the diastolic pressure. Edema is diagnosed as clinically evident generalized swelling. However, fluid retention can also be manifest as a rapid increase in weight without evidence of edema. Proteinuria is defined as a concentration of 0.1 g/L or more in at least two random urine specimens collected 6 hours or more apart or 0.3 g in a 24-hour collection. In mild preeclampsia, the diastolic blood pressure remains below 110 mmHg. The criteria for severe preeclampsia are given in the box below.[4] Eclampsia is the occurrence of seizures not attributable to other causes.

Chronic Hypertension

Chronic hypertension is defined as hypertension present before the pregnancy or that diagnosed before the 20th week of gestation. The Committee defines hypertension as a blood pressure greater than 140/90 mmHg. Hypertension that persists for more than 42 days postpartum is also classified as chronic hypertension.

Chronic Hypertension with Superimposed Preeclampsia

Women with chronic hypertension may also show the development of superimposed preeclampsia. The Committee recommends that the diagnosis be made on

Criteria for Severe Preeclampsia

1. Blood pressure of ≥160 mmHg systolic or ≥110 mmHg diastolic, recorded on at least two occasions at least 6 hours apart with patient at bedrest
2. Proteinuria of ≥5 g in 24 hours (3+ or 4+ on qualitative examination)
3. Oliguria (≤400 ml in 24 hours)
4. Cerebral or visual disturbances
5. Epigastric pain
6. Pulmonary edema or cyanosis
7. Impaired liver function of unclear etiology
8. Thrombocytopenia

(From ACOG,[4] with permission.)

the basis of an elevation of blood pressure (30 mmHg systolic or 15 mmHg diastolic or 20 mmHg mean arterial pressure) together with the appearance of proteinuria or generalized edema.

Transient Hypertension

Transient hypertension is the development of an elevated blood pressure during pregnancy or in the first 24 hours postpartum without other signs of preeclampsia or preexisting hypertension. The blood pressure must return to normal within 10 days after delivery.

Despite these diagnostic criteria, problems remain in classifying the hypertensive disorders of pregnancy.[5] Generalized edema is common in normal pregnancy, although it does not occur as frequently and is not as marked as when associated with preeclampsia. Dexter and Weiss[6] reported edema of the hands, face, or both in 64 of 100 consecutive women examined during the third trimester of normotensive uncomplicated pregnancies. In addition, one-third of eclamptic women never demonstrate the presence of edema.[7] The Nelson[8] classification, widely used in the British Commonwealth, does not include edema as a diagnostic criterion in the classification of preeclampsia. Furthermore, the World Health Organization[9] (Technical Report Series No. 758) and the International Society for the Study of Hypertension in Pregnancy (ISSHP)[10] do not include edema as a diagnostic criterion for preeclampsia. The American College of Obstetricians and Gynecologists (ACOG) did not insist on proteinuria as a diagnostic sign because it usually appears late. For example, proteinuria is reportedly absent in almost 20 percent of eclamptic women.[7] In addition, the renal lesion characteristic of preeclampsia is almost never seen in the absence of proteinuria.[11] Because of its simplicity, the

ACOG classification was recently endorsed and adopted by the National High Blood Pressure Education Working Group.[2] It is interesting to note that some members of the above group were also members of the study committees that wrote the World Health Organization Report and the ISSHP classification.[9,10]

Preeclampsia

Preeclampsia is a form of hypertension that is unique to human pregnancy. Very rarely has it been reported in subhuman primates.[12] The incidence ranges between 10 and 14 percent in primigravidas and between 5.7 and 7.3 percent in multiparas.[13,14] The incidence is significantly increased in patients with twin pregnancies[15] and in those with previous preeclampsia.[16] For patients with a twin pregnancy, both the incidence and severity are significantly higher than in singleton pregnancies.[15]

The etiology of preeclampsia is unknown. Many theories have been suggested, but most of them did not withstand the test of time. Some of the theories that are still under consideration are listed below. In addition, there is an association between preeclampsia and trisomy 13, suggesting a fetal factor in the pathogenesis of preeclampsia.[17,18]

Pathophysiology

During normal pregnancy impressive physiologic changes occur in the uteroplacental vasculature in general and in the cardiovascular system in particular. These changes are most likely induced by the interaction of the fetal (parental) allograft with maternal tissue. The development of mutual immunologic tolerance in the first trimester is thought to lead to important morphologic and biochemical changes in the systemic and uteroplacental maternal circulation.

Theories Associated with the Etiology of Preeclampsia

Abnormal trophoblast invasion

Coagulation abnormalities

Vascular endothelial damage

Cardiovascular maladaptation

Immunologic phenomena

Genetic predisposition

Dietary deficiencies or excesses

Uterine Vascular Changes

The human placenta receives its blood supply from numerous uteroplacental arteries that are developed by the action of migratory interstitial and endovascular trophoblast into the walls of the spiral arterioles. This transforms the uteroplacental arterial bed into a low resistance, low pressure, high flow system. The conversion of the spiral arterioles of the nonpregnant uterus into the uteroplacental arteries has been termed *physiologic changes* by Brosens.[19] In a normal pregnancy, these trophoblast-induced vascular changes extend all the way from the intervillous space to the origin of the spiral arterioles from the radial arteries in the inner one-third of the myometrium. It is suggested that these vascular changes are effected in two stages: "the conversion of the decidual segments of the spiral arterioles by a wave of endovascular trophoblast migration in the first trimester and the myometrial segments by a subsequent wave in the second trimester."[19] This process was reportedly associated with extensive fibrinoid formation and degeneration of the muscular layer in the arterial wall. These vascular changes result in the conversion of approximately 100 to 150 spiral arterioles into distended, tortuous, and funnel-shaped vessels that communicate through multiple openings into the intervillous space.

In contrast, pregnancies complicated by preeclampsia and/or by fetal growth retardation demonstrate inadequate maternal vascular response to placentation. In these pregnancies, the above vascular changes are usually restricted only to the decidual segments of the uteroplacental arteries. Hence, the myometrial segments of the spiral arterioles are left with their musculoelastic architecture, thereby rendering them responsive to hormonal influences.[20] Additionally, the number of well-developed arterioles is smaller than that found in normotensive pregnancies. The authors postulated that this defective vascular response to placentation is due to inhibition of the second wave of endovascular trophoblast migration that normally occurs from about 16 weeks' gestation onward. These pathologic changes may have the effect of curtailing the increased blood supply required by the fetoplacental unit in the later stages of pregnancy, and they may be responsible for the decreased uteroplacental blood flow seen in most cases of preeclampsia. These conclusions were recently supported by Frusca and associates.[21] These authors studied placental bed biopsies obtained during cesarean delivery from normal pregnancies ($N = 14$), preeclamptic pregnancies ($N = 24$), and chronic hypertensive pregnancies only ($N = 5$). Biopsies from the preeclamptic group demonstrated abnormal vascular changes in all of them, with 18 having acute atherosclerotic changes. On the other hand, 13 of the 14 biopsies from normotensive pregnancies had normal vascular physiologic changes, while the biopsies from the hypertensive patients showed all three types of physiologic changes. In addition, they found that the mean birth weight was significantly lower in the group with atherosclerosis than it was in the other group without such findings. However, it is important to note that these vascular changes are not a consistent finding in spiral arterioles of hypertensive pregnancies and were demonstrated in a significant proportion of normotensive pregnancies complicated by fetal growth retardation.[20,22] Furthermore, a recent investigation by Meekins and associates[23] found that endovascular trophoblast invasion was not an all-or-none phenomenon in normal and preeclamptic pregnancies. They also observed that morphological features in one spiral artery may not be representative of all vessels in a placental bed.

Using electron microscopy, Shanklin and Sibai[24] studied the ultrastructural changes in placental bed and uterine boundary vessels in 33 preeclamptic and 12 normotensive pregnancies. They found extensive ultrastructural endothelial injury in both placental site and nonplacental site in all the specimens from preeclamptic women, but not in the normotensive women. The injury appeared to affect the endothelial mitochondria, which suggests a possible metabolic link in the pathophysiology. The endothelial injury ranged from swelling to complete erosion and the swelling was associated with enlargement of endothelial nuclei resulting in reduction of the lumen. In some cases, the erosion was complete with associated deposition of heavy fibrin (Fig. 28-1). In addition, there was no correlation between the type or degree of endothelial damage and the level of maternal hypertension.

Hemostatic Changes

Preeclampsia is associated with vasospasm, activation of the coagulation system, and abnormal hemostasis. There is good evidence from several studies that preeclampsia is accompanied by endothelial injury, increased platelet activation with platelet consumption in the microvasculature, and excessive clotting activity.[25,26] Saleh et al.[25] evaluated the hemostatic system before and 24 to 48 hours after delivery in 26 control pregnancies, 15 with mild preeclampsia and 18 with severe preeclampsia. They found that preeclampsia was associated with high fibronectin, low antithrombin III, and low α_2-antiplasmin levels. They suggested that these findings reflected endothelial injury (high fibronectin), clotting (low antithrombin III), and fibrinolysis (low α_2-antiplasmin). In addition, they found that, after delivery, fibronectin levels decreased in the preeclamptic group while α_2-antiplasmin levels increased in all

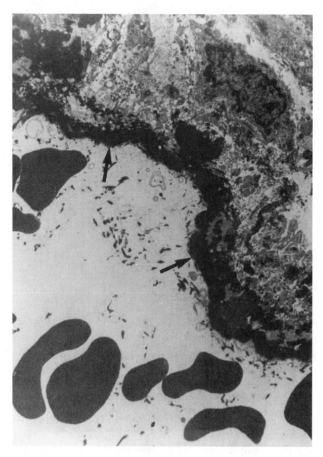

Fig. 28-1 Compacted heavy fibrin deposition (arrows) and loose luminal fibrin replacing extensively eroded endothelium, nonplacental site region, uterine boundary zone, preeclampsia. (Original electron microscopic magnification × 2,500). (From Shanklin and Sibai,[24] with permission.)

groups. They concluded that "vascular endothelial injury plays a central role in the hemostatic changes associated with preeclampsia." In a subsequent report,[26] the authors evaluated hemostasis in various hypertensive disorders of pregnancies. They found elevated fibronectin, low antithrombin III, and reduced α_2-antiplasmin in patients with pure preeclampsia as well as chronic hypertension with superimposed preeclampsia. In addition, they observed that fibronectin levels had better correlation with preeclampsia than either antithrombin III or α_2-antiplasmin. They suggested that fibronectin might be useful for diagnosing superimposed preeclampsia in women with chronic hypertension. In recent reports, elevated fibronectin values were identified in some patients prior to the development of preeclampsia.[27,28] Lockwood and Peters[27] reported that increased plasma levels of ED$^+$ (extra type III domain) cellular fibronectin, almost exclusively localized to endothelium, may precede the clinical signs of preeclampsia. They reported that ED$^+$ fibronectin levels were significantly higher in the preeclamptic

group during the first and second trimesters before clinical evidence of preeclampsia. Taylor and colleagues[28] measured cellular fibronectin levels in plasma of women who ultimately had preeclampsia, hypertension only, or normotensive pregnancies. They found elevated cellular fibronectin levels during the second and third trimesters only in women destined to develop preeclampsia.[28]

Some authors suggested that endothelial cell injury plays a central role in the pathophysiology of preeclampsia.[29–31] Rodgers et al.[29] reported that serum from preeclamptic women is cytotoxic to endothelial cells in vitro. In addition, they found that the cytotoxic activity in serum of preeclamptic women was reduced after 24 to 48 hours following delivery. In a subsequent report,[30] the authors noted that mitogenic activity was significantly increased in the sera of preeclamptic women before delivery compared with normotensive pregnant controls. In addition, the mitogenic activity diminished rapidly postpartum. They suggested that vasospasm in preeclampsia may result from potent vasoconstrictors released at sites of endothelial cell injury. More recently,[31] the same group proposed that "poorly perfused placental tissue releases a factor(s) into the systemic circulation that injures endothelial cells."

Antithrombin III is a plasma proteinase inhibitor and is a major plasma inhibitor of thrombin. Weiner and Brandt[32] reported that the level of plasma antithrombin III activity remains unaltered during normal pregnancy, while it was reduced in patients with preeclampsia. In a subsequent report, Weiner et al.[33] evaluated the use of antithrombin III measurement as a diagnostic test for preeclampsia in pregnancies complicated by hypertension. Women with chronic hypertension only had normal values, while those with either preeclampsia or superimposed preeclampsia had significantly lower levels than the normotensive group. There are currently about 20 reports dealing with this subject in preeclampsia; however, the findings have been inconsistent. In general, the evidence supports reduced antithrombin III activity in preeclampsia that reflects consumption secondary to enhanced clotting.

β-Thromboglobulin and platelet factor 4 are platelet-specific proteins. Their presence in the plasma indicates platelet aggregation and degranulation secondary to platelet activation and aggregation in vivo. Higher levels of plasma β-thromboglobulin have been reported in patients with preeclampsia than in normotensive pregnancies. Socol et al.[34] measured plasma β-thromboglobulin and platelet factor 4 in 11 patients with preeclampsia, 11 with superimposed preeclampsia, and 10 normotensive controls. They found higher plasma levels of β-thromboglobulin, but normal platelet factor 4 in the preeclamptic groups.

Thrombin is an enzyme that converts fibrinogen to

fibrin. It is inactivated by antithrombin III, resulting in generation of thrombin-antithrombin III complexes. An increased level of this complex suggests enhancement of thrombin generation. deBoer et al.[35] investigated plasma levels of the coagulation inhibitors antithrombin III, protein C, protein S, and thrombin-antithrombin III complexes. They observed reduced protein C levels, but normal protein S levels, in preeclampsia compared with normotensive pregnancies. In addition, they observed an increased thrombin-antithrombin III complex level in the preeclamptic group. The level of these complexes correlated with platelet count and antithrombin III levels. Thus, they suggested that enhanced thrombin generation in preeclampsia may result from increased platelet activation and consumption. Gilabert et al.[36] evaluated protein C, protein S, and antithrombin III in normal pregnancy and severe preeclamptic states. They found reduced protein C and antithrombin III levels, but normal protein S in severe preeclampsia.

Changes In Prostanoids

Several studies described the various prostaglandins and their metabolites throughout pregnancy. They have measured the concentrations of these substances in plasma, serum, amniotic fluid, placental tissues, urine, or cord blood. The data have been conflicting and inconsistent, which reflects differences in methodology. This subject was recently reviewed by Friedman.[37] In general, the data suggest that the production of both prostacyclin (PGI_2) and thromboxane A_2 (TXA_2) is increased during pregnancy, with the balance in favor of PGI_2.

Reproductive tissues produce large amounts of both prostanoids, and during pregnancy production increases in both maternal and fetoplacental tissues.[38] Prostacyclin is produced by the vascular endothelium as well as in the renal cortex. It is a potent vasodilator and inhibitor of platelet aggregation. TXA_2 is produced by the platelets and trophoblasts. It is a potent vasoconstrictor and platelet aggregator. Hence, these eicosanoids have opposite effects and play a major role in regulation of vascular tone and vascular blood flow.

Changes in prostaglandin production and/or catabolism in uteroplacental and umbilical tissues have been reportedly associated with the development of preeclampsia, although the reports have been inconsistent.[37] These discrepancies may reflect some of the inherent problems in the measurement of prostaglandins and the diagnosis of preeclampsia. Recently, an imbalance in prostanoid production or catabolism has been suggested as responsible for the pathophysiologic changes in preeclampsia.[39] However, the role of prosta-glandins in the etiology of preeclampsia remains unclear.

Goodman et al.[40] investigated PGI_2 biosynthesis during pregnancy by measuring urinary excretion of various dimer metabolites with the use of specific gas chromatography-mass spectrometry assays. They found that normal pregnant women had a fivefold higher rate of urinary excretion of these dimer metabolites than nonpregnant women. In addition, patients with pregnancy-induced hypertension (PIH) had a significant reduction (50 percent) in urinary dinor excretion compared with normotensive patients. Fitzgerald et al.[41] prospectively determined PGI_2 biosynthesis in pregnant women at risk for developing PIH by measurement of the urinary metabolite 2,3-dinor-6-keto-PGFIα. The study groups included 12 women who developed PIH, 22 women with hypertension during labor, 9 women with chronic hypertension and 24 women with hypertension during labor, 9 women with chronic hypertension, and 24 women who remained normotensive throughout gestation. They found a significant increase in prostacyclin-biosynthesis in all study groups during pregnancy. However, patients who ultimately developed PIH exhibited a lesser increment, and the difference persisted throughout gestation. In addition, they found that measurement of the urinary dinor metabolites was a better predictor of subsequent development of PIH than the more invasive angiotensin infusion test.

In contrast to the above urinary findings in preeclampsia, the data regarding maternal plasma findings of either PGI_2 or TXA_2 metabolites have been highly variable and inconsistent.[37,42] The most consistent finding was an increase in the TXA_2/PGI_2 ratio. In addition, Moodley et al.[43] found significantly lower levels of 6-keto-PGF1α in central venous blood from 21 primigravid women with diagnosed eclampsia.

There are several studies that reported abnormal prostanoid production in either fetal or placental tissues. These findings were recently reviewed by Friedman,[37] as well as by Walsh and Parisi.[42] The evidence suggests that umbilical artery production of PGI_2 is reduced and the capacity of umbilical vessels to synthesize PGI_2 and TXA_2 are impaired. In addition, there is agreement in the literature that in preeclampsia placental production of PGI_2 is reduced while that of TXA_2 is increased, leading to an increased TXA_2/PGI ratio. Walsh[39] and Walsh and Parisi[42] measured the simultaneous production rates of PGI_2 and TXA_2 in normal and preeclamptic patients. They found that the production of TXA_2 by placentas from preeclamptic patients is three times as high as that in placentas from normotensive pregnancies, while PGI_2 production was less than half. In addition, they found that the ratio of the placental production rate of TXA_2 to PGI_2 was seven times higher in preeclamptic than normotensive preg-

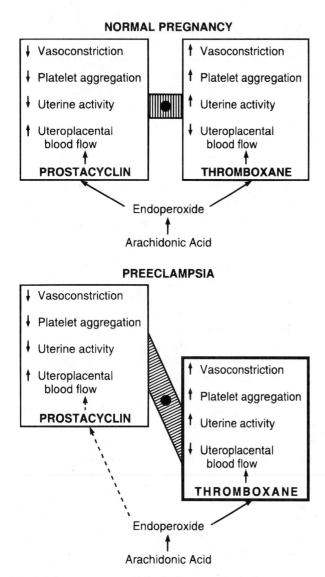

Fig. 28-2 Comparison of the balance in the biologic actions of prostacyclin and thromboxane in normal pregnancy with the imbalance of increased thromboxane and decreased prostacyclin in preeclamptic pregnancy. The heavy type and box for thromboxane suggest an exacerbation of its actions in preeclampsia, whereas the lighter type and box for prostacyclin suggest a diminution of its actions. (From Walsh,[39] with permission.)

nancy. Walsh[39] suggested that this imbalance would account for the major clinical symptoms seen in preeclampsia (Fig. 28-2).

Several investigators compared prostacyclin or TXA_2 levels in the amniotic fluid of normotensive and preeclamptic-eclamptic patients. The findings of six such studies suggest that TXA_2 values are normal while PGI_2 values are abnormal only in patients with severe disease.[44,45] The above data suggest that the pathogenesis of preeclampsia may be related to abnormal prostaglandin production and/or metabolism in the uteroplacental and umbilical vasculature. However, it should be noted that the increased TXA_2/PGI_2 ratio, observed by various investigators in different materials and fetal tissues, may be an effect rather than a cause of preeclampsia.

Changes in Endothelium-Derived Factors

Recent data indicate that endothelium-derived substances such as endothelium-derived relaxing factor (EDRF) and endothelin may play a central role in the pathophysiology of preeclampsia.[46] After its discovery, EDRF was found to be nitric oxide, an extremely potent vasodilator. In contrast, endothelin is an extremely potent vasoconstrictor. Pinto and associates[47] reported a significant reduction in EDRF release from the endothelium of human umbilical blood vessels collected from patients with pregnancy-induced hypertension. In addition, Fickling et al.[48] found higher concentrations of an endogenous inhibitor of nitric oxide synthesis in 8 third trimester patients with preeclampsia than in 9 patients with PIH and 10 women with normotensive pregnancies. Currently, there is extensive research concerning the role of EDRF in the pathogenesis of preeclampsia. There are several reports describing plasma levels of endothelin in patients with preeclampsia. While the majority of these studies report elevated levels in preeclamptic pregnancies compared with normotensive pregnancies,[49–51] a recent study did not find increased levels of endothelin in patients with preeclampsia.[52]

Lipid Peroxide, Free Radicals, and Antioxidants

Evidence is accumulating that lipid peroxides and free radicals may be important in the pathogenesis of preeclampsia.[46,53,54] Superoxide unions may be cytotoxic to the cell by changing the characteristics of cellular membrane and producing membrane lipid peroxidation. Elevated plasma concentrations of free radical oxidation products precede the development of preeclampsia.[55] Uotila et al.[56] demonstrated that lipid peroxidation was significantly higher in 56 women with hypertension in pregnancy than in control subjects. Lipid peroxidation products had a high correlation with the level of hypertension but failed to show a significant relation to perinatal outcome. In contrast, high levels of plasma and platelet glutathione peroxidase (antioxidative compounds) were found to have an association with fetal growth retardation and asphyxia. In addition, several studies reported lower serum antioxidant activity in patients with preeclampsia than in normotensive pregnancies.[57–60]

Diagnosis

Preeclampsia is a clinical syndrome that embraces a wide spectrum of signs and symptoms that have been clinically observed to develop alone or in combination.

Elevated blood pressure is the traditional hallmark for diagnosis of the disease. However, recent evidence suggests that in some patients the disease may manifest itself in the form of either a capillary leak (edema, proteinuria) or a spectrum of abnormal hemostasis with multiple organ dysfunction. These latter patients usually present with clinical manifestations that are not typical of preeclampsia (i.e., hypertension is absent).

The diagnosis of preeclampsia and the severity of the disease process are generally based on maternal blood pressure measurements as ascertained by a variety of medical personnel who regularly measure blood pressure in prenatal clinics, local physicians' offices, and in-hospital units. There are considerable factors that may influence measurement of the blood pressure by means of a sphygmomanometer. These are accuracy of the equipment used, size of cuff, duration of rest period before recording, posture of patient, and the Korotkoff phase used (phase IV or phase V) for diastolic blood pressure measurement.[10,16] Reports on effects of these factors on measurements of blood pressure have been recently summarized by Sibai.[61] In these reports, the authors recommend that all blood pressure values be recorded with the woman in a sitting position (ambulatory patient) or in a semireclining position for hospitalized patients. The right arm should be used consistently, with the arm being in a roughly horizontal position at heart level. For diastolic blood pressure measurements, both phases (muffling sound and disappearance sound) should be recorded. This is very important since the level measured at phase IV is about 5 to 10 mmHg higher than that measured at phase V.[62] Lopez et al.[62] compared Korotkoff phases IV and V in a cohort of 1,194 nulliparous pregnant women who were followed prospectively from the 20th week of pregnancy until delivery. Blood pressure measurements were obtained with random-zero sphygmomanometers and were recorded in supine, lateral, and seated positions. Lopez et al.[62] found that the prevalence of hypertension (diastolic blood pressure [BP] $\geq$90 mmHg on two occasions 6 hours apart) when phase IV was used was double the prevalence when phase V was used. However, phase IV had a better sensitivity in the prediction of complications associated with hypertension (proteinuria, hyperuricemia, and intrauterine growth retardation), but a lower specificity. In addition, the authors found that phase V was easy to obtain during pregnancy. Blank et al.[63] compared diastolic blood pressure values using Korotkoff phases IV and V in 58 pregnant women (42 hypertensive and 16 normotensive) at various stages of pregnancy. They concluded that phase V is a more accurate, reliable, and less variable measurement of diastolic blood pressure in pregnancy than muffling (phase IV). The literature in this area was recently reviewed by Johenning and Barron.[64]

The National High Blood Pressure Education Report recommend the use of phase V.[2]

A rise in blood pressure has been used by several authors as a criterion for the diagnosis of hypertension in pregnancy. This definition is usually unreliable since a gradual increase in blood pressure from second to third trimester is seen in most normotensive pregnancies. MacGillivray et al.[65] reported that 73 percent of primigravid patients with normotensive pregnancies demonstrate an increase in diastolic blood pressure of more than 15 mmHg at some stage during the course of their pregnancies. In addition, 57 percent of these patients demonstrated an increase of more than 20 mmHg during the course of pregnancy. Redman and Jeffries[66] analyzed different thresholds of raised diastolic blood pressure in 16,211 singleton pregnancies to determine the best way of diagnosing preeclampsia. They found that elevation in diastolic blood pressure of at least 25 mmHg and a maximum reading of at least 90 mmHg were the best acceptable criteria. Similar findings were recently reported by Perry and Beevers.[67]

Villar and Sibai[13] prospectively studied blood pressure changes during the course of pregnancy in 700 young primigravidas. One hundred thirty-seven patients (19.6 percent) had preeclampsia. The pregnancy outcome according to blood pressure findings is summarized in Table 28-1. The sensitivity and positive predictive values for preeclampsia of a threshold increase in diastolic blood pressure of at least 15 mmHg on two occasions were 39 and 32 percent, respectively. The respective values for a threshold increase in systolic pressures were 22 and 33 percent. In addition, the use of a threshold increase criterion is dependent on at least two observations during the course of pregnancy that will be influenced by at least three factors: gestational age at time of first observation, frequency of blood pressure measurements, and the two observations to be selected. Thus, these criteria are inadequate to diagnose preeclampsia as such. However, they may be useful if used in association with the presence of pathologic edema, proteinuria, or other associated

Table 28-1 Pregnancy Outcome According to Threshold Increase in Systolic or Diastolic Pressures on Two Occasions During the Third Trimester

Blood Pressure Criteria	Normotensive No. (%)	Preeclampsia No. (%)
Increase in diastolic $\geq$15 mmHg	113 (68)	53 (32)
Increase in systolic $\geq$30 mmHg	60 (67)	30 (33)
Threshold increase in both	32 (58)	23 (42)

(Adapted from Villar and Sibai,[13] with permission.)

Table 28-2 Value of Dipstick Protein in Predicting 24-Hour Urinary Protein Excretion

Urinary Dipstick	Protein Excretion (mg/24 hour)	Sensitivity (%)	Specificity (%)	Positive Predictive Value (%)	Negative Predictive Value (%)
≥1+	≥300	67	74	92	34
≥3+	≥500	75	81	36	96

symptoms of preeclampsia such as persistent headache, visual symptoms, or epigastric pain. It should be emphasized that the presence of these symptoms is more important than the absolute level of blood pressure in establishing the diagnosis of preeclampsia. Indeed, there is more to preeclampsia than the presence of hypertension.[68]

The diagnosis of preeclampsia requires the presence of elevated blood pressure with proteinuria, or edema, or both.[3,4] However, poor perinatal outcome is usually seen in patients who have hypertension plus proteinuria.[69] The presence of proteinuria is usually determined by the use of either dipstick or protein-to-creatinine ratio in random urine samples. The concentration of urinary protein is highly variable. It is influenced by several factors, including contamination, urine-specific gravity, pH, exercise, and posture.[10] In addition, urinary protein-to-creatinine excretion is highly variable in patients with preeclampsia.[70] Moreover, two recent studies found that urinary dipstick determinations correlate very poorly with the amount of proteinuria found in 24-hour urine determinations.[71,72] Therefore, the definitive test for diagnosing proteinuria should be quantitative measurement of total protein excretion over a 24-hour period. For making the diagnosis of severe preeclampsia based on proteinuria, it is recommended that the presence of more than 5 g/24 hours be documented. The diagnosis of severe preeclampsia based on dipstick measurements in urine sample (≥3+) is not adequate for such a diagnosis (Table 28-2).[72]

Prediction of Preeclampsia

A review of the world literature reveals that more than 100 clinical, biophysical, and biochemical tests have been recommended to predict or identify the patient at risk for the future development of the disease.[73] A summary of these clinical tests is listed below. The value of MAP-2 in predicting preeclampsia was investigated by Chesley and Sibai,[74] as well as by Villar and Sibai.[13] The sensitivity of the test in various reports ranged from 0 to 99 percent, and the specificity varied from 53 to 97 percent. The value of the rollover test in predicting preeclampsia was evaluated in 14 reports. The sensitivity ranged from 0 to 93 percent and the specific-

Clinical Tests Used To Predict Preeclampsia

Average mean arterial pressure (MAP) in the second trimester ≥85–90 mmHg

MAP at 20 weeks ≥90 mmHg

Rollover test at 28–32 weeks

Combination of the above

Isometric exercise test

Angiotensin infusion test at 26–30 weeks

Doppler velocimetry of uterine and umbilical vessels at 18–26 weeks

ity ranged from 54 to 91 percent. In addition, the results of the pooled data for the various tests and the lack of agreement between serial tests suggest that none of these clinical tests is sufficiently reliable for use as a screening test in clinical practice.[73] At our institution, none of these tests are used for screening purposes.

There are reports describing the predictive value of substances that can be measured in maternal plasma, serum, or urine. Some of the substances evaluated included cations, hormones, prostaglandin, metabolites, various parameters of coagulation and hemostasis, and uric acid.[73] These reports differed in their methodologies and included a heterogeneous group of patients with all forms of hypertension, parity, and gestational ages at time of sampling. Comparison and evaluation is, therefore, limited, which explains the wide scatter of results and lack of agreement among the findings by various authors. Hence, none of these substances has proven sufficiently reliable to use as a screening test.[73]

Prevention of Preeclampsia

There are numerous reports and clinical trials describing the use of various methods to prevent or reduce the incidence of preeclampsia. Since the etiology of the disease is unknown, these methods were used in an attempt to correct theoretical abnormalities in preeclampsia. Some of the methods used are summarized below.[61] No efficacy of high protein or low salt diets has ever been documented.

Calcium Supplementation

The relationship between dietary calcium intake and hypertension has been the subject of several experimental and observational studies.[75,76] Several authors reported reduced urinary excretion of calcium at the

Methods Used To Prevent Preeclampsia

High protein and low salt diet

Nutritional supplementation
  Calcium
  Magnesium
  Zinc
  Fish and evening primrose oil

Antihypertensive drugs including diuretics

Antithrombotic agents
  Low-dose aspirin
  Dipyridamole
  Combination low-dose aspirin/dipyridamole
  Heparin

(From Sibai,[61] with permission.)

time of preeclampsia, as well as several weeks prior to the onset of PIH or preeclampsia.[77–79] In addition, abnormal intracellular calcium metabolism in both platelets and red blood cells has been demonstrated in women with PIH compared with normotensive pregnancies.[80,81]

It has been shown that there is an inverse association between calcium intake and maternal blood pressure and the incidences of preeclampsia and eclampsia in epidemiologic studies. The findings of these studies were recently reviewed by Belizan and associates.[82] The blood pressure lowering effect of calcium was thought to be mediated by alterations in plasma renin activity and parathyroid hormone. In addition, calcium supplementation during pregnancy was shown to reduce angiotensin II vascular sensitivities in such pregnancies.[83,84]

There are nine clinical studies comparing the use of calcium versus no treatment or a placebo in pregnancy.[83–91] These trials differed regarding the population studied (low-risk or high-risk for hypertensive disorders of pregnancy), study design (randomization, double-blind, or use of a placebo), gestational age at enrollment (20 to 32 weeks' gestation), sample size in each group (range 22 to 588), and dose of elemental calcium used (156 to 2,000 mg/d). In addition, these studies differed regarding the definition of hypertensive disorders of pregnancy. A critical analysis of the design of eight of these studies was recently reported by Levine and associates.[92]

Two of the nine studies compared the use of calcium to no treatment. One investigation by Kawasaki et al.[83] included the use of 156 mg of elemental calcium and

reported a significant reduction in the incidence of PIH (4.5 percent in the calcium group versus 21.2 percent in the placebo group).[83] The other study, by Marya and associates,[85] compared the use of 375 mg of elemental calcium plus 1,200 IU/d of vitamin D to no supplementation. The incidence of preeclampsia in the supplemental group was 6 percent, which was similar to the incidence in the nonsupplemental group (9 percent).[85]

Seven other studies were randomized placebo-controlled.[84,86–91] The dose of elemental calcium used in these trials was 1,500 to 2,000 mg/d. Five of these trials studied healthy pregnant women (low risk),[86–90] and the other two studied pregnant women who had either a positive rollover test[91] or both a positive rollover test and increased sensitivity to angiotensin II infusion.[84] Results of the seven studies are summarized in Table 28-3. The findings suggest that calcium supplementation reduces the overall incidence of hypertensive disorders of pregnancy, with a trend toward reducing the incidence of preeclampsia. Currently, a large multicenter trial is underway to evaluate the benefits and side effects of calcium supplementation to prevent preeclampsia. This trial is being conducted at five medical centers in the United States and is sponsored by the National Institute of Child Health and Human Development. This trial will randomize a total of 4,500

Table 28-3 Randomized Trials of Calcium Versus Placebo in Pregnancy

Authors	Hypertension Only (%)	Preeclampsia (%)	Hypertensive Disorders (%)
Villar et al[86]			
Calcium ($N = 25$)	4.0	0	4.0
Placebo ($N = 27$)	11.0	0	11.1
Lopez-Jaramillo et al[87]			
Calcium ($N = 49$)	n/a	n/a	4.1[a]
Placebo ($N = 43$)	n/a	n/a	27.9
Lopez-Jaramillo et al[91]			
Calcium ($N = 22$)	14	0	14.0[a]
Placebo ($N = 34$)	47	23.5	70.5
Villar and Repke[88]			
Calcium ($N = 90$)	3.3	0	3.3
Placebo ($N = 88$)	5.7	3.3	9.0
Montanaro et al[89]			
Calcium ($N = 84$)	4.8	2.4	7.2[a]
Placebo ($N = 86$)	16.3	10.5	26.8
Belizan et al[82]			
Calcium ($N = 579$)	7.2	2.6	9.8[a]
Placebo ($N = 588$)	10.7	3.9	14.8
Sanchez-Ramus et al[79]			
Calcium ($N = 29$)	17.2	13.8	31.0[a]
Placebo ($N = 34$)	20.6	44.1	64.7

Abbreviations: n/a, not available.
[a] $p < 0.01$ for overall hypertensive disorders.

healthy nulliparous women who will be enrolled prior to 20 weeks' gestation.

Magnesium Supplementation

Serum magnesium levels are usually lower during the pregnant than the nonpregnant state and rapidly return to prepregnancy concentrations after delivery. The relationship between dietary magnesium deficiency and hypertension has been the subject of several experimental and observational studies.[93] Dietary magnesium deficiency during pregnancy has been implicated in the pathogenesis of preeclampsia, fetal growth retardation, and preterm delivery.[94,95] In addition, in patients with preeclampsia, magnesium levels were reported to be lower or similar to those in normotensive pregnancies. Since parenteral magnesium sulfate is the drug of choice in preeclampsia, some authors suggested an etiologic relationship between magnesium deficiency and preeclampsia.[94,95]

In a retrospective study, Conradt et al.[95] compared the pregnancy outcomes in 4,023 low-risk pregnancies with those in 882 high-risk pregnancies. The high-risk group was treated with β-sympathomimetic agents in combination with various doses of magnesium aspartate hydrochloride. The incidence of preeclampsia in the high-risk treated group was 0, and it was 2 percent in the no treatment group. In addition, the incidence of fetal growth retardation was significantly reduced in the treated group. The authors concluded that routine supplementation with magnesium during pregnancy prevents preeclampsia and fetal growth retardation.

Spatling and Spatling[96] reported a double-blind study involving 568 women who were randomized to receive either 14-mmol magnesium aspartate hydrochloride ($N = 278$) or aspartic acid as placebo ($N = 290$). The supplementation was given daily starting at or before 16 weeks' gestation and was continued throughout pregnancy. The incidences of preeclampsia were similar in the two groups; however, the magnesium-supplemented group had a lower incidence of both preterm delivery and number of newborns admitted to the intensive care unit.

Sibai et al.[93] studied 400 young primigravidas who were enrolled at 13 to 24 weeks' gestation to receive either 365 mg of elemental magnesium (as magnesium aspartate hydrochloride) or aspartic acid placebo. The magnesium-supplemented group had significantly higher serum magnesium levels. However, there were no significant differences between the two groups regarding the incidences of preeclampsia, fetal growth retardation, or preterm delivery. In addition, magnesium supplementation did not influence the course of either systolic or diastolic blood pressure during the course of pregnancy.

Zinc Supplementation

Dietary zinc deficiency during pregnancy has been reportedly associated with poor pregnancy outcome.[97] In addition, reduced plasma zinc levels as well as lowered placental zinc levels have been reported in pregnancies complicated by preeclampsia.[98] Hunt et al.[99] studied the effects of zinc supplementation on the outcomes of pregnancy in 213 low-income Mexican women. The patients were randomly allocated in a double-blind fashion to receive either placebo capsules or capsules containing 20 mg zinc/d. The incidence of pregnancy-induced hypertension was significantly reduced in the zinc-supplemented group (2 vs. 16 percent). In addition, there were no other differences in pregnancy outcome between the two groups.

Mohamed and associates[100] studied pregnancy outcome in 494 women who were enrolled in a zinc supplemented trial (246 were given 20 mg/d zinc supplementation, 248 received placebo). They found no differences between the two groups regarding weight gain, blood pressure, or incidence of preeclampsia (4.6 percent in the zinc group vs. 1.3 percent in the control group). In addition, they found no differences regarding neonatal birth weight, fetal growth retardation, or incidence of preterm delivery.

At the present time, there are no adequate data to prove a strong association between prevention of preeclampsia and any nutritional supplementation. Thus, routine supplementation of all pregnant women with these nutrients is not recommended.

Antithrombic Agents

Preeclampsia is associated with vasospasm and activation of the coagulation-hemostasis systems. Enhanced platelet activation plays a central role in the above process with resultant abnormality in the thromboxane/prostacyclin balance. Hence, several authors have used pharmacologic manipulation to alter the above ratio in an attempt to prevent or ameliorate the course of preeclampsia.

Aspirin inhibits the synthesis of prostaglandins by irreversibly acetylating and inactivating cyclooxygenase. In vitro, platalet cyclooxygenase is more sensitive to inhibition by very low doses of aspirin (<80 mg) than vascular endothelial cyclooxygenase. Therefore, treatment with low doses of aspirin could alter the balance between prostacyclin and thromboxane.[101] This biochemical selectivity of low-dose aspirin appears to be related to its unusual kinetics that result in presystemic acetylation of platelets exposed to higher concentrations of aspirin in the portal circulation. Sibai et al.[102] found that effective inhibition of thromboxane generation by platelets (98 percent decrease from baseline) can be achieved after 1 week of therapy with 80 mg of daily aspirin during pregnancy. In addition, they found that a 60-mg dose resulted in a 60 percent decrease in platelet thromboxane generation after 1 week and a 97 percent decrease after 2 weeks of therapy.

There are some studies describing the effects of low-dose aspirin (60 to 81 mg/d) on angiotensin II sensitivity during pregnancy. The results of these studies were reviewed by Dekker and Sibai.[103] Findings from these studies suggest that enhanced vascular responsiveness to angiotensin II infusions may be mediated by an imbalance in thromboxane/PGI_2 production that may be corrected in some women by the use of low-dose aspirin. In addition, several prospective studies have been published that suggest that administration of aspirin in women at high risk for preeclampsia might reduce the incidence of hypertensive disorders of pregnancy, fetal growth retardation, and preterm delivery. These studies included a limited number of patients who were identified to be at high risk for preeclampsia on the basis of a poor obstetric history, chronic hypertension, positive rollover test, increased sensitivity to angiotensin II infusions, or abnormal Doppler studies of the uterine vessels. The findings of these studies were recently reviewed by Dekker and Sibai[103] and thus are not presented here. In general, the findings of these studies suggested that low-dose aspirin was highly effective in the prevention of preeclampsia and fetal growth retardation in women considered at risk for these complications.

Recently, several multicenter randomized prospective studies were reported from various countries. Some of these studies were conducted in healthy nulliparous women,[104,105] whereas others included patients with various obstetric and medical complications.[106–108]

In general, about 75 percent of all preeclampsia cases occur in nulliparous women. Therefore, prevention of preeclampsia in these women has major clinical implications. There are two randomized placebo-controlled trials describing the use of 60 mg/d of aspirin in healthy nulliparous women (Table 28-4). Hauth et al.[104] studied 604 healthy nulliparous women who were randomized at 24 weeks' gestation: 302 women received 60

mg/d of aspirin and 302 women received a matching placebo. The incidence of preeclampsia was significantly lower in the aspirin-treated women; however, there were no differences between the two groups regarding gestational age at delivery, neonatal birth weight, or frequency of fetal growth retardation or preterm delivery.

Sibai and associates[105] reported a multicenter study in 2,985 health nulliparous women who were randomized at 13 to 26 weeks' gestation: 1,485 women received 60 mg/d of aspirin, and 1,500 women received a matching placebo. The women were enrolled at seven medical centers in the United States, and the study was sponsored by the National Institute of Child Health and Human Development. The incidence of preeclampsia was reduced by only 26 percent in the aspirin-treated women; however, there were no differences in mean gestational age at delivery, birth weight, or frequency of fetal growth retardation or preterm delivery. Table 28-4 summarizes pregnancy outcomes for the two randomized studies. It is important to note that, despite a reduction in incidence of preeclampsia with aspirin in both trials, perinatal outcome was not improved with such therapy. In addition, mean gestational age at delivery in women who developed preeclampsia and who received aspirin was similar to the respective group who received placebo (both trials). Moreover, the trial by Sibai and associates[105] found a significantly higher incidence of abruptio placentae in women receiving aspirin (0.7 percent) than in those receiving placebo (0.1 percent).

Viinikka et al.[106] studied 197 women with preexisting chronic hypertension or a history of severe preeclampsia in their previous pregnancies who were randomized at 15 weeks' gestation: 97 received 50 mg/d of aspirin, and 100 received a matching placebo. The incidences of exacerbation of hypertension as well as preeclampsia were similar in the two groups. In addition, the two groups had similar mean gestational ages at delivery. However, patients receiving low-dose aspirin had a higher mean birth weight and a lower frequency of fetal growth retardation (Table 28-5).

Table 28-4 Pregnancy Outcome in Healthy Nulliparous Women Receiving Aspirin or Placebo

	Hauth et al[104]		Sibai et al[105]	
	Aspirin (N = 302)	Placebo (N = 302)	Aspirin (N = 1,485)	Placebo (N = 1,500)
Preeclampsia (%)	1.7	5.6	4.6	6.3
Gestational hypertension (%)	6.3	5.6	6.7	5.9
Mean birth weight (g)	3,249	3,169	3,188	3,189
<10th percentile (%)	5.6	6.3	4.6	5.8
Mean delivery gestational age (wk)	39.1	38.9	38.6	38.7
<37 weeks (%)	6.7	8.0	10.6	9.8

Table 28-5   Low-Dose Aspirin in Hypertensive Women

	Aspirin (N = 97)	Placebo (N = 100)	P Value
Hypertension only	12	14	
Preeclampsia	9	11	
GA at delivery (wk)	38.6 ± 2.1	38.2 ± 2.0	
Birth weight (g)	3,348 ± 707	3,170 ± 665	0.07
≤2 D	4	9	
Admitted to NICU	10	21	
Perinatal deaths	2	0	0.04

The Italian multicenter trial compared the use of 50 mg/d of aspirin to no treatment in a large group of pregnant women considered at risk for preeclampsia.[107] Eligible women were randomly assigned treatment with 50 mg aspirin daily until delivery (N = 583) or no treatment (N = 523); 18 and 46 women, respectively, were lost to follow up. There were no differences between the two groups regarding the incidences of hypertension only, preeclampsia, fetal growth retardation, preterm delivery, abruptio placentae, or perinatal deaths (Table 28-6).

The Collaborative Low-Dose Aspirin Study in Pregnancy (CLASP) is a multinational randomized trial of low-dose aspirin for the prevention and treatment of preeclampsia and intrauterine growth retardation (IUGR).[108] In this trial, 9,364 women were randomly assigned 60 mg aspirin daily or matching placebo. Seventy-four percent were entered for prophylaxis of preeclampsia, 12 percent for prophylaxis of IUGR, 12 percent for treatment of preeclampsia, and 3 percent for treatment of IUGR. Twenty-eight percent were primigravid, 20 percent had chronic hypertension, 5 percent had renal disease, and 3 percent had diabetes. Outcome data were available for 4,659 aspirin-allocated women and 4,650 placebo-allocated women. There were no differences between the two study groups regarding the incidences of preeclampsia, IUGR, abruptio placentae, or perinatal deaths. However, the

Table 28-6   Italian Study of Aspirin in Pregnancy

	No Treatment (N = 477) (%)	Aspirin (N + 565) (%)
Hypertension only	12.5	16.4
Preeclampsia	2.7	2.9
Fetal growth retardation	18.3	19.0
<37 Weeks' gestation	35.6	33.9
≤34 Weeks' gestation	12.4	12.0
Abruptio placentae	1.9	1.2
Perinatal deaths	3.6	2.9

(From the Italian Study of Aspirin in Pregnancy,[107] with permission.)

Table 28-7   The CLASP Trial

	Aspirin (N = 4,659) (%)	Placebo (N = 4,650) (%)
Preeclampsia	6.7	7.6
Eclampsia	0.2	0.2
IUGR	7.8	8.3
<37 Weeks' gestation	19.7	22.2[a]
Abruptio placentae	1.8	1.5
Perinatal deaths	2.7	2.8

[a] $p = 0.003$.

aspirin-treated group had a lower incidence of preterm delivery (Table 28-7). In addition, there was a significant trend ($p = 0.004$) toward progressively greater reductions in preeclampsia, in those leading to the preterm delivery. The study group suggested that low-dose aspirin may be justified in women judged to be at risk for early onset preeclampsia. For such women, the study group recommended that low-dose aspirin be started early during the second trimester.

Currently, a large multicenter clinical trial is underway in which pregnant women with high-risk characteristics (previous preeclampsia eclampsia, chronic hypertension, class B to F diabetes, or multifetal gestation) are being randomized to either aspirin 60 mg/d or matching placebo. This trial is being conducted at 11 centers in the United States and is sponsored by the National Institute of Child Health and Human Development. Thus, the use of low-dose aspirin to prevent preeclampsia in pregnant women with these complications should await the results of this trial. It is important to emphasize that low-dose aspirin in pregnancy was associated with a significant increase in the incidence of abruptio placentae in one study[105] and an increased perinatal mortality due to abruptio placentae in two studies.[105,109]

Laboratory Abnormalities in Preeclampsia

Women with preeclampsia may exhibit a symptom complex ranging from minimal blood pressure elevation to derangements of multiple organ systems. The renal, hematologic, and hepatic systems are most likely to be involved.

Renal Function

Renal plasma flow and glomerular filtration rate (GFR) increase during normal pregnancy.[110] These changes are responsible for the fall in serum creatinine, urea, and uric acid concentrations. In preeclampsia, vasospasm and glomerular capillary endothelial swelling (glomerular endotheliosis) lead to an average reduction in GFR of 25 percent below the rate for normal pregnancy.[111] Serum creatinine is rarely elevated in preeclampsia, but uric acid is commonly increased.[112] In a study of 200 women with mild preeclampsia remote from term, Sibai et al.[112] found the mean serum creatinine to be 0.80 mg/dl, the mean uric acid to be 6.1 mg/dl, and the mean creatinine clearance to be 112 ml/min. In a subsequent study involving 95 women with severe preeclampsia, Sibai and associates[113] reported a mean serum creatinine of 0.91 mg/dl, a mean uric acid of 6.6 mg/dl, and a mean creatinine clearance of 100 ml/min.

The clinical significance of elevated uric acid levels in preeclampsia/eclampsia has been confusing. In a study of 332 women with preexisting hypertension, plasma urate levels were found to be a better indicator of fetal prognosis than blood pressure. Uric acid levels above 5 mg/dl were associated with poor perinatal outcome.[114] However, in a comparison of 69 eclamptic women who had uric acid levels of less than 6.0 mg/dl with those who had values above 10.0 mg/dl, Pritchard and Stone[115] found no significant difference between the two groups for blood pressure, perinatal outcome, or incidence of hypertension in subsequent pregnancies.

Hepatic Function

The liver is not primarily involved in preeclampsia, and hepatic involvement is seen in only 10 percent of women with severe preeclampsia.[116] Fibrinogen deposition has been found along the walls of hepatic sinusoids in preeclamptic patients with no laboratory or histologic evidence of liver involvement.[117] When liver dysfunction occurs in preeclampsia, mild elevation of serum transaminase is most common.[118] Bilirubin is rarely increased in preeclampsia but, when elevated, the indirect fraction predominates. Elevated liver enzymes are part of the syndrome of hemolysis, elevated liver enzymes, and low platelets (HELLP), a variant of severe preeclampsia.

Hematologic Changes

There are numerous studies evaluating the hematologic abnormalities in women with preeclampsia. The findings of these studies were the subject of two recent reviews.[119,120] In general, the findings of these studies reveal that plasma fibrinopeptide-A, D-dimer levels, and circulating thrombin-antithrombin complexes are higher in women with preeclampsia than in normotensive pregnant women. In contrast, plasma antithrombin III activity is decreased in women with preeclampsia. These findings indicate enhanced thrombin generation.[119,120]

Plasma fibrinogen rises progressively during normal pregnancy. When a group of 50 severe preeclamptic women were compared with 50 normotensive women matched by gestational age, no differences in mean plasma fibrinogen levels were found between the two groups.[121] In general, plasma fibrinogen levels are rarely reduced in women with preeclampsia in the absence of abruptio placentae.

Thrombocytopenia is the most common hematologic abnormality in women with preeclampsia. Its incidence will depend on severity of the disease process, definition, and the presence or absence of abruptio placentae. A platelet count of less than 150,000/mm^3 was reported in 32 to 50 percent of women with severe preeclampsia.[121,122] In a study of 1,414 women with hypertension during pregnancy, Burrows and Kelton[123] found a platelet count of less than 150,000/mm^3 in 15 percent of the women.

Recently, Leduc and associates[122] studied the coagulation profile (platelet count, fibrinogen, prothrombin time, and partial thromboplastin time) in 100 consecutive women with severe preeclampsia. A platelet count less than 150,000/mm^3 was found in 50 percent and a count of less than 100,000/mm^3 was found in 36 percent of the women. Thirteen women had a fibrinogen level of less than 300 mg/dl, and two women had prolonged prothrombin and partial thromboplastin times. Interestingly, all of the latter women also had thrombocytopenia on admission. In addition, they found the admission platelet count to be an excellent predictor of subsequent thrombocytopenia. They concluded that fibrinogen levels, prothrombin time, and partial thromboplastin time should be obtained only in women with a platelet count of less than 100,000/mm^3.

The HELLP Syndrome

Recent reports have described the syndrome of hemolysis, elevated liver enzymes, and low platelets (HELLP) in severe preeclampsia. There is considerable debate regarding the definition, diagnosis, incidence, etiology, and management of this syndrome.[124] Patients with such findings were previously described by many investigators. Goodlin[125] labeled this syndrome "EPH gestosis type B"; he claimed that this clinical presentation had been reported in the obstetric literature a century earlier. Weinstein[116] considered it a unique variant of preeclampsia and coined the term "HELLP syndrome" for this entity, while MacKenna and colleagues[126] considered it to be misdiagnosed preeclampsia.[126]

A review of the literature highlights the differences regarding the degree of abnormal laboratory findings and the criteria used to diagnose HELLP syndrome. Thrombocytopenia (platelet count $<100 \times 10^3$/mm^3)

has been the most consistent finding among the various reports. However, some investigators have included only those values determined before delivery, while others have reported platelet counts obtained both antepartum and postpartum. In addition, there are considerable differences regarding what constitutes an abnormal level of serum glutamic-oxaloacetic transaminase (SGOT) or bilirubin. Several reports have not even included these data.[127] Barton and associates[128] performed liver biopsies in patients with preeclampsia and HELLP syndrome. Periportal necrosis and hemorrhage were the most common histopathologic findings. In addition, they found that the degree of laboratory abnormalities in HELLP syndrome (platelet count and liver enzymes) does not correlate with hepatic histopathologic findings.

Martin et al.,[129] in a retrospective review of 302 cases of HELLP syndrome at the University of Mississippi, Jackson, have devised the following classification of subpopulations based on platelet count nadir. Class I HELLP syndrome was defined as a platelet nadir below 50,000/mm^3. Those with platelet nadirs between 50,000 and 100,000/mm^3 were defined as class 2. Class 3 represents a platelet nadir between 100,000 and 150,000/mm^3. These classes have been used to predict the rapidity of postpartum disease recovery, maternal-perinatal outcome, and the need for plasmapheresis.[130] Miles et al.[131] from the same institution reported a strong association between the presence of HELLP syndrome and eclampsia. In that study, the HELLP syndrome was present in 30 percent of patients with postpartum eclampsia and in 28 percent of patients having eclampsia prior to delivery. As a result, they suggested that the presence of HELLP syndrome may be a predisposing factor in the development of eclampsia.[131]

Hemolysis, defined as the presence of microangiopathic hemolytic anemia, is the hallmark of the HELLP syndrome. The role of disseminated intravascular coagulation (DIC) in preeclampsia is controversial. Most authors do not regard HELLP syndrome to be a variant of DIC, since coagulation parameters such as prothrombin time, partial thromboplastin time, and serum fibrinogen are normal. However, the diagnosis of DIC in clinical practice is difficult. When sensitive determinants of this condition are used (such as antithrombin III, fibrinopeptide-A, fibrin monomer, D-dimer, α_2-antiplasmin, plasminogen, prekallikrein, and fibronectin), many patients have laboratory values consistent with DIC.[132,133] Unfortunately, these tests are time consuming and not suitable for routine monitoring. Consequently, less sensitive parameters are often used in clinical practice. Sibai et al.[124] defined DIC as the presence of thrombocytopenia, low fibrinogen levels (plasma fibrinogen <300 mg/dl), and fibrin split products above 40 µg/ml. These authors observed DIC in 38 percent of the 112 patients with HELLP syndrome. In a subsequent report, Sibai et al.[134] noted the present of DIC in 21 percent of 442 patients with HELLP syndrome. They also found that the majority of cases occurred in women who had antecedent abruptio placentae or peripartum hemorrhage and in all four women who had subcapsular liver hematomas. In the absence of these complications, the frequency of DIC was only 5 percent.[134] Aarnoudse et al.[135] diagnosed DIC in HELLP syndrome by light microscopic and immunofluorescence findings in tissue biopsies and laboratory findings of thrombocytopenia, elevated fibrinogen degradation products, reduced antithrombin III levels, and fragmented red blood cells.

In view of the above diagnostic problems, Sibai[127] recommended that uniform and standardized laboratory values be used to diagnose this syndrome. He suggested that low-density lipoprotein and bilirubin values be included in the diagnosis of hemolysis. In addition, the degree of abnormality of liver enzymes should be defined as a certain number of standard deviations from the normal value for each hospital population. Furthermore, the rate of change in either liver enzymes or platelet count may be as important as the absolute value in establishing the diagnosis. Our laboratory criteria to establish the diagnosis are presented in the box below.

The reported incidence of HELLP syndrome in preeclampsia has ranged from 2 to 12 percent.[127] The true incidence remains unknown, however, considering the differences in diagnostic criteria used. The syndrome appears to be most common in white patients. The incidence of HELLP syndrome is also higher in preeclamptic patients who have been managed conservatively.

The patient is usually seen remote from term complaining of epigastric or right upper-quadrant pain (65 percent), some will have nausea or vomiting (50 percent), and others will have nonspecific viral-syndrome-like symptoms. The majority of patients (90 percent)

Criteria To Establish the Diagnosis of HELLP Syndrome

Hemolysis
    Abnormal peripheral blood smear
    Increased bilirubin ≥1.2 mg/dl
    Increased lactic dehydrogenase >600 IU/L

Elevated liver enzymes
    Increased SGOT ≥72 IU/L
    Increased lactic dehydrogenase as above

Low platelets
    Platelet count <100 × 10^3/mm^3

Medical and Surgical Disorders Confused with the HELLP Syndrome

Acute fatty liver of pregnancy

Appendicitis

Diabetes

Gallbladder disease

Gastroenteritis

Glomerulonephritis

Hemolytic uremic syndrome

Hepatic encephalopathy

Hyperemesis gravidarum

Idiopathic thrombocytopenia

Kidney stones

Peptic ulcer

Pyelonephritis

Systemic lupus erythematosus

Thrombotic thrombocytopenic purpura

Viral hepatitis

tion of HELLP syndrome is transient nephrogenic diabetes insipidus. Unlike central diabetes insipidus, which occurs due to diminished or absent secretions of arginine vasopressin by the hypothalamus, transient nephrogenic diabetes insipidus is characterized by a resistance to arginine vasopressin mediated by excessive vasopressinase. It is postulated that elevated circulating vasopressinase may result from impaired hepatic metabolism of the enzyme.

It is important to emphasize that some of these patients may have a variety of signs and symptoms, none of which are diagnostic of severe preeclampsia. Thus, Sibai[127] recommended that all pregnant women having any of these symptoms should have a complete blood count and platelet and liver enzyme determinations irrespective of maternal blood pressure.

Management of preeclamptic patients presenting with the HELLP syndrome is highly controversial. A review of the literature highlights the confusion surrounding the management of this syndrome.[127] Consequently, there are several therapeutic modalities described in the literature to treat or reverse the HELLP syndrome. Most of these modalities are similar to those used in the management of severe preeclampsia remote from term.[127]

Goodlin[137] described five patients with features of HELLP syndrome who were treated conservatively with bedrest in an attempt to increase plasma volume. Three women also received intravenous infusions of 5 or 25

will give a history of malaise for the past few days before presentation; some may present with hematuria or gastrointestinal bleeding. Hypertension and proteinuria may be absent or slightly abnormal.[135,136] Physical examination will demonstrate right upper-quadrant tenderness and significant weight gain with edema.

It is important to appreciate that severe hypertension is not a constant or even a frequent finding in HELLP syndrome. Although 66 percent of the 112 patients studied by Sibai and associates[124] had a diastolic blood pressure of at least 110 mmHg, 14.5 percent had a diastolic blood pressure of less than 90 mmHg. Aarnoudse and colleagues[135] described six women presenting with severe epigastric pain in the third trimester who had significantly elevated liver enzymes, low platelets, and evidence of hemolysis. None of these patients had a blood pressure of 140/90 or higher proteinuria. Thus, these patients may present with a variety of signs and symptoms, none of which are diagnostic of severe preeclampsia. As a result, they are often misdiagnosed as having various medical and surgical disorders. Occasionally the presence of this syndrome is associated with hypoglycemia leading to coma, severe hyponatremia, and cortical blindness. A rare but interesting complica-

Therapeutic Modalities Used To Treat or Reverse HELLP Syndrome

Plasma volume expansion
  Bedrest
  Crystalloids
  Albumin 5 to 25 percent

Antithrombotic agents
  Low-dose aspirin
  Dipyridamole
  Heparin
  Antithrombin III
  Prostacyclin infusions

Immunosuppressive agents
  Steroids

Miscellaneous
  Fresh frozen plasma infusions
  Exchange plasmapheresis
  Dialysis

(From Sibai,[127] with permission.)

percent albumin. Goodlin felt that the efforts at plasma volume expansion were in part beneficial as measured by a fall in hemoglobin concentration, rise in platelet count, and resolution of some of the symptoms of "severe toxemia." Thiagarajah et al.[138] treated five patients with prednisone or betamethasone and reported an improvement in platelet count and liver enzymes.

Heyborne[139] reported five cases where temporary reversal of the HELLP syndrome was achieved using low-dose aspirin (81 mg/d) and corticosteroids. The average prolongation of pregnancy was 4 weeks; however, three pregnancies beginning at 25 weeks or earlier were prolonged for an average of 5.5 weeks. No long-term maternal morbidity occurred, although one patient developed disseminated intravascular coagulation and eclampsia. Criticisms of this study include that three of five patients had platelet counts above 100,000 mm³ at initial diagnosis and hemolysis was not documented in three of five patients.

Clark and associates[140] reported three cases in which temporary reversal of the HELLP syndrome was achieved using bedrest and corticosteroids. Pregnancy prolongation ranged form 4 to 10 days, and all pregnancies resulted in a live birth. It is important to note that two of the patients had a platelet count of more than 100,000/mm³, and one patient had normal liver enzymes.

Recently, Van Assche and Spitz[141] reported on a patient who developed preeclampsia with HELLP syndrome at 32 weeks' gestation. The patient was treated with bedrest, albumin infusion, and 200 mg dazoxiben (a thromboxane synthetase inhibitor) four times a day. All maternal laboratory values returned to normal after 4 days of treatment with dazoxiben; however, the patient had a cesarean delivery 1 week later. Both infant and placenta were small for gestational age. The authors suggested that dazoxiben might have beneficial effects in the management of such patients.

Two recent reports by Magann and associates[142,143] suggested that the use of corticosteriods either antepartum or postpartum results in transient improvement in laboratory values and urine output in some patients diagnosed with HELLP syndrome. It is important to note that in the antepartum group delivery was delayed by an average of 41 hours only and the study was not placebo controlled.[142]

The described conservative management techniques were often associated with the use of inappropriate invasive procedures (various biopsies) and medical and surgical treatments. These confounding variables make it difficult to evaluate any treatment modality proposed for this syndrome. Occasionally, some patients without the "true HELLP" syndrome may demonstrate antepartum reversal of hematologic abnormalities following bedrest, the use of steroids, or plasma volume ex-

pansion. However, the majority of these patients will demonstrate deterioration in either maternal or fetal condition within 1 to 10 days after conservative management. Hence, it is doubtful that such a limited pregnancy prolongation will result in improved perinatal outcome, especially when maternal and fetal risks are substantial.

There is general agreement that pregnancies complicated by preeclampsia and the HELLP syndrome are associated with poor maternal and perinatal outcomes.[124,134,143] The reported perinatal mortality has ranged from 7.7 to 60 percent and maternal mortality from 0 to 24 percent. Maternal morbidity is common. Most of these patients have required transfusions of blood and blood products and are at increased risk for the development of acute renal failure, pulmonary edema, ascites, pleural effusions, and hepatic rupture.[132,134,144–146] Moreover, these pregnancies are associated with high incidences of abruptio placentae and DIC.

Sibai et al.[124] reported on 112 patients with severe preeclampsia eclampsia in which the diagnosis of HELLP syndrome had been made before delivery. The incidence of this syndrome was significantly higher in white women, multigravidas, and those who had been misdiagnosed or treated conservatively. The overall perinatal outcome is summarized in Table 28-8. The incidence of abruptio placentae was 20 percent, and 104 (93 percent) required blood and/or blood products to correct hypovolemia or coagulopathy.

The HELLP syndrome may develop antepartum or postpartum. Analysis of 442 cases studied by Sibai and associates[134] revealed that 309 (70 percent) had evidence of the syndrome antepartum, and 133 (30 percent) developed the manifestations postpartum. There were four maternal deaths, and morbidity was very frequent (Table 28-9).

In the postpartum period, the time of onset of the manifestations ranged from a few hours to 7 days, with the majority developing within 48 hours postpartum. Eighty percent of the postpartum patients had evidence

Table 28-8 Perinatal Outcome in HELLP Syndrome

(N = 114 births)	No.	%
Stillbirths	22	19.3
Neonatal deaths	16	17.4
Perinatal deaths	38	33.3
Gestational age (wk)		
≤30	47	41.2
31–36	46	40.4
>36	21	18.4
SGA	36	31.6

(From Sibai et al,[124] with permission.)

Table 28-9 Serious Maternal Complications in 442 Patients with HELLP Syndrome

Complication	No.	%
Disseminated intravascular coagulopathy	92	21
Abruptio placentae	69	16
Acute renal failure	33	8
Severe ascites	32	8
Pulmonary edema	26	6
Pleural effusions	26	6
Cerebral edema	4	1
Retinal detachment	4	1
Laryngeal edema	4	1
Subcapsular liver hematoma	4	1
ARDS	3	1
Death, maternal	4	1

(From Sibai et al,[134] with permission.)

of preeclampsia prior to delivery, whereas 20 percent had no such evidence either antepartum or intrapartum. It is the author's experience that patients in this group are at increased risk for the development of pulmonary edema and acute renal failure (Table 28-10). The differential diagnosis in these patients should include exacerbation of systemic lupus erythematosus, thrombotic thrombocytopena purpura (TTP), and hemolytic uremic syndrome.

Patients with the HELLP syndrome who are remote from term should be referred to a tertiary care center and initial management should be as for any patient with severe preeclampsia. The first priority is to assess and stabilize maternal condition, particularly coagulation abnormalities. The next step is to evaluate fetal well-being using the nonstress test and biophysical profile. Then, a decision must be made as to whether or not immediate delivery is indicated. Amniocentesis may be performed in patients at less than 34 weeks' gestation without risk of bleeding complications. In the absence of laboratory evidence of DIC and fetal lung maturity, the patient may be given two doses of steroids to accelerate fetal lung maturity and then delivered 24 hours after the last dose. During this time, both maternal and fetal conditions should be monitored very closely. In addition, the presence of this syndrome is not an indication for immediate cesarean delivery. It is the author's opinion that such an approach might prove detrimental for both mother and fetus. Patients presenting with well-established labor should be allowed to deliver vaginally as indicated. In addition, labor may be initiated with oxytocin in those with a favorable cervix.

Patients with delayed resolution of HELLP syndrome (including persistent severe thrombocytopenia) represent a management dilemma. Exchange plasmapheresis with fresh frozen plasma has been advocated as a treatment by some authors.[130,147] Since the majority of these patients will have spontaneous resolution of their disease, however, early initiation of plasmapheresis may result in unnecessary treatment. Schwartz[147] suggested that serial studies indicating a progressive elevation of bilirubin or creatinine associated with hemolysis and thrombocytopenia be considered an indication for plasmapheresis. Martin et al.[130] reported the use of plasma exchange with fresh frozen plasma in seven women in the postpartum period with HELLP syndrome that persisted for more than 72 hours following delivery. All patients had persistent thrombocytopenia, rising lactic dehydrogenase, and evidence of multiorgan dysfunction. Sustained increases in mean platelet count and decreases in LDH concentrations were associated with plasma exchange. The authors recommended that a trial of plasma exchange with fresh frozen plasma be considered in HELLP syndrome that persists past 72 hours from delivery and in which there

Table 28-10 Outcome and Complications of HELLP Syndrome in Relation to Time of Onset

	Antepartum Onset ($N = 309$) (%)	Postpartum Onset ($N = 133$) (%)	Relative Risk	95% Confidence Interval
Delivery at <27 weeks[a]	15	3	4.84	2.0–11.6
Delivery at 37–42 weeks[b]	15	25	0.61	0.41–0.91
Pulmonary edema	5	9	0.50	0.24–1.05
Acute renal failure[b]	5	12	0.46	0.24–0.87
Eclampsia	7	10	0.73	0.38–1.40
Abruptio placentae	16	15	1.05	0.65–1.70
DIC	21	20	1.09	0.73–1.64

Abbreviations: DIC, disseminated intravascular coagulopathy.
[a] $p < 0.0007$.
[b] $p < 0.002$.
(From Sibai et al,[134] with permission.)

is evidence of a life-threatening microangiopathy. Potential adverse effects of this technique are numerous. Ultimately, the question remains how many patients would spontaneously improve without benefit of plasmapheresis. It is the author's experience that plasmapheresis is not needed in the management of such patients.[134]

Subcapsular Hematoma of the Liver in HELLP Syndrome

The diagnosis of a subcapsular hematoma of the liver in pregnancy is often overlooked because of its rarity. Indeed in four recent cases managed at our institution, our initial clinical impression was placental abruption with disseminated intravascular coagulation DIC in three cases and a complication of a postpartum tubal ligation in the fourth patient.[134] The differential diagnosis of an unruptured subcapsular hematoma of the liver in pregnancy should include acute cholecystitis with sepsis, acute fatty liver of pregnancy, ruptured uterus, placental abruption with DIC, and TTP. Most patients present in the third or late second trimester of pregnancy, although cases have been reported in the immediate postpartum period. In addition to the signs and symptoms of preeclampsia, physical examination findings consistent with peritoneal irritation and hepatomegaly may be present. Profound hypovolemic shock with hypotension in a previously hypertensive patient is a hallmark of rupture of the hematoma.

Laboratory evaluation is often consistent with DIC, including low platelet count, low fibrinogen, and prolonged prothrombin and partial thromboplastin times. As a result of hemolysis, total bilirubin and serum lactate dehydrogenase are markedly elevated. Other liver function tests such as aspartate and alanine aminotransferase are also significantly elevated.

Rupture of a subcapsular hematoma of the liver is a life-threatening complication of HELLP syndrome. In most instances, rupture involves the right lobe and is preceded by the development of a parenchymal hematoma. The condition usually presents with severe epigastric pain that may persist for several hours prior to circulation collapse.

Patients frequently present with shoulder pain, shock, or evidence of massive ascites, respiratory difficulty, or pleural effusions, and often with a dead fetus. An ultrasound or computed axial tomography of the liver should be performed to rule out the presence of subcapsular hematoma of the liver and assess for the presence of intraperitoneal bleeding. Paracentesis confirms the presence of intraperitoneal hemorrhage suspected by examination or radiographic imaging.

The presence of ruptured subcapsular liver hematoma resulting in shock is a surgical emergency requiring acute multidisciplinary treatment. Resuscitation should consist of massive transfusions of blood, correction of coagulopathy with fresh frozen plasma and platelets, and immediate laparotomy. Options at laparotomy include packing and drainage (preferred), surgical ligation of the hemorrhaging hepatic segments, embolization of the hepatic artery to the involved liver segment, and loosely suturing omentum or surgical mesh to the liver to improve integrity. Even with appropriate treatment, maternal and fetal mortality is over 50 percent. Mortality is most commonly associated with exsanguination and coagulopathy. Initial survivors are at increased risk for developing adult respiratory distress syndrome, pulmonary edema, and acute renal failure in the postoperative period.[134,145]

Surgical repair has been recommended for hepatic hemorrhage without liver rupture. More recent experience suggests, however, that this complication can be managed conservatively in patients who remain hemodynamically stable.[148,149] Management should include close monitoring of hemodynamics and coagulation status. Serial assessment of the subcapsular hematoma with ultrasound or computed tomography is necessary with immediate intervention for rupture or worsening of maternal status. It is important with conservative management to avoid exogenous sources of trauma to the liver such as abdominal palpation, convulsions, or emesis and to use care in transportation of the patient. Indeed, any sudden increase in intraabdominal pressure could potentially lead to rupture of the subcapsular hematoma.[150]

Smith et al.[151] recently reviewed their management of seven cases of spontaneous rupture of the liver occurring during pregnancy. Of the four survivors, the mean gestational age was 32.8 weeks and the mean duration of hospitalization was 16 days. All the survivors were managed with packing and drainage of the liver, whereas the three patients treated with hepatic lobectomy died. The authors also extracted 28 cases from the literature reported since 1976. From a total of 35 cases analyzed, there was an 82 percent overall survival for the 27 cases managed by packing and drainage, whereas only 25 percent of eight patients undergoing hepatic lobectomy survived. The authors emphasized that hepatic hemorrhage with persistent hypotension unresponsive to transfusion of blood products may be managed surgically with laparotomy, evaluation of the hematoma, packing of the damaged liver, and draining of the operative site. In certain cases where the patient is stable enough to undergo angiography, transcatheter embolotherapy is a reasonable alternative to surgery.[152]

At the University of Tennessee, Memphis, we have managed four patients with HELLP syndrome complicated by ruptured subcapsular hematoma in the last 14 years. Three cases required transfusion of 22 to 40 units of packed red blood cells and multiple units of platelets and fresh frozen plasma. Two of these three cases were complicated by pulmonary edema and acute renal failure, but all survived without any residual deficiency. The fourth case was a patient who presented in profound shock and with disseminated intravascular coagulopathy. This patient subsequently died secondary to a ruptured pulmonary emphysematous bleb during management of adult respiratory distress syndrome.[134]

Any algorithm for the management of a subcapsular hematoma of the liver in pregnancy must emphasize the potential need for large amounts of blood products and the need for aggressive intervention if rupture of the hematoma is suspected. Our algorithm, employed at the University of Tennessee, Memphis, is presented in Fig. 28-3. Our experience is in agreement with the recent observations of Smith et al.[151] in that a stable patient with an unruptured subcapsular hematoma may be managed conservatively. Constant monitoring must continue during this management, however, as patients can rapidly become unstable following rupture of the hematoma.

Survival is clearly associated with rapid diagnosis and medical and surgical stabilization. Coagulopathy must be aggressively reversed, as failure to do so is associated with an increased incidence of renal failure. In addition, these patients should be managed in an intensive care unit with close monitoring of various hemodynamic parameters and fluid states to avoid the potential of pulmonary edema, respiratory compromise, or both.

Postpartum follow up for patients with subcapsular hematoma of the liver should include serial computed tomography or ultrasound until the defect resolves.

Hemodynamic Changes in Preeclampsia

The cardiovascular hemodynamics of preeclampsia have been investigated over the years by many authors using various techniques for measurements of blood pressure, cardiac output, pulmonary capillary wedge pressure (PCWP), and central venous pressure (CVP).[153]

The true hemodynamic findings in patients with preeclampsia are controversial. A review of the English literature demonstrates considerable disagreement regarding one or more of the hemodynamic parameters studied. This lack of agreement has been attributed to differences in the definition of preeclampsia, variable severity and duration of the disease process, presence of underlying cardiac or renal disease, the technique of measuring cardiac output, the technique of measuring blood pressure, and the therapeutic interventions used before obtaining the various measurements. In addition, the dynamic minute-to-minute fluctuation of the various cardiovascular parameters studied makes it difficult to standardize the conditions under which these observations are made and limits the value of a single measurement.

Invasive techniques were used to study the hemodynamic findings in untreated women with severe preeclampsia by many authors.[154–158] The reported cardiac index ranged from a low of 2.8 to a high of 4.8 L/min·m². The reported PCWP ranged from a low of 3.3 to a high of 12 mmHg. The findings suggest that cardiac index and PCWP are either low or normal in severe preeclampsia. The reported CVP values also ranged from 2 to 6 mmHg.

Table 28-11 compares the invasive hemodynamic

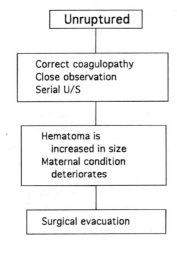

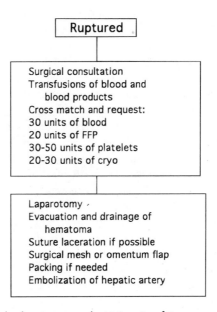

Fig. 28-3 An algorithm for the management of a subcapsular hematoma at the University of Tennessee, Memphis.

Table 28-11   Invasive Hemodynamic Findings in Treated Patients with Severe Preeclampsia/Eclampsia: Comparison of Three Large Series

	Wallenburg[156] (N = 22)[a]	Cotton et al[159] (N = 45)[b]	Mabie et al[160] (N = 41)[c]
Diastolic pressure (mmHg)	110	110 ± 2	106 ± 2
Pulmonary artery pressure (mmHg)	19	17 ± 1	15 ± 0.5
Cardiac index (L/min·m^2)	3.8	4.1 ± 0.1	4.4 ± 0.1
SVRI (dynes·sec·cm^{-5}, M^2)	2,475	2,726 ± 1	2,293 ± 65
PWCP (mmHg)	8	10 ± 1	8.3 ± 0.3
Central venous pressure (mmHg)	2	4 ± 1	4.8 ± 0.4

[a] Values expressed as median.

[b] Values as mean ± SEM; includes two patients with pulmonary edema.

[c] Values as means ± SEM; excludes eight patients with pulmonary edema.

findings in treated patients with severe preeclampsia.[156,159,160] The data for the various parameters are similar among the three studies. The findings demonstrated that treated patients with preeclampsia have normal to high cardiac index, normal to high systemic vascular resistance index, and normal to high PCWP.

In summary, the true hemodynamic findings of preeclampsia remain unknown. The majority of the data indicate that both cardiac output and systemic vascular resistance appear to be elevated in women with severe preeclampsia. This finding suggests that the problem in preeclampsia is a systemic vascular resistance that is inappropriately high for the level of cardiac output. Both the PCWP and the CVP appear to be in the low to normal range; however, there is no correlation between the two values.

Doppler Velocimetry Studies

There are numerous reports describing the use of uteroplacental and umbilical arteries flow velocity waveforms (FVW) in the prediction, diagnosis, and management of preeclampsia. The findings of these reports were the subject of a recent study.[161] Early studies suggested that Doppler ultrasound held great promise as a noninvasive, repeatable, and simple method of predicting hypertension in pregnancy and identifying those hypertensive pregnancies at high risk of maternal and fetal complications.[162–165] However, subsequent studies have emphasized the multiplicity of factors that may influence the Doppler waveform pattern.[161]

Steel et al.[166] screened 1,014 nulliparous women by the recording of Doppler ultrasound waveforms from the uteroplacental circulation at 18 to 20 weeks. One hundred eighteen (12 percent) had persistently abnormal tests at both 18 and 24 weeks' gestation. Incidence of hypertension among these 118 women was 25 percent. Sensitivity was high for hypertension associated with proteinuria (63 percent) or IUGR (100 percent).

Bower and associates[167] screened 2,430 women with continuous wave Doppler ultrasound of both uterine arteries at 18 to 20 weeks' gestation. An abnormal FVW in either uterine artery was used to predict preeclampsia and poor perinatal outcome. By including an early diastolic notch in the definition of an abnormal FVW, the sensitivity for moderate and severe preeclampsia was 79 to 88 percent and the specificity, 2 to 82, was 85 percent. However, the positive predictive value was 4.3 to 6.9 percent.

Trudinger and Cook[168] studied Doppler umbilical and uterine FVW in women with severe hypertension in pregnancy. They found that perinatal complications correlated more closely with umbilical artery indices than uteroplacental indices. More recently, Yoon and associates[169] studied umbilical artery waveforms in 72 women with preeclampsia. The Doppler studies were performed within 7 days of delivery. They found that an abnormal umbilical artery waveform was a strong and independent predictor of adverse perinatal outcome in patients with preeclampsia.

Pattinson and associates[170] reported on a randomized controlled trial evaluating the role for umbilical artery Doppler velocimetry in the management of patients with hypertensive diseases or suspected fetal growth retardation. The Doppler findings were revealed to the managing physicians of 108 patients, and the results were not revealed for 104 patients (control group). Pattinson et al.[170] found that knowledge of Doppler velocimetry results was beneficial in the subset with absent end-diastolic velocities. On the other hand, for women with hypertension whose fetuses had end-diastolic velocities, there was no beneficial or adverse effect.

In summary, the data regarding examination of the uteroplacental circulation for the prediction of preeclampsia indicate that the presence of abnormal tests both at 18 to 20 weeks' and at 24 weeks' gestation and the presence of a diastolic notch may be helpful as a screening test in selected, high-risk populations. However, it is important to note that it is difficult to interpret results obtained from the uteroplacental circulation due to its anatomic complexity.

On the other hand, evaluation of fetal vessels is very helpful in identifying those pregnancies that might require frequent monitoring with traditional tests of fetal well-being such as the nonstress test and biophysical profile. In general, the presence or absence of end-diastolic frequencies or reverse flow patterns in the umbilical artery is usually associated with poor perinatal outcome.[171]

The Management of Preeclampsia

Once the diagnosis of preeclampsia has been made, definitive therapy in the form of delivery is the only cure. The ultimate goals of therapy must always be safety of the mother first and then the delivery of a live, mature newborn who will not require intensive and prolonged neonatal care. However, in some cases such an approach is not in the best interest of the fetus. As a result, the decision between immediately delivery and expectant management will depend on one or more of the following: severity of the disease process, maternal and fetal status at the time of initial evaluation, fetal gestational age, presence of labor, Bishop cervical score, and the wishes of the mother.

Mild Preeclampsia

Patients with diagnosed preeclampsia should ideally be hospitalized at the time of diagnosis for evaluation of maternal and fetal conditions. These pregnancies may be associated with reduced unteroplacental blow flow. In addition, the mother is at slightly increased risk for the development of abruptio placentae or convulsions, particularly in cases remote from term. Thus, women with mild disease who have a favorable cervix at or near term should undergo induction of labor for delivery. The pregnancy should not continue past term (beyond 40 weeks' gestation), even if conditions for induction of labor are unfavorable, because the uteroplacental blood flow becomes suboptimal.

The optimal management of mild preeclampsia remote from term (<37 weeks' gestation) is controversial. In general, there is considerable disagreement regarding the need for hospitalization versus ambulatory management, the use of antihypertensive drugs, and the use of sedatives.

In some medical centers in the United States, management of these patients usually involves bedrest in the hospital for the duration of pregnancy, because this approach enhances fetal survival and diminishes the frequency of progression to severe disease. In many such instances, this treatment arrests the clinical course of the disease or at least improves it long enough to

achieve fetal maturity and reduces maternal morbidity.[172,173]

On the other hand, the benefits of prolonged antepartum hospitalization for women with mild gestational hypertension (without proteinuria) were challenged by several European investigators who reported that most of these women can be safely managed on an ambulatory basis or in a day care facility.

Two studies reported on the pregnancy outcome in women with mild hypertension (without proteinuria) remote from term who were randomized to either bedrest at hospital or normal activity at home.[174,175] Both studies questioned the value of hospitalization and came to the conclusion that management at home is safe and cost effective. Two other studies reported that management of these women can be done safely and efficiently in day care units, thereby diminishing the number of hospitalization days.[176,177] Finally, a recent review analyzing the value of bedrest in severe obstetric complications including mild hypertension suggested that such management is not cost effective and might be potentially harmful.[178]

In contrast, others reported that early and prolonged hospitalization for patients with mild hypertension remote from term had improved perinatal survival and reduced maternal morbidity and was cost effective (Table 28-12).[112,172,173] However, Barton et al.[179] reported that a similar pregnancy outcome can be achieved by monitored outpatient management. This study included 592 patients with mild gestational hypertension remote from term who were monitored with automated blood pressure measurement four times daily and daily assessment of weight, proteinuria, and fetal movement. The authors concluded that such management reduces the number of days of maternal hospitalization with similar maternal and perinatal outcome compared with previously published results from inpatient management.

There are numerous clinical reports (controlled and uncontrolled) describing the use of various drugs in an attempt to prolong gestation and improve perinatal outcome in women with mild preeclampsia remote from term. However, it is almost impossible to evaluate and to compare the results of these studies because of the heterogeneous populations studied (all forms of hypertension), the various parities, and the absence of a control group in most of these studies. It is important to note that these drugs are used overseas and are rarely used in this country for this purpose. In addition, none of these studies have reported a better perinatal outcome than the respective outcomes in studies using hospitalization alone.

There are few controlled studies comparing the use of β-blockers versus either placebo or no treatment in the management of mild preeclampsia remote from

Table 28-12 Inpatient Management of Mild Preeclampsia Remote from Term

	Gilstrap et al,[172] (1978)	Sibai et al,[173] (1987)	Sibai et al,[112] (1992)
Patients (N)	545	200	200
GA enrollment (mean, wks)	Unknown	32.5	33.1
<30 (%)	4.8	18.5	11.7
30–32 (%)	15.8	33.1	22.8
33–36 (%)	47.9	48.4	65.5
≥37 (%)	31.5	None	None
Hospitalization (days)	24	20.7	12.4
GA delivery (mean, wks)	Unknown	35.5	36.7
Pregnancy prolongation (mean, days)		20.7	22.4
Birth weight (g)	2,824	2,258	2,509
Corrected PMR/1,000	9	5	0

Abbreviations: GA, gestational age; PMR, perinatal mortality rate.

term.[173,180–183] Perinatal outcome derived from these studies is summarized in Table 28-13. One of the five studies reported lower neonatal morbidity in the treatment group, and the other four reported no differences in perinatal outcome between treatment and control patients. However, all studies reported a lower incidence of progression to severe hypertension in the treatment group. Of note, the sample was not adequate in any study to evaluate perinatal mortality. In addition, none of these studies showed a better perinatal outcome than studies that included hospitalization only for management of mild preeclampsia.

Recently, Sibai et al.[112] (in a prospective, randomized trial) compared no therapy to the use of nifedipine in the management of mild preeclampsia remote from term. They found that nifedipine was effective in reducing maternal systolic and diastolic blood pressures in women with mild preeclampsia. However, this reduc-

tion in maternal blood pressure was not associated with a reduced number of antepartum hospital days in the nifedipine group. In addition, the use of nifedipine led to a lower incidence of delivery for severe hypertension (9 percent) than no therapy (18 percent). However, such reduction in incidence of severe hypertension in the nifedipine group was not associated with a concomitant improved pregnancy prolongation when compared with the no-therapy group.

Our management plan at the University of Tennessee, Memphis, for patients with mild preeclampsia is summarized in Figure 28-4. All patients with mild preeclampsia are initially hospitalized at the time of their diagnosis. During hospitalization, patients receive regular diet with no salt restriction and no activity limits. Diuretics and antihypertensive drugs are not prescribed, and sedatives are not used. Patients initially undergo evaluation of maternal and fetal well-being.

Table 28-13 Randomized Trials of β-Blockers Versus Placebo or No Treatment in Mild Preeclampsia

Authors	Patients (No.)	GA at Entry	GA at Delivery	Birth Weight (g)	SGA No. (%)	Perinatal Deaths No. (%)
Wichman et al[181]						
Metoprolol	26	33.0	38.0	2,700	N/A	0
Placebo	26	33.0	38.0	2,962	N/A	1
Plouin et al[182]						
Oxprenolol	78	28.0	38.4	3,079	5 (7)	2 (2.6)
No treatment	77	28.2	38.1	3,023	8 (11)	3
Rubin et al[180]						
Atenolol	46	33.8	39.0	2,961	7 (15)	1 (2.2)
Placebo	39	33.8	38.0	3,017	7 (18)	2 (5.1)
Sibai et al[173]						
Labetalol	92	32.6	35.4	2,204	18 (19.1)	1 (1.1)
No treatment	94	32.4	35.5	2,258	9 (9.3)	0
Pickles et al[183]						
Labetalol	70	34.0	37.8	2,948	10 (14)	0
Placebo	74	34.2	37.5	2,913	5 (7)	0

Abbreviations: GA, gestational age; SGA, small-for-gestational age.

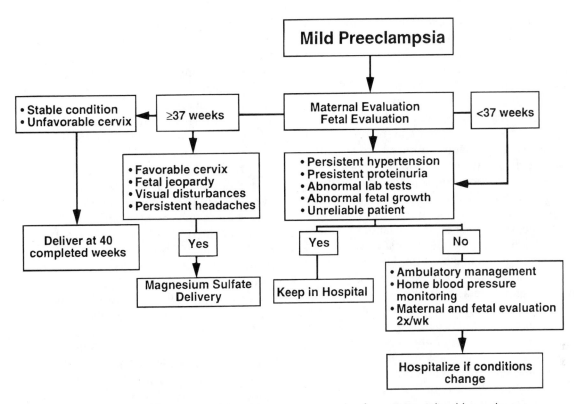

Fig. 28-4 University of Tennessee, Memphis, management plan for patients with mild preeclampsia.

The frequency of subsequent testing usually depends on the fetal gestational age and maternal response following hospitalization. Subsequent fetal evaluation includes serial ultrasonography for fetal growth every 3 weeks, daily fetal movement count, nonstress testing every week, and biophysical profile if needed. Maternal evaluation includes blood pressure monitoring (q 4 h during the day), maternal weight assessment, and checking for the presence of edema daily. In addition, women are questioned regarding symptoms of impending eclampsia (persistent headache, visual disturbances, or epigastric pain). Laboratory evaluation includes measurements of urine protein, hematocrit, and platelet count (every 2 days), and liver function test (one to two times per week). This evaluation is extremely important because patients may develop thrombocytopenia and elevated liver enzymes with minimal blood pressure elevation.[136]

If the patient's blood pressure remains stable in the absence of either significant proteinuria (<500 mg/24 hours) or maternal symptoms (headaches, visual disturbances, or epigastric pain), then outpatient observation may be considered on a selective basis. This form of management is appropriate in a reliable patient only during the early stages of the disease and in the absence of fetal jeopardy (abnormal testing or abnormal fetal growth).[179] These patients are instructed to rest at home, to have daily urine dipstick measurements of proteinuria, and to have blood pressure monitoring (by self or by nurse). The patient is also instructed to keep fetal movement counts and to report any symptoms of impending eclampsia. The patient is then evaluated in the antepartum testing area for maternal and fetal well-being at least two times per week. If there is any evidence of disease progression and if acute hypertension or substantial proteinuria develops, then prompt hospitalization is indicated.

The success rate of outpatient management will depend on fetal gestational age and on maternal status at time of diagnosis. Patients diagnosed with mild hypertension only (diastolic pressure <100 mmHg, absent proteinuria) will have a longer duration of pregnancy prolongation than those diagnosed with moderate elevations of hypertension (diastolic >100 mmHg) and significant proteinuria.[179] If there are any signs of worsening maternal or fetal conditions at any time during outpatient management, then hospitalization is indicated. In addition, after 37 weeks gestation, labor should be induced as soon as the cervix is favorable (Bishop score ≥ −6).

Severe Preeclampsia

The clinical course of severe preeclampsia may be characterized by progressive deterioration in both maternal and fetal conditions, and pregnancies complicated by severe preeclampsia are associated with increased rates of perinatal mortality and increased risks of maternal morbidity and mortality. As a result, there is universal agreement that all such patients should be delivered if the disease develops after 34 weeks' gestation or prior to that time if there is evidence of maternal or fetal distress.[184] There is also agreement on delivery of such patients prior to 35 weeks' gestation in the presence of any of the following: premature rupture of membranes, labor, severe fetal growth retardation (<5th percentile for age). In this situation, appropriate management consists of parenteral medications to prevent convulsions, control of maternal blood pressure within a relatively safe range, and then induction of labor to achieve delivery.[113] If delivery of a preterm infant (<36 weeks' gestation) is anticipated at a level I or level II hospital, the mother should be transferred to a tertiary care center with adequate neonatal intensive facilities.

On the other hand, there is considerable disagreement about management of patients with severe disease prior to 34 weeks' gestation. Some authors consider delivery as the definitive therapy for all cases, regardless of gestational age, whereas others recommend prolonging pregnancy in all severe preeclamptic gestations remote from term until development of fetal lung maturity, fetal or maternal distress, or a gestational age of 34 to 36 weeks is achieved.[185–187] Some of the measures used in these latter cases have included one or more of the following: antihypertensive agents, diuretics, sedatives, chronic parenteral magnesium sulfate, plasma volume expanders, and antithrombotic agents.

Severe Preeclampsia at 28 to 32 Weeks' Gestation

There are several retrospective studies describing expectant management of women with severe preeclampsia at 28 to 32 weeks' gestation. The results of these studies were recently summarized by Schiff and associates.[184] In general, the findings of these studies suggest that expectant management improves outcome in a selective patient population.[184]

There are three randomized trials describing expectant management in patients with severe preeclampsia. In the first recent study, the results of individualized management were reported in 58 women with severe preeclampsia at 28 to 34 weeks' gestation.[188] These patients were treated initially with magnesium sulfate, hydralazine, and corticosteroids for fetal lung immaturity. All received intensive maternal and fetal care in a high-risk obstetric ward. Nonstress tests were done at least three times daily, and laboratory tests were evaluated at least twice weekly. Twenty of the 58 women were delivered because of maternal or fetal reasons within 48 hours after hospitalization. The remaining 38 were

then randomized to either aggressive or expectant management (N = 20). Patients assigned to the aggressive-management group, received steroids and were delivered within 72 hours. Patients assigned to the expectant-management group were treated with hydralazine to maintain blood pressure between 140/90 and 150/100 mmHg. In addition, they received frequent evaluations for maternal and fetal well-being. These patients were delivered at 34 weeks' gestation or before in the presence of maternal or fetal distress. The authors found lower neonatal complications and lower number of days spent in the neonatal intensive care unit in the expectant-management group.[189]

In a second study,[190] the randomized clinical trial was conducted in which patients with severe preeclampsia between 26 and 36 weeks' gestation were assigned to be treated with either nifedipine (N = 24) or hydralazine (N = 25). Patients assigned to the nifedipine group received 10 to 30 mg sublingually initially, then 40 to 120 mg/d orally. Those assigned to the hydralazine group received 6.25 to 12.5 mg intravenously initially. Maternal evaluation included frequent measurements of blood pressure, heart rate, platelet reflexes, urine output, and laboratory tests. Fetal evaluation included daily fetal heart rate monitoring, biophysical profile three times a week, and weekly ultrasonographic assessment of fetal growth. The authors found better control of blood pressure and a lower incidence of fetal distress in the group managed with nifedipine.[190] In addition, the group receiving nifedipine had a better perinatal outcome than those receiving hydralazine. They concluded that nifedipine is a safe and effective drug in the management of patients with severe preeclampsia remote from term.[190]

Sibai et al.[113] studied 95 women with severe preeclampsia at 28 to 32 weeks' gestation who were randomly assigned to either aggressive management (AM) (N = 46) or expectant management (EM) (N = 49).[113] The two groups were similar at the time of randomization with respect to several clinical and laboratory findings.

The average pregnancy prolongation in the EM group was 15.4 ± 6.6 days (range 4 to 36 days), which was significantly higher than the average in the AM group of 2.6 days ($p < 0.0001$, range 2 to 3 days). In the EM group, the average pregnancy prolongation period was not affected by the amount of proteinuria at randomization. Indications for delivery in the EM group were maternal reasons (N = 16), fetal compromise (N = 13), attainment of 34 weeks' gestation (N = 10), preterm labor or rupture of membranes (N = 7), or vaginal bleeding (N = 3). The maternal indications for delivery were thrombocytopenia (N = 5), uncontrolled severe hypertension (N = 3), headache/blurred vision

Table 28-14 Pregnancy Outcome

	Aggressive Management (N = 46)	Expectant Management (N = 49)	Significance
Gestational age at delivery (wk)	30.8 ± 1.7	32.9 ± 1.5	$p < 0.0001$
Placental weight (g)	355 ± 88	435 ± 117	$p < 0.01$
Birth weight (g)	1,233 ± 287	1,622 ± 360	$p = 0.0004$
Cesarean delivery (No., %)	39 (85)	36 (73)	NS
Abruptio placentae (No., %)	2 (4.3)	2 (4.1)	NS
HELLP syndrome (No., %)	1 (2.1)	2 (4.1)	NS
Postpartum stay (d)	5.3 ± 2.1	5.1 ± 1.9	NS

Abbreviations: NS, not significant; HELLP, hemolysis, elevated liver enzymes, and low platelets; d, days.

(N = 3), epigastric pain (N = 2), severe ascites (N = 1), and maternal demand (N = 2).

Table 28-14 compares the pregnancy outcomes in the two groups. Gestational age at delivery, placental weight, and birth weight were significantly higher in the EM group. The two cases of abruptio placentae in the AM group were found at time of cesarean delivery, whereas the two cases in the EM group were suspected because of abnormal fetal heart rate testing and vaginal bleeding. There were no cases of eclampsia, pulmonary edema, renal failure, or disseminated coagulopathy in either group.

No fetal or neonatal deaths occurred in either group. The number of infants admitted to a neonatal care unit (37 vs. 46 percent), average duration of stay in that unit (20 vs. 37 percent), and the frequency of respiratory distress syndrome (22 vs. 50 percent) and necrotizing enterocolitis (0 vs. 11 percent) were significantly lower in the EM group.[113]

Mid-Trimester Severe Preeclampsia

Severe preeclampsia developing in the mid-trimester is associated with high perinatal mortality and morbidity.[191,192] Aggressive management with immediate delivery will result in high neonatal mortality. In addition, all surviving neonates will develop significant neonatal complications and will require prolonged hospitalization in neonatal intensive care units. On the other hand, attempts to prolong pregnancy may result in fetal demise or asphyxiated damage in utero. Moreover, this management may expose the mother to severe morbidity and even mortality. The perinatal survival rate is usually poor when the disease develops before 24 weeks' gestation (2 percent); however, it is good when the disease occurs at or beyond 25 weeks' gestation.[191–193]

Sibai et al.[192] reviewed pregnancy outcome in 60 such patients who had had conservative management over a 7-year period. The mean gestational age at time of management was 24.8 weeks (range 17 to 27), and average days of pregnancy prolongation was 11.4 days

(range 2 to 40). The perinatal outcomes of these pregnancies were poor, with 31 of the 60 resulting in fetal demise and 21 ending in neonatal death, for a total perinatal mortality of 87 percent. In addition, maternal morbidity was significantly high. This study was retrospective, most patients were managed at level 1 hospitals, and few of these pregnancies had antepartum fetal evaluation.

Pattinson et al.[191] described the results of conservative management in 34 patients who had severe preeclampsia before 28 weeks. The patients were managed by bedrest, antihypertensive drugs, and intensive fetal and maternal monitoring. Eleven patients presented before 24 weeks, all of them resulting in perinatal deaths, and the remaining 34 were between 24 and 37 weeks' gestation, with 13 (38 percent) resulting in a surviving infant. Maternal complications included three cases (9 percent) of pulmonary edema and one case (3 percent) of pleural effusion.

Recently, Sibai et al.[193] described a new protocol for managing severe preeclampsia in the mid-trimester. The study included 109 patients with severe preeclampsia at 19 to 27 weeks gestation. All patients were first admitted to labor and delivery and were evaluated carefully for the presence of either maternal or fetal distress. Pregnancy termination was recommended for patients with gestation ages of 24 weeks or less (N = 25), whereas aggressive expectant management was recommended for patients with gestational age over 24 weeks (N = 84). Of the 25 patients with gestational age 24 weeks or less, 10 accepted termination and the other 15 elected to continue with their pregnancies. The latter patients were managed with bedrest, antihypertensive drugs, and frequent evaluation of maternal and fetal well-being. The average days of pregnancy prolongation in these 15 pregnancies was 19.4 days; 11 ended in stillbirths, and 3 resulted in neonatal deaths, for an overall perinatal survival of 6.7 percent. Of the 84 patients with gestational ages more than 24 weeks, 30 had immediate delivery either because of patient's desire or because of attending staff desire. These patients received magnesium sulfate, antihypertensive drugs, and steroids and then were delivered within 48 hours. The other 54 patients were managed conservatively with antihypertensive drugs and daily evaluation of maternal and fetal well-being. The conservative management group had significantly higher perinatal survival (64.5 versus 23.6 percent) and lower neonatal complications. In addition, the two groups had similar frequencies of maternal complications. They concluded that expectant management for women with severe preeclampsia should be selective and done only in a tertiary care center with adequate intensive care facilities.[193]

At the University of Tennessee, Memphis, patients with severe preeclampsia remote from term are admitted initially to the labor and delivery area for continuous evaluation of maternal and fetal conditions for at least 24 hours. Subsequent management is based on gestational age (Fig. 28-5). During observation, they receive continuous infusion of magnesium sulfate to prevent convulsions and bolus doses of hydralazine (5 to 10 mg), labetalol (20 to 40 mg), or oral nifedipine (10 mg) as needed to keep diastolic blood pressure below 110 mmHg. Maternal evaluation includes continuous monitoring of blood pressure, heart rate, urine output, cerebral status, and the presence of epigastric pain. Laboratory evaluation includes a platelet count and liver enzymes. Fetal evaluation includes continuous fetal heart monitoring, a biophysical profile, and ultrasonographic assessment of fetal growth. Patients with resistant severe hypertension or other signs of maternal or fetal deterioration are delivered within 24 hours, irrespective of gestational age or fetal lung maturity.[184] In addition, patients in labor, or those with fetuses with

a gestational age older than 35 weeks, and those with evidence of fetal lung maturity (by amniocentesis) at 33 to 35 weeks also are delivered within 24 hours.[184] Patients at 33 to 35 weeks' gestation with immature fluid receive steroids to accelerate fetal lung maturity and are delivered 24 hours after the last dose of steroids in the absence of any change in maternal or fetal condition.

It is a commonly held clinical impression that fetuses of preeclamptic women have accelerated lung maturation as a result of stress in utero. This phenomenon, however, has never been documented in a well-controlled study. The effect of hypertension during pregnancy on the incidence of neonatal respiratory distress syndrome is highly controversial.[194] Schiff and associates[194] compared fetal lung maturity indices in 127 preterm patients with preeclampsia and 127 normotensive controls matched by gestational age, race, and fetal gender. They found no differences in the incidences of immature result between the two groups. They concluded that fetuses of preeclamptic women do not exhibit accelerated lung maturation.[194]

Corticosteroids have been suggested as safe and effective drugs for preventing respiratory distress syndrome, treating thrombocytopenia, and improving perinatal outcome in severe preeclampsia. A review of the literature reveals substantial differences in methodology and drug selection among investigators who advocate the use of steroids for preeclampsia. This subject was recently reviewed by Sibai.[195] A patient may be considered suitable for steroid therapy if there is no evidence of maternal or fetal jeopardy and if delivery is not expected to occur within 48 hours. Maximum benefit is

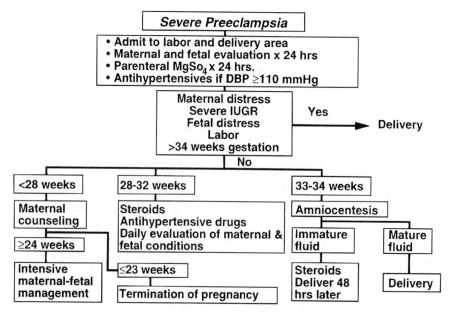

Fig. 28-5 University of Tennessee, Memphis, management plan for patients with severe preeclampsia.

achieved when steroid therapy is given in appropriate doses and the last dose is given at least 24 hours before delivery. Different regimens of steroids have been suggested for preventing respiratory distress syndrome, but we prefer betamethasone given as 12 mg as soon as possible and the dose repeated 24 hours later.

Patients at 28 to 32 weeks' gestation receive individualized management based on their clinical response during the observation period. All of these patients receive steroids to accelerate fetal lung maturity, as there is still benefit even if the delivery occurs less than 24 hours or more than 1 week later. Some demonstrate marked diuresis and improvement in blood pressure during the observation period. If the blood pressure remains below 100 mmHg diastolic (without antihypertensive therapy) after the observation period, magnesium sulfate is discontinued, and the patients are followed closely on the high-risk ward until fetal maturity is achieved. During hospitalization, they receive antihypertensive drugs (usually oral nifedipine 40 to 120 mg/d) to keep their diastolic blood pressure between 90 and 100 mmHg with daily evaluation of maternal and fetal well-being. In general, most of these patients will require delivery within 2 weeks.[113] However, some patients may continue their pregnancies for several weeks. It is important to note that such pregnancies should be managed at tertiary care centers because their courses are very unpredictable.

We believe that all women who meet the blood pressure criteria for preeclampsia should receive intravenous magnesium sulfate to prevent eclamptic convulsions.[196] Our rationale for this approach is the observation that, in most series of eclampsia, 20 percent of the women had only minimal blood pressure elevation, frequently without edema or proteinuria.

Magnesium sulfate is administered by a controlled continuous intravenous infusion with a loading dose of 6 g in 100 ml over 15 to 20 minutes. We believe that the intravenous route for magnesium therapy permits more precise control of the patient's blood level and avoids the pain of intramuscular injections. Maintenance therapy is given at a rate of 2 g in 100 ml of fluid per hour. Serum magnesium levels are obtained 4 to 6 hours later, with the rate of infusion adjusted to keep serum magnesium levels between 4.8 and 9.6 mg/dl (4 to 6 mEq/L). Treatment is continued for 24 hours postdelivery.

The magnesium ion goes beyond intracellular fluid and enters bones and cells as well.[197] Magnesium circulates largely unbound to protein and is excreted in the urine. Therefore, an accurate record of maternal urine output must be maintained. In patients with normal renal function, the half-life for magnesium excretion is about 4 hours. In the therapeutic range (4.8 to 9.6 mg/

Magnesium Toxicity	
Loss of patellar reflex	8–12 mg/dl
Feeling of warmth, flushing	9–12 mg/dl
Somnolence	10–12 mg/dl
Slurred speech	10–12 mg/dl
Muscular paralysis	15–17 mg/dl
Respiratory difficulty	15–17 mg/dl
Cardiac arrest	30–35 mg/dl

dl), magnesium sulfate slows neuromuscular conduction and depresses central nervous system irritability.

For this reason, maternal respiratory rate, deep tendon reflexes, and state of consciousness must be frequently monitored to detect magnesium toxicity. An ampule of calcium gluconate, 1 g (10 ml of 10 percent solution) should be drawn up in a syringe and clearly labeled and be kept at the bedside in case of magnesium toxicity. If magnesium toxicity is suspected, the infusion of magnesium sulfate should be discontinued. If respiratory depression occurs, the calcium gluconate should be given intravenously over 3 minutes. If respiratory arrest develops, the patient should receive mechanical ventilatory support as needed.

We carefully monitor the amount of intravenous fluids used in women with preeclampsia or eclampsia. Intake and output should be assessed hourly. We give a 5 percent dextrose in Ringer's lactate solution at 50 to 125 ml/h. A Foley catheter should be inserted to permit accurate evaluation of urine output. We are particularly cautious with women with chronic hypertension or renal disease. Frequently in the active phase of labor, urine output may drop below 30 ml/h. In those cases in which the cervix is continuing to dilate, we have not given a fluid challenge or diuretics. Typically in these women, urine output will increase to 30 ml/h after 2 to 3 hours. Our goal is to maintain the urine output at 30 ml/h. If urine output drops below 100 ml in 4 hours, the dose of magnesium sulfate and intravenous fluids should be reduced accordingly. Another cause of decreased urine output is a drop in maternal blood pressure due to the repeated injections of hydralazine. Hydralazine has a relatively long duration of action and, when multiple bolus injections of hydralazine are used to control blood pressure, the diastolic blood pressure may be reduced more than intended, that is, below 90 mmHg. This will frequently reduce urine output for 2 to 3 hours. One of the potential problems when attempting to limit intravenous fluids to 125 ml/h is that high concentrations of drugs must be used if the woman is receiving intravenous magnesium sulfate, oxytocin, and hydralazine.

To control severe maternal hypertension intrapartum, we use bolus injections of hydralazine 5 to 10 mg every 20 to 30 minutes to lower the diastolic blood pressure to 90 to 100 mmHg range. This requires monitoring of blood pressure every 5 minutes for at least 30 minutes after the drug is given. Recently, Patterson-Brown and associates reported on 70 women with severe preeclampsia who received bolus injections of hydralazine for the treatment of sustained severe hypertension (mean arterial pressure greater than 125 mmHg for 45 minutes or greater than 140 mmHg for 15 minutes).[198] Each treatment episode consisted of hydralazine 5 mg given as intravenous bolus dose, repeated after 15-minute intervals until the mean arterial pressure fell below 125 mmHg, up to a maximum of three boluses. All women received 400- to 500-ml albumin solution (5 percent) over 20 minutes prior to hydralazine. They found that this protocol was effective in lowering maternal blood pressure in 89 percent of the cases. In addition, they found no significant maternal or fetal side effects from such therapy. They concluded that hydralazine given in 5-mg boluses is a safe and effective method of treating severe hypertension in preeclampsia.[198] An alternative regimen is to use bolus injections of labetalol hydrochloride 20 to 50 mg. Unlike hydralazine, labetalol does not cause maternal tachycardia, flushing, or headaches. We have found this drug to be safe and effective in the management of these patient.[199] Other potent antihypertensive medications such as sodium nitroprusside, diazoxide, or nitroglycerine are rarely needed in the management of these patients. Diuretics such as furosemide are not used except in the presence of pulmonary edema.[200]

Anesthesia in Severe Preeclampsia

Maternal analgesia can be provided by the intermittent use of small doses (25 to 50 mg) of intravenous meperidine or segmental epidural analgesia. Local infiltration anesthesia with or without pudendal block or epidural can be used for all cases of vaginal delivery for patients with mild disease. In addition, continuous epidural anesthesia or balanced general anesthesia can be used for all cesarean deliveries. The use of epidural anesthesia for patients with severe preeclampsia eclampsia is controversial. It is important to emphasize that the administration of epidural requires the availability of personnel with special expertise in obstetric anesthesia. In addition, in selected cases it requires the availability of central hemodynamic monitoring, since infusions of large amounts of crystalloids or colloids are usually used as precautionary measures before its administra-

tion. Moreover, the use of conduction anesthesia is contraindicated in the presence of fetal distress or in the presence of coagulopathy.

On the other hand, significant hypertension and tachycardia are frequently observed after laryngoscopy and endotracheal intubation in patients undergoing general anesthesia. Transient but severe hypertension after tracheal intubation can result in a significant increase in maternal intracranial pressures with the dangers of cerebral edema and hemorrhage and increased afterload with the dangers of pulmonary edema. These responses can be prevented or attenuated by the use of labetalol prior to endotracheal intubation. Labetalol should be used in a dose of 20 mg intravenously followed by 10 mg increments up to a total dose of 1 mg/kg.[201]

Ramanathan and associates[202] conducted a prospective evaluation of the hemodynamic and neuroendocrine stress responses at time of cesarean delivery in 21 women with severe preeclampsia (11 received epidural anesthesia and 10 received general anesthesia). The authors found that epidural anesthesia caused blunting of the hemodynamic and neuroendocrine stress responses to cesarean delivery in women with severe preeclampsia. The findings support the concept that epidural anesthesia should be the method of choice in these women.

For patients with the HELLP syndrome, the use of pudendal block or epidural anesthesia is contraindicated since these patients are at risk of bleeding into these areas. In case of cesarean delivery, platelet transfusions are usually indicated to correct severe thrombocytopenia. Our policy is to transfuse 10 units of platelets in all patients with a platelet count less than $50 \times 10^3/mm^3$ prior to intubation. Generalized oozing from the operative site is very common, and, to minimize the risk of hematoma formation, we recommend that a subfascial drain be used, the bladder flap be left open, and the wound be left open with sutures in situ above the fascia. All these wounds can be successfully closed within 72 hours. Failure to adhere to these recommendations will result in 25 percent incidence of hematoma formation.[127]

Some investigators recommended the use of invasive hemodynamic monitoring in managing patients with severe preeclampsia. Clark and Cotton[203] reported that indications for such monitoring should include pulmonary edema, persistent oliguria unresponsive to fluid challenge, intractable severe hypertension, and in some patients requiring epidural anesthesia. Other authors recommended using Swan-Ganz catheters to monitor fluid therapy and response to antihypertensive drugs. These authors recommended plasma volume expansion with colloid plasma substitute to increase cardiac index and pulmonary capillary wedge pressure prior to the use of epidural or vasodilator drugs in an attempt to avoid the potential of severe hypotension.[156,158]

We believe that the use of invasive hemodynamic monitoring is rarely indicated in the management of these patients. Its use for the above indications is empiric, and its benefit has not been conclusively proven. We believe that only a select group of women with pulmonary edema may benefit from invasive hemodynamic monitoring.[153,204]

Management

If the patient is already in spontaneous labor, continuous electronic fetal heart rate and uterine activity monitoring should be instituted in all cases. If labor is not well established, and in the absence of fetal malpresentation or distress, intravenous oxytocin should be administered to induce labor. This approach is used in all patients with favorable cervix and all patients with gestational age at 30 weeks or more irrespective of cervical status. In patients with unripe cervix and gestation age of less than 30 weeks, elective cesarean delivery is the method of choice for all patients with severe preeclampsia eclampsia. This approach is based on our experience of a high incidence of intrapartum complications such as abruptio placentae, fetal growth retardation, and fetal. distress in these patients. Alternatively, these women may be induced with PGE_2 gel followed by oxytocin, if needed.

At delivery, blood loss may be increased above that expected in normal patients. Magnesium sulfate may impair uterine contractility after delivery. The woman with severe preeclampsia or eclampsia has a contracted blood volume and tolerates blood loss poorly. These patients should have blood typed and cross-matched and available in the delivery area A sudden drop in blood pressure following delivery may be due to hypovolemia.

Following delivery, the patient should be kept in the recovery room under close observation for about 12 to 24 hours, during which magnesium sulfate should be continued. Most patients will show evidence of resolution of the disease process within 24 hours. However, some patients, especially those with the HELLP syndrome or severe disease in the mid-trimester, might require intensive monitoring for several days. Such patients will require magnesium sulfate administration for more than 24 hours. These patients are at increased risk for the development of pulmonary edema from fluid overload, fluid mobilization, and compromised renal function.[146]

Maternal and Perinatal Outcome with Preeclampsia

Perinatal outcome in preeclampsia is usually dependent on one or more of the following factors: gestational age at onset of preeclampsia and at time of delivery, severity of disease process, presence of multiple gestation, and the presence of underlying hypertensive or renal disease. For patients with mild disease at term, the perinatal mortality, incidence of fetal growth retardation, and neonatal morbidity are similar to those of normotensive pregnancies. At the E.H. Crump Women's Hospital in Memphis, the perinatal mortality rate in these pregnancies is 1/1,000, and the incidence of fetal growth retardation is only 4 percent.

Long et al.[14] reported the pregnancy outcome in 2,434 singleton pregnancies with preeclampsia during a 7-year period (1971 to 1978). They found that patients with preterm preeclampsia (<37 weeks) had a worse perinatal outcome than those with preeclampsia at 37 weeks or later. In the preterm group, the perinatal mortality was 10.5 percent, the incidence of fetal growth retardation was 18.2 percent, and the incidence of abruptio placentae was 4.5 percent. In contrast for women with term preeclampsia, the respective incidences were 0.6, 5.6, and 0.4 percent. In a subsequent report, Long and Oats[15] reported that in patients with twin pregnancy preeclampsia tends to develop earlier in gestation, and the maternal disease is usually more severe than it is in singleton pregnancies. Thus, the perinatal outcome for twins in preeclampsia is worse than that in singleton pregnancy.

Severe preeclampsia is a major cause of maternal mortality and morbidity. Complicated or mismanaged cases are responsible for most deaths. Patients with onset in midtrimester and those with the HELLP syndrome and pulmonary edema are at significant risk for maternal mortality and morbidity.[205]

Counseling Women Who Have Had Preeclampsia in Prior Pregnancies

There appears to be a strong familial predisposition for preeclampsia. The incidence of severe preeclampsia was compared in the first pregnancies of sisters of primigravidas with and without preeclampsia.[206] In 273 primigravidas whose sisters did not have preeclampsia, the incidence of severe preeclampsia was 4.5 percent. The incidence of severe preeclampsia was 13.8 percent for women whose sisters had severe preeclampsia during their first pregnancies. The incidence of severe preeclampsia in the mothers and mothers-in-law of women in whom preeclampsia developed during their first pregnancies has been examined as well. The incidence of severe preeclampsia was 15.9 percent in the 126 mothers of primigravidas who had severe preeclampsia compared with a 4.4 percent incidence of severe preeclampsia in the 136 mothers-in-law. The incidence of severe preeclampsia in a control group of primigravidas was 3.1 percent. The incidence of mild preeclampsia was higher in the mothers than in the mothers-in-law of these women, but this difference was not significant.

We have examined the pregnancy outcomes and incidences of preeclampsia in subsequent pregnancies, as well as the incidences of chronic hypertension and diabetes in women who had severe preeclampsia (287 women) or eclampsia (119 women) in their first pregnancies (aged 11 to 25 years) compared with 409 women (aged 12 to 25 years) who remained normotensive during their first pregnancies. Each woman had at least one subsequent pregnancy (range 1 to 11) and was followed for a minimum of 2 years (range 2 to 24). There was no significant difference in the incidences of diabetes mellitus in the two groups (1.3 vs, 1.5 percent). The incidence of chronic hypertension was significantly higher in the preeclampsia group (14.8 vs. 5.6 percent; $p < 0.001$). This difference became even greater for those women followed for more than 10 years (51 vs. 14 percent; $p < 0.001$). The incidence of severe preeclampsia was also significantly higher in the second pregnancies (25.9 to 4.6 percent) as well as in the subsequent pregnancies (12.2 to 5.0 percent) of women with preeclampsia.[207]

In a later report, subsequent pregnancy outcome and long-term prognosis was studied in 108 women who had severe preeclampsia in the second trimester.[208] These women were followed for a minimum of 2 years (range 2 to 12 years) and had a total of 169 subsequent pregnancies. Fifty-nine (35 percent) subsequent pregnancies were normotensive, and 110 (65 percent) were complicated by preeclampsia. Overall, 21 percent of all subsequent pregnancies were complicated by severe preeclampsia in the second trimester. In addition, these women had a high incidence of chronic hypertension on follow-up, with the highest incidence being in those who had recurrent severe preeclampsia in the second trimester (55 percent).

Some women with preeclampsia remote from term may have abruptio placentae. The risk of this complication is increased significantly in those with severe preeclampsia before 34 weeks' gestation and particularly in those who have severe preeclampsia in the second trimester.[209] For patients with preeclampsia complicated by abruptio placentae, the risk of subsequent abruptio ranges from 5 to 20 percent. In addition, these women are at increased risk for subsequent chronic hypertension.[209]

Pregnancy outcome and long-term prognosis were studied in 37 women with severe preeclampsia complicated by pulmonary edema, and 18 of these women had subsequent pregnancies.[200] Ten of the 18 were normotensive, four were complicated by chronic hypertension, and four (22 percent) were complicated by preeclampsia; one of the latter women also had pulmonary edema.

Pregnancy outcome and remote prognosis also were studied in 18 women with severe preeclampsia complicated by acute renal failure.[210] All 18 had acute tubular necrosis, 9 required dialysis, and 2 died within 8 weeks postpartum. All patients had serial evaluation of renal function, urine microscopic testing, and electrolyte studies at the onset of acute renal failure and during follow-up. All 16 surviving patients had normal renal function on long-term follow-up (average 4 years). Four of the 16 women had 7 subsequent pregnancies: 1 ended in miscarriage, 1 was complicated by preeclampsia at 35 weeks, and 5 were term pregnancies without complications.[210]

Patients with preeclampsia and the HELLP syndrome can receive oral contraceptives without any risk of developing the syndrome again.[211] In addition, the recurrence risk for this syndrome in subsequent pregnancies is very small. Sibai and associates[211] followed 152 patients with previous HELLP syndrome through their subsequent pregnancies. Thirteen patients with preexisting chronic hypertension had 20 subsequent pregnancies, whereas 139 normotensive women had 192 subsequent pregnancies following HELLP. The outcomes of these pregnancies are listed in Table 28-15. Overall, the risk for recurrent HELLP syndrome was 5 percent in women with preexisting chronic hypertension and 3 percent in normotensive women.[211] Two women with previous ruptured liver hematomas were followed through three subsequent pregnancies without complications. Two other case reports described successful pregnancy outcomes in women with previous ruptured liver hematomas.[212,213]

Patients with preeclampsia remote from term are reportedly at increased risk for undiagnosed renal disease. In one report, renal function was studied 6 weeks to 6 months postpartum in 84 women who had severe preeclampsia at 24 to 36 weeks' gestation.[214] Maternal evaluation included a 24-hour urine study, urine microscopic testing, intravenous pyelography, and renal biopsy when appropriate. The authors found a high incidence of renal disease and essential chronic hypertension (90 percent) in these women. In two-thirds of the women studied, the renal lesion was glomerulonephritis, mostly of the immunoglobulin A variety. They concluded that women with severe preeclampsia remote from term may have underlying renal disease for which they should be evaluated after delivery.

Eclampsia

Eclampsia is the occurrence of convulsions or coma unrelated to other cerebral conditions with signs and symptoms of preeclampsia. Early writings of both the Egyptians and Chinese warned of the dangers of con-

Table 28-15   Subsequent Pregnancy Outcome after HELLP Syndrome in the Index Pregnancy

	Normotensive (N = 139)	Hypertensive (N = 13)	Significance
Pregnancies (No.)	192	20	
Normotensive (%)[a]	73	—	
Hypertension only (%)	8	25	$p = 0.09$
Preeclampsia (%)	19	75	$p < 0.001$
Mild (%)	11	15	$p = 0.48$
Severe (%)	6	55	$p < 0.001$
HELLP (%)	3	5	$p = 0.45$
Delivery <37 weeks (%)	21	80	$p < 0.001$
IUGR (<10th percentile) (%)	12	45	$p < 0.001$
Abruptio placentae (%)	2	20	$p = 0.002$
Perinatal death (%)	4	40	$p < 0.001$

Abbreviations: HELLP, hemolysis, elevated liver enzymes, low platelets; IUGR, intrauterine growth restriction.

[a] Percentage of pregnancies.

(From Sibai et al,[211] with permission.)

vulsions encountered during pregnancy.[215] Hippocrates noted that headaches, convulsions, and drowsiness were ominous signs associated with pregnancy. The term *eclampsia* appeared in a treatise on gynecology written by Varandaeus in 1619. Clonic spasms in association with pregnancy were described by Pew in 1694. In 1772, De la Motte recognized that prompt delivery of pregnant women with convulsions favored their recovery. Stroganoff, in 1900, reported a 5.4 percent maternal mortality rate compared with 17 to 29 percent for European clinics and 21 to 49 percent for American clinics of the same period.[216] Stroganoff placed his patients in a darkened room and administered chloroform, chloral hydrate, and morphine to produce profound sedation and narcosis. Modifications were made in this regimen; eventually, magnesium sulfate was popularized by Pritchard and Zuspan as the drug of choice for eclampsia.

Pathophysiology

Although great advances have been made in treating eclampsia, the pathophysiologic events leading to convulsions remain unknown. Several theories have been advanced but are unproved. There is a functional derangement of multiple organ systems, such as the central nervous system and hematologic, hepatic, renal, and cardiovascular systems.[217] The degree of dysfunction depends not only on other medical or obstetric factors that may be present but on whether there has been a delay in the treatment of preeclampsia or iatrogenic complicating factors as well. These organ system derangements are summarized below.

Women in whom eclampsia develops exhibit a wide spectrum of signs and symptoms, ranging from extremely high blood pressure, 4+ proteinuria, general-

ized edema, and 4+ patellar reflexes to minimal blood pressure elevation, no proteinuria or edema, and normal reflexes.

Eclampsia usually begins as a gradual process, starting with rapid weight gain and ending with the onset

Organ System Derangements in Eclampsia

Cardiovascular
  Generalized vasospasm
  Increased peripheral vascular resistance
  Increased left ventricular stroke work index
  Decreased central venous pressure
  Decreased pulmonary wedge pressure

Hematologic
  Decreased plasma volume
  Increased blood viscosity
  Hemoconcentration
  Coagulopathy

Renal
  Decreased glomerular filtration rate
  Decreased renal plasma flow
  Decreased uric acid clearance

Hepatic (at autopsy)
  Periportal necrosis
  Hepatocellular damage
  Subcapsular hematoma

Central nervous system (at autopsy)
  Cerebral edema
  Cerebral hemorrhage

of generalized convulsions or coma. Excess weight gain (with or without clinical edema) of more than 2 pounds per week during the last trimester may be the first warning sign. Hypertension is the hallmark of eclampsia and excess weight gain or edema are not necessary for the diagnosis.[7] In about 20 percent of cases, hypertension may be "relative" (130 to 140/80 to 90 mmHg), signified by any rise in blood pressure that is 30 mmHg systolic or 15 mmHg diastolic above the nonpregnant blood pressure reading. Eclampsia is usually associated with significant proteinuria (>2+ on dipstick). In eclamptic women, headache, visual disturbances, and right upper quadrant/epigastric pain are the most common premonitory symptoms before convulsions. Of interest was the absence of edema (32 percent) and proteinuria (19 percent) in 254 eclamptic women studied by the author.[7]

Convulsions may occur antepartum, intrapartum, or postpartum. One-half of cases of eclampsia usually occur before the onset of labor, with the other 50 percent equally divided between the intrapartum and postpartum periods. Analysis of 254 cases of eclampsia managed at our institution revealed that eclampsia developed before delivery in 181 patients (71 percent) and postpartum in 73 (29 percent).[7] Although rare, atypical eclampsia may occur before the 20th week of gestation and more than 48 hours after delivery.[218,219] Table 28-16 summarizes the time of onset of eclampsia among 254 eclamptic women studied by the author.[7]

Eclampsia is primarily a disease of the young primigravida. The incidence of eclampsia has ranged from 1:147 to 1:3,448 pregnancies,[220,221] with an incidence of 3.6 percent in twin gestations.[15] The incidence depends on the socioeconomic status of the patient population and the number of maternal referrals to the hospital. At the University of Mississippi Medical Center, the incidence of eclampsia was 1:147 for 1955 to 1960 and 1:254 for 1971 to mid-1973.[220] Of interest, only 7.2 percent of these patients received prenatal care in the medical center's prenatal clinics. The incidence of eclampsia at the E. H. Crump Women's Hospital is now 1:337 deliveries; however, the hospital has a large number of referrals (approximately 2,000 women annu-

Table 28-17   Incidence of Eclampsia

Institution	Patient Population	Incidence
University of Tennessee (Memphis)		
1960–1970	All	1:300
1977–1992	All	1:337
University of Mississippi		
1955–1960	All	1:147
1971–mid-1973	All	1:254
University of Virginia		
1938–1963	All	1:235
1970–1976	All	1:623
Parkland Memorial Hospital		
1955–1975	All	1:766
Athens General (Athens, GA)		
1966–1975	All	1:1,228

ally).[219] Table 28-17 shows the incidences of eclampsia reported from several institutions.

Cerebral Pathology of Eclampsia

Autoregulation of the cerebral circulation is a mechanism for the maintenance of constant cerebral blood flow during changes in blood pressure and may be altered in eclampsia. Through active changes in cerebrovascular resistance at the arteriolar level, cerebral blood flow normally remains relatively constant when cerebral perfusion pressure ranges between 60 and 120 mmHg. In this normal range, vasoconstriction of cerebral vessels occurs in response to elevations in blood pressure, while vasodilation occurs as blood pressure is lowered. Once cerebral perfusion pressure exceeds 130 to 150 mmHg, however, the autoregulatory mechanism fails. In extreme hypertension, the normal compensatory vasoconstriction may become defective and cerebral blood flow increases. As a result, segments of the vessels become dilated, ischemic, and increasingly permeable. Thus, exudation of plasma occurs, giving rise to focal cerebral edema and compression of vessels, resulting in a decreased cerebral blood flow.[222] Hypertensive encephalopathy (a possible model for eclampsia) is an acute clinical condition that results from abrupt severe hypertension and subsequent severe increases in intracranial pressure. Since this is an acute disturbance in the hemodynamics of cerebral arterioles, morphologic changes in anatomy may not be uniformly evident in pathology material. Several autopsy findings that are relatively constant include cerebral swelling and fibrinoid necrosis of vessel walls. Petechinal hemorrhages and microinfarcts may appear in some cases, not disimilar to those noted in eclampsia.

The mechanisms leading to the development of convulsions or coma in eclamptic patients may include cerebral edema, ischemia, hemorrhage or transient vaso-

Table 28-16   Gestational Age at Onset of Convulsions (N = 254)

Weeks' Gestation	Total Cases No.	%	Postpartum Cases (N)
≤20	6	2.4	0
21–26	8	3.2	1
27–36	125	49.2	32
37–41	115	45.2	40

spasm. However, none of these mechanisms has been conclusively proven.

Computerized Axial Tomography

The introduction of the computerized axial tomography (CT scan) has provided an opportunity to investigate the nature of cerebral abnormalities in eclamptic patients. This technique is considered safe in pregnancy when performed beyond the first trimester. There are several reports describing the CT scan findings in complicated cases of eclampsia. The reported abnormal CT scan findings in complicated eclampsia are summarized in below.[222,223]

Cerebral hemorrhage is a common autopsy finding in patients dying from eclampsia; however, it is an unusual finding on CT scanning. Beck and Menezes[224] reported a case of eclampsia in which CT scan evaluation demonstrated the presence of periventricular subependymal hemorrhage. Colosimo et al.[225] reported abnormal CT scan findings in five eclamptic women, one of whom demonstrated the presence of intracerebral hemorrhage. Will et al.[226] reported on three patients with eclampsia who developed acute neurologic deterioration in the postpartum period. Two patients had subarachoid hemorrhage and one of them had residual neurologic deficit. CT scan demonstrated the presence of infarcts in two cases and intracerebral hemorrhage in the third case. In all three cases, cerebral angiography revealed widespread arterial vasoconstriction. In the one case demonstrating hemorrhage on CT scan, an MRI examination performed 1 week later was reported normal.

Reported CT Scan Findings in Complicated Eclampsia

Cerebral Edema
  Diffuse white matter low-density areas
  Patchy areas of low density
  Occipital white matter edema
  Loss of normal cortical sulci
  Reduced ventricular size
  Acute hydrocephalus

Cerebral hemorrhage
  Intraventricular hemorrhage
  Parenchymal hemorrhage (high density)

Cerebral infarction
  Low-attenuation areas
  Basal ganglia infarctions

(From Barton and Sibai,[222] with permission.)

Sibai et al.[227] studied the CT scan findings in 20 patients with atypical eclampsia. Three patients had transient neurologic deficit, three experienced transient cortical blindness, one was in a deep comatose state, and the others had either late postpartum eclampsia or early onset eclampsia. The CT scan findings were normal in all 20 studies.[227] In contrast, Richards et al.[228] described the cranial CT scan findings in 20 patients remaining in a coma for 6 hours or more after delivery from a total of 192 patients with eclampsia. Scan appearance was normal in five patients (25 percent) while the remaining 15 patients (75 percent) had scans demonstrating low density areas consistent with cerebral edema of varying degrees. A low density pattern diffusely distributed throughout the white matter was regarded as the most severe form of edema. Three of four patients with this specific finding had significantly elevated intracranial pressure during monitoring.

Three large series presenting the CT scan findings in eclampsia were reported. Abnormal CT scan findings were found in 14 (29 percent) of 49 eclamptic patients studied by Brown and associates.[229] These authors noted that the incidence of abnormal CT scan findings significantly increased with the recent use of high resolution CT scan equipment. The CT scans were performed over a 6-year period, with the highest incidence of abnormal findings (50 percent) being present during the final year of the study. This increased sensitivity was attributed to improved "fourth generation" imaging equipment. Furthermore, they noted that 50 to 60 percent of scans performed within 2 days of a seizure were abnormal, implying rapid reversal of abnormalities detected by CT scan. The authors noted, however, that CT scan findings altered the clinical management in only one patient. Milliez et al.[230] reported on cranial CT scans in 44 women with eclampsia performed within 24 hours of seizure. Twenty-six scans (59 percent) were considered normal, while three (7 percent) had evidence of cerebral hemorrhage or thrombosis and six (14 percent) revealed areas of localized hypodensity located in the cortical lobes and the subcortical white matter. Of the remaining nine scans (20 percent), the interpretation was of minimal cerebral atrophy with enlarging cerebral ventricles. Moodley and associates[231] reported on cranial CT scan findings in 31 women with eclampsia. Ten of these women also had focal neurologic findings. Fourteen (45 percent) of the scans were considered abnormal.

Magnetic Resonance Imaging and Eclampsia

Magnetic resonance imaging (MRI) is a recently developed noninvasive technique that appears superior to other processes for defining intracranial anatomy and pathophysiology. The technique provides images in multiple planes, avoids the use of ionizing radiation, and, except for selected contraindications (some aneurysm clips, pace makers), there are no significant health risks associated with MRI when used at present operating conditions.

There are several case reports describing abnormal MRI findings in eclampsia.[232,233] In addition, there are three large series describing MRI findings in eclampsia. Sanders et al.[234] studied MRI findings in eight women with eclampsia. Abnormal findings were reported in seven of the eight women. Digre and associates[233] studied MRI findings in 16 women with severe preeclampsia and 10 women with eclampsia. They found that half of the women with severe preeclampsia had abnormal scans with nonspecific foci of increased signal in the deep cerebral white matter on T_2-weighted images. In contrast, nine women with eclampsia had abnormal findings in the form of either a multifocal area of increased signal at the grey-white matter junction on T_2-weighted images or cortical edema and hemorrhage. Dahmus et al.[223] compared MRI and CT scan findings in 24 women with eclampsia. Forty-six percent of the MRIs were abnormal and 33 percent of the CT scans were abnormal. The authors concluded that cerebral imaging is not necessary in women with uncomplicated eclampsia.[223]

Angiography and Eclampsia

The use of cerebral angiography in the evaluation of eclampsia is limited.[232] Will et al.[226] described the cerebral angiographic findings in three patients with preeclampsia/eclampsia. All were significant for widespread arterial vasoconstriction of the intracranial vessels. Trommer et al.[235] reported cerebral angiography findings in a single eclamptic patient. Similarly, they reported diffuse vasospasm of large- and medium-caliber cerebral vessels. Cranial CT obtained following the angiography revealed diffuse hypodensity throughout the brainstem, thalamus, and internal capsules bilaterally. These few studies support cerebral vasoconstriction as an important cause of neurologic complications in preeclampsia. Similar findings were also reported with the use of cerebral and retinal vascular Doppler flow studies.[236]

EEG Findings

Abnormal electroencephalograms (EEGs) have been reported in women with eclampsia.[222] Most common were changes compatible with a recent convulsive state. We have performed EEGs on 65 women with eclampsia.[227] Initial EEGs were obtained within 48 hours of hospitalization and then serially during the next 6 months. Three women also had normal cerebral arteriograms. Forty-nine of the 65 patients with eclampsia (75 percent) had abnormal findings. We previously reported that 7 of 14 women with preeclampsia (50 percent) and 2 of 13 normotensive women (15 percent) had abnormal EEGs. All patients had adequate serum magnesium levels (4.5 to 11 mg/dl). Five of the 65 women demonstrated seizure activity on EEG with serum magnesium levels in the therapeutic range. It appears that magnesium suppresses seizure activity by a mechanism other than one that alters the EEG. All the abnormalities noted on EEG are nonspecific and have been reported in other conditions such as polycythemia, hypoxia, renal disease, hypocalcemia, hypercalcemia, and water intoxication.[237]

Abnormal EEG findings were also reported in 90 percent of eclamptic women studied by Moodley and associates.[231] EEG abnormalities have been reported to be directly related to the severity of maternal hypertension in eclampsia, with some abnormal EEGs becoming normal after lowering blood pressure to the normotensive range. We found no correlation between the degree of blood pressure elevation and EEG abnormalities and consider it unlikely that these abnormal EEG changes were due to hypertensive encephalopathy alone.[237]

Management of Labor and Delivery in Eclampsia

The woman with eclampsia should undergo continuous intensive monitoring. She should not be left alone in a darkened room. The guard rails should be up on the bed and a padded tongue blade kept at the bedside. A large-bore peripheral intravenous line should be in place. No other anticonvulsants should be left at the bedside except for a syringe containing 2 to 4 g magnesium sulfate. Control of convulsions with magnesium sulfate is outlined below. We agree with Pritchard et al.[238] that no more than 8 g magnesium sulfate should be given over a short period of time to control convulsions.

No single test or set of laboratory determinations is useful in predicting maternal or neonatal outcome in women with eclampsia. Alterations in renal or hepatic function occur frequently. There is unlikely to be a significant disturbance in the integrity of the coagulation system. We previously recommended only a complete blood count (including blood smear and platelet count), clot observation, and serum creatinine in women with eclampsia.[239] Liver function tests were obtained only in women with upper abdominal pain. However, because of an increase in the number of women with HELLP syndrome and eclampsia as well as those with serious medical problems, we have expanded the laboratory tests ordered in eclamptic women to include fibrinogen, electrolytes, and arterial blood gases.

Once convulsions have been controlled and the woman has regained consciousness, her general medical condition is assessed. When she is stable, induction of labor with oxytocin is initiated. Delivery is the treatment for eclampsia. Fetal heart rate and intensity of uterine contractions should be closely monitored. If labor is not well established, and in the absence of fetal malpresentation or fetal distress, oxytocin may be used to induce labor in all patients beyond 30 weeks' gestations irrespective of cervical dilatation or effacement. The same approach is used for patients with a gestational age below 30 weeks if the cervix is favorable for induction. However, women with an unfavorable cervix and a gestational age of 30 weeks or less are stabilized with magnesium sulfate and are then delivered electively by cesarean section. This approach is based on our previous experience with high intrapartum complication rates in eclampsia that develops before 30 weeks gestation.[240] These complications include a high incidence of fetal growth retardation (30 percent), abruption (23 percent), and fetal distress during labor (65 percent).

In a review of 10 women who had undergone electronic internal fetal monitoring during an eclamptic convulsion, six had fetal bradycardia (fetal heart rate below 120 beats/min) that varied in duration from 30 seconds to 9 minutes.[241] The interval from onset of the seizure to the fall in fetal heart rate was 5 minutes. Transitory fetal tachycardia occurred frequently after the prolonged bradycardia. In addition, loss of beat-to-beat variability with transitory late decelerations occurred during the recovery phase.

Uterine hyperactivity demonstrated by both increased uterine tone and increased frequency of uterine contractions occurs during an eclamptic seizure. The duration of the increased uterine activity varies from 2 to 14 minutes.

Fetal outcome is generally good after an eclamptic convulsion. The mechanism for the transitory fetal distress may be a decrease in uterine blood flow caused by intense vasospasm and uterine hyperactivity. The absence of maternal respiration during the convulsion may also be a contributing factor to these fetal heart rate changes. Since the fetal heart rate pattern usually returns to normal after a convulsion, other conditions should be considered if an abnormal pattern persists. It may take longer for the heart rate pattern to return to baseline in an eclamptic woman whose fetus is preterm and growth retarded. Placental abruption may occur after the convulsion and should be considered if uterine hyperactivity remains or the bradycardia persists.

Treatment of Eclamptic Convulsions

Eclamptic convulsions are a life-threatening emergency and require proper care in order to minimize morbidity and mortality. The development of an eclamptic convulsion is frightening to observe. Initially, the patient's face becomes distorted with protrusion of the eyes. This is followed by a congested facial expression. Foam often exudes from the mouth. The woman usually bites her tongue unless it is protected. Respirations are absent throughout the seizure. Typically, the convulsion, which can be divided into two phases, will continue for 60 to 75 seconds. The first phase, which lasts 15 to 20 seconds, begins with facial twitching, proceeding to the body becoming rigid with generalized muscular contractions. The second phase lasts approximately 60 seconds and consists of the muscles of the body alternately contracting and relaxing in rapid succession. This phase begins with the muscles of the jaw and rapidly involves the eyelids, other facial muscles, and then all the muscles of the body. Coma follows the convulsion and the woman usually remembers nothing of the recent events. If she has repeated convulsions, some degree of consciousness returns after each convulsion. She may enter a combative state and be very agitated and difficult to control. Rapid and deep respirations usually begin as soon as the convulsions end. Maintenance of oxygenation is usually not a problem after a single convulsion; the risk of aspiration is low in the well-managed patient.

Several steps should be taken in managing an eclamptic convulsion:

1. *Do not attempt to shorten or abolish the initial convulsion:* Because eclampsia is so frightening, the natural tendency is to do something to abolish the convulsion. Drugs such as diazepam should not be given in an attempt to stop or shorten the convulsion, especially if the patient does not have an intravenous line in place and someone skilled in intubation is not immediately available. Diazepam causes phlebitis and venous thrombosis and should not be given without secure intravenous access. In addition, no more than 5 mg should be given over a 60-second period. Rapid administration of diazepam may lead to apnea or cardiac arrest, or both.[242]

2. *Prevent maternal injury during the convulsion:* A padded tongue blade should be inserted between the patient's teeth to prevent biting of the tongue. Care should be taken to avoid stimulating the gag reflex with the blade. Its only purpose is to prevent the patient from biting her tongue. Place the woman on her left side and then suction the foam and secretions from her mouth. That serious maternal injuries may occur during eclamptic seizures is well demonstrated

in the report from Magee-Women's Hospital.[243] Among the 52 women with eclampsia, one had a dislocated shoulder, fractured humerus, and multiple facial contusions from a fall in the emergency room following a convulsion. Two other women had severe airway obstruction.

3. *Maintain adequate oxygenation:* After the convulsion has ceased, the patient begins to breathe again and oxygenation is rarely a problem. Difficulty with oxygenation may occur in women who have had repetitive convulsions or who have received drugs in an attempt to abolish the convulsions. Such women should have a chest radiograph to rule out aspiration pneumonia.

4. *Minimize the risk of aspiration:* Aspiration should be a rare occurrence with eclamptic convulsions. It may be caused by forcing the padded tongue blade to the back of the throat, stimulating the gag reflex with resultant vomiting and aspiration. At our hospital, all the women who have had aspiration as a result of eclamptic convulsions had received many drugs in an attempt to control their convulsions. The lungs should always be auscultated after the convulsion has ended to ensure they are clear.

5. *Give adequate magnesium sulfate to control the convulsions:* As soon as the convulsion has ended, a large secure IV line should be inserted and a loading dose of magnesium sulfate given intravenously. In our institution, we use a 6-g intravenous loading dose given over *15 to 20 minutes*. In addition to providing a good initial serum magnesium level, the serum magnesium level does not fall below the therapeutic range for several hours after the initial 6-g loading dose as often happens when using a 4-g loading dose. If the patient has a convulsion after the loading dose, another bolus of 2 g magnesium sulfate can be given intravenously over 3 to 5 minutes. Approximately 10 to 15 percent of women will have a second convulsion after receiving the intravenous loading dose of magnesium sulfate. Pritchard et al.[238] reported that 10 of 83 women who had eclampsia treated before delivery again suffered convulsions shortly after an initial injection of magnesium sulfate, 4 g IV and 10 g IM. However, most remained free of seizures after an additional 2 g magnesium sulfate IV.

We use serum magnesium levels in the clinical management of the eclamptic woman. If the initial level, obtained 4 hours after the loading dose, is high (over 10 mg/dl), we reduce the 2-g maintenance dose of magnesium sulfate. This will occasionally occur in women with renal compromise. Similarly, in the rare patient with a brisk urine output, we give a maintenance dose of 3 g to keep levels in the therapeutic range.

In my series of 262 eclamptic women, 36 (14 per-

cent) had an additional convulsion after receiving magnesium sulfate.[244] An occasional patient will have recurrent convulsions while receiving therapeutic doses of magnesium sulfate. In these cases, a short-acting barbiturate such as sodium amobarbital can be given in a dose of up to 250 mg IV over 3 to 5 minutes. We treated one patient who had recurrent convulsions with a serum magnesium level of 9.4 mg/dl and who had also received sodium amobarbital. She was given an intravenous sodium pentothal drip and experienced no further seizures.

Magnesium toxicity was responsible for the only death in the Pritchard et al.[238] series of eclamptic women and nearly led to a maternal death at the University of Tennessee, Memphis.[245] In both cases, the patients were supposed to have received a loading dose of 4 g magnesium sulfate but, because of an error in preparing the drug, received 20 g magnesium sulfate over a few minutes.

Rarely, a woman may have an eclamptic seizure, lapse into a coma, and die. Magnesium toxicity should be considered in those women who do not regain consciousness. A case report of magnesium sulfate toxicity details the features of this serious complication.[245] Within a few minutes of starting what was supposed to be a magnesium loading dose, 4 g magnesium sulfate in 250 ml saline, the patient went into cardiorespiratory arrest. Immediate resuscitation including intubation was performed. Approximately one-half of the loading dose had been given. An intracerebral accident or eclampsia was thought to be the etiology of the coma; the loading dose was continued and maintenance therapy started. Initial blood gases were normal, and the ECG was normal 15 minutes after the arrest. Mechanical ventilatory support was required. The patient's vital signs were stable, but her pupils were nonreactive. Serum electrolytes, glucose, blood urea nitrogen, and creatinine were normal. Computed tomography of the head and cerebral angiograms were normal. A magnesium level of 35 mg/dl was reported 3.5 hours later from a blood sample taken via femoral venipuncture at the time of arrest. The magnesium sulfate infusion was stopped immediately. During the first 5 hours after the cardiorespiratory arrest, 1,344 mg of magnesium were excreted in the urine. Twelve hours after the arrest, an uncomplicated low vertical cesarean delivery was done for a breech presentation. The 3,160-g male infant had Apgar scores of 8 and 9 at 1 and 5 minutes. Maternal and cord blood magnesium level at delivery was 5.8 mg/dl. Both mother and baby were discharged from the hospital with no apparent residual effects. Of interest, the patient reported she could hear and see what was occurring around her, but she could not

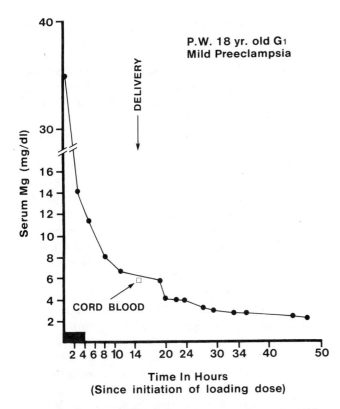

P.W. 18 yr. old G₁
Mild Preeclampsia

Time In Hours
(Since initiation of loading dose)

Fig. 28-6 A patient with magnesium toxicity. (From McCubbin et al.,[245] with permission.)

make any movements while she had the endotracheal tube in place. Figure 28-6 presents the maternal magnesium levels in this case.[245]

6. *Maternal acidemia should be corrected:* We obtain a blood gas reading on every patient who has had an eclamptic convulsion. Blood oxygenation and pH should be in the normal range. Patients who have had repeated convulsions may be acidotic and a low PO_2 may indicate aspiration pneumonitis. Sodium bicarbonate is not given unless the pH is below 7.10. Abnormal blood gases may be the result of respiratory depression.

7. *Avoid polypharmacy:* Polypharmacy is extremely hazardous in the woman with eclampsia, as addition of diazepam or phenytoin may lead to respiratory depression or respiratory arrest.

In many medical centers outside the United States, magnesium sulfate is rarely used to prevent or treat eclamptic convulsions. As a result, the ideal anticonvulsant in these centers is yet to be found.[244] During the past 60 years numerous anticonvulsive drugs have been introduced and replaced due to the dissatisfaction with the results obtained with the use of these drugs. These drugs have included bromethol, chloral, hydrate paraldehyde, phenothiazines, lytic cocktails, barbiturates, diazepam, chlordiazepoxide, and clonazepam. The ov-

erzealous use of these drugs in eclampsia has been associated with significant maternal-neonatal central nervous system and respiratory depression.[247] The use of large doses of diazepam (>30 mg) during labor is associated with loss of beat-to-beat fetal heart rate variability and significant neonatal morbidity (respiratory depression, apnea, hypotonia, cold stress, poor sucking). The use of the barbiturate chlormethiozole (which is commonly used in Europe and Australia) in anticonvulsive doses may depress maternal laryngeal reflexes, thus increasing the likelihood of aspiration during convulsion. In addition, the use of intravenous phenobarbital has the potential of producing laryngospasm and circulatory and respiratory depression. Moreover, none of these drugs has been proven to be superior to or as effective as magnesium sulfate in treating eclamptic convulsions.[2]

Recently, phenytoin has been advocated for the prevention and treatment of eclamptic convulsions. Slater et al.[246] evaluated a regimen of phenytoin based on maternal weight in 26 patients (7 had severe preeclampsia, 17 had mild disease, and 2 had eclampsia). They reported no seizures after the initiation of phenytoin (750 to 1,250 mg IV at a rate of ≤25 mg/min), and they noted no major maternal or neonatal side effects.

Ryan et al.[247] investigated the safety, efficacy, and pharmacokinetics of phenytoin. They reported that an appropriate regimen should include a loading dose of 15 mg/kg pregnancy weight to be administered as 10 mg/kg initially and 5 mg/kg 2 hours later. This loading dose was to be followed by a maintenance dose of 200 mg orally or intravenously every 8 hours to start 12 hours after a second bolus. The maintenance dose is continued for 3 to 5 days after delivery. This regimen requires obtaining frequent monitoring of phenytoin and albumin levels. They reported this regimen to be effective and safe in 80 such patients studied. One of the 80 patients developed convulsions after receiving an inadequate dose. They recommended phenytoin as a logical alternative to magnesium sulfate.

Friedman and associates[248] reported a prospective, randomized clinical trial comparing a standardized regimen of intravenous phenytoin ($N = 45$) to intravenous magnesium sulfate ($N = 60$) as seizure prophylaxis in preeclampsia eclampsia. No seizures occurred in preeclamptic patients who received either drug, but subsequent convulsions developed in the two eclamptic patients assigned to the phenytoin group. The authors noted lower maternal side effects, shorter duration of active phase of labor, and lower amount of estimated blood loss at vaginal delivery in the phenytoin group.

There are three randomized studies comparing the use of $MgSO_4$ to phenytoin or diazepam in eclampsia.[249,250] Dommisse[249] reported on 22 patients with eclampsia who were randomly allocated to receive intravenous phenytoin or intravenous magnesium sulfate. None of 11 patients managed with magnesium sulfate had further convulsions, while 4 of 11 patients treated with phenytoin had further convulsions. All four patients who failed phenytoin therapy subsequently were effectively treated with magnesium sulfate, and the author suggested that magnesium sulfate is a more effective agent in eclampsia. Crowther,[250] in a randomized controlled trial, compared the use of magnesium sulfate and diazepam as an anticonvulsant in 51 eclamptic patients. She noted that the use of magnesium sulfate was associated with less serious morbidity but the difference was not statistically significant. The Eclampsia Trial Collaborative Group studied 1,680 women randomized to receive magnesium sulfate, diazepam, or phenytoin after convulsions. Magnesium sulfate proved superior in preventing recurrent seizures.[251]

On the other hand, the widespread use of phenytoin for severe preeclampsia-eclampsia in the United Kingdom was questioned by Tufnell et al.[252] They reported that 3 (17 percent) of 18 preeclamptic eclamptic women developed a further convulsion after the administration of the recommended dose. Phenytoin serum levels were measured in two of the three patients and were in the therapeutic range in both of them. In addition, the efficacy of phenytoin for the prevention and treatment of eclamptic convulsions was studied by Coyaji and Otiv,[253] as well as by Naidu and associates.[254] Both of these studies reported a relatively high failure rate in controlling eclamptic convulsions.

Atypical Eclampsia

Eclampsia occurring before the 20th week of gestation or after 48 hours postpartum is exceedingly rare and for lack of a better term has been called *atypical eclampsia*. Eclampsia occurring before the 20th week of gestation has usually been reported with molar or hydropic degeneration of the placenta. Chesley et al.[255] observed 35 cases of probable eclampsia associated with molar degeneration of the placenta in a review of the literature through 1944. In 26 of these patients, eclampsia occurred during the first half of gestation. Six of the women had a coexistent fetus. A case report and a review of the literature was recently reported by Newman and Eddy.[256] Two cases of eclampsia have been reported without molar degeneration of the placenta during the first half of gestation.[257,258] In one woman who had Rh isoimmunization, eclampsia developed at 16 weeks' gestation. The placenta revealed cystic hydropic degeneration of the villi. No molar changes were present.

Although rare, eclampsia can occur during the first half of gestation.[7] These women may be misdiagnosed as having hypertensive encephalopathy or a seizure disorder. Women in whom convulsions develop in association with hypertension and proteinuria during the first half of pregnancy should be considered to have eclampsia. They should be treated with parenteral magnesium sulfate to control convulsions, with termination of pregnancy as the definitive goal.

Late postpartum eclampsia is eclampsia that occurs more than 48 hours after delivery. Of the women we have treated for eclampsia during the past 15 years, eclampsia developed in 54 patients more than 48 hours postpartum (16 percent). A review of the clinical course of late postpartum eclampsia has been reported.[219] Thirty of the 54 women described in that report had been treated for preeclampsia and received standard intravenous magnesium sulfate therapy. The mean duration of magnesium sulfate therapy was 32 hours (range 24 to 72 hours). Several women were at home when the convulsions developed. Forty-five of the women had experienced headaches or visual disturbances (blurred vision and scotomas from 2 to 72 hours before the onset of convulsions).[219] The most striking finding in these women was the brisk diuresis that occurred immediately after the convulsion. Urinary outputs of 500 to 1,000 ml during the first hour after the seizure were common. Because of the unusual time of occurrence of eclampsia in these women, neurologic consultations are recommended to rule out abnormalities.[219]

Of interest is the high rate of occurrence of late postpartum eclampsia in Nigerian women. In a report of 25 cases of postpartum eclampsia, 17 (68 percent) occurred more than 48 hours postpartum.[259] Uric acid levels were elevated in these women with eclampsia before delivery or during the immediate postpartum period.

Maternity Morbidity and Mortality in Eclampsia

Pritchard et al.[238] reported only one maternal death in 245 women treated for eclampsia at Parkland Hospital (Dallas, TX) from 1955 to 1983, a maternal mortality rate of 0.4 percent. This death was caused by magnesium toxicity. Endotracheal intubation was not accomplished promptly in this short and very obese woman; as a result, respiratory arrest, cardiorespiratory arrest, and death ensued. Three other women had respiratory depression.

One maternal death occurred in our series of 254 patients with eclampsia.[7] The patient had five convulsions before arriving at our hospital and went into cardiorespiratory arrest in the parking lot. The patient was resuscitated, and her seizures were controlled with magnesium sulfate. However, the patient did not regain consciousness after cardiac arrest. She underwent a cesarean delivery for fetal distress and had a 3,090-g infant with normal Apgar scores. The child had no serious problems in the nursery and was discharged in good condition. DIC developed after the operation. The postoperative course was complicated by sepsis, continuing convulsions, and pulmonary insufficiency. An EEG on the second postoperative day demonstrated absent cortical activity. A CT scan failed to demonstrate either intracerebral hemorrhage or cerebral edema. The patient remained comatose and died 8 weeks' postpartum.

Harbert et al.[260] reported on 168 women treated for eclampsia between 1939 and 1963. Delivery within an arbitrary time limit after control of the convulsion was not an essential part of therapy. Forty-seven of the 83 patients in whom eclampsia occurred before the spontaneous onset of labor were delivered within 48 hours of the first convulsive episode. In the other 36 patients with eclampsia before delivery, the interval between occurrence of the convulsion and spontaneous onset of labor ranged from 93 hours to 43 days. During the first 6 years of the study, eight maternal deaths occurred. From December 1944 to termination of the study in 1963, 108 women with eclampsia were managed without another maternal death. The uncorrected perinatal mortality rate PMR was 216:1,000. The PMR was 28 percent (14 fetal deaths and three neonatal deaths) in 60 patients delivered 72 hours or longer after admission.

Lopez-Llera[261] reviewed 990 cases of eclampsia in Mexican women during a 22-year period ending in 1985. There were 138 deaths, for a mortality rate of 14 percent. Several factors were found to increase the risk of maternal death in eclampsia: gestational age at which eclampsia occurred, maternal age, complications, underlying disease, and multiple gestation.

In our experience, primigravid women with eclampsia have a lower incidence of serious complications than multigravid women. This is probably attributable to the higher incidence of chronic hypertension and underlying renal disease in the multigravid women rather than to any effect of eclampsia per se. In particular, we believe that careful attention should be given to IV fluid therapy in multigravid women with eclampsia. In our experience, pulmonary edema is much more likely to develop. Likewise, the incidence of renal failure is much higher in multigravid women with eclampsia than in primigravid women with eclampsia.

In our series, maternal transfers and patients who had received no prenatal care had higher complication rates. More than 90 percent of women with eclampsia who had no prenatal care were first seen in the emergency room of another hospital. Many were treated by a physician who was seeing his or her first case of eclampsia. Referral often occurred before the women had received adequate treatment with magnesium sulfate.

Perinatal Outcome in Eclampsia

The main risks to the fetus of the eclamptic woman are abruptio placentae, prematurity, intrauterine growth retardation, and hypoxic episodes during the convulsions.[7,238,261]

Sibai et al.[240] followed 28 premature infants and 14 full-term infants of eclamptic mothers for up to 50 months. Eight of the 12 infants who were small for age by weight at birth showed catch-up growth at an average of 20.6 months (range 2 to 48 months). In all, only two of the infants remained growth retarded by weight, height, and head circumference; both were mentally retarded. A total of three infants had major neurologic deficits resulting in cerebral palsy and mental retardation on follow up evaluation. General health continued to be a problem for the premature infants during the first year of life. Several had multiple hospitalizations for either pulmonary or neurologic complications.

Maternal Transport of the Eclamptic Patient

During the past 20 years, there has been a marked reduction in the number of eclamptic patients. Consequently, most obstetricians have little or no experience in the management of eclampsia. A recent survey of a random sample of obstetricians from all 50 states indicated that about 50 percent of obstetricians in private practice had not seen an eclamptic patient during the past year.

Because management of the eclamptic patient requires the availability of neonatal and obstetric intensive care units and personnel with special expertise, we believe that eclamptic patients should not be managed at level I hospitals. We recommend that eclamptic patients with term gestations be cared for only at level II or III hospitals with adequate facilities and with consultants from other specialties, if needed. For those eclamptic patients who are remote from term, referral should be made to a tertiary care center. We recommend that the following steps be taken before transfer of these critically ill patients:

1. The referring physician or nurse should consult with the physician at the perinatal center regarding the referral and appropriate treatment. All maternal records including prenatal data and a detailed summary of the patient's condition should be sent with the patient.
2. Blood pressure should be stabilized and convulsions controlled.

3. Adequate prophylactic anticonvulsive medications should be given. An accepted regimen is 4-g intravenous magnesium sulfate as a loading dose, with a simultaneous intramuscular dose of 10 g.
4. Such patients should be sent in an ambulance with medical personnel in attendance for proper management in case of subsequent convulsions.

Can Eclampsia Be Prevented?

Eclampsia is generally considered a preventable complications of pregnancy. Zuspan[262] believes that the severe forms of preeclampsia should be preventable by appropriate prenatal care. He also contends that convulsions should not occur once the woman with preeclampsia is admitted to the hospital.

We recently reviewed 254 cases of eclampsia treated at the University of Tennessee in an attempt to determine the number of cases of preventable eclampsia.[7] All factors that may have been involved in the development of eclampsia were reviewed. Patients were then grouped into categories of physician error, patient failure, and failure of magnesium sulfate therapy. We found that about 30 percent of cases were nonpreventable.

These findings are in agreement with those of Campbell and Templeton,[263] who studied factors leading to the development of eclampsia in 66 patients. These workers found that in 28 patients (42.4 percent), eclampsia was not preventable.

Counseling Women with Eclampsia and Their Relatives

Bryans et al.,[264] in their long-term follow-up study of women who had eclampsia treated at the Medical College of Georgia, found no increase in hypertension in these patients above that expected in the general female population. They concluded that preeclampsia/eclampsia did not cause hypertensive disease and was not a manifestation of subsequent essential hypertension in pregnant women. Chesley et al.[265] followed women who developed eclampsia at the Margaret Hague Hospital from its opening in 1931 through 1951. They traced all but three of the women who survived to 1974. Chesley et al. also concluded that eclampsia does not cause hypertension. The average annual death rate was 5.11 in 1,000, with 31 deaths in the 187 white women who had eclampsia during their pregnancies. This was not significantly different from the number of deaths expected. However, 33 of 59 white women who had eclampsia as multiparas had died at an average rate of 21.3 in 1,000, which was significantly higher than the expected mortality rate. Eighty-two percent of the remote deaths were due to cardiovascular-renal disease in women who had eclampsia as multiparas.

Chesley et al.[266] reported that the prognosis for future pregnancies after eclampsia was good. Another 409 pregnancies occurred in the 158 women in whom eclampsia developed during their first pregnancy. Preeclampsia/eclampsia recurred in 34.5 percent of the women and in 20.6 percent of their subsequent pregnancies. When hypertension occurred in a future pregnancy, it was usually mild. Eclampsia developed in three women for an incidence of 0.9 percent in pregnancies beyond 20 weeks gestation.

The sisters and daughters of eclamptic women are at increased risk for the development of preeclampsia and eclampsia.[266] Chesley et al.[267] reviewed the incidence of preeclampsia in the first pregnancies of daughters of eclamptic mothers. Preeclampsia developed in 63 of the 257 first pregnancies (24.9 percent). Eclampsia occurred in seven of these pregnancies (2.7 percent). The outcomes of the first pregnancies carried to viability by sisters of eclamptic women were also studied. Preeclampsia occurred in 54 (37 percent) of first pregnancies, and eclampsia developed in 6 women (4.1 percent). Because of the increased risk of preeclampsia/

Table 28-18   Pregnancy After Eclampsia

	Chesley[267]	Lopez-Llera and Horta[268a]	Adelusi and Ojengbeda[269a]	Sibai et al[271]
No. of women	171	110	64	182
No. of pregnancies	398	110	64	366
Preeclampsia (%)	23.1	35.4	26.6	21.9
Eclampsia (%)	1.0	†	15.6	1.9
Abruptio placenta (%)	2.0	†	†	2.5
Preterm delivery (%)	6.5	†	34	13.7
IUGR (%)	†	22	12.5	6.0
Perinatal deaths (%)	4.7	3.6	6.25	2.7

a Followup in only one subsequent pregnancy
† Data not available.
(From Sibai et al,[271] with permission.)

eclampsia in these women, their pregnancies should be closely monitored.

During the past 20 years, there have been four studies describing pregnancy outcomes after eclampsia.[268–270] The findings of these studies are summarized in Table 28-18. It is important to note that the incidence of preeclampsia is much higher in future pregnancies in women who have had eclampsia remote from term.

Sibai and associates[271] studied the long-term effects of eclampsia on maternal blood pressure in 210 women who were normotensive prior to the eclamptic pregnancy. The average duration of follow up in these women was 7.2 years (range 2 to 13 years). The overall incidence of chronic hypertension on follow up was only 9.5 percent.

Chronic Hypertension

Pathophysiology of Chronic Hypertension

Patients with labile or borderline hypertension have several pathophysiologic alterations with elevated cardiac output, central redistribution of blood volume, enhanced activity of the autonomic nervous system, increased left ventricular ejection rate, and a normal total peripheral resistance.[271] However, patients with mild to moderate hypertension have a normal cardiac output.[272] In these cases, the increase in blood pressure is due to an increase in total peripheral resistance. Because vascular resistance and arterial pressure are elevated, ventricular workload is increased. The heart rate may be increased, while stroke volume and left ventricular ejection rate are normal. Over time, the patient with moderate essential hypertension will show evidence of cardiac strain. Stroke volume remains normal or may start to fall. Myocardial contractility remains normal, while ECG studies frequently show an increased thickness of the left ventricular wall. In the absence of renal disease, plasma volume contraction is proportionate to the increase in diastolic blood pressure. When the diastolic blood pressure equals or exceeds 105 mmHg, a decrease in plasma volume becomes more apparent.

Clinical evidence of end organ damage characterizes severe essential hypertension. Cardiac enlargement is evident on chest radiograph and ECG. Total peripheral resistance becomes even higher, and cardiac output may begin to fall. Stroke volume decreases, and intravascular volume decreases still further. With the decrease in cardiac output and intravascular volume, plasma renin activity rises. These changes lead to a great increase in left ventricular tension, making myocardial contractions increasingly difficult. Pulmonary edema will occur if the patient is not treated.

Diagnosis of Chronic Hypertension

The diagnosis of chronic hypertension in pregnancy is usually made on the basis of either of the following:

1. Documented history of high blood pressure antedating pregnancy.
2. Persistent elevation of blood pressure (at least 140/90 mmHg) on two occasions more than 24 hours apart before the 20th week of gestation.

When a solid diagnosis, by both or either of the above findings, cannot be made, other findings might be suggestive of the presence of chronic hypertension:

> Retinal changes on fundoscopic examination
> Cardiac enlargement on chest x-ray and ECG
> Compromised renal function or associated renal disease
> Presence of medical disorders known to lead to hypertension
> Multiparity with previous history of hypertensive pregnancies
> Evidence of persistent hypertension beyond the 42nd day postpartum.

Sometimes the diagnosis is difficult to make because of the marked and variable changes seen with blood pressure during midpregnancy. This becomes problematic in patients with no prior medical care and who are first seen in early third trimester. Chesley and Annitto[273] observed that women with chronic hypertension show greater decreases in their blood pressure during pregnancy than do normotensive patients. They reported a marked decrease in 39 percent of 301 pregnancies studied. They also noted that during midpregnancy the blood pressure was in the normal range in women who were severely hypertensive prior to pregnancy. Similar findings were observed at our institution in the course of pregnancy in 211 patients with mild chronic hypertension.[273]

Etiology and Classification of Chronic Hypertension

Essential hypertension is by far the most common cause of chronic hypertension during pregnancy. A description of all causes of hypertension is beyond the scope of this chapter.

For this review, chronic hypertension in pregnancy is classified as mild or severe depending on the systolic or diastolic blood pressure reading. The hypertension is classified as mild if systolic blood pressure is less than 160 mmHg and the diastolic is less than 110 mmHg. Hypertension is severe if either systolic pressure is more than 160 mmHg or diastolic pressure is above 110 mmHg.

Superimposed preeclampsia is defined as exacerbation of hypertension of at least 30 mmHg in systolic or at least 15 mmHg in diastolic blood pressure, together with the development of generalized edema, or proteinuria during the course of the pregnancy (at least 300 mg/24 hours), or exacerbation of preexisting proteinuria (at least 2 g/24 hours), and elevation of serum uric acid levels (at least 6 mg/dl) during the second half of the pregnancy.

Maternal and Fetal Risks of Chronic Hypertension

Pregnancies complicated by chronic hypertension are at increased risk for the development of superimposed preeclampsia, abruptio placentae, and poor perinatal outcome. The reported incidence of superimposed preeclampsia ranges from 4.7 to 52 percent depending on the severity of hypertension at the onset of pregnancy and on the criteria used to make the diagnosis.[273-276] As for the severity of hypertension in the first trimester, the reported incidence of superimposed preeclampsia ranged from 28.2 to 52 percent in severe chronic hypertension, and this rate was unaffected by the use of antihypertensive medication.[276,277] On the other hand, the reported incidence for patients with mild hypertension in pregnancy was as low as 4.7 percent.[278]

The criteria that were used in these reports to diagnose superimposed preeclampsia included one or more of the following: exacerbation of hypertension, development of edema, appearance of proteinuria, and elevation of serum uric acid levels (>6 mg/dl). In general, the incidence of this complication will be high if only exacerbation of blood pressure was used in the diagnosis, whereas this incidence will be lower if significant proteinuria (>1 g/24 hrs) was added to make such a diagnosis. This incidence was also found to be increased in severe disease (25 to 52 percent).[276] In addition, some pregnant chronic hypertensives may have silent undiagnosed chronic renal disease and may experience urinary protein excretion that increases with advancing gestation, particularly in the third trimester (usually >300 mg, but <1 g/24 hrs); many such women will demonstrate an increase in either their systolic (>30 mmHg) or diastolic (>15 mmHg) blood pressure with advancing gestation. If either of these criteria is used, the incidence of superimposed preeclampsia will be extremely high.[279] Thus, it is recommended that superimposed preeclampsia be diagnosed on the basis of exacerbated hypertension plus the development of either substantial proteinuria (>1 g/24 hrs) or elevated serum uric acid levels. In women on antihypertensive medications where exacerbation of blood pressure is less common, the diagnosis should be based on the development of substantial proteinuria.

In general, pregnancies complicated only by exacerbation of blood pressure have a perinatal outcome similar to those in normotensives, while the appearance of proteinuria is more significant for fetal prognosis since in such pregnancies most of the poor perinatal outcomes are associated with proteinuria. Because many obstetricians consider superimposed preeclampsia as an indication for delivery, it is important to use strict criteria to avoid potential unnecessary preterm delivery.

Likewise, the incidence of abruptio placentae is reportedly increased and ranges between 0.45 and 10 percent depending on the duration and the severity of hypertension. For those with mild uncomplicated disease the incidence has ranged from 0.45 to 1.9 percent,[280,281] while in cases with severe hypertension the incidence was markedly increased from 2.3 to 10 percent.[273,276] This incidence is not influenced by the use of antihypertensive medications.[275] Of note also is the compounding effect of superimposed preeclampsia in cases complicated by abruptio placentae where its presence was associated with higher perinatal mortality than when preeclampsia was absent. Also, this incidence is substantially increased in those with a history of abruption in previous pregnancies.[282]

The above-mentioned complications are responsible for most of the perinatal deaths as well as the increased incidence of fetal growth retardation and premature delivery in such pregnancies. In addition, these pregnancies are reportedly associated with increased frequency of midtrimester losses, particularly in those not receiving antihypertensive therapy.[278,283,284] In general, perinatal mortality and morbidity are not increased in patients with uncomplicated mild chronic hypertension, whereas they are markedly increased in patients with severe disease, in those with renal disease, and in those complicated by superimposed preeclampsia.[275]

Pregnancy Outcome in Relation to Treatment of Chronic Hypertension

There is general agreement that chronic antihypertensive therapy will decrease the incidence of cardiovascular complications and cerebrovascular accidents in nonpregnant patients with diastolic blood pressures exceeding 105 mmHg. In addition, since maternal mortality and morbidity are increased in pregnant women with diastolic blood pressures of 110 mmHg or higher,[275,276] there are potential maternal and fetal benefits from treating severe chronic hypertension during pregnancy.[285] However, it is not clear if antihypertensives are equally beneficial in pregnancies with mild uncomplicated hypertension (about 95 percent of all pregnant women with chronic hypertension). In addition, neither controlled nor uncontrolled studies showed any reduction in the incidence of superimposed preeclampsia or abruptio placentae when antihypertensives were used.[275]

Severe Chronic Hypertension in Pregnancy

There are few reports describing pregnancy outcomes in women with severe chronic hypertension. Three retrospective studies described pregnancy outcomes in untreated women with severe chronic hypertension early in pregnancy.[273,277,286] These studies were conducted during 1931 to 1953, before modern advances in obstetric and neonatal practices. The reported perinatal survival ranged from 19 to 50 percent, and most of the fetal losses occurred in women with superimposed preeclampsia. In addition, the studies reported an increased frequency of maternal mortality and morbidity (acute and long term). As a result, the reported maternal and perinatal outcome was invariably poor. Hence, concerns about the risk of acute renal failure and cerebrovascular accidents have led many obstetricians to recommend early termination of such pregnancies. A recent survey of American obstetricians (Sibai and Watson, unpublished data) found that 20 percent of the respondents recommended termination of such pregnancies regardless of renal function, and 45 percent did so only in the presence of impaired renal function.

In 1966, Kincaid-Smith et al.[285] reported pregnancy outcomes in 32 patients with severe hypertension who were treated with methyldopa during their pregnancy. The perinatal survival was 90.7 percent, and there were no maternal complications. The authors attributed this good outcome to the control of maternal blood pressure with methyldopa. However, only five subjects were started on treatment during the first trimester, while the rest received treatment during the second or third trimester. Recently, Sibai et al.[276] documented pregnancy outcomes in 44 patients with severe hypertension who were seen during the first trimester. Each was treated with methyldopa and oral hydralazine as needed to keep diastolic blood pressure below 110 mmHg. The patients were observed closely throughout pregnancy, with frequent prenatal visits and intensive monitoring of the clinical status of both mother and fetus. Twenty-three women (52 percent) developed superimposed preeclampsia; there were no maternal deaths. The total perinatal survival was 75 percent; 31 infants (70 percent) were delivered preterm and 19 (43 percent) were small for gestational age (Table 28-19). However, among the subjects without superimposed preeclampsia, there were no perinatal deaths and only one infant (5 percent) was small for gestational age.

Table 28-19 Pregnancy Outcome in 44 Women with Severe Hypertension in the First Trimester

	With Preeclampsia (N = 23)	Without Preeclampsia (N = 21)
Gestational age (wk)	28.6 ± 2.4	36.5 ± 2.9
<37 weeks	23 (100%)	8 (38%)
Birth weight (g)	827 ± 314	2632 ± 743
SGA	18 (78%)	1 (5%)
Perinatal deaths	11 (48%)	0
Abruptio placentae	2 (8.7%)	0
Deterioration in renal function	15 (65%)	5 (24%)

These findings argue against the practice of recommending termination of pregnancy for severe hypertension in the first trimester. However, such women should be counseled regarding the potential maternal risks, and they must be observed and managed at a tertiary care center with adequate maternal-neonatal care facilities.

Mild Chronic Hypertension in Pregnancy

There are many reports (retrospective and prospective) describing pregnancy outcome in women with mild-to-moderate hypertension. It is, however, difficult to evaluate or compare the benefits of antihypertensive therapy in the management of these pregnancies because of differences in definition, populations studied, and treatments used. Some of these studies were controlled, and others were selective; some studied chronic hypertension only, yet others included all forms of hypertension. Some compared treatment with no treatment or with placebo, others compared two different antihypertensive drugs, and still others used a combination of drugs. In addition, the gestational ages at treatment and the durations of therapy were highly variable.[275]

Methyldopa is the drug most commonly used to treat chronic hypertension during pregnancy.[274,275] As a result, most clinical trials have compared methyldopa with either no medication or β-blockers. To evaluate the effects of antihypertensive drugs in pregnancy, we will describe only randomized trials in which adequate pregnancy data were available.[278,281,283,287–289]

Five prospective controlled trials compared methyldopa with either no medication or a placebo for the management of mild chronic hypertension in pregnancy, while in the sixth study atenolol was used (Table 28-20). Only two studies included a placebo in a double-blind fashion,[288,289] but the sample size was limited in both trials and the diagnosis of chronic hypertension in one of them was based on an increased blood pressure before 34 weeks' gestation. The other four studies were

Table 28-20 Pregnancy Outcome in Randomized Controlled Trials of Chronic Hypertension

Author(s)	Gestation at Entry (wk)	Gestation at Delivery (wk)	Birth Weight (g)	IUGR (%)	Preeclampsia (%)	Perinatal Death (%)
Leather et al[283]						
Control (N = 24)	<28	36.5	2,520		N/A	8.3[a]
Treated (N = 23)		38.0	2,840	N/A	N/A	0
Redman et al[278]						
Control (N = 107)	20.6 ± 0.5	38.1 ± 0.2	3,130 ± 49		4.7	1.9[a]
Treated (N = 101)	21.9 ± 0.5	38.1 ± 0.2	3,090 ± 60	N/A	6.7	1.0
Arias and Zamora[287]						
Control (N = 29)	16.4 ± 1.1	38.3 ± 0.4	3,011 ± 103	14.2	10.3	3.4
Treated (N = 29)	14.7 ± 1.0	38.1 ± 0.5	2,926 ± 131	14.2	3.4	0
Weitz et al[288]						
Control (N = 12)	<34	37.6 ± 0.5	2,820	25	33.3	0
Treated (N = 13)		39.0 ± 0.4	3,140	0	38.4	0
Sibai et al[281]						
Control (N = 90)	11.3 ± 0.2	39.0 ± 0.2	3,123 ± 69	8.9	15.6	1.1
Treated (N = 173)	11.2 ± 0.2	38.7 ± 0.2	3,060 ± 72	7.5	17.3	1.2
Butters et al[289]						
Control (N = 14)	15.9	39.5	3,530	0	N/A	0
Treated (N = 15)	15.8	38.5	2,620	66	N/A	6

Abbreviations: IUGR, intrauterine growth retardation; preeclampsia, increased blood pressure plus proteinuria; N/A, not available.

Data are presented as mean ± SEM where available.

[a] Excludes second-trimester losses.

not placebo controlled, and only one included subjects who were randomized in the first trimester.[278] It is evident from Table 28-20 that the use of antihypertensive medications did not affect perinatal outcome except for reducing second trimester abortions. There were three second trimester abortions in the control group of Leather et al.[283]; however, it was unclear whether these losses were the result of severe hypertension or were spontaneous abortions. Of the four second trimester abortions in the control group in the study reported

by Redman et al.,[278] none were directly related to hypertension and none had evidence of preeclampsia. These losses might have been due to preterm labor or incompetent cervix. On the other hand, Sibai et al.[281] noted only one second trimester loss, which occurred in the methyldopa group. Also in Butters et al.[289] study, the only stillbirth was in the atenolol group. In the six trials summarized in Table 28-20, there were no maternal benefits from antihypertensive therapy except for a reduction in the frequency of exacerbation of hyper-

Table 28-21 Methyldopa Vs. β-Blockers for Mild Hypertension in Pregnancy[a]

	Gallery et al		Fidler et al[b]		Plouin et al	
	Methyldopa	Oxprenolol	Methyldopa	Oxprenolol	Methyldopa	Labetalol
No.	27	26	22	24	85	91
Initial systolic pressure (mmHg)	151 ± 12	147 ± 14	146 ± 9	151 ± 9	148 ± 13	146 ± 13
Initial diastolic pressure (mmHg)	102 ± 10	102 ± 12	99 ± 3	99 ± 4	96 ± 9	94 ± 8
Initial gestational age (wk)	32 ± 4.2	31 ± 9.1	23.9 ± 6.7	22.5 ± 7.2	26.2 ± 6.8	25.8 ± 7.5
Birth weight (g)	2,654 ± 821	3,051 ± 663	2,992 ± 732	2,715 ± 919	2,897 ± 727	2,860 ± 728
Preeclampsia (%)	7.4	7.6	9.1	8.3	9.4	8.8
Perinatal death (%)	7.4	0	4.5	4.2	4.7	1.1

Data are presented as mean ± SD.

[a] Includes patients with all forms of mild hypertension (diastolic pressure <110 mmHg).

[b] Excludes patients enrolled beyond 32 weeks' gestation.

(Adapted from Sibai,[275] with permission.)

tension. The incidence of perinatal death among the controls ranged from 0 to 8.3 percent; this incidence was particularly low (<2 percent) in the two studies with the largest number of subjects. None of these trials had a sample size sufficient enough to permit direct assessment of the effects of antihypertensive drugs on perinatal death rate.

Three prospective controlled trials compared methyldopa with a β-blocker for mild hypertension in pregnancy (Table 28-21).[290–292] Gallery et al.[290] found greater plasma volume expansion, larger neonatal birth weights, and no perinatal deaths among 26 exprenolol-treated patients. In contrast, Fidler et al.[291] found no difference in pregnancy outcome and neonatal birth weight between 24 women treated with oxprenolol and 22 treated with methyldopa. They also found that the oxprenolol-treated group had a higher incidence of abnormal fetal heart tracings during labor. Plouin et al.[292] found no difference in neonatal heart rate, blood pressure, and respiratory rate between the two treatment groups and concluded that labetalol is as safe as methyldopa for the fetus and newborn. However, all three studies included patients with all forms of hypertension; less than one-third of the subjects had chronic hypertension, and very few were enrolled during the first trimester. In addition, none of these trials had an adequate number of subjects to demonstrate a difference in either preeclampsia or perinatal death. In summary, superimposed preeclampsia and abruptio placentae are responsible for most of the poor perinatal outcome in women with mild chronic hypertension. Antihypertensive drugs do not reduce the frequency of either of these complications. Most patients with mild chronic hypertension will have a good outcome with proper obstetric follow-up without the use of antihypertensive agents.

Antihypertensive Drugs in Pregnancy

Many drugs are available for treating hypertension in pregnancy. Some have been studied extensively (methyldopa, β-blockers); others have been used infrequently or are still under clinical trial (calcium channel blockers, prazosin). The drugs used most often in pregnancy are adrenoreceptor-blocking agents, thiazide diuretics, hydralazine, and recently, calcium channel blockers. There are potential adverse effects from the chronic use of any drug during pregnancy. When using antihypertensives, one must weigh the benefits of such treatment against the potential adverse effects on the mother, fetus, and neonate.

Methyldopa

Methyldopa is the only antihypertensive drug whose long-term safety for the mother and the fetus has been adequately assessed. It is the drug most commonly used to treat hypertension during pregnancy and is the standard against which other agents are compared. It lowers blood pressure by stimulation of central α_2-receptors via α-methylnorepinephrine, which is the active form of α-methyldopa. In addition, it might act as an α_2-peripheral blocker via a false neurotransmitter effect. It reduces systemic vascular resistance without causing physiologically significant changes in heart rate or cardiac output, while renal blood flow is maintained. Maternal side effects include dry mouth, lethargy, and drowsiness. Other side effects include liver function abnormalities, postural hypotension, hemolytic anemia, and a positive Coombs test. The usual oral dosage in women with severe hypertension is an initial loading dose of 1 g followed by a maintenance dose of 1 to 2 g/d given in four divided doses, which can be increased to 4 g as needed. If used in mild hypertension, however, the usual dose is 250 mg three times daily. The plasma half-life is about 2 hours, and peak plasma levels occur within 2 hours after oral administration. The fall in blood pressure is maximal about 4 hours after an oral dose. Most of the drug is excreted via the kidney. It is considered a weak antihypertensive best suited for cases with mild hypertension, and if adequate blood pressure control is not achieved with the maximum dosage, additional antihypertensive agents, such as hydralazine, β-blockers, or nifedipine may be added.

Clonidine

Clonidine is a potent α_2-adrenoceptor central stimulant, used primarily for treatment of mild to moderate hypertension. Approximately 40 to 60 percent of the oral dose is excreted in unaltered form in the urine. Its potential side effects include sedation, dry mouth, and rebound hypertension following abrupt discontinuation. The usual oral dose in pregnancy is 0.1 to 0.3 mg/d given in two divided doses, which can be increased up to 1.2 mg/d as needed. Its safety and efficacy during pregnancy are unknown. Horvath et al.[293] reported a randomized study in 100 pregnant hypertensive women comparing clonidine to methyldopa. They found no significant difference in blood pressure control or maternal and fetal outcome. The authors concluded that clonidine was a safe and effective antihypertensive agent to use in pregnancy.

Prazosin

Prazosin is a selective α_1-postsynaptic blocker. It reduces both systolic and diastolic blood pressures, while producing significantly less tachycardia and sodium retention than methyldopa. It causes vasodilation of both the resistance and capacitance vessels, thereby reducing cardiac preload and afterload without reducing renal blood flow or glomerular filtration rate. In addition, it produces a decrease in plasma renin activity and it is probably the drug of choice for treatment of hypertension characterized by high plasma renin levels. It is metabolized in the liver and excreted almost completely in the bile. The usual dose of prazosin is 1 mg twice daily; however, the drug has been used in doses as high as 20 mg/d. The first dose in some individuals can produce syncope due to exaggerated hypotension "first pass," and this can be avoided by decreasing the first dose. The median time to peak concentration in nonpregnant individuals is 2 hours, and the mean elimination half-life is 2 to 3 hours. Side effects include fluid retention, orthostatic hypotension, and nasal congestion. Lubbe et al.[294] assessed the pregnancy outcomes in 14 women receiving prazosin and exprenolol. They reported no incidence of superimposed preeclampsia, and infant birth weights were higher than those receiving either methyldopa or no medication. Sibai and Tabb (unpublished data, 1984) compared pregnancy outcomes in 80 women with chronic hypertension who were treated with either prazosin ($N = 40$) or methyldopa ($N = 40$). Both drugs were effective in controlling hypertension, and the incidence of superimposed preeclampsia was similar in both groups. There were no differences in perinatal outcome between the two groups. However, patients receiving prazosin had higher plasma volume findings at term than those receiving methyldopa.

Calcium Channel Blockers

Calcium channel blockers act by inhibiting transmembrane calcium ion influx from the extracellular space into the cytoplasm, thus blocking excitation-contraction coupling in smooth muscle fibers and thereby causing vasodilation and reduction in the peripheral resistance. They also have mild tocolytic properties. They have been used extensively in the treatment of hypertensive emergencies and urgencies as monotherapy or as a part of combination therapy. They have rapid onset of action following oral administration. Nifedipine has potent vasodilating properties without reduction in cardiac output. Few reports have described the use of nifedipine in a limited number of women with acute hypertension during pregnancy.[112,113,190,295–297] The drug was effective in controlling maternal blood pressure, and no adverse fetal or neonatal effects were noted. However, there is limited experience with nifedipine treatment of chronic hypertension. Common side effects include headache, flushing, tachycardia, and fatigue. Care should be exercised when using nifedipine with magnesium sulfate (which is a calcium channel blocker itself), since the use of both agents together could potentiate the antihypertensive action.

Angiotensin-Converting Enzyme (ACE) Inhibitors

Three ACE inhibitors are available in the United States: captopril, enalapril, and lisinopril. They induce vasodilation by inhibiting the enzyme that converts angiotensin I to angiotensin II (potent vasoconstrictor), without reflex increase in the cardiac output. In addition, they increase the synthesis of vasodilating prostaglandins and diminish the rate of bradykinin inactivation (potent vasodilator). Because of their efficacy and low side effects, these agents are becoming widely used as first-line therapy for chronic hypertension in the nonpregnant state. In the experimental animal model, captopril causes abortion and fetal death, apparently by reducing the uteroplacental perfusion. In human pregnancy, the chronic use of ACE inhibitors has reportedly been associated with several fetal and neonatal complications: neonatal hypotension, fetal growth retardation, oligohydramnios, neonatal anuria and renal failure, and neonatal death.[298–301] Thus, it is recommended that the use of these agents in pregnancy be avoided.[299]

Hydralazine

Hydralazine is a potent vasodilator that acts directly on the vascular smooth muscle. Hydralazine is the agent most commonly used to control severe hypertension in preeclampsia, where it is given intravenously in bolus injections. After its intravenous use, the hypotensive effect of this drug develops gradually over 15 to 30 minutes, peaking at 20 minutes. The elimination half-life is about 3 hours. The usual bolus dose is 5 to 10 mg to be repeated every 20 to 30 minutes as needed. Its main side effects are fluid retention, tachycardia, palpitation, headache, and a lupus-like syndrome, as well as neonatal thrombocytopenia. About 50 percent of the U.S. population are genetically determined slow acetylators and thus are at higher risk for hypotension. Many of these side effects are common with high chronic doses and are usually minimized when it is used in combination with other antihypertensives. Because oral hydralazine when used as a monotherapy is a weak antihypertensive, it is usually combined with diuretics, methyldopa, or β-blockers; however, the use of multiple agents is discouraged in pregnancy. The usual oral dose is 10 mg given four times daily, but this can be increased up to 300 mg/d.

β-Blockers

The drugs in this category have different hemodynamic effects that depend on their receptor selectivity, the presence of intrinsic sympathomimetic activity (ISA), and their lipid solubility. The mechanisms of action of these drugs are complex and highly controversial.[302–304] Drugs without ISA reduce both cardiac output and heart rate in association with their antihypertensive effects. On the other hand, drugs with ISA reduce mean arterial blood pressure without influencing either cardiac output or heart rate. β-Blockers have been extensively used, since their introduction in the 1960s, to treat thyroid disease, mitral valve prolapse, migraine headache, glaucoma, and chronic hypertension. Side effects in the nonpregnant state include bronchial spasm, hypoglycemia, cold extremities, as well as disturbances in the lipid metabolism. Their use in pregnancy has been reportedly associated with neonatal bradycardia, hypoglycemia, fetal growth retardation, altered adaptation to perinatal asphyxia, and neonatal respiratory depression.[305] However, most of these neonatal effects could be attributed to maternal disease as well.

There are numerous reports describing the management of hypertension during pregnancy with various β-blockers, but only a few are well-controlled. This subject was recently reviewed by Rubin,[305] who concluded that these drugs are safe when used in pregnancy. In addition, he reported that their use was associated with better perinatal outcome than that achieved with either methyldopa or hydralazine. However, we believe it is almost impossible to make any conclusions regarding the safety and efficacy of these drugs from such studies. It is difficult to compare the results of these studies because (1) they involved heterogeneous groups of patients with chronic hypertension, preeclampsia, and chronic hypertension with superimposed preeclampsia; (2) the β-blockers were used in association with other antihypertensive agents such as diuretics, hydralazine, methyldopa, or prazosin; and (3) the blood pressure value at the time of initiating therapy and the duration of treatment were highly variable.

Thiazide Diuretics

Thiazide diuretics are generally the first drugs selected in the treatment of nonpregnant hypertensive patients. Consequently, most women with chronic hypertension become pregnant while on diuretics. Initially, in the first 3 to 5 days of treatment, these drugs result in reduction (5 to 10 percent) in both plasma and extracellular fluid volumes with a concomitant decrease in the cardiac output and lowering of the blood pressure. However, these changes tend to return to pretreatment levels within 4 to 6 weeks. These effects are followed by a long-term reduction in peripheral resistance, which is thought to be related to reduced intracellular sodium concentration in vascular smooth muscle cells. The usual dose is a single 25-mg dose in the morning. Adverse maternal effects reported with diuretics during pregnancy include hypokalemia, hyponatremia, hyper-

glycemia, hyperuricemia, hyperlipidemia, hemorrhagic pancreatitis, and even death. Neonatal adverse effects are electrolyte imbalance, thrombocytopenia, and small size for gestation.

Other harmful maternal and fetal effects were reported from the use of diuretics during pregnancy, including significant plasma volume depletion that may be detrimental to fetal growth.[306,307] Sibai et al.[308] noted that pregnant patients with chronic hypertension treated with diuretics have a marked reduction in plasma volume compared with a control group not receiving these medications. However, plasma volume expansion was normal after the discontinuation of diuretics. In a subsequent report, Sibai et al.[309] measured the plasma volume in 20 hypertensive women who received diuretics before and early in pregnancy. Diuretics were continued in 10 of these subjects but were discontinued in the remainder. In the group whose diuretics were continued, subsequent plasma volume at various stages of gestation were markedly reduced compared with findings in the others. Collins et al.[310] reviewed nine randomized trials of diuretics in pregnancy involving nearly 7,000 women and concluded that prophylactic thiazide therapy does not reduce the incidence of preeclampsia. Similar findings were reported by MacGillivray,[311] who found that patients receiving diuretics delivered infants who weighed less than those born to control pregnant women.

Because the initiation of diuretic therapy causes a decrease in blood volume and cardiac output, adding a diuretic late in pregnancy is probably contraindicated unless it is needed for treatment of pulmonary edema. On the other hand, continuing a diuretic as a part of therapeutic program in patients with chronic hypertension who become pregnant remains an unresolved issue. Our policy is to discontinue thiazide diuretics in such patients at the time of first visit. Since plasma volume depletion is associated with poor perinatal outcome we have cautioned against the use of diuretics in pregnancies complicated by chronic hypertension. Furthermore, when diuretics are discontinued, few patients require additional medications during the remainder of the pregnancy.[309]

Management of Chronic Hypertension

The primary objective in the management of pregnancies complicated with chronic hypertension is to reduce maternal risks and achieve optimal perinatal survival. This objective can be achieved by formulating a rational approach that includes preconceptional evaluation and counseling, early antenatal care, frequent antepartum visits to monitor both maternal and fetal well-being, timely delivery with intensive intrapartum monitoring, and proper postpartum management.

Preconceptional Evaluation of Chronic Hypertension

Management of patients with chronic hypertension should ideally begin before pregnancy, when extensive evaluation is undertaken to assess the etiology and the severity of the hypertension, as well as the presence of other medical illnesses, and to rule out the presence of target organ damage of long standing hypertension.[275]

An in-depth history should delineate in particular the duration of hypertension, the use of antihypertensive medications, their type, and the response to these medications. As some medications that have potentially harmful effects on both the fetus and the mother are frequently used in the nonpregnant state (diuretics, ACE inhibitors, ganglion blockers), it is prudent to change these drugs to others with well-documented safety and to monitor the responses of the patients to these medications. Also attention should be given to the presence of cardiac or renal disease, diabetes, thyroid disease, and a history of cerebrovascular accident or congestive heart failure. A detailed obstetric history should include maternal as well as neonatal outcome of previous pregnancies with stresses on history of development of abruptio placentae, superimposed preeclampsia, preterm delivery, small for gestation infants, intrauterine fetal death, and neonatal morbidity and mortality. A detailed physical examination should include the following:

> General physical examination
> Fundoscopic examination
> Measurement of blood pressure in the four extremities
> Measurement of blood pressure with changes in posture and after rest
> Detailed auscultation of chest and flanks
> Checking of pulses in the four extremities

Laboratory evaluation is obtained in order to assess the functions of different organ systems that are likely to be affected by chronic hypertension, and as a baseline for future assessments; these should include

1. For all patients
   a. Urine analysis
   b. Urine culture and sensitivity
   c. 24-Hour urine evaluation for protein, sodium, potassium, and creatinine clearance
   d. SMAC-20
   e. CBC
   f. Glucose tolerance test
2. Selectively
   a. If hyperglycemia or wide blood pressure swings are evident, a 24-hour urine evaluation for vanil-

lylmandelic acid (VMA) and metanephrines is recommended to rule out pheochromocytoma.
   b. For patients with severe hypertension or significant proteinuria, chest x-ray, ECG, antinuclear antibody, and serum complement studies are indicated.
   c. For patients with severe long-standing hypertension, or if there is a suspicion of heart disease, an echocardiogram is recommended.
   d. Women with a history of poor pregnancy outcome (repetitive midpregnancy losses), and those with recent thromboembolic disease, should be evaluated for the presence of lupus anticoagulants and anticardiolipin antibodies.[312]

Pregnancies in women with chronic hypertension and renal insufficiency are associated with increased perinatal loss and higher incidence of superimposed preeclampsia, preterm delivery, and fetal growth retardation.[313–315] These risks rise in proportion to the severity of the renal insufficiency; women with severe renal insufficiency, particularly primary glomerular disease, risk rapid progression to end-stage renal disease during pregnancy or postpartum.[313–315] Thus, women with renal disease desiring pregnancy should be counseled to conceive before renal insufficiency becomes severe. For women with hypertension and severe renal insufficiency in the first trimester, the decision to continue pregnancy should not be made without extensive counseling regarding the potential maternal and fetal risks, particularly the potential need for dialysis during pregnancy[314,315] Women who elect to continue their pregnancies must be observed and managed at a tertiary care center with adequate maternal-neonatal care facilities.

Initial and Subsequent Prenatal Visits for Patients with Chronic Hypertension

Early prenatal care will ensure accurate determination of gestational age as well as the severity of hypertension in the first trimester, which have prognostic values for the outcome of such pregnancies. At the time of initial and subsequent visits, the patient should be counseled regarding the following aspects as they pertain to her pregnancy:

1. Instruction by a nutritionist regarding nutritional requirements, weight gain, and sodium intake
2. Instruction regarding the negative impact of maternal anxiety, smoking, and caffeine, as well as drugs, on maternal blood pressure and perinatal outcome
3. Instruction regarding the positive impact of adequate bedrest during the day and at night on maternal blood pressure and pregnancy outcome

4. Counsel regarding the possible adverse effects and complications of hypertension during pregnancy
5. Counsel regarding the importance of frequent prenatal visits and their impact on preventing or minimizing the above adverse effects

If the patient is well motivated, she can be instructed in self-determination of blood pressure, as recommended by Zuspan and Rayburn.[316] This approach avoids the phenomenon of "white coat hypertension," which is associated with a visit to the physician's office, and avoids need for starting or increasing the dose of antihypertensive medications. It is recommended that patient-recorded measurements of blood pressure be used to supplement those recorded in the doctor's office.

During the course of pregnancy, the patient should be seen once every 2 to 3 weeks in the first two trimesters and thereafter adjusted based on maternal and fetal conditions. Systolic and diastolic blood pressure readings should be carefully measured at each visit. At each visit, the urine should be checked for protein. Maternal evaluation should include serial measurements of hematocrit, serum creatinine, uric acid, and 24-hour urinary excretion of protein at least once every trimester. Other tests are obtained as needed. The occurrence of one or more of the following is an indication for prompt maternal hospitalization:

1. Pyelonephritis
2. Significant elevations in blood pressure with levels in the range of severe hypertension
3. Significant elevation in serum uric acid level and new onset of substantial proteinuria (>1 g/24 hour). This finding is usually an early sign of developing superimposed preeclampsia
4. Severe fetal growth retardation

Based on the initial assessment, the patient is then classified as having low-risk or high-risk chronic hypertension depending on duration of hypertension, severity of hypertension early in pregnancy, and the extent of cardiovascular and renal involvement at the onset of pregnancy and other factors.

Managing Low-Risk Chronic Hypertension

As stated previously, most patients with uncomplicated mild chronic hypertension will have a good perinatal outcome irrespective of the use of antihypertensive drugs. A recent analysis of pregnancy outcome in 211 patients with mild chronic hypertension managed at our institution[1] suggests that the use of antihypertensive drugs is not necessary to achieve a good pregnancy outcome. The changes in average MAP throughout the course of pregnancy is summarized in Figure 28-7. It is of interest to note that 49 percent of patients will demonstrate a decrease in MAP and an additional 34 percent will demonstrate no change in MAP at 20 to 26 weeks' gestation without the use of antihypertensive medications. Furthermore, only 13 percent of patients will require antihypertensive medications for exacerbation of hypertension during the third trimester. In the same study, we found that most of the poor outcome was related to the development of superimposed preeclampsia in such pregnancies. In addition, in the absence of superimposed preeclampsia, the perinatal outcome in patients with mild chronic hypertension was similar to that in the general obstetric population. We attribute the good perinatal outcome in these pregnancies to early onset of perinatal care, intensive antepartum and intrapartum monitoring, and timely delivery. Thus, it is our policy to discontinue all antihypertensive medications in all such patients at the time of first prenatal visit. Antihypertensive therapy is subsequently started only if the blood pressure exceeds 160 mmHg systolic or 110 mmHg diastolic. These patients are usually treated with methyldopa (750 to 4,000 mg/d) given as needed to keep diastolic blood pressure consistently at or below 105 mmHg. It is important to emphasize that the development of exacerbated hypertension alone is not an indication for delivery. The pregnancy in these patients may be continued until term or till the onset of superimposed preeclampsia. In the absence of superimposed preeclampsia or fetal jeopardy, routine induction before 41 weeks' gestation is not warranted. Superimposed preeclampsia or suspected fetal growth retardation is an indication for hospitalization and close evaluation of maternal and fetal well-being. Subsequent management is similar to that in the high-risk group and will depend on the fetal gestational age and the result of antepartum fetal testing. Mild superimposed preeclampsia is an indication for delivery if the gestational age is at least 37 weeks. Otherwise, the pregnancy can be managed conservatively until the cervix is ripe for induction, onset of labor, or completion of 40 weeks' gestation.

Managing High-Risk Chronic Hypertension

Pregnancies in women at high risk are associated with increased maternal and perinatal complications.[275] As a result, these patients should be managed in consultation with a fetomaternal medicine specialist. Furthermore, patients with chronic renal disease—particularly those with primary glomerular diseases and significant renal function impairment (serum creatinine >2.5 mg/dl)—should be managed in consultation with a nephrologist. All these patients should be hospitalized at the time of first prenatal visit for evaluation of cardio-

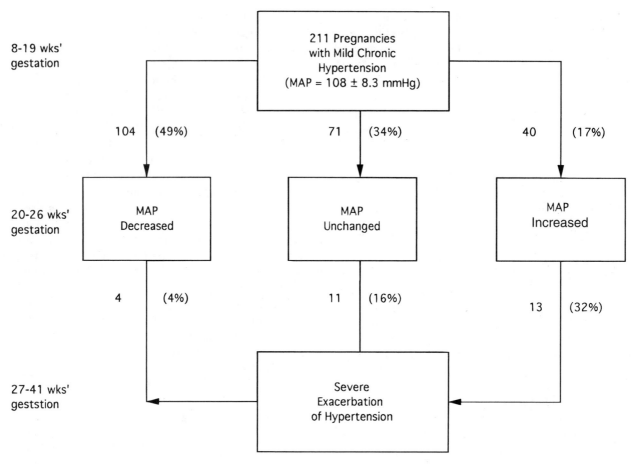

Fig. 28-7 Mean arterial blood pressure (MAP) during pregnancy. (Modified from Sibai et al.,[274] with permission.)

High-Risk Characteristics

Maternal age >40 years

Duration of hypertension >15 years

Blood pressure ≥160/110 mmHg early in pregnancy

Diabetes (class B–F)

Renal disease (all causes)

Cardiomyopathy

Connective tissue disease

Coarctation of the aorta

Presence of lupus anticoagulant

Previous pregnancy with perinatal loss

(From Sibai et al,[275] with permission.)

vascular and renal status and for regulation of antihypertensive medications, as well as other prescribed medications (insulin, thyroid drugs, cardiac drugs). Antihypertensive medications should be used to keep systolic blood pressure between 140 and 160 mmHg and diastolic blood pressure between 90 and 105 mmHg. Maternal blood pressure can be controlled with methyldopa (1 to 4 g/d), labetalol (600 mg to 2,400 mg/d), or nifedipine (40 to 120 mg/d). In some patients, blood pressure may be difficult to control, demanding the use of multiple oral drugs as well as intravenous therapy. Antihypertensives must be used in all women with severe hypertension. In addition, there are short-term maternal benefits from treating women with mild hypertension and target organ damage such as diabetes mellitus, renal disease, and cardiac dysfunction. As a result, we recommend treating mild chronic hypertension in pregnant women with these complications (keeping diastolic blood pressure <90 mmHg). For patients with significant proteinuria in the first trimester, antinuclear antibody and serum complement are performed to rule out the presence of lupus nephritis. Early and frequent prenatal care is the key to a successful outcome for patients with high-risk characteristics. These women need close monitoring throughout pregnancy and may require multiple hospital admissions for control of blood pressure or associated medical complications. Fetal evaluation should be started as early as 26 weeks and repeated as needed. Superimposed preeclampsia is an indication for immediate hospitalization. Subsequent management will depend on the severity of preeclampsia and fetal gestational age. Severe superimposed preeclampsia is an indication for delivery in all patients with gestational age beyond 34 weeks. If preeclampsia develops before this time, the pregnancy may be followed conservatively with daily evaluation of maternal and fetal well-being.

Hypertensive Emergencies in Chronic Hypertension

On rare occasions, pregnant women may present with life-threatening clinical conditions that require immediate control of blood pressure, such as hypertensive encephalopathy, acute left ventricular failure, acute aortic dissection, or increased circulating catecholamines (pheochromocytoma, clonidine withdrawal, cocaine ingestion). Patients at highest risk for these complications include those with underlying cardiac disease, chronic glomerular renal disease, multiple drugs to control their hypertension, superimposed preeclampsia in the second trimester, and abruptio placentae complicated by disseminated intravascular coagulation. Although a diastolic blood pressure of 115 mmHg or greater is usually considered as a hypertensive emergency, this level is actually arbitrary and the rate of change of blood pressure may be more important than absolute level.[317] The association of elevated blood pressure with evidence of new or progressive end-organ damage determines the seriousness of the clinical situation.[318]

Hypertensive Encephalopathy

Untreated essential hypertension progresses to a hypertensive crisis in up to 1 to 2 percent of cases for unknown reasons. Hypertensive encephalopathy is usually seen in patients with systolic blood pressure above 250 mmHg or diastolic blood pressure above 150 mmHg.[318] Patients with acute onset of hypertension may develop encephalopathy at pressure levels that are generally tolerated by those with chronic hypertension. Normally, cerebral blood flow is approximately 50 ml/100 g tissue per minute. When the blood pressure falls, cerebral arterioles normally dilate, whereas, when blood pressure increases, they constrict to maintain constant cerebral blood flow.[319] This mechanism usually remains operative between 60 and 120 mmHg diastolic blood pressure. Hypertensive encephalopathy is

currently considered to be a derangement of the autoregulation of cerebral arterioles, which occurs when the upper limit of autoregulation is exceeded.[318] With severe hypertension (130 to 150 mmHg cerebral perfusion pressure), cerebral blood vessels constrict as much as possible and then reflex cerebral vasodilatation occurs. This results in overperfusion, damage to small blood vessels, cerebral edema, and increased intracranial pressure (breakthrough theory). Others believe that hypertensive encephalopathy results from an exaggerated vasoconstrictive response of the arterioles resulting in cerebral ischemia (over-regulation theory). Patients who have impaired autoregulation involving the cerebral arterioles may experience necrotizing arteriolitis, microinfarcts, petechial hemorrhages, multiple small thrombi, or cerebral edema.[318] Typically, hypertensive encephalopathy has a subacute onset (over 24 to 72 hours).[319]

During a hypertensive crisis, other evidence for end-organ damage may be present: cardiac, renal, or retinal dysfunction secondary to impaired organ perfusion and loss of autoregulation of blood flow.[318] Ischemia of the retina (with flame-shaped retinal hemorrhages, retinal infarcts, or papilledema) may occur—causing decreased visual acuity. Impaired regulation of coronary blood flow and marked increase in ventricular wall stress may result in angina, myocardial infarction, congestive heart failure, malignant ventricular arrhythmia, pulmonary edema, or dissecting aortic aneurysm. Necrosis of the afferent arterioles of the glomerulus results in hemorrhages of the cortex and medulla, fibrinoid necrosis, and proliferative endarteritis (resulting in elevated serum creatinine [>3 mg/dl], proteinuria, oliguria, hematuria, hyaline or red blood cell casts, and progressive azotemia).[318] Severe hypertension may result in abruptio placentae with resultant disseminated intravascular coagulopathy. In addition, high levels of angiotensin II, norepinephrine, and vasopressin accompany ongoing vascular damage. These circulating hormones increase relative efferent arteriolar tone, resulting in sodium pressure diuresis and hypovolemia. Because levels of renin and angiotensin II are increased, the aldosterone level is also elevated. The impact of these endocrine changes may be important in maintaining the hypertensive crisis.

Treatment of Hypertensive Encephalopathy

The ultimate goal of therapy is to prevent the occurrence of a hypertensive emergency. Patients at risk for hypertensive crisis should receive intensive management during labor and for a minimum of 48 hours after delivery. Although pregnancy may complicate the diagnosis, once the life-threatening conditions are recognized, pregnancy should not in any way slow or alter the mode of therapy. The only reliable clinical criterion for confirming the diagnosis of hypertensive encephalopathy is prompt response of the patient to antihypertensive therapy. The headache and sensorium often clear dramatically—sometimes within 1 to 2 hours after the treatment. The overall recovery may be somewhat slower in patients with uremia and in whom the symptoms have been present for a prolonged period before the therapy is given. Sustained cerebrovascular deficits should suggest other diagnoses.[319]

Patients with hypertensive encephalopathy or other hypertensive crisis should be hospitalized for bedrest. Intravenous lines should be inserted for fluids and medications. Although there is a tendency to restrict sodium intake in patients with hypertensive emergency, volume contraction from sodium pressure diuresis may be present. A marked drop in diastolic blood pressure with a rise in heart rate on standing from the supine position is evidence of volume contraction. Infusion of normal saline solution during the first 24 to 48 hours to achieve volume expansion should be considered. Saline infusion may help decrease the activity of the renin-angiotensin-aldosterone axis and result in better blood pressure control. Simultaneous repletion of potassium losses and continuous monitoring of blood pressure, volume status, urinary output, electrocardiographic readings, and mental status is mandatory. An intra-arterial line may provide the most accurate blood pressure information. Laboratory studies include complete blood count, differential, reticulocyte count, platelets, and an SMAC. A urinalysis should be obtained for protein, glucose, blood, cells, casts, and bacteria. Assessment for end-organ damage (central nervous system, retina, renal, cardiovascular) should be done periodically. Antepartum patients should have continuous fetal monitoring.[317,320]

Lowering Blood Pressure

There are risks associated with a too rapid or excessive reduction of elevated blood pressure. The aim of therapy is to lower mean blood pressure by no more than 15 to 25 percent. Small reductions in blood pressure in the first 60 minutes, working toward a diastolic level of 100 to 110 mmHg, have been recommended.[317,321] Although cerebral blood flow is maintained constantly over a wide range of blood pressures, there is a lower (as well as an upper) limit to autoregulation. In chronic hypertensives who have a rightward shift of the cerebral autoregulation curve secondary to medial hypertrophy of the cerebral vasculature, lowering blood pressure too rapidly may produce cerebral ischemia, stroke, or coma. Coronary blood flow, renal perfusion, and uteroplacental perfusion also may deteriorate, resulting in

acute renal failure, myocardial infarction, fetal distress, or death. If the hypertension proves increasingly difficult to control ("blood pressure escapes") this is an indication to end the pregnancy. If the patient's outcome appears to be grave, consideration of perimortem cesarean delivery should be made.[317]

The drug of choice in hypertensive crisis is sodium nitroprusside. Other drugs such as nitroglycerin, diazoxide, trimetaphan, labetalol, and hydralazine can also be used.

Sodium Nitroprusside

Sodium nitroprusside causes arterial and venous relaxation by interfering with both influx and the intracellular activation of calcium. It is given as an intravenous infusion of 0.25 to 8.0 μg/kg/min. The onset of action is immediate, and its effect may last 3 to 5 minutes after discontinuing the infusion. Hypotension caused by nitroprusside should resolve within a few minutes of stopping the infusion, because the drug's half-life is so short. If it does not resolve, other causes for hypotension should be suspected. The effect of nitroprusside on uterine blood flow is controversial. Nitroprusside is metabolized into thiocyanate, which is excreted in the urine. Cyanide can accumulate if there is either increased production due to large doses (>10 μg/kg/min) or prolonged administration (>48 hours), or if there is renal insufficiency or decreased metabolism in the liver. Signs of toxicity include anorexia, disorientation, headache, fatigue, restlessness, tinnitus, delirium, hallucinations, nausea, vomiting, and metabolic acidosis. When it is infused at less than 2 μg/kg/min, cyanide toxicity is unlikely. At a maximum dose rate of 10 μg/kg/min, infusion should never last more than 10 minutes. Animal experiments and the few reported cases of nitroprusside use in pregnancy have revealed that thiocyanate toxicity to mother and fetus rarely occur if it is used in a regular pharmacological dose. Before toxicity manifests, usually tachyphylaxis to nitroprusside effect develops. Whenever toxicity is suspected, therapy should be initiated with 3 percent sodium nitrite at a rate not exceeding 5 ml/min, up to a total dose of 15 ml. Then, infusion of 12.5 g of sodium thiosulfate in 50 ml of 5 percent dextrose in water over a 10-minute period should be started.[321]

Nitroglycerin

Nitroglycerin is an arterial and venous dilator (mostly venous). It is given as an intravenous infusion of 5 μg/min that is gradually increased every 3 to 5 minutes to titrate blood pressure up to a maximum dose of 100 μg/min. It is the drug of choice in preeclampsia associated with pulmonary edema and for control of hypertension associated with tracheal manipulation. Side effects such as headache, tachycardia, and methemoglobinemia may develop. It is contraindicated in hypertensive encephalopathy because it increases cerebral blood flow and intracranial pressure.[318]

Postpartum Management of Hypertension

High-risk chronic hypertensives can develop hypertensive encephalopathy, pulmonary edema, and renal failure in the postpartum period. These risks are particularly increased in women with underlying cardiac disease, chronic glomerular renal disease, superimposed preeclampsia in the second trimester, abruptio placentae complicated by disseminated intravascular coagulation, and those requiring multiple hypertensive agents.[275] Patients with these complications should receive intensive management for a minimum of 48 hours after delivery and intravenous hydralazine or labetalol for control of severe hypertension as needed. Moreover, diuretic therapy should be used in women who are at risk for delayed onset of postpartum circulatory congestion and pulmonary edema (massively obese older women with long-standing hypertension and those with previous antepartum congestive heart failure).

Oral antihypertensive drugs may be needed to control maternal blood pressure after delivery. Some women may wish to breast-feed their infants while receiving these agents. Unfortunately, data are limited concerning the excretion of these drugs into human breast milk and their effects on the infant.[322,323] In addition, there are no published reports describing the long-term effects of antihypertensive agents on infants exposed to these drugs through breast-feeding. Most of the published data have described the milk-plasma ratio after a single measurement of the drug concentration.[322,323] The data in the literature indicate that all studied antihypertensive agents are excreted into human breast milk, although there are differences among these drugs in the milk-plasma ratio.[323] The available data also show that there are no short-term adverse effects on the breast-feeding infant exposed to methyldopa, hydralazine, or β-blockers. However, thiazide diuretics should be avoided during lactation because their use has been reported to decrease or inhibit milk production.[322,323]

Ten Key Points

- Hypertension is the most common medical complication during pregnancy.
- Preeclampsia is a leading cause of maternal mortality and morbidity worldwide.
- The pathophysiologic abnormalities of preeclampsia are numerous, but the etiology is unknown.
- At present, there is no proven method to prevent preeclampsia.
- The HELLP syndrome may develop in the absence of maternal hypertension.
- Expectant management improves perinatal outcome in a select group of women with severe preeclampsia before 32 weeks' gestation.
- Magnesium sulfate is the ideal agent to prevent or treat eclamptic convulsions.
- Rare cases of eclampsia can develop before 20 weeks' gestation and beyond 48 hours postpartum.
- Antihypertensive agents do not improve pregnancy outcome in women with mild uncomplicated chronic hypertension.
- Methyldopa is the drug of choice for the treatment of chronic hypertension; ACE Inhibitors should be avoided.

References

1. Sibai BM: Hypertension in pregnancy. Obstet Gynecol Clin North Am 19:615, 1992
2. National High Blood Pressure Education Program Working Group: Report on high blood pressure in pregnancy. Am J Obstet Gynecol 163:1689, 1990
3. Hughes EC (ed): Obstetric-Gynecologic Terminology. FA Davis, Philadelphia, 1972
4. American College of Obstetricians and Gynecologists: Technical Bulletin No. 91. Management of Preeclampsia. February 1986
5. Zuspan FP: New concepts in the understanding of hypertensive diseases during pregnancy. Clin Perinatol 18:653, 1991
6. Dexter L, Weiss S: Preeclamptic and eclamptic toxemia of pregnancy. Little, Brown, Boston, 1941
7. Sibai BM: Eclampsia VI. Maternal-perinatal outcome in 254 consecutive cases. Am J Obstet Gynecol 163:1045, 1990
8. Nelson TR: A clinical study of preeclampsia. J Obstet Gynaecol Br Emp 62:48, 1955
9. World Health Organization: The hypertensive disorders of pregnancy: report of a WHO study group. Technical Report Series No. 758. WHO, Geneva, 1987
10. Davey DA, MacGillivray I: The classification and definition of the hypertensive disorders of pregnancy. Am J Obstet Gynecol 158:892, 1988

11. Sheehan HL, Lynch JB: Pathology of Toxaemia of Pregnancy. Churchill Livingstone, Edinburgh, 1973

12. Beurel JN Jr: Eclampsia in lowland gorilla. Am J Obstet Gynecol 141:345, 1981

13. Villar MA, Sibai BM: Clinical significance of elevated mean arterial blood in second trimester and threshold increase in systolic or diastolic pressure during third trimester. Am J Obstet Gynecol 60:419, 1989

14. Long PA, Abell DA, Beischer NA: Parity and preeclampsia. Aust NZ J Obstet Gynaecol 19:203, 1979

15. Long P, Oats J: Preeclampsia in twin-pregnancy—severity and pathogenesis. Aust NZ J Obstet Gynaecol 27:1, 1987

16. Campbell DM, MacGillivray I, Carr-Hill R: Preeclampsia in second pregnancy. Br J Obstet Gynaecol 92:131, 1985

17. Boyd PA, Lindenbaum RH, Redman C: Pre-eclampsia and trisomy 13: a possible association. Lancet 2:425, 1987

18. Tuohy JP, James DK: Pre-eclampsia and trisomy 13. Br J Obstet Gynaecol 99:891, 1992

19. Brosens IA: Morphological changes in the uteroplacental bed in pregnancy hypertension. Clin Obstet Gynaecol 4:583, 1977

20. Kong TY, DeWolf F, Robertson WB, Brosens I: Inadequate maternal vascular response to placentation in pregnancies complicated by preeclampsia and by small-for-gestational age infants. Br J Obstet Gynaecol 93:1049, 1986

21. Frusca T, Morassi L, Pecorell S et al: Histological features of uteroplacental vessels in normal and hypertensive patients in relation to birthweight. Br J Obstet Gynaecol 96:835, 1989

22. Sheppard BL, Bonnar J: An ultrastructural study of uteroplacental spiral arteries in hypertensive and normotensive pregnancy and fetal growth retardation. Br J Obstet Gynaecol 88:695, 1981

23. Meekins JW, Pijneborg R, Hanssens M et al: A study of placental bed spiral arteries and trophoblast invasion in normal and severe preeclamptic pregnancies. Br J Obstet Gynaecol 101:669, 1994

24. Shanklin DR, Sibai BM: Ultrastructural aspects of pre-eclampsia. I. Placental bed and uterine boundary vessels. Am J Obstet Gynecol 161:735, 1989

25. Saleh AA, Bottoms SF, Welch RA et al: Preeclampsia, delivery, and the hemostatic system. Am J Obstet Gynecol 157:331, 1987

26. Saleh AA, Bottoms SF, Norman G et al: Hemostasis in hypertensive disorders of pregnancy. Obstet Gynecol 71:719, 1988

27. Lockwood CJ, Peters JH: Increased plasma levels of ED1 + cellular fibronectin precede the clinical signs of preeclampsia. Am J Obstet Gynecol 162:358, 1990

28. Taylor RM, Crombleholme WR, Friedman SA et al: High plasma cellular fibronectin levels correlate with biochemical and clinical features of preeclampsia but cannot be attributed to hypertension alone. Am J Obstet Gynecol 165:895, 1991

29. Rodgers GM, Taylor RN, Roberts JM: Preeclampsia is associated with a serum factor cytotoxic to human endothelial cells. Am J Obstet Gynecol 159:908, 1988

30. Musci TJ, Roberts JM, Rodgers GM, Taylor RN: Mitogenic activity is increased in the sera of preeclamptic women before delivery. Am J Obstet Gynecol 159:1446, 1988

31. Roberts JM, Taylor RN, Musci TJ et al: Preeclampsia: an endothelial cell disorder. Am J Obstet Gynecol 161:1200, 1989

32. Weiner CP, Brandt J: Plasma antithrombin III activity: an aid in the diagnosis of preeclampsia-eclampsia. Am J Obstet Gynecol 142:275, 1982

33. Weiner CP, Kwaan HC, Xu C et al: Antithrombin III activity in women with hypertension with pregnancy. Obstet Gynecol 65:301, 1985

34. Socol ML, Weiner CP, Louis G et al: Platelet activation in preeclampsia. Am J Obstet Gynecol 151:494, 1985

35. deBoer K, Tencate JW, Sturk A et al: Enchanced thrombin generation in normal and hypertensive pregnancy. Am J Obstet Gynecol 160:96, 1989

36. Gilabert J, Fernandez JA, Espana F et al: Physiological coagulation inhibitors (protein S, protein C and antithrombin III) in severe preeclamptic states and in users of oral contraceptives. Thrombos Res 49:319, 1988

37. Friedman SA: Preeclampsia: a review of the role of prostaglandins. Obstet Gynecol 71:122, 1988

38. Ylikorkala O, Makila UM: Prostacyclin and thromboxane in gynecology and obstetrics. Am J Obstet Gynecol 152:318, 1985

39. Walsh SW: Preeclampsia: an imbalance in placenta prostacyclin and thromboxane production. Am J Obstet Gynecol 152:335, 1985

40. Goodman RP, Killam AP, Brash AR, Branch RA: Comparison of production during normal pregnancy and pregnancy complicated by hypertension. Am J Obstet Gynecol 142:817, 1982

41. Fitzgerald DJ, Entmann SS, Mulloy K, Fitzgerald GA: Decreased prostaglandin biosynthesis preceding the clinical manifestation of pregnancy-induced hypertension. Circulation 75:956, 1987

42. Walsh SW, Parisi VM: The role of arachidonic acid metabolites in preeclampsia. Semin Perinatol 10:335, 1986

43. Moodley J, Reddi K, Norman RJ: Decreased central venous concentration of immunoreactive prostaglandins E, F, and 6-keto-PGF1α, in eclampsia. BMJ 288:1487, 1984

44. Brown HL, Klein L, Waitzman M: Plasma and amniotic fluid prostacyclin and thromboxane in mild pregnancy induced hypertension. Am J Perinatol 4:152, 1987

45. Moodley J, Kistnasarny MB, Reddi K et al: Amniotic fluid prostacyclin in African women with eclampsia. Clin Exp Hyper-Hyper Pregnancy B5:29, 1986

46. Zeeman GG, Dekker GA: Pathogenesis of preeclampsia: a hypothesis. Clin Obstet Gynecol 35:317, 1992

47. Pinto A, Sorrentino R, Sorrentino P et al: Endothelial-derived relaxing factor released by endothelial cells of human umbilical vessels and its impairment in pregnancy-induced hypertension. Am J Obstet Gynecol 164:507, 1991

48. Fickling SA, Williams D, Vallance P et al: Plasma con-

centrations of endogenous inhibitor of nitric oxide synthesis in normal pregnancy and pre-eclampsia. Lancet 342:242, 1993

49. Nova A, Sibai BM, Barton JR et al: Maternal plasma levels of endothelin is increased in preeclampsia. Am J Obstet Gynecol 164:794, 1991

50. Branch DW, Dudley DJ, Mitchell MD: Preliminary evidence for homeostatic mechanism regulating endothelin production in preeclampsia. Lancet 337:943, 1991

51. Clark BA, Halvorson L, Sachs B, Epstein FH: Plasma endothelin levels in preeclampsia: elevations and correlation with uric acid and renal impairment. Am J Obstet Gynecol 166:962, 1992

52. Benigni A, Orisio S, Gaspari F et al: Evidence against a pathologic role for endothelin in preeclampsia. Br J Obstet Gynecol 99:798, 1992

53. Hubel CA, Roberts JM, Taylor RN et al: Lipid peroxidation in pregnancy: new perspective on preeclampsia. Am J Obstet Gynecol 161:1025, 1989

54. Walsh SW: Lipid peroxidation in pregnancy. Hypertension in pregnancy. Am J Obstet Gynecol 13:1, 1994

55. Dekker GA, Kraayenbrink AA: Oxygen free radicals in preeclampsia. Am J Obstet Gynecol 164:273, 1991

56. Uotila JT, Tuinaala RJ, Aarnis TM et al: Findings on lipid peroxidation and antioxidant function in hypertensive complications of pregnancy. Br J Obstet Gynaecol 100:270, 1993

57. Wang Y, Walsh SW, Guo J et al: The imbalance between thromboxane and prostacyclin in preeclampsia is associated with an imbalance between lipid peroxides and vitamin E in maternal blood. Am J Obstet Gynecol 167: 946, 1992

58. Davidge ST, Hubel CA, Braden RD et al: Sera antioxidant activity in uncomplicated and preeclamptic pregnancies. Obstet Gynecol 79:897, 1992

59. Wisdom SJ, Wilson R, McKillop JH, Walker JJ: Antioxidant systems in normal pregnancy and in pregnancy-induced hypertension. Am J Obstet Gynecol 165:1701, 1991

60. Mikhail MS, Anyaegbunam A, Garfinkel D et al: Preeclampsia and antioxidant nutrients: decreased plasma levels of reduced ascorbic acid, α-tocopherol, and beta-carotene in women with preeclampsia. Am J Obstet Gynecol 171:150, 1994

61. Sibai BM: Pitfalls in diagnosis and management of preeclampsia. Am J Obstet Gynecol 159:1, 1988

62. Lopez MC, Belizan JM, Villar J, Bergel E: The measurement of diastolic blood pressure during pregnancy: Which Korotkoff phase should be used? Am J Obstet Gynecol 170:574, 1992

63. Blank SG, Heleth G, Pickering TG et al: How should diastolic blood pressure be defined during pregnancy. Hypertension 24:234, 1994

64. Johenning AR, Barron WM: Indirect blood pressure measurement in pregnancy: Korotkoff phase 4 versus phase 5. Am J Obstet Gynecol 167:577, 1992

65. MacGillivray I, Rose GA, Rowe D: Blood pressure survey in pregnancy. Clin Sci 72:395, 1969

66. Redman CWG, Jeffries M: Revised definition of pre-eclampsia. Lancet 1:809, 1988

67. Perry IJ, Beevers DG: The definition of pre-eclampsia. Br J Obstet Gynaecol 101:587, 1994

68. Roberts JM, Redman CWE: Pre-eclampsia is more than pregnancy-induced hypertension. Lancet 341:1447, 1993

69. Ferrazani S, Caruso A, Carolis S et al: Proteinuria and outcome of 444 pregnancies complicated by hypertension. Am J Obstet Gynecol 162:366, 1990

70. Lindow SW, Davey DA: The variability of urinary protein and creatinine excretion in patients with gestational proteinuric hypertension. Br J Obstet Gynaecol 99:869, 1992

71. Kuo VS, Koumantakis G, Gallery EDM: Proteinuria and its assessment in normal and hypertensive pregnancy. Am J Obstet Gynecol 167:723, 1992

72. Meyer NL, Mercer BM, Friedman SA, Sibai BM: Urinary dipstick protein: a poor predictor of absent or severe proteinuria. Am J Obstet Gynecol 170:137, 1994

73. Dekker GA, Sibai BM: Early detection of preeclampsia. Am J Obstet Gynecol 165:160, 1991

74. Chesley LC, Sibai BM: Clinical significance of elevated mean arterial pressure in the second trimester. Am J Obstet Gynecol 159:275, 1988

75. Repke JT, Villar J: The role of dietary calcium in pregnancy-induced hypertension. Clin Nutr 8:169, 1989

76. Hatton DC, McCarron DA: Dietary calcium and blood pressure in experimental models of hypertension: a review. Hypertension 23:513, 1994

77. Taufield PA, Ales KL, Resnick LM et al: Hypocalciuria in preeclampsia. N Engl J Med 316:715, 1987

78. Sanchez-Ramos L, Sandroni S, Andres FL, Kaunitz AM: Calcium excretion in preeclampsia. Obstet Gynecol 77: 510, 1991

79. Sanchez-Ramos L, Jones DC, Cullen MT: Urinary calcium as an early marker for preeclampsia. Obstet Gynecol 77:685, 1991

80. Zemel MB, Zemel PC, Berry S et al: Altered platelet calcium metabolism as an early predictor of increased peripheral vascular resistance and preeclampsia in urban black women. N Engl J Med 323:434, 1990

81. Sowers JR, Zemel MB, Bronsteen RA: Erythrocyte cation metabolism in preeclampsia. Am J Obstet Gynecol 161:441, 1989

82. Belizan JM, Villar J, Repke J: The relationship between calcium intake and pregnancy induced hypertension: up to date evidence. Am J Obstet Gynecol 158:898, 1988

83. Kawasaki N, Matsui K, Nakamura T et al: Effect of caclium supplementation on the vascular sensitivity to angiotensin II in pregnant women. Am J Obstet Gynecol 153:576, 1985

84. Sanchez-Ramos L, Briones DK, Kaunitz AM et al: Prevention of pregnancy-induced hypertension by calcium supplementation in angiotensin-II sensitive patients. Obstet Gynecol 84:349, 1994

85. Marya RK, Rathee S, Manrow M: Effect of calcium and vitamin D supplementation on toxaemia of pregnancy. Gynecol Obstet Invest 24:38, 1987

86. Villar J, Repke J, Belizan JM et al: Calcium supplementation reduces blood pressure during pregnancy: results

from a randomized clinical trial. Obstet Gynecol 70: 317, 1987

87. Lopez-Jaramillo P, Narvaez M, Weigel RM et al: Calcium supplementation reduces the risk of pregnancy-induced hypertension in an Andes population. Br J Obstet Gynaecol 96:648, 1987

88. Villar J, Repke JT: Calcium supplementation during pregnancy may reduce preterm delivery in high-risk populations. Am J Obstet Gynecol 163:1124, 1990

89. Montanaro D, Boscutti G, Mioni G et al: Calcium supplementation decreases the incidence of pregnancy-induced hypertension (PIH) and preeclampsia. Abstract No. 91. p. 267. Proceedings of the VIIth World Congress of Hypertension in Pregnancy, Perugia, Italy. October 1990

90. Belizan JM, Villar J, Gonzalez L et al: Calcium supplementation to prevent hypertensive disorders of pregnancy. N Engl J Med 325:1399, 1991

91. Lopez-Jaramillo P, Narvaez M, Felix C, Lopez A: Dietary calcium supplementation and prevention of pregnancy hypertension. Lancet 335:293, 1990

92. Levine RJ, Raymon E, Der Simonian R, Clemens JD: Preeclampsia prevention with calcium supplementation. Clin Appl Nutr 2:30, 1992

93. Sibai BM, Villar MA, Bray E: Magnesium supplementation during pregnancy: a double-blind randomized controlled clinical trial. Am J Obstet Gynecol 161:115, 1989

94. Altura BM, Altura BT, Carella A: Magnesium deficiency induced spasm of umbilical vessels: relation to preeclampsia, hypertension, growth retardation. Science 221:376, 1983

95. Conradt A, Weidinger H, Algayer H: On the role of magnesium in fetal hypotrophy, pregnancy-induced hypertension and preeclampsia. Mag Bull 6:68, 1984

96. Spatling L, Spatling G: Magnesium supplementation in pregnancy. A double-blind study. Br J Obstet Gynaecol 95:120, 1988

97. Lazebnik N, Kuhnert BR, Kuhnert BM, Thompson KL: Zinc status, pregnancy complications and labor abnormalities. Am J Obstet Gynecol 158:161, 1988

98. Brophy MH, Harris NF, Crawford IL: Elevated copper and lowered zinc in the placentae of preeclampsia. Clin Acta 145:107, 1985

99. Hunt IF, Murphy NJ, Cleaver AE et al: Zinc supplementation during pregnancy: effects on selected blood constituents and on progress and outcome of pregnancy in low-income women of Mexican descent. Am J Clin Nutr 40:508, 1984

100. Mohamed K, James DK, Golding J, McCabe R: Zinc supplementation during pregnancy: a double-blind randomized controlled trial. BMJ 299:826, 1989

101. Spitz B, Magness RR, Cox SM et al: Low-dose aspirin. I. Effect on angiotensin II pressor responses and blood prostaglandin concentration in pregnant women sensitive to angiotensin II. Am J Obstet Gynecol 159:1035, 1988

102. Sibai BM, Mirro R, Chesney CM, Leffer C: Low dose aspirin in pregnancy. Obstet Gynecol 74:551, 1989

103. Dekker GA, Sibai BM: Low-dose aspirin: the prevention of preeclampsia and fetal growth retardation: rationale,

mechanisms, and clinical trials. Am J Obstet Gynecol 168:214, 1993

104. Hauth JC, Goldenberg RL, Parker Jr R et al: Low-dose aspirin therapy to prevent preeclampsia. Am J Obstet Gynecol 168:1083, 1993

105. Sibai BM, Caritis SN, Thom E et al: Prevention of preeclampsia with low-dose aspirin in healthy, nulliparous, pregnant women. N Engl J Med 329:1213, 1993

106. Viinikka L, Hartikainen-Sorri A-L, Lumme R et al: Low dose aspirin in hypertensive pregnant women: effect on pregnancy outcome and prostacyclin-thromboxane balance in mother and newborn. Br J Obstet Gynaecol 100:809, 1993

107. Italian Study of Aspirin in Pregnancy: Low-dose aspirin in prevention and treatment of intrauterine growth retardation and pregnancy-induced hypertension. Lancet 341:396, 1993

108. CLASP: A randomized trial of low-dose aspin for the prevention and treatment of pre-eclampsia among 9364 pregnant women. Lancet 343:619, 1992

109. HAMID R, Robson M, Pearch JM: Low-dose aspirin in women with raised maternal serum alpha-fetoprotein and abnormal Doppler waveform patterns from the uteroplacental circulation. Br J Obstet Gynaecol 101: 481, 1994

110. Dunlop W, Davidson JM: The effect of normal pregnancy on renal handling of uric acid. Br J Obstet Gynaecol 84:13, 1987

111. Cunningham FG, Lindheimer MD: Hypertension in pregnancy. N Engl J Med 326:927, 1992

112. Sibai BM, Barton JR, Akl S et al: A randomized prospective comparison of nifedipine and bed rest versus bed rest alone in the management of preeclampsia remote from term. Am J Obstet Gynecol 167:879, 1992

113. Sibai BM, Mercer BM, Schiff E, Friedman SA: Aggressive versus expectant management of severe preeclampsia at 28 to 32 weeks' gestation: a randomized controlled trial. Am J Obstet Gynecol 171:818, 1994

114. Redman CWG, Beilin LJ, Bonnar J: Plasma urate measurement in predicting fetal death in hypertensive pregnancies. Lancet 1:1370, 1976

115. Pritchard JA, Stone SR: Clinical and laboratory observations on eclampsia. Am J Obstet Gynecol 99:6:754, 1967

116. Weinstein L: Syndrome of hemolysis, elevated liver enzymes, and low platelet count; a severe consequence of hypertension in pregnancy. Am J Obstet Gynecol 142: 159, 1982

117. Arias F, Mancill-Jimenez R: Hepatic fibrinogen deposits in preeclampsia-immunofluorescent evidence. N Engl J Med 11:294, 1976

118. Romero R, Vizosa J, Emamian M et al: Clinical significance of liver dysfunction in pregnancy-induced hypertension. Am J Perinatol 5:146, 1988

119. Weiner C: Preeclampsia-eclampsia syndrome and coagulation. Clin Perinatol 18:713, 1992

120. Perry KG Jr, Martin JN Jr: Abnormal hemostasis and coagulopathy in preeclampsia and eclampsia. Clin Obstet Gynecol 35:338, 1992

121. Sibai BM, Watson DL, Hill GA et al: Maternal-fetal cor-

relations in patients with severe preeclampsia-eclampsia. Obstet Gynecol 62:745, 1983

122. Leduc L, Wheeler JM, Kirshon B et al: Coagulation profile in severe preeclampsia. Obstet Gynecol 79:14, 1992

123. Burrows F, Kelton JG: Fetal thrombocytopenia in relation to maternal thrombocytopenia. N Engl J Med 329:1463, 1993

124. Sibai BM, Taslimi MM, El-Nazer A et al: Maternal-perinatal outcome associated with the syndrome of hemolysis, elevated liver enzymes, and low platelets in severe preeclampsia-eclampsia. Am J Obstet Gynecol 155:501, 1986

125. Goodlin RC: Hemolysis, elevated liver enzymes, and low platelets syndrome. Obstet Gynecol 64:449, 1984

126. MacKenna J, Dover NL, Brame RG: Preeclampsia associated with hemolysis, elevated liver enzymes and low platelets—an obstetric emergency? Obstet Gynecol 62:751, 1983

127. Sibai BM: The HELLP syndrome (hemolysis, elevated liver enzymes, and low platelets): much ado about nothing? Am J Obstet Gynecol 162:311, 1990

128. Barton JR, Riely CA, Adamec TA et al: Hepatic histopathologic condition does not correlate with laboratory abnormalities in HELLP syndrome. Am J Obstet Gynecol 167:1538, 1992

129. Martin JN Jr, Files JC, Black PG et al: Plasma exchange for preeclampsia. I. Postpartum use for persistently severe preeclampsia-eclampsia with HELLP syndrome. Am J Obstet Gynecol 162:126, 1990

130. Martin JN Jr, Blake PG, Lowry SL et al: Pregnancy complicated by preeclampsia-eclampsia with the syndrome of hemolysis, evelvated liver enzymes, and low platelet count: how rapid is postpartum recovery? Obstet Gynecol 76:737, 1990

131. Miles JF Jr, Martin JN Jr, Blake PG et al: Postpartum eclampsia: a recurring perinatal dilemma. Obstet Gynecol 76:328, 1990

132. Van Dam PA, Reiner M, Baeklandt M et al: Disseminated intravascular coagulation and the syndrome of hemolysis, elevated liver enzymes, and low platelets in severe preeclampsia. Obstet Gynecol 73:97, 1989

133. DeBoer K, Buller HR, Ten Cato JW, Treffers PE: Coagulation studies in the syndrome of haemolysis, elevated liver enzymes, and low platelets. Br J Obstet Gynaecol 98:42, 1991

134. Sibai BM, Ramadan MK, Usta I et al: Maternal morbidity and mortality in 442 pregnancies with hemolysis, elevated liver enzymes, and low platelets (HELLP syndrome). Am J Obstet Gynecol 169:1000, 1993

135. Aarnoudse JG, Houthoff HF, Weits J et al: A syndrome of liver damage and intravascular coagulation in the last trimester of normotensive pregnancy. A clinical and histopathological study. Br J Obstet Gynaecol 93:145, 1986

136. Schwartz ML, Brenner WE: Pregnancy-induced hypertension presenting with life-threatening thrombocytopenia. Am J Obstet Gynecol 146:756, 1983

137. Goodlin RC: Beware the great imitator-severe preeclampsia. Contemp Obstet Gynecol 20:215, 1982

138. Thiagarajah S, Bourgeois FJ, Harbert GM, Caudle MR: Thrombocytopenia in preeclampsia: associated abnormalities and management principles. Am J Obstet Gynecol 150:1, 1984

139. Heyborne KD, Burke MS, Porreco RP: Prolongation of premature gestation in women with hemolysis, elevated liver enzyme, and low platelets. A report of 5 cases. J Reprod Med 35:53, 1990

140. Clark SL, Phelan JR, Allen SH, Golde SR: Antepartum reversal of hematologic abnormalities associated with the HELLP syndrome: a report of three cases. J Reprod Med 31:70, 1986

141. Van Assche FA, Spitz B: Thromboxane synthetase inhibition in pregnancy-induced hypertension. Am J Obstet Gynecol 159:1015, 1988

142. Magann EF, Bass D, Chauhan SP et al: Antepartum corticosteroids: disease stabilization in patients with the syndrome of hemolysis, elevated liver enzymes, and low platelets (HELLP). Am J Obstet Gynecol 171:1148, 1994

143. Magann EF, Perry KO Jr, Meydrech EF et al: Postpartum corticosteroids: accelerated recovery from the syndrome of hemolysis, elevated liver enzymes, and low platelets (HELLP). Am J Obstet Gynecol 171:1154, 1994

144. Woods JB, Blake PG, Perry KG Jr et al: Ascites: a portent of cardiopulmonary complications in the preeclamptic patient with the syndrome of hemolysis, elevated liver enzymes, and low platelets. Obstet Gynecol 80:87, 1992

145. Abroug F, Boujdaria R, Nouira S et al: HELLP syndrome: incidence and maternal-fetal outcome: a prospective study. Intensive Care Med 18:274, 1992

146. Sibai BM, Ramadan MK: Acute renal failure in pregnancies complicated by hemolysis, elevated liver enzymes, and low platelets. Am J Obstet Gynecol 168:1682, 1993

147. Schwartz ML: Possible role for exchange plasmapheresis with fresh frozen plasma for maternal indications in selected cases of preeclampsia and eclampsia. Obstet Gynecol 68:136, 1986

148. Goodlin RC, Anderson JC, Hodgson PE: Conservative treatment of liver hematoma in the postpartum period. J Reprod Med 30:368, 1985

149. Manas KJ, Welsh JD, Rankin RA: Hepatic haemorrhage without rupture in preeclampsia. N Engl M Med 312:424, 1985

150. Barton JR, Sibai BM: Care of the pregnancy complicated by HELLP syndrome. Obstet Gynecol Clin North Am 18:165, 1991

151. Smith JG Jr, Moise KJ Jr, Dildy GA et al: Spontaneous rupture of the liver during pregnancy: current therapy. Obstet Gynecol 77:171, 1991

152. Lovinger EH, Lee WM, Andersen MC: Hepatic rupture associated with pregnancy: treatment with transcatheter embolotherapy. Obstet Gynecol 65:281, 1985

153. Sibai BM, Mabie WC: Hemodynamics of preeclampsia. Clin Perinatol 18:727, 1991

154. Groenendijk R, Trimbos JBMJ, Wallenburg HCS: Hemodynamic measurements in preeclampsia. Preliminary observations. Am J Obstet Gynecol 150:812, 1985

155. Cotton DB, Jones MM, Longmire S et al: Role of intravenous nitroglycerin in the treatment of severe preg-

nancy-induced hypertension complicated by pulmonary edema. Am J Obstet Gynecol 143:91, 1986

156. Wallenburg HS: Hemodynamics in hypertensive pregnancy. p. 66. In Rubin PC (ed): Handbook of Hypertension—Hypertension in Pregnancy. Vol. 10. Elsevier, Amsterdam, 1988

157. Belfort MA, Anthony J, Buccimmazza et al: Hemodynamic changes associated with intravenous infusion of the calcium antagonist verapamil in the treatment of severe gestational proteinuric hypertension. Obstet Gynecol 75:970, 1990

158. Belfort MA, Uys P, Dommisse J et al: Hemodynamic changes in gestational proteinuric hypertension: the effects of rapid volume expansion and vasodilator therapy. Br J Obstet Gynaecol 96:634, 1989

159. Cotton DB, Lee W, Huhta JC, Dorman K: Hemodynamic profile of severe pregnancy-induced hypertension. Am J Obstet Gynecol 158:523, 1988

160. Mabie WE, Ratts TE, Sibai BM: The hemodynamic profile of severe preeclamptic patients requiring delivery. Am J Obstet Gynecol 161:1443, 1989

161. Fairlie FC: Doppler flow velocimetry in hypertension in pregnancy. Clin Perinatol 18:749, 1991

162. Fleischer A, Schulman H, Favenakides G et al: Uterine artery Doppler velocimetry in pregnant women with hypertension. Am J Obstet Gynecol 154:806, 1986

163. Ducey J, Schulman H, Farmakides G et al: A classification of hypertension in pregnancy based on Doppler velocimetry. Am J Obstet Gynecol 157:680, 1987

164. Gudmumdsson S, Marsal K: Ultrasound Doppler evaluation of uteroplacental and fetoplacental circulation in preeclampsia. Arch Gynecol Obstet 243:199–206, 1988

165. Cameron AD, Nicholson SF, Nimrod CA et al: Doppler waveforms in fetal aorta and umbilical artery in patients with hypertension in pregnancy. Am J Obstet Gynecol 1988, 158:339, 1988

166. Steel SA, Pearce JM, McParland P, Chamberlain CVP: Early Doppler ultrasound screening in prediction of hypertensive disorders of pregnancy. Lancet 335:1548, 1990

167. Bower S, Schuchter K, Campbell S: Doppler ultrasound screening as part of routine antenatal scanning: prediction of pre-eclampsia and intrauterine growth retardation. Br J Obstet Gynaecol 199:989, 1993

168. Trudinger BJ, Cook CM: Doppler umbilical and uterine flow waveforms in severe pregnancy hypertension. Br J Obstet Gynaecol 97:142, 1990

169. Yoon BH, Lee CM, Kim SW: An abnormal umbilical artery waveform: a strong and independent predictor of adverse perinatal outcome in patients with preeclampsia. Am J Obstet Gynecol 171:713, 1994

170. Pattinson RC, Norman K, Odendaal HJ: The role of Doppler velocimetry in the management of high risk pregnancies. Br J Obstet Gynaecol 101:114, 1994

171. Fairlie FM, Moretti M, Walker JJ, Sibai BM: Umbilical artery and uteroplacental velocimetry in pregnancies complicated by idiopathic low birthweight centile. Am J Perinatol 9:250, 1992

172. Gilstrap LC, Cunningham GR, Whalley PJ: Management of pregnancy induced hypertension in the nullipa-rous patient remote from term. Semin Perinatol 2:73, 1978

173. Sibai BM, Gonzalez AR, Mabie WC et al: A comparison of labetalol plus hospitalization versus hospitalization alone in the management of preeclampsia remote from term. Obstet Gynecol 70:323, 1987

174. Mathews DD: A randomized controlled trial of bed rest and sedation or normal activity and non-sedation in the management of nonalbuminuric hypertension in late pregnancy. Br J Obstet Gynaecol 84:108, 1977

175. Crawther CA, Boumeester AM, Ashwist HM: Does admission to hospital for bedrest prevent disease progression or improve fetal outcome in pregnancy complicated by non-proteinuric hypertension? Br J Obstet Gynaecol 99:13, 1992

176. Soothill PW, Ajayi R, Campbell S et al: Effect of a fetal surveillance unit on admission of antenatal patients to hospital. BMJ 303:269, 1991

177. Tuffnell DJ, Lilford RJ, Buchan PC et al: Randomized controlled trial of day care for hypertension in pregnancy. Lancet 339:224, 1992

178. Goldenberg RL, Cliver SP, Bronstein J et al: Bedrest in pregnancy. Obstet Gynecol 84:131, 1994

179. Barton JR, Stanziano GJ, Sibai BM: Monitored outpatient management of mild gestational hypertension remote from term. Am J Obstet Gynecol 170:765, 1994

180. Rubin PC, Clark DM, Sumner DJ et al: Placebo-controlled trial of atenolol in treatment of pregnancy associated hypertension. Lancet 1:431, 1983

181. Wichman K, Ryden E, Kalberg BE: A placebo controlled trial of metoprolol in the treatment of hypertension in pregnancy. Scand J Clin Lab Invest 44:90, 1984

182. Plouin PF, Breart E, Llado J et al: A randomized comparison of early with conservative use of antihypertensive drugs in the management of pregnancy-induced hypertension. Br J Obstet Gynaecol 97:134, 1990

183. Pickles CJ, Symonds EM, Broughton Pipkin F: The fetal outcome in a randomized double-blind controlled trial of labetalol versus placebo in pregnancy-induced hypertension. Br J Obstet Gynaecol 96:38, 1989

184. Schiff E, Friedman S, Sibai BM: Conservative management of severe preeclampsia remote from term. Obstet Gynecol 84:626, 1994

185. Olah KS, Redman CWG, Gee H: Management of severe early preeclampsia: is conservative management justified? Eur J Obstet Gynaecol Reprod Biol 51:175, 1993

186. Chua S, Redman CWG: Prognosis for preeclampsia complicated by 5 g or more of proteinuria in 24 hours. Eur J Obstet Gynaecol Reprod Biol 43:9, 1992

187. Odendaal HJ, Pattinson RC, DuToit R: Fetal and neonatal outcome in patients with severe preeclampsia delivered before 34 weeks. S Afr Med J 71:555, 1987

188. Moodley J, Koranteng SA, Rout C: Expectant management of early onset of severe preeclampsia in Durban. S Afr Med J 83:584, 1993

189. Odendaal HJ, Pattinson RC, Bam R et al: Aggressive or expectant management of patients with severe preeclampsia between 28–34 weeks' gestation: a randomized controlled trial. Obstet Gynecol 76:1070, 1990

190. Fenakel K, Fenakel E, Appleman Z et al: Nifedipine in

the treatment of severe preeclampsia. Obstet Gynecol 77:331, 1991

191. Pattinson RC, Odendaal HJ, DuToit R: Conservative management of severe proteinuric hypertension before 28 weeks' gestation. S Afr Med J 73:516, 1988

192. Sibai BM, Taslimi M, Abdella TN et al: Maternal and perinatal outcome of conservative management of severe preeclampsia in midtrimester. Am J Obstet Gynecol 1988152:32, 1988

193. Sibai BM, Aki S, Fairlie F, Moretti M: A protocol for managing severe preeclampsia in the second trimester. Am J Obstet Gynecol 163:733, 1990

194. Schiff E, Friedman SA, Mercer BM, Sibai BM: Fetal lung maturity is not accelerated in preeclamptic pregnancies. Am J Obstet Gynecol 169:1096, 1993

195. Sibai BM: Hypertension in pregnancy. Obstet Gynecol Clin N Am 19:615, 1992

196. Lucas MJ, Leveno KJ, Cunningham FG: A comparison of magnesium sulfate with phenytoin for the prevention of eclampsia. N Engl J Med 333:201, 1995

197. Chesley LC: Parenteral magnesium sulfate and the distribution, plasma levels and excretion of magnesium. Am J Obstet Gynecol 133:1, 1979

198. Patterson-Brown S, Robson SC, Redfern N et al: Hydralazine boluses for the treatment of severe hypertension in pre-eclampsia. Br J Obstet Gynaecol 101:409, 1994

199. Mabie WC, Gonzalez AR, Sibai BM et al: A comparative trial of labetalol and hydralazine in the acute management of severe hypertension complicating pregnancy. Obstet Gynecol 70:328, 1987

200. Sibai BM, Mabie WE, Harvey CJ, Gonzalez AR: Pulmonary edema in severe preeclampsia-eclampsia: analysis of 37 consecutive cases. Am J Obstet Gynecol 159:650, 1988

201. Ramanathan J, Sibai BM, Mabie WC et al: The use of labetalol for attenuation of the hypertensive response to endotracheal intubation in preeclampsia. Am J Obstet Gynecol 159:650, 1988

202. Ramanathan J, Coleman P, Sibai B: Anesthestic modification of hemodynamic and neuroendocrine stress responses to cesarean delivery in women with severe preeclampsia. Anesth Analg 73:772, 1991

203. Clark SL, Cotton DB: Clinical indications for pulmonary artery catheterization in the patient with severe preeclampsia. Am J Obstet Gynecol 158:650, 1988

204. Mabie WC, Ratts TE, Ramanathan KB, Sibai BM: Circulatory congestion in obese hypertensive women: a subset of pulmonary edema in pregnancy. Obstet Gynecol 72:553, 1988

205. Sibai BM: Preeclampsia-eclampsia: maternal and prenatal outcomes. Contemp OB/GYN 32:109, 1988

206. Sutherland A, Cooper DW, Howie PW et al: The incidence of severe preeclampsia among mothers and mothers-in-law of preeclamptics and controls. Br J Obstet Gynaecol 88:785, 1981

207. Sibai BM, El-Nazer A, Gonzalez-Ruiz AR: Severe preeclampsia-eclampsia in young primigravid women: subsequent pregnancy outcome and remote prognosis. Am J Obstet Gynecol 155:1011, 1986

208. Sibai BM, Mercer B, Sarinoglu C: Severe preeclampsia in the second trimester: recurrence risk and long-term prognosis. Am J Obstet Gynecol 165:1408, 1991

209. Sibai BM: Management and counseling of patients with preeclampsia remote from term. Clin Obstet Gynecol 2:426, 1992

210. Sibai BM, Villar MA, Mabie BC: Acute renal failure in hypertensive disorders of pregnancy: pregnancy outcome and remote prognosis in thirty-one consecutive cases. Am J Obstet Gynecol 62:777, 1990

211. Sibai BM, Ramadan MK, Chari RS, Friedman SA: Pregnancies complicated by hemolysis, elevated liver enzymes, and low platelets (HELLP): subsequent pregnancy outcome and long-term prognosis. Am J Obstet Gynecol 172:125, 1995

212. Sakala EP, Moore WD: Successful term deliery after previous pregnancy with ruptured liver. Obstet Gynecol 68:124, 1986

213. Alleman JSP, Delarue MWG, Hasaart THM: Successful delivery after hepatic rupture in previous pre-eclamptic pregnancy. Eur J Obstet Gynaecol 47:76, 1992

214. Ihle BU, Long P, Oats J: Early onset preeclampsia: recognition of underlying renal disease. BMJ 294, 1987

215. Chesley LC: History. p. 17. In Chesley LC (ed): Hypertensive Disorders in Pregnancy. 2nd Ed. Appleton-Century-Crofts, New York, 1978

216. Walker VN, Baker WS: A compariosn study of antihypertensive drug therapy and modified Stroganoff method in the management of severe toxemia of pregnancy. Am J Obstet Gynecol 81:1, 1961

217. Sheehan HL, Lunch JB: Pathology of Toxemia of Pregnancy. Churchill Livingstone, Edinburgh, 1973

218. Sibai BM, Abdella TN, Taylor HA: Eclampsia in the first half of pregnancy. Report of three cases and review of the literature. J Reprod Med 27:11, 1982

219. Lubarsky SL, Barton JR, Friedman SA et al: Late postpartum eclampsia revisited. Obstet Gynecol 83:502, 1994

220. Ferraz EM, Sherline DM: Convulsive toxemia of pregnancy (eclampsia). South Med J 69:2, 1976

221. Moller B, Lindmark G: Eclampsia in Sweden, 1976–1980. Acta Obstet Gynaecol Scand 65:307, 1986

222. Barton JR, Sibai BM: Cerebral pathology in eclampsia. p. 891. In Sibai BM (ed): Clinics Perinatolology. Vol. 18. WB Saunders Company, Philadelphia, 1991

223. Dahmus MA, Barton JR, Sibai BM: Cerebral imaging in eclampsia: magnetic resonance imaging versus computed tomography. Am J Obstet Gynecol 167:935, 1992

224. Beck DW, Menezes AH: Intracerebral hemorrhage in a patient with eclampsia. J Am Med Assoc 246:1442, 1981

225. Colosimo C Jr, Fileni A, Moschini M, Guerrini P: CT findings in eclampsia. Neuroradiology 27:313, 1985

226. Will AD, Lewis KL, Hinshaw DB Jr et al: Cerebral vasoconstriction in toxemia. Neurology 37:1555, 1987

227. Sibai BM, Spinnato JA, Watson DL, Anderson GD: Eclampsia. IV. Neurological findings and future outcome. Am J Obstet Gynecol 152:184, 1985

228. Richards AM, Moodley J, Graham DI, Bullock MRR: Active management of the unconscious eclamptic patient. Br J Obstet Gynaecol 93:554, 1986

229. Brown CEL, Purdy P, Cunningham FG: Head computed tomographic scans in women with eclampsia. Am J Obstet Gynecol 159:915, 1988

230. Milliez J, Dahoun A, Boudraa M: Computed tomography of the brain in eclampsia. Obstet Gynecol 75:975, 1990

231. Moodley J, Bobat SM, Hoffman M, Bill PLA: Electroencephalogram and computerized cerebral tomography findings in eclampsia. Br J Obstet Gynaecol 100:984, 1993

232. Royburt M, Seidman DS, Serr DM, Mashiach S: Neurologic involvement in hypertensive disease of pregnancy. Obstet Gynecol Surv 46:656, 1991

233. Digre KB, Varner MW, Osborn AG, Crawford S: Cranial magnetic resonance imaging in severe preeclampsia vs. eclampsia. Arch Neurol 50:399, 1993

234. Sanders TG, Clayman DA, Sanchez-Ramos L et al: Brain in eclampsia: MR imaging with clinical correlation. Radiology 180:475, 1991

235. Trommer BL, Homer D, Mikhael MA: Cerebral vasospasm and eclampsia. Stroke 19:326, 1988

236. Belfort MA, Carpenter RJ, Kirshon B et al: The use of nimodipine in a patient with eclampsia: color flow Doppler demonstration of retinal artery relaxation. Am J Obstet Gynecol 169:204, 1993

237. Sibai BM, Spinnato JA, Watson DL et al: Effects of magnesium sulfate on electroencephalographic findings in preeclampsia-eclampsia. Obstet Gynecol 64:261, 1984

238. Pritchard JA, Cunningham FG, Pritchard SA: The Parkland Memorial Hospital protocol for treatment of eclampsia: evaluation of 245 cases. Am J Obstet Gynecol 148:951, 1984

239. Sibai BM, Anderson GD, McCubbin JH: Eclampsia II. Clinical significance of laboratory findings. Obstet Gynecol 59:153, 1982

240. Sibai BM, Anderson GD, Abdella TN et al: Eclampsia III. Neonatal outcome, growth and development. Am J Obstet Gynecol 146:307, 1983

241. Paul RH, Koh KS, Bernstein SG: Changes in fetal heart rate-uterine contraction patterns associated with eclampsia. Am J Obstet Gynecol 130:165, 1978

242. Medical Economics Data: Physicians' Desk Reference 1994. 48th Ed. p. 1967. Medical Economics Data, Montvale, New Jersey, 1994

243. Gedekoh RH, Hayashi TT, McDonald HM: Eclampsia at Maggee-Women's Hospital, 1970 to 1980. Am J Obstet Gynecol 140:860, 1981

244. Sibai BM: Magnesium sulfate is the ideal anticonvulsant in preeclampsia-eclampsia. Am J Obstet Gynecol 162:1141, 1990

245. McCubbin JH, Sibai BM, Abdella TN et al: Cardiopulmonary arrest due to acute maternal hypermagnesemia, lett. Lancet 1:1058, 1981

246. Slater RM, Wilcox FL, Smith WD et al: Phenytoin infusion in severe preeclampsia. Lancet 1:1417, 1987

247. Ryan G, Lange Ir, Naugler MA: Clinical experience with phenytoin prophylaxis in severe preeclampsia. Am J Obstet Gynecol 161:1297, 1989

248. Friedman SA, Lim KH, Baker CA, Repke JT: Phenytoin versus magnesium sulfate in preeclampsia: a pilot study. Am J Perinatol 10:233, 1993

249. Dommisse J: Phenytoin sodium and magnesium sulphate in the management of eclampsia. Br J Obstet Gynaecol 94:104, 1990

250. Crowther C: Magnesium sulphate versus diazepam in the management of eclampsia: a randomized controlled trial. Br J Obstet Gynaecol 97:110, 1990

251. The Eclampsia Trial Collaborative Group: Which anticonvulsant for women with eclampsia? Evidence from the Collaborative Eclampsia Trial. Lancet 345:1455, 1995

252. Tufnell D, O'Donovan P, Lilfard RJ et al: Phenytoin in preeclampsia. Lancet 2:273, 1989

253. Coyaji KJ, Otiv SR: Single high dose intravenous phenytoin sodium for the treatment of eclampsia. Acta Obstet Gynaecol Scand 69:115, 1990

254. Naidu S, Moodley J, Botha J, McFadyen L: The efficacy of phenytoin in relation to serum levels in severe preeclampsia and eclampsia. Br J Obstet Gynaecol 99:881, 1992

255. Chesley LC, Cosgrove SA, Preece J et al: Hydatidiform mole, with special reference to recurrence and associated eclampsia. Am J Obstet Gynecol 52:311, 1946

256. Newman RB, Eddy GL: Association of eclampsia and hydatidiform mole: case report and review of the literature. Obstet Gynecol Surv 43:185, 1988

257. Lindheimer MD, Spargo BH, Katz AI: Eclampsia during the 16th gestational week. JAMA 230:1006, 1974

258. Speck G: Eclampsia at the sixteenth week of gestation, with Rh isoimmunization and cystic degeneration of the placenta. Obstet Gynecol 15:70, 1960

259. Agobe JT, Adewaze HO: Biochemical studies and delayed postpartum convulsions in Nigeria. p. 501. In Bomar J, MacGillivray I, Symonds EM (eds): Pregnancy Hypertension. University Park Press, Baltimore, 1980

260. Harbert GM, Claiborne HA, McGaughey HS et al: Convulsive toxemia. Am J Obstet Gynecol 10:336, 1968

261. Lopez-Llera M: Main clinical types and subtypes of eclampsia. Am J Obstet Gynecol 166:4, 1992

262. Zuspan FP: Problems encountered in the treatment of pregnancy induced hypertension. Am J Obstet Gynecol 131:591, 1978

263. Campbell DM, Templeton AA: Is eclampsia preventable? p. 483. In Bonnar, MacGillivary I, Symonds EM (eds): Pregnancy Hypertension. University Park Press, Baltimore, 1980

264. Bryans CI, Southerland WL, Zuspan FP: Eclampsia: a long-term followup study. Obstet Gynecol 21:6, 1963

265. Chesley LC, Cosgrove RA, Annitto JE: A followup study of eclamptic women. Am J Obstet Gynecol 83:1360, 1962

266. Chesley LC, Cosgrove RA, Annitto JE: Pregnancy in the sisters and daughters of eclamptic women. Pathol Microbiol (Basel) 24:662, 1961

267. Chesley LC, Annitto JE, Cosgrove RA: The familial factor in toxemia of pregnancy. Obstet Gynecol 32:3, 303, 1968

268. Lopez-Llera M, Horta JLH: Pregnancy after eclampsia. Am J Obstet Gynecol 119:193, 1974

269. Adelusi B, Ojengbeda OA: Reproductive performance after eclampsia. Int J Gynaecol Obstet 24:183, 1986

270. Chesley LC: Remote prognosis. p. 421. In Chesley LC (ed): Hypertensive Disorders in Pregnancy. Appleton-Century-Crofts, East Norwalk, CT, 1978

271. Sibai BM, Sarinoglu C, Mercer BM: Eclampsia VII. Pregnancy outcome after eclampsia and long-term prognosis. Am J Obstet Gynecol 166:1757, 1992

272. Frohlich ED: Hemodynamics of hypertension. In Genest J, Koiw E, Kuchel O (eds): Hypertension. McGraw-Hill, New York, 1977

273. Chesley LC, Annitto JE: Pregnancy in the patient with hypertensive disease. Am J Obstet Gynecol 53:372, 1947

274. Sibai BM, Abdella TN, Anderson GD: Pregnancy outcome in 211 patients with mild chronic hypertension. Obstet Gynecol 61:571, 1983

275. Sibai BM: Diagnosis and management of chronic hypertension in pregnancy. Obstet Gynecol 78:451, 1991

276. Sibai BM, Anderson GD: Pregnancy outcome of intensive therapy in severe hypertension in first trimester. Obstet Gynecol 67:517, 1986

277. Landesman R, Holze W, Scherr L: Fetal mortality in essential hypertension. Obstet Gynecol 6:354, 1955

278. Redman CWE, Beilin LJ, Bonnar J et al: Fetal outcome in trial of antihypertensive treatment in pregnancy. Lancet 2:753, 1976

279. Packham DK, Fairley KF, Ihle BU et al: Comparison of pregnancy outcome between normotensive and hypertensive women with primary glomerulonephritis. Clin Exp Hypertens Pregnancy B6:387, 1987

280. Dunlop JCH: Chronic hypertension and perinatal mortality. Proc R Soc Med 59:838, 1966

281. Sibai BM, Mabie WC, Shamsa F et al: A comparison of no medication versus methyldopa or labetalol in chronic hypertension during pregnancy. Am J Obstet Gynecol 162:960, 1990

282. Abdella TN, Sibai BM, Hays JM et al: Relationship of hypertensive disease to abruptio placentae. Obstet Gynecol 63:365, 1984

283. Leather HM, Humphreys DM, Baker PB et al: A controlled trial of hypertensive agents in hypertension in pregnancy. Lancet 1:488, 1968

284. Silverstone A, Trudinger BJ, Lewis PJ et al: Maternal hypertension and intrauterine fetal death in mid pregnancy. Br J Obstet Gynecol 87:457, 1980

285. Kincaid-Smith P, Bullen M, Mills J: Prolonged use of methyldopa in severe hypertension in pregnancy. BMJ 1:274, 1966

286. Taylor HC Jr, Tillman AJB, Blanchard J: Fetal losses in hypertension and preeclampsia. Part I. Analysis of 4432 cases. Obstet Gynecol 3:225, 1954

287. Arias F, Zamora J: Antihypertensive treatment and pregnancy outcome in patients with mild chronic hypertension. Obstet Gynecol 53:489, 1979

288. Weitz C, Khouzami V, Maxwell K, Johnson JWC: Treatment of hypertension in pregnancy with methyldopa, randomized double-blind study. Int J Gynaecol Obstet 25:35, 1987

289. Butters L, Kennedy S, Rubin PC: Atenolol in essential hypertension during pregnancy. BMJ 301:587, 1990

290. Gallery EDM, Saunders DM, Hunyor DN et al: Randomized comparison of methyldopa and oxprenolol for treatment of hypertension in pregnancy. BMJ 1:1591, 1979

291. Fidler J, Smith V, Fayers P et al: Randomized controlled comparative study of methyldopa and oxprenolol in treatment of hypertension in pregnancy. BMJ 286:1927, 1983

292. Plouin PF, Breart G, Maillard F et al: Comparison of antihypertensive efficacy and perinatal safety of labetalol and methyldopa in the treatment of hypertension in pregnancy: a randomized controlled trial. Br J Obstet Gynaecol 95:868, 1988

293. Horvath JS, Phippard A, Korda A et al Clonidine hydrochloride: a safe and effective antihypertensive agent in pregnancy. Obstet Gynecol 66:634, 1985

294. Lubbe WF, Hodge JV, Kellaway GSM: Antihypertensive treatment and fetal welfare in essential hypertension in pregnancy. NZ Med J 95:1, 1982

295. Walters BNJ, Redman CWG: Treatment of severe pregnancy-associated hypertension with the calcium antagonist nifedipine. Br J Obstet Gynaecol 91:330, 1984

296. Constantine G, Beevers DG, Reynolds AL, Luesley DM: Nifedipine as a second line antihypertensive drug in pregnancy. Br J Obstet Gynaecol 94:1136, 1987

297. Childress CH, Katz VL: Nifedipine and its indications in obstetrics and gynecology. Obstet Gynecol 83:616, 1994

298. Kreft-Jais C, Plouin PF, Tchobroutsky C, Boutroy MJ: Angiotensin-converting enzyme inhibitors during pregnancy: a survey of 22 patients given captopril and 9 given enalapril. Br J Obstet Gynaecol 95:420, 1988

299. Rosa FW, Bosco LA, Graham CF et al: Neonatal anuria with maternal angiotensin-converting enzyme inhibitor. Obstet Gynecol 74: 371, 1989

300. Lumbers ER, Burrell JH, Menzies RI et al: The effects of a converting enzyme inhibitor (captopril) and angiotensin II on fetal renal function. Br J Pharmacol 110:821, 1993

301. Hanssens M, Keirse MJNC, Vankelecom F, Van Assche FA: Fetal and neonatal effects of treatment with angiotensin-converting enzyme inhibitors in pregnancy. Obstet Gynecol 171:128, 1991

302. Veld AJM, Schalekamp MADH: Effects of 10 different beta-adrenoreceptor antagonists on hemodynamics, plasma renin activity, and plasma norepinephrine in hypertension. J Cardiovasc Pharmacol, suppl. 5:1, 1983

303. Svenden TL: Central hemodynamics of beta-adrenoreceptor blocking drugs: beta₁, selectivity versus intrinsic sympathomimetic activity. J Cardiovasc Pharmacol, suppl. 5:1, 1983

304. Van Zweiten PA, Timmermans PBMWM: Differential pharmacological properties of beta-adrenoreceptor blocking drugs. J Cardiovasc Pharmacol, suppl. 5:1, 1983

305. Rubin PC: Beta-blockers in pregnancy. N Engl J Med 305:1323, 1981

306. Schoenfeld A, Segal J, Friedman S et al: Adverse reac-

tions to antihypertensive drugs in pregnancy. Obstet Gynecol Surv 41:67, 1986

307. Sibai BM, Abdella TN, Anderson GD et al: Plasma volume determination in pregnancies complicated by chronic hypertension and intrauterine fetal demise. Obstet Gynecol 60:174, 1982

308. Sibai BM, Grossman RA, Grossman HE: Effects of diuretics on plasma volume in pregnancies with long-term hypertension. Am J Obstet Gynecol 150:831, 1984

309. Sibai BM, Abdella TN, Anderson GD et al: Plasma volume findings in pregnant women with mild hypertension. Therapeutic considerations. Am J Obstet Gynecol 145:539, 1983

310. Collins R, Yusf S, Peto R: Overview of randomized trials of diuretics in pregnancy. BMJ 190:17, 1985

311. McGillivray I: Sodium and water balance in pregnancy hypertension: the role of diuretics. Clin Obstet Gynecol 4:459, 1977

312. Branch DW, Silver RM, Blackwell JL et al: Outcome of treated pregnancies in women with antiphospholipid syndrome: an update of the Utah experience. Obstet Gynecol 80:614, 1992.

313. Abe S, Amagasaki Y, Konishi K et al: The influence of antecedent renal disease on pregnancy. Am J Obstet Gynecol 153:508, 1985

314. Hou SH, Grossman SD, Madias NE: Pregnancy in women with renal disease and moderate renal insufficiency. Am J Med 78:185, 1985

315. Cunningham FG, Cox SM, Harstad TW et al: Chronic renal disease and pregnancy outcome. Am J Obstet Gynecol 163:453, 1990

316. Zuspan FP, Rayburn WF: Blood pressure self-monitoring during pregnancy: practical considerations. Am J Obstet Gynecol 164:2, 1991

317. Barton JR, Sibai BM: Acute life-threatening emergencies in preeclampsia-eclampsia. Clin Obstet Gynecol 35: 402, 1992

318. Prisant LM, Carr AA, Hawkins DW: Treating hypertensive emergencies: controlled reduction of blood pressure and protection of target organs. Postgrad Med 93: 92, 1993

319. Meese R, Ram CVS: Hypertensive cardiovascular emergencies. Compr Ther 11:28, 1985

320. Silver HM: Acute hypertensive crisis in pregnancy. Med Clin North Am 73:623, 1989

321. Gifford R Jr: Management of hypertensive crisis. JAMA 266:829, 1991

322. Committee on Drugs, American Academy of Pediatrics: the transfer of drugs and other chemicals into human milk. Pediatrics 93:137, 194

323. White WB: Management of hypertension during lactation. Hypertension 6:297, 1984

Chapter 29

Cardiac and Pulmonary Disease

Heart Disease

Mark B. Landon

Cardiac disease complicates approximately 1 percent of all pregnancies. It remains a major nonobstetric cause of maternal death in the United States.[1] The cardiovascular changes that accompany pregnancy may impose a tremendous risk on women with certain categories of heart disease. Patients known to have only minimal limitation of their activity while nonpregnant can suddenly experience worsening of their symptoms during gestation. The fetus may also become jeopardized when maternal cardiac status deteriorates. Severe limitations on cardiac performance that result in the delivery of poorly oxygenated blood to the pregnant uterus can critically affect fetal growth and viability. Therefore, the consideration of hemodynamic changes that occur during gestation becomes extremely important when planning therapy for the pregnant patient with heart disease. Before describing specific maternal cardiac diseases, it is best to begin by reviewing some of the basic circulatory adjustments of normal pregnancy.

Blood Volume

Expansion of maternal plasma volume accounts for most of the increase in blood volume found in pregnancy. This increase begins in the first trimester and accelerates to levels that are 50 percent above the nonpregnant mean by 32 weeks' gestation (Table 29-1).[2] Patients with a multiple gestation may show significantly greater increments in their plasma volume. Early investigators believed that plasma volume declined in later pregnancy. However, their studies were performed while patients remained supine. In the supine position, caval compression results in increased pooling of blood in the lower extremities and increased venous pressure. This proportionately increases filtration of plasma into the extracellular space.[3] Studies subsequently performed in the left lateral position have documented that plasma volume remains stable from 32 weeks' gestation until delivery.

Hormonal mechanisms seem to be primarily responsible for the plasma volume expansion of normal pregnancy. Plasma renin activity rises sharply secondary to estrogen-augmented hepatic production of renin substrate. Progesterone competitively blocks the action of aldosterone at the renal tubule. Nevertheless, sodium and water are gradually retained, resulting in a 6- to 8-L expansion of total body water. Two-thirds of this increase, or 4 to 6 L, are distributed extracellularly, which clinically is manifested as edema of normal pregnancy.[4]

Red cell mass increases from 16 weeks' gestation until term and may reach values that are 20 percent above the average nonpregnant mean. A dilutional anemia results during the second trimester because of the proportionately greater rise in plasma volume. Later in pregnancy, hemoglobin levels increase as erythropoiesis continues while plasma volume stabilizes. Blood volume rises an average of 40 percent over nonpregnant levels.[5] The magnitude of this increment in blood volume may be correlated with birth weight in primigravid patients.

After delivery, blood volume declines significantly. Postpartum diuresis as well as the blood loss associated with delivery contribute to a rapid decline in plasma volume. The hematocrit will rise 2 to 3 percent in the week following vaginal delivery. In women who are not

Table 29-1   Circulatory Adjustments During Normal Pregnancy

	Rise	Peak
Blood volume	Early 6 weeks	↑ 40% (avg) by 32 weeks
Plasma volume	Early 6 weeks	↑ 50% (avg) by 32 weeks
Red cell volume	Progressively after first trimester	↑ 20% by term

breast-feeding, blood volume usually returns to nonpregnant levels within 2 months.

Cardiac Output

Cardiac output rises early in pregnancy and reaches levels approximately 30 to 50 percent over baseline by 20 to 24 weeks' gestation.[6] Marked fluctuations in resting output are observed with changes in maternal position. Cardiac output measured in the left lateral position falls slightly during the last trimester of pregnancy.[7] In supine subjects studied during the second half of gestation, cardiac output is significantly decreased, falling to values below those obtained in the immediate postpartum period.[8] This phenomenon is believed to result from venacaval compression by the gravid uterus. Normally, collateral vessels serve to ensure adequate return of blood to the right side of the heart. Women who fail to develop sufficient collateral circulation will experience hypotension should they re-

main supine for a prolonged period of time. This vaso-vagal-like syndrome has been termed the *supine hypotensive syndrome of pregnancy*. The characteristic symptoms of hypotension and bradycardia may be promptly relieved by placing the patient in the left lateral position.

The increased cardiac output observed early in pregnancy can be attributed to a larger stroke volume. Robson and colleagues[7] have documented a rise in stroke volume by the eighth week of pregnancy, with maximal levels reached by midgestation. As pregnancy advances, heart rate rises 10 to 20 percent, while cardiac output remains unchanged or falls. It follows, therefore, that stroke volume exhibits a progressive modest decline (Fig. 29-1). The physiologic mechanism for the early increase in stroke volume has not been well explained. The early rise in cardiac output associated with pregnancy does coincide with a decline in total peripheral vascular resistance.[7] In later pregnancy, the circulation of the pregnant woman has been likened to an arteriovenous fistula, with creation of a low-resistance circulation in the gravid uterus.

Volume changes alone are not responsible for the increased cardiac output found in pregnancy. Studies of the pulmonary vasculature reveal no change in pulmonary artery diastolic pressure during gestation.[9] This important index of cardiac function reflects left ventricular filling pressure. For end-diastolic volume to increase without a change in end-diastolic pressure, left ventricular enlargement must be present. Katz et al., using echocardiographic techniques, have demonstrated that the diameter of the left ventricle increases early in gestation. It has been postulated that ventricu-

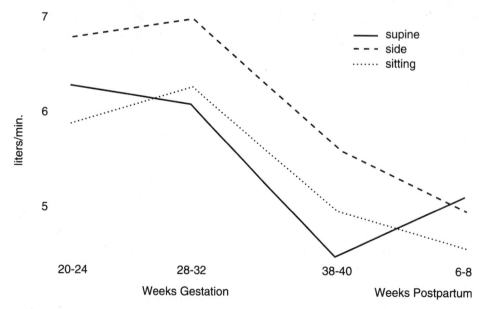

Fig. 29-1 Maternal cardiac output during pregnancy and postpartum. Cardiac output is greatest in the lateral recumbent position, peaking at 28 to 32 weeks' gestation. In supine subjects near term, cardiac output falls to values lower than those obtained during the immediate postpartum period. (From Veland et al,[8] with permission.)

lar distensibility may be affected by elevated levels of steroid hormones.[6] End-diastolic volume can thereby increase without an increased filling pressure, resulting in an increased stroke volume. Estrogens may alter contractile proteins within the myocardium, resulting in improved contractility and further increasing stroke volume and output. Several echocardiographic studies performed during pregnancy demonstrate an increase in left ventricular circumferential fiber shortening, a decrease in the pre-ejection period, and an increase in left ventricular ejection time, reflecting an increase in left ventricular contractility.[11]

Blood Pressure

Normal pregnancy is accompanied by a slight decline in systolic blood pressure and a modest decrease in diastolic values. Mean systemic blood pressure declines to a nadir at midpregnancy and features a somewhat widened pulse pressure. The decline in systemic blood pressure mirrors that of total vascular resistance, which in turn is accompanied by a progressive rise in cardiac output. The low resistance circulation created by midpregnancy is believed to be hormonally modulated and is characterized by a refractoriness to vasopressors such as angiotension (see Chrs. 4, 28). Women who fail to demonstrate a decline in systemic blood pressure in early gestation are more likely to develop pregnancy-induced hypertension.

Labor and Delivery

Labor produces sudden and often profound changes in the cardiovascular system. With each uterine contraction approximately 300 to 500 ml of blood is shifted from the uterus to the maternal circulation. Systemic venous pressure increases as a result of this "autotransfusion" from the engorged uterine veins. Right ventricular pressure rises, and cardiac output increases about 20 percent in the supine position. Mean arterial pressure rises and is followed by a reflex bradycardia. Because uterine contractions may result in significant compression of the aorta and iliac arteries, much of the increase in cardiac output is distributed to the upper extremities and head.

Maternal pain and anxiety result in increased adrenergic stimulation that is accompanied by a rise in blood pressure and heart rate, particularly during the second stage of labor. Thus, anesthesia can greatly influence the hemodynamic changes observed during labor. Epidural anesthesia may attenuate the normal increase in cardiac output and heart rate because it acts as an analgesic as well as a peripheral vasodilator, which reduces venous return to the heart. These changes result in a

diminished preload or ventricular end-diastolic volume. Similar effects may be observed with spinal anesthesia, if a patient is not adequately hydrated prior to its administration. Nonetheless, regional anesthesia may be used effectively in most patients with cardiac disease. For patients undergoing cesarean delivery, consideration of potentiating right to left shunting with diminished preload must be weighed against the risk of myocardial depression of general anesthetic agents, as well as acute hypertension associated with intubation and extubation.

Both epidural and spinal anesthesia may produce a fall in cardiac output and blood pressure prior to elective cesarean delivery. Hypotension is generally corrected by employing left lateral uterine displacement and infusing appropriate intravenous fluids. Correction of hypotension with ephedrine is inadvisable in patients who cannot tolerate tachycardia.

Following vaginal delivery, because of the reduction in caval compression and an increase in blood volume, circulating cardiac output may rise 10 to 20 percent. A bradycardia often ensues that lasts for a few days. After a cesarean delivery that is accompanied by an average blood loss in excess of 1,000 cc, cardiac output and blood pressure may temporarily decrease. Serial measurements of cardiac output performed up to 24 weeks' postpartum have revealed a 33 percent decline, with most of this fall being evident by 2 weeks' postpartum.[12]

Diagnosis and Detection of Cardiac Disease

Pregnancy is often accompanied by physical changes that may be confused with underlying cardiac disease. Symptoms and clinical signs that are associated with heart disease are often present in a normal pregnancy. It is not unusual for patients to experience fatigue, shortness of breath, orthopnea, and peripheral edema, findings similar to those present in congestive heart failure. Palpitations may also be reported by a normal obstetric patient. The following symptoms, however, should alert the obstetrician to the presence of underlying cardiac disease: (1) any progressive limitation of physical activity due to worsening dyspnea, (2) chest pain that accompanies exercise or increased activity, and (3) syncope that is preceded by palpitations or physical exertion.

Physical examination of the heart and cardiovascular system reveals normal physiologic changes that, like many of the symptoms described above, suggest heart disease. Systolic outflow murmurs, believed to represent pulmonic flow, are observed in 90 percent of pregnant women. In addition to this left sternal murmur, other systolic flow murmurs are often auscultated in the neck (brachiocephalic arteries) as well as a continuous

Signs and Symptoms of Cardiac Disease

History
  Progressive or severe dyspnea
  Dyspnea at rest
  Paroxysmal nocturnal dyspnea
  Angina or syncope with exertion
  Hemoptysis
Physical examination
  Loud systolic murmur or click
  Diastolic murmur
  Cardiomegaly including parasternal heave
  Cyanosis or clubbing
  Persistent jugular venous distension
  Features of Marfan syndrome
Electrocardiogram
  Dysrhythmia

mammary souffle over the breast in late pregnancy. Diastolic murmurs are uncommon and, when present, require further evaluation. A third heart sound is often heard and is not a sign of abnormality. Venous distension and accompanying peripheral edema are found in the majority of pregnancies. While neck veins may become pronounced, normal venous pulsations should occur. If absent, further evaluation is required.

Interpreting the results of standard techniques used to investigate cardiac disease may be difficult in pregnancy. Chest radiographs will often demonstrate cardiomegaly and increased pulmonary vascular markings. Therefore, more significant changes must be present to suggest hemodynamically significant cardiac disease. Electrocardiographic findings may aid in the preliminary diagnosis of valvular disease or anatomic defects if chamber hypertrophy is suggested. However, myocardial ischemia must not be confused with the ST-T segment depression and flattening of T waves in the precordial leads, which may be present in normal pregnant women. Premature atrial and ventricular beats are also common in pregnancy.

Because it does not expose the mother and the fetus to radiation, echocardiography has become the preferred technique for detection and management of cardiac abnormalities during pregnancy. Using M-mode echocardiography, several investigators have documented that the internal dimensions of the left ventricle, ejection fraction, and stroke volume are all increased in pregnant women after the first trimester.[13,14] Echocardiography has also confirmed that cardiac output rises later in pregnancy in patients studied in the lateral recumbent position.

General Considerations in Management

The successful management of heart disease in pregnancy requires close cooperation between the cardiologist and the obstetrician. In the best circumstances, cardiac disease is identified *prior* to pregnancy so that appropriate counseling regarding risks and outcome can be undertaken. Certain conditions including Eisenmenger syndrome and primary pulmonary hypertension have been associated with such high maternal mortality rates that pregnancy is not advised. Patients with mitral stenosis may elect to undergo cardiac catheterization and possible valve replacement earlier in their illness if contemplating pregnancy. In such patients, a porcine valve may be preferred since it reduces the need for anticoagulation.

It is important to define precisely the nature of a patient's cardiac disease. This information will enable the physician to assess appropriately the risks of pregnancy not only for the mother but for her fetus as well. A multifactorial pattern of inheritance has been suggested for most congenital heart disease, with risk varying according to the site of the specific lesion.

The specific cardiac lesion present will also determine the need for antibiotic prophylaxis during labor and delivery. Although the efficacy of antibiotic pro-

Maternal Mortality Risk Associated with Specific Cardiac Diseases

Group I, mortality <1%
  Atrial septal defect (uncomplicated)
  Ventricular septal defect (uncomplicated)
  Patient ductus arteriosus (uncomplicated)
  Pulmonic/tricuspid disease
  Corrected tetralogy of Fallot
  Porcine valve
  Mitral stenosis (mild)
Group II, mortality 5 to 15%
  Mitral stenosis with atrial fibrillation
  Artificial valve
  Mitral stenosis (moderate to severe)
  Aortic stenosis
  Coarctation of aorta, uncomplicated
  Uncorrected tetralogy of Fallot
  Previous myocardial infarction
Group III, mortality 25 to 50%
  Pulmonary hypertension
  Coarctation of aorta (complicated)
  Marfan syndrome with aortic involvement

(Adapted from Clark,[78] with permission.)

phylaxis against infective endocarditis has not been proven, the low risk of drug toxicity when weighed against the dangers of endocarditis makes such prophylaxis the recommended practice. Manual removal of the placenta is an absolute indication for antibiotic prophylaxis in patients with structural heart disease. For some patients, including those with prosthetic valves, mortality rates are particularly high should they become infected. Prophylaxis usually includes the intravenous administration of aqueous penicillin G and an aminoglycoside at the start of true labor, with continuation every 8 hours until one dose postdelivery has been given. Vancomycin may be substituted in patients who are allergic to penicillin (Table 29-2).

Antibiotic prophylaxis for rheumatic fever should be used in patients with a positive past history, especially if they demonstrate valvular disease. The American Heart Association recommends a monthly injection of 1.2 million units of benzathine penicillin G. Alternative regimens include daily oral administration of penicillin or erythromycin.

Anticoagulation may be required in individuals with prosthetic valves as well as those with arrhythmias who may be at risk for an arterial embolus. Patients with mitral stenosis and associated atrial fibrillation should also be anticoagulated. Pregnancy will influence the type of anticoagulation therapy to be used. Oral anticoagulants are contraindicated, as fetal exposure to coumadin during the first 2 months of gestation may result in a significant malformation rate. Heparin does not cross the placenta, and it is the preferred anticoagulant.

Careful assessment by both the cardiologist and obstetrician should ensure that the patient's hemodynamic status remains optimal during pregnancy. Monitoring of weight, blood pressure, and pulse as well as

a detailed cardiovascular examination should be performed at each visit. It is important to consider conditions such as anemia and infection that may stress patients with significant cardiac disease. In a patient who demonstrates worsening symptoms, it is often necessary to institute changes in diet, activity, or medication. In doing so, one must carefully consider the effects on the fetus of such therapeutic decisions.

Occasionally, cardiac function in patients with valvular disease may deteriorate, and, when medical management fails, cardiac surgery may become necessary. This decision usually follows conservative treatment, including hospitalization, bedrest, diuresis, and correction of arrhythmias when present. If it must be performed, cardiac surgery should ideally be undertaken early in gestation, but preferably following fetal organogenesis. Open heart surgery has been associated with a low maternal mortality rate.[14] Fetal survival rates appear to be improving, following earlier experience in which fetal mortality was found to be as high as 33 percent. In 68 cases utilizing cardiopulmonary bypass, Becker[15] reported one maternal death and an 80 percent fetal salvage rate. It is recommended that perfusion hypothermia be avoided, as this may be responsible for the fetal bradycardia observed during cardiopulmonary bypass. Fetal heart rate and uterine monitoring have been used sparingly, but may help guide the adjustment of blood flow and pressure while the pregnant patient is maintained on bypass.[16]

Specific Cardiac Diseases

Despite the declining incidence of rheumatic fever in the United States, rheumatic heart disease remains the most common cardiac problem encountered in pregnancy. A review of 519 pregnancies complicated by maternal heart disease at the Royal Maternity Hospital in Dublin revealed 60 percent to be rheumatic, 31 percent to be congenital, with the remaining 9 percent being arrhythmias, ischemic disease, or cardiomyopathy.[17] In Third World countries where congenital lesions often remain uncorrected, rheumatic fever is still common and may result in valvular disease in women of childbearing age. The prognosis for patients with rheumatic disease who receive optimal care is generally good. Prior to 1970, a maternal mortality rate of approximately 1 percent was reported for 2,856 pregnancies managed over a 27-year period.[18] In this series, no maternal deaths were reported after 1960. Patients at greatest risk are those who develop severe congestive failure or atrial arrhythmias.

Chesley[19] has studied the long-term effects of pregnancy in women with severe rheumatic heart disease. He compared the survivals of 38 patients with 51 pregnancies to those of 96 patients who did not become

Table 29-2   Recommended Regimen for Antibiotic Prophylaxis

For labor and delivery	Ampicillin 2.0 g IM or IV plus gentamicin 1.5 mg/kg IM or IV given in active labor; one follow-up dose given 8 hours later and postpartum
Oral regimen for minor or repetitive procedures in low-risk patients	Amoxicillin 3.0 g orally 1 hour before procedure and 1.5 g 6 hours later
Penicillin-allergic patients	Vancomycin 1.0 g IV slowly over 1 hour, plus gentamicin 1.5 mg/kg IM or IV given 1 hour before procedure; repeat once 8 hours later.

(Adapted from Shulman et al.,[78] and Dajani et al.,[53] with permission.)

pregnant after heart disease was diagnosed. Both groups were comparable with respect to mortality statistics, suggesting that in patients who survive pregnancy life expectancy is not shortened.[19]

The improvement in pediatric surgical techniques and neonatal intensive care over the past two decades has allowed more patients with congenital heart disease to become pregnant. Patients who develop right to left shunting with increased pulmonary vascular pressure still exhibit maternal mortality rates approaching 50 percent. Prior surgical repair for patients with congenital heart disease does appear to make a significant difference in the outcome of their pregnancy. Whittemore and colleagues[20] examined this issue by comparing two subgroups of a total of 233 patients with congenital heart defects through 482 pregnancies. The percentage of pregnancies resulting in live births did not differ significantly between the surgically corrected and control groups (average live birth rate, 77 percent). Outcome as determined by birth weight and viability, however, was markedly improved in patients who underwent successful surgery for cyanotic lesions. As expected, the live birth rate was also dependent on the degree of cardiac impairment. This study also demonstrated a significantly higher incidence of congenital heart defects (16.1 percent) in infants born to affected mothers than had been previously reported.

Acquired Valvular Disease

Mitral Stenosis

This lesion is the most common form of rheumatic heart disease found in pregnancy. It can be an isolated lesion or accompany aortic or right-sided valvular lesions. Mitral stenosis is usually a sequel of rheumatic fever. In patients who develop carditis, mitral insufficiency often precedes the development of stenosis. Symptoms may not appear for over a decade, at which time a reduction in cardiac output causes patients to become easily fatigued. Obstruction to left atrial outflow produces a rise in atrial pressure and eventually pulmonary capillary wedge pressure. Pulmonary congestive and right ventricular failure are seen 5 to 10 years after the onset of symptoms.[21] The normal cross-sectional area of the mitral valve is greater than 4 cm^2. Patients generally remain asymptomatic until area decreases to less than 2.5 cm^2. In patients with a valve area of less than 1 cm^2, mild exercise will produce symptoms. In symptomatic patients, the maternal mortality rate during pregnancy is sufficiently high to recommend surgical correction prior to pregnancy.

The augmented cardiac output of pregnancy, including tachycardia and increased circulatory volume, impose a tremendous stress on patients with significant mitral disease. Any condition, such as pregnancy, that increases cardiac output and shortens diastolic filling time may raise the diastolic gradient across the mitral valve, thereby elevating left atrial pressure and pulmonary capillary pressure. Szekely and Snaith[22] estimated that symptoms of pulmonary congestion may develop in 25 percent of pregnant women. Dyspnea is often present by 20 weeks' gestation, when resting cardiac output has reached its maximum.

Symptoms of reduced cardiac output should be treated with limitation of activity and, if the patient is volume overloaded, cautious diuresis. Control of arrhythmias, particularly atrial fibrillation is essential. In hemodynamically stable patients, digitalis is initially used to slow the ventricular rate prior to cardioversion. As the size of the left atrium increases, there is a possibility that mural thrombus formation may occur. Two-dimensional echocardiography is useful to follow atrial size and potential thrombus formation. Transesophageal imaging may be required to best visualize the atrial appendage. Anticoagulation employing heparin therapy should be used in suspected cases or if atrial fibrillation develops.

If medical measures are unsuccessful in the treatment of symptoms, valve commisurotomy or replacement must be considered. Commisurotomy should ideally be performed in patients who do not have significant regurgitation and who have limited calcification of the mitral valve. No other valvular disease should be present. Szekely and Snaith[22] reported 69 cases of mitral commisurotomy in which two maternal deaths occurred. Six fetal deaths also followed the procedure. Recently, percutaneous, mitral balloon valvuloplasty has been performed successfully during pregnancy.[23,24] In pregnant women with pure mitral stenosis characterized by simple commissural or commissural band stenosis, balloon valvuloplasty is a desirable procedure in light of the risks associated with surgery. Ultimately the choice of the procedure for relief of stenosis is determined by the pathologic anatomy of the stenotic valve. Valve replacement has become more popular with improved understanding of maternal and fetal physiology during cardiopulmonary bypass. It does, however, carry a higher risk of maternal and fetal mortality than valvotomy. Becker[15] reported 19 cases of mitral valve replacement during pregnancy in which the major indications for surgery was refractory congestive failure. All mothers survived, as did 15 fetuses (79 percent). This series included four patients with thrombosed prostheses and one case of infective endocarditis.

Labor and delivery is a hazardous process for the patient with mitral stenosis. Patients with significant disease require invasive monitoring (Ch. 18). Pulmonary capillary wedge pressure and cardiac output are determined by the use of the Swan-Ganz catheter. The volume of fluids administered should be monitored carefully during both labor and the immediate postpartum period. Clark et al.[26] emphasized that because pulmonary capillary wedge pressure does not accurately reflect left ventricular filling pressures in women with mitral stenosis, such patients often require high-normal wedge pressure in order to maintain cardiac output. Ducey and Ellsworth[27] have described a 46 percent decline in cardiac output at the peak of uterine contractions in a woman with severe mitral stenosis undergoing invasive hemodynamic monitoring during labor. Patients should be given oxygen and should labor in the semi-Fowler position. Although epidural anesthesia is the preferred anesthetic technique, a decline in cardiac output has been associated with its use.[27] Ventricular rate must be monitored closely to avoid tachycardia, which can result in decreased cardiac output. It should be remembered that stenosis of the mitral valve is accompanied by a relatively fixed stroke volume, which may not rise with an increase in heart rate. Rapid heart rates further decrease diastolic filling time and elevate left atrial pressure. Verapamil or digitalis may be required to slow the ventricular rate in cases of atrial arrhythmias. If sinus tachycardia becomes excessive (> 140 bpm), the use of anesthetics to alleviate pain or cautious use of propranolol may be employed. Patients who receive epidural anesthesia should be carefully observed for hypotension, which may precipitate tachycardia. Systemic vascular resistance is best maintained with the α-agonist metaraminol. The β-agonist component of ephedrine will result in tachycardia, and its use should, therefore, be avoided. In patients delivering vaginally, the second stage of labor, including intense Valsalva efforts, may be shortened by the use of outlet forceps or vacuum extraction. A large bolus of intravenous oxytocin should be avoided, as it may precipitate hypotension.

The most hazardous time for women with mitral stenosis is the postpartum period.[18] A rise in wedge pressure is common, and careful attention must be given to changes in cardiac output that accompany fluid shifts following delivery. In general, a requirement for frequent administration of furosemide is to be anticipated.[27] Antibiotic prophylaxis is required in patients with mitral stenosis.

Aortic Stenosis

Aortic stenosis is a rare complication of pregnancy. Valvular thickening resulting from acute rheumatic disease does not typically occur for several decades following the initial attack. Most patients become symptomatic in the fifth or sixth decade of life. Similarly, many patients with a congenital bicuspid aortic valve do not become symptomatic until after their childbearing years. Once symptoms of angina, dys-

pnea, or syncope arise in patients with aortic stenosis, progressive decompensation follows, with mortality rates approaching 50 percent within 5 years.[22] Prior to conception, the severity of aortic stenosis should be evaluated. Women with significant left ventricular dysfunction and a valve area less than 1 cm^2 should be advised against pregnancy, as clinical deterioration is likely with the hemodynamic stresses encountered. Surgical correction consisting of commisurotomy or heterograft prosthetic valve replacement are options for management.

Obstruction to left ventricular outflow and reduction in cardiac output are responsible for the symptomatology associated with aortic stenosis. Physical exertion may result in relative ischemia of the cerebral and coronary vessels, producing syncope and angina. With long-standing aortic stenosis, left ventricular hypertrophy occurs as a compensatory mechanism. This further increases the oxygen requirements of the heart and the propensity for anginal episodes. A rise in left atrial pressure is needed to fill the hypertrophied left ventricle. This may be reflected in elevated pulmonary vascular pressures, leading to progressive dyspnea. Critical aortic stenosis creates a narrow window of appropriate fluid loading. Small decreases in preload due to hemorrhage or regional anesthesia may result in decreased cardiac output and hypotension.[28] Small increases in intravascular volume may produce significant increases in filling pressures, resulting in pulmonary edema. *The goal of hemodynamic management should be to maintain filling pressures within the narrow therapeutic window and to avoid tachycardia.*[28]

Mortality rates as high as 17 percent have been reported in 23 pregnant patients with aortic stenosis managed prior to 1978.[29] There may not be a clear advantage to pregnancy termination. Arias and Pineda[29] reported two fatalities in five patients whose pregnancies were interrupted. Of note, these patients were probably among the most critically ill in their series. The high mortality rate associated with pregnancy termination may reflect the occurrence of hypovolemia, which decreases venous return and left ventricular filling. This effect is poorly tolerated in patients with aortic stenosis who require an adequate end-diastolic volume in the face of increased filling pressures and a fixed afterload or impedance to outflow. More recent reports emphasize the use of noninvasive techniques to secure a diagnosis and provide physiologic assessment in women with aortic stenosis. Maternal mortality has been rare.[28,30] While mild to moderate stenosis is generally well tolerated during pregnancy, more severe lesions that fix cardiac output may become symptomatic during the second half of gestation. Valve replacement or valvulotomy has been successfully undertaken as has percutaneous balloon aortic valvuloplasty during pregnancy in cases refractory to medical management.[31]

Regional anesthetic techniques that may decrease preload or end-diastolic volume must be used with great caution during labor and delivery. Hypotension is avoided by the use of left lateral uterine displacement and appropriate fluid administration. A fall in blood pressure produces tachycardia, which may aggravate the condition of compromised patients. Tachycardia will decrease the ventricular filling time and further reduce cardiac output. Central monitoring employing a Swan-Ganz catheter is encouraged for all symptomatic patients as well as for those who have physical or diagnostic signs suggesting significant valve obstruction. As hypovolemia poses a greater risk than fluid overload, wedge pressures should be maintained in the 16 to 18 mmHg range to protect against unexpected blood loss.

Antibiotic prophylaxis is recommended in laboring women with aortic stenosis.

Mitral Regurgitation

Mitral regurgitation may follow rheumatic fever or an episode of endocarditis. It is also observed in patients with idiopathic hypertrophic subaortic stenosis (IHSS) and mitral valve prolapse. A floppy mitral valve may be the most common cause of regurgitation in women of childbearing age.

Women with mitral regurgitation develop symptoms of left-sided failure later in life than do patients with pure mitral stenosis. A diminished ventricular output results in symptoms of fatigue and, eventually, dyspnea from pulmonary congestion. Elevation of pressure within the left atrium predisposes to fibrillation and mural thrombus formation. At the end stage of this disease, patients with elevated pulmonary arteriolar pressure will demonstrate signs of right-sided failure, including peripheral edema and hepatomegaly.

The hemodynamic changes of pregnancy are usually well tolerated in patients with minimal mitral insufficiency. Frequently, the typical decrescendo systolic murmur will be diminished during pregnancy as the fall in peripheral vascular resistance reduces the amount of regurgitant flow across the mitral valve. Patients with long-standing disease may develop atrial enlargement and fibrillation. The risk for arrhythmias may be increased during pregnancy.[32] Reduction of left ventricular afterload may therefore become an important therapeutic maneuver in patients with impaired cardiac output. Patients with chronic disease including those with a large left ventricle may require inotropic support if the afterload is substantially reduced.

During labor and delivery, patients with significant mitral insufficiency may benefit from central monitoring to direct fluid and drug therapy. Pain may be associated with an increase in blood pressure that is due to enhanced sympathetic activity. If systemic vascular resistance also rises, pulmonary congestion may follow. Epidural analgesia is recommended to prevent this occurrence. Regional anesthesia may impair venous return to the heart and often requires careful administration of intravenous fluids to maintain filling of the enlarged left ventricle. Patients with this lesion should also receive antibiotic prophylaxis during labor and delivery.

Aortic Regurgitation

Aortic regurgitation occurs approximately 10 years after the onset of rheumatic fever. In this setting, coexistent mitral disease is common. Occasionally, aortic regurgitation is seen with a congenital bicuspid valve or in association with a collagen vascular disease such as rheumatoid arthritis or systemic lupus erythematosus. Dilatation of the aortic root is responsible for regurgitation in patients with Marfan syndrome.

Most patients with aortic insufficiency experience symptoms of failure during the fourth of fifth decade of life. Progressive left ventricular dilatation results from a state of chronic volume overload. In compensated cases, left ventricular end-diastolic pressure remains normal for several years. Pregnancy is complicated by episodes of failure in less than 10 percent of cases.[22] Restriction of activity, treatment with digitalis and diuretics, or afterload reduction is employed should symptoms of cardiac failure develop. Women receiving angiotension-converting enzyme (ACE) inhibitors for afterload reduction should be changed to an agent such as hydralazine, as ACE inhibitors are contraindicated during pregnancy. Patients with aortic regurgitation due to endocarditis may require valve replacement.[33] Heterograft valves are preferred in pregnancy because they do not require anticoagulation.[33]

As with mitral regurgitation, the decrease in systemic vascular resistance observed during pregnancy may reduce the amount of regurgitant flow and the intensity of the murmur. The stress of labor and delivery, however, may precipitate left-sided ventricular dysfunction. Afterload reduction has been successfully employed when vascular resistance remains high. Epidural anesthesia is recommended for vaginal delivery and may serve to prevent peripheral vasoconstriction. Bradycardia is poorly tolerated in patients with significant aortic regurgitation. Slowing of the heart rate increases the duration of ventricular diastole and regurgitation across the valve. Ideally, the maternal heart rate should be maintained between 80 and 100 bpm.[34] Bacterial endocarditis prophylaxis is required for patients with aortic regurgitation.

Congenital Lesions

Left to Right Shunt

Left to right shunting may occur through an atrial septal defect, ventricular septal defect, or patent ductus arteriosus. Surgical correction of these lesions is often performed during infancy and childhood. Patients treated successfully in childhood may be followed for varying periods of time as long as their disease is stable. However, the hemodynamic changes of pregnancy may result in cardiovascular decompensation, even after years of apparently good health.[35] In addition, some patients are first discovered to have such defects when pregnant. During pregnancy, right-sided and left-sided resistances decrease in a similar manner; therefore, the degree of shunting is not significantly altered. Small defects are usually associated with a good pregnancy outcome. In patients who have developed pulmonary hypertension which has led to shunt reversal as in Eisenmenger Syndrome, maternal mortality rates of up to 50% have been reported. During pregnancy, left to right shunting may be increased following the expected increases in intravascular volume and cardiac output.

Ventricular Septal Defect

Small ventricular septal defects (VSD) often close spontaneously in early life, and large defects discovered in childhood are most often surgically repaired. The small group of patients with uncorrected large VSDs are themselves growth-restricted and may experience frequent respiratory infections. Most VSDs involve the membranous septum inferior to the crista supraventricularis. Other congenital lesions including atrial septal defects or transposition of the great arteries may be present.

Patients with small VSDs generally tolerate pregnancy well. The degree of left to right shunting is not significantly altered if baseline pulmonary vascular resistance is normal.[36] Hemodynamic changes of pregnancy, including an increased circulating blood volume and tachycardia, may, however, increase left to right shunting to a critical level. Once pulmonary vascular resistance rises, right ventricular failure develops and reverse shunting with cyanosis may occur.

Increases in systemic vascular resistance, which accompany the stress of labor, may increase the degree of left to right shunting. Continuous epidural anesthesia is an effective method to relieve pain and lower systemic resistance. However, recognition that lowering of systemic pressure may not be tolerated by all patients is essential. Women with significant pulmonary hypertension exhibit a right to left shunt, and a further fall in arterial Po_2 will occur if systemic vascular resistance is markedly reduced. During labor, the development of cyanosis while a good cardiac output is maintained signals right to left shunting. Oxygen should be administered and steps taken to increase vascular resistance. A Swan-Ganz catheter should be inserted, if not already in place. Patients with VSDs do require antibiotic prophylaxis during labor and delivery. Careful assessment of the offspring of affected mothers has revealed a 6 to 21 percent incidence of VSDs. [37]

Atrial Septal Defect

Atrial septal defect (ASD) is the most common congenital heart lesion found in the adult population, accounting for 30 percent of such lesions. The most common defect in the adult population is the ostium secundum defect in the region of the fossa ovalis. This defect is often associated with mitral valve prolapse. Primum defects are generally corrected during childhood, but may have residual mitral regurgitation associated with them. Interatrial shunting, through a typical ASD, produces greater pulmonary blood flow relative to the systemic circulation. This change is generally well tolerated, unless pulmonary hypertension is present. Young women with an ASD are often asymptomatic or may experience mild fatigue. Atrial arrhythmias, pulmonary hypertension, and right-sided failure are complications that are not observed until the fourth or fifth decade of life.

No specific therapy is required for this group of pregnant women. Prophylactic antibiotics are often administered although the risk of bacterial endocarditis is low, and routine anticoagulation is not recommended. Uncomplicated patients may be managed during labor and delivery without invasive monitoring. Epidural anesthesia is a well-accepted analgesic technique. It avoids marked increases in systemic vascular resistance that would augment left to right shunting.[32]

In advanced cases of ASD, shunting increases during pregnancy, right and left atrial pressure may rise, and atrial distention worsens. Associated supraventricular arrhythmias may occur with atrial enlargement. Serial Doppler echocardiographic studies are useful in following these patients. Eventually, marked increases in pulmonary blood flow produce a rise in pulmonary vascular resistance, which leads to right-sided heart failure. With dysfunctional atrial contractions, incomplete atrial emptying occurs, increasing the potential for shunting. Hypotension may follow. These patients will require more intensive monitoring during pregnancy, labor, and delivery. Treatment to correct arrhythmias should be immediately instituted. Supraventricular tachycardia that results in that cardiac failure or hypotension is best treated with direct current cardioversion. Digitalization may also be necessary. The risk of congenital heart disease in the offspring of women with ASD ranges from 4 to 10 percent.

Patent Ductus Arteriosus

The persistence of the ductus arteriosus results in blood flow throughout the cardiac cycle from the higher pressure aorta to the lower pressure pulmonary artery, thereby increasing pulmonary blood flow with resulting enlargement of the pulmonary vasculature and left-sided chambers of the heart. Most patients with patent ductus arteriosus (PDA) have their lesion corrected during childhood. As with an ASD, patients with a small ductus usually have a benign clinical course until middle age. Young patients will tolerate pregnancy well and specifically require only antibiotic prophylaxis during labor and delivery.

Large PDAs are associated with growth restriction, chronic respiratory infections, and congestive heart failure during childhood and early adulthood. These patients develop pulmonary hypertension that is associated with significant mortality during gestation.[22]

The increase in left ventricular volume and work that accompanies pregnancy results in left-sided failure, which further exacerbates pre-existing pulmonary congestion. For this reason, therapeutic termination of pregnancy is generally indicated if significant right to left shunting is detected early in gestation. The risk for congenital heart disease in the offspring of women with PDA ranges from 4 to 11 percent.

Right to Left Shunts

Tetralogy of Fallot

This congenital anomaly consists of right ventricular outflow obstruction, VSD, right ventricular hypertrophy, and an overriding aorta. Right to left shunting is usually present, resulting in cyanosis. In the past, patients with uncorrected tetralogy of Fallot rarely lived past childhood, making pregnancy with this condition extremely uncommon. Spontaneous abortions and intrauterine growth restriction were frequently observed.

The outcome for these patients has improved remarkably following corrective surgery. Singh et al[38] reported 31 pregnancies in 27 patients with completely corrected lesions. All of these pregnancies ended in live births at term, and few maternal complications were reported. There was, however, a 20 percent incidence of growth restriction in the infants studied. Only one neonate was detected to have pulmonary atresia. Few maternal complications were reported in the study group.

Whittemore et al[20] have confirmed both the safety and the improved outcome in pregnancy in patients with corrected cyanotic lesions. They reported an overall 78 percent live birth rate versus 55 percent in the uncorrected group. Cardiovascular complications were more common in the cyanotic group, though overall the incidence of congestive failure was low. Palliative surgery for tetralogy was also effective, and 13 of 18 pregnancies in these patients resulted in a liveborn infant.[20]

As many as 40 percent of patients with an uncorrected tetralogy will experience cardiac failure during pregnancy. Poor prognostic signs include polycythemia and diminished peripheral oxygen saturation. Echocardiographic assessment is utilized to document ventricular function as well as the degree of shunting present. During pregnancy, there is increased right to left shunting due to a decline in systemic vascular resistance. The result is a fall in peripheral oxygen saturation. Thus, the uncorrected lesion can present a challenge to both the cardiologist and the obstetrician. Symptoms of left-sided heart failure and endocarditis should be carefully considered. Obstetric management includes monitoring to detect possible fetal growth restriction. As noted, cyanosis has been associated with miscarriage and preterm birth in these patients.

During labor and delivery, invasive monitoring will permit the prompt recognition of cardiac failure. The increase in cardiac output observed during labor may raise pulmonary vascular tone and increase shunting to the left side of the heart. Venous return should be carefully maintained because a fall in blood volume may limit the ability of the right ventricle to perfuse the lungs. This will also depend on the degree of right ventricular obstruction. Continuous delivery of oxygen to the cyanotic mother is recommended.

In these patients, relief of pain during labor and delivery is best managed with systemic medications, inhalation analgesia, or pudendal block. Epidural or spinal anesthesia should be employed with caution because of the potential for hypotension resulting from decreases in vascular resistance and venous return. Ephedrine should be carefully administered in patients with right-sided failure, as it may produce a rise in pulmonary vascular resistance. In most cases, general anesthesia is preferred for cesarean delivery.

Complications may arise in the postpartum period, particularly if maternal blood volume is contracted. As systemic resistance falls, right to left shunting will be increased, and cyanosis will worsen. For this reason, it is essential that blood be made available for these patients.

Eisenmenger Syndrome

Eisenmenger syndrome is defined as right to left or bidirectional shunting at either the atrial or ventricular level, combined with elevated pulmonary vascular resistance. Maternal mortality ranges from 12 to 70 percent, and fetal mortality approaches 50 percent.[22] Gleicher et al[34] have reported that at least 30 percent of fetuses will be growth restricted. Because of these risks, termination of pregnancy is strongly recommended in patients with Eisenmenger syndrome complicated by significant pulmonary hypertension. Women who continue pregnancy require strict limitation of activity with strong consideration for anticoagulation.

The amount of right to left shunting observed in patients with this disorder will be dependent on the degree of pulmonary hypertension present. It will also be affected by the relationship between pulmonary and systemic vascular resistances. Right ventricular failure will also limit pulmonary blood flow and may increase right to left shunting. Physical signs of Eisenmenger syndrome include cyanosis and digital clubbing. Chest pain, syncope, and hemoptysis are symptoms associated with poor prognosis.

It is imperative that Swan-Ganz monitoring be employed for management during labor and delivery. Efforts should be made to avoid central hypovolemia. This includes the use of uterine displacement to ensure adequate venous return to the heart. Controversy exists regarding the use of epidural anesthesia in patients with Eisenmenger syndrome. Theoretically, a fall in systemic vascular resistance could result in greater right to left shunting and cyanosis. Several authors, however, have failed to demonstrate a change in shunt flow or pulmonary resistance in patients treated with epidural analgesia during labor and delivery.[40,41] Oxygen has proved to be an effective pulmonary vasodilator and can result in increased peripheral oxygen saturation. Abboud and coworkers[42] have described the use of epidural morphine in a patient with pulmonary hypertension. This technique provides good analgesia with little effect on systemic blood pressure. Because the degree of pulmonary vascular reactivity probably varies in patients with Eisenmenger syndrome, it is best to make serial determinations of arterial oxygen concentrations when administering epidural anesthesia. Patients who manifest a fall in Po_2 despite oxygen support should probably not be managed with this anesthetic technique. There appears to be no advantage to cesarean delivery compared with vaginal delivery in women with Eisenmenger syndrome.[39]

Obstructive Lesions

Coarctation of the Aorta

Patients with severe coarctation usually have their defect surgically corrected during infancy. Therefore, this lesion is infrequently encountered in pregnant women. Early studies reported a maternal mortality rate of 17 percent. Fortunately, maternal death is now a rare complication of this lesion.[43]

Patients at greatest risk are those with associated cardiac lesions or aneurysms of the aorta or circle of Willis. Classically, coarctation is recognized when a large difference in blood pressure is found between measurements in the upper extremities and legs. Because the constriction is often located at the level of the left subclavian artery, there may be isolated hypertension when blood pressure is determined in the right arm.

The risk of aortic dissection is probably overstated. However, antihypertensive therapy probably reduces whatever risk is present.[44] In suspected cases of dissection, vaginal delivery is not advised.

Following repair of coarctation, antihypertensive therapy may still be required. Women with repair performed during childhood should be carefully evaluated for potential restenosis. If significant obstruction of the aorta is present, left ventricular compromise may be exacerbated during pregnancy. Stroke volume is relatively fixed in these patients, so that normal compensatory mechanisms such as tachycardia may not be sufficient to maintain an adequate cardiac output. Hypotension during labor and postpartum should therefore be avoided. Appropriate precautions should be taken against infective endocarditis.

Surgical repair during pregnancy should be limited to cases of aortic dissection. Neurologic symptoms should be carefully evaluated as well. As stated earlier, it is not uncommon to find cerebral berry aneurysms in association with coarctation of the aorta. The risk that the newborn will have congenital heart disease varies from 4 to 23 percent.

Developmental Cardiac Lesions

Marfan Syndrome

Marfan syndrome is an autosomal dominant disorder of connective tissue marked by joint deformities, arachnodactyly, dislocations of the ocular lens, and cardiac manifestations, including weakness of the aortic root and wall. Mitral valve prolapse is found in 90 percent of cases. The prevalence of Marfan syndrome is 4 to 6 per 100,000. Certain families with Marfan syndrome appear to have formed frustes of this condition, in which there are significant skeletal deformities present in the absence of disease of the aorta or aortic valve.[45]. Prenatal diagnosis of a mutation of fibrillin, an elastin-associated glycoprotein, has been described in a family with Marfan syndrome.[46]

Patients with Marfan syndrome must receive genetic counseling and be made aware of the risks of pregnancy with their particular condition. The variability in the clinical expression of this disorder makes it imperative to study the cardiovascular system of these patients before counseling them about the dangers of pregnancy. Transesophageal echocardiographic measurement of the width of the aorta has been helpful in selecting patients at greatest risk for aortic dissection, although serial measurements of aortic root diameter may occasionally fail to detect a patient at risk for dissection.[47] Pyeritz[48] has suggested that dilatation of the aorta greater than 40 mm is a contraindication to pregnancy. He reviewed 26 pregnancies complicated by Marfan syndrome in which there was only one maternal death. This resulted from endocarditis in a woman who had congestive heart failure and mitral insufficiency before conception. A review of the literature in this report substantiates that the mortality rates of up to 50 percent that have been associated with Marfan disease in pregnancy reflect cases in which significant maternal cardiovascular disease existed prior to conception.

Aortic dissection occurs frequently during pregnancy and may be influenced by superimposed hypertension. Symptoms of dissection include excruciating chest pain that migrates posteriorly. Occasionally, painless dissection is encountered that may be accompanied by hypertension and tachycardia. β-Blockade and sodium nitroprusside infusion are the preferred medical therapy in such cases. Hypotension follows if the dissection is large or if it ruptures. With ascending aortic arch involvement, a loud murmur of aortic insufficiency may be auscultated. Emergency surgical correction is required in patients with progressive dissection.

The management of patients with Marfan disease includes efforts to minimize hypertension as well as the contractile force transmitted to the aortic wall. β-Blockade using propranolol may be efficacious. Regional anesthesia for labor and delivery is generally well tolerated.[49] If a patient requires surgical treatment for her cardiovascular disease, a cesarean delivery is recommended. Cardiac surgery is preferably performed at a later date.[50] When administering general anesthesia, avoidance of agents that promote hypertension during induction is recommended. Antibiotic prophylaxis is suggested during labor and delivery.

Mitral Valve Prolapse

Mitral valve prolapse (MVP) is the most common congenital heart lesion found in young women of child-bearing age. The incidence in this population is approximately 12 percent.[51] While there appears to be a genetic predisposition influencing development of this lesion, no clear pattern of inheritance exists. Histologic examination of the mitral valve leaflets reveals myxomatous degeneration. MVP is associated with skeletal deformities including pectus excavatum and a high arched palate, and it is observed in Marfan syndrome, as noted above, and the Ehler-Danlos syndrome. The dysfunctional characteristic of MVP is abnormal prolapse of one or both mitral leaflets into the left atrium during ventricular systole; while most women with MVP are asymptomatic, others experience palpitations, atypical chest pain, and syncope.

Most women with MVP have uneventful pregnancies.

It is possible that the increased intravascular volume of pregnancy that increases left ventricular end-diastolic volume results in less prolapse of the mitral valve leaflets. Rayburn and Fontana[52] reviewed the outcomes in 42 pregnancies among 25 patients diagnosed by auscultatory and echocardiographic findings.[52] In their series, cardiovascular complications were limited to one case of congestive heart failure, which occurred in a preeclamptic patient treated with intravenous β-mimetics as well as glucocorticoids.

Debate still exists as to whether routine antibiotic prophylaxis is warranted during pregnancy in patients with MVP. The American Heart Association has advised that antibiotics are not necessary in most patients undergoing routine vaginal or cesarean delivery.[53] Other authors suggest treating only those patients who have mitral regurgitation. However, in pregnancy, defining a normal physiologic ejection murmur may not be possible, particularly in patients presenting during labor and delivery. Moreover, the click and murmur of MVP may vary with both left ventricular volume and contractility. Therefore, because of the relative safety of therapy, it is recommended that prophylactic antibiotics be administered until this issue is further resolved.

Idiopathic Hypertrophic Subaortic Stenosis

IHSS, or asymmetric septal hypertrophy (ASH), is an autosomal dominant cardiac lesion with variable penetrance. As such, genetic counseling should be undertaken in affected individuals. Prenatal ultrasonographic diagnosis has been reported.[54] IHSS manifests as obstruction to left ventricular flow secondary to the hypertrophied interventricular septum and outflow tract. The symptoms at presentation with this lesion include dyspnea, angina, and syncope.

During ventricular systole, contraction of the myocardium results in narrowing of the outflow tract. Conditions that increase left ventricular end-diastolic volume will improve this condition. Pregnancy, which is marked by an increased circulating blood volume, may initially result in improvement in outflow tract obstruction. As gestation advances, the fall in systemic vascular resistance and diminished preload due to reduced venous return resulting from compression of the vena cava may exacerbate the symptoms of patients with IHSS. Complications arising in pregnancy include ventricular failure and supraventricular tachycardias.[55] These may be found in association with left atrial distention resulting from coexisting mitral regurgitation. Two maternal deaths have been reported in patients with IHSS.[56,57]

Management of patients with IHSS should include (1) avoidance of inotropic agents such as digitalis, which may exacerbate obstruction and precipitate failure; (2) maintenance of the left lateral decubitus position during labor; (3) restriction of the use of diuretics or drugs that decrease systemic vascular resistance; and (4) prompt recognition and treatment of arrhythmias.[58] Kolibash et al[58] have suggested that β-blockade can be helpful when symptoms arise during pregnancy or labor. They advocated the use of forceps to minimize Valsalva efforts, which might increase outflow obstruction.

Other Cardiac Diseases

Peripartum Cardiomyopathy

Peripartum cardiomyopathy has classically been defined as congestive failure with cardiomyopathy found in the last month of pregnancy or in the first 5 months postpartum.[59,60] Symptoms of left-sided failure occur in association with a dilated hypocontractile heart in patients who have no previous history of cardiac disease. The overwhelming majority (82 percent) of patients present with cardiac failure in the first 3 months postpartum.[59] Most reports have documented the higher frequency of this lesion among older black multiparas, particularly in association with twins or preeclampsia.

The etiology of this disease is unknown despite multiple theories suggesting an autoimmune process, viral infections, and genetic predisposition. Histologic examination of the myocardium reveals muscular hypertrophy surrounded by interstitial edema and chronic inflammatory infiltrate.[61] These findings, which are suggestive of an infectious or immune-mediated myocarditis, have led investigators to believe that an acute viral infection possibly from Coxsackie B may be responsible for this disorder.[62] Melvin and associates[62] studied endomyocardial biopsies obtained in three patients with postpartum congestive cardiomyopathy and found acute myocardial inflammatory changes. Two of the patients had histories of influenza-like infections, and one patient had antibody to Coxsackie B virus. The authors postulated that viral myocardial infections could trigger an autoimmune myocarditis. They therefore treated these patients with steroids and azathioprine and later found that two of the patients had no residual fibrosis on biopsy. This management should probably be restricted to cases in which the diagnosis has been established by endomyocardial biopsy.

It is unclear whether peripartum cardiomyopathy is a distinct entity from idiopathic dilated cardiomyopathy. Van Hoeven and colleagues[63] compared clinicopathologic features of women with peripartum cardiomyopathy and 14 women with nonpregnancy-associated cardiomyopathy. While no presenting clinical or pathologic variable distinguished these groups, 11 of 13 patients with idiopathic dilated cardiomyopathy experienced persistent heart failure or death compared with 5 of 13 women who had peripartum disease. The higher reported incidence of myocarditis in peripartum cardiomyopathy has been suggested as an explanation for the improved outcome in this group. However, a recent retrospective review of endomyocardial biopsy specimens from 34 patients fulfilling the criteria for a diagnosis of peripartum cardiomyopathy indicated a lower incidence of myocarditis (8.8 percent; 3 of 34) than that reported in other studies.[64] This incidence is similar to that found in age- and sex-matched controls with dilated cardiomyopathy undergoing cardiac transplantation.

Primary therapy of peripartum cardiomyopathy should include bedrest, sodium restriction, digitalis, and diuretics.[65] Thromboembolic complications stemming from mural thrombi are not uncommon. Anticoagulation may be necessary, particularly in patients with massively enlarged cardiac chambers.

It is generally accepted that the clinical course of this disease can be predicted by the size of the heart several months after the diagnosis has been made. Approximately 50 percent of affected women will continue to have symptoms of failure and cardiomegaly beyond 6 months. These women should be advised against pregnancy as the incidence of recurrent disease is high, with mortality rates approaching 100 percent.[66] Based on data from two studies, persistent cardiomegaly has been associated with a 5-year mortality rate exceeding 50 percent.[59,60] If a viral etiology has been established with return to normal size and function, the recurrence risk is believed to be minimal.[67]

Ischemic Cardiac Disease

Coronary artery disease is uncommon in women during the reproductive years. However, more women are delaying childbearing, and more are smoking. For these reasons, the frequency of ischemic cardiac disease during pregnancy may be increasing. The incidence of myocardial infarction during pregnancy has been estimated to be 1 in 10,000.[68] This is likely to be an overestimate as less than 100 cases have been published.[69] Arterial hypertension has been documented in one-third of women who suffer a myocardial infarction during pregnancy; however, mortality rates for these women do not appear to be greater than those without an elevation in blood pressure.[70] Whereas cigarette smoking and diabetes mellitus are other recognized risk factors for atherosclerosis, maternal age exceeding 35 years is the most consistent characteristic in pregnant women suffering a myocardial infarction.[71]

Coronary atherosclerosis is the predominant finding in pregnant women with a myocardial infarction; however, other causes of limited coronary blood flow may be observed. Coronary artery spasm and embolism may also limit oxygen availability to the myocardium and can produce angina as well as infarction. Beary et al[72] noted normal coronary anatomy in two of five women who sustained an infarction and subsequently underwent coronary angiography during the postpartum period. Acute myocardial infarction has been described following ergonovine administration for uterine bleeding.[73]

Chest pain suggesting myocardial ischemia requires medical attention, even in seemingly low-risk pregnant women. Anginal episodes should be evaluated with electrocardiography and exercise stress testing, if clinical suspicion is high. Thallium nucleotide imaging of coronary blood flow is generally not performed during pregnancy because of the associated radiation exposure (estimated 780 mrad) with this procedure.[74] Two-dimensional echocardiography may be of some value in detecting wall motion abnormalities during chest pain. If myocardial ischemia is strongly suggested, then interruption of pregnancy should be considered. In women less than 24 weeks, this may provide rapid symptomatic improvement.[70] If pregnancy is continued and symptoms do not abate with cessation of smoking and prescribed rest, then medical therapy to prevent coronary artery spasm including nitrates, β-adrenergics, or calcium channel blockers should be initiated. Repeated severe anginal episodes may necessitate coronary angiography with consideration for angioplasty or even bypass surgery during pregnancy.[76]

Myocardial infarction is usually suggested by prolonged chest pain associated with diaphoresis, nausea, and dyspnea. It may or may not be related to physical exertion. Electrocardiographic changes and a rise in the serum creatinine phosphokinase MB fraction have been documented in most cases during gestation.[48] Approximately two-thirds of women have had their infarction during the third trimester. In these women, the mortality rate has been reported to be 45 percent compared to 23 percent suffering an infarction during the first two trimesters.[71] Hankins and colleagues[71] have reported that approximately 20 percent of pregnant women die at the time of infarction, and mortality occurs in 50 percent of patients who deliver within 2 weeks of the event. In contrast, these authors found no deaths among 34 women without recurrent infarction who delivered more than 2 weeks postinfarction. Unexplained fetal death was reported in five of these cases. The preponderance of infarctions during the third trimester and the increased risk of maternal mortality when delivery occurs within 2 weeks of infarction suggest that the hemodynamic burdens of late pregnancy and delivery are particularly hazardous to women with coronary artery disease.[71]

The management of myocardial infarction during pregnancy is essentially the same as in the nonpregnant individual. Patients are admitted to the coronary or medical intensive care unit. Oxygen is administered, and pain should be minimized. Careful observation is undertaken for signs of congestive failure, arrhythmias, and further chest pain. These complications warrant consideration of pregnancy termination in women less than 24 weeks' gestation. As stated above, an effort should be made to allow a period of healing and recovery before initiating labor. In women with no symptoms, pregnancy can be allowed to progress to fetal maturity. During labor and delivery, pain should be minimized in order to decrease myocardial oxygen consumption. Conduction anesthesia is recommended and may reduce the normal anticipated increase in cardiac output.[71] Invasive hemodynamic monitoring is often employed, but may not be necessary in the absence of unstable angina, recent infarction, or impaired ventricular function.[75] Cesarean delivery is reserved for obstetric indications, as it does not improve maternal survival rates. There is continued debate as to whether women with a previous myocardial infarction should attempt pregnancy. A recent report suggests favorable outcomes in selected cases.[77] Careful evaluation including thallium scanning and angiography may identify women at greatest risk, although there are insufficient data available with which to counsel this group of patients.

Key Points

- The presence of underlying cardiac disease should be suspected in any pregnant woman with (1) a progressive limitation of physical activity due to worsening dyspnea, (2) chest pain that accompanies exercise or increased activity, and (3) syncope that is preceded by palpitations or physical exertion.

- Women who develop right to left shunting with increased pulmonary vascular pressure (Eisenmenger syndrome) may exhibit maternal mortality rates approaching 50 percent.

- Treatment of mitral stenosis involves limitation of activity, cautious diuresis, and control of arrhythmias. Tachycardia is poorly tolerated as stroke volume is relatively fixed. If medical treatment fails to control symptoms, valvuloplasty or replacement must be considered.

- Marfan syndrome, when accompanied by a significantly dilated aortic root (>40 mm), is associated with mortality rates up to 50 percent. Pregnancy is contraindicated with significant aortic root dilatation.

- Peripartum cardiomyopathy is a congestive cardiomyopathy found in the last month of pregnancy or in the first 5 months postpartum. It is more common in African Americans and twin gestations. Half of affected women will continue to have failure or cardiomegaly beyond 6 months.

- Myocardial infarction, when it occurs during pregnancy, is often observed in older gravidas with a history of chronic hypertension. Mortality rates are highest during the third trimester and when delivery occurs within 2 weeks of the event. Cesarean delivery is reserved for obstetric indications.

References

1. Hibbard LT: Maternal mortality due to cardiac disease. Clin Obstet Gynecol 18:27, 1975
2. Scott DE: Anemia in pregnancy. Obstet Gynecol Annu 1:219, 1972
3. Chesley LC, Duffus GM: Posture and apparent plasma volume in late pregnancy. J Obstet Gynaecol Br Commonw 78:406, 1971
4. Lindheimer MD, Katz AI: Sodium and diuretics in pregnancy. N Engl J Med 288:891, 1973
5. Metcalfe J, Ueland K: Maternal cardiovascular adjustment to pregnancy. Prog Cardiovasc Dis 16:363, 1974
6. Metcalfe J, McAnulty JH, Ueland K: Cardiovascular physiology. Clin Obstet Gynecol 24:693, 1981
7. Robson S, Hunter S, Boys RJ et al: Serial study of factors influencing changes in cardiac output during human pregnancy. Am J Physiol 256:H-1060, 1989
8. Ueland K, Novy MJ, Peterson EN, Metcalfe J: Maternal cardiovascular dynamics. IV. The influence of gestational age on the maternal cardiovascular response to posture and exercise. Am J Obstet Gynecol 104:856, 1969
9. Barry WH, Crossman W: Cardiac catheterization. In Braunwald E (ed); Heart Disease: A Textbook of Cardiovascular Medicine Vol. I WB Saunders, Philadelphia, 1980
10. Katz R, Karliner JS, Resnik R: Effects of a natural volume overload state (pregnancy) on left ventricular performance in normal human subjects. Circulation 58:434, 1978
11. Sadaniantz A, Kocheril AG, Emans S et al: Cardiovascular changes in pregnancy evaluated by two-dimensional and Doppler echocardiography. Am J Soc Endocardiol 2:253, 1992
12. Robson SC, Hunter S, Moore M et al: Hemodynamic changes during the puerperium: a Doppler and M-mode echocardiographic study. Br J Obstet Gynaecol 94:1028, 1987
13. Rubler S, Damini PM, Pinto ER: Cardiac size and performing during pregnancy estimated with echocardiography. Am J Cardiol 40:534, 1977
14. Vered Z, Poler SM, Gibson P et al: Non-invasive detection of the morphologic and hemodynamic changes during normal pregnancy. Clin Cardiol 14:327, 1991
15. Becker RM: Intracardiac surgery in pregnant women. Ann Thoracic Surg 36:463, 1983
16. Strickland RA, Oliver WC, Chatigian RC et al: Anesthesia cardiopulmonary bypass and the pregnant patient. Mayo Clin Proc 66:411, 1991
17. McFaul PB, Dornan JC, Lamki H et al: Pregnancy complicated by maternal heart disease. A review of 519 women. Br J Obstet Gynecol 95:861, 1988
18. Szekely P, Turner R, Snaith L: Pregnancy and the changing pattern of rheumatic heart disease. Br Heart J 35:1293, 1973
19. Chesley LC: Severe rheumatic cardiac disease and pregnancy: the ultimate prognosis. Am J Obstet Gynecol 136:552, 1980
20. Whittemore R, Hobbins JC, Engle MA: Pregnancy and its outcome in women with and without surgical treatment of congenital heart disease. Am J Cardiol 50:641, 1982
21. Rapaport E: Natural history of aortic and mitral valve disorders. Am J Cardiol 35:221, 1982
22. Szekely P, Snaith L: Heart Disease and Pregnancy. Churchill Livingstone, Edinburgh, 1974
23. Ribeiro PA, Fawzy ME, Awad M: Balloon valvotomy for pregnant patients with severe pliable mitral stenosis using the Inoue technique with total abdominal and pelvic shielding. Am Heart J 125:1558, 1992
24. Kultursay H, Turkoglu C, Akin P et al: Mitral balloon valvuloplasty with transesophageal echocardiography without using fluoroscopy. Cathet Cardiovasc Diagn 27:317, 1992
25. Stephen JJ: Changing patterns of mitral stenosis in childhood and pregnancy in Sri Lanka. J Am Coll Cardiol 19:1276, 1992
26. Clark SL, Phelan J, Greenspoon J: Labor and delivery

in the presence of mitral stenosis: central hemodynamic observations. Am J Obstet Gynecol 152:984, 1985

27. Ducey JP, Ellsworth SM: The hemodynamic effects of severe mitral stenosis and pulmonary hypertension during labor and delivery. Intensive Care Med 15:192, 1989

28. Easterling TR, Chadwick HS, Otto CM, Benedetti TJ: Aortic stenosis in pregnancy. Obstet Gynecol 72:113, 1988

29. Arias F, Pineda J: Aortic stenosis and pregnancy. J Reprod Med 20:229, 1978

30. Lao TT, Sermer M, MaGee L et al: Congenital aortic stenosis and pregnancy—a reappraisal. Am J Obstet Gynecol 169:540, 1993

31. Angel JL, Chapman C, Knuppel RA et al: Percutaneous balloon aortic valvuloplasty in pregnancy. Obstet Gynecol 72:438, 1988

32. Sullivan JM, Ramanathan KB: Management of medical problems in pregnancy—severe cardiac disease. N Engl J Med 313:304, 1985

33. Westaby S, Parry AJ, Forfar JC: Reoperation for prosthetic valve endocarditis in the third trimester of pregnancy. Ann Thoracic Surg 53:263, 1992

34. Mangano DT: Anesthesia for the pregnant cardiac patient. In Shnider SM, Levinson G (eds); Anesthesia for Obstetrics, Williams & Wilkins, Baltimore, 1987 pp 180–223

35. Jackson GM, Dildy GA, Varner MW et al: Severe pulmonary hypertension in pregnancy following successful repair of ventricular septal defect in childhood. Obstet Gynecol 82:6805, 1993

36. Pitkin RM, Perloff JK, Boos BJ et al: Pregnancy and congenital heart disease. Ann Intern Med 112:445, 1990

37. Nora JJ, Nora AH: Update on counseling the family with a first-degree relative with a congenital heart defect. Am J Med Genet 29:137, 1988

38. Singh H, Bolton PJ, Oakley CM: Pregnancy after surgical correction of Tetralogy of Fallot. BMJ 285:168, 1982

39. Gleicher N, Midwall J, Hockberger D: Eisenmenger's syndrome and pregnancy. Obstet Gynecol Surv 34:721, 1979

40. Midwall J, Jaffin H, Herman MV, Kupersmith J: Shunt flow and pulmonary hemodynamics during labor and delivery in the Eisenmenger syndrome. Am J Cardiol 42:299, 1978

41. Smedstad KG, Cramb R, Morison DH: Pulmonary hypertension and pregnancy: a series of eight cases. Can J Anaesth 41:502, 1994

42. Abboud JK, Raya J, Noueihed R: Intrathecal morphine for relief of labor pain in a parturient with severe pulmonary hypertension. Anesthesiology 59:477, 1983

43. Deal K, Wooley CF: Coarctation of the aorta and pregnancy. Ann Intern Med 78:706, 1973

44. Benny PS, Prasao J, MacVicar J: Pregnancy and coarctation of the aorta. Case report. Br J Obstet Gynaecol 87:1159, 1980

45. Pyeritz RE, McKusick VA: The Marfan syndrome: diagnosis and management. N Engl J Med 300:722, 1979

46. Godfrey M, Vandemark N, Wang M et al: Prenatal diagnosis and a donor slice mutation in fibrillin in a family with Marfan syndrome. Am J Hum Genet 53:472, 1993

47. Rosenblum N, Grossman A, Gabbe SG: Failure of serial echocardiographic studies to predict dissection in a pregnant woman with Marfan's syndrome. Am J Obstet Gynecol 146:470, 1983

48. Pyeritz RE: Maternal and fetal complications of pregnancy in the Marfan syndrome. Am J Med 71:784, 1982

49. Gordon CF, Johnson MD: Anesthetic management of the pregnant patient with Marfan syndrome. J Clin Anesth 5:248, 1993

50. Mor-Yosef S, Younis J, Granat M et al: Marfan's syndrome in pregnancy. Obstet Gynecol Surv 43:382, 1988

51. Devereuz RB, Kramer-Fox R, Kligfield P: Mitral valve prolapse: causes, clinical manifestations, and management. Ann Intern Med 111:305, 1989

52. Rayburn WF, Fontana ME: Mitral valve prolapse and pregnancy. Am J Obstet Gynecol 141:9, 1981

53. Dajani AS, Bisno A, Chung KJ: Prevention of bacterial endocarditis. JAMA 264:2919, 1990

54. Stewart PA, Buis-Lein T, Verivey RA, Wladimiroff JW: Prenatal ultrasonic diagnosis of familial asymmetric septal hypertrophy. Prenat Diagn 6:249, 1986

55. Turner GD, McGarry K, Oakley CM: Management of pregnancy with hypertrophic cardiomyopathy. BMJ 1:1749, 1979

56. Shah DM, Sunderji SG: Hypertrophic cardiomyopathy and pregnancy: report of a maternal mortality and review of literature. Obstet Gynecol Surv 40:444, 1985

57. Pellicca F, Cianfrocca C, Gaudio C et al: Sudden death during pregnancy in hypertrophic cardiomyopathy. Eur Heart J 13:241, 1992

58. Kolibash AJ, Ruiz DE, Lewis RP: Idiopathic hypertrophic subaortic stenosis in pregnancy. Ann Intern Med 82:791, 1975

59. Walsh JJ, Burch GE: Postpartal heart disease. Arch Intern Med 108:817, 1961

60. DeMakis JG, Rahimtoola SH: Peripartum cardiomyopathy. Circulation 44:964, 1971

61. DeMakis JG, Rahimtoola SH, Sutton GC: Natural course of peripartum cardiomyopathy. Circulation 44:1053, 1971

62. Melvin KR, Richardson PJ, Olsen EGJ et al: Peripartum cardiomyopathy due to myocarditis. N Engl J Med 307:731, 1982

63. VanHoeven KH, Kitsis RN, Katz SD et al: Peripartum versus idiopathic dilated cardiomyopathy in young women—a comparison of clinical, pathologic, and prognostic features. Int J Cardiol 40:57, 1993

64. Rizeo MN, Rickenbacher PR, Fowler MB et al: Incidence of myocarditis in peripartum cardiomyopathy. Am J Cardiol 74:474, 1994

65. Julian DG, Szekely P: Peripartum cardiomyopathy. Prog Cardiovasc Dis 27:223, 1985

66. St. John Sutton M, Cole P, Plappert M: Effects of subsequent pregnancy on left ventricular function in peripartum cardiomyopathy. Am Heart J 121:1776, 1991

67. Carvalho A, Brandao A, Martinez EE et al: Prognosis in peripartum cardiomyopathy. Am J Cardiol 64:540, 1989

68. Ginz B: Myocardial infarction in pregnancy. J Obstet Gynaecol Br Commonw 77:610, 1970

69. Gordon MC, Landon MB, Boyle J et al: Myocardial infarction during pregnancy in a patient with Class R/F diabetes: a case report and review of the literature on Class H IDDM. Obstet Gynecol Surv (in press)

70. Hussaini MH: Myocardial infarction during pregnancy: report of two cases with a review of the literature. Postgrad Med J 47:660, 1971

71. Hankins GDV, Wendel GD, Leveno KJ et al: Myocardial infarction during pregnancy; a review. Obstet Gynecol 65:139, 1985

72. Beary JF, Summer WR, Bulkley BH: Postpartum acute myocardial infarction: a rare occurrence of uncertain etiology. Am J Cardiol 43:158, 1979

73. Liao JK, Cockrill BA, Yurchak PM: Acute myocardial infarction after ergonovine administration for uterine bleeding. Am J Cardiol 68:823, 1991

74. Sheikh AU, Harper MA: Myocardial infarction during pregnancy: management and outcome of two pregnancies. Am J Obstet Gynecol 169:279, 1993

75. Goldmann ME, Mueller J: Coronary artery disease in pregnancy. p. 141. In Elkayam U, Gleicher N (eds): Cardiac Problems in Pregnancy. Alan R. Liss, New York, 1982

76. Majdan JF, Walinsley P, Cowchock SF et al: Coronary artery bypass surgery during pregnancy. Am J Cardiol 52:1145, 1983

77. Frenkel Y, Barkai G, Brisin L et al: Pregnancy after myocardial infarction: are we playing safe? Obstet Gynecol 77:822, 1991

78. Clark SL: Structural cardiac disease in pregnancy. In Clark SL, Phelan JP, Cotton DB (eds): Critical Care Obstetrics. Medical Economics Books, 1987

79. Shulman ST, Amren DP, Bisno AL et al: Prevention of bacterial endocarditis. Circulation 70:1125A, 1984

Pulmonary Disease

Philip Samuels

Tuberculosis

Tuberculosis is a pulmonary infection caused by the acid-fast bacillus *Mycobacterium tuberculosis*. There has been a decline in the frequency of tuberculosis in the United States over the past 50 years. Most obstetricians do not consider this diagnosis when a pregnant patient presents with lethargy and respiratory symptoms. However, as more women enter the United States from developing nations, there has been a resurgence of tuberculosis in the pregnant population, primarily in urban areas. Furthermore, the increasing number of pregnant women with HIV has also led to an increase in tuberculosis complicating pregnancy.

Pregnancy should not be a deterrent to the accurate diagnosis and treatment of tuberculosis. Tuberculin skin testing with subcutaneous administration of intermediate strength purified protein derivative (PPD) is the mainstay of testing for tuberculosis in the United States. In high-risk areas and populations, it should be administered at the first prenatal visit. Carter and Mates[1] found that most women with tuberculosis were asymptomatic and would have escaped diagnosis and thus treatment if they had not undergone PPD testing. A positive PPD only means that the patient has been previously exposed to tuberculosis and that there are dormant organisms present. Less than 10 percent of patients with a positive PPD and an intact immune system will progress to active disease. This method, however, has several drawbacks. Only 80 percent of patients with a reactivation of tuberculosis will have positive skin tests. In addition, any patient who has previously received the bacillus Calmette-Guèrin (BCG) vaccine will retain a positive tuberculin skin test for life. Although this vaccine is rarely used in the United States, it is administered routinely in countries where tuberculosis is endemic.

If a differential diagnosis of tuberculosis is entertained in a patient presenting with respiratory symptoms and lethargy, a chest x-ray with abdominal shielding should be obtained without hesitation. A chest x-ray should also be taken without delay if the patient's previously negative tuberculin skin test becomes positive, if it cannot be determined when a patient's skin test became positive, or if a patient has persistent respiratory or constitutional symptoms.[2] Many obstetricians are fearful and hesitate too long before obtaining chest x-rays during pregnancy. Without abdominal shielding, the radiation exposure to the fetus from a single chest x-ray is minimal, approximately 2.5 mrad. With abdominal shielding, the exposure is even less.[3,4] Nonetheless, chest x-rays should be delayed until after the first trimester if there is not a pressing indication.

The definitive diagnosis of tuberculosis is based on identifying *M. tuberculosis* by culture or by acid-fast or fluorescent stain of the sputum. First-morning sputum specimens obtained on 3 consecutive days are usually the best source for cultures and stain. If the patient is not able to produce a sputum sample voluntarily, production can be elicited by having the patient inhale aerosolized hypertonic saline. Any patient having a positive smear for acid-fast bacilli should be started on antituberculous chemotherapy while awaiting the results of cultures and drug sensitivity tests. One must often wait up to 6 weeks before final culture results are available.

When adequate treatment is implemented, tuberculosis appears to have no adverse effect on pregnancy, and, conversely, pregnancy does not alter the natural history of the disease.[5–7] This differs sharply from studies earlier in the century that allegedly showed that pregnancy had a deleterious effect on the course of tuberculosis. One controversial study did find a 10-fold increase in spontaneous first-trimester pregnancy losses in patients with active tuberculosis.[8] In that study, however, the control group had a first-trimester miscarriage rate of only 2 percent, which is excessively low. Early in this century, abortion was recommended for patients with tuberculosis. Current data, however, strongly suggest that there is no maternal or fetal indication for pregnancy termination in the gravida with tuberculosis.[9]

Highly effective chemotherapeutic agents have been developed for the treatment of tuberculosis (Table 29-3). Although the prognosis for tuberculosis during pregnancy is excellent, severe complications such as miliary, renal, and meningeal tuberculosis have developed.[10] Treatment has become more complex as resistant strains of *M. tuberculosis* have developed. It is paramount that cultures and sensitivities be obtained on all patients. Treatment should be started empirically when the diagnosis is strongly suspected, but should be individualized when sensitivities are available. Current standard therapy for pregnancy is isoniazid in a single daily dose of 300 mg and rifampin, 600 mg/day.[11] If a resistant strain is suspected, ethambutol should be added.[11] This therapy should be continued for 9 months.

Isoniazid prophylaxis is often recommended for patients under the age of 35 years who have recently converted their tuberculin skin test but do not have active disease and do have normal liver function. Such prophylaxis is discouraged during pregnancy but may be begun during the postpartum period. The major adverse effects of isoniazid include toxic hepatitis, peripheral neuropathy, and hypersensitivity reactions. Transient elevations of the serum transaminases are seen in approximately 20 percent of patients. Transaminase levels should therefore be monitored monthly. If they reach five times the upper limit of normal, the drug should be discontinued. If these guidelines are followed, serious isoniazid hepatitis can be avoided.[12]

Peripheral neuropathy appears to be related to a deficiency of pyridoxine, vitamin B_6. Patients taking isoniazid should receive a 25 to 50-mg supplement of pyridoxine daily to prevent this complication. Hypersensitivity reactions to isoniazid may take the form of an antinuclear antibody-positive, drug-induced systemic lupus erythematosus. Other less serious hypersensitivity manifestations may also be seen. Isoniazid has been studied extensively during pregnancy, and there appears to be no increase in congenital malformations.[13] Only one study noted a small excess of nonspecific congenital anomalies in patients taking this drug, but certainly no associated syndrome was observed.[14]

Ethambutol also appears safe for use during gestation and has not been associated with an increase in congenital anomalies.[13] In doses higher than those usually recommended (>15 mg/kg/day), ethambutol can produce retrobulbar neuritis. This finding has not been observed in abortuses or in neonates of mothers receiving this medication.[15,16]

If possible, streptomycin should be avoided during pregnancy. In one report, more than 10 percent of the offspring of patients treated with streptomycin during pregnancy showed damage to cranial nerve VIII.[13] This could also hold true for kenamycin, capreomycin, and

Table 29-3 Antituberculosis Agents

Drug	Dosage	Maternal Side Effects
Isoniazid	300 mg/day (single dose) PO	Toxic hepatitis, peripheral neuropathy (prevented with pyridoxine)
Ethambutol	15 mg/kg/day (single dose) PO	Optic neuritis
p-Aminosalicylic acid	10–12 g/day (two or three divided doses) PO	Gastrointestinal disturbance
Rifampin	600 mg/day (single dose) PO	Orange discoloration of body secretions, gastrointestinal disturbance, liver toxicity
Pyrazinamide	15 mg/kg PO	Hepatitis, hyperuricemia
Streptomycin	15 mg/kg/day (single dose) IM	Cranial nerve VIII toxicity, nephrotoxicity
Cycloberine	15 mg/kg PO	Headache, drowsiness, seizures
Kenamycin	20 mg/kg IM	Cranial nerve VIII toxicity, nephrotoxicity
Viomycin	20 mg/kg IM	Cranial nerve VIII toxicity, nephrotoxicity
Ethionamide	15 mg/kg PO	Gastrointestinal disturbance, hepatotoxicity

viomycin. While other studies have also shown severe hearing loss as well as abnormal caloric tests and audiograms, none has found auditory nerve damage in as many as 10 percent of cases.[17] Drug levels were not meticulously monitored in the patients in those studies. The drugs are probably much safer today, as drug levels of aminoglycosides are routinely measured.

Rifampin inhibits DNA-dependent RNA polymerase. It readily crosses the placenta and could theoretically injure the fetus. One study reported a 3 to 4 percent incidence of severe congenital malformations associated with the use of rifampin during pregnancy.[13] This figure, however, is not significantly higher than the expected background rate of malformations. Nevertheless, rifampin should be used with caution during gestation.

p-Aminosalicylic acid was once commonly used during pregnancy. Because it is associated with severe gastrointestinal side effects, it is no longer recommended for the gravida who is already prone to nausea and vomiting. Its use has not been associated with congenital malformations.

Transplacental passage of tuberculosis is extremely rare. Most perinatal infections occur when a mother with active tuberculosis handles her neonate.[18] The risk to the child of contracting tuberculosis from a mother with active disease during the first year of life may be as high as 50 percent.[19] Daily administration of isoniazid chemoprophylaxis can be given to the newborn for the length of the mother's treatment.[20] This therapy, however, requires a great deal of compliance and motivation on the part of the parent to make certain that the child receives the medication. Another alternative is to administer BCG vaccine to the neonate.[19] After vaccination, the child must then be separated from the mother until he or she develops a positive PPD skin test. This approach, however, has the drawback of rendering the child tuberculin positive for life. This vaccine is also recommended if the child will be exposed to individuals with drug-resistant tuberculosis.

Sarcoidosis

Sarcoidosis is a granulomatous disease that can involve many organ systems. It most commonly affects the lungs and lymph nodes but may also affect the skin, eyes, liver, central nervous system, and heart. The hallmark histologic finding is the noncaseating granuloma. While the etiology of the disease is unknown, patients demonstrate excessive immunoglobulin levels and impaired delayed hypersensitivity, suggesting an immune cause. The disease is most commonly diagnosed between the ages of 20 and 40 years. The usual clinical presentation includes symmetric bilateral hilar lymphadenopathy discovered on a routine chest x-ray and

palpable cervical adenopathy. The differential diagnosis must include Hodgkin's disease, other lymphomas, and tuberculosis. The only method for definitive diagnosis is lymph node biopsy usually performed during bronchoscopy or mediastinoscopy. In more advanced cases of sarcoidosis, there is a constant nonproductive cough and interstitial pulmonary disease. The Kveim test is positive in most patients with sarcoidosis presenting with lymphadenopathy. This test, however, is rarely used today and is mentioned here for historical purposes. Most patients with sarcoidosis will also have abnormal levels of angiotensin-converting enzyme.

Many patients with sarcoidosis require no treatment. Approximately two-thirds will improve spontaneously within 2 to 3 years of the initial diagnosis. These women usually have no clinical evidence of disease and only minor residual findings on chest x-ray. Of the remaining patients, most will experience a slow progression of the disease over many years with both exacerbations and remissions. Very few will suffer a rapid downhill course. It has been estimated that 0.05 percent of pregnancies are associated with sarcoidosis.[20] This means that in a large hospital that delivers 5,000 infants annually, two or three pregnant women may have sarcoidosis.

Pregnancy has no long-term adverse effect on the course of sarcoidosis. Similarly, sarcoidosis does not have a deleterious effect on perinatal outcome in asymptomatic patients. Therefore, sarcoidosis is not a contraindication to pregnancy. Most patients appear to improve during gestation.[21-23] This amelioration may be due to increased circulating levels of cortisol. During the puerperium, however, there may be a relapse of the illness, but such relapses are usually not serious.[23,24] Haynes de Regt[25] reviewed 15 cases of proven sarcoidosis during a 10-year period at Downstate Medical Center. Eleven patients remained stable during pregnancy, while two experienced progression of the disease and two others died of complications. Factors that appear to indicate a poor prognosis include pulmonary parenchymal lesions on chest x-ray, advanced roentgenologic staging, advanced maternal age, low inflammatory activity, requirement of drugs other than steroids, and presence of extrapulmonary sarcoidosis.[25]

In patients with known sarcoidosis, an attempt must be made early in gestation to identify renal or hepatic involvement. A report by Warren et al highlights a case in which sarcoidosis first presented as acute renal failure during pregnancy.[26] This evaluation should include a 24-hour urine collection for creatinine clearance and total protein excretion, liver function studies, and an ECG. Any patient presenting with an unknown skin rash and pulmonary symptoms should be evaluated for the possibility of sarcoidosis, as a case report demonstrated that sarcoidosis first appeared as pruritic white papules in a pregnant woman.[27] The pregnant patient with sarcoidosis should also undergo pulmonary function testing early in pregnancy and again near term. Arterial blood gas evaluation is necessary only when clinically indicated.

When medical treatment is necessary, glucocorticoids are the mainstay for sarcoidosis. Progressive deterioration of pulmonary function testing is the major indication for corticosteroids. Patients are usually started on 60 mg of prednisone daily. The dose is tapered once a remission has been established. During pregnancy, the amount of corticosteroid can often be reduced because of the aforementioned increased levels of circulating cortisol. The risk of postpartum relapse, however, requires that these women receive parenteral steroids during labor and increased doses of steroids immediately after delivery.

Pneumonia

Most bacterial pneumonia in pregnant women is due to *Streptococcus pneumoniae*. Most of these patients are smokers.[28] The clinical hallmarks of pneumococcal pneumonia include sudden onset, productive cough, purulent sputum, tachypnea, and fever with shaking chills. The diagnosis should be made on the basis of chest x-ray, Gram stain of the sputum, and cultures of blood and sputum. The chest x-ray usually reveals lobar consolidation and air bronchograms. Gram stain shows numerous leukocytes and gram-positive diplococci.

Patients with pneumococcal pneumonia complicating pregnancy should be initially hospitalized and receive 600,000 units of aqueous penicillin G intravenously four times daily. Parenteral treatment should continue for several days after defervescence. The therapy can then be changed to an oral penicillin or ampicillin (500 mg four times daily). The treatment should be continued for a total of 10 to 14 days. For patients who are allergic to penicillin, either a cephalosporin or erythromycin can be used. It should be noted, however, that 10 to 15 percent of patients who are allergic to penicillin will also react to cephalosporins. A vaccine consisting of the capsular antigens from *S. pneumoniae* has been used to prevent pneumococcal infections. It should be used during pregnancy in special circumstances, such as the patient about to undergo splenectomy[29] and in the immunosuppressed patient.

Mycoplasma pneumonia is caused by *Mycoplasma pneumoniae*, a small organism lacking a cell wall. It therefore does not respond to therapy with penicillin or cephalosporins. This form of pneumonia is common in young adults. In contrast to the sudden onset of pneumococcal pneumonia, patients with mycoplasma pneumonia usually have a slow, gradual onset of symptoms with a nonproductive cough. The diagnosis is usu-

ally made clinically. On chest x-ray, infiltrates are diffuse and patchy and can be either unilateral or bilateral. Antibodies to mycoplasma can be used to confirm the clinical diagnosis of this disease. One must consider the diagnosis of mycoplasma pneumonia in any patient whose clinical symptoms are not responding to penicillin or to cephalosporins. During pregnancy, the treatment of mycoplasma pneumonia consists of the administration of erythromycin for 10 to 14 days. Azithromycin and clarithromycin can also be used. These medications may cause less gastrointestinal distress than erythromycin but are considerably more expensive. Tetracycline and its derivatives should be avoided.

In immunocompromised patients, patients with alcoholism, and heavy smokers, pneumonia secondary to *Hemophilus influenzae* and *Klebsiella pneumoniae* can be seen. Pneumonia caused by these organisms require immediate hospitalization and therapy with the appropriate antibiotics.

In recent years, there has been a resurgence of pneumonia due to influenza A. It is uncertain whether this is due to a true increase in the disease or to an increased ability to diagnosis it. Maternal deaths have been reported.[30,31] Patients need supportive therapy if they develop this complication of influenza A. The routine use of influenza vaccine in pregnancy is not recommended. It is, however, a killed vaccine and should theoretically not cause any adverse effects in pregnancy. It should certainly be routinely administered to immunosuppressed patients and should probably be considered in pregnant women who work in a health care environment where they are often exposed to respiratory illnesses. Amantidine should be administered to those with known exposures to patients with influenza A. The prophylactic dose is 200 mg in a single or divided dose daily for ten days. It must be administered immediately after exposure. If given prophylactically, it can prevent 70 to 90 percent of infections. Some believe that it can decrease the duration of illness and severity of symptoms if used within 48 hours of the onset of symptoms. In this instance, the patient should take 200 mg daily until symptoms have been gone for 24 hours.[32] If a patient develops influenza A pneumonia, the physician must be surveillant for the development of a superinfection with *Staphylococcus aureus*.

Varicella affects very few adults, but up to 25 percent of those exposed may develop varicella pneumonia.[33,34] The mortality rate of varicella pneumonia in pregnancy may approach 30 percent.[35] The likelihood of developing pneumonia during primary varicella infection during pregnancy appears to be increased in the third trimester and in smokers. It should be treated aggressively with supportive therapy and acyclovir in an intravenous dose of 7.5 mg/kg every 8 hours. The use of this medication has been shown to decrease mortality rates by one half.[35] The live attenuated varicella vaccine that was released in 1995 may help or hurt obstetricians in the future. If the immunity is long lived, it may prevent much varicella during pregnancy. If, however, young women who were vaccinated in childhood begin to lose their immunity when they reach the childbearing years, we may see an increase in this disease in the future.

Even with improved technology and antibiotics, Madinger and coworkers[36] believe that the maternal and fetal outcomes are not considerably improving in patients with pneumonia. They retrospectively reviewed 250 cases of pneumonia during pregnancy that occured among 32,179 deliveries. Medical complications included bacteremia in 16 percent, empyema in 8 percent, atrial fibrillation in 4 percent, and respiratory failure necessitating intubation and ventilation in 20 percent. Preterm labor occurred in 44 percent of the patients and preterm delivery in 36 percent. One patient with cystic fibrosis died. Perinatal mortality included one stillbirth and two neonatal deaths. There is a significant correlation between underlying maternal disease, maternal medical complications, and preterm delivery in the gravida with pneumonia.[36]

Asthma

Asthma is the most common obstructive pulmonary disease that coexists with pregnancy. It is observed in 0.4 to 1.3 percent of pregnant women.[37,38] A study at Johns Hopkins Hospital reported a 1 percent incidence of asthma complicating pregnancy and a 0.15 percent incidence of severe asthma during gestation requiring hospitalization.[39] Pregnancy can have a varying effect on the course of asthma. Data compiled from nine studies published between 1953 and 1976 revealed that 49 percent of pregnant patients had no change in the course of their asthma, 29 percent showed improvement, and 22 percent showed exacerbation of their disease.[40–43] A 1989 study from the United Kingdom demonstrated that asthma improved in 69 percent of pregnant women, worsened in 9 percent, and showed no change in 22 percent.[44] Juniper and colleagues[45] examined reasons for improvement of asthma during pregnancy. They studied airway compliance in asthmatic women at 3-month intervals prior to pregnancy and subsequently in each trimester of pregnancy. A twofold improvement in airway responsiveness during pregnancy was observed.[45] This improvement was not statistically related to changes in levels of progesterone or estriol.

Nonetheless, asthma continues to be a major problem for adolescents who become pregnant. Apter and coinvestigators[46] studied 28 pregnancies in 21 adolescents at Northwestern University Medical School.

There were 56 exacerbations of asthma, including 22 hospitalizations and 20 emergency room visits. In 64 percent of the pregnancies, systemic corticosteroids had to be administered on an inpatient or outpatient basis.[46] These investigators found that the two most frequent factors associated with exacerbations of asthma included respiratory tract infections (59 percent) and noncompliance with medical regimens (27 percent). Williams[47] noted that approximately one-third of patients with asthma reacted differently in subsequent pregnancies irrespective of the sex of the fetus.

Older studies have suggested that intrauterine growth restriction (IUGR), preterm birth, and perinatal morbidity and mortality occurred more commonly in pregnancies associated with asthma.[43,48] No study demonstrates an increase in the rate of fetal malformations in the asthmatic patient. More recent data indicate that the risk of perinatal morbidity and mortality is minimally increased in the asthmatic patient, especially if adequate medical care is received. Sims and coworkers[49] observed a small increase in the number of small for gestational age newborns in mothers receiving oral steroid therapy. In the study of Apter et al.[46] there was only one premature infant and no cases complicated by IUGR.

Mabie and coworkers[50] investigated outcomes in 200 pregnancies in 142 asthmatics compared with a control group of 22,651 nonasthmatics. In this 1992 study, they found no difference in prematurity, IUGR, or perinatal mortality. Most of the patients had mild asthma, and 12 percent experienced exacerbations during labor. They also found that the rate of postpartum exacerbations was higher in those who had undergone cesarean delivery.

In another study, Perlow and colleagues[51] retrospectively studied 183 asthmatics. Steroid-dependent asthmatics showed a higher incidence of gestational diabetes, preterm labor, premature rupture of the membranes, and preterm delivery. Cesarean delivery, growth restriction, and birthweight below 1,000 g were not increased. These factors were also increased somewhat in nonsteroid-dependent asthmatics on chronic medications. They concluded that perinatal outcome is compromised in asthmatics taking chronic medications.

Schatz et al[52] recently published a prospective case–control study of 486 asthmatics in 1995. They found that in well-controlled, actively managed patients there was no increase in perinatal complications. They attribute this to aggressive management of the asthma.

The goals in treating asthma during pregnancy are (1) reduction in the number of asthmatic attacks, (2) prevention of severe asthmatic attacks (status asthmaticus), and (3) assurance of adequate maternal and fetal oxygenation. Patients receiving allergen desensitization may continue this treatment throughout pregnancy.[53] The Centers for Disease Control and Prevention (CDC) recommends that patients with chronic bronchial asthma receive yearly influenza immunization.[54] This is a killed vaccine and can be administered safely during pregnancy.

Asthma therapy in pregnancy has undergone significant change since the last edition of this text was published. Inhaled β-agonists have become the mainstay of acute and chronic therapy for asthma in pregnancy. This has been true for the nonpregnant asthmatic for years, but has only become the main therapy during pregnancy in the past 5 years, replacing theophylline. The most widely used of these agents are albuterol and metaproterenol. This therapy can be used on an as needed basis for mild cases or on a scheduled basis for severe patients. In a fairly large study, no adverse pregnancy outcome was seen in women who used β-agonist inhalers in the first trimester.[55] The most common side effects seen with these agents include cardiac arrhythmias and tachyphylaxis.

In addition to inhaled β-agonists, many patients require inhaled glucocorticoids. This therapy has helped control asthma on an outpatient basis over the past few years.[56,57] Beclomethasone is the most commonly used inhaled corticosteroid, but triamcinolone and flunisolide are also available. The main side effect is oropharyngeal candidiasis, but this is minimized if a spacer device is used in the inhaler. Cromolyn is another anti-inflammatory agent that may be used during pregnancy. It prevents mast cell degranulation. It is not as powerful as glucocorticoids and works more slowly. It is usually used as adjunctive therapy and may be used with both β-agonists and glucocorticoids.

The use of aminophylline has declined during pregnancy, but many obstetricians still use it because of their familiarity with this agent. cAMP, which produces relaxation of the bronchi, is released when β_2-receptors are stimulated by agonists. cAMP is metabolized by phosphodiesterase. Aminophylline derivatives inhibit phosphodiesterase and therefore increase circulating levels of cAMP. Aminophylline crosses the placenta but has shown no harmful fetal effects.[58–60] Similarly, aminophylline will appear in breast milk but will not have significant effects on the neonate. Smoking increases the clearance of aminophylline, and a higher dose is needed for these patients. If this therapy is used, the goal is to keep the theophylline level between 10 and 20 μg/ml. Theophylline toxicity is commonly manifested by nausea and vomiting, but increased levels of theophylline may also cause tachycardia and cardiac arrhythmias.

Oral or parenteral corticosteroids should be employed when the aerosolized forms are inadequate. Although administration of glucocorticoids to pregnant rabbits has been associated with cleft palate,[61] these medications are safe for use during pregnancy when indicated. In one literature review, 2 of 260 infants born to mothers taking steroids before 14 weeks' gestation developed a cleft palate.[62] Many studies have since clearly demonstrated that the use of glucocorticoids is safe during gestation and is not associated with congenital anomalies.[63–66] An increased incidence of IUGR in fetuses born to women taking 10 mg prednisone daily throughout pregnancy for a history of infertility has been reported.[67] Presumably these women were nonsmokers who did not have underlying chronic diseases that would be associated with IUGR.

Although fetal adrenal suppression may occur after maternal glucocorticoid ingestion, it is extremely rare. Schatz and colleagues[68] found no evidence of neonatal adrenal suppression in 71 infants born to mothers receiving a daily average of 8.2 mg of prednisone during gestation. In another report, neonatal adrenal insufficiency was not observed in infants whose mothers received up to 60 mg of prednisone daily throughout pregnancy.[69]

The lack of fetal and neonatal effects associated with maternal glucocorticoid ingestion is probably due to the small amount of administered glucocorticoid that actually reaches the fetal compartment. A fetus is exposed to only 10 to 30 percent of the prednisone ingested by the mother.[70,71] Most of the drug is inactivated by placental 11-β-ol-dehydrogenase. Of the small amount of prednisone that actually reaches the fetus, even a smaller fraction will be metabolized by the fetus to the active form of the drug, prednisolone. Ballard and coworkers[72] reported that one-sixth of a dose of hydrocortisone reaches the fetus and one-third of a dose of betamethasone enters the fetal circulation. It is apparent therefore that prednisone is the oral glucocorticoid of choice to treat maternal asthma while minimizing fetal exposure. When selecting a corticosteroid for use during pregnancy, it is important to look at the ratio of glucocorticoid to mineralocorticoid activity as well as the amount of drug that crosses the placenta. Prednisone and methylprednisolone are excellent choices. They have minimal mineralocorticoid effects and cross the placenta poorly.

Status asthmaticus requires immediate therapeutic intervention. During this period of acute treatment, the patient should receive a 30 to 40 percent concentration of humidified oxygen and should be well hydrated. Subcutaneous catecholamines should be administered. Because it has both α- and β-agonist activities, epinephrine can theoretically decrease uterine blood flow and thus decrease fetal oxygenation during this critical period. In a pregnant sheep model, while epinephrine did reduce uterine blood flow, it did not impair fetal oxygenation. In humans, there is no evidence that using epinephrine for the treatment of acute asthma has deleterious effects on the fetus. Terbutaline, a β_2-agonist that is more selective than epinephrine, is a better first-line drug in pregnancy. In the emergent situation, however, epinephrine can be used if terbutaline is not immediately available. If the patient does not improve rapidly after the subcutaneous administration of catecholamines, intravenous corticosteroids should be administered. Methylprednisolone in a dose of 100 mg every 6 to 8 hours or hydrocortisone in a dose of 100 mg every 4 hours is usually administered until the asthma attack clears. Nebulized β-agonists should also be used. Rarely, intravenous aminophylline in a loading dose of 5 mg/kg followed by 0.6 mg/kg/hr can be used in the poorly responsive patient.

In the unusual patient who is resistant to these measures and has a falling P_{O_2}, endotracheal intubation should be considered. This procedure should only be undertaken under the guidance of a pulmonary specialist or anesthesiologist. Schreier and colleagues[73] reported two pregnant women who required intubation for respiratory failure complicating asthma during the third trimester. They demonstrated that maintenance of an adequate P_{O_2} was an essential component of therapy in these cases. In addition, they utilized a warm solution of metaproterenol in saline for bronchial irrigation and suction. They found that this served as a bronchoalveolar lavage and facilitated recovery.[73]

Acute asthma attacks are unusual during labor. Should they occur, however, they are treated in the usual fashion. Epidural anesthesia is preferred for labor, vaginal delivery, and cesarean delivery. General anesthesia carries the risks of atelectasis and subsequent chest infection.[74] If the patient has been receiving oral corticosteroids during pregnancy, intravenous dosages should be used for labor and delivery. Generally, 100 mg of hydrocortisone every 4 to 6 hours or 100 mg of methylprednisolone administered intravenously at 6- to 8-hour intervals during labor and for 24 hours after delivery should suffice. Thereafter the patient should resume her maintenance dose of oral glucocorticoids.

Pulmonary Embolus

Pulmonary embolus complicates between 0.09 and 0.7 per 1,000 pregnancies.[75,76] Prompt diagnosis and treatment are imperative, as untreated pulmonary emboli during pregnancy carry a 12.8 percent mortality rate, while treatment lowers this to 0.7 percent.[77] If untreated, more than one-third of these patients will have recurrent emboli.[78] The vast majority of pulmonary emboli arise from thrombophlebitis of the deep femoral and pelvic veins. The reported incidence of deep venous thrombosis during pregnancy is 0.4 per 1,000.[75] This figure is six times more frequent than in nonpregnant women.[79] In a review by Weiner,[80] the incidence of deep vein thrombosis in pregnancy was 0.36 percent.

It is now common for patients in preterm labor to be aggressively treated with prolonged bedrest. This approach places these patients at an increased risk for thrombophlebitis and pulmonary embolism. Gurz and Heiselman[81] report a case of a fatal pulmonary embolus that occurred during tocolysis. It is prudent therefore to administer prophylactic, low-dose heparin to patients who are at prolonged bedrest.

The patient with an acute pulmonary embolus usually presents with chest pain and dyspnea. Occasionally, a pleural friction rub may be auscultated. The chest x-ray is often normal, but arterial blood gas values usually show a decreased P_{O_2} and a slightly more decreased P_{CO_2}. Hypercapnea, however, bodes a poor outcome.[81] Massive pulmonary emboli are easily diagnosed. Hypotension and cardiovascular collapse often complicate such cases. In contrast, patients with small emboli may only have subtle signs and symptoms. It is imperative to establish the proper diagnosis in affected patients, as these small clots may be the harbinger of a massive embolus. Two reports show that the sudden onset of blindness may be due to hypotension caused by pulmonary embolus in the absence of other symptoms.[82,83]

Certain acquired disorders of coagulation place the patient at increased risk of developing thrombophlebitis and pulmonary emoblism. Congenital deficiency of antithrombin III is an autosomal dominant trait. The prevalence is approximately 1 in 3,500 individuals. Pregnancy in these patients is often complicated by thrombophlebitis.[84] Protein C deficiency is another autosomal dominant trait. During pregnancy, there may be up to 25 percent risk of deep venous thrombosis in those with a protein C deficiency.[84] In congenital deficiencies of protein S, a vitamin K-dependent inhibitor of hemostasis, there is a high incidence of thrombophlebitis.[84] In patients with a prior history of deep venous thrombosis, levels of protein C, protein S, and antithrombin III should be checked prior to pregnancy, as gestation causes changes that may make the results confusing or unreliable.

Although impedance plethysmography is still occasionally used to detect lower extremity thrombosis, Doppler studies with compression sonography have made testing much more accurate. Its positive predictive value is 94 percent compared with 83 percent for impedance plethysmography. A recent study by Spritzer et al[86] shows the utility and excellent sensitivity of magnetic resonance imaging in detecting thrombosis above the knee.

The diagnosis of pulmonary embolus must be established radiographically. Adequate technique is essential so that fetal exposure to ionizing radiation is minimized. Pulmonary ventilation and perfusion (V/Q) scans are useful in diagnosing pulmonary embolism only if the chest x-ray is normal. Calculations have shown that maximum fetal radiation exposure from this type of study is 50 mrem.[87] These isotopes are excreted through the maternal urinary tract. The fetus receives 85 percent of its radiation exposure from the maternal bladder. Brisk diuresis and frequent micturition should therefore theoretically lower fetal exposure.[87] If necessary, a Foley catheter can be used to empty the bladder. A large study showed that "high probability" V/Q scans with clinical symptoms carried a high likelihood that the patient actually had a pulmonary embolus.[88]

If the ventilation/perfusion scan is equivocal or if the patient's chest x-ray is abnormal, selective pulmonary angiography should be immediately undertaken. In experienced hands, the procedure carries a morbidity of less than 1 percent. Abdominal shielding should be used during the procedure. The increased plasma volume and vasodilatation that occur during pregnancy should make the procedure faster and technically easier than in the nonpregnant patient. Ginsburg and colleagues[89] have carefully looked at radiation exposure from various procedures during pregnancy. Their review suggests that there is a small increase in the risk of childhood cancer following radiation exposures of less than 5 rads.[89] They believe that, with careful use of available procedures, the diagnosis of venous thrombosis is possible with fetal exposure below 0.5 rads. Furthermore, in diagnosing pulmonary embolism, it is possible to keep fetal radiation exposure below 0.05 rads.[89] Because the risk to the fetus from such exposure is small in both relative and absolute terms, the diagnostic procedure should be undertaken without hesitation when necessary.

Once the diagnosis is established, therapy should be initiated without delay. Anticoagulation with heparin is the treatment of choice. Heparin, a large negatively charged protein with a molecular weight of 20,000 daltons, does not cross the placenta.[90] The main complication of heparin therapy is maternal bleeding. This can be reduced, however, with meticulous attention to dosage and frequent monitoring of the activated partial thromboplastin time (APTT). Hemorrhage, nevertheless, appears to complicate the course of between 8 and 33 percent of patients anticoagulated with heparin.[91-93] Heparin works by binding to antithrombin III. The anticoagulant activity of heparin can be quickly reversed with protamine sulfate. Other potential complications of heparin therapy include osteoporosis, alopecia, urticaria, bronchoconstriction secondary to histamine release, and profound thrombocytopenia.[94] Platelet counts should be checked twice weekly during the first 2 weeks of therapy. Bone demineralization can occur if more than 22,000 units of heparin is administered daily for more than 20 weeks.

An initial heparin loading dose of 70 units/kg is administered intravenously, followed by a continuous infusion of 1,000 units per hour. This dose must be adjusted to keep the APTT approximately twice normal or the heparin titer at 0.2 to 0.4 units/ml. The required maintenance dose of heparin can show large interpatient variation. This regimen is continued for approximately 10 days in clinically stable patients.

Low molecular weight heparin is gaining in popularity because there are fewer bleeding complications and no reason to follow the APTT. It can be administered in a fixed or weight-adjusted dose once or twice daily. Even though it is low molecular weight, it does not cross the placenta because it is still strongly negatively charged. Low molecular weight heparin has not been used in pregnancy and probably should be reserved for those patients with an allergy or hypersensitivity to the base (beef or pork) from which the heparin was prepared. When the next edition of this text is printed, low molecular weight heparin will probably be used more commonly during pregnancy.

For the remainder of pregnancy, patients should receive a moderate dose of subcutaneous heparin. A dose of 7,500 to 10,000 units of heparin administered every 8 to 12 hours is usually sufficient to keep the APTT about 1.5 times normal and the heparin titer approximately 0.1 to 0.2 units/ml.[96] Continuous subcutaneous pumps can also be used for this purpose on an outpatient basis. One must realize that the dosage must be individualized until the desired APTT is reached. With the increases in Factor VIII and most other coagulation factors that are normally seen in pregnancy, the subcutaneous dose may need to be increased rather frequently during gestation.[97] In the stable patient, therapy should be discontinued during labor and delivery but can be restarted several hours postpartum. If delivery is imminent and the patient is fully anticoagulated, protamine can be carefully administered to reverse the heparin. This is especially necessary if a cesarean delivery is anticipated. During the postpartum period, the patient can be given coumadin, even if breast-feeding. Although coumadin does not appear in breast milk in significant amounts, its use during breast-feeding has been controversial. Anticoagulant therapy should be continued for 6 to 10 weeks' postpartum, at which time coagulation factors should have returned to prepregnant levels. After that time, the duration of therapy should be individualized.

Oral anticoagulants should not be used during gestation. These drugs are vitamin K antagonists that readily cross the placenta and are teratogenic when used in early pregnancy. In the first trimester, these drugs are associated with facial dysmorphisms, hypoplastic digits, stippled epiphyses, and mental retardation.[98-100] In midtrimester, optic atrophy, faulty brain development, and developmental retardation may occur.[98] In addition, the fetus is anticoagulated by these drugs, which can result in severe fetal hemorrhage in the event of trauma or preterm labor.

Currently, heparin used throughout pregnancy appears to be safer than switching to oral anticoagulants during the second and early third trimesters. Even though it is more expensive and more inconvenient, the benefits of heparin therapy appear to outweigh the risks of using oral anticoagulants during gestation.

Several studies have advocated the use of a surgical approach to thrombophlebitis and pulmonary emboli during pregnancy. Mogensen and coworkers[79] treated eight pregnant women with acute iliofemoral venous thrombosis by thrombectomy. All of the women did well and were treated with heparin postoperatively. These researchers surmised that even when thrombophlebitis occurs in early pregnancy there is no need for pregnancy termination. Blegvad and coinvestigators[101] performed a pulmonary embolectomy successfully on a woman during the second trimester. The patient had severe right ventricular failure caused by obstruction of 85 percent of the pulmonary arterial circulation. Three months after embolectomy, she delivered a normal infant. Splinter and colleagues[102] report an open pulmonary embolectomy that was performed after cesarean delivery. Both mother and child recovered fully. In both cases, the embolectomy was carried out with the mother on cardiopulmonary bypass.[101,102] While these cases present interesting options, the role of surgical intervention in thromboembolic disease during pregnancy needs to be further delineated.

There is no consensus on treatment of the patient with thrombophlebitis in a prior pregnancy. If the patient had never experienced an embolus, many individuals would give the patient prophylactic heparin beginning with a dose of 5,000 units twice daily and increasing the dose each trimester until the patient is receiving 10,000 units twice daily. The lower doses actually may not be enough heparin, even when used prophylactically, to have any impact on the coagulation system. Many believe that some form of anticoagulant therapy is necessary, because the incidence of recurrence of thromboembolic disease after it occurred in a prior pregnancy is 4 to 12 percent.[103,104] There is also no consensus whether women with a pulmonary embolus in the distant past need heparin prophylaxis or actual anticoagulation. In general, we tend toward anticoagulation under careful supervision.

Cystic Fibrosis

Cystic fibrosis is an autosomal recessive disorder whose gene was first cloned in 1989. It is a disease of mucous glands of the digestive, respiratory, and reproductive tracts. With advances in antibiotic therapy and respirator care, the life span of patients with cystic fibrosis has increased greatly over the last 20 years; therefore, many of these patients are reaching the reproductive age.

Because it is a disease of the mucous glands, some patients have infertility problems. Often patients, because of digestive tract problems, have poor nutrition and delayed menarche or anovulatory cycles. Others have decreased cervical mucous. Once patients become pregnant, it is imperative to maintain a good nutritional status to help them throughout the pregnancy. Patients need approximately an additional 300 Kcal/day to meet the energy needs of pregnancy.[105] It is important to stress a healthy diet to these patients.

Many patients who have progressive deterioration of their pulmonary status, with hypoxemia and/or hypercapnia, may not be good candidates for pregnancy. In a case report of two patients, their pulmonary function declined greatly during pregnancy.[106] Cohen et al[107] reported congestive heart failure in 13 percent of 129 pregnancies in 100 women with cystic fibrosis. In that series, 18 percent of the women died within 24 months of delivery. However, this study occurred almost 20 years ago; with the changes in antibiotic therapy and respiratory care, the current risk is not nearly as high.

It is most important that the patient understand her needs during pregnancy. Her pulmonary status, as well as her cardiovascular status, must be monitored constantly. Because these patients have many respiratory infections, especially with *Pseudomonas aeruginosa*, with chronic bronchiectasis, they often must undergo repeated antibiotic therapy throughout the pregnancy. They also have a propensity toward infections with *S. aureus*. Therefore, aminoglycosides and antistaphylococci penicillins, or cephalosporins, are often used during pregnancy. Although toxicity is a theoretical risk with aminoglycosides, with the ability to measure levels this risk should be minimized. As noted above, the patients need extra calories during pregnancy and sometimes may require enteral or parenteral nutrition in order to gain them. Because of these needs, patients with cystic fibrosis may have permanent central lines placed. Furthermore, aggressive respiratory therapy is needed in these patients.

In summary, with careful attentiveness to cardiac and pulmonary status, as well as proper nutritional counseling, patients with cystic fibrosis can carry to term with minimal difficulty if their disease is not too severe. It will take careful cooperation between pulmonary care specialists and maternal-fetal medicine specialists to make this occur. Furthermore, the patient must realize that she may be hospitalized several times throughout the pregnancy in order to receive the appropriate antibiotic therapy. Also, because of recurrent infections and poor nutritional status, the fetus is at risk for growth restriction. Serial sonography, therefore, is indicated in these patients.

Key Points

- Tuberculosis is making a reappearance in the pregnant population in this country and any patient with systemic or pulmonary symptoms of tuberculosis should be tested.

- Any pregnant individual with a newly converted PPD test should also be tested for HIV.

- Smokers are at the highest risk of developing pneumococcal pneumonia during pregnancy.

- Nebulized betamimetics have become the keystone for treating asthma in pregnancy. Nebulized steroids should be used as second line therapy.

- If a pregnant patient is suspected of having a pulmonary embolus, heparin therapy should be immediately instituted while awaiting definitive testing.

References

1. Carter EJ, Mates S: Tuberculosis during pregnancy: the Rhode Island experience, 1987–1991. Chest 106:1466, 1994

2. Weinstein L, Murphy T: The management of tuberculosis during pregnancy. Clin Perinatol 1:395, 1974

3. Bonebarak CR, Noller KL, Loehnen CP et al: Routine chest roentgenography in pregnancy. JAMA 240:2747, 1978

4. Swartz HM, Reichling BA: Hazards of radiation exposure for pregnant women. JAMA 239:1907, 1978

5. Schaefer G, Zervoudakis IA, Fuchs FF, David S: Pregnancy in pulmonary tuberculosis. Obstet Gynecol 46:706, 1975

6. De March AP: Tuberculosis in pregnancy: five to ten year review of 215 patients in their fertile age. Chest 68:800, 1975

7. Maccato ML: Pneumonia and pulmonary tuberculosis in pregnancy. Obstet Gynecol Clin North Am 16:417, 1989

8. Bjerkedal T, Bahna SL, Lehmann EH: Course and outcome of pregnancy in women with pulmonary tuberculosis. Scand Respir Dis 56:245, 1975

9. Hamadeh MA, Glassroth J. Tuberculosis in pregnancy. Chest 101:1114, 1992

10. Golditch IM: Tuberculous meningitis in pregnancy. Am J Obstet Gynecol 110:1144, 1971

11. Centers for Disease Control and Prevention: Initial therapy for tuberculosis in the era of multi-drug resistance: recommendations of the Advisory Council for the Elimination of Tuberculosis. MMWR 42:1, 1993

12. Byrd RB, Horn BR, Solomon DA, Griggs GA: Toxic effects of isoniazid in tuberculosis chemoprophylaxis. JAMA 241:1239, 1979

13. Sider DF, Layde PM, Johnson MW, Lyle HA: Treatment of tuberculosis during pregnancy. Am Rev Respir Dis 122:65, 1980

14. Heinonen OP, Slone D, Shapiro S: Birth Defects and Drugs in Pregnancy. Publishing Sciences Croup, Littleton, MA, 1977

15. Sewitt T, Nebel L, Terracina S, Ankarman S: Ethambutol in pregnancy: observations on embryogenesis. Chest 66:25, 1974

16. Brobowitz ID: Ethambutol in pregnancy. Chest 66:20, 1974

17. Robinson GC, Cambon KG: Hearing loss in infants of tuberculous mothers treated with streptomycin in pregnancy. N Engl J Med 271:949, 1964

18. Editorial: Perinatal prophylaxis of tuberculosis. Lancet 336:1479, 1990

19. Kendig EL Jr: The place of BCC vaccine in the management of infants born of tuberculous mothers. N Engl J Med 281:520, 1969

20. Grossman JH III, Littner MD: Severe sarcoidosis in pregnancy. Obstet Gynecol 50(Suppl):81, 1976

21. Dines DE, Banner EA: Sarcoidosis during pregnancy: improvement in pulmonary function. JAMA 200:726, 1967

22. Mayock RL, Sullivan RD, Greening RR, Jones R: Sarcoidosis in pregnancy. JAMA 164:158, 1957

23. O'Leary JA: Ten year study of sarcoidosis in pregnancy. Am J Obstet Gynecol 84:462, 1962

24. Weinberger SE, Weiss ST, Cohen WR et al: Pregnancy and the lung. Am Rev Respir Dis 121:559, 1980

25. Haynes de Regt R: Sarcoidosis and pregnancy. Obstet Gynecol 70:369, 1987

26. Warren GV, Sprague SM, Corwin HL: Sarcoidosis presenting as acute renal failure during pregnancy. Am J Kidney Dis 12:161, 1988

27. Sahn EE: Pruritic white papules in pregnant women: sarcoidosis. Arch Dermatol 123:1559, 1987

28. Hopwood HG: Pneumonia in pregnancy. Obstet Gynecol 25:875, 1965

29. Austrian R: Pneumococcal vaccine: development and prospects. Am J Med 67:546, 1979

30. McKinney P, Volkert P, Kaufman R: Fatal swine influenza pneumonia during late pregnancy. Arch Intern Med 150:213, 1990

31. Kort BA, Cefalo RC, Baker VV. Fatal influenza A pneumonia in pregnancy. Am J Perinatol 3:179, 1986

32. Mostow SR: Prevention, management and control of influenza. Role of amantadine. Am J Med 82(Suppl 6a):35, 1987

33. Cox SM, Cunningham FG, Luby J: Management of varicella pneumonia complicating pregnancy. Am J Perinatol 7:100, 1990

34. Esmonde TF, Herdman G, Anderson G: Chickenpox pneumonia: an association with pregnancy. Thorax 44:812, 1989

35. Haake DA, Zakowski PC, Haake DL, Bryson YJ: Early treatment with acyclovir for varicella pneumonia in otherwise healthy adults: retrospective controlled study and review. Rev Infect Dis 12:788, 1990

36. Madinger NE, Greenspoon JS, Ellrodt AG: Pneumonia during pregnancy: has modern technology improved maternal and fetal outcome? Am J Obstet Gynecol 161:657, 1989

37. Greenberger PA, Patterson R: Management of asthma during pregnancy. N Engl J Med 312:897, 1985

38. De Swiet M: Diseases of the respiratory system. Clin Obstet Cynecol 4:287, 1977

39. Hernandez E, Angle CS, Johnson JWC: Asthma in pregnancy: current concepts. Obstet Gynecol 55:739, 1980

40. Turner ES, Greenberger PA, Patterson R: Management of the pregnant asthmatic patient. Ann Intern Med 93:905, 1980

41. Hiddleson HJH: Bronchial asthma and pregnancy. NZ Med J 63:521, 1964

42. Gordon M, Niswander KR, Berendes H, Kantor AG: Fetal morbidity following potentially anoxigenic obstetric conditions. VII. Bronchial asthma. Am J Obstet Gynecol 106:421, 1970

43. Schaefer G, Silverman F: Pregnancy complicated by asthma. Am J Obstet Gynecol 82:182, 1961

44. White RJ, Coutts II, Gibbs CJ, MacIntyre C: A prospective study of asthma during pregnancy and the puerperium. Respir Med 83:103, 1989

45. Juniper EF, Daniel EE, Roberts RS et al: Improvement in airway responsiveness and asthma severity during pregnancy: a prospective study. Am Rev Respir Dis 140:924, 1989

46. Apter AJ, Greenberger PA, Patterson R: Outcomes of pregnancy in adolescents with severe asthma. Arch Intern Med 149:2571, 1989

47. Williams DA: Asthma in pregnancy. Acta Allergy 22:311, 1967

48. Gordon M, Niswander KR, Berendes H, Kantor AG: Fetal morbidity following potentially anoxigenic obstetric conditions. VII. Bronchial asthma. Am J Obstet Gynecol 106:421, 1970

49. Sims CD, Chamberlin CVP, DeSwiet M: Lung function tests in bronchial asthma during and after pregnancy. Br J Obstet Gynaecol 88:434, 1976

50. Mabie WC, Barton JR, Wasserstrum N, Sibai BM: Clinical observations on asthma in pregnancy. J Mat Fet Med 1:45, 1992

51. Perlow JH, Montgomery D, Morgan MA et al: Severity of asthma and perinatal outcome. Am J Obstet Gynecol 167:963, 1992

52. Schatz M, Zeiger RS, Hoffman CP et al: Perinatal outcomes in the pregnancies of asthmatic women: a prospective controlled analysis. Am J Resp Crit Care Med 151:1170, 1995

53. Metzger WJ, Turner E, Patterson R: The safety of immunotherapy during pregnancy. J Allergy Clin Immunol 61:268, 1978

54. Centers for Disease Control and Prevention: Prevention and control of influenza. MMWR 33:253, 1984

55. Schatz M, Zeiger RS, Harden KM et al: The safety of inhaled beta-agonist bronchodilators during pregnancy. J Allergy Clin Immunol 82:686, 1988

56. Barnes PJ: A new approach to the treatment of asthma. N Engl J Med 221:1517, 1989

57. Kerstjens JAM, Brand PLP, Hughes MD et al: A comparison of bronchodilator therapy with or without inhaled corticosteroid therapy for obstructive airways disease. N Engl J Med 327:1413, 1992

58. Greenberger P, Patterson R: Safety of therapy for allergic systems during pregnancy. Ann Intern Med 89:234, 1978

59. Weinstein AM, Dubin BD, Podleski WK et al: Asthma in pregnancy. JAMA 241:1161, 1979

60. Nelson MM, Forfar JO: Associations between drugs administered during pregnancy and congenital abnormalities of the fetus. BMJ 1:523, 1971

61. Fainstat TP: Cortisone-induced congenital cleft palate in rabbits. Endocrinology 55:502, 1954

62. Bongiovanni AM, McPadden AJ: Steroids during pregnancy and possible fetal consequences. Fertil Steril 2:181, 1960

63. Greenberger PA, Patterson R: Beclomethasone dipropionate for severe asthma during pregnancy. Ann Intern Med 98:478, 1983

64. Schatz M, Patterson R, Zeitz S et al: Corticosteroid therapy for the pregnant asthmatic patient. JAMA 233:804, 1975

65. Turner ES, Greenberger PA, Patterson R: Management of the pregnant asthmatic patient. Ann Intern Med 93:905, 1980

66. Greenberger P, Patterson R: Safety of therapy for allergic symptoms during pregnancy. Ann Intern Med 89:234, 1978

67. Reinisch JM, Simon NG, Karow WG, Gandelman R: Prenatal exposure to prednisone in humans and animals retards intrauterine growth. Science 202:436, 1978

68. Schatz M, Patterson R, Zeitz S et al: Corticosteroid therapy for the pregnant asthmatic patient. JAMA 233:804, 1975

69. Weinberger SE, Weiss ST, Coatan WR et al: Pregnancy and the lung. Am Rev Respir Dis 121:559, 1980

70. Beitins R, Baynard F, Ances IG et al: The transplacental passage of prednisone and prednisolone in pregnancy near term. J Pediatr 81:936, 1972

71. Levitz M, Jansen V, Dancis J: The transfer and metabolism of corticosteroids in the perfused human placenta. Am J Obstet Gynecol 132:363, 1978

72. Ballard PL, Granberg P, Ballard RA: Glucocorticoid levels in maternal and cord serum after prenatal beclomethasone therapy to prevent respiratory distress syndrome. J Clin Invest 56:1548, 1975

73. Schreier L, Cutler RM, Saigal V: Respiratory failure in asthma during the third trimester: report of two cases. Am J Obstet Gynecol 160:80, 1989

74. Marx GF: Obstetric anesthesia in the presence of medical complications. Clin Obstet Gynecol 17:165, 1974

75. Aaro LA, Jjergens JL: Thrombophlebitis associated with pregnancy. Am J Obstet Gynecol 109:1128, 1971

76. Treffers BL, Fluiderkoper GH, Weehink GH, Kloosterman GJ: Epidemiological observations of thromboembolic disease during pregnancy and in the puerperium in 56,022 women. Int J Gynaecol Obstet 21:327, 1983

77. VillaSanta U: Thromboembolic disease in pregnancy. Am J Obstet Gynecol 93:142, 1965

78. Barritt DW, Jorden SC: Anticoagulant drugs in the treatment of pulmonary embolism: a controlled trial. Lancet 1:1309, 1960

79. Mogensen K, Skibsted L, Wadt J, Nissen F: Thrombectomy of acute iliofemoral venous thrombosis during pregnancy. Surg Gynecol Obstet 169:50, 1989

80. Weiner CP: Diagnosis and management of thromboembolic disease during pregnancy. Clin Obstet Gynecol 28:107, 1985

81. Girz BA, Heiselman DE: Fatal intrapartum pulmonary embolus during tocolysis. Am J Obstet Gynecol 158:145, 1988

82. Stiller RJ, Leone-Tomaschoff S, Cuteri J, Beck L: Postpartum pulmonary embolus as an unusual cause of cortical blindness. Am J Obstet Gynecol 162:696, 1990

83. Stein LB, Robert RI, Marx J, Rossoff L: Transient cortical blindness following an acute hypotensive event in the postpartum period. NY State J Med 89:682, 1989

84. Conrad J, Horellou MJ, Van Dreden P et al: Thrombosis and pregnancy in congenital deficiencies in AT-III protein C or protein S: study of 78 women. Thromb Haemost 63:319, 1990

85. Heijboer H, Buller HR, Lensing AW et al: A comparison of real-time compression ultrasonography with impedance plethysmography for the diagnosis of deep vein thrombosis in symptomatic patients. N Engl J Med 329:1365, 1993

86. Spritzer CE, Evans AC, Kay JJ: Magnetic resonance imaging of deep venous thrombosis in pregnant women with lower extremity edema. Obstet Gynecol 85:603, 1995

87. Macus CS, Mason GR, Kuperus JH, Mena I: Pulmonary imaging in pregnancy: maternal risk and fetal dosimetry. Clin Nucl Med 10:1, 1985

88. The PIOPED Investigators: Value of the ventilation/perfusion scan in acute pulmonary embolism: results of the prospective investigation of pulmonary embolism diagnosis (PIOPED). JAMA 273:2753, 1990

89. Ginsberg JS, Hirsh J, Rainbow AJ, Coates G: Risks to the fetus of radiologic procedures used in the diagnosis of maternal venous thromboembolic disease. Thromb Haemost 61:189, 1989

90. Qaso LA, Juergens JL: Thrombophlebitis associated with pregnancy. Am J Obstet Gynecol 109:1128, 1971

91. Gervin AS: Complications of heparin therapy. Surg Gynecol Obstet 140:789, 1975

92. Hall JG, Pauli RM, Wilson KM: Maternal and fetal sequelae of anticoagulation during pregnancy. Am J Med 68:122, 1978

93. Walker AM, Jick H: Predictors of bleeding during heparin therapy. JAMA 244:1209, 1980

94. Merrill LK, VerBurg DJ: The choice of long term anticoagulants for the pregnant patient. Obstet Gynecol 47:711, 1976

95. DeSwiet M, Dorrington-Ward P, Fidler J et al: Prolonged heparin therapy in pregnancy causes bone demineralization (heparin induced osteopenia). Br J Obstet Gynaecol 90:1129, 1983

96. Baskin HF, Murray JM, Harris RE: Low dose heparin for the prevention of thromboembolic disease in pregnancy. Am J Obstet Gynecol 129:590, 1977

97. Spearing GS, Fraser I, Turner G, Dixon G: Long term self administered subcutaneous heparin in pregnancy. BMJ 1:1457, 1978

98. Stevenson R, Burton DM, Ferlavto GJ, Taylor HA: Hazards of oral anticoagulants during pregnancy. JAMA 243:1549, 1980

99. Shavi WL, Hall JG: Multiple congenital anomalies associated with oral anticoagulants. Am J Obstet Gynecol 127:191, 1977

100. Harrod MJE, Sherrod PS: Warfarin embryopathy in siblings. Obstet Gynecol 57:673, 1981

101. Blegvad S, Lund O, Nielsen TT, Guldholt I: Emergency embolectomy in a patient with massive pulmonary embolism during second trimester pregnancy. Acta Obstet Gynecol Scand 68:267, 1989

102. Splinter WM, Dwane PD, Wigle RD, McGrath MJ: Anaesthetic management of emergency cesarean section followed by pulmonary embolectomy. Can J Anaesth 36:689, 1989

103. Howell R, Fidler J, Letsky E et al: The risks of antenatal subcutaneous heparin prophylaxis: a controlled trial. Br J Obstet Gynaecol 90:1124, 1983

104. Lao TT, Deswiet M, Letsky E et al: Prophylaxis of thromboembolism in pregnancy: an alternative. Br J Obstet Gynaecol 92:202, 1985

105. Rush D, Johnstone FD, King JC: Nutrition and pregnancy. In Burrows GN, Ferris TF (eds): Medical Complications During Pregnancy, 3rd Ed WB Saunders, Philadelphia, 1988

106. Corkey CW, Newth CJ, Corey M et al: Pregnancy in cystic fibrosis: a better prognosis in patients with pancreatic function? Am J Obstet Gynecol 140:737, 1981

107. Cohen LF, deSant' Agnese PA, Friedlander J: Cystic fibrosis and pregnancy: a national survey. Lancet 2:842, 1980

Chapter 30

Renal Disease

Philip Samuels

Altered Renal Physiology in Pregnancy

Renal plasma flow (RPF) increases greatly during pregnancy.[1] It peaks in the first trimester and, although it decreases near term, remains higher than in the nonpregnant patient. This change is due in part to increased cardiac output and decreased renal vascular resistance. The glomerular filtration rate (GFR) increases by 50 percent during a normal gestation.[2] It rises early in pregnancy and remains elevated through delivery. The percentage increase in GFR is greater than the percentage increase in RPF. This elevation of the filtration fraction leads to a fall in the blood urea nitrogen (BUN) and serum creatinine values.

Because GFR increases to such a great degree, electrolytes, glucose, and other filtered substances reach the renal tubules in greater amounts. The kidney handles sodium efficiently, reabsorbing most of the filtered load in the proximal convoluted tubule. Glucose reabsorption, however, does not increase proportionately during pregnancy. The average renal threshold for glucose is reduced to 155 mg/dl from 194 mg/dl in the nonpregnant individual.[3] Glycosuria therefore can be seen in the normal gravida.

Urate is handled by filtration and secretion. Its clearance increases early in pregnancy, leading to lower serum levels of uric acid. In late pregnancy, urate clearance and serum urate levels return to their prepregnancy values. Serum urate levels are elevated in patients with preeclampsia. Whether this is due to decreased RPF, hemoconcentration, renal tubular dysfunction, or other renal circulatory changes remains uncertain.

Asymptomatic Bacteriuria and Acute Pyelonephritis

The diagnosis of asymptomatic bacteriuria (ASB) is based on a clean catch voided urine culture revealing greater than 100,000 colonies/ml of a single organism.[4] Some investigators have suggested that two consecutively voided specimens should contain the same organism before making the diagnosis of bacteriuria.[5,6] Between 1.2 and 5 percent of young girls will demonstrate ASB at some time before puberty.[7] After puberty, with the onset of sexual activity, the prevalence of ASB may increase to 10 percent.[7] Of women with ASB, approximately 35 percent have bacteria arising from the kidneys rather than from the lower urinary tract.

It is important to diagnose and treat ASB in pregnancy. Left untreated, a symptomatic urinary tract infection (UTI) will develop in up to 40 percent of these patients.[8,9] Recognition and therapy for ASB can eliminate 70 percent of acute UTIs in pregnancy. Nonetheless, 2 percent of pregnant women with negative urine cultures develop symptomatic cystitis or pyelonephritis. This group accounts for 30 percent of the cases of acute UTI that develop during gestation. We advocate screening of all women for ASB at their first prenatal visit.

Escherichia coli is the organism responsible for most cases of ASB. Patients can therefore be safely treated with nitrofurantoin, ampicillin, cephalosporins, and short-acting sulfa drugs. Sulfa compounds should be avoided near term, as they compete for bilirubin-binding sites on albumin in the fetus and newborn and could cause kernicterus. Nitrofurantoin should not be used in patients with glucose-6-phosphate dehydrogenase deficiency, as there is a risk for hemolytic crisis. If the fetus has this enzyme deficiency, it may also experience hemolysis. Therapy for ASB should be continued for 10 to 14 days. The patient should have another culture performed 1 to 2 weeks after discontinuing therapy. Approximately 15 percent of patients will experience a reinfection and/or will not respond to initial therapy. Therapy should be reinstituted after careful microbial sensitivity testing. Patients with recurrent UTI during pregnancy and those with a history of pyelonephritis should undergo radiographic evaluation of the upper urinary tract. This procedure should be delayed until the patient is 3 months postpartum so that the anatomic and physiologic changes of pregnancy can regress. Of the women in the above categories, 20 percent will show a structural abnormality, but most will be insignificant.

Occasionally it is difficult to distinguish severe cystitis from pyelonephritis. Although the drugs used for treatment are similar, pyelonephritis requires intravenous antibiotics. Sandberg and coinvestigators[10] studied symptomatic UTI in 174 women. They found that C-reactive protein was elevated in 91 percent of pregnant women with acute pyelonephritis and only 5 percent of women with cystitis. They also noted that the urine-concentrating ability was lower in women with acute pyelonephritis. Because the erythrocyte sedimentation rate is normally elevated in pregnancy, they found that this was not a useful parameter for distinguishing pyelonephritis from cystitis.

Occurring in approximately 1 to 2 percent of all pregnancies, pyelonephritis is an important source of maternal morbidity. Pyelonephritis is the most common nonobstetric cause of hospitalization during pregnancy.[11] Recurrent pyelonephritis has been implicated as a cause of fetal death and intrauterine growth restriction (IUGR). There appears to be an association between acute pyelonephritis and preterm labor.[12,13] Fan and coworkers,[14] however, have shown that if pyelonephritis is aggressively treated, it does not increase the likelihood of preterm labor, premature delivery, or low-birth-weight infants.

Acute pyelonephritis should be initially treated on an inpatient basis, utilizing intravenous antibiotics. Empiric therapy should be begun as soon as the presumptive diagnosis is made. Therapy can be tailored to the specific organism after sensitivities have been obtained approximately 48 hours later. Because septicemia may occasionally result from pyelonephritis, blood cultures should be obtained if patients do not respond rapidly to initial antibiotic therapy. *E. coli* is the most common organism isolated in pyelonephritis. During gestation, the right side is most often affected, as engorged blood vessels may inhibit ureteral drainage of the kidney. Generally, a broad-spectrum first-generation cephalosporin is the initial therapy of choice. Fan and coinvesti-

gators[14] reviewed 107 cases of pyelonephritis in 103 pregnant women. They report that 33 percent were resistant to ampicillin and 13 percent to first-generation cephalosporins. As this study was reported 9 years ago and the data are probably even older, the resistance for ampicillin and first-generation cephalosporins is probably even higher. That is why it is so important to treat these women initially as inpatients. If resistance to more common therapies is encountered, a later generation cephalosporin or an aminoglycoside can safely be administered. Peak and trough aminoglycoside levels, however, should be monitored. The serum creatinine and BUN levels should be followed as well. During the febrile period, acetaminophen should be employed to keep the patient's temperature below 38°C. Small doses of acetaminophen will not mask the fever and symptoms of a patient who is unresponsive to treatment.

Intravenous antibiotic therapy should be continued for 24 to 48 hours after the patient becomes afebrile and costovertebral angle tenderness disappears. After the cessation of intravenous therapy, treatment with appropriate oral antibiotics should be continued for 2 to 3 weeks. Upon termination of therapy, urine cultures should be obtained on a regular basis for the remainder of gestation. After an episode of acute pyelonephritis, antibiotic suppression should be implemented and continued for the remainder of the pregnancy. Nitrofurantoin 100 mg once or twice daily is an acceptable regimen for suppression. In a study by van Dorsten and colleagues,[15] the overall frequency of positive urine cultures following hospitalization for pyelonephritis was 38 percent. Nitrofurantoin suppression reduced the rate to 8 percent. Nitrofurantoin did not lower the rate of positive cultures if the inpatient antibiotic selection was inappropriate or if the culture was positive at time of discharge.[15] Today, there is increased pressure to treat pyelonephritis as an outpatient condition. Although this is discouraged, it is possible if daily nursing contact is maintained during the acute phase of the disease and appropriate laboratory parameters are followed.

Cunningham and coworkers[16] point out that pulmonary injury resembling adult respiratory distress syndrome (ARDS) can occur in patients with acute pyelonephritis. Clinical manifestations of this complication usually occur 24 to 48 hours after the patient is admitted for pyelonephritis.[16,17] Some of these patients will require endotracheal intubation, mechanical ventilation,[18] and positive end expiratory pressure (PEEP). In Cunningham's series, there was no evidence that pulmonary edema was caused by intravenous fluid overload.[16] This ARDS-type picture probably results from endotoxin-induced alveolar capillary membrane injury. Towers et al found pulmonary injury in 11 of 130 patients with pyelonephritis. A fever of greater than 103°F, a maternal heart rate above 110, and a gestation further than 20 weeks placed the patient at increased risk for pulmonary injury. The most predictive factors were fluid overload and tocolytic therapy.[18a]

Austenfeld and Snow[19] studied 64 pregnancies in 30 women who had previously undergone ureteral reimplantation for vesicoureteral reflux. During pregnancy, 57 percent of these women had one or more UTIs, and 17 percent had more than one UTI or an episode of pyelonephritis.[19] More frequent urine cultures and aggressive therapy during pregnancy are recommended for this group of patients.

Urolithiasis

The prevalence of urolithiasis during pregnancy is 0.03 percent, with an incidence no higher than that of the general population.[20] Colicky abdominal pain, recurrent UTI, and hematuria suggest urolithiasis. If the diagnosis is suspected, intravenous pyelography should be undertaken, limiting this study to the minimum number of exposures necessary to make the diagnosis. Ultrasound can often be used to establish the diagnosis without radiation exposure. Newer ultrasound flow studies can actually follow flow from the ureter to the bladder and detect obstruction without the use of ionizing radiation. Urine microscopy can often detect crystals and help distinguish the type of stone before it is passed. For any patient suspected or proved to have renal stones, serum calcium and phosphorous levels should be measured to rule out hyperparathyroidism. Serum urate should also be determined.

Because of the physiologic hydroureter characteristic of pregnancy, most patients with symptomatic urolithiasis will spontaneously pass their stones. Treatment should be conservative, consisting of hydration and narcotic analgesia for pain relief.[21] Epidural anesthesia has been advocated to establish a segmental block from T11 to L2. While this approach may promote passage of the stone, it remains controversial. Lithotripsy is contraindicated during pregnancy.

Recurrent UTI with urease-containing organisms causes precipitation of calcium phosphate in the kidney that may lead to the development of staghorn calculi. Surgery is rarely indicated in these patients, especially during gestation. Patients with staghorn calculi should have frequent urine cultures, and bacteriuria should be treated aggressively. Recurrent infections can lead to chronic pyelonephritis with resultant loss of kidney function.

Glomerulonephritis

Acute glomerulonephritis is an uncommon complication of pregnancy, with an estimated incidence of 1 per 40,000 pregnancies.[22] Poststreptococcal glomerulonephritis rarely occurs in adults. In this disorder, renal function tends to deteriorate during the acute phase of the disease, but usually later recovers.[23] Acute glomerulonephritis can be difficult to distinguish from preeclampsia. Periorbital edema, a striking clinical feature of acute glomerulonephritis, is often seen in preeclampsia. Hematuria, red blood cell (RBC) casts in the urine sediment, and depressed serum complement levels indicate glomerular disease. In poststreptococcal acute glomerulonephritis, antistreptolysin O titers rise.

Treatment of acute glomerulonephritis in pregnancy is similar to that for the nonpregnant patient. Blood pressure control is essential, and careful attention to fluid balance is imperative. Sodium intake should be restricted to 500 mg/day during the acute disease. Serum potassium levels must also be carefully monitored.

Packham and coworkers[24] extensively reviewed 395 pregnancies in 238 women with primary glomerulonephritis. Only 51 percent of infants were born after 36 weeks' gestation. Excluding therapeutic abortion, 20 percent of fetuses were lost, 15 percent after 20 weeks' gestation. IUGR was noted in 15 percent of the fetuses. Maternal renal function deteriorated in 15 percent of pregnancies and failed to resolve postpartum in 5 percent.[24] Hypertension was recorded in 52 percent of the pregnancies, developing before 32 weeks' gestation in 26 percent. This blood pressure elevation was not an exacerbation of previously diagnosed hypertension, as in only 12 percent of pregnancies was there noted to be antecedent hypertension. Eighteen percent of the women who developed de novo hypertension in pregnancy remained hypertensive postpartum. Increased proteinuria was recorded in 59 percent of these pregnancies and was irreversible in 15 percent.[24] The highest incidence of fetal and maternal complications occurred in patients with primary focal and segmental hyalinosis and sclerosis. The lowest incidence of complications was observed in non-IgA diffuse mesangial proliferative glomerulonephritis.[24] The presence of severe vessel lesions on renal biopsy was associated with a significantly higher rate of fetal loss after 20 weeks' gestation. Packham and coworkers[25] also studied 33 pregnancies in 24 patients with biopsy-proven membranous glomerulonephritis. Fetal loss occurred in 24 percent of pregnancies, preterm delivery in 43 percent, and a term liveborn in only 33 percent of patients. Hypertension was noted in 46 percent of these pregnant women. Thirty percent of patients had proteinuria in the nephrotic range in the first trimester.[25] The presence of heavy proteinuria during the first trimester correlated with a poor fetal and maternal outcome.[25] Jungers et al[26] described 69 pregnancies in 34 patients with IgA glomerulonephritis. The fetal loss rate in this group was 15 percent. Preexisting hypertension was statistically associated with poor fetal outcome. Hypertension at the time of conception also correlated with a deterioration of maternal renal function during pregnancy. Hypertension in the first pregnancy was highly predictive of recurrence of hypertension in a subsequent pregnancy.[26] Kincaide-Smith and Fairley[27] analyzed 102 pregnancies in 65 women with IgA glomerulonephritis. They noted that hypertension occurred in 63 percent of pregnancies, with 18 percent being severe. They also observed a decrease in renal function in 22 percent of these women.[27] Abe[28] retrospectively studied 240 pregnancies in 166 women with preexisting glomerular disease between 1976 and 1988. Eight percent of the pregnancies resulted in a spontaneous abortion, 6 percent resulted in stillbirth, and 86 percent were liveborn. Most losses occurred in women with a GFR less than 70 ml/min and preexisting hypertension. Even though the majority of women with renal insufficiency had good pregnancy outcomes, the long-term prognosis of the kidney disease was worse if the GFR was less than 50 ml/min and the serum creatinine was more than 1.5 mg/dl.[28] Renal complications were worse in patients with membranoproliferative glomerulonephritis, with 29 percent developing hypertension and 33 percent developing a long-term decrease in renal function.

Imbasciati and Ponticelli[29] summarized six studies containing a total of 906 pregnancies in 558 women with preexisting glomerular disease. This review, of course, has the limitations of including patients from a wide span of years and varying geographic locations. Nonetheless, broad generalizations can be made. The overall perinatal mortality was 13 percent. Hypertension, renal insufficiency, and nephrotic range proteinuria were the strongest prognostic factors for a poor pregnancy outcome. Having two of these factors was a particularly strong harbinger of fetal loss. The histologic type of glomerulonephritis had little correlation with pregnancy outcome. Hypertension persisted in 3 to 12 percent of patients who developed hypertension for the first time during pregnancy. In 25 percent of patients, hypertension worsened during pregnancy and corrected postpartum.[29] This is very suspicious for superimposed preeclampsia, but that diagnosis is very difficult to make in a patient who already has hypertension and proteinuria. In 3 percent of these 166 women, the course of their glomerular disease accelerated after pregnancy.

CHRONIC RENAL DISEASE

Diagnosis

Chronic renal disease can be silent until its advanced stages. Because obstetricians routinely examine the patient's urine for the presence of protein, glucose, and ketones, they may be the first to detect chronic renal disease.

Any gravida with more than trace proteinuria should collect a 24-hour urine specimen for creatinine clearance and total protein excretion. This test is safe, inexpensive, and of only minor inconvenience to the patient. Creatinine clearance is elevated in pregnancy and, during the first trimester, may exceed 140 ml/min. Before pregnancy, 24-hour urinary protein excretion should not exceed 0.2 g. During gestation, quantities up to 0.3 g per day may be normal. Moderate proteinuria (less than 2 g per day) is seen in glomerular disease, most commonly lipoid nephrosis, systemic lupus erythematosus, and glomerulonephritis.

Microscopic examination of the urine can reveal much about the patient's renal status. If renal disease is suspected, a catheterized specimen should be obtained. More RBCs than one to two per high-power field or RBC casts are indicative of renal disease. RBCs usually indicate glomerular disease or collagen vascular disease. Less frequently, they suggest trauma or malignant hypertension. Increased numbers of white blood cells (WBCs) (more than one to two per high-power field) or the appearance of WBC casts is usually indicative of acute or chronic infection. Cellular casts are found in the presence of renal tubular dysfunction, and hyaline casts suggest significant proteinuria. A single bacterium seen in an unspun catheterized urine specimen is suggestive of significant bacteriuria, and a follow-up culture should be performed.

The obstetrician can easily be misled when relying solely on the BUN and serum creatinine to assess renal function. A 70 percent decline in creatinine clearance, an indirect measure of GFR, can be seen before a significant rise in the BUN or serum creatinine occurs. In fact, little change in the serum creatinine or the BUN is seen until the creatinine clearance falls to 50 ml/min. Below that level, small decrements in creatinine clearance can lead to large increases in the BUN and creatinine. A single creatinine clearance value less than 100 ml/min is not diagnostic of renal diseases. An incomplete 24-hour urine collection is the most frequent cause of this finding. An abnormal clearance rate should therefore be restudied.

Serum urate is an often overlooked but helpful parameter in detecting renal dysfunction. Excretion of uric acid is dependent not only on glomerular filtration but also on tubular secretion. An elevated serum urate in the presence of a normal BUN and serum creatinine may therefore implicate tubular disease. A solitary increase in uric acid may also signify impending or early preeclampsia.

Effect of Pregnancy on Renal Function

Although baseline creatinine clearance is decreased in patients with chronic renal insufficiency, it should still increase during gestation. A moderate fall in creatinine clearance is often observed during late gestation in patients with renal disease. This decrease is typically more severe in patients with diffuse glomerular disease. It usually reverses after delivery.

The long-term effect of pregnancy on renal disease remains controversial. If the patient's serum creatinine is less than 1.5 mg/dl, pregnancy should have little effect on the long-term prognosis of the patient's kidney disease. Pregnancy, however, is associated with an increased incidence of pyelonephritis in patients with chronic renal disease. There are few data concerning the long-term effect of pregnancy on renal disease in women with true renal insufficiency. Occasionally, some patients with a baseline serum creatinine of more than 1.5 mg/dl will experience a significant decrease in renal function during gestation that does not improve during the postpartum period.[29–31] This deterioration occurs more frequently in women with diffuse glomerulonephritis. It is not possible, however, to predict which patients with renal insufficiency will experience a permanent reduction in renal function. If renal function significantly deteriorates during gestation, termination of pregnancy may not reverse the process. Abortion therefore cannot be routinely recommended for patients who become pregnant and whose baseline serum creatinine level exceeds 1.5 mg/dl. Ideally, patients with chronic renal disease should be thoroughly counseled before conception about the possible consequences of pregnancy.

Severe hypertension is the greatest threat to the pregnant patient with chronic renal disease. Left uncontrolled, hypertension can lead to intracerebral hemorrhage as well as deteriorating renal function. In most pregnancies complicated by chronic renal dysfunction, some degree of hypertension is present.[30,32] Approximately 50 percent of these patients will have worsening hypertension as pregnancy progresses, and diastolic blood pressures of 110 mmHg or greater will develop in about 20 percent of cases.[33] Those patients with diffuse proliferative glomerulonephritis and nephrosclerosis are at greatest risk for the development of severe hypertension. Blood pressure control is the cornerstone of successful treatment of chronic renal disease in pregnancy.

Worsening proteinuria is common during pregnancy complicated by chronic renal disease and often reaches the nephrotic range.[33] In general, massive proteinuria does not indicate an increased risk for mother or fetus.[34] Low serum albumin, however, has been correlated with low birth weight.[35] The development of massive proteinuria is not necessarily a harbinger of preeclampsia. Nevertheless, in late pregnancy it is often difficult to differentiate impending preeclampsia from worsening chronic renal disease.

Effect of Chronic Renal Disease on Pregnancy

More than 85 percent of women with chronic renal disease will have a surviving infant if renal function is well preserved. Earlier reports were more pessimistic, citing a 5.8 percent incidence of stillbirth, a 4.9 percent incidence of neonatal deaths, and an increase in second trimester losses.[33] If hypertension is not controlled and if renal function is not well preserved, there is still a high likelihood of pregnancy loss.[24] Antepartum fetal surveillance and advances in neonatal care have made great strides in improving perinatal outcome in these patients. One study reported a total fetal loss rate of 13.8 percent, including miscarriage, stillbirths, and neonatal deaths.[32] This is not very different from the general population.

The outlook for women with severe renal insufficiency whose baseline serum creatinine level is more than 1.5 mg/dl is less clear. This is due in part to the limited number of pregnancies in such patients as well as to the large number who undergo elective abortion. One study reported no surviving infants when the maternal BUN was greater than 60 mg/dl.[34] Other investigations, however, have found that about 80 percent of such pregnancies resulted in surviving infants.[32,36] Preterm births and IUGR remain important problems in these pregnancies. The reported incidence of preterm birth ranges from 20 to 50 percent.[33,37]

Imbasciati and Ponticelli[29] summarize three studies containing 81 pregnancies in 78 women with serum creatinine concentrations less than 1.4 mg/dl.[29] The perinatal loss rate was only 9 percent. However, 33 percent of the infants were growth restricted, and 50 percent were born preterm secondary to either maternal or fetal indications. Disturbingly, 33 percent of the women showed acceleration of their renal disease after delivery. Some researchers believe that growth restriction may be due to the lack of plasma volume increase as the pregnancy progresses. In one study, Cunningham et al[38] showed that women with moderate renal dysfunction did have increased creatinine clearances and plasma volumes during gestation, whereas women with severe renal dysfunction did not.[38]

Surveillance and Treatment

A 24-hour urine collection for creatinine clearance and total protein excretion should be obtained as soon as the pregnancy is confirmed. These parameters should be monitored monthly. The patient should be seen once every 2 weeks until 32 weeks' gestation and weekly thereafter. These are general guidelines, and more frequent visits may be necessary in individual cases.

Control of hypertension is critical in managing patients with chronic renal disease. β-Blockers, calcium channel blockers, and hydralazine can be used to treat blood pressure effectively as long as the dosages are monitored carefully. Clonidine is occasionally useful in refractory patients. Doxazosin and prazosin may be used if necessary. Angiotensin-converting enzyme inhibitors should be avoided during pregnancy. These drugs have been associated with fetal and neonatal oliguria/anuria.[39,40] In one study, 1 of 19 infants had anuria and required dialysis.[39] In another study, an infant required peritoneal dialysis.[40] Furthermore, congenital anomalies, including microcephaly and encephalocele,[39] have been associated with the use of angiotensin-converting enzymes inhibitors.

The use of diuretics in pregnancy is controversial.[41-43] For massive debilitating edema, a short course of diuretics can be helpful. Electrolytes must be monitored carefully. Salt restriction does not appear to be beneficial once edema has developed. Salt restriction, however, should be instituted without hesitation in pregnant women with true renal insufficiency.

Fetal growth should be assessed with serial ultrasonography, because growth restriction is common in women with chronic renal disease. Antepartum fetal heart rate testing should be started at 28 weeks' gestation.[44]

Obstetricians should have a low threshold for hospitalizing patients with chronic renal disease. Increasing hypertension and decreasing renal function warrant immediate hospitalization. A sudden deterioration of renal function may be due to infection, dehydration, electrolyte imbalance, or obstruction.

The timing of delivery must be individualized. Maternal indications for delivery include uncontrollable hypertension, the development of superimposed preeclampsia, and decreasing renal function after fetal viability has been reached. Fetal indications are dictated by the assessment of fetal growth and fetal well-being.

Renal biopsy is rarely indicated during pregnancy. It is never indicated after 34 weeks' gestation, when delivery of the fetus and subsequent biopsy would be a safer alternative. Excessive bleeding secondary to the greatly increased renal blood flow has been reported by some[45] but not all[46] observers. If coagulation indices are normal and blood pressure is well controlled, morbidity should be no greater than that observed in the nonpregnant patient.[47] Packham and Fairley[48] report a series of 111 renal biopsies performed in 104 pregnant women over 20 years. The complication rate was 4.5 percent. The most likely clinical dilemma necessitating renal biopsy in a pregnant woman would be the development of nephrotic syndrome and increasing hypertension between 22 and 32 weeks' gestation. In this case, renal biopsy may distinguish chronic renal disease from preeclampsia and impact significantly on the treatment plan.

Hemodialysis in Pregnancy

Patients with chronic hemodialysis can have successful pregnancies.[49-55] Many women with chronic renal failure, however, experience oligomenorrhea, and their fertility is often impaired.[56] These women commonly fail to use a method of contraception. It is therefore important that a serum β-hCG level be assessed whenever pregnancy is suspected.

As in all patients with impaired renal function, the most important aspect of care is meticulous control of blood pressure. During dialysis, wide fluctuations in blood pressure often occur. One case report describes fetal distress associated with hypotension during dialysis.[57] Sudden volume shifts therefore should be avoided.[55] In late pregnancy, continuous fetal heart rate monitoring should be carried out during dialysis. If possible, the patient should be positioned on her left side with the uterus displaced from the vena cava. During dialysis, one must pay particular attention to electrolyte balance. Pregnant patients are in a state of chronic compensated respiratory alkalosis, and large drops in serum bicarbonate should be prevented. Dialysates containing glucose and bicarbonate are preferred, and those containing citrates should be avoided.[55]

Patients should be counseled that a successful pregnancy will require longer and more frequent periods of dialysis.[50,55,57] Patients must also follow a careful diet, ingesting at least 70 g of protein and 1.5 g of calcium daily. Weight gain should be limited to 0.5 kg between dialysis sessions.

Chronic anemia is often a problem in hemodialysis patients. The hematocrit should be kept above 25 percent, and transfusion with packed RBCs or erythropoietin therapy may be necessary to accomplish this objective.[50] Polyhydramnios appears to be a frequent complication in pregnant patients undergoing hemodialysis.[55,58]

The point at which to initiate hemodialysis is controversial. Cohen and coinvestigators[52] believe that the early initiation of regular hemodialysis in patients with moderate renal insufficiency may improve pregnancy outcome. In two cases, when regular hemodialysis was begun in the second trimester, both patients carried to term, although the infants were growth restricted.[52] Redrow and coworkers[53] report 14 pregnancies in 13 women undergoing dialysis. Ten of those pregnancies were successful. Five of eight pregnancies managed with chronic ambulatory peritoneal dialysis or chronic cycling peritoneal dialysis were successful. The investigators hypothesize several advantages for peritoneal dialysis. These include a more constant chemical and extracellular environment for the fetus, higher hematocrit levels, infrequent episodes of hypotension, and no heparin requirement. They also postulate that intra-peritoneal insulin facilitates the management of blood glucose in diabetic patients and that intraperitoneal magnesium used in the dialysate reduces the likelihood of preterm labor.

Preterm birth does occur more frequently in patients undergoing dialysis.[59] Progesterone is removed during dialysis and at least one group has advocated that par-enteral progesterone therapy should be administered to the patient undergoing dialysis.[60] In their review, Yasin and Doun[55] report a 40.7 percent incidence of premature contractions. Although it is tempting to con-sider cesarean delivery when the patient approaches term, this method should not be routine for these pa-tients. Its use should be based only on obstetric indica-tions.

The Europeans have compiled a registry of pregnant women requiring dialysis. There has been a 23 percent pregnancy success rate in 70 women with end-stage renal disease requiring dialysis.[58] The mean gestational age was 33.2 weeks. Most preterm births were due to growth restriction, hypertension, preterm labor, and abruption. These findings suggest that more frequent dialysis results in more uniform control of uremia and less fluctuation in blood volume, which should result in better pregnancy outcomes.

Pregnancy in the Renal Transplant Recipient

Pregnancy following renal transplantation has become increasingly common. Many previously anovulatory pa-tients begin ovulating postoperatively and regain fertil-ity as renal function normalizes.[61] As in the case of women on hemodialysis, many transplant recipients have failed to realize they are pregnancy until well into the second trimester.

Upon learning they are pregnant, many women stop taking all medications. The importance of continuing immunosuppressive therapy cannot be emphasized strongly enough to renal allograft recipients. Glucocor-ticoids, especially prednisone, are metabolized in the placenta by 11 β-ol-dehydrogenase, with only limited amounts reaching the fetus. No studies have docu-mented an increased rate of malformations. Adreno-cortical insufficiency has been rarely reported in infants born to mothers taking glucocorticoids.[62] Nevertheless, a pediatrician should be present at the delivery and should be aware of this possibility.

Azathioprine cannot be activated in the fetus because of its lack of inosinate pyrophosphorylase.[63] Azathio-prine has been shown to cause decreased levels of IgG and IgM as well as a smaller thymic shadow on chest x-ray in these neonates.[64] Chromosomal aberrations, which cleared within 20 to 32 months, have also been demonstrated in lymphocytes of infants exposed to aza-thioprine in utero.[65] The long-term implications of this treatment are not yet known. IUGR has been reported in infants born to mothers receiving azathioprine.[66] These risks are outweighed, however, by the disastrous consequences of allograft rejection that may occur if the patient stops her medication.

Cyclosporin A appears to be relatively safe for use during gestation, but does hold some risks. Patients may develop arterial hypertension secondary to its in-terference with the normal hemodynamic adaptation to pregnancy.[67] Cyclosporin crosses the placenta, but there is no evidence of teratogenesis.[68,69] Intrauterine growth restriction, in the absence of maternal hyper-tension, has been reported in a patient taking cyclosporin A during pregnancy.[70] Most women taking cyclosporin have had no complications attributable to the drug, and the risk of allograft rejection certainly outweighs the fetal risk of the medication. Therefore, the medication should be continued throughout gesta-tion.

Davison[71] reviewed 1,569 renal transplants in 1,009 women. He found that 22 percent of the women elected to abort their pregnancies, 16 percent had a sponta-neous abortion, and 8 percent experienced perinatal deaths. Furthermore, he observed that 45 percent of the surviving pregnancies were delivered preterm and 22 percent were complicated by intrauterine growth restriction.[71] Three percent of the infants were born with major malformations, a rate no different from ex-pected in the background population. Preeclampsia complicated 30 percent of the pregnancies, but, as pre-viously noted, the diagnosis is difficult to make in a patient who may already have hypertension and pro-teinuria. The allograft rejection rate in these women was 9 percent, no different from that expected in a nonpregnant population.[71] Also, the long-term rejec-tion rate was the same as for women who had not expe-rienced a pregnancy.

During pregnancy, renal allograft recipients must be carefully watched for signs of rejection. As previously mentioned, significant episodes of rejection may occur in as many as 9 percent of transplant recipients during gestation. This figure is no greater than that expected in the nonpregnant population. Unfortunately, the clinical hallmarks of rejection—fever, oliguria, tender-ness, and decreasing renal function—are not always ex-hibited by the pregnant patient. Occasionally, rejection may mimic pyelonephritis or preeclampsia, which oc-curs in approximately one-third of renal transplant pa-tients. In these cases renal biopsy is indicated to distin-guish rejection from preeclampsia. Rejection has been known to occur during the puerperium, when maternal immune competence returns to its prepregnancy level.[72] Therefore, it may be advisable to increase the dose of immunosuppressive medications in the immediate postpartum period.

Infection can be disastrous for the renal allograft. Therefore, urine cultures should be obtained at least monthly during pregnancy, and any bacteriuria should be aggressively treated. It is crucial to remember that the allograft is denervated, and the patient may experience no pain with pyelonephritis. The only symptoms may be fever and nausea.

Renal function, as determined by 24-hour creatinine clearance and protein excretion, should be assessed monthly. Approximately 15 percent of transplant recipients will exhibit a significant decrease in renal function in late pregnancy.[73] This condition usually, but not always, reverses after pregnancy. Proteinuria develops in about 40 percent of patients near term, but most often disappears soon after delivery unless significant hypertension is present.

As for patients with chronic renal disease, serial ultrasonography should be used to assess fetal growth, and antepartum fetal heart rate testing should be started at 28 weeks' gestation. Approximately 50 percent of renal allograft recipients will deliver preterm. Preterm labor, preterm rupture of membranes, and IUGR are common. Vaginal delivery should be accomplished when possible, with cesarean delivery reserved for obstetric indications. Allograft recipients may have an increased frequency of cephalopelvic disproportion from pelvic osteodystrophy,[74] resulting from prolonged renal disease with hypercalcemia or extended steroid use. The transplanted kidney, however, rarely obstructs vaginal delivery despite its pelvic location.

Although there have been many successful pregnancies in renal allograft recipients, no group has really devised criteria for when it is safe to conceive after

Table 30-1   Guidelines for Renal Allograft Recipients Who Wish To Conceive

Absolute criteria
  Wait 2 years after cadaver transplant or 1 year after graft from living donor
  Immunosuppression should be at maintenance levels.
Relative criteria
  Plasma creatinine <1.5 mg/dl
  Absent or easily controlled hypertension
  No or minimal proteinuria
  No evidence of active graft rejection
  No pelvicalyceal distension on a recent ultrasound or intravenous pyelogram
  Prednisone dose ≤15 mg/day
  Azathioprine dose ≤2 mg/kg/day
  Cyclosporin A dose 2–4 mg/kg (available data on the use of this drug in pregnancy includes <150 patients)

(Adapted from Lindheimer and Katz,[74] with permission.)

transplantation. In a recent editorial, Lindheimer and Katz,[75] the leading authorities on renal disease in pregnancy, have suggested some guidelines, which are summarized in Table 30-1.

Acute Renal Failure in Pregnancy

Acute renal failure (ARF) is defined as a urine output of less than 400 ml in 24 hours. To make the diagnosis, ureteral and urethral obstruction must be excluded. The incidence of ARF during pregnancy is approximately 1 per 10,000. It is seen most frequently in septic first trimester abortions and in cases of sudden severe volume depletion resulting from hemorrhage caused by placenta previa, placental abruption, or postpartum uterine atony.[76] It is also observed in the marked volume contraction associated with severe preeclampsia[77] and with acute fatty liver of pregnancy.[77,78]

The incidence of ARF in pregnancy has decreased over the years. Stratta and colleagues[79] reported 81 cases of pregnancy-related ARF between 1958 and 1987, accounting for 9 percent of the total number of ARF cases needing dialysis during that interval. In three successive 10-year periods (1958–1967, 1968–1977, and 1978–1987), the incidence of pregnancy-related ARF fell from 43 to 2.8 percent of the total number of cases of ARF. The incidence changed from 1 in 3,000 to 1 in 15,000 pregnancies over the study period.[79] In these 81 ARF cases, 11.6 percent experienced irreversible renal damage, the majority of which involved severe preeclampsia/eclampsia.[79]

Renal ischemia is the common denominator in all cases of ARF. With mild ischemia, quickly reversible prerenal failure results. With more prolonged ischemia, acute tubular necrosis occurs. This process is also reversible, as glomeruli are not affected. Severe ischemia, however, may produce acute cortical necrosis. This pathology is irreversible, although on occasion a small amount of renal function is preserved.[80] Stratta and colleagues[81] have reported 17 cases of ARF occurring over 15 years, and all were due to preeclampsia/eclampsia. Cortical necrosis occurred in 29.5 percent of the cases.[81] Whether or not ARF was associated with cortical necrosis did not appear to be related to chronologic age, parity, gestational age at which preeclampsia commenced, duration of preeclampsia prior to delivery, or eclamptic seizures. The only statistically significant factor associated with the appearance of cortical necrosis was placental abruption.[81] In another study, Turney and coworkers[82] demonstrated that acute cortical necrosis, which occurred in 12.7 percent of their patients with ARF, carried a 100 percent mortality within 6 years.

Sibai and colleagues[83] studied the remote prognosis in 31 consecutive cases of ARF in patients with hypertensive disorders of pregnancy. Eighteen of the 31 patients had "pure" preeclampsia, while 13 pregnancies had other hypertensive disorders and renal disease. Five percent of the 18 patients with pure preeclampsia required dialysis during hospitalization, and all 18 patients had acute tubular necrosis. Of the other 13 women, 42 percent required dialysis and three patients had bilateral cortical necrosis. The majority of pregnancies in both groups were complicated by placental abruption and hemorrhage.[83] All 16 surviving patients in the pure preeclampsia group had normal renal function on long-term follow-up. Conversely, 9 of the 11 surviving patients in the other group required long-term dialysis, and four ultimately died of end-stage renal disease.[83] Turney and colleagues[82] also performed follow-up examinations of their patients. They found that maternal survival was adversely affected by increasing age. Their 1-year maternal survival rate was 78.6 percent. Follow-up of survivors showed normal renal function up to 31 years after ARF.[82]

Clinically, patients with reversible ARF first experience a period of oliguria of variable duration. Polyuria then occurs. It is important to recognize that BUN and serum creatinine levels continue to rise early in the polyuric phase. During the recovery phase, urine output approachs normal. In these patients, it is important to monitor electrolytes frequently and to treat any imbalance carefully. The urine to plasma osmolality ratio should be determined early in the course of the disease. If the ratio is 1.5 greater, prerenal pathology is likely, and the disorder tends to be of shorter duration and less severity. A ratio near 1.0 suggests acute tubular necrosis.

The main goal of treatment is the elimination of the underlying cause. Volume and electrolyte balance must receive constant scrutiny. To assess volume requirements, invasive hemodynamic monitoring is useful and lessens the need for clinical guesswork. This is especially true during the polyuric phase. Central hyperalimentation may also be required if renal failure is prolonged.

Acidosis frequently occurs in cases of ARF. Arterial blood gases therefore should be followed regularly. Acidosis must be treated promptly to prevent hyperkalemia, which may develop rapidly and can be fatal. Absolute restriction of potassium intake should be instituted immediately. Sodium bicarbonate, used to treat acidosis, may overload the patient with sodium and water. In this case, peritoneal or hemodialysis may be instituted. The main indications for dialysis in ARF of pregnancy are hypernatremia, hyperkalemia, severe acidosis, volume overload, and worsening uremia.

Hemolytic Uremic Syndrome

The postpartum hemolytic uremic syndrome is a rare idiopathic disorder that must be considered when a patient shows signs of hemolysis and decreasing renal function in the postpartum period. This idiopathic syndrome was first described in 1968 and may occur as early as the first trimester and up to 2 months postpartum.[84–87] In fact, it has even been reported following an ectopic pregnancy.[88] Most patients have no predisposing factors. Prodromal symptoms include vomiting, diarrhea, and a flu-like illness. Forty-nine cases have been reported with 61 percent mortality rate.[86] These cases date back to 1968; with improved intensive care monitoring and treatment, the prognosis is now probably much better. Coratelli and coworkers[84] reported a case of hemolytic uremic syndrome that was diagnosed at 13 weeks' gestation and confirmed by renal biopsy. Circulating endotoxin was detected and was progressively reduced by hemodialysis performed daily from the third to the ninth days of the disease. Complete normalization of renal function occurred by day 34. These investigators propose that initiation of early dialysis may play an important role in supporting patients through the disease process. They also feel that endotoxins are key pathogenic factors in the disorder.[84] Conversely, Li and coworkers[89] discovered hemolytic uremic syndrome in a patient recovering from an uncomplicated cesarean delivery. No endotoxins were found in the patient's serum, stool, or renal biopsy material. The patient underwent dialysis and recovered.[89] Conte and coworkers[90] suggest that plasma exchange in cases of acute renal failure caused by the postpartum hemolytic uremic syndrome can play a vital role in supporting a patient through the illness. This does appear to be the key to therapy today.

Disseminated intravascular coagulation (DIC) with hemolysis usually accompanies the renal failure. However, DIC is not the cause of the syndrome. Microscopically, the kidney shows thrombotic microangiopathy. The glomerular capillary wall is thick, and biopsy specimens taken later in the course of the disease show severe nephrosclerosis and deposition of the third component of complement (C_3).

Some researchers believe that this syndrome is due to decreased production of prostacyclin in the kidneys.[91,92] Prostacyclin infusions have been used to treat patients, but this therapy still remains experimental. One observer noted a decrease in antithrombin III in a patient with postpartum hemolytic uremic syndrome. This patient was successfully treated with an infusion of antithrombin III concentrate.[93] This concentrate is readily available today.

Miscellaneous Renal Problems That May Coexist with Pregnancy

Adult polycystic kidney disease is an autosomal dominant disorder that usually begins to manifest itself in the fifth decade of life. Patients may occasionally begin displaying symptoms earlier. Hypertension is part of this disorder. If a patient with adult polycystic kidney disease becomes pregnant, hypertension may be exacerbated and not improve postpartum.[29] The overall prognosis for the disorder does not appear to worsen with an increasing number of pregnancies.

Vesicoureteral reflux increases with pregnancy. It usually does not cause problems unless the reflux is severe. If it is severe enough to warrant surgery, this should be done before pregnancy. Even with surgical correction, patients with ureterovesical reflux are at increased risk for pyelonephritis and should have cultures performed frequently.[29] If an individual was receiving antibiotic prophylaxis prior to pregnancy, this should be continued. If an individual was not on prophylaxis, the obstetrician may wish to begin prophylaxis with nitrofurantoin, depending on the clinical situation.

Brandes and Fritsche[94] report a case of acute renal failure due to obstruction of the ureters by a gravid uterus. Only 13 other cases have been reported prior to their case, a twin pregnancy complicated by polyhydramnios at 34 weeks' gestation. The serum creatinine level peaked at 12.2 mg/dl, but resolved immediately after amniotomy.[94] In cases remote from term, ureteral stenting or dialysis may be necessary.

Renal artery stenosis is an extremely rare complication of pregnancy. Heyborne et al[95] reviewed the literature on this subject. This disorder may present as chronic hypertension with superimposed preeclampsia or as recurrent isolated preeclampsia. Although Doppler flow studies may be suggestive, renal angiography is the most specific and sensitive diagnostic procedure. Percutaneous transluminal angioplasty can be carried out at the time of angiography. Heyborne et al[95] present a case in which this procedure was accomplished at 26 ½ weeks' gestation.

Key Points

- Asymptomatic bacteriuria complicates 10 percent of pregnancies and if left untreated will result in symptomatic urinary tract infections in 40 percent of patients.

- Pyelonephritis complicates 1 to 2 percent of pregnancies, making it the most frequent nonobstetric cause of hospitalization during pregnancy.

- Patients with glomerulonephritis can have successful pregnancies, but pregnancy loss rates increase greatly if the patient has preexisting hypertension.

- Creatinine clearance can decline 70 percent before significant increases are seen in the BUN or serum creatinine level. Therefore, a 24-hour urine specimen for creatinine clearance should be collected from any patient in whom renal disease is suspected.

- The chance of successful pregnancy is reduced if the creatinine clearance is less than 50 ml/min or if the serum creatinine level is more than 1.5 mg/dl.

- Severe hypertension is the greatest threat to the pregnant woman with chronic renal disease.

- Growth restriction and preeclampsia are common in women with chronic renal disease. These patients should have frequent sonograms and should start antepartum fetal surveillance at 28 weeks' gestation.

- Patients with chronic renal disease are often anovulatory. After transplantation, as renal function returns, they ovulate and may become pregnant unexpectedly.

- Patients should wait 2 years after receiving a cadaver renal allograft and 1 year after receiving a living allograft before contemplating pregnancy. Furthermore, there should be no signs of allograft rejection.

- Renal transplant patients should remain on their immunosuppressive medications throughout gestation.

References

1. DeAlvarez R: Renal glomerulotubular mechanisms during normal pregnancy. I. Glomerular filtration rate, renal plasma flow and creatinine clearance. Am J Obstet Gynecol 75:931, 1958
2. Davidson J: Changes in renal function and other aspects of homeostasis in early pregnancy. J Obstet Gynaecol Br Commonw 81:1003, 1974
3. Christensen P: Tubular reabsorption of glucose during pregnancy. Scand J Clin Lab Invest 10:364, 1958
4. Kass E: Asymptomatic infections of the urinary tract. Trans Assoc Am Physicians 60:56, 1956
5. Norden C, Kass E: Bacteriuria of pregnancy—a critical reappraisal. Annu Rev Med 19:431, 1968
6. McFadyen I, Eykryn S, Gardner N et al: Bacteriuria of

pregnancy. J Obstet Gynaecol Br Commonw 80:385, 1973

7. Kunin C: The natural history of recurrent bacteriuria in schoolgirls. N Engl J Med 282:1443, 1970

8. Savage W, Hajj S, Kass E: Demographic and prognostic characteritics of bacteriuria in pregnancy. Medicine (Baltimore) 46:385, 1967

9. Whalley P: Bacteriuria of pregnancy. Am J Obstet Gynecol 97:723, 1967

10. Sandberg T, Likin-Janson G, Eden CS: Host response in women with symptomatic urinary tract infection. Scand J Infect Dis 21:67, 1989

11. Plattner MS: Pyelonephritis in pregnancy. J Perinatol Neonat Nursing 8:20, 1994

12. Brumfitt W: The significance of symptomatic and asymptomatic infection in pregnancy. Contrib Nephrol 25:23, 1981

13. Gilstrap L, Leveno K, Cunningham F et al: Renal infection and pregnancy outcome. Am J Obstet Gynecol 141:709, 1981

14. Fan YD, Pastorek JG II, Miller JM Jr, Mulvey J: Acute pyelonephritis in pregnancy. Am J Perinatol 4:324, 1987

15. Van Dorsten JP, Lenke RR, Schifrin BS: Pyelonephritis in pregnancy: the role of in-hospital management and nitrofurantoin suppression. J Reprod Med 32:895, 1987

16. Cunningham FG, Lucas MJ, Hankins GD: Pulmonary injury complicating antepartum pyelonephritis. Am J Obstet Gynecol 156:797, 1987

17. Pruett K, Faro S: Pyelonephritis associated with respiratory distress. Obstet Gynecol 69:444, 1987

18. Goorman G, Schlaeffer E, Kopernic G: Adult respiratory distress syndrome as a complication of acute pyelonephritis during pregnancy. Eur J Obstet Gynecol Rep Biol 36:75, 1990

18a.Towers CV, Kaminskas CM, Garite TJ, et al: Pulmonary injury associated with antepartum pyelonephritis: Can at risk patients be identified? Am J Obstet Gynecol 164:974, 1991

19. Austenfeld MS, Snow BW: Complications of pregnancy in women after reimplantation for vesicoureteral reflux. J Urol 140:1103, 1988

20. Harris R, Dunnihoo D: The incidence and significance of urinary calculi in pregnancy. Am J Obstet Gynecol 99:237, 1967

21. Strong D, Murchison R, Lynch D: The management of ureteral calculi during pregnancy. Surv Gynecol Obstet 146:604, 1978

22. Nadler N, Salinas-Madrigal L, Charles A, Pollack V: Acute glomerulonephritis during late pregnancy. Obstet Gynecol 34:277, 1969

23. Wilson C: Changes in renal function. p. 177. In Morris N, Browne J (eds): Nontoxemic Hypertension in Pregnancy. Little, Brown, Boston, 1958

24. Packham DK, North RA, Fairley KF et al: Primary glomerulonephritis and pregnancy. Q J Med 71:537, 1989

25. Packham DK, North RA, Fairley KF et al: Membranous glomerulonephritis and pregnancy. Clin Nephrol 30:487, 1988

26. Jungers P, Forget D, Houillier P et al: Pregnancy in IgA nephropathy, reflux nephropathy, and focal glomerular sclerosis. Am J Kidney Dis 9:334, 1987

27. Kincaid-Smith P, Fairley KF: Renal disease in pregnancy:

three controversial areas: mesangial IgA nephropathy, focal glomerular sclerosis (focal and segmental hyalinosis and sclerosis), and reflux nephropathy. Am J Kidney Dis 9:328, 1987

28. Abe S: An overview of pregnancy in women with underlying renal disease. Am J Kidney Dis 17:112, 1991

29. Imbasciati E, Ponticelli C: Pregnancy and renal disease: predictors for fetal and maternal outcome. Am J Nephrol 11:353, 1991

30. Bear R: Pregnancy in patients with renal disease: a study of 44 cases. Obstet Gynecol 48:13, 1976

31. Hou S: Pregnancy in women with chronic renal disease. N Engl J Med 312:839, 1985

32. Hou S, Grossman S, Madias N: Pregnancy in women with renal disease and moderate renal insufficiency. Am J Med 78:185, 1985

33. Katz A, Davison J, Hayslett J et al: Pregnancy in women with kidney disease. Kidney Int 18:192, 1980

34. Mackay E: Pregnancy and renal disease: a ten-year study. Aust NZ J Obstet Gynaecol 3:21, 1963

35. Studd J, Blainey J: Pregnancy and the nephrotic syndrome. BMJ 1:276, 1969

36. Kincaid-Smith P, Fairley K, Bullen M: Kidney disease and pregnancy. Med J Aust 11:1155, 1967

37. Surian M, Imbasciati E, Banfi G et al: Glomerular disease and pregnancy. Nephron 36:101, 1984

38. Cunningham FG, Cox SG, Harstad TW et al: Chronic renal disease and pregnancy outcome. Am J Obstet Gynecol 163:453, 1990

39. Piper JM, Ray WA, Rosa FW: Pregnancy outcome following exposure to angiotensin-converting enzyme inhibitors. Obstet Gynecol 80:429, 1992

40. Hulton SA, Thompson PD, Cooper PA, Rothberg AD: Angiotensin-converting enzyme inhibitors in pregnancy may result in neonatal renal failure. S Afr Med J 78:673, 1990

41. Sibai B, Grossman R, Grossman H: Effects of diuretics on plasma volume in pregnancies with long term hypertension. Am J Obstet Gynecol 150:831, 1984

42. Crosland D, Flowers C: Chlorothiazide and its relationship to neonatal jaundice. Obstet Gynecol 22:500, 1963

43. Rodriguez S, Leikin S, Hiller M: Neonatal thrombocytopenia associated with antepartum administration of thiazide drugs. N Engl J Med 270:881, 1964

44. Sanchez-Casajuz A, Famos I, Santos M: Monitorization fetal en el transcurso de hemodialissi durante el embarazo. Rev Clin Esp 149:187, 1978

45. Schewitz L, Friedman E, Pollak V: Bleeding after renal biopsy in pregnancy. Obstet Gynecol 26:295, 1965

46. Lindheimer M, Spargo B, Katz A: Renal biopsy in pregnancy-induced hypertension. J Reprod Med 15:189, 1975

47. Lindheimer M, Fisher K, Spargo B, Katz A: Hypertension in pregnancy: a biopsy study with long term follow-up. Contrib Nephrol 25:71, 1981

48. Packham D, Fairley KF: Renal biopsy: indications and complications in pregnancy. Br J Obstet Gynaecol 94:935, 1987

49. Ackrill P, Goodwin F, Marsh F et al: Successful pregnancy in patient on regular dialysis. BMJ 2:172, 1975

50. Kobayashi H, Matsumoto Y, Otsubo O et al: Successful pregnancy in a patient undergoing chronic hemodialysis. Obstet Gynecol 57:382, 1981

51. Savdie E, Caterson R, Mahony J, Clifton-Bligh P: Successful pregnancies in women treated by haemodialysis. Med J Aust 2:9, 1982

52. Cohen D, Frenkel Y, Maschiach S, Eliahou HE: Dialysis during pregnancy in advanced chronic renal failure patients: outcome and progression. Clin Nephrol 29:144, 1988

53. Redrow M, Cherem L, Elliott J et al: Dialysis in the management of pregnant patients with renal insufficiency. Medicine 67:199, 1988

54. Hou S: Pregnancy in women requiring dialysis for renal failure. Am J Kidney Dis 9:368, 1987

55. Yasin SY, Doun SWB: Hemodialysis in pregnancy. Obstet Gynecol Surv 43:655, 1988

56. Lim V, Henriquez C, Sievertsen G, Prohman L: Ovarian function in chronic renal failure: evidence suggesting hypothalamic anovulation. Ann Intern Med 57:7, 1980

57. Nageotte MP, Grundy HO: Pregnancy outcome in women requiring chronic hemodialysis. Obstet Gynecol 72:456, 1988

58. EDTA Registration Committee: Successful pregnancies in women treated by dialysis and kidney transplantation. Br J Obstet Gynaecol 87:839, 1980

59. Fine L, Barnett E, Danovitch G et al: Systemic lupus erythematosus in pregnancy. Ann Intern Med 94:667, 1981

60. Johnson T, Lorenz R, Menon K, Nolan G: Successful outcome of a pregnancy requiring dialysis: effects on serum progesterone and estrogens. J Reprod Med 22:217, 1979

61. Merkatz I, Schwartz G, David D et al: Resumption of female reproductive function following renal transplantation. JAMA 216:1749, 1971

62. Penn I, Makowski E, Harris P: Parenthood following renal transplantation. Kidney Int 18:221, 1980

63. Saarikoski S, Sappala M: Immunosuppression during pregnancy: transmission of azathioprine and its metabolites from mother to the fetus. Am J Obstet Gynecol 115:1100, 1973

64. Cote C, Meuwissen H, Pickering R: Effects on the neonate of prednisone and azathioprine administered to the mother during pregnancy. J Pediatr 85:324, 1974

65. Price H, Salaman J, Laurence K, Langmaid H: Immunosuppressive drugs and the fetus. Transplantation 21:294, 1976

66. Scott J: Fetal growth retardation associated with maternal administration of immunosuppressive drugs. Am J Obstet Gynecol 128:668, 1977

67. Ponticelli C, Montagnino G: Causes of arterial hypertension in kidney transplantation. Contrib Nephrol 54:226, 1987

68. Derfler K, Schuller A, Herold C et al: Successful outcome of a complicated pregnancy in a renal transplant recipient taking cyclosporin A. Clin Nephrol 29:96, 1988

69. Salamalekis EE, Mortakis AE, Phocas I et al: Successful pregnancy in a renal transplant recipient taking cyclosporin A: hormonal and immunological studies. Int J Gynaecol Obstet 30:267, 1989

70. Pickerell MD, Sawers R, Michael J: Pregnancy after renal transplantation: severe intrauterine growth retardation during treatment with cyclosporin A. BMJ 1:825, 1988

71. Davison J: Renal transplantation and pregnancy. Am J Kidney Dis 9:374, 1987

72. Parsons V, Bewick M, Elias J et al: Pregnancy following renal transplantation. J R Soc Med 72:815, 1979

73. Davison J, Lindheimer M: Pregnancy in women with renal allografts. Semin Nephrol 4:240, 1984

74. Huffer W, Kuzela D, Popovtzer M: Metabolic bone disease in chronic renal failure. II. Renal transplant patients. Am J Pathol 78:385, 1975

75. Lindheimer MD, Katz AI: Pregnancy in the renal transplant patient. Am J Kidney Dis 19:173, 1992

76. Davison J: Renal disease. p. 236. In deSwiet M (ed): Medical Disorders in Obstetric Practice. Blackwell, Oxford, 1984

77. Pertuiset N, Grunfeld JP: Acute renal failure in pregnancy. Baillieres Clin Obstet Gynaecol 1:873, 1987

78. Grunfeld JP, Pertuiset N: Acute renal failure in pregnancy: 1987. Am J Kidney Dis 9:359, 1987

79. Stratta P, Canavese C, Dogliani M et al: Pregnancy-related acute renal failure. Clin Nephrol 32:14, 1989

80. Grunfeld J, Ganeval D, Bournerias F: Acute renal failure in pregnancy. Kidney Int 18:179, 1980

81. Stratta P, Canavese C, Colla L et al: Acute renal failure in preeclampsia-eclampsia. Gynecol Obstet Invest 24:225, 1987

82. Turney JH, Ellis CM, Parsons FM: Obstetric acute renal failure 1956–1987. Br J Obstet Gynaecol 96:679, 1989

83. Sibai BM, Villar MA, Mabie BC: Acute renal failure in hypertensive disorders of pregnancy: pregnancy outcome and remote prognosis in thirty-one consecutive cases. Am J Obstet Gynecol 162:777, 1990

84. Coratelli P, Buongiorno E, Passavanti G: Endotoxemia in hemolytic uremic syndrome. Nephron 50:365, 1988

85. Robson J, Martin A, Burkley V: Irreversible postpartum renal failure: a new syndrome. Q J Med 37:423, 1968

86. Seconds A, Louradour N, Suc J, Orfila C: Postpartum hemolytic uremic syndrome: a study of three cases with a review of the literature. Clin Nephrol 12:229, 1979

87. Wagoner R, Holley K, Johnson W: Accelerated nephrosclerosis and postpartum acute renal failure in normotensive patients. Ann Intern Med 69:237, 1968

88. Creasey GW, Morgan J: Hemolytic uremic syndrome after ectopic pregnancy: postectopic nephrosclerosis. Obstet Gynecol 69:448, 1987

89. Li PK, Lai FM, Tam JS, Lai KN: Acute renal failure due to postpartum haemolytic uraemic syndrome. Aust NZ J Obstet Gynaecol 28:228, 1988

90. Conte F, Mewroni M, Battini G et al: Plasma exchange in acute renal failure due to postpartum hemolytic-uremic syndrome: report of a case. Nephron 50:167, 1988

91. Remuzzi G, Misiani R, Marchesi D et al: Treatment of hemolytic uremic syndrome with plasma. Clin Nephrol 12:279, 1979

92. Webster J, Rees A, Lewis P, Hensby C: Prostacyclin deficiency in haemolytic uraemic syndrome. BMJ 281:271, 1980

93. Brandt P, Jesperson J, Gregerson G: Post-partum haemolytic-uraemic syndrome successfully treated with antithrombin III. BMJ 281:449, 1980

94. Brandes JC, Fritsche C: Obstructive acute renal failure by a gravid uterus: a case report and review. Am J Kidney Dis 18:398, 1991

95. Hayborne KD, Schultz MF, Goodlin RC, Durham JD: Renal artery stenosis during pregnancy: a review. Obstet Gynecol Survey 46:509, 1991

Chapter 31

Diabetes Mellitus and Other Endocrine Diseases

Mark B. Landon

Diabetes Mellitus

Prior to the introduction of insulin therapy 75 years ago, pregnancy in the diabetic woman was uncommon and was likely to be accompanied by fetal mortality and a substantial risk for maternal death as well. Through improved understanding of the pathophysiology of diabetes in pregnancy as well as the development of techniques to prevent these complications, perinatal mortality has been reduced from approximately 65 percent before the discovery of insulin to 2 to 5 percent at the present time. This dramatic improvement in perinatal outcome has been largely attributed to clinical efforts to establish improved maternal glycemic control. (Fig. 31-1). If optimal care is delivered to the diabetic woman, the perinatal mortality rate excluding major congenital malformations is equivalent to that observed in normal pregnancies.

While the benefit of careful regulation of maternal glucose levels is generally well accepted, failure to establish optimal glycemic control as well as other factors continue to result in significant perinatal morbidity. For this reason, both clinical and basic laboratory investigations concerning the etiology of congenital malformations and intrauterine death have become a focus in recent years. Fortunately, the outlook for most diabetic women considering pregnancy remains excellent. Clinicians have recently developed a more realistic appreciation of the impact that vascular complications can have on pregnancy, as well as the complications that pregnancy may have on these disease processes. With modern management techniques and an organized team approach, successful pregnancies have become the norm for women with complicated diabetes. Before considering these clinical issues, it is important to have an understanding of carbohydrate metabolism as it relates to the pathophysiology of diabetes during pregnancy.

Pathophysiology

During normal pregnancy, maternal metabolism adjusts to provide adequate nutrition for both the mother and the growing fetoplacental unit. Early in pregnancy, glucose homeostasis is affected by increases in estrogen and progesterone that lead to β-cell hyperplasia and increased insulin secretion.[1] The heightened peripheral utilization of glucose results in a 10 percent reduction in maternal glucose levels by the end of the first trimester. At the same time, glycogen deposition increases in peripheral tissues, accompanied by a decrease in hepatic glucose production. Insulin-dependent diabetic women therefore commonly experience periods of hypoglycemia in the first trimester. Additionally, availability of gluconeogenic amino acids such as alanine are reduced, whereas levels of fatty acids, triglycerides, and ketones are increased. This state of "accelerated starvation" during fasting marked by increased fat catabolism and a decline in maternal glucose production allows utilization of fat stores for energy and protects against muscle mass breakdown.[2] As pregnancy progresses, fasting levels of insulin rise from approximately 5 to 8 mU/L at term.[3] Fasting hypoglycemia may appear more rapidly in late pregnancy as the conceptus increases its glucose utilization coupled with a reduction in maternal gluconeogenic substrates and hepatic glucose production.

Lipids continue as an important maternal fuel as pregnancy advances. Despite the "accelerated starvation" of the fasting state, early in pregnancy fat storage increases. With the rise of human placental lactogen

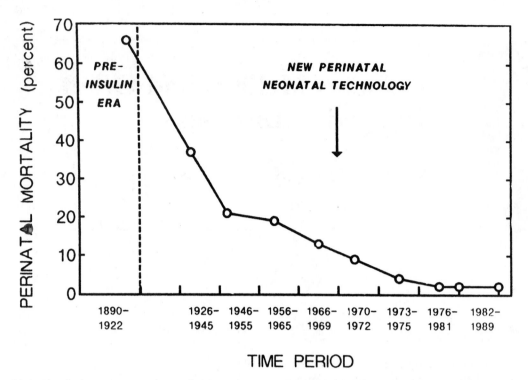

Fig. 31-1 The decline in perinatal mortality from the preinsulin era until 1989. At present, perinatal mortality in pregnancies complicated by diabetes is minimally elevated compared with the nondiabetic population if optimal care is provided. (From Hollingsworth,[278] with permission.)

(hPL), a polypeptide hormone produced by the syncytiotrophoblast, lipolysis is stimulated in adipose tissue. The release of glycerol and fatty acids reduces both maternal glucose and amino acid utilization and in doing so spares these fuels for the fetus.

Rising levels of hPL and other "contra-insulin" hormones modify maternal utilization of glucose and amino acids. The actions of hPL are responsible, in part, for the "diabetogenic state" of pregnancy. The blood glucose response to an oral or intravenous carbohydrate load is greater than in the nonpregnant state. In the normal pregnant woman, glucose hemostasis is maintained by an exaggerated rate and amount of insulin release, which accompanies decreased sensitivity to insulin.[4] (Fig. 31-2).[4] Resistance to insulin action during pregnancy has been documented by a reduction in glucose required to maintain euglycemia with insulin infusion (clamp technique) as well as with intravenous glucose tolerance testing with frequent sampling and simultaneous determination of insulin and glucose levels (minimal model technique).[5,6] Normal pregnancy has been observed to result in a 44 percent decline in insulin sensitivity by the late third trimester.[5] The mechanism responsible for insulin resistance involves hPL, progesterone, cortisol, and prolactin, which all impair glucose uptake by insulin-sensitive cells.[7] As insulin binds in a normal fashion to maternal cells, it has

been proposed that a postreceptor defect is responsible for insulin resistance during gestation.[8]

The resulting modest deterioration in glucose tolerance observed during normal pregnancy has been described as advantageous to both mother and fetus. Elevation of maternal glucose levels in the fed state serve to increase glucose supply to the fetus and placenta. The greater insulin resistance in skeletal muscle compared with adipose tissue preferentially diverts glucose as a substrate toward fat accretion and thus facilitates maternal anabolism.

With placental growth, larger amounts of these contra-insulin factors are synthesized. A woman with overt diabetes cannot respond to this stress and requires additional insulin therapy as pregnancy progresses. Her increased insulin requirement, approximately 30 percent over the prepregnancy dose, is roughly equivalent to the endogenous increase seen in a normal gestation. If the pregnant woman has borderline pancreatic reserve, it is possible that her endogenous insulin production will be inadequate, particularly late in gestation. Diabetes will then be revealed for the first time. Unlike known insulin-requiring patients, obese gestational diabetics with limited β-cell reserve but presumed peripheral insulin resistance may experience large increases in both their insulin secretion and requirement during pregnancy. The pathophysiology of insulin resistance

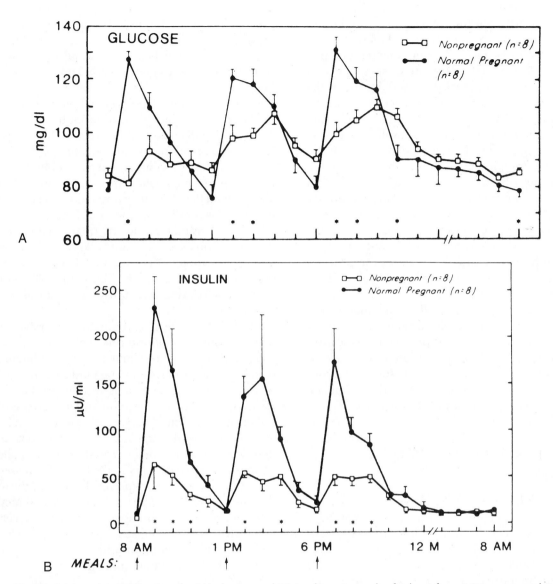

Fig. 31-2 Mean (± SEM) values for (A) glucose and (B) insulin at intervals of 1 hour from 8:00 A.M. to midnight and 2 hours thereafter in eight nonpregnant and eight normal pregnant women in the third trimester. Mealtimes are indicated by arrows along the abscissa. Pregnant women demonstrate a greater amplitude in plasma glucose excursion after meals. The increased postprandial insulin secretion is apparent. (From Phelps et al[279] with permission.)

in gestational diabetes mellitus (GDM) has been evaluated using the hyperinsulinemia euglycemic clamp technique.[5] Catalano and coworkers[5] performed longitudinal metabolic studies in obese women with GDM prior to conception, at 12 to 14 weeks, and at 34 to 36 weeks' gestation. An exaggerated fall in insulin sensitivity was noted across the three time periods in GDM subjects compared with normal controls. The differences in insulin-stimulated glucose uptake were greatest prior to conception and early gestation, and, by the later third trimester, the differences in insulin sensitivity were less pronounced. Normal pregnancy was observed to result in a 44 percent decline in insulin sensitivity compared with a 56 percent decline in preg-

nancies complicated by GDM. Insulin suppression of hepatic glucose production was also diminished in late pregnancy in women with GDM, indicating that, in GDM, hyperglycemia results from insulin resistance arising from several metabolic changes.

The placenta not only produces hormones that alter maternal metabolism, but also controls the transport of nutrients to the fetal compartment. Substrate supply to the fetus depends on the specific modes of transfer. Glucose transport across the placenta occurs by carrier-mediated facilitated diffusion. Therefore, glucose levels in the fetus are directly proportional to maternal plasma glucose concentrations. Glucose is the primary fuel utilized by the fetus for protein and fat synthesis.

The degree of placental transfer of glucose and other fuels is also affected by placental metabolism. In the sheep model, the placenta uses approximately one-half of the glucose delivered to the uterus to support its own metabolic processes.[9] Further modification of the transfer of carbohydrate may be influenced by placental insulin receptors. The placenta is essentially impermeable to protein hormones such as insulin, glucagon, growth hormone, and hPL. Although maternal insulin does not cross the placenta, it may enhance placental glucose transport by affecting the glucose carrier.[9] In addition to glucose transfer, many amino acids are actively transported across the placenta to the fetal compartment. This process contributes to the maternal hypoaminoacidemia observed in the fasting state. Ketoacids appear to diffuse freely across the placenta and may serve as a fetal substrate during periods of maternal starvation.

Fetal glucose levels are normally maintained within narrow limits because maternal carbohydrate homeostasis is so well regulated. During pregnancy in the insulin-dependent diabetic woman, periods of hyperglycemia lead to fetal hyperglycemia. Persistent elevations of glucose and perhaps amino acids may then stimulate the fetal pancreas, resulting in β-cell hyperplasia and fetal hyperinsulinemia.[10]

Perinatal Morbidity and Mortality

Fetal Death

In the past, sudden and unexplained stillbirths occurred in 10 to 30 percent of pregnancies complicated by insulin-dependent diabetes mellitus (IDDM).[11] Although relatively uncommon today, such losses still plague the pregnancies of patients who do not receive optimal care. Stillbirths have been observed most often after the 36th week of pregnancy in patients with vascular disease, poor glycemic control, hydramnios, fetal macrosomia, or preeclampsia. Women with vascular complications may develop fetal growth retardation and intrauterine demise as early as the second trimester. In the past, prevention of intrauterine death led to a strategy of scheduled preterm deliveries for IDDM women. This empiric approach reduced the number of stillbirths, but errors in estimation of fetal size and gestational age as well as the functional immaturity characteristic of the infant of the diabetic mother (IDM) contributed to many neonatal deaths from hyaline membrane disease.

The precise cause of the excessive stillbirth rate in pregnancies complicated by diabetes remains unknown. Because extramedullary hematopoiesis is frequently observed in stillborn IDMs, chronic intrauterine hypoxia has been cited as a likely cause of these intrauterine fetal deaths. Recent studies of fetal umbilical cord blood samples in IDDM pregnancy have demonstrated "relative fetal erythremia and lactic acidemia."[12] Maternal diabetes may also produce alterations in red blood cell oxygen release and placental blood flow.[13]

Reduced uterine blood flow is thought to contribute to the increased incidence of intrauterine growth restriction (IUGR) observed in pregnancies complicated by diabetic vasculopathy. Investigations using radioactive tracers have also suggested a relationship between poor maternal metabolic control and reduced uteroplacental blood flow.[14] Ketoacidosis and preeclampsia, two factors known to be associated with an increased incidence of intrauterine deaths, may further decrease uterine blood flow. In diabetic ketoacidosis, hypovolemia and hypotension caused by dehydration may reduce flow through the intervillous space, while in preeclampsia narrowing and vasospasm of spiral arterioles may result.

Alterations in fetal carbohydrate metabolism also may contribute to intrauterine asphyxia.[15–17] There is considerable evidence linking hyperinsulinemia and fetal hypoxia. Hyperinsulinemia induced in fetal lambs by an infusion of exogenous insulin produces an increase in oxygen consumption and a decrease in arterial oxygen content.[18] Persistent maternal–fetal hyperglycemia occurs independent of maternal uterine blood flow, which may not be increased enough to allow for enhanced oxygen delivery in the face of increased metabolic demands. Thus, hyperinsulinemia in the fetus of the diabetic mother appears to increase fetal metabolic rate and oxygen requirement in the face of several factors such as hyperglycemia, ketoacidosis, preeclampsia, and maternal vasculopathy, which can reduce placental blood flow and fetal oxygenation.

Congenital Malformations

With the reduction in intrauterine deaths and a marked decrease in neonatal mortality related to hyaline membrane disease and traumatic delivery, congenital malformations have emerged as the most important cause of perinatal loss in pregnancies complicated by IDDM. In the past, these anomalies were responsible for approximately 10 percent of all perinatal deaths. At present, however, malformations account for 30 to 50 percent of perinatal mortality.[11] Neonatal deaths now exceed stillbirths in pregnancies complicated by IDDM, and fatal congenital malformations account for this changing pattern.

Most studies have documented a two- to sixfold increase in major malformations in infants of insulin-dependent diabetic mothers. In The Ohio State University Diabetes in Pregnancy Program, we have observed 29 congenital anomalies in 289 (10 percent) IDDM

Congenital Malformations in Infants of Diabetic Mothers

Cardiovascular
>   Transposition of the great vessels
>   Ventricular septal defect
>   Atrial septal defect
>   Hypoplastic left ventricle
>   Situs inversus
>   Anomalies of the aorta

Central nervous system
>   Anencephaly
>   Encephalocele
>   Meningomyelocele
>   Holoprosencephaly
>   Microcephaly

Skeletal
>   Caudal regression syndrome
>   Spina bifida

Genitourinary
>   Absent kidneys (Potter syndrome)
>   Polycystic kidneys
>   Double ureter

Gastrointestinal
>   Tracheoesophageal fistula
>   Bowel atresia
>   Imperforate anus

Table 31-1. Frequency of Congenital Malformations in Infants of Diabetic Mothers

Study	Incidence	
	No. Patients	Percentage
Ylinen et al.[155]	11/142	7.7
Mills et al.[21]	25/279	9.0
Greene[156]	35/451	7.7
Steel et al.[178]	12/239	7.8
Fuhrmann et al.[153]	22/292	7.5
Simpson et al.[20]	9/106	8.5
Albert et al.[19]	29/289	10.0

found 200 to 400 times more often in offspring of diabetic women (Fig. 31-3). However, this defect is not pathognomonic for diabetes since it occurs in nondiabetic pregnancies.

Impaired glycemic control and associated derangement in maternal metabolism appear to contribute to abnormal embryogenesis. The notion of excess glucose as the single teratogenic agent in diabetic pregnancy has thus been replaced with the view of a multifactorial etiology.[26]

Maternal hyperglycemia has been proposed by most investigators as the primary teratogenic factor, but hyperketonemia, hypoglycemia, somatomedin inhibitor excess, and excess free oxygen radicals have also been suggested.[22] The profile of a woman most likely to produce an anomalous infant would include a patient with poor periconceptional control, long-standing diabetes, and vascular disease.[23] Genetic susceptibility to the teratogenic influence of diabetes may be a factor. Koppe and Smoremberg-School[24] as well as Simpson and colleagues[25] have suggested that certain maternal HLA types may be more often associated with anomalies.

Several mechanisms have been proposed by which the above teratogenic factors produce malformations. Freinkel et al[27] suggested that anomalies might arise from inhibition of glycolysis, the key energy-producing

women enrolled from 1987 through 1993.[19] In a prospective analysis, Simpson and Elias[20] observed an 8.5 percent incidence of major anomalies in the IDDM population, while the malformation rate in a small group of concurrently gathered control subjects was 2.4 percent. Similar figures were obtained in the Diabetes in Early Pregnancy Study in the United States.[21] The incidence of major anomalies was 2.1 percent in 389 control patients and 9.0 percent in 279 IDDM women. In general, the incidence of major malformations in worldwide studies of offspring of IDDM mothers has ranged from 5 to 10 percent (Table 31-1).

The insult that causes malformations in IDM impacts on most organ systems and must act before the seventh week of gestation.[22] Central nervous system malformations, particularly anencephaly, open spina bifida, and, possibly, holoprosencephaly, are increased 10-fold.[23] Cardiac anomalies, especially ventricular septal defects and complex lesions such as transposition of the great vessels, are increased fivefold. The congenital defect thought to be most characteristic of diabetic embryopathy is sacral agenesis or caudal dysplasia, an anomaly

Proposed Factors Associated With Teratogenesis in Pregnancy Complicated by Diabetes Mellitus

Hyperglycemia

Ketone body excess

Somatomedin inhibition

Arachidonic acid deficiency

Free oxygen radical excess

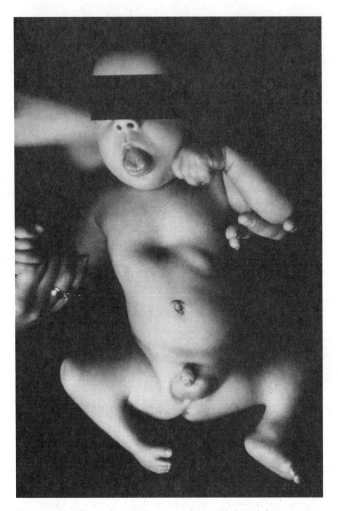

Fig. 31-3 Infant of a diabetic mother with caudal regression syndrome. The mother of this infant presented with class F diabetes at 26 weeks, in poor glycemic control. Ultrasound examination revealed absent lower lumbar spine and sacrum and hypoplastic lower extremities.

process during embryogenesis. They found that D-mannose added to the culture medium of rat embryos inhibited glucolysis and produced growth retardation and derangement of neural tube closure. Freinkel et al[27] stressed the sensitivity of normal embryogenesis to alterations in these key energy-producing pathways, a process they labeled "fuel-mediated" teratogenesis. Goldman et al[28] have suggested that the mechanism responsible for the increased incidence of neural tube defects in embryos cultured in a hyperglycemic medium may involve a functional deficiency of arachidonic acid, because supplementation with arachidonic acid or myoinositol will reduce the frequency of neural tube defects in this experimental model. Pinter and Reece[29] and Pinter et al[30] have confirmed these studies and demonstrated that hyperglycemia-induced alterations in neural tube closure include disordered cells, decreased mitoses, and changes indicating premature

maturation. These authors have further demonstrated that hyperglycemia during organogenesis has a primary deleterious effect on yolk sac function with resultant embryopathy.

Altered oxidative metabolism from maternal diabetes may cause increased production of free oxygen radicals in the developing embryo, which are likely teratogenic. Supplementation of oxygen radical scavenging enzymes, such as superoxide dismutase, to culture medium of rat embryos protects against growth delay and excess malformations.[31] It has been suggested that excess free oxygen radicals may have a direct effect on embryonic prostaglandin biosynthesis. Free oxygen radical excess may enhance lipid peroxidation, and in turn generated hydroperoxides might stimulate thromboxane biosynthesis and inhibit prostacyclin production, an imbalance that could have profound effects on embryonic development.[22]

Macrosomia

Excessive growth may predispose the IDM to shoulder dystocia, traumatic birth injury, and asphyxia. Newborn adiposity also may be associated with a significant risk for obesity in later life (Fig. 31-4).[32]

Some have defined macrosomia as a birth weight in excess of 4,000 to 4,500 g, but others prefer categorizing infants as large for gestational age (a birth weight above the 90th percentile) using population-specific growth curves. According to these definitions, macrosomia has been observed in as many as 50 percent of pregnancies complicated by GDM and 40 percent of IDDM pregnancies. Delivery of an infant weighing greater than 4,500 g occurs *10 times* more often in diabetic women than in a nondiabetic control population.[33]

Fetal macrosomia in the IDM is reflected by increased adiposity, muscle mass, and organomegaly. The disproportionate increase in the size of the trunk and shoulder compared with the head may contribute to the likelihood of a difficult vaginal delivery.[34] An increase in total body fat in the IDM has been supported by direct measurements as well as by assessment of subcutaneous stores using skinfold thickness measurements.[35] The amount of subcutaneous fat present in the IDM may be an indication of the quality of diabetic control achieved during gestation.[36]

The concept that maternal hyperglycemia leading to fetal hyperglycemia and hyperinsulinemia results in excessive fetal growth and adipose deposition was first advanced by the Danish internist Pedersen.[37] Increased β-cell mass may be identified as early as the second trimester.[38] Evidence supporting the Pedersen hypothesis also has come from studies of amniotic fluid (AF) and cord blood insulin and C-peptide levels. Both are

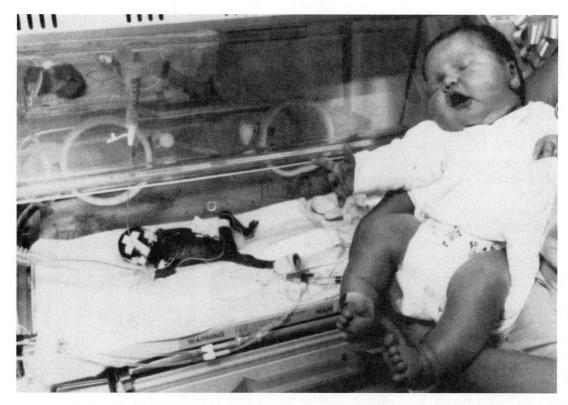

Fig. 31-4 Two extremes of growth abnormalities in infants of diabetic mothers. The small growth-retarded infant on the left weighed 470 g and is the offspring of a woman with nephropathy and hypertension, delivered at 28 weeks' gestation. The neonate on the right is the 5,100-g baby of a woman with suboptimally controlled class C diabetes.

increased in the AF of insulin-treated diabetic women at term.[39] In addition to glucose, other substrates can modify the fetal insulin secretory response. Of the major nutrients, it is likely that amino acids are important regulators of fetal insulin secretion.[40]

The results of several clinical series have validated the Pedersen hypothesis inasmuch as good maternal glycemic control has been associated with a decline in the incidence of macrosomia. In a series of 260 insulin-dependent women achieving fasting plasma glucose levels between 109 and 140 mg/dl, Gabbe et al[41] observed 58 (22 percent) macrosomic infants. Kitzmiller and Cloherty[42] reported that 11 percent of 134 women achieving fasting levels between 105 and 121 mg/dl were delivered of an infant with a birth weight in excess of 4,000 g. A more dramatic reduction in the rate of macrosomia has been reported when more physiologic control is achieved. Roversi and Gargiulo[43] instituted a program of "maximally tolerated" insulin administration and observed macrosomia in only 6 percent of cases, while Jovanovic and coworkers[44] eliminated macrosomia in 52 women who achieved mean glucose levels of 80 to 87 mg/dl throughout gestation. Landon and colleagues,[45] using daily capillary glucose values obtained during the second and third trimesters in in-

sulin-dependent women, reported a rate of 9 percent macrosomia when mean values were less than 110 mg/dl compared with 34 percent when less optimal control was achieved. Jovanovic et al[46] have suggested that 1-hour postprandial glucose measurements correlate best with the frequency of macrosomia. After controlling for other factors, these authors noted the strongest prediction for birth weight was third trimester nonfasting glucose measurements. Not surprisingly, glycosylated hemoglobin in well-controlled IDDM does not correlate closely with fetal macrosomia.[47] The persistent high frequency of macrosomia in diabetic pregnancy is likely explained by the inability of any diabetic population to achieve true physiologic glucose levels particularly in the postprandial state. Alternatively, individual fetal response including the possibility of varying glucose transport activity and thus β-cell stimulus may explain why macrosomia continues to occur in seemingly well-controlled patients.[47]

Hypoglycemia

Neonatal hypoglycemia, a blood glucose below 35 to 40 mg/dl during the first 12 hours of life, results from a rapid drop in plasma glucose concentrations following clamping of the umbilical cord. Hypoglycemia is particularly common in macrosomic newborns, in which rates exceed 50 percent. With near physiologic control of maternal glucose levels during pregnancy, overall rates of 5 to 15 percent have been reported.[43,44] The degree of hypoglycemia may be influenced by at least two factors: (1) maternal glucose control during the latter half of pregnancy and (2) maternal glycemia control during labor and delivery. Maternal blood glucose levels greater than 90 mg/dl during delivery have been found to increase significantly the frequency of neonatal hypoglycemia.[48] Presumably, prior poor maternal glucose control can result in fetal β-cell hyperplasia, leading to exaggerated insulin release following delivery. IDMs exhibiting hypoglycemia have elevated cord C-peptide and free insulin levels at birth and an exaggerated pancreatic response to glucose loading.[49]

Respiratory Distress Syndrome

The precise mechanism by which maternal diabetes affects pulmonary development remains unknown. Experimental animal studies have focused primarily on the effects of hyperglycemia and hyperinsulinemia on pulmonary surfactant biosynthesis. An extensive review of the literature confirms that both of these factors are involved in delayed pulmonary maturation in the IDM.[50]

In vitro studies have documented that insulin can interfere with substrate availability for surfactant biosynthesis.[51,52] Smith[52] has postulated that insulin interferes with the normal timing of glucocorticoid-induced pulmonary maturation in the fetus. Cortisol apparently acts on pulmonary fibroblasts to induce synthesis of fibroblast-pneumocyte factor, which then acts on type II cells to stimulate phospholipid synthesis.[53] Carlson and coworkers[54] have shown that insulin blocks cortisol action at the level of the fibroblast by reducing the production of fibroblast-pneumocyte factor.

Clinical studies investigating the effect of maternal diabetes on fetal lung maturation have produced conflicting data. With the introduction of protocols that have emphasized glucose control and antepartum surveillance until lung maturity has been established, respiratory distress syndrome has become a less common occurrence in the IDM. Several studies agree that in well-controlled diabetic women delivered at term, the risk of respiratory distress syndrome is no higher than that observed in the general population.[55,56] Kjos and Walther studied the outcome of 526 diabetic gestations delivered within 5 days of AF fetal lung maturation testing and reported hyaline membrane disease in 5 neonates (0.95 percent), all of whom were delivered prior to 34 weeks' gestation.[56] Mimouni et al[57] compared the outcomes of 127 IDMs with those of matched controls

and have concluded that diabetes in pregnancy as currently managed is not a direct risk factor for the development of respiratory distress syndrome. Yet, cesarean delivery not preceded by labor and prematurity, both of which are increased in diabetic pregnancies, clearly increase the likelihood of neonatal respiratory disease.[57]

Calcium and Magnesium Metabolism

Neonatal hypocalcemia, serum levels below 7 mg/dl, occurs at an increased rate in the IDM when one controls for predisposing factors such as prematurity and birth asphyxia.[58] Hypocalcemia in the IDM has been associated with a failure to increase parathyroid hormone synthesis following birth.[58] Decreased serum magnesium levels have also been documented in pregnant diabetic women as well as in their infants. Mimouni et al[59] described reduced AF magnesium concentrations in women with IDDM. These findings may be explained by a drop in fetal urinary magnesium excretion, which would accompany a relative magnesium-deficient state. Magnesium deficiency paradoxically then may inhibit fetal parathyroid hormone secretion.

Hyperbilirubinemia and Polycythemia

Hyperbilirubinemia is frequently observed in the IDM. Neonatal jaundice has been reported in as many as 53 percent of pregnancies complicated by IDDM and 38 percent of pregnancies with GDM.[60,61] Although several mechanisms have been proposed to explain these clinical findings, the pathogenesis of hyperbilirubinemia remains uncertain. In the past, the jaundice observed in the IDM often was attributed to prematurity. Studies that have analyzed morbidity carefully, according to gestational age, however, have rejected this concept.[62]

Although severe hyperbilirubinemia may be observed independent of polycythemia, a common pathway for these complications most likely involves increased red blood cell production, stimulated by increased erythropoietin in the IDM. Presumably, the major stimulus for red cell production is a state of relative hypoxia in utero, as described previously. Although cord erythroprotein levels generally are normal in IDMs whose mothers demonstrate good glycemic control during gestation, Shannon et al[63] and Ylinen et al[61] found that HbA1c values in late pregnancy were significantly elevated in mothers of hyperbilirubinemic infants.

Maternal Classification and Risk Assessment

Priscilla White[64] first noted that the patient's age at onset of diabetes, the duration of the disease, and the presence of vasculopathy significantly influenced peri-

Table 31-2. Modified White Classification of Pregnant Diabetic Women

Class	Diabetes Onset Age (Year)		Duration (Year)	Vascular Disease	Insulin Need
Gestational diabetes					
A$_1$	Any		Any	0	0
A$_2$	Any		Any	0	+
Pregestational diabetes					
B	> 20		< 10	0	+
C	10–19	or	10–19	0	+
D	< 10	or	> 20	+	+
F	Any		Any	+	+
R	Any		Any	+	+
T	Any		Any	+	+
H	Any		Any	+	+

(Modified from White,[64] with permission.)

natal outcome. Her pioneering work led to a classification system that has been widely applied to pregnant women with diabetes.[64] A modification of this scheme is presented in Table 31-2. Counseling a patient and formulating a plan of management requires assessment of both maternal and fetal risks. The White classification facilitates this evaluation.

Class A$_1$ diabetes mellitus includes those patients who have demonstrated carbohydrate intolerance during a 100-g 3-hour oral glucose tolerance test (GTT); however, their fasting and 2-hour postprandial glucose levels are less than 105 mg/dl and 120 mg/dl, respectively. These patients are generally managed by dietary regulation alone. If the fasting value of the GTT is elevated (≥ 105 mg/dl) or 2-hour postprandial glucose levels exceed 120 mg/dl, patients are designated class A$_2$. Insulin is most often required for these women.

The Second and Third International Workshop Conferences on Gestational Diabetes sponsored by the American Diabetes Association in cooperation with the American College of Obstetricians and Gynecologists recommended that the term *gestational diabetes* rather than *class A diabetes* be used to describe women with carbohydrate intolerance of variable severity with onset or recognition during the present pregnancy.[65,66] The term *gestational diabetes* fails to specify whether the patient requires dietary adjustment alone or treatment with diet and insulin. This distinction is important because those patients who are normoglycemic while fasting have a significantly lower perinatal mortality rate.[67] They do not appear to experience an increased incidence of intrauterine deaths in late pregnancy. Gestational diabetics who require insulin are at greater risk for a poor perinatal outcome than are those controlled by diet alone. This observation probably reflects more marked maternal hyperglycemia and, in some cases, a delay in the institution of insulin therapy.

Patients requiring insulin are designated by the letters B, C, D, R, F, and T. Class B patients are those whose onset of disease occurs after age 20. They have had diabetes less than 10 years and have no vascular complications. Included in this subgroup of patients are those who have been previously treated with oral hypoglycemic agents.

Class C diabetes includes patients who have the onset of their disease between the ages of 10 and 19 or have had the disease for 10 to 19 years. Vascular disease is not present.

Class D represents women whose disease is of 20 years duration or more, or whose onset occurred before age 10, or who have benign retinopathy. The latter includes microaneurysms, exudates, and venous dilatation.

Nephropathy

Renal disease develops in 25 to 30 percent of women with insulin-dependent diabetes mellitus with a peak incidence after approximately 16 years of diabetes.[68] Women with diabetic nephropathy have earlier deaths than those without this complication. Class F describes the 5 to 10 percent of pregnant patients with underlying renal disease. This includes those with reduced creatinine clearance or proteinuria of at least 400 mg in 24 hours measured during the first 20 weeks of gestation. Two factors present prior to 20 weeks' gestation appear to be predictive of perinatal outcome in these women (e.g., preterm delivery, low birth weight, or preeclampsia). These are (1) proteinuria above 3.0 g/24 h and (2) serum creatinine above 1.5 mg/dl.

In our series of 45 class F women, 12 had such risk factors.[69] Preeclampsia developed in 92 percent with a mean gestational age at delivery of 34 weeks compared with an incidence of preeclampsia of 36 percent in 33

Table 31-3. Comparative Studies in Outcomes in Class F Diabetes Mellitus

	Kitzmiller et al.[70]	Grenfel[277]	Reece et al.[71]	Gordon et al.[69]
n	26	20	31	45
Chronic HTN	31%	27%	22%	26%
Initial creat. > 1.9 mg/dl	38%	10%	22%	11%
Initial proteinuria > 3.0 g/24 h	8.3%	—	22%	13%
Preeclampsia	15%	55%	35%	53%
Cesarean delivery	—	72%	70%	80%
Perinatal survival (%)	88.9	100	93.5	100
Major anomalies	3 (11.1%)	1 (4.3%)	3 (9.7%)	2 (4%)
IUGR (%)	20.8	NA	19.4	11.0
Delivery				
< 34 weeks (%)	30.8	27	22.5	15.5
34–36 weeks (%)	40.7	23	32.3	35.5
> 36 weeks (%)	28.5	50	45.2	49

women without these risk factors who reached an average gestational age of 36 weeks. Remarkably, perinatal survival was 100 percent in this series, and no deliveries occurred prior to 30 weeks' gestation. Comparable series detailing perinatal outcomes in class F patients are presented in Table 31-3.

The management of the diabetic women with nephropathy requires great expertise. Limitation of dietary protein, which may reduce protein excretion in nonpregnant patients, has not been adequately studied during pregnancy. Although controversial, some nephrologists recommend a modified reduction in protein intake for pregnant women with nephropathy. Control of hypertension in pregnant women with diabetic nephropathy is crucial to prevent further deterioration of kidney function and to optimize pregnancy outcome. Although the efficacy is debatable, some cautiously use diuretics when patients are extremely nephrotic, as this group may be prone to volume-dependent forms of hypertension. Angiotension-converting enzyme inhibitors, which reduce intraglomerular pressure and improve proteinuria in nonpregnant diabetic patients, should be avoided during pregnancy as these agents affect fetal urine production and may also be teratogenic.

Several studies have failed to demonstrate a permanent worsening of diabetic renal disease as a result of pregnancy.[69–71] Kitzmiller and colleagues[70] reviewed 35 pregnancies complicated by diabetic nephropathy. Proteinuria increased in 69 percent, and hypertension developed in 73 percent. Following delivery, proteinuria declined in 65 percent of cases. In only two patients did protein excretion increase after gestation. In the series of Gordon et al,[69] 26 women (58 percent) had more than a 1 g increase in proteinuria, and by the third trimester 25 (56 percent) excreted more than 3.0 g/24 h. In the vast majority of cases, protein excretion returned to baseline levels following gestation. Changes in creatinine clearance during pregnancy are variable in class F patients. Kitzmiller,[72] in reviewing 44 patients from the literature, noted that about one-third of women had an expected rise in creatinine clearance during gestation compared with one-third who had a decline of more than 15 percent by the third trimester. In the series of Gordon's et al, 12 of 16 women in this category developed preeclampsia. Of interest, most patients with a severe reduction in creatinine clearance (< 50 ml/min) did not demonstrate a further reduction in first trimester clearance during pregnancy.[72] However, a decline in renal function can be anticipated in 20 to 30 percent of cases. Several authors have suggested that any deterioration of renal function after pregnancy is probably consistent with the natural course of diabetic nephropathy and is not related to pregnancy per se.[73] Thus, women with early stage nephropathy (less than 1 g/24 h of proteinuria and normal creatinine clearance) entering pregnancy are unlikely to manifest a decline in renal function in 1 to 2 years of follow-up.[69]

With improved survival of diabetic patients following renal transplantation, a small group of kidney recipients have now achieved pregnancy (class T). Nine cases of pregnancy complicated by diabetes and prior renal transplantation have recently been described.[74] In this series, there was no episode of renal allograft rejection. Prednisone and azathioprine were administered throughout gestation. A single maternal death and two fetal deaths did occur in patients with pre-existing peripheral vascular disease. Superimposed preeclampsia occurred in six patients. All seven surviving infants were delivered prior to term, with fetal compromise evident in six of these cases.

Retinopathy

Class R diabetes designates patients with proliferative retinopathy. There is no difference in the prevalence of retinopathy in women who have or have not been pregnant.[75] Klein and colleagues[76] prospectively evaluated 171 pregnant diabetic woman, comparing them with 298 nonpregnant controls. They found that pregnancy conveyed greater than a twofold independent risk for progression of retinopathy.[76] Retinopathy may worsen significantly during pregnancy in spite of the major advances that have been made in diagnosis and treatment. Laser photocoagulation therapy during pregnancy with careful follow-up has helped to maintain many pregnancies to a gestational age at which neonatal survival is likely.

In a large series of 172 patients, including 40 cases with background retinopathy and 11 with proliferative changes, only one patient developed new onset proliferative retinopathy during pregnancy.[77] A review of the literature by Kitzmiller et al[78] confirms the observation that progression to proliferative retinopathy during pregnancy rarely occurs in women with background retinopathy or in those without any eye ground changes. Of the 561 women in these two categories, only 17 (3.0 percent) developed neovascularization during gestation.[78] In contrast, 23 of 26 (88.5 percent) with untreated proliferative disease experienced worsening retinopathy during pregnancy.

Moloney and Drury[79] have reported that pregnancy may increase the prevalence of some background changes. These authors noted a characteristic increase in streak-blob hemorrhages and soft exudates, which often resolved between examinations. Retinopathy progressed despite strict metabolic control. Phelps and colleagues[80] have related worsening retinal disease to plasma glucose at the first prenatal visit as well as the magnitude of improvement in glycemia during early pregnancy. Chew and colleagues[81] have recently confirmed the development of both nonproliferative and proliferative changes with rapid normalization of glucose control in early pregnancy. In a subset of 140 women without proliferative retinopathy at baseline followed in the Diabetes in Early Pregnancy Study, progression of retinopathy was seen in 10.3, 21.1, 18.8, and 54.8 percent of patients with no retinopathy, microaneurysms only, mild nonproliferative retinopathy, and moderate-to-severe nonproliferative retinopathy at baseline, respectively. Elevated glycosylated hemoglobin at baseline and the magnitude of improvement of glucose control through week 14 was associated with higher risk of progression of retinopathy.[81] Women with an initial glycohemoglobin of more than 6 SD above the control mean compared with those within 2 SD of the mean were nearly three times as likely to experience worsening retinopathy. Whether improving control or simply suboptimal control itself contributes to a deterioration of background retinopathy remains uncertain. Fortunately, most patients who require laser photocoagulation will respond to this therapy and should therefore be promptly treated. However, those women who demonstrate severe florid disc neovascularization that is unresponsive to laser therapy during early pregnancy may be at great risk for deterioration of their vision. Termination of pregnancy should be considered in this group of patients.

In addition to background and proliferative eye disease, Sinclair and colleagues[82] have described vaso-occlusive lesions associated with the development of macular edema during pregnancy. Cystic macular edema is most often found in patients with proteinuric nephropathy and hypertensive disease leading to retinal edema. Macular capillary permeability is a feature of this process. The degree of macular edema is directly related to the fall in plasma oncotic pressure present in these women. In the series of Sinclair et al,[82] seven women with minimal or no retinopathy before becoming pregnant developed severe macular edema associated with preproliferative or proliferative retinopathy during the course of their pregnancies. Although proliferation was controlled with photocoagulation, the macular edema worsened until delivery in all cases and was often aggravated by photocoagulation.[82] While both macular edema and retinopathy regressed after delivery in some patients, in others these pathologic processes persisted, resulting in significant visual loss.

Coronary Artery Disease

Class H diabetes refers to the presence of diabetes of any duration associated with ischemic myocardial disease. There is evidence that the small number of women who have coronary artery disease are at an increased risk for mortality during gestation, particularly true of women who suffer an infarction during pregnancy.[83] For these cases, the maternal mortality rate is approximately 50 percent.[84] A high index of suspicion for ischemic heart disease should be maintained in women with long-standing diabetes, since anginal symptoms may be minimal and infarction may thus present as congestive heart failure.[84] While there are a few reports of successful pregnancies following myocardial infarction in diabetic women, cardiac status should be carefully assessed early in gestation or preferably prior to pregnancy. If electrocardiogram abnormalities are encountered, echocardiography may be employed to assess ventricular function or modified stress testing may be performed. The decision of a woman with IDDM and coronary artery disease to undertake a pregnancy needs to be made only after serious consideration. The potential for morbidity and mortality must be thoroughly reviewed with the patient and her family. The management of myocardial infarction during pregnancy is discussed in Chapter 29.

Detection of Diabetes in Pregnancy

It has been estimated that 2 to 3 percent of pregnancies are complicated by diabetes mellitus and that 90 percent of the cases represent women with GDM.[85] The detection of GDM is, therefore, an important diagnostic challenge. Patients with GDM represent a group with significant risk for developing glucose intolerance later in life. O'Sullivan[86] has projected that 50 percent of these patients will become diabetic in 22 to 28 years.[86] The likelihood for subsequent diabetes apparently increases when GDM is diagnosed in early pregnancy or when fasting hyperglycemia is present.

As noted above, GDM is a state restricted to pregnant women whose impaired glucose tolerance is discovered during pregnancy. Because in most cases patients with GDM have normal fasting glucose levels, some challenge of glucose tolerance must be undertaken. Traditionally, obstetricians relied on historical and clinical risk factors to select those patients most likely to develop GDM. This group included patients with a family history of diabetes or those whose past pregnancies were marked by an unexplained stillbirth or the delivery of a malformed or macrosomic infant. Obesity, hypertension, glycosuria, and maternal age over 25 were other indications for screening. Glycosuria is common in pregnancy and reflects a relative decrease in the tubular reabsorption of glucose. This finding is more likely to signal true carbohydrate intolerance if noted on a second voided fasting urine specimen. Interestingly, over half of all patients who exhibit an abnormal GTT lack the risk factors mentioned above. Coustan and colleagues[87] reported that in a series of 6,214 women the historical risk factors and an arbitrary age cut-off of 30 years for screening would miss 35 percent of cases of GDM.

The American Diabetes Association (ADA)[88] has recommended that *all* pregnant women be screened for gestational diabetes with a 50-g oral glucose load followed by a glucose determination 1 hour later (Table 31-4).

In contrast, the American College of Obstetricians and Gynecologists (ACOG)[89] has suggested that whereas selective screening for GDM may be appropriate in some clinical settings such as teen clinics (low-risk populations), universal screening may be more appropriate in other settings (high-risk populations). It should be noted that in some countries experts have questioned the benefit of GDM screening programs altogether.[90] The fact that O'Sullivan's original work es-

Table 31-4. Detection of Gestational Diabetes—Upper Limits of Normal

Screening Test (50 g) 1 hour Oral GTT[a]	Plasma (mg/dl) (130–140)	
	NDDG[276]	Carpenter[280] and Coastan
Fasting	105	95
1-hour	190	180
2-hour	165	155
3-hour	145	140

[a] Diagnosis of gestational diabetes is made when any two values are met or exceeded.

tablishing the criteria used for the diagnosis of GDM failed to evaluate an association between mild carbohydrate tolerance and perinatal outcome has led many to question the overall significance of this diagnosis. It has been further suggested that the criteria for the diagnosis of GDM are conceptually flawed in that they represent a dichotomous definition of normal and abnormal gestational glucose tolerance, when the risk of adverse fetomaternal outcomes and later diabetes should be logically graded upward with higher values on the oral glucose tolerance test (OGTT) and with the degree of fasting hyperglycemia.[91] Two studies have in fact addressed the relationship between mild degrees of carbohydrate tolerance and rates of neonatal macrosomia. In a study of 3,637 women without GDM, Sermer and colleagues[92] demonstrated a graded increase in adverse outcomes (including large infants) with increasing maternal carbohydrate intolerance. Similarly, Sacks et al[93] identified fasting and 2-hour glucose values as independent risk factors for macrosomia in a multivariate analysis of over 3,500 pregnant women. However, as no clinically meaningful glucose threshold could be identified, Sacks et al[93] concluded that the criteria for GDM will likely be established by consensus.

The 50-g glucose challenge may be performed in the fasting or fed state; sensitivity is improved if the test is performed in the fasting state.[94,95] A plasma value between 135 and 140 mg/dl is commonly used as a threshold for performing a 3-hour OGTT. Coustan et al[87] have demonstrated that 10 percent of GDM women will have screening test values between 130 and 139 mg/dl. This study indicated that the sensitivity of screening would be increased from 90 percent to nearly 100 percent if universal screening were employed using a threshold of 130 mg/dl. The prevalence of positive screening tests requiring further diagnostic testing increases from 14 percent (140 mg/dl) to 23 percent (130 mg/dl), which is accompanied by an approximately 12 percent increase in the overall cost to diagnose each case of GDM.

Few false-negative results are obtained when the 50-g screening test is performed at 24 to 28 weeks' gestation.[96] Utilizing the plasma cut-off of 140 mg/dl, one can expect approximately 15 percent of patients with an abnormal screening value to have an abnormal 3-hour OGTT. Patients whose 1-hour screening value exceeds 190 mg/dl (10.5 mmol/L) rarely exhibit a normal OGTT.[97] In these women, it is preferable to check a fasting blood glucose level before administering a 100-g carbohydrate load. If the fasting glucose is 105 mg/dl or greater, the patient is treated for GDM.

The OGTT rather than the intravenous test is favored because it is probably more physiologic and assesses the gastrointestinal factors involved in insulin secretion. The oral test also appears to be more sensitive and has been well standardized. The criteria for establishing the diagnosis of gestational diabetes are listed in Table 31-4. The US National Diabetes Data Group criteria represent a theoretic conversion of O'Sullivan's threshold in whole blood. Carpenter and Coustan[97] prefer to use another modification of these data, which is supported by a comparison of the old Somogyi-Nelson method and current plasma glucose oxidase assays.[98] Recently, Magee and colleagues[99] confirmed that patients diagnosed according to the less stringent Carpenter criteria experience as much perinatal morbidity and fetal macrosomia as subjects diagnosed by the National Diabetes Data Group Criteria.[99] With either set of criteria, the patient must have a normal fasting value and two abnormal postprandial glucose determinations to be designated as class A_1. In a patient who demonstrates a normal OGTT despite significant risk factors, including obesity, advanced maternal age, or a previous history of GDM, a repeat test may be performed at 32 to 34 weeks' gestation.

The criteria used to establish the diagnosis of GDM are based on the data of O'Sullivan et al,[100] who examined the likelihood of subsequent development of overt diabetes mellitus. As these criteria are unrelated to pregnancy outcome, there remains a need to better define the level of glycemia that poses a risk for fetal and neonatal complications such as macrosomia. Tallarigo et al[101] have suggested that subtle degrees of maternal hyperglycemia, levels below those that would classify an individual as a gestational diabetic, can have a detrimental effect on perinatal outcome. In their study, women with a 2-hour plasma glucose value between 120 and 165 mg/dl (6.7 and 9.2 mmol/L) during a 3-hour OGTT were more likely to have a macrosomic infant than were women with lower 2-hour values. Women with an abnormal 50-g screening value and normal 3-hour OGTT may also be more likely to produce a large infant when controlling for factors such as obesity.[102] Similarly, women who demonstrate one abnormal value on the diagnostic 3-hour GTT are at apparent increased risk for fetal macrosomia.[103] Langer and colleagues[103] prefer to identify and treat such patients as GDM. Other authors have suggested repeating the GTT later in pregnancy in women who initially demonstrate one abnormal value and reserving the diagnosis for women with two subsequent abnormal values. In a study of 106 women with one abnormal GTT value at approximately 30 weeks' gestation and in whom the GTT was repeated 1 month later, 34 percent developed gestational diabetes.[104]

Treatment of the Insulin-Dependent Patient

As fetal glucose levels reflect those of the mother, it is not surprising that clinical efforts aimed at optimizing maternal control are considered paramount in the decline in perinatal death seen in IDDM pregnancies over the last few decades.[44] Self-monitoring of blood glucose levels combined with aggressive insulin therapy has made the maintenance of maternal normoglycemia (levels of 60 to 120 mg/dl) a therapeutic reality (Table 31-5). In most institutions, patients are taught to monitor their glucose control using glucose-oxidase impregnated reagent strips and a glucose reflectance meter.[105]

To achieve the best glycemic control possible for each patient, during pregnancy conventional insulin therapy often needs to be abandoned in favor of intensive therapy. Insulin regimens have classically included one to two injections of insulin usually prior to breakfast and the evening meal, complimented by self-monitoring of blood glucose level and adjustment of insulin dose according to glucose profiles. Patients are instructed on dietary composition, insulin action, recognition and treatment of hypoglycemia, adjusting insulin dosage for exercise and sick days, as well as monitoring for hyperglycemia and potential ketosis. These principles form the foundation for intensive insulin therapy in which an attempts is made to simulate physiologic insulin requirements. Insulin administration is provided for both basal needs and meals, and rapid adjustments are made in response to glucose measurements. The treatment regimen often involves three to four daily injections or the use of continuous subcutaneous infusion devices. With either approach, frequent self-monitoring of blood glucose is fundamental to achieve the therapeutic objective of physiologic glucose control. Glucose determinations are made in the fasting state and before lunch, dinner, and bedtime.

Table 31-5. Target Plasma Glucose Levels in Pregnancy

Time	mg/dl
Before breakfast	60–90
Before lunch, supper, bedtime snack	60–105
Two hours after meals	≤ 120
2 a.m. to 6 a.m.	> 60

Postprandial and nocturnal values are also helpful. Patients are instructed on an insulin dose for each meal and at bedtime if necessary. Meal-time insulin needs are determined by the composition of the meal, the premeal glucose measurement, and the level of activity anticipated following the meal. Basal or intermediate acting insulin requirements are determined by periodic 2 A.M. to 4 A.M. glucose measurements as well as late afternoon values that reflect morning Neutral Protamine Hagedorn or lente action. During pregnancy, many diabetic women develop the self-management skills that are essential to an intensive insulin therapy regimen.

For patients who are not well controlled, a brief period of hospitalization is often necessary for the initiation of therapy. Individual adjustments to the regimens implemented can then be made. It is gratifying for many patients to take charge of their own diabetic control. Women who have previously followed a prescribed dosage regimen for years gain confidence in making adjustments in their insulin dosage after a short period of time. Patients are encouraged to contact their physician at any time if questions should arise concerning the management of their diabetes. During early pregnancy, patients are instructed to report their glucose values by telephone on a minimum weekly basis.

Insulin therapy must be individualized with dosage determinations tailored to diet and exercise. Beef and pork insulin have largely been replaced by semisynthetic human insulin preparations. Since human insulin is far less immunogenic than animal insulin, it is preferred for pregnant women and especially for those receiving insulin for the first time. Human insulin may have a more rapid onset and shorter duration of action, factors that must be considered when changing patients to these preparations.

Insulin is generally administered in two to three injections. We prefer a three-injection regimen, although most patients present taking a combination of intermediate acting and regular insulin before dinner and breakfast. As a general rule, the amount of intermediate acting insulin will exceed the regular component by a two-to-one ratio. Patients usually receive two-thirds of their total dose with breakfast and the remaining third in the evening as a combined dose with dinner or split into components with regular insulin at dinner time and then intermediate acting insulin at bedtime in an effort to minimize periods of nocturnal hypoglycemia. These episodes frequently occur when the mother is in a relative fasting state while placental and fetal glucose consumptions continue. Finally, some women may require a small dose of regular insulin before lunch, thus constituting a four-injection daily regimen.

There has now been considerable experience with open-loop continuous subcutaneous insulin infusion pump therapy during pregnancy. The pump is a battery-powered unit that can be worn during most daily activities like a beeper. These systems provide continuous short-acting insulin therapy via a subcutaneous infusion. The basal infusion rate and bolus doses to cover meals are determined by frequent self-monitoring of blood glucose level. The basal infusion rate is generally close to 1 unit per hour.

Pregnant patients will often require hospitalization before initiation of pump therapy. Women must be educated regarding the strategy of continuous infusion and have their glucose levels stabilized over several days. This requires that multiple blood glucose determinations be made for the prevention of periods of hyper- and hypoglycemia. Glucose values may become normalized with minimal amplitude of daily excursions in most patients.

Episodes of hypoglycemia are not uncommon with pump therapy. These are usually secondary to errors in dose selection or failure to adhere to the required diet. The risk of nocturnal hypoglycemia, which is increased in the pregnant state, necessitates that great care be undertaken in selecting patients for pump therapy. Patients who fail to exhibit normal counterregulatory responses to hypoglycemia should probably be discouraged from using an insulin pump.

The mechanics of the continuous subcutaneous insulin infusion pump systems are relatively simple. A fine-gauge butterfly needle device is attached by connecting tubing to the pump. This cannula is reimplanted every 2 to 3 days at a different site in the anterior abdominal wall. Short acting (regular insulin) is stored in the pump syringe. Infusion occurs at a basal rate, which can be fixed or altered for specific time of day by a computer program. For example, the basal rate can be programmed for a lower dose at night. Similarly, preprandial boluses can be delivered manually or by computer preset. Half of the total daily insulin is usually given as the basal rate and the remainder as premeal boluses infused 15 to 45 minutes before each meal. The largest bolus (30 to 35 percent) is administered with breakfast, followed by 25 percent before dinner and 15 to 20 percent before snacks.

Patients without any pancreatic reserve may have rapid elevations in blood glucose level if there is pump failure or intercurrent infection. Since the advent of buffered insulin, insulin aggregation leading to occlusion of the silastic infusion tubing is uncommon. Failure of the pump is associated with a steady rise in ketonemia in the nonpregnant patient. Initial experience with insulin pumps suggested a high risk for ketoacidosis with pump failure or intercurrent infection. The necessity of using continuous infusion pumps to achieve glycemic control has been challenged. In the largest study of pregnant women, Coustan and colleagues[106] randomized 22 patients to intensive conventional therapy with multiple injections versus pump therapy. There were no differences between the two treatment groups with respect to outpatient mean glucose levels, glycosylated hemoglobin levels, or glycemic excursions.

To summarize, the limitations of pump therapy outlined above as well as the complications of this method have decreased enthusiasm for its use during pregnancy. Additionally, serious concern exists regarding abrupt initiation of tight glycemic control in nonpregnant patients beginning pump therapy that may adversely affect established diabetic retinopathy. In the Ohio State University Diabetes in Pregnancy Program, over the last 9 years we have found it necessary to institute pump therapy to achieve good glycemic control in only one patient. It must be appreciated that pump therapy does not guarantee improved glucoregulation. However, it is recommended that women who have demonstrated good glycemic control using continuous infusion devices prior to pregnancy be maintained on this therapy.

Diet therapy is critical to successful regulation of maternal diabetes. A program consisting of three meals and several snacks is employed for most patients. Dietary composition should be 50 to 60 percent carbohydrate, 20 percent protein, and 25 to 30 percent fat with less than 10 percent saturated fats, up to 10 percent polyunsaturated fatty acids, and the remainder derived from monosaturated sources.[107] Caloric intake is established based on prepregnancy weight and weight gain during gestation. Weight reduction is not advised. Patients should consume approximately 35 Kcal/kg ideal body weight. Obese women may be managed with an intake as low at 1,600 calories per day, although if ketonuria develops this allowance may be increased.

The presence of maternal vasculopathy should be thoroughly assessed early in pregnancy. The patient should be evaluated by an ophthalmologist familiar with diabetic retinopathy. Ophthalmologic examinations are performed during each trimester and repeated more often if retinopathy is detected. Baseline renal function is established by assaying a 24-hour urine collection for creatinine clearance and protein. An electrocardiogram and urine culture are also obtained.

Most patients with IDDM are followed with outpatient visits at 1 to 2 week intervals. At each visit, control is assessed and adjustments in insulin dosage are made. However, patients should be instructed to call at any time if periods of hypoglycemia (< 50 mg/dl) or hyperglycemia (> 200 mg/dl) occur. The increased risk of hypoglycemia in pregnant individuals may be related to defective glucose counterregulatory hormone mechanisms.[108] Both epinephrine and glucagon appear to be suppressed in pregnant diabetic women during hypoglycemia.[108] For these reasons, family members should be instructed on the technique of glucagon injection for the treatment of severe reactions.

Ketoacidosis

With the implementation of antenatal care, programs stressing strict metabolic control of blood glucose levels for insulin-dependent women, diabetic ketoacidosis has fortunately become a less common occurrence. Kilvert and colleagues[109] reported 11 cases of ketoacidosis in 635 insulin-treated pregnancies between 1971 and 1990. One fetal loss and one spontaneous miscarriage complicated the pregnancies affected by diabetic ketoacidosis.[109]

Diabetic ketoacidosis can occur in the newly diagnosed diabetic patient, and the hormonal milieu of pregnancy may become the background for this phenomenon. As pregnancy is a state of relative insulin resistance marked by enhanced lipolysis and ketogenesis, diabetic ketoacidosis may develop in a pregnant woman with glucose levels barely exceeding 200 mg/dl (11.1 mmol/L). Thus, diabetic ketoacidosis may be diagnosed during pregnancy with minimal hyperglycemia accompanied by a fall in plasma bicarbonate and a pH value less than 7.30. Serum acetone is positive at a 1:2 dilution.

Early recognition of signs and symptoms of diabetic ketoacidosis will improve both maternal and fetal outcome. As in the nonpregnant state, clinical signs of volume depletion follow the symptoms of hyperglycemia, which include polydipsia and polyuria. Malaise, headache, nausea, and vomiting are common complaints. Occasionally, diabetic ketoacidosis may present in an undiagnosed diabetic woman receiving β-mimetic agents to arrest preterm labor. Because of the risk of hyperglycemia and diabetic ketoacidosis in insulin-dependent women receiving intravenous medications such as a ritodrine, magnesium sulfate has become the preferred tocolytic for preterm labor in these cases.

Once the diagnosis of diabetic ketoacidosis is established and the patient is stabilized, she should be transported to a facility where tertiary care in both perinatology and neonatology is available. Therapy hinges on the meticulous correction of metabolic and fluid abnormalities. An attempt to treat any underlying cause for ketoacidosis, such as infection, should be instituted as well. The general management of diabetic ketoacidosis in pregnancy is outlined in the box below . Diabetic ketoacidosis does represent a substantial risk for fetal compromise. However, successful fetal resuscitation will often accompany correction of maternal acidosis. Every effort should therefore be made to correct mater-

Management of Diabetic Ketoacidosis During Pregnancy

1. Laboratory assessment
   Obtain arterial blood gases to document degree of acidosis present; measure glucose, ketones, electrolytes, at 1 to 2 hours intervals
2. Insulin
   Low dose, intravenous (IV)
   Loading dose: 0.2–0.4 units/kg
   Maintenance: 2.0–10.0 units/h
3. Fluids
   Isotonic NaCl
   Total replacement in first 12 hours = 4–6 L
   1 L in first hour
   500–1,000 ml/h for 2–4 hours
   250 ml/h until 80% replaced
4. Glucose
   Begin 5% D/NS^a when plasma level reaches 250 mg/dl (14 mmol/L)
5. Potassium
   If initially normal or reduced, an infusion rate up to 15–20 mEq/h may be required; if elevated, wait until levels decline into the normal range, then add to IV solution in a concentration of 20–30 mEq/L
6. Bicarbonate
   Add one ampule (44 mEq) to 1 L of 0.45 NS if pH is <7.10

^{a} D/NS, Dextrose in normal saline.

nal condition before intervening and delivering a preterm infant.

Antepartum Fetal Evaluation

Over the past 15 years, protocols for antepartum fetal assessment in pregnancies complicated by diabetes mellitus have shifted the focus of care during the third trimester to an outpatient setting. During this time period, when the risk of sudden intrauterine death increases, a program of fetal surveillance is initiated. The improved understanding of the importance of maternal control in relation to fetal outcome has played a major role in reducing perinatal mortality in diabetic pregnancies. Therefore, antepartum fetal monitoring tests have been used primarily to reassure the obstetrician and avoid unnecessary premature intervention. These techniques have few false-negatives results, and, in a patient who is well controlled and exhibits no vascu-

lopathy or significant hypertension, reassuring antepartum testing allows the fetus to benefit from further maturation in utero.

Maternal assessment of fetal activity serves as a screening technique in a program of fetal surveillance. To date, few studies have applied this method to a large number of women with diabetes mellitus. Patients with a variety of high-risk antepartum conditions including diabetes appear to have an increased incidence of alarming fetal activity patterns.[110] While the false-negative rate with maternal monitoring of fetal activity is low (about 1 percent), the false-positive rate may be as high as 60 percent. Maternal hypoglycemia, while generally believed to be associated with decreased fetal movement, may actually stimulate fetal activity.[111]

Sadovsky and coworkers[112] reported that fetal movement at 25 to 33 weeks' gestation in 67 diabetic pregnancies was lower than in controls, while in the final 2 months of pregnancy activity levels were similar to those in the nondiabetic population. In this series, there were four cases of cessation of fetal movement. Two fetuses died in utero 10 and 11 hours after maternal perception that activity had stopped, an interval shorter than that seen in other complications of pregnancy.

The nonstress test (NST) has become the preferred method to assess antepartum fetal well-being in the patient with diabetes mellitus.[113] If the NST is nonreactive, a contraction stress test (CST) or biophysical profile (BPP) is then performed (Fig. 31-5). Heart rate monitoring is begun early in the third trimester, usually by 32 weeks' gestation. Barrett et al[114] documented 6 antepartum deaths in 425 patients having weekly tests, a significantly greater fetal death rate than in other high-risk pregnancies. Other studies have also demonstrated an increased fetal death rate within 1 week of a reactive NST in pregnancies complicated by IDDM when compared with other high-risk gestations.[115] If the NST is to be used as the primary method of antepartum heart rate testing, we prefer that it be done at least twice weekly once the patient reaches 32 weeks' gestation. In patients with vascular disease or poor control, in whom the incidence of abnormal tests and intrauterine deaths is greater, testing is often performed earlier and more frequently.

The fetal BPP rather than the CST is often employed to evaluate the significance of a nonreactive NST result. In a series of diabetic women, Golde and colleagues[116] observed that 430 of 434 BPPs performed after a reactive NST were associated with reassuring scores of 8 or greater. Of 25 BPPs performed after a nonreactive NST result, 21 had scores of 8, and 4 had lower scores. In this series, even patients with low scores had good perinatal outcomes. The BPP did not appear to add more information about fetal condition if the NST result was reac-

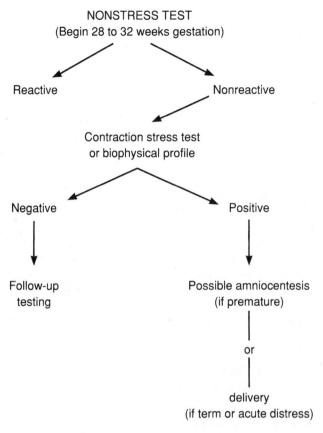

NONSTRESS TEST
(Begin 28 to 32 weeks gestation)

Reactive   Nonreactive

Contraction stress test
or biophysical profile

Negative   Positive

Follow-up
testing

Possible amniocentesis
(if premature)

or

delivery
(if term or acute distress)

Fig. 31-5 Scheme for antepartum fetal testing in pregnancy complicated by diabetes mellitus.

tive, but a score of 8 based on ultrasound parameters was as reliable in predicting good fetal outcome as was a reactive NST. In a study of 98 patients, Dicker and colleagues[117] confirmed that a normal BPP predicts normal Apgar scores in 99 percent of patients. In their series, only 2.9 percent of 978 BPPs were abnormal. Importantly, a total of 10 patients had an abnormal BPP just before delivery. In six of these cases, neonatal asphyxia or depression was present. Unfortunately, these authors did not describe the metabolic status of their patients.

Johnson and associates[118] have also described their experience with the BPP in diabetic women. These authors performed twice-weekly tests in 50 women with insulin-dependent diabetes and weekly examinations in 188 women with GDM. There were no stillbirths in this series. The incidence of abnormal BPPs was low—only 8 of 238 tests (3.3 percent). The 230 fetuses with a normal score before delivery experienced minimal morbidity. In contrast, of 8 patients with an abnormal score, 37.5 percent suffered significant neonatal morbidity. Although this study did not demonstrate the superiority of the BPP over the NST alone, it did establish that the BPP may also be used for fetal surveillance with few unnecessary interventions, thereby allowing

prolongation of pregnancy beyond 37 weeks in most of the patients studied.

Doppler umbilical artery velocimetry has been proposed as a clinical tool for antepartum fetal surveillance in pregnancies at risk for placental vascular disease. We have found that Doppler studies of the umbilical artery may be predictive of fetal outcome in diabetic pregnancies complicated by vascular disease.[119] Elevated placental resistance as evidenced by an increased systolic-diastolic ratio is associated with fetal growth restriction and preeclampsia in these high-risk patients.[119] In contrast, well-controlled patients without vascular disease rarely demonstrate abnormal fetal umbilical artery waveforms.

Recently, Johnstone and colleagues[120] reported their experience with serial Doppler umbilical waveforms in 128 pregnancies complicated by diabetes. Significant abnormal flow patterns were observed in 9 cases. Three of these woman had nephropathy and three preeclampsia. All of these pregnancies had normal outcomes. Importantly, several cases of fetal distress as defined by abnormal biophysical testing were accompanied by normal Doppler studies. Therefore, it appears that undue reliance should *not* be placed on normal waveform values in the diabetic pregnancy.[120]

It is important not only to include the results of antepartum fetal testing but also to weigh all the clinical features involving mother and fetus before a decision is made to intervene for suspected fetal distress, especially if this decision may result in a preterm delivery (Tables 31-6 and 31-7). In reviewing nine series involving 993 diabetic patients, an abnormal test of fetal condition led to delivery 5 percent of the time.[121] It appears that outpatient testing protocols work well in insulin-dependent patients. Whether such testing is required for all patients with IDDM remains controversial.[122] Certainly those women whose diabetes is poorly controlled, who have hypertension, or who have significant vasculopathy that may be associated with fetal growth restriction require a program of antepartum fetal surveillance.

Ultrasound is an extremely valuable tool in evaluating fetal growth, estimating fetal weight, and detecting hydramnios and malformations. A determination of maternal serum α-fetoprotein level at 16 weeks' gestation should be employed in association with a detailed ultrasound study at 18 weeks in an attempt to detect neural tube defects and other anomalies. Normal values of maternal α-fetoprotein for diabetic women are lower than for the nondiabetic population.[123] A lower threshold for the upper limit of normal may thus be preferable in pregnancies complicated by diabetes mellitus in order to help detect spina bifida and other major malformations that are increased in this population. Fetal echocardiography is performed at 20 to 22

Table 31-6.   Antepartum Fetal Surveillance in Low-Risk Insulin-Dependent Diabetes Mellitus[a]

Study	
Ultrasonography at 4–6 week intervals	Yes
Maternal assessment of fetal activity, daily at 28 weeks	Yes
Nonstress test (NST) weekly at 28 weeks	Yes
	Twice weekly at 34 weeks
Contraction stress test or biophysical profile if NST nonreactive, L/S, lung profile	Yes, if elective delivery planned prior to 39 weeks

[a] Low-risk IDDM: excellent control (60–120 mg/dl), no vasculopathy (classes B, C), no stillbirth.

weeks' gestation for the investigation of possible cardiac anomalies. Using such an approach, Greene and Benacerral[124] detected 18 of 32 malformations in a series of 432 diabetic pregnancies. The specificity was in excess of 99 percent, and the negative predictive value was 97 percent. Spina bifida was identified in all cases; however, ventricular septal defects, limb abnormalities, and facial clefts were missed. A review of the prenatal diagnosis experience in 289 IDDM women in The Ohio State University Diabetes in Pregnancy Program revealed 29 anomalies in which 12 were cardiac, 14 were noncardiac, and 3 were combined.[19] Twelve of 15 (80 percent) cardiac and 10 of 17 (59 percent) noncardiac lesions were identified prenatally. When considering cardiac defects alone, we could not identify a glycosylated hemoglobin cut-off for these anomalies. Therefore, we believe detailed cardiac imaging should be offered to all IDDM women to assist in the detection of cardiac lesions, especially those of the great vessels and cardiac septum.

Ultrasound examinations should be repeated at 4 to 6 week intervals to assess fetal growth. The detection of fetal macrosomia, the leading risk factor for shoulder dystocia, is important in the selection of patients who are best managed by cesarean delivery. An increased rate of cephalopelvic disproportion and shoulder dystocia accompanied by significant risk of traumatic birth injury and asphyxia have been consistently associated with the vaginal delivery of large infants. The risk of such complications rises exponentially when birth weight exceeds 4 kg and is greater for the fetus of a diabetic mother than for the fetus with similar weight whose mother does not have diabetes.[125] Sonographic

measurements of the fetal abdominal circumference have proved most helpful in predicting fetal macrosomia.[126] The abdomen is likely to be large because of increased glycogen deposition in the fetal liver and subcutaneous fat deposition. Using serial sonographic examinations, accelerated abdominal growth can be identified by 32 weeks' gestation.[127] Subcutaneous fat stores may also be estimated by upper arm fetal soft tissue measurements made during the third trimester of gestation. This measurement is sensitive for detecting macrosomia in the IDM and may distinguish the asymmetrically large fetus of a diabetic mother from symmetrically large fetuses.[128]

Timing and Mode of Delivery

Delivery should be delayed until fetal maturation has taken place, provided that the patient's diabetes is well controlled and antepartum surveillance remains normal. In our practice, elective induction of labor is often planned at 38 to 40 weeks' gestation in well-controlled patients without vascular disease. Patients with vascular disease are delivered prior to term only if hypertension worsens or fetal growth restriction mandates early delivery. Before elective delivery prior to 39 weeks' gestation, an amniocentesis may be performed to document fetal pulmonary maturity. Although the value of the lecithinsphingomyelin (L/S) ratio has been questioned in pregnancies complicated by diabetes mellitus, as mentioned earlier, many series report a low incidence of respiratory distress syndrome is observed with a mature ratio of 2.0 or greater (Table 31-8).[56]

The presence of the acidic phospholipid phosphati-

Table 31-7.   Antepartum Fetal Surveillance In High-Risk Insulin-Dependent Diabetes Mellitus[a]

Study	
Ultrasonography at 4–6-week intervals	Yes
Maternal assessment of fetal activity, daily at 28 weeks	Yes
Nonstress test (NST)	Minimum twice weekly
Contraction stress test or biophysical profile if NST nonreactive, L/S, lung profile at 37–38 weeks	Yes

[a] High-risk IDDM: poor control (macrosomia, hydramnios), vasculopathy (classes D, F, R), prior stillbirth.

Table 31-8. Frequency of RDS in Diabetic Pregnancy
(Mature L/S Ratio)

Author	M	RDS
Gabbe et al[174]	210	3 (3%)
Tabsh et al[175]	77	3 (1.5%)
Dudley and Black[55]	104	0 (0)
Amon et al[176]	24	0 (0)
Kjos and Walther[56]	493	0 (0)

dylglycerol (PG) is the final marker of fetal pulmonary maturation. Several authors have suggested that fetal hyperinsulinemia may be associated with delayed appearance of PG and an increased incidence of respiratory distress syndrome. Landon et al[45] have correlated the appearance of PG in AF with maternal glycemic control during gestation. Respiratory distress syndrome may occur in the IDM with a mature L/S ratio but absent PG. Caution should be used, therefore, in planning the delivery of patients with an L/S ratio of 2.0 and absent PG. Most important, the clinician must be familiar with the laboratory analysis of AF in his or her institution and the neonatal outcome for the IDM at various L/S ratios in the presence or absence of PG.

When antepartum testing suggests fetal compromise, delivery must be considered. If AF analysis yields a mature L/S ratio, delivery should be accomplished promptly. In the presence of an immature L/S ratio, the decision to proceed with delivery should be based on confirmation of deteriorating fetal condition by several abnormal tests. For example, if the NST and the CST indicate fetal compromise, delivery is indicated. Finally, there remain several maternal indications for delivery, including preeclampsia, worsening renal function, or deteriorating vision secondary to proliferative retinopathy.

The route of delivery for the diabetic patient remains controversial. Cousins,[129] in reviewing over 1,600 (White classes B, C, D, and R) patients in the literature between 1965 and 1985, noted a cesarean delivery rate of approximately 45 percent. This figure is likely to represent the practice trends of most US obstetricians and perinatologists.[113] Cesarean delivery usually is favored when fetal distress has been suggested by antepartum heart rate monitoring. If a patient reaches 38 weeks' gestation with a mature fetal lung profile and is at significant risk for intrauterine demise because of poor control or a history of a prior stillbirth, an elective delivery is planned. Elective cesarean delivery is performed if the cervix is not favorable for induction or if the infant is believed to be macrosomic.

During labor, continuous fetal heart rate monitoring is mandatory. Labor is allowed to progress as long as normal rates of cervical dilatation and descent are doc-umented. Acker et al[125] have reported that the overall risk for shoulder dystocia in the macrosomic IDM is greater than for the large, normal infant. In their series of diabetic women, the risk for shoulder dystocia with a fetal weight greater than 4,000 g was approximately 30 percent. Despite attempts to select patients with obvious fetal macrosomia for elective cesarean delivery, arrest of dilatation or descent should alert the physician to the possibility of cephalopelvic disproportion. About 25 percent of macrosomic infants (≥4,000 g) delivered after a prolonged second stage will have shoulder dystocia.[130] It follows that cesarean delivery is preferred for a patient who demonstrates significant protracted labor or failure of descent.

Glucoregulation During Labor and Delivery

As neonatal hypoglycemia is in part related to maternal glucose levels during labor, it is important to maintain maternal plasma glucose levels at approximately 100 mg/dl. The patient is given nothing by mouth after midnight of the evening before induction or elective cesarean delivery. The usual bedtime dose of insulin is administered. Upon arrival to labor and delivery, early in the morning the patient's capillary glucose level is assessed with a bedside reflectance meter. Continuous infusion of both insulin and glucose are then administered based on maternal glucose levels.) Ten units of

---

Insulin Management During Labor and Delivery

Usual dose of intermediate acting insulin is given at bedtime.

Morning dose of insulin is withheld.

Intravenous infusion of normal saline is begun.

Once active labor begins or glucose levels fall below 70 mg/dl, the infusion is changed from saline to 5 percent dextrose and delivered at a rate of 2.5 mg/kg/min.

Glucose levels are checked hourly using a portable reflectance meter allowing for adjustment in the infusion rate.

Regular (short acting) insulin is administered by intravenous infusion if glucose levels exceed 140 mg/dl.

(Adapted from Jovanovic and Peterson,[46] with permission.)

regular insulin may be added to 1,000 ml of solution containing 5 percent dextrose. An infusion rate of 100 to 125 ml/h (1 unit/h) will, in most cases, result in good glucose control. Insulin may also be infused from a syringe pump at a dose of 0.25 to 2.0 units/h and adjusted to maintain normal glucose values. Glucose levels are recorded hourly, and the infusion rate is adjusted accordingly. Jovanovic and Peterson[131] have noted that well-controlled patients will often be euglycemic once active labor begins and will then require glucose at an infusion rate of 2.5 mg/kg/min. It may be necessary to increase the insulin infusion during the second stage of labor with increased catecholamine secretion.

When cesarean delivery is to be performed, it should be scheduled for early morning. This simplifies intrapartum glucose control and allows the neonatal team to prepare for the care of the newborn. The patient is given nothing by mouth, and her usual morning insulin dose is withheld. If her surgery is not performed early in the day, one-third to one-half of the patient's intermediate acting dose of insulin may be administered. Epidural anesthesia is preferred because an awake patient permits earlier detection of hypoglycemia. Following surgery, glucose levels are monitored every 2 hours and an intravenous solution of 5 percent dextrose is administered.

Following delivery, insulin requirements are usually significantly lower than were pregnancy or prepregnancy needs. The objective of "tight control" used in the antepartum period is relaxed, and glucose values of 150 to 200 mg/dl are acceptable. Patients delivered vaginally who are able to eat a regular diet are given one-third to one-half of their end of pregnancy dose of neutral protamine Hagedorn (NPH) insulin the morning of the first postpartum day. Frequent glucose determinations are used to guide insulin dosage. If the patient has been given supplemental regular insulin in addition to the morning NPH dose, the amount of NPH insulin on the following morning is increased in an amount equal to two-thirds of the additional regular insulin. Most patients are stabilized on this regimen within a few days after delivery.

Women with diabetes are encouraged to breast-feed. The additional 500 kcal required daily are given as approximately 100 g of carbohydrate and 20 g of protein.[132] The insulin dose may be somewhat lower in lactating diabetic women. Hypoglycemia appears to be common in the first week following delivery and immediately after nursing.

Management of the Patient with GDM

The mainstay of treatment of GDM is nutritional counseling and dietary intervention. The optimal diet should provide caloric and nutrient needs to sustain pregnancy without resulting in significant postprandial hyperglycemia.[133] Women with GDM generally do not need hospitalization for dietary instruction and management. Once the diagnosis is established, patients are begun on a dietary program of 2,000 to 2,500 kcal daily.[132] This represents approximately 35 kcal/kg present pregnancy weight. Jovanovic-Peterson and Peterson[134] have noted that such a diet composed of 50 to 60 percent carbohydrate will cause excessive weight gain and postprandial hyperglycemia and 50 percent of patients will require insulin therapy.

For this reason, several groups have studied the use of calorie-restricted diets. Algert and colleagues[135] have reported that obese women with GDM may be managed on as little as 1,700 to 1,800 kcal/day with less weight gain and no apparent reduction in fetal size. Magee et al[136] designed a study to evaluate strict caloric restriction as a treatment for obese subjects with GDM. They randomized patients to a 2,400 kcal/d diet compared to a 1,200 kcal/d group. Average glucose levels and fasting insulin levels were reduced in the hypocaloric group. However, fasting glucose levels and post-challenge glucose levels were not significantly different. Significant ketonuria did develop in the restricted group, which may have a detrimental effect on fetal neurologic development. The authors thus went on to study a 1,800 kcal diet, which improved glycemia and did not increase serum ketone levels.[137] Similar results have been reported by Jovanovic-Peterson and Peterson,[138] who recommend 30 kcal/kg present pregnant weight for normal weight women, 24 kcal/kg for overweight women, and 12 kcal/kg for morbidity obese women. These authors indicate that moderate caloric restriction with modification of the carbohydrate component may be advised in obese GDM women.

Once the patient with GDM is placed on an appropriate diet, surveillance of blood glucose levels is necessary to be certain that good glycemic control has been established. At a minimum, practitioners have performed weekly assessment of fasting or postprandial glucose levels or both at clinic or office visits. Some clinicians prefer to have patients perform daily self-monitoring of blood glucose level, which in two retrospective studies has been associated with a decline in macrosomia at the expense of nearly half of all women requiring insulin therapy.[139] A practical approach may be to provide women with GDM with a reflectance meter; however, if after a few weeks both fasting and postprandial measurements are within the normal range, the frequency of testing can be reduced accordingly.

Both ADA and ACOG have recommended that fasting plasma glucose levels be maintained below 105 mg/dl and 2-hour postprandial values be less than 120 mg/dl in women with GDM. If a patient repetitively exceeds these thresholds, then insulin therapy is suggested. The use of the above cut-offs for initiating insulin are based on data regarding increased perinatal morbidity when such values are exceeded in women with pre-existing diabetes. However, are these thresholds appropriate for instituting insulin in women with GDM?

In a national survey of both perinatologists and maternal–fetal subspecialists, only 50 percent followed ACOG recommendations, whereas 50 percent of care providers used higher or lower threshold criteria.[113] The recommended postprandial value of 120 mg/dl was applied by only 22 percent of those surveyed, indicating that a wide degree of variation exists in practice with regard to insulin therapy for GDM.

Langer et al[140] have critically evaluated thresholds for insulin therapy in GDM and concluded that to evaluate the effect of therapy appropriate endpoints should include fetal macrosomia or LGA infants and neonatal metabolic complications. Langer and colleagues[142] evaluated insulin secretion patterns in women with GDM and non-GDM during an OGTT. Patients with fasting plasma glucose less than 95 mg/dl had significantly greater insulin production than those with a glucose level greater than or equal to 95 mg/dl. To test whether the assignment to insulin therapy for a patient with a fasting value of 95 mg/dl or higher was appropriate, Langer et al[140] compared rates of delivery of LGA infants among women with GDM grouped according to their fasting plasma glucose levels and whether diet or diet and insulin were used. He found that patients with a fasting glucose level between 96 and 105 mg/dl had a greater incidence of LGA infants (28.6 percent) when receiving diet therapy alone versus obese women with GDM receiving both diet and insulin.

Whereas Langer and coworkers[140] have documented a relationship between maternal glycemia and macrosomia in GDM, which would establish guidelines for insulin therapy, some authors have suggested that estimation of glycemia alone may be insufficient to prescribe insulin therapy optimally in these cases. Coustan and Imrah[143] reported that prophylactic insulin given to women who would normally be treated by diet alone may also reduce the frequency of macrosomia, cesarean delivery, and birth trauma. It has been suggested that insulin may reduce maternal levels of other fetal insulin secretagogues such as branched chain amino acids. Other studies have also suggested a potential role for prophylactic insulin therapy in obese GDM, although the lack of glucose surveillance data have failed to establish whether insulin was truly prophylactic in these cases. A recent study of 102 women with GDM treated to achieve a 1-hour postprandial glucose level of less than 130 mg/dl, in essence a prophylactic insulin regimen, reduced morbidity in the offspring to control

rates, but insulin was required in 86 percent of women.[143] In a well-designed prospective randomized study, Persson et al[145] noted similar rates of neonatal macrosomia and skinfold thickness amount, diet, and diet plus insulin-treated women with GDM. Until large prospective randomized studies indicate the benefit of prophylactic insulin, insulin should be reserved for women who demonstrate significant fasting or postprandial hyperglycemia.

In addition to aggressive insulin therapy and hypocaloric diet regimens, exercise has recently been studied as an alternative primary treatment for GDM. Such an approach is beneficial for noninsulin-dependent nonpregnant diabetic patients in whom physical training increases insulin sensitivity. Fasting and postprandial insulin concentrations and glucose excursions are lowered in both obese and physically fit individuals who exercise. This effect apparently is sustained up to 5 to 7 days after the last training session.

Jovanovic-Peterson and colleagues[146] have studied exercise in regimens in women with GDM and concluded that a rowing arm ergometer is associated with the fewest complications such as maternal hypotension and excessive uterine activity. These investigators randomized 20 women with GDM into two groups: one group receiving intensive dietary therapy and the other group receiving similar therapy in addition to a supervised arm ergometry exercise regimen of three times per week for 20 minutes over a period of 6 weeks. Glycemic levels were significantly different between the two groups by week 4 of the study. By week 6, the post-50-g challenge glucose levels in the exercise-plus-diet group were 106 ± 19.8 mg/dl compared with 187 ± 2.90 mg/dl in the diet intervention group. Fasting glucose levels were also lower in the exercise group, reflecting enhancement of insulin action on hepatic glucose production.

Bung and colleagues[147] also conducted a prospective study of the utility of exercise in the treatment of GDM. These authors randomized 41 women with GDM who manifested elevated fasting glucose levels, which would normally require insulin therapy. In the final analysis, 17 women completed a supervised bicycle ergometry training program compared with 17 women receiving insulin treatment. No statistical differences were observed in weekly blood glucose determinations between study groups. All fetal heart rate patterns were reactive before and after exercise. Thus exercise programs for the treatment of GDM appear to be safe and may obviate the need for insulin therapy in some individuals.

Patients with GDM who are well controlled are at low risk for an intrauterine death. For this reason, we do not routinely institute antepartum fetal heart rate testing in uncomplicated diet-controlled GDM patients unless the patient has a hypertensive disorder or a history of a prior stillbirth.[148] Women who require insulin treatment of GDM undergo twice-weekly heart rate testing at 32 weeks' gestation. Using such a protocol at The Ohio State University Hospital Diabetes in Pregnancy Program, only two intrauterine deaths in over 1,000 uncomplicated GDM have been observed in the last 9 years. Thus, it appears that the third-trimester stillbirth rate in these patients is no higher than that of the general obstetric population. A recent study of 389 women with GDM documented an antepartum stillbirth rate of 7.7 per 1,000, which was not significantly different from the rate of 4.8 per 1,000 observed in nondiabetic low-risk patients.[149] In this study, because 7 percent of fetuses were delivered on the basis of a low BPP score, the benefit of testing all GDM pregnancies remains in question. Without a large prospective study comparing outcomes in monitored and nonmonitored GDM women without other risk factors, it is not possible to determine if any benefit exists to antepartum fetal surveillance in this seemingly low-risk population. Instituting a program of fetal surveillance once these pregnancies reach 40 weeks' gestation does, however, seem prudent.

Because many obstetricians have extrapolated the increased risk for stillbirth in IDDM women to those with GDM, a remarkable number of these pregnancies are subject to scheduled delivery at term. If glycemic control is suboptimal, or maternal hypertension or a previous stillbirth exists, such an approach seems warranted. As with antepartum fetal testing, should elective induction be the standard approach for uncomplicated GDM pregnancies? Lurie and coworkers[150] have in part addressed this issue by retrospectively comparing the outcomes of 124 GDM women delivered beyond 40 weeks' gestation with the same number of GDM women delivered before their expected date of confinement. Antepartum fetal surveillance was not routinely begun until 40 weeks' gestation. No significant differences in perinatal outcome, cesarean delivery rates, or shoulder dystocia were found between study groups. A vaginal delivery rate of 75.8 percent was achieved in GDM women delivering beyond 40 weeks' gestation. These authors concluded that elective induction before 40 week's gestation should be avoided, and every attempt should be made to allow women with GDM, both diet and insulin treated, to proceed to spontaneous labor.

Kjos and colleagues[151] have conducted a prospective randomized trial of active induction of labor at 38 weeks' gestation versus expectant management in a series that included 187 insulin-requiring women with GDM. The cesarean delivery rate was not significantly different in the expectant management group (31 percent) from the active-induction group (25 percent). However, an increased prevalence of LGA infants (23 percent vs. 10 percent) was observed in the expectant management group. Moreover, the frequency of shoulder dystocia was 3 percent in this group, with no cases reported in those undergoing induction at 38 weeks' gestation. These data led the authors to conclude that elective delivery be considered in insulin-requiring patients with GDM because it does not increase the risk of cesarean delivery and does lower the risk for fetal death. In patients managed expectantly, careful monitoring of fetal growth should be performed because of an apparent increasing risk for macrosomia with advancing gestational age in this population.

Counseling the Diabetic Patient

Anomalies of the cardiac, renal, and central nervous systems arise during the first 7 weeks of gestation, a time when it is most unusual for patients to seek prenatal care. Therefore, the management and counseling of women with diabetes in the reproductive age group should begin prior to conception. Unfortunately, it has been estimated that less than 20 percent of diabetic women in the United States obtain prepregnancy counseling.[113]

A reduced rate of major congenital malformations in patients optimally managed before conception is observed in special diabetes clinics (Table 31-9). In Copenhagen, the rate of malformations fell from 19.4 to 8.5 percent in class D and F patients who attended a prepregnancy clinic.[152] Fuhrmann et al[153] found that intensive treatment begun prior to conception in 307 East German diabetic women reduced the malformation rate to 1 percent. Nearly 90 percent of women in this study maintained mean glucose levels less than 100 mg/dl (5.6 mmol/l). In contrast, the incidence of anomalies in the offspring of 593 diabetic women who registered for care after 8 weeks' gestation was 8.0 percent (47/593). Only 205 of those women had mean daily glucose levels of less than 100 mg/dl (5.6 mmol/l). Mills et al[21] have reported that diabetic women registered prior to pregnancy had fewer infants with anomalies than late registrants (4.9 vs. 9.0 percent). While the incidence of 4.9 percent remains higher than that in a normal control population (2 percent), normalization of glycemia was not established in the early entry group.

Glycosylated hemoglobin levels obtained during the first trimester may be used to counsel diabetic women regarding the risk for an anomalous infant. In a respective study of 116 women at the Joslin Clinic, Miller and colleagues[154] observed that elevated hemoglobin A_{1c} concentrations early in pregnancy correlated with an increased incidence of malformations. In 58 patients with elevated glycosylated hemoglobin levels, 13 (22 percent) malformed infants were noted. This is in contrast to a 3.4 percent incidence of major malformations in 58 women whose glycosylated hemoglobin levels

Table 31-9. Comparative Rates of Major Malformations in Offspring of IDDM Women Receiving Preconceptional Counseling

Study	With Preconceptional Counseling	Without Preconceptional Counseling
Fuhrmann et al[153]	1/128 (0.8%)	22/292 (7.5%)
Steel et al[178]	2/143 (1.4%)	10/96 (10.4%)
Kitzmiller et al[159]	1/84 (1.2%)	12/110 (10.9%)
Whillhoite et al[177]	1/62 (1.6%)	8/123 (6.5%)

were in the normal range. Their findings have been confirmed by Ylinen et al[155] who measured glycosylated hemoglobin before the 15th week of gestation in 142 pregnancies. In pregnancies complicated by fetal malformations, mean values were significantly higher than in pregnancies without malformations. In the subgroup of patients with glycosylated hemoglobin values greater than 10 percent (normal < 8 percent), fetal malformations were present in 6 of 17 cases. Overall, the risk of a major fetal anomaly may be as high as 1 in 4 or in 5 when the glycosylated hemoglobin level is several percent above normal values. Greene[156] has reported that 14 of 35 pregnancies with a glycosylated hemoglobin exceeding 12.8 percent were complicated by major malformations. In his series from the Joslin Clinic, the risk for major anomalies did not become evident until glycosylated hemoglobin values exceeded 6 SD above the mean. In contrast to the studies cited above is the DIEP study[21] in which malformation rates in IDMs were not correlated with first trimester maternal glycosylated hemoglobin levels. The authors suggested that more sensitive measures are needed to identify teratogenic mechanisms or that not all malformations can be prevented by good glycemic control. Further review of these data, which included glycosylated hemoglobin levels only in the early entry patients, demonstrates that these women were a relatively homogeneous group with respect to glycemic control; 93 percent had glycosylated hemoglobin levels less than 7 SD below the mean, a level of control that barely increases the risk for anomalies according to Greene's data.[156] Regardless of the glycosylated hemoglobin value obtained, all patients require a careful program of surveillance, as outlined earlier, to detect fetal malformations. The risk for spontaneous abortion also appears to be increased with marked elevations in glycosylated hemoglobin. However, for diabetic women in good control, there appears to be no greater likelihood of miscarriage.[157]

With the increasing evidence that poor control is responsible for the congenital malformations seen in pregnancies complicated by diabetes, it is apparent that preconception counseling involving the patient and her family should be instituted.[158,159] Physicians who care for young women with diabetes must be aware of the importance of such counseling (Table 31-9). At this time, the nonpregnant patient may be taught techniques for self-monitoring of glucose level as well as proper dietary management. Folic acid dietary supplementation at a dose of at least 0.4 mg daily should be prescribed as there is increasing evidence that this vitamin may reduce the frequency of neural tube defects, although it has not specifically been studied in the diabetic population.[160,161] During counseling, questions may be answered regarding risk factors for complications and the plan for general management of diabetes in pregnancy. Planning for pregnancy should optimally be accomplished over several months. Glycosylated hemoglobin measurements are performed to aid in the timing of conception. As a conservative recommendation, the patient should attempt to achieve a glycosylated hemoglobin level within 2 SD of the mean for the reference laboratory.[162]

Contraception

There is no evidence that diabetes mellitus impairs fertility. Family planning is thus an important consideration for the diabetic woman. A careful history and complete gynecologic examination and counseling are required before selecting a method of contraception. Barrier methods continue to be a safe and inexpensive method of birth control. The diaphragm, used correctly with a spermicide, has a failure rate of less than 10 percent. Because there are no inherent risks with the diaphragm or other barrier methods, these have become the preferred interim method of contraception for women with IDDM. The intrauterine device may also be used by diabetic women without an increased risk of infection compared to nondiabetic controls.[163]

Combined oral contraceptives (OCs) are the most effective reversible method of contraception, with failure rates generally less than 1 percent. There is, however, continued controversy regarding their use by the diabetic woman. The serious side effects of pill use, including thromboembolic disease and myocardial infarction, may be increased in diabetic women using combined OCs. In a retrospective study, Steel and Duncan[164] observed five cardiovascular complications in 136 diabetic women using primary low-dose pills. Three patients had cerebrovascular accidents, one had a myocardial infarction, and one an axillary vein thrombosis. In a recent retrospective case–control study, despite diabetes increasing the risk for cerebral thromboembolism fivefold compared with controls, this risk was not enhanced by use of combined OCs.[165]

In Steel and Duncan's report,[164] several women exhibited rapid progression of retinopathy. Klein and colleagues[166] studied OC use in a cross-sectional study of 384 insulin-dependent women and reported no association between OCs and progression of vascular complications. For physicians who prescribe low-dose OCs to diabetic women, their use should probably be restricted to patients without vascular complications or additional risk factors such as a strong family history of myocardial disease. The lowest dose of estrogen and progesterone should be employed. Patients should have blood pressure monitoring after the first cycle and quarterly with baseline and follow-up lipid levels as well.

Women using OCs may demonstrate increased resistance to insulin as a result of a dimished concentration of insulin receptors.[167] Despite the fact that carbohydrate metabolism may be affected by the progestin component of the pill, disturbances in diabetic control are actually uncommon with its use. In another study by Steel and Duncan,[168] 81 percent of patients using the pill did not require a change in insulin dose. Triphasic OCs may also be used safely in former GDM women without other risk factors. Skouby et al[169] have demonstrated that normal glucose tolerance and lipid levels can be expected in nonobese former GDM women followed after 6 months of therapy. Kjos and colleagues[170] performed a prospective randomized study of 230 woman with recent GDM. OC users were randomized to low-dose norethindrone or levonorgestrel preparations in combination with ethinyl estradiol. The rate of subsequent diabetes in OC users was 15 to 20 percent after 1 year follow-up. This rate was not significantly different from that in non-OC users (17 percent). Importantly, no adverse effects on total cholesterol, low- or high-density lipoprotein, (LDL, HDL), or triglycerides were found with OC use.

At present, there is little information available concerning long-acting progestins in women with diabetes or previous GDM. A statistically significant, yet clinically limited deterioration in carbohydrate tolerance has been reported in healthy depomedroxyprogesterone acetate (Depo-Provera; DMPA) users.[171] The progestin effect of lowering serum triglyceride and HDL-C levels, but not total cholesterol or LDL-C, has also been demonstrated with Depo-Provera.[172] Similarly, the subdermal implant Norplant, which releases levonorgestrel, has been associated with elevated glucose and insulin levels in the nondiabetic population.[173] For these reasons, neither DMPA nor Norplant is recommended as first-line methods of contraception for women with diabetes. The progestin-only OC would be preferred, as it does not produce significant metabolic effects in diabetic women. For those choosing long-acting progestins, periodic lipid assessment in all diabetic women and glucose monitoring in former GDM is indicated.

Thyroid Disease

Thyroid disorders are commonly found in women of childbearing age and have been estimated to occur in 0.2 percent of all pregnancies. While the euthyroid state appears to benefit pregnancy, the precise role of the thyroid gland in reproduction is poorly understood. In most series, untreated hypothyroidism has been associated with impaired fertility and pregnancy loss.[179] Successful management of the pregnant woman with thyroid disease requires an understanding of the potential effects on the mother and fetus of these disorders and their treatment.

Thyroid Function During Pregnancy and Laboratory Assessment

The thyroid gland appears to be functioning maximally during normal pregnancy. Basal metabolic rate, which in the past was employed as an indirect measurement of thyroid function, is elevated in pregnancy women.

The activity of the thyroid gland as measured by radioactive uptake studies depends on the pool of circulating inorganic iodine. A greater uptake of radioactive iodine is observed in states such as pregnancy in which circulating levels of iodine are reduced. Early in pregnancy, increased glomerular filtration and renal excretion of iodine result in a decreased plasma inorganic iodine concentration.[180] Enlargement of the thyroid gland during gestation is believed to represent a compensatory mechanism to maintain gland activity despite the decrease in plasma inorganic iodine. This observation may explain the discrepancies between studies contrasting the appearance of goiter in pregnancy in different geographic locations.[181] Presumably, the availability of iodine in the diet can influence the incidence of goiter in pregnancy. Placental production of independent thyroid stimulators such as human chorionic thyrotropin (hCT) is not believed to contribute greatly to increase in gland size or activity.

Laboratory assessment of thyroid function is dramatically altered by the hormonal changes of pregnancy. The most significant finding is a rise in thyroxine-binding globulin (TBG) to levels twice that of normal by the 12th week of gestation. Hyperestrogenic states, including use of OCs, also induce hepatic biosynthesis of TBG. The majority of thyroid hormone (> 99 percent) is bound to TBG. Measurements of total serum thyroxine (T4) by radioimmunoassay or competitive protein-binding techniques include bound as well as the minute fraction of free T4. It is this free fraction that exerts its biologic activity. Minor elevations of free T4 and T3 can be demonstrated in the first trimester, which correlate directly with human chorionic gonadotropin (hCG) levels and indirectly with serum thyroxine-stimulating hormone (TSH).[182] Measurements of free T4 and free T3 reveal a fall in levels later in pregnancy associated with a minor rise in TSH.[183] Relative iodine deficiency is unlikely to be the sole explanation for these findings, since they are observed in iodine-replete areas. Wiersinga[184] has speculated that resetting of the thyrostat leading to lower tissue concentrations of thyroid hormone is a normal physiologic response to a situation where preservation of energy and protein synthesis represents an adaptive advantage, such as that which occurs in late pregnancy.

Despite the above findings, serum levels of free T4, free T3, and TSH remain in the normal nonpregnant range during gestation.[185] Direct measurement of free levels of T3 and T4 is the most accurate method for assessing thyroid function in the face of increased TBG concentrations. When assays for free T3 and T4 are not available, an estimate of free hormone activity is generally obtained by employing the T3 resin uptake test (T3RU).

The T3RU serves as an indirect measurement of thyroid-binding globulin concentration. The patient's serum is incubated along with radioiodine labeled T3 as well as an ion exchange resin. The resin competes with TBG binding sites in the patient's serum for the tracer labeled T3. Pregnancy and other conditions in which TBG is elevated produce more unoccupied binding sites and therefore *decreases* resin uptake of the radioiodine labeled T3. In pregnancy complicated by hyperthyroidism, the T3RU is higher than normal. This reflects greater saturation of the patient's TBG with thyroid hormone, allowing the resin to bind more tracer (Table 31-10).

It is useful to calculate the free thyroxine index (FT4I) based on the results obtained by the T3RU and total T4. The use of this formula attempts to correct for states of altered TBG concentrations, yet this index is not directly proportional to free hormone concentration. In clinical practice, an elevated FT4I is, however, consistent with hyperthyroidism just as a low value reflects hypothyroidism:

$$\text{Free thyroxine index (FT4I)} = \text{Total T4} \times (\text{patient T3RU/normal T3RU})$$

The most sensitive test for the detection of primary hypothyroidism is a measurement of serum TSH concentration. Elevated values in the presence of a normal FT4I value reflect pituitary stimulation of a marginally active gland. In this case, early thyroid failure may be diagnosed and treated. Normal TSH values in the face of a low FT4I most often reflect secondary hypothyroidism of central (hypothalamic-pituitary) origin.

Fetal and Neonatal Thyroid Function

The fetal thyroid gland develops by the 7 weeks' gestation. However, synthesis of thyroid hormone does not begin until approximately 10 weeks, when colloid and follicle formation may be demonstrated and the gland begins to concentrate iodide. It is at this time that the fetal thyroid may become vulnerable to both exogenous iodide such as I[131], as well as antithyroid medications.

The fetal hypothalamic-pituitary-thyroid system appears to function independently from that of the mother. The role of maternal thyroid hormone in early fetal development is unknown. Thyroxine and T3 and TSH do not cross the placenta in significant amounts (Table 31-11). Therefore, fetal levels of these hormones do not correspond to maternal levels. Fetal TSH can be measured after the first trimester, and, by 20 weeks, rises abruptly, causing an increase in fetal T4 production.[186] Fetal T3 levels are quite low during the first

Table 31-10   Effects of Pregnancy and Hyperthyroidism on Tests Commonly Used to Evaluate Thyroid Status

Test	Normal Pregnancy	Hyperthyroidism
TSH	No change	Decreased[a]
TBG	Increased	No change
Total T4	Increased	Increased
Free T4	No change	Increased
Total T3	Increased	Increased
Free T3	No change	Increased
Radioiodine Uptake	Increased	Increased
T3RU	Decreased	Increased

[a] In rare cases may be increased from pituitary hypersecretion or tumor
(Adapted from ACOG Technical Bulletin,[281] with permission.)

Table 31-11   Placental Transfer of Thyroid-Related Hormones and Medications

	Transfer
Iodide	Yes
Thioamides	Yes
TSIG	Yes
TRH	Yes
T3	Minimal
T4	Minimal
TSH	None

two trimesters and then rise during the third trimester. This change probably reflects maturity of the enzyme systems that deiodinate T4. Interestingly, prior to the third trimester fetal thyroxine is principally metabolized to 3, 3', 5'-triiodothyronine or reverse T3. This hormone is found in large concentrations in the amniotic fluid, with peak levels occurring by midgestation.[187] The reason for this augmented production of reverse T3 remains unclear.

Following delivery, there is an abrupt increase in neonatal TSH concentration, which is believed to be secondary to a rise in hypothalamic TRH secretion.[188] T4 and T3 levels increase as a result of TSH secretion and enhanced monodeiodination of T4 to T3. Reverse T3 levels then decline sharply. Peak T4 activity occurs by the second day of life, returning to normal adult concentrations by the end of the first week after delivery.[189]

Hyperthyroidism

Thyrotoxicosis is encountered in approximately 0.2 percent of pregnancies.[185] While menstrual irregularities have been observed in hyperthyroid women, fertility is generally not impaired. Most women with mild to moderate disease appear to tolerate pregnancy well. There is no clear evidence that pregnancy worsens the disease or makes it more difficult to treat. However, thyroid storm is a serious complication that can be encountered in undiagnosed or undertreated patients. Control of hyperthyroidism is essential for both fetal and maternal well-being (Table 31-12). Uncontrolled

disease is associated with an increased incidence of neonatal morbidity resulting from preterm birth and low birth weight.[190] There is debate as to whether pregnancy-induced hypertension is more common in hyperthyroid women.

Graves' disease is the most frequent cause of hyperthyroidism in pregnancy. Toxic nodular goiter, thyrotoxicosis factitia, and gestational trophoblastic disease are far less common etiologies. Patients with Hashimoto's disease may experience periods of hyperactive thyroid secretion before manifesting overt hypothyroidism.

The clinical diagnosis of hyperthyroidism in pregnancy may be difficult because of confusion with symptoms normally present during gestation. Pregnancy is a hypermetabolic state in which heat intolerance, nervousness, and mild tachycardia are common. In contrast, a resting tachycardia in excess of 100 bpm or weight loss despite good dietary intake should alert the physician to the possibility of hyperthyroidism. Ophthalmologic signs of Graves' disease, including exophthalmos, and lid lag (von Graefe's sign) are also helpful in making the diagnosis. The presence of hyperactive deep tendon reflexes, tremor, and eye signs, coupled with an obvious goiter, usually correlate with a positive laboratory diagnosis.

Patients with hyperemesis may also have underlying biochemical hyperthyroidism.[191] It is unusual for such women to have clinical signs of hyperthyroidism.[192] Elevated free T4 associated with suppressed TSH levels may be present in up to 60 percent of women presenting with severe hyperemesis gravidavium.[192,193] These biochemical abnormalities generally return to normal by 18 weeks' gestation. Goodwin and colleagues[192] suggest that elevated hCG stimulates thyroxine biosynthesis, and vomiting may be secondary to an hCG-induced increase in estradiol. There appears to be a correlation of free T4 with hCG level that corresponds to symptoms of hyperemesis.

As noted earlier, laboratory testing for hyperthyroidism, particularly during pregnancy, requires calculation of the FT4I. In rare cases, hyperthyroidism will be

Table 31-12   Perinatal Outcome According to Treatment in Pregnancy Complicated by Hyperthyroidism[a]

Therapy	Medical	Surgical	None
n	265	43	34
Abortions	20 (8)	4 (9)	3 (9)
Stillbirths	13 (5)	3 (7)	8 (24)
Term birth	211 (80)	34 (79)	6 (18)
Preterm birth	29 (11)	4 (9)	18 (53)
Thyroid crisis	5 (2)	1 (2)	7 (21)

[a] Numbers in parentheses are percentages.
(Adapted from Davis et al,[203] with permission.)

present with a normal FT4I but elevated free T3 levels (T3 thyrotoxicosis). This condition can be demonstrated by calculating the free triiodothyronine index (FT3I).

Treatment of hyperthyroidism during pregnancy involves either antithyroid medications or surgery. Radioactive ablation employing I^{131} is contraindicated. By 10 weeks' gestation, the fetus may concentrate this radioisotope, resulting in hypothyroidism. A careful review of the patient's menstrual history and contraception practices should be undertaken before administering I^{131} to any young woman.

Medical therapy for hyperthyroidism is generally preferred in the pregnant patient because it presents less risk than surgery. Propylthiouracil (PTU) and methimazole (Tapazole) are equally effective drugs that block thyroid hormone synthesis. Methimazole has been used less commonly because of a reported association with aplasia cutis of the scalp in newborns. Recent studies of offspring exposed to methimazole do not support this association.[194,195] Nonetheless, Mandel and colleagues,[196] reporting another case of aplasia cutis in a methimazole-treated pregnancy, caution that there is insufficient evidence to establish or eliminate a direct causal relationship between methimazole use and this complication. These authors thus consider PTU the preferred thioamide for treatment of hyperthyroidism during pregnancy. It is recommended that the minimal amount of thiomide necessary to maintain the patient in a euthyroid state be used during pregnancy. The usual starting dose of PTU is approximately 300 mg/day in two or three divided doses. Patients must be closely followed for improvement in their symptoms, including weight gain and normalization of pulse, as well as a decline in serum T4-levels. These therapeutic effects do not usually occur until 2 to 4 weeks after the initiation of treatment. At that time, if the FT4I is falling, the dose of PTU may be reduced. Subsequent determinations of thyroid activity are made every 2 weeks, and in one-third of cases the medication can be discontinued during the second half of pregnancy.[197] Because disease may flare in the postpartum period, it is important to determine thyroid hormone levels prior to discharge from the hospital.

Minor side effects are frequently noted in patients receiving antithyroid medications. Approximately 5 percent will develop a purpuric rash, pruritus, or drug fever. Agranulocytosis is the most serious complication. Patients taking antithyroid drugs are instructed to seek immediate medical attention if early signs of neutropenia such as a sore throat and fever develop. In this setting, a leukocyte count should be performed immediately.

A major concern when using antithyroid medications during gestation is transplacental passage of these drugs and their effects to the fetus. However, fetal goiter and neonatal hypothyroidism appear to be rare complications of maternal therapy. In the past, T4 or T3 was given to mothers receiving PTU in the hope that these drugs would protect the fetus from developing hypothyroidism. This practice is now discouraged, since transplacental passage of T4 and T3 is minimal. In addition, administration of thyroid hormones may make maternal thyrotoxicosis more difficult to control. In infants born to mothers receiving antithyroid medications, early diagnosis and treatment of hypothyroidism probably prevents neurologic sequelae. Transient mild hypothyroxinemia and elevated TSH values have been observed in neonates exposed to antithyroid medication in utero.[198,199] Therefore, it is important to repeat abnormal neonatal blood studies several days after birth in this group of infants. Burrow and colleagues[200] have examined intellectual development in 28 children whose mothers received PTU during gestation. They compared intelligence quotients with siblings not exposed to antithyroid medication and found no difference among the groups.

Careful evaluation of the neonate for hyperthyroidism is equally important. It is estimated that 1 percent of pregnant women with Graves' disease gave birth to an infant with neonatal hyperthyroidism.[201] The onset of neonatal thyrotoxicosis may be delayed in women treated with antithyroid medication. The mother may not necessarily be hyperthyroid during pregnancy, as cases have been described of patients treated years before their pregnancy for Graves' disease. Thyroid stimulation of the fetus is believed to result from maternal passage of a thyroid-stimulating antibody. Fetal thyrotoxicosis secondary to transplacental passage of maternal thyroid-stimulating antibodies has been reported as a cause of fetal demise.[202] Fortunately, most cases of neonatal hyperthyroidism are transient, although, if progressive and unrecognized, central nervous system development may be impaired.

Thyroid Storm

Thyroid storm is an uncommon endocrinologic emergency that can occur in the undiagnosed as well as the partially treated hyperthyroid patient. In pregnancy, rare cases may follow infection or surgery or may accompany labor and delivery. This clinical state of exaggerated hypermetabolism is characterized by hyperpyrexia (> 103°F), tachycardia, and agitation. Tachycardia is often out of proportion to the fever present. Blood pressure is generally normal, although a widened pulse pressure is the norm. Cardiovascular complications in addition to sinus tachycardia include atrial dysrhythmia and occasionally congestive heart failure.[203] Hypotension and cardiovascular collapse may ensue if the entity is not promptly recognized and properly treated. Peripheral catecholamine-mediated effects of thyroid excess are responsible for the presentation of this disorder, which may resemble amphetamine-induced psychosis. Treatment with propranolol is usually successful in counteracting the catecholamine excess present. This drug may be administered orally or intravenously in association with careful cardiac monitoring. Following stabilization of the patient's pulse, an oral maintenance dose of 20 to 80 mg every 6 hours is prescribed. Because large amounts of insensible water loss from perspiration may be present, adequate hydration is an essential component of the therapy for thyroid storm.

Reduction in thyroid hormone production is achieved initially by the administration of either intravenous sodium iodide (1 g in two divided doses of 500 mg over 24 hours) or oral SSKI solution (5 drops every 6 hours). It should be remembered that these compounds may cross the placenta and block fetal thyroid hormone synthesis. PTU is begun immediately in doses up to 1,800 mg/day (600 to 1,000 mg initial dose) and is then tapered to a maintenance dosage. An additional benefit of PTU therapy is a reduction in the peripheral conversion of T4 to T3. Methimazole lacks this property and is, therefore, generally not used in the treatment of thyroid storm. Since there is some evidence that ACTH secretion is inadequate during this crisis, parenteral steroids (dexamethasone 2 mg q 6h × 4 doses) have been advocated as well.[204] Glucocorticoids act synergistically with iodide and PTU to inhibit T4 release as well as peripheral conversion of T4 to T3.

Hypothyroidism

Hypothyroidism is rare in pregnancy because women with markedly reduced thyroid gland function are often infertile. Hypothyroidism is usually secondary to Hashimoto's disease, thyroid gland ablation by I[196], surgery, or antithyroid medications. Iodine deficiency is rare in the United States. Secondary hypothyroidism from hypothalamic or pituitary failure is also uncommon.

The effect of hypothyroidism on pregnancy outcome has been widely debated. The rate of stillbirth and miscarriage appears to be increased in hypothyroid women. Davis and colleagues[205] have reported an increased incidence of preeclampsia, abruption, and fetal growth restriction in the setting of maternal hypothyroidism. Normalization of thyroid function may prevent gestational hypertension and its attendant complications in hypothyroid patients.[206] Early studies demonstrated a higher incidence of mental retardation and congenital anomalies in children whose mothers were believed to be hypothyroid during pregnancy.[207,208] In these reports, the diagnosis of hypothy-

roidism was made on the basis of "hypothyroxinemia" as reflected by lower butanol-extractable iodine levels during pregnancy. These findings have not been supported by more recent investigators.[208] Today, the diagnosis of true hypothyroidism is confirmed by the presence of a low free thyroxine index and an elevated serum TSH level.

The clinical diagnosis of hypothyroidism may be extremely difficult. Nonspecific symptoms such as lethargy and weakness are often present. Weight gain and cold sensitivity may accompany physical findings that include myxedematous changes, hair loss, and cool, dry skin.

Since the advent of radioimmunoassay, more documented cases of hypothyroidism in pregnancy have been reported. The outcomes of such pregnancies generally appear to be good provided replacement therapy is instituted and patients are carefully followed. In one report of 11 pregnancies occurring in nine hypothyroid women, pregnancy outcome was not altered by the disease, and newborn follow-up at 2.7 years failed to reveal any developmental abnormalities.[209]

Therapy consists of sufficient replacement of thyroid medication to achieve a euthyroid state. The patient is generally begun on 0.05 to 0.1 mg daily of L-thyroxine (Synthroid) with the dose increased to a maximum of 0.2 mg daily over several weeks. Ideal replacement may be titrated by following the serum TSH concentration, which may take as long as 2 months to return to baseline.

Occasionally, a pregnant patient may present who is already taking thyroid replacement but does not have well-documented hypothyroidism. Proper evaluation of such patients would require discontinuing thyroid replacement for a period of at least 1 month before assaying serum TSH levels. The hypothalamic-pituitary-thyroid axis takes at least this long to recover after a period of chronic thyroid therapy. Because hypothyroidism may present a risk to mother and fetus, replacement therapy is generally not interrupted during pregnancy. In this setting, it is most appropriate to follow TSH and free thyroxine indices to determine the amount of medication required to keep the patient euthyroid. Recent studies have revealed that there may be a 50 to 100 percent increase in T4 requirements during pregnancy.[210] Patients maintained on a modest dose of Synthroid such as 0.1 mg daily demonstrate elevations of TSH as early as the first trimester. Patients who are hypothyroid after ablation require higher T4 doses than those with Hashimoto's disease, who presumably have some thyroid reserve.[211]

Postpartum Thyroid Dysfunction

Postpartum exacerbations of subclinical thyroid disease have been found in several studies. During pregnancy, a relative suppression of both humoral and cellular immunity may occur. Therefore, autoimmune thyroid disease may improve early in gestation. However, this condition, like many autoimmune disorders, may worsen after delivery.[212-214] The usual pattern of postpartum thyroid dysfunction is hyperthyroidism followed by transient hypothyroidism with subsequent recovery.[215] Histologically, postpartum thyroid dysfunction is characterized by a destructive lymphocytic thyroiditis. During the first few postpartum months, transient thyrotoxicosis develops abruptly in association with a small painless goiter. Fatigue and palpitations are often present. Thyrotoxicosis develops as a result of destructive thyroiditis and glandular release rather than stimulation by antibody present in Graves' disease. Thus, PTU is ineffective, and treatment consists of peripheral β-blockade if symptoms are severe. Approximately two-thirds of women who develop transient hyperthyroidism return to a euthyroid state, whereas one-third develop hypothyroidism.[216] Amino and colleagues[214] reported that 5.5 percent (28/507) of postpartum women experienced transient thyrotoxicosis or hypothyroidism 3 to 8 months after delivery. Most of the patients studied had antithyroid microsomal antibodies present in their serum, although they did not have a previous history of a thyroid disorder. Transient hyperthyroidism alone occurred in 2.5 percent of this patient population. Interestingly, the presentation of some of these patients mimicked postpartum psychosis. Approximately one-third of patients with transient thyrotoxicosis later developed hypothyroidism, confirming that Graves' disease and Hashimoto's thyroiditis may present as a spectrum of thyroid disorders. In those patients documented to have postpartum hypothyroidism, the disease persisted in only one of eight cases. However, these patients were followed no longer than 1 year. In another series of six cases of primary hypothyroidism (lymphocytic thyroiditis) presenting in the postpartum period, chronic thyroid dysfunction was documented in all cases followed up to 2 years after delivery.[214] Postpartum thyroiditis may recur with subsequent pregnancies.[215]

Solitary Thyroid Nodule

Because they are potentially malignant, solitary thyroid nodules require evaluation. Since small masses in the thyroid gland are common and most often benign, a complete evaluation is recommended before surgical excision. The suspicion of malignancy is heightened if the patient's past history includes neck irradiation or inherited medullary carcinoma. Most often, however, there are no predisposing factors.

Because radioisotope scanning is contraindicated during pregnancy, ultrasound is the preferred method for evaluating a thyroid nodule. Cystic lesions are usu-

ally benign. Thyroid function tests may be helpful in the evaluation of solid lesions, as these may occasionally represent a toxic adenoma. Fine-needle aspiration has been shown to be a safe and reliable technique that may distinguish between benign and malignant disease with a high degree of accuracy.[217] If needle aspiration fails to reveal a malignancy, suppression therapy with thyroxine may be utilized. Many nodules will diminish in size when TSH production is inhibited. If this does not occur or if enlargement is observed, a malignancy is more likely. Definite enlargement of the mass or the presence of suspicious palpable nodes requires prompt surgical attention. Fortunately, most papillary adenocarcinomas of the thyroid are limited to the gland and are cured by surgical excision. As a several month delay in treatment does not often significantly alter prognosis in these cases, definitive surgery is often withheld until following pregnancy. In cases of medullary or anaplastic carcinoma, prompt treatment is recommended.

Parathyroid Disease

Calcium Metabolism During Pregnancy

During pregnancy, daily calcium intake must be increased to 1,200 mg/day, approximately one-third greater than the nonpregnant requirement. An increase in calcium intake is necessary during gestation to preserve maternal homeostasis while fetal and placental growth occurs. At term, it is estimated that 25 to 30 g of calcium will have accumulated in the fetus. The fetal uptake of calcium is greatest late in gestation.

Levels of ionized calcium do not change appreciably in pregnancy. However, the total calcium concentration does fall progressively, reaching its nadir during the middle of the third trimester. Serum magnesium and phosphorus levels also decline during pregnancy (Fig. 31-6).[218] The decrease in total serum calcium is believed to reflect principally a fall in the protein-bound portion of the ion. Almost half of all plasma calcium is bound to protein, albumin being the greatest carrier. Ionized or free amounts of calcium account for up to 45 percent, with the remainder forming complexes with phosphate and other anions. As albumin levels decrease and plasma volume expansion takes place, calcium levels decline to an average of 5 percent lower than nonpregnant values by the end of pregnancy. Increased glomerular filtration leading to greater calcium excretion as well as active placental transfer may also contribute to the fall in calcium levels observed during normal gestation.

Maternal gastrointestinal absorption of calcium is enhanced by increased levels of 1,25-dihydroxyvitamin D.[219] The mechanism responsible for this rise in vitamin D is uncertain, although it may result from the

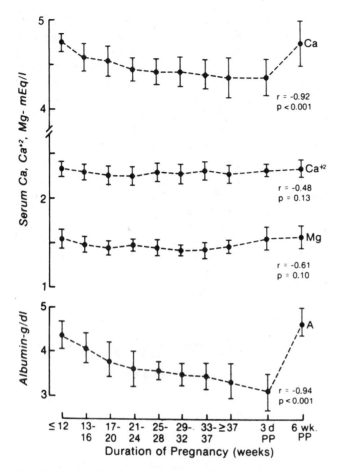

Fig. 31-6 Mean (± SD) serum levels of total and ionic calcium, magnesium, and albumin during pregnancy and the puerperium. The total calcium concentration in maternal serum declines during gestation, reaching a nadir during the third trimester and rising thereafter. (From Pitkin et al[220] with permission.)

elevated parathyroid hormone secretion that accompanies pregnancy. Pitkin et al[220] have demonstrated a progressive increase in parathyroid hormone levels in 30 patients studied longitudinally during pregnancy. A more recent study, using a specific radioimmunoassay for parathyroid hormone actually demonstrated a fall in levels during midpregnancy and a return to baseline by the late third trimester.[221] Thus, debate continues as to whether a "physiologic hyperparathyroidism of pregnancy" exists, and, if so, is it secondary to the decline in maternal serum ionized calcium levels or primary in response to fetal demands for calcium? If the latter is true, then these maternal adjustments precede that period of pregnancy when fetal requirements are greatest. Nonetheless, a rise in maternal parathyroid hormone would facilitate both calcium reabsorption from bone and renal hydroxylation of 25-hydroxyvitamin D. The placenta may also contribute to increased levels of vitamin D.[222] The pregnancy requirement for vitamin D is roughly 400 IU/day, the same as that of the

nonpregnant woman. Studies on calcitonin secretion during pregnancy have produced conflicting data. A rise in calcitonin secretion during pregnancy might be protective against maternal osteopenia from excess parathyroid hormone production. However, increased levels of this hormone have not been uniformly observed.[221,223]

The placenta plays an important role in calcium and phosphorus metabolism. Active transport of calcium to the fetus probably occurs, since newborn levels are in excess of those measured in the mother by 1 or 2 mg/dl.[224] While it has been suggested that parathyroid hormone may facilitate placental transfer of calcium to the fetal compartment, it is important to note that parathyroid hormone and calcitonin do not cross the placenta. While 25-hydroxyvitamin D is transferred across the placenta, passage of 1,25-dihydroxyvitamin D is unlikely.[225]

Parathyroid hormone has been identified in the fetus as early as 10 weeks' gestation. However, most reports suggest that the state of chronic hypercalcemia in utero suppresses parathyroid hormone and stimulates calcitonin during fetal life. At birth, with cessation of the maternal supply of calcium, fetal calcium levels begin to fall. Both parathyroid hormone and 1,25-dihydroxyvitamin D levels increase and are probably involved in the stabilization of neonatal calcium levels by the first week of life.[226]

Hyperparathyroidism

Hyperparathyroidism occurs infrequently during pregnancy, with fewer than 90 cases reported prior to 1982.[227] More cases are now being detected through the widespread use of automated assays for serum calcium determinations. Primary hyperparathyroidism usually results from a parathyroid adenoma, although hyperplasia of the glands is found in 10 to 20 percent of cases. This condition does not seem to affect fertility and is more common in women than men by a 3:1 ratio. Approximately one-fourth of all cases are found in the reproductive age group.

Patients with hyperparathyroidism and mild hypercalcemia may present with rather nonspecific symptoms, including generalized fatigue, muscle weakness, constipation, and abdominal or back pain. Hypercalcemia may impair renal concentrating ability, leading to polyuria and polydipsia. The presence of bone pain and fractures, as well as nephrolithiasis, usually signifies progressive disease. Rarely, patients may present with pancreatitis or peptic ulcer disease.

Establishing the laboratory diagnosis of hyperparathyroidism during pregnancy may be difficult. As noted above, total serum calcium is reduced in a normal pregnancy. However, serum calcium is usually elevated and

Clinical Features of Hyperparathyroidism

Fatigue

Muscle weakness

Abdominal pain

Bone pain, fractures

Polyuria

Polydipsia

Nephrolithiasis

Pancreatitis

Peptic ulcer disease

Hypocalcemic tetany of the newborn

Constipation

phosphate levels reduced in hyperparathyroidism. Occasionally, it may be helpful to measure the serum level of ionized calcium. Marked phosphaturia secondary to a reduction in tubular reabsorption of phosphate when accompanied by hypercalcemia suggests hyperparathyroidism. Parathyroid hormone levels, which normally increase in pregnancy, are usually elevated out of proportion to the serum calcium level.[218] When parathyroid hormone levels are not elevated, other causes of hypercalcemia, including malignancy, hypervitaminosis D, sarcoidosis, milk alkali syndrome, and thyroid disease must be considered.

Hyperparathyroidism during pregnancy is associated with increased perinatal morbidity and mortality. The review of Shangold et al[228] of 159 pregnancies in 63 perinatal women revealed that 84 resulted in normal liveborn term infants, 7 were interrupted by elective abortion, 13 terminated in spontaneous abortion, and 11 ended in intrauterine fetal death. The incidence of preterm births and growth restriction did not appear greater than that in the normal population. All four neonatal deaths followed episodes of tetany. Overall, some morbidity was observed in 45 percent of these infants, including 35 cases of neonatal tetany. Recent analysis of collected case reports has revealed a decline in the frequency of stillbirths, neonatal deaths, and tetany during the past three decades. In the last 10 years, the incidence of stillbirths and neonatal deaths has fallen to 2 percent. Neonatal tetany is observed in 15 percent of cases. The fall in perinatal mortality probably reflects detection and better management of maternal disease.

Hypocalcemic tetany in the newborn often leads to the diagnosis of maternal hyperparathyroidism. Reduced serum calcium levels in the neonatal period are believed to result from chronic maternal hypercalcemia and resultant fetal hypercalcemia that suppresses fetal parathyroid hormone synthesis. After delivery, the fetus exhibits relative hypoparathyroidism and is unable to mobilize calcium. Neonatal tetany may occur at birth or appear after a period of several days. Severe hypocalcemia may also lead to seizures in the newborn. It is possible that other factors such as diminished end-organ response to parathyroid hormone or defective 1,25-dihydroxyvitamin D synthesis may also be responsible for some cases of neonatal tetany.[228] In any event, the neonatologist must be informed of the birth of potentially affected infants.

Because of the high rate of perinatal complications observed in hyperparathyroidism, many authorities recommend prompt surgical excision of abnormal parathyroid tissue at the time of diagnosis. Parathyroidectomy, although traditionally performed in the second trimester, may in selected cases be a reasonable treatment option in late pregnancy.[229] In the review cited above, surgery was performed in 16 cases. Fourteen women were cured by the procedure, and 12 of these subsequently had a successful pregnancy. Surgical therapy is indicated in patients with severe disease (i.e., those with markedly elevated levels of serum calcium and progressive symptoms including bone disease and nephrocalcinosis). Occasionally, such patients will present in hypercalcemic crisis (calcium $\geq$ 12 mg/dl), requiring emergency medical intervention. In these cases, medical control of hypercalcemia should be undertaken prior to surgery. Therapy includes careful administration of intravenous isotonic saline along with a loop diuretic such as furosemide, which inhibits tubular reabsorption of calcium. Thiazides should be avoided, as they result in calcium retention. Mithramycin, which has been used effectively in hypercalcemic cancer patients, is contraindicated during pregnancy, as its effects are not fully known.

The treatment of hyperparathyroidism during pregnancy must be individualized. The patient's symptoms, the severity of her disease, and the gestational age are factors that will influence therapy. Medical treatment may be successfully employed for short periods of time, particularly if delivery can be accomplished. Montoro et al[230] reported two pregnant patients treated with oral phosphate whose infants remained normocalcemic throughout the neonatal period. Patterson[227] described a case treated with oral phosphosoda in which the mother became profoundly hypokalemic in the absence of diarrhea. Phosphate therapy is best reserved for patients with relatively mild disease and normal renal function. It should be remembered that soft tissue calcification may develop in patients with renal insufficiency whose excretion of phosphate is reduced.

Hypoparathyroidism

Hypoparathyroidism is an uncommon entity that usually results from inadvertent removal of the parathyroid gland during thyroid surgery. It has also been found in association with various autoimmune endocrine diseases, including Addison's disease, chronic lymphocytic thyroiditis, and premature ovarian failure. Pseudohypoparathyroidism refers to a condition in which the glands are normal. However, end-organ refractoriness to parathyroid hormone is observed.

The diagnosis of hypoparathyroidism is usually suggested by a history of prior neck surgery and is confirmed by the presence of low serum calcium levels and elevated serum phosphate. Hypocalcemia produces nonspecific symptoms of weakness, lethargy, and bone pain. With severe depression of serum calcium, however, irritability and tetany may develop. Tetany may be demonstrated by the appearance of carpopedal spasm (Trousseau's sign) following the inflation of the blood pressure cuff above the systolic pressure for a period of several minutes. It may also be elicited by tapping the facial nerve, which causes twitching of the upper lip (Chvostek's sign).

In pregnancy, the principal concern associated with this disorder is inadequate transfer of calcium to the fetus, with the subsequent development of secondary hyperparathyroidism in the fetus and newborn. Bone demineralization and subperiosteal resorption, as well as osteitis fibrosa cystica, have been described in infants born to hypoparathyroid mothers.[231,232]

Therapy is aimed at supplying adequate calcium to elevate maternal concentration to the normal range. Maternal treatment consists of supplemental calcium in daily doses of 1 to 4 g, as well as 100,000 to 150,000 IU of vitamin D. During pregnancy, because of profound physiologic changes in calcium homeostasis, careful monitoring of maternal calcium levels must be performed. The short-acting vitamin D, 1,25-dihydroxycholicalciferol (Calcitrol), has been found to be fairly predictable in its response in pregnant women. The recommended dose is 2 to 3 µg/day.[233] However, during pregnancy, the dosage of Calcitrol must often be increased to maintain normal serum calcium levels.

During labor and delivery, calcium levels, if low, may be normalized by an intravenous infusion of calcium gluconate. Hyperventilation, which results in tetany, may aggravate this condition and should therefore be discouraged. Since maternal transfer of calcium to the fetus ceases following delivery, it is important to lower the dose of supplemental calcium to prepregnancy levels. In nonlactating women, levels of calcium may rise dramatically if calcium and Calcitrol intake is not reduced. In women who breast-feed, however, little adjustment in the amount of the vitamin D supplementation appears necessary. There is a single report of a woman with hypoparathyroidism who experienced significant reduction in vitamin D requirements with lactation.[234]

Pituitary Disease

Prolactin-Producing Adenomas

With widely available radioimmunoassays for serum prolactin level determination and improved techniques for radiologic diagnosis, an increasing number of prolactin-secreting pituitary adenomas are now being detected in women. Spontaneous ovulation is uncommon when a pituitary tumor is present. Therefore, most patients with this disorder will present with amenorrhea-galactorrhea or anovulatory cycles and infertility. With the use of ovulation induction and suppression of prolactin synthesis by dopaminergic agents such as bromocriptine, pregnancy has become increasingly common in patients with prolactinomas.

The pituitary gland normally increases in size during pregnancy. Much of the gland enlargement is thought to be secondary to hyperplasia of the lactotrophic cells of the anterior pituitary, which are stimulated by estrogen. Although this stimulus may result in the enlargement of adenomas during pregnancy,[235] most patients with a microadenoma, a pituitary tumor less than 1 cm in size, have an uneventful pregnancy.[236–238] In those few patients who do become symptomatic, regression usually follows delivery.

The vast majority of women with prolactin-secreting adenomas will require ovulation induction to conceive. Nonpregnant patients who present with amenorrhea-galactorrhea and hyperprolactinemia (a prolactin level ≥20 ng/ml) should be investigated for the presence of a pituitary adenoma. While serum prolactin levels have been correlated with the presence of pituitary adenomas, in a patient considering pregnancy with hyperprolactinemia of any degree a thorough radiologic investigation is warranted. Computerized axial tomography and magnetic resonance imaging have replaced coned down sella turcica radiographs and polytomography as the procedure of choice to evaluate the size of the pituitary gland.

Once a pituitary tumor is diagnosed, it may be prudent to re-evaluate the gland for growth after several months before attempting ovulation induction. Macroadenomas, tumors measuring 1 cm or more, should probably be treated with surgery, as over one-third of these patients may develop symptoms during pregnancy.[235,238] Radiotherapy is reserved for patients who do not respond to either medical or surgical treatment.[239]

Evaluation for possible prolactin-secreting tumors is made difficult during pregnancy by the physiologic rise in serum prolactin that accompanies normal gestation. At term, serum prolactin levels may reach values 20 times normal. Furthermore, prolactin levels do not always rise during pregnancy in women with prolactinomas, nor do they always rise with pregnancy-induced tumor enlargement.[240] Therefore, radiologic diagnosis is necessary for the pregnant patient who develops severe headaches or a visual field defect.

Management of the pregnant patient with a previously diagnosed prolactinoma requires careful attention by a team of physicians, including the obstetrician, endocrinologist, and ophthalmologist. The development of headaches may reflect tumor enlargement and impingement on the diaphragmatic sella or adjacent dura. Visual disturbances result from optic nerve compression. If the optic chiasm is compressed by superior extension, bitemporal hemianopsia may develop. Visual field and ophthalmologic examinations should, therefore, be performed in symptomatic patients.[238] While the limitations of serum prolactin levels have been discussed, marked elevations outside of the pregnant range for a given gestational age may signal rapid tumor enlargement.

Gemzell and Wang[235] reviewed the course of 85 women during 91 pregnancies with previously untreated microadenomas and reported that only 5 percent experienced complications. Four of the five pregnancies associated with symptoms of headache and visual disturbance showed resolution following delivery. One patient who had a visual field defect noted early in pregnancy subsequently underwent a transphenoidal hypophysectomy after a cesarean delivery for a triplet gestation at 36 weeks.

Maygar and Marshal[236] report that symptoms seem to occur more frequently in the first trimester than in the second or third, noting a median time at onset of 10 weeks' gestation. However, the likelihood of developing visual symptoms did not differ in each trimester. In their series, symptoms requiring therapy occurred in over 20 percent of the 91 patients who had untreated tumors, but in only 1 percent of women with previously treated adenomas.

Kupersmith and colleagues[237] recently reported their experience monitoring visual loss in 65 consecutive women with pituitary adenomas during 11 pregnancies not previously treated with surgery or radiation. None of the 57 patients with a microadenoma experienced visual loss, whereas 6 of 8 primiparous women with adenomas greater than 1.1 cm did develop either field or acuity loss.

Molitch[238] has reviewed 16 series of 246 cases of pregnancy and prolactin secreting pituitary microadenomas. Only 4 of the 246 women (1.6 percent) had symptoms of tumor enlargement and 11 (4.5 percent) had asymptomatic enlargement on radiologic examination. In no case was surgical intervention necessary. Molitch[239] also reviewed 45 cases of women with macroadenomas, of which 7 (15.5 percent) experienced symptomatic tumor enlargement. Surgery was required in four of these women during pregnancy. The risk of developing symptoms is probably related to the size of the tumor at the onset of pregnancy. Further data will be necessary to define which group of patients with a microadenoma should be treated with bromocriptine for a prolonged period of time prior to conception.

Therapy for complications arising during pregnancy is influenced by both gestational age and the severity of symptoms. If fetal maturity is present, induction of labor or cesarean delivery should be accomplished. Cesarean delivery is generally performed for obstetric indications. Earlier in gestation, if radiologic evidence suggests tumor enlargement, therapy should not be delayed. Treatment employing bromocriptine has been successful in several symptomatic patients and has become the preferred therapy during pregnancy.[240] This drug appears to be safe in early pregnancy, as evidenced by its use for induction of ovulation in large groups of hyperprolactinemic women without an increased incidence of congenital malformations.[241] Other treatment modalities employed during pregnancy include transphenoidal surgery and, in one case, hydrocortisone therapy.[237] Complications of transphenoidal surgery are infection, hypopituitarism, hemorrhage, and transient diabetes insipidus. The risk of these complications is probably not increased during pregnancy.

Following delivery, radiologic assessment of tumor size and a serum prolactin assay should be performed at the first postpartum visit. Breast-feeding is not contraindicated in the presence of a prolactin-secreting microadenoma.[242] Furthermore, treatment with bromocriptine appears safe as well and is apparently not causally related to cases of stroke or seizure during the postpartum period.[243] Since serum prolactin levels may remain elevated while nursing, caution must be used in interpreting these results. Counseling patients regarding future pregnancies requires establishing that progression of tumor growth has not occurred. Contraceptive choices for the woman with a microadenoma include oral contraceptives. Their use has not been associated with growth of pre-existing microadenomas or their development.[244] Regarding subsequent pregnancies, Gemzell and Wang[235] concluded that, in 16 patients with untreated pituitary adenomas, symptoms did not seem to occur with increasing frequency.

Diabetes Insipidus

Diabetes insipidus is a rare disorder, with fewer than 100 cases complicating pregnancy reported in the literature. The disease results from inadequate or absent arginine vasopressin (AVP) production by the posterior pituitary gland. The etiology of diabetes insipidus is often unknown, although in most cases it follows pituitary surgery or destruction by tumor of the normal pituitary architecture. Massive polyuria, resulting from failure of the renal tubular concentrating mechanism, and a dilute urine, specific gravity less than 1.005, are characteristic of diabetes insipidus. To combat dehydration and the intense thirst produced by this syndrome, patients consume large quantities of fluid. The diagnosis of diabetes insipidus relies on the demonstration of continued polyuria and relative urinary hyposmolarity when a patient is water restricted. The administration of intramuscular vasopressin to such a patient will result in water retention and an appropriate increase in urine osmolality. This responses is not observed in patients with nephrogenic diabetes insipidus, a state in which free water clearance is increased because of the renal tubule's insensitivity to AVP. Other conditions that cause polyuria such as diabetes mellitus, hyperparathyroidism with hypercalcemia, and chronic renal tubular disease must also be considered in the differential diagnosis. However, these can usually be distinguished from central diabetes insipidus by appropriate laboratory investigation.

Hime and Richardson[245] reviewed 67 cases of diabetes insipidus complicating pregnancy and noted that 58 percent of cases seemed to deteriorate during gestation. In an attempt to explain this phenomenon, Durr[246] has suggested that the increased glomerular filtration rate seen in pregnancy may increase the requirement of AVP. Patients with mild disease may also worsen during pregnancy because of a diminished response of the renal tubule to AVP, possibly as a result of progesterone antagonism.[247] Recent descriptions of transient diabetes insipidus or disease with first onset during pregnancy have prompted further explanations. While believed by some to be associated with excessive placental vasopressinase activity, deterioration of central diabetes insipidus is more likely a combination of physiologic vasopressin secretion coupled with reduced AVP secretory capacity and reduction in the thirst threshold that accompanies normal pregnancy. Impaired liver function including fatty liver of pregnancy has also been observed with diabetes insipidus during pregnancy, suggesting that several factors may explain worsening of this condition.[247,248]

Synthetic vasopressin, in the form of L-deamino-8-D-arginine vasopressin (DDAVP) is the treatment of choice. This drug is given intranasally in doses of approximately 0.1 mg up to three times daily. Oxytocic activity is rarely observed. Burrow and colleagues[248] have reported the successful use of DDAVP in pregnancy and the puerperium and suggest that this drug is safe for both mother and fetus.

Spontaneous labor and lactation seem to occur in most cases of diabetes insipidus. While older reports suggest an increased number of dysfunctional labors in affected patients, oxytocin release appears to be independent of vasopressin secretion.[249]

Pituitary Insufficiency

In 1937, Sheehan[250] described postpartum ischemic necrosis of the anterior pituitary. This form of hypopituitarism is usually observed in patients who have experienced severe postpartum hemorrhage with hypotensive shock. Lymphocytic hypophysitis may also occur during the postpartum period, giving rise to various degrees of hypopituitarism.[251,252] Destruction of the pituitary from tumor invasion, surgery, or radiotherapy may also accompany pregnancy, although fertility is often compromised in such patients. Anterpartum pituitary infarction has been described as a rare complication of IDDM.[253] In these cases, insulin requirements may fall dramatically.

The acute form of Sheehan syndrome is characterized by hypotension, tachycardia, failure to lactate, and hypoglycemia.[254,255] This form of the disease is potentially lethal, so consideration of this diagnosis is important for women who experience postpartum hemorrhage and shock. Treatment consisting of intravenous corticosteroids and fluid replacement should be initiated pending endocrinologic confirmation of the diagnosis. Patients with a history of Sheehan syndrome or chronic disease may exhibit varying degrees of hypopituitarism; thus specific assays of tropic hormones as well as stimulation and suppression tests may be necessary to establish the diagnosis.[255] During pregnancy, because of normal physiologic changes, adjustments must be made in interpreting both hormone levels and responses to various stimuli. An average delay of 7 years has been observed between the onset and the diagnosis of this disorder. A history of hypovolemic shock and antecedent postpartum hemorrhage has been recorded as a precipitating event in up to 79 percent of cases.[255] CT of the pituitary generally reveals empty or partially empty sella turcica, which may correlate with hormonal secretory capacity.[256] The characteristic clinical picture begins with failure to lactate. However, this may not be observed in all cases. Some patients may present with late onset disease and progress to loss of axillary and pubic hair, oligomenorrhea, or amenorrhea with senile vaginal atrophic changes, and loss of libido, as well as signs and symptoms of hypothyroidism. Patients with these findings are usually infertile, although the frequency of pregnancy with this disorder is difficult to ascertain. In a review of 19 patients with Sheehan syndrome documented by endocrinology studies or postmortem examination, 39 pregnancies occurred after the onset of hypopituitarism.[255] Eleven of these women required hormonal therapy to establish a pregnancy, and replacement therapy was used during 15 (38 percent) of the 39 pregnancies. The treated group had a live birth rate of 87 percent compared with 54 percent in untreated patients, suggesting that early diagnosis and proper therapy result in a more favorable outcome.

The treatment of pituitary insufficiency involves replacement of those hormones necessary to maintain normal metabolism and response to stress. Thyroid hormone may be provided as L-thyroxine in doses of 0.1 to 0.2 mg daily. Corticosteroids are essential for those patients who manifest any degree of adrenal insufficiency. The maintenance dosage of cortisone acetate is provided as 25 mg every morning and 12.5 mg every evening or as prednisone 5 mg and 2.5 mg, respectively. Mineralocorticoid replacement is rarely necessary because adrenal production of aldosterone is not solely dependent on ACTH stimulation. The dose of glucocorticoids should be increased during the stress of labor and delivery.

Adrenal Disease

Cushing Syndrome

Cushing syndrome, which is characterized by excess glucocorticoid production, is usually secondary to inappropriate hypersecretion of ACTH by a pituitary adenoma. Primary adrenal disease resulting from an adrenal tumor has been reported to be more common during pregnancy than in the nonpregnant state. However, adrenal hyperplasia still causes most cases of Cushing syndrome in pregnancy.[257] Other etiologies include neoplastic ectopic ACTH production, nodular adrenal hyperplasia, or excessive doses of exogenous corticosteroids.[258]

Women with Cushing syndrome are usually infertile, making de novo cases rare in pregnancy. Most occur in patients who have been previously or partially treated. The clinical features of this disorder may be difficult to distinguish from many signs and symptoms that accompany normal pregnancy. Weakness, weight gain, edema, striae, hypertension, and impaired glucose tolerance may be observed both during gestation and in Cushing syndrome. The early onset of hypertension with easy bruising and proximal myopathy should strongly suggest the diagnosis and prompt further evaluation.

Laboratory diagnosis includes the demonstration of

elevated serum cortisol levels without diurnal variation, as well as a failure to suppress cortisol secretion with the administration of dexamethasone. Assays for ACTH are normal or elevated and may confuse the diagnosis. Normal rather than suppressed levels of ACTH in patients with adrenal adenomas may be a result of placental production of ACTH or pituitary stimulation by placental corticotrophin-releasing hormone. During gestation, there is normally a rise in total and free cortisol. Therefore, laboratory results must be compared with established norms for pregnancy. Importantly, diurnal variation in cortisol production is maintained in normal pregnancy, although free plasma cortisol levels at term may be twice those of nonpregnant women. Furthermore, even in normal pregnant patients, cortisol secretion may not be suppressed with low doses (1 mg) of dexamethasone.[257] Most patients with adrenocortical hyperplasia will demonstrate a reduction in plasma and urinary corticosteroids with an 8-mg dose (2 mg every 6 hours for 2 days). If such suppression fails, adrenal tumor, autonomous adrenal nodule, or ectopic ACTH production must be considered.

Pregnancy outcome in Cushing syndrome is marked by a high rate of preterm delivery and stillbirths in cases not electively terminated.[257–262] It has been suggested that maternal hyperglycemia may be a contributing factor to the intrauterine deaths observed.

Koerten and colleagues[262] reviewed 33 cases of Cushing syndrome in pregnancy and concluded that maternal complications are more common with adrenal adenomas than with hyperplasia. In this review, every patient with an adenoma developed hypertension if the pregnancy progressed beyond the first trimester. Seven of 16 patients (47 percent) developed pulmonary edema, and one died. In contrast, only 1 of the 12 patients with adrenal hyperplasia demonstrated hypertensive disease. The overall prematurity rate (delivery after 20 weeks) was 20 of 33 cases (61 percent); stillbirths occurred in four cases.

Management of the pregnant patient with cortisol excess includes first identifying the source of the hormone production and then instituting proper therapy. Patients with pituitary disease are most often treated surgically if a tumor can be well defined. Metyrapone therapy has been successfully employed to treat primary adrenal hyperplasia during pregnancy.[263] Surgical removal of adrenal adenomas is recommended and can be accomplished through a posterior incision.[264] Bevan and colleagues[265] have examined maternal and fetal outcomes based on the timing of surgical therapy. Fetal loss occurred in 1 of 11 patients (9 percent) treated during gestation versus 8 of 26 (31 percent) in whom definitive therapy was delayed. Buescher and colleagues[261] noted similar high rates of fetal loss (38 percent) in cases where treatment was delayed. Because the incidences of adrenal adenoma and carcinoma appear to be increased in pregnant patients with Cushing syndrome, prompt investigation employing abdominal CT or magnetic resonance imaging is warranted, particularly if failure to suppress excess cortisol production with high levels of dexamethasone is observed. Again, surgery is indicated if an adrenal tumor is discovered.

Primary Aldosteronism

Few cases of primary aldosteronism during pregnancy have been reported. The diagnosis is suggested in a patient with hypertension, hypokalemia, and metabolic alkalosis. Because aldosterone secretion is increased during pregnancy, the diagnosis can be difficult to establish. However, in cases of pathologic hyperaldosteronism, renin activity should be reduced in comparison to elevated levels accompanying normal pregnancy. Failure to replete serum potassium may also suppress aldosterone secretion, thus obscuring the diagnosis.[266] Amelioration of hypertension and hypokalemia during gestation has been attributed to high levels of progesterone, which may block the action of aldosterone. In spite of this, patients often present with severe hypertension and superimposed preeclampsia. The management of patients without toxemia is controversial. While prompt surgical excision of underlying adrenal adenomas has been suggested by early case reports, Lotgering and associates[267] have described successful medical therapy from midgestation, consisting of spironolactone, an aldosterone antagonist, as well as other antihypertensive medications.

Adrenal Insufficiency

Adrenal insufficiency may be a primary autoimmune disorder (Addison's disease) or secondary to pituitary failure or adrenal suppression resulting from steroid replacement. Adrenal crisis, an acute life-threatening condition, may accompany stressful conditions such as labor, the puerperium, or surgery. Unfortunately, the diagnosis of hypoadrenalism is often made with difficulty, particularly in those patients who possess enough adrenal reserve to sustain normal daily activity. In pregnancy, adrenal crisis during the postpartum period may lead to the diagnosis of adrenal insufficiency for the first time.[268]

The clinical presentation of Addison's disease during gestation is similar to that in the nonpregnant state. Fatigue, weakness, anorexia, nausea, hypotension, hypoglycemia, and increased skin pigmentation are hallmarks for this endocrinopathy. Mineralocorticoid deficiency leads to renal sodium loss with resultant depletion of the intravascular volume. A small cardiac silhouette on chest x-ray is often associated with a state of reduced cardiac output and, eventually, circulatory collapse. Hypoglycemia, which occurs frequently in early pregnancy, may be exacerbated by glucocorticoid deficiency.

The diagnosis of adrenal insufficiency is based on specific laboratory findings. Plasma cortisol levels are decreased. However, since cortisol-binding globulin is elevated in pregnancy, even low normal cortisol values may actually reflect a state of adrenal insufficiency.[269]

Stimulation of the adrenal gland by synthetic ACTH may be helpful in establishing a diagnosis.[270]Following the intravenous administration of 0.25 mg of Cortrosyn, plasma cortisol should be increased at least twofold over baseline values. Failure to respond to this stimulus suggests primary adrenal insufficiency. This test may be used in pregnancy since little ACTH crosses the placenta. Measurement of serum ACTH may also be of benefit in distinguishing primary adrenal insufficiency from hypopituitarism.

Pregnancy usually proceeds normally in treated patients, although there is an increased risk for fetal growth restriction.[270] Maintenance replacement of adrenocortical hormones is provided by either hydrocortisone, in doses of 20 mg in the morning and 10 mg in the evening, or cortisone acetate 25 mg orally each morning and 12.5 mg in the evening. As an alternative, prednisone may be substituted in doses of 5 mg and 2.5 mg, respectively. Mineralocorticoid deficiency is treated with fludrocortisone acetate (Florinef) in a dose of 0.05 to 0.1 mg/day. The use of a mineralocorticoid necessitates careful observation for symptoms of fluid overload. The presence of edema, excess weight gain, and electrolyte imbalance often requires an adjustment in the dose of mineralocorticoid.

Adrenal crisis is a rare, life-threatening disturbance that demands immediate medical attention. Treatment in an intensive care setting is recommended. As noted, women with undiagnosed Addison's disease may present with a crisis during the puerperium. Symptoms include nausea, vomiting, and profound epigastric pain accompanied by hypothermia and hypotension. Treatment initially consists of glucocorticoid and fluid replacement. Baseline blood studies for cortisol and ACTH should be obtained. Intravenous hydrocortisone should then be given in a dose of 100 mg, followed by repeat doses every 6 hours for a period of up to several days. Mineralocorticoid replacement is indicated in cases of refractory hypotension or hyperkalemia.

All patients with adrenal insufficiency should wear an identifying bracelet. Emergency medical kits have also been prepared to help these patients when they travel. Women with Addison's disease require an increase in steroid replacement during periods of infection or stress and during labor and delivery.

Pheochromocytoma

Pheochromocytoma is a rare catecholamine-producing tumor that is uncommonly associated with pregnancy. The tumors arise from chromaffin cells of the adrenal medulla or sympathetic nervous tissue, including remnants of the organs of Zuckerkandl, neural crest tissue that lies along the abdominal aorta. In pregnancy, as in the nonpregnant states, the tumor is located in the adrenal gland in 90 percent of cases.[271] The incidence of malignancy, which can be diagnosed only when metastases are present, is approximately 10 percent. Pheochromocytoma may be associated with medullary carcinoma of the thyroid as part of the multiple endocrine adenomatosis type II syndrome. Schenker and Granat[272] have reported mortality rates of 55 percent with postpartum diagnosis versus 11 percent if diagnosed during pregnancy. Fetal loss can exceed 50 percent.

In pregnancy, pheochromocytoma may present as a hypertensive crisis marked by cerebral hemorrhage or severe congestive heart failure. Pheochromocytoma can be easily confused with other medical diseases. The signs and symptoms of pheochromocytoma can mimic those of severe pregnancy-induced hypertension. Hypertension, headache, abdominal pain, and blurring of vision are common to both entities (Table 31-13). Sustained hypertension may be observed; however, the presence of paroxysmal hypertension, particularly before 20 weeks' gestation, and the absence of significant proteinuria and edema may be helpful in the differential diagnosis. Thyrotoxicosis may also resemble this disease. However, significant diastolic hypertension is rarely observed with hyperthyroidism. Unexplained circulatory collapse following induction of anesthesia or that occurs after delivery should also warrant evaluation for a possible pheochromocytoma.

The definitive diagnosis depends on laboratory measurement of norepinephrine and epinephrine as well as their metabolites in a 24-hour urine collection. Elevated metanephrine excretion appears to be the most sensitive and specific finding, although isolated elevated vanillylmandelic acid excretion may also be present.[271] The use of certain medications such as α-methyldopa (Aldomet) will interfere with these assays. Plasma assays for catecholamines may also be helpful if obtained during a hypertensive episode.

Pharmacologic testing may establish this diagnosis in the nonpregnant patient. The phentolamine (Regitine) test is based on the observation that marked α-adrenergic blockade will produce a fall in blood pressure in many patients with pheochromocytoma. This test is *not* advised during pregnancy, as it has been associated with both maternal and fetal deaths.[273] Nonetheless, it is of extreme importance that the diagnosis be established. Approximately 90 percent of maternal deaths due to pheochromocytoma occur in those patients who were undiagnosed prior to delivery. In patients with symptoms suggesting pheochromocytoma and with laboratory findings that support the diagnosis, an effort should be made with radiologic techniques to localized the tumor. CT of the abdomen or magnetic resonance imaging is the procedure of choice. If necessary, selective venous catheterization of the adrenals may be performed. I^{131} metaiodobenzylguanidine (MIBG) scanning has also proved helpful in locating these tumors. The fetal risk of this isotope study may be outweighed by the benefit of tumor localization. Pheochromocytoma is bilateral in about 10 percent of cases, including those encountered during gestation.

Prior to surgery, the patient should be stabilized on either oral doses of phenoxybenzamine or intravenous phentolamine in an effort to reduce the catecholamine-mediated effects. Volume repletion with careful evaluation of hemodynamic status employing central monitoring is essential when using these preparations. β-Blockade employing propranolol or similar agents should be reserved for treatment of tachyarrhythmias and should not be instituted prior to α-blockade, as hypertensive crisis may ensue.

Schenker and Crowers[271] have recommended prompt surgical removal of any pheochromocytoma detected during pregnancy, regardless of gestational age. In their series, fetal loss exceeded 50 percent and was not improved with early diagnosis. In patients detected during the third trimester, maternal stabilization with medical therapy has been successfully accomplished, thereby allowing further fetal maturation.[273,274] Cesarean delivery is preferred as it minimizes the potential catecholamine surges associated with labor and vaginal delivery. Adrenal exploration may also be performed at the time of cesarean delivery. Careful follow-up of these patients is advised since the tumors may recur in subsequent pregnancies and are potentially malignant.[275]

Table 31-13　Symptoms and Signs in 89 Cases of Pheochromocytoma in Pregnancy

	Percent
Paroxysmal or sustained hypertension	82
Headaches	66
Palpitation	36
Sweating	30
Blurred vision	17
Anxiety	15
Convulsion dyspnea	10

(Adapted from Schenker and Crowers,[271] with permission.)

Key Points

- During pregnancy in the insulin-dependent diabetic woman, periods of maternal hyperglycemia lead to fetal hyperglycemia and thus fetal pancreatic stimulation. The resulting fetal hyperinsulinemia is associated with excessive fetal growth and other morbidities.

- Congenital malformations are two to four times more common in the offspring of insulin-dependent diabetic women. Cardiac, central nervous system, and skeletal malformations are most commonly observed. Poor glycemic control during organogenesis is associated with an increased risk for malformations.

- Women with diabetic nephropathy are at increased risk for preeclampsia, fetal growth retardation, and early delivery. Management involves control of maternal hypertension and intensive fetal surveillance.

- Screening for gestational diabetes, a disorder of carbohydrate intolerance discovered during pregnancy, should be undertaken at 24 to 28 weeks' gestation using a 1-hour 50-g oral glucose challenge.

- Delivery of the insulin-dependent diabetic should be delayed until fetal maturation has taken place, provided that the patient is well controlled and that antepartum fetal surveillance remains reassuring.

- Uncontrolled maternal hyperthyroidism is associated with an increased incidence of neonatal morbidity resulting from preterm birth and low birth weight.

- The rates of stillbirth, miscarriage, preeclampsia, and growth restriction appear to be increased in hypothyroid women.

- The usual pattern of postpartum thyroid dysfunction is hyperthyroidism followed by transient hypothyroidism with subsequent recovery.

- Uncontrolled hyperparathyroidism is associated with an increased risk of stillbirth. Hypocalcemic tetany in the newborn may lead to a diagnosis of maternal hyperparathyroidism.

- The vast majority of women with a prolactin-secreting pituitary microadenoma have uneventful pregnancies. Women with pituitary macroadenomas are more likely to experience symptomatic tumor enlargement during pregnancy. Breast-feeding is not contraindicated in the presence of a prolactin-secreting macroadenoma.

- Pheochromocytoma is associated with a 55 percent maternal mortality rate with postpartum diagnosis versus 11 percent if diagnosed during pregnancy. Cesarean delivery is preferred, as it minimizes the potential catecholamine surges associated with labor and vaginal delivery.

References

1. Kuhl C: Glucose metabolism during and after pregnancy in normal and gestational diabetic woman: I. Influence of normal pregnancy on serum glucose and insulin concentration during basal fasting conditions and after a challenge with glucose. Acta Endocrinol 79:709, 1995
2. Freinkel N, Metzger BE, Mitzan M et al: Accelerated starvation and mechanisms for the conservation of maternal nitrogen during pregnancy. Isr J Med Sci 8:426, 1972
3. Kuhl C, Holst JJ: Plasma glucagon and insulin: glucagon ratio in gestational diabetes. Diabetes 25:16, 1976
4. Yen SSC: Endocrine regulation of metabolic homeostasis during pregnancy. Clin Obstet Gynecol 16:130, 1973
5. Catalano P, Tyzbir E, Roman NM et al: Longitudinal changes in insulin release and insulin resistance in nonobese pregnant women. Am J Obstet Gynecol 165:1667, 1991
6. Buchanan TA, Metzger GE, Freinkel N, Bergman RN: Insulin sensitivity and B-cell responsiveness to glucose during late pregnancy in lean and moderately obese women with normal glucose tolerance or mild gestational diabetes. Am J Obstet Gynecol 162:1009, 1990
7. Ryan EA, Erns L: Role of gestational hormones in the induction of insulin resistance. J Clin Endocrinol Metab 67:341, 1988
8. Puavalai G, Drobry EC, Domont LA et al: Insulin receptors and insulin resistance in human pregnancy: evidence for a post receptor defect in insulin action. J Clin Endocrinol Metab 54:247, 1982
9. Hay WW, Sparks JW: Placental, fetal and neonatal carbohydrate metabolism. Clin Obstet Gynecol 28:473, 1985
10. Metzger BE: Biphasic effects of maternal metabolism on fetal growth. Quitessential expression of fuel-mediated metabolism. Diabetes 40(suppl 2):99, 1991
11. Perinatal mortality and congenital malformations in infants born to women with insulin dependent diabetes. MMWR 39:363, 1990
12. Salversen DR, Brudenell MJ, Nicholaides KH: Fetal polycythemia and thrombocytopenia in pregnancies complicated by maternal diabetes. Am J Obstet Gynecol 166:1987, 1992
13. Madsen H: Fetal oxygenation in diabetic pregnancy. Dan Med Bull 33:64, 1986
14. Nyland L, Lunell NO et al: Uteroplacental blood flow in diabetic pregnancy: measurements with indium 113m and a computer linked gamma camera. Am J Obstet Gynecol 144:298, 1982
15. Kitzmiller JL, Phillippe M et al: Hyperglycemia hypoxia, and fetal acidosis in rhesus monkeys, abstracted. Presented in 28th Annual Meeting of The Society for Gynecologic Investigation, St. Louis, MO, March 1981
16. Phillips AF, Dubin JW, Matty PJ et al: Arterial hypoxemia and hyperinsulinemia in the chronically hyperglycemia fetal lamb. Pediatr Res 16:653, 1982
17. Shelley JH, Bassett JM et al: Control of carbohydrate

metabolism in the fetus and newborn. Br Med Bull 31: 37, 1975

18. Carson BS, Phillips AF et al: Effects of a sustained insulin infusion upon glucose uptake and oxygenation of the ovine fetus. Pediatr Res 14:147, 1980

19. Albert TJ, Landon MB, Wheller JJ et al: Prenatal detection of fetal anomalies in pregnancies complicated by insulin-dependent diabetes mellitus. Am J of Obstet Gynecol (in press)

20. Simpson JL, Elias S et al: Diabetes in pregnancy, Northwestern University Series (1977–1981). I. Prospective study of anomalies in offspring of mothers with diabetes mellitus. Am J Obstet Gynecol 146:263, 1983

21. Mills JL, Knopp RH, Simpson JP et al: Lack of relations of increased malformation rates in infants of diabetic mothers to glycemic control during organogenesis. N Engl J Med 318:671, 1988

22. Eriksson U: The pathogenesis of congenital malformations in diabetic pregnancy. Diabetes/Metab Rev 11:63, 1995

23. Reece EA, Hobbins JC: Diabetic embryopathy: pathogenesis, prenatal diagnosis and prevention. Obstet Gynecol Surv 41:325, 1986

24. Koppe J, Smoremberg-School M: Diabetes, congenital malformations and HLA types. p. 15. In Listen E, Band H, Frus-Hansen B (eds): Intensive Care in the Newborn. Vol. 4, Masson Publishing, Newark, 1983

25. Simpson JL, Mills J, Ober C et al: DR3+ and DR4+ diabetes women have increased risk for anomalies. Presented at the 37th Annual Meeting of the Society for Gynecologic Investigation. Abstract 3901. St. Louis, Missouri, 1990

26. Styrud J, Thunberg L, Nybacka O et al: Correlations between maternal metabolism and deranged development in the offspring of normal and diabetic rats. Pediatr Res 37:343, 1995

27. Freinkel N, Lewis NJ et al: The honeybee syndrome: implication of the teratogenicity of mannose in rat-embryo culture. N Engl J Med 310:223, 1984

28. Goldman AS, Baker L et al: Hyperglycemia-induced teratogenesis is mediated by a functional deficiency of arachidonic acid. Proc Natl Acad Sci USA 82:8227, 1985

29. Pinter E, Reece EA: Arachidonic acid prevents hypreglycemia-associated yolk sac damange and embryopathy. Am J Obstet Gynecol 166:691, 1986

30. Pinter E, Reece EA, Leranth CZ et al: Yolk sac failure in embryopathy due to hyperglycemia ultrastructural analysis of yolk sac differentiation associated with embryopathy in rat conceptuses under hyperglycemic conditions. Teratology 33:73, 1986

31. Eriksson NJ: Protection by free oxygen radical scavenging enzymes against glucose-induced embryonic malformations in vitro. Diabetologia 34:325, 1991

32. Silverman BL, Rizzo T, Green OC et al: Longterm prospective evaluation of offspring of diabetic mothers. Diabetes 40(suppl 2):121, 1991

33. Spellacy WN, Miller S et al: Macrosomia—maternal characteristics and infant complications. Obstet Gynecol 66:185, 1985

34. Modanlou HD, Komatsu G et al: Large-for-gestational age neonates: anthropometric reasons for shoulder dystocia. Obstet Gynecol 60:417, 1982

35. Brans YW, Shannon DL et al: Maternal diabetes and neonatal macrosomia. II. Neonatal anthropometric measurements. Early Hum Dev 8:297, 1983

36. Whitelaw A: Subcutaneous fat in newborn infants of diabetic mothers: an indication of quality of diabetic control. Lancet 1:15, 1977

37. Pedersen J: The Pregnant Diabetic and Her Newborn. 2nd Ed. Williams & Wilkins, Baltimore, 1977

38. Reiher H, Fuhrmann K et al: Age-dependent insulin secretion of the endocrine pancreas in vitro from fetuses of diabetic and nondiabetic patients. Diabetes Care 6: 446, 1983

39. Falluca F, Garguilo P et al: Amniotic fluid insulin, C-peptide concentrations and fetal morbidity in infants of diabetic mothers. Am J Obstet Gynecol 153:534, 1985

40. Milner RD, Hill DH: Fetal growth control: the role of insulin and related peptides. Clin Endocrinol 21:415, 1984

41. Gabbe SG, Mestman JH, Freeman RK et al: Management and outcome of pregnancy in diabetes mellitus, classes B–R. Am J Obstet Gynecol 129:723, 1977

42. Kitzmiller JL, Cloherty JP: Diabetic pregnancy and perinatal morbidity. Am J Obstet Gynecol 131:560, 1978

43. Roversi GD, Gargiulo M: A new approach to the treatment of diabetic pregnant women. Am J Obstet Gynecol 135:567, 1979

44. Jovanovic L, Druzin M, Peterson CM: Effect of euglycemia on the outcome of pregnancy in insulin-dependent diabetic women as compared with normal control subjects. Am J Med 72:921, 1981

45. Landon MB, Gabbe SG, Piana R et al: Neonatal morbidity in pregnancy complicated by diabetes mellitus: predictive value of maternal glycemic profile. Am J Obstet Gynecol 156:1089, 1987

46. Jovanovic-Peterson L, Peterson CM, Reed GF et al: Maternal postprandial glucose levels and infant birthweight: The Diabetes in Early Pregnancy Study. Am J Obstet Gynecol 164:103, 1991

47. Schwartz R, Gruppuso PA, Petzold K: Hyperinsulinemia and macrosomia in the fetus of the diabetic mother. Diabetes Care 17:540, 1994

48. Soler NG, Soler SM et al: Neonatal morbidity among infants of diabetic mothers. Diabetes Care 1:340, 1978

49. Kuhl C, Anderson GE et al: Metabolic events in infants of diabetic mothers during first 24 hours after birth. Acta Paediatr Scand 71:19, 1982

50. Bourbon JR, Farrell PM: Fetal lung development in the diabetic pregnancy. Pediatr Res 19:253, 1985

51. Smith BT, Giroud CJP et al: Insulin antagonism of cortisol action on lecithin synthesis by cultures of fetal lung cells. J Pediatr 87:953, 1975

52. Smith BT: Pulmonary surfactant during fetal development and neonatal adaptation: hormonal control. p. 357. In Robertson B, Van Golde LMB, Batenburg JJ (eds): Pulmonary Surfactant Amsterdam, Elsevier, New York, 1985

53. Post M, Barsoumian A et al: The cellular mechanisms

of glucocorticoid acceleration of fetal lung maturation. J Biol Chem 261:2179, 1986

54. Carlson KS, Smith BT et al: Insulin acts on the fibroblast to inhibit glucocorticoid stimulation of lung maturation. J Appl Physiol 57:1577, 1984

55. Dudley DKL, Black DM: Reliability of lecithin/ sphingo-myelin ratios in diabetic pregnancy. Obstet Gynecol 66: 521, 1985

56. Kjos SL, Walther F: Prevalence and etiology of respiratory distress in infants of diabetic mothers: predictive value of lung maturation tests. Am J Obstet Gynecol 163:898, 1990

57. Mimouni F, Miodovnik M, Whittset J et al: Respiratory distress syndrome in infants of diabetic mothers in the 1980s: no direct adverse effect of maternal diabetes with modern management. Obstet Gynecol 69:191, 1987

58. Tsang RC, Chen I-W et al: Parathyroid function in infants of diabetic mothers. J Pediatr 86:399, 1975

59. Mimouni F, Miodovnik M et al: Decreased amniotic fluid magnesium concentration in diabetic pregnancy. Obstet Gynecol 69:12, 1987

60. Widness JA, Cowett RM et al: Neonatal morbidities in infants of mothers with glucose intolerance in pregnancy. Diabetes 34(suppl 2):61, 1985

61. Ylinen K, Raivio K et al: Haemoglobin A1c predicts the perinatal outcome in insulin-dependent diabetic pregnancies. Br J Obstet Gynaecol 88:961, 1981

62. Stevenson DK, Bartoletti AL et al: Pulmonary excretion of carbon monoxide in the human infants as an index of bilirubin production. II. Infants of diabetic mothers. J Pediatr 94:956, 1979

63. Shannon K, Davis JC et al: Erythropoiesis in infants of diabetic mothers. Pediatr Res 30:161, 1986

64. White P: Pregnancy complicating diabetes. Am J Med 7:609, 1949

65. Summary and Recommendations of the Second International Workshop–Conference on Gestational Diabetes, Diabetes 34(suppl 2):123, 1985

66. Proceedings of the Third International Workshop-Conference on Gestational Diabetes Mellitus, Diabetes 40(suppl 2), 197–201, 1991

67. Gabbe SG, Mestman JH, Freeman RK et al: Management and outcome of class A diabetes mellitus. Am J Obstet Gynecol 127:465, 1977

68. Selby JV, Fitzsimmons SC, Newman JM et al: The natural history and epidemiology of diabetic nephropathy. JAMA 263:1954, 1990

69. Gordon M, Landon MB, Samuels P et al: Perinatal outcome and long-term follow-up associated with modern management of diabetic nephropathy. Obstet Gynecol 87:401, 1996

70. Kitzmiller JL, Brown ER, Phillippe M et al: Diabetic nephropathy and perinatal outcome. Am J Obstet Gynecol 141:741, 1981

71. Reece EA, Coustan DR, Hayslett JP et al: Diabetic nephropathy: pregnancy performance and fetomaternal outcome. Am J Obstet Gynecol 159:56, 1988

72. Kitzmiller JP: Diabetic nephropathy. p. 489. In Reece EA, Coustan DR (eds): Diabetes Mellitus in Pregnancy. Principles and Practice. Churchill Livingstone, New York, 1988

73. Hayslett JP, Reece EA: Effects of diabetic nephropathy on pregnancy. Am J Kidney Dis 9:344, 1987

74. Ogburn PL Jr, Kitzmiller JL, Hare JW et al: Pregnancy following renal transplantation in class T diabetes mellitus. JAMA 255:911, 1986

75. Carstensen LL, Frost-Lansen K, Fulgeberg S, Nerup J: Does pregnancy influence the prognosis of uncomplicated insulin-dependent diabetes? Diabetes Care 5:1, 1982

76. Klein BEK, Moss Klein R: Effect of pregnancy on the progression of diabetic retinopathy. Diabetes Care 13: 34, 1990

77. Horvat M, Maclear H, Goldberg L, Crock CW: Diabetic retinopathy in pregnancy: a 12 year prospective study. Br J Ophthalmol 64:398, 1980

78. Kitzmiller JL, Gavin LA, Gin GD et al: Managing diabetes and pregnancy. Curr Probl Obstet Gynecol Fertil 11:113, 1988

79. Moloney JBM, Drury MI: The effect of pregnancy on the natural course of diabetic retinopathy. Am J Ophthalmol 93:745, 1982

80. Phelps RL, Sakol P, Metzger BE et al: Changes in diabetic retinopathy during pregnancy, correlations with regulation of hyperglycemia. Arch Ophthalmol 104: 1806, 1986

81. Chew EY, Mills JL, Metzger BE et al: Metabolic control and progression of retinopathy. The diabetes in early pregnancy study. Diabetes Care 18:631, 1995

82. Sinclair SH, Nesler C, Foxman B et al: Macular edema and pregnancy in insulin dependent diabetes. Am J Ophthalmol 97:154, 1984

83. Gordon MC, Landon MB, Boyle J et al: Myocardial infarction during pregnancy in a patient with class R/F diabetes mellitus: a case report and review of literature on class H IDDM. Obstet Gynecol Survey (in press)

84. Hare JW: Maternal complications. p. 96. In Hare JW (ed): Diabetes Complicating Pregnancy. The Joslin Clinic Method. Alan R. Liss, New York, 1989

85. Freinkel N: Gestational diabetes 1979: philosophical and practical aspects of a major health problem. Diabetes Care 3:399, 1980

86. O'Sullivan JB: Body weight and subsequent diabetes mellitus. JAMA 248:949, 1982

87. Coustan DR, Nelson C, Carpenter NW et al: Maternal age and screening for gestational diabetes: a population based study. Obstet Gynecol 73:557, 1989

88. Summary and Recommendations of the Third International Workshop–Conference on Gestational Diabetes. Diabetes 40:197, 1991

89. ACOG Technical Bulletin Number 200. Diabetes and Pregnancy, December 1994

90. Periodic health examination, 1992 update: 1. Screening for gestational diabetes mellitus. Can Med Assoc J 147: 435, 1992

91. Naylor CD: Diagnosing gestational diabetes mellitus: is the gold standard valid? Diabetes Care 12:565, 1989

92. Sermer M, Naylor CD, Gore DJ et al: Impact of increasing carbohydrate intolerance on maternal-fetal out-

comes in 3637 women without gestational diabetes. Am J Obstet Gynecol 173:146, 1995

93. Sacks DA, Greenspoon JS, Abu-Fadil S et al: Toward universal criteria for gestational diabetes: the 75-gram glucose tolerance test in pregnancy. Am J Obstet Gynecol 172:607, 1995

94. Coustan DR, Widness JA, Carpenter NW et al: Should the fifty-gram, one-hour plasma glucose screening test be administered in the fasting or fed state? Am J Obstet Gynecol 154:1031, 1986

95. Sermer M, Naylor CD, Gare DJ et al: Impact of time since last meal on the gestational glucose challenge test. Am J Obstet Gynecol 171:607, 1994

96. Landon MB: Gestational diabetes mellitus: screening and diagnosis. Lab Med 21:527, 1990

97. Carpenter MW, Coustan DR: Criteria for screening tests of gestational diabetes. Am J Obstet Gynecol 144:768, 1982

98. Sacks DA, Abu-Fadil S, Greenspoon J et al: Do the current standards for glucose tolerance testing in pregnancy represent a valid conversion of O'Sullivan's original criteria? Am J Obstet Gynecol 161:638, 1989

99. Magee MS, Walden CE, Benedetti TJ et al: Influence of diagnostic criteria on the incidence of gestational diabetes and perinatal morbidity. JAMA 269:609, 1993

100. O'Sullivan JB, Mahan CM, Boston AB: Criteria for the oral glucose tolerance test in pregnancy. Diabetes 13:278, 1964

101. Tallarigo L, Giampietro O, Penna G et al: Relation of glucose tolerance to complications of pregnancy in nondiabetic women. N Engl J Med 315:889, 1986

102. Leikin EL, Jenkins JH, Pomerantz GA et al: Abnormal glucose screening tests in pregnancy: a risk factor for fetal macrosomia. Obstet Gynecol 69:570, 1987

103. Langer O, Anyaegbunam A, Brustman L et al: Management of women with one abnormal oral glucose tolerance test value reduces adverse outcome in pregnancy. Am J Obstet Gynecol 161:593, 1989

104. Neiger R, Coustan DR: The role of repeat glucose tolerance tests in the diagnosis of gestational diabetes. Am J Obstet Gynecol 165:787, 1991

105. Landon MB, Gabbe SG: Insulin treatment p. 173. In Reece FA, Coustan DR (eds): Diabetes Mellitus in Pregnancy, Churchill Livingstone, New York 1995

106. Coustan DR, Reece EA, Sherwin RS et al: A randomized clinical trial of the insulin pump versus intensive conventional therapy in diabetic pregnancy. JAMA 255:631, 1986

107. The American Diabetes Association: Principles of nutrition and dietary recommendations for individuals with diabetes mellitus. Diabetes 28:1027, 1979

108. Diamond MP, Reece EA, Caprio S et al: Impairment of counterregulatory hormone responses to hypoglycemia in pregnant women with insulin-dependent diabetes mellitus. Am J Obstet Gynecol 166L:70, 1992

109. Kilvert JA, Nicholson HO, Wright AD: Ketoacidosis in diabetic pregnancy. Diabetic Medicine 10:278, 1993

110. Rayburn WF, McKean HE: Maternal perception of fetal movement and perinatal outcome. Obstet Gynecol 56:161, 1980

111. Holden KP, Jovanovic L, Druzin M et al: Increased fetal activity with low maternal blood glucose levels in pregnancies complicated by diabetes. Am J Perinatol 1:161, 1984

112. Sadovsky E, Brjejinski A, Mor-Yosef S et al: Fetal activity in diabetic pregnancy. J Fetal Med 3:1, 1983

113. Landon MB, Gabbe SG, Sachs L: Management of diabetes mellitus and pregnancy: a survey of obstetricians and maternal–fetal specialists. Obstet Gynecol 75:635, 1990

114. Barrett JM, Salyer SL, Boehm FH: The non-stress test: an evaluation of 1000 patients. Am J Obstet Gynecol 141:153, 1981

115. Miller JM, Horger EO: Antepartum heart rate testing in diabetic pregnancy. J Reprod Med 30:515, 1985

116. Golde SH, Montoro M, Good-Anderson B et al: The role of non-stress tests, fetal biophysical profile, and CSTs in the outpatient management of insulin-requiring diabetic pregnancies. Am J Obstet Gynecol 148:269, 1984

117. Dicker D, Feldberg D, Yeshaya A et al: Fetal surveillance in insulin-dependent diabetic pregnancy: predictive value of the biophysical profile. Am J Obstet Gynecol 159:800, 1988

118. Johnson JM, Lange IR, Harman CR et al: Biophysical profile scoring in the management of the diabetic pregnancy. Obstet Gynecol 72:841, 1988

119. Landon MB, Gabbe SG, Bruner JP, Ludmir J: Doppler umbilical artery velocimetry in pregnancy complicated by insulin dependent diabetes mellitus. Obstet Gynecol 73:961, 1989

120. Johnstone FD, Steel JM, Haddad NG et al: Doppler umbilical artery flow velocity waveforms in diabetic pregnancy. Br J Obstet Gynaecol 99:135, 1992

121. Landon MB, Gabbe SG: Fetal surveillance in the pregnancy complicated by diabetes mellitus. Clin Perinatol 20:549, 1993

122. Landon MB, Langer O, Gabbe SG et al: Fetal surveillance in pregnancies complicated by insulin dependent diabetes mellitus. Am J Obstet Gynecol 167:617, 1992

123. Milunsky A, Alpert E, Kitzmiller JL et al: Prenatal diagnosis of neural tube defects VIII. The importance of serum alpha-fetoprotein screening in diabetic pregnant women. Am J Obstet Gynecol 142:1030, 1982

124. Greene MF, Benacerraf B: Prenatal diagnosis in diabetic gravidas: utility of ultrasound and MSAFP screening. Obstet Gynecol 77:420, 1991

125. Acker DB, Sachs BP, Friedman EA: Risk factors for shoulder dystocia. Obstet Gynecol 66:762, 1985

126. Tamura RK, Shabbagha RE, Depp R et al: Diabetic macrosomia: accuracy of third trimester ultrasound. Obstet Gynecol 67:828, 1986

127. Landon MB, Mintz MG, Gabbe SG: Sonographic evaluation of fetal abdominal growth: predictor of the large-for-gestational age infant in pregnancies. Am J Obstet Gynecol 160:45, 1989

128. Landon MB, Sonek J, Foy P et al: Sonographic measurement of fetal humeral soft tissue thickness in pregnancy complicated by GDM. Diabetes 40(suppl 2):66, 1991

129. Cousins L: Pregnancy complications among diabetic

women: review 1965–1985. Obstet Gynecol Surv 42: 140, 1987

130. Benedetti TJ, Gabbe SG: Shoulder dystocia: a complication of fetal macrosomia and prolonged second stage of labor tiwh midpelvic delivery. Obstet Gynecol 52:526, 1978

131. Jovanovic L, Peterson CM: Management of the pregnant, insulin-dependent diabetic woman. Diabetes Care 3:63, 1980

132. Hollingsworth DR, Ney DM: Dietary management of diabetes during pregnancy. p. 285. In Reece EA, Coustan DR (eds): Diabetes Mellitus in Pregnancy: Principles and Practice. Churchill Livingstone, New York, 1988

133. Mumford MI, Jovanovic-Peterson L, Peterson CM: Alternative therapies for the management of gestational diabetes. Clin Perinatol 20:619, 1993

134. Jovanovic-Peterson L, Peterson CM: Nutritional management of the obese gestational diabetic pregnant women. J Am Coll Nutr 11:246, 1992

135. Algert S, Shragg P, Hollingsworth DR: Moderate caloric restriction in obese women with gestational diabetes. Obstet Gynecol 65:487, 1985

136. Magee MS, Knopp RH, Benedetti TJ: Metabolic effects of 1200 kcal diet in obese pregnant women with gestational diabetes. Diabetes 39:324, 1990

137. Knopp RH, Magee MS, Raisys V et al: Hypocaloric diets and ketogenesis in the management of obese gestational diabetic women. J Am Coll Nutr 10:649, 1991

138. Peterson CM, Jovanovic-Peterson L: Percentage of carbohydrate and glycemia response to breakfast, lunch, and dinner in women with gestational diabetes. Diabetes 40(suppl 2):172, 1991

139. Goldberg J, Franklin B, Lasser L et al: Gestational diabetes: impact of home glucose monitoring on neonatal birth weight. Am J Obstet Gynecol 154:546, 1986

140. Langer O, Rodriguez DA, Xenakis E MJ et al: Intensified versus conventional management of gestational diabetes. Am J Obstet Gynecol 170:1036, 1994

141. Langer O: Management of gestational diabetes. Clin Perinatol 20:603, 1993

142. Langer O, Brustman L, Anyaegbunam A et al: Glycemic control in gestational diabetes mellitus—how tight is tight enough; small for gestational age versus large for gestational age? Am J Obstet Gynecol 161:645, 1989

143. Coustan DR, Imrah J: Prophylactic insulin treatment of gestational diabetes reduced the incidence of macrosomia, operative delivery, and birth trauma. Am J Obstet Gynecol 150:836, 1984

144. Drexell H, Bichler A, Saller S et al: Prevention of perinatal morbidity by tight metabolic control of gestional diabetes. Diabetes Care 11:761, 1988

145. Persson B, Stangenberg M, Hasson U, Nordlander E: Gestational diabetes mellitus: comparative evaluation of two treatment regimens, diet versus insulin and diet. Diabetes 34(suppl 2):101, 1985

146. Jovanovic-Peterson L, Durak EP, Peterson CM: Randomized trial of diet versus diet plus carbohydrate conditioning on glucose levels in gestational diabetes. Am J Obstet Gynecol 161:415, 1989

147. Bung P, Artal R, Khodiguian N, Kjos S: Exercise in gestational diabetes: an optional therapeutic approach? Diabetes 40(suppl 2):182, 1991

148. Landon MB, Gabbe SG: Antepartum fetal surveillance in gestational diabetes mellitus. Diabetes 34(suppl 2): 50, 1985

149. Girz BA, Divon MY, Merkatz IR: Sudden fetal death in women with well controlled, intensively monitored gestational diabetes. J Perinatol 12:229, 233, 1992

150. Lurie S, Matzkel A, Weissman A et al: Outcome of pregnancy in class A1 and A2 gestational diabetic patients delivered beyond 40 weeks gestation. Am J Perinatal 9: 484, 1992

151. Kjos S, Henry O, Montoro M et al: Insulin-requiring diabetes in pregnancy: a randomized trial of active induction of labor and expectant management. Am J Obstet Gynecol 169:611, 1993

152. Molsted-Pedersen L: Pregnancy and diabetes, a survey. Acta Endocrinol 238:13,1980

153. Fuhrmann K, Reiher H, Semmler K et al: Prevention of congenital malformations in infants of insulin-dependent diabetic mothers. Diabetes Care 6:219, 1983

154. Miller E, Hare JW, Cloherty JP et al: Elevated maternal HbA$_1$ in early pregnancy and major congenital anomalies in infants of diabetic mothers. N Engl J Med 304: 1331, 1981

155. Ylinen K, Aula P, Stnman UH et al: Risk of minor and major fetal malformations in diabetics with high haemoglobin A$_{1c}$ values in early pregnancy. BMJ 289:345, 1984

156. Greene MF: Prevention and diagnosis of congenital anomalies in diabetic pregnancies. Clin Perinatol 20: 533, 1993

157. Mills J, Simpson JL, Drisoll SG et al: Incidence of spontaneous abortion among normal and insulin-dependent diabetic women whose pregnancies were identified within 21 days of conception. N Engl J Med 319:1617, 1988

158. Whillhoite MB, Bennert HW, Palomaki GE et al: The impact of preconception counseling on pregnancy outcomes. The experience of the Maine Diabetes in Pregnancy Program. Diabetes Care 16:450, 1993

159. Kitzmiller JL, Gavin LA, Gin GD et al: Preconception management of diabetes continued through early pregnancy prevents the excess frequency of major congenital anomalies in infants of diabetic mothers. JAMA 265: 731, 1991

160. Centers for Disease Control and Prevention: Recommendations for the use of folic acid to reduce the number of cases of spina bifida and other neural tube defects. MMWR 417:1, 1992

161. MRC Vitamin Study Research Group: Prevention of neural tube defects; results of the medical research council vitamin study. Lancet 338:131, 1991

162. Freinkel N: Diabetic embryopathy and fuel-mediated organ teratogenesis: lessons from animal models. Horm Metab Res 20:463, 1988

163. Skouby S, Molsted-Pederson LL, Kuhl C et al: Consequences of intrauterine contraception in diabetic women. Fertil Steril 42:568, 1984

164. Steel JM, Duncan LJP: Serious complications of oral

contraceptives in insulin-dependent diabetes. Contraception 17:291, 1978

165. Lidegard O: Oral contraceptives, pregnancy, and the risk of cerebral thromboembolism: the influence of diabetes, hypertension, migraine and previous thrombotic disease. Br J Obstet Gynaecol 102:153, 1995

166. Klein BEK, Moss SE, Klein R: Oral contraceptives in women with diabetes. Diabetes Care 13L895, 1990

167. DePiaro R, Forte F, Bertoli A et al: Changes in insulin receptors during oral contraception. J Clin Endocrinol Metab 52:29, 1981

168. Steel JM, Duncan LJP: The effect of oral contraceptives on insulin requirements in diabetes. Br J Fam Plan 3:77, 1978

169. Skouby S, Kuhl C, Molsted-Pederson L et al: Triphasic oral contraception: metabolic effects in normal women and those with previous gestational diabetes. Am J Obstet Gynecol 163:495, 1985

170. Kjos SL, Shoupe D, Dougan S et al: Effect of low-dose oral contraceptives on carbohydrate and lipid metabolism in women with recent gestational diabetes: results of a controlled randomized prospective study. Am J Obstet Gynecol 163:1822, 1990

171. Liew DFM, Ng CSA, Yong YM et al: Long term effects of Depo-Provera on carbohydrate and lipid metabolism. Contraception 31:51, 1985

172. DeSlypere JP, Thiery N, Vermeulen A: Effect of long-term hormonal contraception on plasma lipids. Contraception 31:633, 1985

173. Konje JC, Otolorin EO, Ladipo AO: The effect of continuous subdermal levonorgestrel on carbohydrate metabolism. Am J Obstet Gynecol 166:15, 1992

174. Gabbe SG, Lowenshon RI, Mestman JH et al: Lecithin/sphingomyelin ratio in pregnancies complicated by diabetes mellitus. Am J Obstet Gynecol 128:575, 1977

175. Tabsh KM, Brinkman CR, Bashore RA et al: Lecithin/sphingomyelin ratio in pregnancies complicated by insulin-dependent diabetes mellitus. Obstet Gynecol 59:353, 1982

176. Amon E, Lipshitz J, Sibai B et al: Quantitative analysis of amniotic fluid phospholipids in diabetic pregnant women. Obstet Gynecol 68:373, 1986

177. Whillhoite MB, Bennert HW, Palomarki GE et al: The impact of preconception counseling on pregnancy outcome. The experience of the Maine Diabetes in Pregnancy Program. Diabetes Care 16:450, 1993

178. Steel JM, Johnstone FD, Hepbum DA, Smith AF: Can prepregnancy care of diabetic women reduce the risk of abnormal babies? BMJ 301:1070, 1990

179. Potter JD: Hypothyroidism and reproductive failure. Surg Gynecol Obstet 150:251, 1980

180. Mestman JH: Thyroid and parathyroid disease in pregnancy. pp 489–532. In Quilligan EJ, Kretchmer N (eds); Fetal and Maternal Medicine. Wiley, New York, 1980

181. Burrow GN, Polackwich R, Donabedian R: The hypothalamic-pituitary-thyroid axis in normal pregnancy. In Fisher DA, Burrow GN (eds); Perinatal Thyroid Physiology and Disease. Raven Press, New York, 1975

182. Glinoer D: The thyroid function during pregnancy: maternal and neonatal aspects. p. 35. In Beckers C, Reinwein D (eds): The Thyroid and Pregnancy. Schattnauer, Stuttgart, 1991

183. Hall R: The clinical and technical background to the use of free hormone measurements in thyroid disease. Kodak Clinical Diagnostics, Monograph Z. Kodak Thyroid Information Service, Kodak Clinical Diagnostics, Ltd. Amersham, UK, 1992

184. Wiersinga WM: Serum free thyroxine during pregnancy: a meta-analysis. p. 79. In Beckers C, Reinwein D (eds): The Thyroid and Pregnancy. Schattnauer, Stuttgart, 1991

185. Burrow GN: The management of thyrotoxicosis in pregnancy. N Engl J Med 313:562, 1985

186. Greenberg AH, Czernichow P, Reba RC et al: Observations on the maturation of thyroid function in early fetal life. J Clin Invest 49:1790, 1970

187. Landau H, Sack J, Fruch TH et al: Amniotic fluid 3, 3', 5'-triiodothyroidism. J Clin Endocrinol Metab 50:799, 1980

188. Lombardi G, Lupoli G, Scopasca F et al: Plasma immunoreactive thyrotropin releasing hormone (TRH) values in normal newborns. J Endocrinol Invest 1:69, 1978

189. Oddie TH, Fisher DA, Bernard B, Lam RW: Thyroid function at birth in infants 30 to 45 weeks gestation. J Pediatr 90:803, 1977

190. Mestman JH, Manning PR, Hodgman J: Hyperthyroidism and pregnancy. Arch Intern Med 134:434, 1974

191. Swaminathan R, Chin RK, Lao TTH et al: Thyroid function in hyperemesis gravidarum. Acta Endocrinol 120:155, 1989

192. Goodwin TM, Montoro M, Mestman JH: Transient hyperthyroidism and hyperemesis gravidarum: clinical aspects. Am J Obstet Gynecol 167:648, 1992

193. Goodwin TM, Montoro M, Mestman JH et al: The role of chorionic gonadotropin in transient hyperthyroidism of hyperemesis gravidarum. J. Clin Endocrinol Metab 75:1333, 1992

194. Van Dyke CP, Heydendael RJ, DeKleine MJ: Methimazole carbimazote, and congential skin defects. Ann Intern Med 106:60, 1987

195. Wing DA, Millar LK, Koonings PP et al: A comparison of prophythiouracil versus methimazole in the treatment of hyperthyroidism in pregnancy. Am J Obstet Gynecol 170:90, 1994

196. Mandel SJ, Brent GA, Larsen PR: Review of antithyroid drug use during pregnancy and report of a case of aplasia cutis. Thyroid 4:129, 1994

197. Hamburger DI: Diabosis and management of Graves disease in pregnancy. Thyroid 2:219, 1992

198. Momotani N, Jaeduk N, Oyanagi H et al: Antithyroid drug therapy for Graves' disease during pregnancy: optimal regimen for fetal status. N Engl J Med 315:1, 1986

199. Cheron RG, Kaplan MG, Larsen PR et al: Neonatal thyroid function after propylthiouracil therapy for maternal Graves' disease. N Engl J Med 304:525, 1981

200. Burrow GN, Klatskin EH, Genel M: Intellectual development in children whose mothers received propylthiouracil during pregnancy. Yale J Biol Med 51:151, 1978

201. Munro DS, Dirmikis SM, Humphries H et al: The role

of thyroid stimulating immunoglobulin of Grave's disease in neonatal thyrotoxicosis. Br J Obstet Gynaecol 85:837, 1988

202. Houck JA, Davis RE, Sharm HM: Thyroid-stimulating immunoglobulin as a cause of recurrent intrauterine fetal death. Obstet Gynecol 71:1018, 1988

203. Davis LE, Lucas MJ, Hankins GDV et al: Thyrotoxicosis complicating pregnancy. Am J Obstet Gynecol 160:63, 1989

204. Lowy C: Endocrine emergencies in pregnancy. Clin Endocrinol Metab 9:569, 1989

205. Davis LE, Leveno KL, Cunningham FG: Hypothyroidism complicating pregnancy. Obstet Gynecol 72:108, 1988

206. Leung AS, Millar LK, Koonings PP et al: Perinatal outcome in hypothyroid pregnancies. Obstet Gynecol 81: 349, 1993

207. Man EB, Holden RH, Jones WS: Thyroid function in human pregnancy. VII. Development and retardation of four year old progeny of euthyroid and hypothyroxinemic women. Am J Obstet Gynecol 109:12, 1971

208. Man EB, Jones WS, Holden RH, Mellita ED: Thyroid function in human pregnancies. VIII. Retardation of progeny aged 7 years; relationships to maternal age and maternal thyroid function. Am J Obstet Gynecol 111: 905, 1971

209. Montoro MN, Collea JA, Frasier SN, Mestman JH: Successful outcome of pregnancy in women with hypothyroidism. Am Intern Med 94:31, 1981

210. Mandel SJ, Larsen PR, Seely EW et al: Increased need for thyroxine during pregnancy in women with primary hypothyroidism. N Engl J Med 323:91, 1990

211. Kaplan MM: Monitoring thyroxine treatment during pregnancy. Thyroid 2:137, 1992

212. Amino N, Miyai K, Kuro R et al: Transient postpartum hypothyroidism: fourteen cases with autoimmune thyroiditis. Ann Intern Med 87:155, 1977

213. Fein HG, Goldman JM, Weintraub BD: Postpartum lymphocytic thyroiditis in American women: a spectrum of thyroid dysfunction. Am J Obstet Gynecol 138:504, 1980

214. Amino N, Mori H, Iwatani Y et al: High prevalence of transient postpartum thyrotoxicosis and hypothyroidism. N Engl J Med 306:849, 1982

215. Walfish PG, Chan JYC: Postpartum hyperthyroidism. Clin Endocrinol Metab 14:417, 1985

216. Lazarus JH, Othman S: Review: thyroid disease in relation to pregnancy. Clin Endocrinol 34:91, 1991

217. VanHerk AJ, Rich P, Ljung BE et al: The thyroid nodule. Ann Intern Med 96:221, 1982

218. Pitkin RM: Calcium metabolism in pregnancy and the perinatal period: a review. Am J Obsted Gynecol 151: 99, 1985

219. Reddy GS, Norman AW, Willis DM: Regulation of vitamin D metabolism in normal human pregnancy. J Clin Endocrinol Metab 56:363, 1983

220. Pitkin RM, Reynolds WA, Williams GA, Harris GK: Calcium metabolism in pregnancy: a longitudinal study. Am J Obstet Gynecol 133:781, 1979

221. Seki K, Makimuar N, Mitsui C et al: Calcium-regulating hormone and osteocalcium levels during pregnancy: a longitudinal study. Am J Obstet Gynecol 164:1888, 1991

222. Turner M, Barre PE, Benjamin A et al: Does the maternal kidney contribute to the increased circulating 1, 25-dihydroxyvitamin D concentrations during pregnancy. Miner Electrolyte Metab 14:246, 1988

223. Whitehead M, Lane G, Young O: Interrelationships of calcium-regulating hormones during normal pregnancy. BMJ 3:10, 1981

224. Schauberger CW, Pitkin RM: Maternal–perinatal calcium relationships. Obstet Gynecol 53:75, 1979

225. Delvin EE, Glorieux FH, Salle BL et al: Control of vitamin D metabolism in preterm infants: fetomaternal relationships. Arch Dis Child 57:754, 1982

226. Steichen JJ, Tsang RC, Gratton TL et al: Vitamin D homeostasis in the perinatal period: 1, 25 dihydroxyvitamin D in maternal, cord, and neonatal blood. N Engl J Med 302:315, 1989

227. Shangold MM, Dor N, Welt SI et al: Hyperparathyroidism and pregnancy: a review. Obstet Gynecol Surv 37: 217, 1982

228. Monteleone JA, Lee JB, Tashjean AH, Cantor HE: Transient neonatal hypocalcemia, hypomagnesemia, and high serum parathyroid hormone with maternal hyperparathyroidism. Ann Intern Med 82:670, 1975

229. Patterson R: Hyperparathyroidism in pregnancy. Obstet Gynecol 70:457, 1987

230. Montoro MM, Collea JV, Mestman JH: Management of hyperparathyroidism in pregnancy with oral phosphate therapy. Obstet Gynecol 55:431, 1989

231. Stuart C, Aceto T, Kuhn JP, Terplan K: Intrauterine hyperparathyroidism. Am J Dis Child 133:67, 1979

232. Graders D, LeRoit HD, Karplus M et al: Congenital hyperparathyroidism and rickets secondary to maternal hypoparathyroidism and vitamin D deficiency. Isr J Med Sci 17:705, 1981

233. Salle BL, Berthezene F, Glorieux FH: Hypoparathyroidism during pregnancy: treatment with Calcitriol. J Clin Endocrinol Metab 52:810, 1981

234. Cundy T, Haining SA, Guilland-Cumming DF et al: Remission of hypoparathyroidism during lactation: evidence for a physiological role for prolactin in the regulation of vitamin D metabolism. Clin Endocrinol 26: 667, 1987

235. Gemzell C, Wang CF: Outcome of pregnancy in women with pituitary adenoma. Fertil Steril 31:363, 1979

236. Maygar DM, Marshall JR: Pituitary tumors and pregnancy. Am J Obstet Gynecol 132:739, 1978

237. Kupersmith MJ, Rosenberg C, Kleinberg D: Visual loss in pregnant women with pituitary adenomas. Ann Intern Med 121:473, 1994

238. Molitch ME: Pregnancy and the hyperprolactinemic women. N Engl J Med 312:21, 1985

239. Molitch ME: Pathologic hyperprolactinemia. Endocrinol Metab Clin North Am 21:877, 1992

240. Divers W, Yen SSC: Prolactin producing microadenomas in pregnancy. Obstet Gynecol 62:425, 1983

241. Turkalj I, Braun P, Krup P: Surveillance of bromocriptine in pregnancy. JAMA 247:1589, 1982

242. Jewelewicz R, VanDeWiele RL: Clinical course and outcome of pregnancy in twenty-five patients with pituitary microadenomas. Am J Obstet Gynecol 136:339, 1980

243. Jewelewicz R, Zimmerman EA, Carmel PW: Conservative management of a pituitary tumor during pregnancy following induction of ovulation with gonadotropins. Fertil Steril 28:35, 1977

244. Corenblum B, Donovan L: The safety of physiological estrogen plus progestin replacement therapy and with oral contraceptive therapy in woman with pathological hyperprolactinemia. Fertil Steril 59:671, 1993

245. Hime MC, Richardson JA: Diabetes insipidus and pregnancy. Cases report, incidence and review of the literature. Obstet Gynecol Surv 33:375, 1978

246. Durr JA: Diabetes insipidus in pregnancy. Am J Kidney Dis 9:276, 1978

247. Barron WM, Cohen LM, Ulland LA et al: Transient vasopressin-resistant diabetes insipidus of pregnancy. N Engl J Med 310:442, 1984

248. Burrow GN, Wassenaar W, Robertson GL, Sehl H: DDAVP treatment of diabetes insipidus during pregnancy and the postpartum period. Acta Endocrinol 97:23, 1981

249. Shangold MM, Freeman R, Kumaresan P et al: Plasma oxytocin concentrations in a pregnant woman with total vasopressin deficiency. Obstet Gynecol 61:662, 1983

250. Sheehan HL: Postpartum necrosis of the anterior pituitary. J Pathol Bacteriol 45:189, 1937

251. McGrail KM, Beyer BD, Black P et al: Lymphocytic adenohypophysitis of pregnancy with complete recovery. Neurosurgery 20:791, 1987

252. Hyashi H, Yamada K, Kuroki T et al: Lymphocytic hypophysitis and pulmonary sarcoidosis. Report of a case. Am J Clin Pathol 95:506, 1991

253. Dorfman SG, Dillaplain RP, Gambrell RD: Antepartum pituitary infarction. Obstet Gynecol 53:215, 1979

254. Molitch ME: Endocrine emergencies in pregnancy. Ballieres Clin Endocrinol Metab 6:167, 1992

255. Grimes HG, Brooks MH: Pregnancy in Sheehan's Syndrome. Report of a case and review. Obstet Gynecol Surv 35:8, 481, 1980

256. Lee HC, Lee EJ, Lee KW et al: Computed tomographic correlation with pituitary function in Sheehan's syndrome. Korean J Int Med 7:48, 1992

257. Anderson KJ, Walters WAW: Cushing's syndrome and pregnancy. Obstet Gynecol 42:550, 1973

258. Aron DC, Schnall AM, Sheeler LR: Cushing's syndrome and pregnancy. Am J Obstet Gynecol 162:244, 1990

259. Grimes EM, Fayez JA, Miller GL: Cushing's syndrome and pregnancy. Obstet Gynecol 42:550, 1973

260. Cook DJ, Riddell RH, Booth JD: Cushing's syndrome in pregnancy. Can Med Assoc J 141:1059, 1989

261. Buescher MA, McClamrock HD, Adashi EY: Cushing's syndrome in pregnancy. Obstet Gynecol 79:130, 1992

262. Koerten JM, Morales WJ, Washington SR, Castaldo TW: Cushing's syndrome in pregnancy: a case report and literature review. Am J Obstet Gynecol 154:626, 1986

263. Close CF, Mann MC, Watt JF, Taylor KG: ACTH-independent Cushing's syndrome in pregnancy with spontaneous resolution after delivery: control of the hypercortisolism with metyrapone. Clin Endocrinol 39:375, 1993

264. Pricolo VE, Monchik JM, Prinz RA et al: Management of Cushing's syndrome secondary to adrenal adenoma during pregnancy. Surgery 108:1072, 1990

265. Bevan JS, Gough MH, Gillmer MDG et al: Cushing's syndrome in pregnancy: the timing of definitive treatment. Clin Endocrinol 27:225, 1987

266. Merrill RH, Dombroski RA, MacKenna JM: Primary hyperaldosteronism during pregnancy. Am J Obstet Gynecol 160:785, 1984

267. Lotgering FK, Derkx FMH, Wallenburg HCS: Primary hyperaldosteronism in pregnancy. Am J Obstet Gynecol 155:986, 1986

268. Brent F: Addison's disease and pregnancy. Am J Surg 79:645, 1950

269. Carr BR, Parker CR, Madden JD et al: Maternal plasma adrenocorticotropin and cortisol relationships throughout human pregnancy. Am J Obstet Gynecol 139:416, 1981

270. O'Shaughnessy RW, Hackett KJ: Maternal Addison's disease and fetal growth retardation. J Reprod Med 29:752, 1984

271. Schenker JG, Crowers I: Pheochromocytoma and pregnancy. Review of 89 cases. Obstet Gynecol Surv 26:739, 1971

272. Schenker JG, Granat M: Pheochromocytoma and pregnancy—an update and appraisal. Aust NZ J Obstet Gynaecol 22:1, 1982

273. Venuto R, Burstein P, Schmeider R: Pheochromocytoma: antepartum diagnosis and management with tumor resection in the puerperium. Am J Obstet Gynecol 150:431, 1984

274. Freier DT, Thompson NW: Pheochromocytoma and pregnancy: the epitome of high risk. Surgery 114:1148, 1993

275. Sweeney WJ, Katz VL: Recurrent pheochromocytoma during pregnancy. Obstet Gynecol 835:829, 1994

276. National Institutes of Health Diabetes Data Group: Classification and diagnosis of diabetes mellitus and other categories of glucose intolerance. Diabetes 28:1039, 1979

277. Grenfel A, Brudenell JM, Doddridge MC, Watkins PJ. Pregnancy in diabetic woman who have proteinuria. Q J Med, New Series 59, 228:379, 1986

278. Hollingsworth: Pregnancy, Diabetes, and Birth. Williams & Wilkins, Boston, 1992

279. Phelps RL, Metzger BE, Freinkel N: Carbohydrate metabolism in pregnancy. Am J Obstet Gynecol 140:730, 1981

280. Carpenter MW, Coustan DR: Criteria for screening tests of gestational diabetes. Am J Obstet Gynecol 144:768, 1982

281. ACOG Technical Bulletin No. 181: Thyroid Disease in Pregnancy, June, 1993

Chapter 32

Hematologic Complications of Pregnancy

Philip Samuels

Pregnancy-Associated Thrombocytopenia

The widespread use of automated blood counts has led to the increased diagnosis of thrombocytopenia co-existing with pregnancy. Affecting approximately 4 percent of pregnancies, thrombocytopenia is the most frequent hematologic complication of pregnancy resulting in consultation. Hospital laboratories vary on their lower limit of a normal platelet count, but it is usually between 135,000 and 150,000/mm^3. Platelet counts generally fall slightly, due to hemodilution and increased turnover, as gestation progresses. Platelet counts, however, should not fall below the normal range. In pregnancy, the vast majority of cases of mild to moderate thrombocytopenia are caused by gestational thrombocytopenia.[1] This form of thrombocytopenia has little chance of causing maternal or neonatal problems.[2] The obstetrician, however, is obliged to rule out other forms of thrombocytopenia that are associated with severe maternal or perinatal morbidity. The common and rare causes of thrombocytopenia in the gravida at term are shown in Table 32-1. Until the late 1980s, it was assumed that all patients with an unexplained low platelet count carried a diagnosis of immune thrombocytopenic purpura (ITP), a recognized cause of neonatal thrombocytopenia. Unfortunately, traditional platelet antibody testing cannot distinguish among ITP, thrombocytopenia accompanying preeclampsia, and gestational thrombocytopenia.[3,4] Yet, the distinction between these disorders is important because each of these diagnoses carries distinct maternal and neonatal implications.

Gestational Thrombocytopenia

Patients with gestational thrombocytopenia usually present with mild (platelet count = 100,000 to 149,000/mm^3) to moderate (platelet count = 50,000 to 99,000/mm^3) thrombocytopenia.[5] These patients usually require no therapy, and the fetus appears to be at little, if any, risk of being born with profound thrombocytopenia (platelet count less than 50,000/mm^3) or a bleeding diathesis. This distinct entity was first suggested but not specifically defined in a study published in 1986 by Hart et al[6] In this study, 28 of 116 pregnant women (24 percent) who were evaluated prospectively during an 8-month period in 1983 had platelet counts less than 150,000/mm^3 at least once during pregnancy. In all 17 patients who were followed after delivery, platelet counts returned to normal. Platelet-associated IgG (a positive direct test) was present in 79 percent of these 28 women, and 61 percent had serum antiplatelet IgG (a positive indirect test). None of these women had positive antibodies after delivery. Hart et al[6] were actually describing gestational thrombocytopenia before the condition had been recognized as a distinct entity. They, furthermore, were the first to demonstrate that conventional platelet antibody testing cannot distinguish gestational thrombocytopenia from ITP.[6] Samuels et al[3] also investigated 74 mothers with gestational thrombocytopenia. Forty-six (62 percent) of these patients had circulating antiplatelet IgG in their plasma (a positive indirect test); these women gave birth to two neonates with thrombocytopenia, both having platelet counts above 50,000/mm^3. Burrows and Kelton[5,7,8] have further shown, in a large series, that there is little risk to the mother or neonate in cases of gestational thrombocytopenia. In one study no mother or infant, in a group of 334 women with gestational thrombocytopenia, experienced bleeding complications.[8] In their earlier study of 1,357 healthy, pregnant women, 112 (8.3 percent) had platelet counts less than 150,000/mm^3.[5] The lowest platelet count was 97,000/mm^3. The incidence of thrombocytopenia (platelet count less than 150,000/mm^3) in the infants

Table 32-1 Pregnancy-Associated Thrombocytopenia

Major causes
    Gestational thrombocytopenia
    Severe preeclampsia
        HELLP syndrome
    Immune thrombocytopenic purpura (ITP)
    Disseminated intravascular coagulation
        Abruptio placenta
        Sepsis
        Following severe hemorrhage
        Retained dead fetus
Rare causes
    Human immunodeficiency virus (HIV) infection
    Lupus anticoagulant/antiphospholipid antibody syndrome
    Systemic lupus erythematosus (SLE)
    Thrombotic thrombocytopenic purpura (TTP)
    Hemolytic uremic syndrome (HUS)
    Type IIB von Willebrand's disease
    Other autoimmune diseases
    Folic acid deficiency

of these 112 women was 4.3 percent, not statistically significantly different from infants born to healthy pregnant women without thrombocytopenia (1.5 percent). None of these infants had platelet counts less than 100,000/mm³. Indeed, the works by Samuels et al[3] and Burrows and Kelton[5,7] have convincingly demonstrated that gestational thrombocytopenia is an entity distinct from ITP.

The decrease in platelet count, occurring in gestational thrombocytopenia, is not merely due to dilution of platelets with increasing blood volume. It appears to be due to an acceleration of the normal increase in platelet destruction that occurs during pregnancy.[1] The increase in platelet-associated IgG seen in these patients may merely reflect immune complexes adhering to the platelet surface rather than specific antiplatelet antibodies. Pregnant women who have gestational thrombocytopenia do not require any special therapy during the puerperium unless their platelet counts fall below 20,000/mm³ or if there is clinical bleeding. These complications, however, are rare, and it is difficult to determine whether these patients, with profound thrombocytopenia, have gestational thrombocytopenia or new onset of immune thrombocytopenic purpura.

Immune Thrombocytopenic Purpura

Although it only affects 1 to 3 per 1,000 pregnancies, ITP has received much attention in the obstetrics literature because of the potential for profound neonatal thrombocytopenia in infants born to mothers with this condition.

In 1954, Peterson and Larson[9] were the first to recognize that profound thrombocytopenia (platelet count below 50,000/mm³) may develop in infants born to women with ITP. A subsequent report confirmed this observation.[10] In 1973, Territo et al[11] made the first effort to predict which infants were at increased risk of being born with profound thrombocytopenia. They demonstrated, in a small number of patients, that fetuses born to mothers with platelet counts less than 100,000/mm³ were at highest risk. Many larger studies have since shown that this arbitrary cut-off, while generally true, is not useful in individual cases. Subsequently a number of efforts have been made to use noninvasive parameters to assess the risk of severe neonatal thrombocytopenia, including the use of maternal glucocorticoids, whether or not the mother had undergone splenectomy, and the presence of maternal antiplatelet antibodies. None of these, however, has shown the desired positive or negative predictive values.[12–16]

In general, pregnancy has not been determined to cause ITP or to change its severity. Other studies, however, have demonstrated that in individual patients ITP exacerbations often occur during pregnancy and improve postpartum.[3,17,18] Harrington et al[19] were the first to demonstrate that this disorder was humorally mediated. Shulman et al[20] showed that the mediator of this disorder was IgG. These findings were confirmed when Cines and Schreiber[21] developed the first platelet antiglobulin test, a radioimmunoassay, in 1979. This test is now mostly performed by enzyme-linked immunoassays (ELISA) or flow cytometry. New assays have shown that these autoantibodies may be directed against specific platelet surface glycoproteins, including the IIb/IIIa and Ib/IX complexes.[22] After the platelets are coated with antibody they are removed from circulation by binding to the F_c receptors of macrophages in the reticuloendothelial system, especially the spleen. Approximately 90 percent of women with ITP will have platelet-associated IgG.[21] Unfortunately, this is not specific for ITP, as studies have shown that these tests are also positive in women with gestational thrombocytopenia and preeclampsia.[3,4] Studies concerning the use of antibodies to specific epitopes on platelet surface glycoproteins are ongoing, and these tests eventually may be useful to distinguish among the various disorders.

To make the issue more confusing, the pathogenesis of ITP in children and adults usually differs. Childhood ITP usually follows a viral infection and clinically presents with petechiae and bleeding.[23] This form of ITP is generally self-limited and disappears over time. Adults, conversely, have milder bleeding and easy bruisability and are often diagnosed after a prolonged period of subtle symptoms. Adult ITP usually runs a chronic course, and long-term therapy is often eventually needed. Many pregnancies occur in women in their late teens and early twenties. In these women, with a history of ITP, it may be difficult to ascertain whether the patient has childhood ITP or early adult ITP. Also, no study has shown whether the risk of neonatal thrombocytopenia is similar in both forms of ITP.

ITP is different from other causes of thrombocytopenia in pregnancy because of the aforementioned risk of profound neonatal thrombocytopenia. This has further been confounded by the fact that before 1990 it was assumed that all patients with unexplained thrombocytopenia during gestation had ITP. It was only after 1990 that gestational thrombocytopenia became recognized as a distinct entity.[2,3] This, therefore, has confounded studies because cases of gestational thrombocytopenia have diluted many studies, making it difficult to determine the true incidence of neonatal thrombocytopenia in women with ITP.

Table 32-2 lists several studies in which all patients had true ITP and delineates the rates of profound neonatal thrombocytopenia. Even these carefully performed studies show wide ranges in the rates of profound neonatal thrombocytopenia.

In 1980, Scott et al[24] were the first to institute direct fetal platelet determination in a series of women with ITP by utilizing fetal scalp sampling. This procedure, however, requires operator skill, an engaged fetal vertex, a dilated cervix, ruptured membranes, and the ability to obtain a pure sample of fetal blood without any contamination with maternal blood or amniotic fluid. The procedure has proven to be technically difficult in the hands of many practicing obstetricians who do not perform fetal scalp sampling on a regular basis. In many cases, amniotic fluid in the vagina contaminates the specimen. Amniotic fluid contains procoagulants, which cause fetal platelet clumping and spurious thrombocytopenia.

With the development and increased use of ultrasound-guided cordocentesis in the mid-1980s, accurate in utero sampling of fetal platelets has become feasible. Some authors advocate routine use of this technique in mothers with ITP.[25-27] Some maternal-fetal specialists believe that there is minimal risk involved with the cordocentesis. Ghidini and colleagues,[28] however, reviewed cordocentesis complications at medical centers where more than 100 procedures had been performed. They found a 1.4 percent risk of perinatal death in low risk fetuses at more than 28 weeks' gestation undergoing the procedure. The complication rate may be appreciably higher when larger numbers of severely thrombocytopenic neonates have been studied. Bleeding may occur in up to 41 percent of cases, but most stop in less than 60 seconds. Complication rates will become higher as this procedure is increasingly performed by less experienced operators. Furthermore, cordocentesis is expensive when including the price of the procedure, the physician consultation fee, the ultrasound guidance, and the fetal monitoring that must accompany the procedure. Indeed, the risks, associated costs, and low yield with which profoundly thrombocytopenic infants are identified do not justify the routine use of cordocentesis in all thrombocytopenic mothers.

The major reason why invasive testing has identified so few thrombocytopenic neonates is that many women with gestational thrombocytopenia were included in these series. Gestational thrombocytopenia, previously cited as the most common cause of thrombocytopenia in the third trimester, was not recognized until 1986. It was first alluded to by Hart et al.[6] In 1990, Burrows and Kelton[8] as well as Samuels et al[3] firmly established thrombocytopenia as an entity distinct from ITP. In the latter study, Samuels et al[3] showed that roughly 50 percent of women referred to two major medical centers over 10 years with presumptive ITP actually had gestational thrombocytopenia. It is likely that the inclusion of large numbers of women with gestational thrombocytopenia in recent studies of maternal "ITP" has led to the spurious impression that the natural history of ITP has changed.

In a meta-analysis by Burrows and Kelton,[29] a 14.6 percent incidence of profound thrombocytopenia in infants born to mothers with ITP was reported. This meta-analysis did not, however, take into account that many of the studies included did not exclude patients

Table 32-2   Incidence of Profound Neonatal Thrombocytopenia in Mothers Known to Have Immune Thrombocytopenic Purpura

Reports	Total Patients with ITP	Infants with Platelet Count < 50,000/mm³	95% Confidence Interval
Karapatkin et al.[15]	19	6 (31.6%)	20.9%–52.5%
Burrows and Kelton[8]	60	3 (5%)	0%–10.5%
Noriega-Guerra et al.[13]	21	8 (38.1%)	17.3%–58.9%
Samuels et al.[3]	88	18 (20.5%)	12.0%–28.9%
Pooled (Crude)	*188*	*35 (18.6%)*	*13%–24%*

with gestational thrombocytopenia. Therefore, the risks of profound thrombocytopenia may very well be greater than this reported incidence. These authors, also, reported a neonatal morbidity rate of 24 per 1,000 with few serious complications. This may only be low for the reasons mentioned above.

Samuels et al[3] reported a neonatal morbidity rate of 278 per 1,000 infants born to mothers with true ITP. The sample size, however, was too small to determine if mode of delivery or degree of neonatal thrombocytopenia made an impact on this morbidity. This rate may be overly high as these were patients referred to two large teriary care centers. Nonetheless, this study does point out that ITP does not always carry a benign course for the neonate. The neonatal morbidities included intraventricular hemorrhage, hemopericardium, gastrointestinal bleeding, and extensive cutaneous manifestations of bleeding.[3]

Thrombotic Thrombocytopenic Purpura and Hemolytic Uremic Syndrome

These two conditions are characterized by microangiopathic hemolytic anemia and severe thrombocytopenia. Pregnancy does not predispose a patient to these conditions, but these conditions should be considered when evaluating the gravida with severe thrombocytopenia. Thrombotic thrombocytopic purpura (ITP) is characterized by a pentad of findings, which are shown in Table 32-3.[30,31] The complete pentad only occurs in approximately 40 percent of patients, but approximately 75 percent present with a triad of microangiopathic hemolytic anemia, thrombocytopenia, and neurologic changes.[32] Pathologically, these patients have thrombotic occlusion of arterioles and capillaries.[30] These occur in multiple organs, and there is no specific clinical manifestation for the disease. The clinical picture will reflect the organs that are involved. The pathophysiology of TTP remains elusive, but diffuse endothelial damage and impaired fibrinolytic activity are hallmarks of this disorder.[33] In many ways, the pathophysiology mirrors that of severe preeclampsia.

Table 32-3 Pentad of Findings in Thrombotic
Thrombocytopenic Purpura (TTP)[a]

Microangiopathic hemolytic anemia[b]

Thrombocytopenia[b]

Neurologic abnormalities[b]—confusion, headache, paresis, visual hallucinations, seizures

Fever

Renal dysfunction

---

[a]The classic pentad is only found in 40% of patients.
[b]These three findings are present in 74% of patients.[32]

Weiner[34] has published the most extensive literature review concerning TTP. In this series of 45 patients, 40 developed the disease antepartum, with 58 percent occurring before 24 weeks' gestation. The mean gestational age at onset of symptoms was 23.5 weeks.

This finding may be helpful when trying to distinguish TTP from other causes of thrombocytopenia and microangiopathic hemolytic anemia occurring during gestation. In Weiner's review, the fetal and maternal mortality rates were 80 and 44 percent, respectively.[34] This series included many patients who contracted the disease before plasma infusion/exchange therapy was used for treating TTP. This disorder may be confused with rarely occurring early onset severe preeclampsia. In preeclampsia, antithrombin III levels are frequently low, and this is not the case with TTP.[35] This test, therefore, may be a useful discriminator between these two disorders.

Although the hemolytic uremic syndrome (HUS) has many features in common with TTP, it usually has its onset in the postpartum period. Patients with HUS display a triad of microangiopathic hemolytic anemia, acute nephropathy, and thrombocytopenia. HUS is rare in adults, and the thrombocytopenia is usually milder than that seen in TTP, with only 50 percent of patients having a platelet count less than 100,000/mm³ at time of diagnosis. The thrombocytopenia worsens as the disease progresses.[36] A major difference between TTP and HUS is that 15 to 25 percent of patients with the latter develop chronic renal disease.[31] HUS often follows infections with verotoxin-producing enteric bacteria.[37] Cyclosporine therapy, cytoxic drugs, and oral contraceptives may predispose adults to develop HUS.[38–40] The majority of cases of HUS occurring in pregnancy develop at least 2 days after delivery.[31,33] In fact, in one series, only 9 of 62 cases (6.9 percent) of pregnancy-associated HUS occurred antepartum.[34] Four of those nine developed symptoms on the day of delivery. The mean time from delivery to development of HUS in patients in this series was 26.6 days. Maternal mortality may exceed 50 percent in postpartum HUS.

Evaluation of Thrombocytopenia During Pregnancy and the Puerperium

Before deciding on a course to follow in treating the patient with thrombocytopenia, the obstetrician must evaluate the patient and attempt to ascertain the etiology of her low platelet count. Important management decisions are dependent on arriving at an accurate diagnosis. A complete medical history, although time consuming, is critically important. It is essential to learn whether the patient has previously had a depressed platelet count or bleeding diathesis. It is also important to know whether these clinical conditions occur coincidentally with pregnancy. A complete medication history should be elicited, as certain medications, such as heparin, can result in profound maternal thrombocytopenia. The obstetric history should focus on whether there have been any maternal or neonatal bleeding problems in the past. Excessive bleeding from an episiotomy site or cesarean delivery incision site, a need for blood component therapy, easy bruising, or bleeding from intravenous sites during labor should alert the physician to the possibility of thrombocytopenia in the previous pregnancy. The obstetrician should also question whether the infant had any bleeding diathesis or if there was any problem following a circumcision. The obstetrician should also ask pertinent questions to determine whether severe preeclampsia or HELLP syndrome is the cause of her thrombocytopenia. The treatment of preeclampsia and HELLP is not discussed in this chapter, as they are covered elsewhere (Ch. 28). Importantly, all thrombocytopenic pregnant women should be carefully evaluated for the presence of risk factors for human immunodeficiency virus (HIV) infection, as this infection can cause an ITP-like syndrome.

An accurate assessment of the gestational age should also be carried out. This is important as some of the etiologies of thrombocytopenia in pregnancy are dependent on the gestational age. A thorough physical examination of the patient should also be performed. The physician should look for the presence of ecchymoses or petechiae. Blood pressure should be determined to ascertain whether the patient has impending preeclampsia. If the patient is developing HELLP syndrome, scleral icterus may be present. The eye grounds should be examined for evidence of arteriolar spasm or hemorrhage.

It is imperative that a peripheral blood smear be examined by an experienced hematologist or pathologist whenever a case of pregnancy-associated thrombocytopenia is diagnosed. This individual must determine if microangiopathic hemolysis is present. This will help in establishing a diagnosis. This specialist can also rule out platelet clumping, which will result in a factitious thrombocytopenia. Other laboratory evaluation should be performed as necessary to rule out preeclampsia and/or HELLP syndrome, as well as disseminated intravascular coagulopathy. If a diagnosis of ITP is entertained, appropriate platelet antibody testing should be performed.

After determining the etiology of thrombocytopenia, the physician can better determine whether imminent delivery is necessary, if the thrombocytopenia should be treated before initiating delivery, or if the low platelet count should be ignored.

THERAPY OF THROMBOCYTOPENIA DURING PREGNANCY

Gestational Thrombocytopenia

Gestational thrombocytopenia, the most common form encountered in the third trimester, requires no special therapy. The most important therapeutic issue is to refrain from therapies and testing that may be harmful to the mother or fetus. In these patients, with mild to moderate thrombocytopenia and no antenatal or antecedent history of thrombocytopenia, the patient should be treated like a normal pregnant patient. If the maternal platelet count drops below 75,000/mm^3, the patient may still have gestational thrombocytopenia, but there are not enough data on mothers with counts this low to determine if there are any maternal or fetal risks. These patients, therefore, should be treated as if they have de novo ITP. Although approximately 4 percent of patients have gestational thrombocytopenia, less than 1 percent of patients with gestational thrombocytopenia have platelet counts less than 100,000/mm^3.[8]

Immune Thrombocytopenic Purpura

Treatment of the gravida with ITP during pregnancy and the puerperium requires attention to both mother and fetus. As in other cases of thrombocytopenia, maternal therapy only needs to be instituted if there is evidence of a bleeding diathesis or to prevent a bleeding complication if surgery is anticipated. Again, there is usually no spontaneous bleeding unless the platelet count falls below 20,000/mm^3. Surgical bleeding does not usually occur until the platelet count is less than 50,000/mm^3. The conventional forms of raising a platelet count in the patient with ITP include glucocorticoid therapy, intravenous gammaglobulins, platelet transfusions, and splenectomy.

If the patient is having a bleeding diathesis or if the platelet count is below 20,000/mm^3, there is usually a need to raise the platelet count in a relatively short period of time. Although oral glucocorticoids can be used, intravenous glucocorticoids may work more rapidly. Any steroid that has a glucocorticoid effect can be used. However, hematologists have the most experience with methylprednisolone. It can be given intravenously, and it has very little mineralocorticoid effect. It is important to avoid steroids with strong mineralocorticoid effects because these agents can disturb electrolyte balance, cause fluid retention, and result in hypertension. The usual dose of methylprednisolone is 1.0 to 1.5 mg/kg of *total body weight* intravenously daily in divided doses. It usually takes about 2 days to see a response, but it may take up to 10 days to see a maximum response. Even though it does have very little mineralocorticoid effect, there is some present. Because of the large dose that is being administered, it is important to follow the patient's electrolytes. There is little chance methylprednisolone will cause neonatal adrenal suppression because very little crosses the placenta. It is metabolized by placental 11-β-ol-dehydrogenase to an inactive 11-keto metabolite.

After the platelet count has risen satisfactorily using intravenous methylprednisolone, the patient can be switched to oral prednisone. The usual dose is 60 to 100 mg/day. It can be given in a single dose, but there is less gastrointestinal upset with divided doses. The physician can rapidly taper the dose to 30 or 40 mg/day, but slowly thereafter. Since the patient did have a very low platelet count before (or otherwise she would not be undergoing therapy), the physician should titrate the dose to keep the platelet count around 100,000/mm³. If the physician begins therapy with oral prednisone, the usual initial daily dose is 1 mg/kg total body weight. The response rate to glucocorticoids is about 70 percent. It is important to realize that if the patient has been taking glucocorticoids for a period of at least 2 to 3 weeks, she may have adrenal suppression and should undergo increased doses of steroids during labor and delivery in order to avoid an adrenal crisis. Tapering should be slowly thereafter. Also, if the patient has been on glucocorticoids for some time, she may experience significant side effects, including fluid retention, hirsutism, acne, striae, poor wound healing, and monilia vaginitis. In rare circumstances, patients on long-term steroids during gestation can develop osteoporosis or cataract formation. The chance of any fetal or neonatal side effects from the glucocorticoids, however, is remote.

Although glucocorticoids are the mainstays of treating maternal thrombocytopenia, up to 30 percent of patients will not respond to these medications. In this instance, the next medication to use is intravenous immunoglobulin. This agent probably works by binding to the Fc receptors on reticuloendothelial cells and preventing destruction of platelets. It may also adhere to receptors on platelets and prevent antiplatelet antibodies from binding to these sites. Liquid and lyophilized forms of this medication are available. The usual dose is 0.4 g/kg/day for 3 to 5 days. However, it may be necessary to use as much as 1 g/kg/day. The response usually begins in 2 to 3 days and usually peaks in 5 days. The length of this response is variable, and the timing of the dose is extremely important. If the obstetrician wants a peak platelet count for delivery, he or she should institute therapy about 5 to 8 days before the planned delivery.

Intravenous immunoglobulin is a blood product, but its method of preparation makes it safe for use. Plasma is thawed and pooled. After the cryoprecipitate is removed, it undergoes Cohn-Oncley cold ethanol fractionation.[41] This inactivates viruses.[42] Furthermore, the liquid form is incubated for 21 days at pH 4.25. This removes and inactivates both enveloped and non-enveloped model viruses,[43,44] including the human immunodeficiency virus, hepatitis C virus, hepatitis B virus, cytomegalovirus virus, Epstein-Barr virus, and herpes simplex virus. It has also been tested against RNA and DNA nonenveloped viruses.[45,46] A recent review of the literature uncovered no cases of viral transmission with the liquid formula of immunoglobulin that had been incubated at pH 4.25. Although intravenous immunoglobulin is very expensive, it should be used before contemplating splenectomy, as some patients with ITP will experience remission after delivery.[47]

In midtrimester, splenectomy can also be used to raise the maternal platelet count. This procedure is reserved for those who do not respond to medical management, with the platelet count remaining below 20,000/mm³. It can be performed postpartum if the patient does not respond to medical management. In extremely emergent cases of life-threatening bleeding or nonresponse, splenectomy can be safely performed at the time of cesarean section after extending a midline incision cephalad.

Platelet transfusions are indicated when there is clinically significant bleeding and while awaiting other therapies to become effective. Platelets can be given if the maternal platelet count is less than 50,000/mm³ before or during splenectomy, or before or during cesarean delivery. They can be used before a vaginal delivery if the mother's platelet count is less than 20,000/mm³. Each "pack" of platelets will increase the platelet count by approximately 10,000/mm³. The half-life of these platelets is extremely short because the same antibodies and reticuloendothelial cell clearance rates that affect the mother's endogenous platelets will also affect the transfused platelets. However, if these platelets are transfused at the time the skin incision is made, it will allow enough hemostasis to carry out the surgical procedure.

If the patient with profound thrombocytopenia undergoes cesarean delivery, certain surgical precautions should be taken. The obstetrician should use electrocautery liberally. The bladder flap may be left open in order to avoid hematoma formation. When the parietal peritoneum is closed, subfascial drains are helpful if hemostasis is imperfect. Some physicians choose to employ delayed primary closure of the skin, but this is controversial.

While treating maternal thrombocytopenia is fairly straightforward, the need for evaluation of the fetal platelet count and how this information should alter patient management remain controversial. Although papers by Cooke[49] and Burrows and Kelton[29] have attempted to show that there is no risk in delivering a profoundly thrombocytopenic fetus vaginally, these meta-analyses are only generalizations. There is no one series large enough from which to draw adequate conclusions concerning mode of delivery of the profoundly thrombocytopenic fetus. There are no randomized studies concerning delivery of these patients. It is not our purpose to recommend a mode of delivery for the profoundly thrombocytopenic fetus, but to outline which fetuses are at risk of being born with thrombocytopenia and to allow the obstetrician to make decisions concerning delivery after discussion with the patient. As previously shown (Table 32-2), anywhere from 5 to 38 percent of fetuses born to mothers with ITP will have platelet counts less than 50,000/mm^3. Several studies have tried to determine if administering glucocorticoids to the mother may have an effect on raising the fetal platelet count in utero.[12,13,15]

Although the study by Karapatkin et al[15] was promising, other studies have not corroborated these findings. Furthermore, studies have shown that splenectomy has no bearing on neonatal platelet counts. The study by Samuels et al[3] showed that 19.2 percent of ITP patients undergoing no therapy gave birth to profoundly thrombocytopenic infants compared with 22.7 percent of those receiving prednisone alone, 23 percent of those who had undergone a splenectomy and received prednisone, and 17.8 percent of those having undergone only splenectomy. The rate of profound neonatal thrombocytopenia was not significantly different among any of these groups. Even if there is not a difference in perinatal morbidity between vaginal and cesarean delivery, there are advantages of knowing whether a fetus is at risk of being born with a platelet count less than 50,000/mm^3. The use of scalp electrodes and vacuum extractors are examples of interventions that may be avoided in the profoundly thrombocytopenic fetus. A prolonged second stage of labor in the nulliparous patient who is carrying a severely thrombocytopenic fetus should probably be avoided. Furthermore, because of the potential neonatal morbidity, it might be safest if the profoundly thrombocytopenic infant were delivered in a tertiary care setting. In the study by Samuels et al[3], there were cases of severe gastrointestinal bleeding, hemopericardium, intraventricular hemorrhage, and severe cutaneous manifestations of bleeding in infants born to mothers with ITP.

The only method currently available to determine the fetal platelet count accurately before the onset of labor (cordocentesis) is both expensive and invasive. Furthermore, it carries an inherent risk of an adverse fetal outcome. Fear of an adverse outcome in the setting of a neonate with an unknown platelet count has led obstetricians to overutilize this invasive testing as well as surgical deliveries. Cordocentesis should be reserved for those patients with true ITP and not those with gestational thrombocytopenia. Because of the risk of complications, cordocentesis should be carried out in close proximity to the labor and delivery unit. If the fetal platelet count is below 50,000/mm^3, the obstetrician should discuss potential ramifications with the patient. The patient and obstetrician should together decide upon an appropriate place and mode of delivery.

In summary, the treatment of thrombocytopenia during gestation is dependent on the etiology. The obstetrician need not act on the mother's platelet count unless it is below 20,000/mm^3 or, if it is below 50,000/mm^3 with evidence of clinical bleeding or if surgery is anticipated. In these cases, the treatment will depend upon the diagnosis. Furthermore, whether delivery needs to be expedited or can be delayed is also dependent on the etiology of thrombocytopenia. The fetal/neonatal platelet count need only be considered if the mother carries a true diagnosis of ITP or, in the case of presumed gestational thrombocytopenia, when the platelet count is less than 75,000/mm^3, as this may actually be de novo ITP. The key to managing these patients is to arrive at an accurate etiology for the thrombocytopenia and to approach the patient and her fetus rationally.

Management of Thrombotic Thrombocytopenic Purpura and Hemolytic Uremic Syndrome

Before the use of plasma exchange, maternal and fetal outcomes in cases complicated by TTP were uniformly poor.[34] The first cases treated with plasma exchange for TTP during pregnancy were reported in 1984.[50] One report described a patient who had previous fetal deaths from chronic TTP and experienced a successful pregnancy when treated with aspirin, dipyridamol, and plasma infusion.[51] There are no large series of patients with TTP in pregnancy. It does appear, however, through case reports, that the prognosis has improved greatly with plasma infusion and plasma exchange.

HUS has been much more difficult to treat. Only a few case reports have appeared. Supportive therapy remains the mainstay of these treatments.[34,50] Dialysis is often necessary with close attention to fluid management. Platelet function inhibitors have also been used in two cases during pregnancy.[52,53] Plasma infusion and plasma exchange can be attempted, but the results have not been as good as in cases of TTP.[54] Vincristine has been used with some success in nonpregnant patients but has not been tried with pregnancy, and prostacyclin infusion has been effective in children but has not been used during pregnancy.[53,55]

Neonatal Alloimmune Thrombocytopenia

In neonatal alloimmune thrombocytopenia, a rare disorder, the mother lacks a specific platelet antigen and develops antibodies to this antigen. The disease is somewhat analogous to Rh isoimmunization, but involves platelets. If the fetus inherits this antigen from its father, maternal antibody can cross the placenta, resulting in severe neonatal thrombocytopenia. The mother, however, will have a normal platelet count. Deaver and coinvestigators[56] reviewed 58 cases of neonatal alloimmune thrombocytopenia. The overall mortality rate was 9 percent, and the total incidence of suspected intracranial hemorrhage was 28 percent. The mortality rate was 24 percent for the firstborn infant and only 5 percent for subsequent offspring. The improved outcome in the latter group appeared to be related to more frequent utilization of cesarean delivery and to earlier use of corticosteroids in these children because obstetricians and pediatricians were expecting the disease.[56] The most common antibodies noted in these patients are anti-PLA 1 and BAK antibodies.[57] Transfusion of maternal platelets into the neonate also improved outcome in these cases. After birth or in utero the child can be transfused with the mother's platelets since she lacks the antigen that would lead to platelet destruction by circulating antibodies. Bussel and colleagues[58] have demonstrated that the antenatal use of intravenous immunoglobulin may help to prevent thrombocytopenia in infants at risk for neonatal alloimmune thrombocytopenia. These investigators administered 1 g/kg per week to at risk mothers and observed no toxicity. The concomitant use of glucocorticoids has not necessarily been shown to boost the effect of the intravenous immunoglobulin.[59] Because of the frequency with which very low platelet counts are encountered in these fetuses, there is a risk of fetal exsanguination with cordocentesis.[60]

Iron Deficiency Anemia

During a singleton pregnancy, maternal plasma volume gradually expands by approximately 50 percent (1,000 ml). The total red blood cell (RBC) mass also increases, but only by approximately 300 ml (25 percent), and this starts later in pregnancy.[61] It is not surprising, therefore, that hemoglobin and hematocrit levels usually fall during gestation. These changes are not necessarily pathologic but usually represent a physiologic alteration of pregnancy. By 6 weeks postpartum, in the absence of excessive blood loss during the puerperium, hemoglobin and hematocrit levels have returned to normal.

Approximately 50 percent of pregnant women are anemic, with a hematocrit less than 32 percent. The incidence of anemia changes with epidemiologic differences in the population studied. Approximately 75 percent of anemias that occur during pregnancy are secondary to iron deficiency.[61] Ho and coinvestigators[62] performed elaborate hematologic evaluations of 221 normal full-term gravidas in Taiwan. None of the studied patients received an added hematinic during gestation. Of the previously nonanemic patients, 23 (10.4 percent) developed clinical anemia after a full-term pregnancy. Of the 23, 11 (47.8 percent) developed florid iron deficiency anemia, while another 11 developed moderate iron depletion. In 22 of 23 anemic patients, therefore, the anemia was secondary to iron deficiency.[62] The remaining patient was diagnosed as having folate deficiency. Among the 198 nonanemic gravidas at term, 92 (46.5 percent) showed evidence of iron depletion even though they had a normal hematocrit.[62]

To distinguish the normal physiologic changes of pregnancy from those of pathologic iron deficiency anemia, one must understand the iron requirements of pregnancy (Table 32-4) and the proper use of hematologic laboratory parameters. In the adult woman, iron stores are located in the bone marrow, liver, and spleen in the form of ferritin. Ferritin comprises approximately 25 percent (500 mg) of the 2-g iron stores found in the normal woman. Approximately 65 percent of stored iron is in the circulating RBCs.[61,63–65] If the dietary iron intake is poor, the interval between pregnancies is short, or delivery is complicated by hemorrhage, iron deficiency anemia readily develops.

The first pathologic change to occur in iron deficiency anemia is the depletion of bone marrow, liver, and spleen iron stores. The serum iron level falls, as does the percentage saturation of transferrin. The total iron-binding capacity rises, as this is a reflection of unbound transferrin. A fall in the hematocrit follows. Microcytic hypochromic RBCs are released into the circulation. Should iron deficiency be combined with folate deficiency, normocytic and normochromic RBCs will be observed on peripheral smear.

Care must be taken when using laboratory parameters to establish the diagnosis of iron deficiency anemia during gestation. A serum iron concentration less than 60 mg/dl with less than 16 percent saturation of

Table 32-4 Iron Requirements for Pregnancy and the Puerperium

Event	Elemental Iron
Increased red blood cell mass	450 mg
Fetus and placenta	360 mg
Vaginal delivery	190 mg
Lactation	1 mg/day

transferrin is suggestive of iron deficiency. An increase in total iron-binding capacity, however, is not reliable, as 15 percent of pregnant women without iron deficiency will show an increase in this parameter.[66] Serum ferritin levels normally decrease mildly during pregnancy. A significantly reduced ferritin concentration is also indicative of iron deficiency anemia and is the best parameter with which to judge the degree of iron deficiency. Ferritin levels, however, can change 25 percent from one day to the next.[67] If a patient has been iron deficient for an extended period of time and begins taking iron, her serum iron level can rise before she has repleted her iron stores. The ferritin level will indicate the status of her iron stores. If hematologic parameters remain confusing, bone marrow aspirations, which can be performed safely during gestation, will usually provide the definitive diagnosis. This procedure, however, is rarely necessary.

Whether all women should receive prophylactic iron during pregnancy remains controversial. Long[68] believes that physiology is responsible for much of the decrease in hematocrit, and, unless the patient is symptomatic or the hematocrit level is very low, iron supplementation is unnecessary. In pregnancy, iron absorption from the duodenum increases, providing 1.3 to 2.6 mg of elemental iron daily in patients with ideal dietary habits.[69,70] In patients who do not show clear signs of iron deficiency anemia, it is uncertain whether prophylactic iron leads to increased hemoglobin levels at term. Iron prophylaxis is safe, and, with the exception of dyspepsia and constipation, side effects are few. One 325-mg tablet of ferrous sulfate daily provides adequate prophylaxis. It contains 60 mg of elemental iron, 10 percent of which is absorbed. If the iron is not needed, it will not be absorbed and will be excreted in the stool. The standard generic iron tablets and the amount of elemental iron they provide are listed in Table 32-5.

One iron tablet three times daily is recommended for the pregnant patient with iron deficiency anemia. To ensure maximum absorption, iron should be ingested about 30 minutes before meals. When taken in this manner, however, dyspepsia and nausea are more common. Therapy, therefore, must be individualized to maximize patient compliance. If isolated iron deficiency anemia is present, one should see a dramatic reticulocytosis approximately 2 weeks after the initiation of therapy. Because iron absorption is pH dependent, taking iron with ascorbic acid (vitamin C) may increase duodenal absorption. Conversely, taking iron with antacids will decrease absorption.

It is controversial whether anemia results in an increase in adverse pregnancy outcomes. In a literature review, Scholl and Hediger[71] concluded that anemia diagnosed in early pregnancy is associated with preterm delivery and low birth weight. Women with iron deficiency anemia had twice the risk of preterm delivery and thrice the risk of delivering a low-birth-weight infant. Preterm labor is a multifactorial problem, and there were many confounders in this study. Despite this study, it is still uncertain whether iron deficiency is an independent causative agent of preterm delivery. In fact, Hemminki and Starfield[72] reviewed controlled trials and concluded that routine iron administration did not decrease preterm labor or raise birth weight.

Folate Deficiency

Folic acid, a water-soluble vitamin, is found in green vegetables, peanuts, and liver. Folate stores are located primarily in the liver and are usually sufficient for 6 weeks. After 3 weeks of a diet deficient in folate, the serum folate level falls. Two weeks later, hypersegmentation of neutrophils occurs. After 17 weeks without folate ingestion, RBC folate levels drop. In the next week a megaloblastic bone marrow develops. During pregnancy, folate deficiency is the most common cause of megaloblastic anemia, as vitamin B_{12} deficiency is extremely rare. The daily folate requirement in the nonpregnant state is approximately 50 µg, but this rises three- to fourfold during gestation.[73] Fetal demands increase the requirement, as does the decrease in the gastrointestinal absorption of folate during pregnancy.[74]

Clinical megaloblastic anemia seldom occurs before the third trimester of pregnancy. If the patient is at risk for folate deficiency or has mild anemia, an attempt should be made to detect this disorder before megaloblastosis occurs. Serum folate and RBC folate levels are the best tests for folate deficiency.[75]

Folate deficiency rarely occurs in the fetus and is not a cause of significant perinatal morbidity. Maternal morbidity, however, may result from the anemia, especially if the patient additionally suffers significant blood loss during the puerperium. Prenatal vitamins that require physician prescription contain 1 mg of folic acid. Most nonprescription prenatal vitamins contain 0.8 mg of folic acid. These amounts are more than adequate to prevent and treat folate deficiency. Women with significant hemoglobinopathies, patients ingesting phenytoin or other anticonvulsants, women carrying a mul-

Table 32-5 Elemental Iron Available from Common Iron Preparations

Preparation	Elemental Iron (mg)
Ferrous gluconate, 325 mg	37–39
Ferrous sulfate, 325 mg	60–65
Ferrous fumarate, 325 mg	107

tiple gestation, and women with frequent conception may require more than 1-mg supplemental folate daily. If the patient is folic acid deficient, her reticulocyte count will be depressed. Within 3 days after the administration of sufficient folic acid, reticulocytosis usually occurs. In fact, folic acid deficiency should be considered when a patient has unexplained thrombocytopenia. (Leukopenia and thrombocytopenia, which accompany megaloblastosis, are rapidly reversed.) The hematocrit level may rise as much as 1 percent per day after 1 week of folate replacement.

Iron deficiency is frequently concomitant with folic acid deficiency. If a patient with folate deficiency does not develop a significant reticulocytosis within 1 week after administration of sufficient replacement therapy, appropriate tests for iron deficiency should be performed.

Hemoglobinopathies

Hemoglobin is a tetrameric protein composed of two pairs of polypeptide chains with a heme group attached to each chain.[76] The normal adult hemoglobin A_1 comprises 95 percent of hemoglobin. It consists of two α-chains and two β-chains. The remaining 5 percent of hemoglobin usually consists of hemoglobin A_2 (containing two α-chains and two δ-chains) and/or hemoglobin F (with two α-chains and two γ-chains). In the fetus, hemoglobin F (fetal hemoglobin) declines during the third trimester of pregnancy, reaching its permanent nadir several months after birth. Hemoglobinopathies arise when there is a change in the structure of a peptide chain or a defect in the ability to synthesize a specific polypeptide chain. The patterns of inheritance are often straightforward. The prevalences of the most common hemoglobinopathies is listed in Table 32-6.

Hemoglobin S

Hemoglobin S, an aberrant hemoglobin, is present in patients with sickle cell disease (hemoglobin SS) and sickle cell trait (hemoglobin AS). A single substitution of valine for glutamic acid at the sixth position in the

Table 32-6 Hemoglobinopathies

Hemoglobinopathy	Frequency in Adult Blacks
Sickle cell trait	1:12
Sickle cell disease	1:708
Hemoglobin C trait	1:41
Hemoglobin C disease	1:4,790
Hemoglobin SC disease	1:757
Hemoglobin S/β-thalassemia	1:1,672

β-polypeptide chain causes a significant change in the physical characteristics of this hemoglobin. At low oxygen tensions, RBCs containing hemoglobin S assume a sickle shape. Sludging in small vessels occurs, resulting in microinfarction of the affected organs. Sickle cells have a life span of 5 to 10 days, compared with 120 days for a normal RBC. Sickling is triggered by hypoxia, acidosis, or dehydration. Infants with sickle cell anemia show no signs of the disease until the concentration of hemoglobin F falls to adult levels. Some patients do not experience symptoms until adolescence.

Approximately 1 of 12 adult blacks in the United States is heterozygous for hemoglobin S and, therefore, has sickle cell trait (hemoglobin AS) and carries the affected gene. These individuals generally have 35 to 45 percent hemoglobin S and are asymptomatic. The child of two individuals with sickle cell trait has a 50 percent probability of inheriting the trait and a 25 percent probability of actually having sickle cell disease. One of every 625 black children born in the United States is homozygous for hemoglobin S, and the frequency of sickle cell disease among adult blacks is 1 in 708.[77] All at-risk patients should be screened for hemoglobin S at their first prenatal visit. Patients with a positive screen should undergo hemoglobin electrophoresis. Women identified as having sickle cell trait (hemoglobin AS) are not at increased risk for poor perinatal outcome. The spouse, however, should be tested, and if both are carriers of a hemoglobinopathy prenatal diagnosis should be offered. Prenatal diagnosis can be performed by DNA analysis with the polymerase chain reaction (PCR) and Southern blotting.[78,79] PCR amplification of DNA fragments can allow a more rapid laboratory diagnosis. Hemoglobin S can also be identified by hemoglobin electrophoresis and DNA analysis of fetal blood.[80] Wang et al[81] reported on 500 prenatal diagnoses of sickle cell disease, 196 utilizing only Southern blotting and 304 utilizing PCR. PCR greatly shortened the time interval from sampling to diagnosis and resulted in an overall fourfold increase in diagnoses. They showed that a diagnosis made prior to 20 weeks' gestation increased the likelihood that the patient would elect pregnancy termination.[81] The odds ratio of termination in cases with earlier relative to later diagnosis was 4.7.

Painful vasoocclusive episodes involving multiple organs are the clinical hallmark of sickle cell anemia. The most common sites for these episodes are the extremities, joints, and abdomen. Vasoocclusive episodes can also occur in the lung, resulting in pulmonary infarction. Analgesia, oxygen, and hydration are the clinical foundations for treating these painful crises.

Sickle cell disease can affect virtually all organ systems. Osteomyelitis is common, and osteomyelitis caused by *Salmonella* is found almost exclusively in these patients. The risk of pyelonephritis is increased. Sickling may also occur in the renal medulla, where oxygen tension is reduced, resulting in papillary necrosis. These patients also exhibit renal tubular dysfunction and hyposthenuria. Because of chronic hemolysis and decreased RBC survival, patients with sickle cell anemia often demonstrate some degree of jaundice. Biliary stasis commonly occurs during crises, and cholelithiasis is seen in about 30 percent of cases.[82,83] Because of chronic anemia, high output cardiac failure can occur. Left ventricular hypertrophy and cardiomegaly are not uncommon.

Many pregnancies complicated by sickle cell anemia are associated with poor perinatal outcomes. The rate of spontaneous abortion may be as high as 25 percent.[84–86] Perinatal mortality rates of up to 40 percent were reported in the past, but the current estimate is approximately 15 percent.[85–90] Powars and coworkers[91] studied 156 pregnancies in 79 women with sickle cell anemia. In this group, the perinatal mortality rate was 52.7 percent before 1972 and 22.7 percent after that time. In a recent report by Seoud and coworkers,[92] the perinatal mortality rate was 10.5 percent. Much of this poor perinatal outcome is related to preterm birth. Approximately 30 percent of infants born to mothers with sickle cell disease have birth weights below 2,500 g.[85] In the Seoud et al[92] report, the mean birth weight was 2,443 g.[92] In a multicenter study, Smith et al[93] reported that 21 percent of infants born to mothers with sickle cell disease were small for gestational age. It has been hypothesized that sickling in the uterine vessels may lead to decreased fetal oxygenation and intrauterine growth restriction.[94] Classic teaching is that increased levels of hemoglobin F in the mother spared her from increased painful crises during pregnancy and may also have a protective effect on the neonate. In a study by Anyaegbunam and colleagues,[95] hemoglobin F levels, however, were inversely correlated with birth weight percentile. In contrast, Morris et al[96] studied 270 singleton pregnancies in 175 women with sickle cell disease. The overall fetal wastage rate was 32.2 percent. Mothers with high hemoglobin F levels had a significantly lower perinatal mortality rate.

Stillbirth rates of 8 to 10 percent have been described in patients with sickle cell anemia.[85] These fetal deaths happen not only during crises but also unexpectedly. Careful antepartum fetal testing must therefore be utilized, including serial ultrasonography to assess fetal growth. In another study, Anyaegbunam and coworkers[97] studied Doppler flow velocimetry in patients with hemoglobinopathies. They showed abnormal systolic/diastolic ratios for the uterine or umbilical arteries in 88 percent of patients with hemoglobin SS compared with 7 percent with hemoglobin AS and 4 percent with

hemoglobin AA. However, only 8 patients with hemoglobin SS were studied compared with 40 patients with hemoglobin AS and 48 women with hemoglobin AA.[97] Howard et al[98] showed that maternal exchange transfusions did not change uteroplacental Doppler blood flow velocimetry in these patients.[8] This demonstrates that although maternal well being may be improved, there is no change in uteroplacental pathology.

Although maternal mortality is rare in patients with sickle cell anemia, maternal morbidity is great. Infections are common, occurring in 50 to 67 percent of women with hemoglobin SS. Most are UTIs, which can be detected by frequent urine cultures. Patients with hemoglobin AS are also at greater risk for a UTI and should be screened as well. Pulmonary infection and infarction are also common. Patients with sickle cell anemia should receive pneumococcal vaccine before pregnancy. Any infection demands prompt attention, because fever, dehydration, and acidosis will result in further sickling and painful crises. The incidence of pregnancy-induced hypertension is increased in patients with sickle cell anemia and may complicate almost one-third of pregnancies in these patients.[88,93] Painful crises also appear to be more common during gestation.[99,100] This was not true, however, in one study.[93]

The care of the pregnant patient with sickle cell anemia must be individualized and meticulous. These patients will benefit from care in a medical center experienced in treating the multitude of problems that can complicate such pregnancies. From early gestation, good dietary habits should be promoted. A folate supplement of at least 1 mg/day should be administered as soon as pregnancy is confirmed. Although hemoglobin and hematocrit levels are decreased, iron supplements need not be routinely given. Serum iron and ferritin levels should be checked monthly and iron supplementation started only when these levels are diminished. Abudu and coworkers[101] found that serum ferritin values were significantly higher in pregnant women with hemoglobin SS disease than in those with hemoglobin AA. They concluded that the physiologic changes of pregnancy in patients with hemoglobin SS did not result in an iron deficiency state and that the use of prophylactic iron supplementations in these patients appears unjustified.

The role of prophylactic transfusions in the gravida with sickle cell anemia is controversial. This therapy, which replaces the patient's sickle cells with normal RBCs, can both improve oxygen carrying capacity and suppress the synthesis of sickle hemoglobin. A previous study showed a sevenfold reduction in perinatal mortality in patients receiving prophylactic transfusions.[102] In the same group of patients, there was a significant decrease in fetal growth restriction and preterm births. Morrison and coworkers[103] have also previously reported reduced perinatal wastage and maternal morbidity using a regimen of exchange transfusion. In contrast, workers at Johns Hopkins believe that meticulous prenatal care gives results as favorable as those obtained with prophylactic transfusion.[84] Many patients in that series, however, did require transfusion for painful crises and anemia. Koshy and coinvestigators[104] followed 72 pregnant patients with sickle cell anemia, one-half of whom received prophylactic transfusions and one-half transfusions only for medical or obstetric emergencies. There was no significant difference in perinatal outcome between the offspring of mothers who received prophylactic transfusions and those who did not. Two risk factors were identified as harbingers of an unfavorable outcome: (1) the occurrence of a perinatal death in a previous pregnancy and (2) twins in the present pregnancy. Even though there was no difference in perinatal morbidity and mortality, prophylactic transfusion did appear to decrease significantly the incidence of painful crises. The investigators concluded that the omission of prophylactic RBC transfusion will not harm pregnant patients with sickle cell disease or their offspring.[104]

Keidan and coworkers[105] performed a prospective study to see which patients might benefit most from transfusion. Although the number of patients was small, the conclusions reached in this study are interesting. These investigators devised a "sicklecrit," which was the product of the hematocrit and the percentage of hemoglobin S. They also looked at erythrocyte filterability through pores of 5 μm diameter. Using these methods, they hoped to assess blood rheology in large and small vessels, respectively, to monitor the effects of exchange transfusion in sickle cell disease.[105] This preliminary work may prove helpful in deciding which patients will benefit from prophylactic transfusion. Tuck and coworkers[106] delineated the risks involved with exchange transfusion. In a study of 51 pregnancies transfused between 1978 and 1984, 22 percent developed atypical red cell antibodies and 14 percent had immediate minor transfusion reactions. These data showed no significant difference in maternal or fetal outcomes among patients who were transfused prophylactically and those who were not.[106] The studies did not show fetal benefits from exchange transfusion. They did not, however, attempt to quantify changes in maternal well-being. This needs to be carefully evaluated before stating that prophylactic transfusions should be eliminated from the care of the pregnant patient with sickle cell disease.

If one chooses to perform prophylactic transfusion, the goal is to maintain a percentage of hemoglobin A above 20 percent at all times and preferably above 40 percent, as well as to maintain the hematocrit above 25 percent. Morrison et al[103] recommend that prophylactic transfusion begin at 28 weeks' gestation. Buffy-coat-poor washed RBCs are used to reduce the risk of isosensitization. Other risks of transfusion therapy include hepatitis, acquired immunodeficiency syndrome (AIDS), transfusion reactions, and hemochromatosis. Human immunodeficiency virus (HIV) antibody testing and new tests for hepatitis C have made transfusions much safer.

Either booster or exchange transfusions can be used. Exchange transfusions are preferable because they result in less stress on the cardiovascular system, thus decreasing the possibility of congestive heart failure. Exchange transfusions also raise the percentage of hemoglobin A more efficiently. If only booster transfusions are utilized, diuretics should probably be administered to prevent fluid overload. Exchange transfusion can easily be performed by the pheresis unit of the hospital. This is faster and safer than older techniques. The patient should be positioned on her left side during the procedure to maximize uterine blood flow.

Vaginal delivery is preferred for patients with sickle cell disease. Cesarean delivery should be reserved for obstetric indications. Patients should labor in the left lateral recumbent position and receive supplemental oxygen. While adequate hydration should be maintained, fluid overload must be avoided. Conduction anesthesia is recommended, as it provides excellent pain relief and can be used for cesarean delivery, if necessary.

Hemoglobin SC Disease

Hemoglobin C is another β-chain variant in which lysine is substituted for glutamic acid in the sixth position. Clinically significant hemoglobin SC disease occurs in 1 in 833 adult blacks in the United States.[77] Women with both S and C hemoglobin suffer less morbidity in pregnancy than do patients with only hemoglobin S.[81,84,86] As in sickle cell disease, however, there is an increased incidence of early spontaneous abortion and pregnancy-induced hypertension.[84–87]

Because patients with SC disease can have only mild symptoms, the hemoglobinopathy may remain undiagnosed until they suffer a crisis during pregnancy. These crises may be marked by sequestration of a large volume of RBCs in the spleen accompanied by a dramatic fall in hematocrit.[107,108] Because these patients have increased splenic activity, they may be mildly thrombocytopenic throughout pregnancy. During gestation, patients with hemoglobin SC should receive the same program of prenatal care outlined for women with hemoglobin SS.

Thalassemia

Thalassemia results from a defect in the rate of globin chain synthesis. Any of the polypeptide chains can be affected. The disease may range from minimal suppression of synthesis of the affected chain to its complete absence. Either α- or β-thalassemia can occur. Heterozygous patients are often asymptomatic. Thalassemia can be detected by prenatal diagnosis. Wainscoat and coworkers[109] were able to offer prenatal diagnosis to 19 of 25 families with a potential for β-thalassemia using linkage analysis of restriction fragment length polymorphisms (RFLP). Cao and colleagues[110] reported their experience with prenatal diagnosis of β-thalassemia in 1,000 pregnancies followed at least 12 months after birth. Fetal blood sampling was carried out by placental aspiration, which yielded a sufficient amount of blood in 99 percent of cases. The fetal mortality rate associated with the fetal blood sampling, however, was 6.3 percent. Focharoen and coworkers[111] have been able to diagnose β-thalassemia in the second trimester by in vitro protein synthesis. They detect α-thalassemia by gene amplification in the first trimester.

Homozygous α-thalassemia results in the formation of tetramers of β-chains known as hemoglobin Bart. This hemoglobinopathy can result in hydrops fetalis. Ghosh and coinvestigators[112] reported their experience with 26 Chinese women who were at risk of giving birth to a fetus with homozygous α-thalassemia. Six of the 26 fetuses were affected. In two of the six cases, progressive fetal ascites appeared before 24 weeks' gestation. These pregnancies were terminated and the diagnoses confirmed. In the remaining four cases, there was evidence of intrauterine growth restriction by 28 weeks' gestation. At later gestational ages, an increase in the transverse cardiac diameter was seen in the affected fetuses.[112] Woo and colleagues[113] reported that umbilical artery velocimetry reveals a hyperdynamic circulatory state in fetuses that are hydropic because of α-thalassemia. In a study from Taiwan, Hsieh et al[114] demonstrated that umbilical vein blood flow measurements can help to distinguish hydrops fetalis caused by hemoglobin Bart from hydrops fetalis having other causes. The umbilical vein diameter, blood velocity, and blood flow in fetuses with hemoglobin Bart were usually higher than those in fetuses with hydrops fetalis having other etiologies.

β-Thalassemia is the most common form of thalassemia. Patients with the heterozygous state are usually asymptomatic. They are detected by an increase in their level of hemoglobin A_2. In the homozygous state, synthesis of hemoglobin A_1 may be completely suppressed. This condition is characterized by an increase in both hemoglobin F and hemoglobin A_2. The homozygous state of β-thalassemia is known as thalassemia major,

or Cooley's anemia. Patients with this disorder are transfusion dependent and have marked hepatosplenomegaly and bone changes secondary to increased hematopoiesis. These individuals usually die of infectious or cardiovascular complications before they reach childbearing age. Successful full-term pregnancies have been reported.[115] The few patients who do become pregnant generally exhibit severe anemia and congestive heart failure. Prenatal care is dependent on transfusion therapy similar to that used in the care of the patient with sickle cell disease.

Heterozygous β-thalassemia has different forms of expression. Patients with thalassemia minima have microcytosis but are asymptomatic. Those with thalassemia intermedia exhibit splenomegaly and significant anemia and may become transfusion dependent during pregnancy. Their anemia can be significant enough to produce high-output cardiac failure.[116] If these patients have not undergone splenectomy, they are at risk for a hypersplenic crisis.[117] Also, extramedullary hematopoiesis may impinge upon the spine, resulting in neurologic symptoms.[118]

These patients should be managed with a treatment program similar to that followed for patients with sickle cell disease. As in the case of sickle hemoglobinopathies, iron supplementation should only be given if necessary, as indiscriminate use of iron can lead to hemochromatosis. White and coworkers[119] have shown that patients with a β-thalassemia usually have a much higher ferritin concentration than normal patients and those who are α-thalassemia carriers. In β-thalassemia carriers, the incidence of iron deficiency anemia is four times less common than it is in α-thalassemia carriers and normal patients.[119] Van der Weyden and coworkers[120] have convincingly shown that red cell ferritin and plasma ferritin can be used in combination to determine if a patient has a potential for iron overload. Although iron is not necessary, folic acid supplementation appears important in β-thalassemia carriers. Leung and coinvestigators[121] showed that the daily administration of folate significantly increased the predelivery hemoglobin concentration in both nulliparous and multiparous patients.

As in the case of sickle cell disease, antepartum fetal evaluation is essential in patients with thalassemia who are anemic. Asymptomatic thalassemia carriers need no special testing. However, patients with thalassemia should undergo frequent ultrasonography to assess fetal growth, as well as nonstress testing to evaluate fetal well-being.

Occasionally, individuals will inherit two hemoglobinopathies, such as sickle cell thalassemia (hemoglobin S thal). The prevalence of this disorder among adult blacks in the United States is 1:1,672.[122] The clinical course is variable. If minimal suppression of β-chains occurs, patients may be free of symptoms. However, with total suppression of β-chain synthesis, a clinical picture similar to that of sickle cell disease will develop. The course of these patients during pregnancy is quite variable, and their therapy must be individualized.

Von Willebrand's Disease

von Willebrand's disease is an inherited disorder of co-agulation and has a prevalence of 1/10,000. Type I is an autosomal dominant disorder, while type III and occasionally type II are autosomal recessive.[123] von Willebrand's disease is characterized by a decrease or defect in the von Willebrand's portion of the Factor VIII complex. von Willebrand's factor, also known as the *ristocetin cofactor*, plays a significant role in platelet aggregation. There are several variants of von Willebrand's disease. These are delineated by the portion of von Willebrand's factor that is decreased or absent. The most common form, type I, is characterized by a quantitative decrease in the entire von Willebrand's factor. In type IIB, the only clinical symptom in pregnancy may be thrombocytopenia. This diagnosis, therefore, should be considered in the gravida presenting with isolated thrombocytopenia during pregnancy.[124,125] The assays used to diagnose von Willebrand's disease are listed in Table 32-7.

The clinical severity of von Willebrand's disease is quite variable. Menorrhagia, easy bruising, gingival bleeding, and epistaxis are common. Some patients may be entirely asymptomatic until they have severe bleeding after surgery or trauma.

Classically the bleeding time is prolonged in patients with von Willebrand's disease as a result of diminished platelet aggregation. Occasionally, the activated partial thromboplastin time (APTT) will also be abnormal. In pregnancy, clotting factors including the Factor VIII complex increase, and the patient's bleeding time may improve as gestation progresses.[126,127] This is especially true for type IA von Willebrand's disease. In type IB, the patient may not correct her bleeding time.[128]

Table 32-7   Diagnosis of von Willebrand's disease

Template bleeding time
Activated partial thromboplastin time
von Willebrand's factor antigen
Ristocetin cofactor activity
Factor VIII coagulant activity
Ristocetin-induced platelet aggregation
Multimeric analysis

In type IIB, the platelet count will decrease. There will, however, be an improvement in the von Willebrand's factor multimeric pattern.[129] Heavy bleeding may be encountered in patients with von Willebrand's disease undergoing elective or spontaneous first trimester abortion because the levels of Factor VIII have not yet risen. von Willebrand's disease does not appear to affect fetal growth or development. Postpartum hemorrhage may be a serious problem. The concentration of Factor VIII C appears to determine the risk of hemorrhage. If the Factor VIII C level is greater than 50 percent of normal and the patient has a normal bleeding time, she should not bleed excessively at vaginal delivery.[127,128,130–132] The clinical course during labor is quite variable. In a study by Chediak and coworkers,[133] bleeding complications were seen in six of eight (75 percent) pregnancies. Five of the newborns had von Willebrand's disease, one of whom was born with a scalp hematoma. Conti and associates,[134] conversely, reported no bleeding complications during the puerperium in five women with von Willebrand's disease. Ieko and colleagues[135] demonstrated that Factor VIII concentrate could raise the platelet levels in patients with type IIB von Willebrand's disease.

Cryoprecipitate was, for many years, the treatment of choice, as it contains all forms of both Factor VIII C and the ristocetin cofactor. Virucidal methods cannot, however, be applied to cryoprecipitate. In those not responding to desmopressin, plasma-derived Factor VIII/von Willebrand's factor concentrates should be used.[123] The medium-purity and high-purity forms should be used, as they contain the most variety of multimers. Desmopressin (DDAVP) is the treatment of choice in all types of von Willebrand's disease except type IIB.[123] It elicits the release of von Willebrand's factor from endothelial cells. Intranasal preparations of 300 μg are usually used. In emergent or preoperative situations, 0.3 μg/kg can be given intravenously over 30 minutes.[123] It can rarely cause hyponatremia and fluid retention.

Bleeding during pregnancy is rare. Patients with classic type I von Willebrand's disease usually need no treatment with the increase in Factor VIII levels during pregnancy. Those with a history of postpartum hemorrhage should be given an intravenous dose of desmopressin immediately after delivery, and the dose should be repeated 24 hours later. For those with type II disease, Factor VIII/von Willebrand's factor concentrates are occasionally needed. Before a cesarean delivery, bleeding time should be measured. If it is prolonged, type I patients should be given desmopressin and type II patients should be given Factor VIII/von Willebrand's factor concentrate.

Key Points

- 4 percent of pregnancies will be complicated by maternal platelet counts of less than 150,000/mm^3. The vast majority of these patients will have gestational thrombocytopenia with a benign course and will need no intervention.

- Surgical bleeding occurs if the platelet count falls below 50,000/mm^3 and spontaneous bleeding occurs if the platelet count falls below 20,000/mm^3.

- If the platelet count falls below 75,000/mm^3, the patient still may have gestational thrombocytopenia, but it is the physician's responsibility to rule out other serious causes of thrombocytopenia before making this diagnosis.

- Glucocorticoids are the first line medication used to raise a low platelet count.

- Iron deficiency anemia is the most common cause of anemia in pregnancy and serum ferritin is the single best test to diagnose it.

- If a patient with presumed iron deficiency does increase her reticulocyte count with iron therapy, she may also have a concomitant folic acid deficiency.

- Patients pregnant with twins, those on anticonvulsant therapy, those with a hemoglobinopathy, and those who conceive frequently need supplemental folic acid during gestation.

- Most hereditary hemoglobinopathies can be detected in utero and prenatal diagnosis should be offered to the patient early in pregnancy.

- As in the nonpregnant patient, analgesia, hydration, and oxygen are the key factors in treating pregnant women with sickle cell crisis.

- Patients with sickle cell disease are at high risk of having a fetus with growth restriction and adverse fetal outcomes. Therefore, they warrant frequent sonography and antepartum fetal evaluation.

References

1. McRae KR, Samuels P, Schreiber AD: Pregnancy-associated thrombocytopenia: pathogenesis and management. Blood 80:2697, 1992
2. Aster RH: Gestational thrombocytopenia. A plea for conservative management. N Engl J Med 323:264, 1990
3. Samuels P, Bussel JB, Braitman LE et al: Estimation of the risk of thrombocytopenia in the offspring of pregnant women with presumed immune thrombocytopenia purpura. N Engl J Med 323:229, 1990
4. Samuels P, Main EK, Tomaski A et al: Abnormalities in platelet antiglobulin tests in preeclamptic mothers and their neonates. Am J Obstet Gynecol 107:109, 1987
5. Burrows RF, Kelton JG: Incidentally detected thrombocytopenia in healthy mothers and their infants. N Engl J Med 319:142, 1988
6. Hart D, Dunetz C, Nardi M et al: An epidemic of maternal thrombocytopenia associated with elevated antiplatelet antibody in 116 consecutive pregnancies: Relationship to neonatal platelet count. Am J Obstet Gynecol 154:878, 1986
7. Burrows RF, Kelton JG: Fetal thrombocytopenia and its relation to maternal thrombocytopenia. N Engl J Med 329:1463, 1993
8. Burrows RF, Kelton JG: Low fetal risks in pregnancies associated with idiopathic thrombocytopenia purpura. Am J Obstet Gynecol 163:1147, 1990
9. Peterson OH Jr, Larson P: Thrombocytopenic purpura in pregnancy. Obstet Gynecol 4:454, 1954
10. Tancer ML: Idiopathic thrombocytopenic purpura and pregnancy: report of 5 new cases and review of the literature. Am J Obstet Gynecol 79:148, 1960
11. Territo J, Finkelstein J, Oh W et al: Management of autoimmune thrombocytopenia in pregnancy and in the neonate. Obstet Gynecol 51:590, 1973
12. Carloss HW, MacMillan R, Crosby WH: Management of pregnancy in women with immune thrombocytopenic purpura. JAMA 244:2756, 1980
13. Noriega-Guerra L, Aviles-Miranda A, de la Cadena OA et al: Pregnancy in patients with autoimmune thrombocytopenic purpura. Am J Obstet Gynecol 133:439, 1979
14. Heys RFI: Child bearing and idiopathic thrombocytopenic purpura. J Obstet Gynaecol Br Commonw 73:205, 1966
15. Karapatkin M, Porges RF, Karapatkin S: Platelet counts in infants of women with autoimmune thrombocytopenia: effects of steroid administration to the mother. N Engl J Med 305:936, 1981
16. Cines DB, Dusak B, Tomaski A et al: Immune thrombocytopenic purpura and pregnancy. N Engl J Med 306:826, 1982
17. Cines DB: Idiopathic thrombocytopenic purpura complicating pregnancy. Medical Grand Rounds 3:344, 1984
18. Kelton JG, Inwood MJ, Narr RM et al: The prenatal prediction of thrombocytopenia in infants of mothers with clinically diagnosed immune thrombocytopenia. Am J Obstet Gynecol 144:449, 1982
19. Harrington WJ, Minnich V, Arimura G: The autoimmune thrombocytopenias. p. 166. In Tascantins LM (ed): Progress in Hematology. Grune and Stratton, New York, 1956
20. Shulman NR, Marder VJ, Weinrach RS: Similarities between known antiplatelet antibodies and the factor responsible for thrombocytopenia in idiopathic purpura. Ann NY Acad Sci 124:499, 1965
21. Cines DB, Schreiber AD: Immune thrombocytopenia: use of a Coombs antiglobulin test to detect IgG and C3 on platelets. N Engl J Med 300:106, 1979
22. He R, Reid DM, Jones CE, Shulman NR: Spectrum of Ig classes, specificities, and titers of serum antiglycopro-

teins in chronic idiopathic thrombocytopenic purpura. Blood 83:1024, 1994

23. Yeager AM, Zinkham WH: Varicella-associated thrombocytopenia: clues to the etiology of childhood idiopathic thrombocytopenic purpura. Johns Hopkins Med J 146:270, 1980

24. Scott JR, Cruikshank DR, Kochenour NK et al: Fetal platelet counts in the obstetric management of immunologic thrombocytopenic purpura. Am J Obstet Gynecol 136:495, 1980

25. Moise KJ, Carpenter RJ, Cotton DB et al: Percutaneous umbilical cord blood sampling in the evaluation of fetal platelet counts in pregnant patients with autoimmune thrombocytopenic purpura. Obstet Gynecol 160:427, 1989

26. Kaplan C, Daffos F, Forstier F et al: Fetal platelet counts in thrombocytopenic pregnancy. Lancet 336:979, 1990

27. Sciosia AL, Grannum PA, Copel JA, Hobbins JC: The use of percutaneous umbilical blood sampling in immune thrombocytopenic purpura. Am J Obstet Gynecol 159:1066, 1988

28. Ghidini A, Sepulveda W, Lockwood CJ, Romero R: Complications of blood sampling. Am J Obstet Gynecol 168:1339, 1993

29. Burrows RF, Kelton JG: Pregnancy in patients with idiopathic thrombocytopenic purpura: assessing the risks for the infant at delivery. Obstet Gynecol Survey 458:781, 1993

30. Moschcowitz E: Hyaline thrombosis of the terminal arterioles and capillaries: a hitherto undescribed disease. Proc NY Pathol Soc 24:21, 1924

31. Miller JM, Pastorek JG: Thrombotic thrombocytopenic purpura and the hemolytic uremic syndrome in pregnancy. Clin Obstet Gynecol 34:64, 1991

32. Ridolfi RL, Bell WR: Thrombotic thrombocytopenic purpura: report of 25 cases and a review of the literature. Medicine 60:413, 1981

33. Kwaan HC: Clinicopathologic features of thrombotic thrombocytopenic purpura. Semin Hematol 24:71, 1987

34. Weiner CP: Thrombotic microangiopathy in pregnancy and the postpartum period. Semin Hematol 24:119, 1987

35. Weiner CP, Kwaan HC, Xu C et al: Antithrombin III activity in women with hypertension during pregnancy. Obstet Gynecol 65:301, 1985

36. Nield GH: Haemolytic uraemic syndrome. Nephron 59:194, 1991

37. Karmali MA, Petrie M, Lim C et al: The association between idiopathic hemolytic uraemic syndrome and infection by verocytotoxin producing *Escherichia coli*. J Infect Dis 151:775, 1985

38. Shulman H, Striker G, Deeg HJ et al: Nephrotoxicity of cyclosporine A after allogeneic marrow transplantation: glomerular thromboses and tubular injury. N Engl J Med 305:1392, 1981

39. Giroux L, Bettez P: Mitomycin C nephrotoxicity: a clinicopathologic study of 17 cases. Am J Kidney Dis 6:28, 1985

40. Brown CG, Robson AP, Robson JG et al: Haemolytic

uraemic syndrome in a woman taking oral contraceptives. Lancet 1:1479, 1973

41. Rousell RH: A new intravenous immunoglobulin in adult and childhood idiopathic thrombocytopenic purpura: a review. J Infect 15:59, 1987

42. Mitra G, Wong MF, Mozen MM et al: Elimination of infectious retroviruses during preparation of immunoglobulins. Transfusion 26:394, 1986

43. Schwartz RS: Overview of the biochemistry and safety of a new native intravenous gammaglobulin, IGIV, pH 4.25. Am J Med 83:46, 1987

44. Schwartz RS: Biochemistry and safety of native intravenous gammaglobulin (IGIV, pH 4.25). J Clin Apheresis 4:89, 1988

45. Rousell RH, Budinger MD, Pirofsky B, Schiff RI: Prospective study on the hepatitis safety of intravenous immunoglobulin, pH 4.25. Vox Sang 60:65, 1991

46. Rousell RH, Good RA, Pirofsky B, Schiff RI: Non-A non-B hepatitis and the safety of intravenous immunoglobulin pH 4.25: a retrospective survey. Vox Sang 54:6, 1988

47. Kelton JG, Inwood MJ, Barr RM et al: The prenatal prediction of thrombocytopenia in infants of mothers with clinically diagnosed immune thrombocytopenia. Am J Obstet Gynecol 144:449, 1982

48. Moise KF Jr: Autoimmune thrombocytopenic purpura in pregnancy. Clin Obstet Gynecol 34:51, 1991

49. Cooke RL, Miller RC, Katz VL, et al: Immune thrombocytopenic purpura in pregnancy: A reappraisal of management. Obstet Gyncol 78:578, 1991

50. Lian ECY, Byrnes JJ, Harkness DR: Two successful pregnancies in a woman with chronic thrombotic thrombocytopenic purpura. Int J Obstet Gynecol 29:359, 1989

51. Ezra Y, Mordel N, Sadovsky E et al: Successful pregnancies of two patients with relapsing thrombotic thrombocytopenic purpura. Int J Obstet Gynecol 29:359, 1989

52. Ponticelli C, Rivolta E, Imbasciatti E et al: Hemolytic uremic syndrome in adults. Arch Int Med 140:353, 1980

53. Beattie TJ, Murphy AV, Willoughby MLN, Belch JJF: Prostacyclin infusion in haemolytic-uraemic syndrome of children. BMJ 283:470, 1981

54. Olah KS, Gee H: Postpartum haemolytic uraemic syndrome precipitated by antibiotics. Br J Obstet Gynaecol 97:83, 1990

55. Gutterman LA, Levin DM, George BS, Sharma HM: The hemolytic-uremic syndrome: recovery after treatment with vincristine. Ann Intern Med 98:612, 1983

56. Deaver JE, Leppert PC, Zaroulis CG: Neonatal alloimmune thrombocytopenic purpura. Am J Perinatol 3:127, 1986

57. Okada N, Oda M, Sano T et al: Intracranial hemorrhage in utero due to fetomaternal Bak(a) incompatibility. Nippon Ketsueki Gakkai Zasshi 51:1086, 1988

58. Bussel JB, McFarland JG, Berkowitz R: Antenatal treatment of fetal alloimmune cytopenias. Blut 59:136, 1989

59. Menell JS, Bussel JB: Antenatal management of thrombocytopenias. Clin Perinatol 21:591, 1994

60. Paidas AH, Berkowitz RL, Lynch L et al: Alloimmune

thrombocytopenia: fetal and neonatal losses related to cordocentesis. Am J Obstet Gynecol 172:475, 1995

61. Pitkin RM: Nutritional influences during pregnancy. Med Clin North Am 61:3, 1977

62. Ho CH, Yuan CC, Yeh SH: Serum ferritin, folate and cobalamin levels and their correlation with anemia in normal full-term pregnant women. Eur J Obstet Gynecol Reprod Biol 26:7, 1987

63. DeLeeuw NKM, Lowenstein L, Hsieh YS: Iron deficiency and hydremia of normal pregnancy. Medicine 45:291, 1966

64. Chopa J, Noe E, Matthew J et al: Anemia in pregnancy. Am J Public Health 57:857, 1967

65. Holly RG: Dynamics of iron metabolism in pregnancy. Am J Obstet Gynecol 93:370, 1965

66. Carr MC: Serum iron/TIBC in the diagnosis of iron deficiency anemia during pregnancy. Obstet Gynecol 38:602, 1971

67. Boued JL: Iron deficiency: assessment during pregnancy and its importance in pregnant adolescents. Am J Clin Nutr 59:5025, 1994

68. Long PJ: Rethinking iron supplementation during pregnancy. J Nurse Midwifery 40:36, 1995

69. Zuspan FP, Long WN, Russell JK et al: Anemia in pregnancy. J Reprod Med 6:13, 1971

70. Pritchard JA: Changes in the blood volume during pregnancy and delivery. Anesthesiology 26:393, 1965

71. Scholl TO, Hediger ML: Anemia and iron-deficiency anemia: compilation of data on pregnancy outcome. Am J Clin Nutr 59:4925, 1994

72. Hemminki E, Starfield B: Routine administration of iron and vitamins during pregnancy: review of controlled clinical trials. Br J Obstet Gynaecol 85:404, 1978

73. Rothman D: Folic acid in pregnancy. Am J Obstet Gynecol 108:49, 1970

74. Giles C, Ball EW: Iron and folic acid deficiency in pregnancy. BMJ 1:656, 1965

75. Ek J: Plasma and red cell folate values in newborn infants and their mothers in relation to gestational age. J Pediatr 97:288, 1980

76. Lambert EK, Bloom RN, Kosby M: Pregnancy in patients with hemoglobinopathies and thalassemias. J Reprod Med 19:193, 1977

77. Motulsky AG: Frequency of sickling disorders in US blacks. N Engl J Med 288:31, 1973

78. Lynch JR, Brown JM: The polymerase chain reaction: current and future clinical applications. J Med Genet 27:2, 1990

79. Husain SM, Kalavathi P, Anandraj MP: Analysis of sickle cell gene using polymerase chain reaction and restriction enzyme Bsu 361. Ind J Med Res 101:273, 1995

80. Posey YF, Shah D, Ulm JE et al: Prenatal diagnosis of sickle cell anemia: hemoglobin electrophoresis versus DNA analysis. Am J Clin Pathol 92:347, 1989

81. Wang X, Seeman C, Chen T et al: Experience with 500 prenatal diagnoses of sickle cell disease. Prenat Diagn 14:851, 1994

82. Barret-Connor E: Cholelithiasis in sickle cell anemia. Am J Med 45:889, 1968

83. Cameron JL, Moddrey WC, Ziridema GD et al: Biliary tract disease in sickle cell anemia: surgical considerations. Ann Surg 174:702, 1971

84. Charache S, Scott J, Niebyl J, Bonds D: Management of sickle cell disease in pregnant patients. Obstet Gynecol 55:407, 1980

85. Fort AT, Morrison JC, Berreras L et al: Counseling the patient with sickle cell disease about reproduction: pregnancy outcome does not justify the maternal risk. Am J Obstet Gynecol 111:391, 1971

86. Freeman MG, Ruth GJ: SS disease and SC disease—obstetric considerations and treatment. Clin Obstet Gynecol 12:134, 1969

87. Curtis EM: Pregnancy in sickle cell anemia, sickle cell-hemoglobin C disease, and variants thereof. Am J Obstet Gynecol 77:1312, 1959

88. Horger EO III: Sickle cell and sickle cell-hemoglobin disease during pregnancy. Obstet Gynecol 39:873, 1972

89. Milner PF, Jones BR, Dobler J: Outcome of pregnancy in sickle cell anemia and sickle cell-hemoglobin C disease. Am J Obstet Gynecol 138:239, 1980

90. Fessas P, Loukopoulos D: Beta thalassaemias. Clin Hematol 3:411, 1974

91. Powars DR, Sandhu M, Niland-Weiss J et al: Pregnancy in sickle cell disease. Obstet Gynecol 67:217, 1986

92. Seoud MA, Cantwell C, Nobles G, Levy OL: Outcome of pregnancies complicated by sickle cell disease and sickle-c hemoglobinopathies. Am J Perinatol 11:187, 1994

93. Smith JA, England M, Bellevue R et al: Pregnancy in sickle cell disease: experience of the cooperative study of sickle cell disease. Obstet Gynecol 87:199, 1996

94. Fiakpui EF, Moron EM: Pregnancy in sickle hemoglobins. J Reprod Med 11:28, 1973

95. Anyaegbunam A, Billet HH, Langer O et al: Maternal hemoglobin F levels may have an adverse effect on neonatal birth weight in pregnancies with sickle cell disease. Am J Obstet Gynecol 161:654, 1989

96. Morris JS, Dunn DT, Poddorr D, Serjeant GR: Hematological risk factors for pregnancy outcome in Jamaican women with homozygous sickle cell disease. Br J Obstet Gynaecol 101:770, 1994

97. Anyaegbunam A, Langer O, Brustman L et al: The application of uterine and umbilical artery velocimetry to the antenatal supervision of pregnancies complicated by maternal sickle hemoglobinopathies. Am J Obstet Gynecol 159:544, 1988

98. Howard RJ, Tuck SM, Pearson TC: Blood transfusion in pregnancy complicated by sickle cell disease: effects on blood rheology and uteroplacental Doppler velocimetry. Clin Lab Haematol 16:253, 1994

99. Perkins RP: Inherited disorders of hemoglobin synthesis and pregnancy. Am J Obstet Gynecol 111:130, 1971

100. Baum KF, Dunn DT, Maude GH, Serjeant GR: The painful crisis of homozygous sickle cell disease: a study of the risk factors. Arch Intern Med 147:1231, 1987

101. Abudu OO, Macaulay K, Oluboyede OA: Serial evaluation of iron stores in pregnant Nigerians with hemoglobin SS or SC. J Natl Med Assoc 82:41, 1990

102. Cunningham FG, Pritchard JA, Mason R: Pregnancy and sickle cell hemoglobinopathies: results with and

without prophylactic transfusions. Obstet Gynecol 62: 419, 1983

103. Morrison JC, Schneider JM, Whybrew WD et al: Prophylactic transfusions in pregnant patients with sickle hemoglobinopathies: benefit versus risk. Obstet Gynecol 56:274, 1980

104. Koshy M, Burd L, Wallace D et al: Prophylactic red-cell transfusions in pregnant patients with sickle cell disease: a randomized cooperative study. N Engl J Med 319:1447, 1988

105. Keidan AJ, Marwah SS, Bareford D et al: Laboratory tests for monitoring prophylactic exchange transfusion in pregnancy. Clin Lab Haematol 10:243, 1988

106. Tuck SM, James CE, Brewster EM et al: Prophylactic blood transfusion in maternal sickle cell syndromes. Br J Obstet Gynecol 94:121, 1987

107. Fullerton WT, Hendrickse J, Williams W et al: Hemoglobin SC: clinical course. p. 215. In Jonxis JHP (ed): Abnormal hemoglobins in Africa: A Symposium. Blackwell Scientific Publications, Oxford, 1965

108. Solanki DL, Kletter GG, Castro O: Acute splenic sequestration crises in adults with sickle cell disease. Am J Med 80:985, 1986

109. Wainscoat JS, Work S, Sampietro M et al: Feasibility of prenatal diagnosis of beta thalassaemia by DNA polymorphisms in an Italian population. Br J Haematol 62: 495, 1986

110. Cao A, Falchi AM, Tuveri T et al: Prenatal diagnosis of thalassemia major by fetal blood analysis: experience with 1,000 cases. Prenat Diagn 6:159, 1986

111. Focharoen S, Winichagoon P, Thonglairoam V. Prenatal diagnosis of thalassemia and hemoglobinopathies in Thailand: Experience from 100 pregnancies. Southeast Asian J of Trop Med & Pub Hlth 22:16, 1991

112. Ghosh A, Tan MH, Liang ST et al: Ultrasound evaluation of pregnancies at risk for homozygous alpha-thalassaemia-1. Prenat Diagn 7:307, 1987

113. Woo JS, Liang ST, Lo RL, Chan FY: Doppler blood flow velocity waveforms in alpha-thalassemia hydrops fetalis. J Ultrasound Med 6:679, 1987

114. Hsieh FJ, Chang FM, Huang HC et al: Umbilical vein blood flow measurement in nonimmune hydrops fetalis. Obstet Gynecol 71:188, 1988

115. Mordel N, Birkenfeld A, Goldfarb AN, Rachmilewitz EA: Successful full-term pregnancy in homozygous beta-thalassemia major: case report and review of the literature. Obstet Gynecol 73:837, 1989

116. Necheles T: Obstetric complications associated with haemoglobinopathies. Clin Hematol 2:497, 1973

117. Savona-Ventura C, Bonello F. Betathalassemia syndromes in pregnancy. Obstet Gynecol Survey 49:129, 1994

118. Singounas EG, Sakas DE, Hadley OM. Paraplegia in a pregnant thalassemic woman due to extramedullary hematopoesis: Successful management with transfusions. Surgical Neurol 36:210, 1991

119. White JM, Richards R, Jelenski G et al: Iron state in alpha and beta thalassaemia trait. J Clin Pathol 39:256, 1986

120. Van der Weyden MB, Fong H, Hallam LJ, Harrison C: Red cell ferritin and iron overload in heterozygous beta-thalassemia. Am J Hematol 30:201, 1989

121. Leung CF, Lao TT, Chang AM: Effect of folate supplement on pregnant women with beta-thalassaemia minor. Eur J Obstet Gynecol Reprod Biol 33:209, 1989

122. Schmidt RM: Laboratory diagnosis of hemoglobinopathies. JAMA 224:1276, 1973

123. Castaman G, Rodeghiero F. Current management of von Willebrand's disease. Drugs 50:602, 1995

124. Giles AR, Hoogendoorn H. Benford K: Type IIB von Willebrand's disease presenting as thrombocytopenia during pregnancy. Br J Haematol 67:349, 1987

125. Rick ME, Williams SB, Sacher RA, McKeown LP: Thrombocytopenia associated with pregnancy in a patient with type IIB von Willebrand's disease. Blood 69: 786, 1987

126. Kasper CK, Hoags MS, Aggeler PM, Stone S: Blood clotting factors in pregnancy: Factor VIII concentrations in normal and AHF-deficient women. Obstet Gynecol 24:242, 1984

127. Telfer MC, Chediak J: Factor VIII-related disorders and their relationship to pregnancy. J Reprod Med 19:211, 1972

128. Takahashi H, Hayashi N, Shibata A: Type IB von Willebrand's disease and pregnancy: comparison of analytical methods of von Willebrand factor for classification of von Willebrand's disease subtypes. Thromb Res 50: 409, 1988

129. Casonato A, Sarrori MT, Bertomoro A, et al Pregnancy-induced worsening of thrombocytopenia in a patient with type IIB von Willebrand's disease. Blood Coag Fibrinolysis 2:33, 1991

130. Noller KL, Bowie EJW, Kempers RD, Owen CA: von Willebrand's disease in pregnancy. Obstet Gynecol 41: 865, 1973

131. Evans P: Obstetric and gynecologic patients with von Willebrand's disease. Obstet Gynecol 38:37, 1971

132. Lipton RA, Ayromlooi J, Coller BS: Severe von Willebrand's disease during labor and delivery. JAMA 248: 1355, 1982

133. Chediak JR, Alban GM, Maxey B: von Willebrand's disease and pregnancy: management during delivery and outcome of offspring. Am J Obstet Gynecol 155:618, 1986

134. Conti M, Mari D, Conti E et al: Pregnancy in women with different types of von Willebrand disease. Obstet Gynecol 68:282, 1986

135. Ieko M, Sakurama S, Sagan A et al: Effect of Factor VIII concentrate on type IIB von Willebrand's disease-associated thrombocytopenia presenting during pregnancy in identical twin mothers. Am J Hematol 35:26, 1990

Chapter 33

Collagen Vascular Diseases

Philip Samuels

With the exception of rheumatoid arthritis, autoimmune diseases are associated with an increased risk of poor pregnancy outcome. Many of these diseases have a predisposition for women in their childbearing years. In fact, autoimmune diseases are occasionally first diagnosed during gestation. Often patients with recurrent pregnancy complications show evidence of autoimmunity but without significant criteria to allow a specific diagnosis. These diseases are characterized by the production of autoantibodies—antibodies synthesized by an individual against a component of her own body. Increasingly sensitive and specific laboratory tests are being developed to aid in the diagnosis of these disorders (Tables 33-1 and 33-2).

Systemic Lupus Erythematosus

Systemic lupus erythematosus (SLE) is a chronic disease with a great diversity of clinical and laboratory manifestations. Its onset is frequently insidious, and its diagnosis is often elusive and delayed. The course of SLE is characterized by chronic exacerbations and remissions. The prevalence of SLE is approximately 1 per 1,000 in the general population. The prevalence of the disease in women 15 to 64 years of age is estimated to be 1 per 700,[1] but in black women of the same age group the prevalence is 1 per 245.[2] The diagnosis of SLE is based on a patient meeting at least four of the diagnostic criteria accepted by the American Rheumatism Association.

Clinical Manifestations

Approximately 80 percent of patients with SLE demonstrate skin lesions. These may include the classic malar (butterfly) rash, alopecia, or discoid lesions. Photosensitivity is common. Arthralgias with some arthritis will be evident in 90 percent of patients. Nephritis and neurologic or psychiatric features are found in approximately 50 percent of cases.

The renal lesions of SLE include focal proliferative glomerulonephritis, membranous glomerulonephritis, mesangial nephritis, and diffuse proliferative glomerulonephritis. Patients with glomerulonephritis will excrete varying quantities of protein. The amount of proteinuria may range widely within the same individual, depending on disease activity. Those patients with focal and diffuse proliferative glomerulonephritis tend to have a worse long-term prognosis. Women with SLE may also present with seizures, peripheral neuropathy, or a psychotic episode. It is important to note that a recurrent fever of unknown etiology may also be the earliest manifestation of SLE.

Laboratory Diagnosis

More than 90 percent of patients with SLE will exhibit significant titers of antinuclear antibodies. In 80 to 90 percent of patients, an autoantibody directed against double-stranded DNA will be detected. Anti-double-stranded DNA antibodies can be divided into subclasses. The high-affinity antibodies are seen more commonly in patients with renal involvement of their SLE, while the low-affinity antibodies are seen in milder forms of the disease. Extractable nuclear antibodies can be subdivided into antibodies against ribonuclear protein (anti-RNP, anti-SM), anti-SSA (Ro), and anti-SSB (La). Anti-RNP antibodies are seen in 26 percent of patients with SLE; anti-SM antibodies are found in 28 percent of patients with SLE and can be correlated with renal involvement. Anti-SSA and anti-SSB antibodies, which are found in 25 and 12 percent of patients with

Table 33-1 Autoantibodies of Diagnostic Significance

Autoantibody	Associated Disease
Antinuclear antibodies (ANA)	Most collagen vascular diseases
Antineutrophil cytoplasmic antibodies (ANCA)	70%–90% of patients with Wegner's granulomatosis, polyarteritis nodosa, crescentic glomerulonephritis
Anti-double-stranded DNA antibodies	80%–90% of SLE patients
High-affinity anti-DNA antibodies	Lupus nephritis
Antihistone antibodies	30%–60% of SLE patients, 95% of drug-induced lupus patients, 20% of rheumatoid arthritis patients
Antimitochondrial antibody	85%–95% of patients with primary biliary cirrhosis, 25%–30% of patients with chronic active hepatitis
Anti-Jo-1	Polymyositis, dermatomyositis
Anti-Ki	10% of SLE patients, especially with arthritis, percarditis, and pulmonary hypertension
Anti-PM-1	Polymyositis
Antiscleroderma (SCL)-70 antibodies	20% of patients with scleroderma or progressive systemic sclerosis
Antiextractable nuclear antibodies (anti-Sm, anti-RNP, anti-SSA, anti-SSB)	SLE, Sjögren syndrome, other collagen vascular diseases
Anti-RANA	Rheumatoid arthritis

SLE, respectively, have been associated with fetal and neonatal heart block. Anti-SSA antibodies are generally associated with manifestations of neonatal lupus. The extractable nuclear antibodies are usually seen in patients who have a speckled pattern of antinuclear antibodies.

Antihistone antibodies are seen in 30 to 60 percent of patients with SLE. They are seen in over 90 percent of patients with drug-induced lupus and are therefore useful in making this diagnosis. Anti-Ki antibodies are found in only 10 percent of patients with SLE, but correlate strongly with arthritis and with serious lupus systemic involvement such as pericarditis and pulmonary hypertension.

The Effects of Pregnancy on SLE

Pregnancy does not appear to affect or alter the long-term prognosis of patients with SLE.[3] Several studies, however, have documented increased flares of SLE dur-

Table 33-2 Antinuclear Antibody Patterns in Rheumatologic Disease

Pattern	Disease State
Homogeneous	SLE, drug-induced lupus, chronic active hepatitis, many collagen vascular diseases
Speckled	SLE, Sjögren syndrome, mixed connective tissue disease, rheumatoid arthritis
Nucleolar	Progressive systemic sclerosis, scleroderma, Sjögren syndrome, subcutaneous SLE, SLE
Centromere	Scleroderma, CREST syndrome

ing pregnancy and particularly during the puerperium.[3,4] It is difficult to compare and corroborate these studies, because there is no uniform definition of a lupus flare. Garsenstein et al[3] predicted that the probability of a flare was three times greater during the first half of pregnancy, 1.5 times greater in the second half, and six times greater in the puerperium.[3] Meehan and Dorsey[5] examined the effects of pregnancy on the course of SLE in patients receiving glucocorticoids or azathioprine at conception. They found no statistically significant difference in the number of flares in pregnant women and nonpregnant controls when matched by disease duration and prior organ involvement. Lockshin[6] and Lockshin et al[7] studied a variety of clinical markers of disease activity in 33 pregnancies in 28 women with SLE. They also demonstrated an absence of exacerbation during or after pregnancy. In a prospective study of 80 women, Lockshin[8] showed that exacerbation occured in less than 13 percent of pregnant patients. He concluded, therefore, that there is no need for prophylactic glucocorticoids in the gravid patient with SLE. Derksen and coworkers[9] found that SLE patients who were in remission at the time of conception did not have any serious flares postpartum. In 82 percent of the 29 prospectively studied pregnancies, the disease remained quiescent throughout gestation.[9]

Conversely, Mintz and colleagues[10] showed an increase in SLE activity during pregnancy. This group studied 102 pregnancies in 75 women during a 10-year period. In this report, 59.7 percent of pregnancies that began with quiescent SLE experienced an exacerbation during pregnancy or the postpartum period. More than one-half of these flares occurred in the first trimester and 20 percent during the puerperium. Most of

Revised Criteria for the Classification of Systemic Lupus Erythematosus (1982)[a]

Malar rash

Discoid rash

Photosensitivity

Oral ulcers

Arthritis, nonerosive, involving two or more peripheral joints

Serositis

    Pleuritis

    OR

    Pericarditis

Renal disorder

    Persistent proteinuria >0.5 g/day

    OR

    Cellular casts

Neurologic disorder

    Seizures

    OR

    Psychosis

Hematologic disorder

    Hemolytic anemia with reticulocytosis

    OR

    Leukopenia, <4,000/mm^3

    OR

    Lymphopenia, <1,500/mm^3

    OR

    Thrombocytopenia, <100,000/mm^3

Immunologic disorder

    Positive lupus erythematosus cell preparation

    Antibody to native DNA

    Anti-SM antibody

    False-positive serologic test for syphilis

Antinuclear antibodies in abnormal titers

---

[a] Four criteria necessary for diagnosis.
(Adapted from Tan et al.,[164] with permission.)

the patients, however, readily responded to increased doses of glucocorticoids. Le Thi Huong and coworkers[11] in Paris found similar findings. Of 75 patients with inactive lupus at conception, 27 relapsed in pregnancy and 7 experienced postpartum flares.[11]

Although it remains debatable whether SLE is exacerbated by pregnancy, there is no dispute that there is a risk of major maternal morbidity and potentially of mortality in the gravida with SLE. Most maternal deaths occur during the puerperium as a result of pulmonary hemorrhage or lupus pneumonitis.[12,13] Rubin and colleagues[14] reported a case of pulmonary vasculitis resulting in pulmonary hypertension and death in a pregnant patient with SLE. Averbuch and coworkers[15] reported a case of cardiac tamponade occurring in the postpartum period caused by SLE. Marabani and coworkers[16] described a case of transverse myelitis during a pregnancy complicated by SLE. This complication responded quickly to steroids. In the study by Le Thi Huong et al,[11] two women had nephrotic syndrome postpartum requiring high doses of steroids. They died of opportunistic infection secondary to immune suppression.[11] Gimovsky and associates[17] reviewed 108 pregnancies in 39 women affected with SLE and found that morbidity was rare in the immediate postpartum period. However, there was increased morbidity and mortality in the first few years after delivery.[17]

Most perinatologists advise their patients not to conceive during a time of increased lupus activity, as this is associated with flares during pregnancy. Although this seems logical, the volume of the literature to support this assertion is small.[18] The work by Mintz and colleagues[10] does, however, seem to favor this postulate. In general, a patient's disease should be quiescent for 5 to 7 months before conception. This recommendation is based on work by Hayslett and Lynn,[19] who observed that pregnancy outcome was good in 92 percent of women whose lupus had been in remission for at least 6 months prior to conception. This concept is also confirmed in the study of 35 pregnancies in 25 women observed by Derksen et al[9] between 1987 and 1993.

Women with lupus nephritis must be aware that there is a small but significant risk of permanent deterioration of renal function during pregnancy. Fine and coworkers[20] noted that in 9.6 percent of their patients renal function remained depressed for 3 to 12 months after delivery. Others have suggested that permanent renal deterioration during pregnancy is more frequent, perhaps as high as 50 percent.[21,22] In these studies, however, sample sizes were small. Conversely, Hayslett and Lynn[19] demonstrated no permanent change in renal function in pregnant patients with lupus nephritis. A summary of six studies reviewing 242 pregnancies in 156 patients revealed a 7.1 percent incidence of permanent renal dysfunction and a 30.2 percent incidence of transient renal dysfunction during gestation.[22] In this review, transient deterioration usually occurred in the third trimester. Poor pregnancy outcome is associated with active lupus nephropathy,[23] a serum creatinine level of at least 1.5 mg/dl, a BUN more than 50 mg/dl, and a creatinine clearance rate less than 50 ml/min.[19,23,24]

A lupus flare and preeclampsia present a difficult differential diagnosis, because they have similar signs and symptoms. Both disorders often present with hypertension, edema, and proteinuria. To confound the issue, patients with lupus nephropathy are at an increased risk for developing superimposed preeclampsia during gestation. It is difficult, but very important, to make the distinction between these two phenomena. The treatment for preeclampsia is delivery, while the treatment for lupus nephritis is increased glucocorticoids and possibly azathioprine therapy. Buyon and coworkers[25] found that serum complement levels (C_3 and C_4) are valuable in differentiating between heightened lupus activity and preeclampsia. In normal pregnancy, complement levels tend to rise. They are, therefore, high or normal in the SLE patient with pure preeclampsia. Conversely, these levels fall with an exacerbation of lupus. If a patient develops hypertension and proteinuria in the second trimester, it is imperative to distinguish between preeclampsia and a lupus flare. If the diagnosis of preeclampsia is made, mandatory obstetric intervention could result in neonatal death or major morbidity from prematurity, depending on the gestational age. If serologic and chemical testing cannot make the distinction between the two conditions, a renal biopsy rarely may be indicated.

The Effects of SLE on Pregnancy

Although fertility is not impaired, SLE can have an adverse effect on pregnancy outcome in each trimester.[26] There is an increase in the spontaneous abortion rate, with the estimated incidence between 16 and 40 percent.[10,17,26–29] The risk of miscarriage is not necessarily related to disease activity. Mintz and coworkers[10] reported a 16 percent spontaneous abortion rate regardless of disease activity.

In a study by Julkunen and colleagues,[30] patients with Sjögren syndrome were compared with patients with SLE, and both were compared with controls. The relative risk of fetal loss was elevated in both patients with Sjögren syndrome and SLE. Clinically significant intrauterine growth restriction was found more frequently in patients with SLE than in patients with Sjögren syndrome.[30] Le Thi Huong et al[11] examined 117 cases of SLE in pregnancy between 1987 and 1993. Twenty-eight infants were delivered full-term, while 48 were delivered prematurely. There were also 13 first trimester losses, 2 second trimester spontaneous abortions, and 3 third trimester stillbirths, statistics above the expected rate of pregnancy loss. In this study, prematurity was related to a history of fetal loss, active SLE at onset of pregnancy, hypertension, and SLE requiring the patient to take at least 20 mg prednisone daily.[11] Growth restriction correlated with hypertension, low complement levels, and absence of anti-SSA antibodies.

In the study of Derksen et al[9] of 35 pregnancies in 25 women, there were 8 first trimester spontaneous abortions, no second trimester losses, and 1 stillbirth. In a study by Ramsey-Goldman et al[31] a previous poor

pregnancy outcome was the best predictor of a poor outcome in the present pregnancy.

In a large retrospective study, Petri and Albritton[32] reviewed 481 pregnancies in 203 women with SLE and used friends and family members without SLE as a control group. They found a 21 percent spontaneous abortion rate in women with SLE compared with 14 percent in friends and 8 percent in family members. Preterm delivery was found in 12 percent of lupus patients compared with 4 percent from each control group.[32] Hypertension requiring therapy, Raynaud's phenomenon, and not finishing high school were found to be significantly correlated with preterm delivery.[32]

In contrast to the study of Le Thi Huong et al[11] Leu and Lan[33] found anti-SSA antibodies were associated with growth restriction in pregnancies complicated by SLE. The presence of these antibodies, however, did not affect perinatal mortality.

Preterm birth is more frequent in women with SLE. Johnson et al[34] attempted to determine the etiology of this preterm birth. In their study of 66 women in 58 pregnancies, they found that 39 percent of those delivering prematurely had experienced preterm premature rupture of the membranes.[34] This was not related to whether the patient was taking prednisone, the level of disease activity, or serologic studies. It appeared that rupture of the membranes was the single most frequent cause of preterm delivery in these patients.

Since the late 1980s, the lupus inhibitor and anticardiolipin antibodies have been the subject of concentrated research relating to recurrent miscarriage and SLE. The diagnosis of the lupus inhibitor is often confusing. There is no single assay that is used to identify this phenomenon, and different assays have different sensitivities and specificities. Some clinicians and researchers rely solely on a prolongation of the activated partial thromboplastin time (APTT) using platelet-poor plasma. A sensitive reagent must be used. Otherwise there will be many false-negative results. Other commonly used tests include the tissue thromboplastin inhibition test (TTI), kaolin clotting time (KCT), dilute Russell viper venom time, and platelet neutralization procedure. The hexagonal antibody has shown promising results. This variety of tests makes it difficult for the critical reader to compare different studies concerning the role of the lupus inhibitor in pregnancy outcome.

There is confusion concerning the difference between anticardiolipin antibodies and antiphospholipid antibodies. Antiphospholipid antibodies encompass many phospholipids, of which cardiolipin is only one. Nonetheless, these terms are often used interchangeably in the obstetrics literature.

The similarities and differences between the lupus inhibitor and anticardiolipin antibodies are also quite confusing. While many clinicians use the assays interchangeably, Rosove et al[35] showed that the correlation between the two is not perfect, and both assays should be performed in order to maximize sensitivity.

Before concluding that the lupus inhibitor and anticardiolipin antibodies are a cause of poor pregnancy outcome, one must look at the prevalence of these phenomena in a normal pregnant population. Lockwood and coworkers,[36] in a study of 737 low-risk pregnancies, were the first to address this issue. Two of the 737 patients (0.27 percent) had a lupus inhibitor documented by a prolonged APTT that did not correct after mixing with normal plasma. Both patients experienced a pregnancy loss. Elevated titers of IgM or IgG anticardiolipin antibodies were found in 16 patients (2.2 percent). Twelve of these 16 patients experienced an adverse pregnancy outcome. This study suggests that, while these phenomena are not widespread, the presence of the lupus inhibitor and anticardiolipin antibodies can be related to poor pregnancy outcome and placental infarction.[37-39] As shown by Lubbe et al[40,41] in New Zealand, Branch et al[42] in the United States, and Unander et al[43] in Sweden, the lupus inhibitor and anticardiolipin antibodies are associated with recurrent spontaneous abortions even when there is no other evidence of collagen vascular disease. Also, in the absence of SLE, anticardiolipin antibodies can be associated with an increased risk for early preeclampsia, intrauterine growth restriction (IUGR), and fetal death.[42,44] Druzin et al[45] and Lockshin and Druzin[46] have observed that patients with elevated anticardiolipin antibodies who have SLE are at significant risk to develop fetal distress in the second trimester with subsequent fetal death. Kutteh et al[47] found that anticardiolipin antibodies were predictors of poor fetal outcome in patients with SLE. In their study, they found that the fetal loss rate was 39 percent in the patients with anticardiolipin antibodies and only 11 percent in those SLE patients without the antibodies.[47] Julkunen and colleagues[48] in Helsinki found that antiphospholipid antibodies were more sensitive in predicting fetal loss, but lupus inhibitor was more specific. Also, in this study, antiphospholipid antibodies did not correlate with prematurity or growth restriction.[48] Birdsall et al[49] also found that antiphospholipid antibodies were present in 41 percent of women with recurrent miscarriage and 29 percent of women with a history of recent stillbirth. Their results were significant even in patients without signs suggestive of a collagen vascular disease.

Treatment of patients with the lupus inhibitor and anticardiolipin antibodies remains controversial and has not been evaluated in a controlled fashion. Several studies report increased fetal survival and decreased morbidity and mortality in patients receiving prednisone in doses of 20 to 60 mg daily and low dose aspirin.[42,50] It appears that this regimen will normalize a prolonged APTT or other coagulation assay, but will have little effect on the level of anticardiolipin antibodies. These investigations, however, have not been controlled for the gestational age at which therapy was initiated. There have been no studies comparing prednisone alone to prednisone and aspirin.

Unander and colleagues[43] showed that 8 of 42 patients with elevated anticardiolipin antibodies conceived and carried a pregnancy to term without specific therapy. Two of these eight patients had high levels of anticardiolipin antibodies, constituting 20 percent of the patients in their study who had this abnormality. Mintz and coinvestigators,[51] in a prospective study of 44 women with idiopathic habitual abortion, found that two of three patients who had anticardiolipin antibodies had subsequent successful pregnancies without therapy. Furthermore, Lockshin and coworkers[52] believe that prednisone may actually increase the incidence of fetal death in women with anticardiolipin antibodies. In their study of 21 women with a prior history of fetal death and a high titer of IgG anticardiolipin antibody, 11 were treated with prednisone. In the 11 treated women, 82 percent of the pregnancies ended in fetal death. In the untreated group, only 50 percent of pregnancies resulted in fetal death, a statistically significant difference. In patients treated with aspirin, there was no statistical difference in the outcomes of the groups. Based on these findings, Lockshin et al[52] concluded that prednisone may actually worsen fetal outcome of the current pregnancy. Karp et al[53] studied the outcomes of 27 pregnancies in 19 patients treated with prednisone and antiaggregants for the lupus inhibitor. There were only 13 successful outcomes, leading them to conclude that prednisone and antiaggregants may prevent second and third trimester losses but have only limited success in treating primary habitual abortion.[53] Nonetheless, there are other data that do support the use of prednisone and low dose aspirin in treating patients with the lupus inhibitor and the anticardiolipin antibody syndrome.[43,50,54-56] Landy and coworkers[57] followed 53 pregnancies complicated by lupus inhibitor or antiphospholipid antibodies. Thirty-three of these patients were treated with glucocorticoids and aspirin. They found that this therapy resulted in a 90.9 percent livebirth rate, higher than that achieved in patients only taking one medication.

Gatenby et al[58] showed a dramatic improvement in patients receiving only aspirin therapy for elevated anticardiolipin antibodies. In patients with elevated antibodies and SLE, the pregnancy wastage rate dropped from 88 to 55 percent. In those with elevated antibodies alone, the rate of loss fell from 79 to 25 percent.[58] In their series, however, some of the patients were also receiving prednisone. Balasch and coworkers[59] studied 65 consecutive women with two or more spontaneous miscarriages. Seven (10.7 percent) were found to have anticardiolipin antibodies. Four of the seven women (57.1 percent) carried to term after being treated with low-dose aspirin alone. While the number of patients treated with aspirin alone is small, it does appear that this therapy might be beneficial in patients who have anticardiolipin antibodies.

Because infarctions are often found in the placentas of patients with anticardiolipin antibodies, researchers have begun using heparin therapy in this group. Rosove et al[60] initiated heparin therapy at a mean gestational age of 10.3 weeks in 14 women with adverse pregnancy outcomes. The daily dosage ranged from 10,000 to 36,000 units. Live births occurred in 14 of 15 pregnancies (93.3 percent) with a mean gestational age of 36.1 weeks and a mean birth weight percentile of 57.[60] Heparin is now frequently used to treat patients with antiphospholipid antibodies. Low dose heparin has less side effects than prednisone. Prednisone can be associated with increased striae, iduction of gestational diabetes mellitus, poor wound healing, increased candidiasis, fluid retention, aseptic necrosis, cataracts, and other complications, especially when used in high doses. Branch et al[61] found equivalent fetal survival when using heparin and aspirin; prednisone and aspirin; or heparin, prednisone, and aspirin. The maternal side effects were much less with a regimen that incorporated only heparin and low dose aspirin. These authors advocate using 10,000 to 20,000 units of heparin daily. This study included 82 pregnancies in 54 women. It showed that the diagnosis of SLE, a history of preeclampsia, a history of thrombosis, a false-positive test for syphilis, and the titer of IgG anticardiolipin antibody made no difference regarding outcome of the current pregnancy.[61] The number of previous fetal deaths did correlate significantly with outcome in the current pregnancy.

Intravenous immunoglobulin is currently being studied for use in treating patients with lupus inhibitor and/or antiphospholipid antibodies. Its mechanism of action is not entirely understood, but it may bind to receptors, preventing the binding of these deleterious antibodies. The correct dosage and dosage interval have not been elucidated. Branch et al[61] have used intravenous immunoglobulin with some success. Kaaja et al.[62] used high dose immunoglobulin in conjunction with low dose aspirin in four patients with good results. This therapy, however, remains experimental.

Anticardiolipin antibodies and the lupus inhibitor are associated with in vitro anticoagulation, but in vivo they are associated with thrombosis. These patients, therefore, are probably at some risk for thrombosis during gestation.[43,63–65] Mizoguchi et al[64] described a 34-year-old woman with lupus inhibitor who had had six recurrent pregnancy losses without an intervening live

birth. During her subsequent pregnancy, she developed multiple brain infarctions and hemiparesis. Rallings and coworkers[65] reported a 28-year-old primigravida who developed an acute anteroseptal myocardial infarction and died during gestation. She had a past history of thromboembolism. The only serologic abnormality noted was an elevated level of IgG anticardiolipin antibody.

We currently individualize our therapy of patients with lupus inhibitor and antiphospholipid antibodies. We take the patient's history and laboratory results into account when making decisions regarding therapy. Unfortunately, patients are occasionally tested for this syndrome after only having one spontaneous abortion. If this patient has equivocal or weakly positive testing, we discourage therapy. For the patient whom we feel truly has this syndrome, we usually prescribe low dose aspirin and heparin. We start the heparin dosing at 5,000 units twice daily and increase to 10,000 units twice daily by term. If the patient has an aversion to administering injections or carries the diagnosis of a collagen vascular disease, we may use prednisone and low dose aspirin. We usually administer the prednisone in a dose of 15 mg daily. This dose is adequate to cause immunosuppression and may cause less side effects than higher doses. There appears to be no advantage to administer all three medications to a patient, and such therapy may truly increase adverse side effects. The use of alternate-day glucocorticoids has never been evaluated in treating these patients. I project that by the time the next edition of this text is published, there will be reports of using low-molecular-weight heparin to treat this disorder. The true key in treating these patients is to make certain they understand the potential side effects of the prescribed medication regimen and that they undergo the proper fetal and maternal surveillance throughout pregnancy.

Neonatal Manifestations of SLE

Complete congenital heartblock, an infrequent complication of SLE, can be diagnosed prenatally. In the midtrimester, a fetal heart rate of about 60 bpm with no baseline variability is indicative of congenital heartblock. The patient should immediately undergo fetal echocardiography to rule out associated congenital cardiac malformations. Doppler studies can also locate the atrial ventricular disassociation. Fetal echocardiography can usually be carried out at 20 to 24 weeks' gestation and earlier in the asthenic patient. Affected fetuses usually show no evidence of congestive heart failure or hydrops. Nonetheless, they should be followed with serial ultrasonography every 1 to 2 weeks to ascertain if any evidence of anasarca has developed. Complete congenital heartblock in the patient with

SLE appears to be the result of immune complex deposition in fetal cardiac tissue as demonstrated by Litsey and coworkers.[66] This process leads to endocardiofibroelastosis and fibrosis of the conduction system.[67,68] Scott and colleagues[69] identified the anti-SSA (Ro) antibody in 83 percent of mothers delivering infants with complete congenital heartblock. Anti-SSB (La) antibodies were found in a smaller but significant number of these mothers. Scheib and Waxman[70] have shown that these antibodies do bind to fetal cardiac tissue. They have described two successive pregnancies in a mother with anti-SSA antibody who gave birth to two antibody-positive children with complete congenital heartblock. Derksen and Meilof[71] found that the level of anti-SSA antibody did not correlate with the development of complete congenital heart block. Le Thi Huong[11] found manifestations of neonatal lupus in 3 of 22 infants whose mothers had anti-SSA antibody. Two had cutaneous manifestations and one had complete heart block.[11] The titer of antibody did not appear to be related to the disease course. Conversely, Leu and Lan[33] found that patients with high titer anti-SSA antibody had a greater chance of having a neonate with manifestations of lupus. Three of 257 women with this antibody gave birth to an infant with complete congenital heart block.[33] All three had high antibody titers.

In most studies, mothers have had no symptoms of collagen vascular disease at the time of delivery. In the study of Vetter and Rashkad,[72] a large proportion of these women later developed SLE. According to Esscher and Scott,[73] the mother of a child born with complete congenital heartblock has a 30 to 60 percent chance of developing a collagen vascular disease. Therefore, patients who deliver an infant with complete congenital heartblock but who do not have SLE should have a careful clinical examination and undergo appropriate serologic tests on a routine basis. In future pregnancies, they should be treated as high-risk patients and undergo fetal echocardiography at the appropriate gestational age.

In the absence of structural cardiac anomalies, the neonatal mortality rate for infants born with complete congenital heartblock is approximately 5 percent. In the studies of Vetter and Rashkad and Esscher and Scott[73] the mortality rate was 20 to 30 percent if a structural abnormality was also found. With recent advances in pediatric cardiac surgery, the mortality rate is probably considerably lower now. Buyon and coworkers[74] aggressively treated a fetus with presumptive fetal myocarditis and heartblock in a mother with SLE. They administered high doses of dexamethasone and performed plasmapheresis three times weekly. The patient responded well to therapy, showing a significant decrease in the titer of anti-SSB antibody. The infant was delivered at 31 weeks, and the heartblock persisted.

Infants born to mothers with SLE may exhibit erythematous skin lesions of the face, scalp, and upper thorax.[11,75,76] These lesions usually disappear by 12 months of age. It appears that there is a higher incidence of anti-SSA antibodies in mothers giving birth to children with these skin lesions.[77]

Surveillance

Because of the increased risk of miscarriage, stillbirth, preterm delivery, and IUGR, the obstetrician caring for the patient with SLE should maintain close maternal and fetal surveillance. Any patient with a history of SLE should undergo preconceptual counseling and should have tests performed for the presence of the lupus inhibitor, anticardiolipin antibodies, anti-SSA (Ro) antibodies, and anti-SSB (La) antibodies. As previously described, these findings are associated with a poorer pregnancy outcome. If indicated, therapy should be initiated after fully informing the patient of risks and benefits to both her and the fetus. If anti-SSA or anti-SSB antibodies are present, fetal echocardiography should be performed in the second trimester to rule out complete congenital heartblock. Because of the risks of IUGR and preterm birth, accurate gestational dating is imperative in the patient with SLE. Patients should also have an examination of their urine sediment and a 24 hour urine collection for creatinine clearance and total protein excretion in early pregnancy to determine if there is any renal involvement of their SLE. Menstrual dating should be confirmed by ultrasonography at the first prenatal visit. At 18 to 20 weeks' gestation an additional ultrasound examination should be performed to confirm gestational age, ascertain appropriate fetal growth, and make certain that fetal anatomy is normal. IUGR in patients with SLE is usually asymmetric.[11] Fine et al,[20] however, showed that symmetric IUGR can also occur. Because of the risk of IUGR and stillbirth, serial ultrasound examinations should be performed monthly after 20 weeks' gestation, with special attention to growth of the fetal abdomen, head, and femur.[77] The obstetrician should also be attentive to the volume of amniotic fluid, as decreased amniotic fluid can be the harbinger of fetal compromise and stillbirth.

At 28 weeks' gestation, weekly antepartum fetal heart rate testing should be initiated using the nonstress test. Antepartum fetal heart rate testing has been shown to improve fetal outcome in patients with systemic lupus erythematosus.[78] At 34 weeks, the frequency of testing should be increased to twice weekly. There are, however, no controlled studies showing that biweekly testing after 34 weeks improves perinatal outcome in the patient with SLE. Carroll[79] has shown that Doppler blood flow velocimetry might be useful in following the gravida with the lupus inhibitor. In that study, abnormal umbilical artery systolic/diastolic ratios were found in five of six women with the lupus inhibitor who delivered growth-restricted fetuses. Only two of these patients demonstrated abnormally elevated uterine artery systolic/diastolic ratios. Ariyuki et al[80] have demonstrated similar findings. Doppler may be a useful adjuvant in caring for the patient with SLE, but more research needs to be done before it can be considered a routine part of the care of these patients.

Despite the sophisticated array of laboratory studies that are available to follow patients with SLE, the patient's clinical status remains of prime importance. There is no substitute for careful monitoring of maternal blood pressure and weight gain. These can be the earliest signs of superimposed preeclampsia, which is common in patients with SLE. They can also be the harbinger of a lupus flare.[81] Twenty-four-hour urine collections for creatinine clearance and total protein excretion should be carried out monthly. Serum creatinine, BUN, and uric acid levels should be determined whenever these urine collections are performed. A rise in serum uric acid can be a sign of impending preeclampsia. During a normal pregnancy, complement levels rise. A fall in the third or fourth components of complement (C_3 or C_4) or a fall in total hemolytic complement (CH_{50}) has been associated with impending exacerbations of SLE[82–84] Devoe and Aloy[85] found that a decrease in serum complement levels was also associated with a poor perinatal outcome. Because complement levels tend to rise during pregnancy, a single complement determination is of no value. A downward trend in complement levels, however, is significant, even though the level may fall within normal limits. Although some investigators have questioned the predictive value of complement levels,[19,86] we follow complement levels every 6 weeks in patients with SLE and more frequently if the clinical situation warrants.

The timing of delivery is important and should be individualized. All too often, preterm delivery is performed merely to allay physician and patient anxiety. The obstetrician should strive for a vaginal delivery. If delivery is indicated near term and the patient's cervix is not favorable, cervical ripening agents may be employed. If the patient is taking glucocorticoids or if there is any evidence of lupus exacerbation, peripartum steroids should be administered parenterally in stress doses. In the patient who undergoes cesarean delivery, intravenous steroids should be continued for 48 hours postoperatively, because adequate gastrointestinal absorption cannot be guaranteed until normal bowel function returns. Steroids should be tapered slowly and with great care in the postpartum period to prevent an exacerbation of SLE.[21,82]

Drug Therapy for SLE During Pregnancy

Patients with SLE are often hesitant to take their prescribed medications during pregnancy for fear of fetal effects. Many obstetricians are also reluctant to prescribe these medications for similar reasons. It is important for the obstetrician to be aware of the benefits and risks of medications used to treat SLE. Pregnancy is accompanied by a 40 to 50 percent increase in intravascular volume and an increase in interstitial fluid. Any steroid that has mineralocorticoid activity exacerbates interstitial fluid retention. This additive effect can cause maternal discomfort. The obstetrician should therefore choose a steroid with minimal mineralocorticoid activity and maximum glucocorticoid activity. Steroids in combination with pregnancy may worsen acne and striae. Corticosteroid administration can also lead to gastrointestinal discomfort and ulceration. We therefore suggest that patients on chronic corticosteroid therapy use antacids after meals and at bedtime.

Chronic corticosteroid administration has been associated with bone demineralization and with an increased risk of hip fractures. For the gravida who is taking increased corticosteroids only during pregnancy, the actual risk is unknown. There is also a risk of cataract formation with long-term corticosteroid administration.

The induction of gestational diabetes from glucocorticoid administration is a distinct possibility. Approximately 3 percent of all pregnancies are complicated by gestational diabetes.[87] We perform 1-hour, 50-g oral glucose screening tests at 20, 28, and 32 weeks' gestation in patients on long-term corticosteroids. We also test for diabetes later in gestation if there is any evidence of fetal macrosomia.

Pregnant women are often more concerned about the effects of the medication on their fetus than they are about the effects on themselves. The chronic ingestion of corticosteroids has not been associated with teratogenesis in humans.[88] An increase in the background incidence of cleft palate has been seen in rats and rabbits exposed to chronic corticosteroids but never in humans.[88–90] Neonatal adrenal suppression is a theoretical consideration in patients taking corticosteroids, but it has only rarely been reported. Nonetheless, the pediatrician should be informed when a mother has been taking corticosteroids antenatally. Rolbin et al[91] have shown an increase in the incidence of IUGR in infants born to mothers who were chronically taking steroids. These patients received 10 mg of prednisone daily because of infertility and remained on this dose throughout gestation.

Only a fraction of the steroids ingested by a pregnant woman reach the fetus. Prednisone, the most widely used glucocorticoid during gestation, is metabolized by the mother to its active form prednisolone. An 11-β-

OH radical is responsible for prednisolone's physiologic activity. The placenta has an abundance of the metabolizing enzyme 11-β-ol dehydrogenase, which converts the active glucocorticoid to an inactive 11-keto metabolite. Depending on the study, only 10 to 50 percent of a dose of prednisone and only one-sixth of a dose of hydrocortisone reach the fetus.[92-94] Levitz et al[95] performed placental perfusion studies showing that steroids are rapidly cleared from the fetus. Beitins and coworkers[96] found that the maternal:fetal concentration gradient after intravenous administration of prednisolone was 10:1.

Dexamethasone and betamethasone cross the placenta more freely and for this reason are used to enhance fetal lung maturity. Blanford et al[97] observed little conversion of dexamethasone or betamethasone to inactive forms. Work by Ballard et al[92] and by Osathanondh et al[94] demonstrate a maternal:fetal concentration gradient of 1:1 for dexamethasone and betamethasone.

To minimize potential fetal effects, prednisone should be the oral glucocorticoid of choice.[98] Both methylprednisolone and hydrocortisone are satisfactory for intravenous use when needed. Methylprednisolone has less mineralcorticoid effect and should create fewer maternal side effects.

Occasionally, azathioprine, a derivative of 6-mercaptopurine, will be required to control a patient's SLE. This medication readily crosses the placenta. In a study by Scott,[99] 64 to 93 percent of an administered dose appeared in fetal blood between 2.5 and 6 hours after intravenous administration. Azathioprine has not been shown to be teratogenic in humans, although congenital malformations have been observed in animal models.[100] Chronic azathioprine use during pregnancy has been associated with neonatal lymphopenia, lower serum IgG and IgM levels, and decreased thymic shadow on x-ray.[101] All of these changes have reversed with time. Scott[99,102] reports an increased incidence of IUGR in infants born to mothers who took azathioprine during pregnancy. As yet, no long-term information is available on immunologic development and later infection rates in children who were exposed to this medication in utero. Before administering azathioprine during pregnancy, however, the benefits and risks should be weighed carefully.

Rheumatoid Arthritis

Rheumatoid arthritis is an autoimmune disease with a prevalence of approximately 2 percent. Its crippling chronic form occurs in about 0.35 percent of the population.[103] The onset of the disease is usually between the ages of 20 and 60 years, and women are two to three times more likely to be affected than are men.[104]

Diagnosis

The diagnosis of rheumatoid arthritis is based on guidelines set forth by the American Rheumatism Association. A list of exclusions has also been devised to make the diagnosis more precise.

Clinical Manifestations

Articular involvement is the hallmark of rheumatoid arthritis. The most common finding is an erythematous, warm, swollen metacarpophalangeal joint. The proximal interphalangeal and wrist joints may also be involved. Less frequently, metatarsophalangeal and shoulder joints are affected. Over time, cartilage destruction and pannus formation occur.[105] Carpal tunnel syndrome is often seen in patients with rheumatoid arthritis.[106]

Extra-articular features of rheumatoid arthritis are found in patients with the most joint involvement and the highest titers of rheumatoid factor.[107,108] Rheumatoid nodules, which occur in 20 percent of patients with rheumatoid arthritis, can appear in the heart and lungs and along any extremity.[109] Pericarditis, myocarditis, and endocarditis are occasionally seen in patients with rheumatoid arthritis. Vasculitis may result secondary to immune complex deposition and may affect the skin, peripheral nerves, and blood vessels.[110] Unlike SLE, rheumatoid arthritis rarely involves the kidneys. It is important to note that after 10 years of disease more than 50 percent of patients are still able to work, and 15 percent will have a complete remission.[111]

Pathophysiology

Rheumatoid arthritis is characterized by proliferation and inflammation of synovial membranes. The membranes characteristically show a dense collection of lymphocytes in a diffuse nodular pattern.[112] T-cell function appears to be impaired, and there is an excessive number of T-suppressor cells.[113] Immune complexes, which activate the complement cascade, have been demonstrated in the blood, synovial fluid, and synovial membranes of patients with rheumatoid arthritis.[114,115] There appears to be a genetic predisposition to rheumatoid arthritis. A strong association between the histocompatibility antigen HLA-DR4 and rheumatoid arthritis has been shown.[116]

Laboratory Findings

Rheumatoid factors, IgM and IgG antibodies directed against the Fc fragment of IgG, are the hallmark laboratory finding of rheumatoid arthritis, but are not pathognomonic for this disorder. More severe disease is seen with higher titers of rheumatoid factor. Antinu-

American Rheumatism Association Diagnostic Criteria for Rheumatoid Arthritis (RA)

Morning stiffness
Pain on motion or tenderness in at least one joint
Soft tissue swelling in at least one joint
Swelling in at least one other joint
Simultaneous symmetric joint swelling
Subcutaneous nodules
Radiologic changes typical of rheumatoid arthritis
Positive rheumatoid factor
Poor mucin precipitate from synovial fluid
Characteristic histologic changes in synovium
Characteristic histologic changes in subcutaneous nodules

A. Classic RA: 7 criteria
B. Definite RA: 5 criteria
C. Probable RA: 3 criteria
D. Signs and symptoms must persist for at least 6 weeks
E. No exclusions can be present

(Adapted from Rodman and Schumacher,[165] with permission.)

clear antibodies are also found in approximately 20 percent of patients with rheumatoid arthritis.

Effects of Pregnancy on Rheumatoid Arthritis

In 1938, Hench[117] observed that many patients with rheumatoid arthritis experienced remissions during pregnancy. Persellin[118] noted that in pregnant women with rheumatoid arthritis 74 percent underwent remission during the first trimester, 20 percent in the second trimester, and 5 percent in the third trimester. In this series, however, 90 percent of patients experienced a postpartum exacerbation of their disease. Approximately 25 percent of these flares occurred in the first 4 weeks postpartum.[118] In a review, Klipple and Cecere[119] reported that approximately 70 percent of patients with rheumatoid arthritis experienced substantial improvements in disease activity during pregnancy including extra-articular symptoms. Most of these patients no longer required medications. This remission, however, was short lived, with more than 90 percent of women relapsing within 6 to 8 months postpartum. Klipple and Cecere[119] also found that in approximately 30 percent of patients with rheumatoid arthritis the course remained unchanged or worsened during gestation.

Quinn and colleagues[120] studied 24 pregnant women with rheumatoid arthritis, 21 of whom had quiescent disease activity during pregnancy. Nineteen of these 21 women had significant flares during the puerperium. These researchers noted that IgM rheumatoid factor levels increased during these flares while pregnancy-associated α_2-glycoprotein levels decreased. IgA rheumatoid factor was unaffected. These authors suggest that pregnancy-associated α_2-glycoprotein may be responsible for modulating the improvement in clinical symptoms in rheumatoid arthritis patients during gestation.[120] Nelson and colleagues[121] investigated HLA antigens in patients with rheumatoid arthritis and their offspring, as this autoimmune disorder has a known HLA class II antigen association. They found that amelioration of rheumatoid arthritis during gestation is associated with a disparity in HLA class II antigens between mother and fetus. They think that the maternal immune response to paternal HLA antigens may play a role in the remission in this disease that is often seen during pregnancy.[121] Lasink and coworkers[122] looked at the onset of rheumatoid arthritis in relation to pregnancy in 135 patients. They concluded that pregnancy may delay the clinical onset of disease in patients who will develop rheumatoid arthritis.

Exclusions From Rheumatoid Arthritis

Typical rash of systemic lupus erythematosus
Strongly positive lupus erythematosus cell preparation
Histologic evidence of periarteritis
Proximal muscle weakness consistent with dermatomyositis
Definite scleroderma
Clinical rheumatic fever
Clinical gouty arthritis
Tophi
Infectious arthritis
Tuberculous arthritis
Reiter syndrome
Clinical picture of shoulder-hand syndrome
Hypertrophic osteoarthropathy
Neuroarthropathy
Homogentisic aciduria
Sarcoidosis or positive Kveim test
Multiple myeloma
Erythema nodosum
Leukemia or lymphoma
Agammaglobulinemia

(Adapted from Rodman and Schumacher,[165] with permission.)

Effect of Rheumatoid Arthritis on Pregnancy

Rheumatoid arthritis appears to have no adverse effects on pregnancy.[119,123,124] Silman et al[125] reported an increase in perinatal deaths in pregnancies complicated by rheumatoid arthritis. In that study, however, there was no significant difference between patients and controls in the rate of spontaneous abortion. Spector and Silman[126] examined pregnancy outcomes in 195 women with rheumatoid arthritis and 462 controls. They found no increase in spontaneous abortions or stillbirths in patients with rheumatoid arthritis. They also concluded that a prior history of poor reproduction did not put the patient at risk for developing rheumatoid arthritis in the future.[126] A theoretical risk of uteroplacental insufficiency and IUGR does exist for patients with advanced extra-articular rheumatoid arthritis, and a case of IUGR attributed to vasculitis associated with severe disease has been described.[127]

To avoid pain and joint damage, care should be taken when positioning the patient with severe articular involvement on the delivery table. This is especially true if the patient has epidural or spinal anesthesia, because a joint can be damaged without the patient feeling pain. Obstetric anesthesiologists must also be cautious during rapid sequence induction of general anesthesia and intubation of patients with spinal involvement of rheumatoid arthritis. Subluxation of the atlanto-occipital joint is possible with devastating consequences.

Effects of Medications Used to Treat Rheumatoid Arthritis

Salicylates

Acetylsalicylic acid (aspirin) is the mainstay for the treatment of rheumatoid arthritis in pregnancy. The desired therapeutic blood level is 15 to 20 mg/dl. To achieve this the patient must take 3.6 to 4 g of acetylsalicylic acid daily in three divided doses. Because salicylism, tinnitus, and deafness usually occur at levels of approximately 25 mg/dl, salicylate levels should be monitored regularly. Salicylate used throughout pregnancy may be associated with a prolonged gestation, long labor, increased blood loss at delivery, and postpartum hemorrhage.[128,129] These effects appear to be related to the inhibition of prostaglandin synthetase.[130] These drugs also block platelet aggregation, and there are rare reports of clotting disorders in the newborn.[131] Neonatal hemostasis should therefore be closely monitored. When a mother has been taking large doses of aspirin, a bleeding time should be performed on the neonate before circumcision is performed. Salicylates have been shown to be teratogenic in animals but not in humans. Despite these potential problems, acetylsalicylic acid remains the drug of choice in treating the pain and stiffness associated with rheumatoid arthritis during gestation.

Other Nonsteroidal Anti-Inflammatory Agents

Therapeutic agents such as indomethacin, ibuprofen, naproxen, and ketoprofen are used in the treatment of rheumatoid arthritis. They have both analgesic and anti-inflammatory properties. Indomethacin, when used in late pregnancy, can cause premature closure of the fetal ductus arteriosus leading to pulmonary hypertension. Closure of the ductus arteriosus appears to be gestation-age dependent. These drugs, therefore, should be discontinued before 32 weeks' gestation if possible. Nonsteroidal anti-inflammatory agents can also cause changes in the fetal renal blood flow, resulting in oligohydramnios. It is unclear how long it takes these changes to occur. Physicians caring for patients taking these medications, therefore, should check the amniotic fluid index frequently.

Gold Therapy

Gold therapy has been utilized for many years in the treatment of rheumatoid arthritis. Although the precise mechanism of its action is unknown, gold has been shown to lower the titer of rheumatoid factor.

Bone marrow suppression can occur during gold therapy. A complete blood count and platelet count should therefore be performed before each injection.[132] Because proteinuria secondary to immune complex nephritis is an infrequent consequence of gold injections, urine should be checked for protein before each dose.[133] Gold compounds are protein bound and have poor placental passage. Chrysotherapy, however, cannot be recommended for routine use during pregnancy because of the limited clinical experience with this agent.[123]

Penicillamine

Penicillamine has been used successfully to treat rheumatoid arthritis in patients who are either resistant or have allergic reactions to gold. Like gold, penicillamine will reduce the titer of rheumatoid factor. Penicillamine freely crosses the placenta, and its use during pregnancy should be curtailed unless the benefits clearly outweigh the potential risks.

Scleroderma and Progressive Systemic Sclerosis

Progressive systemic sclerosis (PSS) and scleroderma are related collagen vascular diseases of unknown etiology. They affect females four times more frequently than males, with onset usually between the ages of 30 and 50 years. The reported incidence is about 5 new cases per 1 million population per year. *Scleroderma*, the term used to describe the disorder when it is localized to the skin, is characterized by tight and bound down skin, sclerodactyly, and Raynaud's phenomenon. Clinical signs may precede development of the overt disease by several years.

In PSS, there is systemic involvement, including the gastrointestinal viscera as well as pulmonary vascular and parenchymal changes. Pulmonary hypertension with resultant right-sided heart failure is often the fatal consequence of PSS. With cardiac involvement, left-sided heart failure is occasionally seen.

Laboratory Manifestations

Speckled-pattern antinuclear antibodies are observed in about 50 percent of patients, and 40 percent will demonstrate a rheumatoid factor. Anti-Scl-70, an extractable nuclear antibody, appears in the serum of 40 percent of patients with scleroderma and PSS. It appears to be fairly specific for this disease. Anti-Jo-1 antibodies are also occasionally seen in patients with scleroderma.

Effects of Pregnancy on Scleroderma and PSS

Johnson and coworkers[134] reported 18 cases of scleroderma and PSS complicating pregnancy. None of the women exhibited visceral involvement. In 39 percent of the patients, the disease showed no change or progressed at the same rate as prior to pregnancy. In an additional 39 percent the disease worsened, but no patient developed visceral involvement. In the remaining 22 percent some improvement was noted, but regression occurred after delivery. Several studies have described the onset of fatal renal involvement during pregnancy in patients with scleroderma and PSS.[135–138] In these reports, it is unclear whether visceral involvement antedated the pregnancy. Altieri and Cameron[139] reported a case of renal failure occurring in a pregnant woman with PSS. Partial recovery did follow the pregnancy. A successful pregnancy has been described in a patient with scleroderma complicated by renal disease and pulmonary hypertension who was treated with angiotensin-converting enzyme inhibitors.[140] The use of these agents during pregnancy is not recommended, but, because of the severity of the illness, they were used in this instance. Furthermore, Spiera et al[141] reported a successful pregnancy in a patient with a previous hypertensive renal crisis caused by PSS. The patient was actually withdrawn from angiotensin-converting enzyme inhibitors when she became pregnant and had no renal complications during the pregnancy.[141] In a large review, Maymon and Fejgin[147] conducted a detailed literature search of scleroderma in pregnancy. Of 94 patients, 14 died during the course of pregnancy secondary to renal and cardiopulmonary involvement. It is important to note that this literature review covered many years. With more sophisticated maternal monitoring and therapy, the maternal mortality rate is probably much lower today.

Effects of Scleroderma on Pregnancy

Many theoretical complications exist, but few have been documented properly because of the rarity with which scleroderma and PSS coexist with pregnancy. Preterm birth, premature rupture of membranes, and stillbirth seem to be more common in patients with scleroderma and PSS.[143,144] Surviving infants show no evidence of scleroderma.[143,145] Recently, Silman and Black[146] found that patients who eventually develop scleroderma have an increased risk of spontaneous abortion and infertility. Furthermore, Freeman and coworkers[147] reported a case of early spontaneous abortion and a circulating "lupus" anticoagulant in a patient with scleroderma. Steen et al[148] examined pregnancy outcomes in 48 women with scleroderma and in two control groups matched for age and race. One control group contained normal patients and the other a group of women with rheumatoid arthritis. No difference was observed in the frequencies of miscarriage or perinatal death. Preterm births and infants with IUGR were found more frequently in patients with scleroderma and PSS. These data are favorable compared with those from the older literature reviewed by Maymon and Fejgin.[142]

Management During Pregnancy

If visceral involvement, especially pulmonary, cardiac, or renal, is documented, counseling should be undertaken before a patient attempts pregnancy. As previously mentioned, patients with renal involvement can carry to term, but gestation is often much more complicated. If a patient with PSS becomes pregnant, pregnancy termination should be considered but is certainly not mandatory. If scleroderma with only skin involvement exists, the patient may be followed expectantly. She should be aware that renal or cardiac involvement may be fatal.

Myasthenia Gravis

Although its prevalence is 1 per 25,000 in the general population, myasthenia gravis frequently coexists with pregnancy.[149] Women are twice as frequently affected as men and have an earlier onset of the disease, with a peak incidence occurring between the ages of 20 and 30 years. Even though 60 percent of patients with myasthenia gravis have enlargement of the thymus, only 8 percent have a malignant thymoma.[150] Thymectomy improves symptoms in up to two-thirds of patients, but most still need additional medical therapy.[151] If the patient presents for prepregnancy counseling and is symptomatic despite large doses of medication, thymectomy should be undertaken before attempting pregnancy. Myasthenia gravis in pregnancy has been extensively studied by Plauché.[152] In a review of 314 pregnancies in 217 patients with myasthenia, he found no change in the myasthenic status throughout pregnancy, the puerperium, or the postpartum period in 31.5 percent of patients. In that review, exacerbations occurred in 40.8 percent of patients during pregnancy, including 30.6 percent during the puerperium. Another 28 percent showed a remission of their myasthenia during gestation.[152] Historically, there is a 25 to 60 percent preterm birth rate among patients with myasthenia gravis.[153,154] These are retrospective studies covering more than 40 years. With modern surveillance and therapy for preterm labor, this rate has probably decreased. Anti-acetylcholinesterase agents, which are used to treat myasthenia gravis, have an oxytocic action. It has been postulated that this could be the explanation for preterm labor observed in patients with myasthenia gravis.[155]

A team approach is necessary for proper treatment of the patient with myasthenia gravis. The neurologist and rheumatologist are not always familiar with the medications used by the obstetrician in treating complications of pregnancy. Conversely, because of the infrequency with which obstetricians see myasthenia gravis, they may be unfamiliar with the interactions between these medications and the disease.

Magnesium sulfate, for example, is absolutely contraindicated in the myasthenic patient. It further interferes with the neuromuscular blockade that is characteristic of the disease.[156] According to Castillo and Engbaek,[156] magnesium reduces the stimulating effect of acetylcholine on the muscle. It affects the amplitude of the end-plate potential without affecting the muscle's resting potential. Cohen and coworkers[157] reported a near maternal death from administration of magnesium to a myasthenic patient. Catanzarite and coinvestigators[155] described a respiratory arrest in a myasthenic patient with preterm labor who was treated with ritodrine and dexamethasone. They thought that the respiratory arrest was due to glucocorticoids. Although glucocorticoids generally ameliorate myasthenic symptoms, they may initially result in increased weakness in 25 to 80 percent of patients. Catanzarite and colleagues[155] proposed that this paradoxic effect, coupled with the hypokalemia caused by the ritodrine, led to the crisis.

Patient Management

Most patients with myasthenia gravis will be taking acetylcholinesterase inhibitors when they become pregnant. These medications are generally safe during gestation. The most commonly used medication, pyridostigmine, does not readily cross the placenta. Dosage adjustments, however, are frequently necessary because of the physiologic changes in vascular volume, renal blood flow, and hepatic function during pregnancy. Because myasthenia gravis is a disease of striated muscle, the smooth muscle of the uterus is generally not affected. The first stage of labor progresses at a normal pace. The second stage of labor involves voluntary pushing and the use of skeletal and pelvic girdle musculature.[158] These maternal expulsive efforts may be impaired because of the myasthenia gravis, and the obstetrician must be prepared to perform an operative vaginal delivery. Cesarean delivery should be reserved for obstetric indications. Patients are apt to undergo myasthenic crisis during labor, and the oral medications normally used have variable gastrointestinal absorption during this time. The obstetrician should therefore be prepared to use parenteral acetylcholinesterase inhibitors during labor and must be able to differentiate between an overdose of these medications and a myasthenic crisis.

Anesthesia and analgesia during labor present special challenges for the patient with myasthenia gravis. Although they are extremely sensitive to narcotics, patients with myasthenia gravis may be given these medications if carefully monitored.[159] Epidural anesthesia decreases the requirements for parenteral narcotics, prevents fatigue, and provides excellent anesthesia.[24] If, however, general anesthesia is elected for cesarean section, nondepolarizing muscle relaxants should be used with great care, if at all. Myasthenics are sensitive to these agents, and a prolonged response is usually seen.[158] It is also imperative to remember that certain inhalation agents may potentiate these agents. If general anesthesia is elected, the patient and her family should be warned that she may need ventilatory support for a period of time after the surgery.

If the patient develops a puerperal infection, aminoglycosides should be used with extreme caution. These agents can block the motor end-plate and cause a myasthenic crisis.[24]

Occasionally myasthenia will be exacerbated during pregnancy. In such cases, therapy with extremely large doses of acetylcholinesterase inhibitors yields little response. These patients can be treated with plasmapheresis. The procedure may need to be repeated as needed, but dramatic results can be seen. After plasmapheresis, symptoms improve and the dose of acetylcholinesterase inhibitors can often be temporarily reduced. The procedure should be carried out with the patient in the left lateral position and with the uterus tilted off the inferior vena cava. It should be performed relatively slowly, with careful attention to maternal blood pressure. If plasmapheresis is being performed after 24 weeks' gestation, continuous fetal monitoring should be employed.

Neonatal Myasthenia Gravis

Neonatal myasthenia occurs in 10 to 25 percent of infants born to mothers with myasthenia gravis.[160–163] In his review series, Plauché[152] reported a 20.2 percent incidence of neonatal myasthenia, with a 2.1 percent stillbirth rate and a 3.8 percent neonatal mortality rate. Again, that study reviewed cases over a 40-year period. With modern neonatal care, the neonatal mortality rate is probably considerably lower. Neonatal myasthenia does not begin at birth but is usually evident within the first 2 days of life. For this reason, mothers with myasthenia gravis are not candidates for early discharge even if their disease is well controlled. It lasts an average of 3 weeks but can persist up to 15 weeks.[163] Symptoms usually include a weak cry, poor sucking effort, and, rarely, respiratory distress. Neonatal myasthenia is thought to be secondary to transplacental passage of IgG antibodies directed against acetylcholine receptors.

Key Points

- Systemic lupus erythamatosus is associated with an increase in poor pregnancy outcome (i.e., from IUGR, stillbirth, and spontaneous abortion).
- The rate of pregnancy complications is decreased if patients with SLE have quiescent disease for 6 months prior to conception.
- Glucocorticoids are safe to use in pregnancy for treating patients with SLE.
- The lupus inhibitor and anticardiolipin antibodies are found in 50 percent of patients with SLE. They are associated with an increased risk of pregnancy loss, including second and third trimester losses.
- Anti-SSA (Ro) and anti-SSA (La) antibodies are associated with complete congenital heart block and other manifestations of neonatal lupus.
- Low dose heparin and low dose aspirin are the therapies of choice for patients with lupus inhibitor/ antiphospholipid antibodies who do not have active SLE.
- Rheumatoid arthritis tends to improve during pregnancy but may relapse in the postpartum period.
- Rheumatoid arthritis does not appear to have a major deleterious effect on pregnancy.
- Pyridostigmine can be safely used to treat patients with myasthenia gravis in pregnancy.
- Infants born to mothers with myasthenia gravis can have muscle weakness and even problems feeding. This usually manifests itself after the second day of life.

REFERENCES

1. Fessel WJ: Systemic lupus erythematosus in the community. Incidence, prevalence, outcome and first symptoms: the high prevalence in black women. Arch Intern Med 134:1027, 1974
2. Estes D, Christian CL: The natural history of systemic lupus erythematosus by prospective analysis. Medicine 50:85, 1971
3. Garsenstein M, Pollak VE, Karik RM: Systemic lupus erythematosus and pregnancy. N Engl J Med 276:165, 1962
4. Zurier RB: Systemic lupus erythematosus and pregnancy. Clin Rheum Dis 1:613, 1975
5. Meehan RT, Dorsey JK: Pregnancy among patients with systemic lupus erythematosus receiving immuno-suppressive therapy. J Rheumatol 14:252, 1987
6. Lockshin MD: Lupus erythematosus and allied disorders in pregnancy. Bull NY Acad Med 63:797, 1987
7. Lockshin MD, Reinitz E, Druzin ML et al: Lupus pregnancy; case–control prospective study demonstrating

absence of lupus exacerbation during or after pregnancy. Am J Med 77:893, 1984

8. Lockshin MD: Pregnancy does not cause systemic lupus erythematosus to worsen. Arthritis Rheum 32:665, 1989

9. Derksen FH, Bruinse HW, deGroot PG, Kater L: Pregnancy in systemic lupus erythematosus: a prospective study. Lupus 3:149, 1994

10. Mintz G, Nitz J, Gutierrez G et al: Prospective study of pregnancy in systemic lupus erythematosus: results of a multidisciplinary approach. J Rheumatol 13:732, 1986

11. Le Thi Huong D, Wechsler B, Piette JC et al: Pregnancy and its outcome in systemic lupus erythematosus. Q J Med 87:721, 1994

12. Ainslie WH, Britt K, Moshipur JA: Maternal death due to lupus pneumonitis in pregnancy. Mt Sinai J Med 46:494, 1979

13. Leikin JB, Arof HM, Pearlman LM: Acute lupus pneumonitis in the postpartum period: a case history and review of the literature. Obstet Gynecol 68:295, 1986

14. Rubin LA, Geran A, Rose TH, Cohen H: A fatal complication of lupus in pregnancy. Arthritis Rheum 38:710, 1995

15. Averbuch M, Bojko A, Levo Y: Cardiac tamponade in the early postpartum period as the presenting and predominant manifestation of systemic lupus erythematosus. J Rheumatol 13:444, 1986

16. Marabani M, Zoma A, Hadley D, Sturrock RD: Transverse myelitis occurring during pregnancy in a patient with systemic lupus erythematosus. Ann Rheum Dis 48:160, 1989

17. Gimovsky ML, Montoro M, Paul RH: Pregnancy outcome in women with systemic lupus erythematosus. Obstet Gynecol 63:686, 1984

18. Devoe L, Taylor RL: Systemic lupus erythematosus in pregnancy. Am J Obstet Gynecol 135:473, 1979

19. Hayslett JP, Lynn RI: Effect of pregnancy in patients with lupus nephropathy. Kidney Int 18:207, 1980

20. Fine LG, Barnett EV, Danovitch GM et al: Systemic lupus erythematosus in pregnancy. Ann Intern Med 94:667, 1981

21. Mackey E: Pregnancy and renal disease: a ten-year study. Aust NZ J Obstet Gynaecol 3:21, 1963

22. Ramsey-Goldman R: Pregnancy in systemic lupus erythematosus. Rheum Dis Clin North Am 14:1988

23. Houser MT, Fish AJ, Tagatz GE et al: Pregnancy and systemic lupus erythematosus. Am J Obstet Gynecol 138:409, 1980

24. Foldes FF, McNall PG: Myasthenia gravis: a guide for anesthesiologists. Anesthesiology 23:837, 1962

25. Buyon JP, Cronstein BN, Morris M et al: Serum complement values (C_3 and C_4) to differentiate between systemic lupus activity and preeclampsia. Am J Med 81:194, 1986

26. Fraga A, Mintz G, Orozco J et al: Sterility and fertility rates, fetal wastage and maternal morbidity in systemic lupus erythematosus. J Rheumatol 1:1293, 1974

27. Castillo JD, Engbaek L: The nature of the neuromuscular block produced by magnesium. J Physiol 124:370, 1954

28. Kitzmiller JL: Autoimmune disorders: maternal, fetal and neonatal risks. Clin Obstet Gynecol 21:385, 1978

29. Zurier RG, Argyros T, Urman J et al: Systemic lupus erythematosus: management during pregnancy. Obstet Gynecol 51:178, 1978

30. Julkunen H, Kaaja R, Kurki P et al Fetal outcome in women with primary Sjögren's syndrome. A retrospective case-control study. Clin Exp Rheumatol 13:65–71, 1995

31. Ramsey-Goldman R, Kutzer JE, Kuller LH et al Pregnancy outcome and anticardiolipin antibody in women with systemic lupus erythematosus. Am J Epidemiol 138:1057–1069, 1993

32. Petri M, Albritton J. Fetal outcome of lupus pregnancy: a retrospective case-control study of the Hopkins Lupus Cohort. J Rheumatol 20:650–656, 1993

33. Leu LY, Lan JL. The influence on pregnancy of anti-SSA/Ro antibodies in systemic lupus erythematosus. Chi Mien I Hsueh Tsa Chih 25:12–20, 1992

34. Johnson MJ, Petri M, Witter FR, Repke JT. Evaluation of preterm delivery in a systemic lupus erythematosus pregnancy clinic. Obstet Gynecol 86:396–399, 1995

35. Rosove MH, Brewer PM, Runge A, Hirji K: Simultaneous lupus anticoagulant and anticardiolipin assays and clinical detection of antiphospholipids. Am J Hematol 32:148, 1989

36. Lockwood CJ, Romero R, Feinber RF: The prevalence and biologic significance of lupus anticoagulant and anticardiolipin antibodies in a general obstetric population. Am J Obstet Gynecol 161:369, 1989

37. Hanly JG, Gladman DD, Rose TH et al: Lupus pregnancy, a prospective study of placental changes. Arthritis Rheum 31:358, 1988

38. Hedfors E, Lindahl G, Lindblad S: Anticardiolipin antibodies during pregnancy. J Rheumatol 14:160, 1987

39. Hokkanen E: Myasthenia gravis. Ann Clin Res 1:94, 1969

40. Lubbe WF, Butler WS, Palmer SJ et al: Lupus anticoagulant in pregnancy. Br J Obstet Gynaecol 97:357, 1984

41. Lubbe WF, Butler WS, Liggins GC: The lupus-anticoagulant: clinical and obstetric implications. NZ Med J 97:398, 1984

42. Branch DW, Scott JR, Kochenour NK et al: Obstetric complications associated with the lupus anticoagulant. N Engl J Med 313:1322, 1985

43. Unander AM, Norberg R, Hahn L et al: Anticardiolipin antibodies and complement in ninety-nine women with habitual abortion. Am J Obstet Gynecol 156:114, 1987

44. Lubbe WF, Walkom P, Alexander CJ: Hepatic and splenic haemorrhage as a complication of toxaemia of pregnancy in a patient with circulating lupus anticoagulant. NZ Med J 95:842, 1982

45. Druzin ML, Lockshin M, Edersheim TG et al: Second-trimester fetal monitoring and preterm delivery in pregnancies with systemic lupus erythematosus and/or circulating anticoagulant. Am J Obstet Gynecol 157:1503, 1987

46. Lockshin MD, Druzin ML, Goei S et al: Antibody to cardiolipin as a predictor of fetal distress or death in pregnant patients with systemic lupus erythematosus. N Engl J Med 313:152, 1985

47. Kutteh WH, Lyda EC, Abraham SM, Wacholtz MC: As-

sociation of anticardiolipin antibodies and pregnancy loss in women with systemic lupus erythematosus. Fertil Steril 60:449, 1993

48. Juikunen H, Jouhikainen T, Kaaja R et al: Fetal outcome in lupus pregnancy: a retrospective case–control study of 242 pregnancies in 112 patients. Lupus 2:125, 1993

49. Birdsall M, Pattison N, Chamley L: Antiphospholipid antibodies in pregnancy. Aust NZ J Obstet Gynecol 32: 328, 1992

50. Lubbe WF, Palmer SJ, Butler WS et al: Fetal survival after prednisone suppression of maternal lupus-anticoagulant. Lancet 1:1361, 1983

51. Mintz G, Nitz J, Gutierrez G et al: Prospective study of pregnancy in systemic lupus erythematosus: results of a multidisciplinary approach. J Rheumatol 13:732, 1986

52. Lockshin MD, Druzin ML, Qamar T: Prednisone does not prevent recurrent fetal death in women with antiphospholipid antibody. Am J Obstet Gynecol 160:439, 1989

53. Karp HJ, Frenkel Y, Many A et al: Fetal demise associated with lupus anticoagulant: clinical features and results of treatment. Gynecol Obstet Invest 28:178, 1989

54. Farquharson RG, Compston A, Bloom AL: Lupus anticoagulant: a place for prepregnancy treatment? Lancet 1:842, 1985

55. Gardlund B: The lupus inhibitor in thromboembolic disease and intrauterine death in the absence of systemic lupus. Acta Med Scand 215:293, 1984

56. Ordi J, Barquinero J, Vilardell M et al: Fetal loss treatment in patients with antiphospholipid antibodies. Ann Rheum Dis 48:798, 1989

57. Landy HJ, Kessler C, Kelly WK, Weingold AB: Obstetric performance in patients with the lupus anticoagulant and/or anticardiolipin antibodies. Am J Perinatol 9:146, 1992

58. Gatenby PA, Cameron K, Shearman RP: Pregnancy loss with phospholipid antibodies: improved outcome with aspirin containing treatment. Aust NZ J Obstet Gynaecol 29:294, 1989

59. Balasch J, Font J, Lopez-Soto A et al: Antiphospholipid antibodies in unselected patients with repeated abortion. Hum Reprod 5:43, 1990

60. Rosove MH, Tabsh K, Wasserstrum N et al: Heparin therapy for pregnant women with lupus anticoagulant or anticardiolipin antibodies. Obstet Gynecol 75:630, 1990

61. Branch DW, Silver RM, Blackwell JL et al: Outcome of treated pregnancies in women with antiphospholipid syndrome: an update of the Utah experience. Obstet Gynecol 80:614, 1992

62. Kaaja R, Julkunen H, Ammala P, et al: Intravenous immunoglobulin treatment of pregnant patients with recurrent pregnancy losses associated with antiphospholipid antibodies. Acta Obstet Gynaecol Scand 72:63, 1993

63. Chamley LW, Pattison NS, McKay EJ: IgM lupus anticoagulants can be associated with recurrent fetal loss of thrombic episodes. Thromb Res 58:343, 1990

64. Mizoguchi K, Kakisako S, Tanaka M et al: Lupus antico-

agulant as a risk factor for cerebral infarction and habitual abortions. Kurume Med J 36:113, 1989

65. Rallings P, Exner T, Abraham R: Coronary artery vasculitis and myocardial infarction associated with antiphospholipid antibodies in a pregnant woman. Aust NZ J Med 19:347, 1989

66. Litsey S, Noonan J, O'Connor W et al: Maternal connective tissue disease and congenital heart block. N Engl J Med 312:98, 1985

67. Draznin TH, Easterly NB, Fureu N et al: Neonatal lupus erythematosus. J Am Acad Dermatol 1:437, 1979

68. McCue C, Mantakas M, Tingelstad JB et al: Congenital heart block in newborns of mothers with connective tissue disease. Circulation 56:82, 1977

69. Scott JS, Maddison PJ, Tayler PV et al: Connective-tissue disease, antibodies to ribonucleoprotein and congenital heart block. N Engl J Med 309:209, 1983

70. Scheib JS, Waxman J: Congenital heart block in successive pregnancies: a case report and evaluation of risk with therapeutic consideration. Obstet Gynecol 73:481, 1989

71. Derksen RH, Meilof JF. Anti-Ro/SS-A and anti La/SS-B autoantibody levels in relation to systemic lupus erythematosus disease activity and congenital heart block. A longitudinal study comprising two consecutive pregnancies in a patient with systemic lupus erythematosus. Arthritis Rheum 45:953–959, 1992

72. Vetter VL, Rashkad WJ: Congenital complete heart block and connective tissue disease. N Engl J Med 309: 236, 1983

73. Esscher E, Scott JS: Congenital heart block and maternal systemic lupus erythematosus. BMJ 1:1235, 1979

74. Buyon JP, Swersky SH, Fox HE et al: Intrauterine therapy for presumptive fetal myocarditis with acquired heart block due to systemic lupus erythematosus. Arthritis Rheum 39:1, 1987

75. Lockshin MD, Gibofsky A, Peebles CL et al: Neonatal lupus erythematosus with heart block: family study of a patient with anti-SS-A and SS-B antibodies. Arthritis Rheum 26:210, 1983

76. McCuiston CH, Schoch EP: Possible discoid lupus erythematosus in a newborn infant: report of case with subsequent development of acute systemic lupus erythematosus in mother. Arch Dermatol Syphilol 70:782, 1954

77. McGee CD, Makowski EL: Systemic lupus erythematosus in pregnancy. Am J Obstet Gynecol 107:1008, 1970

78. Adams D, Druzin MI, Edersheim T et al: Condition specific antepartum testing: systemic lupus erythematosus and associated serologic abnormalities. Am J Reprod Immunol 28:159, 1992

79. Carroll BA: Obstetric duplex sonography in patients with lupus anticoagulant syndrome. J Ultrasound Med 9:17, 1990

80. Ariyuki Y, Hata T, Kitao M: Reverse end-diastolic umbilical artery velocity in a case of intrauterine fetal death at 14 weeks gestation. Am J Obstet Gynecol 169:1621, 1993

81. Buyon JP, Cronstein BN, Morris M et al: Serum complement values (C_3 and C_4) to differentiate between systemic lupus activity and pre-eclampsia. Am J Med 81: 194, 1986

82. Tozman ECS, Urowitz MB, Gladman DD: Systemic lupus erythematosus and pregnancy. J Rheumatol 7: 624, 1980

83. Zulman MI, Talal N, Hoffman GS et al: Problems associated with the management of pregnancies in patients with systemic lupus erythematosus. J Rheumatol 7:37, 1980

84. Zurier RG, Argyros T, Urman J et al: Systemic lupus erythematosus: management during pregnancy. Obstet Gynecol 51:178, 1978

85. Devoe LD, Aloy GL: Serum complement levels and perinatal outcome in pregnancies complicated by systemic lupus erythematosus. Obstet Gynecol 63:796, 1984

86. Lockshin MD, Qamar T, Levy RA, Druzin ML: Pregnancy in systemic lupus erythematosus. Clin Exp Rheumatol 7:S195, 1989

87. Freinkel N: Gestational diabetes, 1979: philosophical and practical aspects of a major health problem. Diabetes Care 3:399, 1980

88. Bongiovanni AM, McPadden AJ: Steroids during pregnancy and possible fetal consequences. Fertil Steril 11: 181, 1960

89. Fainstat T: Cortisone-induced congenital cleft palate in rabbits. Endocrinology 55:502, 1954

90. Giannopoulos G, Tulchinsky D: The influence of hormones on fetal lung development. p. 310. In Ryan KJ, Tulchinsky D (eds): Maternal-Fetal Endocrinology. WB Saunders, Philadelphia, 1988

91. Rolbin SH, Levinson G, Shnider SM et al: Anesthetic considerations for myasthenia gravis and pregnancy. Anesth Analog 57:441, 1978

92. Baliard PL, Granberg P, Ballard RA: Glucocorticoid levels in maternal and cord serum after prenatal betamethasone therapy to prevent respiratory distress syndrome. J Clin Invest 56:15, 1975

93. Blanford AT, Pearson-Murphy BE: In vitro metabolism of prednisolone, dexamethasone, betamethasone, and cortisol by the human placenta. Am J Obstet Gynecol 137:264, 1977

94. Osathanondh R, Tulchinsky D, Kamali H et al: Dexamethasone levels in treated pregnant women and newborn infants. J Pediatr 90:617, 1977

95. Levitz M, Jansen V, Dancis J: The transfer and metabolism of corticosteroids in the perfused human placenta. Am J Obstet Gynecol 132:363, 1978

96. Beitins IZ, Bayard F, Ances IG et al: The transplacental passage of prednisone and prednisolone in pregnancy near term. J Pediatr 81:936, 1972

97. Blanford AT, Pearson Murphy BE: In vitro metabolism of prednisolone, dexamethasone, betamethasone, and cortisol by the human placenta. Am J Obstet Gynecol 127:264, 1977

98. Gabbe SG: Drug therapy in autoimmune disease. Clin Obstet Gynecol 26:635, 1983

99. Scott JR: Fetal growth retardation associated with maternal administration of immunosuppressive drugs. Am J Obstet Gynecol 128:668, 1977

100. Davison JM, Lindheimer MD: Pregnancy in renal transplant recipients. J Reprod Med 27:613, 1982

101. Cote CJ, Meuwissen HJ, Pickering RJ: Effects on the neonate of prednisone and azathioprine administered to the mother during pregnancy. J Pediatr 85:324, 1974

102. Scott JR: Immunologic diseases in pregnancy. Prog Allergy 23:321, 1977

103. Turnam GR: Rheumatoid arthritis. Clin Obstet Gynecol 26:560, 1983

104. Masi AT, Maldonade-Cocco JA, Kaplan SB et al: Prospective study of the early course of rheumatoid arthritis in young adults: comparison of patients with and without rheumatoid factor positivity at entry and identification of variables correlating with outcome. Semin Arthritis Rheum 5:299, 1976

105. Baum J, Ziff M: Laboratory findings in rheumatoid arthritis. p. 491. In McCary D (ed): Arthritis and Allied Conditions. 9th Ed. Philadelphia, Lea & Febiger, 1979

106. Harris ED Jr: The proliferative lesion in rheumatoid arthritis: manifestation and pathophysiology. p. 374. In Harris ED Jr (ed): Rheumatoid Arthritis. Medcom, New York, 1974

107. Gordon DA, Stein JL, Broder I: The extraarticular features of rheumatoid arthritis: a systemic analysis of 127 cases. Am J Med 54:445, 1973

108. Hurd ER: Extraarticular manifestations of rheumatoid arthritis. Semin Arthritis Rheum 8:151, 1979

109. Hollingsworth JW, Saykaly RJ: Systemic complications of rheumatoid arthritis. Med Clin North Am 61:217, 1977

110. Williams RC: Adult and juvenile rheumatoid arthritis. p. 184. In Parker GW (ed): Clinical Immunology. WB Saunders, Philadelphia, 1980

111. Rodman GP (ed): Primer on the rheumatic diseases. JAMA, suppl 224:661, 1973

112. Robbins SL, Cotran RS: The musculoskeletal system—joints and related structures. p. 1452. In Robbins SL, Cotran RS (eds): Pathologic Basis of Disease. 2nd Ed. WB Saunders, Philadelphia, 1979

113. Yu DTY, Peter JB: Cellular immunological aspects of rheumatoid arthritis. Semin Arthritis Rheum 4:24, 1974

114. McDuffie FC: Immune complexes in the rheumatic disease. J Allergy Clin Immunol 62:37, 1978

115. Paget S, Gibofsky A: Immunopathogenesis of rheumatoid arthritis. Am J Med 67:961, 1979

116. Stobo JD: Rheumatoid arthritis restriction maps. West J Med 137:109, 1982

117. Hench PS: The ameliorating effect of pregnancy on chronic atrophic (infectious) rheumatoid arthritis, fibrositis and intermittent hydrarthrosis. Proc Mayo Clin 13:161, 1938

118. Persellin RH: The effect of pregnancy on rheumatoid arthritis. Bull Rheum Dis 27:922, 1977

119. Klipple GL, Cecere FA: Rheumatoid arthritis and pregnancy. Rheum Dis Clin North Am 15:213, 1989

120. Quinn C, Mulpeter K, Casey EB, Feighery CF. Changes in levels of IgM RF and alpha 2 PAG correlate with increased disease activity in rheumatoid arthritis during the puerperium. Scand J Rheumatol 22:273, 1993

121. Nelson JL, Hughes KA, Smith AG et al: Maternal-fetal disparity in HLA class II alloantigens and the pregnancy-induced amelioration of rheumatoid arthritis. N Engl J Med 329:466, 1993

122. Lasink M, de Boer A, Kijkmans BA et al: The onset of rheumatoid arthritis in relation to pregnancy and childbirth. Clin Exp Rheumatol 11:171, 1993

123. Kaplan D, Diamond H: Rheumatoid arthritis and pregnancy. Clin Obstet Gynecol 8:286, 1965

124. Betson JR, Dorn RV: Forty cases of arthritis and pregnancy. J Int Coll Surgeons 42:521, 1964

125. Silman AJ, Roman E, Beral V, Brown A: Adverse reproductive outcomes in women who subsequently develop rheumatoid arthritis. Ann Rheum Dis 47:979, 1988

126. Spector TD, Silman AJ: Is poor pregnancy outcome a risk factor in rheumatoid arthritis? Ann Rheum Dis 49:12, 1990

127. Duhring JL: Pregnancy, rheumatoid arthritis, and intrauterine growth retardation. Am J Obstet Gynecol 108:325, 1970

128. Bulmash JM: Rheumatoid arthritis and pregnancy. Obstet Gynecol Annu 8:223, 1979

129. Bulmash JM: Systemic lupus erythematosus and pregnancy. Obstet Gynecol Annu 7:153, 1978

130. Lewis RB, Shulman JD: Influence of acetylsalicylic acid, an inhibitor of prostaglandin synthesis, on the duration of human gestation and labour. Lancet 2:1159, 1973

131. Bleyer WA, Breckenridge RT: The effect of prenatal aspirin on newborn hemostasis. JAMA 213:2049, 1970

132. Silverberg DS, Kidd EG, Shnitka TK, Ulan RA: Gold nephropathy: a clinical and pathologic study. Arthritis Rheum 13:812, 1970

133. Vaamonde CA, Hunt FR: The nephrotic syndrome as a complication of gold therapy. Arthritis Rheum 13:826, 1970

134. Johnson TR, Banner EA, Winkelmann RK: Scleroderma and pregnancy. Obstet Gynecol 23:467, 1964

135. Fear RE: Eclampsia superimposed on renal scleroderma: a rare cause of maternal and fetal mortality. Obstet Gynecol 31:69, 1968

136. Sood SV, Kohler HG: Maternal death from systemic sclerosis. J Obstet Gynaecol Br Commonw 77:1109, 1970

137. Karlsen JR, Cook WA: Renal scleroderma and pregnancy. Obstet Gynecol 44:349, 1974

138. Ehrenfeld M, Licht A, Stersman J et al: Postpartum renal failure due to progressive systemic sclerosis treated with chronic hemodialysis. Nephron 18:175, 1977

139. Altieri P, Cameron JS: Scleroderma renal crisis in a pregnant woman with late partial recovery of renal function. Nephrol Dial Transplant 3:677, 1988

140. Baethge BA, Wolf RE: Successful pregnancy with scleroderma renal disease and pulmonary hypertension in a patient using angiotensin converting enzyme inhibitors. Ann Rheum Dis 48:776, 1989

141. Spiera H, Krakoff L, Fishbane-Mayer J: Successful pregnancy after scleroderma hypertensive renal crisis. J Rheumatol 16:1597, 1989

142. Maymon R, Fejgin M: Scleroderma in pregnancy. Obstet Gynecol Surv 44:530, 1989

143. Spellacy WN: Scleroderma and pregnancy. Obstet Gynecol 23:297, 1964

144. Slate WG, Graham AR: Scleroderma and pregnancy. Am J Gynecol 101:335, 1968

145. Jones WR, Storey B: Perinatal aspects of maternal autoimmune disease. Aust Paediatr J 8:306, 1972

146. Silman AJ, Black C: Increased incidence of spontaneous abortion and infertility in women with scleroderma before disease onset: a controlled study. Ann Rheum Dis 47:441, 1988

147. Freeman WE, Lesher JL Jr, Smith JG Jr: Connective tissue disease associated with sclerodermoid features, early abortion, and circulating anticoagulant. J Am Acad Dermatol 19:932, 1988

148. Steen VD, Conte C, Day N et al: Pregnancy in women with systemic sclerosis. Arthritis Rheum 32:151, 1989

149. Kurtzke JF: Epidemiology of myasthenia gravis. Adv Neurol 19:545, 1978

150. Hokkanen E: Myasthenia gravis. Ann Clin Res 1:94, 1969

151. Havard CW, Fonseca V: New treatment approaches to myasthenia gravis. Drugs 39:66, 1990

152. Plauché WC: Myasthenia gravis. Clin Obstet Gynecol 26:594, 1983

153. Petri M, Golbus M, Anderson R et al: Antinuclear antibody, lupus anticoagulant and anticardiolipin antibody in women with idiopathic habitual abortion. Arthritis Rheum 30:601, 1987

154. Plauché WC: Myasthenia gravis in pregnancy: an update. Am J Obstet Gynecol 135:691, 1979

155. Catanzarite VA, McHargue AM, Sandberg EC et al: Respiratory arrest during therapy for premature labor in a patient with myasthenia gravis. Obstet Gynecol 64:819, 1984

156. Castillo JD, Engbaek L: The nature of the neuromuscular block produced by magnesium. J Physiol 124:370, 1954

157. Cohen BA, London RS, Goldstein PJ: Myasthenia gravis and pre-eclampsia. Obstet Gynecol 48:35, 1976

158. McNall PG, Jafarnia MR: Management of myasthenia gravis in obstetrical patient. Am J Obstet Gynecol 92:518, 1965

159. Rolbin SH, Levinson G, Shnider SM et al: Anesthetic considerations for myasthenia gravis and pregnancy. Anesth Analog 57:441, 1978

160. Barlow CF: Neonatal myasthenia gravis. Am J Dis Child 135:209, 1981

161. Donaldson JO, Penn AS, Lisak RP et al: Antiacetylcholine receptor antibody in neonatal myasthenia gravis. Am J Dis Child 135:222, 1981

162. Namba T, Brown SB, Grob D: Neonatal myasthenia gravis: report of two cases and review of the literature. Pediatrics 45:488, 1970

163. Scott JR: Immunologic diseases in pregnancy. Prog Allergy 23:321, 1977

164. Tan EM, Cohen AS, Fries JF et al: The 1982 revised criteria for the classification of systemic lupus erythematosus. Arthritis Rheum 25:1274, 1982

165. Rodman GP, Schumacher HR: Appendix 2. p. 207. In Primer on the Rheumatic Diseases. 9th Ed. Arthritis Foundation, New York, 1988

Chapter 34

Hepatic Disease

Philip Samuels and Mark B. Landon

Liver dysfunction and disease occasionally complicate pregnancy. The most commonly seen problems include the liver dysfunction associated with preeclampsia and hepatitis. These topics are covered in detail elsewhere in this text. This chapter focuses on acute fatty liver, intrahepatic cholestasis of pregnancy, and gallbladder disease associated with gestation (Table 34-1).

Acute Fatty Liver

Acute fatty liver is a rare condition of unknown etiology that has an incidence of between 1 in 6,692 and 1 in 15,900 pregnancies.[1-3] Before 1970, the published mortality rate for both mother and infant was approximately 85 percent.[4] Since 1975, maternal survival has increased to 72 percent, with neonatal survival slightly lower. These improved outcomes have been attributed to early recognition of the disorder followed by prompt delivery.[1,5-7] Usually beginning late in the third trimester, acute fatty liver often presents with nausea and vomiting[1,7,8] followed by severe abdominal pain and headache. The right upper quadrant is generally tender, but the liver is not enlarged to palpation. Within a few days jaundice appears, and the patient becomes somnolent and eventually comatose. Hematemesis and spontaneous bleeding result when the patient develops hypoprothrombinemia and disseminated intravascular coagulation (DIC). Oliguria, metabolic acidosis, and eventually anuria occur in approximately 50 percent of patients with acute fatty liver of pregnancy.[9] Diabetes insipidus may also accompany the disease, but may not manifest itself until postpartum.[7,10] These patients may respond to desamino-cys-1-D-arginine-8-vasopressin (DDAVP) after delivery.[10] If the disease is allowed to progress, labor begins and the patient delivers a stillborn infant. Although the etiology of these fetal losses has not been convincingly demonstrated. Moise and Shali[2] suggest that uteroplacental insufficiency may be the cause of fetal distress and fetal death in acute fatty liver. During the immediate postpartum period, the mother becomes febrile, comatose, and, without therapy, dies within a few days. Rather than liver failure, DIC, renal failure, profound hypoglycemia, and occasionally pancreatitis are the most often cited immediate causes of death.[2,8,9] Two cases of liver rupture associated with acute fatty liver have also been reported.[11,12] In one case, a patient receiving intravenous heparin for thrombophlebitis suddenly expired as a result of rupture of a subcapsular hematoma of the liver.[12] The diagnosis of acute fatty liver in pregnancy was confirmed microscopically.

The primary differential diagnoses in cases of acute fatty liver include fulminant hepatitis and the liver dysfunction associated with the HELLP syndrome (hemolysis, elevated liver enzymes, and low platelet count) or preeclampsia (Table 34-1).[13-15] Several researchers have suggested a spectrum of diseases between acute fatty liver of pregnancy and preeclampsia.[13,15] Although it is often difficult, physicians are usually able to differentiate between these disorders based on physical and laboratory findings.

Etiology

The cause of acute fatty liver remains elusive. Brown et al[16] think that there is a spectrum of diseases that includes the whole range from mild preeclampsia to acute fatty liver of pregnancy. Grimbert and colleagues[17] investigated the effects of estradiol and progesterone on liver mitochondria in mice. Administration of these hormones resulted in decreased β-

Table 34-1 Differential Diagnosis of Liver Disease in Pregnancy

	Serum Transaminase Levels (IU/L)	Bilirubin Level (mg/dl)	Coagulopathy	Histology	Other Features
Acute hepatitis B	>1,000	>5	−	Hepatocellular necrosis	Potential for perinatal transmission
Acute fatty liver	<500	<5	+	Fatty infiltration	Coma, renal failure, hypoglycemia
Intrahepatic cholestasis	<300	<5, mostly direct	−	Dilated bile canaliculi	Pruritus, increased bile acids
HELLP	>500	<5	+	Variable periportal necrosis	Hypertension, edema, thrombocytopenia

Abbreviations: HELLP, hemolysis, elevated liver enzymes, low platelets; −, absent; +, present.

oxidation of palmitic acid and decreased activity of the tricarboxylic acid cycle. These mitochondrial changes are similar to what has been seen in acute fatty liver of pregnancy, leading the authors to conclude that imbalances of these hormones may contribute to the development of this pregnancy complication.

Treem and coworkers[18] note the similarities in clinical presentation and histologic appearance of the liver in pregnant women with acute fatty liver and in children with metabolic defects in the intramitochondrial β-oxidation pathway.[18] These authors report a case of a woman who had acute fatty liver whose infant at 4 months of age had hypoglycemia, coma, and profound hepatic steatosis. The infant had a defect of fatty acid oxidation, a deficiency of long-chain 3-hydroxyacyl-coenzyme A dehydrogenase. The mother was found to be heterozygous for this condition. This suggests that acute fatty liver may be a result of a defect in fatty acid oxidation. Sims et al[19] found the same defect in affected children from three families, all of whose mothers had experienced acute fatty liver of pregnancy. Schoeman et al[20] discuss a similar case in which a mother had acute fatty liver in two successive pregnancies and delivered two healthy infants. Both infants died at around 6 months of age with fatty infiltration of the liver, with similar disorders of fatty acid oxidation. Much research remains to be done, but it does appear that a disorder of fatty acid oxidation, perhaps precipitated by the hormones of pregnancy, may play a role in the etiology of this uncommon complication of pregnancy.

Clinical Diagnosis

Malaise, nausea with vomiting, and epigastric and/or right upper quadrant pain are usually present. The duration of these prodromal symptoms and signs is variable. In a study of 14 cases over 8 years. Usta et al[7] reported a mean gestational age of 34.5 weeks, with a range of 28 to 39 weeks. Four patients had hepatic encephalopathy, three had pulmonary edema, and three had ascites.[7] Reyes et al[3] report lethargy and jaundice as main presenting symptoms and signs in 11 patients with acute fatty liver of pregnancy in Chile. Unusual findings included seven patients with pruritus, two of whom experienced it weeks before the clinical onset of disease, and nine with polydypsia.[3] This is consistent with the occasional finding of diabetes insipidus previously mentioned.[7,10] Patients may also be febrile or present with hepatorenal syndrome.[21] By the time diagnosis is made, patients often have a clinically manifested coagulopathy. Rarely, acute fatty liver may occur concomitantly with other diseases such as severe preeclampsia,[21] chronic active hepatitis,[22] and pregnancy-induced cholestasis.[3,23]

Laboratory Diagnosis

In acute fatty liver of pregnancy, serum transaminase levels are elevated but usually remain below 500 IU/L.[5] In acute hepatitis, however, these levels are frequently above 1,000 IU/L. In liver dysfunction associated with preeclampsia or the HELLP syndrome, the transaminases are often in the same range as in acute fatty liver of pregnancy, but are occasionally higher. As a result of DIC, the prothrombin time and activated partial thromboplastin times (APTT) are often prolonged. The prothrombin time is usually increased before the APTT because it reflects the vitamin K-dependent clotting factors synthesized in the liver. A decreased fibrinogen level is accompanied by an elevation in fibrin degradation products, the D-dimer, and prothrombin 1.2. Although the serum bilirubin level is elevated, it usually remains below 5 mg/dl and rarely rises as high as 10 mg/dl, a level lower than one would expect in acute hepatitis. A liver biopsy specimen will reveal pericentral microvesicular fatty change. There is little inflammatory cell infiltration or hepatic necrosis. Periportal areas are usually preserved.[6,24] This picture is very different from fulminant hepatitis in which hepatocellular necrosis is significant. Special staining and electron microscopy yield no evidence of viral particles in acute fatty liver of pregnancy. The diagnosis can be made on frozen section of the liver biopsy material using oil red O stain.[6] This staining is very sensitive but not specific for acute fatty liver of pregnancy. Similar staining is also seen in patients with severe preeclampsia and the HELLP syndrome. Barton and colleagues[25] believe that electron microscopy is more beneficial in establishing a definitive diagnosis. Reyes et al[3] showed mega-mitochondria with paracrystalline inclusions in all patients who underwent liver biopsy. Because of the coagulopathy associated with acute fatty liver of pregnancy, liver biopsy is not advisable in most cases. If biopsy is essential to make the diagnosis and establish a plan of treatment, fresh frozen plasma can be administered to correct the coagulopathy before performing the procedure. Goodacre and colleagues[26] and Mabie and colleagues[27] believe that diagnosis of acute fatty liver of pregnancy can occasionally be made using computed tomography (CT). The finding of decreased attenuation over the liver is compatible with fatty infiltration. Usta et al[7] found that CT resulted in a large number of false-negative diagnoses. Thus, a negative scan does not rule out fatty liver of pregnancy. This finding was corroborated by Van Le and Podrasky.[28] In their study of five patients with acute fatty liver, none had an abnormal CT scan, and only one had an abnormal right upper quadrant ultrasound examination.

Management

Once the diagnosis has been established, delivery should be accomplished as quickly as is safely possible.[29] Important supportive measures must first be undertaken to ensure maternal well-being. The patient's coagulopathy must be corrected with fresh frozen plasma. If more concentrated fibrinogen is needed, cryoprecipitate can be administered. In a study by Castro et al,[1] 28 patients with acute fatty liver were identified at the University of Southern California Medical Center. All 28 had evidence of persistent DIC, and 23 had a markedly depressed level of antithrombin III. Although some patients received antithrombin III concentrate, it did not appear to make a difference in the clinical course. Although antithrombin III concentrate may eventually play a role in treating patients with acute fatty liver and severe preeclampsia, its use is still considered experimental, and more research needs to be performed. Intravenous fluids containing adequate glucose should be given. This will prevent hypoglycemia, which can be fatal in this disorder. If there is not a severe coagulopathy or the coagulopathy has been corrected, invasive hemodynamic monitoring may be instituted if necessary before delivery. This technique will allow the anesthesiologist and obstetrician to monitor the patient's fluid status. Delivery soon after diagnosis is paramount. Vaginal delivery is preferable. If the patient's cervix is not ripe, cervical ripening agents may be employed to maximize the likelihood of a vaginal delivery. Cesarean delivery, however, is warranted if it appears that delivery cannot be effected in a timely fashion, and the patient is deteriorating. If the patient's coagulopathy has been corrected, epidural anesthesia is the best choice. Spinal anesthesia can also be used. Regional anesthesia is preferable, because it allows adequate assessment of the patient's level of consciousness. General anesthesia should be avoided if possible because of the hepatotoxicity of some anesthetic agents. Narcotic doses must be adjusted, as these drugs are metabolized by the liver.

Early diagnosis and delivery afford both mother and neonate an excellent chance for survival.[5,6] If delivery is effected before hepatic encephalopathy and renal failure develop, patients usually improve rather rapidly.[5–7,9,13] However, Ockner and colleagues[30] have reported a case in which the patient did not improve postpartum. After orthotopic liver transplantation, the multisystem failure rapidly reversed.[30] In that case, the diagnosis of acute fatty liver was documented histopathologically. Southern blot analysis for viral DNA was also negative, ruling out hepatitis. Amon et al[21] also reported as successful postpartum liver transplant in a patient with acute fatty liver and severe preeclampsia. There is little risk of recurrence of acute fatty liver in subsequent pregnancies.[9] Barton and colleagues,[25] described the first case of recurrent acute fatty liver in pregnancy confirmed by biopsy. Schoeman et al[20] also reported a case of a mother who had acute fatty liver in two successive pregnancies. Nonetheless, if the diagnosis is certain in the first pregnancy, patients should be reassured that they can carry a pregnancy in the future with little chance for recurrence.

Intrahepatic Cholestasis of Pregnancy

Intrahepatic cholestasis is characterized by pruritus and mild jaundice during the last trimester of pregnancy. It can, however, occur earlier in gestation.[31,32] The disease is reported to affect up to 10 percent of pregnancies in Chile.[33] In a recent study, Gonzalez et al.[34] determined the prevalence of intrahepatic cholestasis of pregnancy in Chile to be 4.7 percent in singleton pregnancies. In twin pregnancies, the incidence was 20.9 percent. The disease is also common in the Swedish population.[35,36] Berg et al[36] reported the incidence in Sweden to be between 1 and 1.5 percent. In their study, the incidence of intrahepatic cholestasis of pregnancy had a distinct seasonal variation, peaking in November. This disorder is much less common in the United States. In 1987, Wilson[37] reported the first case of intrahepatic cholestasis of pregnancy in an American-born black patient. Intrahepatic cholestasis tends to recur in subsequent pregnancies, but the severity may vary from one pregnancy to the next. In their Chilean study, Gonzalez et al[34] found a recurrence rate of 70.5 percent in singleton pregnancies.

Clinical Manifestations

Patients with intrahepatic cholestasis usually begin having pruritus at night. It progresses, and the patient is soon experiencing bothersome pruritus continuously. Approximately 2 weeks later, clinical jaundice will develop in 50 percent of cases. The jaundice is usually mild, soon plateaus, and remains constant until delivery. The pruritus worsens with the onset of jaundice, and the patient's skin can become excoriated. The symptoms usually abate within 2 days after delivery. The differential diagnosis must include viral hepatitis and gallbladder disease. There is usually no fever or abdominal discomfort, as in hepatitis, or nausea or vomiting, as seen in hepatitis and gallbladder disease.

Laboratory Diagnosis

Serum alkaline phosphatase levels are increased 5- to 10-fold in intrahepatic cholestasis of pregnancy. Alkaline phosphatase, however, is normally increased in pregnancy. This is due to the fact that the placenta produces this enzyme. Upon fractionation, most of the alkaline phosphatase is hepatic in origin rather than placental. Unfortunately, fractionation of alkaline phosphatase may not be readily available, making it impossible to separate the hepatic and placental contributions. Serum 5′-nucleotidase levels are also increased. Bilirubin is elevated, but usualy not above 5 mg/dl. Most is the direct, conjugated form. If intrahepatic cholestasis lasts for several weeks, liver dysfunction may result in decreased vitamin K reabsorption or decreased prothrombin production, leading to a prolongation of the prothrombin time. Serum transaminase levels are usually normal or moderately elevated, remaining well below the levels associated with viral hepatitis. Serum cholesterol and triglyceride levels may also be markedly elevated.

The serum bile acids (chenodeoxycholic acid, deoxycholic acid, and cholic acid) are increased. The levels are often more than 10 times the normal concentration. These acids are deposited in the skin and probably cause the extreme pruritus.[38] The degree of pruritus, however, is not always related to the serum level of bile acids.[39] To make the diagnosis of intrahepatic cholestasis of pregnancy, the fasting levels of serum bile acids should be at least three times the upper limit of normal. Elevation of serum bile acids alone cannot be used to make the diagnosis. The patient must also have clinical symptoms. Wojcicka-Jagodzinska and colleagues[40] re-

ported that carbohydrate metabolism is disturbed in patients with intrahepatic cholestasis of pregnancy. These patients should therefore be screened for gestational diabetes when the diagnosis of cholestasis is made.

Histologically, the periportal areas show no change, and the hepatocellular architecture remains undisturbed. The centrilobular areas, however, reveal dilated bile canaliculi, many containing bile plugs. Ultrastructurally, there appears to be some destruction and atrophy of microvilli in the bile canaliculi.[41] These changes tend to regress after pregnancy.

Perinatal Outcome

The risk of preterm birth and fetal death may be increased in patients suffering from intrahepatic cholestasis of pregnancy.[31,42] While the preterm birth rate has been reported to be between 30 and 60 percent by some investigators, another study noted no increase in preterm delivery or fetal loss.[43] Fisk and Storey[44] studied 83 pregnancies complicated by intrahepatic cholestasis over a 10-year period. Meconium staining occurred in 45 percent of the pregnancies, spontaneous preterm labor occurred in 44 percent, and intrapartum fetal distress complicated 22 percent. Of the 86 infants, two were stillborn and one died soon after birth. The overall perinatal mortality in this group of patients was 35 per 1,000. Nonstress tests, serial ultrasonography to assess amniotic fluid volume, and estriol determinations failed to predict fetal compromise.[44] Early intervention was indicated in 49 pregnancies, 12 because of suspected fetal distress. In light of this study, antepartum fetal heart rate testing and intense surveillance should be undertaken in gravidas with intrahepatic cholestasis of pregnancy. It may also be prudent to induce labor at term or when amniotic fluid studies indicate fetal lung maturity.[44] Over the past 8 years, we have also observed 2 unexplained stillbirths in 14 cases of pregnancy-induced cholestasis.

Management

Treatment is aimed at reducing the intense pruritus. Diphenhydramine, hydroxyzine, and other antihistamines are of little use, but cholestyramine resin has proven highly effective. Cholestyramine is an anion-binding resin that interrupts the enterohepatic circulation, reducing the reabsorption of bile acids. A total of 8 to 16 g per day in three to four divided doses is often helpful in relieving pruritus. It is most effective if started as soon as the pruritus is noted, before it becomes severe. It often takes up to 2 weeks to work. Because cholestyramine also interferes with vitamin K absorption, the prothrombin time should be checked at least weekly. If prolonged, parenteral vitamin K should be administered. When the prothrombin time returns to normal, the frequency of injections can be decreased. Cholestyramine causes a sensation of bloating and often results in constipation. If the patient cannot tolerate cholestyramine, antacids containing aluminum may be used to bind bile acids. These medications are usually not as effective as cholestyramine. An occasional patient may not respond to cholestyramine therapy. In those cases, phenobarbital, in a dose of 90 mg daily given at bedtime, can be helpful. Phenobarbital induces hepatic microsomal enzymes, increasing bile salt secretion and bile flow.[45-47] This medication usually takes more than 1 week to be effective. It is important to remember that phenobarbital must not be given within 2 hours of cholestyramine, or the phenobarbital will be bound and excreted without being absorbed. The key to treating pregnancy-induced cholestasis is to begin therapy as soon as the diagnosis is made.

Low doses of dexamethasone have also been used with some success in treating pregnancy-induced cholestasis. When pruritus is intolerable, delivery may be undertaken as soon as fetal lung maturity has been documented. Jaundice usually disappears within 2 days after delivery. The patient should be counseled that the condition may recur during subsequent pregnancies.[34] It is also important to note that some patients may manifest symptoms of intrahepatic cholestasis when taking oral contraceptives.[36]

Pregnancy and Liver Transplantation

At present, pregnancy in the liver transplant patient is a rare occurrence. As the procedure becomes more widespread, more liver transplant recipients will become pregnant. Laifer and colleagues[48] reported the results of eight pregnancies in women with liver transplants. Seven of the eight patients conceived between 3 weeks and 24 months after transplantation. Six had live births, and one electively terminated her pregnancy. Five patients developed pregnancy-induced hypertension, including three with severe preeclampsia. The six infants born to these women were delivered between 26 and 37 weeks.[48] Five of the six infants survived, and none had structural anomalies. One patient underwent orthotopic liver transplantation at 26 weeks' gestation after presenting in hepatic coma from fulminant hepatitis B. She was delivered on postoperative day 7 because of fetal distress. Laifer et al[48] concluded that pregnancy does not appear to have a deleterious effect on hepatic graft function or survival. All eight of the patients in their series survived without permanent sequelae. As in the case of patients with a renal allograft, liver transplant recipients should continue their immunosuppressive medications throughout pregnancy. Furthermore, they should wait several years before conception to make certain that liver function is acceptable and there are no signs of rejection.

Gallbladder Disease

Cholelithiasis is responsible for approximately 7 percent of cases of jaundice occurring during gestation.[49] Pregnancy appears to increase the likelihood of gallstone formation but not the risk of developing acute cholecystitis.[50-52]

Pregnancy markedly alters gallbladder function. Ultrasound studies performed after 14 weeks' gestation have shown that fasting gallbladder volume is twice normal, the rate of gallbladder emptying is decreased, and the percentage of emptying is lower, thus leaving a higher residual than in the nonpregnant patient.[51] Cholecystokinin is the major stimulus for gallbladder contraction. It appears that estrogen and/or progesterone may make these contractions less effective, leading to an increased residual volume.

Once the diagnosis is confirmed, attacks of biliary colic should be treated symptomatically during gestation. Ultrasound examination of the gallbladder will aid in the evaluation and diagnosis of these patients. Hiatt and colleagues[53] report that ultrasound successfully confirmed the presence of gallstones in 18 of 26 patients. In the same series, ultrasound also demonstrated dilated intrahepatic ducts in one of two patients with surgically proven choledocholithiasis. Before resorting to surgery, attempts should be made to treat these patients medically. Attacks usually respond to intravenous hydration, analgesics, nasogastric suction, and antibiotics. Lockwood and associates[54] have also utilized total parenteral nutrition. Their patient did well with no fetal or maternal morbidity.

If possible, cholecystectomy should be postponed until after delivery. In their study of 26 patients, Hiatt and coworkers[53] found it necessary to perform cholecystectomy and cholangiography on 19 women, with four requiring common bile duct explorations. They noted that only two of seven patients who presented in the first trimester with cholecystitis carried their pregnancies to term.

If ascending cholangitis develops, cholecystectomy should not be postponed. Cholecystectomy should also be performed if common bile duct obstruction occurs or severe pancreatitis develops. Certainly, surgery should not be delayed if an acute abdomen develops. In these instances temporizing will only increase perinatal and maternal risks.[50] If cholecystectomy is performed in the second or third trimester, fetal mortality is less than 5 percent.[52] If pancreatitis secondary to biliary tract stones remains untreated, however, the fetal mortality approaches 60 percent.[52]

Dixon and colleagues,[55] reviewing their experience

with 44 patients, found that conservative management of cholecystitis was followed by recurrent episodes of biliary tract symptoms requiring multiple hospitalizations. Cholecystectomy performed in the second trimester was associated with little maternal morbidity, no fetal loss, and a substantial reduction of total hospital days. Baille and colleagues[56] demonstrated that they were able to avoid cholecystectomy in five women by performing endoscopic sphincterotomy. Four of these patients had acute cholangitis, and one had pancreatitis. All five women delivered healthy infants at term. Their experience indicates that endoscopic retrograde cholangiopancreatography and sphincterotomy can be safely performed in pregnancy.[56] Before recommending such treatment on a widespread basis, more studies need to be conducted with this technique.

Laparoscopic cholecystectomy has successfully been performed in early pregnancy.[57] If the uterus is below the umbilicus, the procedure should be safe. However, the abdomen should be insufflated to the lowest possible pressure, and fetal heart tones should be auscultated intermittently during the case, especially if surgery is prolonged.

Gallbladder rupture has been reported as a rare complication of pregnancy.[58,59] This may occur because gastrointestinal symptomatology is often confusing in pregnancy, thus delaying appropriate diagnosis. In one of the reported cases, the patient died from complications.[58] Surgeons may be reluctant to operate on a pregnant patient even though her gallbladder disease warrants intervention. Such delays can have devastating consequences. As obstetricians, it is our duty to help establish the proper diagnosis and, if therapy is out of our field, to encourage our colleagues to undertake appropriate therapy in a manner that is most beneficial to mother and fetus.

References

1. Castro MA, Goodwin TM, Shaw KJ et al: Disseminated intravascular coagulation and antithrombin III depression in acute fatty liver of pregnancy. Am J Gynecol 174:211, 1996
2. Moise KJ Jr, Shah DM: Acute fatty liver of pregnancy: etiology of fetal distress and fetal wastage. Obstet Gynecol 69:482, 1987
3. Reyes H, Sandoval L, Wainstein A et al: Acute fatty liver of pregnancy: a clinical study of 12 episodes in 11 patients. Gut 35:101, 1994
4. Nash DT, Dale JT: Acute yellow atrophy of liver in pregnancy. NY State J Med 71:458, 1971
5. Hou SH, Levin S, Ahola S et al: Acute fatty liver of pregnancy: survival with early cesarean section. Dig Dis Sci 29:449, 1984
6. Ebert EC, Sun EA, Wright SH et al: Does early diagnosis and delivery in acute fatty liver of pregnancy lead to improvement in maternal and infant survival? Dig Dis Sci 29:453, 1984
7. Usta IM, Barton JR, Amon EA et al: Acute fatty liver of pregnancy: an experience in the diagnosis and management of fourteen cases. Am J Obstet Gynecol 171:1342, 1994
8. Purdie JM, Walters BN: Acute fatty liver of pregnancy: clinical features and diagnosis. Aust NZ J Obstet Gynaecol 28:62, 1988
9. Shaffer EA: Liver disease in pregnancy. Curr Probl Obstet Gynecol 7:15, 1984
10. Kennedy S, Hall PM, Seymour AE, Hague WM: Transient diabetes insipidus and acute fatty liver of pregnancy. Br J Obstet Gynaecol d101:387, 1994
11. Minuk GY, Lui RC, Kelly JK: Rupture of the liver associated with acute fatty liver of pregnancy. Am J Gastroenterol 82:457, 1987
12. Roh LS: Subcapsular hematoma in fatty liver of pregnancy. J Forensic Sci 31:1509, 1986
13. Riley CA, Romero R, Duffy TP: Hepatic dysfunction with disseminated intravascular coagulation in toxemia of pregnancy: a distinct clinical syndrome. Gastroenterology 80:1346, 1981
14. Brown MS, Reddy KR, Hensley GT et al: The initial presentation of fatty liver of pregnancy mimicking acute viral hepatitis. Am J Gastroenterol 82:554, 1987
15. Riley CA, Latham PS, Romero R, Duffy TP: Acute fatty liver of pregnancy: a reassessment based on observations in nine patients. Ann Intern Med 106:703, 1987
16. Brown MA, Pasaris G, Carlton MA. Pregnancy-induced hypertension and acute fatty liver of pregnancy: atypical presentations. Am J Obstet Gynecol 164:154, 1990
17. Grimbert S, Fisch C, Deschamps D et al: Effects of female sex hormones on mitochondria: possible role of acute fatty liver of pregnancy. Am J Physiol 268:6107, 1995
18. Treem WR, Rinaldo P, Hale DE et al: Acute fatty liver of pregnancy and long-chain 3-hydroxyacyl-coenzyme A dehydrogenase deficiency. Hepatology 19:339, 1994
19. Sims HF, Brackett JC, Powell CK et al: The molecular basis of pediatric long chain 3-hydroxyacyl-CoA dehydrogenase deficiency associated with maternal acute fatty liver of pregnancy. Proc Natl Acad Sci USA 92:841, 1995
20. Schoeman MN, Batey RG, Wilcken B: Recurrent acute fatty liver of pregnancy associated with a fatty-acid oxidation defect in the offspring. Gastroenterology 100:544, 1991
21. Amon E, Allen SR, Petrie RH, Belew JE: Acute fatty liver of pregnancy associated with preeclampsia: management of hepatic failure with postpartum liver transplantation. Am J Perinatol 8:278, 1991
22. Minton D, Yancey MK, Dolson DJ, Duff P: Acute fatty liver of pregnancy in a patient with chronic active hepatitis and associated hepatocyte alpha 1-antrypsin inclusions. Obstet Gynecol 81:819, 1993
23. Vanjak D, Moreau R, Roche-Sicot J et al: Intrahepatic cholestasis of pregnancy and acute fatty liver of pregnancy: an unusual, but favorable association? Gastroenterology 100:1123, 1991
24. Snyder RR, Hankins GD: Etiology and management of

acute fatty liver of pregnancy. Clin Perinatol 13:813, 1986

25. Barton JR, Sibai BM, Mabie WC, Shanklin DR: Recurrent acute fatty liver of pregnancy. Am J Obstet Gynecol 163: 534, 1990

26. Goodacre RL, Hunter DJ, Millward S et al: The diagnosis of acute fatty liver of pregnancy by computed tomography. J Clin Gastroenterol 10:680, 1988

27. Mabie WC, Dacus JV, Sibai BM et al: Computed tomography in acute fatty liver of pregnancy. Am J Obstet Gynecol 158:142, 1988

28. Van Le L, Podrasky A: Computed tomographic and ultrasonographic findings in women with acute fatty liver of pregnancy. J Reprod Med 35:815–817, 1990

29. Bacq Y, Riely CA: Acute fatty liver of pregnancy: the hepatologist's view. Gastroenterologist 1:257, 1993

30. Ockner SA, Brunt EM, Cohn SM et al: Fulminant hepatic failure caused by acute fatty liver of pregnancy treated by orthotopic liver transplantation. Hepatolos 11:59, 1990

31. Furhoff AK, Hellstrom K: Jaundice in pregnancy: follow-up study of the series of women originally reported by L. Thorling. I. The pregnancies. Acta Med Scand 193: 259, 1973

32. Rencoret R, Aste H: Jaundice during pregnancy. Med Aust 1:167, 1973

33. Reyes H, Gonzalez MC, Rabalta J et al: Prevalence of intrahepatic cholestasis of pregnancy in Chile. Ann Intern Med 88:487, 1978

34. Gonzalez MC, Reyes H. Arrese M et al: Intrahepatic cholestasis of pregnancy in twin pregnancies. J Hepatol 9: 84, 1989

35. Rannevik G, Jeppsson S, Kullinder S: Effect of oral contraceptives on the liver in women with recurrent cholestasis during previous pregnancies. J Obstet Gynaecol Br Commonw 79:1128, 1972

36. Berg B, Helm G, Petersohn L, Tryding N: Cholestasis of pregnancy: clinical and laboratory studies. Acta Obstet Gynecol Scand 65:107, 1986

37. Wilson JA: Intrahepatic cholestasis of pregnancy with marked elevation of transaminases in a black American. Dig Dis Sci 32:665, 1987

38. Engstrom J, Hellstrom J, Posse N, Sjoball J: Recurrent cholestasis of pregnancy: treatment with cholestyramine of one case with an unusually early onset. Acta Obstet Gynecol Scand 49:29, 1970

39. Ghent CN, Bloomer JR, Koatska G: Elevations in skin tissue levels of bile acids in humans with cholestasis: relation to serum levels and to pruritus. Gastroenterology 73:125, 1977

40. Wojcicka-Jagodzinska J, Kuczynska-Sicinska J, Czajkowski K, Smolarczyk R: Carbohydrate metabolism in the course of intrahepatic cholestasis in pregnancy. Am J Obstet Gynecol 161:959, 1989

41. Adlercreutz H, Svanbor A, Anber A: Recurrent jaundice in pregnancy. I. A clinical and ultrastructural study. Am J Med 42:335, 1967

42. Johnson WG, Baskett TF: Obstetric cholestasis: a 14 year review. Am J Obstet Gynecol 143:299, 1979

43. Johnson P, Samsioe G, Gustafsson A: Studies in cholestasis of pregnancy with special reference to clinical aspects and liver function tests. Acta Obstet Gynecol Scand, Suppl 54:77, 1975

44. Fisk NM, Storey GN: Fetal outcome in obstetric cholestasis. Br J Obstet Gynaecol 95:1137, 1988

45. Espinoza J, Barnaf L, Schnaidt E: The effect of phenobarbital on intrahepatic cholestasis of pregnancy. Am J Obstet Gynecol 119:234, 1974

46. Bloomer JR, Bower JL: Phenobarbital effects in cholestasis liver disease. Ann Intern Med 82:310, 1975

47. Laatikinen T: Effect of cholestiramine and phenobarbital on pruritis and serum bile acid levels in cholestasis of pregnancy. Am J Obstet Gynecol 132:501, 1978

48. Laifer SA, Darby MJ, Scantlebury VP et al: Pregnancy and liver transplantation. Obstet Gynecol 76:1083, 1990

49. Riley CA, Romero R, Duffy TP: Hepatic dysfunction with disseminated intravascular coagulation in toxemia of pregnancy: a distinct clinical syndrome. Gastroenterology 80:1346, 1981

50. Kammerer WS: Nonobstetric surgery during pregnancy. Med Clin North Am 63:1157, 1979

51. Bennion LJ, Grundy SM: Risk factors for the development of cholelithiasis in man. N Engl J Med 299:1221, 1978

52. Printen KJ, Ott RA: Cholecystectomy during pregnancy. Am Surg 44:432, 1978

53. Hiatt JR, Hiatt JC, Williams RA, Klein SR: Biliary disease in pregnancy: strategy for surgical management. Am J Surg 151:263, 1986

54. Lockwood C, Stiller RJ, Bolognese RJ: Maternal total parenteral nutrition in chronic cholecystitis: a case report. J Reprod Med 32:785, 1987

55. Dixon NP, Faddis DM, Silberman H: Aggressive management of cholecystitis during pregnancy. Am J Surg 154:292, 1987

56. Baillie J, Cairns SR, Putman WS, Cotton PB: Endoscopic management of choledocholithiasis during pregnancy. Surg Gynecol Obstet 171:1, 1990

57. Penton ON, Nagy AG, Scudamore CH, Panton RJ: Laparoscopic cholecystectomy: a continuing plea for routine cholangiography. Surg Laparosc Endosc 5:43, 1995

58. Petrozza JC, Mastrobattista JM, Monga M: Gallbladder perforation in pregnancy. Am J Perinatol 12:339, 1995

59. Behera A, Gupta NM: Haemoperitoneum and haemobilia due to cystic artery tear associated with gall bladder perforation in acute cholecystitis complicating pregnancy: case report. Eur J Surg 157:619, 1991

Gastrointestinal Disease

Mark B. Landon

Peptic Ulcer Disease

The symptoms and complications of peptic ulcer seem to decrease during pregnancy. This observation, which remained anecdotal for many years, has been supported by Clark,[1] who interviewed pregnant women with a previous history of peptic ulcer disease and found that, in 313 pregnancies, 44 percent became asymptomatic and 44 percent demonstrated a marked improvement in symptoms. Only 12 percent remained the same or experienced worsening symptoms during gestation. There were no serious complications reported in this series. Of note, nearly half of the patients relapsed by 3 months' postpartum, and 75 percent of the patients questioned had experienced recurrent symptoms by 6 months after delivery. Vessey and colleagues have also reported a low rate of hospitalization for peptic ulcer disease in pregnant women and users of the contraceptive pill.[2] Of 175 woman hospitalized for advanced symptoms of ulcer disease, none were pregnant.

Several factors that might improve the clinical course of patients with peptic ulcer disease during pregnancy have been investigated. It is well known that patients with duodenal ulcer have higher levels of basal and stimulated acid secretion. It has been suggested that the amelioration of symptoms during pregnancy may in part be secondary to progesterone-induced lower gastric acid output as well as increased mucus production. The latter may exert a protective effect on the intestinal mucosa. In addition, the placenta is rich in histaminase, which may inactivate histamine or block its action at the level of the parietal cell. Plasma levels of histaminase increase dramatically during pregnancy and may be responsible for a decline in gastric acid output in patients who exhibit hyperacidity in the non-pregnant state.[3]

Studies investigating gastric acid secretion during pregnancy have presented conflicting data. Spiro et al[4] obtained serial gastric aspirates on one woman with a previous history of duodenal ulcer and reported a diminution in pepsin output and an associated elevation of pH during the last 4 months of gestation. In contrast, VanThiel et al[5] reported no significant differences in basal and peak acid outputs at 12, 24, and 36 weeks' gestation and at 1 to 4 weeks' postpartum in four women without a previous history of peptic ulcer disease.

The interplay of acid secretion and mucosal resistance is believed to be important in the pathogenesis of peptic ulceration. Recently, infection of the stomach and duodenum with *Helicobacter pylori* has been implicated as a significant factor, as well. This organism is found in nearly all patients with duodenal ulceration.

Most physicians, when evaluating pregnant women with dyspepsia, attribute this complaint to gastric reflux in the lower esophagus. Heartburn is most often observed in the second and third trimesters. It usually responds to antacid therapy, and reflux can be minimized by having the mother assume a semirecumbent position when she is supine. This regimen will often bring relief to patients with underlying peptic ulcer disease as well, and further diagnostic procedures are rarely needed. In patients with profound pain that is unresponsive to antacid regimens, panendoscopic examination of the stomach and upper duodenum may be performed. These procedures, performed with appropriate analgesia, are generally well tolerated during pregnancy. Barium studies of the upper gastrointestinal tract should, in most cases, be avoided in a gravid woman, as they present a potential risk to the developing fetus.

The primary medical treatment for the symptomatic patient with peptic ulcer disease during pregnancy remains antacid therapy and diet. Administration of 15 to 30 cc of antacid 1 hour after meals and at bedtime usually provides relief of symptoms and promotes ulcer healing. In refractory cases, a dose may be added at 3 hours after meals. It is important to be aware that potential side effects of antacid therapy exist (Table 34-2). Patients with peptic ulcer disease should be maintained on a normal diet, avoiding caffeine, salicylates, ethanol, and any gastric stimulant that aggravates their condition. Because basal acid output may normally rise

Table 34-2 Potential Side Effects of Antacid Therapy

Agent	Side Effect
Sodium bicarbonate	May yield large amount of absorbed sodium
Magnesium hydroxide	Hypermagnesemia in renal insufficiency: laxative effect
Calcium carbonate	Constipation, hypercalcemia, milk alkali syndrome
Aluminum hydroxide	Constipation, phosphate binding and depletion

during evening hours, it follows that patients should avoid bedtime snacks.

At the present time, H_2 antagonists (cimetidine and ranitidine) remain a second line choice for therapy in pregnancy. If possible, these agents should be reserved for use during the second and third trimesters.[6] Cimetidine has antiandrogenic activity, as demonstrated by feminization of male rat pups exposed in utero.[7] As adults, these animals had diminished weights of androgen-sensitive tissues and reduced libido. Because antiandrogenic effects have not been associated with ranitidine use, this agent is preferred during gestation. Omeprazole, a recently introduced powerful inhibitor of acid secretion, is not recommended for use during pregnancy. This compound blocks hydrogen potassium ATPase in gastric parietal cells. Preliminary studies have suggested a potential for teratogenesis.[8] Elective treatment of *H. Pylori* with antibiotics and bismuth subsalicylate is generally recommended following delivery and breastfeeding.[8]

Fewer than 100 cases of pregnant women who develop serious complications from peptic ulcer disease have been reported in the literature.[9] Bleeding, perforation, and obstruction should be treated as they would be in nonpregnant patients. Becker-Andersen and Husfelt,[9] in reviewing 30 cases of hemorrhage from peptic ulcer during pregnancy, clearly demonstrated a decrease in maternal and fetal mortality rates with prompt surgical exploration. The only two maternal deaths in their series occurred in patients who were in shock at the time of operation. However, a 44 percent fetal mortality rate was recorded in cases that were first managed conservatively. The authors stressed that perforation and hemorrhage must be treated surgically using the same indications as for nonpregnant patients. If a partial gastrectomy is to be performed in the third trimester, it may be advisable to begin the procedure with a cesarean section. The fetus appears to be quite sensitive to maternal circulatory failure due to hypovolemia, and, in addition, gastric surgery may be facilitated after the gravid uterus has been evacuated.

Acute Pancreatitis

The true incidence of pancreatitis complicating pregnancy is difficult to ascertain. In a review of 500 cases of acute pancreatitis, only 7 patients developed the disease while pregnant.[10] Corlett and Mishell[11] reported an incidence of 1 in 1,066 pregnancies, while Wilkinson[12] noted 1 in 2,888 deliveries over a 5-year period. Review of the literature prior to 1972 reveals maternal mortality rates approaching 50 percent in some series. Maternal death is now uncommon, especially if the diagnosis is established promptly.[11] There appears to be a greater association of gallstones with the development of pancreatitis during gestation. McKay et al[10] noted that 18 of 20 patients who developed pancreatitis while pregnant or within 5 months' postpartum had cholelithiasis. In a 22-year study, Block and Kelly[13] reported that all 21 cases of pancreatitis during pregnancy in their institution were associated with gallstones. In nonpregnant individuals, alcoholism is by far the most common etiologic factor. Other causes for pancreatitis include idiopathic factors, infection, previous surgery, preeclampsia, hyperparathyroidism, thiazide ingestion, and penetrating duodenal ulcer. The normal hypertriglyceridemia of pregnancy may be exaggerated in patients with hyperlipidemia, thereby inducing acute pancreatitis.[14] These rare cases have been treated with either hyperalimentation or lipoprotein apheresis when dietary fat restriction failed to improve symptoms during pregnancy.[14,15]

The clinical presentation of pancreatitis is not significantly altered in pregnancy. The disease may occur at any stage of gestation, but is more common in the third trimester and the puerperium. Epigastric pain, which may radiate to the flanks or shoulders, along with abdominal tenderness should prompt appropriate laboratory investigation. Occasionally, a patient will present with nausea and vomiting as her only complaints. Mild fever and leukocytosis may be present. Radiographic examination of the abdomen may simply reveal an adynamic ileus. Ultrasound imaging of the pancreas can be difficult. Therefore, if significant pancreatic necrosis is suspected, computed tomographic (CT) imaging becomes preferable. Such images should be limited to reduce fetal exposure. In most cases, this type of radiologic study is unnecessary.

In evaluating the pregnant patient with suspected pancreatitis, the differential diagnosis includes most causes of abdominal pain in young women. These are principally peptic ulcer disease, including perforation, acute cholecystitis, biliary colic, and intestinal obstruction. Specific tests employed to corroborate the diagnosis of pancreatitis rely on the measurement of pancreatitic enzymes, principally amylase. Elevated values should suggest pancreatitis, although they may be present with other conditions such as cholecystitis, intestinal obstruction, peptic ulcer disease, hepatic trauma, and ruptured ectopic pregnancy. There is controversy as to whether serum amylase values are affected during gestation. DeVore et al[16] noted that amylase levels were lower in pregnancy, although this difference was not statistically significant. They have utilized the amylase/creatinine clearance ratio to diagnose pancreatitis in pregnancy. This ratio is normally lowered during gestation as a result of an increased creatinine clearance. In the experience of DeVore et al,[16] all patients with pancreatitis demonstrated an increased ratio, including two with preeclampsia and hyperemesis gravidarum.

In most cases, acute pancreatitis resolves spontaneously within several days. However, in some 10 percent of cases, the illness is complicated and such patients are best managed in an intensive care environment. Pancreatic secretory activity should be reduced by keeping the patient NPO. Nasogastric suction is reserved for those with nausea and vomiting. Meperidine is the drug of choice for analgesia as, unlike morphine, it does not constrict the sphincter of Oddi. Fluid, electrolyte replacement, and serial laboratory assays of hemoglobin, white blood cell count, amylase, liver function enzymes, glucose, and calcium are essential. In advanced cases, hypocalcemia may be present, and calcium replacement is necessary. Patients who have been unable to eat for periods of longer than 1 week may benefit from intravenous alimentation.

Percutaneous aspiration of pancreatic exudate is important in refractory cases. This CT-guided procedure may be necessary to distinguish between sterile and infected pancreatic necrosis. For infected cases, surgical drainage of the pancreatic exudate is necessary. Jacobs et al[17] found that profoundly ill patients survived twice as often if they underwent surgical drainage. Of course, laparotomy, carries with it the added risks of preterm labor and delivery. Patients who relapse may also develop a pseudocyst. This complication requires surgical intervention after a period of time in which an adequate drainage procedure can be accomplished. In spite of the high rate of preterm labor even in conservatively managed cases, the fetal salvage rate, in cases of maternal pancreatitis, has been reported to be as high as 89 percent.[12]

Inflammatory Bowel Disease

The inflammatory bowel diseases ulcerative colitis (UC) and Crohn's disease (CD) or regional enteritis are idiopathic disorders that have their peak incidence in the reproductive age group. UC is a disease of the colon or rectum, marked by acute attacks of bloody stools, diarrhea, cramping, abdominal pain, weight loss, and dehydration. The histologic findings include a decreased number of goblet cells, crypt abscesses, ulcerations, and an inflammatory infiltrate consisting of lymphocytes, plasma cells, and polymorphonuclear cells. The prevalence of UC in the female population under 40 years of age is 40 to 100/100,000.[18] CD is considerably less common than UC, with an incidence of 2 to 4/100,000. The average age of onset is between 20 and 30 years. CD, in contrast to UC, tends to run a more subacute and chronic course, with symptoms including fever, diarrhea, and cramping abdominal pain.[19] CD may be found anywhere from mouth to anus, including

the perineum. However, the distal ileum, colon, and anorectal region are most frequently involved. Histologically, the inflammation is focal, with fissuring, ulcerations, and prominent lymphoid aggregates present. The hallmark of the histologic diagnosis is transmural involvement of the bowel coupled with the presence of multiple noncaseating granulomas. Because CD may involve only the colon, histologic differentiation from UC becomes important.

Ulcerative Colitis

Most studies have failed to provide adequate information on the specific effects of UC on fertility. Early reports suggested a fertility rate of 15 to 31 percent; however, few data were provided about method of fertility assessment of these women as well as their partners.[20,21] Subsequently, Willoughby and Truelove[22] provided data that suggested that UC had little if any effect on fertility. Of 137 women desiring pregnancy, 119 (87 percent) conceived, a rate similar to that in most normal populations. This study, however, spanned 10 years and may not reflect periods of impaired fertility related to increased activity of the disease.

Data describing the influence of UC on pregnancy outcome is more conclusive. Prior to 1948, UC was believed to have a deleterious effect on pregnancy. Subsequently, Felsen and Wolarsky[23] reported 34 women who experienced 43 full-term deliveries in 50 pregnancies. There were three spontaneous abortions, two therapeutic abortions, and one ectopic pregnancy in this early series. Because the women who suffered a miscarriage did not have active disease, Felsen and Wolarsky[23] concluded that UC did not adversely affect pregnancy.

Abramson et al[24] first described the pregnancy outcome of patients with UC according to their disease during gestation. In their report, group I consisted of women with inactive disease at the start of pregnancy; group II patients had active disease in early pregnancy; group III patients had onset of disease during gestation; and group IV patients had disease that developed during the puerperium.[24] The data revealed that patients in group I had the best prognosis, as 18 of 20 had full-term pregnancies, with seven experiencing exacerbation of disease during gestation or in the postpartum period. Of 12 patients in group II, all had term pregnancies marked by exacerbation of disease during pregnancy or the puerperium. Of five women in group III whose disease commenced during pregnancy, three fetal deaths occurred. It should be remembered, however, that this report antedated the use of steroids and other medications presently available to control active disease.

In 1956, Crohn et al[25] published their experience with UC in pregnancy. They analyzed the perinatal outcomes in 110 women during 150 pregnancies using the Abramson et al classification. Group I contained 74 pregnancies in which 62 were successful. The disease was reactivated in 54 percent of cases, including all six spontaneous abortions. Group II patients suffered reactivation of disease during pregnancy or postpartum in nearly 75 percent of cases. Pregnancy was successful in 84 percent of women (32 of 38) in this group. The Crohn et al[25] data suggested that patients with reactivation of quiescent disease during pregnancy had higher rates of abortion. However, their 19 group III patients with new onset disease experienced only one stillbirth and no spontaneous losses. The data of De-Dombal et al[21] support the view that women with quiescent UC that becomes active during pregnancy are not at increased risk for miscarriage. In their series, only 1 of 17 patients with active disease in the first 6 months miscarried. In contrast, a Danish study demonstrated a higher probability of miscarriage in women with active disease at conception. Seven of 19 women in this category versus 9 of 133 with quiescent disease suffered a miscarriage.[26]

Willoughby and Truelove[22] have confirmed that a good outcome can generally be expected in pregnancies complicated by UC. Furthermore, their study included a group of 102 patients treated with modern therapies, including either steroids or sulfasalazine, or both. They recorded a spontaneous abortion rate of only 11 percent in 216 women followed over a 20-year period.[22] Women with quiescent disease at conception had a slightly greater chance of successfully reaching term when compared with patients whose disease was active during pregnancy. The proportion of low-birth-weight babies and the incidence of anomalies were similar to those of the general population. This study also examined the effect of pregnancy on UC. Of the 129 pregnancies in which colitis was quiescent at the time of conception, 90 (70 percent) of the patients remained free of symptoms throughout pregnancy and the puerperium. This figure compares favorably the data of Crohn et al,[25] in which 46 percent remained free of active disease (Table 34-3). The results of DeDombal et al[23] also confirmed that pregnancy had little adverse effect on UC. In the reproductive age group, they found a 45 percent chance of developing recurrent disease in any given year. This figure seems appropriate to apply to pregnant patients from the data currently available.

Crohn's Disease

As in studies of UC, it has been difficult to determine the effect of CD on fertility. In studies that lacked full evaluation and follow-up, Crohn et al[27] and Fielding and Cooke[28] reported infertility rates of 38 and 26 percent, respectively. Interestingly, Fielding and Cooke's study revealed a much higher infertility rate (67 percent) if CD involved the colon. DeDombal et al[29] have confirmed that a high proportion of patients with large bowel disease are "subfertile." They suggest that temporary infertility may be related to the activity of the disease.[29] Khosla et al[30] described infertility in 112 patients with CD and reported a 12 percent rate, similar to that seen in the general population. In a more recent case–control study, the number of offspring of women with CD was 57 percent of that of paired controls. This study concluded that disease location had no influence on fertility.[31]

Studies describing the effect of CD on pregnancy suggest minimal if any increased risk to both mother and fetus. In the original report,[27] 53 patients with regional ileitis had 84 pregnancies, and 75 infants (89 percent) survived. Seventy-one of these deliveries occurred at term.[27] However, the three patients who developed CD during pregnancy suffered two stillbirths and one preterm delivery. The only maternal death occurred in this group. Fielding and Cooke[28] also reported favorable outcomes in a series of patients with both regional ileitis and Crohn's colitis. Their study described an 85 percent live birth rate among 52 women in 98 pregnancies. More recent studies confirm these excellent results, with full-term delivery rates of 73 to 83 percent (Table 34-4).[32,33]

Table 34-3   Effect of Pregnancy on Ulcerative Colitis

Investigators	No. of Pregnancies	Exacerbation During Gestation[a]	Active Disease in Pregnancy[a]
Quiescent disease at conception			
Abramson et al (1951)[24]	20	7 (35)	—
Crohn et al (1956)[25]	74	40 (54)	—
DeDombal et al (1965)[21]	80	27 (33)	—
Willoughby and Truelove (1980)[22]	129	39 (30)	—
Active disease at conception			
Abramson et al (1951)[24]	12	—	12 (100)
Crohn et al (1956)[25]	38	—	29 (76)
Willoughby and Truelove (1980)[22]	55	—	29 (53)

[a]Percentages in parentheses.

Table 34-4   Live Birth Rate in Pregnancies Complicated by Crohn's Disease

Investigators	No. of Pregnancies[a]	Early Active Disease		Disease in Remission		Total	
		No.	Percent	No.	Percent	No.	Percent
Crohn et al (1956)[27]	75	28/30	93	36/45	80	64/75	85
Felding and Cooke (1970)[28]	98	—		—		82/98	85
DeDombal et al (1972)[29]	57	—		—		53/57	93
Khosla et al (1984)[30]	74	12/20	60	36/54	66[b]	48/74	65
Woolfson et al (1990)[33]	78	13/16	81	56/62	90	69/78	88

[a]Excludes terminations.
[b]One patient had nine successive miscarriages (patients included were diagnosed before conception).

Three recent investigations suggest that active CD carries with it a greater risk of spontaneous miscarriage.[30,32,33] Khosla et al[30] reported a spontaneous loss rate of 35 percent in patients with active disease at the time of conception and 50 percent in patients with severe disease. These data are supported by Danish and Canadian studies in which the risk of both preterm delivery and spontaneous abortion were found to be significantly higher in women with active disease at conception.[32,33]

A subgroup of patients deserves further mention, those who first develop disease during pregnancy. The caution[27] about unfavorable outcomes in such patients has been supported by Martimbeau et al[34] They reported 10 patients including one with twins in whom infant deaths occurred. Four of these neonatal deaths followed an operative procedure. However, tocolytics and neonatal intensive care were unavailable in most of these cases.

The effect of pregnancy on CD is similar to that reported for patients with UC. DeDombal et al[29] reported that 73 percent of patients had no change in disease activity during pregnancy, 15 percent improved, and 10 percent worsened. If a woman conceives while CD is in remission, she is just as likely to remain in remission as a nonpregnant patient. In the study of Woolfson et al,[33] 18 of 73 women (25 percent) with quiescent CD at conception relapsed during pregnancy. Maintenance on medication did not affect the relapse rate. In the study of Khosla et al,[30] postpartum flare-ups were virtually absent in contrast to the DeDombal et al.[29] report of a 40 percent postpartum recurrence rate. Khosla et al[30] also noted that patients with clinically active disease at the time of conception usually continue to have symptoms during pregnancy. Only 7 of 20 patients (35 percent) in this category went into remission or had slight improvement with pregnancy. Overall, the risk of exacerbation during pregnancy is not higher than that in the nonpregnant population.[31]

Treatment of Inflammatory Bowel Disease During Pregnancy

The medical treatment of inflammatory bowel disease is not altered greatly by pregnancy. All patients should be followed closely so that the activity of their disease may be assessed and psychological support can be provided. Since emotional tension may adversely affect both UC and CD, it is important that patients with inflammatory bowel disease have the opportunity to discuss the stress of pregnancy openly. Dietary counseling for patients with UC should emphasize proper nutritional intake. Patients with mild disease may respond to a low roughage diet or to the exclusion of milk products if they are lactose intolerant. In contrast, patients with CD often benefit from low residue diets, presumably because the caliber of their small bowel may be limited by inflammation.

The initial therapy for episodes of diarrhea generally includes narcotics such as codeine and diphenoxylate. Chronic use of narcotics should be avoided as it may incite toxic megacolon in patients with UC. When simple measures are unsuccessful in quieting an attack, sulfasalazine and steroid therapy should be strongly considered. The safety of both of these drugs has been well established in pregnancy. Sulfasalazine (Azulfidine) is most effective in maintaining remission and preventing further attacks. Patients who present early in pregnancy on sulfasalazine for a recent flare of their disease should probably be maintained on this therapy as active colitis may develop if the drug is discontinued. Recently, the active metabolite of sulfasalazine, 5-amniosalicylic acid, and its N-acetyl derivative have become available for treatment.[35] Concerns about the use of sulfasalazine in late pregnancy centered on its ability to cross the placenta, displace bilirubin, and cause kernicterus. However, the active fetal metabolite sulfapyridine, has weak bilirubin-displacing activity, and the actual risk is small. Jaundice was not increased in 209 neonates of women treated with Azulfidine. The safety of sulfasalazine in breast-feeding has raised some concern. The concentration of sulfapyridine in breast milk is approximately 45 percent that in maternal serum.[32] Similarly, concentrations of 5-aminosalicylic acid are lower in fetal plasma and breast milk than in maternal serum.[35] Thus, sulfasalazine and 5-aminosalicylic acid can be given safely to nursing mothers.[36]

Steroids are indicated in patients who fail to respond to simple supportive measures. Steroid retention enemas may be effective for mild to moderate distal colitis or proctitis. Patients with severe disease are initially treated with high doses of intravenous hydrocortisone or its equivalent. Oral prednisone can then be substituted and tapered as the attack subsides. The safety of corticosteroids and sulfasalazine in pregnancy associated with inflammatory bowel disease was addressed in a national survey by Mogadam et al[36] In examining 287 pregnancies in which either or both drugs were employed versus 244 untreated patients, they found no adverse effects that were attributable to these drugs. The higher complication rates associated with severe CD in this study seemed to be more related to disease activity than to the use of medication.[36]

Occasionally, patients with inflammatory bowel disease may be receiving azathioprine for treatment. The safety of this medication during pregnancy remains controversial. Alstead and colleagues[37] recently reported 16 pregnancies in 14 women receiving azathioprine for inflammatory bowel disease. There was one infectious complication of pregnancy (hepatitis B infection), but no congenital abnormalities or health problems in the offspring.[37] The decision to utilize this medication must be made after consultation with the patient, including weighing the risk of exacerbation of disease upon discontinuation.

Patients with severe disease who become profoundly dehydrated require hospitalization and intravenous fluids. The development of significant hypoalbuminemia coupled with inadequate caloric intake may require the institution of parenteral hyperalimentation. The benefits of such nutritional therapy include diminished gastrointestinal secretion and motility, potential relief of partial obstruction, closure of fistulas, and renewal of immunocompetence. Anemia should also be treated aggressively by transfusion, although mild anemias will generally respond to oral iron therapy.

Surgical Treatment

Although most acute episodes of inflammatory bowel disease respond to medical treatment, operative intervention will occasionally be necessary to treat perforation, obstruction, or patients unresponsive to standard therapies. While elective surgery for medically intractable disease or recurrent dysplastic lesions of the colon is best accomplished following pregnancy, patients who have undergone definitive surgical procedures for UC seem to fare well during pregnancy. Surgery during pregnancy does carry a significant risk of preterm delivery, probably due to the amount of uterine manipulation required during efforts to reach the distal colon. Surgery should not be delayed, however, in cases of perforation or complete obstruction. Anderson and colleagues[38] have reported three cases of emergency colectomy during pregnancy for toxic megacolon in women with fulminant UC. There were no maternal deaths; however, two stillbirths occurred as well as one preterm delivery.[38]

Ileostomy function during pregnancy is normal in most cases. Of 84 term pregnancies reported by Hudson,[39] intestinal obstruction occurred in just 7 cases. Of 17 cesarean deliveries in his series, all were done for obstetric indications. Similarly, Gopal and colleagues[40] described 82 pregnancies in 66 women following colostomy or ileostomy. Stomal dysfunction responded to conservative measures in all but three women who required surgery for intestinal obstruction. Complications from an episiotomy have been uncommon in patients previously operated on for UC. Data are not available for CD. However, the higher rate of perineal involvement in these patients should warrant a thorough evaluation before contemplating vaginal delivery.

Surgery for CD, unlike UC, is generally not curative. It is estimated that 40 percent of patients with ileitis will require surgery at some time for obstruction, perforation, extensive fistulas, or perirectal suppuration.[19] Most surgical procedures must limit the amount of bowel resection because of the diffuse nature of this disease. Prior bowel resection has been associated with increased risk of preterm delivery and spontaneous miscarriage.[32]

Patients with Crohn's colitis who have undergone proctocolectomy are at substantial risk for recurrent disease, including persistent perineal wounds in up to 60 percent of cases.[41] Cesarean delivery should be considered for patients with perianal disease who have been diverted to promote healing. Those patients with CD who require surgery during pregnancy are usually operated on for obstruction.[42] As with UC, there may be a high incidence of fetal loss. The decision to perform a simultaneous cesarean delivery must be individualized according to the type of procedure involved, its indications, and the gestational age of the pregnancy.

Key Points

- Acute fatty liver of pregnancy is a medical emergency requiring stabilization of the patient and timely delivery. Almost all cases will be complicated by disseminated intravascular coagulation.

- Liver transaminase levels in acute fatty liver of pregnancy are lower than what one would see in acute hepatitis.

- Profound hypoglycemia is a frequent concomitant of acute fatty liver and can cause death if untreated.

- Pregnancy-induced cholestasis usually occurs in the third trimester, causing intense pruritus and jaundice. Elevated serum bile acids are the best laboratory test for making the diagnosis in symptomatic patients.

- Cholecystectomy can be successfully accomplished during pregnancy in patients with recurrent cholecystitis or acute ascending cholangitis. It is best carried out in the second trimester if possible.

- Women with peptic ulcer disease usually have improvement in symptoms during pregnancy. Primary medical treatment for symptomatic cases is antacid therapy and diet.

- Most cases of pancreatitis during pregnancy are associated with gallstones. Conservative supportive care aimed at decreasing pancreatic secretion is generally successful therapy.

- Women with active ulcerative colitis in early pregnancy usually have recurrent flare-ups during gestation and postpartum.

- The onset of ulcerative colitis or Crohn's disease during pregnancy is associated with increased miscarriage and fetal loss rates.

- Sulfasalazine (Azulfidine) may be safely used to treat inflammatory bowel disease during pregnancy and in lactating women.

References

1. Clark DH: Peptic ulcer in women. BMJ 1:1259, 1953
2. Vessey MP, Villard-Mackintoch L, Painter R: Oral contraceptives and pregnancy in relation to peptic ulcer. Contraception 46:349, 1992
3. Clark DH, Tankel HI: Gastric acid and plasma histaminase during pregnancy. Lancet 2:886, 1954
4. Spiro HM, Schwartz RD, Pilot ML: Peptic ulcer in pregnancy. A serial study of gastric secretion during pregnancy. Am J Dig Dis 4:289, 1959
5. VanThiel DH, Gavaler JS, Joshi SN et al: Heartburn of pregnancy. Gastroenterology 72:666, 1977
6. Lewis JH, Weingold AB: The use of gastrointestinal drugs during pregnancy and lactation. Am J Gastroenterol 80:912, 1985
7. Parker S, Schade R, Pohl C et al: Prenatal and neonatal exposure of male rats to cimetidine but not ranitidine adversely affect subsequent sexual functioning. Gastroenterology 86:675, 1984
8. Baron TH, Ramirez B, Richter JE: Gastrointestinal motility disorders during pregnancy. Ann Intern Med 118:306, 1993
9. Becker-Anderson H, Husfelt V: Peptic ulcer in pregnancy. Acta Obstet Gynaecol Scand 59:391, 1971
10. McKay AJ, O'Neill J, Imrie CW: Pancreatitis, Pregnancy, and Gallstones. Br J Obstet Gynaecol 87:47, 1980
11. Corlett RC, Mishell DR: Pancreatitis in pregnancy. Am J Obstet Gynecol 113:281, 1972
12. Wilkinson EJ: Acute pancreatitis in pregnancy: a review of 98 cases and a report of 8 new cases. Obstet Gynecol Surv 28:5,281, 1973
13. Block P, Kelly TR: Management of gallstone pancreatitis during pregnancy and the postpartum period. Surg Gynecol Obstet 168:426, 1989
14. Achard JM, Westeel PF, Morniere P et al: Pancreatitis related to severe acute hypertryglyceridemia during pregnancy: treatment with lipoprotein apheresis. Intensive Care Med 17:236, 1991
15. Sanderson SL, Iverius PH, Wilson DE: Successful hyperlipemic pregnancy. JAMA 265:1858, 1991
16. DeVore GR, Bracken M, Berkowitz RL: The amylase/creatinine clearance ratio in normal pregnancy and pregnancies complicated by pancreatitis, hyperemesis grandarum, and toxemia. Am J Obstet Gynecol 136:747, 1980
17. Jacobs ML, Daggett WM, Civetta JM: Acute pancreatitis: analysis of factors influencing survival. Ann Surg 185:43, 1977
18. Kirsner JB, Shorter RG: Recent developments in "nonspecific" inflammatory bowel disease. N Engl J Med 306:775, 1982
19. Sorokin JJ, Levine SM: Pregnancy and inflammatory bowel disease: a review of the literature. Obstet Gynecol 62:247, 1983
20. MacDougall I: Ulcerative colitis and pregnancy. Lancet 271:641, 1956
21. DeDombal FT, Watts JM, Watkinson G, Goligher JC: Ulcerative colitis and pregnancy. Lancet 2:599, 1965
22. Willoughby CP, Truelove SC: Ulcerative colitis and pregnancy. Gut 21:469, 1980
23. Felsen J, Wolarsky W: Chronic ulcerative colitis and pregnancy. Am J Obstet Gynecol 56:751, 1948
24. Abramson D, Jankelson IR, Milner LR: Pregnancy in idiopathic ulcerative colitis. Am J Obstet Gynecol 6:121, 1951
25. Crohn BB, Yarnis H, Cohen EB et al: Ulcerative colitis and pregnancy. Gastroenterology 30:391, 1956
26. Nielson OH, Andreasson B, Dondesen S et al: Pregnancy in ulcerative colitis. Scand J Gastroenterol 18:735, 1986
27. Crohn BB, Yarnis H, Korelitz BI: Regional ileitis complicating pregnancy. Gastroenterology 31:615, 1956
28. Fielding JF, Cooke WT: Pregnancy and Crohn's disease. BMJ 2:76, 1970
29. DeDombal FT, Burton IL, Goligher JC: Crohn's disease and pregnancy. BMJ 3:550, 1972

30. Khosla R, Willoughby CP, Jewell DP: Crohn's disease and pregnancy. Gut 25:52, 1984

31. Mayberry JF, Weterman IT: European survey of fertility and pregnancy in women with Crohn's disease: a case control study by European collaborative group. Gut 27:821, 1986

32. Haagen Nielsen O, Andreasson B, Bondesen B et al: Pregnancy in Crohn's disease. Scand J Gastroenterol 19:724, 1984

33. Woolfson K, Cohen Z, McLeod RS: Crohn's disease and pregnancy. Dis Colon Rectum 33:869, 1990

34. Martimbeau PW, Welch JS, Weiland LH: Crohn's disease and pregnancy. Am J Obstet Gynecol 122:746, 1975

35. Christensen LA, Rasmussen SN, Hansen SH: Disposition of 5-aminosalicylic acid and N-acetyl-5-aminosalicylic acid in fetal and maternal body fluids during treatment with different 5-aminosalicylic acid preparation. Acta Obstet Scand 73:399, 1994

36. Mogadam M, Dibbins MO, Korelitz BI, Ahmed SW: Pregnancy and inflammatory bowel disease: effect of sulfasalazine and corticosteroids on fetal outcome. Gastroenterology 80:72, 1981

37. Alstead EM, Ritchie JK, Lennard-Jones JE et al: Safety of azathioprine in pregnancy in inflammatory bowel disease. Gastroenterology 99:443, 1990

38. Anderson JB, Turner GM, Williamson RCN: Fulminant ulcerative colitis in late pregnancy and the puerperium. Proc R Soc Med 80:492, 1987

39. Hudson CN: Ileostomy in pregnancy. Proc R Soc Med 65:281, 1972

40. Gopal KA, Amshel AL, Shonberg IL et al: Ostomy and pregnancy. Dis Colon Rectum 28:912, 1985

41. Block GE: Surgical management of Crohn's colitis. N Engl J Med 302:1068, 1980

42. Davis MR, Bohon CJ: Intestinal obstruction in pregnancy. Clin Obstet Gynecol 26:832, 1983

Chapter 35

Neurologic Disorders

Philip Samuels

Seizure Disorders

Affecting approximately 1 percent of the general population, seizure disorders are the most frequent major neurologic complication encountered in pregnancy.Seizure disorders may be divided into those that are acquired and those that are idiopathic. Acquired seizure disorders, which account for less than 15 percent of all seizures, may result from trauma, infection, space occupying lesions, or metabolic disorders. Over 85 percent of seizure disorders are classified as idiopathic, meaning that no etiologic agent or inciting incident can be identified. Idiopathic seizures can be divided into types such as tonic-clonic, partial complex with or without generalization, myoclonic, focal, or absence.

In general, initial therapy is based on the type of seizure disorder experienced by the patient. There are, however, many crossovers, and patients may respond differently to each medication despite their seizure type. It is, therefore, not unusual to encounter a patient with any seizure type who may be taking any of the major antiepileptic medications. Furthermore, patients may be placed on a certain medication because they did not tolerate the side effect profile of another anticonvulsant (Table 35-1). Because of the prevalence of this group of disorders in women of childbearing age, the stigmata surrounding epilepsy, and the misguided fears many patients and physicians have surrounding epilepsy in pregnancy, the treatment of the pregnant patient with a seizure disorder can create quite a challenge for the obstetrician. In addition, many patients with epilepsy have done very well on their medications so they have not been evaluated by a neurologist in many years. Some patients have been seizure free for many years and have stopped their medications, while others have been seizure free for many years but have continued to take their medication without being re-evaluated. Still others have poorly controlled seizures, and it is unclear whether this is due to noncompliance with or ineffectiveness of their medication regimen. The obstetrician and neurologist must work closely together to guide the patient through her pregnancy and find the safest and most effective medical therapy for the patient. Through this cooperation, the vast majority of pregnant women with seizure disorders can have a successful pregnancy with minimal risk to mother and fetus.

Effects of Epilepsy on Reproductive Function

Women with seizure disorders should seek care from an obstetrician/gynecologist as soon as they become sexually active. Contraception may present a challenge to women with epilepsy, and the use of oral contraceptives may require special adjustments. Certain antiepileptic medications have been associated with contraceptive failure. Carbamazepine, phenobarbital, and phenytoin enhance the activities of hepatic microsomal oxidative enzymes.[1] The cytochrome P450 system is shared by these medications as well as by the steroid hormones. This increased enzymatic activity may lead to rapid clearance of these hormones, which may allow ovulation to occur. Therefore, medicated patients taking low dose oral contraceptives may have more breakthrough bleeding[2] and may be at increased risk for unplanned pregnancy.[3,4] This rapid clearance does not appear to be induced by valproate or benzodiazepines.[1]

Fertility rates may be lower in patients with epilepsy. A retrospective study by Webber and colleagues[5] reviewed fertility rates in individuals with epilepsy over

Table 35-1 Common Side Effects of Anticonvulsants

Drug	Maternal Effects	Fetal Effects
Phenytoin	Nystagmus, ataxia, hirsutism, gingival hyperplasia, megaloblastic anemia	Possible teratogenesis and carcinogenesis, coagulopathy, hypocalcemia
Phenobarbital	Drowsiness, ataxia	Possible teratogenesis, coagulopathy, neonatal depression, withdrawal
Primidone	Drowsines, ataxia, nausea	Possible teratogenesis, coagulopathy, neonatal depression
Carbamazepine	Drowsiness, leukopenia, ataxia, mild hepatotoxicity	Possible craniofacial and neural tube defects
Valproic acid	Ataxia, drowsiness, alopecia, hepatotoxicity, thrombocytopenia	Neural tube defects and possible craniofacial and skeletal defects
Trimethadione	Drowsiness, nausea	Strong teratogenic potential
Ethosuximide	Nausea, hepatotoxicity, leukopenia, thrombocytopenia	Possible teratogenesis

a 50-year period. They found that fertility rates were significantly lower in both men and women with epilepsy and that this could not be explained solely by the rate of marriage in these patients. Men appeared to be more adversely affected than women. Women with epilepsy had fertility rates 85 percent of the expected. Furthermore, in this retrospective review, women with partial seizures seemed to have lower fertility rates than those with generalized seizures. In a study by Dansky et al,[6] fertility rates appeared to be lower in those women with early onset epilepsy than those with late onset. Cramer and Jones[1] also reviewed a study published in Poland in 1979 that investigated the fertility rate in 263 unselected patients with epilepsy. They found that the fertility rate was half that of the general population, and 25 percent of married patients had no children.[1] All of these cited studies concerning lower fertility rates have many methodologic problems. Yet, even in these studies, the majority of patients with epilepsy were able to conceive without difficulty. Nonetheless, the practicing obstetrician/gynecologist should be prepared to undertake an infertility evaluation of these patients or to refer them to an infertility specialist should the need arise.

Effect of Pregnancy on Epilepsy

It has been taught that between 30 percent and 50 percent of patients will show an increase in seizure frequency during pregnancy. This was confirmed in the classic study of Knight and Rhind[7] of 153 pregnancies in 59 patients between 1953 and 1973. In that study, 45 percent of patients showed an increase in seizure frequency during pregnancy, while 50 percent had no change and 4.8 percent experienced a decrease. It is very important to note that anticonvulsant levels could not be readily measured until the mid 1970s. When the study of Knight and Rhind[7] was performed, anticonvulsant doses were usually only increased by physicians

when patients had breakthrough seizures. An important finding from that study, however, was that patients with more frequent seizures tended to have exacerbations during pregnancy.[8] In fact, virtually all patients who had more than one seizure each month experienced worsening of their epilepsy during pregnancy, whereas only about 25 percent of patients who had not had a seizure in over 9 months experienced exacerbation of epilepsy during pregnancy. With the introduction of new medications and the ability to monitor anticonvulsant levels, these absolute numbers are no longer true. The relationship, however, does remain. Patients with more frequent seizures tend to have exacerbations of seizures during pregnancy. In a large study by Schmidt et al,[8] 63 percent of patients had no change or a decrease in seizure frequency during pregnancy, while only 37 percent of patients had an increase of seizures during pregnancy. Importantly, in 34 of the 50 patients who showed an increase in seizure frequency during pregnancy, the increase was associated with noncompliance with their drug regimen or sleep deprivation. Conversely, in 7 of the 18 pregnancies in which improvement of seizure frequency was shown, this was related to improved compliance with the drug regimen or a correction of sleep deprivation for the 9 months preceding pregnancy. In a study by Tanganelli and Regesta,[9] seizure frequency did not change or improved in 82.6 percent of pregnancies. As has been shown in other studies, increases in seizure frequency were often due to noncompliance with medication regimens as well as frequent seizures in the preconception period.

In summary, we now have the means to monitor anticonvulsant levels in patients frequently, and we have the medications to control seizures. We also understand that sleep deprivation can be a catalyst for seizures. With patient cooperation and close surveillance, seizure frequency should remain the same or even improve in most epileptic patients during pregnancy.

Effects of Pregnancy on the Disposition of Anticonvulsant Medications

It is well known that the levels of anticonvulsant medications can change dramatically during pregnancy. They usually decrease in total concentration as pregnancy progresses. Many factors including altered protein binding, delayed gastric emptying, nausea and vomiting, changes in plasma volume, and changes in the volume of distribution can affect the levels of anticonvulsant medications. It is beyond the scope of this Chapter to elucidate these mechanisms. Without some understanding of this subject, however, it is difficult to manage the patient with epilepsy correctly. Therefore, some of the salient points of this topic are covered.

As phenytoin is one of the most widely prescribed anticonvulsant medications, its metabolism and elimination are discussed. Landon and Kirkley[10] and Kochenour et al[11] showed that the serum concentration of phenytoin tends to fall during pregnancy and rise again during the puerperium and postpartum periods. Several factors can account for this. In early gestation, patients often have nausea and vomiting. Phenytoin is usually administered on a once daily basis. If the patient vomits the medication, the drug levels will be highly variable. Furthermore, an increase in calcium intake during pregnancy, as well as the use of antacids, will lead to the formation of insoluble complexes with phenytoin, resulting in lower total drug levels. Also, with delayed gastric emptying in pregnancy, the time to peak drug level will be lengthened. Phenytoin is inactivated in the liver. Its rate of conversion may increase greatly during pregnancy, as the activity of oxidative enzymes increases. This is due to increased progesterone levels, which induce enzyme activity. This may also be enhanced by increased folic acid, which serves as a cofactor in these metabolic processes. Outside of pregnancy, approximately 90 percent of phenytoin is protein bound. Plasma albumin levels decrease during pregnancy while other protein levels may rise. This will cause changes in the total phenytoin level that do not necessarily reflect the free, active phenytoin concentrations. This effect is also enhanced by free fatty acids displacing phenytoin from albumin. In a recent study by Yerby et al,[12] free levels of phenobarbital, carbamazepine, and phenytoin rose significantly throughout pregnancy while total levels fell. Therefore, the nonpregnant relationship between total drug and free (active) drug is not maintained. Free phenytoin levels, therefore, should be measured if possible. If free levels are unavailable, drug doses should be adjusted according to the total serum level and the clinical picture. If the patient has increased seizure activity, medication doses should be increased as long as the patient is not showing signs of toxicity. Likewise, if the medication level is low but the patient is seizure free, no adjustment in dosing is necessary.

Similar pharmacokinetic changes occur in phenobarbital and carbamazepine, but to different degrees. Both of these drugs also show changes in protein binding and increased hepatic clearance during pregnancy. With phenobarbital, the protein binding is considerably less than phenytoin, and changes in plasma protein are less likely to be clinically significant. Primidone is an anticonvulsant medication that is metabolized to phenobarbital and another active metabolite, phenylethylmalonic acid diamide. When checking primidone levels, one must also check levels of phenobarbital. Infants born to mothers who have been taking barbiturates during pregnancy may exhibit some withdrawal symptoms that begin about 1 week after birth and usually last 1 to 2 weeks.[13] These symptoms usually involve minor irritability but may occasionally be more serious.

Carbamazepine also has an active metabolite, carbamazepine 10,11-epoxide. Carbamazepine is not as highly protein bound as phenytoin and is therefore not subject to as wide a fluctuation due to changes in protein levels. Carbamazepine also induces its own metabolic enzymes in the liver, so the half-life changes as the dose increases.[11]

All anticonvulsants interfere with folic acid metabolism. Patients on anticonvulsants may actually become folic acid deficient and develop macrocytic anemia. Folic acid deficiency has been associated with neural tube defects and other congenital malformations.[14,15] Because organogenesis occurs during the first weeks after conception, folic acid supplementation should be begun before pregnancy if possible. A dose of 4 mg daily is more than sufficient. As previously stated, increasing folic acid ingestion may increase the activity of hepatic microsomal enzymes and thus the clearance of anticonvulsant medications. Levels should be checked frequently, therefore, after folic acid therapy is implemented. Furthermore, therapy with phenytoin may result in increased metabolism of vitamin D, leading to decreased vitamin D levels. This has been shown to cause neonatal hypocalcemia in one case report.[16] The patient should be reminded to take her prenatal vitamins, which include an adequate amount of vitamin D to prevent problems.

Neonatal hemorrhage, due to decreased vitamin K-dependent clotting factors (II, VII, IX, X), has been seen in infants born to mothers taking phenobarbital, phenytoin, and primidone.[17] In one series,[17] 8 of 16 infants exposed to these medications had a cord blood coagulation pattern similar to that of a vitamin K deficiency. This occurred earlier than the customary hemorrhagic disease of the newborn. These infants responded to vitamin K infusion. Bleyer and Skinner[18] reviewed a case of their own and another 21 cases of hemorrhagic disease following anticonvulsant therapy that have appeared in the literature. They reached similar conclusions that these cases are vitamin K-dependent clotting factors deficiencies and that, at birth, infants should be given 1 mg of vitamin K intramuscularly.

Effect of Epilepsy on Pregnancy

The majority of women with seizure disorders who become pregnant will have an uneventful pregnancy with an excellent outcome. There appear, however, to be several pregnancy complications that are more prevalent in the mother with epilepsy than in the general population. In a review of all birth certificates for infants born in the state of Washington in 1980–81, Yerby and coworkers[19] identified 200 births to mothers with seizure disorders. Although birth certificate studies are often limited, these researchers controlled for many variables including previous adverse pregnancy outcome and socioeconomic status.[19] They found that mothers with seizure disorders were 2.66 times more likely to have had a previous fetal death after 20 weeks' gestation than the control population. Because of the retrospective nature of this study, the authors were unable to correlate this with growth restriction or other fetal problems. This increased incidence of stillbirth is confirmed in other studies.[7,20,21] It is unclear in any of these studies what type of fetal surveillance was utilized and if there were any predictors that these fetuses were at risk. Because of the long duration of many of these studies, many patients were pregnant during the 1970s and early 1980s. With the increased use of ultrasound to identify fetal growth restriction, malformations, and oligohydramnios, many of the stillborn fetuses may have been identified as being at risk and might have undergone antepartum fetal testing and intervention before the fetal demise occurred. These studies also were not stratified by medications taken, dosages, drug levels, or seizure activity during pregnancy.

Hiilesmaa et al,[22] in a study of 150 pregnant women with seizure disorders, found no difference in perinatal mortality between patients and controls. There were, however, three third trimester stillbirths in the epileptic group and two in the control group. Yerby and colleagues[19] also found an increased incidence of preeclampsia in women with seizure disorders. This has also been identified in other large retrospective studies.[7,20] Hiilesmaa et al,[22] however, found no difference in the rate of preeclampsia between pregnant women with epilepsy and controls. Yerby et al[19] also showed a 2.79-fold increase in low-birth-weight infants. In a carefully performed study in Italy, Mastroiacovo and coworkers[23] found that the mean birth weight in neonates born to women with epilepsy was 107 g lower than controls.

The mean birth weight in the epilepsy group, however, still fell within the normal range for gestational age. The clinical significance of this finding, therefore, is questionable. When considering all commonly used anticonvulsants, this decrease in neonatal weight appeared to be more common in infants exposed in utero to phenobarbital.

Mastroiacovo et al[23] also found a decrease in head circumference in infants of mothers with epilepsy. This effect was seen both in untreated women with epilepsy and in those receiving medications.[23] Although this change was statistically significant, the mean head circumferences of both study and control infants still fell within the normal range. These authors found no difference in neonatal length comparing groups of mothers with epilepsy and control populations. Hiilesmaa et al[24] also found a decrease in head circumference in neonates born to women with epilepsy. This decrease was most marked in women taking carbamazepine both alone or in combination with phenobarbital. Again, the mean head circumferences, however, were still within the expected normal range.[24] In the follow-up of this study, head circumferences were still smaller at 18 months of age.

Yerby and colleagues[19] found a sixfold increased rate of maternal herpes in women with epilepsy. There is no readily available explanation for this, and it has not been seen in other studies, although it is doubtful that anyone has looked for this as an endpoint. They further found a significant decrease in 1- and 5-minute Apgar scores. This may be attributed to fetal effect of maternal depressant medications such as phenobarbital. Conversely, Hiilesmaa et al[22,24] found no increase in pregnancy complications in women with epilepsy. They found no increase in preterm labor, bleeding, pregnancy-induced hypertension, operative vaginal delivery, or cesarean delivery rates. These authors imply that the lack of increased operative deliveries in their study is due to the comfort of the obstetrician in caring for patients with seizure disorders. However, Yerby et al[19] found an increased rate of cesarean deliveries in their review. For uncertain reasons, they also found an unexplained increase in third trimester amniocentesis and labor inductions. This may be construed as insecurity on the part of the obstetrician in caring for the patient with a seizure disorder and the desire to effect a delivery as soon as fetal pulmonary maturity could be documented.

In summary, there appears to be an increased risk of stillbirths in women with seizure disorders. The cause of this is not readily apparent but may be due to factors that are easily detectable today (such as intrauterine growth restriction) that were not detected when these studies were carried out. It also appears that infants born to mothers with seizure disorders, on average, are smaller than their control counterparts. It is uncertain whether the incidence of actual intrauterine growth restriction is higher. Furthermore, the incidence of preeclampsia may be higher in mothers with seizure disorders. The vast majority of pregnancies, however, will be uncomplicated with no increase in complications over the expected rate. Nonetheless, because of these few potential problems, the obstetrician should be more surveillant for pregnancy-related complications in pregnant women with seizure disorders.

Effects of Anticonvulsant Medications on the Fetus

There is little doubt that anticonvulsant medications are associated with an increase in congenital malformations, but the magnitude of this risk and the association of certain anomalies with specific drugs remain debatable. Although there was some evidence for teratogenicity related to phenytoin in the 1960s, Hanson and Smith[25] identified a specific fetal hydantoin syndrome in 1975. They noted growth and performance delays, craniofacial abnormalities (including clefting), and limb anomalies (including hypoplasia of nails and distal phalanges). They first reported this syndrome in five infants exposed to phenytoin in utero. Hanson et al[26] later reported that 7 to 11 percent of infants exposed to phenytoin had this recognizable pattern of malformations. They furthermore found that 31 percent of exposed fetuses had some aspects of the syndrome. Yet in 1988 Gaily et al[27] reported no evidence of the hydantoin syndrome in 82 women exposed in utero to phenytoin. Some of the patients had hypertelorism and hypoplasia of the distal phalanges, but none had the full hydantoin syndrome.

Since the original reports by Hanson and colleagues, many studies have reported congenital malformations in infants born to mothers taking anticonvulsant medications. These reports typify the discrepancies that fill the medical literature concerning this subject. There are studies that report each of the commonly used anticonvulsant medications (phenytoin, phenobarbital, carbamazepine, valproate, and primidone) is the worst teratogen, yet there are other studies that report each of these medications has a weak teratogenic potential. It remains of prime importance, therefore, to treat the patient with the medication that best controls her seizures. Another example of discrepancies and the need for more research involves the incidence of facial clefting among infants born to mothers with epilepsy. This is one of the most common anomalies found in these neonates. In a study by Friis et al,[28] untreated epileptics had an incidence of facial clefting 2.7 times the expected rate, whereas infants of mothers treated with anticonvulsants had 4.7 times the expected rate of

clefting. All of the observed clefts in these groups were cleft lip with or without cleft palate. There was no increased incidence of isolated cleft palate. These authors concluded that epilepsy itself may increase the risk for cleft lip, with anticonvulsant medications increasing the risk even more.[28] A study by Kelly et al[29] demonstrated that the association between epilepsy and facial clefting is in large part due to shared causal determinants that are probably both genetic and environmental in origin. They believe that the role of anticonvulsant medications in this association seems to be overestimated and probably represents only a modest additive influence. In contrast, however, Hecht et al,[30] in an epidemiologic study, found no evidence for familial association between epilepsy and clefting disorders.

Nakane and colleagues[31] published the first major, multi-institutional study investigating the teratogenecity of antiepileptic medications. This study, carried out between 1974 and 1977, examined 902 pregnancies in mothers with idiopathic epilepsy. The overall rate of congenital malformations was 7.2 percent. This included 8.7 percent in the mothers who received anticonvulsant medications during pregnancy and 1.9 percent in nonmedicated mothers. Looking only at liveborn infants, 9.9 percent had malformations (11.5 percent in the medicated group and 2.3 percent in the nonmedicated group). The incidence of malformations in mothers receiving anticonvulsant therapy was therefore about five times that of the nonmedicated group.[31] The predominant malformations were cleft lip/palate (3.14 percent) and cardiovascular malformations (2.95 percent). These authors also noted that as the number of anticonvulsant medications used in combination during pregnancy increased, the incidence of fetal malformations rose dramatically.[31] The malformation rate was less than 5 percent when one medication (monotherapy) was used and was greater than 20 percent when four medications were used. Of note, 537 patients were taking two or more medications while 93 patients were only taking one medication. This is fairly reflective of the prescribing patterns for anticonvulsant medications in the 1970s and shows why many of the studies and case reports from the 1970s are not relevant today, as many more patients are receiving monotherapy. In this study, only 15 percent of patients were treated with a single antiepileptic medication.[31] Congenital heart disease was significantly higher in infants born to mothers taking phenobarbital, and cleft lip/palate was more common in infants born to women taking primidone.

Kaneko and colleagues performed a prospective study to determine primary factors responsible for the increased incidence of malformations in infants born to mothers being treated with anticonvulsants.[32] They specifically looked at various drug combinations. The overall malformation rate was 14 percent. In the 16.1 percent of patients who were receiving a single medication, the malformation rate was 6.5 percent.[32] The malformation rate for those treated with multiple medications was 15.6 percent. There was no dose-dependent increase in the incidence of malformations associated with any individual medication. In this study there was also no relationship between the type of defect and the individual anticonvulsant. This contrasts with the study by Nakane et al[31]. In that study, polypharmacy including valproate had a significantly higher risk of causing congenital malformations than other medications.[26]

Kaneko et al[33] published a follow-up study looking at malformations in infants exposed in utero to anticonvulsant medications. They compared these results with their previous study.[32] The first study looked at infants born between 1978 and 1984, while the later study looked at infants born between 1985 and 1989. Whereas 14 percent of infants had some malformation in the previous study, the malformation rate was only 6.3 percent in the second group.[33] Again, there was no relationship between the medication taken and the type of malformation found.[33] The lower rate of malformations may be attributable to the increase in patients receiving monotherapy. In the earlier study 16.1 percent of patients received a single medication, whereas 63.4 percent received a single medication in the later study.[33] This confirms the impression that more neurologists are treating patients with a single agent. Now that blood levels of anticonvulsant medications can be easily measured, single medications can be given at higher doses to make certain that therapeutic levels are achieved. This has lessened the need for multiple medications in the same patient. Prior to the ability to measure these levels, empiric doses of medication were given. If the patient continued to have seizures, another medication was often added rather than increasing the dose of the initial medication.

The same concept was verified in a study by Lindhout et al[34] They compared the pattern of malformations in the offspring of two cohorts of women with seizure disorders, one from 1972 to 1979 and one from 1980 to 1985. In the earlier cohort, 15 of 151 (10 percent) of liveborn infants had at least one congenital anomaly. The most common anomalies were those most frequently reported for anticonvulsant medications: congenital heart defects, facial clefts, facial dysmorphism, and developmental retardation. In the later cohort, 13 of 172 infants (7.6 percent) exposed in utero to anticonvulsant medications had congenital malformations.[37] The most frequent anomalies in this group were spinal defects and hypospadias. All of these were associated with maternal therapy with valproate, carbamazepine, or both.[34] In the earlier cohort of patients, the mean number of drugs used during gestation was 2.2 compared with 1.7 in the later cohort. Whereas only 28 percent of women in the earlier cohort received only one medication, 47 percent of the women received monotherapy in the second group of patients. The lower overall rate of malformations in the latter cohort appeared to be due to the reduction in the number of pregnancies during which a combination of medications was used.[34] It is also apparent in this study that neither the duration of maternal epilepsy nor the maternal age was associated with malformations in the infants born to these mothers.

Dravet et al[35] studied 227 women participating in a prospective study between 1984 and 1988. In that study there was a 7 percent malformation rate among infants born to mothers taking antiepileptic medications compared with 1.36 percent in the control group. Therefore, fetuses exposed in utero to anticonvulsants had a relative risk of 6.9 of being born with a congenital malformation. In this study, the frequency of spina bifida was 17 times more than would be expected in the general population, and heart defects were 9.6 times greater than expected. Cleft lip with or without cleft palate was 8.4 times more frequent than expected in the general population. Using logistic regression, these authors concluded that valproate and phenytoin were the two most teratogenic medications.[35] Also in this study, there was a high correlation with congenital heart defects and maternal ingestion of phenobarbital.[35] The cases of neural tube defect and congenital heart defect were studied carefully and could not be related to a familial disposition to these defects. As other studies have shown, there was a higher incidence of malformations in infants born to mothers receiving polytherapy (16 percent) than in those receiving monotherapy (6 percent).

A study by Koch et al[36] however, shows no difference between the rate of malformations in mothers receiving polytherapy and mothers receiving a single medication. Furthermore, they found that the infants born to mothers with epilepsy, regardless of therapy, had only twice as many major malformations as infants born to the control population. The number of minor anomalies, however, was approximately three times greater in infants born to mothers receiving anticonvulsant medication than in the control group. In the mothers receiving monotherapy, those taking valproate had the highest rate of minor malformations.[36] In this study, there appeared to be a link between the dose of valproate and the rate of malformations.

Gaily and Granstrom[37] also investigated minor anomalies in children of mothers with epilepsy. These authors point out that many of the supposedly specific syndromes resulting from intrauterine exposure to certain medications have many common features. They argue that specific syndromes and their association with specific drugs, as well as the frequencies of these syndromes, have not been confirmed in epidemiologic studies. They found that many of the minor anomalies that are thought to be specific features of a medication appear to be genetically linked with epilepsy.[37] Indeed, this is in contrast to many of the other published studies. In this study only distal digital hypoplasia appeared to be a specific marker for phenytoin teratogenicity. Again, this points out that there is no uniform consensus concerning the teratogenicity of anticonvulsant medications.

Yerby and colleagues[38] also looked prospectively at malformations in infants born to mothers with epilepsy. They further investigated whether pure folate deficiency might to be responsible for the malformations. None of the women in their study had deficient folate levels. There was no difference in major malformations between patients and controls in this study.[38] The infants born to mothers taking anticonvulsant medications, however, had a higher mean number of minor anomalies. They found no difference in the number of minor anomalies whether the child was exposed in utero to one anticonvulsant medication or to several.[38] The only specific minor anomaly that was found statistically more frequently in infants born to mothers with epilepsy than in the control population was a prominent occiput. The authors also confirm the great overlap in minor anomalies and various medications, further casting doubt upon whether individual medications cause specific syndromes.[38]

Teenagers are often treated with valproate as the anticonvulsant of choice because of its low side effect profile in this age group. It has, however, been reported to be associated with specific anomalies. DiLiberti et al,[39] in 1984, reported a specific fetal valproate syndrome. This was based on seven infants. They found a consistent facial phenotype in all seven children and other birth defects in four. This syndrome phenotype was confirmed by Ardinger and colleagues[40] in 1988. Jager-Roman et al,[41] in 1986, reported fetal distress in 50 percent of 14 infants receiving valproate. Furthermore, 28 percent had low Apgar scores. They also found the same craniofacial defects as reported by DiLiberti et al.[39] Lindhout and Schmidt[42] confirmed the association between neural tube defects and valproate exposure in utero. They contend that there is a 1.5 percent risk of an infant being born with a neural tube defect if the mothers took valproate in the first trimester. Lindhout et al[43] also studied 34 cases of neural tube defects in mothers taking anticonvulsant medications. In 33 of the 34 cases, mothers were exposed to either valproate or carbamazepine. Most of the cases of neural tube defects were lumbosacral. There was only one case of anencephaly. This implies that these medications have a predisposition to cause lumbosacral defects, since in the general population spina bifida and anencephaly are equally distributed. In only two cases were other major malformations found. The development of neural tube defects in these infants of mothers taking valproate also appeared to be a dose-dependent phenomenon. Wegner and Nau[44] have shown, in a mouse model, that valproate alters folic acid metabolism in embryos. This could account for the increased risk of neural tube defects in infants born to mothers who have taken valproate.

Until recently, it was felt that carbamazepine was safer than the other anticonvulsant medications for use in pregnancy. In 1989, Jones et al[45] reported a pattern of minor cranio-facial defects, fingernail hypoplasia, and developmental delay in infants exposed in utero to carbamazepine. Rosa[46] has also shown that there is a 1 percent risk of spina bifida in infants of mothers taking carbamazepine. Because this spectrum of defects (except spina bifida) is similar to that in the fetal hydantoin syndrome, Jones et al[45] hypothesized that, as both drugs are metabolized through an arene oxide pathway, perhaps an epoxide intermediary is the teratogenic agent. Those fetuses with low levels of epoxide hydrolase are exposed to higher levels of epoxide intermediaries, and this may lead to an increase in malformations. Conversely, fetuses with high enzyme levels clear epoxides rapidly, minimizing exposure to the potential teratogens. Phenytoin, phenobarbital, and, to a lesser extent, carbamazepine are metabolized through this pathway.[47] Much work in this area is being performed by Finnell et al,[47] who believe that low levels of epoxide hydrolase activity may be the common link explaining why only certain fetuses exposed to anticonvulsant medications in utero develop congenital malformations.

There has been much debate over whether epilepsy itself and/or the use of antiepileptic medications is associated with psychomotor delays or mental retardation. In the landmark study by Nelson and Ellenberg,[20] an IQ below 70 was seen in 65.2 per 1,000 7-year-old children in the seizure group compared with 34 per 1,000 in the age-matched control group, a statistically significant difference. Before generalizations can be made, many confounding factors must be evaluated including other anomalies and social environment. In a review by Granstrom and Gaily,[48] none of the major antiepileptic medications appeared to carry special risk for mental retardation. They suggest, however, that polytherapy and inherited deviations in antiepileptic medication metabolism in the fetus increase the risk for mental retardation. This study is important because these researchers stress that other factors associated with maternal epilepsy such as seizures during pregnancy, inherited brain disorders, and a nonoptimal psychosocial environment can also affect a child's psychomotor development.[48] These factors are hard to control in any study. In a recent study by Gaily et al,[49] 2 of 48 (4.1 percent) infants of mothers with epilepsy had mental retardation, and two additional infants had borderline intelligence. The mean IQ of the infants exposed in utero to anticonvulsant medications was statistically lower than the control group. When these four children were excluded from the analysis, the difference in mean IQ disappeared.[49] There was no increased risk of low intelligence attributable to fetal exposure either to antiepileptic medications below toxic levels or to brief maternal convulsions. No particular medication appeared to be associated with a lower IQ. Social class also appeared to play a role in the differences in IQs in these patients.[49]

In short, there appears to be a small, undefined risk of a slightly lower IQ in infants born to mothers with epilepsy. It does not appear that any particular medication results in a higher risk of this outcome.

Preconceptual Counseling for the Reproductive Age Woman with a Seizure Disorder

Although not always possible, it is preferable to counsel the patient with epilepsy before she becomes pregnant. A detailed history should be taken to see if there are any seizure disorders or congenital malformations in the family. This could provide a clue for fetal risks. The obstetrician must stress that the patient has greater than a 90 percent chance of having a successful pregnancy resulting in a normal newborn. A detailed history of medication use and seizure frequency should be obtained. The patient must be informed that if she has frequent seizures before conception, this pattern will probably continue. If she has frequent seizures, she should delay conception until control is better, even if this entails a change of medication. The obstetrician must stress that controlling seizures is of primary importance and that the patient will need to take whatever medication(s) are necessary to achieve this goal throughout her pregnancy. If the patient has had no seizures during the past 2 to 5 years, an attempt may be made to withdraw her from anticonvulsant medications. This is usually done over a 1- to 3-month period, slowly reducing the medication. Up to 50 percent of patients will relapse and need to start their medications again. This withdrawal should be attempted only if the patient is completely seizure-free and only with the help of a neurologist. During the period of withdrawal from medications, patients should refrain from driving.

Furthermore, as previously shown, it is best to have the patient taking a single medication during pregnancy. If the patient is on multiple medications, the patient can be changed to monotherapy (over a several month period). The drug of choice for the specific type of epilepsy should be the one chosen for monotherapy. As the other medications are gradually withdrawn, levels of the remaining medication should be monitored frequently to make certain that the level remains therapeutic. When other medications are withdrawn, the level of the primary medication often increases without a dose increment. If it does not, however, the dose of the primary medication may need to be increased. The patient should refrain from conceiving until seizures have been well controlled for several months on the single medication. The patient must also be counseled that she should get adequate rest and sleep during pregnancy, as sleep deprivation is associated with increased seizure frequency.

The choice of antiepileptic medication depends on the seizure type. As the foregoing literature review has shown, there are studies claiming teratogenesis for each of the major anticonvulsant medications, yet there are also studies showing that each medication individually may not be particularly teratogenic. The most important point is to control maternal seizures. There may be some additional concern for using valproate in pregnancy due to the reported high incidence of fetal distress.[41] It is important to note that this finding has not been corroborated in other studies. Therefore, if valproate is the anticonvulsant that works best for the patient, it should be used without hesitation. If valproate is used, the dose should be divided over three to four administrations daily to avoid high peak plasma levels.

In the past, it was thought that carbamazepine was the anticonvulsant of choice and had the least teratogenic effect. As has been shown in the foregoing literature review, there are studies that report malformations with the use of carbamazepine.[39,40] It is important to stress again that the anticonvulsant that does the best job of controlling seizures is the one that should be used for the patient.

Folic acid supplementation should be begun before or early in pregnancy. Folic acid supplementation may help to prevent neural tube defects, which are more common in treatment with carbamazepine and valproate but have been reported in women taking other anticonvulsants. Studies have shown that folic acid may decrease the incidence of neural tube defects in at-risk women.[15] It is important that this be implemented early in pregnancy, as open neural tube defects occur by the end of the fifth week of gestation. Furthermore, low folate levels have been associated with an increase in adverse pregnancy outcomes in women taking anticonvulsants.[50] Anticonvulsant levels should be checked frequently after implementing or increasing folic acid administration, as it leads to lower anticonvulsant levels.[50] A daily dose of 4 mg/day should be more than ample. Patients should also be encouraged to take their prenatal vitamins, which contain vitamin D. This is because anticonvulsants may interfere with the conversion of 25-hydroxycholecalciferol to 1-25-dihydroxycholecalciferol, the active form of vitamin D.

Whether or not they ask, all mothers with idiopathic epilepsy wonder if their child will develop epilepsy. There is a surprising paucity of studies in this area. Children of parents without seizures have a 0.5 to 1 percent risk of developing epilepsy. It appears that the infant born to a mother with a seizure disorder of unknown etiology has a four times greater chance of developing idiopathic epilepsy than the general population.[51] Furthermore, it appears that epilepsy in the father does not increase a child's risk of developing a seizure disorder. Many of the rare seizure disorders have a stronger genetic component.[52]

Care of the Patient During Pregnancy

Once the patient becomes pregnant, it is of the utmost importance to establish accurate gestational dating. This will prevent any confusion over fetal growth in later gestation. The patient's anticonvulsant level should be followed frequently and dosages adjusted accordingly to keep the patient seizure free. It is a common pitfall to monitor levels too frequently and adjust dosages in a likewise frequent manner. It is important to remember that it takes several half-lives for a medication to reach a steady state (Table 35-2). Drugs like phenobarbital have extremely long half-lives, and the levels should not be checked too frequently. If levels are measured before the drug reaches a steady state and the dosage is increased, the patient will eventually become toxic from the medication. Drug levels should be drawn immediately before the next dose (trough levels) in order to assess if dosing is adequate. If the patient is showing signs of toxicity, a peak level may be obtained.

At approximately 16 weeks' gestation, the patient should undergo blood testing for maternal serum α-fetoprotein in an attempt to detect neural tube defect. This coupled with ultrasonography gives a more than 90 percent detection rate for open neural tube defects. If the patient is difficult to scan or if she wants to be even more certain that there is no neural tube defect, amniocentesis can be undertaken. This should be considered if the patient is taking valproate or carbamazepine, as these medications appear to carry almost the same risk as if the patient had a family history of a neural tube defect.[42,43,46] At 18 to 22 weeks, the patient should undergo a comprehensive ultrasound examination by an experienced obstetric sonographer to look for congenital malformations. A fetal echocardiogram can be obtained at 20 to 22 weeks to look for cardiac malformations, which are among the more common malformations of women taking any antiepileptic medications. This is helpful, but certainly not mandatory, as an adequate "four-chamber view" of the heart on ultrasound will identify 68 to 95 percent of major cardiac anomalies.[53,54]

As previously noted, there appears to be an increased risk for intrauterine growth restriction for fetuses exposed in utero to anticonvulsant medications. If the patient's weight gain and fundal growth appear appropriate, regular ultrasound examinations for fetal weight assessment are probably unnecessary. If, however, there is a question of fundal growth or if the patient's habitus precludes adequate assessment of this clinical parameter, serial ultrasonography for fetal weight assessment can be performed.

In older and retrospective studies, there appears to be an increased risk of stillbirth in mothers taking anticonvulsant medications.[7,19-21] In a recent prospective study, however, this complication was not seen.[22] As previously noted, in the studies that showed an increase in stillbirths, factors such as intrauterine growth restriction or oligohydramnios were not prenatally identified. With modern surveillance and the more common use of ultrasonography, many of these risk factors can be detected before the fetus faces imminent risk. Nonstress testing, therefore, is not necessary in all mothers with seizure disorders. It should be limited to those who have other medical or obstetric complications that place the patient at increased risk of stillbirth.

If at all possible, the patient should be maintained on a single medication, and drug levels should be drawn at appropriate intervals to make certain that the patient

Table 35-2 Anticonvulsants Commonly Used During Pregnancy

Drug	Therapeutic Level (mg/L)	Usual Nonpregnant Dosage	Half-Life
Carbamazepine	4–10	600–1,200 mg/day in three or divided doses	Initially 36 hours, chronic therapy 16 hours
Phenobarbital	15–40	90–180 mg/day in two or three divided doses	100 Hours
Phenytoin	10–20, total; 1–2, free	300–500 mg/day in single or divided doses[a]	Avg 24 hours
Primidone	5–15	750–1,500 mg/day in three divided doses	8 Hours
Valproic acid	50–100	550–2000 mg/day in three or divided doses	Avg 13 hours

[a] If a total dose of more than 300 mg is needed, dividing the dose will result in a more stable serum concentration.

is receiving enough medication. If possible, free levels of the anticonvulsant medication should be measured, especially in the case of phenytoin. This is usually not readily available. A drug dosage should not be increased only because the total level of drug is falling. The free level of drug may still be therapeutic. If, however, the patient develops any seizure activity, dosages should then be adjusted upward. A brief seizure during pregnancy does not appear to be deleterious to the fetus.[23] It is best to use the lowest dose of a single medication possible that will keep the patient seizure free. This, however, must be individualized. For instance, if the patient usually experiences seizures during the day and drives, it is important to make certain that the patient remains seizure free. For this type of patient, drug dosages should be increased if levels fall. If, on the other hand, the patient only has brief partial complex seizures that do not generalize and occur only during her sleep, it is optimal to keep the medications at the lowest serum concentration that will keep her seizure free. An occasional seizure of this type would not harm either patient or fetus. The key to managing anticonvulsants in pregnancy is individualization of therapy.

Early hemorrhagic disease of the newborn can occur in infants exposed to anticonvulsants in utero, and this appears to be a deficiency of the vitamin K-dependent clotting factors II, VII, IX, and X. The use of vitamin K in the third trimester to prevent hemorrhagic disease is somewhat controversial. Although some advocate administering 10 to 20 mg of vitamin K orally, daily, to mothers during the final 1 or 2 months of pregnancy, this is certainly not the standard of care. There appears to be no adverse effect of administering this vitamin, but, on the other hand, its utility has not been clearly demonstrated. Very little hemorrhagic disease of the newborn is seen today, and this is probably because most infants receive 1 mg of vitamin K intramuscularly at birth. This certainly should be given to all infants of mothers receiving anticonvulsants. Because of early discharges and the shortened time of neonatal observation, it might be prudent to check a prothrombin time on the cord blood at birth. This can be done by taking fresh cord blood and placing it in a citrated blood tube and having it sent immediately for prothrombin time. This might be especially prudent if the child is to undergo a very early circumcision.

Labor and Delivery

Vaginal delivery is the route of choice for the mother with a seizure disorder. If the mother has frequent seizures brought on by the stress of labor, she may undergo cesarean delivery after stabilization. Furthermore, seizures during labor may cause transient fetal bradycardia.[22] The fetal heart rate should be given time to recover. If it does not, then one must assume fetal distress and/or placental abruption and deliver by cesarean section. Because stress often exacerbates seizure disorders, an epidural anesthetic can benefit many laboring patients with epilepsy.

Management of anticonvulsant medications during a prolonged labor presents a challenge. During labor, oral absorption of medications is erratic and, if the patient vomits, almost negligible. If the patient is taking phenytoin or phenobarbital, these medications may be administered parenterally. An anticonvulsant level should be obtained first to help ascertain the appropriate dosage. Phenobarbital may be given intramuscularly, and phenytoin may be given intravenously. If the patient's phenytoin level is normal, the usual daily dose may be administered intravenously. The medication may only be mixed in normal saline and must be administered at a rate no faster than 50 mg/min. Because of the long half-life of phenobarbital, if the patient's serum level is therapeutic, a 60- to 90-mg intramuscular dose will probably be sufficient to maintain the patient throughout labor and delivery. The main problem arises if the patient is taking carbamazepine. This medication is not manufactured in a parenteral form. Oral administration may be attempted, but, if the patient has seizures or a pre-seizure aura, she may be loaded with a therapeutic dose of phenytoin to carry her through labor. The usual loading dose is 10 to 15 mg/kg administered intravenously at a rate no faster than 50 mg/min. This should be effective in controlling seizures. Benzodiazepines may also be used for acute seizures, but one must remember that they can cause early neonatal depression as well as maternal apnea.[55] Prenatal diagnostic techniques are not perfect. Even if the infant appears to have no anomalies, an experienced pediatrician should be present at the delivery of the infant born to a mother taking anticonvulsant medications.

New Onset of Seizures in Pregnancy and the Puerperium

Occasionally, seizures will be diagnosed for the first time during pregnancy. This may present a diagnostic dilemma (Table 35-3). If the seizures occur in the third trimester, they are eclampsia until proven otherwise and should be treated as such until the attending physician can perform a proper evaluation. The treatment of eclampsia is delivery, but the patient must first be stabilized. It is often difficult, however, to distinguish eclampsia from an epileptic seizure. The patient may be hypertensive initially after an epileptic seizure and may exhibit some myoglobinuria secondary to muscle breakdown. The diagnosis becomes clearer over time, but in either case, rapid, thoughtful action must be un-

Table 35-3   Differential Diagnosis of Peripartum Seizures

	Blood Pressure	Proteinuria	Seizures	Timing	CSF	Other Features
Eclampsia	+ + +	+ + +	+ + +	Third trimester	Early: RBC, 0–1,000; protein, 50–150 mg/dl Late: grossly bloody	Platelets normal or ↓ RBC normal
Epilepsy	Normal	Normal to +	+ + +	Any trimester	Normal	Low anticonvulsant levels
Subarachnoid hemorrhage	+ to + + + (labile)	0 to +	+	Any trimester	Grossly bloody	
Thrombotic thrombocytopenic purpura	Normal to + + +	+ +	+ +	Third trimester	RBC 0–100	Platelets ⇊ RBC fragmented
Amniotic fluid embolus	Shock	−	+	Intrapartum	Normal	Hypoxia, cyanosis Platelets ⇊ RBC normal
Cerebral vein thrombosis	+	−	+ +	Postpartum	Normal (early)	Headache Occasional pelvic phlebitis
Water intoxication	Normal	−	+ +	Intrapartum	Normal	Oxytocin infusion rate >45 mU/min Serum Na <124 mEq/L
Pheochromocytoma	+ + + (labile)	+	+	Any trimester	Normal	Neurofibromatosis
Autonomic stress syndrome of high paraplegics	+ + + with labor pains	−	−	Intrapartum	Normal	Cardiac arrhythmia
Toxicity of local anesthetics	Variable	−	+ +	Intrapartum	Normal	

(Modified from Donaldson,[127] with permission.)

dertaken. The first physician to attend a patient after a seizure may not be an obstetrician/gynecologist, and magnesium sulfate may not be started acutely. This should be remedied as soon as possible.

If the patient at an earlier gestational age develops seizures for the first time, she should be evaluated and started on the proper medication. The physician must be alert to look for acquired causes of seizures including trauma, infection, metabolic disorders, space occupying lesions, central nervous system bleeding, and ingestion of drugs such as cocaine and amphetamines. The patient must be stabilized, and the physician must make certain that an adequate airway is established for the protection of both mother and fetus. The physician should also look for focal signs that may be more suggestive of a space occupying lesion, central nervous system bleeding, or abscess.

Blood should be obtained for electrolytes, glucose, calcium, magnesium, renal function studies, and toxi-

cologic studies, while intravenous access is being established. If the patient had a tonic-clonic seizure, and the attending physician feels that this is probably new onset epilepsy, she should be started on the appropriate anticonvulsant medication while awaiting results of laboratory studies. If she is not in status epilepticus, this medication may be given orally.

If the patient presents with recurrent generalized seizures, status epilepticus, immediate therapeutic action must be taken. The drug of choice is intravenous phenytoin, as it is highly effective, has a long duration of action, and a low incidence of serious side effects. This medication should be administered in a loading dose of 18 to 20 mg/kg at a rate not exceeding 50 mg/min. Rapid infusion may cause transient hypotension and heart block. If possible, the patient should be placed on a cardiac monitor while receiving a loading dose of phenytoin. Also, this medication must be given in a glucose-free solution to avoid precipitation.[56] If phenytoin is unavailable, phenobarbital or diazepam may be used as a first line drug for status epilepticus. These drugs, however, cause respiratory depression, and the physician must have the ability to intubate the patient if necessary when these medications are used. If these measures are ineffective, an anesthesiologist and neurologist should be immediately consulted if they are not already involved in the patient's care.

Any patient experiencing seizures for the first time during pregnancy without a known cause should undergo an EEG and some type of intracranial imaging. In looking only at eclamptic patients, Sibai et al[57] found that EEGs were initially abnormal in 75 percent of patients but normalized within 6 months in all patients studied. While this group found no uniform computed tomography (CT) abnormalities in this set of eclamptics, they did find that 46 and 33 percent of eclamptics had some abnormalities in the magnetic resonance imaging (MRI) and CT, respectively. Most of the findings were nonspecific and were not helpful in diagnosis or treatment. If the physician is not certain that the patient has eclampsia, an imaging study should be part of the evaluation described above.

Postpartum Period

The levels of anticonvulsant medications must be monitored frequently during the first few weeks postpartum, as they can rapidly rise. If the patient's medication dosages were increased during pregnancy, they will need to be decreased rather rapidly after delivery to prepregnancy levels. All of the major anticonvulsant medications cross into breast milk. The levels vary in breast milk from 18 to 79 percent of the plasma levels.[55,58] The use of these medications, however, is not a contraindication to breast-feeding. Primidone, phenobarbital, and benzodiazepines may have a sedative effect on the fetus with later withdrawal symptoms. Should the infant exhibit these types of symptoms, breast-feeding should be discontinued.

All methods of contraception are available to women with idiopathic seizure disorders. The majority of women are able to take oral contraceptives without any adverse side effects.[59] Oral contraceptive failures are more common in women taking anticonvulsants. This is due to the fact that all of the major anticonvulsant medications induce hepatic enzymes, which metabolize estrogen faster.[59,60] These patients may, therefore, require oral contraceptives with higher dosages of estrogens. The amount of enzyme induction, however, varies and oral contraceptive doses must be individualized.

In conclusion, the majority of women with idiopathic epilepsy will have an uneventful pregnancy with an excellent outcome. To optimize neonatal outcome, the patient should take only one medication and, when possible, use the lowest dose effective in keeping her free of seizures. It is important, though, for the patient to realize that prevention of seizures is the most important goal during pregnancy. Simple interventions such as taking folic acid from the time of conception, taking prenatal vitamins containing vitamin D, and giving the infant vitamin K at birth will help to optimize the outcome. There is an increase in congenital malformations in infants exposed to anticonvulsant medications in utero. The majority of infants exposed to these medications, however, will have no malformations. With modern techniques for prenatal diagnosis, including ultrasound and α-fetoprotein determination, many of these malformations can be detected early. The majority of women with epilepsy will labor normally and have spontaneous vaginal deliveries. In short, with close cooperation and excellent communication among the obstetrician, neurologist, and pediatrician, the vast majority of these patients will have a safe pregnancy with an excellent outcome.

Migraine

Headaches are extremely common in women, and the majority of migraine headaches occur in women of childbearing age. Between 15 and 20 percent of pregnant women are affected by migraine headaches.[61] This statistic is difficult to confirm, as many patients without classic migraine symptoms claim to have migraine headaches. Migraines can be classified as those with aura (other neurologic signs and symptoms) and those without aura. The headaches, which are associated with vasodilation of the cerebral vasculature, last a variable amount of time. They are often accompanied by photosensitivity and nausea. Migraines with aura may be accompanied by sensations in the extremities and other lateralizing signs, sometimes making them difficult to distinguish from transient ischemic attacks.

Migraine symptoms tend to improve during pregnancy.[62–64] Friedman and Merritt[63] found that more than 80 percent of their patients reported improvement of migraine symptoms, with some experiencing no headache at all during pregnancy. Granella and coworkers[65] found that migraines disappeared during pregnancy in 67 percent of cases. Lance and Anthony[64] noted that those patients who experience severe migraines near the time of their menses actually improve most during pregnancy. Granella et al[65] also confirmed this. Chen and coworkers[66] identified 508 women with a history of migraine from the Collaborative Perinatal Project of the National Institute of Neurological and Communicative Disease Disorders and Stroke. They found that patients with migraines smoke more heavily and had a longer smoking history than did their headache-free peers. They also found that in nonsmokers migraine was often associated with allergies.[66]

Chancellor and colleagues[67] followed nine patients whose migraines first occurred during pregnancy at various gestational ages. They were followed for more than 4 years after pregnancy, and the prognosis for headache was excellent. Four of the nine patients developed complications of pregnancy, including preeclampsia in two.[67] It is unknown if the headaches were caused by developing preeclampsia. It is important to rule out other severe complications of pregnancy before assigning a new diagnosis of migraine to a pregnant patient. Jacobson and Redman[68] reported a patient who actually lost consciousness during pregnancy because of a basilar migraine.

Supportive therapy is recommended for patients who experience migraine attacks during gestation. Both narcotic and non-narcotic analgesics can be used as necessary. The use of nonsteroidal anti-inflammatory agents should be limited in late pregnancy, because when used over a long period they can cause premature closure of the ductus arteriosus and/or oligohydramnios. Nonetheless, they can be used for brief periods under physician supervision. When pain is severe, parenteral narcotics and appropriate antiemetic therapy may be used. β-Blockers may be safely administered during pregnancy. The calcium channel blockers used in the treatment of migraine can also be safely administered during gestation. Fluoxetine is occasionally successfully used to treat migraines and is generally safe for use during pregnancy.

Ergotamine is best avoided during pregnancy. Previous reports have suggested it may cause birth defects that have a vascular disruptive etiology. Hughes and Goldstein[69] report a case in which an infant showed evidence of early arrested cerebral maturation and paraplegia. They hypothesize that ergotamine, acting either alone or in synergy with propranolol and caffeine, produced fetal vasoconstriction resulting in tissue ischemia and subsequent malformation.[69] It is important to note that this etiology is strictly theoretical. In addition, ergots are uterotonic and have an abortifacient potential. They should be avoided during pregnancy. Sumatriptan, a serotonin receptor agonist, is very successful in treating migraines. It has a potential for vasoconstriction and has not been studied in pregnancy. It should only be used if the physician feels that the potential benefit clearly outweighs the potential risk.

Dietary factors may precipitate migraine attacks. Careful history may uncover foods that should be avoided, including foods containing monosodium glutamate, red wine, cured meats, and strong cheeses containing tyramine. Relative hypoglycemia and alcohol can also trigger migraine attacks.

Cerebrovascular Diseases

Arterial Occlusion

Twelve percent of arterial occlusions occur in women between the ages of 15 and 45 years, and approximately one-third of these patients may be pregnant.[70] In a study from India, 37 percent of patients affected with cerebrovascular disease were under the age of 40 years, with a significant number of thromboses occurring during pregnancy and the puerperium.[71] Overall, the incidence of cerebral arterial occlusion in pregnancy is approximately 1 per 20,000 live births.[70,72] The mortality rate for pregnant women with cerebral arterial occlusion is twice that of men and three times that of nonpregnant women. According to Jennett and Cross,[70] middle cerebral artery occlusion is most common during pregnancy, whereas internal carotid artery occlusion is observed most often in the puerperium. Hemiplegia and dysphasia are frequent findings.[72] Predisposing factors such as preeclampsia, chronic hypertension, or hypotensive episodes can be demonstrated in about one-third of these patients. Brick and Riggs[73] have shown that oral contraceptives also raise the risk of ischemic cerebral vascular disease. One-half of the pregnancy-related cases occur during the immediate postpartum period and the remainder during the second and third trimesters. In a recent study, Lidegaard[74] concluded that pregnancy was associated with an elevated odds ratio of only 1.3 for cerebral thromboembolism. Brick[75] reported the case of a woman who had a documented partial obstruction of the left middle cerebral artery during the third trimester of pregnancy. Following delivery, her symptoms abated, and angiography 11 weeks later revealed complete resolution of the obstruction. Brick[75] therefore thought that this lesion was the result of reversible intimal hyperplasia from the increased estrogen and progesterone levels of pregnancy.

In cases of cerebral arterial occlusion, care must be taken to avoid increased intracranial pressure. If signs of increased intracranial pressure develop, parenteral dexamethasone should be administered. Osmotic diuresis can be used if needed. Supportive measures are also necessary, including close monitoring of electrolytes to detect inappropriate secretion of antidiuretic hormone. Physical and rehabilitative therapy should be started as soon as possible. These patients can progress normally through pregnancy and deliver vaginally.

A case of maternal death from carotid artery thrombosis associated with the HELLP syndrome (hemolysis, elevated liver enzymes, and low platelet count) has been reported by Katz and Cefalo.[76] They proposed that the infarction occurred because the patient experienced a rebound thrombocytosis leading to a hypercoagulable state. They stress the importance of closely following patients with HELLP syndrome so that those who develop a reactive thrombocytosis can be monitored for signs and symptoms of cerebral thrombosis.

Cortical Venous Thrombosis

The chief symptoms in patients with cortical venous thrombosis are headache, lethargy, and vomiting. Hemiplegia has a gradual onset, and seizure activity is common (Table 35-3).[77,78] This disorder occurs most frequently during the immediate postpartum period and may be attributed to a hypercoagulable state.[79] An incidence of 1 in 10,000 pregnancies was suggested in one study.[80] With the availability of CT and MRI, accurate diagnosis is possible. The actual incidence may be higher if patients are asymptomatic. Many patients with cortical venous thrombosis show signs of seizure activity, and prophylactic anticonvulsants were once routinely given.[77] The drug of choice is phenytoin. The patient should be given a loading dose of 10 mg/kg followed by 300 to 500 mg orally each day. Phenytoin levels should be checked frequently to make certain that they are therapeutic and that the patient does not develop phenytoin toxicity. Some neurosurgeons are advocating expectant management and do not routinely give anticonvulsants.

Suborachnoid Hemorrhage

The rate of subarachnoid hemorrhage complicating pregnancy is approximately 1 per 10,400.[81] With the increase in cocaine abuse occurring across the country, this incidence may rise over the next few years, as the associated increase in vasospasm associated with this drug is bleeding from preexisting berry aneurysms and arterial-venous (A-V) malformations.[82] Most subarachnoid hemorrhages occurring in pregnant patients are caused either by rupture of a berry aneurysm or bleeding from a congenital A-V malformation. Most berry aneurysms are thought to be due a congenital defect in the elastic and smooth muscle layers of cerebral blood vessels. They are usually located in the vessels of the circle of Willis or those arising from it. Robinson and coworkers[83] evaluated 26 patients with spontaneous subarachnoid hemorrhage during pregnancy and found that approximately one-half were caused by berry aneurysms and one-half by A-V malformations. They observed that A-V malformations are more common in patients below the age of 25 years and usually bleed before 20 weeks' gestation. Conversely, berry aneurysms occur in patients over the age of 30 years and usually bleed in the third trimester.[83] Pregnancy appears to increase the risk of bleeding from an A-V malformation. The maternal mortality rate associated with an untreated A-V malformation is reported to be 33

percent. This figure, however, is based on old data, and the rate is significantly lower today.

Diagnosis and Treatment

Any patient with localized signs of cerebral or meningeal irritation must be thoroughly evaluated. If the clinical examination dictates that further evaluation is necessary, MRI or a CT scan should be performed. If necessary, contrast dyes may be used. The dyes employed in CT scanning do contain nonradioactive iodine, but when used judiciously the chance of inducing a fetal goiter is small. Cerebral angiography can be safely used to pinpoint the origin of cerebral bleeding. Subarachnoid hemorrhages, whether caused by A-V malformations or berry aneurysms, should be treated surgically when possible. Surgery under hypothermia or hypotension appears to cause no adverse fetal effects. The fetal heart rate should be monitored. If fetal bradycardia occurs, blood pressure should be raised sufficiently to normalize the fetal heart rate.[84] Kawasaki and colleagues[85] report a case of cerebellar hemorrhage in a 32-week primigravida. She was treated conservatively until term and was delivered by elective cesarean section. Her surgery, which was delayed until after delivery, was successful.

If the patient has undergone corrective surgery for an aneurysm or A-V malformation, she should be allowed to deliver vaginally. Because the Valsalva maneuver can increase intracranial pressure,[83] epidural anesthesia is recommended. Interestingly, Szabo and colleagues[86] have reported that moderate increases in blood pressure do not cause spontaneous hemorrhage in nonpregnant patients with intracranial A-V malformations. If the aneurysm or A-V malformation has not been surgically corrected, elective cesarean delivery should be performed when fetal lung maturity has been documented.[83] Laidler and colleagues[87] discussed the advantages of regional anesthesia in these patients. Buckley and coworkers[88] have described a case of simultaneous cesarean delivery and ablation of a cerebral A-V malformation.

As pregnancy has a deleterious effect on A-V malformations, those patients with inoperable lesions should be counseled about the dangers of future childbearing. Previously, permanent sterilization was encouraged.[83] With improved imaging techniques, the patient should be thoroughly evaluated before any recommendations are made for permanent sterilization.

Venous-venous (V-V) malformations are low-pressure phenomena. Patients should progress to term and deliver vaginally without any hemorrhagic event or complications.

Multiple Sclerosis

Multiple sclerosis (MS) is a demyelinating disease that attacks men and women equally. The onset of symptoms usually occurs between the ages of 20 and 40 years. In the United States, the disease is more common in those residing above 40 degrees north latitude. The prevalence for those living in the southern United States is 10 per 100,000, while it is approximately 50 per 100,000 in those living in the northern states.[89] The disease may also cluster within a community.[90] MS has no clear genetic predisposition.

The diagnosis of MS is often made years after the initial onset of sensory symptoms. The onset is usually subtle. Common presenting symptoms include weakness of one or both lower extremities, visual complaints, and loss of coordination. Because the disease primarily affects the white matter of the central nervous system, symptoms attributable to disruption of gray matter are uncommon. The disease is characterized by exacerbations and remissions. Less than one-third of patients show steady progression of their disease after its onset.

It is impossible to predict the long-range prognosis of a patient with MS. About one-half of patients are still able to work at their usual profession 10 years after the onset of the illness. After 20 years, however, only about one-third remain employed. In a study of 185 women with MS, Weinshenker and colleagues[91] showed that there was no association between long-term disability and (1) total number of term pregnancies, (2) the timing of pregnancy relative to the onset of MS, or (3) the worsening of MS in relation to a pregnancy. The average life expectancy in patients with MS is also impossible to predict. Patients may live with the disease for more than 25 years. When death does occur, it is usually attributable to infection.

MS and pregnancy can coexist without unusual complications. Leibowitz and colleagues[92] found no decrease in fertility and no increase in perinatal mortality in patients with MS. Their study suggested that pregnancy does not predispose a patient to MS but that patients with "premorbid" disease are more likely to have the onset of early symptoms during pregnancy.

In fact, Runmarker and Andersen[93] demonstrated that the risk of onset of MS is reduced during gestation while the risk of onset during the postpartum period was no different than for the nonpregnant state. Furthermore, these investigators demonstrated a lower risk of onset of MS in parous than in nulliparous patients. Of 170 pregnant patients with MS studied by Millar and coworkers,[94] relapses occurred in only 45, the majority during the puerperium and postpartum periods. Birk and co-investigators[95] carefully followed pregnancies in eight women with MS. None of the women worsened during pregnancy. Six of the eight women, however, experienced relapses within the first 7 weeks after delivery. They also reported that there were differences in suppressor T cell levels during pregnancy, but these were not predictive of changes in clinical disease.[95] Frith and McLeod[96] studied 85 pregnancies and found no increased risk of relapse during pregnancy. They noted that most of the relapses that did occur during pregnancy took place in the third trimester. In another series, Frith and McLeod[97] reported that relapses occur most frequently in the last trimester and also in the first 3 months postpartum. In a large study, Nelson and colleagues[98] analyzed 191 pregnancies in women with nonprogressive MS. The exacerbation rate during the 9-month postpartum period was 34 percent, three times that of the 9 months during pregnancy. The rate was highest in the 3 months immediately following delivery and stabilized after postpartum month 6.[98] The exacerbation rates were the same in breast-feeding and non-breast-feeding women. The average time to flare was also similar in both groups. This study verifies that it is safe for women with MS to breast-feed their newborns.[98]

Conversely, in a recent study, Bernardi and colleagues showed a decreased risk of relapse during the 9 months of pregnancy and the first 6 months postpartum.[99] In this study of 52 women, these researchers concluded that pregnancy, as a whole, is a protective event. Worthington et al,[100] however, found more frequent relapses in the first 6 months postpartum, but not after that. Long-term prognosis was unaffected by pregnancy.[100] Vendro et al[101] demonstrated that pregnancy delays the onset of long-term disability. As an index of progression, they used the length of time from onset of disease until wheel chair dependence. In patients with at least one pregnancy after onset, the mean time to wheel chair dependence was 18.6 years compared with 12.5 years for other women.[101]

Paraplegic patients are more susceptible to urinary tract infections during pregnancy but may feel no symptoms. Therefore, they should be screened routinely. If the patient has become paraplegic as a result of MS, there may be little pain associated with labor. It might be difficult therefore for the patient to discern when labor begins. Uterine contractions occur normally, but voluntary expulsive efforts may be hindered in the second stage of labor. Delivery by forceps or vacuum extraction therefore may be indicated. Bader and colleagues[103] report that women with MS who receive epidural anesthesia for vaginal delivery do not have a significantly higher incidence of exacerbation of their MS than those receiving only local anesthesia.

Corticosteroids and immunosuppressive agents are occasionally used to treat multiple sclerosis. In one case report, plasmapheresis was used with dramatic improvement in a woman with rapidly progressive MS.

Carpal Tunnel Syndrome

The medial border of the carpal tunnel consists of the pisiform and hamate bones, and its lateral border consists of the scaphoid and trapezium bones. They are covered on the palmar surface by the flexor retinaculum. The median nerve and flexor tendons pass through this carpal tunnel, which has little room for expansion. If the wrist is extremely flexed or extended, the volume of the carpal tunnel is reduced. In pregnancy, weight gain and edema can produce the carpal tunnel syndrome that results from compression of the median nerve. Wallace and Cook[104] first reported the association between carpal tunnel syndrome and pregnancy in 1957. Although 20 percent of pregnant women complain of pain on the palmar surface of the hand, few actually have the true carpal tunnel syndrome.[105] Commonly, the syndrome consists of pain, numbness, and/or tingling in the distribution of the median nerve in the hand and wrist. This includes the thumb, index finger, long finger, and radial side of the ring finger on the palmar aspect. Compressing the median nerve and percussing the wrist and forearm with a reflex hammer, the Tinel maneuver, often exacerbates the pain. In severe cases, weakness and decreased motor function can occur.

McLennan and coworkers[106] studied 1,216 consecutive pregnancies. Of these patients, 427 (35 percent) reported hand symptoms. Fewer than 20 percent of these 427 affected women described the classic carpal tunnel syndrome. No patient required operative intervention. Most symptoms were bilateral and commenced in the third trimester of pregnancy. Ekman-Ordeberg et al[107] found a 2.3 percent incidence of carpal tunnel syndrome in a prospective study of 2,358 pregnancies. The syndrome appeared to be more common in primigravidas with generalized edema. Conservative therapy with splinting of the wrist at night completely relieved symptoms in 46 of 56 patients. Of the remaining 10, three required surgery before delivery. Wand[108] retrospectively studied 40 women with carpal tunnel syndrome developing in pregnancy and 18 women with carpal tunnel syndrome that developed in the puerperium. He confirmed that the syndrome occurs most frequently in primigravidas over the age of 30 years. All cases that developed before delivery occurred during the third trimester and resolved within 2 weeks after delivery. In those cases developing during the puerperium in women who breast-fed their infants, the symptoms lasted longer, a mean of 5.8 months.[108] In another series, Wand[109] studied 27 women who developed carpal tunnel syndrome during the puerpe-

rium. The condition was associated with breast-feeding in 24 of these women. Symptoms lasted an average of 6.5 months in the breast-feeding women. Only two of these patients required surgical decompression.[109]

Supportive and conservative therapies are usually adequate for the treatment of carpal tunnel syndrome. Symptoms usually subside in the postpartum period as total body water returns to normal.[110] Splints placed on the dorsum of the hand, which keep the wrist in a neutral position and maximize the capacity of the carpal tunnel, often provide dramatic relief. Local injections of glucocorticoids may also be used in severe cases. Although diuretics may help to control carpal tunnel syndrome symptoms over a short period of time, their use is not recommended because the symptoms return rather rapidly after the cessation of treatment. In an uncontrolled series, Ellis[111] reported that pyridoxine in a dose of 100 to 200 mg daily for 12 weeks can provide relief in a large percentage of patients with carpal tunnel syndrome. Before this can be recommended, controlled trials need to be undertaken.

Surgical correction of this syndrome should not be delayed in patients with deteriorating muscle tone and motor function. Decompression surgery for carpal tunnel syndrome is a simple procedure that can be safely carried out during pregnancy using local anesthesia, an axillary block, or a Bier block. With new endoscopic procedures, the procedure is even less invasive. It is important to warn patients that carpal tunnel syndrome can recur in future pregnancies.[112]

Pseudotumor Cerebri

Pseudotumor cerebri may complicate as many as 1 in 870 births.[113] It is seen more frequently in pregnant women, particularly those who are obese.[114–116] However, in a study by Ireland and colleagues[117] the incidences in pregnant women and in oral contraceptive users were no higher than in control groups. More than 95 percent of these patients present with headaches, and 15 percent have diplopia. Papilledema is found in virtually all patients.[114,118] To establish the diagnosis, one must demonstrate elevated cerebrospinal fluid (CSF) pressure, normal CSF composition, and the absence of an intracranial mass on MRI or CT scan.[119]

The pathogenesis of this disorder is unknown. Bates and colleagues[120] found CSF prolactin to be markedly elevated in cases of pseudotumor cerebri. Prolactin appears to have an affinity for receptors in the choroid plexus, where CSF is produced. Prolactin has osmoregulatory functions and therefore may have a role in the increased CSF production found in pseudotumor cerebri.[114] Some believe that reduced CSF reabsorption is the etiology of pseudotumor cerebri. Ahlskog and O'Neill[121] noted an association between the occurrence of pseudotumor cerebri and the following conditions: corticosteroid therapy and its withdrawal, nalidixic acid therapy, nitrofurantoin therapy, tetracycline therapy, hypoparathyroidism, deficiencies or excesses of vitamin A, and iron deficiency anemia.

Pregnancy outcome appears to be unaffected by the illness.[114,118] There is no increase in fetal wastage or congenital anomalies.[114] Koppel and colleagues[122] reported a case of pseudotumor cerebri that presented in a 15-year-old primigravida following eclampsia. It lasted for 3 weeks. Wheatley and colleagues[123] noted a case of pseudotumor cerebri occurring in a diabetic pregnancy. They caution that it is important to make the distinction between symptoms of pseudotumor cerebri and visual impairment caused by diabetic retinopathy, as the treatments are different.[123] Thomas[124] described a case of pseudotumor cerebri occurring in two consecutive pregnancies in a woman with hemoglobin SC. In both instances, symptoms resolved following delivery and both infants were born at term.

Most patients respond well to conservative management.[113] The main objectives of treatment are relief of pain and preservation of vision. The patient should be followed closely with visual acuity and visual field determinations at intervals indicated by the clinical condition. In patients with mild disease, analgesics may be adequate. If pain persists, diuretics may be used. Acetazolamide, a carbonic anhydrase inhibitor, will reduce CSF production in many patients.[125] The usual dose is 500 mg twice daily. In more difficult cases, prednisone in doses of 40 to 60 mg daily usually provides good results.[113] Patients may be treated for 2 weeks, with the dose being tapered over the next month.[114] Serial lumbar punctures to reduce CSF pressure are rarely necessary today. Surgical approaches are reserved for refractory patients in whom rapid visual deterioration occurs.

Pseudotumor cerebri is not an indication for cesarean delivery. A review of the literature reveals that 73 percent of the reported patients delivered vaginally.[114] Cesarean delivery should be undertaken only for obstetric indications. Both epidural and spinal anesthesia, when expertly administered, can be safely used in patients with pseudotumor cerebri.[126] Bearing down, which can increase CSF pressure, should be avoided when possible. The second stage of labor should therefore be shortened by outlet forceps or by vacuum extraction.

The recurrence rate for pseudotumor cerebri appears to be between 10 and 12.3 percent in nonpregnant patients.[115,116] Pregnancy does not appear to predispose to a recurrence.[114]

Key Points

- Idiopathic seizures affect approximately 1 percent of the general population and are the most frequent neurologic complication of pregnancy.

- Prepregnancy counseling is imperative in the patient with a seizure disorder, and preconceptual folic acid therapy should be implemented under the direction of an obstetrician and a neurologist.

- Those with seizures occurring less than once each month will have the best control during pregnancy.

- The anticonvulsant medication that best controls the patient's seizures should be used during pregnancy.

- Because of the changes in plasma volume, drug distribution, and metabolism that occur during pregnancy, anticonvulsant levels should be checked frequently and dosages adjusted accordingly.

- Patients taking anticonvulsants have an increased risk of giving birth to an infant with both major and minor anomalies, but this risk is probably less than 10 percent. Therefore, the majority of patients with epilepsy will give birth to healthy infants.

- Carbamazepine and valproate are associated with neural tube defects, and these patients should receive 4 mg folic acid daily before and during early pregnancy.

- The vasocontrictor drugs used to treat migraines should be avoided during pregnancy and lactation.

- Carpal tunnel syndrome is common in pregnancy and usually responds to conservative splinting. Surgery can be safely undertaken if indicated during pregnancy.

- Pregnancy does not hasten the onset of multiple sclerosis, nor does it hasten the onset of disability from multiple sclerosis.

References

1. Cramer JA, Jones EE: Reproductive function in epilepsy. Epilepsia 32(Suppl 6):S19, 1991
2. Back DJ, Bates M, Bowden A et al: The interaction of phenobarbital and other anticonvulsants with oral contraceptive steroid therapy. Contraception 22:495, 1980
3. Coulam CB, Annegers JF: Do anticonvulsants reduce the efficacy of oral contraceptives? Epilepsia 20:519, 1979
4. Janz D, Schmidt D: Anti-epileptic drugs and failure of oral contraceptives. Lancet 1:1113, 1974
5. Webber MP, Hauser WA, Ottman R, Annegers JF: Fertility in persons with epilepsy: 1935–1974. Epilepsia 27:746, 1986
6. Dansky LV, Anderman E, Anderman F: Marriage and fertility in epileptic patients. Epilepsia 21:261, 1980

7. Knight AH, Rhind EG: Epilepsy and pregnancy: a study of 153 pregnancies in 59 patients. Epilepsia 16:99, 1975

8. Schmidt D, Canger R, Avanzini G et al: Change of seizure frequency in pregnant epileptic women. J Neurol Neurosurg Psychiatry 46:751, 1983

9. Tanganelli P, Regesta G: Epilepsy, pregnancy, and major birth anomalies: an Italian prospective, controlled study. Neurology 42(Suppl 5):89, 1992

10. Landon MJ, Kirkley M: Metabolism of diphenylhydantoin (phenytoin) during pregnancy. Br J Obstet Gynaecol 86:125, 1979

11. Kochenour NK, Emery MG, Sawohuck RJ: Phenytoin metabolism in pregnancy. Obstet Gynecol 56:577, 1980

12. Yerby MS, Friel PN, McCormick K et al: Pharmacokinetics of anticonvulsants in pregnancy: alterations in plasma protein binding. Epilepsy Res 5:223, 1990

13. Desmond MM, Schwanecke RP, Wilson GS et al: Maternal barbiturate utilization and neonatal withdrawal symptomatology. J Pediatr 80:190, 1972

14. Ogawa Y, Kaneko S, Otani K, Fukushima Y: Serum folic acid in epileptic mothers and their relationship to congenital malformations. Epilepsy Res 8:75, 1991

15. Milunsky A, Jick H, Jick SS et al: Multivitamin/folic acid supplementation in early pregnancy reduces the prevalence of neural tube defects. JAMA 262:2847, 1989

16. Friis B, Sardemann H: Short reports: neonatal hypocalcaemia after intrauterine exposure to anticonvulsant drugs. Arch Dis Child 52:239, 1977

17. Mountain KR, Hirsh J, Gallus AS: Neonatal coagulation defect due to anticonvulsant drug treatment in pregnancy. Lancet 1:265, 1970

18. Bleyer WA, Skinner AL: Fatal neonatal hemorrhage after maternal anticonvulsant therapy. JAMA 235:626, 1976

19. Yerby M, Koepsell T, Daling J: Pregnancy complications and outcomes in a cohort of women with epilepsy. Epilepsia 26:631, 1985

20. Nelson KB, Ellenberg JH: Maternal seizure disorder, outcome of pregnancy, and neurologic abnormalities in the children. Neurology 32:1247, 1982

21. Kallen B: A register study of maternal epilepsy and delivery outcome with special reference to drug use. Acta Neurol Scand 73:253, 1986

22. Hiilesmaa VK, Bardy A, Teramo K: Obstetric outcome in women with epilepsy. Am J Obstet Gynecol 152:499, 1985

23. Mastroiacovo P, Bertollini R, Licata D: Fetal growth in the offspring of epileptic women: results of an Italian multicentric cohort study. Acta Neurol Scand 78:110, 1988

24. Hiilesmaa VK, Teramo K, Granstrom ML: Fetal head growth retardation associated with maternal antiepileptic drugs. Lancet 1:165, 1981

25. Hanson JW, Smith DW: The fetal hydantoin syndrome. J Pediatr 87:285, 1975

26. Hanson JW, Myrianthopoulos NC, Sedgwick Harvey MA, Smith DW: Risks to the offspring of women treated with hydantoin anticonvulsants, with emphasis on the fetal hydantoin syndrome. J Pediatr 89:662, 1976

27. Gaily E, Granstrom ML, Hiilesmaa V, Bardy A: Minor anomalies in offspring of epileptic mothers. J Pediatr 112:520, 1988

28. Friis ML, Holm NV, Sindrup EH et al: Facial clefts in sibs and children of epileptic patients. Neurology 36:346, 1986

29. Kelly TE, Rein M, Edwards P: Teratogenicity of anticonvulsant drugs. Am J Med Genet 19:451, 1984

30. Hecht JT, Annegers JF, Kurland LT: Epilepsy and clefting disorders: lack of evidence of a familial association. Am J Med Genet 33:244, 1989

31. Nakane Y, Okuma T, Takahashi R et al: Multi-institutional study on the teratogenicity and fetal toxicity of antiepileptic drugs: a report of a collaborative study group in Japan. Epilepsia 21:663, 1980

32. Kaneko S, Otani K, Fukushima Y et al: Teratogenicity of antiepileptic drugs: analysis of possible risk factors. Epilepsia 29:459, 1988

33. Kaneko S, Otani K, Kondo T et al: Malformation in infants of mothers with epilepsy receiving antiepileptic drugs. Neurology 42(Suppl 5):68, 1992

34. Lindhout D, Meinardi H, Meijer JWA, Nau H: Antiepileptic drugs and teratogenesis in two consecutive cohorts: changes in prescription policy paralleled by changes in pattern of malformations. Neurology 42(Suppl 5):94, 1992

35. Dravet C, Julian C, Legras C et al: Epilepsy, antiepileptic drugs, and malformations in children of women with epilepsy: a French prospective cohort study. Neurology 42(Suppl 5):75, 1992

36. Koch S, Losche G, Jager-Roman E et al: Major and minor birth malformations and antiepileptic drugs. Neurology 42(Suppl 5):83, 1992

37. Gaily E, Granstrom ML: Minor anomalies in children of mothers with epilepsy. Neurology 42(Suppl 5):128, 1992

38. Yerby MS, Leavitt A, Erickson M et al: Antiepileptics and the development of congenital anomalies. Neurology 42(Suppl 5):132, 1992

39. DiLiberti JH, Farndon PA, Dennis NR, Curry CJR: The fetal valproate syndrome. Am J Med Genet 19:473, 1984

40. Ardinger HH, Atkin JF, Blackston RD et al: Verification of the fetal valproate syndrome phenotype. Am J Med Genet 29:171, 1988

41. Jager-Roman E, Deichl A, Jakob S et al: Fetal growth, major malformations, and minor anomalies in infants born to women receiving valproic acid. J Pediatr 108:997, 1986

42. Lindhout D, Schmidt D: In-utero exposure to valproate and neural tube defects. Lancet 2:1392, 1986

43. Lindhout D, Omtzigt JGC, Cornel MC: Spectrum of neural-tube defects in 34 infants prenatally exposed to antiepileptic drugs. Neurology 42(Suppl 5):111, 1992

44. Wegner C, Nau H: Alteration of embryonic folate metabolism by valproic acid during organogenesis: implications for mechanism of teratogenesis. Neurology 42(Suppl 5):17, 1992

45. Jones KL, Lacro RV, Johnson KA, Adams J: Pattern of malformations in the children of women treated with

carbamazepine during pregnancy. N Engl J Med 320: 1661, 1989

46. Rosa FW: Spina bifida in infants of women treated with carbamazepine during pregnancy. N Engl J Med 324: 674, 1991

47. Finnell RH, Buehler BA, Kerr BM et al: Clinical and experimental studies linking oxidative metabolism to phenytoin-induced teratogenesis. Neurology 42(Suppl 5):25, 1992

48. Granstrom ML, Gaily E: Psychomotor development in children of mothers with epilepsy. Neurology 42(Suppl 5):144, 1992

49. Gaily E, Kantola-Sorsa E, Granstrom ML: Intelligence of children of epileptic mothers. J Pediatr 113:677, 1988

50. Dansky LV, Andermann E, Rosenblatt D et al: Anticonvulsants, folate levels, and pregnancy outcome: a prospective study. Ann Neurol 21:176, 1987

51. Annegers JF, Hauser WA, Elveback LR et al: Epilepsia 17:1, 1976

52. Blandfort M, Tsuboi T, Vogel F: Genetic counseling in the epileptics. Hum Genet 76:303, 1987

53. Bronshtein M, Zimmer EZ, Gerlis LM et al: Early ultrasound diagnosis of fetal congenital heart defects in high-risk and low-risk pregnancies. Obstet Gynecol 82: 225, 1993

54. Wigton TR, Sabbagha RE, Tamura RK et al: Sonographic diagnosis of congenital heart disease: comparison between the four-chamber view and multiple cardiac views. Obstet Gynecol 82:219, 1993

55. Yerby MS: Problems and management of the pregnant woman with epilepsy. Epilepsia 28(Suppl 3):S29, 1987

56. Orland MJ, Saltman RJ: Seizures. Washington Manual of Medical Therapeutics, 25th Ed. 1986

57. Sibai BM, Spinnato JA, Watson DL et al: Eclampsia IV. Neurological findings and future outcome. Am J Obstet Gynecol 152:184, 1985

58. Kaneko S, Sato T, Suzuki K: The levels of anticonvulsants in breast milk. Br J Clin Pharmacol 7:624, 1974

59. Mattson RH, Cramer JA, Darney PD, Naftolin F: Use of oral contraceptives by women with epilepsy. JAMA 256:238, 1986

60. Orme MLE: The clinical pharmacology of oral contraceptive steroids. Br J Clin Pharmacol 14:31, 1982

61. Callaghan P: The migraine syndrome in pregnancy. Neurology 18:197, 1968

62. Somerville B: A study of migraine in pregnancy. Neurology 22:824, 1972

63. Friedman AP, Merritt HH: Headache, Prognosis and Treatment. FA Davis, Philadelphia, 1959

64. Lance JW, Anthony MD: Some clinical aspects of migraine. Arch Neurol 15:356, 1966

65. Granella F, Sances G, Zanferrar C, et al. Migraine without aura and reproductive life events: a clinical epidemiological study of 1300 women. Headache 33: 385–384,1993

66. Chen TC, Leviton A, Edelstein S, Ellenberg JH: Migraine and other diseases in women of reproductive age: the influence of smoking on observed associations. Arch Neurol 44:1024, 1987

67. Chancellor AM, Wroe SJ, Cull RE: Migraine occurring for the first time in pregnancy. Headache 30:224, 1990

68. Jacobson SL, Redman CW: Basilar migraine with loss of consciousness in pregnancy: case report. Br J Obstet Gynaecol 96:494, 1989

69. Hughes HE, Goldstein DA: Birth defects following maternal exposure to ergotamine, beta blocker, and caffeine. J Med Genet 25:396, 1988

70. Jennett WB, Cross JN: Influence of pregnancy and oral contraception on the incidence of strokes in women of childbearing age. Lancet 1:1019, 1967

71. Banerjee AK, Varma M, Vasista RK, Chopra JS: Cerebrovascular disease in north-west India: a study of necropsy material. J Neurol Neurosurg psychiatry 52:512, 1989

72. Cross JN, Castro PO, Jennett WB: Cerebral strokes associated with pregnancy in the puerperium. Br Med J 3: 214, 1968

73. Brick JF, Riggs JE: Ischemic cerebrovascular disease in the young adult: emergence of oral contraceptive use and pregnancy as the major risk factors in the 1980s. WV Med J 85:7, 1989

74. Lidegaard O. Oral contraceptives, pregnancy and the risk of cerebral thromboembolism: the influence of diabetes, hypertension, migraine, and previous thrombotic disease. Br J Obstet Gynaecol 102:153–159, 1995

75. Brick JF: Vanishing cerebrovascular disease of pregnancy. Neurology 38:804, 1988

76. Katz VL, Cefalo RC: Maternal death from carotid artery thrombosis associated with the syndrome of hemolysis, elevated liver function, and low platelets. Am J Perinatol 6:360, 1989

77. Estanol B, Rodriguez A, Counte G et al: Intracranial venous thrombosis in young women. Stroke 10:680, 1979

78. Krayenbuhl HA: Cerebral venous and sinus thrombosis. Clin Neurosurg 14:1, 1967

79. Bansal BC, Prakash C, Gupta RR, Brahmanandam KRV: Study of serum lipid and blood fibrinolytic activity in cases of cerebral venous/venous sinus thrombosis during the puerperium. Am J Obstet Gynecol 119:1079, 1974

80. Abraham J, Rios PS, Inbaraj SG et al: An epidemiological study of hemiplegia due to stroke in south India. Stroke 1:477, 1970

81. Miller HJ, Hinkley CM: Berry aneurysms in pregnancy: a ten year report. South Med J 63:279, 1970

82. Henderson CE, Torbey M: Rupture of intracranial aneurysm associated with cocaine use during pregnancy. Am J Perinatol 5:142, 1988

83. Robinson JL, Hall CJ, Sevzimer CB: Arterial venous malformations, aneurysms, and pregnancy. J Neurosurg 41:63, 1974

84. Minielly R, Yuzpe AA, Drake CC: Subarachnoid hemorrhage secondary to ruptured cerebral aneurysm in pregnancy. Obstet Gynecol 53:64, 1979

85. Kawasaki N, Uchida T, Yamada M et al: Conservative management of cerebellar hemorrhage in pregnancy. Int J Gynaecol Obstet 31:365, 1990

86. Szabo MD, Crosby C, Sundaram P et al: Hypertension

does not cause spontaneous hemorrhage of intracranial arteriovenous malformations. Anesthesiology 70:761, 1989

87. Laidler JA, Jackson IJ, Redfern N: The management of caesarean section in a patient with an intracranial arteriovenous malformation. Anaesthesia 44:490, 1989

88. Buckley TA, Yau GH, Poon WS, Oh T: Caesarean section and ablation of a cerebral arteriovenous malformation. Anaesth Intensive Care 18:248, 1990

89. McAlpine D, Lunisden CE, Acheson ED: Multiple Sclerosis, a Reappraisal. 2nd Ed. Williams & Wilkins, Baltimore, 1972

90. Eastman R, Sheridan J, Poskanzer DA: Multiple sclerosis clustering in a small Massachusetts community. N Engl J Med 289:793, 1973

91. Weinshenker BG, Hader W, Carriere W et al: The influence of pregnancy on disability from multiple sclerosis: a population-based study in Middlesex County, Ontario. Neurology 39:1438, 1989

92. Liebowitz U, Antonovosky A, Katz R et al: Does pregnancy increase the risk of multiple sclerosis? J Neurol Neurosurg Psychiatry 30:354, 1967

93. Runmanker B, Andersen O: Pregnancy is associated with a lower risk of onset and a better prognosis in multiple sclerosis. Brain 118:253, 1995

94. Millar JHD, Allison RS, Cheeseman EA: Pregnancy as a factor influencing relapse in disseminated sclerosis. Brain 82:417, 1959

95. Birk K, Ford C, Smeltzer S et al: The clinical course of multiple sclerosis during pregnancy and the puerperium. Arch Neurol 47:738, 1990

96. Frith JA, McLeod JC: Pregnancy and multiple sclerosis. J Neurol Neurosurg Psychiatry 51:495, 1988

97. Frith JA, McLeod JG: Pregnancy and multiple sclerosis: an Australian perspective. Clin Exp Neurol 24:1, 1987

98. Nelson LM, Franklin GM, Jones MC: Risk of multiple sclerosis exacerbation during pregnancy and breastfeeding. JAMA 259:3441, 1988

99. Bernardi S, Grasso MG, Bertollini R et al: The influences of pregnancy on relapses of multiple sclerosis: a cohort study. Acta Neurol Scand 84:403, 1991

100. Worthington J, Jones R, Crawford M, Forti A: Pregnancy and multiple sclerosis—a 3-year prospective study. J Neurol 241:228, 1994

101. Verdru P, Theys P, Beartrijs M et al: Pregnancy and multiple sclerosis: the influence on longterm disability. Clin Neurol Neurosurg 96:38, 1994

102. Khatri BO, D'Cruz O, Preissler G et al: Plasmaphoresis in a pregnant patient with multiple sclerosis. Arch Neurol 47:11, 1990

103. Bader AM, Hunt CO, Datta S et al: Anesthesia for the obstetric patient with multiple sclerosis. J Clin Anesth 1:21, 1988

104. Wallace JT, Cook AW: Carpal tunnel syndrome in pregnancy. Am J Obstet Gynecol 73:1333, 1957

105. Nicholas CG, Noone RB, Graham WP: Carpal tunnel syndrome in pregnancy. HAND 3:80, 1971

106. McLennan HG, Oats JN, Walstab JE: Survey of hand symptoms in pregnancy. Med J Aust 147:542, 1987

107. Ekman-Ordeberg G, Salgeback S, Ordeberg G: Carpal tunnel syndrome in pregnancy: a prospective study. Acta Obstet Gynecol Scand 66:233, 1987

108. Wand JS: Carpal tunnel syndrome in pregnancy and lactation. J Hand Surg 15:93, 1990

109. Wand JS: The natural history of carpal tunnel syndrome in lactation. J R Soc Med 82:349, 1989

110. Massey EW: Carpal tunnel syndrome in pregnancy. Obstet Gynecol Surv 33:145, 1978

111. Ellis JM: Treatment of carpal tunnel syndrome with vitamin B6. South Med J 80:882, 1987

112. Tobin SM: Carpal tunnel syndrome in pregnancy. Am J Obstet Gynecol 97:493, 1967

113. Katz VL, Peterson R, Cefalo RC: Pseudotumor cerebri and pregnancy. Am J Perinatol 6:442, 1989

114. Peterson CM, Kelly JV: Pseudotumor cerebri in pregnancy: case reports and literature reviewed. Obstet Gynecol Surv 40:323, 1985

115. Weisberg LA: Benign intracranial hypertension. Medicine (Baltimore) 54:197, 1975

116. Johnston I, Paterson A: Benign intracranial hypertension. II. CSF pressures and the circulation. Brain 97:301, 1974

117. Ireland B, Corbett JJ, Wallace RB: The search for causes of idiopathic intracranial hypertension: a preliminary case–control study. Arch Neurol 47:315, 1990

118. Koontz WL, Herbert WNP, Cefalo R: Pseudotumor cerebri in pregnancy. Obstet Gynecol 62:325, 1983

119. Donaldson JO: Neurology in Pregnancy. WB Saunders, Philadelphia, 1978

120. Bates GW, Whiteworth NS, Parker JL et al: Elevated cerebrospinal fluid prolactin concentration in women with pseudotumor cerebri. South Med J 75:807, 1982

121. Ahlskog JE, O'Neill BP: Pseudotumor cerebri. Ann Intern Med 97:249, 1982

122. Koppel BS, Kaunitz AM, Tuchman AJ: Pseudotumor cerebri following eclampsia. Eur Neurol 30:6, 1990

123. Wheatley T, Clark JD, Edwards OM, Jordan K: Retinal haemorrhages and papilloedema due to benign intracranial hypertension in a pregnant diabetic. Diabetic Med 3:482, 1986

124. Thomas E: Recurrent benign intracranial hypertension associated with hemoglobin SC disease in pregnancy. Obstet Gynecol 67:7S, 1986

125. Rubin RC, Henderson ES, Ommaya AK et al: The production of cerebrospinal fluid in man and its modification by acetazolamide. J Neurosurg 25:430, 1966

126. Palop R, Choed-Amphai E, Miller R: Epidural anesthesia for delivery complicated by benign intracranial hypertension. Anesthesiology 50:159, 1979

127. Donaldson JO: Peripartum convulsions. p. 312. In Donaldson JO (ed): Neurology of Pregnancy. WB Saunders, Philadelphia, 1989

Chapter 36

Malignant Diseases and Pregnancy

Larry J. Copeland and Mark B. Landon

The juxtaposition of life and death presents numerous emotional and ethical conflicts to the patient, her family, and her physicians. The diagnosis of cancer for anyone is understandably frightening. To deal with cancer in the context of a pregnancy is particularly burdensome since the patient may need to, or may perceive that she needs to, choose between her life or the life of her unborn. Cancer in pregnancy complicates the management of both the cancer and the pregnancy. Both diagnostic and therapeutic interventions must carefully address the associated risks to both the patient and the fetus. Informed decisions will require evaluation of a number of factors, and after careful counseling these considerations will be the foundation upon which treatment decisions will be made. Over recent years there has been an evolution in the philosophy of care from one of total disregard of the pregnancy with frequent immediate termination to a more thoughtful approach in which management decisions attempt to balance the maternal and fetal interests ideally to limit risk of death or injury to both.

While cancer is the second most common cause of death for women in their reproductive years, only about 1 in 1,000 pregnancies[1] is complicated by cancer. Since there are no large prospective studies that address cancer treatment in pregnancy, physicians tend to base treatment strategies on small retrospective studies or anecdotal reports that occasionally present conflicting information.[2]

A successful outcome is dependent on a cooperative multidisciplinary approach. The management plan must be formulated within a medical, moral, ethical, legal, and religious framework acceptable to the patient and guided by and dependent on the communication and education resources of the health care team.

The malignancies most commonly encountered in the pregnant patient are, in descending order, breast cancer, cervical cancer, melanoma, ovarian cancer, thyroid cancer, leukemia, lymphoma, and colorectal cancer.[3] The frequencies of these diseases may increase secondary to the trend to delay childbearing. Before specific malignancies are discussed, some of the general issues are reviewed.

Chemotherapy During Pregnancy

Pharmacology of Chemotherapy During Pregnancy

Since pregnancy alters physiology, there is the potential for altered pharmokinetics of the chemotherapy. Orally administered medications will be subjected to altered gastrointestinal motility. Peak drug concentrations will be decreased due to the 50 percent expansion in plasma volume, producing a longer drug half-life unless there is a concurrent increase in metabolism or excretion. The increase in plasma proteins and fall in albumin may alter drug availability, and amniotic fluid may act as a pharmacologic third space, potentially increasing toxicity due to delayed metabolism and excretion. Hepatic oxidation and renal blood flow are both elevated during pregnancy and may influence the metabolism and excretion of most drugs.[4] However, since pharmacologic studies in the pregnant woman are lacking, we currently assume that initial drug dosages are similar to the nonpregnant woman and adjustments to dose are based on toxicity on a course by course basis.

Since antineoplastic agents can be found in breast milk, breast-feeding is contraindicated.[5]

Factors Impacting Management of the Pregnant Patient with a Malignancy

1. The gestation of the pregnancy—fetal viability
2. The stage of the cancer and associated prognosis
3. The potential for the cancer treatment to have adverse effects on the fetus, including the potential for long-term occult problems.
4. The risk to the mother of delaying therapy to permit fetal viability
5. The risk to the fetus of early delivery to allow more timely cancer therapy
6. The possible need to terminate an early pregnancy to allow an optimal opportunity to treat and cure the malignancy

Drug Effects on the Fetus

Acute Effects

Because antineoplastic agents are targeted for the rapidly dividing malignant cell, one would expect the fetus with its accelerated growth pattern to be particularly subject to a high rate of serious toxicities. Clear documentation of such is not the case. Spontaneous abortions, fetal organ toxicity, premature birth, and low birth weight are potential risks in the pregnant patient receiving chemotherapy. Excluding the intentional use of abortifacients, it is difficult to demonstrate clearly that the use of chemotherapy results in an increase in the spontaneous abortion rate over the expected 15 to 20 percent. Fetal organ toxicity has not been reported as a major problem, although neonatal myelosuppression[6] and hearing loss in a 1 year old[7] have been reported. Since early induction of labor or surgical delivery is often a component of the overall treatment plan, it is difficult to identify premature birth as a specific

result of the chemotherapy. On the other hand, it appears that low birth weight is associated with the administration of chemotherapy in the second and third trimesters.[8]

Teratogenicity

All drugs undergo animal teratogenicity testing, and based on these results the drugs are assigned risk categories (Table 36-1) by the Food and Drug Administration (FDA). Based on this system, most chemotherapeutic agents are rated as C, D, or X. However, animal teratogenicity testing cannot always be reliably extrapolated to the human. For example, a drug (e.g., aspirin) may show teratogenic effects in animals and not affect humans. The opposite is also true and as such has serious potential to do harm; for example, a drug may show no animal teratogenicity (e.g., thalidomide) but cause serious human anomalies (see Chs. 8 and 10).

While the literature addressing chemotherapy administration during pregnancy is somewhat limited and dated, reviews by Nicholson[9] and Doll and colleagues[4] provide us with some information regarding the frequency of affected offspring. Nicholson reported that first trimester exposure resulted in about a 10 percent frequency of major fetal malformations. For a similar situation, Doll and colleagues reported 17 and 25 percent frequencies for single agent chemotherapy and combination chemotherapy, respectively. However, some of the patients from the later study also received irradiation, and exclusion of these cases drops the malformation rate to 6 percent. The risk of fetal malformation varies with the drug classification and specific drug (Table 36-2). In general, antimetabolites and the alkalating agents appear to carry the highest risk.

Antimetabolites

Historically, aminopterin was used as an abortifacient, and in cases of failed abortion the risk of fetal malformation was about 50 percent. Methotrexate has replaced aminopterin for chemotherapeutic purposes,

Table 36-1   FDA Risk Categories for Drug Use During Pregnancy

Category	Definition
A	Controlled studies have demonstrated no risk, and the possibility of fetal harm appears remote
B	*Either* animal studies have failed to identify a risk but there are no controlled studies in women, *or* animal studies have shown an adverse effect that was not confirmed in controlled studies in women
C	*Either* animal studies have revealed adverse effects and there are no controlled studies in women, *or* studies in women and animals are not available. Use drugs only if the potential benefit justifies the potential risk to the fetus
D	There is evidence of fetal risk, but the benefits may be acceptable despite the risk in either a life-threatening situation or a serious disease for which safer drugs are ineffective
X	Studies in animals or humans have demonstrated fetal abnormalities, and the risk of the drug in pregnant women clearly outweighs any possible benefit

(Adapted from Briggs et al.,[196] with permission.)

Table 36-2　Malformations and Exposure to Chemotherapeutic Agents During Early Pregnancy[a]

Class and Drug	Total Exposed	Total Deformed (%)	FDA Category
Antimetabolites			
Aminopterin	34	18 (53)	X
Azauridine	15	11 (73)	X
Cytarabine	13	2 (15)	D
5-Fluouracil	6	1 (17)[b]	D
6-Mercaptopurine	31	1[c]	D
Methotrexate	48	3 (7)	D
Thioguanine	6	1[c]	D
Total	153	37 (24)	
Alkylating agents			
Busulfan	28	3 (11)	C
Carmustine	1	0	C
Chlorambucil	5	3 (60)	D
Cyclophosphamide	18	4 (22)	D
Mechlorethamine	6	2 (33)	D
Total	58	12 (21)	
Antibiotics			
Dactinomycin	6	0	C
Daunorubicin	4	0	D
Doxorubicin	7	0	D
Bleomycin[15–17]	3	0	D
Total	20	0	D
Miscellaneous			
Cisplatinum[7,15–23]	10	0	D
Asparaginase	2	0	D
Procarbazine	4	2[c]	D
Vinblastine	3	1[c]	D
Vincristine	12	1[c]	D

[a] Summarized by Schardein et al.[10] Additional cases in the literature since their summary was published are added.
[b] This patient also received irradiation.
[c] Attributed to another drug.

and, while similar types of anomalies occur, the 7 percent frequency is much reduced.[10] The use of low dose methotrexate for systemic diseases (e.g., rheumatic disease and psoriasis) does not appear to produce teratogenicity.[11]

Alkylating Agents

The alkylating agents are a commonly used group of drugs for the management of malignancies. Unfortunately, most of the alkylating agents have demonstrated some teratogenic potential. Since these drugs are frequently given in combination with other nonalkylating agents, it is often difficult to identify the risk specific to the alkylating agent.

Because detailed ultrasonography may fail to identify subtle anatomic but serious functional abnormalities prior to 20 weeks' gestation, patients may want to consider the option of pregnancy termination if first trimester chemotherapy is planned or administered.

The risk of teratogenicity during the second and third trimesters is significantly reduced, possibly no different from that for pregnant women who are not exposed to chemotherapy.[4]

Antitumor Antibiotics

Even when administered in early pregnancy, antitumor antibodies appear to be associated with a low risk of teratogenicity. There is conflicting information in the literature as to whether the anthracyclines cross the placenta.[12–14] There is no evidence of bleomycin or dactinomycin teratogenicity.[15–17]

Vinca Alkaloids

Vincristine and vinblastine, while potent teratogens in animals, do not appear to be as teratogenic in humans. Of the two cases reported, other concurrent agents were thought to be more active in each.

Miscellaneous

Cisplatinum has been used in at least 10 pregnancies[7,15–23] without fetal malformation or toxicity. Henderson and colleagues[7] report bilateral sensorineural hearing loss at age 1 following in utero second trimester exposure to carboplatinum. However, there were other potential causes of the hearing loss in this patient, including prematurity, prior cisplatin exposure, and neonatal gentamicin. Procarbazine and asparginase have both been associated with subsequent fetal malformations.[4,9,24]

Combination Chemotherapy

There is no convincing evidence that there is a synergistic increase in malformations with the use of multiple agent regimens when compared with single agent therapy.[4,9]

National Registry

In 1985 the National Cancer Institute established a national registry for in utero exposure to chemotherapy.[25] The registry is currently located at the Pittsburgh Genetics Institute and is under the direction of Dr. John J. Mulvihill. Through June 1994 the registry had summaries of approximately 250 patients. Of the first 210 case studies there were 29 abnormal outcomes with a total of 52 defects. Only two abnormal outcomes were associated with exposure after the first trimester.

Delayed Effects

While second malignancies, impaired growth and development, intellectual impairment, and infertility have been reported after chemotherapy administration to children, the delayed effects of in utero exposure are less well documented.[6,26]

In summary, the risks of exposing a fetus to chemotherapy correlate highly with the gestational age at the time of the exposure. Most organogenesis occurs between 3 and 8 weeks of embryonic life, and it is during this time that major morphologic abnormalities are most likely to occur from exposure to any chemotherapeutic agent. Second and third trimester chemotherapy exposure does not appear to carry a significantly increased risk of major fetal anomalies.

Radiation, Diagnostic and Therapeutic

The potential for fetal injury arises from exposure to ionizing radiation, both the low dose diagnostic procedures and the more intense doses associated with radiation therapy. This subject is discussed in Chapter 8.

Surgery and Anesthesia, General Factors

While aspects of surgery are addressed below under the specific cancer sites, there are some general considerations worthy of review. Although complications of surgery can threaten the fetus, extraperitoneal surgery is not related to spontaneous abortion or preterm labor. Abdominal or pelvic surgery, if timing flexibility exists, is best performed in the second trimester to limit the risk of first trimester spontaneous abortion or preterm labor. In the first trimester, progesterone therapy is indicated (weeks 7 to 12) following a bilateral oophorectomy. Perioperative cautions include attention to the relative safety of all drugs administered. Fever secondary to either infection or atelectasis should be treated promptly since it may be associated with fetal abnormalities.

There is no evidence that there are significant risks of anesthesia independent of coexisting disease.[27] In the second and third trimesters careful attention to positioning is required so as to avoid vena cava compression from the enlarged uterus.

Pregnancy Following Cancer Treatment

With improved survival rates for many childhood and adolescent malignancies, one must be prepared to offer prenatal counseling to the young woman who presents with a personal cancer history. Issues worthy of review and in need of clarification for the obstetrician and the patient are listed in the box.

While previous abdominal irradiation for a Wilm's tumor appears to adversely affect the risk of pregnancy complications, including increased perinatal mortality,

---

Counseling Issues for Pregnancy Following Cancer Treatment

1. What is the risk of recurrence of the malignancy?
2. If a recurrence was diagnosed, depending on the most likely sites, what would be the nature of the probable treatment? How would such treatment compromise both the patient and the fetus?
3. Will prior treatments—pelvic surgery, radiation to pelvis or abdomen, or chemotherapy—affect fetility or reproductive outcome?
4. Will the hormonal milieu of pregnancy adversely affect an estrogen-receptor-positive tumor?

---

low birth weight, and abnormal pregnancy, a review of pregnancies following treatment for Hodgkin's lymphoma revealed no increased poor pregnancy outcome.[28] However, the rate of ovarian failure following the multiple drug combinations is over 50 percent in recent reports.[29] Also, a combination of pelvic irradiation and chemotherapy for Hodgkin's disease results in an even higher rate of ovarian failure.

Will a pregnancy increase the risk of recurrence or accelerate recurrence? Even in women with estrogen receptor-positive breast cancer, there is no evidence that pregnancy adversely affects survival. In addition to the altered hormonal milieu, concern is also directed toward the potential for accelerated tumor activity associated with alterations in the pregnant patient's immune system. There are no data to support this concern. Long-term follow-up studies of children with in utero exposure to antineoplastic agents have not demonstrated any impairment in growth, despite an increased frequency of intrauterine growth restriction.[6,26] In those children who have been tested for intellectual development, no impairment has been identified.[30]

Cancer During Pregnancy

General Considerations

The risk of having a coincident malignant tumor during pregnancy is approximately 0.1 percent. Approximately one-third of recorded maternal deaths are secondary to a coexisting malignancy. Delays in diagnosis of the cancer during pregnancy are common for a number of reasons: (1) many of the presenting symptoms of cancer are often attributed to the pregnancy; (2) many of the physiologic and anatomic alterations of pregnancy can compromise the physical examination; (3) many serum tumor markers (β-hCG, α-fetoprotein, CA 125, and others) are increased during pregnancy; and (4) our ability to perform either imaging studies or invasive diagnostic procedures is often altered during pregnancy.

Since the gestational age is significant when evaluating the risks of treatments, it is important to determine gestational age accurately. An ultrasound evaluation may be useful in this regard.

Breast Cancer

The predicted number of breast cancer cases in women in the United States for 1996 is 184,300, and the predicted number of related deaths is 44,300.[31] Approximately 2 to 3 percent of all breast cancers in women under age 40 occur concurrent with pregnancy or lactation, and approximately 1 in 1,360 to 3,330 pregnancies is complicated by breast cancer.[32] However, there may be an increase in the frequency of breast cancer complicating other forms of cancer due to delayed childbearing.[33]

In general, the risk of breast cancer is directly related to the duration of ovarian function. Therefore, both early menarche and late menopause appear to increase the likelihood of developing breast cancer. However, interruption of the normal cyclic ovarian function by pregnancy appears protective. This apparent protective effect may be secondary to the normal hormonal milieu of pregnancy that produces epithelial proliferation, followed by marked differentiation and mitotic rest. Multiparity and in particular multiparous patients who breast feed have a lower risk of developing breast cancer than does the nulliparous woman. Based on a recent study of almost 90,000 women, breast-feeding may not be an independent protective factor.[34]

Diagnosis and Staging

Breast abnormalities should be evaluated in the same manner as if the patient were not pregnant. The most common presentation of breast cancer in pregnancy is a painless lump discovered by the patient. Despite the striking physiologic breast changes of pregnancy, including nipple enlargement and increases in glandular tissue resulting in engorgement and tenderness, breast cancer should be screened for during pregnancy. Since the breast changes become more pronounced in later pregnancy, it is important to perform a thorough breast examination at the initial visit. Diagnostic delays are often attributed to physician reluctance to evaluate breast complaints or abnormal findings in pregnancy.[35] While bilateral serosanguinous discharge may be normal in late pregnancy, masses require prompt and definitive evaluation. The lengths of delays in diagnosis of breast cancer in pregnancy are commonly 3 to 7 months or longer.[36]

A case–control study from Princess Margaret Hospital suggested that pregnant patients are at higher risk of presenting with advanced disease because pregnancy impedes early detection.[37] Mammography in pregnancy is controversial. While the radiation exposure to the fetus is negligible,[38, 39] the hyperplastic breast of pregnancy is characterized by increased tissue density, making interpretation more difficult.[40]

Fine-needle aspiration (FNA) of a mass for cytologic study is recommended. FNA is reliable for a diagnosis of carcinoma (false-positive results are rare), but if a solid mass is negative for tumor it should be evaluated by excisional biopsy. Similar to the nonpregnant patient, approximately 20 percent of breast biopsies performed in pregnancy reveal cancer.[35] Tissue biopsies should be submitted for estrogen receptor (ER) and progesterone receptor (PR) analyses. Consistent with the fact that these patients are young, the majority are receptor negative.[41] There is concern that false-negative ER results performed by the ligand-binding method may occur in pregnancy because of either competitive inhibition by high levels of estrogens or by down regulation.[42] Immunologic assays that use monoclonal antibody recognize both occupied and unoccupied receptors and therefore may more accurately reflect the receptor status.

Prior to proceeding with treatment, the patient requires staging. All draining lymph nodes areas should be evaluated. The contralateral breast must be carefully assessed. Laboratory tests should include baseline liver function tests and serum tumor markers, carcinoembryonic antigen (CEA), and CA 15–3. A chest x-ray is indicated, and, if the liver function tests are abnormal, the liver can be evaluated by ultrasound. With precautions of good hydration and insertion of a urinary bladder catheter, a bone scan can be performed in pregnancy. However, in an asymptomatic patient with normal blood tests, the yield is low, and therefore it is not usually performed in those circumstances. In a symptomatic patient, radiographs of the specific symptomatic bones are advised.

While one report suggests an increased incidence of inflammatory breast cancer in pregnancy,[43] other reviews have not confirmed this observation, and it is generally thought that breast cancers in pregnancy are histologically identical to the nonpregnant patient of the same age. Because inflammatory breast cancer can be mistaken for mastitis, a biopsy of breast tissue should be performed when a breast suspected of being infected is incised and drained.

Treatment

The treatment of breast carcinoma at any time is often overshadowed by psychologic and emotional factors. Because of potential risks to the developing fetus, treatment decisions carry an additional burden. Patients with advanced disease and a poor prognosis may consider termination on this basis alone. Therapy, however, must be individualized in accordance with present knowledge and with the specific desires of the patient.

Local Therapy

The usual criteria for breast-preserving therapy versus modified radical mastectomy pertain to the patient with breast cancer, stages I to III.[44] However, the option of lumpectomy, axillary node dissection, and irradiation is complicated by the presence of the pregnancy. Consideration should be given to the delay of irradiation until after delivery. Experimetal calculations suggest that a tumor dose of 5,000 cGy will expose the fetus to 10 to 15 cGy while the fetus is within the true pelvis. Later in pregnancy parts of the fetus may receive as much as 200 cGy.[45] Brent[46] has suggested that 5 cGy is a relatively safe upper limit of fetal exposure. While the potential for teratogenesis is reduced later in pregnancy, radiation can affect fetal growth and may carry a risk for future carcinogenesis or secondary birth defects.

Pregnancy Termination

Since early studies suggested a poorer outcome in the pregnant patient, it was assumed that the hormonal changes of pregnancy contributed to rapid growth.

Therefore therapeutic abortion was frequently advised. At present, a harmful effect of continuing pregnancy has not been demonstrated in most published series (Table 36-3). However, it is difficult to evaluate the potential bias toward performing abortion in patients with advanced disease. Since young women tend to have hormone-receptor negative tumors,[47] it is difficult to make an argument, based on hormonal concerns, for either termination of pregnancy or oophorectomy as an adjunct to therapy.[48–50]

Patients who present with either metastatic breast carcinoma or rapidly progressive inflammatory carcinoma frequently elect pregnancy termination. In general, delays of therapy should be avoided, especially for the patient with inflammatory breast cancer. Immediate initiation of chemotherapy is critical to providing the patient with inflammatory carcinoma with any chance for long-term survival. In the patient with a clinical indication for adjuvant chemotherapy, other than inflammatory carcinoma, the delay of instituting chemotherapy and awaiting fetal pulmonary maturity should be considered in select third trimester situations.

Prognosis

As with any malignant disease, the prognosis best correlates with the anatomic extent of disease at the time of diagnosis. The presence and extent of nodal involvement is especially predictive of prognosis in both nonpregnant and pregnant patients. Table 36-4 provides 5- and 10-year survival data by nodal status.[35,43,48,51–55] While nodal status is of prognostic significance, the number of positive nodes is also important. In the pregnant patient, the 5-year survival rate is 82 percent for patients with three or fewer positive nodes and 27

Table 36-3   Survival from Breast Cancer in Patients Undergoing Therapeutic Abortion Compared to Those Not Undergoing Abortion

Authors	Delivered		Therapeautic Abortion		Comments
	No. Patients	5-Yr Survival	No. Patients	5-Yr Survival	
Adair (1953)	36	44	23	70	25 pregnant at diagnosis, 34 pregnant after treatment for cancer. Only node-positive patients benefited from abortion
Holleb and Farrow (1962)	12	33	12	17	Surgery during first trimester
Rissanen (1968)	20	50	7	43	4 patients (1 aborted; 3 delivered) were stage IV
Clark and Reid (1978)	93	29	13	15	12% spontaneous abortion; 1 stillbirth. Abortion was not biased for more advanced disease
King et al. (1985)	35	67	18	53	For stage I patients: delivery vs. abortion: 18 vs. 4 patients; 5-year survival is 88% vs. 33%

(Modified from Holmes,[197] with permission.)

Table 36-4 5- and 10-Year Survival Rates, by Nodal Status, of Pregnant or Lactating Patients Treated for Breast Cancer

Investigators	No. Patients	Overall		Node Negative		Node Positive	
		5-Yr (%)	10-Yr (%)	5-Yr (%)	10-Yr (%)	5-Yr (%)	10-Yr (%)
White and White[51]	806	13	9	21	13	7	6
Holleb and Farrow[48]	117	31	—	65	—	17	—
Byrd et al.[35]	29	55	—	100	80	28	6
Applewhite et al.[36]	48	25	15	56	22	18	13
Riberio and Palmer[53]	59	31	24	90	90	37	21
Clark et al.[54]							
Pregnant	121	—	22	—	35	—	22
Lactating	80	—	32	—	69	—	18
King et al.[43]	63	53	49	82	71	36	36
Petrek[55]	56	61	45	82	77	47	25

percent if greater than three nodes contain tumor.[43] Pregnancy, probably due to the associated delays in diagnosis, appears to increase the frequency of nodal disease, with 60 to 85 percent of patients exhibiting axillary nodal disease at diagnosis.[43,56]

When controlled for age and stage, pregnancy does not seem to affect prognosis adversely.[37,55,57,58] Some have suggested a worse prognosis if the cancer is diagnosed in the second trimester.[57]

Subsequent Pregnancy

While the general consensus is that subsequent pregnancies do not adversely affect survival, there are recommendations regarding the timing of a subsequent pregnancy.[59] It is generally advised that women with node-negative disease wait for 2 to 3 years, and this interval should be extended to 5 years for patients with positive nodes. Others have advised that no delay is indicated for the patient with good prognostic disease who does not receive postoperative adjuvant chemotherapy.[60] It has been advised that patients should undergo a complete metastatic work-up prior to a subsequent pregnancy.

While no studies indicate that subsequent pregnancy adversely affects survival, the retrospective reports that suggest a potential favorable affect of subsequent pregnancy are too small to draw firm conclusions.[57,61] The trend to better survival is also noted in patients who received adjuvant chemotherapy and subsequently became pregnant.[62]

Lactation and Breast Reconstruction

Lactation is possible in a small percentage of patients after breast-conserving therapy for early stage breast cancer.[63,64] Lumpectomy using a radial incision rather than the cosmetically preferred circumareolar incision is less likely to disrupt ductal anatomy. Disruption of the ductal system may increase the rate of mastitis. Breast-feeding is contraindicated in women receiving chemotherapy since significant levels can be found in breast milk.

Breast reconstruction with the use of autologous tissue has increased secondary to questions about the use of silicone-filled implants. The transverse rectus myocutaneous flap (TRAM) is one popular method of breast reconstruction. Since the donor site is a portion of the anterior abdominal wall, there is potential concern when the patient develops abdominal distention from pregnancy. In one case report and review of the literature nine cases of pregnancy following breast reconstruction experienced no problem with anterior abdominal wall integrity.[65]

Hodgkin's Disease and Non-Hodgkin's Lymphoma

Hodgkin's Disease

Hodgkin's disease, commonly encountered in patients in their late teens and twenties, occurs at a mean age of 32 years. Non-Hodgkin's lymphomas occur at a mean age of 42 and therefore are reported less frequently in association with pregnancy. Lymphomas complicate approximately 1 in 6,000 pregnancies. Spontaneous abortion, stillbirth rates, and preterm births do not appear to be increased.[66,67] A retrospective cohort study supports the conclusions from earlier small series that pregnancy does not appear to affect adversely the course of the disease.[68] Routine termination of pregnancy should not be advised. While some advocate therapeutic abortion for the patient with a first trimester pregnancy and Hodgkin's disease to allow complete staging, others, probably more appropriately, have limited the role of therapeutic abortion to those women requiring infradiaphragmatic irradiation or those with systemic symptoms or visceral disease, which are best managed with multiagent chemotherapy.

Hodgkin's disease frequently presents with enlarged cervical or axillary lymph nodes. The diagnosis is established by biopsy of the suspicious nodes. The presence of systemic symptoms such as night sweats, pruritis, or weight loss suggests more extensive disease. Two histologic variants, nodular sclerosis and lymphocyte predominant, have a better prognosis than mixed cellularity and lymphocyte-depleted tumors.

Clinical staging for lymphoma necessitates the systemic evaluation by history, laboratory findings, bone marrow, and radiographic imaging. Clinical treatment and staging should be individualized. Pathologic staging for Hodgkin's disease may involve laparotomy and splenectomy; however, this is not usually necessary for non-Hodgkin's lymphoma, as disseminated disease can usually be documented without surgery. The minimal staging for Hodgkin's disease during pregnancy includes roentgenographic examination of the chest, liver function tests, bone marrow biopsy, complete blood count, and urinalysis. Chest tomography or computed tomography (CT) scan of the mediastinum may be necessary to evaluate nodal enlargement in the chest. Evaluation of the abdomen is compromised by the gravid uterus, and some consideration should be given to delaying abdominal imaging until after the first trimester. Magnetic resonance imaging (MRI) may be the safest technique for demonstrating intra-abdominal adenopathy. Isotope scans of the liver and bone are best avoided during pregnancy. A single shot lymphangiogram results in an exposure of less than 1 rad to the fetus and is probably safe after the first trimester.[69] Ultrasonography is safe and may provide useful information.

Disease stage (Table 36-5) is the most important fac-

tor in treatment planning and prognosis. Survival for early-stage Hodgkin's disease exceeds 90 percent, whereas patients with disseminated nodal disease have a 5-year survival rate of about 50 percent. As expected, patients with stage IV disease have poor survival rates. While radiation therapy is the mainstay of treatment for early- stage Hodgkin's disease, combination chemotherapy is employed for the treatment of advanced stage disease with organ involvement. The MOPP regimen (nitrogen mustard, vincristine, procarbazine, and prednisone) in combination with radiation is often used to treat patients with bulky, large mediastinal masses or disseminated nodal disease. Most investigators agree that treatment should not be withheld during pregnancy except in early stage disease, particularly if the diagnosis is made in late gestation. Radiotherapy to the supradiaphragmatic regions may be performed with abdominal shielding after the first trimester. Thomas and Peckham[69] reported three cases of mantle field irradiation with abdominal shielding for supradiaphragmatic disease. The estimated radiation exposures to the fetus for these patients at 10, 15, and 16 weeks were 2.5, 4.4, and 10.4 rad, respectively. While these pregnancies went to term with apparent normal outcomes, long-term follow-up on these infants was not presented. Spontaneous abortion has been reported with an estimated first trimester fetal dose of 9 rad secondary to scatter from delivering 4,400 rad to the chest of a patient receiving treatment for a recurrence.[70] Another patient in the same report received 3,300 rad to a mantle field at 16 weeks' gestation, and no adverse affects were noted. In general, if the estimated exposure to a first trimester fetus is expected to exceed 10 rads or if combination chemotherapy is planned for the first trimester, therapeutic abortion should be considered because of the risk of fetal malformation.[71] Asymptomatic early stage disease presenting in the second half of pregnancy may be followed closely while preparations are made for early delivery.[70] The use of steroids and single agent chemotherapy has been proposed for the patient with systemic symptoms.

Subdiaphragmatic or advanced disease requires chemotherapy. Since many of the most commonly used chemotherapeutic agents are known teratogens, such treatment is best avoided in the first trimester. Similar treatments should also be approached with caution later in pregnancy, although most case reports have documented only intrauterine growth restriction and neonatal neutropenia as complications. Long-term follow-up toxicity studies are lacking.

Following therapy for Hodgkin's disease, it has been suggested that pregnancy planning should take into consideration that about 80 percent of recurrences will manifest within 2 years. Treatments for Hodgkin's dis-

Table 36-5   Staging Classification of Hodgkin's Disease[a]

Stage	Description
I	Involvement of a single lymph node region (I) or of a single extralymphatic organ site (I_E)
II	Involvement of two or more lymph node regions on the same side of the diaphragm (II) or localized involvement of an extralymphatic organ site and of one or more lymph node regions on the same side of the diaphragm (II_E)
III	Involvement of lymph node regions on both sides of the diaphragm (III), which also may be accompanied by localized involvement of an extralymphatic organ or site (III_E), of the spleen (III_S), or of both (III_{SE})
IV	Diffuse or disseminated involvement of an extralymphatic organ with or without localized lmph node involvement (liver, bone marrow, lung, skin)

[a] Symptoms of unexplained fever, night sweats, and unexplained weight loss of 10 percent of normal body weight results in classification of patients as B; absence of these symptoms is denoted as a A.

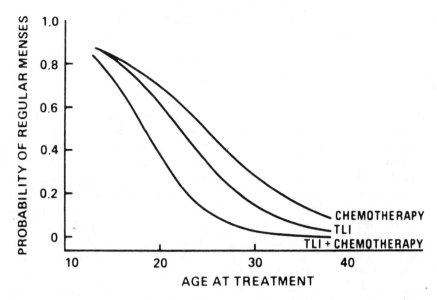

Fig. 36-1 Probability of regular menses after chemotherapy, total lymphoid irradiation (TLI), and TLI and chemotherapy in patients with Hodgkin's disease. The synergistic effect is more apparent in younger women. (From Horning et al,[73] with permission.)

ease may compromise the reproductive potential of young patients.[29,72]

As reflected in Figure 36-1, ovarian failure is more likely to occur in older patients, even if treated with fewer courses of chemotherapy.[73] Some studies have reported a rate of only 12 percent of normal ovarian function following therapy for Hodgkin's disease.[74] Combined treatment with irradiation and chemotherapy provides the highest risk of ovarian failure.

Bilateral midline oophoropexy at staging laparotomy has been advocated for the patient requiring pelvic node irradiation.[73] Even with this technique the ovaries may be exposed to a significant dose of irradiation, ranging from 600 to 3,500 rad.[69] Additionally, there are concerns of adhesions and ovum pick-up and transport. While combined oral contraceptives have been advocated to preserve ovarian function, there is no evidence that the gonads are protected.[75] Depending on their availability, new reproductive technologies, including oocyte donation and embryo cryopreservation, can be considered for select situations.[76]

In patients who are able to become pregnant after treatment for Hodgkin's lymphoma, there does not appear to be an increase in adverse perinatal outcomes such as fetal wastage, term birth, and birth defects when compared with sibling controls.[77,78] While fetal anomalies have occurred after treatment for Hodgkin's disease,[79] chromosomal abnormalities or a new gene mutation have not been diagnosed.[72] The absence of a repetitive pattern of malformations makes it difficult to imply a casual relationship between any birth defects observed and previous therapy for Hodgkin's disease.

Non-Hodgkin's Lymphoma

Non-Hodgkin's lymphoma occurs at a mean age of 42 years and therefore is reported less frequently than Hodgkin's disease in association with pregnancy. In general, non-Hodgkin's disease is more likely to affect a pregnancy adversely because patients usually have an aggressive histology and advanced stage disease. Burkitt's lymphoma is usually rapidly progressive and may involve the breast and ovary. Lymphoma of the breast has a particularly poor prognosis, and it has been speculated that there may be a hormonal influence on this malignancy in pregnant patients.[80]

In a report by Ward and Weiss,[81] over 70 percent (15 of 21) of second and third trimester cases resulted in surviving infants. The perinatal mortality rate associated with patients who were either not treated or treated by surgery was almost 40 percent (5 of 13), while almost 90 percent (7 of 8) of infants of mothers treated by chemotherapy survived. Of the mothers treated with chemotherapy, 50 percent (4 of 8) survived. Of the 13 patients who were not treated or who were treated with surgical resection, 5 (38 percent) survived. The nature of the presenting disease probably played a preselection role regarding the treatments. Including additional, more recent, reports, it is evident that about 60 to 70 percent of patients and about 75 percent of infants survive.

Adult T cell leukemia/lymphoma, caused by the human T cell lymphotropic virus type I, is found in Japan, the Caribbean, and the southern United States. The virus is present in familial clusters and is transmitted by sexual intercourse, blood transfusions, and breast milk. Infants seroconvert between 12 and 19 months of age at a rate of 20 to 25 percent.[82,83]

Acute Leukemia

While the incidence of leukemia in pregnancy is not specifically known, it is estimated to occur in less than 1 in 75,000 pregnancies. Acute leukemia represents about 90 percent of leukemias coexisting with pregnancy. Acute myeloid leukemia accounts for about 60 percent and acute lymphoblastic leukemia (ALL) for about 30 percent of cases. Over three-fourths of the cases are diagnosed after the first trimester.[6,84]

The prognosis for acute leukemia in pregnancy is guarded.[6,84–87] In adults, acute leukemia in the non-pregnant patient, if untreated, has a median survival of about 2 months.[88] In the treated patient, the median survival is between 1 and 2 years. Immediate and aggressive therapeutic intervention will yield complete remission rates of about 75 percent, and 40 percent of these are sustained. While there is no evidence that pregnancy adversely affects the prognosis of acute leukemia, it is noted that a 1987 report identified a median survival of 16 months in the pregnant patient,[6] and another study in 1988 reported a median survival of 27.5 months in a nonpregnant population.[89] However, the differences in patient populations (the latter study was a report on the more favorable ALL) and the varied treatments precludes any reliable comparison.[88] Optimal care of the pregnant patient with acute leukemia necessitates a team effort and is best achieved in a cancer referral center.

The diagnosis of acute leukemia is rarely difficult. The signs and symptoms of anemia, granulocytopenia, and thrombocytopenia, including fatigue, fever, infection, and easy bleeding or petechiae, usually prompt a complete blood count. A normal or elevated white blood cell count is present in up to 90 percent of patients with ALL. Counts in excess of 50,000 are found in only one-fourth of patients. In contrast, patients with acute nonlymphocytic leukemia (ANLL) may present with markedly elevated white blood cell counts, although one-third will present with leukopenia.[90] The diagnosis of leukemia should be confirmed by bone marrow biopsy and aspirate. The biopsy material is usually hypercellular with leukemic cells. The smear of the aspirate reveals decreased erythocyte and granulocytic precursors as well as megakaryocytes. Leukemic cells comprise greater than one-half of the marrow's cellular elements in most patients. The morphology of the marrow and the peripheral leukemic cells help to distinguish between lymphocytic and nonlymphocytic leukemias. This latter group includes acute myelocytic (granulocytic), promyelocytic, monocytic, and myelo-

monocytic leukemias, and erythroleukemia. Acute myelocytic leukemia is the most common form of ANLL. Patients who develop ANLL as a result of previous chemotherapy have a particularly poor response to treatment.

There are numerous reports of successful pregnancies in patients aggressively treated with combination chemotherapy for acute leukemia. Acute leukemia and its therapy are associated with an increase in stillbirths (approximately 15 percent), prematurity (approximately 50 percent), and growth restriction.[85,88] In 1988 and 1991, reports by Aviles and colleagues,[30,91] no serious long-term effects of in utero exposure to chemotherapy were reported. The first report included 17 children, aged 4 to 22, whose mothers received treatment for acute leukemia.[91] In the second report, 43 children who were born to mothers with a variety of hematologic malignancies were examined at 3 to 19 years of age.[30] In both studies, greater than 40 percent of the cases involved exposure during the first trimester.

If the mother is exposed to cytotoxic drugs within 1 month of delivery, the newborn should be monitored closely for evidence of granulocytopenia or thrombocytopenia.

Chronic Leukemia

Chronic leukemia accounts for approximately 10 percent of cases of leukemia during pregnancy, with the majority of these being patients with chronic myelocytic leukemia (CML).[88] Chronic lymphocytic leukemia has a median age of onset of about 60 years, making cases during pregnancy rare. The median age of patients with CML is 35 years. CML is characterized by excessive production of mature myeloid cell elements, with granulocyte counts averaging 200,000/dl. Most patients have thrombocytosis and a mild normochromic normocytic anemia. Platelet function is often abnormal, although hemorrhage is usually limited to patients with marked thrombocytopenia. CML tends to be indolent, and normal hematopoiesis is only mildly affected in the early stages of disease. Therefore, delay of aggressive treatment is a more feasible option than with acute leukemia. Unless complications such as severe systemic symptoms, autoimmune hemolytic anemia, recurrent infection, or symptomatic lymphatic enlargement occur, treatment for chronic leukemia should be withheld until after delivery. Therapy, when necessary, usually includes prednisone and an alkylating agent such as chlorambucil or cyclophosphamide. High dose steroids alone may be used to treat autoimmune hemolytic anemia. Currently, the median survival for CML is over 60 months, with survivals up to 10 years common.

Often, the diagnosis of CML antedates the pregnancy. While pregnancy does not appear to affect CML adversely, therapy does increase the frequency of preterm birth and low birth weight. Information about contemporary management and prognosis is scarce secondary to the fact that few recent cases of CML during pregnancy have been reported. There are reports of CML treatment with leukapheresis during pregnancy. This treatment appears to be both safe and effective. Leukapheresis results in improvement of blood counts, systemic symptoms, and splenomegaly. Also, this treatment, although costly and involved, offers less risk of teratogenesis than cytotoxic treatments.[84,92] Other treatment regimens reported include biologic modifiers, such as α-interferon[93,94] and hydroxyurea.[94–97]

Hairy cell leukemia during pregnancy is rare, with only six reported cases. A predilection for men and the older age groups is the reason for the infrequency. α-Interferon treatment has been used in two cases with no adverse fetal effects.[93]

Melanoma

The incidence of malignant melanoma is increasing in the childbearing years, and it is estimated that 1 percent of the population will develop this disease.[98] Since the median age at onset is approximately 50 years, the disease is relatively uncommon. However, one study reported malignant melanoma in 2.8 per 1,000 deliveries.[99] The understanding of the natural history of melanoma has been advanced by the identification of prognostic variables.[100] Prognostic features of the primary tumor include tumor thickness, Clark's level of invasion, Breslow's modifications, and Chung's modifications (Fig. 36-2), ulceration, and body location.

A topic of continued debate is whether pregnancy exerts a negative effect on the course of malignant melanoma. Reports from the 1950s suggested that melanoma arising during pregnancy is associated with an aggressive clinical course.[101,102] Subsequent reports, some being controlled studies, suggest melanoma diagnosed during pregnancy is more likely to be diagnosed at an advanced stage.[103–105] Most of the more recent studies are limited to patients with stage I disease and thus do not address this issue.[106,107] While many studies suggest that melanoma developing during pregnancy is more likely to appear in locations associated with a poor prognosis,[103–107] others show no increase in poor prognostic location of lesions in the pregnant patient.[108,109]

The World Health Organization (WHO) 1991 study examined the relevant prognostic features of melanoma in the childbearing years and in pregnancy.[107] This report suggested that patients who were diagnosed during pregnancy had tumors demonstrating

Table 36-6 WHO Stages I and II Study of Malignant Melanoma

Relationship to Time of Pregnancy	No. of Patients	Mean Tumor Thickness (mm)
Before	85	1.29
During	92	2.38[a]
After all	143	1.96
Between	68	1.78

[a] $p < 0.004$. When corrected for tumor thickness, survival rates were not different. Multivariate analysis identified tumor thickness as an independent prognostic variable, not pregnancy.

significantly greater tumor thickness (Table 36-6). However, after correcting for tumor thickness, survival rates were similar. Additional studies from Massachusetts General Hospital and Duke University have supported the observation of greater tumor thickness in patients diagnosed during pregnancy (Table 36-7). Other investigators have found no difference in lesion thickness in pregnancy.[110] The issue remains unsettled, and explanations for the increased tumor thickness include hormonal stimulation, growth factor stimulation, immunologic alterations of pregnancy, and delays in diagnosis. Delays in diagnosis are understandable since it is not uncommon for pigmentation changes to take place during pregnancy. Therefore, tissue sampling is often delayed secondary to abnormalities being dismissed as a normal change of pregnancy.

Surgery remains the most effective modality for the treatment of melanoma. For patients with stage I or II tumors, the standard surgical excision with margins appropriate for tumor thickness should be performed. Regional lymph node dissection can be done in the patient with regional (stage III) disease. Since adjuvant chemotherapy is experimental and has not demonstrated improved survival, it is not recommended for the pregnant patient because of the potential risk to the fetus. Adjuvant interferon and vaccines for the nonpregnant patient are also under evaluation. These treatments hold more promise for the pregnant patient, based on fetal considerations. Advanced metastatic disease carries a poor prognosis. Since chemotherapy with dacarbazine results in a clinical response, usually of short duration, in no more than 30 percent of patients, it is usually most appropriate to plan for

Table 36-7 Primary Melanoma Tumor Thickness in Pregnant and Nonpregnant Patients

Study	Tumor Thickness (mm)		p Value
	Pregnant	Nonpregnant	
Singluff et al.[109]	2.7	1.5	0.052
MacKie et al.[107]	2.3	1.7	0.002
Travers et al.[198]	2.3	1.2	0.0001

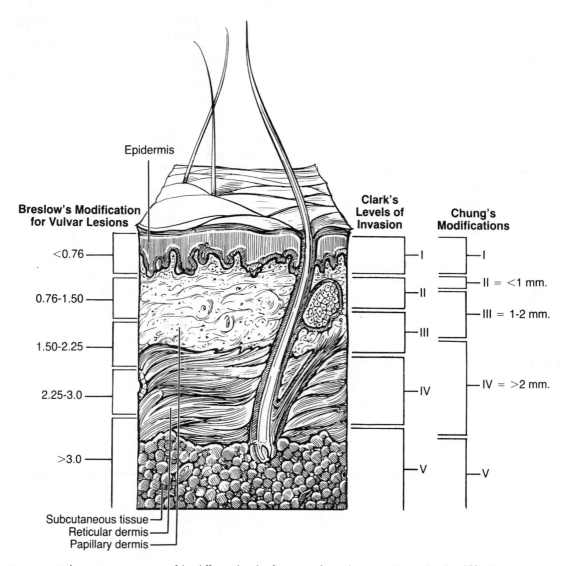

Epidermis

**Breslow's Modification
for Vulvar Lesions**

**Clark's
Levels of
Invasion**

**Chung's
Modifications**

<0.76 — I — I

0.76-1.50 — II — II = <1 mm.

1.50-2.25 — III — III = 1-2 mm.

2.25-3.0 — IV — IV = >2 mm.

>3.0 — V — V

Subcutaneous tissue
Reticular dermis
Papillary dermis

Fig. 36-2 Schematic comparison of the different levels of invasion for melanoma. (From Gordon,[199] with permission.)

early delivery in cases of disseminated disease presenting late in pregnancy.

Is there a role for therapeutic abortion? Despite rare reports of regression after delivery, no studies support any therapeutic benefit associated with therapeutic abortion.[111,112] However, given the aggressive nature of the current therapies available for metastatic disease, it is not inappropriate to consider abortion when managing advanced disease presenting in the first trimester.[112]

The patient who has undergone apparent successful treatment for a malignant melanoma may express concern about the safety of a future pregnancy. No adverse impact on recurrence or survival has been identified in the majority of the literature on this issue.[104,107,108] However, the timing of the subsequent pregnancy deserves some consideration. The probability of survival of a specific cancer should be evaluated based on the known prognostic variables. The 5-year survival rate for the patient with a melanoma less than 1.5 mm thick is 90 percent. For a tumor of intermediate thickness (1.5 to 4 mm) the 5-year survival rate is 50 to 75 percent, and for a more deeply invasive tumor survival is less than 50 percent. While some report that approximately 60 to 70 percent of patients will develop their recurrence within 2 years and 80 to 90 percent within 5 years, the WHO study claimed that 83 percent of recurrences develop within the first 2 years.[112] Based on this information, it is generally recommended that patients wait 2 to 3 years before attempting another pregnancy, especially with nodal disease.[107] There are insufficient data on the select group of patients who develop their initial melanoma during pregnancy to make recommendations regarding the safety of a subsequent pregnancy.

Another issue of concern is which form of birth control should be used. The use of oral contraceptives has not been demonstrated to affect adversely the natural history of a previously treated melanoma.[113,114]

Cervical Cancer

Approximately 3 percent of all invasive cervical cancers occur during pregnancy. Cervical cancer is the most common gynecologic malignancy associated with pregnancy, occurring in approximately 1 per 2,200 pregnancies.[115–117]

However, the true incidence is difficult to ascertain due to the reporting biases associated with the reports originating from large referral centers. Also various reports may include patients who have preinvasive lesions as well as patients who are diagnosed postpartum.

All pregnant patients should be evaluated on their initial obstetric visit with visualization of the cervix and cervical cytology, including an endocervical brush. The general principles of screening for cervical neoplasia apply to the pregnant patient. The Papanicolaou smear is used to screen the normal-appearing cervix. If the cervix appears friable, cervical cytology alone may not be sufficient to alert the physician to the presence of a malignant tumor. False-negative cervical cytology is at increased risk in pregnancy due to excess mucous and bleeding from cervical eversion. Therefore it is necessary to obtain a biopsy to ensure that tissue friability is not secondary to tumor. Also, an ulcerative or exophytic lesion must have histologic sampling performed. While approximately one-third of pregnant patients with cervical cancer are asymptomatic at the time of diagnosis, the most common symptoms are vaginal bleeding or discharge. Evaluation for the possibility of neoplastic disease of the lower genital tract is required in the evaluation of vaginal bleeding in the pregnant as well as the nonpregnant patient.

Considering the routine practice of performing cervical cytology in early pregnancy, one would expect there to be a preponderance of early stage disease diagnosed in the first trimester. Surprisingly, this is not the situation. The diagnosis of cervical cancer is commonly made postpartum rather than during pregnancy and, while stage IB disease is the most commonly diagnosed stage, all stages are represented in significant numbers. Both patient and physician factors, including lack of prenatal care, failure to obtain cervical cytology or to biopsy gross cervical abnormalities, false-negative cytology, and failure to evaluate abnormal cytology or vaginal bleeding properly, contribute to the delays in diagnosis. Unfortunately, the complaint of spotting or bleeding during pregnancy is common and usually secondary to pregnancy-related conditions.

Cervical cytology suggestive of a squamous intraepithelial lesion or a report of atypical glandular cells during pregnancy requires appropriate clinical evaluation (Fig. 36-3). The colposcopic evaluation of the pregnant cervix is altered by the physiologic changes of pregnancy, and, since most practicing physicians will diagnose invasive cervical cancer associated with pregnancy only once or twice in their careers, it may be prudent to consult a gynecologic oncologist. While colposcopy during pregnancy is usually enhanced by the physiologic eversion of the lower endocervical canal, vascular changes and redundant vagina may alter or obscure normal visualization. During pregnancy, failure to visualize the entire transformation zone and squamocolumnar junction is uncommon. While endocervical curettage is not generally recommended during pregnancy, lesions involving the lower endocervical canal can often be directly visualized and biopsied. While the pregnant cervix is hypervascular, serious hemorrhage from an out-patient biopsy is uncommon, and the risk of bleeding is offset by the risk of missing an early invasive cancer. Following a coloposcopic evaluation with appropriate tissue sampling, most patients with preinvasive lesions can be followed with repeat colposcopy at 6- to 8-week intervals to delivery.[118,119]

Patients then require a careful and complete colposcopic evaluation 6 weeks' postpartum. Cone biopsy during pregnancy, when necessary, should ideally be performed during the second trimester to reduce the risks of first trimester abortion and rupture of membranes or premature labor in the third trimester.[120–122] Complications from conization of the pregnant cervix are common Therapeutic conization for intraepithelial squamous lesions is contraindicated during pregnancy. Diagnostic cone biopsy in pregnancy is reserved for patients whose colposcopic-directed biopsy has shown superficial invasion (suspect microinvasion) or in other situations where an invasive lesion is suspected but cannot be confirmed by biopsy. When a cone biopsy is necessary during pregnancy, one should keep in mind the anatomic alteration of the cervix secondary to pregnancy. A shallow disk-like cone is usually satisfactory to clarify the diagnosis with a minimum of morbidity. It should be kept in mind that patients who have had a conization during pregnancy are at higher risk for residual disease. Therefore close follow-up is essential.

Following the diagnosis of invasive cervical cancer, a staging evaluation is indicated. The standard cervical staging is clinical and usually based on the results of physical examination, cystoscopy, proctoscopy, chest x-ray, and intravenous pyelogram. CT or, in some centers, lymphangiography is often performed to identify lymph node metastasis. In the pregnant patient the standard staging evaluation is modified. The chest radiograph is performed with abdominal shielding. Sonography is used to detect hydronephrosis, and, if additional retroperitoneal imaging is desired for the

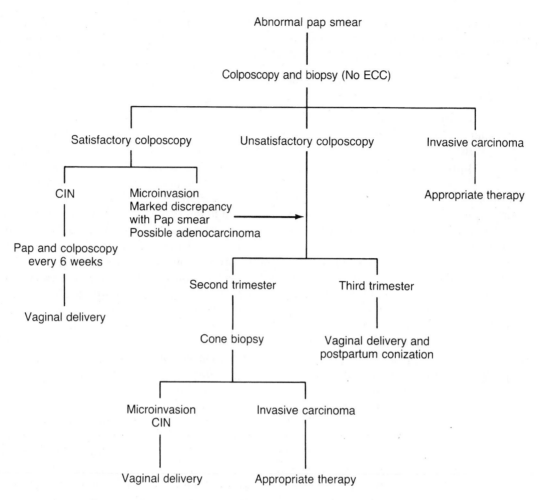

Fig. 36-3 Suggested protocol for evaluation of abnormal cervical cytology in pregnancy. ECC, endocervical curettage. CIN, cervical intraepithelial neoplasia (From Hacker et al,[115] with permission.)

Microinvasion

In patients with a microinvasive squamous carcinoma with negative margins on cone biopsy, consideration can be given to conservative management until delivery. The risk of occult metastatic disease is predominantly dependent on two pathologic features: (1) the depth of invasion and (2) the presence or absence of lymphovascular space involvement.[123] Whether the cone biopsy can be considered sufficient long-term therapy or whether a postpartum hysterectomy with or without lymphadenectomy should be performed is also based on the detailed analysis of the pathologic features of the cone biopsy. In these cases, consultation with a gynecologic oncologist is appropriate.

Before evaluation of lymphadenopathy, consideration should be given to using magnetic resonance imaging (MRI). While the use of MRI during pregnancy is not approved, there have been no reported sequelae and the theoretical risks are less than the risks associated with ionizing radiation techniques.

Invasive, Early Stage Disease

Since the definitive treatment of invasive cervical cancer is not compatible with pregnancy continuation, the clinical question that must be addressed is when to conclude the pregnancy so that therapy can be completed. Considering this requirement, treatment options will be influenced by gestational age, tumor stage and metastatic evaluation, and maternal desires and expectations regarding the pregnancy. The management of early invasive cervical cancer (stages IB and IIA) in the young patient is usually by radical hysterectomy, pelvic lymphadenectomy, and aortic lymph node sampling.[124] The primary advantage over radiation therapy for these patients is preservation of ovarian function. For the patient with a high probability of having a poor prognostic lesion and therefore requiring postoperative irradiation, consideration can be given to performing a unilateral or bilateral oophoropexy at the time of the hysterectomy. The ovarian suspension should be intraperitoneal, as retroperitoneal placement seems to predispose to subsequent ovarian cyst formation. In the first trimester this surgery is usually carried out with the fetus in utero. In the third trimester the radical hysterectomy and pelvic lymphadenectomy are performed after completion of a high classic cesarean delivery. Delays in therapeutic intervention have not been reported to increase recurrence rates for patients with small-volume stage I disease.[125] While the pelvic vessels are large, the dissection is enhanced by more easily defined tissue planes.[126,127]

Second trimester situations are more problematic. Serious consideration should be given to administering one to three cycles of platinum-based chemotherapy and thereby allowing an additional 7 to 15 weeks of fetal maturation. In one study, maturation from the 26 to 27 weeks' gestation compared with 34 to 35 weeks increased fetal viability from 67 to 97 percent.[128] The neoadjuvant chemotherapy approach (chemotherapy prior to either surgery or irradiation) would unlikely compromise and may enhance the overall efficacy of treatment. Also, having passed the primary interval of organogenesis, it is unlikely that serious fetal sequelae will occur secondary to the chemotherapy. Certainly in terms of general fetal salvage and outcome, the risk of extreme prematurity would far outweigh the risk of the chemotherapy exposure. While this management of second trimester cervical cancer presentations seems logical, there is scant information about this treatment approach. However, neoadjuvant chemotherapy with platinum-based chemotherapy for ovarian cancers has been reported with no fetal sequelae identified.[17,19]

Invasive, Locally Advanced Disease

The management of the patient with more advanced local disease is based on treatment with irradiation, both external beam to treat the regional nodes and shrink the central tumor and brachytherapy to complete the delivery of a tumoricidal dose to the cervix and adjacent tissues.[124] Coordinating a radiation treatment plan for pregnant patients with stages IIB, stage III, and stage IVA is challenging. The patient with a first trimester pregnancy can usually be treated in the standard fashion with initiation of external therapy to the pelvis or extended field, as dictated by standard treatment guidelines. Most of these patients will proceed to abort spontaneously within 2 to 5 weeks of initiating the radiation. Patients in the late first trimester are least likely to abort spontaneously, and it may be necessary to perform a uterine evacuation on the completion of external therapy in some patients. Following either spontaneous abortion or uterine evacuation, the brachytherapy component of the radiation therapy can proceed in the standard fashion. Patients in either their second or third trimester should have a high classical cesarean delivery prior to starting standard irradiation.

Again, it would seem appropriate to strongly consider neoadjuvant chemotherapy for this group of patients, especially the patient with a second trimester or early third trimester presentation, when the opportunity for fetal maturation could be provided.

Invasive, Distant Metastasis

Metastatic disease to extrapelvic sites carries a poor prognosis. While a select few patients with aortic node metastasis may receive curative therapy, it is unlikely for the patient with pulmonary metastasis, bone metastasis, or supraclavicular lymph node metastasis to be cured. Personal patient choices and ethical considerations will be the major factors guiding treatment in these situations.

Small cell neuroendocrine tumors of the cervix associated with pregnancy are rare. Neoadjuvant or adjuvant chemotherapy with cisplatin, etoposide, and doxorubicin is recommended.[129]

Method of Delivery

Controversy continues to surround the issue of the method of delivery for the term patient with cervical cancer. It seems heroic and unjustifiably risky to encourage vaginal delivery of a patient with a large, firm, barrell-shaped tumor or a large friable and hemorrhagic exophytic tumor. However, many small-volume stage IB, IIA, and early IIB tumors are potential candidates for vaginal delivery. Whether vaginal delivery promotes systemic dissemination of tumor cells is unknown. While the general opinion is that survival rates are not influenced by the mode of delivery,[115,138] a recent multivariate analysis "showed a possible trend ($p = 0.08$) toward a negative outcome after vaginal delivery."[117]

Although systemic tumor dissemination secondary to vaginal delivery has not been documented, there are reports of episiotomy implants for both squamous carcinoma and adenocarcinoma following vaginal delivery.[131-133] Episiotomy implants are sufficiently rare that the risk should not be a determining factor for a given patient. However, the episiotomy should be carefully followed in a cervical cancer patient who delivers vaginally. Episiotomy nodules in these patients must be promptly evaluated by biopsy, as an early diagnosis may permit curative therapy.[131] Diagnostic delays secondary to suspicion of the nodules representing stitch abscess should be avoided.

Survival

While some authors have suggested that the survival of patients with cervical cancer associated with pregnancy is compromised,[134] most reports indicate that the prognosis is not altered.[115-117,134]

Ovarian Cancer

With the increased use of diagnostic ultrasound, ovarian cysts and masses are more frequently encountered in early pregnancy.[135] While adnexal masses are frequently encountered in pregnancy, only 2 to 5 percent are malignant ovarian tumors.[136,137] Ovarian cancer occurs in approximately 1 in 18,000 to 1 in 47,000 pregnancies.[138,139]

While the three major categories of ovarian tumors—epithelial, germ cell, and stromal—occur during pregnancy, there is a disproportionate number of patients with germ cell tumors compared with the nonpregnant patient. A review of the literature since 1984 reveals 40 patients having malignant primary ovarian tumors during pregnancy. Germ cell tumors account for 45 percent (Fig. 36-4); 37.5 percent are epithelial tumors, 10 percent are stromal tumors, and 7.5 percent are categorized as miscellaneous. This distribution is undoubtedly skewed by the reporting bias associated with rare tumors. Characteristic of epithelial tumors in young patients who are not pregnant, the majority of epithelial ovarian tumors complicating pregnancy are of low grade (grade 1 or low malignant potential) or early stage, not uncommonly both low grade and stage I.

Management of the adnexal mass in pregnancy is the subject of some controversy. The risks of surgical intervention may favor a conservative approach.[140] Serial sonograms may be of some value in determining the nature and biologic potential of the tumor. If the clinical presentation is consistent with torsion, rupture, or hemorrhage, immediate surgical intervention is indicated. Prompt surgical exploration is also performed for the mass associated with ascites or when there is

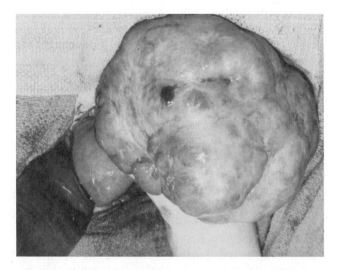

Fig. 36-4 Dysgerminoma, the most common malignant ovarian neoplasm found in pregnancy, characterized by a lobulated solid gross appearance. (From Copeland,[193] with permission.)

evidence of metastatic disease. Since surgical exploration during pregnancy is associated with an increase in pregnancy loss and neonatal morbidity, it is ideal to delay surgical intervention until term or after delivery. A number of opposing risks require consideration prior to following a conservative approach. The risk of greatest concern is that a delay of surgical intervention could permit a malignant ovarian tumor to spread, resulting in a decreased opportunity for cure. However, considering the rarity of advanced-stage poorly differentiated epithelial tumors in this age group, this risk is relatively small. There does appear to be an increased probability that an adnexal mass during pregnancy will undergo torsion or rupture,[141,142] and surgical intervention for these events is associated with higher fetal loss than an elective procedure.[136,143] While ovarian tumors may be the cause of obstructed labor,[136] this is uncommon. Serial sonographic evaluations will identify the rare tumor that remains pelvic as the gestation progresses. Since most ovarian masses relocate to the abdomen as the pregnancy advances, other explanations should be considered for persistent pelvic masses, including pelvic kidney, uterine fibroids, and colorectal or bladder tumors.

When a malignant ovarian tumor is encountered at laparotomy, surgical intervention should be similar to that for the nonpregnant patient. If the patient is preterm and the tumor appears confined to one ovary, consideration should be given to limiting the staging to removal of the ovary, cytologic washings, and a thorough manual exploration of the abdomen and pelvis. The potential benefit of more extensive staging, including aortic node sampling, may be offset by higher pregnancy loss or neonatal morbidity. Prior to surgery, a comprehensive discussion with the patient should guide the extent of surgery if metastatic disease, especially a high grade epithelial lesion, is encountered. Depending on the gestational age and the patient's desires, limited surgery followed by chemotherapy and additional extirpative surgery following delivery must be offered in select cases.

Preoperative serum tumor markers are of limited value during pregnancy secondary to the physiologic increases in hCG, α-fetoprotein, and CA 125. Kobayashi and colleagues[144] have reported the mean CA 125 levels during pregnancy. CA 125 increases during the first trimester (mean, 72 U/ml) and then normalizes during the second trimester. CA 125 values tend to be significantly elevated following second trimester abortion (mean, 447 U/ml) and term delivery (mean, 204 U/ml). Following diagnostic confirmation of a malignant ovarian tumor, the appropriate serum markers are useful to monitor the course of the disease.

Virilizing ovarian tumors during pregnancy are most commonly secondary to theca-lutein cysts, and their evaluation and management should be conservative.[145] These benign exaggerated physiologic "tumors" may redevelop with subsequent pregnancies.[146]

Postoperative Adjuvant Therapy

Postoperative adjuvant therapy should follow the treatment guidelines for the nonpregnant patient. Following tumor debulking, patients with advanced epithelial tumors should receive combination chemotherapy. Until 1995, the standard therapy was a platinum and alkylating combination. However, with the recent demonstration of the superior effectiveness of the combination of cisplatinum and taxol,[147] these agents may offer the patient a better survival. Unfortunately, there is no information available regarding the potential toxic effects of taxol on a developing fetus. There are favorable case reports on the treatment of stage III serous ovarian carcinoma with postoperative platinum-based chemotherapy.[148–150]

Young and colleagues[162] reviewed their collective experience with stromal ovarian tumors in pregnancy. One-third of the patients presented with tumor rupture. Since the role of adjuvant chemotherapy for stromal tumors is complex and controversial, consultation with a gynecologic oncologist is recommended. Virilizing ovarian tumors during pregnancy are most commonly secondary to theca-lutein cysts. In these cases, management should be conservative.[145]

Vulvar and Vaginal Cancer

Since vulvar and vaginal cancers usually occur after age 40, the diagnosis of either disease concurrent with pregnancy is rare. Fewer than 20 cases of vulvar carcinoma diagnosed and treated during pregnancy have been reported.[163–165]

Vulvar carcinoma in pregnancy is usually stage I or II disease. The diagnosis is based on biopsy, and neither pregnancy nor the young age of a patient should discourage the biopsy of a vulvar mass. Since verrucous squamous carcinoma tends to be misdiagnosed as condyloma, it is important to inform the pathologist of the clinical characteristics of unusually large or aggressive condyloma-like lesions. Surgical management is similar to that used in the nonpregnant patient, with the preference being to perform surgery in the second trimester to avoid the fetal risks of anesthesia exposure in the first trimester and the maternal risks associated with operating on the hypervascular vulva in third trimester. The surgical management of vulvar carcinoma is trending to more conservative procedures.[166] Vaginal delivery has been reported following surgical resection of vulvar cancers during pregnancy.[163,164]

Vaginal carcinoma is less common than vulvar carci-

noma. The same limitations apply to vaginal cancer as locally advanced cervical cancer in pregnancy. The cornerstone of treatment is irradiation therapy. Clear cell adenocarcinoma of the vagina has been reported in 16 patients, and 13 were long-term survivors.[167]

Gastrointestinal Cancers

Upper Gastrointestinal Cancers

The diagnostic delay in detecting an upper gastrointestinal cancer is often attributable to the frequency and duration of gastrointestinal symptoms in pregnancy. In the United States, stomach cancer is rarely diagnosed in women during the reproductive years. During pregnancy, persistent severe upper gastrointestinal symptoms are best evaluated by gastroduodenoscopy rather than radiologic studies. Since curative resection of localized stomach cancer is possible in only approximately 30 percent of patients, it is imperative that treatment not be delayed.

Malignant hepatic tumors are rare during the reproductive years. Hepatocellular tumors detected during pregnancy should be resected since the maternal and fetal mortality associated with subcapsular hemorrhage and liver rupture during pregnancy is high. Elevated steroid levels may predispose the tumor to rupture during pregnancy. There is no increase in the vascularity of the liver during pregnancy. In patients with unresectable hepatomas, therapeutic abortion may be considered to decrease the risk of subsequent rupture and bleeding.

Colon and Rectal Cancer

The incidence of colon cancer during pregnancy is about 1 in 13,000 liveborn deliveries.[168] Colorectal carcinoma is usually found in women beyond childbearing age, with only 8 percent of patients diagnosed before age 40. Over 200 cases of colorectal cancer in pregnancy have been reported.[169]

Since pregnancy is often accompanied by constipation and exacerbations of hemorrhoids and anal fissures, the symptoms of colorectal carcinoma, namely, rectal bleeding, constipation, pain, and backache, tend to be attributed to the pregnancy, and diagnostic delays occur. The majority of colorectal carcinomas during pregnancy are rectal and palpable on rectal examination, contrary to what is found in the nonpregnant patient (Table 36-8).[170] Patients with unexplained hypochromic microcytic anemia should be evaluated with stool guaiac testing. If a colorectal lesion is suspected, endoscopic methods of evaluation are preferred to radiologic imaging studies. Unfortunately, most cases of colorectal cancer are not diagnosed until late preg-

Table 36-8 Distribution of Colon and Rectal Carcinomas in Nonpregnant and Pregnant Populations

Patient Group	Total	Colon	Rectum
General population	1,704	1,244 (73%)	460 (27%)
Age under 40 years	186	127 (68%)	59 (32%)
Pregnant	244	41 (17%)	203 (83%)

(From Medich and Fazio,[170] with permission.)

nancy or at the time of delivery. Delays in diagnosis are probably responsible for a higher likelihood of advanced stage colorectal cancer in pregnancy and an associated poor prognosis. The hormonal effect of pregnancy on tumor development is unknown.[169] A report by Woods and colleagues[168] suggests that colorectal carcinoma in pregnancy adversely affects the pregnancy. Only 78 percent of their cases resulted in healthy liveborn infants.[168]

Management of colon cancer is determined by gestational age at diagnosis and tumor stage. During the first half of pregnancy colon resection with anastomosis is indicated for colon cancers.[171] Abdominoperineal resection or low anterior resection has been accomplished up to 20 weeks' gestation without disturbing the gravid uterus. In some cases, access to the rectum may be impossible without a hysterectomy or uterine evacuation.

In late pregnancy, a diverting colostomy may be necessary to relieve a colonic obstruction and allow the development of fetal maturity before instituting definitive therapy. Some patients with a diagnosis after 20 weeks may opt to continue the pregnancy to fetal viability. Vaginal delivery is planned unless the tumor is obstructing the pelvis or is located on the anterior rectum. If cesarean delivery is performed, tumor resection can be accomplished immediately. Neoadjuvant chemotherapy or radiation therapy for colorectal carcinoma in the pregnant patient has not demonstrated sufficient response to risk fetal exposure.

In the most recent report, the stage-specific survival rates for pregnant patients with rectal cancer were 83, 27, and 0 percent for stages B, C, and D, respectively.[169] The corresponding survivals rates for the same stages of colon cancer were 75, 33, and 0 percent.[169] No Dukes A classification rectal or colon cancer was reported, consistent with the frequency of diagnostic delays.[169]

Urinary Tract Cancers

Fewer than 50 cases of renal cell carcinoma and less than 10 cases of bladder cancer have been reported during pregnancy. Urethral carcinoma during pregnancy is also rare. The hallmark of urinary tract cancers is hematuria. The initial evaluation of hematuria in pregnancy should be urethrocystoscopy, urinary cytol-

ogy, and renal ultrasonography. The primary therapy for renal cell carcinoma is surgery, and the survival rate for localized disease may exceed 50 percent. While preoperative arterial embolization may facilitate surgery on hypervascular tumors, improved survival rates have not been conclusively demonstrated. Adjuvant radiotherapy or chemotherapy tends to have minimal impact on long-term outcomes.

Transitional carcinoma of the bladder can be managed by local fulguration or resection if it is well differentiated and superficial. Less differentiated, deeply invasive, and recurrent tumors may require a partial or complete cystectomy. Urethral carcinoma treatment varies with the size and location. Distal urethral tumors are usually treated with excision and interstitial brachytherapy implants.

Central Nervous System Tumors

The spectrum of central nervous system tumors found in pregnant patients is similar to that of the nonpregnant patient.[172] In pregnancy, 32 percent of brain tumors are gliomas, 29 percent meningiomas, 15 percent acoustic neuromas, and the other 24 percent are divided among other more rare subtypes. Spinal tumors account for only about one eighth of the central nervous system tumors. Vertebral hemangiomas comprise 61 percent of the spinal tumors and meningiomas, 18 percent. Unfortunately, the presenting symptoms of headache and nausea and vomiting are often attributed to normal complaints of pregnancy, and delays in diagnosis result. Meningiomas, pituitary adenomas, acoustic neuromas, and vertebral hemangiomas may demonstrate rapid enlargement during pregnancy. This may be secondary to fluid retention, increase in blood volume, or hormonal stimulation.[173] MRI is the most common form of imaging used to diagnose intracranial neoplasms.

Since painful contractions and pushing increase intracranial pressure, it is recommended that labor be as pain free as possible, and the second stage of labor should be assisted with forceps to reduce the risk of herniation.[173] The anesthetic management of labor and delivery for patients with intracranial neoplasms has been reviewed by Finfer.[174]

While high grade glial tumors should undergo prompt diagnosis and treatment, low grade glial tumors such as astrocytomas and oligodendrogliomas do not usually require immediate intervention. Adjuvant cranial radiotherapy with abdominal shielding should be considered for patients with high grade tumors. Adjuvant chemotherapy is not usually effective and therefore should probably be delayed until after delivery.

Successful surgical removal of a variety of central nervous system tumors has been reported.[173,175–179] Corticosteroids are recommended to reduce the surrounding edema of intracranial masses.

The use of bromocriptine in pregnancy is controversial. A report of no adverse fetal effects in over 1,400 pregnancies in which bromocriptine was taken in the first trimester supports the use of bromocriptine during pregnancy if expansion of a prolactinoma is detected.

Miscellaneous Tumors

Similar to the management for small cell neuroendocrine tumors of the cervix,[129] neuroendocrine tumors or neuroblastomas of other primary sites tend to demonstrate excellent response to chemotherapy.[180]

Fetal-Placental Metastasis

Metastatic spread of a maternal primary tumor to the placenta or fetus is rare. One review identified 45 cases of placental metastases and 7 cases of fetal metastases.[181] Malignant melanoma is the most frequently reported tumor metastatic to the placenta. Hematologic malignancies are the second most common tumor to spread to the placenta. Placental and fetal dissemination of lymphomas have been reported.[182–185] One case of vertical transmission of a mother's leukemia cell line was demonstrated through identification of a leukemia clone.[186] There is one case report of a central nervous system tumor metastatic to the placenta.[187]

Gestational Trophoblastic Disease and Pregnancy-Related Issues

It is uncommon for a normal viable pregnancy to be complicated by gestational trophoblastic disease (GTD). A comprehensive summary of the evaluation and management of the complete spectrum of GTD is beyond the spectrum of this textbook. However, the aspects of GTD related to the general obstetric and postpartum care are reviewed.

Hydatidiform Mole (Complete Mole)

The incidence of hydatidiform mole has great geographic variability. In the United States it occurs in approximately 1 in 1,000 to 1 in 1,500 pregnancies. The two clinical risk factors that carry the highest risk of a molar pregnancy are (1) the extremes of the reproductive years (age 50 or older carries a relative risk of over 500)[188] and (2) the history of a prior hydatidiform mole (the risk for development of a second molar pregnancy is 1 to 2 percent,[189–191] and the risk of a third after two is approximately 25 percent.)[192] Patients with these risk factors should have an ultrasound evaluation of uterine

contents in the first trimester. While historically approximately 50 percent of patients were not diagnosed with a molar pregnancy prior to vaginal expulsion of molar tissue, currently in developed countries most patients are diagnosed either by ultrasound while asymptomatic or by ultrasound for the evaluation of vaginal spotting or cramping symptoms. Approximately 95 percent of complete hydatidiform moles have a 46XX paternal homologous chromosomal pattern.

The safest technique of evacuating a hydatidiform mole is with the suction aspiration technique. Oxytocin should not be initiated until the patient is in the operating room and evacuation is imminent in order to minimize the risk of embolization of trophoblastic tissue. The alternative management for the elderly patient who requests concurrent sterilization is hysterectomy. Following either evacuation or hysterectomy, weekly β-hCG is drawn until the hCG titer is within normal limits for 3 weeks. The titers are then observed at monthly intervals for 6 to 12 months. Figure 36-5 illustrates an algorithm for molar pregnancy management.[193]

For the patient with a complete molar pregnancy, the risk of requiring chemotherapy for persistent GTD is approximately 20 percent. Clinical features that increase this risk include delayed hemorrhage, excessive uterine enlargement, theca-lutein cysts, serum hCG greater than 100,000 mIU/ml, and maternal age over 40. It is obviously particularly important not to misinterpret a rising β-hCG due to a new intervening pregnancy, as persistent GTD as intervention with chemotherapy would be a significant risk to a new gestation, inducing either abortion or possible teratogenic defects.

Invasive Mole (Chorioadenoma Destruens)

Since invasion of the myometrium by molar tissue is clinically occult, it is difficult to assess the true incidence, estimated to be between 5 and 10 percent. The clinical hallmark of invasive mole is hemorrhage, often severe, either vaginal or intraperitoneal.

Partial Hydatidiform Mole

Most partial moles have a triploid karyotype, and the next most common is a trisomy 16. A minority of partial moles exhibit normal diploidy. Karyotype analysis of the accompanying fetus is important in planning therapeutic intervention. A partial mole associated with a nonviable fetal chromosomal abnormality will require either mechanical or medically induced uterine evacuation (Fig. 36-6). In the presence of an abundance of hydropic tissue, there is always the concern that trophoblastic tissue embolization may occur during uterine contractions induced to evacuate molar tissue. The

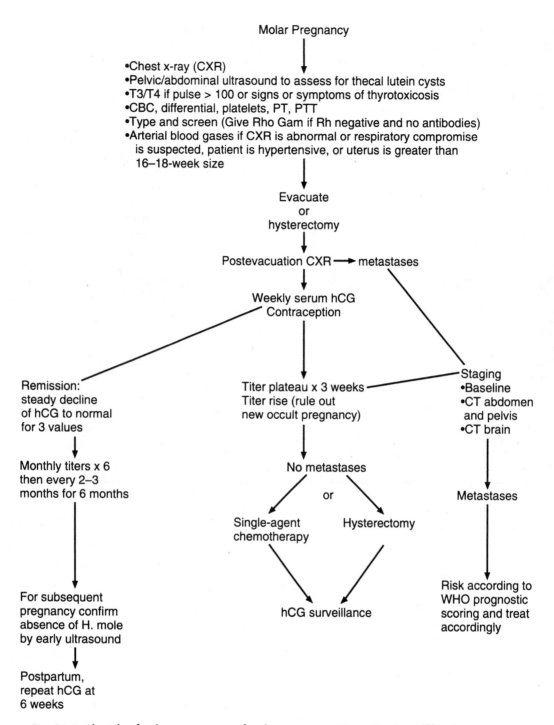

Fig. 36-5 Algorithm for the management of molar pregnancy. (From Copeland,[193] with permission.)

management of a patient with sonographic findings suggestive of a diagnosis of a partial mole is particularly challenging if the karyotype analysis of the fetus is diploid, especially if the diagnosis is made in the second or third trimester. When a normal karyotype exists, it is appropriate to consider diagnostic possibilities other than partial mole, such as a twin gestation—one normal-developing fetus and one molar pregnancy. Also

degenerative changes (hydropic villi), retroplacental hematomas, placental abnormalities (chorioangiomas), degenerative uterine myomas, and aborted tissue, sometimes referred to as a "transitional mole," may lead to imaging abnormalities that are difficult to interpret.

Approximately 2 to 6 percent of patients develop persistent GTD after a partial molar pregnancy.[194,195]

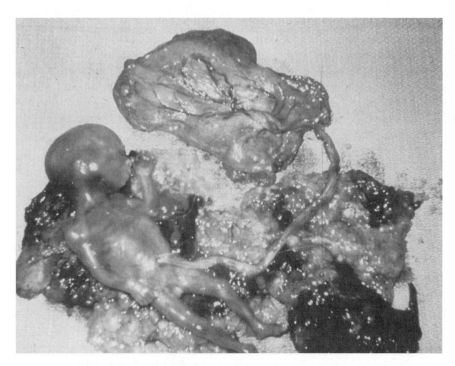

Fig. 36-6 Partial mole with dead fetus of abnormal karyotype. (From Copeland,[193] with permission.)

Therefore, these patients require the same postevacuation surveillance and management as the patient with a complete mole.

Placental Site Trophoblastic Tumor

Less than 1 percent of all patients with GTD have placental site trophoblastic tumor. While this tumor usually presents with abnormal vaginal bleeding following a term pregnancy, it can also be a sequelae to a molar pregnancy or abortion. The postpartum presentation is characterized by a slightly enlarged uterus, persistent bleeding or, occasionally, amenorrhea, and a slightly elevated β-hCG level. The hCG may not reliably reflect disease progression. The histologic diagnosis may be obtained by uterine curettage, possibly hysteroscopically directed. Since this disease tends to metastasize late and be somewhat resistant to chemotherapy, surgical excision (hysterectomy) should be considered. If the patient is desirous of future childbearing, management considerations that have been reported with some success include systemic chemotherapy, regional infusion chemotherapy, and uterine curettage.

Choriocarcinoma

Choriocarcinoma develops in approximately 1 in every 40,000 term pregnancies and represents about one-fourth of all cases of choriocarcinoma. The other cases follow molar disease or an abortion (spontaneous, therapeutic, or ectopic). GTD following a term pregnancy is always either choriocarcinoma or a placental site trophoblastic tumor, assuming a singleton pregnancy.

Choriocarcinoma is notorious for masquerading as other diseases. This is secondary to hemorrhagic metastases producing symptoms such as hematuria, hemoptysis, hematemesis, hematochezia, stroke, or vaginal bleeding. The common sites for metastatic disease are listed in Table 36-9. The diagnosis of choriocarcinoma is based on history, imaging studies, and a serum β-hCG level. Histologic confirmation is neither necessary for the diagnosis nor a prerequisite to initiate therapy. Again, it is necessary to exclude the presence of a new gestation as the source of a rising β-hCG level prior to extensive diagnostic imaging or therapeutic intervention.

Table 36-9 Common Sites for Metastatic Choriocarcinoma[a]

Site	Percent
Lung	60–95
Vagina	40–50
Vulva/cervix	10–15
Brain	5–15
Liver	5–15
Kidney	0–5
Spleen	0–5
Gastrointestinal	0–5

[a] Frequencies vary, depending on whether data are based on autopsy studies or are obtained from pretreatment imaging.
(From Copeland,[193] with permission.)

The complexities of the general treatment approach or treatment for special situations is beyond the scope of this textbook. It is recommended that the reader refer to a gynecology or gynecologic oncology resource for discussions of the therapeutic subtleties and pitfalls. Choriocarcinoma should be managed by a gynecologic oncologist, preferably one with a special interest in the disease.

Key Points

- Since many of the common complaints of pregnancy are also early symptoms of metastatic cancer, pregnant women with cancer are at risk for delays in diagnosis and therapeutic intervention.

- The safest interval for most cancer therapies in pregnancy is the second trimester, thereby avoiding induction of teratogenic risks or miscarriage in the first trimester and avoiding neonatal morbidity associated with preterm delivery in the third trimester.

- Antimetabolites and alkylating agents present the greatest hazard to the developing fetus.

- Diagnostic delays of breast cancer in pregnancy are often attributed to physician reluctance to properly evaluate breast complaints or abnormal findings in pregnancy.

- Treatment for Hodgkin's disease may compromise the reproductive potential, and combined treatment with irradiation and chemotherapy provides the highest risk of ovarian failure.

- If a mother is exposed to cytotoxic drugs within 1 month of delivery, the newborn should be monitored closely for evidence of granulocytopenia or thrombocytopenia.

- The effect of pregnancy on the clinical course of melanoma has been the subject of debate. When corrected for tumor thickness, pregnancy does not appear to be an independent prognostic variable for survival.

- After stratifying for stage and age, patients with pregnancy-associated cervical carcinoma have survival rates similar to the nonpregnant patient.

- Since most malignant ovarian tumors found in pregnancy are either germ cell tumors or low grade, early stage epithelial tumors, the therapeutic plan will usually permit continuation of the pregnancy and preservation of fertility.

- While rare, most colorectal carcinomas in pregnancy are detectable on rectal examination, underscoring the need for a rectal examination at the patient's first prenatal visit.

References

1. Donnegan WL: Cancer and pregnancy. Cancer 33:194, 1983
2. Koren G, Weiner L, Lishner M et al: Cancer in pregnancy: identification of unanswered questions on maternal and fetal risks. Obstet Gynecol Surv 45:509, 1990
3. Doll DC, Ringenberg QS, Yarbro JW: Management of cancer during pregnancy. Arch Intern Med 148:2058, 1988

4. Doll DC, Ringenberg QS, Yarbro JW: Antineoplastic agents and pregnancy. Semin Oncol 16:337, 1989

5. Ben-Baruch G, Menczer J, Goshen R et al: Cisplatin excretion in human milk. J Natl Cancer Inst 84:451, 1992

6. Reynoso EE, Shepherd FA, Messner HA et al: Acute leukemia during pregnancy: the Toronto leukemia study group experience with long term follow-up in children exposed in utero to chemotherapeutic agents. J Clin Oncol 5:1098, 1987

7. Henderson CE, Elia G, Garfinkel D et al: Platinum chemotherapy during pregnancy for serious cystadenocarcinoma of the ovary. Gynecol Oncol 49:92, 1993

8. Zemlickis D, Lishner M, Degendorfer P et al: Fetal outcome after in utero exposure to cancer chemotherapy. Arch Intern Med 152:573, 1992

9. Nicholson HO: Cytotoxic drugs in pregnancy. J Obstet Gynaecol Br Commonw 75:307, 1968

10. Schardein: Cancer chemotherapeutic agents. pp. 457–508. In Schardein JL (ed.) Chemically Induced Birth Defects, 2nd ed. Marcel Dekker, New York, 1993

11. Kozlowski RD, Steinbrunner JV, Mackenzie AH et al: Outcome of first-trimester exposure to low-dose methotrexate in eight patients with rheumatic disease. Am J Med 88:589, 1990

12. Roboz J, Gleichner N, Wu K et al: Does doxorubicin cross the placenta? Lancet 2:2691, 1979

13. Barni S, Ardizzola A, Zanetta G et al: Weekly doxorubicin chemotherapy for breast cancer in pregnancy: a case report. Tumori 78:349, 1992

14. Karp GI, Von Oeyen P, Valone F et al: Doxorubicin in pregnancy: possible transplacental passage. Cancer Treat Rep 67:773, 1983

15. Malone JM, Gershenson DM, Creasy RK et al: Endodermal sinus tumor of the ovary associated with pregnancy. Obstet Gynecol 68:86, 1986

16. Kim DS, Park MI: Maternal and fetal survival following surgery and chemotherapy of endodermal sinus tumor of the ovary during pregnancy: a case report. Obstet Gynecol 73:503, 1989

17. Christman JE, Teng NNH, Lebovic GS, Sikic BI: Case report: delivery of a normal infant following cisplatin, vinblastine, and bleomycin chemotherapy for malignant teratoma of the ovary during pregnancy. Gynecol Oncol 37:292, 1990

18. Metz SA, Day TG, Pursell SH: Adjuvant chemotherapy in a pregnant patient with endodermal sinus tumor. Gynecol Oncol 32:371, 1989

19. Malfetano JH, Goldkrand JW: Cisplatinum combination chemotherapy during pregnancy for advanced epithelial ovarian carcinoma. Obstet Gynecol 75:545, 1990

20. King LA, Nevin PC, Williams PP et al: Treatment of advanced epithelial ovarian carcinoma in pregnancy with cisplatin-based chemotherapy. Gynecol Oncol 41:78, 1991

21. van der Zee AGJ, de Bruijn HWA, Bouma J et al: Endodermal sinus tumor of the ovary during pregnancy: a case report. Am J Obstet Gynecol 164:504, 1991

22. Farahmand SH, Marchetti DL, Asirwatham JE, Dewey MR: Case report: ovarian endodermal sinus tumor associated with pregnancy: review of the literature. Gynecol Oncol 41:156, 1991

23. Horbelt D, Delmore J, Meisel R et al: Mixed germ cell malignancy of the ovary concurrent with pregnancy. Obstet Gynecol 84:662, 1994

24. Gilland J, Weinstein L: The effects of cancer chemotherapeutic agents on the developing fetus. Obstet Gynecol Surv 38:6, 1983

25. Randall T: National registry seeks scarce data on pregnancy outcomes during chemotherapy. JAMA 269:323, 1993

26. Garber JE: Long-term follow-up of children exposed in utero to antineoplastic agents. Semin Oncol 16:437, 1989

27. Mazze RI, Kallen B: Reproductive outcome after anesthesia and operation during pregnancy: a registry study of 5405 cases. Am J Obst Gynecol 161:1178, 1989

28. Aisner J, Weirnik PH, Pearl P: Pregnancy outcome in patients treated for Hodgkin's disease. J Clin Oncol 11:507, 1993

29. Clark ST, Radford JA, Crowther D et al: Gonadal function following chemotherapy for Hodgkin disease: a comparative study of MVPP and a seven-drug hybrid regimen. J Clin Oncol 13:134, 1995

30. Aviles A, Diaz-Maqueo JC, Talavera A et al: Growth and development of children and mothers treated with chemotherapy during pregnancy; current status of 43 children. Am J Hematol 36:243, 1991

31. Parker SL, Tong T, Bolden S, Wingo PA: Cancer statistics. Cancer 65:5, 1996

32. Lewison EF: Breast cancer and pregnancy or lactation. Surg Gynecol Obstet 99:417, 1954

33. White E: Projected changes in breast cancer incidence due to the trend toward delayed childbearing. Am J Public Health 77:495, 1987

34. Michels KB, Willett WC, Rosner BA et al: Prospective assessment of breastfeeding and breast cancer incidence among 89,877 women. Lancet 347:431, 1996

35. Byrd BF Jr, Bayer DS, Robertson JC, Stephenson SE: Treatment of breast tumors associated with pregnancy and lactation. Ann Surg 155:940, 1962

36. Applewhite RR, Smith LR, DiVincenti F: Carcinoma of the breast associated with pregnancy and lactation. Ann Surg 39:101, 1973

37. Zemlickis D, Lishner M, Degendorfer P et al: Maternal and fetal outcomes after breast cancer in pregnancy. Am J Obstet Gynecol 166:781, 1992

38. Wagner LK, Lester RG, Saldana LR: The amount of radiation absorbed by the conceptus. p. 52. In Exposure of the Pregnant Patient to Diagnostic Radiation. A Guide to Medical Management. JB Lippincott, Philadelphia, 1985

39. Parente JT, Amsel M, Lerner R, Chinea F: Breast cancer associated with pregnancy. 71:861, 1988

40. Max MH, Lamer TW: Breast cancer in 120 women under 35 years old. Ann Surg 50:23, 1984

41. Clark GM, Osborne CK, McGuire WL: Correlations between estrogen receptor, progesterone receptor, and patient characteristics in human breast cancer. J Clin Oncol 2:1102, 1984

42. Sarrif WM, Durant JR: Evidence that estrogen-receptor negative and progesterone-receptor negative breast and ovarian carcinoma contain estrogen receptors. Cancer 48:1215, 1981

43. King RM, Welch JS, Martin JK Jr, Coul CB: Carcinoma of the breast associated with pregnancy. Surg Gynecol Obstet 160:228, 1985

44. Kinne DW: Primary treatment of breast cancer. p. 356 In Harris JR, Hellman S, Henderson IC, Kinne DW, (eds): Breast Diseases, 2nd Ed. JB Lippincott, Philadelphia, 1991

45. van der Vange N, van Donegan JA: Breast cancer and pregnancy. Eur J Surg Oncol 17:1, 1991

46. Brent RL: The effect of embryonic and fetal exposure to x-ray, microwaves, and ultrasound: counseling the pregnant and nonpregnant patient about these risks. Semin Oncol 16:347, 1989

47. Elledge RM, Ciocca DR, Langione DR et al: Estrogen receptor, progesterone receptor, and HER-2/neu protein in breast cancers from pregnant patients. Cancer 71:2499, 1993

48. Holleb AI, Farrow JH: The relationship of carcinoma of the breast and pregnancy in 283 patients. Surg Gynecol Obstet 115:65, 1962

49. Lee TN, Horz JM: Significance of ovarian metastases in therapeutic oophorectomy for advanced breast cancer. Cancer 27:1374, 1971

50. Ravdin RG, Lewison EF, Slack NH: The results of a clinical trial concerning the worth of prophylactic oophorectomy for breast cancer. Surg Gynecol Obstet 131:1055, 1970

51. White TT, White WC: Breast cancer and pregnancy: report of 49 cases followed five years. Ann Surg 144:384, 1956

52. Applewhite RR, Smith LR, DiVencenti F: Carcinoma of the breast associated with pregnancy and lactation. Ann Surg 39:101, 1973

53. Riberio GG, Palmer MK: Breast carcinoma associated with pregnancy: a clinician's dilemma. BMJ 2:1524, 1977

54. Clark RM, Reid J: Carcinoma of the breast in pregnancy and lactation. Int Radiat Oncol Biol Phys 4:693, 1978

55. Petrek JA, Dukoff R, Rogatko A: Prognosis of pregnancy-associated breast cancer. Cancer 67:869, 1991

56. Donegan WL: Breast cancer and pregnancy. Obstet Gynecol 50:244, 1977

57. Peters MV: The effect of pregnancy in breast cancer. p. 120. In Forrest APM, Kunkler PB (eds): Prognostic Factors in Breast Cancer. Williams & Wilkins, Baltimore, 1968

58. Nugent P, O'Connell TX: Breast cancer and pregnancy. Arch Surg 120:1221, 1985

59. Danforth DN Jr: How subsequent pregnancy affects outcome in women with a prior breast cancer. Oncology 11:21, 1991

60. Epstein RJ, Henderson IC: The Danforth article reviewed: the jury is in. Oncology 11:30,31, 1991

61. Cooper DR, Butterfield J: Pregnancy subsequent to mastectomy for cancer of the breast. Ann Surg 171:429, 1970

62. Sutton R, Buzdar AU, Hortobagyi GN: Pregnancy and offspring after adjuvant chemotherapy in breast cancer patients. Cancer 71:2499, 1990

63. Higgins S, Haffty B: Pregnancy and lactation after breast-conserving therapy for early-stage breast cancer. Cancer 73:2175, 1994

64. Tralins A: Is lactation possible after breast irradiation? Proc Am Soc Clin Oncol 12:77, 1993

65. Miller MJ, Ross ME: Case report: pregnancy following breast reconstruction with autologous tissue. Cancer Bull 45:546, 1993

66. Barry RM, Diamond HD, Craver LF: Influence of pregnancy on the course of Hodgkin's disease. Am J Obstet Gynecol 84:445, 1962

67. Sweet DL Jr: Malignant lymphoma: implications during the reproductive years and pregnancy. J Reprod Med 17:198, 1976

68. Lishner M, Zemlickis D, Degendorfer P et al: Maternal and fetal outcome following Hodgkin's disease in pregnancy. Br J Cancer 65:114, 1992

69. Thomas PRM, Peckham MJ: The investigation and management of Hodgkin's disease in the pregnant patient. Cancer 38:1443, 1976

70. Jacobs C, Donaldson SS, Rosenberg SA, Kaplan HS: Management of the pregnant patient with Hodgkin's disease. Ann Intern Med 95:649, 1981

71. Friedman E, Jones GW: Fetal outcome after maternal radiation treatment of supradiaphragmatic Hodgkin's disease. Can Med Assoc J 149:1281, 1993

72. Dein RA, Mennuti MT, Kovach P, Gabbe SG: The reproductive potential of young men and women with Hodgkin's disease. Obstet Gynecol Surv 39:474, 1984

73. Horning SJ, Hoppe RT, Kaplan HS: Female reproduction after treatment for Hodgkin's disease. N Engl J Med 304:1377, 1981

74. Chapman RM, Sutcliffe SB, Malpas JS: Cytotoxic induced ovarian failure in women with Hodgkin's disease. I. Hormone function. J Am Med Assoc 242:1877, 1979

75. Chapman, RM, Sutcliffe SB, Lees LH: Cyclical combination chemotherapy and gonadal function. Lancet 1:285, 1979

76. Jarrell JJ: Reproductive toxicology. p. 363. In Copeland LJ (ed): Textbook of Gynecology. WB Saunders, Philadelphia, 1993

77. Holmes GE, Holmes FF: Pregnancy outcome of patients treated for Hodgkin's disease. Cancer 41:1317, 1978

78. Janov AJ, Anderson J, Cella DF et al: Pregnancy outcome in survivors of advanced Hodgkin's disease. Cancer 70:688, 1992

79. McKeen EA, Mulvill JJ, Rosner F, Zarrari MH: Pregnancy outcome in Hodgkin's disease. Lancet 2:590, 1979

80. Selvais PL, Mazy G, Gosseye S et al: Breast infiltration by acute lymphoblastic leukemia during pregnancy. Am J Obstet Gynecol 169:1619, 1993

81. Ward FT, Weiss RB: Lymphoma and pregnancy. Semin Oncol 16:397, 1989

82. Ohba T, Matusuo I, Katabuchi H et al: Adult T-cell leukemia/lymphoma in pregnancy. Obstet Gynecol 72:445, 1988

83. Manns A, Blattner WA: The epidemiology of the human T-cell lymphotropic virus type I and type II: etiologic role in human disease. Transfusion 31:67, 1991

84. Caligiuri MA, Mayer RJ: Pregnancy and leukemia. Semin Oncol 16:338, 1989

85. Catanzarite VA, Ferguson JE: Acute leukemia and preg-

nancy: a review of management and outcome, 1972–1982. Obstet Gynecol Surv 39:663, 1984

86. Juarez S, Cuadrado JM, Feliu J et al: Association of leukemia and pregnancy: clinical and obstetric aspects. Am J Clin Oncol 11:159, 1988

87. Zuazu J, Julia A, Sierra J et al: Pregnancy outcome in hematologic malignancies. Cancer 61:703, 1991

88. Antonelli NM, Dotters DJ, Katz VL, Kuller JA: Cancer in pregnancy: a review of the literature. Part II. Obstet Gynecol Surv 51:135, 1996

89. Hoelzer D, Thiel E, Loffler H et al: Prognostic factors in a multicenter study for treatment of acute lymphoblastic leukemia in adults. Blood 71:123, 1988

90. Wiernik PH: Acute leukemias of adults. p. 302. In DeVita VT Jr, Hellman S, Rosenberg SA (eds): Cancer: Principles and Practice of Oncology. JB Lippincott, Philadelphia, 1982

91. Aviles A, Niz J: Long term follow-up of children born to mothers with acute leukemia during pregnancy. Med Pediatr Oncol 16:3, 1988

92. Bazarbashi MS, Smith MR, Karanes C et al: Successful management of Ph chromosome chronic myelogenous leukemia with leukapheresis during pregnancy. Am J Hematol 38:235, 1991

93. Baer MR, Ozer H, Foon KA: Interferon-alpha therapy during pregnancy in chronic myelogenous leukemia and hairy cell leukemia. Br J Haematol 81:167, 1992

94. Delmer A, Rio B, Baudner F et al: Pregnancy during myelosuppressive treatment for chronic myelogenous leukemia. Br J Haematol 82:783, 1992

95. Jackson N, Shukri A, Ali K: Hydroxyurea treatment for chronic myeloid leukemia during pregnancy. Br J Haematol 85:203, 1993

96. Patel M, Dukes IAF, Hill JC: Use of hydroxyurea in chronic myeloid leukemia during pregnancy: a case report. Am J Obstet Gynecol 165:565, 1991

97. Tertian G, Tchernia G, Papiernik E et al: Hydroxyurea and pregnancy. Am J Obst Gynecol 166:1868, 1992

98. Friedman RJ, Rigel DS, Kopf AW: Early detection of malignant melanoma: the role of the physician examination and self examination of the skin. Ca 35:130, 1985

99. Smith RS, Randall P: Melanoma during pregnancy. Obstet Gynecol 34:825, 1969

100. Balch CM, Soong SJ, Milton GW et al: A comparison of prognostic factors and surgical results in 1,786 patients with localized (stage I) melanoma treated in Alabama, USA, and New South Wales, Australia. Ann Surg 146:677, 1982

101. Pack GT, Scharnagel IM: The prognosis for malignant melanoma in the pregnant woman. Cancer 4:324, 1951

102. Byrd BF, McGanty WJ: The effect of pregnancy on the normal course of malignant melanoma. South Med 47:324, 1951

103. George PA, Fortner JG, Pack GT: Melanoma with pregnancy: a report of 115 cases. Cancer 13:854, 1960

104. Shiu MH, Schottenfeld D, Maclean B, Fortner JG: Adverse effect of pregnancy on melanoma. Cancer 37:181, 1976

105. Houghton AN, Flannery J, Viola MV: Malignant mela-

noma of the skin occurring during pregnancy. Cancer 48:407, 1981

106. Wong DJ, Stassner HT: Melanoma in pregnancy. Clin Obstet Gynecol 33:782, 1990

107. MacKie RM, Bufalino R, Morabito A et al: Lack of effect on pregnancy outcome of melanoma. Lancet 337:653, 1991

108. McManamny DS, Moss ALH, Pocock PV et al: Melanoma and pregnancy: a long-term follow-up. Br J Obstet Gynaecol 96:1419, 1989

109. Slingluff CL Jr, Reintgen D, Vollmer RT et al: Malignant melanoma arising during pregnancy: a study of 100 patients. Ann Surg 211:552, 1990

110. Lederman JS, Sober AJ: Effect of prior pregnancy on melanoma survival. Arch Dermatol 121:716, 1985

111. Colburn DS, Nathanson L, Belilos E: Pregnancy and malignant melanoma. Semin Oncol 16:377, 1989

112. Ross MI: Melanoma and pregnancy: prognostic and therapeutic considerations. Cancer Bull 46:412, 1994

113. Ostelind A, Tucker MA, Stone BJ et al: The Danish case control study of cutaneous malignant melanoma III: hormonal and reproductive factors in women. Int J Cancer 42:821, 1988

114. Lederman JS, Lew RA, Koh HK, Sober AJ: Influence of estrogen administration on tumor characteristics and survival in women with cutaneous melanoma. J Natl Cancer Inst 74:981, 1985

115. Hacker NF, Berek JS, Lagasse LD et al: Carcinoma of the cervix associated with pregnancy. Obstet Gynecol 59:735, 1982

116. Zemlickis D, Lishner M, Degendorfer P et al: Maternal and fetal outcome after invasive cervical cancer in pregnancy. J Clin Oncol 9:1956, 1991

117. Nevin D, Soeters R, Dehaeck K et al: Cervical carcinoma associated with pregnancy. Obstet Gynecol Surv 50:228, 1995

118. Benedet JL, Selke PA, Nickerson KG: Colposcopic evaluation of abnormal Papanicolaou smears in pregnancy. Am J Obstet Gynecol 157:932, 1987

119. Economos K, Perez Veridiano N, Delke I et al: Abnormal cervical cytology in pregnancy: a 17-year experience. Obstet Gynecol 81:915, 1993

120. Averette HE, Nasser N, Yankow SL: Cervical conization in pregnancy. Am J Obstet Gynecol 106:543, 1970

121. Hannigan EV, Whitehouse III HH, Atkinson WD et al: Cone biopsy during pregnancy. Obstet Gynecol 60:450, 1982

122. Hannigan EV: Cervical cancer in pregnancy. Clin Obstet Gynecol 33:837, 1990

123. Copeland LJ, Silva EG, Gershenson DM et al: Superficially invasive squamous cell carcinoma of the cervix. Gynecol Oncol 45:307, 1992

124. Lewandowski GS, Copeland LJ, Vaccarello L: Surgical issues in the management of carcinoma of the cervix in pregnancy. Surg Clin North Am 75:89, 1995

125. Duggan B, Muderspach LI, Roman LD et al: Cervical cancer in pregnancy: reporting on planned delay in therapy. Obstet Gynecol 82:598, 1993

126. Monk BJ, Montz FJ: Invasive cervical cancer complicat-

ing intrauterine pregnancy. Treatment with hysterectomy. Obstet Gynecol 80:199, 1992

127. Sivanesaratnam V, Javalakshmi P, Loo C: Surgical management of early invasive cancer of the uterine cervix associated with pregnancy. Gynecol Oncol 48:68, 1993

128. Greer BE, Easterling TR, McLennan DA et al: Fetal and maternal considerations in the management of stage IB cervical during pregnancy. Gynecol Oncol 34:61, 1989

129. Lewandowski GS, Copeland LJ: A potential role for invasive chemotherapy in the treatment of small cell neuroendocrine tumors of the cervix. Gynecol Oncol 48:127, 1993

130. Shingleton HM, Orr JW. Cervical cancer complicating pregnancy. p. 284. In Cancer of the Cervix. Churchill Livingstone, Edinburgh, 1983

131. Copeland LJ, Saul PB, Sneige N: Cervical adenocarcinoma: tumor implantation in the episiotomy sites of two patients. Gynecol Oncol 28:230, 1987

132. Gordon AN, Jensen R, Jones HW III: Squamous carcinoma of the cervix complicating pregnancy: recurrence in episiotomy after vaginal delivery. Obstet Gynecol 73:850, 1989

133. Cliby WA, Dodson WA, Podratz KC: Cervical cancer complicated by pregnancy: episiotomy site recurrences following vaginal delivery. Obstet Gynecol 84:179, 1994

134. Hopkins MP, Morley GW: The prognosis and management of cervical cancer associated with pregnancy. Obstet Gynecol 80:9, 1992

135. Fleischer AC, Shah DM, Entman SS: Sonographic evaluation of maternal disorders during pregnancy. Radiol Clin North Am 28:51, 1990

136. Hess LW, Peaceman A, O'Brien W et al: Adnexal mass occurring with intrauterine pregnancy: a report of 54 patients requiring laparotomy for definitive management. Am J Obstet Gynecol 158:1029, 1988

137. El Yahia AR, Rahman J, Rahman MS et al: Ovarian tumors in pregnancy. Aust NZ J Obstet Gynecol 31:327, 1991

138. Munnell EW: Primary ovarian cancer associated with pregnancy. Clin Obstet Gynecol 6:983, 1963

139. Dgani R, Shoham Z, Atar E et al: Ovarian carcinoma during pregnancy: a study of 23 cases in Israel between the years of 1960 and 1984. Gynecol Oncol 33:326, 1989

140. Platek DN, Henderson CE, Goldberg GL: The management of a persistent adnexal mass in pregnancy. Am J Obstet Gynecol 173:12236, 1995

141. Jacob JH, Stringer CA: Diagnosis and management of cancer during pregnancy. Semin Perinatol 14:79, 1990

142. Jolles CJ: Gynecologic cancer associated with pregnancy. Semin Oncol 16:417, 1989

143. Katz VL, Watson WJ, Hansen WF et al: Massive ovarian tumor complicating pregnancy: a case report. J Reprod Med 38:907, 1993

144. Kobayashi F, Sagawa N, Nakamura K et al: Mechanism and clinical significance of elevated CA 125 levels in the sera of pregnant women. Am J Obstet Gynecol 160:563, 1989

145. Manganiello PD, Adams LV, Harris RD, Ornvold K: Virilization during pregnancy with spontaneous resolution postpartum: a case report and review of the English literature. Obstet Gynecol Surv 50:404, 1995

146. VanSlooten AJ, Rechner SF, Dods WG: Recurrent maternal virilization during pregnancy caused by benign androgen-producing ovarian lesions. Am J Obstet Gynecol 167:1342, 1992

147. McGuire WP, Hoskins WJ, Brady MF et al: Cyclophosphamide and cisplatin compared with paclitaxel and cisplatin in patients with stage III and stage IV ovarian cancer. N Engl J Med 334:1, 1996

148. Malfetano JH, Goldkrand JW: Cisplatinum combination chemotherapy during pregnancy for advanced epithelial ovarian carcinoma. Obstet Gynecol 75:545, 1990

149. King LA, Nevin PC, Williams PP, Carson LF: Case report of treatment of advanced epithelial ovarian carcinoma in pregnancy with cisplatin-based chemotherapy. Gynecol Oncol 41:78, 1991

150. Henderson CE, Giovanni E, Garfinkel D et al: Case report: platinum chemotherapy during pregnancy for serous cystadenocarcinoma of the ovary. Gynecol Oncol 49:92, 1993

151. Buller RE, Darrow V, Manetta A et al: Conservative surgical management of dysgerminoma concomitant with pregnancy. Obstet Gynecol 79:887, 1992

152. Weed JC, Roh RA, Mendenhall HW: Recurrent endodermal sinus tumor during pregnancy. Obstet Gynecol 54:653, 1979

153. Petrucha RA, Ruffolo E, Messina AM et al: Endodermal sinus tumor: report of a case associated with pregnancy. Obstet Gynecol, suppl 55:90, 1980

154. Schwartz RP, Chatwani AJ, Strimel W, Putong PB: Endodermal sinus tumors in pregnancy: report of a case and review of the literature. Gynecol Oncol 15:434, 1983

155. Ito K, Teshima K, Suzuki H, Noda K: A case of ovarian endodermal sinus tumor associated with pregnancy. Tohoku J Exp Med 142:183, 1984

156. Malone JM, Gershenson DM, Creasy RK et al: Endodermal sinus tumor associated with pregnancy. Obstet Gynecol 68:86, 1984

157. Kim DS, Park MI: Maternal and fetal survival following surgery and chemotherapy of endodermal sinus tumor of the ovary during pregnancy: a case report. Obstet Gynecol 73:503, 1989

158. Metz SA, Day TG, Pursell SH: Adjuvant chemotherapy in a pregnant patient with endodermal sinus tumor. Gynecol Oncol 32:371, 1989

159. van der Zee AGL, de Bruijn HWA, Bouma J et al: Endodermal sinus tumor of the ovary during pregnancy: a case report. Am J Obstet Gynecol 164:504, 1991

160. Farahmand SH, Marchetti DL, Asirwatham JE, Dewey MR: Case report: ovarian endodermal sinus tumor associated with pregnancy: review of the literature. Gynecol Oncol 41:156, 1991

161. Horbelt D, Delmore J, Meisel R et al: Mixed germ cell malignancy of the ovary concurrent with pregnancy. Obstet Gynecol 84:662, 1994

162. Young RH, Dudley AG, Scully RE: Granulosa cell, Sertoli-Leydig cell and unclassified sex-cord stromal tumors associated with pregnancy: a clinical pathological analysis of 36 cases. Gynecol Oncol 18:181, 1984

163. Collins CG, Barclay DL: Cancer of the vulva and cancer of the vagina in pregnancy. Clin Obstet Gynecol 6:927, 1973

164. Lutz MH, Underwood PB, Rozier JC et al: Genital malignancy in pregnancy. Am J Obstet Gynecol 129:536, 1977

165. Moore DH, Fowler WC, Currie JL, Walton LA: Squamous cell carcinoma of the vulva in pregnancy. Gynecol Oncol 41:74, 1991

166. Burke TW, Stringer CA, Gershenson DM et al: Radical wide excision and selective inguinal node dissection for squamous cell carcinoma of the vulva. Gynecol Oncol 38:328, 1990

167. Senekjian EK, Hubby M, Bell DA et al: Clear cell adenocarcinoma of the vagina and cervix in association with pregnancy. Gynecol Oncol 24:207, 1986

168. Woods JB, Martin JN Jr, Ingram FH et al: Pregnancy complicated by carcinoma of the colon above the rectum. Am J Perinatol 9:102, 1992

169. Bernstein MA, Madoff RD, Caushaj PF: Colon and rectal cancer in pregnancy. Dis Colon Rectum 36:172, 1993

170. Medich DS, Fazio VW: Hemorrhoids, anal fissure, and carcinoma of the colon, rectum, and anus during pregnancy. Surg Clin North Am 75:77, 1995

171. Nesbitt JC, Moise KJ, Sawyers JL: Colorectal carcinoma in pregnancy. Arch Surg 120:636, 1985

172. Roelvink NCA, Kamphorst W, van Alphen HAM et al: Pregnancy-related primary brain and spinal tumors. Arch Neurol 44:209, 1987

173. DeAngelis LM: Central nervous system neoplasms in pregnancy. Adv Neurol 64:139, 1994

174. Finfer SR: Management of labor and delivery in patients with intracranial neoplasms. Br J Anaesth 67:784, 1991

175. Lunardi P, Rizzo A, Missori P et al: Pituitary apoplexy in an acromegalic woman operated on during pregnancy by transsphenoidal approach. Int J Gynecol Obstet 34:71, 1990

176. Coyne TJ, Atkinson RL, Prins JB: Adrenocorticotropic hormone-secreting pituitary tumor associated with pregnancy. Case report. Neurosurgery 31:953, 1992

177. Johnson RJ Jr, Voorhies RM, Witkin M et al: Fertility following excision of a symptomatic craniopharyngioma during pregnancy: case report. Surg Neurol 39:257, 1993

178. Tokuda Y, Hatayama T, Sakoda K: Metastasis of malignant struma ovarii to the cranial vault during pregnancy. Neurosurgery 33:515, 1993

179. Doyle KJ, Luxford WM: Acoustic neuroma in pregnancy. Am J Otol 15:111, 1994

180. Arango HA, Kalter CS, Decesare SL et al: Management of chemotherapy in a pregnancy complicated by a large neuroblastoma. Obstet Gynecol 84:665, 1994

181. Dildy GA III, Moise KJ Jr, Carpenter RJ Jr et al: Maternal malignancy metastatic to the products of conception: a review. Obstet Gynecol Surv 44:535, 1989

182. Rothman LA, Cohen CJ, Astarola J: Placental and fetal involvement by maternal malignancy: a report of rectal carcinoma and a review of the literature. Am J Obstet Gynecol 116:1023, 1973

183. Kurtin PJ, Gaffney TA, Haberman TM: Peripheral T cell lymphoma involving the placenta. Cancer 70:2963, 1992

184. Pollack RN, Sklarin NT, Rao S et al: Metastatic placental lymphoma associated with maternal human immunodeficiency virus infection. Obstet Gynecol 81:856, 1993

185. Tsujimura T, Matsumoto K, Aozasa K: Placental involvement by maternal non-Hodgkin's lymphoma. Arch Pathol Lab Med 117:325, 1993

186. Osada S, Horibe K, Oiwa K et al: A case of infantile acute monocytic leukemia caused by vertical transmission of the mother's leukemic cells. Cancer 65:1146, 1990

187. Pollack RN, Pollak M, Rochon L: Pregnancy complicated by medulloblastoma with metastases to the placenta. Obstet Gynecol 81:858, 1993

188. Bandy LC, Clarke-Pearson DL, Hammond CB: Malignant potential of gestational trophoblastic disease at the extreme age of reproductive life. Obstet Gynecol 64:395, 1984

189. Matalon M, Modan B: Epidemiologic aspects of hydatidiform mole in Israel. Am J Obstet Gynecol 112:107, 1972

190. Lurain JR, Brewer JI, Turok EE, Halpern B: Gestational trophoblastic disease: treatment results at the Brewer Trophoblastic Disease Center. Obstet Gynecol 60:354, 1982

191. Berkowitz RS, Goldstein DP, Bernstein MR, Sablinska B: Subsequent pregnancy outcomes in patients with molar pregnancies and gestational trophoblastic tumors. J Reprod Med 32:680, 1987

192. Sand PK, Lurain JR, Brewer JI: Repeat gestational trophoblastic disease. Obstet Gynecol 63:140, 1984

193. Copeland LJ: Gestational trophoblastic neoplasia. p. 1137. In Copeland LJ (ed): Textbook of Gynecology. WB Saunders, Philadelphia, 1993

194. Rice LW, Berkowitz, RS, Lage JM, Goldstein DP: Persistent gestational trophoblastic tumor after partial molar pregnancy. Gynecol Oncol 48:165, 1993

195. Goto S, Yamada A, Ishizuka T, Tomoda Y: Development of post molar trophoblastic disease after partial molar pregnancy. Gynecol Oncol 48:165, 1993

196. Briggs GG, Freeman RK, Yaffe SJ: Instructions for use of the reference guide. p. xix. In A Reference Guide to Fetal and Neonatal Risk: Drugs in Pregnancy and Lactation. 3rd Ed. Briggs GG, Freeman RK, Yaffe SJ (eds): Williams & Wilkins, Baltimore, 1990

197. Holmes FA: Breast cancer during pregnancy. Cancer Bull 46:405, 1994

198. Travers R, Sober A, Barnhill R et al: Increased thickness of pregnancy-associated melanoma: a study of the MGH pigmented lesion clinic. Melanoma Res 3(suppl):44, 1993

199. Gordon AN: Vulvar tumors. p. 1110. In Copeland LJ (ed): Textbook of Gynecology. WB Saunders, Philadelphia, 1993

Dermatologic Disorders

Michael C. Gordon and Mark B. Landon

Skin Changes During Normal Pregnancy

Physiologic changes in the skin during gestation can result in hyperpigmentation, hirsutism, hair loss, and several vascular abnormalities. Some of these conditions are believed to result from alterations in the hormonal milieu of pregnancy. Yet, for most skin changes in pregnancy there is little information concerning the precise etiologic factors involved in these processes. The obstetrician must be able to distinguish common skin changes of pregnancy from primary cutaneous diseases that antedate or develop during pregnancy.

Hyperpigmentation

Hyperpigmentation can be found in approximately 90 percent of pregnancies.[1] Women with a dark complexion are more likely to manifest hyperpigmentation during gestation. The hyperpigmentation maybe generalized or be localized only to areas of increased melanocyte density. Darkening of the areolae, umbilicus, vulva, and perianal skin may occur as early as the first trimester. The linea alba often becomes the hyperpigmented linea nigra. Pigmented nevi, freckles, and recent scars may also deepen in color. Hyperpigmentation on the face, known as *melasma* or *chloasma*, will often prompt complaints from pregnant women. Chloasma is usually manifested by well-defined hyperpigmented centrofacial patches and appears in various shades of brown, depending on the site of melanin distribution. Chloasma occurs in at least 70 percent of women and affects all races equally.[2] In addition to pregnancy, chloasma can occur with oral contraceptive use, liver disease, hyperthyroidism, and as a phototoxic reaction to certain cosmetics. Sunlight is thought to be necessary

for the development of chloasma. The role of hormonal factors such as melanocyte-stimulating hormone (MSH) is unclear. Levels of estrogen, which, like MSH, can stimulate melanogenesis, are not consistently elevated in women with chloasma.[3] During pregnancy, women with chloasma should avoid excessive sun exposure. Sunscreens may be helpful in retarding progression and recurrence postpartum. Chloasma normally regresses or disappears in the majority of women; however, nearly 30 percent of patients will have persistent hyperpigmentation at 10 year follow-up.[1] Women with persistent chloasma may be treated with 2 to 4 percent hydroquinone cream, 0.5 percent retinoic acid cream, or corticosteroid creams.[4]

During pregnancy, some nevi may increase in size, and new nevi may develop. This may necessitate the need to perform a biopsy if there is clinical suspicion for melanoma. In general, no evidence exists that pregnancy causes malignant transformation of nevi to melanoma.[5] However, a special subgroup of women with the familial dysplastic nevus syndrome appear to be at an increased risk for dysplastic changes during pregnancy. These women have a family history of melanoma and multiple clinically atypical nevi.[6] They should have careful dermatologic examination during gestation, and any changes in the shape, configuration, pigmentation, or elevation of a nevus should lead to a biopsy.

HAIR CHANGES

Hirsutism

Mild degrees of hirsutism are common during pregnancy. The face is frequently affected, although hair growth may be pronounced on the extremities as well. Abdominal hair growth is less common but may be exacerbated in women with a prominent male pattern escutcheon. Hirsutism is believed to be primarily an endocrinologic phenomenon. During normal pregnancy, the proportion of hair in the anagen (growing) phase is higher than that in the telogen (resting) phase. Hirsutism and elevated levels of cortisol may result from placental androgen production during normal pregnancy. Mild hirsutism rarely requires therapy. It normally regresses following delivery, but does recur with subsequent pregnancies. Excessive hirsutism with virilization should warrant investigation for an androgen-secreting tumor.

Telogen Effluvium

Telogen effluvium, or hair loss after a shift of anagen follicles to telogen, is often seen during the postpartum period. Because the telogen phase may last several months, patients may report hair loss for 3 to 4 months following delivery. Patients should be reassured that normal hair growth will occur 6 to 15 months postpartum, but in rare circumstances the hair may never be as thick as it was before pregnancy. The shedding actually represents reactivation of the hair follicle, which is followed by new growth.

Striae Distensae

Striae distensae begin to appear in the late second trimester in up to 90 percent of pregnant women.[3] Striae are thin atrophic pink or purple linear bands on the abdomen, breasts, and thighs. Striae are believed to result from a combination of two factors. Stretching is necessary to produce striae; however, adrenocorticosteroids and estrogen also promote tearing in the collagen matrix of the dermis and weakening of elastic fibers.[1] While many creams and ointments have been employed to treat striae distensae, these therapies are not believed to be of any benefit. Striae are permanent, yet the purplish color most often fades with time.

Vascular Changes

Vascular changes are evident within the skin of most pregnant women. High levels of estrogen are believed to be responsible for proliferation of blood vessels and congestion. Vasomotor instability may also produce pallor, flushing, and mottling of the skin in response to temperature changes. Increased capillary fragility is common in late pregnancy. Scattered petechiae are often seen on the lower extremities due to increased capillary hydrostatic pressure and capillary fragility.

Spider angiomata may be observed in up to 70 percent of white women during pregnancy. These lesions consist of a central red arteriole with tortuous radiating branches resembling a spider. Also common to liver disease, spider angiomata are found on the face, trunk, and upper extremities in the areas drained by the superior vena cava. Most lesions fade during the postpartum period within 3 months.

Similar to spider angiomata, palmar erythema is more common in white than black women, with nearly two-thirds of pregnancies affected. Erythema of the midpalm, hypothenar, and thenar eminences may occur as early as the first trimester as a result of a sixfold increase in blood flow to the hands.[7] This lesion is also seen with cirrhosis, systemic lupus erythematosus, and hyperthyroidism. When observed as a manifestation of pregnancy, it typically resolves following delivery.

Small capillary hemangiomas may be found during the second and third trimesters in up to 5 percent of pregnant women.[1] Unlike spider angiomata, these lesions do not necessarily blanch with compression. Most small hemangiomas will involute after delivery. Large hemangiomas may persist and can be associated with arteriovenous shunting and high-output cardiac failure.

During gestation the gingiva swells, giving rise to so-called pregnancy gingivitis.[8] Pyogenic granuloma or granuloma gravidarum of pregnancy may be seen in 2 percent of pregnancies.[3] Hypertrophy with capillary proliferation produces an elevated red-purple mass arising from the gingiva. The lesion consists of granulation tissue and an inflammatory infiltrate composed of various leukocytes and histiocytes. It is thought to be an abnormal tissue response to trauma. Although these masses usually remit during the postpartum period, surgical excision may be required if the lesion fails to resolve.

Specific Dermatologic Conditions Associated with Pregnancy (Table 37-1)

Pruritus

Pruritus is a common symptom in pregnancy, occurring in 3 to 14 percent of all women.[9] In a prospective study by Roger et al of 3,192 pregnant women, 1.6 percent suffered from persistent pruritus severe enough to warrant treatment. Pruritus is the common symptom of the majority of pregnancy-specific dermatologic diseases as well as nonpregnancy-specific disorders. It can also be caused by systemic entities such as liver disease, thyroid dysfunction, diabetes mellitus, drug eruptions, parasites, and malignancy. Cholestasis of pregnancy, which occurs in 0.5% of pregnancies, is one of the most common causes of pruritus. It is caused by intrahepatic cholestasis leading to increased levels of serum bile salts.[9,10] Itching, a result of the increased deposition of

Table 37-1 Pruritic Dermatoses of Pregnancy

Disease	Onset	Degree of Pruritus	Types of Lesions	Distribution	Increased Incidence of Fetal Morbidity or Mortality
Herpes gestationis	1st month to postpartum	Moderate to severe	Erythematous papules, vesicles, bullae	Abdomen, extremities, generalized	Unresolved
Prurigo gestationis	4th to 9th month	Moderate	Excoriated papules	Extensor surfaces of extremities	No
Impetigo herpetiformis	1st to 9th month	Minimal	Pustules	Genitalia, medial thighs umbilicus, breasts, axillas	Yes
Pruritic urticarial papules and plaques of pregnancy	3rd trimester	Severe	Erythematous urticarial papules and plaques	Abdomen, thighs, buttocks, occasionally arms and legs	No
Cholestasis of pregnancy	3rd trimester	Moderate to severe	None or excoriations	Generalized	Unresolved

bile salts found in the skin, occurs in the third trimester of pregnancy.

The differential diagnosis of dermatologic disorders specific to pregnancy that present with pruritus as a common symptom include herpes gestationis, pruritic urticarial papules and plaques of pregnancy (PUPPP), prurigo gestationis, and pruritic folliculitis of pregnancy. The difficulty in diagnosing these disorders can be attributed to a confusing nomenclature and to the lack of specific diagnostic criteria for each of the disorders with the exception of herpes gestationis. Different terms have been used to classify similar skin lesions. Recently an attempt was made to simplify the classification scheme into fewer entities if no clear clinical, biologic, histologic, immunologic, or hormonal differences exist that can be used to differentiate between the lesions.[10–12] Roger et al proposed a routine laboratory evaluation in all cases of pruritic dermatoses of pregnancy, including a skin biopsy of all lesions with direct immunofluorescence testing as well as serum bile salts and/or transaminase levels. Other authors have argued that this workup is not cost effective.[13]

Herpes Gestationis

Herpes (pemphigoid) gestationis is a pruritic, autoimmune, bullous disease of the skin that occurs during pregnancy and the puerperium.[14] It has been reported only in female patients and occurs only if placental tissue is present. Herpes gestationis has been reported in women with choriocarcinomas and hydatiform moles. The disease has a reported incidence of 1 per 1,700 to 50,000 pregnancies.[10,14,15] In a prospective study in which all pregnant women with pruritic skin lesions had skin biopsies, the incidence of herpes gestationis was found to be 1 per 7,000.[16] A hormonal influence seems to be operable as this disorder can recur with menses

and oral contraceptive use. A genetic predisposition is also suggested by an increased frequency of certain HLA antigens. Up to 85 percent of women with herpes gestationis have HLA-DR3 and 45 percent have the combination of DR3 and DR4.[14,17] An increased frequency of these HLA antigens has been found in association with other autoimmune disorders.

Clinically, the disease presents with lesions that initially may closely resemble PUPPP and later, when bullae or vesicles develop, may closely resemble dermatitis herpetiformis and pemphigus vulgaris (Fig. 37-1).[18,19] The initial symptom is pruritus, characteristically extreme, followed by erythema and edema of the subcutaneous tissue. Within days or weeks, papules and plaques form that have been described as having an urticarial quality. The lesions are often present on the trunk, back, buttocks, forearms, palms, and soles and initially develop around the umbilicus in 50 percent of patients. The face, scalp, and mucosa are infrequently involved (less than 10 percent of women). Vesicles and tense serum-filled bullae develop at the margins of the edematous, erythematous plaques or can appear de novo in otherwise clinically uninvolved skin within 2 to 4 weeks of the initial onset of the disease. This represents the final stage of the disease and does not always develop.[14] The lesions tend to heal without scarring if secondary infection is prevented. The onset is usually during the second or third trimester, with a mean onset of 21 weeks' gestation, although patients may present with recurring crops of blisters at any time during pregnancy. Herpes gestationis occurs for the first time during the early postpartum period (less than 4 days) in about 20 percent of cases.[14] An inconsistent clinical finding is the tendency for spontaneous improvement during the last 6 to 8 weeks of pregnancy. However, the puerperium is often marked by exacerbation of this condition within 24 to 48 hours of delivery. The dura-

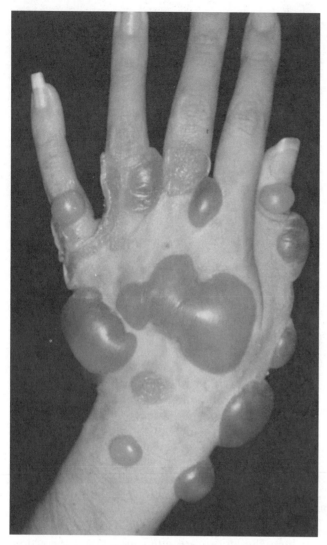

Fig. 37-1 Herpes gestationis during the third trimester. This patient developed erythematous macules on the chest and hands that progressed to bullae formation. Biopsy revealed a heavy linear complement deposition at the basement membrane zone, consistent with herpes gestationis. (Courtesy of Dr. Steven Wolverton, Division of Dermatology, Department of Medicine, The Ohio State University.)

tion postpartum is variable, with the bullous lesions persisting 5 to 24 weeks and the urticarial lesions even longer, depending on a number of factors such as use of steroids, levels of antibasement membrane zone antibody, and whether the woman nurses.[14] Herpes gestationis may be recurrent and is usually more severe with an earlier onset in subsequent pregnancies.

The diagnosis of herpes gestationis can be made with reasonable assurance if there is a typical clinical presentation and recurrence with pregnancy, as well as peripheral eosinophilia. Absolute confirmation is made by biopsy and immunopathologic studies that reveal complement, C_3, in a band-like distribution along the basement membrane between the epidermis and der-

mis.[20] This complement deposition is now accepted as the sine qua non of herpes gestationis and is demonstrable in essentially 100 percent of cases.[14] The importance of biopsy with immunofluorescent staining to confirm the diagnosis may be in providing a better ability to counsel women as to the risk of recurrence in future pregnancies. IgG is found at the basement membrane in a minority of cases. Histology reveals extensive necrosis of the basal cell layer and edema of the papillary dermis. A chronic inflammatory response with infiltrates of eosinophils admixed with lymphocytes is present around the bullae in a perivascular distribution. Herpes gestationis is IgG mediated and the so-called herpes gestationis factor (HG factor) is a circulating IgG1 autoantibody with complement-fixing capability.[12] In recent years, significant advances have been made in understanding the pathophysiology of the herpes gestationis factor. The antigen involved in herpes gestationis is a 180 kD transmembrane collagenous protein found in the cellular matrix of the epidermis and mediates the attachment of the keratinocytes to the underlying basement membrane.[12,21] Circulating HG factor has not been isolated from the sera of all affected women and when found rarely exceeds a titer of 1:16.[14] The HG factor crosses the placenta, binds with the basement membrane of amnion and chorion laeve[22] and can be deposited in fetal skin.[14] It is currently hypothesized that the expression of molecules of the major histocompatibility complex (MHC) in the placenta triggers an allogenic reaction between maternal lymphocytes and the paternal-derived MHC molecules. This then results in the formation of the HG factor against a placental antigen that cross reacts with the normal maternal basement membrane and causes the skin lesions.[12]

The treatment for herpes gestationis is aimed at controlling pruritus, suppressing the formation of new vesicles and bullae and preventing secondary infection of skin lesions. Topical steroids and antihistamines may be used initially if the symptoms are mild. Most patients will, however, require systemic corticosteroid therapy. Prednisone is often begun in doses of 40 to 60 mg/day. The dose of steroid can be tapered to 10 to 20 mg/day if clinical improvement is noted. Azathioprine, dapsone, and, rarely, plasmapheresis have been employed in cases that fail to respond to corticosteroids.[14] Herpes gestationis does not increase the risk of maternal mortality.

Prior to the development of immunologic techniques that permitted an accurate diagnosis, herpes gestationis was believed to have minimal adverse effects on pregnancy.[23] In 1969, Kolodny[15] reported no increase in preterm births, stillbirths, or abortions. However, Lawley et al[24] subsequently reviewed 40 immunologically proven cases and documented serious fetal morbidity and mortality: the preterm birth rate was 22 percent and three stillbirths were noted. Lawley et al[24] suggested that high levels of circulating antibasement membrane antibody and peripheral eosinophilia were the cause of the increased fetal risk. More recently, Shornick and Black[25] described 74 patients with herpes gestationis confirmed by immunofluorescence studies. They found an increased frequency of fetal growth restriction and prematurity but not stillbirth or miscarriage.[25] The increased risk of adverse outcomes has been thought to be secondary to possible abnormal immunologic response within the placenta due to the HG factor. For this reason, antepartum testing is currently recommended. Transient newborn herpes gestationis has also been reported, along with the presence of circulating HG factor in 10 percent of newborns. Neonatal herpes gestationis is usually mild and may be marked only by erythematous papules or frank bullae.[26] Presumably, passive transfer of antibody is the stimulus for this process, which generally resolves within a short period of time.[27]

PUPPP Syndrome

In 1979, Lawley et al[28] described seven patients with severe pruritic eruption that first occurred during the third trimester of pregnancy. It was initially felt this eruption could be differentiated by clinical presentation and histologic findings from any other previously described dermatologic condition associated with pregnancy. In the United Kingdom, the term *polymorphic eruptions of pregnancy* was developed by Holmes and Black[11] in an attempt to better describe the polymorphic features of this skin disease. The incidence of PUPPP is uncertain, although Holmes et al,[29] suggested a figure of 1 in 240 pregnancies and Roger et al[10] found an incidence of 1 in 200 women. PUPPP is the most common dermatosis of pregnancy, but the etiology and pathogenesis are unknown.[19] No hormonal or autoimmune abnormalities have been found in women with PUPPP.[30] Since the majority of women affected by PUPPP are primigravidae with prominent striae or have uterine distention with twins or hydramnios, it has been hypothesized that increased skin tension resulting in skin damage may play a role in the etiology of PUPPP.[12]

The lesions of PUPPP typically begin on the abdomen and initially consist of 1 to 2 mm erythematous papules surrounded by a narrow pale halo that coalesce into urticarial plaques.[31] Small vesicles can also develop on the plaques. They usually spread to the thighs and possibly the buttocks and arms within 2 to 3 days. In contrast to herpes gestationis, the periumbilical area is uninvolved in PUPPP. The face is not affected. Most patients complain of intense pruritus that improves

rapidly following delivery with resolution in 1 to 2 weeks. The average onset of the skin lesions is 36 weeks' gestation, and PUPPP rarely develops postpartum (Fig. 37-2).[31] There are limited data concerning recurrence risk with subsequent pregnancies; however, it is thought not to recur.

Histologic findings in this disorder consist of a normal epidermis accompanied by a superficial perivascular infiltrate of lymphocytes and histiocytes associated with edema of the papillary dermis.[28] Another pattern is that of a spongiotic epidermis with a dermal perivascular and interstitial lymphohistiocytic infiltrate revealing marked edema and the presence of eosinophilia. Immunofluorescence studies are negative for both immunoglobulins and complement. These histologic findings are nonspecific and may be associated with any urticarial allergic response as well as several viral exanthems. It is essential, therefore, to obtain a complete drug history and to consider skin biopsy with immunofluorescence studies to exclude early or atypical herpes gestationis before making the diagnosis of PUPPP and starting treatment.

Therapy employing topical steroids is generally successful in the vast majority of women, but some will require systemic steroids.[31] Antipruritic drugs such as hydroxyzine or diphenhydramine may be helpful. The response to treatment may be difficult to evaluate, as abatement of cutaneous lesions and pruritus typically accompanies delivery.[28] Some authors have recommended use of antepartum testing in pregnancies with PUPPP, but the few reported series of women with PUPPP have failed to reveal an adverse effect on fetal or maternal outcome. The main goal of therapy is symptomatic relief of the intense pruritus.[31] In some women, the pruritus will be significant enough to warrant induction of labor once fetal lung maturity is ensured.

Prurigo Gestationis (Papular Dermatitis)

This disorder consists of pruritic excoriated papules usually limited to the extensor surfaces of the extremities. The disease is said to occur in 1 per 50 to 200 pregnancies.[32] Lesions generally appear during the second half of gestation. They are small, 1 to 2 mm papules that are distributed symmetrically. Vesicle or bullae formation does not occur. The disease usually resolves following delivery. Maternal and fetal conditions are not affected, and recurrence during subsequent gestations is uncommon. Papular dermatitis probably represents a more severe and widespread form of this condition. In the past, papular dermatitis was considered a separate skin disorder due to the original reports of increased fetal risk and abnormal biochemical findings of elevations of urinary chorionic gonadotropin and decreased plasma levels of hydro-

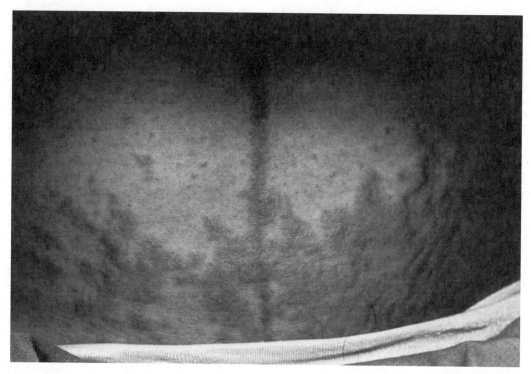

Fig. 37-2 Pruritic urticarial papules and plaques of pregnancy (PUPPP syndrome). Erythematous urticarial plaques and small papules erupted on the abdomen of this patient during the third trimester.

cortisone.[33,34] Because of the inadequate assessment of the fetal risk, the absence of adequate controls of the biochemical findings, and the lack of further reports of this specific skin rash, the majority of current authors do not recognize this as a separate disorder.[10–12]

Nurse[35] has described two types of prurigo of pregnancy. The early form, which presents between 25 and 29 weeks' gestation, is marked by intensely pruritic papules of the proximal extremities and trunk. The late form typically appears close to term with abdominal papules often located in abdominal striae. No laboratory or biological abnormalities have been consistently found in these women, and the etiology and pathogenesis of these papular lesions are unknown, although there is some evidence of an atopic diathesis.[10] The histological findings show a nonspecific dermal perivascular lymphohistiocytic infiltrate. The diagnosis of prurigo gestationis is made by the clinical appearance of a primary papular eruption in a woman without laboratory evidence of cholestasis of pregnancy. Due to the lack of a major clinical, biologic, histologic, or hormonal features that can be used to distinguish this dermatitis, Roger et al[10] suggest this condition cannot be reliably differentiated from PUPPP. The pruritus responds to calamine lotion and oral antipruritics. Corticosteroid therapy is rarely necessary for the treatment of prurigo gestationis.

Pruritic Folliculitis of Pregnancy

In 1981, Zoberman and Farmer[36] described six pregnant women with a disseminated erythematous, excoriated papular rash of the hair follicles and surrounding dermis. In the study by Roger et al,[10] the incidence of this skin disease was found to be 1 per 3,000. The lesions consist of multiple 2 to 4 mm follicular papules or pustules on the shoulders, upper back, arms, chest, and abdomen and clinically resemble acne. The exact etiology is unknown but could be hormonally induced since the lesions disappear following delivery.[11] Histopathologic findings show acute folliculitis with a neutrophilic infiltrate of the follicle and the surrounding dermis.[4] The disorder is not associated with maternal or fetal morbidity. Treatment is similar to that of mild acne, consisting of 10 percent benzoyl peroxide and 1 percent hydrocortisone if severe pruritus exists.

Impetigo Herpetiformis

Although not a typical cause of pruritus, impetigo herpetiformis is a rare pustular skin disease that has been reported in less than 100 pregnancies. There is disagreement among various authors as to whether impetigo herpetiformis is a distinct entity caused by pregnancy or simply a form of pustular psoriasis triggered by pregnancy.[37] In the typical woman with impetigo herpetiformis, there is no prior history of skin disease, no family history of psoriasis, and, following the pregnancy, the lesions do not recur except with subsequent pregnancies. The disorder usually occurs is the second half of gestation and begins with the appearance of groups of painful sterile pustules on an erythematous base typically in the groin and inner thighs. These lesions coalesce and spread to the trunk and extremities and may become secondarily impetiginized. Bullae formation is uncommon. Unlike may of the dermatoses of pregnancy, the mucous membranes are frequently affected. Painful, oral, grayish white plaques may resemble the oral lesions of pemphigus vulgaris.[18] Histologically, these lesions reveal spongioform pustules that are intradermal and subcorneal in location. A dense inflammatory exudate surrounds dermal blood vessels. The histopathologic features are indistinguishable from pustular psoriasis.[37] Impetigo herpetiformis must be differentiated from impetigo, herpes gestationis, and pemphigus.

Impetigo herpetiformis may be accompanied by systemic symptoms, including fever, chills, arthralgias, vomiting, diarrhea, and lymphadenopathy.[37] Prostration with septicemia may follow. Cardiac and renal failure have occurred in severe cases. Hypocalcemia and hyperphosphatemia are not uncommon in this setting and have led investigators to postulate that hypoparathyroidism is associated with this disorder. Successful treatment of impetigo herpetiformis includes the administration of systemic corticosteroid and antibiotics for secondary infection, although most authors report only a moderate response to the corticosteroid treatment.[37] The disease usually remits following delivery but may recur in future pregnancies at an earlier gestational age. Maternal fatalities and increased fetal wastage have been observed in the few reported cases. Therefore, fetal surveillance and elective delivery after fetal maturity has been documented are recommended.[38]

Specific Dermatologic Conditions Affected by Pregnancy

Pemphigus Vulgaris

Pemphigus vulgaris is an uncommon autoimmune, intraepidermal, bullous dermatitis that is similar in appearance and pathogenesis to herpes gestationis but is not unique to pregnancy. It normally occurs in the fourth to sixth decades of life and therefore is rarely encountered in pregnancy, with less than 30 reported cases.[39] Pemphigus vulgaris is caused by a circulating IgG autoantibody directed against the cell surface of keratinocytes, which causes disruption of the cohesive forces between these epidermal cells. This results in numerous vesicles, flaccid bullous lesions, and subsequent erosions of the skin and the mucous membranes. Areas typically affected include the groin, scalp, face, neck, axilla, trunk, periumbilical area, and genitalia. The lesions develop on previously normal-appearing skin and heal without scarring unless they become secondarily infected. Before the advent of steroids, mortality was near 100 percent due to sepsis and electrolyte abnormalities. Treatment options now include steroids, immunosuppressants, and plasmapheresis. With such therapies mortality has been decreased.[40]

Histologically, pemphigus vulgaris is characterized by acantholysis with intraepithelial blisters.[40] Immunofluorescence studies of the skin reveal deposits of IgG on the cell surfaces of keratinocytes with or without complement deposits. The majority of patients with active disease have circulating antiepithelial IgG antibody. Since the clinical appearance of herpes gestationis and pemphigus vulgaris are similar, and because pemphigus vulgaris can occur for the first time in pregnancy, the use of skin biopsies with immunofluorescence studies is necessary to differentiate these two bullous disease.

Like herpes gestationis, the antibody in pemphigus vulgaris can cross the placenta and cause neonatal skin eruptions.[39] Neonatal illness has been reported in 14 of 23 reported pregnancies and resolves in 2 to 6 weeks without treatment. In addition, pemphigus vulgaris has been reported to cause stillbirths in 4 fetuses and low birth weight in 3 neonates in the 23 reported cases. The fetal risks, but not the risks of neonatal skin disease, seem to be directly related to the severity of the maternal illness.[39]

Erythema Nodosum

Another uncommon skin disorder that is sometimes associated with pregnancy is erythema nodosum.[41] The exact pathogenesis of this apparently autoimmune skin disease is unknown but is associated with malignant disorders, infections, drugs, and pregnancy. The peak incidence of this disease occurs at 20 to 30 years of age, with more women than men affected.[42] Clinically, individuals present with a sudden onset of an erythematous, warm, tender nodule on the extensor surface of the lower extremities. These nodules then progress to ecchymotic lesions that resemble a bruise and resolve without scarring over 3 to 6 weeks. The nodules are 1 to 15 cm in diameter, multiple, and usually bilateral. Histologically erythema nodosum is a nodular inflammation of the subcutaneous tissue that leads to a granulomatous infiltrate.

In the 1960s the association between the hormonal changes of pregnancy and erythema nodosum was first reported. Pregnancy appears to provide a hormonal environment that promotes the development of erythema nodosum.[41] Effective treatment of erythema nodosum involves a rapid investigation for the associated cause. Treatment is then directed specifically at the underlying disorder. With treatment of the primary illness or discontinuation of the offending medication, the skin lesions resolve. Although the clinical presentation of erythema nodosum is frequently classic, a skin biopsy to confirm the diagnosis is usually recommended. In the few reported cases involving pregnancy, no adverse effects upon the pregnancy or fetal outcome were noted.[43]

KEY POINTS

- Pregnancy is associated with several physiologic changes of the skin that may concern the pregnant woman, and these concerns can be quickly resolved if the health care provider is aware of such changes. These include hyperpigmentation, mild hirsutism, striae distensae, and vascular changes.

- During pregnancy, some nevi may increase in size, and new nevi may develop. This may necessitate the need to perform a biopsy if there is clinical suspicion for melanoma.

- Pruritus is a relatively common symptom in pregnancy (3 to 14 percent), but infrequently is due to a serious dermatologic disease and usually resolves postpartum. In addition to evaluating the pregnant woman for dermatologic diseases that occur unassociated with pregnancy, the health care provider must evaluate for pregnancy-specific dermatologic diseases.

- The most common causes of pruritic rashes in pregnancy are PUPPP, prurigo gestationis, and cholestasis of pregnancy.

- Rare dermatologic lesions associated with pregnancy are herpes gestationis, pruritic folliculitis of pregnancy, and impetigo herpetiformis.

- The only dermatologic diseases of pregnancy that have been shown to cause fetal morbidity are herpes gestationis and impetigo herpetiformis. Antepartum testing for fetal well-being should be utilized in these women. Transient newborn herpes gestationis has also been reported along with the presence of circulating HG factor in 10 percent of newborns in women with herpes gestationis.

- Herpes (pemphigoid) gestationis is a pruritic, autoimmune, bullous disease of the skin that occurs during pregnancy and the puerperium. Clinically, the disease presents with lesions that initially may closely resemble PUPPP and later, when bullae or vesicles develop, may closely resemble dermatitis herpetiformis and pemphigus vulgaris.

- In the majority of cases PUPPP and herpes gestationis can be diagnosed by the appearance of the rash, but occasionally a skin biopsy with immunofluorescence studies will be needed to differentiate the two disorders.

- The treatment for herpes gestationis is aimed at controlling pruritus, suppressing the formation of new vesicles and bullae, and preventing secondary infection of skin lesions. Topical steroids and antihistamines may be used initially if the symptoms are mild. Most patients will, however, require systemic corticosteroid therapy.

- Therapy employing topical steroids is generally successful in the vast majority of women with PUPPP, but some will require systemic steroids. Antipruritic drugs such as hydroxyzine or diphenhydramine may be helpful. The main goal of therapy is symptomatic relief of the intense pruritus. In some women, the pruritus will be significant enough to warrant induction of labor once fetal lung maturity is ensured.

References

1. Wong RC, Ellis CN: Physiologic skin changes in pregnancy. J Am Acad Dermatol 10:929, 1984
2. Sanchez NP, Pathak MA, Sato S et al: Melasma: a clinical, light microscopic, ultrastructural, and immunofluorescence study. J Am Acad Dermatol 4:698, 1981
3. Winston GB, Lewis CW: Dermatoses of pregnancy. J Am Acad Dermatol 6:977, 1982
4. Murray JC: Pregnancy and the skin. Dermatol Clin 8:327, 1990
5. Lerner AB, Nordlund JJ, Kirkwod JM: Effects of oral contraceptives and pregnancy on melanoma. N Engl J Med 301:47, 1979
6. Ellis DL: Pregnancy and sex steroid hormone effects on nevi of patients with the dysplastic nevus syndrome. J Am Acad Dermatol 25:467, 1991
7. Mattison MD: Transdermal drug absorption during pregnancy. Clin Obstet Gynecol 33:718, 1990
8. Parmley T, O'Brien TJ: Skin changes during pregnancy. Clin Obstet Gynecol 33:713, 1990
9. Dacus JV: Pruritus in pregnancy. Clin Obstet Gynecol 33:738, 1990
10. Roger D, Vaillant L, Fignon A et al: Specific pruritus diseases of pregnancy, a prospective study of 3,192 pregnant women. Arch Dermatol 130:734, 1994
11. Holmes RC, Black MM: The specific dermatoses of pregnancy. J Am Acad Dermatol 8:405, 1983
12. Borradori L, Saurat J: Specific dermatoses of pregnancy, toward a comprehensive view? Arch Dermatol 130:778, 1994
13. Goodall J: Immunofluorescence biopsy for pruritic urticarial papules and plaques of pregnancy. J Am Acad Dermatol 22:322, 1990
14. Shornick JK: Herpes gestationis. J Am Acad Dermatol 17:539, 1987
15. Kolodny R: Herpes gestationis: a new assessment of incidence, diagnosis, and fetal prognosis. Am J Obstet Gynecol 104:39, 1969
16. Zurn A, Celebi CR, Bernard P et al: A prospective immunofluorescence study of 111 cases of pruritic dermatosis of pregnancy: IgM anti-basement membrane zone antibodies as a novel finding. Br J Dermatol 126:474, 1992
17. Homes RC, Black MM: Herpes gestationis. Dermatol Clin 1:195, 1987
18. Wade TR, Wade SL, Jones HE: Skin changes and diseases associated with pregnancy. Obstet Gynecol 52:233, 1978
19. Alcalay J, Wolf JE: Pruritic urticarial papules and plaques of pregnancy: the enigma and the confusion. J Am Acad of Dermatol 19:1115, 1988
20. Jordon ER, Heine KG, Tappeiner G et al: The immunopathology of herpes gestationis: immunofluorescence studies and characterization of "HG factor." J Clin Invest 57 1426, 1976
21. Morrison LH, Labib RS, Zone JJ et al: Herpes gestationis autoantibodies recognize a 180-kD human epidermal antigen. J Clin Invest 81:2023, 1988
22. Ortonne JP, Hsi BL, Verrando P et al: Herpes gestationis factor reacts with amniotic epithelial basement membrane. Br J Dermatol 117:147, 1987
23. Carruthers JA: Herpes gestationis: clinical features of immunologically proven cases. Am J Obstet Gynecol 131:865, 1978
24. Lawley TJ, Stingl G, Katz SI: Fetal and maternal risk factors in herpes gestationis. Arch Dermatol 114:552, 1978
25. Shornick JK, Black MM: Fetal risks in herpes gestationis. J Am Acad Dermatol 26:63, 1992
26. Bonifazi E, Meneghini CL: Herpes gestationis with transient bullous lesions in the newborn. Pediatr Dermatol 34:715, 1984
27. Chorzelski TP, Jablonska S, Beutner EH et al: Herpes gestationis with identical lesions in the newborn: passive transfer of disease? Arch Dermatol 112:129, 1976
28. Lawley TJ, Hertz KC, Wade TR et al: Pruritic urticarial papules and plaques of pregnancy. JAMA 241:1696, 1979
29. Holmes RC, Black MM, Dann J et al: A comparative study of toxic erythema of pregnancy and herpes gestationis. Br J Dermatol 106:499, 1982
30. Alcalay J, Ingber A, Kafri B et al: Hormonal evaluation and autoimmune background in pruritic urticarial papules and plaques of pregnancy. Am J Obstet Gynecol 158:417, 1988
31. Yancey KB, Hall RP, Lawley TJ: Pruritic urticarial papules and plaques of pregnancy. Clinical experience in 25 patients. J Am Acad Dermatol 10:473, 1984
32. Ware M, Swinscow TDV, Thwaites JG: Pregnancy prurigo. BMJ 1:397, 1969
33. Spangler AS, Reddy W, Bardawil WA: Papular dermatitis of pregnancy: a new clinical entity? JAMA 181:577, 1962
34. Spangler AS, Emerson K: Estrogen levels and estrogen therapy in papular dermatitis of pregnancy. Am J Obstet Gynecol 110:435, 1971
35. Nurse DS: Prurigo of pregnancy. Aust J Dermatol 9:258, 1968
36. Zoberman E, Farmer ER: Pruritic folliculitis of pregnancy. Arch Dermatol 117:20, 1981
37. Lotem M, Katzenelson V, Rotem A et al: Impetigo herpetiformis: a variant of pustular psoriasis or a separate entity. J Am Acad Dermatol 20:338, 1989
38. Oumeish OY, Farraj SE, Bataineh A: Some aspects of impetigo herpetiformis. Arch Dermatol 118:103, 1982
39. Rauch M, Ohel G, Rahav D, Samueloff A: Pemphigus vulgaris and pregnancy. Obstet Gynecol Surv 50:755, 1995
40. Stanley JR: Pemphigus. p. 606. In Fitzpatrick TB, Eisen AZ, Wolff K et al: (eds): Dermatology in General Medicine. 4th eD. McGraw-Hill, New York, 1993

41. Bartelsmeyer JA, Petrie RH: Erythema nodosum, estrogens, and pregnancy. Clin Obstet Gynecol 33:777, 1990

42. Bondi EE, Lazarus GS: Disorders of subcutaneous tissue. p. 1329. In Fitzpatrick TB, Eisen AZ, Wolff K et al: (eds): Dermatology in General Medicine. 4th eD. McGraw-Hill, New York, 1993

43. Larger L, Bukovsky I, Ariely S, Capsi E: Erythema nodosum associated with pregnancy. Case reports. Eur J Obstet Gynecol 9:399, 1979

Chapter 38

Maternal and Perinatal Infection

Patrick Duff

Infection is the single most common complication encountered by the obstetrician. Some infections such as puerperal endometritis, candidiasis, trichomoniasis, and lower urinary tract infections are of principal concern to the mother and pose little or no risk to the fetus or neonate. Others, such as rubella, cytomegalovirus infection, and parvovirus infection cause minimal maternal morbidity but devastating fetal injury. Still others, for example, chorioamnionitis, gonorrhea, syphilis, toxoplasmosis, pyelonephritis, group B streptococcal infection, rubeola, and human immunodeficiency virus (HIV) infection, may cause serious morbidity, and even mortality, for the mother, fetus, or neonate.

The purpose of this chapter is to review in detail the major maternal and perinatal infections that the obstetrician confronts in clinical practice. The first portion of the chapter focuses primarily on bacterial infections of the lower and upper genital tract. The second portion considers the infections that pose special risks to the fetus. The principal features of these infections are summarized in Tables 38-1 and 38-2.

Vaginal Infections

Bacterial Vaginosis

Epidemiology

Bacterial vaginosis (BV) is responsible for approximately 45 percent of cases of vaginitis. It is a polymicrobial infection, and the predominant pathogens are anaerobes, *Gardnerella vaginalis*, *Mobiluncus* species, and genital mycoplasmas.[1] BV usually results from disturbances in the normal vaginal ecosystem caused by hormonal changes, pregnancy, or antibiotic adminis-

tration. The principal feature of this alteration in vaginal flora is a marked decrease in the lactobacilli species that produce hydrogen peroxide and a corresponding increase in anaerobic organisms. In some instances, BV can result from sexual contact with an infected partner. In contrast to trichomoniasis and candidiasis, symptomatic BV in pregnancy has been associated with several serious maternal complications, including preterm labor, preterm premature rupture of membranes, chorioamnionitis, and puerperal endometritis.[2-4]

Diagnosis

The most prominent clinical manifestation of BV is a thin, gray, homogeneous, malodorous vaginal discharge. The odor is often accentuated after intercourse. Vulvar or vaginal pruritus is uncommon, and the vaginal pH is characteristically more than 4.5. When vaginal secretions are mixed with several drops of a 10 percent potassium hydroxide (KOH) solution, a pungent fishy odor is produced ("whiff test" or amine test). On microscopic examination of a saline preparation, the normal lactobacilli flora is largely replaced by multiple small bacilli and cocci. Motile, comma-shaped *Mobiluncus* species and clue cells are present (Fig. 38-1). Culture of vaginal secretions is not indicated in routine clinical practice.[1,5]

Treatment

Because of the potential serious sequelae associated with BV, *pregnant* patients should be screened for this condition and treated once the diagnosis is established. Concurrent treatment of the woman's sexual partner(s) has not been shown to improve outcome or prevent recurrences.

Table 38-1   Etiology, Diagnosis, and Management of Major Obstetric Infections

Condition	Microbiology	Confirmatory Diagnostic Test	Treatment[a]
Vaginal Infection			
Bacterial vaginosis	*Gardnerella vaginalis, Mobiluncus* species, anaerobes, mycoplasmas	Saline preparation	Topical or oral clindamycin or metronidazole
Candidiasis	*Candida albicans, C. tropicalis, C. glabrata*	KOH preparation	Topical antifungal cream
Trichomoniasis	*Trichomonas vaginalis*	Saline preparation	Oral metronidazole
Endocervical infection			
Gonorrhea	*Neisseria gonorrhoeae*	Endocervical culture	Oral cefixime or intramuscular ceftriaxone
Chlamydia	*C. trachomatis*	Endocervical culture, antigen detection	Oral erythromycin, azithromycin, or amoxicillin
Urinary tract infection			
Urethritis	*N. gonorrhoeae*	Culture of urethral discharge	Oral cefixime or intramuscular ceftriaxone
	C. trachomatis	Culture of urethral discharge or antigen detection	Oral erythromycin, azithromycin, or amoxicillin
Asymptomatic bacteriuria or cystitis	*E. coli, Klebsiella pneumoniae, Proteus* species	Urinalysis, culture	Sulfisoxazole, nitrofurantoin macrocrystals, trimethoprim-sulfamethoxazole
Pyelonephritis	As above	As above	Intravenous cefazolin and/or gentamicin or aztreonam
Chorioamnionitis	Group B streptococci, coliforms, anaerobes	Clinical examination; amniotic fluid leukocyte esterase, glucose, gram stain, and culture	Intravenous ampicillin plus gentamicin; add clindamycin or metronidazole if cesarean delivery is required
Puerperal endometritis	Group B streptococci, coliforms, anaerobes	Clinical examination	Intravenous clindamycin plus gentamicin or extended spectrum cephalosporin or penicillin

[a] See text for detailed prescribing information.

Both oral clindamycin, 300 mg twice daily for 7 days, and metronidazole, 500 mg twice daily for 7 days, result in microbiologic and clinical cure in approximately 90 percent of women.[6–8] These drugs also are highly effective when administered for short courses in topical form. However, the latter preparations are more expensive. Concerns about metronidazole's possible mutagenicity and carcinogenicity support a recommendation for use of topical clindamycin vaginal cream (2 percent) for treatment of BV in early pregnancy (one applicatorful daily for 7 days). Once the period of organogenesis is complete, oral metronidazole may be used because it offers a distinct cost savings with respect to either topical medication or oral clindamycin.

Candidiasis

Epidemiology

Candidiasis is responsible for approximately 25 to 30 percent of all cases of vaginitis. The three principal organisms that cause symptomatic infection are, in descending order of frequency: *Candida albicans, C. tropicalis,* and *C. glabrata.*[9] Candidiasis is not usually a sexually transmitted disease. Yeast are part of the normal vaginal flora in many women, and symptoms develop only when overgrowth of these organisms occurs. Several conditions predispose to symptomatic moniliasis, including recent antibiotic or corticosteroid therapy, diabetes, use of oral contraceptives, pregnancy, and im-

Table 38-2 Summary of Etiology, Diagnosis, and Management of Major Perinatal Infections

Condition	Complications		Diagnosis		Management[a]	
	Maternal	Fetal/Neonatal	Maternal	Fetal/Neonatal	Maternal	Fetal/Neonatal
CMV	Chorioretinitis, pneumonia in immunocompromised patient	Congenital infection	Detection of antibody	Amniocentesis—culture of amniotic fluid, ultrasound	Ganciclovir for severe infection	Consider pregnancy termination when mother has primary infection
Group B streptococci	UTI, chorioamnionitis, endometritis, wound infection, preterm labor, PROM	Sepsis, pneumonia, meningitis	Culture	Culture	Intrapartum antibiotic prophylaxis	Treatment with antibiotics
Hepatitis A	Rare	None	Detection of antibody	NA	Supportive care	Administer immunoglobulin to neonate if mother acutely infected at delivery
B	Chronic liver disease	Neonatal infection	Detection of surface antigen	NA	HBIG + HBV for susceptible household contacts	HBIG + HBV immediately after delivery
C	Chronic liver disease	Neonatal infection	Detection of antibody	NA	Supportive care	No immunoprophylaxis available
D	Chronic liver disease	Neonatal infection	Detection of antigen and antibody	NA	Supportive care	HBIG + HBV immediately after delivery
E	Increased mortality	None	Detection of antibody	NA	Supportive care	None
Herpes simplex	Disseminated infection in immunocompromised patient	Neonatal infection	Clinical examination, culture, PCR	Clinical examination, culture	Acyclovir for severe primary infection	Cesarean delivery when mother has overt infection
HIV infection	Opportunistic infection, malignancy	Congenital or perinatal infection	Detection of antibody or antigen	Same	Zidovudine for prevention of vertical transmission	Zidovudine
Parvovirus infection	Rare	Anemia → hydrops	Detection of antibody	Ultrasound	Supportive care	Intrauterine transfusion for severe anemia
Rubella	Rare	Congenital infection	Detection of antibody	Ultrasound	Supportive care	Pregnancy termination for affected fetus
Rubeola	Otitis media, pneumonia, encephalitis	Abortion, preterm delivery	Detection of antibody	N/A	Supportive care	N/A
Syphilis	Aortitis, neurosyphilis	Congenital infection	Darkfield examination or serology	Ultrasound	Penicillin	Penicillin
Toxoplasmosis	Chorioretinitis, CNS infection	Congenital infection	Detection of antibody	Cordocentesis, detection of fetal antibody	Sulfadiazine, pyrimethamine, spiramycin	Treatment of mother prior to delivery prevents fetal infection
Varicella	Pneumonia, encephalitis	Congenital infection	Clinical examination, detection of antibody	Amniocentesis, detection of organism with PCR Ultrasound	VZIG, acyclovir for prophylaxis or treatment	VZIG, acyclovir for prophylaxis or treatment of neonate

Abbreviations: HBIG, hepatitis B immune globulin; HBV, hepatitis B vaccine; PCR, polymerase chain reaction.
[a] See text for detailed discussion of patient management.

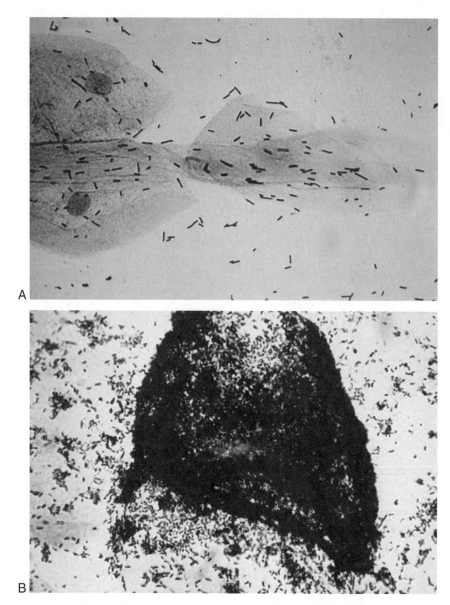

Fig. 38-1 (A) Gram stain of normal vaginal secretions. Note the predominance of lactobacilli and the clear borders of the vaginal epithelial cells. (B) Gram stain of vaginal secretions in a patient with BV. Note the absence of lactobacilli, the abundance of other cocci and bacilli, and the epithelial cell studded with bacteria (clue cell). (Courtesy of Sharon L. Hillier, Ph.D., University of Pittsburgh.)

munodeficiency states. Although isolated cases of chorioamnionitis due to *Candida* species have been reported, serious systemic infections are uncommon unless the patient is receiving hyperalimentation or is immunocompromised.

Diagnosis

Infected patients usually report vaginal and vulvar pruritus and a white, curd-like vaginal discharge. The vaginal pH is typically below 4.5. The vaginal mucosa and vulva may be erythematous and edematous, and punc-

tate, erythematous satellite lesions may be present on the lateral aspect of the vulva and medial aspect of the thighs.[9]

The simplest test for confirmation of diagnosis is microscopic examination of a KOH preparation for hyphae, pseudohyphae, and budding yeast. Cultures are indicated only for patients who have persistent clinical findings and a negative microscopic examination and for those with recurrent infections who have had poor responses to treatment. Sabouraud's medium is the optimal medium for culture and may permit identification of a species of *Candida* with an unusual pattern of sensitivity to antimicrobial compounds.

Treatment

For uncomplicated *Candida* infections, topical therapy for 3 to 7 days with agents such as miconazole, terconazole, clotrimazole, and butoconazole is usually highly effective. Treatment of women with persistent or recurrent infection is more problematic. These patients should be counseled about preventive measures such as avoidance of bubble baths, use of cotton undergarments, and close attention to perineal hygiene.[9,10] In particularly refractory cases, administration of systemic antimicrobials such as ketoconazole or fluconazole should be considered because of their greater activity against reservoirs of yeast in the gastrointestinal tract.[11–13] Neither drug has been studied extensively in pregnancy. However, fluconazole appears to have a more favorable toxicity profile. The appropriate oral dose of this compound for treatment of a refractory infection is 150 mg in a single dose.

Trichomoniasis

Epidemiology

Trichomoniasis is a sexually transmitted disease caused by the protozoan *Trichomonas vaginalis*. Trichomonas is responsible for approximately 25 percent of cases of vaginitis. It is an extremely contagious infection; virtually 100 percent of women who have sexual contact with an infected partner contract the disease.[1] Trichomoniasis has not been *conclusively* associated with serious maternal or neonatal complications.

Diagnosis

The usual symptoms of trichomoniasis are vaginal pruritus, superficial dyspareunia, frequency, dysuria, and a malodorous, yellow-green, frothy vaginal discharge. On physical examination, the vaginal mucosa is typically erythematous, and punctate hemorrhages may be present on the cervix ("strawberry cervix"). The pH of the vagina is usually in the range of 5 to 7.[1]

The most useful test for rapid confirmation of infection is direct visualization of the flagellated organisms in a saline preparation (wet mount). The sensitivity of this test is 60 to 80 percent, depending on the size of the inoculum and the thoroughness with which the slide is inspected. The Papanicolaou smear has similar sensitivity, but it is not as readily available to the office-based practitioner. *T. vaginalis* can be cultured on specialized media such as Hollander's medium or Feinberg-Whittington medium. However, culture is a more expensive and time-consuming diagnostic test, and, accordingly, it is rarely indicated in clinical practice.[1]

Treatment

Metronidazole is the only antibiotic with uniform activity against *T. vaginalis*. Treatment efficacy is at least 95 percent if the patient is compliant and her sexual partner is treated concurrently. Absolute resistance of the organism to metronidazole is uncommon, and relative resistance can usually be overcome by administering the drug in higher doses for longer periods of time.[2,3]

Metronidazole can be given in three oral dosage regimens: a single dose of 2 g; 250 mg three times daily for 7 days; or 500 mg twice daily for 7 days. The former dosage schedule improves compliance and reduces expense.

In laboratory models, metronidazole has been associated with both mutagenicity and carcinogenicity. Although these effects have not been documented in humans, use of the drug in pregnancy, especially the first trimester, still raises theoretical concerns.[4] Accordingly, if the patient is relatively asymptomatic, treatment should be delayed until organogenesis is complete.

Endocervical Infections

Chlamydia

Epidemiology

Chlamydia trachomatis is the most common sexually transmitted pathogen in Western nations. The organism can cause localized infection of the urethra, endocervix, and rectum. It also is the most common cause of perihepatitis (Fitz-Hugh-Curtis syndrome) and an occasional cause of pneumonia. In addition, in the developing nations of the world, *C. trachomatis* is responsible for inclusion conjunctivitis, a leading cause of blindness. Infants delivered to infected women may develop conjunctivitis or pneumonia. The former complication occurs in up to 50 percent of infants delivered to infected mothers; the latter complication affects 3 to 18 percent of infants.[17,18]

Diagnosis and Clinical Management

C. trachomatis may be grown in tissue culture. However, this methodology is relatively expensive and time-consuming. Fortunately, less expensive, rapid identification tests such as the monoclonal antibody test (Microtrak), enzyme-linked immunosorbent assay (ELISA, Chlamydiazyme), and DNA probe are sufficiently sensitive to justify their clinical use for identification of chlamydial infection. In high-risk populations, the sensitivity and specificity of these tests is approximately 90 and 95 percent, respectively.[17,19]

Although tetracycline and doxycycline have the greatest activity against *C. trachomatis*, these drugs should not be used in pregnancy because of their harmful effects on fetal teeth. The agent of choice in pregnancy is erythromycin base 500 mg orally four times daily for 7 days. Erythromycin estolate should not be used in pregnancy because of possible hepatotoxicity.[20] For patients who cannot tolerate erythromycin, azithromycin, 1,000 mg orally in a single dose,[21] and amoxicillin, 500 mg orally three times a day for 7 days, are acceptable alternatives.[22]

In view of the fact that 5 to 10 percent of patients do not respond to the initial course of treatment, a culture for test of cure should be performed approximately 2 weeks after therapy is completed. In addition, infected patients should be screened for other sexually transmitted diseases like gonorrhea, syphilis, hepatitis B, and HIV infection. Neonates delivered to infected mothers should receive prophylaxis with tetracycline or erythromycin ophthalmic preparations and observed for evidence of an ensuing respiratory tract infection.

Gonorrhea

Epidemiology

Gonorrhea is caused by the gram-negative, intracellular diplococcus *Neisseria gonorrhoeae*. The infection is transmitted primarily by sexual contact. Gonorrhea also may be transmitted perinatally from mother to infant and cause serious ophthalmic injury.

In pregnant women, gonorrhea may be manifested as an asymptomatic to mildly symptomatic localized infection of the urethra, endocervix, or rectum. Local infection may increase the risk of preterm labor and preterm premature rupture of membranes and predispose to intrapartum and postpartum infection. Gonorrhea also may present as a disseminated infection.[17] The most common manifestation of disseminated gonococcal infection is arthritis, typically affecting several small- to medium-sized joints. The next most common manifestation is a diffuse violaceous, papular skin rash. Less common, but potentially more serious, sequelae of disseminated infection include meningitis, pericarditis, endocarditis, and perihepatitis (Fitz-Hugh-Curtis syndrome).[23]

Diagnosis and Management

The most reliable test for confirmation of gonococcal infection is culture of the organism on selective agar such as Thayer-Martin or VCN medium. Gram stain and nucleic acid probes are helpful when positive, but their sensitivity varies widely.

The drugs of choice for treating *localized* gonococcal infections in pregnancy are ceftriaxone (125 to 250 mg IM in a single dose) and cefixime (400 mg PO once). The former drug is the preferred agent for treatment of *disseminated* infection and should be administered in a dose of 1 g IV or IM every 24 hours until a clinical response has been achieved.[17] Tetracyclines and quinolones should not be used in pregnancy because of their injurious effects on fetal teeth and cartilage. Patients who are allergic to β-lactam antibiotics may be treated with a single 2-g intramuscular dose of spectinomycin.[17] Treatment of the neonate with either silver nitrate or tetracycline ophthalmic preparations is effective in preventing most cases of ophthalmia neonatorum.

Patients who test positive for gonorrhea should be screened for other sexually transmitted diseases. Because of the uniformly excellent activity of ceftriaxone and cefixime against *N. gonorrhoeae*, tests of cure are not routinely indicated when patients are treated with these agents.

Urinary Tract Infections

Acute Urethritis

Acute urethritis (acute urethral syndrome) is usually caused by one of three organisms: coliforms (principally *Escherichia coli*), *N. gonorrhoeae*, and *C. trachomatis*. Coliform organisms are part of the normal vaginal and perineal flora and may be introduced into the urethra during intercourse or when wiping after defecation. *N. gonorrhoeae* and *C. trachomatis* are sexually transmitted pathogens.[24]

Affected patients typically experience frequency, urgency, and dysuria. Hesitancy, dribbling, and a mucopurulent urethral discharge may be present. On microscopic examination the urine usually has white blood cells, but bacteria are not consistently present. Urine cultures may have low colony counts of coliform organisms, and cultures of the urethral discharge may be positive for gonorrhea and chlamydia. Rapid diagnostic tests, such as the ELISA, fluorescent monoclonal antibody test, and DNA probe may be used in lieu of cultures for *C. trachomatis*.[24]

Most patients with acute urethritis warrant empiric treatment before the results of urine or urethral cultures are available. Infections caused by coliforms will usually respond to the antibiotics described below for treatment of asymptomatic bacteriuria and cystitis. If gonococcal infection is suspected, the patient should be treated with either oral cefixime (400 mg in a single dose) or intramuscular ceftriaxone (125–250 mg in a single dose).[17] The former is approximately one-third the cost of the latter. If the patient is allergic to β-lactam antibiotics, an effective alternative is spectinomycin, administered intramuscularly in a single dose of 2 g. If chlamydial infection is suspected or confirmed, appropriate treatment regimens include erythromycin base (500 mg PO four times daily for 7 days), amoxicillin (500 mg PO three times daily for 7 days), or azithromycin (1,000 mg PO in a single dose).[17,21] The latter drug is a long-acting derivative of erythromycin and is presently the only antibiotic that is effective in a single dose against *C. trachomatis*. It is now available in a powdered formulation, which is only slightly more expensive than generic erythromycin or amoxicillin. Doxycycline or tetracycline should not be used in pregnancy because of their adverse effects on fetal bone and teeth.

Asymptomatic Bacteriuria and Acute Cystitis

The prevalence of asymptomatic bacteriuria in pregnancy is 5 to 10 percent, and the vast majority of cases antedate the onset of pregnancy. The frequency of acute cystitis in pregnancy is 1 to 3 percent. Some cases of cystitis arise de novo; others develop as a result of failure to identify or treat asymptomatic bacteriuria.[25]

E. coli is responsible for 80 to 90 percent of cases of *initial* infections and 70 to 80 percent of recurrent cases. *Klebsiella pneumoniae* and *Proteus* species also are important pathogens, particularly in patients who have a history of recurrent infection. Approximately 3 to 7 percent of infections will be caused by gram-positive organisms such as group B streptococci, enterococci, and staphylococci.[24,25]

All pregnant women should have a urine culture at their first prenatal appointment to detect pre-existing asymptomatic bacteriuria. If the culture is negative, the likelihood of the patient subsequently developing an *asymptomatic* infection is 5 percent or less. If the culture is positive (defined as at least 10^5 colonies/ml urine from a midstream, clean catch specimen), prompt treatment is necessary to prevent ascending infection.[25]

Patients with acute cystitis usually have symptoms of frequency, dysuria, urgency, suprapubic pain, hesitancy, and dribbling. Gross hematuria may be present, but fever and systemic symptoms are uncommon. In symptomatic patients, microscopic examination of the urine shows white cells and bacteria. The leukocyte esterase and nitrate tests will usually be positive if urine has been incubating in the bladder for several hours. When a urine culture is obtained, a catheterized sample is preferred because it minimizes the probability that urine will be contaminated by vaginal flora. With a catheterized specimen, a colony count of at least 10^2/ml is considered indicative of infection.[26]

Asymptomatic bacteriuria and acute cystitis characteristically respond well to short courses of oral antibiotics. Single dose therapy is not as effective in pregnant women as in nonpregnant patients. However, a 3-day course of treatment appears to be comparable to a 7 to 10 day regimen for an initial infection.[24] The longer courses of therapy are most appropriate for patients with recurrent infections. Table 38-3 lists several antibiotics of value for treatment of asymptomatic bacteriuria and cystitis.

When sensitivity tests are available (e.g., in patients with asymptomatic bacteriuria), they may be used to guide antibiotic selection. When empiric treatment is indicated, the choice of antibiotics must be based on established patterns of susceptibility. In recent years, 20 to 30 percent of strains of *E. coli* have developed resistance to ampicillin; thus, this drug should not be used when the results of sensitivity tests are unknown.[27]

When choosing among the drugs listed in Table 38-

Table 38-3 Antibiotics for Treatment of Asymptomatic Bacteriuria and Acute Cystitis

Drug	Strength of Activity	Oral Dose × 3 Days	Relative Cost
Amoxicillin	Some *E. coli*, most *Proteus* species, group B streptococci, enterococci, some staphylococci	250 mg TID	Low
Amoxicillin-clavulanic acid (Augmentin)	Most gram-negative aerobic bacilli and gram-positive cocci	250 mg TID	High
Ampicillin	Some *E. coli*, most *Proteus* species, group B streptococci, enterococci, some staphylococci	250–500 mg QID	Low
Cephalexin (Keflex)	Most *E. coli*, most *Klebsiella* and *Proteus* species, group B streptococci, staphylococci	250 mg QID	Low
Nitrofurantoin macrocrystals—sustained release preparation (Macrobid)	Most gram-negative aerobic bacilli	100 mg BID	Moderate
Sulfisoxazole (Gantrisin)	Most gram-negative aerobic bacilli	2 g × 1 dose, then 1 g QID	Low
Trimethoprim-sulfamethoxazole-DS (Bactrim, Septra)	Most gram-negative aerobic bacilli	800 mg/160 mg BID	Low

Abbreviations: BID, twice daily; TID, three times daily; QID, four times daily.
(Modified from Duff,[24] with permission.)

3, the clinician should consider the following factors. First, the sensitivity patterns of ampicillin, amoxicillin, and cephalexin will be the most variable.[27] Second, these drugs, along with amoxicillin-clavulanic acid, will also have the most pronounced effect on normal bowel and vaginal flora and thus be the most likely to cause diarrhea or monilial vulvovaginitis. Third, amoxicillin-clavulanic acid and trimethoprim-sulfamethoxazole will usually be the best empiric agents for treatment of patients with suspected drug-resistant pathogens.[28] In this situation, the latter drug offers a major cost advantage over the former. Finally, because of theoretical concerns about their effect on protein binding of bilirubin, sulfonamide drugs should probably be avoided near the time of delivery.

For patients who have an initial infection and experience a prompt response to treatment, a urine culture for test of cure is probably unnecessary.[29] Cultures during, or immediately after, treatment are indicated for patients who have a poor response to therapy or who have a history of recurrent infection. During subsequent clinic appointments, the patient's urine should be screened for nitrites and leukocyte esterase. If either of these tests is positive, repeat urine culture and re-treatment are indicated.[30]

Acute Pyelonephritis

The incidence of pyelonephritis in pregnancy is 1 to 2 percent.[25] The vast majority of cases develop as a consequence of undiagnosed or inadequately treated lower urinary tract infection. Two major physiologic changes occur during pregnancy that predispose to ascending infection of the urinary tract. First, the high concentration of progesterone secreted by the placenta has an inhibitory effect on ureteral peristalsis. Second, the enlarging gravid uterus often compresses the ureters, particularly the right, at the pelvic brim, thus creating additional stasis. Stasis, in turn, facilitates migration of bacteria from the bladder into the ureters and renal parenchyma (Fig. 38-2).

Approximately 75 to 80 percent of cases of pyelonephritis occur on the right side. Ten to 15 percent are left sided, and a slightly smaller percentage are bilateral.[25] *E. coli* is again the principal pathogen.[25,27] *K. pneumoniae* and *Proteus* species also are important causes of infection, particularly in women with recurrent episodes of pyelonephritis.[27] Highly virulent gram-negative bacilli, such as *Pseudomonas, Enterobacter,* and *Serratia,* are unusual isolates except in immuno-compromised patients. Gram-positive cocci do not usually cause upper tract infection. Anaerobes also are unlikely pathogens unless the patient is chronically obstructed or instrumented.

The usual clinical manifestations of acute pyelo-

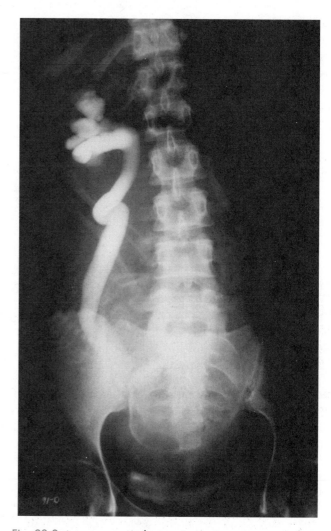

Fig. 38-2 Intravenous pyelogram in a pregnant woman shows marked dilatation of the right ureter and mild dilation of renal collecting system.

phritis in pregnancy are fever, chills, flank pain and tenderness, frequency, urgency, hematuria, and dysuria. Patients also may have signs of preterm labor, septic shock, and adult respiratory distress syndrome (ARDS). Urinalysis is usually positive for white cell casts, red blood cells, and bacteria. Urine colony counts greater than 10^2 colonies/ml, in samples collected by catheterization, confirm the diagnosis of infection.

Pregnant patients with pyelonephritis may be considered for outpatient therapy if their disease manifestations are mild, they are hemodynamically stable, and they have no evidence of preterm labor. If an outpatient approach is adopted, the patient should be treated with agents that have a high level of activity against the common uropathogens. Acceptable oral agents include amoxicillin-clavulanic acid, 500 mg three times daily, or trimethoprim-sulfamethoxazole-DS, one twice daily for 7 to 10 days. Alternatively, a visiting home nurse may be contracted to administer a parenteral agent, such as ceftriaxone, 2 g IM or IV, once daily.

Pregnant patients who appear to be moderately to severely ill or who show any signs of preterm labor should be hospitalized for intravenous antibiotic therapy. They should receive appropriate supportive treatment and be monitored closely for complications, such as sepsis, (ARDS), and preterm labor. One of the best choices for empiric intravenous antibiotic therapy is cefazolin, 1 to 2 g every 8 hours.[27] For hospitalized patients, this drug is less expensive to administer than the newer broader spectrum cephalosporins or penicillins and has an equivalent spectrum of activity against the coliform organisms most likely to be responsible for infection. If the patient is critically ill or is at high risk for a resistant organism, a second antibiotic, such as gentamicin (1.5 mg/kg every 8 hours) or aztreonam (500 mg to 1 g every 8 to 12 hours) should be administered, along with cefazolin, until the results of susceptibility tests are available.

Once antibiotic therapy is initiated, approximately 75 percent of patients defervesce within 48 hours. By the end of 72 hours, almost 95 percent of patients will be afebrile and asymptomatic.[31] The two most likely causes of treatment failure are a resistant microorganism or obstruction. The latter condition is best diagnosed with renal ultrasonography or intravenous pyelography and typically results from a stone or physical compression of the ureter by the gravid uterus.

Once the patient has begun to defervesce and her clinical examination has improved, she may be discharged from the hospital. Oral antibiotics should be prescribed to complete a total of 7 to 10 days of therapy. Selection of a specific oral agent should be based on considerations of efficacy, toxicity, and expense.

Approximately 20 to 30 percent of pregnant patients with acute pyelonephritis will develop a recurrent urinary tract infection later in pregnancy.[25] The most cost-effective way to reduce the frequency of recurrence is to administer a daily prophylactic dose of an antibiotic, such as sulfisoxazole, 1 g, or nitrofurantoin macrocrystals, 100 mg. Patients receiving prophylaxis should have their urine screened for bacteria at each subsequent clinic appointment. They also should be questioned about recurrence of symptoms. If symptoms recur, or the dipstick test for nitrite or leukocyte esterase is positive, a urine culture should be obtained to determine if retreatment is necessary.

Chorioamnionitis

Epidemiology

Chorioamnionitis (amnionitis, intra-amniotic infection) occurs in approximately 1 to 5 percent of term pregnancies.[32] In patients with preterm delivery, the frequency of clinical or subclinical infection may approach 25 percent.[33] Although chorioamnionitis may result from hematogenous dissemination of microorganisms, it more commonly is an ascending infection caused by organisms that are part of the normal vaginal flora. The principal pathogens are *Bacteroides* and *Prevotella* species, *E. coli*, anaerobic streptococci, and group B streptococci.[34] Several clinical risk factors for chorioamnionitis have been identified. The most important are young age, low socioeconomic status, nulliparity, extended duration of labor and ruptured membranes, multiple vaginal examinations, and pre-existing infections of the lower genital tract.[32]

Diagnosis

In most situations the diagnosis of chorioamnionitis can be established on the basis of the clinical findings of maternal fever and maternal and fetal tachycardia, in the absence of other localizing signs of infection. In more severely ill patients, uterine tenderness and purulent amniotic fluid may be present.[32] The disorders that should be considered in the differential diagnosis of chorioamnionitis include upper respiratory infection, bronchitis, pneumonia, pyelonephritis, viral syndrome, and appendicitis.

Laboratory confirmation of the diagnosis of chorioamnionitis is not routinely necessary in term patients who are progressing to delivery. However, in preterm patients who are being evaluated for tocolysis or corticosteroids, laboratory assessment may be of value in excluding or establishing the diagnosis of intrauterine infection. In this clinical context, amniotic fluid should be obtained by transabdominal amniocentesis. Table 38-4 summarizes the abnormal laboratory findings that may be present in infected patients.[32,35–40]

Management

Both the mother and infant may experience serious complications when chorioamnionitis is present. Bacteremia occurs in 3 to 12 percent of infected women. When cesarean delivery is required, up to 8 percent of women develop a wound infection and approximately 1 percent develop a pelvic abscess. Fortunately, maternal death due to infection is exceedingly rare.[32]

Five to 10 percent of neonates delivered to mothers with chorioamnionitis have pneumonia or bacteremia. The predominant organisms responsible for these infections are group B streptococci and *E. coli*. Meningitis occurs in 1 percent or less of term infants and in a slightly higher percentage of preterm infants. Mortality due to infection ranges from 1 to 4 percent in term neonates but may approach 15 percent in preterm infants because of the confounding effects of other com-

Table 38-4 · Diagnostic Tests for Chorioamnionitis

Test	Abnormal Finding	Comment
Maternal white blood cell count (WBC)[32]	≥15,000 cells/mm³ with preponderance of leukocytes	Labor and/or corticosteroids may result in elevation of WBC
Amniotic fluid glucose[35-37]	≤10–15 mg%	Excellent correlation with positive amniotic fluid culture and clinical infection
Amniotic fluid interleukin-6[38]	≥7.9 ng/ml	Excellent correlation with positive amniotic fluid culture and clinical infection
Amniotic fluid leukocyte esterase[39]	≥1⁺ reaction	Good correlation with positive amniotic fluid culture and clinical infection
Amniotic fluid Gram stain[32]	Any organism in an oil immersion field	Allows identification of particularly virulent organism such as group B streptococci. However, the test is very sensitive to inoculum effect. In addition, it cannot identify pathogens such as mycoplasmas
Amniotic fluid culture[32]	Growth of aerobic or anaerobic microorganism	Results are not immediately available for clinical management
Blood cultures[32,40]	Growth of aerobic or anaerobic microorganism	Will be positive in 5–10% of patients. However, will usually not be of value in making clinical decisions unless patient is at increased risk for bacterial endocarditis, is immunocompromised, or has a poor response to initial treatment

plications such as hyaline membrane disease and intraventricular hemorrhage.[32]

To prevent maternal and neonatal complications, parenteral antibiotic therapy should be initiated as soon as the diagnosis of chorioamnionitis is made, unless delivery is imminent. Three separate investigations have demonstrated that mother-infant pairs who receive prompt intrapartum treatment have better outcomes than patients treated after delivery.[41-43] The principal benefits of early treatment include decreased frequency of neonatal bacteremia and pneumonia and decreased duration of maternal fever and hospitalization.

The most extensively tested intravenous antibiotic regimen for treatment of chorioamnionitis is the combination of ampicillin (2 g every 6 hours) or penicillin (5 million units every 6 hours) plus gentamicin (1.5 mg/kg every 8 hours).[15,32] These antibiotics specifically target the two organisms most likely to cause neonatal infection: group B streptococci and *E. coli*. With rare exceptions, gentamicin is preferred to tobramycin or amikacin because it is available in an inexpensive generic formulation. Amikacin should be reserved for immunocompromised patients who are particularly likely to be infected by highly virulent, drug-resistant aerobic gram-negative bacilli. In patients who are allergic to β-lactam antibiotics, vancomycin (500 mg every 6 hours or 1 g every 12 hours), erythromycin (1 g every 6 hours), or clindamycin (900 mg every 8 hours) can be substituted for ampicillin.

If a patient with chorioamnionitis requires cesarean delivery, a drug with activity against anaerobic organisms should be added to the antibiotic regimen. Either clindamycin (900 mg every 8 hours) or metronidazole (500 mg every 6 hours) is an excellent choice for this purpose. Failure to provide effective coverage of anaerobes may result in treatment failures in 20 to 30 percent of patients.

Extended spectrum cephalosporins, penicillins, and carbapenems also provide excellent coverage against the bacteria that cause chorioamnionitis. Dosages and dose intervals for several of these agents are listed in Table 38-5.[44] Less information is available concerning

Table 38-5 · Single Agents of Value in Treatment of Chorioamnionitis

Drug	Dosage and Dose Interval	Relative Cost to the Pharmacy[a]
Extended Spectrum Cephalosporins		
Cefotaxime	2 g q8–12h	Intermediate
Cefotetan	2 g q12h	Low
Cefoxitin	2 g q6h	High
Ceftizoxime	2 g q12h	Intermediate
Extended Spectrum Penicillins		
Ampicillin-sulbactam	3 g q6h	Low
Mezlocillin	3–4 g q6h	Intermediate
Piperacillin	3–4 g q6h	Intermediate
Piperacillin-tazobactam	3.375 g q6h	Intermediate
Ticarcillin-clavulanic acid	3.1 g q6h	Low
Carbapenem		
Imipenem-cilastatin	500 mg q6h	High

[a] Cost estimates do not include dose preparation fees and administration charges.

the effectiveness of these drugs compared with the ampicillin-gentamicin regimen. In addition, the toxicity profile for the fetus and neonate has not been as well delineated.

As a general rule, parenteral antibiotics should be continued until the patient has been afebrile and asymptomatic for approximately 24 hours. Once an adequate clinical response has been achieved, antibiotics may be discontinued and the patient discharged. A course of oral antibiotics administered as an outpatient is rarely indicated.[15,32,44]

There are two principal exceptions to the above rule. First, a patient with a documented staphylococcal bacteremia may require a longer period of intravenous therapy and, subsequently, an extended course of oral antibiotics. Second, the patient who has a vaginal delivery and then experiences a rapid defervescence may be a suitable candidate for a short course of oral antibiotics administered as an outpatient. In this situation, amoxicillin-clavulanic acid (500 mg every 8 hours) provides effective coverage against most of the organisms responsible for chorioamnionitis and is usually very well tolerated.

Patients with chorioamnionitis are at increased risk for dysfunctional labor. Approximately 75 percent require oxytocin for augmentation of labor, and up to 30 to 40 percent require cesarean delivery, usually for failure to progress in labor. While chorioamnionitis by itself should not be regarded as an indication for cesarean delivery, affected patients need close monitoring during labor to ensure that uterine contractility is optimized. In addition, the fetus also needs close surveillance. Fetal heart rate abnormalities such as tachycardia and decreased variability (Fig. 38-3) occur in over three-fourths of cases, and additional tests such as vibroacoustic stimulation, scalp stimulation, or scalp pH assessment may be necessary to evaluate fetal well-being.[32,45]

Puerperal Endometritis

Epidemiology

The frequency of puerperal endometritis in women having vaginal delivery is approximately 1 to 3 percent. In women having a scheduled cesarean prior to the onset of labor and rupture of membranes, the frequency of endometritis ranges from 5 to 15 percent. When cesarean delivery is performed after an extended period of labor and ruptured membranes, the incidence of infection is 30 to 35 percent without antibiotic prophylaxis and 15 to 20 percent with prophylaxis. In

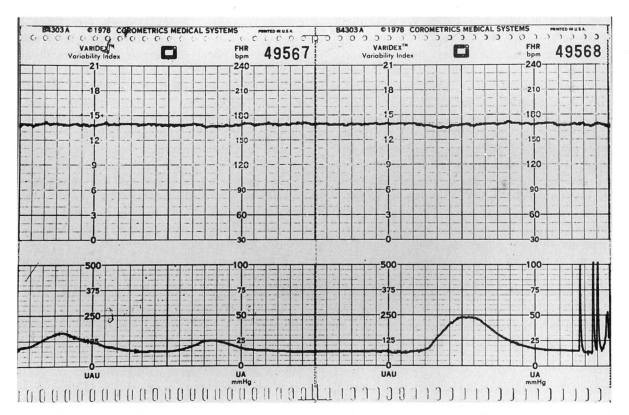

Fig. 38-3 Fetal heart tracing from a patient with chorioamnionitis. Note the tachycardia of 170 bpm and the decrease in both short- and long-term variability.

highly indigent patient populations, the frequency of infection may be almost double the figures cited above.[46]

Endometritis is a polymicrobial infection caused by microorganisms that are part of the normal vaginal flora. These bacteria gain access to the upper genital tract, peritoneal cavity, and, occasionally, the bloodstream as a result of vaginal examinations during labor and manipulations during surgery. The most common pathogenic bacteria are group B streptococci, anaerobic streptococci, aerobic gram-negative bacilli (predominantly *E. coli, K. pneumoniae,* and *Proteus* species), and anaerobic gram-negative bacilli (principally *Bacteroides* and *Prevotella* species). *C. trachomatis* is not a common cause of early onset puerperal endometritis but has been implicated in late onset infection. Similarly, the genital mycoplasmas are uncommon pathogens in patients with puerperal endometritis.[46]

The principal risk factors for endometritis are cesarean delivery, young age, low socioeconomic status, extended duration of labor and ruptured membranes, and multiple vaginal examinations. In addition, preexisting infection or colonization of the lower genital tract (gonorrhea, group B streptococci, bacterial vaginosis) also predisposes to ascending infection.[46]

Clinical Presentation and Diagnosis

Affected patients typically have a fever of 38°C or higher within 36 hours of delivery. Associated findings include malaise, tachycardia, lower abdominal pain and tenderness, uterine tenderness, and discolored, malodorous lochia. A small number of patients also may have an inflammatory mass in the broad ligament, posterior cul de sac, or retrovesicle space.

The initial differential diagnosis of puerperal fever should include endometritis, atelectasis, pneumonia, viral syndrome, pyelonephritis, and appendicitis. Distinction among these disorders usually can be made on the basis of physical examination and a limited number of laboratory tests such as white blood cell count (WBC), urinalysis and culture, and, in select patients, chest x-ray. Endometrial cultures are of primary value in evaluating patients who have a poor initial response to antibiotic treatment. When these cultures are obtained, they should be collected with a double-lumen instrument to prevent contamination by lower genital tract flora.[47] Blood cultures also are indicated in such patients and in those who are immunocompromised or at increased risk for bacterial endocarditis.[46]

Management

Patients who have mild to moderately severe infections, particularly after vaginal delivery, can be treated with short intravenous courses of single agents such as the extended spectrum cephalosporins and penicillins or

Table 38-6 Combination Antibiotic Regimens for Treatment of Puerperal Endometritis

Antibiotics	Intravenous Dose	Relative Cost to the Pharmacy[a]
Regimen 1		
Clindamycin	900 mg q8h	Intermediate
Gentamicin	1.5 mg/kg q8h	Low
Regimen 2		
Clindamycin	900 mg q8h	Intermediate
Aztreonam	1–2 g q8h	High
Regimen 3		
Metronidazole	500 mg q6h	Low
Penicillin or	5 million units q6h	Low
ampicillin	2 g q6h	Low
Gentamicin	1.5 mg/kg q8h	Low

[a] Cost estimate does not include dose preparation fees and administration charges.

imipenem-cilastatin. Table 38-6 lists several antibiotics that have acceptable breadth of coverage against the polymicrobial genital tract flora. Combination antibiotic regimens should be considered for more severely ill patients, particularly those who are indigent and in poor general health and those who have had cesarean deliveries. Table 38-6 lists several antibiotic combinations of proven value in treatment of puerperal endometritis.[15,44]

Once antibiotics are begun, approximately 90 percent of patients will defervesce within 48 to 72 hours. When the patient has been afebrile and asymptomatic for approximately 24 hours, parenteral antibiotics should be discontinued and the patient should be discharged. As a general rule, an extended course of oral antibiotics is not necessary following discharge.[18] There are at least two notable exceptions to this rule. First, patients who have had a vaginal delivery and who defervesce within 24 hours are candidates for early discharge. In these individuals, a short course of an oral antibiotic such as amoxicillin-clavulanate (500 mg every 8 hours) may be substituted for continued parenteral therapy. Second, patients who have had a staphylococcal bacteremia require a more extended period of administration of parenteral and oral antibiotics with specific antistaphylococcal activity.[49]

Patients who fail to respond to the antibiotic therapy outlined above usually have one of two problems. The first is a resistant organism. Table 38-7 lists possible weaknesses in coverage of selected antibiotics and indicates the appropriate change in treatment. The second major cause of treatment failure is a wound infection. Infected wounds should be opened completely to provide drainage. If extensive cellulitis at the margin of the incision is present, an antibiotic with specific coverage against staphylococci, such as nafcillin, should be added to the treatment regimen.

When changes in antibiotic therapy do not result in

Table 38-7   Treatment of Resistant Microorganisms in Patients with Puerperal Endometritis

Initial Antibiotic(s)	Principal Weakness in Coverage	Modification of Therapy
Extended spectrum cephalosporins	Some aerobic and anaerobic gram-negative bacilli Enterococci	Change treatment to clindamycin or metronidazole plus penicillin or ampicillin plus gentamicin
Extended spectrum penicillins	Some aerobic and anaerobic gram-negative bacilli	As above
Clindamycin plus gentamicin or aztreonam	Enterococci Some anaerobic gram-negative	Add ampicillin Consider substitution of metronidazole for clindamycin

(From Duff,[15] with permission.)

clinical improvement and no evidence of wound infection is present, several unusual disorders should be considered. The differential diagnosis of persistent puerperal fever is summarized in Table 38-8.[46]

Prevention of Puerperal Endometritis

Prophylactic antibiotics are clearly of value in reducing the frequency of postcesarean endometritis, particularly in women having surgery after an extended period of labor and ruptured membranes.[50] The most appropriate agent for prophylaxis is a limited spectrum (first generation) cephalosporin, such as cefazolin. Cefazolin should be administered in an intravenous dose of 1 to 2 g immediately after the neonate's umbilical cord is clamped. A second dose is indicated approximately 4 hours after the first dose in high-risk patients, especially when operating time is prolonged beyond 1 hour. Although extended spectrum penicillins and cephalosporins are effective for prophylaxis, they offer no advantage over cefazolin and are severalfold more expensive. Moreover, widespread use of these drugs for prophylaxis may ultimately limit their usefulness for treatment of established infections.

Patients who have an immediate hypersensitivity to β-lactam antibiotics pose a special problem. One alternative is to administer metronidazole, 500 mg IV. Another alternative is to administer a single dose of clindamycin (900 mg) plus gentamicin (1.5 mg/kg). Although these antibiotics are commonly used for treatment of overt infections, their administration is still warranted in penicillin-allergic patients who are at high risk for postoperative infection.

Serious Sequelae of Puerperal Infection

Wound Infection

Wound infection after cesarean delivery typically occurs in association with endometritis. Approximately 3 to 5 percent of patients with the latter disorder subsequently are found to have an incisional infection.[46] The major risk factors for wound infection are listed below. The principal causative organisms are *Staphylococcus aureus*, aerobic streptococci, and aerobic and anaerobic bacilli.[51]

The diagnosis of wound infection always should be considered in patients who have a poor clinical response to antibiotic therapy for endometritis.[46] Clinical

Table 38-8   Differential Diagnosis of Persistent Puerperal Fever

Condition	Diagnostic Test(s)	Treatment
Resistant microorganism	Endometrial culture, blood culture	Modify antibiotic therapy
Wound infection	Physical examination, needle aspiration, ultrasound	Incision and drainage, antibiotics
Pelvic abscess	Physical examination, ultrasound, CT, MRI	Drainage, antibiotics
Septic pelvic vein thrombophlebitis	Ultrasound, CT, MRI	Heparin anticoagulation, antibiotics
Recrudescence of connective tissue disease	Serology	Corticosteroids
Drug fever	Inspection of temperature graph, WBC—identify eosinophilia	Discontinue antibiotics
Mastitis	Physical examination	Modify antibiotic treatment to provide coverage of staphylococcal organisms

(From Duff,[15] with permission.)

Principal Risk Factors for Postcesarean Wound Infection

Poor surgical technique

Low socioeconomic status

Extended duration of labor and ruptured membranes

Pre-existing infection such as chorioamnionitis

Obesity

Insulin-dependent diabetes

Immunodeficiency disorder

Corticosteroid therapy

Immunosuppressive therapy

examination characteristically shows erythema, induration, and tenderness at the margins of the abdominal incision. When the wound is probed with either a cotton-tipped applicator or a fine needle, pus usually exudes. Some patients, however, may have an extensive cellulitis without harboring frank pus in the incision. Clinical examination should be sufficient to establish the correct diagnosis. Gram stain and culture of the wound exudate are not routinely needed since the results of these tests rarely influence selection of antibiotics or duration of antibiotic treatment.

When pus is present in the incision, the wound must be opened and drained completely. Antibiotic therapy should be modified to provide coverage against staphylococci since some regimens for endometritis may not specifically target this organism. Nafcillin, 2 g IV every 6 hours, would be a suitable drug for this purpose. In a patient who is allergic to β-lactam antibiotics, vancomycin, 1 g IV every 12 hours, is an acceptable alternative.[44]

Once the wound is opened, a careful inspection should be made to be certain that the fascial layer is intact. If it is disrupted, surgical intervention will be necessary to reapproximate the fascia. Otherwise, the wound should be irrigated two to three times daily with a solution such as warm saline, a clean dressing should be maintained, and the incision should be allowed to heal by secondary intention. Antibiotics should be continued until the base of the wound is clean and all signs of cellulitis have resolved. Patients usually can be treated at home once the acute signs of infection have subsided.

Necrotizing fasciitis is an uncommon, but extremely serious, complication of abdominal wound infection.[52]

It also has been reported in association with infection of the episiotomy site.[53] This condition is most likely to occur in patients with insulin-dependent diabetes, cancer, or an immunosuppressive disorder. Multiple bacterial pathogens, particularly anaerobes, have been isolated from patients with necrotizing fasciitis.

Necrotizing fasciitis should be suspected when the margins of the wound become discolored, cyanotic, and devoid of sensation. When the wound is opened, the subcutaneous tissue is easily dissected free of the underlying fascia, but muscle tissue is not affected. If the diagnosis is uncertain, a tissue biopsy should be performed and examined by frozen section.

Necrotizing fasciitis is a life-threatening condition and requires aggressive medical and surgical management. Broad spectrum antibiotics with activity against all potential aerobic and anaerobic pathogens should be administered. Intravascular volume should be maintained with infusions of crystalloid, and electrolyte abnormalities should be corrected. Finally, and most importantly, the wound must be debrided and all necrotic tissue removed. In many instances, the dissection must be quite extensive and may be best managed in conjunction with an experienced general or plastic surgeon.[52]

Pelvic Abscess

With the advent of modern antibiotics, pelvic abscesses after cesarean or vaginal delivery have become extremely rare. One percent or less of patients with puerperal endometritis develop a pelvic abscess.[46] When present, abscess collections are typically located in the anterior or posterior cul de sac, most commonly the latter, or the broad ligament. The usual bacteria isolated from abscess cavities are coliforms and anaerobic gram-negative bacilli, particularly *Bacteroides* and *Prevotella* species.[54]

Patients with an abscess typically experience a persistent fever despite initial therapy for endometritis. In addition, they usually have malaise, tachycardia, lower abdominal pain and tenderness, and a palpable pelvic mass anterior, posterior, or lateral to the uterus. The peripheral WBC count is usually elevated, and there is a shift toward immature cell forms. Ultrasound, computerized tomographic (CT) scan, and magnetic resonance imaging (MRI) may be used to confirm the diagnosis of pelvic abscess.[55] Although the latter two tests may be slightly more sensitive, the former offers the advantages of decreased expense and ready availability.

Patients with a pelvic abscess require surgical intervention to drain the purulent collection. When the abscess is in the posterior cul de sac, colpotomy drainage may be possible. For abscesses located anterior or lateral to the uterus, drainage may be accomplished by

CT or ultrasound-guided needle aspiration.[66] When needle access is limited or the abscess is extensive, open laparotomy is indicated.

Patients with a pelvic abscess must receive antibiotics with excellent activity against coliform organisms and anaerobes.[54] One regimen that has been tested extensively in obstetric patients with serious infections is the combination of penicillin (5 million units IV every 6 hours) or ampicillin (2 g IV every 6 hours) plus gentamicin (1.5 mg/kg IV every 8 hours) plus clindamycin (900 mg IV every 8 hours) or metronidazole (500 mg IV every 6 hours). If a patient is allergic to lactam antibiotics, vancomycin (500 mg IV every 6 hours or 1 g IV every 12 hours) can be substituted for penicillin or ampicillin. Aztreonam (1 to 2 g IV every 8 hours) also can be used in lieu of gentamicin when the patient is at risk for nephrotoxicity. Alternatively, the single agent imipenem-cilastatin (500 mg IV every 6 hours) provides excellent coverage against the usual pathogens responsible for an abscess. Antibiotics should be continued until the patient has been afebrile and asymptomatic for a minimum of 24 to 48 hours.[46]

Septic Pelvic Vein Thrombophlebitis

Like pelvic abscess, septic pelvic vein thrombophlebitis is extremely rare, occurring in 1:2,000 pregnancies overall and in 1 percent of less of patients who have puerperal endometritis.[57] Intrauterine infection may cause seeding of pathogenic microorganisms into the venous circulation; in turn, these organisms may damage the vascular endothelium and initiate thrombosis.

Septic pelvic vein thrombophlebitis occurs in two distinct forms.[57] The most commonly described disorder is acute thrombosis of one (usually the right), or both, ovarian veins (*ovarian vein syndrome*).[58] Affected patients typically develop a moderate temperature elevation in association with lower abdominal pain in the first 48 to 96 hours postpartum. Pain usually localizes to the side of the affected vein but may radiate into the groin, upper abdomen, or flank. Nausea, vomiting, and abdominal bloating may be present.

On physical examination, the patient's pulse is usually elevated. Tachypnea, stridor, and dyspnea may be evident if pulmonary embolization has occurred. The abdomen is tender, and bowel sounds are often decreased or absent. Most patients demonstrate voluntary and involuntary guarding, and 50 to 70 percent have a tender, rope-like mass originating near one cornua and extending laterally and cephalad toward the upper abdomen. The principal conditions that should be considered in the differential diagnosis of ovarian vein syndrome are pyelonephritis, nephrolithiasis, appendicitis, broad ligament hematoma, adnexal torsion, and pelvic abscess.

The second presentation of septic pelvic vein thrombophlebitis is termed *enigmatic fever*.[59] Initially, affected patients have clinical findings of endometritis and receive systemic antibiotics. Subsequently, they experience subjective improvement, with the exception of temperature instability. They do not appear to be seriously ill, and positive findings are limited to persistent fever and tachycardia. Disorders that should be considered in the differential diagnosis of enigmatic fever are drug fever, viral syndrome, collagen vascular disease, and pelvic abscess.

The diagnostic tests of greatest value in evaluating patients with suspected septic pelvic vein thrombophlebitis are CT scan and MRI (Fig. 38-4). These tests are most sensitive in detecting large thrombi in the major pelvic vessels. They are not as useful in identifying thrombi in smaller vessels. In such cases, the ultimate diagnosis may depend on the patient's response to an empiric trial of heparin.[60,61]

Patients with septic pelvic vein thrombophlebitis should be treated with therapeutic doses of intravenous heparin.[57,60] The dose of heparin should be adjusted to maintain the activated partial thromboplastin time (aPTT) at two times normal or to achieve a serum heparin concentration of 0.2 to 0.7 IU/ml. Therapy should be continued for 7 to 10 days. Long-term anticoagulation with oral agents in probably unnecessary unless the patient has massive clotting throughout the pelvic venous plexus or has sustained a pulmonary embolism. Patients should be maintained on broad spectrum antibiotics throughout the period of heparin administration.

Once medical therapy is initiated, the patient should

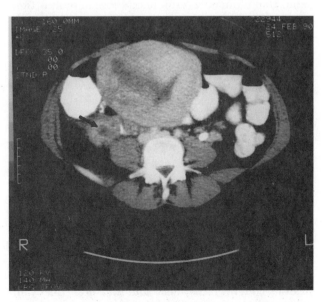

Fig. 38-4 CT scan shows a thrombus (*arrow*) in right ovarian vein.

have objective evidence of a response within 48 to 72 hours. If no improvement is noted, surgical intervention may be necessary.[57,60] The decision to perform surgery should be based on clinical assessment and the relative certainty of the diagnosis. The surgical approach, in turn, should be tailored to the specific intraoperative findings. In most instances, treatment requires only ligation of the affected vessel(s). Extension of the thrombosis along the vena cava to the point of origin of the renal veins may necessitate embolectomy. Excision of the infected vessel and removal of the ipsilateral adnexa and uterus is indicated only in the presence of a well-defined abscess. Whenever any of the above procedures are being considered, consultation with an experienced vascular surgeon is imperative.

Septic Shock

Septic shock in obstetric patients is usually associated with four specific infections: septic abortion, acute pyelonephritis, and severe chorioamnionitis or endometritis.[13] Fortunately, fewer than 5 percent of patients with any of these infections develop septic shock. The most common organisms responsible for septic shock are the aerobic gram-negative bacilli, principally *E. coli, K. pneumoniae,* and *Proteus* species. Highly virulent, drug-resistant coliforms such as *Pseudomonas, Enterobacter,* and *Serratia* species are uncommon except in immunosuppressed patients.[62]

Aerobic gram-negative bacilli have a complex lipopolysaccharide in their cell wall that is termed *endotoxin.* When released into the systemic circulation, endotoxin is capable of causing a variety of immunologic, hematologic, neurohormonal, and hemodynamic derangements that ultimately result in multiorgan dysfunction. Figure 38-5 presents a simplified summary of the pathophysiology of endotoxic shock.[62]

In the early stages of septic shock, patients usually are restless, disoriented, tachycardic, and hypotensive. Although hypothermia is occasionally present, most patients have a relatively high fever. Their skin may be warm and flushed due to an initial phase of vasodilation (*warm shock*). Subsequently, as extensive vasoconstriction occurs, the skin becomes cool and clammy. Cardiac arrhythmias may be present, and signs of myocardial ischemia may occur. Jaundice, often due to hemolysis, may be evident. Urinary output typically decreases, and frank anuria may develop. Spontaneous bleeding from the genitourinary tract or venipuncture sites may occur as a result of disseminated intravascular coagulation (DIC). ARDS is a common complication of severe sepsis and is associated with manifestations such as dyspnea, stridor, cough, tachypnea, and bilateral rales and wheezing (Fig. 38-5).[63] In addition to these systemic signs and symptoms, affected patients also may have findings related to their primary site of infection such as purulent lochia, uterine tenderness, peritonitis, or flank tenderness.

The differential diagnosis of septic shock in obstetric patients includes hypovolemic and cardiogenic shock, diabetic ketoacidosis, anaphylactic reaction, anesthetic reaction, and amniotic fluid or venous embolism.[62] Distinction among these disorders usually can be made on the basis of a thorough history and physical examination and a limited number of laboratory studies. The WBC initially may be decreased but subsequently is elevated in the majority of patients. A large percentage of bands is usually evident. The hematocrit may be decreased if blood loss has occurred. Tests of coagulation such as platelet count, serum fibrinogen concentration, serum concentration of fibrin degradation products, prothrombin time, and partial thromboplastin time are frequently abnormal. Serum concentrations of the transaminase enzymes and bilirubin are often increased. Similarly, increased concentrations of blood urea nitrogen and creatinine reflect deterioration of renal function. Chest x-ray in patients with septic shock is indicated to determine if pneumonia or ARDS is present. In addition, CT scan, MRI, and ultrasound may be of value in localizing an abscess.[55] Affected patients also require electrocardiographic monitoring to detect arrhythmias or signs of ischemic injury.

The first goal of treatment of septic shock is to correct the hemodynamic derangements precipitated by endotoxin. Two large-bore intravenous catheters and a urinary catheter should be inserted. An isotonic crystalloid such as Ringer's lactate solution or normal saline should be administered and the infusion titrated in accordance with the patient's pulse, blood pressure, and urine output. Application of the military antishock garment also may be helpful in stabilizing the patient's blood pressure, especially when bleeding is occurring.

If the initial fluid infusion is not successful in restoring hemodynamic stability, a right heart catheter should be inserted to monitor pulmonary artery wedge pressure. In addition, dopamine should be administered.[64] In low doses, this vasopressor stimulates myocardial contractility and improves perfusion of central organs. In higher doses, the drug has primarily vasoconstrictive effects and may actually compromise tissue perfusion.

Corticosteroids no longer are recommended for treatment of septic shock. Although these drugs may initially improve hemodynamic instability, they ultimately promote superinfection with resistant microorganisms and do not improve overall mortality.[65,66] In selected patients with refractory hypotension, intravenous administration of the narcotic antagonist naloxone has led to reversal of the shock state.[67] The dose

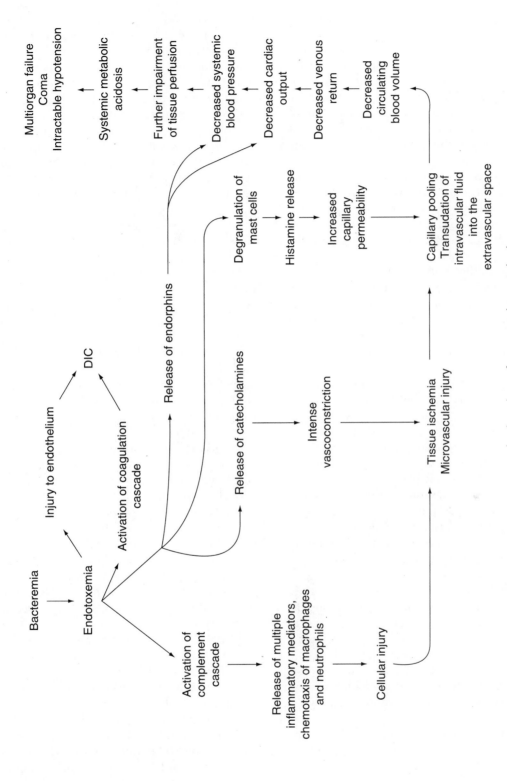

Fig. 38-5 Pathophysiology of septic (endotoxic) shock.

and duration of administration of naloxone have not been standardized.

The second objective of treatment is to administer broad spectrum antibiotics targeted against the most likely pathogens.[62] For genital tract infections, the combination of penicillin or ampicillin plus clindamycin or metronidazole plus an aminoglycoside or aztreonam is an appropriate regimen. Alternatively, imipenem-cilastatin can be administered as a single agent. Patients also may require surgery, for example, to evacuate infected products of conception, drain a pelvic abscess, or remove badly infected pelvic organs. Indicated surgery never should be delayed because a patient is unstable, for operative intervention may be precisely the step necessary to reverse the hemodynamic derangements of septic shock.

Other adjuncts in the treatment of infection include infusion of granulocytes and administration of antisera to the major antigens of coliform bacteria.[62,68] The former modality has its greatest application in treatment of neutropenic patients. The second intervention has appeared promising in some investigations but remains experimental.

Patients with septic shock require meticulous supportive care. Core temperature should be maintained as close to normal as possible by use of antipyretics and a cooling blanket. Coagulation abnormalities should be identified promptly and treated by infusion of platelets and coagulation factors, as indicated. Finally, patients should be given oxygen supplementation and observed closely for evidence of ARDS, one of the major causes of mortality in cases of severe sepsis.[14] Oxygenation should be monitored by means of a pulse oximeter or radial artery catheter. At the first sign of respiratory failure, the patient should be intubated and supported with mechanical ventilation.

The prognosis in patients with septic shock clearly depends on the severity of the patient's underlying illness. In patients with "rapidly fatal illnesses," such as hematopoietic malignancies, mortality approaches 80 percent. In patients with "ultimately fatal illnesses," such as solid tumors, mortality decreases to 40 to 50 percent. However, in otherwise healthy patients, mortality rarely exceeds 15 percent.[69] Fortunately, most obstetric patients are in the latter category. Therefore, the prognosis for complete recovery is excellent provided that the patient receives competent, timely intervention.

Cytomegalovirus Infection

Epidemiology

Cytomegalovirus (CMV) is a double-stranded DNA virus that replicates within the nucleus of an infected cell. Humans are its only known host. Like herpes simplex virus, CMV may remain latent in host cells after the initial infection. Recurrent infection is usually due to reactivation of endogenous latent virus rather than reinfection with a new strain of virus. Cell-mediated immunity is more important than humoral mechanisms in controlling infection.[70]

CMV is not highly contagious, and, therefore, close personal contact is required for infection to occur. *Horizontal transmission* may result from receipt of an infected organ or blood, from sexual contact, or from contact with contaminated saliva or urine. *Vertical transmission* may occur as a result of transplacental infection, exposure to contaminated genital tract secretions during delivery, or breast-feeding. The incubation period of the virus ranges from 28 to 60 days, with a mean of 40 days.[70–72]

Among young children, the most important risk factor for infection is close contact with playmates, particularly in the setting of day care. In an early report, Pass and coworkers[73] surveyed 70 children attending a day care center in Birmingham, Alabama. Investigators obtained mouth swabs from 29 children and urine specimens from 68. Forty-five percent of mouth swabs and 53 percent of urine cultures were positive for CMV. Nine percent of infants less than 1 year of age shed virus in either saliva or urine; 83 percent of children 1 to 2 years of age shed virus.

Jones et al.[74] conducted a similar survey in a regular day care center and a facility for developmentally delayed children. Twenty-two percent of children in both centers were viruric, and 11 percent shed virus in their saliva. Hutto and coworkers[75] surveyed 47 toddlers attending day care. Fourteen (30 percent) shed virus in saliva. The highest rate of salivary excretion (80 percent) occurred in children 12 to 24 months of age. Forty percent of the children were viruric.

Infected children clearly pose a risk of transmitting virus to adult day care workers. Adler[76] recently examined the rate of seroconversion to CMV among day care employees. At the time of initial assessment, 202 workers were seronegative. Within 10 months, 19 (11 percent) had seroconverted. The rate of seroconversion was greatest among employees who cared for children under 2 years of age.

Small children also pose a risk to members of their own family. Taber et al.[77] performed a serologic study and identified 68 families in which both parents were seronegative for CMV. Over a 3-year period, seroconversion occurred in one or more members of 37 families (53 percent). Mean annual seroconversion rates were approximately 10 percent for fathers, mothers, and children. The index case was usually a child.

In addition to acquiring infection from young children, adolescents and adults may develop infection as a result of sexual contact. CMV infection is endemic among homosexual men and heterosexuals with multiple partners.[70,78] Additional risk factors for infection include lower socioeconomic status, history of abnormal cervical cytology, birth outside of North America, first pregnancy at less than 15 years, and coinfection with other sexually transmitted diseases such as trichomoniasis.[79]

Clinical Manifestations in Children and Adults

Most children who acquire CMV infection are asymptomatic. When clinical manifestations are present, they usually are mild and include malaise, fever, lymphadenopathy, and hepatosplenomegaly. Similarly, most adults with either primary or recurrent CMV are asymptomatic. Symptomatic patients typically have findings suggestive of mononucleosis. Respiratory infection is uncommon in adults with normal immune function, but an increasing number of cases of serious CMV infection are likely to occur as a consequence of the rising prevalence of HIV infection in women.

Diagnosis of Infection in Adults and Children

The diagnosis of CMV infection can be confirmed by isolation of virus in tissue culture. The highest concentration of CMV is usually present in urine, seminal fluid, saliva, and breast milk. Several different cell lines have been used to support viral growth, and techniques such as the viral shell assay, immunofluorescent staining, monoclonal antibody, and polymerase chain reaction permit identification of viral antigen within 24 hours.[80-83]

Serologic methods also are helpful in establishing the diagnosis of CMV infection provided that the reference laboratory is skilled in performing such tests. In the acute phase of infection, viral-specific IgM antibody is present in serum. IgM titers decline rapidly over a period of 30 to 60 days. There is no absolute IgG titer that clearly will differentiate acute from recurrent infection. However, a fourfold or greater change in the IgG titer is consistent with recent acute infection.[70] Other laboratory tests suggestive of CMV infection include a differential WBC showing atypical lymphocytes, low platelet count, and elevated serum transaminase concentrations.

Congenital and Perinatal Infection

As a result of exposure to either young children or an infected sexual partner, approximately 50 to 80 percent of adult women in the United States have serologic evidence of past CMV infection. Unfortunately, the presence of antibody is not perfectly protective against

vertical transmission, and, thus, pregnant women with both recurrent and primary infection pose a special risk to their fetus. Fetal and neonatal CMV infection may occur at three distinct times: antepartum, intrapartum, and postpartum. Antepartum or congenital infection is the greatest risk to the fetus and is perhaps the most difficult to understand because of the often bewildering array of statistics reported in epidemiologic surveys.

Congenital (Antepartum) Infection

Congenital CMV infection results from hematogenous dissemination of virus across the placenta. Dissemination may occur with both primary and recurrent (reactivated) infection but is much more likely in the former setting. From 1 to 4 percent of uninfected women seroconvert during pregnancy.[84] In women who acquire primary infection, 40 to 50 percent of the fetuses will be infected. Based on work with a guinea pig model, Kumar and Prokay[85] have concluded that the overall risk of congenital infection is greatest when maternal infection occurs in the third trimester, but the probability of severe fetal injury is highest when maternal infection occurs in the first trimester.

Of fetuses with congenital infection, 5 to 18 percent will be overtly symptomatic at birth. The most common clinical manifestations are hepatosplenomegaly, intracranial calcifications, jaundice, growth restriction, microcephaly, chorioretinitis, and hearing loss. The most frequent laboratory abnormalities are thrombocytopenia, hyperbilirubinemia, and elevated serum transaminase concentrations. Approximately 30 percent of severely infected infants die. Eighty percent of the survivors have severe neurologic morbidity, ocular abnormalities, or sensorineural hearing loss.[86,87] Approximately 85 to 90 percent of infants delivered to mothers with primary infection will be asymptomatic at birth. Ten to 15 percent subsequently develop hearing loss, chorioretinitis, or dental defects within the first 2 years of life.

Pregnant women who experience recurrent CMV infection are much less likely to transmit infection to their fetus. Recurrent infection occurs predominantly as a result of reactivation of latent infection rather than reinfection with a new viral strain. The most recent, and probably clearest, delineation of fetal risk in this situation is the report by Fowler et al.[87] In an excellent epidemiologic investigation, these authors studied 125 women with serologic evidence of primary infection and 64 with recurrent infection. In the former group, 18 percent of infants were symptomatic at birth. An additional 7 percent developed at least one major sequela within 5 years of follow-up. Two percent died, 15 percent had sensorineural hearing loss, and 13 percent had IQs less than 70. In contrast, none of the infants delivered to mothers with recurrent infection were symptomatic at birth. During the period of surveillance, 8 percent had at least one sequela, but none had multiple defects. The most common sequela was hearing loss. The authors concluded that maternal antibody provided substantial, but not complete, protection against serious fetal infection.

Overall, approximately 1 percent of infants (40,000) born in the United States each year have congenital CMV infection. Approximately 3,000 to 4,000 infants are symptomatic at birth, and an additional 4,000 to 6,000 subsequently have neurologic or developmental problems in the first years of life. CMV infection is now the principal cause of hearing deficits in children. Public health officials estimate that the annual cost of caring for children with congenital CMV is $1.86 billion.[88]

Perinatal (Intrapartum and Postpartum) Infection

Perinatal infection may occur *during delivery* as a result of exposure to infected genital tract secretions. At the time of delivery, up to 10 percent of pregnant women may be shedding CMV in cervical secretions or urine. Twenty to 60 percent of exposed fetuses may subsequently shed virus in their pharynx or urine. The incubation period for this form of infection ranges from 7 to 12 weeks, with an average of 8 weeks. Fortunately, infected infants rarely have serious sequelae of infection acquired during delivery.[86,89]

Perinatal infection also may develop as a *result of breast-feeding*. Stagno et al.[90] surveyed 278 women who had recently delivered and who agreed to provide samples of breast milk. Thirty-eight (13 percent) had CMV isolated at least once from colostrum or milk. Twenty-eight of these women were shedding CMV only in breast milk. Nineteen of their neonates were breast-fed, and 11 (58 percent) acquired CMV infection, despite the presence of neutralizing antibody in breast milk. Fortunately, serious sequelae did not occur in infected infants.

Diagnosis of Fetal Infection

In recent years, much attention has focused on analysis of amniotic fluid and fetal serum as a means to diagnose congenital infection. Several authors have compared the relative value of the following diagnostic tests: viral culture of amniotic fluid and fetal serum, determination of total IgM concentration in fetal serum, identification of anti-CMV IgM in fetal serum, and assessment of fetal liver function tests. These reports uniformly have supported the superiority of amniotic fluid culture in confirming the diagnosis of congenital CMV infection.

Lange and coworkers[91] were the first to report suc-

cessful diagnosis of congenital infection by sampling of fetal blood. They performed cordocentesis on a hydropic fetus at 25 weeks' gestation, and the fetal blood smear showed severe erythroblastosis. Total IgM concentration was normal, but viral-specific IgM antibody to CMV was detected by radioimmunoassay. Hohlfeld et al.[80] subsequently described their assessment of 15 women with documented primary CMV infection in pregnancy. Eight fetuses were infected, and all were correctly identified by detection of antigen in amniotic fluid by the shell viral assay. In each instance, the subsequent viral culture was positive. Only four fetuses (50 percent) had increased total IgM concentrations and abnormal liver function tests. Two fetuses had thrombocytopenia, and none had positive viral blood cultures. The finding of a negative amniotic fluid culture was 100 percent specific in predicting the absence of congenital infection.

Lynch and coauthors[82] recently described their experience with assessment of 12 patients, 7 of whom had serologically confirmed primary infection and 5 of whom were evaluated because of abnormal sonographic findings. Eleven of the patients had an amniocentesis and cordocentesis. Of the seven women with serologically confirmed primary CMV infection, only one fetus was infected. This fetus had a normal hematocrit and platelet count, negative IgM-specific antibody, elevated γ-glutamyltranspeptidase (GGTP) concentration, and positive amniotic fluid culture. In the group of five women with abnormal sonograms, all of the fetuses were infected. Four (80 percent) had positive amniotic fluid cultures, and none had a positive blood culture. One had thrombocytopenia, three had elevated GGTP, and four had elevated total IgM.

In the most recent and largest series of invasive diagnostic testing for congenital CMV infection, Donner et al.[83] assessed 52 fetuses at risk for congenital CMV. Sixteen fetuses were infected, 13 of whom were diagnosed antenatally. Thirteen of 16 (81 percent) had at least one abnormal test. Detection of virus in amniotic fluid by culture or polymerase chain reaction methodology correctly identified 12 (75 percent) infected fetuses. Four patients required two amnioceteses to establish the diagnosis. Nine of 16 fetuses (56 percent) had viral-specific IgM antibody in cord blood. Six of 11 (55 percent) fetuses who had hematologic assays were thrombocytopenic. A negative amniotic fluid culture was 100 percent specific in identifying an uninfected fetus.

Although identification of virus in amniotic fluid appears to be the most sensitive and specific test for diagnosing congenital infection, it does not necessarily identify the *severity* of fetal injury. This issue is obviously of great importance in counseling parents about the prognosis for their infant. Fortunately, detailed sonography can be invaluable in providing information about severity of fetal impairment. The principal sonographic findings suggestive of serious fetal injury include microcephaly, ventriculomegaly, intracerebral calcifications, hydrops, growth restriction, and oligohydramnios.[92] In addition, unusual findings that may also indicate a severely infected infant include fetal heart block,[93] intra-abdominal echodensities,[94] meconium peritonitis,[95] and isolated serous effusions.[92] Clinicians should be aware that the ultrasound examination may be normal early in the course of fetal infection. Therefore, fetuses at risk should have repeat examinations to determine if anomalies are apparent.

Treatment and Prevention

At the present time, a vaccine for CMV is not available. Antiviral agents such as gancyclovir and foscarnet have moderate activity against CMV, but their use is limited primarily to treatment of severe infections in immunocompromised patients. Accordingly, obstetrician-gynecologists should focus most of their attention on educating patients about preventive measures.

One of the most important interventions is helping patients understand that CMV infection can be a sexually transmitted disease and that sexual promiscuity significantly increases an individual's risk of acquiring the infection. Individuals who have multiple sexual partners should be counseled that latex condoms provide an effective barrier to transmission of CMV.[96] Another important intervention is educating health care workers, day care workers, elementary school teachers, and mothers of young children about the importance of simple infection control measures such as handwashing and proper cleansing of environmental surfaces. Obstetricians and pediatricians must be consistently aware of the importance of transfusing only CMV-free blood products to fetuses, neonates, pregnant women, and immunocompromised patients and of screening potential donors of organs and semen for CMV infection.[71] Finally, health care workers must adhere to the principles of universal precautions when treating patients and handling potentially infected body fluids.[84]

For several reasons, routine prenatal screening for CMV infection is not recommended. First, laboratory resources may be overwhelmed if all pregnant women were screened. Second, if laboratories do not ensure a high level of quality control, the interpretation of serologic tests may be confusing and may lead to incorrect, and irreversible, interventions such as pregnancy termination. Third, neither antiviral chemotherapy nor immunoprophylaxis is available to protect the fetus or neonate. Accordingly, screening should be limited to women who have symptoms suggestive of acute CMV infection, who have had definite occupational exposure to CMV, or who are immunocompromised.

Group B Streptococcal Infection

Epidemiology

Streptococcus agalactiae is a gram-positive encapsulated coccus that produces β-hemolysis when grown on blood agar. Fifteen to 40 percent of pregnant women harbor group B streptococci in their lower genital tract or rectum. The group B streptococcus is one of the most important causes of early onset neonatal infection. The prevalence of neonatal group B streptococcal infection is 1 to 2 per 1,000 live births, and approximately 10,000 to 12,000 cases of neonatal streptococcal septicemia occur each year in the United States.[97,98]

Neonatal group B streptococcal infection can be divided into *early onset* and *late onset* infection. Approximately 80 to 85 percent of cases of neonatal group B streptococcal infection are early in onset and result almost exclusively from vertical transmission from a colonized mother. Early onset infection presents primarily as a severe pneumonia or overwhelming septicemia. In preterm infants, the mortality from early onset group B streptococcal infection approaches 25 percent. In term infants, the mortality is lower, averaging approximately 5 percent in recent investigations. Late onset neonatal group B streptococcal infection occurs as a result of both vertical and horizontal transmission. It is manifested by bacteremia, meningitis, and pneumonia. The mortality from late onset infection is approximately 5 to 10 percent for both preterm and term infants.[97,98]

Unfortunately, obstetric interventions have proven ineffective in preventing late onset neonatal infection. Therefore, the remainder of this discussion will focus on early onset infection. Major risk factors for early onset infection include preterm labor, especially when complicated by preterm premature rupture of membranes (PROM); intrapartum maternal fever (chorioamnionitis); prolonged rupture of membranes, defined as more than 12 to 18 hours; and previous delivery of an infected infant.[97,99,100] Approximately 25 percent of pregnant women have at least one risk factor for group B streptococcal infection. The neonatal attack rate in colonized patients is 40 to 50 percent in the presence of a risk factor and 5 percent or less in the absence of a risk factor. In infected infants, neonatal mortality approaches 30 to 35 percent when a maternal risk factor is present but is 5 percent or less when a risk factor is absent.[97–99]

Maternal Complications

Several obstetric complications occur with increased frequency in pregnant women who are colonized with group B streptococci.[97] The organism is a major cause of chorioamnionitis and postpartum endometritis. It also may cause postcesarean wound infection, usually in conjunction with other aerobic and anaerobic bacilli and staphylococci. Group B streptococci also are responsible for approximately 2 to 3 percent of lower urinary tract infections in pregnant women but usually do not cause pyelonephritis. Group B streptococcal urinary tract infection, in turn, is a risk factor for preterm labor. Thomsen et al.[101] recently reported a study of 69 women at 27 to 31 weeks' gestation who had streptococcal urinary tract infections. Patients were assigned to treatment with either penicillin or placebo. Treated patients had a significant reduction in the frequency of both preterm PROM and preterm labor. Other investigations have confirmed the association between group B streptococcal colonization, preterm labor, and preterm PROM. Women with the latter complication who are colonized with group B streptococci tend to have a shorter latent period and higher frequency of chorioamnionitis and puerperal endometritis than noncolonized women.[102]

Diagnosis

The gold standard for the diagnosis of group B streptococcal infection is bacteriologic culture. Todd-Hewitt broth or selective blood agar is the preferred medium. Specimens for culture should be obtained from the lower vagina, perineum, and perianal area, using a simple cotton swab. In recent years, considerable research has been devoted to assessment of rapid diagnostic tests for the identification of colonized women. Table 38-9 summarizes the results of several investigations of rapid diagnostic tests. The information in this table is based on the review by Yancey et al.,[103] who noted that, although the rapid diagnostic tests had reasonable sensitivity in identifying heavily colonized patients, they had poor sensitivity in identifying lightly and moderately colonized patients. This latter finding severely limits the usefulness of the rapid diagnostic tests in clinical practice.

Prevention of Group B Streptococcal Infection

Several different strategies have been proposed for the prevention of neonatal group B streptococcal infection. One of the first interventions provided for antepartum screening early in pregnancy and treatment of colonized patients at the time of identification of a positive culture. Abundant evidence now indicates that this strategy is clearly ineffective.[98] Screening remote from term is not predictive of colonization status at the time of delivery. Women treated early in gestation frequently recolonize. Early treatment exposes up to 40 percent of pregnant women to antibiotics and yet has no significant impact on the frequency of neonatal infection.

Another early approach to the problem of neonatal streptococcal infection was described by Siegel and associates.[104] These investigators conducted a prospective study of 18,738 neonates delivered during a 25-month period at Parkland Hospital in Dallas, Texas. One group of infants received a single intramuscular dose of aqueous penicillin G after delivery, and the second group received only tetracycline ophthalmic ointment. The overall prevalence of maternal streptococcal colonization was 27 percent. The incidence of disease caused by all penicillin-susceptible organisms was decreased in the infants treated with penicillin. However, the incidence of disease caused by resistant organisms was increased in the infants treated with penicillin. This latter effect is a sufficiently serious problem to make universal penicillin prophylaxis a risky preventive strategy.

A third preventive approach is the strategy recently proposed by the American Academy of Pediatrics.[106] This organization recommended universal screening of all pregnant women at 26 to 28 weeks' gestation and selective intrapartum treatment of colonized women who have risk factors for group B streptococcal infection. This approach is based on a series of investigations that have been published during the last 15 years. One

Table 38-9   Reliability of Rapid Diagnostic Tests for Group B Streptococci

Test	Test Performance			
	SENS. (%)	SPEC. (%)	PV⁺ (%)	PV⁻ (%)
Gram stain	34–100	60–70	13–33	86–100
Growth in starch medium	93–98	98–99	65–98	89–99
Antigen detection (coagglutination, latex particle agglutination, enzyme immunoassay)	4–88[a]	92–100	15–100	76–99
DNA probe[b]	71	90	61	94

[a] Sensitivities for identification of heavily colonized women ranged from 29 to 100%.
[b] Specimens were grown in culture for 3.5 hours before DNA probe was used.
(Data from Yancey et al.[103])

of the first of these was the report by Yow and coworkers in 1979.[105] These authors treated 34 colonized women with ampicillin during labor; 24 colonized women received no treatment. None of the infants delivered to treated mothers were colonized compared with 58 percent of infants delivered to untreated women (*p* < 0.001). In a subsequent investigation, Boyer and associates[106] studied the effect of intrapartum treatment with ampicillin in a much larger series of 575 colonized women. This study included several subsets of women, and treatment was not randomized in all subsets. However, treatment with ampicillin significantly reduced the frequency of vertical transmission in patients with, and without, risk factors.

The most highly publicized investigation was reported by Boyer and Gotoff in 1986.[99] These investigators screened a population of over 13,000 women. Twenty-three percent of women had positive cultures for group B streptococci. At the time of presentation in labor, colonized patients were enrolled in the study if they had preterm labor or ruptured membranes for more than 12 hours. Patients were randomly assigned to no treatment or to ampicillin, 2 g IV every 4 hours, until delivery. Normal infants delivered to treated mothers received four doses of intramuscular ampicillin until surveillance cultures were available. Healthy infants delivered to untreated mothers received no antibiotics. Infants with clinical evidence of respiratory distress syndrome, sepsis, or asphyxia were treated with ampicillin plus gentamicin. As noted in Table 38-10, intrapartum prophylaxis with ampicillin was effective in decreasing the overall prevalence of neonatal colonization, colonization at multiple sites, and bacteremia.

Several problems may occur during an effort to implement universal screening. First, this approach requires a major commitment of both financial and logistic resources. Second, universal screening at 26 to 28 weeks' gestation may not reliably identify all patients who will actually be colonized at term. Third, depending on the organization of the laboratory, results of antenatal cultures may not be readily available to physicians at all hours of the day and night. Despite these caveats, universal screening clearly will be cost effective in most populations.[98] The Centers for Disease Control

and Prevention estimate that universal screening and selective treatment will prevent approximately 3,300 cases of neonatal infection each year and save approximately $16 million.[107] Approximately 4 to 5 percent of all pregnant women will be treated with antibiotics under this protocol. This estimate is based on the assumptions that approximately 20 percent of pregnant women are colonized and that approximately 25 percent of colonized patients have at least one risk factor for infection.

An alternative to universal screening is the intervention strategy suggested by Tuppurainen and Hallman.[108] These investigators recently screened approximately 9,000 Finnish patients with a latex agglutination test at the time of admission for delivery. One hundred ninety-nine women who were heavily colonized were accurately identified by the latex agglutination test. These women were randomly assigned to receive 5,000,000 units of penicillin during labor or no treatment. Of the 88 colonized women who received intrapartum penicillin, only 1.1 percent of the neonates developed early onset infection compared with 9 percent of neonates in the no treatment group (p < 0.01).

Certain pitfalls also exist with this approach. As noted previously, rapid slide tests have poor sensitivity in identifying lightly colonized women, and yet some cases of neonatal sepsis still occur in infants delivered to these women. Not all rapid tests are easy to perform; some are not well adapted for use in a labor and delivery suite. Moreover, rapid tests may not be readily available in all hospitals on a 24-hour a day basis.[103]

Another theoretical solution to the problem of neonatal group B streptococcal infection is universal antibiotic prophylaxis for all women in labor. In an elaborate decision analysis, Rouse et al.[109] recently demonstrated that this strategy was, in fact, the most cost effective of all interventions considered. However, extensive administration of broad spectrum antibiotics clearly has the potential to exert selective pressure for emergence of drug-resistant strains of bacteria. Therefore, this strategy should not be widely adopted until the risk of superinfection in mother and infant resulting from universal prophylaxis has been precisely delineated.

Yet another strategy for prevention of neonatal group B streptococcal infection is that proposed by the American College of Obstetricians and Gynecologists (ACOG).[110] ACOG does not endorse universal screening; rather, it recommends selective screening of patients who have specific risk factors such as preterm labor and preterm PROM. Colonized patients with risk factors are then targeted for intrapartum antibiotic prophylaxis. Intrapartum treatment is also recommended for women whose colonization status is unknown but who develop a risk factor, such as extended duration of rupture of membranes, during labor. The approach

Table 38-10 Effect of Intrapartum Chemoprophylaxis on Neonatal Outcome

End Point	Ampicillin (N = 85)	No Treatment (N = 79)	p
Neonatal colonization	9%	51%	<0.001
Colonization at ≥3 sites	4%	30%	<0.001
Bacteremia	0	6%	0.02

(Data from Boyer and Gotoff.[99])

Table 38-11   Antibiotics with Activity Against
             Group B Streptococci

Drug	Dose for Intrapartum Prophylaxis
Ampicillin	2 g q4–6h
Penicillin	2–5 million units q6h
Erythromycin	1–2 g q6h
Clindamycin	600 mg q6h or 900 mg q8h
Vancomycin	500 mg q6h or 1,000 mg q12h

suggested by ACOG avoids some of the problems associated with universal screening. Approximately 10 to 20 percent of women will be candidates for treatment under this protocol, which is a figure greater than that cited for the American Academy of Pediatrics' protocol. However, in two recent decision analyses, this approach compared favorably with that of universal screening.[98,109]

Antibiotics with specific activity against group B streptococci are listed in Table 38-11. Ampicillin and penicillin are the antibiotics that have been tested most extensively. The other antibiotics noted in Table 38-11 should be reserved for patients who have immediate hypersensitivity reactions to β-lactam antibiotics. Prophylactic antibiotics should be administered intravenously as soon as a risk factor is identified. They should be continued until delivery is completed but do not need to be administered in the postpartum period. Only patients who have overt chorioamnionitis require antibiotic treatment beyond delivery.

Hepatitis

Hepatitis is one of the most common and most highly contagious viral infections. At present, five distinct types of hepatitis virus have been identified: A, B, C, D, and E. Each type of hepatitis has a slightly different clinical implication for the pregnant woman and her fetus.

Hepatitis A

Hepatitis A is responsible for approximately 30 to 35 percent of cases of hepatitis in the United States. It is caused by a 27-nm RNA virus that is a member of the picornavirus family. The virus is transmitted by person to person contact through fecal-oral contamination. Poor hygiene, poor sanitation, and intimate personal or sexual contact facilitate transmission. Epidemics frequently result from common exposure to contaminated food and water. In the United States, individuals at particular risk for hepatitis A are those who have recently immigrated from, or traveled to, developing nations of the world where the disease is endemic.[111] Drug abusers, homosexual men, and children in day care centers also are at increased risk of acquiring hepatitis A.[112,113]

The incubation period of hepatitis A ranges from 15 to 50 days, with a mean of 28 to 30 days. The highest concentration of viral particles is in fecal material. The virus is not normally excreted in urine or other body fluids.

Some patients with hepatitis A are relatively asymptomatic. When symptoms do occur, they usually include malaise, fatigue, anorexia, nausea and vomiting, and right upper quadrant pain. The characteristic physical findings of acute hepatitis A are jaundice, hepatic tenderness, darkened urine, and acholic stools.

The most useful diagnostic test for hepatitis A is detection of IgM-specific antibody. IgM antibody usually is detectable 25 to 30 days following the initial exposure and persists in the serum for up to 6 months. IgG antibody is detectable within 35 to 40 days of exposure and persists indefinitely, thus conferring lifelong immunity. In addition, the serum concentration of alanine aminotransferase (ALT), aspartate aminotransferase (AST), and bilirubin are usually moderately to markedly elevated. Liver biopsy is rarely indicated to confirm the diagnosis of viral hepatitis.[114] When performed, it characteristically shows extensive hepatocellular injury and a prominent inflammatory infiltrate (Fig. 38-6).

Fortunately, acute hepatitis A is usually a self-limited illness, and only supportive care is required for the vast majority of patients. Recovery is typically complete within 4 to 6 weeks. Fewer than 0.5 percent of affected patients develop fulminant hepatitis, coagulopathy, or encephalopathy. Infected patients should be advised of the need for sound nutrition. Physical activity should be limited to prevent upper abdominal trauma. Drugs with potential hepatotoxicity should be avoided. Sexual and household contacts should receive immunoprophylaxis with a single intramuscular dose of immunoglobulin, 0.02 ml/kg within 2 weeks of exposure. In addition, they also should receive the formalin-inactivated hepatitis A vaccine, in a single IM dose of 0.06 ml. The vaccine is highly immunogenic and is safe for use in pregnancy.[115,116]

As a general rule, unless the pregnant mother becomes severely ill, hepatitis A does not pose a serious risk to the fetus. Perinatal transmission of infection does not occur, and a chronic carrier state does not exist. An infant delivered to an acutely infected mother should receive immunoglobulin to prevent horizontal transmission of infection after delivery. In addition, mothers who develop evidence of encephalopathy, coagulopathy, or severe debilitation should be hospitalized for supportive care.[114]

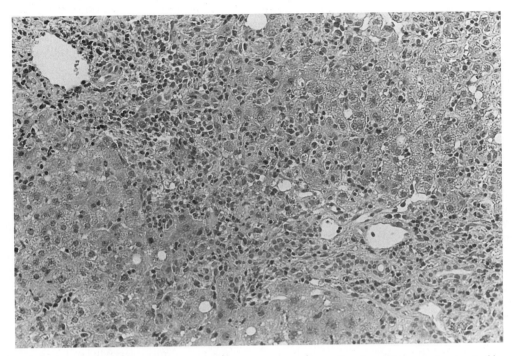

Fig. 38-6 Photomicrograph of liver biopsy specimen shows characteristic histologic changes of acute viral hepatitis. Note the intense inflammatory infiltrate.

Hepatitis B

Approximately 40 to 45 percent of all cases of hepatitis in the United States are caused by hepatitis B virus. Over 300,000 new cases of hepatitis B occur annually, and about 1 million Americans are chronic viral carriers. The frequencies of acute and chronic hepatitis B in pregnancy are 1 to 2/1,000 and 5 to 15/1,000, respectively.[117]

Hepatitis B is caused by a DNA virus, and the intact virus is termed the *Dane particle*. The virus has three major structural antigens: surface antigen (HB$_s$Ag), core antigen (HB$_c$Ag), and e antigen (HB$_e$Ag). Transmission of hepatitis B occurs primarily as a result of parenteral injection, sexual contact, and perinatal exposure.[114] Certain population groups have an increased prevalence of hepatitis B: Asians, Eskimos, drug addicts, transfusion recipients, dialysis patients, residents and employees of chronic care residencies, prisoners, and recipients of tatoos.

Following an acute infection caused by hepatitis B virus, less than 1 percent of patients develop fulminant hepatitis and die. Eighty-five to 90 percent experience complete resolution of their physical findings and develop protective levels of antibody. Ten to 15 percent of patients become chronically infected. Of these, 15 to 30 percent subsequently develop chronic active or persistent hepatitis or cirrhosis, and a small percentage develop hepatocellular carcinoma. Chronic liver disease is particularly likely to occur in patients who re-

main seropositive for HB$_e$Ag and who become superinfected with the hepatitis D virus.[114]

The diagnosis of *acute* hepatitis B is confirmed by detection of the surface antigen and IgM antibody to the core antigen. Identification of HB$_e$Ag is indicative of an exceptionally high viral inoculum and active viral replication. Patients who have *chronic* hepatitis B infection have persistence of the surface antigen in the serum and liver tissue. Some individuals, particularly Asians, also remain seropositive for HB$_e$Ag.[114,115,118]

Patients with acute and chronic hepatitis B infection pose a major threat of transmission to other household members, especially their sexual partner. In addition, infected women also may transmit infection to their fetus. Perinatal transmission occurs primarily as a result of the infant's exposure to infected blood and genital secretions during delivery. In the absence of immunoprophylaxis for the neonate, perinatal transmission occurs in 10 to 20 percent of women who are seropositive for HB$_s$Ag. The frequency of perinatal transmission increases to almost 90 percent in women who are seropositive for both HB$_s$Ag and HB$_e$Ag.[114,115,119]

Fortunately, a combination of passive and active immunization is highly effective in preventing both horizontal and vertical transmission of hepatitis B infection. All individuals who have had household or sexual exposure to another person with hepatitis B infection should be tested to determine if they have antibody to the virus. If they are seronegative, they should immediately receive immunoprophylaxis with hepatitis B immunoglobulin (HBIG), 0.06 ml/kg IM. They then should receive the hepatitis B vaccination series. Similarly, infants who are delivered to seropositive mothers should receive HBIG, 0.5 ml IM, immediately after birth. They then should begin the hepatitis B vaccination series within 12 hours of birth. At the present time, two recombinant hepatitis B vaccines are available, Recombivax-HB and Engerix-B.[114,115] Both products are composed of inactivated portions of the surface antigen and are prepared by recombinant DNA technology. Neither poses a risk of transmission of a blood-borne pathogen, and both are safe for administration during pregnancy to patients at risk.

Neonatal immunoprophylaxis is approximately 85 to 95 percent effective in preventing neonatal hepatitis B infection. In view of the extremely favorable results of immunoprophylaxis, the Centers for Disease Control and Prevention (CDC) recently recommended universal hepatitis B vaccination for all infants.[120] Dosage recommendations vary depending on the mother's serostatus. Infants born to seronegative mothers require only the vaccine. Infants born to seropositive mothers should receive both the vaccine and HBIG. Therefore, obstetricians must continue to screen *all* of their patients for hepatitis B at some point during pregnancy. Selective screening on the basis of acknowledged risk factors will fail to identify 30 to 50 percent of seropositive women.[114]

Patients infected with hepatitis B virus also may transmit infection to medical and nursing personnel who care for them. Each year approximately 12,000 American health care workers contract hepatitis B as a result of an occupational injury such as a needle stick or splash to a mucous membrane. Of these, approximately 200 develop fulminant hepatitis and subsequently die.[115,121] Health care workers can protect themselves from hepatitis in three principal ways. First, they should be vaccinated for hepatitis B. Second, they should encourage *all* young adults and other individuals who have a specific risk factor to receive the hepatitis B vaccine. Third, they should consistently follow universal precautions to prevent sharp injuries and splashes to exposed mucous membrane or skin surfaces.

Conversely, health care workers who are infected with hepatitis B also pose a risk to others. They, too, must observe safeguards to prevent horizontal transmission of infection to their patients. Infection is most likely to occur as a consequence of direct blood-to-blood exposure during invasive surgical procedures. Unless the patient has documented immunity to hepatitis B, the infected health care worker has an ethical obligation to inform her that some risk of transmission exists. The attendant should then perform the procedure only if the patient explicitly consents. During the actual procedure, the operator must take every precaution, including double gloving, to ensure that a sharp injury does not occur.

Non-A, Non-B Hepatitis

Non-A, non-B hepatitis accounts for 10 to 20 percent of cases of hepatitis in the United States. Non-A, non-B hepatitis occurs in two forms: parenterally transmitted hepatitis C and enterically transmitted hepatitis E.

Hepatitis C

Hepatitis C is a 30- to 38-nm, single-stranded RNA virus, that is similar in structure to flaviviruses and pestiviruses. Its incubation period is 5 to 10 weeks. The principal risk factors for hepatitis C are intravenous drug abuse, transfusion, and sexual intercourse.[122] In a recent survey by Osmond and coworkers,[123] two-thirds of a selected population of drug abusers were seropositive for hepatitis C. In a similar survey of patients attending a sexually transmitted disease (STD) clinic in San Francisco, Weinstock et al.[124] found the prevalence of hepatitis C to be 7.7 percent. Approximately 90 percent of all cases of post-transfusion hepatitis are due to hepatitis C, and 2.5 to 15 percent of patients who receive multiple transfusions become infected with this virus. Hepatitis C is particularly likely to result in chronic liver disease. Approximately 50 percent of infected patients develop biochemical evidence of hepatic dysfunction. Of these, about 20 percent subsequently develop chronic active hepatitis or cirrhosis.[114]

Approximately 75 percent of patients with hepatitis C are asymptomatic. The diagnosis of hepatitis C infection is confirmed by identification of anti-C antibody. Initial screening for this antibody should be performed with an enzyme immunoassay (EIA). A positive EIA should be followed with a recombinant immunoblot assay (RIBA). The present RIBA is able to detect four specific viral antigens. If at least two antigens are identified, the test is considered positive. If only one antigen is identified, the test is considered indeterminant. The present generation of laboratory assays does not precisely discriminate between IgM and IgG antibody. Moreover, antibody may not be detectable until up to 22 weeks after the onset of clinical illness. Direct detection of antigen also is possible with polymerase chain reaction methodology, although this test is not yet widely available.[114]

In a general obstetric population, the prevalence of hepatitis C is 1 to 3 percent. The principal risk factors that identify an obstetric patient at high risk for hepatitis C include concurrent STDs, such as hepatitis B and HIV infection; multiple sexual partners; history of recent multiple transfusions; and history of intravenous drug abuse.[125] In selected series, the frequency of perinatal transmission of hepatitis C infection has ranged from 10 to 44 percent,[122,126] but the epidemiology of perinatal transmission has not been completely delineated. Many of the infected neonates in these series were coinfected with HIV.

At the present time, a vaccine for hepatitis C is not available. Passive immunization with immunoglobulin (0.06 ml/kg IM) should be administered following percutaneous exposure to a person with hepatitis C. The benefit of immunoprophylaxis for the neonate has not been proven in controlled clinical trials. Although α-interferon has shown some activity against the virus, relapses occur in 44 to 80 percent of patients within 6 to 12 months of discontinuation of therapy.[114]

Hepatitis E

The hepatitis E virus is an RNA virus that is closely related to the calicivirus family. It may present in both an icteric and anicteric form. The virus is transmitted by the fecal/oral route, and, therefore, the epidemiology of hepatitis E is similar to that of hepatitis A. The incubation period ranges from 2 to 9 weeks, with a mean of 45 days.[127,128] Hepatitis E is rare in the United States but is endemic in developing countries.[129–131] In these countries, maternal mortality has been alarmingly high, ranging from 10 to 20 percent. Extreme poverty, coexisting medical illnesses, malnutrition, and poor prenatal care are at least partially responsible for the poor maternal prognosis. The only cases of hepatitis E in the United States have occurred in patients who traveled to countries where the disease was endemic.[132]

Three new diagnostic tests are available for confirmation of hepatitis E infection. Viral-like particles can be identified in the stool of infected patients by electron microscopy. These particles will agglutinate when combined with serum from the patient. In addition, a fluorescent antibody blocking assay and Western blot assay are now available for use.[114,133]

Patients with acute hepatitis E should be treated as described previously for patients with hepatitis A. Once a patient has recovered from the acute illness, a chronic carrier state does not develop, and perinatal transmission does not occur. If the mother survives the acute stage of infection, fetal outcome is not adversely affected.

Hepatitis D

Hepatitis D, or delta hepatitis, is caused by an RNA virus that is dependent on coinfection with the hepatitis B virus for replication. Hepatitis D has an external coat of hepatitis B surface antigen and an internal delta antigen that is encoded by its own genome. The epidemiology of hepatitis D is essentially identical to that of hepatitis B.[134]

Acute hepatitis D occurs in two forms: *coinfection* and *superinfection*. Coinfection represents the simultaneous occurrence of acute hepatitis B and D. It is usually a self-limited disorder and rarely leads to *chronic* liver disease. Superinfection occurs when *acute* hepatitis D develops in a patient who is a *chronic* hepatitis B carrier. Approximately 20 to 25 percent of patients with chronic hepatitis B ultimately become superinfected with the delta virus, and about 80 percent of these individuals subsequently develop chronic hepatitis. Of those who have chronic hepatitis, 70 to 80 percent develop cirrhosis and portal hypertension, and, unfortunately, almost 25 percent ultimately die of hepatic failure.[134–136]

The clinical manifestations of acute hepatitis D are similar to those of any acute viral hepatitis. The diagnosis of *acute coinfection* can be confirmed by detection of delta antigen in hepatic tissue or serum and IgM-specific antibody in serum. In addition, the tests for HBsAg-IgM and HBcAb are positive. In patients with *superinfection,* serologic tests reflect acute hepatitis D (positive antigen, positive IgM antibody) and chronic hepatitis B infection (positive surface antigen, negative HBcAb-IgG). Patients with *chronic* hepatitis D usually have detectable serum levels of IgG-specific antibody for the delta virus and are seropositive for HBsAg. Unfortunately, IgG antibody does not eradicate the delta viremia, and the antigen still can be identified in serum and hepatic tissue.[114,134,135]

Patients with acute hepatitis D should receive the general supportive care outlined for hepatitis A. Patients with chronic infection should be monitored periodically for worsening hepatic function or coagulopathy. At present, there is no specific antiviral agent or immunotherapy that is curative for either acute or chronic delta infection. Perinatal transmission of hepatitis D virus has been reported. Fortunately, transmission is uncommon because the neonatal immunoprophylaxis for hepatitis B is almost uniformly effective against hepatitis D.[114]

Herpes Simplex Virus Infection

Epidemiology

Herpes simplex (HSV), a double-stranded DNA virus, is transmitted by direct, intimate contact. Following the initial infection, the virus remains dormant in neuronal ganglia and may reactivate at later times. Two strains of the virus have been identified: HSV-1 and HSV-2. The former causes primarily oropharyngeal infection and the latter, genital tract infection. Approximately 0.5 to 1.0 percent of women have an overt herpetic

Table 38-12 Classification of Herpes Simplex Virus Infection

Classification	Criteria
Primary	First clinical infection No preexisting antibody
Nonprimary, first episode	No history of genital tract infection Positive antibody for HSV-1 or HSV-2
Recurrent	Prior history of clinical infection Positive antibody for HSV-2

Table 38-13 Comparison of Primary Vs. Recurrent Herpes Simplex Virus Infection

Stage of Illness	Type of Infection	
	Primary	Recurrent
Incubation period and/or prodrome (days)	2–10	1–2
Vesicle, pustule (days)	6	2
Wet ulcer (days)	6	3
Dry crust (days)	8	7
Total	22–30	13–14

infection during pregnancy. About 400 cases of neonatal herpes occur annually in the United States, and the estimated incidence of neonatal infection ranges from 1:7,500 to 1:30,000 livebirths.[137,138]

HSV infections are classified as primary, non-primary-first episode, and recurrent on the basis of historical and clinical findings and serologic testing.[137–140] Table 38-12 summarizes the criteria for each diagnosis. Approximately 20 to 40 percent of Americans are seropositive for HSV. Up to 80 percent of these individuals do not have a history of an overt primary infection.

Clinical Manifestations

The onset of HSV infection is usually heralded by a prodrome of neuralgias, paresthesias, and hypesthesias, followed by an eruption of painful vesicles in either the orolabial area or genitalia. The vesicles typically rupture, forming a shallow based ulcer (Fig. 38-7), and then form a dry crust. Some vesicles become secondarily infected and evolve into frank pustules. Ultimately, the vesicles heal without scarring[137,138]

In patients experiencing a primary HSV infection, vesicles may be present for up to 3 weeks. Systemic symptoms may be moderately severe, and local complications such as urinary retention may occur. In recurrent infections, overt vesicles are fewer in number and less painful and typically persist for 14 days or less. Table 38-13 compares the incubation period and clinical features of primary and recurrent HSV infection.[137]

In some patients, particularly those who are immunocompromised, HSV infection may be widely disseminated, affecting extensive areas of skin, mucosal membranes, and visceral organs. HSV also may cause a severe ocular infection, meningitis, encephalitis, and ascending myelitis.

Diagnosis

Several laboratory tests may be used to confirm the diagnosis of HSV infection. Cytologic preparations show characteristic multinucleated giant cells and intranuclear inclusions.[137,138] Polymerase chain reaction PCR assays are extremely sensitive in detecting low concen-

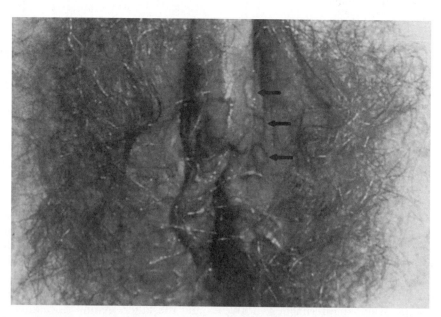

Fig. 38-7 Ulcerated lesions (*arrow*) characteristic of herpes simplex infection. (From Duff et al.,[229] with permission.)

Table 38-14	Frequency of Isolation of Herpes Simplex Virus from Skin Lesions

Type of Lesion	Approximate Frequency of Viral Isolation (%)
Vesicle	90
Pustule	85
Ulcer	70
Crust	25

trations of viral DNA, but such assays are not yet widely available.[141] Serology is especially useful in classifying the initial herpetic episode as *primary* versus *non-primary-first episode*.[137,138] However, serologic testing is rarely indicated in patients who experience recurrent HSV infection.

Until the advent of polymerase chain reaction, viral isolation in tissue culture was considered the standard for confirmation of diagnosis. Viral isolation is usually possible within 72 to 96 hours of inoculation of the tissue culture. The highest rate of isolation is achieved when clinical specimens are obtained from fresh vesicles or pustules (Table 38-14). Vesicular fluid should be aspirated with a fine needle into a tuberculin syringe. Ulcers should be scraped vigorously with a wooden spatula or cotton-tipped applicator.[137,138]

Obstetric and Perinatal Complications

Severe primary HSV infection has been associated with spontaneous abortion, preterm delivery, and intrauterine growth restriction. Isolated case reports also have been published documenting in utero infection even in the presence of intact membranes.[137,138,142] However, the greatest risk to the fetus occurs when overt HSV infection is present at the time of labor. In this situation, the principal mechanism of infection is direct contact with infected vesicles during the process of vaginal birth. The frequency of neonatal infection clearly is dependent on whether the mother has a primary or recurrent HSV infection. In the setting of a primary infection, the viral inoculum in the genital tract is high, and maternal antibody is not present. Approximately 40 percent of neonates delivered vaginally to such women will become infected. In the absence of antiviral chemotherapy, almost half of these infants die, and 35 to 40 percent experience severe neurologic morbidity such as chorioretinitis, microcephaly, mental retardation, seizures, and apnea. In women who have recurrent *symptomatic* HSV infection, the risk of neonatal infection following vaginal delivery is 5 percent or less. In women who have a history of recurrent HSV infection but no prodromal symptoms or overt lesions, the risk of neonatal infection with vaginal delivery is 1:1,000 or less.[137,138,140,143–145]

Neonatal HSV infection may take many forms. In its simplest manifestation, it may appear as a localized abscess at the site of attachment of a scalp electrode or as isolated mucocutaneous lesions. In its more severe forms, neonatal HSV infection may present as widely disseminated mucocutaneous lesions, visceral infection, meningitis, and encephalitis. In such instances, mortality may approach 50 to 60 percent, and up to half of the survivors may have persistent morbidity.[137,138,140,142,143,146]

Management During Pregnancy

Clinical management of HSV infection has changed dramatically in recent years. For several reasons, surveillance cultures of the genital tract in patients with a history of HSV infection have been ineffective in preventing neonatal HSV infection.[147–149] First, cultures are not perfectly sensitive. In a recent report, Cone, et al.[141] detected HSV DNA by polymerase chain reaction in 9 of 100 asymptomatic pregnant women who had negative viral cultures. Second, culture results are not always readily available at the time a patient is admitted for delivery. Third, most children with neonatal HSV infection are actually born to women who do not have a history of prior infection and who, hence, would not be targeted for surveillance cultures.[145,147–150]

Accordingly, the following simplified guidelines have now been recommended by the Infectious Diseases Society for Obstetrics and Gynecology and endorsed by ACOG.[138,144] At the time of the patient's initial prenatal appointment, she should be questioned about a prior history of HSV infection. If her history is positive, she should be screened for other sexually transmitted diseases such as gonorrhea, chlamydia, syphilis, hepatitis B, and HIV infection. When the patient ultimately is admitted for delivery, she should be asked about prodromal symptoms and examined thoroughly for cervical, vaginal, and vulvar lesions. If no prodromal symptoms or overt lesions are present, vaginal delivery should be anticipated. If symptoms or lesions are present, cesarean delivery should be performed. Cesarean is indicated even in the presence of ruptured membranes of extended duration since operative delivery significantly decreases the size of the viral inoculum to which the infant is exposed.

Mothers with symptomatic infection do not need to be isolated from their infants or other patients. They should wash their hands carefully before handling the infant and shield the baby from any contact with vesicular lesions. Breast-feeding is permissible as long as no skin lesions are present on the breast.

In addition to the guidelines outlined above, clinicians should be aware of possible indications for use of acyclovir during pregnancy. Immunocompromised patients with disseminated infections require hospitalization for treatment with intravenous acyclovir. Oral acyclovir, 200 mg five times daily or 400 mg three times daily for 5 to 7 days, should be considered for immunocompetent patients who have *severe* herpetic infection (e.g., prominent systemic symptoms and urinary retention), especially near term.[151] In addition, prophylactic treatment with acyclovir, 400 mg twice daily, may be appropriate in women with frequent recurrent infections in pregnancy, particularly near term.[151] Acyclovir is classified by the FDA as a category C drug. To date, the Acyclovir Registry has reported no increase in the frequency of adverse effects in infants exposed in utero to this antiviral agent.[153,154]

Human Immunodeficiency Virus Infection

Epidemiology

HIV infection is caused by an RNA retrovirus. The principal viral strain responsible for disease in the United States is HIV-1. HIV-2 is a related strain that is endemic in Africa, Portugal, and France. HIV-2 infection is uncommon in the United States except in individuals who have traveled to endemic areas or had sexual contact or shared needles with persons from endemic areas.[155,156]

HIV has a unique propensity to attack and infect CD4 lymphocytes. Upon entering the host cell, the virus uses its reverse transcriptase enzyme to synthesize DNA from RNA. It then integrates the DNA into the host genome. Subsequently, as the host cell replicates its nucleic acid, it also unwittingly replicates new viral nucleic acid. As viral replication continues, the CD4 lymphocyte is progressively weakened and ultimately destroyed, thus rendering the host susceptible to an extensive variety of opportunistic infections and malignancies.[155]

HIV infection occurs in a continuum that can be divided arbitrarily into four stages. Stage one of the disease is the acute retroviral infection that develops several weeks after exposure to the virus. In this stage, the patient has symptoms similar to mononucleosis. Over a period of several weeks, the acute episode resolves, and the patient enters the latent phase of illness. During the latent phase, the patient is asymptomatic, but viral replication occurs, albeit slowly, in lymphatic tissue. The duration of the latent phase is approximately 5 to 10 years. Inexorably, the viral inoculum progressively increases, and the patient enters stage three. This stage is characterized by mild to moderately severe symptoms and debilitating, but usually not life-threatening, opportunistic infections. Ultimately, the patient develops full-blown acquired immunodeficiency syndrome (AIDS). Once symptomatic HIV infection develops, the patient's life expectancy is usually 3 to 5 years.[157]

At the present time, approximately 350,000 to 400,000 Americans have AIDS or have died from AIDS. An additional 1 million are infected with the virus but are not yet in the terminal stage of their illness. In the United States, approximately 12 percent of all cases of HIV infection occur in women. Almost 75 percent of infected women are black or Hispanic. In women, the two most important mechanisms of HIV infection are intravenous drug abuse and heterosexual contact with a high-risk male. In the general obstetric population in the United States, the frequency of HIV infection is approximately 1 per 1,000. However, in some inner city populations, the prevalence of infection is as high as 1 to 1.5 percent.[158–160]

Heterosexual transmission is increasing in importance as a mechanism of spread of HIV infection.[161] Several sexual practices have been shown to increase substantially the risk of transmission of infection. Of these, the most important is unprotected intercourse with multiple partners. Receptive anal intercourse is a particularly dangerous practice because the columnar epithelium of the anus and rectum is more susceptible to trauma than the stratified squamous epithelium of the vagina. The presence of other sexually transmitted diseases that cause genital ulcers, such as herpes, syphilis, and chancroid, also is an important risk factor for HIV infection. Concurrent use of illicit intravenous drugs and crack cocaine and contact with a noncircumcised male also are independent risk factors for HIV infection.

Clinical Manifestations

Symptomatic patients with HIV infection typically have fever, malaise, fatigue, anorexia, nausea, vomiting, diarrhea, weight loss, and generalized lymphadenopathy. Neurologic manifestations may be quite prominent and debilitating, specifically peripheral neuropathy and dementia. These neurologic manifestations result both from direct injury of the central nervous system by HIV and the effects of opportunistic infections such as toxoplasmosis.[155,157]

Opportunistic infections, of course, are the hallmark of HIV infection.[162] Among the most common are *Pneumocystis carinii* pneumonia, tuberculosis, toxoplasmosis, candidiasis, and CMV infection. Genital herpes, hepatitis B, C, and D, and syphilis are common concurrent STDs. Unusual malignancies occur with disturbing regularity in patients with HIV infection.[163] The two most common are Kaposi's sarcoma and non-Hodgkin's lymphoma. The latter disorder appears to have an alarming propensity for early invasion of the central nervous system.

Diagnosis

The diagnosis of HIV infection can be confirmed by direct culture of virus from peripheral blood lymphocytes and monocytes. The diagnosis also can be established by detection of viral antigen by the polymerase chain reaction. Infected patients usually have a decreased number of CD4 cells and an inverted CD4:CD8 ratio. Serum immunoglobulin levels also are elevated.[164]

The principal diagnostic test at present is identification of viral-specific antibody.[164] The initial serologic screening test should be an ELISA or EIA. These tests are highly sensitive, inexpensive, and readily suited for screening large numbers of patients. If the initial ELISA or EIA test is positive, the test should be repeated. If the second test is positive, a confirmatory Western blot assay should be performed. This test detects specific viral antigens, and it is considered positive when any two of the following three antigens are identified: p24 (viral core), gp-41 (envelope), and gp-120/160 (envelope). If a patient has two positive ELISAs or EIAs, followed by a confirmatory Western blot, the likelihood of a false-positive test is less than 1 in 10,000.[165,166]

As a general rule, patients in the United States should be routinely tested only for HIV-1 infection. Testing for HIV-2 infection is indicated if the patient has had sexual contact, or has shared needles, with a partner from an area of the world where HIV-2 infection is endemic. Testing also should be done if the patient has recently traveled to an endemic area or received a blood transfusion or nonsterile injection in such a locale. In addition, testing also should be performed in individuals who have clinical evidence of HIV infection, but in whom serologic tests for HIV-1 are nonconfirmatory. Screening for HIV-2 infection may be done with a specific EIA and Western blot. In addition, a commercial EIA is now available that simultaneously screens for HIV-1 and HIV-2.[156]

Perinatal Transmission

Approximately 90 percent of all cases of HIV infection in children are due to perinatal transmission. Perinatal transmission occurs as a result of hematogenous dissemination and as a result of intrapartum exposure to infected maternal blood and genital tract secretions. The relative importance of each mechanism has not been precisely delineated.[157,159]

The frequency of vertical transmission of HIV infection varies from a low of 5 to 10 percent to a high of 50 to 60 percent. The average in most investigations has been 20 to 30 percent.[167,168] Factors that increase

Table 38-15 Factors That Increase the Risk of Vertical Transmission of HIV Infection

Risk Factor	Presumed Mechanism
HIV-1 vs. HIV-2	Risk is much greater with HIV-1, presumably as a result of greater virulence of HIV-1
History of previous child with HIV infection	Higher viral inoculum in mother
Mother with AIDS	Higher viral inoculum, decreased immunocompetence of the mother
Preterm delivery	Decreased neonatal immunocompetence
Decreased maternal CD_4 count	Impaired maternal immunity
p24 antigenemia in mother	Denotes higher rate of viral replication and greater infectivity
Firstborn twin	With vaginal delivery, firstborn twin has more prolonged exposure to infected blood and genital tract secretions
Chorioamnionitis	Placental vasculitis facilitates hematogenous dissemination of virus
Intrapartum blood exposure, e.g., episiotomy, vaginal laceration, forceps delivery	Greater contact with infected blood and genital secretions

the likelihood of vertical transmission are summarized in Table 38-15.

Obstetric Complications

Studies of obstetric outcome in patients with HIV infection are difficult to interpret because affected patients have so many confounding conditions that may complicate pregnancy. Such conditions include drug addiction, poor nutrition, limited access to prenatal care, poverty, and concurrent sexually transmitted diseases. When investigators have tried to control for these confounding variables, infected women appear to be at increased risk for several major complications: preterm delivery, preterm PROM, intrauterine growth restriction, increased perinatal mortality, and postpartum endometritis. Pregnancy per se probably does not significantly accelerate the progression of HIV infection.[157,159]

Management

All obstetric patients should be offered voluntary screening for HIV infection at the time of their first prenatal appointment. Selective screening only in patients presumed to be high risk will fail to identify approximately 50 percent of seropositive women.[169] Infected women should be counseled about the risk of perinatal transmission of infection and about potential obstetric complications. They should then be offered the option of pregnancy termination. In addition, arrangements should be made for patients to obtain assistance from appropriate support personnel such as social workers, nutritionists, and psychologists. Patients also should be advised to discontinue smoking since this practice appears to accelerate the course of the disease.[157,159]

Infected patients should be screened for other sexually transmitted diseases such as gonorrhea, chlamydia, herpes, hepatitis B, C, and D and syphilis. They should be tested for antibody to CMV and toxoplasmosis because both of these infections can cause severe chorioretinitis and central nervous system disease, and both are amenable to treatment with antimicrobial agents. Patients also should have a tuberculin skin test; if this test is positive, a chest x-ray should be performed to identify active pulmonary disease. In addition, patients should receive vaccinations for hepatitis B, pneumococcal infection, hemophilus B influenza, and viral influenza. Finally, patients should have a Papanicolaou smear to determine if cervical intraepithelial neoplasia is present.

Patients who are symptomatic and those who have CD4 counts below 200 cells/mm^3 should be offered treatment with zidovudine. Zidovudine should be administered in a dosage of 100 mg PO five times daily. The principal toxicity of this drug is marrow suppression, and patients receiving this agent should have periodic assessment of hematocrit, white cell count, and platelet count. Patients receiving zidovudine for these indications also should receive prophylaxis against *P. carinii* infection. The prophylactic agent of choice in pregnant women is trimethoprim-sulfamethoxazole, one double-strength tablet daily. This regimen also provides protection against toxoplasmic encephalitis. If a patient's CD4 count falls below 50/mm^3 she also should receive prophylaxis against cryptococcal infection. The appropriate drug for prophylaxis is fluconazole, 100 to 200 mg PO, daily.[157,159,170,171]

In addition to these indications, a new rationale for administration of zidovudine has recently been delineated. Connor and coworkers[172] have now published the results of the AIDS Clinical Trials Group Protocol 076. This study was conducted in both the United States and France and included a select group of obstetric patients: asymptomatic women beyond the first trimester of pregnancy who had CD4 counts greater than 200/mm^3. millimeter. Women were randomized to receive active antiviral treatment or placebo. Antiviral therapy consisted of zidovudine, 100 mg PO, five times daily

during the antepartum period. Patients then received intravenous zidovudine during labor, in a loading dose of 2 mg/kg over 1 hour, followed by 1 mg/kg/hr throughout labor. Following delivery, infants in the active treatment group received oral zidovudine, 2 mg/kg every 6 hours, for 6 weeks postpartum. At the first interim data analysis, information was available for 363 infants. The independent safety monitor recommended that the study be discontinued because the frequency of perinatal transmission was 25.5 percent in the placebo arm versus 8.3 percent in the active treatment arm, representing a 67 percent reduction in the risk of vertical transmission ($p = 0.00006$).

The results of this investigation are clearly impressive. However, several questions remain to be answered. First, in this investigation, zidovudine was not administered until the end of the first trimester. Although no harmful fetal effects were noted, the safety of the drug when administered in the first trimester has not been established. Second, all patients in this investigation were asymptomatic and had CD4 counts greater than 200/mm^3. The efficacy of zidovudine may not be as high in a population of women who are more seriously ill. Third, and perhaps most important, the key intervention in this particular trial has not been conclusively identified (i.e., is it the antepartum, intrapartum, or postpartum arm that is of most importance in reducing the risk of perinatal transmission?). Multicenter trials currently are underway to try to determine which part of the treatment protocol is of most importance.

When the physician is caring for the HIV-positive patient intrapartum, every effort must be made to avoid instrumentation that would increase the neonate's exposure to infected maternal blood and secretions. Specifically, whenever feasible, the fetal membranes should be left intact until delivery. In addition, application of the fetal scalp electrode and scalp pH sampling should be avoided. In the postpartum period, the mother should be advised to avoid any contact between her body fluids and an open area on the skin or mucous membranes of the neonate. She also should be cautioned against breast-feeding. Initially, the risk of HIV transmission through breast milk was regarded as low. Recently, however, a report by Dunn et al.[173] called this original assumption into serious question. In this investigation of African women, the authors divided subjects into two groups, those who acquired HIV infection postnatally and those who were infected prenatally. In the former group, 29 percent of breast-fed infants became infected. In the latter group, the added risk of infection from breast-feeding (i.e., above the inherent risk associated with perinatal transmission) was 14 percent. Finally, infected patients should be urged to use secure contraception and adopt responsible sexual practices to prevent spread of infection to their partners.

Parvovirus Infection

Epidemiology

Human parvovirus B19 is a member of the Parvoviridae family. It is a single-stranded DNA virus that codes for only a small number of proteins. Its reproductive capability is limited: therefore, it can only replicate in cells that are dividing rapidly.[174,175] The virus is distributed worldwide, and infection may occur in both a sporadic and an epidemic form. Humans are the only known host for the B19 virus. The organism is transmitted by respiratory droplets and infected blood components, and the incubation period is 4 to 20 days. Serum and respiratory secretions become positive for the virus several days before clinical symptoms develop. Once symptoms appear, respiratory secretions and serum are usually free of the virus.[174,175] Prevalence of antibody to parvovirus increases with age. In children aged 1 to 5 years, approximately 2 to 15 percent are seropositive for antibody. In adolescents and adults the seroprevalence increases to more than 60 percent.[174,175]

Clinical Manifestations

The most common clinical presentation of parvovirus infection is erythema infectiosum or fifth disease. This illness typically occurs in elementary school and day care populations in the late winter and early spring. Patients usually have low-grade fever, malaise, adenopathy, and polyarthritis, affecting the hands, wrists, and knees. In addition, they have a characteristic pruritic, erythematous "slapped cheek" rash on the face and a finely reticulated erythematous rash on the trunk and extremities (Fig. 38-8). The rash may wax and wane over a period of several months in response to stress, exercise, sunlight, or bathing. Erythema infectiosum is a self-limited illness. Complete recovery is the norm, and serious long-term sequelae rarely occur.[174,175]

The second major clinical presentation of parvovirus infection is transient aplastic crisis. This disorder occurs almost exclusively in individuals who have an underlying hemoglobinopathy and results from viral infection of the bone marrow, with resultant destruction of red blood cell precursors. Affected patients have prodromal symptoms similar to erythema infectiosum. One to 7 days after the onset of the prodrome, signs of anemia develop, such as pallor, weakness, and lethargy. Patients with transient aplastic crisis usually do not have a skin rash. Full recovery without sequelae is the usual outcome, provided the patient receives appropriate supportive care.[174,175]

Fetal Infection

The risk that a susceptible mother will acquire infection from an infected household member is 50 to 90 percent.[174–176] The risk of transmission in a day care setting or classroom is lower, ranging from 20 to 30 percent.[176–178] Published information regarding subsequent risk of transmission to the fetus is based on one principal endpoint, namely, fetal hydrops. Hydrops appears to result primarily from viral infection of fetal erythroid stem cells, leading to an aplastic anemia and high output congestive heart failure. Hydrops may also be due, at least in part, to direct infection of the myocardium by the virus.

The reported frequency of fetal hydrops or other adverse outcome following maternal infection has varied from 0 to 38 percent, with most authors citing frequencies in the range of 5 to 15 percent.[174–176,179–181] The risk of fetal infection is greatest when maternal illness occurs in the first trimester, as noted in Table 38-16.[176] Parvovirus does not typically cause a structural defect in the fetus.

Diagnosis of Maternal Infection

Parvovirus can be grown in tissue culture consisting of fresh bone marrow supplemented with erythropoietin. The virus also can be detected by DNA hybridization assays using serum, leukocytes, respiratory secretions, urine, or tissue. In addition, infection can be documented by characteristic histologic changes in infected cells, such as eosinophilic inclusion bodies, marginated chromatin, and direct detection of viral particles by electron microscopy.[174–176]

However, the mainstay of laboratory diagnosis is serologic testing. Antibody to parvovirus can be measured by ELISA, RIA, and Western blot. IgM-specific antibody is usually positive by the third day after symptoms develop. It typically disappears within 30 to 60 days, but may persist for up to 120 days. IgG antibody is detectable by the seventh day of illness and persists for life.[174–176] Table 38-17 summarizes the interpretation of serologic tests for parvovirus.

Diagnosis of Fetal Infection

The most valuable test for diagnosis of fetal parvovirus infection is ultrasound. Severely affected fetuses typically have evidence of hydrops. Since the incubation period of the virus may be longer in the fetus than in the child or adult, the patient should be followed with serial ultrasound examinations for up to 10 weeks after her acute illness. If the fetus shows no signs of hydrops, additional diagnostic studies are unnecessary. If hydropic changes appear and the fetus is at an appropriate gestational age, cordocentesis is indicated (see below).[174–176,182]

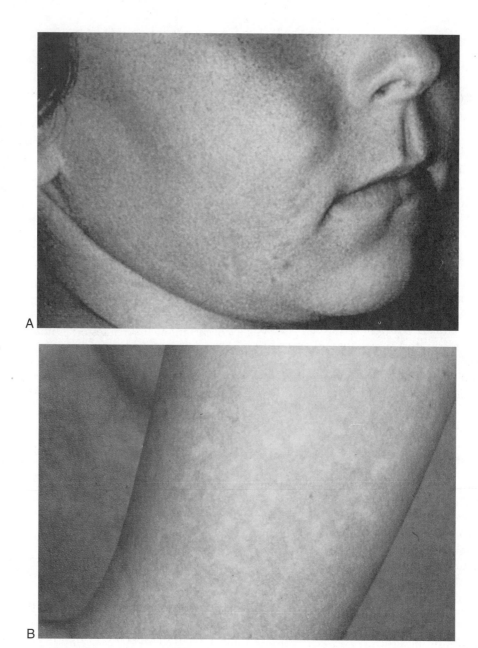

Fig. 38-8 Characteristic "slapped cheek" rash of erythema infectiosum (A). Note lace-like rash on upper extremity (B). (Courtesy of Phillip Mead, M.D., University of Vermont.)

Table 38-16 Association Between Gestational Age at Time of Exposure and Risk of Fetal Parvovirus Infection

Time of Exposure (Weeks' Gestation)	Frequency of Severely Affected Fetuses (%)
1–12	19
13–20	15
>20	6

Table 38-17 Interpretation of Serologic Tests for Maternal Parvovirus Infection

Condition	Maternal Antibody	
	IgM	IgG
Susceptible	−	−
Immune—infection >120 days ago	−	+
Infection within 7 days	+	−
Infection within 7–120 days	+	+

Maternal Management

Following a documented exposure to parvovirus, the mother should immediately have a serologic test to determine if she is immune or susceptible to the virus. If pre-existing IgG antibody is present, the patient can be reassured that second infections are extremely unlikely and that her fetus is not at risk. If the patient is susceptible, she should have a repeat serologic test in approximately 3 weeks to determine if she has seroconverted. If seroconversion is detected, serial ultrasound examinations should be performed over the ensuing 10 weeks to evaluate fetal well-being.

No antiviral agent or vaccine is presently available for treatment of parvovirus infection, but patients with erythema infectiosum rarely need more than simple supportive care. Patients with transient aplastic crisis may require red cell transfusion during the acute phase of their illness. As a general rule, isolation of patients with erythema infectiosum is not of value in reducing transmission of infection since spread by respiratory droplets has already occurred by the time the patient has clear signs of clinical disease. Conversely, if patients with transient aplastic crisis are isolated early in the course of their illness, horizontal transmission to other susceptible individuals may be reduced.[174–176]

Fetal Management

If fetal hydrops is documented by ultrasound, cordocentesis should be performed. Fetal blood should be collected for determination of hematocrit and detection of IgM-specific antibody.[182] Although case reports have described spontaneous resolution of hydrops in infected fetuses, criteria predictive of such a good outcome are not well established.[183,184] Therefore, if severe anemia is present, intrauterine transfusion should be performed.[185,186]

Until recently, most authors had reported normal long-term development in surviving infants. However, in 1993, Conry and coworkers[187] described three children with persistent neurologic morbidity following parvovirus infection that occurred at 21 to 24 weeks' gestation. Neurologic abnormalities included hypotonia, arthrogryposis, motor developmental delay, infantile spasms, intracranial calcifications, and ventriculomegaly. One child died on the sixth day of life. In 1994, Brown et al.[188] described three infants with persistent severe anemia following intrauterine transfusion for parvovirus infection. One of the children died, and autopsy demonstrated widespread viral infection. The other children required regular transfusions. In view of these recent unfavorable reports, clinicians should be cautious in counseling parents regarding the long-term prognosis in affected infants.

Rubella

Epidemiology

Rubella is an RNA virus that is a member of the togavirus family. Only a single serotype is known. The virus has three principal structural proteins: hemagglutinin (E_1), which is located on the surface of the virus; envelope glycoprotein (E_2), also located on the surface of the virus; and the nucleocapsid, located in the interior of the organism.[189]

Rubella occurs primarily in young children and adolescents. The disease is most common in the springtime. Major epidemics of rubella occurred in the United States in 1935 and 1964; minor sporadic epidemics occurred approximately every 7 years until the late 1960s. With licensure of an effective rubella vaccine in 1969, the frequency of this infection has declined by almost 99 percent.[190] In 1992, a new low of 160 cases was reported to the CDC.[191] The persistence of this infection appears to be due to failure to vaccinate susceptible individuals rather than to lack of immunogenicity of the vaccine.

The rubella virus enters the host through the upper respiratory tract. From this site, the virus travels quickly to the cervical lymph nodes and then is disseminated hematogenously throughout the body. The incubation period of the virus is approximately 2 to 3 weeks. The virus is present in blood and nasopharyngeal secretions for several days before appearance of the characteristic rash. The virus also is shed from the nasopharynx for several days after appearance of the exanthem. Therefore, the patient can be contagious for an extended period of time.[189,192]

Antibody against rubella does not normally appear in the serum until after the rash has developed. Acquired immunity to rubella is usually lifelong. Second infections have occurred after both natural primary infections and vaccination. However, recurrent infections generally are not associated with serious illness, viremia, or congenital infection.

Clinical Manifestations

Most children and adults with rubella have mild constitutional symptoms such as malaise, headache, myalgias, and arthralgias. The principal clinical manifestation of this illness, of course, is a widely disseminated, nonpruritic, erythematous, maculopapular rash (Fig. 38-9). Postauricular adenopathy and mild conjunctivitis also are common. These clinical manifestations usually are short lived and typically resolve within 3 to 5 days. The differential diagnosis of rubella includes rubeola, roseola, other viral exanthems, and drug reaction.[189]

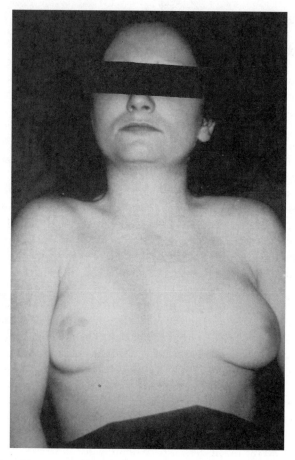

Fig. 38-9 Typical erythematous, maculopapular rash of rubella.

Diagnosis

The diagnosis of rubella can usually be established on the basis of the patient's physical examination. If necessary, serologic tests can be used to confirm the diagnosis. IgM antibody usually reaches a peak 7 to 10 days after the onset of illness and then declines over a period of 4 weeks. The serum concentration of IgG antibody usually rises more slowly, but antibody levels persist throughout the lifetime of the individual. Several different types of antibody detection tests are available, including EIA, indirect immunofluorescence, and latex agglutination. In a recent comparative study, Sautter et al.[193] found that the EIA and latex agglutination tests were the most rapid and convenient methods for screening for antibody to rubella.

Congenital Rubella Syndrome

Because of the success of rubella vaccination campaigns, the incidence of congenital rubella syndrome in the United States has declined dramatically over the past 25 years.[189-191] In 1991, 31 cases of congenital rubella syndrome were reported to the CDC; in 1992,

only five cases were reported.[191] Unfortunately, however, approximately 10 to 20 percent of women in the United States remain susceptible to rubella and, hence, their fetuses are at risk for serious injury should the mother become infected during pregnancy.

The rubella virus crosses the placenta by hematogenous dissemination, and the frequency of congenital infection is critically dependent on the time of exposure to the virus.[189,194,195] Approximately 50 percent of infants exposed to the virus within 4 weeks of conception will manifest signs of congenital infection. When maternal infection occurs in the second 4 week period after conception, approximately 25 percent of fetuses will be infected. When infection develops in the third month, approximately 10 percent of fetuses will be infected. When maternal infection occurs beyond this point in time, less than 1 percent of babies will be infected.

An entire spectrum of anomalies has been associated with congenital rubella syndrome. The four most common abnormalities are deafness (affecting 60 to 75 percent of fetuses), eye defects (10 to 30 percent), central nervous system defects (10 to 25 percent), and cardiac malformations (10 to 20 percent). The most common cardiac abnormality associated with congenital rubella is patent ductus arteriosus, although supravalvular pulmonic stenosis is perhaps the most pathognomonic. Other possible abnormalities include microcephaly, mental retardation, pneumonia, intrauterine growth restriction, hepatosplenomegaly, hemolytic anemia, and thrombocytopenia.[194,195]

A variety of tests have been proposed for the diagnosis of congenital rubella syndrome. Cordocentesis can be performed to determine the total serum IgM concentration in fetal blood and to detect viral-specific antibody. However, fetal immunoglobulin production usually cannot be detected prior to 19 to 22 weeks of gestation. Some authors have proposed chorionic villus sampling (CVS) as a diagnostic test because placental tissue infected with rubella virus produces a cytopathic effect when grown in tissue culture. Viral antigen also can be identified rapidly in tissue culture by RNA-DNA hybridization techniques, and amniotic fluid can be cultured for rubella virus. Unfortunately, although the tests outlined above can demonstrate that rubella virus is present in the fetal compartment, they do not indicate the degree of fetal injury. Accordingly, detailed ultrasound examination is the best test to determine if serious fetal injury has occurred. Abnormalities that can be identified accurately by ultrasound include intrauterine growth restriction, microcephaly, and cardiac malformations.

The prognosis for infants with congenital rubella syndrome is guarded.[194-196] Approximately 50 percent of affected individuals have to attend schools for the hearing impaired. An additional 25 percent of infected children require at least some special schooling because of hearing impairment, and only 25 percent are able to attend mainstream regular schools. Some affected individuals develop insulin-dependent diabetes later in life, presumably secondary to in utero infection of the pancreas. The estimated lifetime cost of caring for a child with congenital rubella syndrome is approximately $200,000 to $300,000.

Obstetric Management

Ideally, women of reproductive age should have a preconception appointment when they are contemplating pregnancy. At this time, they should be evaluated for immunity to rubella. If serologic testing demonstrates that they are susceptible, they should be vaccinated with rubella vaccine prior to conception.[189] When preconception counseling is not possible, all obstetric patients should have a test for rubella at the time of their first prenatal appointment. Women who are susceptible to rubella should be counseled to avoid exposure to other individuals who may have viral exanthems.

If a susceptible patient is subsequently exposed to rubella, serologic tests should be obtained to determine whether acute infection has occurred. If acute infection is documented, patients should be counseled about the risk of congenital rubella syndrome. Obviously, specific counseling should be based on the time in gestation when maternal infection occurred. The diagnostic tests for detection of in utero infection should be reviewed. Patients should be offered the option of pregnancy termination based on the assessed risk of serious fetal injury.[192]

Susceptible patients who are fortunate enough to escape infection during pregnancy should be vaccinated immediately postpartum. The present rubella vaccine is the RA 27/3 preparation. It is much more immunogenic than the earlier HPV-77 and Cendehill vaccines and is available in a monovalent form, bivalent form (measles-rubella, MR), and trivalent form (measles-mumps-rubella, MMR). Approximately 95 percent of patients who receive rubella vaccine seroconvert. Antibody levels persist for at least 18 years in more than 90 percent of vaccinees.

There are few adverse effects of vaccination, even in adults. Less than 25 percent of patients experience mild constitutional symptoms such as low-grade fever and malaise. Less than 10 percent experience arthralgias, and less than 1 percent develop frank arthritis. Interestingly, when the vaccine is administered in the immediate postpartum period, these adverse effects are often delayed for up to 21 days. Women who have received the vaccine cannot transmit infection to susceptible contacts, such as younger children in the home. Breast-feeding is not a contraindication to vaccination.

In addition, the vaccine can be administered in conjunction with other immunoglobulin preparations such as Rh-immune globulin.

Women who receive rubella vaccine should practice secure contraception for a minimum of 3 months after vaccination. For a number of years, the CDC maintained a registry of women who received the rubella vaccine within 3 months of conception. That registry included almost 400 patients, and, fortunately, there were no instances in which congenital rubella syndrome resulted from vaccination.[197] However, there were cases in which women elected to have abortions following vaccination and rubella virus was isolated from the products of the conception. The maximum theoretical risk of congenital rubella resulting from rubella vaccine in early pregnancy is 1 to 2 percent.

Rubeola (Measles)

Virology

The measles virus is a paramyxovirus that is closely related to the canine distemper virus. The organism was first successfully isolated by Enders and Peebles in 1954. The wild virus is pathogenic only for primates, and humans are the only natural host. The organism is a single-stranded RNA virus and is composed of six major structural proteins. Three are complexed with the nucleid acid component of the organism, and three are associated with the envelope (M,H,F). The M protein is part of the inner lipid bilayer of the organism. The H glycoprotein is responsible for adsorption of the virus to receptors on the host cell and for hemagglutination. The F glycoprotein is responsible for fusion between the virus and host cell. The virus is quite labile and is extremely sensitive to acid, proteolytic enzymes, strong light, and drying.[198,199]

Epidemiology

Measles virus is spread primarily by respiratory droplets, and it is highly contagious. Seventy-five to 90 percent of susceptible contacts become infected after exposure. The incubation period is 10 to 14 days. Before a vaccine was available, virtually all children acquired measles. In 1963, however, inactivated and live attenuated vaccines were licensed. The inactivated vaccine was subsequently discontinued in 1967. The current vaccine (Moraten) used in the United States is a further attenuated preparation that was licensed in 1968.[198–200]

Since licensure of the measles vaccine, the reported incidence of measles has decreased by almost 99 percent. As expected, children less than 10 years of age have shown the greatest decline in incidence of measles. During the mid-1980s, almost 60 percent of reported cases of measles affected children greater than 10 years of age compared with only 10 percent during the period 1960 to 1964.[198–200] In recent years, two major types of measles outbreaks have been reported in the United States. One type has occurred among unvaccinated preschoolers, including children less than 15 months of age. Another has occurred among previously vaccinated school age children and college students. Approximately one-third of the cases in the latter type of outbreak have been in individuals who previously were vaccinated. Presumably, these cases result from either *primary failure* to respond to the first vaccine or *secondary failure*, a situation in which an adequate serologic response initially develops but immunity wanes over time.[201,202]

Clinical Manifestations

The clinical manifestations of measles usually appear within 10 to 12 days of exposure. The most common are fever, malaise, coryza, sneezing, conjunctivitis, cough, and photophobia. All patients typically develop a generalized maculopapular rash, and the majority also have Koplik's spots, which are blue-gray specks on a red base that develop on the buccal mucosa opposite the second molars. The skin exanthem typically begins on the face and neck and then spreads to the trunk and extremities. It usually lasts for approximately 5 days and then recedes in the order in which it appeared. The duration of illness is approximately 7 to 10 days. Patients are contagious from 1 to 4 days before the onset of coryza. Immunity to measles should be lifelong following wild virus infection and is mediated by both humoral and cell-mediated mechanisms.

Although measles is typically a minor illness, some patients develop serious sequelae. Otitis media occurs in 7 to 9 percent of infected patients; bronchiolitis and pneumonia affect 1 to 6 percent. A severe form of hepatitis also may occur. In a recent report by Atmar and associates,[203] 7 of 13 (54 percent) pregnant women with measles developed hepatitis.

Encephalitis occurs in approximately 1 in 1,000 cases of measles. It results from both viral infection of the central nervous system and a hypersensitivity reaction to the systemic viral infection. Measles encephalitis may result in permanent neurologic impairment, including mental retardation; the mortality rate from this complication is approximately 15 to 33 percent.[198–200] Another unusual but extremely serious complication of measles is subacute sclerosing panencephalitis (SSPE). This complication occurs in 0.5 to 2 per 1,000 cases. The manifestations of SSPE typically develop approximately 7 years after the acute measles infection. SSPE is more common in children who had measles before the age of 2 years. The disorder is characterized by progressive neurologic debilitation and a virtually uniformly fatal outcome.

A final complication is an unusual condition termed *atypical measles*. This disorder is a severe form of measles reinfection that affects young adults previously vaccinated with the formalin-inactivated killed measles vaccine that was distributed in the United States from 1963 to 1967. Affected patients have extremely high antibody titers to measles. They typically experience high fever, pneumonitis, pleural effusion, and a coarse, maculopapular, hemorrhagic, or urticarial rash. Although the disease is usually self-limited, atypical measles can lead to hepatic, cardiac, and renal failure. Interestingly, affected patients are not contagious to others. The risk of perinatal transmission with atypical measles has not been defined precisely.[199]

Diagnosis

Five clinical criteria should be present to establish the diagnosis of measles: fever of 38.3°C or higher, characteristic rash lasting longer than 3 days, cough, coryza, and conjunctivitis.[2] Although the virus can be cultured, the mainstay of diagnostic tests is detection of antibody to measles. Four types of antibody assays are presently available.[198–201] The advantages and disadvantages of each assay are summarized in Table 38-18. The confirmation of acute measles virus infection is based on detection of IgM-specific antibody or a fourfold change in the IgG titer in acute and convalescent sera. The acute titer for IgG antibody should be obtained within 3 days of the onset of the rash and the convalescent titer, 10 to 20 days later.

The differential diagnosis of measles can be difficult. A variety of other infections must be considered, includ-

Table 38-18   Serologic Tests for Detection of Antibody to Rubeola (Measles) Virus

Test	Remarks
Neutralizing antibody	Sensitive test, but requires propagation of the virus in vitro. Therefore, the assay is infrequently used
Complement fixing (CF) antibody	Relatively insensitive. Adequate for diagnosis of acute measles infection. Not useful for determining immune status
Hemaglutination inhibition (HI) antibody	Sensitive. Easy to perform. Useful for diagnosis of acute infection and for determination of immune status
Enzyme linked immunosorbent assay (ELISA)	Sensitive and easier to perform than HI assay

ing rubella, scarlet fever, Rocky Mountain spotted fever, toxoplasmosis, enterovirus infection, mononucleosis, meningococcemia, and serum sickness.

Complications of Measles During Pregnancy

Several reports have described an increase in maternal mortality associated with measles infection during pregnancy. Most fatalities have been due to pulmonary complications. In one of the earliest reports, Christensen et al.[204] described a serious epidemic of measles in Greenland in 1951. Four of 83 pregnant women (4.8 percent) who developed measles died. An unspecified number of these women also had active tuberculosis. In the report by Atmar et al.,[203] 1 of 13 pregnant women (8 percent) with measles died because of severe respiratory infection. In another recent report, Eberhart-Phillips and coworkers[205] evaluated 58 pregnant women with measles. Thirty-five (60 percent) required hospitalization. Fifteen (26 percent) developed pneumonia, and two (3 percent) died.

Early reports described a slight increase in the frequency of preterm delivery and spontaneous abortion when women developed measles during pregnancy. In the report by Eberhart-Phillips et al.,[205] 13 of 50 (26 percent) women with continuing pregnancies delivered preterm. The frequency of congenital anomalies is not significantly increased in women who have measles during pregnancy, although Ekbom and associates[206] recently reported a possible association between perinatal measles infection and subsequent Crohn's disease.

Infants of mothers who are acutely infected at the time of delivery are at risk for neonatal measles. This infection typically develops within the first 10 days of life and results from transplacental viral dissemination. In some reports, the mortality in preterm and term infants with neonatal measles has been as high as 60 and 20 percent, respectively.[198–201,203,205,207] Of importance is the fact that these alarmingly high mortality figures were published prior to the era of skilled NICU care and the availability of broad spectrum antibiotics for treatment of secondary bacterial infectious.

Management of Measles During Pregnancy

Pregnant women with measles should be observed carefully for evidence of serious complications such as otitis media, hepatitis, encephalitis, and pneumonia. Secondary bacterial infections should be treated promptly with antibiotics. Administration of aerosolized ribavirin may be of benefit to patients with severe viral pneumonitis.[203] The affected patient should be counseled that the risk of injury to her fetus is very low. Probably the most effective method for evaluating the fetus for in utero infection is detailed ultrasound examination. Findings suggestive of in utero infection include microcephaly, growth restriction, and oligohydramnios. Neonates delivered to a mother who has developed measles within 7 to 10 days of delivery should receive intramuscular immunoglobulin in a dose of 0.25 mg/kg. These infants should subsequently receive the live measles vaccine when they are 15 months of age.[199,201]

Prevention of Infection

All children should receive measles vaccine when they are 15 months of age. The immunization should be administered as part of the trivalent measles-mumps-rubella (MMR) vaccine. The appropriate initial dose for young children is 0.5 ml subcutaneously. The original public health recommendations provided for only a single dose of measles vaccine. However, as noted previously, recent outbreaks of measles have occurred in individuals who received only one dose of the vaccine. Accordingly, the CDC now recommends that all individuals who have not been infected with the wild measles virus receive a second dose of vaccine. Children who receive their first dose at age 15 months should receive a second dose at 4 to 6 years of age. Children who are vaccinated with the live vaccine before their first birthday should be considered unvaccinated and should receive the full two-dose series. Individuals who received "further attenuated vaccine," accompanied by immunoglobulin or measles immunoglobulin, should be considered unvaccinated and receive two doses of the vaccine. Individuals who were given the inactivated vaccine during the period 1963 to 1967 are at risk for developing severe atypical measles syndrome if they are exposed to the natural virus. Accordingly, these individuals also should receive two doses of the live vaccine. Women of reproductive age who have only one documented measles vaccination also are candidates for a second immunization. The seroconversion rate with the new live virus vaccine is at least 95 percent.[199,201]

There are three specific contraindications to vaccination: pregnancy, severe febrile illness, and history of anaphylaxis to egg protein or neomycin. The vaccine should not be given for 3 months after a person has received immunoglobulin, whole blood, or other antibody-containing blood products. However, the vaccine can be administered concurrently with Rh-immune globulin in the immediate postpartum period. Although no cases of congenital infection have been described as a result of the measles vaccine, patients receiving the vaccine should practice effective contraception for 3 months following inoculation.[199,201]

Very few adverse effects are associated with measles vaccination. Approximately 5 to 15 percent of vaccinees develop a low grade fever. Five percent or less develop a rash. Less than 1 percent have febrile seizures, and less than 1 per 1 millon cases develops encephalitis.

When an outbreak of measles does occur, susceptible individuals should be targeted for postexposure prophylaxis. If they are not pregnant, they should receive the live measles vaccine within 72 hours of exposure. They also should receive immunoglobulin within 6 days of exposure. The appropriate dose of immunoglobulin is 0.25 ml/kg for immunocompetent patients and 0.5 ml/kg for immunocompromised individuals. The maximum dose of the immunoglobulin preparation is 15 ml. Pregnant patients should receive only immunoglobulin.[199,201]

Syphilis

Epidemiology

Syphilis is caused by the spirochete, *Treponema pallidum*. Infection occurs primarily as a result of sexual contact. The organism penetrates mucosal barriers and is highly contagious. Infection develops in 10 percent of contacts after a single exposure and in 70 percent after multiple exposures.[208,209] Syphilis also may be transmitted perinatally, with devastating consequences for the fetus.

The prevalence of syphilis in the United States has increased dramatically in recent years, coincident with the upsurge in cases of HIV infection and the growing epidemic of drug abuse. The greatest increase has been in females, aged 15 to 24 years, and a disproportionate number of cases have occurred in blacks and Hispanics living in urban areas.[208,209]

Clinical Manifestations and Staging

Syphilis can be divided into four *clinical* categories: primary, secondary, tertiary, and neurosyphilis. In addition, syphilis can present as a latent infection. Latent syphilis is subdivided into early latent (<1 year duration) and late latent (>1 year) infection.[208–210] The incubation period of syphilis ranges from 10 to 90 days. At the end of this period, the characteristic raised, painless chancre appears. In women, the chancre is usually on the cervix or vaginal wall and may not be apparent except on close inspection (Fig. 38-10). In some patients, the chancre may be present in extragenital sites such as the fingers, oropharynx, nipples, or anus. The chancre usually heals in 3 to 6 weeks even without specific antimicrobial treatment. The principal disorders that must be considered in the differential diagnosis of primary syphilis are HSV infection, chancroid, trauma, scabies, Behcet syndrome, Stevens Johnson syndrome, and carcinoma.

Patients who receive either no treatment or inadequate treatment may develop secondary syphilis 2 to 6 months after their primary infection. The principal clinical manifestation of this stage of the infection is a generalized maculopapular rash that is most obvious on the palms of the hands and soles of the feet (Fig. 38-11). This rash may be confused with disseminated gonococcal infection, measles, rubella, scabies, psoriasis, and drug eruption. Other findings associated with secondary syphilis include mucous patches (Fig. 38-12), of the oropharynx and condylomata lata which

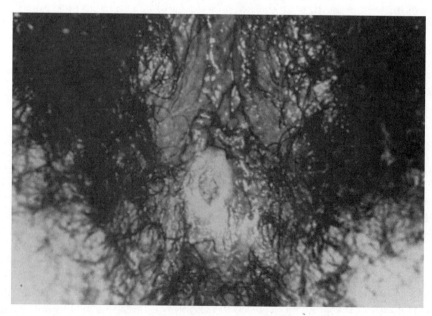

Fig. 38-10 Painless chancre characteristic of primary syphilis. (From Duff et al.,[229] with permission.)

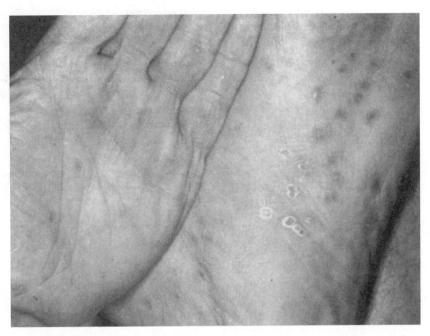

Fig. 38-11 Maculopapular rash characteristic of secondary syphilis. (From Duff et al.,[229] with permission.)

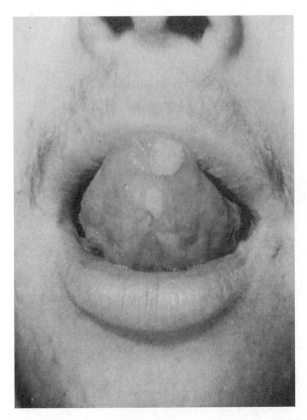

Fig. 38-12 Mucous patch, characteristic of secondary syphilis. (From Duff et al.,[229] with permission.)

are gray, raised papules that appear on the vulva and near the anus. In addition, bone tenderness, iritis, alopecia, and generalized lymphadenopathy also may be present. The lesions of secondary syphilis usually resolve spontaneously in 3 to 6 weeks, even without treatment. Untreated patients then enter a latent phase of their illness. In this phase, infected women pose only a small risk of horizontal transmission of infection to their sexual partner. However, vertical transmission to the fetus still can occur.[208–210]

Approximately one-third of patients with untreated secondary disease ultimately develop tertiary syphilis after an interval of several years. Tertiary syphilis is distinguished by three principal findings: gumma formation, cardiac lesions, and central nervous system abnormalities (neurosyphilis). The characteristic cardiac lesions are aortic insufficiency and dissecting aortic aneurysm. Neurologic manifestations include meningovascular syphilis, cranial nerve palsies, generalized paresis, tabes dorsalis, optic atrophy, uveitis, and Argyll-Robertson pupils. Four to 9 percent of patients with untreated syphilis ultimately develop neurosyphilis. In some individuals, particularly those with concurrent HIV infection, neurologic manifestations may occur early in the course of syphilis and can cause severe morbidity.[208–210]

Diagnosis

T. pallidum cannot be cultured. It can be identified from overt lesions such as the chancre by darkfield microscopy and fluorescent antibody staining. However, most

Table 38-19   Frequency of Vertical Transmission of Syphilis

Stage of Maternal Infection	Approximate Frequency of Congenital Syphilis (%)
Primary	50
Secondary	50
Early latent	40
Late latent	10
Tertiary	10

cases of infection, particularly those in the latent stage, are diagnosed by serology. The initial screening test for syphilis should be a nontreponemal assay such as the Venereal Disease Research Laboratory test (VDRL) or Rapid Plasma Reagin (RPR) test. Several factors can cause biologically false-positive test results such as collagen vascular disease, bacterial and viral infections, multiple myeloma, advanced cancer, chronic liver disease, intravenous drug use, multiple blood transfusions, and pregnancy. Accordingly, a positive screening test must be confirmed by a specific treponemal assay such as the fluorescent treponemal antibody absorption test (FTA-ABS) or microhemagglutination assay (MHA-TP). Biologic false-positive treponemal tests have been reported in patients with Lyme disease, leprosy, malaria, mononucleosis, and collagen vascular disease.

Lumbar puncture is indicated when neurosyphilis is suspected and in all patients who are coinfected with syphilis and HIV. Cerebrospinal fluid abnormalities include a mononuclear pleocytosis (10 to 400 cells/mm^3), elevated protein (>45 mg/dl), and a positive VDRL test.[208-210]

Virtually 100 percent of patients will have a positive serologic test within 4 weeks of their primary infection. With appropriate antibiotic treatment, quantitative nontreponemal tests usually decrease fourfold within 3 months in patients with primary or secondary syphilis. When this decline does not occur, patients should be re-evaluated and considered for a second course of treatment. Antibody titers may decline more slowly in patients with more advanced stages of disease. Specific treponemal tests typically remain positive for life even after adequate treatment, although 13 to 24 percent of patients may ultimately become seronegative.[208-210] Ideally, patients should be followed with quantitative titers for up to 12 to 18 months after their initial infection to determine if they become seronegative.

Perinatal Complications

Syphilis in pregnancy may be associated with an increased risk of fetal demise, intrauterine growth restriction, and preterm delivery.[211] It also may accelerate the course of HIV infection in pregnant women. However, the most frequent, and potentially ominous, complication of syphilis in pregnancy is congenital infection. *T. pallidum* can cross the placenta and infect the fetus *at any stage of gestation*. Up to one-third of fetuses with congenital syphilis are stillborn.[4] The frequency of vertical transmission varies primarily with the stage of maternal disease, as noted in Table 38-19. The many possible clinical manifestations of congenital syphilis are summarized in Table 38-20 and illustrated in Figures 38-13 and 38-14.

T. pallidum has been recovered from fetal blood and amniotic fluid in cases of congenital infection.[212] However, the prenatal diagnostic test with the greatest po-

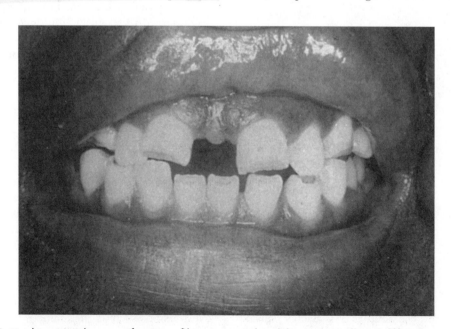

Fig. 38-13 Hutchinson teeth, a manifestation of late congenital syphilis. (From Duff et al.,[229] with permission.)

Table 38-20 Clinical Manifestations of Congenital Syphilis

Early	Late
Maculopapular rash	Hutchinson teeth
Snuffles (syphilitic rhinitis)	Mulberry molars
Mucous patches	Interstitial keratitis
Hepatosplenomegaly	Deafness
Jaundice	Saddle nose
Pneumonia	Rhagades
Lymphadenopathy	Saber shins
Osteochondritis	Mental retardation
Chorioretinitis	Hydrocephalus
Iritis	Generalized paresis
	Optic nerve atrophy
	Clutton joints (hydrarthosis)

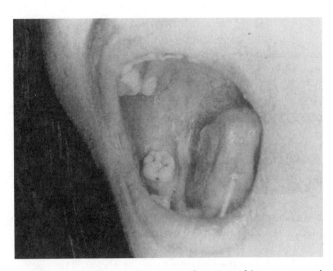

Fig. 38-14 Mulberry molar, a manifestation of late congenital syphilis. (From Duff et al.,[229] with permission.)

tential for identifying the severely infected fetus is ultrasound. Ultrasound findings suggestive of in utero infection include placentomegaly, intrauterine growth restriction, microcephaly, hepatosplenomegaly, and hydrops.

Treatment

The treatment of syphilis in pregnancy is summarized in Table 38-21.[208–210] Clearly, penicillin is the drug of choice for this infection because of its proven ability to prevent congenital infection in most cases. Patients who have a previous history of an allergic reaction to penicillin should be skin tested to determine if their allergy persists.[208–210] In point of fact, only approximately 10 percent of patients who report a history of severe allergy to penicillin remain allergic throughout life. They can be reliably identified by testing with major and minor penicillin determinants. If allergy is confirmed,

patients should be desensitized with either oral or intravenous regimens.[206,210,213] Desensitization can usually be completed within 4 hours. It is best accomplished in consultation with an allergist and performed in an area of the hospital with immediate access to emergency resuscitative equipment. A simple regimen for densitization is outlined by Ziaya et al.[213] Alternative antibiotic regimens are not of proven value for prevention of congenital syphilis or treatment of advanced stages of disease. Accordingly, they should be used only if desensitization is unsuccessful.

Pregnant women receiving penicillin for treatment of syphilis may develop uterine contractions and decreased fetal movement as a result of a Jarisch-Herxheimer reaction. In a recent report, Klein and coworkers[214] observed this reaction in 15 of 33 women (45

Table 38-21 Recommendations for Treatment of Syphilis in Pregnancy

Stage of Disease	Principal Treatment	Alternate Treatment if Allergic to Penicillin[a]
Primary, secondary, or latent syphilis <1 year's duration	Benzathine penicillin G, 2.4 million units IM × 1[b]	Erythromycin, 500 ng PO QID × 15 days; ceftriaxone, 250 mg IM QD × 10 days
Latent syphilis >1 year's duration or cardiovascular syphilis	Benzathine penicillin G, 2.4 million units IM weekly × 3	Erythromycin, 500 mg QID × 30 days
Neurosyphilis	Aqueous crystalline penicillin G, 2–4 million units Q4h × 10–14 days, followed by benzathine penicillin G, 2.4 million units IM × 1	No regimen of proven value other than penicillin
	Aqueous procaine penicillin G, 2.4 million units IM daily with probenecid, 500 mg PO QID, both for 10–14 days, followed by benzathine penicillin G, 2.4 million units IM × 1	

[a] These regimens should be administered only if desensitization to penicillin is unsuccessful.
[b] In patients who are concurrently infected with HIV, treat as outlined below for late latent or tertiary syphilis. Patients also should have a lumbar puncture to determine if neurosyphilis is present.

percent). The reaction was particularly likely in those patients who had primary and secondary syphilis, and the abnormalities typically appeared 2 to 8 hours after treatment and resolved within 24 hours. There are no reliable clinical or laboratory assessments that predict which patients will develop the Jarisch-Herxheimer reaction, and no specific treatment is available.

Toxoplasmosis

Epidemiology

Toxoplasma gondii is a protozoan that has three distinct forms: trophozoite, cyst, and oocyst (Fig. 38-15). The life cycle of *T. gondii* is dependent on wild and domestic cats, which are the only host for the oocyst. The oocyst is formed in the cat intestine and subsequently excreted in the feces. Mammals, such as cows, then ingest the oocyst, which is disrupted in the animal's intestine, releasing the invasive trophozoite. The trophozoite then is disseminated throughout the body, ultimately forming cysts in brain and muscle.

Human infection occurs when infected meat is ingested or when food is contaminated by cat feces (e.g., via flies, cockroaches, or fingers). Infection rates are highest in areas of poor sanitation and crowded living conditions. Stray cats and domestic cats that eat raw meat are most likely to carry the parasite. The cyst is destroyed by heat, and the practice of eating rare or raw meat in France may explain the high prevalence of infection in that country.[215]

Approximately 40 to 50 percent of adults in the United States have antibody to this organism, and the

prevalence of antibody is highest in lower socioeconomic populations. The frequency of seroconversion during pregnancy is 5 percent or less, and approximately 3:1,000 infants show evidence of congenital infection. Clinically significant congenital toxoplasmosis occurs in approximately 1:8,000 pregnancies. Toxoplasmosis is more common in Western Europe, particularly France. More than 80 percent of women of childbearing age in Paris have antibody to *T. gondii*, and congenital toxoplasmosis is about twice as frequent there as in the United States.[215,216]

Clinical Manifestations

The ingested organism invades across the intestinal epithelium and spreads hematogenously throughout the body. Intracellular replication leads to cell destruction. Clinical manifestations of infection are the result of direct organ damage and the subsequent immunologic response to parasitemia and cell death. Host immunity is mediated primarily through T lymphocytes.

Most infections in humans are asymptomatic. Even in the absence of symptoms, however, patients may have evidence of multiorgan involvement, and clinical disease can follow a long period of asymptomatic infection. Symptomatic toxoplasmosis usually presents as an illness similar to mononucleosis.[215,216]

In contrast to infection in the immunocompetent host, toxoplasmosis can be a devastating infection in the immunosuppressed patient. Because immunity to *T. gondii* is cell mediated, patients with HIV infection and those treated with chronic immunosuppressive therapy after organ transplantation are particularly susceptible to new or reactivated infection. In these patients, central nervous system dysfunction is the most common manifestation of infection. Findings typically include encephalitis, meningoencephalitis, and intracerebral mass lesions. Pneumonitis, myocarditis, and generalized lymphadenopathy also commonly occur.[215,216]

Diagnosis

The diagnosis of toxoplasmosis can be confirmed by serologic and histologic methods. Serologic tests that suggest an acute infection include detection of IgM-specific antibody, demonstration of an extremely high IgG antibody titer, and documentation of IgG seroconversion from negative to positive.[215,216] Clinicians should be aware that serologic assays for toxoplasmosis are not well standardized. When initial laboratory tests appear to indicate that an acute infection has occurred, repeat serology should be performed in a well-recognized reference laboratory.

The best tissue for identification of *T. gondii* is a lymph node or brain biopsy specimen. Histologic

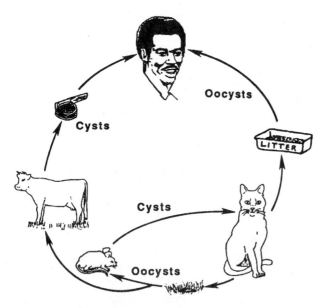

Fig. 38-15 Life cycle of *Toxoplasma gondii*. (From Duff et al.,[229] with permission.)

preparations can be examined by light and electron microscopy. For light microscopy, specimens should be stained with either Giemsa or Wright stain.[215–218]

Congenital Toxoplasmosis

Congenital infection can occur if a woman develops *acute* toxoplasmosis during pregnancy. Chronic or latent infection is unlikely to cause fetal injury except perhaps in an immunosuppressed patient. Approximately 40 percent of neonates born to mothers with acute toxoplasmosis show evidence of infection. Congenital infection is most likely to occur when maternal infection develops in the third trimester. Less than half of affected infants are symptomatic at birth. The clinical manifestations of congenital toxoplasmosis are quite varied and are summarized below.[216–218]

The most valuable tests for antenatal diagnosis of congenital toxoplasmosis are ultrasound, cordocentesis, and amniocentesis. Ultrasound findings suggestive of infection include ventriculomegaly, intracranial calcifications, microcephaly, ascites, hepatosplenomegaly, and growth restriction. Fetal blood samples can be tested for IgM-specific antibody after 20 weeks' gestation. Fetal blood and amniotic fluid can be inoculated into mice, and the organism can subsequently be recovered from the blood of infected animals. In addition, Hohlfeld et al.[219] have now identified a specific gene of *T. gondii* in amniotic fluid using a polymerase chain reaction test. In their investigation, 34 of 339 infants had congenital toxoplasmosis confirmed by serologic testing or autopsy. All amniotic fluid samples from affected pregnancies were positive by polymerase chain reaction. Test results were available within 1 day of specimen collection.

Clinical Manifestations of Congenital Toxoplasmosis

Rash

Hepatosplenomegaly

Ascites

Fever

Chorioretinitis

Periventricular calcifications

Ventriculomegaly

Seizures

Mental retardation

Uveitis

Management

Toxoplasmosis in the immunocompetent adult is usually an asymptomatic or self-limited illness and does not require treatment. Immunocompromised patients, however, should be treated, and the regimen of choice is a combination of oral sulfadiazine (4 g loading dose, then 1 g four times daily) plus pyrimethamine (50 to 100 mg initially, then 25 mg daily). In such patients, extended courses of treatment may be necessary to cure the infection.

Treatment also is indicated when acute toxoplasmosis occurs during pregnancy. Treatment of the mother clearly has been shown to reduce the risk of congenital infection and decrease the late sequelae of infection.[217,218] Pyrimethamine is not recommended for use during the first trimester of pregnancy because of possible teratogenicity. Sulfonamides can be used alone, but single agent therapy appears to be less effective than combination therapy. In Europe, spiramycin, a macrolide antibiotic, has been used extensively in pregnancy with excellent success.[217,218] It is available for use in the United States through the CDC.

Aggressive early treatment of infants with congenital toxoplasmosis is indicated and consists of combination therapy with pyrimethamine, sulfadiazine, and leucovorin for 1 year.[220] Early treatment reduces, but does not eliminate, the late sequelae of toxoplasmosis such as chorioretinitis.

In the management of the pregnant patient, *prevention* of acute toxoplasmosis is of paramount importance. Pregnant women should be advised to avoid contact with stray cats or cat litter. They should always wash their hands after preparing meat for cooking and should never eat raw or rare meat. Fruits and vegetables also should be washed carefully to remove possible contamination by oocysts.

Varicella

Epidemiology

The varicella-zoster virus (VZV) is a DNA organism, which is a member of the herpes virus family. Humans are the only known source of infection. Natural varicella infection occurs primarily during early childhood. Less than 10 percent of cases occur in individuals over 10 years of age; however, older patients account for more than 50 percent of all fatalities due to varicella. Varicella is transmitted by direct contact and respiratory droplets. The virus is highly infectious, and approximately 95 percent of susceptible household contacts become infected following exposure. The incubation period is 10 to 14 days. Patients are infectious from 1 day before the outbreak of the rash until all of the cutaneous lesions have dried and crusted over. Immunity to varicella is usually lifelong.[221]

Herpes zoster infection occurs as a result of reactivation of latent virus infection in a patient who already has had varicella. Because of the presence in the host of viral-specific antibody, herpes zoster is usually a much less serious disorder than varicella and rarely poses a major risk to either the mother or her baby unless the former is immunocompromised. However, susceptible patients may develop acute varicella when exposed to individuals with herpes zoster, and, therefore, they must be counseled appropriately about this risk.[221]

Clinical Manifestations

The usual clinical manifestations of varicella are fever, malaise, and a skin rash. The characteristic skin lesions usually begin as pruritic macules, which appear in crops. The macules progress to papules, then to vesicles, and finally to crusts. The lesions initially appear on the trunk and then spread centripetally to the extremities.

In immunocompetent children serious complications of varicella are exceedingly rare. However, in adults, two life-threatening sequelae may develop: encephalitis and pneumonia. The former occurs in 1 percent or less of pregnant women; the latter may develop in up to 20 percent of patients. Prior to the development of acyclovir, the mortality associated with varicella pneumonia in pregnancy approached 40 percent.[221,222]

Diagnosis

The diagnosis of varicella is usually made by clinical examination alone. In problematic cases, the virus can be isolated in tissue culture, and cytologic preparations may show multinucleated giant cells and eosinophilic intranuclear inclusions. Serologic assays are of primary value in assessing a patient's susceptibility to varicella immediately following exposure. The two most useful antibody assays are the fluorescent antimembrane antibody test (FAMA) and the ELISA. Both assays show sustained elevations, usually lifelong, following natural infection.[221,223]

Management of Maternal Infection

The optimal approach to maternal varicella infection is *prevention*. All women of reproductive age should be assessed for immunity to varicella, ideally before they attempt pregnancy. Susceptible patients, particularly those who are likely to be exposed to varicella either at home or in the workplace, should be offered the new varicella vaccine. Varivax (Merck) is a live attenuated

vaccine and is highly immunogenic, and it is approximately 70 to 80 percent effective in protecting the patient against natural infection. Individuals older than 12 years should receive two subcutaneous doses of the vaccine, 4 to 8 weeks apart. Vaccine recipients should use effective contraception for 3 months after immunization. The vaccine can be administered simultaneously with the MMR immunization, but it should not be given in conjunction with blood or blood products. In addition, the vaccine is contraindicated in patients who are pregnant, who have immunodeficiency disorders, or who have received high-dose systemic steroids within 30 days of vaccination.[224]

If the patient first presents for medical care when she is pregnant, she should be questioned about varicella immunity at the time of her first prenatal appointment. If she is uncertain about prior infection, an IgG varicella serology should be performed. If the serology is positive, the patient can be reassured that she is immune and that she and her fetus are not at risk should subsequent exposure occur. If the serology is negative, the patient should be counseled to avoid exposure to individuals who may have varicella or herpes zoster.

Unfortunately, however, the more common situation that the obstetrician encounters is a pregnant patient who has been exposed acutely to an individual who "may have had chickenpox." The clinician's first step in the approach to this situation is to verify that the index patient actually has varicella. If infection is confirmed, the pregnant woman should then be questioned about immunity to varicella. If immunity cannot be documented by history, an IgG varicella serology should be obtained, and the result should be reviewed within 24 to 48 hours of exposure. If the serology is positive, the patient can be reassured that her fetus is not at risk. If the serology is negative, the patient should receive varicella-zoster immunoglobulin (VZIG). This preparation is 60 to 80 percent effective in preventing infection if given within 96 hours of exposure. The dose of VZIG is one vial (125 units) per 10 kg of actual body weight, up to a maximum of five vials. In problematic cases, if waiting for the varicella serology will delay administration of VZIG for more than 96 hours after exposure, the immunization should be given without confirmatory serology.[221,225,226]

Patients who receive VZIG, as well as those who present for care too late for passive immunoprophylaxis, should be counseled about the clinical signs and symptoms of varicella. In particular, they must be advised to report immediately if early manifestations of varicella encephalitis or pneumonia develop. If serious sequelae occur, the patient should be admitted to the hospital for intravenous therapy with acyclovir. The recommended dose of acyclovir is 500 mg/m^2 every 8 hours, and treatment should be continued until the patient's systemic symptoms have resolved and the cutaneous lesions have begun to crust. Immunocompromised patients should be treated with acyclovir immediately at the onset of clinical illness because they are at such increased risk for serious complications.[221,222]

Congenital Infection

Congenital varicella results primarily from hematogenous dissemination of virus across the placenta. Ascending infection following rupture of membranes is possible but extremely unlikely. Congenital infection may lead to spontaneous abortion, intrauterine fetal demise, and varicella embryopathy. The latter disorder is manifested by multiple abnormalities such as cutaneous scars, limb hypoplasia, muscle atrophy, malformed digits, psychomotor retardation, microcephaly, cortical atrophy, cataracts, chorioretinitis, and microophthalmia.[221]

Fortunately, two recent investigations have demonstrated a relatively low frequency of anomalies even following exposure in the first half of pregnancy. Pastuszak et al.[227] reported a study of 106 women with varicella in the first 20 weeks of gestation. The frequency of varicella embryopathy was 1.2 percent, and the prevalence of preterm birth was 14 percent. Subsequently, Enders and coworkers[228] published the largest prospective study of varicella in pregnancy. They observed a 2 percent incidence of congenital infection when maternal varicella occurred at 13 to 20 weeks' gestation. The frequency of congenital infection was only 0.4 percent when maternal infection occurred before 13 weeks' gestation.

The presence of varicella virus in the fetal compartment can be identified by detection of viral-specific IgM antibody and elevated total IgM antibody in cord blood. Virus also can be cultured in amniotic fluid and identified by polymerase chain reaction in placental tissue. Unfortunately, identification of viral DNA, viral-specific antibody, or even the virus itself does not accurately predict the degree of fetal injury. For this purpose ultrasonography is the preferred diagnostic modality. Sonographic findings suggestive of fetal varicella include polyhydramnios; hydrops; hyperechogenic foci in the abdominal organs, particularly the liver; cardiac malformations; limb deformities; microcephaly; and intrauterine growth restriction.[221]

Neonatal Infection

The final major complication of varicella infection in pregnancy is neonatal varicella. Infection of the neonate occurs in 10 to 20 percent of infants whose mothers have acute varicella within the period from 5 days before to 2 days after delivery.[221] Infection usually results from hematogenous dissemination of virus across the placenta at a time when no maternal antibody is present to provide passive immunity to the fetus. Less commonly, neonatal varicella results from postnatal exposure to the mother or another infected person.

The clinical course of neonatal varicella can be variable in progression and severity. The infant usually becomes symptomatic within 5 to 10 days of delivery. Some neonates have only scattered skin lesions and no systemic signs of illness. Others have a biphasic course, initially presenting with a cluster of skin lesions, followed by more widespread dissemination. Still others have a more severe acute illness associated with extensive cutaneous lesions and visceral infection. The most common life-threatening complication is pneumonia. In reports published before the widespread availability of acyclovir, the mortality associated with neonatal varicella was 20 to 30 percent.[221]

To prevent neonatal varicella, an effort should be made to delay delivery until 5 to 7 days after the onset of maternal illness. If delay is not possible, the neonate should receive VZIG (one vial, 125 units) immediately after birth. An important additional preventive measure is isolation of the infant from the mother until all vesicular lesions likely to come in contact with the infant have crusted over.[221,226]

Occasionally herpes zoster is present in the newborn. This condition is usually a manifestation of intrauterine varicella that occurs in the second half of pregnancy. The clinical course is typically benign, but, in rare instances, encephalitis has been documented.

Key Points

- Vaginal infections occur commonly in pregnancy. Moniliasis is best treated with topical antifungal compounds such as miconazole, terconazole, or chlortrimazole. Metronidazole is the only antibiotic with uniform efficacy against trichomonas. Clindamycin and metronidazole, administered either orally or topically, are effective for treatment of bacterial vaginosis.

- Urinary tract infections in pregnancy are caused primarily by *E. coli*, *K. pneumoniae*, and *Proteus* species. Pyelonephritis is a particularly serious infection in pregnancy because it may be complicated by preterm labor, bacteremia, and ARDS.

- Chorioamnionitis and puerperal endometritis are caused by multiple aerobic and anaerobic organisms. Antibiotic therapy should be directed against group B streptococci, aerobic gram-negative bacilli, and *Bacteroides* and *Prevotella* species.

- Primary maternal CMV infection during pregnancy is associated with a 40 percent risk of fetal infection. Ten to 15 percent of infected infants are severely affected at birth. Ultrasonography and amniotic fluid viral culture are the best methods for diagnosing fetal infection.

- All pregnant women should be screened for hepatitis B infections. Infants delivered to seropositive mothers should receive both HBIG and HBV shortly after birth.

- HSV infection may be classified as *primary*, *initial*, *nonprimary*, and *recurrent*. *Primary infection* poses the major risk of perinatal transmission. Women with prodromal symptoms or visible lesions should be delivered by cesarean; asymptomatic women may deliver vaginally.

- All pregnant women should be screened for HIV infection. Prophylactic treatment of seropositive women with zidovudine significantly reduces the risk of perinatal transmission of infection.

- Maternal parvovirus infection may result in fetal hydrops. Intrauterine transfusion may be a lifesaving intervention for the hydropic fetus.

- Primary maternal toxoplasmosis poses a serious risk of fetal infection. Fetal infection is best diagnosed by DNA analysis of amniotic fluid. Spiramycin is effective in treating both maternal and fetal infection.

- Varicella in pregnancy presents serious risk to both the mother and her infant. Susceptible women exposed to varicella should be treated with VZIG. Neonates delivered to mothers with acute varicella also should receive immunoprophylaxis with VZIG. Following delivery, susceptible women should be vaccinated with the new live virus vaccine, provided they are willing to use effective contraception for 3 months.

References

1. Eschenbach DA, Hillier S, Critchlow C et al: Diagnosis and clinical manifestations of bacterial vaginosis. Am J Obstet Gynecol 158:819, 1988
2. Gravett MG, Hummel D, Eschanbach DA, Holmes KK: Preterm labor associated with subclinical amniotic fluid infection and with bacterial vaginosis. Obstet Gynecol 67:229, 1986
3. Martius J, Krohn MA, Hillier SL et al: Relationships of vaginal *Lactobacillus* species, cervical *Chlamydia trachomatis*, and bacterial vaginosis to preterm birth. Obstet Gynecol 71:89, 1988
4. Clark P, Kurtzer TA, Duff P: The role of bacterial vaginosis in peripartum infections. Infect Dis Obstet Gynecol 2:179, 1994
5. Thomasen JL, Gelbart SM, Anderson RJ et al: Statistical evaluation of diagnostic criteria for bacterial vaginosis. Am J Obstet Gynecol 162:155, 1990
6. Greaves WL, Chungafung J, Morris B et al: Clindamycin versus metronidazole in the treatment of bacterial vaginosis. Obstet Gynecol 72:799, 1988
7. Hillier S, Krohn MA, Watts H et al: Microbiologic efficacy of intravaginal clindamycin cream for the treatment of bacterial vaginosis. Obstet Gynecol 76:407, 1990
8. Hillier SL, Lipinski C, Briselden AM, Eschenbach DA: Efficacy of intravaginal 0.75% metronidazole gel for the treatment of bacterial vaginosis. Obstet Gynecol 81:963, 1993
9. Friedrich EG: Vaginitis. Am J Obstet Gynecol. 152:247, 1985
10. American College of Obstetrics and Gynecologists: Vulvovaginitis. ACOG Tech. Bull. No. 135, November 1989
11. Sobel JD: Recurrent vulvovaginal candidiasis. N Engl J Med 315:1455, 1986
12. Multicentre Study Group: Treatment of vaginal candidiasis with a single oral dose of fluconazole. Eur J Clin Microbiol Infect Dis 7:364, 1988
13. Andersen GM, Barrat J, Bergan T et al: A comparison of single-dose oral fluconazole with 3-day intravaginal clotrimazole in the treatment of vaginal candidiasis. Br J Obstet Gynecol 96:226, 1989
14. Thomason JL, Gelbart SM: Trichomonas vaginalis. Obstet Gynecol 74:536, 1989
15. Duff P: Antibiotic selection for infections in obstetric patients. Semin Perinatol 17:367, 1993
16. Robbie M, Sweet RL: Metronidazole use in obstetrics and gynecology: a review. Am J Obstet Gynecol 145:865, 1983
17. Centers for Disease Control: 1993 Sexually transmitted diseases treatment guidelines. MMWR 42:1, 1993
18. Alexander ER, Harrison HR: Role of *Chlamydia trachomatis* in perinatal infection. Rev Infect Dis 5:713, 1983
19. Baselski VS, McNeeley SG, Ryan G, Robison M: A comparison of nonculture-dependent methods for detec-

tion of *Chlamydia trachomatis* infections in pregnant women. Obstet Gynecol 70:47, 1987

20. Schachter J, Sweet RL, Grossman M et al: Experience with the routine use of erythromycin for chlamydial infections in pregnancy. N Engl J Med 314:276, 1986

21. Martin DH, Mroczkowski TF, Dalu ZA et al: A controlled trial of a single dose of azithromycin for the treatment of chlamydia urethritis and cervicitis. N Engl J Med 327:921, 1992

22. Magat AH, Alger LS, Nagey DA et al: Double-blind randomized study comparing amoxicillin and erythromycin for the treatment of Chlamydia trachomatis in pregnancy. Obstet Gynecol 81:745, 1993

23. Al-Suleiman SA, Grimes EM, Jonas HS: Disseminated gonococcal infections. Obstet Gynecol 61:48, 1983

24. Duff P: Urinary tract infections. Prim Care Update Ob/Gyn 1:12, 1994

25. Duff P: Pyelonephritis in pregnancy. Clin Obstet Gynecol 27:17, 1984

26. Stamm WE, Counts GW, Running KR et al: Diagnosis of coliform infection in acutely dysuric women. N Engl J Med 307:463, 1982

27. Dunlow S, Duff P: Prevalence of antibiotic-resistant uropathogens in obstetric patients with acute pyelonephritis. Obstet Gynecol 76:241, 1990

28. Stamm WE, Hooton TM: Management of urinary tract infections in adults. N Engl J Med 329:1328, 1993

29. MacMillan MC, Grimes DA: The limited usefulness of urine and blood cultures in treating pyelonephritis in pregnancy. Obstet Gynecol 78:745, 1991

30. Robertson AW, Duff P: The nitrite and leukocyte esterase tests for the evaluation of asymptomatic bacteriuria in pregnant patients. Obstet Gynecol 71:878, 1988

31. Cunningham FG, Morris GB, Mickal A: Acute pyelonephritis of pregnancy: a clinical review. Obstet Gynecol 43:112, 1973

32. Gibbs RS, Duff P: Progress in pathogenesis and management of clinical intraamniotic infection. Am J Obstet Gynecol 164:1317, 1991

33. Armer TL, Duff P: Intraamniotic infection in patients with intact membranes and preterm labor. Obstet Gynecol Surv 46:589, 1991

34. Gibbs RS, Blanco JD, St. Clair PJ et al: Quantitative bacteriology of amniotic fluid from women with clinical intraamniotic infection at term. J Infect Dis 145:1, 1982

35. Romero R, Jimenez C, Lohda AK et al: Amniotic fluid glucose concentration: a rapid and simple method for the detection of intraamniotic infection in preterm labor. Am J Obstet Gynecol 163:968, 1990

36. Kirshon B, Rosenfeld B, Mari G, Belfort M: Amniotic fluid glucose and intraamniotic infection. Am J Obstet Gynecol 164:818, 1991

37. Gauthier DW, Meyer WJ, Bieniarz A: Correlation of amniotic fluid glucose concentration and intraamniotic infection in patients with preterm labor or premature rupture of membranes. Am J Obstet Gynecol 165:1105, 1991

38. Romero R, Yoon BH, Mazor M et al: The diagnostic and prognostic value of amniotic fluid white blood cell count, glucose, interleukin-6, and Gram stain in pa-

tients with preterm labor and intact membranes. Am J Obstet Gynecol 169:805, 1993

39. Hoskins IA, Johnson TRB, Winkel CA: Leukocyte esterase activity in human amniotic fluid for the rapid detection of chorioamnionitis. Am J Obstet Gynecol 157:730, 1987

40. Locksmith G, Duff P: The value of routine blood cultures in patients with chorioamnionitis: An outcome analysis. Infect Dis Obstet Gynecol 2:111, 1994

41. Sperling RS, Ramamurthy RS, Gibbs RS: A comparison of intrapartum versus immediate postpartum treatment of intra-amniotic infection. Obstet Gynecol 70:861, 1987

42. Gilstrap LC, Leveno KJ, Cox SM et al: Intrapartum treatment of acute chorioamnionitis: Impact on neonatal sepsis. Am J Obstet Gynecol 159:579, 1988

43. Gibbs RS, Dinsmoor MJ, Newton ER et al: A randomized trial of intrapartum versus immediate postpartum treatment of women with intra-amniotic infection. Obstet Gynecol 72:823, 1988

44. Duff P: Antibiotics for pelvic infections. p. 577. In Rayburn WF, Zuspan FP (eds): Drug Therapy in Obstetrics and Gynecology. 3rd Ed. Mosby Year Book, St. Louis, 1992

45. Duff P, Sanders R, Gibbs RS: The course of labor in term patients with chorioamnionitis. Am J Obstet Gynecol 147:391, 1983

46. Duff P: Pathophysiology and management of postcesarean endomyometritis. Obstet Gynecol 67:269, 1986

47. Duff P, Gibbs RS, Blanco JD et al: Endometrial culture techniques in puerperal patients. Obstet Gynecol 61:217, 1983

48. Milligan DA, Brady K, Duff P: Short-term parenteral antibiotic therapy for puerperal endometritis. J Mat Fetal Med 1:60, 1992

49. Duff P: Staphylococcal infections. p. 518. In Gleicher N (ed): Principles and Practice of Medical Therapy in Pregnancy. 2nd Ed. Appleton & Lange, New York, 1992

50. Duff P: Prophylactic antibiotics for cesarean delivery: a simple cost-effective strategy for prevention of postoperative morbidity. Am J Obstet Gynecol 157:794, 1987

51. Gibbs RS, Blanco JD, St. Clair PJ: A case–control study of wound abscess after cesarean delivery. Obstet Gynecol 62:498, 1983

52. Golde S, Ledger WJ: Necrotizing fasciitis in postpartum patients. Obstet Gynecol 50:670, 1977

53. Shykk, Eschenbach DA: Fatal perineal cellulitis from an episiotomy site. Obstet Gynecol 54:292, 1979

54. Weinstein WM, Onderdonk AB, Bartlett JG, Gorbach SL: Experimental intra-abdominal abscesses in rats: development of an experimental model. Infect Immun 10:1250, 1974

55. Knochel JQ, Koehler PR, Lee TG, Welch DM: Diagnosis of abdominal abscesses with computed tomography, ultrasound, and ^{111}In leukocyte scans. Radiology 137:425, 1980

56. Gerzof SG, Robbins AH, Johnson WC et al: Percutaneous catheter drainage of abdominal abscesses. A five-year experience. N Engl J Med 305:653, 1981

57. Duff P, Gibbs RS: Pelvic vein thrombophlebitis: diagnostic dilemma and therapeutic challenge. Obstet Gynecol Surv 38:365, 1983

58. Brown TK, Munsick RA: Puerperal ovarian vein thrombophlebitis: a syndrome. Am J Obstet Gynecol 109:263, 1971

59. Dunn LJ, Van Voorhis LW: Enigmatic fever and pelvic thrombophlebitis. N Engl J Med 276:265, 1967

60. Duff P: Septic pelvic vein thrombophlebitis. p. 104–108. In Charles D (ed): Obstetric and Perinatal Infections. Mosby Year Book, St. Louis, 1993.

61. Brown CEL, Lowe TE, Cunningham FG, Weinreb JC: Puerperal pelvic vein thrombophlebitis: impact on diagnosis and treatment using x-ray computed tomography and magnetic resonance imaging. Obstet Gynecol 68:789, 1986

62. Duff P, Gibbs RS: Maternal sepsis. In Berkowitz RL (ed): Critical Care of the Obstetric Patient. Churchill Livingstone, New York, 1983

63. Kaplan RL, Sahn SA, Petty TL: Incidence and outcome of the respiratory distress syndrome in gram-negative sepsis. Arch Intern Med 139:867, 1979

64. Goldberg LI: Dopamine—Clinical uses of an endogenous catecholamine. N Engl J Med 291:707, 1974

65. The Veterans Administration Systemic Sepsis Cooperative Study Group: Effect of high-dose glucocorticoid therapy on mortality in patients with clinical signs of systemic sepsis. N Engl J Med 317:659, 1987

66. Sprung CL, Caralis PV, Marcial EH et al: The effects of high dose corticosteroids in patients with septic shock. A prospective controlled study. N Engl J Med 311:1137, 1984

67. Holaday JW, Faden AI: Nalaxone reversal of endotoxin hypotension suggests role of endorphins in shock. Nature 275:450, 1979

68. Ziegler EJ, McCutchan JA, Fierer J et al: Treatment of gram-negative bacteremia and shock with human antiserum to a mutant Escherichia coli. N Engl J Med 307:1125, 1982

69. Freid MA, Vosti KL: The importance of underlying disease in patients with gram-negative bacteremia. Arch Intern Med 121:418, 1968

70. Betts RF: Cytomegalovirus infection epidemiology and biology in adults. Semin Perinatol 7:22, 1983

71. Wilhelm JA, Malter L, Schopfer K: The risk of transmitting cytomegalovirus to patients receiving blood transfusions. J Infect Dis 154:169, 1986

72. Stagno S, Pass RF, Dworsky ME, Alford CA: Congenital and perinatal cytomegalovirus infections. Semin Perinatol 7:31, 1983

73. Pass RF, August AM, Dworsky M, Reynolds DW: Cytomegalovirus infection in a day care center. N Engl J Med 307:477, 1982

74. Jones LA, Duke-Duncan PM, Yeager AS: Cytomegaloviral infections in infant-toddler centers: centers for the developmentally delayed versus regular day care. J Infect Dis 151:953, 1985

75. Hutto C, Little EA, Ricks R et al: Isolation of cytomegalovirus from toys and hands in a day care center. J Infect Dis 154:527, 1986

76. Adler SP: Cytomegalovirus and child day care. N Engl J Med 321:1290, 1989

77. Taber LH, Frank AL, Yow MD, Bagley A: Acquisition of cytomegaloviral infections in families with young children: a serological study. J Infect Dis 151:948, 1985

78. Demmler GJ, Schydlower M, Lampe RM: Texas, teenagers, and CMV. J Infect Dis 152:1350, 1985

79. Chandler SH, Alexander ER, Holmes KK: Epidemiology of cytomegaloviral infection in a heterogeneous population of pregnant women. J Infect Dis 152:249, 1985

80. Hohlfeld P, Vial Y, Maillard-Brignon C et al: Cytomegalovirus fetal infection: prenatal diagnosis. Obstet Gynecol 78:615, 1991

81. Lamy ME, Mulongo KN, Gadisseaux JF et al: Prenatal diagnosis of fetal cytomegalovirus infection. Am J Obstet Gynecol 166:914, 1992

82. Lynch L, Daffos F, Emanuel D et al: Prenatal diagnosis of fetal cytomegalovirus infection. Am J Obstet Gynecol 165:714, 1991

83. Donner C, Liesnard C, Content J et al: Prenatal diagnosis of 52 pregnancies at risk for congenital cytomegalovirus infection. Obstet Gynecol 82:481, 1993

84. Adler SP: Cytomegalovirus and pregnancy. Curr Opin Obstet Gynecol 4:670, 1992

85. Kumar ML, Prokay SL: Experimental primary cytomegalovirus infection in pregnancy: timing and fetal outcome. Am J Obstet Gynecol 145:56, 1983

86. Stagno S, Pass RF, Dworsky ME et al: Congenital cytomegalovirus infection. N Engl J Med 306:945, 1982

87. Fowler KB, Stagno S, Pass RF et al: The outcome of congenital cytomegalovirus infection in relation to maternal antibody status. N Engl J Med 326:663, 1992

88. Dobbins JG, Stewart JA, Demmler GJ: Surveillance of congenital cytomegalovirus disease, 1990–1991. MMWR 41:35, 1992

89. Reynolds DW, Stagno S, Hosty TS et al: Maternal cytomegalovirus excretion and perinatal infection. N Engl J Med 289:15, 1973

90. Stagno S, Reynolds DW, Huang ES et al: Congenital cytomegalovirus infection. N Engl J Med 296:1254, 1977

91. Lange I, Rodeck CM, Morgan-Capner P, Simmons A: Prenatal serological diagnosis of intrauterine cytomegalovirus infection. BMJ 284:1673, 1982

92. Grose C, Weiner CP: Prenatal diagnosis of congenital cytomegalovirus infection: two decades later. Am J Obstet Gynecol 163:447, 1990

93. Lewis PE, Cefalo RC, Zaritsky AL: Fetal heart block caused by cytomegalovirus. Am J Obstet Gynecol 136:967, 1980

94. Forouzan I: Fetal abdominal echogenic mass: an early sign of intrauterine cytomegalovirus infection. Obstet Gynecol 80:535, 1992

95. Pletcher BA, Williams MK, Mulivor RA et al: Intrauterine cytomegalovirus infection presenting as fetal meconium peritonitis. Obstet Gynecol 78:903, 1991

96. Katznelson S, Drew WL, Mintz L: Efficacy of the condom as a barrier to the transmission of cytomegalovirus. J Infect Dis 150:155, 1984

97. American College of Obstetrics and Gynecologists: Group B streptococcal infections in pregnancy. ACOG Tech Bull No. 170, July 1992

98. Yancey MK, Duff P: An analysis of the cost-effectiveness of selected protocols for the prevention of neonatal group B streptococcal infection. Obstet Gynecol 83:367, 1994

99. Boyer KM, Gotoff SP: Prevention of early-onset neonatal group B streptococcal disease with selective intrapartum chemoprophylaxis. N Engl J Med 314:1665, 1986

100. Committee on Infectious Diseases and Committee on Fetus and Newborn: Guidelines for prevention of group B streptococcal (GBS) infection by chemoprophylaxis. Pediatrics 90:775, 1992

101. Thomsen AC, Morup L, Hansen KB: Antibiotic elimination of group-B streptococci in urine in prevention of preterm labor. Lancet 1:591, 1987

102. Newton ER, Clark M: Group B streptococcus and preterm rupture of membranes. Obstet Gynecol 71:198, 1988

103. Yancey MK, Armer T, Clark P, Duff P: Assessment of rapid identification tests for genital carriage of group B streptococci. Obstet Gynecol 80:1038, 1992

104. Siegel JD, McCracken GH, Threlkeld N et al: Single-dose penicillin prophylaxis against neonatal group B streptococcal infections. N Engl J Med 303:769, 1980

105. Yow MD, Mason EO, Leeds LJ et al: Ampicillin prevents intrapartum transmission of group B streptococcus. JAMA 241:1245, 1979

106. Boyer KM, Gadzala CA, Kelly PD, Gotoff SP: Selective intrapartum chemoprophylaxis of neonatal group B streptococcal early-onset disease. III. Interruption of mother-to-infant transmission. J Infect Dis 148:810, 1983

107. Mohle-Boetani JC, Schuchat A, Plikaytis BD et al: Comparison of prevention strategies for neonatal group B streptococcal infection. JAMA 270:1442, 1993

108. Tuppurainen N, Hallman M: Prevention of neonatal group B streptococcal disease: intrapartum detection and chemoprophylaxis of heavily colonized parturients. Obstet Gynecol 73:583, 1989

109. Rouse DJ, Goldenberg RL, Cliver SP et al: Strategies for the prevention of early-onset neonatal group B streptococcal sepsis: a decision analysis. Obstet Gynecol 83:483, 1994

110. American College of Obstetrics and Gynecologists: Group B streptococcal infections in pregnancy: ACOG Techn Bull No. 170, July 1992

111. Shapiro CN, Coleman PJ, McQuillan GM et al: Epidemiology of hepatitis A: seroepidemiology and risk groups in the USA. Vaccine, Suppl. 10:S59, 1992

112. Centers for Disease Control: Hepatitis A among drug abusers. MMWR 37:297, 1988

113. Hepatitis A among homosexual men—United States, Canada, and Australia. MMWR 41:155, 1992

114. American College of Obstetricians and Gynecologists: Hepatitis in pregnancy. ACOG Tech Bull 174:1, 1992

115. Centers for Disease Control: Protection against viral hepatitis. Recommendations of the Immunization Practices Advisory Committee. MMWR 39:1, 1990

116. Werzberger A, Mensch B, Kuter B et al: A controlled trial of a formalin-inactivated hepatitis: a vaccine in healthy children. N Engl J Med 327:453, 1992

117. Syndman DR: Hepatitis in pregnancy. N Engl J Med 313:1398, 1985

118. Hoofnagle JH: Chronic hepatitis B. N Engl J Med 323:337, 1990

119. Sweet RL: Hepatitis B infection in pregnancy. Obstet Gynecol Rep 2:128, 1990

120. Centers for Disease Control: Hepatitis B virus: a comprehensive strategy for eliminating transmission in the United States through universal vaccination: recommendations of the Immunization Practices Advisory Committee (ACIP). MMWR 40:1, 1991

121. Jagger J, Hunt EH, Brand-Elnaggar J et al: Rates of needle-stick injury caused by various devices in a university hospital. N Engl J Med 319:284, 1988

122. Lynch-Salamon DI, Combs CA: Hepatitis C in obstetrics and gynecology. Obstet Gynecol 79:621, 1992

123. Osmond DH, Padian NS, Sheppard HW et al: Risk factors for hepatitis C virus positivity in heterosexual couples. JAMA 269:361, 1993

124. Weinstock HS, Bolan G, Reingold AL et al: Hepatitis C virus infection among patients attending a clinic for sexually transmitted diseases. JAMA 269:392, 1993

125. Bohman VR, Stettler RW, Little BB et al: Seroprevalence and risk factors for hepatitis C virus antibody in pregnant women. Obstet Gynecol 80:609, 1992

126. Lau JY, Davis GL, Kniffen J et al: Significance of serum hepatitis C virus RNA levels in chronic hepatitis C. Lancet 341:1501, 1993

127. Chauhan A, Jameel S, Chawla YK et al: Common aetiological agent for epidemic and sporadic non-A, non-B hepatitis. Lancet 339:1509, 1992

128. Bradley DW, Maynard JE. Etiology and natural history of post-transfusion and enterically transmitted non-A, non-B hepatitis. Semin Liver Dis 6:56, 1986

129. Velazquez O, Stetler HC, Avila C et al: Epidemic transmission of enterically transmitted non-A, non-B hepatitis in Mexico, 1986–1987. JAMA 263:3281, 1990

130. Wong DC, Purcell RH, Sreenivasan MA et al: Epidemic and endemic hepatitis in India: evidence for a non-A, non-B hepatitis virus aetiology. Lancet 2:876, 1980

131. Thomas DL, Mahley RW, Badur S et al: Epidemiology of hepatitis E virus infection in Turkey. Lancet 341:1561, 1993

132. Centers for Disease Control: Hepatitis E among U.S. travelers, 1989–1992. MMWR 42:1, 1993

133. Favorov MO, Fields HA, Purdy MA et al: Serologic identification of hepatitis E virus infections in epidemic and endemic settings. J Med Virol 36:246, 1992

134. Rizzetto M: The delta agent. Hepatology 3:729, 1983

135. Hoofnagle JH: Type D (delta) hepatitis. JAMA 261:1321, 1989 erratum to JAMA 261:3552, 1989

136. Jacobson IM, Dienstag JL, Werner BG et al: Epidemiology and clinical impact of hepatitis D virus (delta) infection. Hepatology 5:188, 1985

137. Cook CR, Gall SA: Herpes in pregnancy. Infect Dis Obstet Gynecol 1:298, 1994

138. American College of Obstetrics and Gynecologists: Herpes simplex virus infection. ACOG Tech Bull No. 102, March 1987

139. Brown ZA, Vontver LA, Benedetti J et al: Effects on infants of a first episode of genital herpes during pregnancy. N Engl J Med 317:1246, 1987

140. Brown ZA, Benedetti J, Ashley R et al: Neonatal herpes simplex virus infection in relation to asymptomatic maternal infection at the time of labor. N Engl J Med 324:1247, 1991

141. Cone RW, Hobson AC, Brown Z et al: Frequent detection of genital herpes simplex virus DNA by polymerase chain reaction among pregnant women. JAMA 272:792, 1994

142. Stone KM, Brooks CA, Guinan ME, Alexander ER: National surveillance for neonatal herpes simplex virus infections. Sex Transm Dis 16:152, 1989

143. Prober CG, Sullender WM, Yasukawa LL et al: Low risk of herpes simplex virus infections in neonates exposed to the virus at the time of vaginal delivery to mothers with recurrent genital herpes simplex virus infections. N Engl J Med 316:240, 1987

144. Gibbs RS, Amstey MS, Sweet RL et al: Management of genital herpes infection in pregnancy. Obstet Gynecol 71:779, 1988

145. Gibbs RS, Mead PB: Preventing neonatal herpes—current strategies. N Engl J Med 326:946, 1992

146. Whitley R, Arvin A, Prober C et al: Predictors of morbidity and mortality in neonates with herpes simplex virus infections. N Engl J Med 324:450, 1991

147. Kulhanjian JA, Soroush V, Au DS et al: Identification of women at unsuspected risk of primary infection with herpes simplex virus type 2 during pregnancy. N Engl J Med 326:916, 1992

148. Prober CG, Hensleigh PA, Boucher FD et al: Use of routine viral cultures at delivery to identify neonates exposed to herpes simplex virus. N Engl J Med 318:887, 1988

149. Arvin AM, Hensleigh PA, Prober CG et al: Failure of antepartum maternal cultures to predict the infant's risk of exposure to herpes simplex virus at delivery. N Engl J Med 315:796, 1986

150. Randolph AG, Washington AE, Prober CG: Cesarean delivery for women presenting with genital herpes lesions. Efficacy, risks, and costs. JAMA 270:77, 1993

151. Brown ZA, Baker DA: Acyclovir therapy during pregnancy. Obstet Gynecol 73:526, 1989

152. Goldberg LH, Kaufman R, Kurtz TO et al: Long-term suppression of recurrent genital herpes with acyclovir. Arch Dermatol 129:582, 1993

153. Centers for Disease Control: Pregnancy outcomes following systemic prenatal acyclovir exposure—June 1, 1984–June 30, 1993. MMWR 42:806, 1993

154. Whitley RJ, Gramm JW: Acyclovir: a decade later. N Engl J Med 327:782, 1992

155. Pantaleo G, Graziosi C, Fauci AS: The immunopathogenesis of human immunodeficiency virus infection. N Engl J Med 328:327, 1993

156. O'Brien TR, George JR, Holmberg SD: Human immunodeficiency virus type 2 infection in the United States. JAMA 267:2775, 1992

157. American College of Obstetricians and Gynecologists: Human immunodeficiency virus infections. ACOG Tech Bull No. 165, March 1992

158. Curran JW, Morgan WM, Hardy AM et al: The epidemiology of AIDS: current status and future prospects. Science 229:1352, 1985

159. Minkoff HL, DeHovitz JA: Care of women infected with the human immunodeficiency virus. JAMA 266:2253, 1991

160. Guinan ME, Hardy A: Epidemiology of AIDS in women in the United States. JAMA 257:2039, 1987

161. Padian NS: Heterosexual transmission of acquired immunodeficiency syndrome: International perspectives and national projections. Rev Infect Dis 9:947, 1987

162. Glatt AE, Chirgwin K, Landesman SH: Treatment of infections associated with human immunodeficiency virus. N Engl J Med 318:1439, 1988

163. MacMahon EME, Glass JD, Hayward SD et al: Epstein-Barr virus in AIDS-related primary central nervous system lymphoma. Lancet 338:969, 1991

164. Sloand EM, Pitt E, Chiarello RJ et al: HIV testing. State of the art. JAMA 266:2861, 1991

165. Centers for Disease Control: Interpretation and use of the Western blot assay for serodiagnosis of human immunodeficiency virus type 1 infections. MMWR 38:1, 1989

166. McNeil JG, Brundage JF, Wann ZF et al: Direct measurement of human immunodeficiency virus seroconversions in a serially tested population of young adults in the United States Army, October 1985 to October 1987. N Engl J Med 320:1581, 1989

167. Italian Multicenter Study: Epidemiology, clinical features, and prognostic factors of paediatric HIV infection. Lancet 2:1043, 1988

168. European Collaborative Study: Mother-to-child transmission of HIV infection. Lancet 2:1039, 1988

169. Duff P: Prenatal screening for human immunodeficiency virus infection: purpose, priorities, protocol, and pitfalls. Obstet Gynecol 74:403, 1989

170. Sperling RS, Stratton P, O'Sullivan MJ et al: Treatment options for human immunodeficiency virus–infected pregnant women. Obstet Gynecol 79:443, 1992

171. Sperling RS, Stratton P, O'Sullivan MJ: A survey of zidovudine use in pregnant women with human immunodeficiency virus infection. N Engl J Med 326:857, 1992

172. Connor EM, Sperling RS, Gelber R et al: Reduction of maternal-infant transmission of human immunodeficiency virus type[1] with zidovudine treatment. N Engl J Med 331:1173, 1994

173. Dunn DT, Newell ML, Ades AE et al: Risk of human immunodeficiency virus type 1 transmission through breastfeeding. Lancet 340:585, 1992

174. Kumar ML: Human parvovirus B_{19} and its associated diseases. Clin Perinatol 18:209, 1991

175. Thurn J: Human parvovirus B_{19}: historical and clinical review. Rev Infect Dis 10:1005, 1988

176. Centers for Disease Control: Risks associated with human parvovirus B$_{19}$ infection. MMWR 38:81, 1989

177. Cartter ML, Farley TA, Rosengren S et al: Occupational risk factors for infection with parvovirus B$_{19}$ among pregnant women. J Infect Dis 163:282, 1991

178. Gillespie SM, Cartter ML, Asch S et al: Occupation risk of human parvovirus B$_{19}$ infection for school and day-care personnel during an outbreak of erythema infectiosum. JAMA 263:2061, 1990

179. Rodis JF, Hovick TJ, Quinn DL et al: Human parvovirus infection in pregnancy. Obstet Gynecol 72:733, 1988

180. Rodis JF, Quinn DL, Gary W et al: Management and outcomes of pregnancies complicated by human B$_{19}$ parvovirus infection: a prospective study. Am J Obstet Gynecol 163:1168, 1990

181. Public Health Laboratory Service Working Party on Fifth Disease: Prospective study of human parvovirus (B$_{19}$) infection in pregnancy. BMJ 300:1166, 1990

182. Peters MT, Nicolaides KH: Cordocentesis for the diagnosis and treatment of human fetal parvovirus infection. Obstet Gynecol 75:501, 1990

183. Pryde PG, Nugent CE, Pridjian G et al: Spontaneous resolution of nonimmune hydrops fetalis secondary to human parvovirus B$_{19}$ infection. Obstet Gynecol 79:859, 1992

184. Humphrey W, Magoon M, O'Shaughnessy R: Severe nonimmune hydrops secondary to parvovirus B$_{19}$ infection: spontaneous reversal in utero and survival of a term infant. Obstet Gynecol 78:900, 1991

185. Sahakian V, Weiner CP, Naides SJ et al: Intrauterine transfusion treatment of nonimmune hydrops fetalis secondary to human parvovirus B$_{19}$ infection. Am J Obstet Gynecol 164:1090, 1991

186. Owen M, McGuffin P: Intrauterine blood transfusion for non-immune hydrops fetalis due to parvovirus B$_{19}$ infection. Lancet 336:121, 1990

187. Conry JA, Torok T, Andrews I: Perinatal encephalopathy secondary to in utero human parvovirus B-19 (HPV) infection, abstracted. Neurology 43:A346, 1993

188. Brown KE, Green SW, deMayolo JA et al: Congenital anaemia after transplacental B$_{19}$ parvovirus infection. Lancet 343:895, 1994

189. American College of Obstetricians and Gynecologists: Rubella and pregnancy. ACOG Tech Bull. No. 171, August 1992

190. Centers for Disease Control: Rubella prevention: recommendations of the Immunization Practices Advisory Committee (ACIP). MMWR 39:1, 1990

191. Centers for Disease Control: Rubella and congenital rubella syndrome—United States, January 1, 1991–May 7, 1994

192. Mann JM, Preblud SR, Hoffman RE et al: Assessing risks of rubella infection during pregnancy. JAMA 245:1647, 1981

193. Sautter RL, Crist AE, Johnson LM, LeBar WD: Comparison of five methods for the determination of rubella immunity. Infect Dis Obstet Gynecol 1:188, 1994

194. Miller E, Cradock-Watson JE, Pollock TM: Consequences of confirmed maternal rubella at successive stages of pregnancy. Lancet 2:781, 1982

195. Munro ND, Smithells RW, Sheppard S et al: Temporal relations between maternal rubella and congenital defects. Lancet 2:201, 1987

196. McIntosh EDG, Menser MA: A fifty-year follow-up of congenital rubella. Lancet 340:414, 1992

197. Bart SW, Stetler HC, Preblud SR et al: Fetal risk associated with rubella vaccine: an update. Rev Infect Dis 7:S95, 1985

198. National Vaccine Advisory Committee: The measles epidemic. The problems, barriers, and recommendations. JAMA 266:1547, 1991

199. Centers for Disease Control: Measles prevention: recommendations of the Immunization Practices Advisory Committee (ACIP). MMWR 38:1, 1989

200. Hersh BS, Markowitz LE, Maes EF et al: The geographic distribution of measles in the United States, 1980 through 1989. JAMA 267:1936, 1992

201. Centers for Disease Control: Measles prevention: supplementary statement. MMWR 38:11, 1992

202. Atkinson WL, Hadler SC, Redd SB, Orenstein WA: Measles surveillance—United States, 1991. MMWR 41:1, 1992

203. Atmar RL, Englund JA, Hammill H: Complications of measles during pregnancy. Clin Infect Dis 14:217, 1992

204. Christensen PE, Schmidt H, Bang HO et al: An epidemic of measles in Southern Greenland, 1951. Acta Med Scand 144:430, 1953

205. Eberhart-Phillips JE, Frederick PD, Baron RC, Mascola L: Measles in pregnancy: a descriptive study of 58 cases. Obstet Gynecol 82:797, 1993

206. Ekbom A, Wakefield AJ, Zack M, Adami HO: Perinatal measles infection and subsequent Crohn's disease. Lancet 344:508, 1994

207. Stein SJ, Greenspoon JS: Rubeola during pregnancy. Obstet Gynecol 78:925, 1991

208. Hook EW, Marra CM: Acquired syphilis in adults. N Engl J Med 326:1060, 1992

209. Rolfs RT, Nakashima AK: Epidemiology of primary and secondary syphilis in the United States, 1981 through 1989. JAMA 264:1432, 1990

210. Centers for Disease Control: 1993 Sexually transmitted diseases treatment guidelines. MMWR 42:1, 1993

211. Ricci JM, Fojaco RM, O'Sullivan MJ: Congenital syphilis: the University of Miami/Jackson Memorial Medical Center experience, 1986–1988. Obstet Gynecol 74:687, 1989

212. Wendel GD, Sanchez PJ, Peters MT et al: Identification of *Treponema pallidum* in amniotic fluid and fetal blood from pregnancies complicated by congenital syphilis. Obstet Gynecol 78:890, 1991

213. Ziaya PR, Hankins GDV, Gilstrap LC, Halsey AB: Intravenous penicillin desensitization and treatment during pregnancy. JAMA 256:2561, 1986

214. Klein VR, Cox SM, Mitchell MD, Wendel GD: The Jarisch-Herxheimer reaction complicating syphilotherapy in pregnancy. Obstet Gynecol 75:375, 1990

215. Krick JA, Remington JS: Toxoplasmosis in the adult—an overview. N Engl J Med 298:550, 1978

216. Sever J: The dangers of toxoplasmosis in pregnancy. Contemp Obstet Gynecol 10:29, 1977

217. Daffos F: Prenatal management of 746 pregnancies at risk for congenital toxoplasmosis. N Engl J Med 318: 271, 1988

218. Desmonts G, Couvreur J: Congenital toxoplasmosis. A prospective study of 378 pregnancies. N Engl J Med 290:1110, 1974

219. Hohlfeld P, Daffos F, Costa JM et al: Prenatal diagnosis of congenital toxoplasmosis with a polymerase-chain reaction test on amniotic fluid. N Engl J Med 331:695, 1994

220. Guerina NG, Hsu HW, Meissner HC et al: Neonatal serologic screening and early treatment for congenital *Toxoplasma gondii* infection. N Engl J Med 330:1858, 1994

221. Chapman S, Duff P: Varicella in pregnancy. Semin Perinatol 17:403, 1993

222. Smego R, Asperilla MO: Use of acyclovir for varicella pneumonia during pregnancy. Obstet Gynecol 78: 1112, 1991

223. McGregor JA, Mark S, Crawford GP, Levin MJ: Varicella zoster antibody testing in the care of pregnant women exposed to varicella. Am J Obstet Gynecol 157: 281, 1987

224. Varicella vaccine. Med Lett 37:55, 1995

225. Duff P: Varicella in pregnancy: five priorities for clinicians. Infect Dis Obstet Gynecol 1:163, 1994

226. Centers for Disease Control: Varicella-zoster immune globulin for the prevention of chickenpox. MMWR 33: 83, 1984

227. Pastuszak AL, Levy M, Schick B et al: Outcome after maternal varicella infection in the first 20 weeks of pregnancy. N Engl J Med 330:901, 1994

228. Enders G, Miller E, Cradock-Watson J et al: Consequences of varicella and herpes zoster in pregnancy: prospective study of 1739 cases. Lancet 343:1547, 1994

229. Duff P, Christian JF, Yancey MK: Infections associated with pregnancy. p. 578. In Coulam CB, Faulk WP, McIntyre JA (eds): Immunologic Obstetrics. WW Norton, New York, 1992

Pregnancy Termination

Chapter 39

Pregnancy Termination

P.G. Stubblefield

Fertility Control and Health

Voluntary control of fertility is essential to the health of women. Every pregnancy carries a risk for illness and a risk for death. Presently in the United States the national maternal mortality rate is about 9 per 100,000 live births; however, careful surveillance in state programs identifies an equal number of deaths that are not reported nationally. This risk for women with pre-existing illnesses such as diabetes, hypertension, and renal and cardiac disease is much greater. The mother's age has a profound effect on the risk of maternal mortality. Women in their 40s are seven times more likely to die in pregnancy than are women in their early 20s, the safest time to have a baby.[1] Fertility control, or lack of it, also impacts on child health. When pregnancies are too close together, the risk of prematurity and perinatal mortality increase.[2] Higher order births to young mothers are at great risk. Second births to a mother under 20 are more likely to be premature and to die than are first born children, and the risk is still higher for a third infant born to a woman under 20.[3,4] The advantages for both mother and child of delaying childbearing until the mother is fully grown, of spacing children, and of avoiding pregnancy toward the end of the reproductive years are obvious.

Legal Abortion and Voluntary Control of Fertility

Properly used, modern methods of contraception are highly effective, and, in the context of formal studies, low pregnancy rates are achieved. In general use, contraceptive methods fail more often than we usually appreciate. Failure rates for present methods from a large national study in the United States are shown in Table 39-1. While no national data are available for the copper T380A intrauterine device (Paragard), levonorgestrel subcutaneous implants (Norplant), or injectable depomedroxyprogesterone acetate (DepoProvera), these contraceptives appear to have greater efficacy. Because they are more fertile and because they are more likely to have intercourse without contraception,[5] young people are more likely to experience contraceptive failure. At the individual level, it is extremely likely that any normal couple will experience at least one unwanted pregnancy sometime during their reproductive years. Contraception is preventive medicine and as such requires advance motivation. Abortion, on the other hand, is sought when pregnancy has occurred, and the individual knows she has a problem. For all of these reasons, access to induced abortion is essential if a high level of voluntary control of fertility is to be achieved.

Finally, societies can and do limit access to contraception. In this country the group most affected by societal limitations on access is young people; hence, that they frequently resort to abortion should be no surprise. Societies cannot prevent abortion, but can determine whether it will be illegal and dangerous or legal and safe.

Approximately 1,400,000 abortions are reported to the Centers for Disease Control and Prevention each year in the United States, a number that has been stable since 1980. In 1991 the national abortion ratio was 339 abortions for every 1,000 live births, and the national abortion rate was 24 per 1,000 women aged 15 to 44.[6] The majority of women who obtain abortions are unmarried, 79.7 percent in 1991, and the ratio of abortions to live births is almost 10 times higher for unmarried women than for married women. Utilization of abortion varies markedly with age. Twenty-one percent

Table 39-1 Percentage of Women Who Experience Contraceptive Failure Within the First Year of Contraceptive Use, by Method, Standardized by Intention, Income, and Age. July 1, 1970 to January 1, 1976

Method	Percent
Pill	2.4
Intrauterine device	4.6
Condom	9.6
Spermicides	17.9
Diaphragm	18.6
Rhythm	23.7
Other	11.9

(From Schirm et al,[123] with permission.)

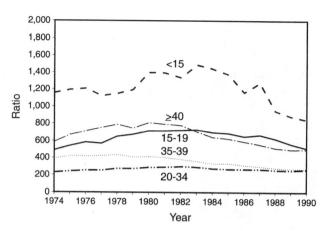

Fig. 39-2 Abortion ratio (per 1,000 live births), by age group and by year—United States, 1974–1989. (From Koonin et al.,[7] with permission.)

of women obtaining abortions were 19 or younger, and 55.2 percent were 24 or younger in 1991. In 1990, the last year for which detailed information is available, the abortion ratio for women under 15 was 844/1,000 live births, almost as many abortions as births (Fig. 39-1).[7] Abortion ratios reached their highest in the early 1980s and have declined somewhat since, especially for the youngest women (Fig. 39-2). The need for abortion is especially a problem for young, sexually active women. If legal abortion were not available, births to teenage women and unmarried women would increase markedly, and women suffering the complications of illegal abortion would once again fill the gynecology beds. Abortion ratios for black women are about double those for whites, although nationally white women have two-thirds of all abortions.[6]

History of Abortion

Some means for attempting abortion occur in all cultural groups and are evident in the artifacts of ancient civilizations.[8,9] Folk methods in use throughout the

world today include various plant substances that are ingested and more direct methods such as the insertion of an object through the cervix into the uterus. In Asia, forceful massage of the uterus to produce abortion is widely practiced.[10] Abortion was common in the 19th century in the United States. The complications from these procedures and the competition from lay abortionists so concerned the "regular" physicians that medical societies carried out intensive campaigns that resulted in the passage of laws making abortion illegal in most states by the end of the 19th century.[11] These laws remained until 1973, when humanitarian efforts to provide for medically necessary abortions culminated in the Supreme Court's decision that legalized abortion throughout the country.[11]

Duty of Health Professionals

Induced abortion continues to excite great controversy; however, as health professionals, we have a duty "to put health first, to do so by respecting the best available scientific evidence, and to be frank when we put aside such evidence for other considerations, be they moral, or religious, or economic, or simply expedient."[12] Whatever our personal feeling about the ethics of interrupting pregnancy, we have a duty to know the medical facts and to share them with our patients. We are not required to perform abortions against our ethical principles, but we have a duty to our patients to help them assess pregnancy risks and make appropriate referrals.

Legal Abortion in the United States: An Overview

Organization of Services

The legalization of abortion did not make the service available in all areas. Hospitals were very resistant to the sudden demand for large numbers of procedures,

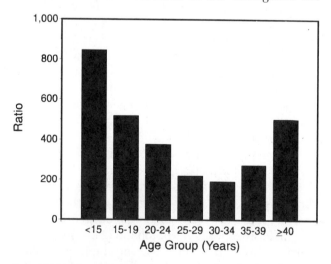

Fig. 39-1 Abortion ratio (per 1,000 live births), by age group—United States, 1989. (From Koonin et al.,[7] with permission.)

Table 39-2 Death to Case Rates for Legal Abortion Mortality by Weeks of Gestation, United States, 1972–1987

Weeks of Gestation	Deaths	Abortions	Rate[a]	Relative Risk
≤8 weeks	33	8,673,759	0.4	Referent
9–10	39	4,847,321	0.8	2.1
11–12	33	2,360,768	1.4	3.7
13–15	28	962,185	2.9	7.7
16–20	74	794,093	9.3	24.5
≥21	21	175,395	12.0	31.5

[a] Legal abortion deaths per 100,000 procedures; excludes deaths from ectopic pregnancies or pregnancy with gestation length unknown.
(From Lawson et al,[14] with permission.)

and a new institution sprang up, the free-standing abortion clinic. The majority of U.S. abortions are presently performed out of hospital, in these clinics or in doctors' offices. For the most part, the clinics follow high medical standards[13] and provide an excellent service at a cost far below other kinds of surgical care. Nationally, the risk of illness or death from legal abortion is 0.4 per 100,000 induced abortions. The risk of death from legal abortion prior to 16 weeks is 5 to 10-fold less than that from continuing the pregnancy. Legal abortion is far safer for women than illegal abortion. As shown in Table 39-2, the risk of death increases with gestational age.[14] For individual women with high-risk conditions, for example, cyanotic heart disease, even late abortion is undoubtedly a safer alternative. Because of the availability of low-cost, out-of-hospital first trimester abortion, 87 percent of legal abortions are performed in the first trimester, when abortion is the safest.[7] Type of procedure is another determinant of risk. First trimester abortions are virtually all performed by vacuum curettage; however, in mid-trimester, a variety of techniques can be used. Risks of death from abortion by the various techniques at different gestational ages are given in Table 39-3. The data clearly show the greater safety of instrumental evacuation of the uterus (dilatation and evacuation) performed in early mid-trimester. Another determinant of risk is anesthesia. Use of general anesthesia increases the risk for perforation of the uterus, visceral injury, hemorrhage, hysterectomy, and death.[15–17] The preferred alternative is paracervical block with local anesthetic, augmented with conscious sedation when needed.

Benefits of Legal Abortion

Death from illegal abortion used to be a major component of maternal mortality, and hospital gynecology wards were filled with women suffering from septic "spontaneous abortion." With legalization, septic "spontaneous abortion" is uncommon. In the 1940s more than 1,000 women died each year from abortion complications.[18] In 1987, the last year for which complete data are available, there were 12 deaths from spontaneous abortion, 6 deaths from abortion legally induced, and only 2 deaths from illegal abortion (abortion induced by a nonprofessional) in the entire United States.[14] The American Medical Association's Council on Scientific Affairs has reviewed the impact of legal abortion and attributes the decline in deaths during this century to the introduction of antibiotics to treat sepsis; the widespread use of effective contraception beginning in the 1960s, which reduced the number of unwanted pregnancies; and, more recently, the shift from illegal to legal abortion.[19] Much of the continued decline in nonabortion maternal mortality of recent years can be attributed to choice of legal abortion by women at high risk for pregnancy mortality. In the United States, the high rate of teenage pregnancy is a serious problem. Without legal abortion, there would be twice as many teenage births each year. For millions of women, legal abortion has provided an important alternative, a second chance, a chance to complete their education and achieve other personal goals prior to childbearing.

Table 39-3 Death to Case Rates[a] for Legal Abortions by Type of Procedure and Weeks of Gestation, United States, 1974–1987

Procedure	Weeks of Gestation					
	≤8	9–10	11–12	13–15	16–20	≥21
Vacuum Curettage[b]	0.3	0.7	1.1	NA	NA	NA
D & E	NA	NA	NA	2.0	6.5	11.9
Instillation[c]	—	—	—	3.8	7.9	10.3
Hysterectomy/hysterotomy	18.3	30.0	41.2	28.1	103.4	274.3

[a] Legal induced abortion deaths per 100,000 legal induced abortions.
[b] Includes all suction and sharp curettage procedures.
[c] Includes all instillation methods (saline, prostaglandin, other).
(From Lawson et al,[14] with permission.)

Table 39-4 Fetal Indications for Termination of a Desired Pregnancy

Category	Examples
Known major fetal malformation	Anencephaly, myelomeningocele, severe hydrocephaly, porencephaly, severe cardiac disease, bilateral cystic kidney disease
Chromosomal abnormality	Down syndrome
Inherited metabolic defect	
Autosomal recessive	Tay-Sachs disease
X-linked recessive	Classic hemophilia
	Duchenne's muscular dystrophy
Fetal exposure to known teratogen	
Infectious illness	Maternal infection with rubella, cytomegalovirus, toxoplasmosis
Drugs	Folate antagonists, warfarin, thalidomide, ethanol in high doses
Irradiation	X-ray exposure of 15 rads or more
Preterm premature rupture of the membranes prior to 24 weeks	
Fetal death in utero	

(Modified from Stubblefield,[20] with permission.)

Indications for Abortion

Prior to 1973, abortion was permitted in many states, but only if certain medical/social criteria were met, such as rape or life-threatening illness. With legalization, the only legal condition necessary for abortion in the first trimester is that the woman consult with her physician. However, there remains the much more difficult question of determining when abortion of a desired pregnancy should be recommended on medical grounds. In some situations, as, for example, congenital heart disease with pulmonary hypertension, the risk of death in late pregnancy is so great that any prudent physician would have to recommend abortion. Similarly, if a major fetal malformation leaves no hope for a meaningful life, most would recommend abortion. However, in the majority of cases of both maternal illness or fetal malformation, there is a strong place for the woman and her husband to determine how much risk they are willing to take. A woman who badly wants a child may decide to accept a significant risk for herself from pregnancy, while another woman with the same illness would find this risk unacceptable and seek abortion. In the author's opinion, this is as it should be, with abortion available as the safer alternative should the couple decide after medical consultation to terminate the pregnancy. Some of the fetal and maternal indications for abortion of a desired pregnancy are listed in Tables 39-4 and 39-5.[20] This list is meant as a guide for thought and is by no means all inclusive.

First Trimester Abortion

Dilatation and curettage is an ancient procedure.[8] Vacuum curettage is of more recent origin and was described for the first time in the literature by two Chinese physicians in 1954.[21] The vacuum technique was intro-

Table 39-5 Maternal Indications for Termination of a Desired Pregnancy

Category	Examples
Cardiovascular disease	Pulmonary hypertension, Eisenmenger syndrome, history of myocardial infarction, history of pregnancy cardiomyopathy, severe hypertensive disease
Genetic disease	Marfan syndrome
Hematologic disease	Thrombotic thrombocytopenic purpura
Infection	Human immunodeficiency virus
Metabolic disease	Proliferative diabetic retinopathy
Neoplastic disease	Invasive carcinoma of the cervix, any neoplasm in which maternal survival depends on prompt treatment with chemotherapy with teratogenic agents or in which the fetus will receive a dangerous dose of radiation
Neurologic disease	Untreated cerebrovascular malformation or berry aneurysm
Renal disease	Deterioration of renal function in early pregnancy
Pregnancy-specific disorder in present pregnancy	Intrauterine infection, severe preeclampsia or eclampsia

(Modified from Stubblefield,[20] with permission.)

duced in England in the 1960s and then brought to the United States by Burdick. After 1973 it quickly became the procedure of choice. Subsequent comparative trials have demonstrated that vacuum curettage is quicker, less traumatic, and safer than sharp curettage.[22]

Minisuction (Menstrual Regulation)

In 1972, Karman and Potts[23], described a small-bore, flexible vacuum cannula that, used with a 50-cc syringe as a vacuum source, allows termination of pregnancy through 7 menstrual weeks with only minimal cervical dilatation. Initially viewed as an alternative to true abortion because it could be performed even before pregnancy could be diagnosed with certainty, the procedure was described as "menstrual regulation" and performed without confirmation of pregnancy. Properly done, the minisuction procedure has many advantages, but, where abortion is legal, the procedure should be delayed until pregnancy is diagnosed. With the sensitive pregnancy tests now available, many women are able to obtain this form of early abortion within 1 or 2 weeks after the menstrual period is missed. The procedure is readily accomplished in the physician's office. The only instruments required in addition to speculum and tenaculum are the Karman cannula and modified 50-ml syringe (Fig. 39-3).

Technique for Minisuction Abortion

After examination to determine shape and position of the uterus and to be sure that pregnancy is 7 weeks or less, the cervix is exposed with a speculum, infiltrated with local anesthetic, and grasped with a tenaculum placed vertically at 12 o'clock (see Fig. 39-4). 4- and 5-mm diameter cannula are passed through the cervical canal as dilators, and then a 6-mm cannula is inserted and attached to the evacuated 50-ml syringe to establish suction. The 4- and 5-mm cannula are not large enough to evacuate the uterus dependably in pregnancy, but are useful as atraumatic dilators and for endometrial biopsies in the nonpregnant state. The 6-mm cannula is rotated and pushed in and out with gentle strokes, taking care to rotate the cannula only on the out stroke so as to avoid twisting off the flexible tip by rotating it when it is pressed against the uterine fundus. When no more tissue comes through, the cannula is withdrawn, its tip is cleared in a sterile fashion, and it is reinserted and vacuum re-established for a final, check curettage to prove the uterus empty. The operator must then carefully examine the aspirated tissue to identify the gestational sac to prevent failed abortion, to diagnose molar pregnancy, and to detect ectopic pregnancy.[24] The fresh examination is best accomplished by floating the aspirated tissue in a clear plastic dish over a light source. Figure 39-5 demonstrates the appearance of an early pregnancy.

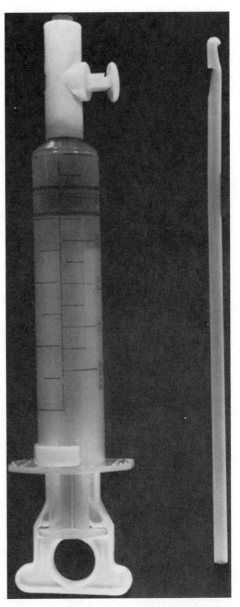

Fig. 39-3 Instruments for early abortion: 6-mm Karman cannula and modified 50-ml plastic syringe. (Photo courtesy of International Projects Assistance, Chapel Hill, NC.)

Technique for Standard Vacuum Curettage

Standard vacuum curettage applies essentially the same technique as minisuction, but utilizes larger cannula, from 7 to 12 mm, and uterine aspirators of greater capacity than the 50-mm syringe. After establishing a paracervical block as above, the operator dilates the cervical canal, utilizing serial insertion of tapered rods that increase progressively in size. We favor the Denniston dilators pictured in Figure 39-6 for their blunt tips, gentle taper, and semirigid "feel." Dilatation is continued to a diameter 1 mm less than the estimated length of gestation in menstrual weeks, and then a vac-

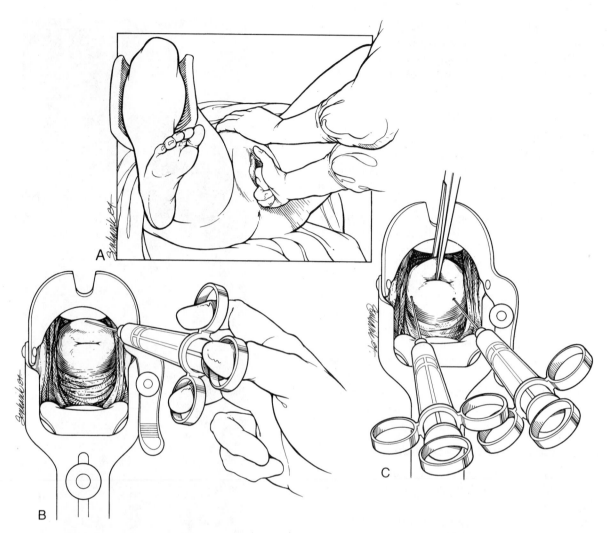

Fig. 39-4 Early vacuum curettage abortion. (A) Examining the patient. (B) Administering paracervical block and superficial injection into the cervix at 12 o'clock to anesthetize tenaculum site. (C) Completing paracervical block and injecting local anesthetic superficially, just under the vaginal mucosa, at the lateral margins of the cervix, 4 and 8 o'clock. *(Figure continues.)*

uum cannula of that same outside diameter is inserted. After aspiration is complete, a sharp curette is gently inserted and used as a finger to explore the cavity gently and prove it empty. Finally, the suction cannula is reintroduced for a final few seconds to remove any additional tissue remaining. Again, as with minisuction, the operator must perform a careful fresh examination of the aspirated tissue. An instrument kit sufficient for all first trimester procedures is pictured in Figure 39-7.

Pain Control for First Trimester Abortion

Most first trimester abortions are performed out of hospital, without a major anesthetic. This practice has contributed to the remarkable safety record of U.S. abortion services. The standard anesthetic involves some variation of local anesthesia injected around or into the cervix to produce paracervical block. There is residual pain in spite of this. Pain is increased for women who exhibit preprocedure anxiety, for the youngest women, and for procedures done prior to 8 weeks or at the end of the first trimester.[25] Premedication with naproxen[26] or ibuprofen[27] is helpful. In a series of studies Wiebe and Rawling[27] explored the effects of variations of technique upon patient pain response as assessed with objective pain scales. Lidocaine, chloroprocaine, and bupivicaine are equally effective for paracervical anesthesia. Lidocaine is most widely used because it is least expensive. Buffering the lidocaine solution by adding 2 ml of 8.4 percent sodium bicarbonate to 18 ml of 1 percent lidocaine reduces the pain of injection.[27]

Where the local anesthetic is injected is more important than what is injected. Glick[28] described a combination superficial and deep injection technique at multi-

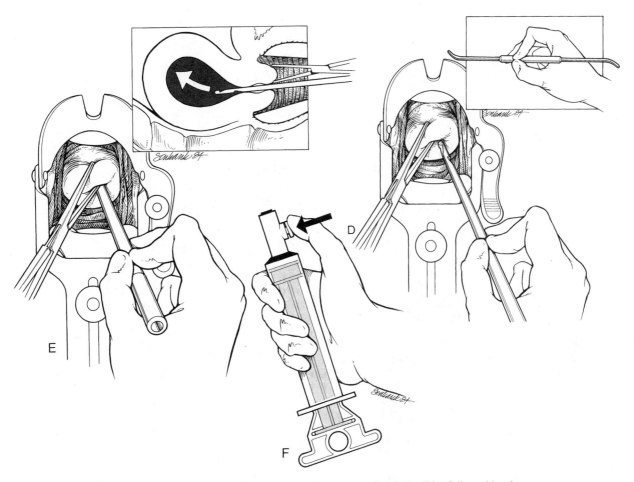

Fig. 39-4 *(Continued).* (D) Dilatation, using a 4-mm Karman cannula. This will be followed by the 5-mm Karman and then the 6-mm cannula. Alternatively, the Denniston dilators 4, 5, and 6 can be used (inset). (E) Insertion of the 6-mm Karman cannula, as far as the top of the cavity (inset). (F) Preparing the syringe by closing the pinch valve. *(Figure continues.)*

ple sites around the cervix. Wiebe[29] demonstrated the superior pain relief of injections deep into the cervical stroma compared with superficial submucosal injection. Slow injection (60 seconds on each side) compared with rapid injection (less than 30 seconds on each side) reduced the pain from injection.[27] With the deep injection technique, waiting 5 to 10 minutes after injection does not improve the efficacy of the block.

I use a modification of Glick's technique. The cervix is infiltrated superficially at 12 o'clock with 2 to 3 ml of the anesthetic solution. The needle is then advanced through the anesthetized area for 3 cm to reach the junction of cervix and lower uterine segment, where an additional 3 ml are injected. The tenaculum is placed in the anesthetized area and used to steady the cervix for placement of an additional anesthetic at 4 and 8 o'clock, again injecting first superficially and then advancing the needle 3 cm into the cervical stroma for the deep injection (Fig. 39-8).[30] Aspiration is performed prior to each injection to prevent intravascular

injection. This is important, as death has been reported with paracervical block.

To avoid systemic toxicity, the initial dose of lidocaine should not exceed 200 mg of average weight patient (20 ml of 1 percent solution). If the patient experiences inadequate pain relief on one side, an additional 5 to 6 ml can be injected after a few minutes. I add 0.5 mg of atropine to the paracervical anesthetic or give it intravenously to block vagal effects that may otherwise be seen with dilatation under paracervical block.

Conscious Sedation

Many patients will benefit from conscious sedation, the use of drugs to reduce pain while maintaining consciousness, the ability to respond to commands, and protective airway reflexes. We use midazolam 2 mg given as two 1-mg IV doses 1 minute apart, then a short-acting narcotic analgesic, either 0.050 mg of fentanyl IV repeated in a few minutes as needed or the ultra-short-acting agent alfentanyl given as boluses of 0.200

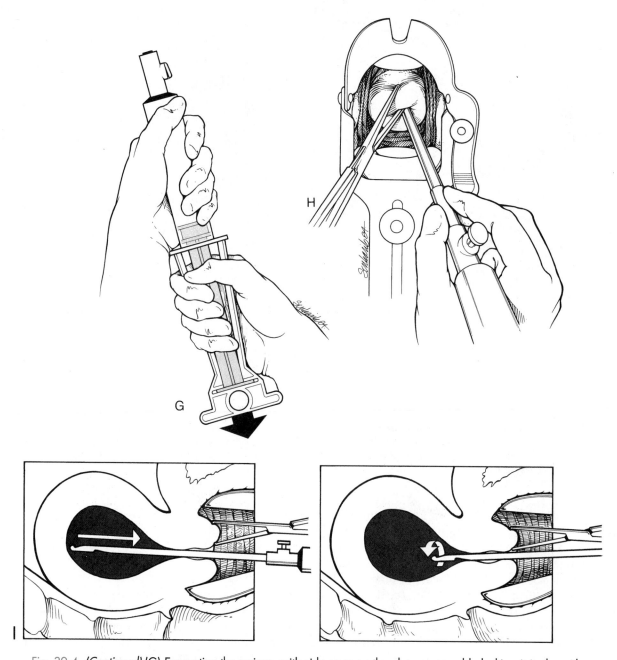

Fig. 39-4 *(Continued).*(G) Evacuating the syringe, with side arms on the plunger assembly locking it in the withdrawn position, maintaining vacuum. (H) Uterine evacuation through the Karman cannula into the syringe. (I) The cannula is rotated and is slid in and out of the cavity in a pistonlike fashion. Care must be taken to rotate only on the out stroke, when the cannula tip is withdrawn away from the top of the uterus. Rotation when the cannula is pressed against the top of the fundus may cause the tip of the cannula to break off inside the uterine cavity. *(Figure continues.)*

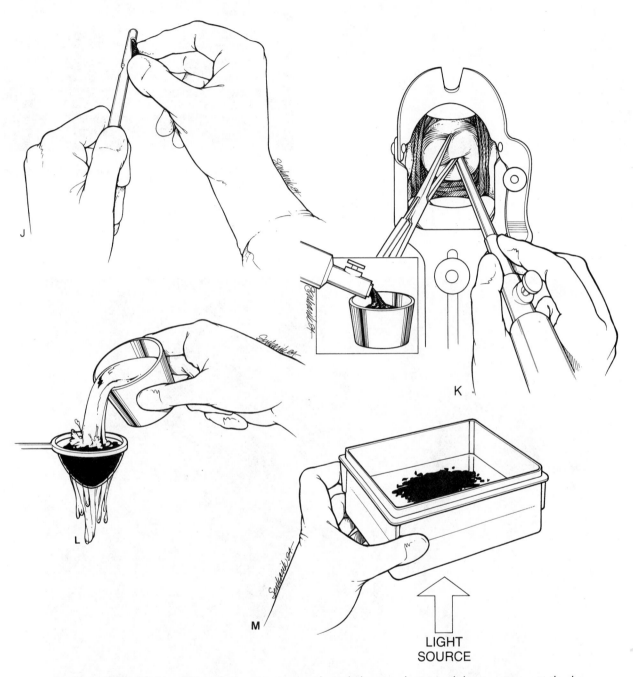

LIGHT
SOURCE

Fig. 39-4 *(Continued).* (J) When no further tissue comes through the cannula, it is withdrawn; using a sterile glove, the tip is cleared. (K) Repeat aspiration. After clearing the tip, the cannula is reinserted, the syringe emptied (inset) and re-evacuated, and vacuum established for a final check to ensure that the uterus is empty. Omission of this step results in incomplete abortion. (L) Preparing the tissue for examination. The tissue is emptied into a tea strainer and washed with saline. (M) Fresh examination. The tissue is floated in saline in a clear plastic dish over a light source. The gestational sac must be identified.

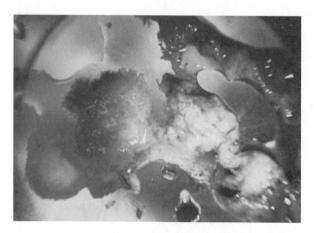

Fig. 39-5 Tissue specimen in a 6-week pregnancy, as seen without magnification. The conceptus is on the left, and to the right is the decidual lining of the uterus. (From Stubblefield,[124] with permission.)

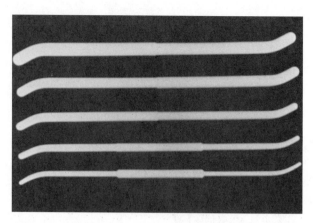

Fig. 39-6 Denniston dilators. (Photo courtesy of International Projects Assistance, Chapel Hill, NC.)

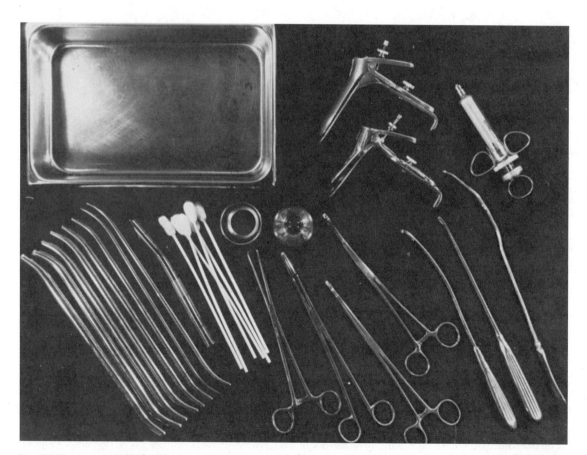

Fig. 39-7 Instrument kit for vacuum curettage abortion. Clockwise (left to right): sterile tray, Graves speculum, Moore speculum, control syringe, uterine sound, No. 1 curette, No. 3 curette, curved Foerrester forcep, straight Forrester forcep, Moore avum forcep, single-toothed tenaculum, medicine glasses, cotton swabs, plastic vacurette, Pratt cervical dilators. (From Stubblefield, with permission.)[124]

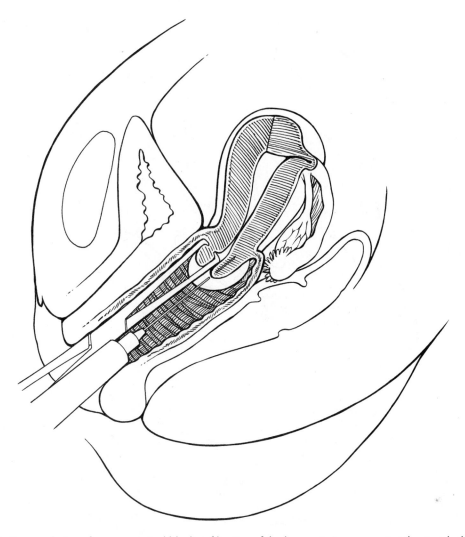

Fig. 39-8 Deep technique for paracervical block. Infiltration of the lower uterine segment at the 4 o'clock position.

mg repeated every few minutes as needed. Respiratory depression occurs with both drugs at higher doses,[31] and we routinely employ a pulse oximeter for monitoring. If oxygen saturation falls, it is usually only necessary to tell the patient to take a deep breath. Occasionally supplemental oxygen is briefly required. Patients who receive intravenous sedation must be under constant observation until fully recovered. If more than minimal doses of sedatives are used, the patient should be monitored as for general anesthesia.

Cervical Dilatation

Forcible dilatation with tapered rods is the standard, and skilled operators have performed large numbers of procedures with rates of uterine perforation as low as 1 in 10,000.[32] We place a single tooth tenaculum vertically, with one branch inside the cervical canal to provide traction near the internal os, the region of greatest resistance. Traction straightens the angle between cervix and

uterus, helping to avoid perforation (Fig. 39-9). We use a uterine sound to gently determine the direction of the cervical canal and depth of the cavity. Then gently tapered dilators, the Pratt or the Denniston plastic modification of the Pratt dilator, are used. Each dilator is inserted slowly and carefully. The dilator tip must negotiate a curve where cervix and uterus join, and, to guide the dilator properly with an anteflexed uterus, the operator's hand must follow a downward curve (Fig. 39-10). The direction is reversed if the uterus is retroverted.

Osmotic Dilators

Even the most accomplished surgeon will have an occasional perforation. Osmotic dilators reduce the risk of perforation, though do not completely prevent it. A fivefold reduction in cervical lacerations[33] and in uterine perforations was seen when *Laminaria* were used instead of forcible dilatation in a large national study.[34] *Laminaria* use has been thought to increase postabortal

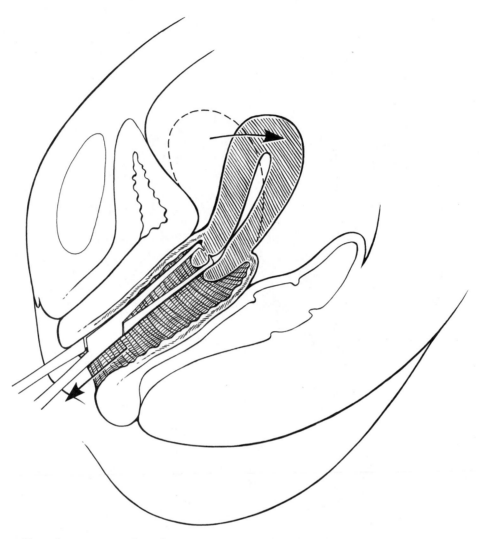

Fig. 39-9 Effect of proper tenaculum placement in straightening the angle between the cervix and uterus by traction.

infection. Indeed, *laminaria* was widely used in obstetrics and gynecology in the last century, but was abandoned because of concerns about infection.[35] The risk appears to be very low with modern methods for sterilization. In a Centers for Disease Control and Prevention study, the *Laminaria*-treated group had no increase in postabortal infection.[36]

Laminaria is a genus of seaweed. The stems are inserted into the cervical canal as small dry sticks. They take up water and swell, exerting gentle pressure (Fig. 39-11) Over several hours this produces softening of the cervix and considerable dilatation. If the *laminaria* are left in place overnight, additional forcible dilatation will not be needed. Two species of *Laminaria* are used for medical purposes: *L. japonicum* and *L. digitatum*. Tents of *L. digitata* become gelatinous as they swell, are easily entrapped in the cervical canal, and may fragment with attempts at removal. *L. japonicum* tents are preferred as they retain their integrity when wet. The

main drawbacks of *Laminaria* are the need for insertion by a skilled practitioner and the requirement of several hours for dilatation to be accomplished. Other osmotic dilators include the magnesium sulfate sponge (Lamicel) and synthetic tents of polyacrilonitrile (Dilapan). Lamicel acts more quickly to pull water from the cervix and cause softening, but exerts little force.[37] Dilapan swells more rapidly than natural *Laminaria* and exerts more force on the cervix. The labeling of Dilapan appears to limit their use to a few hours. This is unfortunate advice, and must be ignored. Left in place only a few hours, a Dilapan tent may swell more rapidly than the cervix can accommodate and be difficult to remove, but left in place overnight each Dilapan produces dilatation comparable to two medium *Laminaria* tents and is usually easily removed with gentle traction. Analogues of prostaglandins will produce some cervical dilatation, but, when used in doses sufficient to produce useful dilatation, prostaglandins produce significant

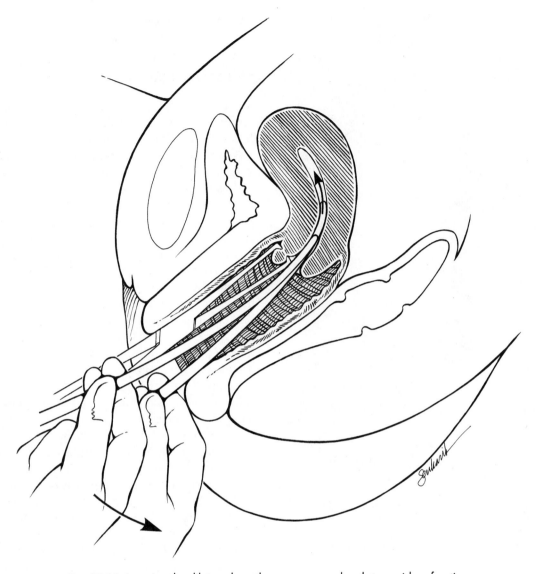

Fig. 39-10 Inserting the dilator along the proper curved path to avoid perforation.

gastrointestinal side effects. Darney and Dorward[38] compared the natural *Laminaria* tents to Dilapan and a prostaglandin analogue in a three-way randomized trial. Dilapan produced more dilatation than *Laminaria,* while the prostaglandin analog produced less dilatation but caused more side effects of vomiting and pain.[38]

Rh Prophylaxis

Risk of Rh sensitization is said to be 2 percent after spontaneous abortion and 4 to 5 percent after induced abortion.[39] Risk could be expected to be influenced by gestational age, since the amount of fetal blood increases markedly as pregnancy proceeds, but this appears not to have been quantified. All Rh-negative women should receive 50 μg of Rh-immune globulin within 72 hours of induced or spontaneous first trimes-

ter abortion. Patients in the mid-trimester, 13 weeks or more, are routinely given a full dose, 300 μg. If administration of Rh-immune globulin is accidentally delayed, it should still be given, even as late as 2 weeks because partial protection will still be provided.

Medical Means for First Trimester Abortion

Historically, a number of plant substances have been ingested in attempts to produce abortion. Extracts of the yew tree were widely used in England and the United States in the last century.[8] Some of the ancient Chinese herbal remedies are truly effective abortifacients. The substance tricocanthin does appear to cause abortion, although there apparently can be some toxicity.[40]

The prostaglandins were the first systemic agents

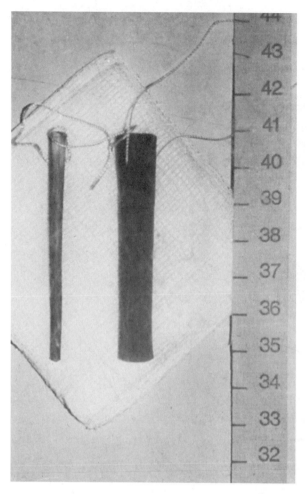

Fig. 39-11 Tents of *Laminaria japonicum*. Dry tent (left) as it would be just before insertion. Wet tent (right) as it would be after several hours exposed to water. (Photo courtesy of Mildred Hanson, M.D., Mount Sinai Hospital, Minneapolis, MN.)

proven truly effective and safe for pharmacologic induction of abortion,[41] but they have a high incidence of vomiting and diarrhea. Two prostaglandins are approved for pregnancy termination in the United states: dinoprostone (prostaglandin F_2 [PGE_2]) as vaginal suppositories and carboprost, the 15 methyl analogue of prostaglandin $F_{2\alpha}$ ($PGF_{2\alpha}$), for intramuscular injection. Though intended for mid-trimester abortion or for inducing labor after fetal death in utero, either could be used in the first trimester but are not because are they are much less convenient than the alternative, vacuum curettage. Given in sufficient doses to produce abortion, side effects of vomiting, diarrhea, and fever are common. It takes several hours of uterine pain before the abortion is produced, and the abortion is frequently incomplete, necessitating a curettage procedure after all.[42] Misoprostol, an analog of PGE_1, is available in the United States for the prevention of ulcers in the gastrointestinal tract, has many fewer side effects than

other prostaglandins, and, as described below, is being studied for use in pregnancy.

Mifepristone (RU486)

Mifepristone (RU486) is an analogue of the progestin norethindrone, first synthesized and studied in France. It has strong affinity for the progesterone receptor, but acts as an antagonist, blocking the effect of natural progesterone.[43] A single oral dose given to women 5 weeks or less from last menses produced complete abortion in 85 percent of cases. The drug was less effective at more advanced gestational ages and more likely to result in incomplete abortion with bleeding. Addition of a low dose of prostaglandin improves efficacy.[44] The standard French protocol is as follows: women with amenorrhea of less than 50 days and pregnancy confirmed by serum β-hCG (human chorionic gonadotropin) or ultrasonography receive an oral dose of 600 mg of mifepristone on day 1. On day 3 the patient returns for the prostaglandin: sulprostone (a PGE_2 analogue) or gemeprost (a PGE_1 analogue), and Rh-immune globulin if she is Rh negative. Patients remain in the clinic for 4 hours during which expulsion of the pregnancy often occurs. They return 8 to 15 days later for measurement of β-hCG or ultrasonography.[43,45,46] If treatment fails or if the patient bleeds excessively, vacuum curettage is performed. In a series of almost 17,000 cases, 600 mg of mifepristone orally followed in 36 to 48 hours by either sulprostone or gemeprost produced complete abortion in 95 percent of cases.[45,46] Three myocardial infarctions and one death have occurred with mifepristone/prostaglandin in a total of 60,000 women treated.[47,48] The myocardial infarctions were attributed to coronary artery spasm from sulprostone. All were in women over 35 who were smokers. An age over 35 and smoking or a history of cardiovascular disease are now considered contraindications to mifepristone/sulprostone for abortion. No myocardial infarctions have occurred with the PGE_1 analogue gemeprost. Misoprostol, another E_1 analogue, seems to have fewer side effects and a greater margin of safety than sulprostone. It is very effective when combined with mifepristone.[47] Mifepristone can also be used to trigger cervical softening and dilatation before surgical abortion.[49]

In spite of fierce political opposition from antichoice groups, mifepristone may soon be available in the United States. Its greatest benefit would be availability in the Third World, where it could revolutionize abortion services and spare the lives of tens of thousands of women who currently die each year from the complications of badly done abortions.

Methotrexate and Misoprostol

The antifolate methotrexate provides another medical approach to pregnancy termination. Widely used to treat ectopic pregnancies without surgery,[50] it can also be used with intrauterine gestations. In a preliminary study, Creinin and Darney[51] administered methotrexate, 50 mg/m^2 IM, followed by misoprostol 800 µg given vaginally. Abortion was induced in 6 women up to 56 days from last menstrual period (LMP).[51] In a subsequent study, 10 patients at 42 days or less from LMP were given methotrexate alone without the misoprostol. Abortion was successfully induced, and, though bleeding did not begin until an average of 24 days after treatment, the amount and duration of bleeding was less than that observed in patients who received both drugs.[52] These inexpensive drugs are already marketed in the United States, where they are approved by the Food and Drug Administration (FDA) for other indications.

Selective Termination of Anomalous Twins and Reduction of Multifetal Pregnancies

Multifetal pregnancies are likely to lead to extreme prematurity with resultant perinatal loss or serious neonatal handicap. Reduction of multifetal pregnancies in the first trimester and selective termination of second trimester anomalous twins have become standard practice in many Medical centers.[53–57] One technique is transabdominal intracardiac instillation of potassium chloride. Injection of air into the heart has also been used. A 22-gauge spinal needle is advanced through the maternal abdominal and uterine walls toward the fetal cardiac echo under guidance with high resolution ultrasound. In the first trimester 0.2 mg to 0.4 ml of a 2-mmol solution of potassium chloride is injected at a time until cardiac asystole is seen. The amount required is 0.2 to 1.8 ml.[54] Observation is continued for 2 minutes and the needle then redirected into another gestational sac. In the second trimester, 0.5 ml is injected at a time, and 0.5 to 3 ml is needed. Cardiac activity resumed 30 minutes later in 2 of 42 first trimester cases, and 1 of 4 second trimester cases in the Wapner et al.[54] series and were successfully reinjected the same day. Multifetal pregnancies are usually reduced to two gestations, since the morbidity of diamniotic twins is acceptable.

Evans and colleagues[55] described 183 completed cases of selective termination for fetal anomalies treated at nine medical centers in four countries. One hundred sixty-nine were twins, 11 were triplets, and 3 were quadruplets. Termination of the affected fetus was successful in all cases. Twelve percent of the pregnancies subsequently miscarried before 24 weeks, and 83 percent of viable pregnancies delivered after 33 weeks. Coagulopathy or ischemic damage did not occur in survivors, and there was no maternal morbidity. Injection of potassium chloride was safer for the pregnancies than air embolization, producing an 8.3 percent rate of loss compared with 41.7 percent, respectively. In monoamniotic twins attempted termination of one twin resulted in loss of both in all three cases where this was tried.[55] The same group reported their experience with termination for the indication of multifetal gestation. Four hundred sixty-three pregnancies were studied.[56] There were no failed procedures. The rate of fetal loss after procedure was 3.9 percent at 2 weeks or less and 4.6 percent at 4 weeks or less. A total of 16.2 percent were lost before 24 weeks of gestation. Eighty-three percent of the pregnancies delivered at 33 weeks or later. Gestational age at delivery was principally determined by the number of fetuses remaining. There was no evidence of damage to the surviving fetuses.

Whether selective reduction should be offered for triplet pregnancies has been argued. In a comparative study, Lipitz and colleagues[57] found that reduction of triplets to twins improved rates of prematurity, low birth weight, very low birth weight, neonatal morbidity, neonatal mortality, and pregnancy complications.

Selective reduction should not be tried with monoamniotic twins or for twin–twin transfusion syndrome, as embolization or exsanguination through the shared circulation to the remaining twin is likely. Maternal serum α-fetoprotein remains elevated into the second trimester after first trimester procedures.[54]

First Trimester Abortion Complications and Their Prevention

Complications of Local Anesthesia

Intravascular injection or an overdose of the medication can produce a severe systemic response: convulsions, cardiorespiratory arrest, and death.[58] Management requires endotracheal intubation and support of respiration plus anticonvulsive therapy. Care must be taken to aspirate before injecting each dose of the local anesthetic to guard against intravascular injection. Epinephrine-containing solutions should not be used for paracervical block. Fatal anaphylaxis from allergy to the metabisulphite preservative in epinephrine solutions can occur in asthmatic patients.[59]

Cervical Shock

Vasovagal syncope produced by stimulation of the cervical canal can be seen even after paracervical block. Although brief tonic clonic activity is observed, it is distinguished from a true seizure by the presence of a very slow pulse, the patient's rapid recovery, and the absence of any postictal state. Routine use of atropine with the paracervical anesthetic prevents "cervical shock."

Cervical Lacerations

Minor lacerations are common during forcible dilatation when the cervical tenaculum pulls off, but more serious injury can also be inflicted with actual full thickness tearing of the cervical wall. A superficial laceration that is bleeding minimally may not need to be sutured if bleeding stops with pressure. If bleeding persists in spite of pressure or the tear is full thickness, then it should be sutured. A long laceration extending through the internal os may well be a partial or complete perforation and, if lateral, may involve the descending branch of the uterine artery. Cervical lacerations are prevented by use of gently tapered dilators and by a firm grasp with a single toothed tenaculum placed vertically with one branch inside the cervical canal so that the full thickness of the cervical wall is held. Osmotic dilators help prevent cervical tears.

Perforation

Perforation can cause injury to major blood vessels, bowel, or bladder and endanger the patient's life. In a study of U.S. national data from 67,175 abortions, the rate of perforation was 0.9 per 1,000.[60] *Laminaria* use reduced the risk of perforation to less than one-fifth, and performance by a resident as opposed to an attending physician was associated with a fivefold increase in risk.[60] Each 2-week increase in gestational age was associated with a 1.4-fold increase in risk of perforation. A much lower rate of perforation (1 in 10,625) in a series of 170,000 abortions was accomplished without *Laminaria* by a small group of very experienced clinicians with predominantly first trimester procedures.[32]

Management of Perforation

The best management is immediate laparoscopy to determine the extent of the injury and complete the abortion under laparoscopic guidance.[61] Perforations of the cervix, either at the junction of the cervix and lower uterine segment or lower down the canal produce two different clinical syndromes, depending on the precise anatomic location of the perforation (Fig. 39-12).[62] Perforations at the junction of the cervix and lower uterine segment can lacerate the ascending branch of the uterine artery within the broad ligament, giving rise to severe pain, a broad ligament hematoma, and intra-abdominal bleeding. These perforations are usually recognized at the time. They are managed by laparoscopy to confirm the injury and then by laparotomy to ligate the severed vessels and repair the uterine injury.

Hysterectomy should not be required to manage such an injury.

Low cervical perforations, on the other hand, may injure the descending branch of the uterine artery within the dense collagenous substance of the cardinal ligaments. In this case there is no intra-abdominal bleeding; the bleeding is only outward, through the cervical canal, and may subside temporarily as the artery goes into spasm. Deaths have occurred when a low cervical perforation was not appreciated and the patient bled again later. If low cervical perforation is suspected, bleeding can be controlled by inflating the balloon of a Foley catheter in the cervical canal while the patient is transferred for x-ray arteriography with selective embolization of the injured vessel. Otherwise, hysterectomy may be needed.

Bowel Injury

If perforation is not recognized, the bowel may be grasped with the vacuum cannula or forceps and lacerated or stripped off its mesentery. A suspected bowel injury must be completely visualized. An experienced operator may accomplish this at laparoscopy, but laparotomy is indicated if the site of injury cannot be completely visualized. Small areas of injury can be managed by oversewing the lesion, irrigating thoroughly, and leaving a large intra-abdominal drain. Full thickness injury or stripping of the mesentery will require segmental resection and anastomosis. High dose antibiotics are given prophylactically. Larger injuries to the colon will require diverting colostomy after anastomosis.

Bladder Injury

The evaluation of a major perforation includes catheterization of the bladder to look for gross hematuria, a sign of bladder laceration. The injury is confirmed at laparoscopy, but laparotomy is required for management. Injuries to the dome are closed in two layers with catheter drainage for 7 days. Injuries to the trigone must not be repaired directly, but require an ample cystotomy incision on the dome for good visualization of the injury, catheterization of the ureters, and then closure in two layers. The best possible operative consultation with an experienced surgical specialist is advised for management of these more extensive injuries. Inadequate initial management of major injury adds markedly to the patient's problems and may jeopardize survival.

Hemorrhage

Excessive bleeding during vacuum curettage may indicate uterine atony, uterine trauma, cervical pregnancy, or a pregnancy of more advanced gestational age than anticipated. Bleeding from atony is common with gen-

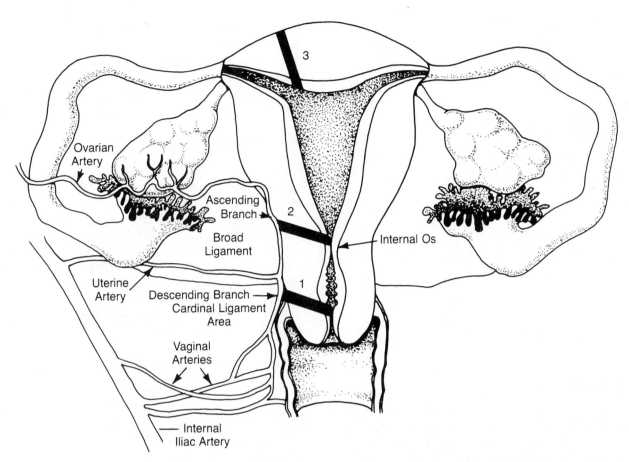

Fig. 39-12 Possible sites of uterine perforation at abortion. 1, Low cervical perforation with laceration of descending branches of uterine artery; 2, perforation at junction of cervix and lower uterine segment with laceration of ascending branch of uterine artery; 3, fundal perforation. (Redrawn from Berek and Stubblefield, with permission.)[62]

eral anesthesia using halothane or enfluorane. Management requires a rapid reassessment of gestational age by examination of the fetal parts already extracted and gentle exploration of the uterine cavity with curette or forceps to confirm that there is no perforation. Intravenous oxytocin is administered and the abortion completed. The uterus is then massaged between two hands to ensure contraction. When these measures fail, adequate fluid resuscitation is begun, and the patient is transferred immediately to the hospital. Insertion of a Foley urinary catheter into the uterine cavity and inflating the 30-cc balloon may be an effective temporizing measure. As an additional emergency measure, IM carboprost (0.250 mg), or vaginal or rectal misoprostol (0.800 mg), can be given. Persistent postabortal bleeding suggests retained tissue or clot (hematometra), cervical or uterine laceration or perforation, uterine atony, or (rarely in the first trimester) disseminated intravascular coagulopathy.

Postabortal Syndrome (Hematometra)

This syndrome is a type of uterine atony.[63] In the classic presentation, the patient begins to complain of increasing lower abdominal pain a half hour or so after abor-

tion and may develop tachycardia and diaphoresis. On examination the uterus is large, globular, and tense and could be mistaken for a broad ligament hematoma except that the mass is midline and arises from the cervix. The treatment is immediate re-evacuation. The uterus will then contract to its normal postabortal size. Sands et al.[63] have reported that pretreatment with ergot, 0.1 mg IM, reduces the incidence of the this phenomenon.

Failed Abortion, Continued Pregnancy, and Ectopic Pregnancy

Failure to interrupt the pregnancy is more often a problem with very early abortions. Pregnancy may continue in spite of the aspiration of histologically proven chorionic villi. The problem is prevented by insistence on identification of the gestational sac in the fresh examination of the aborted tissue.[64] When no chorionic villi are found in the fresh examination, ectopic pregnancy is a risk. Death from ectopic is five times more likely when the ectopic is associated with attempted abortion than when it is not, presumably because the history of apparent induced abortion delays diagnosis.[65] Various plans of management to reduce risk from ectopic preg-

Table 39-6 Findings at Repeat Uterine Evacuation in 53 Consecutive Cases of Patients Presenting With Pain, Bleeding, and Low-Grade Fever After First Trimester Abortion

Findings	No.
Retained tissue	24
Scant fragments of gestational tissue or decidua	4
Clot and gestational tissue mixture	10
Blood clot only (hematometra)	9
Continued pregnancy (intact gestational sac)	6
Total	53

(From Stubblefield,[97] with permission.)

nancy have been proposed.[24] Evaluation with quantitative β-hCG levels and vaginal probe ultrasound are essential. Women with unruptured ectopics of diameter 3.5 cm or less can be treated with methotrexate, 50 mg/m^{2}IM.[50] Patients with larger ectopics or peritoneal signs indicating rupture are offered immediate laparoscopy.

Postabortal Triad

The most common postabortal problem is the triad of pain, bleeding, and low grade fever. While these symptoms may be managed successfully by oral antibiotics and ergot preparations, the great majority of cases will exhibit some retained gestational tissue or clot in the uterine cavity. The best management is repeat uterine evacuation, performed under local anesthesia in the ambulatory setting. Results obtained in 54 consecutive reaspirations done for these symptoms are displayed in Table 39-6.

Incomplete Abortion

Retained tissue will produce increased postabortal bleeding and places the patient at risk for infection. Management is by repeat curettage. If the uterus is larger than 12 weeks, it is wise to obtain a preoperative ultrasound to determine the amount of tissue remaining. When fever is present, a cervical Gram stain and appropriate cultures are taken. Then high dose intravenous antibiotic therapy is initiated and the curettage performed shortly thereafter. Formerly it was taught that in cases of sepsis with retained tissue one should wait a day or more after starting antibiotic therapy before instrumenting the uterus. There is no merit to this theory. Women have gone into septic shock in spite of antibiotic therapy while awaiting curettage.[66]

Endometritis, myometritis, and pelvic peritonitis can be seen postabortally without any retained tissue. This is probably most likely in patients with pre-existing cervical colonization with gonorrhea, *Chlamydia*, or *Myco-*

plasma. A small, firm uterus on pelvic examination suggests that the uterus is empty and the curettage will not be needed. Where there is a question as to retained tissue, we have found ultrasound useful in making the decision whether to perform curettage or to treat with antibiotics alone.

Management of Septic Abortion

American obstetricians once were experts at managing septic abortion, but with legalization the problem has all but gone away. Since delay in initiating adequate therapy may result in preventable death, we review management in Table 39-7.[66] Clostridial sepsis, not uncommon as a complication of illegal abortion, is occasionally seen as a complication of legal abortion. This should be suspected from the presence of large grampositive rods on Gram stain of the cervical secretions or curetted tissue, when tachycardia seems out of proportion to the fever, and especially when hematuria

Table 39-7 Management of Septic Abortion

1. Be suspicious when a woman of childbearing age presents with unexplained fever, vaginal bleeding, and a history of amenorrhea
2. Make the diagnosis with a sensitive pregnancy test and pelvic examination
3. Eradicate the infection
   Obtain cultures by endometrial biopsy or uterine evacuation
   Start high dose broad spectrum antibiotics
4. Empty the uterus
   First trimester: vacuum curettage under local anesthesia with conscious sedation
   Mid-trimester: D & E, with ultrasound guidance or prostaglandin induction (carboprost 250 μg IM q2h or misoprostol 200 μg vaginally q12h) or high dose oxytocin regimen
5. Laparotomy if no response to uterine evacuation and adequate medical therapy, or perforation with suspected bowel injury, pelvic abscess, or clostridial myometritis. Hysterectomy, bilateral salpingoophorectomy for severe myometritis. Copious irrigation of abdominal cavity, drainage, closure with Smead-Jones or similar stay sutures, delayed primary closure
6. Supportive care
   Severe sepsis and septic shock require intensive care unit management
   Provide cardiovascular support to restore close to normal blood pressure. Monitor with arterial line, balloon-flotation right heart catheter. Fluid resuscitation plus dopamine and dobutamine as needed if pulmonary wedge pressure becomes elevated before target mean arterial pressure is reached.
   Manage adult respiratory distress syndrome. Monitor tissue oxygenation and begin ventilation if oxygen saturation falls below 90% or if pulmonary compliance begins to decrease

(After Stubblefield and Grimes,[66] with permission.)

and shock develop rapidly. These patients can rapidly develop a severe adult respiratory distress syndrome.

Initial treatment requires high dose penicillin, vacuum aspiration of the uterus, and fluid management. A superficial clostridial infection will respond to these measures, but, if hemolysis is present, indicating systemic release of clostridial toxins, prompt hysterectomy and bilateral salpingoophorectomy will probably be necessary.[67,68] Hyperbaric oxygenation may play a role in addition to effective surgical and medical management of clostridial sepsis.[69]

Choice of Antibiotics for Postabortal Infection

A number of different species of bacteria, *Chlamydia*, and *Mycoplasma* have been implicated in postabortal sepsis. No one agent or even pair of agents is effective against all possible organisms. Modern therapy requires the use of a drug highly effective against the anaerobic bacteria, and therefore antibiotic regimens will include clindamycin, tetracycline, metronidazole, or one of the newer cefalosporins. In practice, when the patient is seriously ill, I use three drugs: ampicillin (2 to 3 g IV every 6 hours), clindamycin (900 mg IV every 8 hours), and an aminoglycoside, either gentamicin or tobramycin (loading dose of 2 mg/kg of body weight, followed by 1.5 mg/kg every 8 hours, depending on the blood level and renal status).[66]

Prophylactic Antibiotics

The use of perioperative antibiotics with induced abortion is advisable.[70,71] Grimes and colleagues[71] evaluated published studies as of 1985 and concluded that a perioperative tetracycline regimen was advisable. This was confirmed by a subsequent analysis of 26,332 abortions from the Joint Program for Abortion.[72] Any perioperative antibiotic regimen was associated with a reduction in postabortal febrile morbidity to one-third

Table 39-8 Rates of Postabortal Pelvic Infection (PID) in a Placebo-Controlled Trial of Prophylactic Doxycycline

	Doxycycline		Placebo	
	No.	%	No.	%
In women with negative *Chlamydia* screening				
PID Yes	2	0.4	15	3.0
PID No	500	99.6	482	97.3
$p = 0.001$				
In women with positive *Chlamydia* screening				
PID Yes	1	3.0	11	26.2
PID No	32	97.0	31	73.8

(Data from Levellois and Rioux,[74] with permission.)

that seen in untreated group. Sonne-Holme et al.[73] found the benefit to be limited to those patients with a history of pelvic inflammatory disease, but the recent randomized study of Levallois and Rioux[74] showed benefit from perioperative oral doxycycline for all patients. Their results are summarized in Table 39-8. Treated patients had one-tenth the risk of developing postabortal infection.

Second Trimester Abortion

Definitions

Conventionally the second trimester has been assumed to begin after 12 menstrual weeks. Because this date is widely used it will be used here, even though it imposes a distortion of reality.* The distinction between first and second trimester abortion was magnified because of the practice, now outmoded, of considering 12 menstrual weeks the outer limit for curettage procedures and of using major surgery or labor induction techniques for abortion at 13 weeks and beyond. How this practice came to be is not clear. By 1972, Tietze and Lewis[75] demonstrated that abortion by curettage at 13 to 14 weeks was only marginally less safe than the same procedure at 11 to 12 weeks and a great deal safer than abortion by saline infusion at later gestational ages. The safety of mid-trimester curettage techniques was subsequently confirmed in a series of publications from the Centers for Disease Control and Prevention.[76] Presently, dilatation and evacuation (D & E) is the most commonly used method through 20 menstrual weeks, with labor induction methods favored only for those procedures performed after 20 weeks.[14]

The Need for Mid-Trimester Abortion

The great majority of legal abortions are performed prior to 13 menstrual weeks. Abortions performed later include those done because of fetal defects, medical or psychiatric illness that had not manifested earlier in pregnancy, and changed social circumstances such as abandonment by the spouse. However, the single greatest determinant of need for late abortion is a young age.[77] In 1990, 22.3 percent of abortions for women under age 15 years were mid-trimester, while 16 percent of abortions for women 15 to 19 and only 8.0 percent of abortions for women 30 to 34 were performed after 12 weeks.[7] Lack of ready access to abortion ser-

---

*On the average, human pregnancy lasts 38 weeks from conception or 40 weeks from the beginning of the last normal menstrual period. One-third of 38 is 12.67 weeks; thus a more correct definition for the beginning of the second trimester would be 12.67 weeks from conception or 14.67 weeks from the beginning of the last menses.

vices still accounts for the delay in many cases and is most acute for young people, especially in states that require parental notification or parental consent prior to abortion. A strategy to reduce the need for mid-trimester abortion must include education of young women to the early signs of pregnancy, early diagnosis of pregnancy by free pregnancy tests, good nonjudgmental counseling, and readily available, low cost abortion services without mandatory parental approval.

D & E in the Mid-Trimester

The variety of techniques that have been employed by different authorities are summarized elsewhere.[78,79] These differ primarily in the preparatory steps that precede the evacuation, whether one stage, with forcible dilatation followed by forceps evacuation of the fetus[80,81]; two stage, with initial dilatation of the cervix using *Laminaria* tents, followed by instrumental evacuation[83]; or multistage, with several sets of *Laminaria* over 40 to 48 hours.[79]

Choice of technique becomes more important as gestational age advances. Pregnancies at 13 to 14 menstrual weeks are readily evacuated using the 12-mm vacuum cannula.[83] Dilatation of this amount is usually readily accomplished with a Pratt or a Denniston dilator. However, unless ultrasound is routinely used, the pregnancy thought preoperatively to be only 14 weeks can easily turn out to be 16, requiring larger instruments and greater cervical dilatation. For this reason, I advise the routine use of *Laminaria* tents after 13 weeks. The actual evacuation of the uterine content is usually accomplished with long, heavy forceps and the vacuum curette is used as an adjunct to rupture the fetal membranes and drain amniotic fluid and then to ensure evacuation is complete at the end of the procedure. The 16-mm vacuum system* allows standard vacuum curettage to be performed through 16 menstrual weeks and facilitates the procedure, especially for new operators.[83]

Anesthesia for D & E

With good psychological support from trained counselors, mid-trimester D & E can be performed under paracervical block with conscious sedation. The necessary psychological support may be difficult to provide in the operating rooms of a busy general hospital, oriented toward major anesthetics. In a multicenter study, general anesthesia increased the risk for cervical laceration and hemorrhage with D & E.[84] On the other hand,

large series have been reported with very low rates of uterine injury with general anesthesia.[85,86] When general anesthesia will be used, it is all the more critical to have adequate preparation of the cervix with *Laminaria* or Dilapan tents. If general anesthesia is used, full compliance with current standards for monitoring tissue oxygen levels, end-expiratory CO_2, and frequent vital signs is mandatory.[87] When these procedures will take place out of hospital, more stringent patient selection is required. Combinations of short-acting intravenous barbiturates and inhaled nitrous oxide/oxygen mixtures or intravenous propofol combined with small doses of short-acting intravenous narcotic agents with inhaled air/oxygen mixtures are preferred regimens. Potent inhalant agents are avoided altogether or are used in very low concentrations to avoid uterine relaxation. Close observation during recovery is essential. Use of intravenous sedation or general anesthesia requires personnel trained in cardiorespiratory support.

An Approach to D & E

Most patients perceive the procedure as relatively minor, especially compared with the alternatives of labor or major surgery.[85] When all goes well, as it usually does, the procedure takes only 10 to 20 minutes, the patient recovers for an hour or two, and goes home. Yet the potential for sudden, life-threatening complications is always there: perforation and intestinal or bladder injury, amniotic fluid embolism, disseminated intravascular coagulopathy. The D & E procedure must be approached with caution and gentleness in the handling of instruments, and the patient must know that serious injury is possible, although not likely.

I describe the technique I use in hopes it will help others to prevent complications. For a more detailed description, the reader is referred to Hern's excellent book.[79] After adequate counseling, complete medical history, and physical examination with attention to uterine size and menstrual history, osmotic dilators are inserted into the cervical canal and held in place with two 4 × 4 gauze sponges tucked into the fornices. At menstrual ages 13 to 15 weeks, two *Laminaria* tents will suffice; at 16 to 20 weeks we insert 4 or more tents and use 8 to 10 tents after 20 weeks. One Dilapan tent will substitute for two *Laminaria*.

Paracervical anesthesia is produced with 10 ml of 1 percent lidocaine for the insertion. The patient is kept lying down for a few minutes after insertion to avoid syncope and then goes home. For gestations of 13 to 20 menstrual weeks, the abortion procedure will be performed the following day. At menstrual ages 20 weeks and beyond the *Laminaria* may be left in place for 48 hours. The additional dilatation greatly facilitates the procedure (P.D. Darney, personal communication,

---

*Sixteen-millimeter vacuum systems are available from Rocket of London, Inc., Branford, CT, and Medispec of Lafayette, CA.

1988). A narcotic analgesic is prescribed, as approximately half of the patients will experience significant cramping during *Laminaria* dilatation. Doxycycline is given routinely, 100 mg after the insertion, an additional 100 mg with food before sleep, and then 100 mg twice a day after the procedure for two days. Occasionally the fetal membranes rupture a few hours after *Laminaria* insertion. The *Laminaria* are left in place and the abortion performed as scheduled the following day. Ultrasound examination is performed during initial evaluation if there is a discrepancy between menstrual dates and uterine size or an abnormality on bimanual examination and for all cases 16 weeks and beyond. Ultrasound guidance during the surgery is helpful for the more advanced cases and has been found to reduce the risk of perforation on a teaching service.[88]

Uterine evacuation is performed as follows. An intravenous line is established, and the anesthetic of choice is begun. The patient is placed in lithotomy position, avoiding the Trendelenburg, or head down, position, which might increase negative pressure in the uterine veins and increase risk for an embolic phenomenon. The previously placed vaginal sponges and *Laminaria* are removed. Occasionally, especially in the young, primigravid patient at 13 to 15 weeks, the cervix is quite resistant to dilatation and the *Laminaria* tents may be entrapped. This is more often a problems when a single large *Laminaria* or Dilapan has been used and is obviated by using two or more tents. If the *Laminaria* cannot be removed with gentle traction, it is best to stop and wait 6 hours for additional cervical softening to occur. Next, the vagina and cervix are cleansed with povidone iodide and paracervical block established with 20 ml of lidocaine 1 percent with 10 U of vasopressin injected deeply into the cervix at 12, 4, and 8 o'clock positions.[89] If general anesthesia is used, the xylocaine is omitted and the vasopressin is diluted in 10 ml of saline and injected into the cervix as above. Two single toothed tenaculi are placed vertically, each with one branch inside the cervical canal. Intravenous infusion of oxytocin, 40 U/1,000 ml is begun at 150 to 200 ml/hr. A large dilator is gently inserted to confirm dilatation. The vacuum cannula is then inserted and vacuum established briefly to rupture membranes and drain amniotic fluid. The cannula is then removed and replaced with an ovum forceps of appropriate size: Forester forceps for 13- to 15-week procedures and Bierer, Sopher, or Kelly placental forceps for more advanced procedures (Fig. 39-13). The forceps are manipulated within the lower uterine segment to remove the pregnancy tissue. The vacuum cannula is reinserted as needed to pull tissue downward where it can be grasped with the forceps. When the procedure feels complete, a large, sharp curette is inserted and used to explore the cavity. If any additional tissue is encountered, the

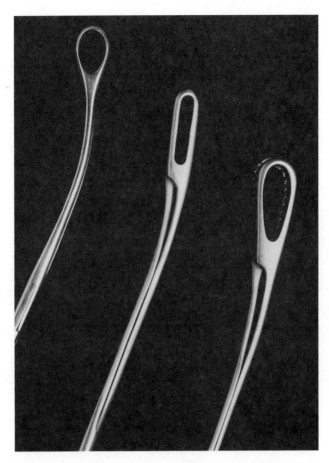

Fig. 39-13 Instruments for D & E. Kelly placental forceps, Sopher forceps, and Bierer forceps (left to right).

forceps or cannula is reinserted to remove it. After the procedure, the operator carefully examines the fetal parts to be sure all have been evacuated. On occasion the fetal calvarium is retained in the uterus. If gentle attempts at extraction fail, operative ultrasound is used. If ultrasound is not available, it is best to stop, administer an oxytocin infusion for 2 hours, and then try again. By then the remaining fetal parts will have been pushed down to the internal os where they can be easily extracted.

Attempting evacuation of a pregnancy of gestational age beyond the operators' skill and experience poses serious risk. The chance that this will occur is reduced by frequent use of preoperative ultrasound. However, if the procedure has begun, the operator can tell gestational age by the size of the fetal parts (Table 39-9). When multiple *Laminaria* tents have been used and the cervix is widely dilated, a surgeon familiar with D & E can satisfactorily extract a pregnancy up to 20 or 21 weeks. Beyond this I believe the procedure should be abandoned unless the surgeon routinely performs these more advanced procedures. The patient can be treated instead with intravenous oxytocin or systemic

Table 39-9 Recommended Values for Fetal Measurements, by Menstrual Age

Weeks	Foot Length (mm)	Fetal Weight (g)	Placental Weight (g)	Sonographic BPD (mm)
10	6			
11	7			
12	8	14	26	18
13	10	18	38	23
14	14	36	63	25
15	18	66	87	30
16	21	97	105	34
17	23	122	117	35
18	25	150	130	38
19	30	234	160	43
20	33	294	178	46
21	35	338	191	47
22	39	434	215	50

(From Hern,[125] with permission.)

prostaglandins. Perforation with mid-trimester D & E is more likely to result in major visceral injury than in perforation in first trimester procedures and will usually require a laparotomy.

Facilitating D & E

Modifications of technique are often used to facilitate D & E in the late mid-trimester. Wright[86] inserts multiple *Laminaria* or four Dilapan tents into the cervix and injects 1.5-mg digoxin into the fetal heart to produce fetal death. The D & E is carried out under brief general anesthesia the following day. Oxytocin is administered as 50 to 100 U/1,000 ml during the procedure. In his series of 2,400 cases at 19 to 23 weeks there were no perforations.[86] Hern et al.[90] described a personal series of gestations with anomalies at 15 to 34 weeks managed as outpatients with a similar technique. After multistage *Laminaria* treatment and ultrasound-guided intrafetal injection of 1.5 to 2.0 mg digoxin, membranes are ruptured on day 3, intravenous oxytocin (167 mlU/min) is started, and assisted delivery is performed after a few hours.

Labor Induction Methods

Hypertonic Saline

Amnioinfusion of hypertonic saline is historically important as one of the oldest of the labor induction methods for abortion. There are serious hazards unique to hypertonic saline: cardiovascular collapse, pulmonary and cerebral edema, and renal failure occur if the solution is injected intravenously, and all patients are at risk for serious disseminated intravascular coagulopathy. However, attention to proper technique for

amnioinfusion with instillation of the saline by gravity flow through connecting tubing from a single dose bottle under ultrasound guidance makes such mishaps very infrequent.

Administered by itself, hypertonic saline produces mean times from instillation to abortion of 33 to 35 hours.[91,92] When intravenous oxytocin is begun within 8 hours of instillation and infused at 17 to 67 mlU/min, the mean time to abortion is reduced to 25 to 26 hours.[92] Augmentation with oxytocin improves efficacy. Not only is the instillation to abortion time shortened, but there are fewer failed abortions, fewer retained placentas, less blood loss, and less risk of infection. Unfortunately, the addition of oxytocin increases the rate of occurrence of disseminated intravascular coagulopathy and adds risk for water intoxication. Higher rates of oxytocin infusion increase risk more. Kerenyi et al.[91] used 100 to 200 mlU/min, thus reducing the interval from injection to abortion to 20 to 21 hours, but reported two uterine ruptures and "a few" cases of annular detachment of the cervix.

Hypertonic Urea

Hypertonic urea is attractive as an alternative to saline because of its greater safety, but the interval from injection to abortion is prolonged. In a series of papers, a group from Johns Hopkins explored this method, augmenting it at first with intravenous oxytocin and subsequently with low does of $PGF_{2\alpha}$. The combination of 5 mg of $PGF_{2\alpha}$ and 80 g of urea instilled into the amniotic sac produces abortion in a mean time of 17.5 hours, with 80 percent of the patients aborting within 24 hours.[93] Fetal survival appears to be very rare with abortion by this method. In a comparative study, urea-prostaglandin produced shorter times from instillation to abortion and fewer serious complications than hypertonic saline.[94]

Intra-Amniotic Prostaglandin Combined with Urea or Saline

The addition of 50 ml of hypertonic saline to intra-amniotic $PGF_{2\alpha}$ shortens the interval from injection to abortion and reduces transient fetal survival prior to 20 weeks.[95]

Prostaglandins

Prostaglandins, oxygenated metabolites of C_{20} carboxylic acid, are found naturally in most biologic tissues where they act as modulators of cell function. They act via specific receptors of the G-protein family that are coupled to a variety of intracellular signaling mechanisms that may stimulate or inhibit adenyl cyclase or phosphatidylinositol.[96] Prostaglandins of the E and F series can cause uterine contraction at any stage of gestation. Pioneering work by Karim[41] demonstrated that intravenous infusion of prostaglandins produced abortion, but this route proved not to be practical because of associated vomiting and diarrhea. Side effects were much reduced when $PGF_{2\alpha}$ was given by the intra-amniotic route and a clinically useful means for mid-trimester abortion developed.

Intra-Amniotic Prostaglandins

Though initially hailed as a better alternative than intra-amniotic saline, acceptance of intra-amniotic $PGF_{2\alpha}$ was limited because of problems with incomplete abortion, the need for a second injection in many cases, the risk for cervical rupture in the primigravida, and the lack of a direct toxic effect on the fetus. Results with intra-amniotic $PGF_{2\alpha}$ are much improved if overnight treatment with *Laminaria* is used prior to infusion: mean times to abortion are reduced from 29 hours to 14 hours, fewer patients require a second dose, and cervical rupture becomes rare.[98] $PGF_{2\alpha}$ was withdrawn by the manufacturer after intense picketing by antichoice extremists, but can be replaced with the analogue 15(s)-15-methyl prostaglandin $F_{2\alpha}$ (carboprost tromethamine, Hemabate). An extensive experience with mid-trimester abortion induced by intra-amniotic carboprost has been reported by Osathanondh[98] from Brigham and Womens' Hospital in Boston. Patients are pretreated overnight with multiple intracervical *Laminaria* tents packed around one Lamicel tent. The following morning the tents are removed and an intra-amniotic injection is given of 2 mg of carboprost combined with 64 mg of 23.4 percent sodium chloride. Four hours later, the membranes are artificially ruptured, and, unless the cervix is found to be well effaced and dilated, a PGE_2 suppository is placed into the cervical canal on the end of a Dilapan tent. Subsequently, vaginal suppositories of the PGE_2 are given at 3-hour intervals. All patients have a brief exploration of the uterine cavity and curettage under low dose intravenous sedation after expulsion of the placenta. If the patient has not aborted by 14 hours, a D & E procedure is performed. The Boston group reports a mean time from instillation to abortion of 8 hours and no cervical lacerations or uterine rupture in over 4,000 consecutive cases treated with this protocol. Another recent series is that of Ferguson and colleagues,[99] who place *Laminaria* in the cervical canal and then immediately administer 80 g of urea and 2.0 mg of caroboprost by the intra-amniotic route. The mean time to abortion was 13 hours for a group of 62 patients. One patient sustained a transverse cervical laceration.

Systemic Prostaglandins

Dinoprostone (PGE_2) by vaginal suppository and intramuscular carboprost (15 S-15-methyl $PGE_{2\alpha}$) are approved by the FDA for induction of abortion. Both are easy to administer and are highly effective. With vaginal dinoprostone, 20 mg every 3 hours, the mean time to abortion is 13.4 hours, with 90 percent of patients aborting by 24 hours.[100] When carboprost is given as 250 μg IM every 2 hours the mean times to abortion are 15 to 17 hours, with about 80 percent aborting by 24 hours.[101] Gastrointestinal side effects are common, with 39 percent of dinoprostone—treated patients experiencing vomiting and 25 percent experiencing diarrhea in one large trial.[100] These side effects are more common with carboprost: 83 percent had vomiting and 71 percent had diarrhea in the trial cited above.[101] Fever is more common with dinoprostone than with carboprost. About one-third of patients treated with dinoprostone 20 mg every 3 hours will have a temperature elevation of 1°C or more. In abortions induced by prostaglandins of the F series, pretreatment with overnight placement of osmotic dilators shortens the length of prostaglandin treatment, reduces the dose of the drug required, and hence reduces the prostaglandin—related side effects.[102] Whether there is benefit from *Laminaria* for abortion induced by E prostaglandins appears not to have been demonstrated, although *Laminaria* are commonly used prior to dinoprostone treatment.

Misoprostol for Mid-Trimester Abortion

A randomized comparison of vaginal dinoprost suppositories, 20 mg every 3 hours, and vaginally administered misoprostol (200 μg every 12 hours) in patients 12 to 22 weeks pregnant showed equal efficacy. The patients receiving misoprostol had fewer side effects of fever, uterine pain, vomiting, and diarrhea. The misoprostol cost much less and was easier to administer.[103] Fifty-seven percent of patients treated with misoprostol aborted after a single 200-μg vaginal dose. Both patient groups included women with fetal death and intact gestations. The mean time intervals from start of treatment to fetal expulsion for fetal death and intact pregnancies were 9.1 and 13.2 hours, respectively, for those receiving dinoprost and 10.4 and 15.4 hours for those receiving misoprostol. More than half of patients in both groups needed manual or instrumental extraction for retained placentae, as is the usual with prostaglandin abortions. If larger trials confirm this favorable experience, misoprostol could become the method of choice for labor induction abortion in the mid-trimester.

High Dose Oxytocin

Oxytocin is usually ineffective in the mid-trimester. This is because inadequate doses have been used. Winkler and colleagues[104] compared dinoprost suppositories to a high dose oxytocin protocol at 17 to 24 weeks and found equal efficacy with fewer side effects from the oxytocin. Patients initially received an infusion of 50 U oxytocin in 500 ml of 5 percent dextrose and normal saline over 3 hours, 1 hour of no oxytocin, followed by 100 U/500 ml solution over 3 hours, another hour of rest, then a 150 U/500 ml solution over 3 hours, etc., alternating 3 hours of oxytocin with 1 hour of rest, increasing the oxytocin by 50 units in each successive time period until a final concentration of 300 U/500 ml was reached. Fifty-nine percent of the oxytocin patients had either fetal death or ruptured membranes, which could be expected to make the uterus more responsive to induction.

Complications of Labor Induction Abortions and Their Management

The labor induction methods share common hazards: failure of the primary procedure to produce abortion within a reasonable time, incomplete abortion, retained placenta, hemorrhage, infection, and embolic phenomena. Failed abortion can lead to serious infection and continued blood loss. Intramuscular injections of carboprost or vaginal suppositories of PGE_2 are important second-line therapies when the primary method has not produced abortion within a reasonable time period.

If dinoprost vaginal suppositories have been used initially and the patient does not abort by 14 to 16 hours, it is reasonable to change to intramuscular carboprost. Also, blood or amniotic fluid may dilute vaginally administered prostaglandin and limit efficacy; hence, early change to intramuscular carboprost is advised. Formerly, hysterotomy was used to manage these cases, but experienced physicians can safely employ D & E techniques, sparing the patient major surgery.[105] Failed saline or prostaglandin abortions are technically easier to manage by D & E than is a primary procedure at the same gestational age, because the cervix is usually widely dilated, the uterus is well contracted, and the fetus and placenta are compacted into the lower uterine segment. All labor induction methods can lead to fetal expulsion through a rent in the cervix above the external os, a cervicovaginal fistula, or even annular detachment of the lower cervix. Use of *Laminaria* tents helps protect the cervix. The protection is greatest with 12 or more hours exposure to *Laminaria* prior to uterine stimulation. Uterine rupture may occur when saline, urea, or prostaglandins are augmented with high dose oxytocin infusion.[106] Easy availability of a treatment room outfitted with a uterine aspirator to allow for early instrumental removal of retained placenta using conscious sedation improves care and avoids the need for an operating room and a major anesthetic.

Prostaglandin abortions are frequently incomplete and hence associated with late bleeding. If the placenta has not delivered within 1 hour after fetal expulsion, further waiting is not advised. Routine exploration of the uterus with ring forceps and vacuum curettage after all abortions, whether apparently complete or not, appears to reduce rates of postabortal hemorrhage and infection to low levels. Oxytocin should be used with caution in prostaglandin-treated patients in order to avoid uterine rupture.[106]

Disseminated intravascular coagulopathy (DIC) is rare after first trimester vacuum curettage where the incidence is 8 per 100,000 procedures.[107] The incidence is higher after mid-trimester D & E, 191 per 100,000, and highest for saline instillation procedures, 658 per 100,000. DIC must be considered whenever postabortal hemorrhage is seen and, if present, must be managed aggressively with infusions of fresh frozen plasma and packed red cells. Heparin therapy is not helpful in these cases.

With increasing use of D & E for the early mid-trimester, labor induction methods primarily are reserved for late procedures, when concerns about fetal viability and transient fetal survival are the greatest. In our experience with prostaglandins, 7 to 10 percent of fetuses exhibit some transient survival. For this reason, and to improve efficacy, $PGF_{2\alpha}$ has been combined with either hypertonic saline or urea. Fetal intracardiac injection of digoxin, performed under ultrasound guidance, prior to the use of vaginal and intra-amniotic prostaglandins to produce abortion has been utilized in some centers.[108]

Choice of Mid-Trimester Procedure

Many different procedures are available in the United States for mid-trimester abortion. Resident physicians on our service have been able to terminate 16- to 20-week pregnancies consistently and safely by D & E under the following conditions: overnight placement of multiple *Laminaria* tents, use of the 16-mm vacuum cannula system, good nursing support, and direct hands-on supervision by a small group of experienced faculty.[109] Robbins and Surrago[110] found D & E to be safer and more effective than vaginal prostaglandin. Therefore, we see little indication for any procedure other than D & E prior to 17 menstrual weeks.

When the entire mid-trimester is considered, D & E appears safer than the alternatives, but, as noted by Kafrissen et al.[111] in their comparison of D & E to urea-$PGF_{2\alpha}$, the advantage of D & E is for procedures done at 13 to 16 weeks. Thereafter, the risks for major complications and death are comparable. Urea, prostaglandins, and saline infusion all involve overnight hospitalization, which greatly increases expense. As documented by Kaltreider et al.,[85] the psychological impact on the patient is much greater with amnioinfusion abortion than with D & E. In my practice, I offer D & E through 22 menstrual weeks. Several skilled surgeons offer D & E techniques to 24 weeks and beyond. Indeed, the lowest reported rate of complications for any late abortion technique is that of Hern et al.[90]: serial multiple *Laminaria* to achieve wide cervical dilatation, amniotomy, intravenous oxytocin, and then D & E. For the operator faced with the need to perform an occasional abortion in the mid-trimester, I suggest intra-amniotic injection of 1.5 mg of digoxin and then vaginal suppositories of dinoprostone or vaginal misoprostol.

Induced Abortion and Subsequent Reproduction

Opponents of legal abortion cite complications in later reproduction as a reason to ban abortion. For the most part, the sources cited are older European authorities. Hogue et al.[112] reviewed the current literature on this topic and concluded that legal abortion as currently practiced in the United States has no measurable adverse effect on later reproduction. A single induced abortion appears safe as far as later reproduction. There is still controversy as to whether multiple induced abortions have some cumulative adverse effect; however, a large Hawaiian study found that even two or more induced abortions had no detectable adverse effect.[113] Studies of reproductive outcome are difficult because of the need to control for multiple confounding factors that are frequently present among women who report multiple abortions. Our group found that women with two or more induced abortions appeared at greater risk for later first or second trimester spontaneous loss, even after appropriate control for other factors.[114] In a separate study, women who reported two or more induced abortions prior to their present pregnancy appeared initially to have more pregnancy complications. However, statistical control by multiple logistic regression analysis found multiple abortions to be associated only with first trimester bleeding, abnormal presentations, and premature rupture of the membranes prior to labor, but not with low birth weight, prematurity, or increased perinatal loss.[115] Concerns about infertility as a result of induced abortion seem largely unfounded, except for the rare severe complication managed by hysterectomy. A prospective follow-up study found no reduction in subsequent pregnancy rates when an abortion group was compared with two control groups.[116] Indeed, the multivariate analysis of these data found that women who reported three or more induced abortions had high rates of pregnancy subsequently, suggesting that their frequent resort to abortion may have reflected greater than average fertility. The lack of adverse effects on later pregnancy probably reflects the safety of current abortion technology in the United States: most abortions are performed by vacuum curettage under local anesthesia in the first trimester. The safety of mid-trimester methods for subsequent pregnancy remains to be demonstrated and unquestionably varies with the method. Forcible dilatation of the cervix to large diameters for D & E in the late mid-trimester may well increase the risk of prematurity later.[117] We have shown that by 2 weeks following *Laminaria* dilatation the cervical canal has recovered to an internal diameter smaller than that found prior to abortion.[118] We feel strongly that *Laminaria* tents, their synthetic alternative, or low dose prostaglandins should be used to prepare the cervix prior to late abortion and that forcible dilatation to large diameters should be avoided.

Pregnancy Termination After Fetal Death in Utero

While fetal death in utero can be managed exactly as induced abortion in the first and second trimesters, there are some differences. Induction of labor within 24 hours from *Laminaria* placement in cases of fetal death is rare. This is not a problem if the patient knows this may happen and has been instructed to return to the hospital. DIC is more common following D & E or induction of labor after a fetal death. The amniotic sac may be more permeable after fetal death, and intra-amniotic injection becomes technically more difficult. For this reason, systemic reactions from hypertonic saline or intra-amniotic prostaglandin are more common in these cases. Indeed, it was this experience that spurred the development of vaginal PGF_2 suppositories to treat fetal death. In cases of fetal death, the response to prostaglandins is faster than with intact gestations. Treatment to expulsion times are shorter.

Special caution is required for managing fetal death after 28 weeks with prostaglandins. A full dose of 20 mg of PGE_2 has produced fatal uterine rupture. Our protocol, used successfully for many years, is to cut the suppository into fourths and treat the patient with one-fourth of the suppository (approximately 5 mg of PGE_2) at 2-hour intervals. The same protocol allows safe and effective treatment for women with severe asthma.

The Limit to Mid-Trimester Abortion

Women must have access to legal abortion. Efforts to ban abortion by making it illegal do not reduce the number of abortions performed but rather results in expensive and dangerous procedures with many complications and high rates of maternal mortality.[119] However, our society will not countenance infanticide.

Inevitably, there must be a gestational age limit for abortion. The U.S. Supreme Court used viability as the limit for abortion based on the decision of the women and allowed states to limit abortion thereafter.[120] With the use of surfactant treatment and current U.S. neonatal intensive care practice, 23-week infants that survive to reach the nursery have approximately a 30 percent probability of survival to leave the hospital, and 24-week infants have approximately a 60 percent probability of survival, but infants born prior to 23 weeks almost never survive (D. Dransfield, MD, personal communication, 1994). In my opinion, 23 weeks should be considered the threshold of viability. I would avoid performing abortion after 22 weeks unless the mother's life were endangered or unless the fetus had major malformations so severe as to preclude prolonged survival. Current ultrasound techniques combine measurements of several fetal dimensions to give more reliable estimates of gestational age than previous techniques that relied on the biparietal diameter alone (Table 39-9).[121] When abortion is performed just prior to viability, a method that ensures fetal demise should be selected to avoid the anguished decisions occasioned by the live birth of a fetus of borderline viability. When termination of pregnancy will be undertaken at or after 23 weeks because of serious risk to maternal health, the fetus must be considered as well. Each case must be managed individually, based on the mother's status, and intervention delayed until survival of the fetus is probable if maternal condition permits.

The ethics of abortion after viability have been explored by Annas and Elias (see Ch. 40) and by Chervanak and colleagues.[122] They conclude that abortion should be considered ethical in cases of fetal conditions with no prospect for prolonged survival after birth and when there is a completely accurate means for diagnosing the conditions. Fetal anencephaly was cited as such as condition.

Key Points

- The risk of death from legal abortion in the United States performed prior to 16 weeks is 5- to 10-fold less than that of continuing the pregnancy.

- Early vacuum curettage abortion is easily performed in an office setting with simple instruments—the Karman cannula and a modified 50-ml syringe.

- General anesthesia adds risk to abortion procedures. Conscious sedation and paracervical block are safer.

- Mifepristone (RU486) and low dose prostaglandin provide a medical means for terminating early pregnancy, producing complete abortion in 95 percent of cases.

- Small scale studies of methotrexate or methotrexate plus misoprostol indicate similar efficacies for termination of early pregnancy.

- Selective termination of multifetal pregnancies and anomalous twin gestations is practical and improves perinatal outcome.

- Mid-trimester abortion prior to 20 weeks is most often accomplished in the United States with D & E as opposed to labor induction methods. Safety with D & E requires close attention to procedural details.

- A variety of techniques for labor induction abortions exist. Dinoprostone and carboprost are the best known. Vaginally administered misoprostol appears equally effective and is much less expensive.

- Intravenous oxytocin will produce abortion in the mid-trimester provided a sufficient infusion rate is used.

- Induced abortion as currently practiced in the United States does not increase the risk of loss in later pregnancies.

References

1. Tietze C: New estimates of mortality associated with fertility control. Fam Plan Perspect 9:74, 1977
2. Eisner V, Brazie JV, Pratt MW, Hexter AC: The risk of low birth weight. Am J Public Health 69:887, 1979
3. Puffer RR, Serrano CV: Birth weight, maternal age and birth order: three important determinants in infant mortality. Pan Am Health Organization, Scientific Publ. No. 294, 1975
4. Bakketieg LS, Hoffman HJ: Epidemiology of preterm birth: results from a longitudinal study of births in Norway. p. 17. In Elder MG, Hendricks CH (eds): Preterm Labour. Butterworths, London, 1981
5. Forrest JD, Henshaw SK: What U.S. women think and do about contraception. Fam Plan Perspect 15:157, 1983
6. Centers for Disease Control and Prevention: Abortion

surveillance: Preliminary data—United States, 1991. MMWR 43:42, 1994

7. Koonin LM, Smith JC, Ramick M: Abortion surveillance—United States, 1990. MMWR 42:29, 1993

8. Potts M, Diggory P, Peel J: Abortion. Cambridge University Press, Cambridge, 1977

9. Deveraux G: A Study of Abortion in Primitive Societies. International Universities Press, New York, 1976

10. Narkavonnakit T, Bennett T: Health consequences of induced abortion in rural Northeast Thailand. Stud Fam Plan 12:58, 1981

11. Mohr JC: Abortion in America: The Origins and Evolution of National Policy. Oxford University Press, New York, 1978

12. Susser M: Induced abortion and health as a value. Am J Public Health 82:1323, 1992

13. Standards for Abortion Facilities. The National Abortion Federation, Washington, DC, 1984

14. Lawson HW, Frye A, Atrash HK et al: Abortion mortality, United States, 1972–1987. Am J Obstet Gynecol 171(5):1365, 1994

15. Peterson HB, Grimes DA, Cates W Jr et al: Comparative risk of death from induced abortion at 12 weeks or less gestation performed with local versus general anesthesia. Am J Obstet Gynecol 141:763, 1981

16. Atrash HK, Cheek TG, Hogue CJ: Legal abortion mortality and general anesthesia. Am J Obstet Gynecol 158: 420, 1988

17. Osborn JF, Arisi E, Spinelli A et al: General anesthesia, a risk factor for complications following induced abortion. Eur J Epideliol 6:419, 1989

18. Cates W Jr, Rochat RW: Illegal abortions in the United States: 1972–1974. Fam Plan Perspect 8:86, 1976

19. Council on Scientific Affairs, American Medical Association: Induced termination of pregnancy before and after Roe v Wade: trends in the mortality and morbidity of women. JAMA 268:3231, 1992

20. Stubblefield PG: Induced abortion: indications, counseling, and services. p. 2. In Sciarra JJ, Zatuchni GI, Daly MJ (eds): Gynecology and Obstetrics. Vol. 6. Philadelphia, Harper & Row, 1982

21. Wu YT: Suction in artificial abortion: 300 cases. Chin J Obstet Gynecol 6:447, 1958

22. Andolsek L (ed): The Ljubljana Abortion Study, 1971–1973. Bethesda, National Institutes of Health, Center for Population Research, 1974

23. Karman H, Potts M: Very early abortion using syringe as vacuum source. Lancet 1:7759, 1972

24. Burnhill MS, Armstead JW: Reducing the morbidity of vacuum aspiration abortion. Int J Gynecol Obstet 16: 204, 1978

25. Smith GM, Stubblefield PG, Chirchirillo L et al: Pain of first trimester abortion: its quantification and relations with other variables. Am J Obstet Gynecol 133:489, 1979

26. Suprato K, Reed S: Naproxen sodium for pain relief in first trimester abortion. Am J Obstet Gynecol 150:1000, 1984

27. Wiebe ER, Rawling M: Pain control in abortion: A comparison of various local anesthetics, preoperative analgesics and techniques. Presented at National Abortion Federation Risk Management Seminar: Pain Management: Reducing patient discomfort and provider anxiety. Philadelphia, PA, September 18, 1994

28. Glick E: Paracervical and lower uterine field block anesthesia for therapeutic abortion and office D & C. Paper presented at the 11th annual Convention of the National Abortion Federation, Salt Lake City, Utah, May 18, 1987

29. Wiebe ER: Comparison of the efficacy of different local anesthetics and techniques of local anesthesia in therapeutic abortion. Am J Obstet Gynecol 167:131, 1992

30. Stubblefield PG: Control of pain for women undergoing abortion. Int J Gynecol Obstet 3:131, 1989

31. Bell GP, Morden A, Coady T et al: A comparison of diazepam and midazolam as endoscopy premedication: assessing changes in ventilation and oxygen saturation. Br J Clin Pharmacol 26:595, 1988

32. Hakim-Elahi E, Tovell HMM, Burnhill MS: Complications of first trimester abortion: A report of 170,000 cases. Obstet Gynecol 76:129, 1990

33. Schulz KF, Grimes DA, Cates W Jr: Measures to prevent cervical injury during suction curettage abortion. Lancet 1:1182, 1983

34. Grimes DA, Schulz KF, Cates W Jr: Prevention of uterine perforation during curettage abortion. JAMA 25: 2108, 1984

35. Hale RW, Pion RJ: *Laminaria:* an underutilized clinical adjunct. Clin Obstet Gynecol 15:829, 1972

36. Gold J, Schulz KR, Cates W Jr, Tyler CW: The safety of *Laminaria* and rigid dilators for cervical dilatation prior to suction curettage for first trimester abortion: a comparative analysis. p. 363. In Naftolin F, Stubblefield PG (eds): Dilatation of the Uterine Cervix: Connective Tissue Biology and Clinical Management. Raven Press, New York, 1980

37. Wheeler RG, Schneider K: Properties and safety of cervical dilators. Am J Obstet Gynecol 164:597, 1983

38. Darney PD, Dorward K: Cervical dilatation before first-trimester election abortion: a controlled comparison of meteneprost, *Laminaria* and hypan. Obstet Gynecol 70: 397, 1987

39. Bowman JM: Controversies in Rh prophylaxis. Am J Obstet Gynecol 151:289, 1985

40. Chen P, Kols A: Population and birth planning in the People's Republic of China. Popul Rep J 10:J-504, 1982

41. Karim SMM: The use of prostaglandins in abortion. p. 68. In Lewit S (ed): Abortion Techniques and Services. Excerpta Medica, Amsterdam, 1972

42. MacKenzue IZ, Embrey MP, Davis AJ, Guillebaud J: Very early abortion by prostaglandins. Lancet 1:1223, 1978

43. Couzinet B, LeStrat N, Ulman A et al: Termination of early pregnancy by the progesterone antagonist RU 486 (mifepristone). N Engl J Med 315:1565, 1986

44. Bygdeman M, Swahm ML: Progesterone receptor blockage: effect on uterine contractility and early pregnancy. Contraception 32:45, 1985

45. Silvestre L, Dubois C, Renault M et al: Voluntary inter-

ruption of pregnancy with mifepristone (RU486) and a prostaglandin analogue. N Engl J Med 322:645, 1990

46. Ulmann A, Silvestre L, Chemama L et al: Medical termination of early pregnancy with mifepristone (RU486) followed by a prostaglandin analogue: study in 16,639 women. Acta Obstet Scand 71:278, 1992

47. Peyron R, Aubeny E, Targosz V et al: Early termination of pregnancy with mifepristone (RU486) and the orally active prostaglandin misoprostol. N Engl J Med 328:1509, 1993

48. A death associated with mifepristone/sulprostone. Lancet 337:969, 1991

49. LeFebre Y et al: The effects of RU38486 on cervical ripening. Am J Obstet Gynecol 161:61, 1990

50. Stovall TG, Ling FW: Single dose methotrexate: an expanded clinical trial. Am J Obstet Gynecol 168:1759, 1993

51. Creinin MD, Darney PD: Methotrexaate and misoprostol for early abortion. Contraception 48:339, 1993

52. Creinin MD, Darney PD: Methotrexate for abortion at ≤42 days gestation. Contraception 48:519, 1993

53. Berkowitz RL, Lynch L, Chitkara U et al: Selection reduction of multifetal pregnancies in the first trimester. N Engl J Med 318:1043, 1988

54. Wapner RJ, Davis GH, Johnson A et al: Selective reproduction of multifetal pregnancies. Lancet 335:90, 1990

55. Evans MI, Goldberg JD, Dommergues M et al: Efficacy of second trimester selective termination for fetal anomalies: International collaborative experience among the world's largest centers. Am J Obstet Gynecol 171:90, 1994

56. Evans MI, Dommergues M, Wapner RJ et al: Efficacy of transabdominal multifetal pregnancy reduction: collaborative experience among the world's largest centers. Obstet Gynecol 82:616, 1993

57. Lipitz S, Reichman B, Uval J et al: A prospective comparison of the outcome of triplet pregnancies managed expectantly or by multifetal reduction to twins. Am J Obstet Gynecol 170:874, 1994

58. Grimes DA, Cates W: Deaths from paracervical anesthesia used for first trimester abortion, 1972–1975. N Engl J Med 295:1397, 1976

59. U.S. Food and Drug Administration: Warning for prescription drugs containing sulfite. Drug Bull 17:2, 1987

60. Grimes DA, Schulz KF, Cates WJ: Prevention of uterine perforation during curettage abortion. JAMA 251:2108, 1984

61. Lauersen NJ, Birnbaum S: Laparoscopy as a diagnostic and therapeutic technique in uterine perforations during first-trimester abortions. Am J Obstet Gynecol 117:522, 1973

62. Berek JS, Stubblefield, PG: Anatomical and clinical correlations of uterine perforations. Am J Obstet Gynecol 135:181, 1979

63. Sands RX, Burnhill MS, Hakim Elahi E: Post-abortal uterine atony. Obstet Gynecol 43:595, 1974

64. Fielding WL, Lee WY, Borten N, Friedman EA: Continued pregnancy after failed first trimester abortion. Obstet Gynecol 63:421, 1984

65. Rubin GL, Peterson EB, Dorfman SF et al: Ectopic pregnancy in the United States, 1970 through 1978. JAMA 249:1725, 1983

66. Stubblefield PG, Grimes DA: Septic abortion. N Engl J Med 331:310, 1994

67. Hoyme UB, Eschenback DA: Postoperative infection. p. 821. In Iffy L, Charles D (eds): Operative Perinatology. MacMillan, New York, 1984

68. Faro S, Pearlman M: Infections and Abortion. New York, Elsevier, 1992

69. Grimm PS, Gottlieb LJ, Bodie A et al: Hyperbaric oxygen therapy. JAMA 263:2216, 1990

70. Hodgson JE, Major B, Portman K et al: Prophylactic use of tetracycline for first trimester abortions. Obstet Gynecol 45:574, 1975

71. Grimes DA, Schulz KF, Cates W: Prophylactic antibiotics for curettage abortion. Am J Obstet Gynecol 150:689, 1984

72. Park TK, Flock M, Schulz KF et al: Preventing febrile complications of suction curettage abortion. Am J Obstet Gynecol 152:252, 1985

73. Sonne-Holme S, Heisterberg L, Hebjorn S et al: Prophylactic antibiotics in first trimester abortion: a clinical controlled trial. Am J Obstet Gynecol 139:693, 1981

74. Levallois P, Rioux JE: Prophylactic antibiotics for suction curettage abortion: results of a clinical controlled trial. Am J Obstet Gynecol 158:100, 1988

75. Tietze C, Lewis S: Joint Program for the Study of Abortion (JPSA): early medical applications for legal abortion. Stud Fam Plan 3:96, 1972

76. Grimes DA, Schulz KF, Cates W Jr, Tyler CW: Midtrimester abortion by dilatation and evacuation: a safe and practical alternative. N Engl J Med 296:1141, 1977

77. Cannon-Bonventre K: Educational Methodologies to Decrease Second Trimester Abortions. American Institutes for Research, Cambridge, MA, Contract 200-77-0701. Centers for Disease Control, Dept. of Health, Education and Welfare, Washington, DC

78. Stubblefield PG: Midtrimester abortion by curettage procedures: an overview. p. 277. In Hodgson JE (ed): Abortion and Sterilization: Medical and Social Aspects. Academic Press, San Diego, CA 1981

79. Hern WM: Abortion Practice. JB Lippincott, Philadelphia, 1984

80. Finks AI: Midtrimester abortion. Lancet 1:263, 1973

81. Peterson W: Dilatation and evacuation: patient evaluation and surgical techniques. p. 184. In Zatuchni GI, Sciarra JJ, Spiedel JJ (eds): Pregnancy Termination: Procedures, Safety, and New Developments. Harper & Row, Hagerstown, MD, 1979

82. Hanson MS: D & E midtrimester abortion preceded by *Laminaria*. Presented at the 16th Annual Meeting of the Association of Planned Parenthood Physicians, San Diego, CA, October 26, 1978

83. Stubblefield PG, Albrecht BH, Koos B et al: A randomized study of 12 mm vs. 15.9 mm vacuum cannulas in midtrimester abortion *Laminaria* and vacuum curettage. Fertil Steril 29:512, 1978

84. MacKay HT, Schulz KR, Grimes DA: The safety of local versus general anesthesia for second trimester dilata-

tion and evacuation abortion. Obstet Gynecol 66:661, 1985

85. Kaltreider NB, Goldsmith S, Margolis AJ: The impact of midtrimester abortion techniques on patients and staff. Am J Obstet Gynecol 135:235, 1979

86. Wright PC: Late midtrimester abortion by dilatation and evacuation using dilapan and digoxin. Paper presented at the 13th Annual Meeting of the National Abortion Federation, San Francisco, CA, April 4, 1989

87. Eichorn JH, Cooper JB, Cullen DJ et al: Standards for patient monitoring during anesthesia at Harvard Medical School. JAMA 256:1017, 1986

88. Darney PD, Sweet RL: Routine intraoperative ultrasonography for second trimester abortion reduces incidence of uterine perforation. J Ultrasound Med 8:715, 1989

89. Schulz KF, Grimes DA, Christensen DD: Vasopressin reduces blood loss from second trimester dilatation and evacuation abortion. Lancet 2:353, 1985

90. Hern WM, Ferguson KA, Hart V et al: Outpatient abortion for fetal anomaly and fetal death from 15–34 menstrual weeks' gestation: techniques and clinical management. Obstet Gynecol 81:3016,1993

91. Kerenyi TD, Mandelman N, Sherman DH: Five thousand consecutive saline abortions. Am J Obstet Gynecol 116:593, 1973

92. Berger GS, Edelman DA: Oxytocin administration, instillation to abortion time, and morbidity associated with saline installation. Am J Obstet Gynecol 121:941, 1975

93. Burkeman RT, King TM, Atienza MF: Hyperosmolar urea. In Berger GS, Brenner WE, Keith LG (eds): Second Trimester Abortion: Perspectives After a Decade of Experience. John Wright, PSG, Inc., Boston, 1981

94. Binkin NJ, Schulz KF, Grimes DA, Cates W Jr: Urea-prostaglandin versus hypertonic saline for instillation abortion. Am J Obstet Gynecol 146:947, 1983

95. Borten M: Use of combination prostaglandin $F_{2\alpha}$ and hypertonic saline for midtrimester abortion. Prostaglandins 12:625, 1976

96. Negishi M, Sugimoto YL, Ichikawa A: Prostanoid receptors and their biological actions. Prog Lipid Res 32:417, 1993

97. Stubblefield PG: Current technology for abortion. Curr Probl Obstet Gynecol 2:1, 1978

98. Osathanondh R: Conception control. p. 480. In Ryan KJ, Barbieri R, Berkowitz RS (eds): Kistner's Gynecology. 5th Ed. Year Book Medical Publishers, Chicago, 1989

99. Ferguson JE, Burkett BU, Pinkerton JV et al: Intraamniotic 15(s)-15-methyl prostaglandin $F_{2\alpha}$ and termination of middle and late second trimester pregnancy for genetic indications: a contemporary approach. Am J Obstet Gynecol 169:332, 1993

100. Surrago EJ, Robins J: Midtrimester pregnancy termination by intravaginal administration of prostaglandin E_2. Contraception 26:285, 1976

101. Robins J, Mann LI: Second generation prostaglandins: midtrimester pregnancy termination by intramuscular injection of a 15-methyl analog of prostaglandins $F_{2\alpha}$

for midtrimester pregnancy termination. Prostaglandins 10:413, 1975

102. Stubblefield PG, Naftolin F, Lee EY et al: Combination therapy for midtrimester abortion: *Laminaria* and analogues of prostaglandin. Contraception 13:723, 1976

103. Jain JK, Mishell DR: A comparison of intravaginal misoprostol with prostaglandin E_2 for termination of second trimester pregnancy. N Engl J Med 331:290, 1994

104. Winkler CL, Gray SE, Hauth JC et al: Mid-second-trimester labor induction: concentrated oxytocin compared with prostaglandin E_2 suppositories. Obstet Gynecol 77:297, 1991

105. Burkeman RT, Atienza M, King TM, Burnett LS: The management of midtrimester abortion failures by vaginal evacuation. Obstet Gynecol 49:233, 1977

106. Propping D, Stubblefield PG, Golub J: Uterine rupture following midtrimester abortion by *Laminaria*, prostaglandin $F_{2\alpha}$ and oxytocin: report of two cases. Am J Obstet Gynecol 128:689, 1977

107. Kafrissen ME, Barke MW, Workman P et al: Coagulopathy and induced abortion methods: rates and relative risks. Am J Obstet Gynecol 147:344, 1983

108. Waters JL, Hames M: Digoxin induction abortion. Paper presented at the 8th Annual Meeting of the National Abortion Federation, Los Angeles, CA, May 14, 1984

109. Altman A, Stubblefield PG, Parker K et al: Midtrimester abortion by *Laminaria* and evacuation (L & E) on a teaching service: a review of 789 cases. Adv Plan Parent 16:1, 1981

110. Robbins J, Surrago EJ: Early midtrimester pregnancy termination: a comparison of dilatation and evacuation and intravaginal prostaglandins $F_{2\alpha}$. J Reprod Med 27:415, 1982

111. Kafrissen ME, Schulz KR, Grimes DA et al: A comparison of intraamniotic instillation of hyperosmolar urea and prostaglandin $F_{2\alpha}$ vs dilatation and evacuation for midtrimester abortion. JAMA 251:916, 1984

112. Hogue CJR, Cates W Jr, Tietze C: The effects of induced abortion on subsequent reproduction. Epidemiol Rev 4:66, 1982

113. Chung CS, Steinhoff PG, Smith RG et al: The effects of induced abortion on subsequent reproductive function and pregnancy. Papers of the East–West Population Institute, No. 86, East–West Institute, Honolulu, Hawaii, June 1983

114. Levin AA, Schoenbaum SC, Monson RR et al: The association of induced abortion with subsequent pregnancy loss. JAMA 243:2395, 1980

115. Linn S, Schoenbaum SC, Monson RR et al: The relationship between induced abortion and outcome of subsequent pregnancies. Am J Obstet Gynecol 146:136, 1983

116. Stubblefield PG, Monson RR, Schoenbaum SC et al: Fertility after induced abortion: a prospective follow-up study. Obstet Gynecol 63:186, 1984

117. Hogue CJR, Peterson WF: Late effects of late D&E. Paper presented at the National Abortion Federation Postgraduate Symposium on D & C. San Francisco, CA, September 20, 1981

118. Stubblefield PG, Altman AM, Goldstein SP: Randomized trial of one versus two days of *Laminaria* treatment

prior to late midtrimester abortion by uterine evacuation: a pilot study. Am J Obstet Gynecol 143:481, 1982

119. The Alan Guttmacher Institute: Clandestine abortion: a Latin American Reality. The Alan Guttmacher Institutes, New York, 1994

120. Roe v. Wade. 410 U.S. 113, 1973

121. Hohler CW: Ultrasound estimation of gestational age. Clin Obstet Gynecol 27:314, 1984

122. Chervenak FA, Farley MA, Walters L et al: When is termination of pregnancy during the third trimester morally justifiable? N Engl J Med 310:501, 1984

123. Schirm AL, Trussell J, Menken J, Grady WR: Contraceptive failure in the United States: the impact of social, economic, and demographic factors Fam Plan Perspect 14:68, 1982

124. Stubblefield PG: Surgical techniques for first trimester abortion. p. 12. In Sciarra JJ, Zatuchni GI, Daly MJ (eds): Gynecology and Obstetrics. Vol. 6. Harper & Row, Hagerstown, MD, 1982

125. Hern WM: Correlation of fetal age and measurements between 10–26 weeks of gestation. Obstet Gynecol 63: 26, 1984.

Legal and Ethical Issues in Perinatology

Chapter 40

Legal and Ethical Issues in Obstetric Practice

George J. Annas and Sherman Elias

Society has great expectations that modern medical technologies will improve longevity and quality of human life, and nowhere are these expectations higher than in the practice of obstetrics. Along with the rapidly expanding capabilities in diagnosis and treatment, physicians find themselves facing numerous ethical dilemmas with confusion and uncertainty while practicing in a climate in which malpractice suits can threaten even the most competent and conscientious practitioner.

We cannot address in a single chapter the seemingly infinite ethical and legal controversies facing contemporary obstetric practice and research. Instead, we focus on several topics we believe are timely and of particular relevance to the practicing obstetrician.

Abortion

Feelings, beliefs, and opinions are strong and divided on the 1973 U.S. Supreme Court decision in *Roe v. Wade*, the Court's 1989 decision in *Webster* that signaled a retreat from *Roe*, and the Court's 1992 compromise decision in *Casey*.[1-4] Opinion polls on abortion since 1973 show that Americans are deeply ambivalent on the issue. A consistent majority believe abortion is immoral in most cases. Nonetheless, overwhelming majorities believe abortion should be available in cases of rape, incest, and severe genetic handicap, and more than two-thirds consistently say even though they believe abortion is either "wrong" or "immoral" the ultimate decision should be made by a woman and her physician rather than by government decree.[5,6]

Physicians' opinions seem to mirror those of society generally. For example, a 1985 survey of 1,300 members of the American College of Obstetricians and Gynecologists found that 90 percent believed fetal ab-normalities were a legitimate reason for first trimester abortions (84 percent for second trimester abortions); this was followed by agreeing to abortions because of a woman's physical health (75 percent), rape or incest (68 percent), a woman's mental health (65 percent), economic difficulties (36 percent), and personal choice (36 percent). Only about 25 percent of the public and 35 percent of obstetricians/gynecologists support "elective" abortions for whatever reason the woman might have.[7]

In 1989, when President George Bush was asked whether he would wait for the U.S. Supreme Court to reconsider *Roe v. Wade* before taking presidential initiatives on abortion replied: "Wait. I think probably wait. . . . But I'd like to see the Supreme Court decision as soon as possible."[8] Then Attorney General Richard Thornburgh also wanted *Roe* overruled, saying: "My guess is that [the U.S. Supreme Court] will return the regulations of abortions, like many health and safety questions, to the states. . . . The decisions will be made by state legislators and state governors and not by the federal government."[9]

Neither the President nor his Attorney General was ever willing or able to discuss the core issue involved in *Roe v. Wade* in public. The President, for example, said in the 1988 presidential debates that he had not thought through the penalties. Later he said the women were co-victims, implying that only the physicians who perform abortions should be considered criminals. And the Attorney General was simply wrong: The shift in decision-making will not be from the federal government to state legislatures, but, rather, from decisions made by individual women and their physicians to decisions made by state legislatures. The core issue is what role the government should play in using the criminal law to restrict access to abortions that are sought by women and agreed to by their physicians.

Roe v. Wade

In *Roe v. Wade*,[10] and in all of the abortion cases that followed it (other than the financing cases), the Court has been faced with a *criminal* statute designed to limit access to abortion. In *Roe*, the Texas statute it was reviewing made it a crime to perform or attempt to perform an abortion, except to save the life of the mother. Justice Harry Blackmum, formerly legal counsel to the Mayo Clinic, wrote the opinion of the Court. One of the major goals was to prevent the government from interfering with the practice of medicine and in the doctor–patient relationship.[11]

The decision was 7 to 2, with Justices William Rehnquist and Byron White dissenting. Building on a series of cases, including a leading one dealing with contraception that had described a "right to personal privacy or a guarantee of certain areas or zones of privacy," the Court determined that a fundamental "right to privacy" existed "in the Fourteenth Amendment's concept of personal liberty and restrictions upon state action." The Court went on to hold that this fundamental right "is broad enough to encompass a woman's decision whether or not to terminate her pregnancy":

> The detriment that the State would impose upon the pregnant woman by denying this choice altogether is apparent. Specific and direct harm medically diagnosable even in early pregnancy may be involved. Maternity, or additional offspring, may force upon the woman a distressful life and future. Psychological harm may be imminent. Mental and physical health may be taxed by child care. . . . All these are factors the woman and her responsible physician necessarily will consider in consultation.

Although granting the abortion decision a very high degree of constitutional protection, the Court stopped short of declaring that a woman's right to an abortion was absolute, that she had a right to "abortion on demand." Instead the Court recognized that the state also has interests that may at times be "compelling" enough to limit abortion. The Court identified two such interests: the protection of maternal health and the protection of fetal life. The protection of maternal health has always been a legitimate state interest. In the case of abortion, however, the Court ruled that this interest could never be so "compelling" as to prohibit abortion prior to the stage in pregnancy when it is less dangerous for the woman to carry the fetus to term than to have an abortion (about the end of the first trimester in 1973). The Court decided that during the first trimester the state could only regulate abortions to protect the woman's health by requiring that they be performed by a physician. Thereafter it could only regulate to protect

women in ways reasonably calculated to enhance the woman's personal health rather than in ways really designed to protect the fetus or simply to discourage abortions.

The second state interest the Court identified was that of "protecting the potentiality of human life." The Supreme Court did not decide that the fetus is not human, but only that a fetus is not a "person" as that term is used in the Fourteenth Amendment. The Court also properly noted that "the pregnant woman cannot be isolated in her privacy"; her interests in privacy must be weighed against the state's interest in the life of the fetus. The question is: When does the state's interest become so "compelling" that the state can justifiably interfere with the woman's constitutional right to have an abortion? No satisfactory answer to this question can be garnered from science, and any line of demarcation during pregnancy is inherently arbitrary. The Court decided to choose fetal viability, the interim point between conception and birth at which the fetus "is potentially able to live outside the woman's womb, albeit with artificial aid," apparently because at this point the fetus is biologically identical to a premature infant.

After viability, which continues to occur near the end of the second trimester, but whose actual determination is a function of medical technology and skill, the state "may, if it chooses, regulate, and even proscribe, abortion except where it is necessary, in appropriate medical judgment, for the preservation of the life or health of the mother." Although states can regulate abortions after fetal viability (or, more accurately, restrict premature birth inductions), by 1990 only 13 states had enacted post-*Roe* laws that attempt to restrict such abortions.[12]

Efforts To Modify Roe

Efforts to amend the U.S. Constitution to change or overturn the decision were unsuccessful and have been all but abandoned. A parallel strategy is ongoing: the passage of state abortion statutes that are as restrictive as possible under the *Roe v. Wade* framework in the hope that the Supreme Court will permit some state restrictions and ultimately modify or abandon *Roe* altogether.

In this exercise, the states of Missouri and Pennsylvania have always been leaders. Missouri's post-*Roe* restrictive abortion statute, for example, was the first to reach the U.S. Supreme Court. In 1976, the Court declared most of its provisions unconstitutional, holding *inter alia* that a state *may not* outlaw a method of abortion that is safer than carrying a child to term, require the consent of a husband before an abortion, or require the consent of a minor's parent before an abortion.[13] In the years before *Casey*, the Court had struck down state statutory provisions that restrict abortion access by requiring any of the following: detailed "informed" consent provisions; second trimester hospitalization; a 24-hour waiting period; the physician personally to obtain consent; record keeping not related to maternal health; reporting the basis for determining that a fetus is not viable; and the balancing of maternal health versus fetal life when physicians perform a postviable abortion. Regulations that had been approved, on the other hand, include requiring a pathologic examination of fetal tissue, record keeping related to maternal health, general informed consent requirements, and the mandatory presence of a second physician at postviability abortions (provided there is an exception for emergencies).

Leonard Glantz derived six "not necessarily independent tests" that the Court had used in various combinations to invalidate or uphold regulations on abortions[14]:

1. Has the state placed an obstacle in front of the woman or otherwise significantly burdened the pregnant woman's ability to choose an abortion?
2. Is abortion treated differently than similar medical or surgical procedures?
3. Does the regulation interfere with the exercise of professional judgment by the attending physician?
4. Does the regulation conflict with, or is it stricter than, accepted medical and scientific standards?
5. Is the regulation reasonably designed to protect maternal health in an area where no less restrictive or less expensive regulation will do?
6. Does the regulation protect the fetus without putting the mother in jeopardy (if it is a postviability requirement)?

The four approved restrictions all produce a positive answer to one of the last two questions and a negative answer to all of the first four questions. A similar, converse, observation can be made of the restrictions the Court has struck down: all produce a negative answer to one or both of the last two questions and a positive answer to at least one of the first four questions. It also appears that the more "yes" answers to the first four questions, the more likely the regulation will be struck down. It is "quite remarkable how consistent the Court has been in protecting a woman's right to obtain an abortion and a physician's right to perform one."[15]

Perhaps because the U.S. Supreme Court had been so consistent in upholding and expanding the rights recognized in *Roe,* opposition to *Roe* continued. One's position on abortion rights became a "litmus test" for judicial appointments. Under President Reagan, who personally said he considered abortion "murder," judges were appointed to the U.S. Supreme Court who were openly opposed to the *Roe v. Wade* decision. By 1989, with the addition of three Reagan appointees to the Court (Justices Sandra Day O'Connor, Antonin

Scalia, and Anthony Kennedy) who joined the two original dissenters in *Roe* who were still on the Court, there first developed a possibility that a five-Justice majority might retreat from *Roe v. Wade* or overrule it entirely. This is why both sides in the abortion rights debate were so hopeful and fearful of the Court's decision in *Webster* and why more friend-of-the-court briefs were filed in that case than in any other case in the history of the United States.

Challenging Another Missouri Statue

In 1986, Missouri enacted a statute that, among other things, provided that "The life of each human being begins at conception" (when a sperm of a man is united with an egg of a woman); "Unborn children (from conception) have protectable interests in life, health, and well-being"; the attending physician must obtain the woman's informed consent personally and so certify; she must be informed by the physician "whether she is or is not pregnant"; all abortions performed after 16 weeks' gestation must be done in a hospital; a detailed examination to determine viability is required after 20 weeks' gestation; and the use of public funds, public employees, and public facilities "to perform or assist an abortion not necessary to save the life of the mother or for the purpose of encouraging or counseling a woman to have an abortion not necessary to save her life" are prohibited. A federal trial court declared all of these provisions unconstitutional and permanently enjoined Missouri officials from enforcing them.[16] The 8th Circuit Court of Appeals affirmed as to all but one provision.[17]

The U.S. Supreme Court Opinion in *Webster*

Because of the way it was argued, only three of the statute's provisions were actually ruled on by the Court.[18] The Court ruled that Missouri *could* constitutionally prohibit state-employed physicians from performing abortions not necessary to save the life of a woman, could prohibit abortions in state facilities, and could require physicians to determine fetal viability at or after 20 weeks' gestation.

None of these three statutory restrictions are inconsistent with *Roe,* although the first two, like the previous Medicaid funding decisions, make it more difficult for poor women to obtain abortions. If this technical holding was all the case did, it would have occasioned almost no comment. The reason it is so important is that five of the Justices, writing three separate opinions, made it clear that they no longer believe that the "trimester" scheme of *Roe* is tenable, and four of them were ready to permit states to heavily regulate, and perhaps even prohibit outright, most abortions at any point in pregnancy.

Roe v. Wade was based on two conceptual foundations: first, that there is a fundamental constitutional right of privacy that is broad enough to encompass a woman's decision to have an abortion and, second, that the state's interests in abridging the exercise of this right are related to the stage of pregnancy. The plurality opinion in *Webster* (which only three Justices agreed on) ignored the right of privacy altogether. Although the scope of the constitutional right of privacy was the issue on which most *amici* who filed briefs argued this case, the Court did not seek to contract this right in areas other than abortion. Instead, the plurality concentrated exclusively on *Roe's* trimester scheme. The plurality said, for example, that "the key elements of the *Roe* framework—trimesters and viability—are not found in the text of the Constitution." Rather than having to balance individual rights and state interests, the plurality concluded that states have a compelling interest "in protecting human life throughout pregnancy." If this is true, of course, then the fact that women have a fundamental constitutional right to make an abortion decision does not help them in a state that wants to outlaw abortion to protect fetal life, because compelling state interests trump individual rights.

Four Justices indicated that they would uphold any state restriction on abortion that "permissibly furthers the state's interest in protecting potential human life." Four other Justices would continue to uphold a *Roe* balancing scheme. The Justice with the ability to make a 5 to 4 majority by joining either side of this debate was Justice O'Connor. She had previously indicated her displeasure with the trimester scheme and suggested that the Court should instead determine the unconstitutionality of state abortion laws on the basis of whether they "unduly burden" the woman's right to have an abortion.[19] However, because she believed that the three provisions in the Missouri law were consistent with *Roe*, she refused to use *Webster* as an opportunity to reverse or restrict *Roe*.

This is why constitutional law on abortion before *Webster* remained the same after *Webster*. On the other hand, anyone who could count knew that one more change in the U.S. Supreme Court's membership or a shift in Justice O'Connor's thinking, could result in *Roe's* reversal and wide powers to restrict abortions being given to the individual state governments. This is the central reason why the appointments of Justices David Souter and Clarence Thomas to replace Justices Brennan and Marshall were viewed with such dismay by the supporters of *Roe*.

What Is at Stake in Abortion Rights

The scope of the constitutional right of privacy is analytically the most challenging and ultimately the most central issue at stake in the abortion debate. The plurality in *Webster* simply ignored it, even though, as Justice Blackmum properly noted in dissent:

These are questions of unsurpassed significance in this Court's interpretation of the Constitution, and mark the battleground upon which this case was fought, by the parties, by the Solicitor General . . . and by an unprecedented number of *amici*. On these grounds, abandoned by the plurality, the Court should decide this case.

"Privacy" has come to be simply a one-word legal description of individual liberty (or self-determination) to make decisions that involve marriage, sterilization, contraception, and abortion. As Ronald Dworkin has aptly described the core of self-determination in the privacy right, decisions that affect marriage and childbirth are "so important, so intimate and personal, so crucial to the development of personality and sense of moral responsibility" that individuals must be allowed to make them, "consulting their own conscience, rather than allowing society to thrust its collective decision on them." Abortion, the Court has consistently reaffirmed, is substantially identical to these decisions. In Dworkin's words:[20]

In many ways it is more private, because the decision involves a woman's control not just of her connections to others, but of the use of her own body, and the Constitution recognizes in a variety of ways the special intimacy of a person's connection to her own physical integrity.

The real constitutional issue is defining the boundaries of this right. If abortion is removed from the compass of this cluster of privacy rights, is there an alternative principle that explains why the abortion decision is not constitutionally protected, but marriage, contraception, and sterilization decisions are? Some contraceptives, such as the intrauterine device, operate to prevent the embryo from implanting. Protection of the embryo from conception on would prohibit not only abortion, but methods of contraception that prevent the implantation of embryos as well. And if an embryo can be protected immediately after fertilization, why cannot the act of fertilization itself be protected by prohibiting the use of contraceptives? Why should the line be drawn at the point where the sperm enters the egg? What *constitutional* principle tells us why we can require women to protect and nurture all embryos, but cannot prohibit women (or men) from taking steps to prevent embryos from being formed in the first place? Because the *Webster* plurality had no answer to this question, and was not eager to provoke a constitutional crisis over contraception, it simply ignored the core issue of the boundaries of the right of privacy.

Compromise on *Roe*

In 1992, reviewing the Pennsylvania Control Act, the Court surprised almost all observers by refusing to reverse *Roe*. Three Reagan-Bush appointees joined together to reinterpret and uphold *Roe*, making it clear that the 12-year attempt to overturn *Roe* by packing the Court with ultraconservative, anti-*Roe* Justices had failed. In the 20 years since *Roe* was decided, only two Justices willing to vote to reverse *Roe* had been appointed (Scalia and Thomas). In this regard, the decision in *Planned Parenthood of Southeastern Pennsylvania v. Casey*,[21] which was condemned by activists on both extremes of the abortions rights debate,[22,23] is extremely important.

Like *Roe v. Wade*, to which it is faithful in spirit if not in letter, *Casey* recognizes the constitutional right of pregnant women to make the ultimate decision about continuing or terminating a pregnancy prior to viability free of substantial government interference. There *are* real differences between *Roe* and *Casey*, but Justice Blackmun is correct in observing, "now, just when so many expected the darkness to fall [on *Roe*], the flame has grown bright."

The Pennsylvania Statue

At issue in *Casey* were a series of provisions of the Pennsylvania Abortion Control Act of 1982 (as amended in 1988 and 1989). These provisions require that all women seeking an abortion give informed consent after being told, at least 24 hours before the abortion, by the referring physician or the physician who will perform the abortion, of the nature, risks, and alternatives of the procedure; the probable gestational age of the "unborn child" at the time the abortion will be performed; and the medical risks of carrying "her child" to term. Either the physician or an assistant must also inform the woman (again, 24 hours before the abortion) that the state has prepared printed materials that describe the "unborn child" and agencies that offer alternatives to abortion; that medical assistance may be available for prenatal care, childbirth, and neonatal care; and that the father of the "unborn child" is liable to assist in the support of her child. The printed material must be made available to the woman, and she must certify in writing that she has been given the above information orally and given a chance to view the printed materials if she so chooses.

There are also provisions in the Pennsylvania law for parental consent, spousal notice, and reporting requirements. As a general rule, an unmarried, financially dependent pregnant woman under the age of 18 must have the consent of either one parent or a guardian or certification of maturity or a best-interest finding by a judge. A married woman must give notice to her husband about her intention to have an abortion (unless the spouse is not the father, cannot be located, has criminally assaulted her, or she fears bodily injury as a result of notice). As with informed consent, any physician who fails to obtain a written confirmation from the woman that she has so notified her husband, or meets an exception, shall be guilty of "unprofessional conduct" and subject to license revocation. In addition, the physician shall be civilly liable to the spouse "who is the father of the aborted child" for any damages caused and for punitive damages in the amount of $5,000 and for reasonable attorney fees. Required reports on each abortion must include such information as the name of the physician performing the abortion, the facility where it was performed, the name of the referring physician, agency, or service, the county and state where the woman resides, the woman's age, the number of prior pregnancies and abortions, the gestational age of the "unborn child," the type of procedure used, and the weight "of the aborted child." Finally, all these requirements are waived in a "medical emergency."

The Joint Opinion in *Casey*

In a very unusual move, three Justices, Sandra Day O'Connor, Anthony Kennedy, and David Souter, wrote a joint opinion reframing *Roe* and, under *Roe's* new contours, upheld the constitutionality of all the provisions of the Pennsylvania law except spousal notification. Since Justices Harry Blackmun and John Paul Stevens agreed that the aspects of *Roe* that these three justices retained should be retained (they would have retained it all), there were five votes for retaining what the joint opinion called the "essential holding" of *Roe*. As recast by the joint opinion's authors, *Roe* now stands for the proposition that pregnant women have a "personal liberty" right to choose to terminate their pregnancies prior to viability that the state cannot "unduly burden."

The nature of the constitutional right to choose an abortion is seen as not only being derived from the "right of privacy" regarding family and personal decision-making, but also from cases restricting the government's power to mandate medical treatment or to bar its rejection. Such post-*Roe* medical treatment cases protecting bodily integrity "accord with *Roe's* view that a state's interest in the protection of life falls short of justifying any plenary override of individual liberty claims" and prohibit the state from forcing either continuing pregnancy or abortion on a pregnant woman.

The joint opinion concludes this substantive due process approach by holding that a woman's constitutional "right to choose to terminate her pregnancy" continues until fetal viability. Viability is chosen because it was the most important line drawn in *Roe*, because "there is no line other than viability which is more workable," and because at viability "the independent existence of the second life can in reason and all fairness be the object of state protection (although *not* a person under the constitution) that now overrides the rights of the woman." The joint opinion continues:

> The woman's right to terminate her pregnancy before viability is the most central principle in *Roe v. Wade*. It is a rule of law and a component of liberty we cannot renounce.

The joint opinion, however, rejects the Court's post-*Roe* cases that struck down most attempts by states to ensure "that a woman's choice contemplates the consequences for the fetus" as misconceiving "the nature of the pregnant woman's interest; and . . . Undervalu[ing] the state's interest in potential life. . . ." In this regard, the joint opinion insists that not every law that makes a right more difficult to exercise "is, *ipso facto*, an infringement on that right," even if such laws make the actual exercise of the right more difficult by increasing its expense or even decreasing the availability of the procedure. "Only where state regulation imposes an *undue burden* on the woman's ability to make this decision does the power of the State reach into the heart of the liberty protected by the Due Process Clause" (emphasis added). The phrase "undue burden" is "a shorthand for the conclusion that a state regulation has the *purpose* or *effect* of placing a substantial obstacle in the path of a woman seeking an abortion of an nonviable fetus" (emphasis added).

Applying the Undue Burden Test

As to informed consent, the joint opinion held that it is not unconstitutional to require physicians to present *"truthful, non-misleading information"* (emphasis added) not only needed to gain consent to the abortion, but also as to the probable gestational age of the fetus, to attempt "to ensure that a woman apprehends the full consequences of her decision. . . ." Making available additional materials relating to the fetus is also acceptable, much the way the joint opinion believes it would be acceptable "for the State to require that in order for there to be informed consent to a kidney transplant operation the recipient must be supplied with information about risks to the donor as well as risks to himself or herself." None of these requirements present a "substantial obstacle to obtaining an abortion, and, it follows, there is no undue burden."

The 24-hour waiting period was found by the lower court to be burdensome for poor, rural women who must travel long distances to a clinic. The joint opinion, however, concluded that a "particular burden is not of necessity a substantial obstacle" and the waiting period, as part of the right to choose, is not an undue burden on the exercise of that right. Likewise, the requirements of having one parent consent or judicial review for a woman under 18 years of age and of requiring the reporting of certain information to the Department of Health were found not to be undue burdens on the woman's right to choose.

On the other hand, the joint opinion found that the requirement of spousal notification could not meet the undue burden test. Because its exceptions were so narrow (not including, for example, psychological abuse, and assault not reported to the police), it would "likely prevent a significant number of women from obtaining an abortion." This is because "the significant number of women who fear for their safety and the safety of their children are likely to be deterred from procuring an abortion as surely as if the Commonwealth had outlawed abortion in all cases." As to the husband's undoubted interest in the pregnancy (when he is the father), the joint opinion concluded: "A State may not give to a man the kind of dominion over his wife that parents exercise over their children. . . ." Women do not lose their constitutionally protected liberty when they marry."

The Concurring/Dissenting Opinions

Justices John Paul Stevens and Harry Blackmun both wrote opinions concurring in the affirmation of *Roe* but dissenting from the approval of the provisions of the Pennsylvania law. The remaining four justices all would have overturned *Roe* and upheld all of the provisions of the Pennsylvania law. They expressed themselves in two opinions, one by Chief Justice William Rehnquist and the other by Justice Antonin Scalia, each of which was concurred in by the four dissenting Justices (the two authors and Justices Byron White and Clarence Thomas). Of these two opinions, the most illuminating portions are their remarks on *Roe* and on the undue burden test. In the Rehnquist opinion, the four dissenters say bluntly:

> We believe that *Roe* was wrongly decided, and that it can and should be overruled consistently with our traditional approach to *stare decisis* in constitutional cases.

In their view, the state should be able to prohibit abortion, or to regulate it in any "rational" way, throughout pregnancy. The undue burden test is dealt with in detail in Justice Scalia's opinion. He argues that the test is ultimately "standardless" and "has no principled or coherent legal basis," noting that "defining an 'undue burden' as an 'undue hindrance' (or a 'substantial obstacle') hardly 'clarifies' the test." Justice Scalia then tries to define the test operationally. He concludes that as applied in the joint opinion the undue burden standard means that "a State may not regulate abortion in such a way as to reduce significantly its incidence."

The Current State of the Law

Justice Scalia's reading of the undue burden test seems correct: under *Casey*, states cannot regulate abortion in ways that will prevent a significant number of women from obtaining them. It is in this sense that the Court affirmed *Roe v. Wade* in *Casey*. In addition, the always problematic emphasis in *Roe* on the right of the physician to practice medicine has been replaced by emphasis on the pregnant woman and her right to make the abortion decision. In *Roe*, for example, the Court had said:

> The decision [*Roe*] vindicates the *right of the physician* to administer medical treatment according to his professional judgment [prior to viability;] the abortion decision in all its aspects is inherently and primarily, a *medical decision*, and basic responsibility for it must rest with the physician. (emphasis added)

It is primarily for this reason, we believe, that the Court had previously consistently struck down detailed informed consent requirements, waiting periods, and reporting requirements: they interfered with the physician's judgment and discretion.

Casey properly focuses on the pregnant woman. It is *her* decision that the constitution protects, not her physician's. This makes requiring an informed consent conversation with the physician perfectly reasonable:

> Whatever constitutional status the doctor–patient relationship may have as a general matter, in the present context it is derivative of the woman's position. The doctor–patient relation does not underlie or override the two more general rights under which the abortion right is justified: the right to make family decisions and the right to physical autonomy.

This shift in emphasis, from doctor to patient, should be applauded by physicians. It *is* the woman, not the physician, who is pregnant, the woman who is making the decision, and the woman who is responsible for the decision. The problem with the joint opinion is not its emphasis on women, but its view of women. The Pennsylvania "informed consent" requirements are based on the supposition that women who decide to have abortions do not think very much about their decision, and if they had some additional information about the procedure and the development of the fetus, as well as 24 hours to think about it, many would continue their pregnancies to term. This view is extraordinarily patronizing to pregnant women, has no empirical support, and the consent requirements are likely to have little effect on the actual number of abortions in Pennsylvania. If they do affect a significant number of women, the Court will hear a further challenge to the restrictions on the basis of their practical impact on obtaining abortions, rather than, as here, solely on theory.

The Court's approval of the Pennsylvania informed consent requirements highlights two major flaws in the approach of the joint opinion. First, the joint opinion seems to rest on the proposition that it is acceptable for the state to require physicians to "inform" women that childbirth is much preferable to abortion, as long as this does not inhibit many women from actually choosing abortion. This suggests that this value judgment and inculcation of guilt feelings based on it is a legitimate state function in the abortion arena—an inconsistent, bureaucratic, and pointless position. Second, the Pennsylvania rules *will* affect some women—notably the rural poor and the very young. This is, however, consistent with prior abortion-related opinions of the Court: government action that in its application is restrictive only to the poor and disadvantaged will be assumed to be constitutionally acceptable absent very specific evidence of its impact on this group. The only way out of this discriminatory impact on the poor is to ensure that birth control services as well as abortion are fully covered in any national system of health care.

Casey has many implications for physicians. The most important one is that states cannot outlaw abortion prior to viability, although they can increase the "hassle factor" for patients and their physicians significantly. Record keeping and consent requirements for abortion, like those approved in *Casey*, will be enacted in other states and could be required for *any* medical procedure. This is because no other medical procedure is as constitutionally protected as abortion, and thus any restriction a state can place on a physician who performs an abortion, it can place on a physician who performs any other medical procedure. Physicians who believe these and similar record-keeping requirements are bureaucratic, burdensome, and nonbeneficial must oppose them both in state legislatures and in Congress.

Ultimately, abortion must remain a moral decision for the individual woman unless gender inequality is to be governmentally enforced. *Roe* is to a large extent a technologically based decision, relying as it does on viability the constitutionally relevant boundary. Thus it will be perfectly fitting if technology, in the form of a drug like RU 486, ultimately makes early abortion readily available to all women in a way that is *de facto* unregulatable by government. The danger is that this will make abortion seem like birth control and thus less morally troubling. The advantage is that it will eliminate governmental involvement in this personal, moral decision.

Genetic Counseling, Screening, and Prenatal Diagnosis

Any woman who employs a physician for prenatal care should have the right to have the physician fully inform her of any reason the physician has to believe that her fetus might be handicapped and to inform her further of the existence of diagnostic tests that might identify the precise genetic condition. The physician incurs this duty to disclose because it is this type of information that the pregnant woman seeks prenatal care to discover (i.e., to learn all she can to help her have a healthy child). It is therefore entirely reasonable for the pregnant woman to expect her physician to apprise her of any relevant information regarding her fetus and options she might have so that she and the child's father can determine what action to take.[24]

A wrongful birth suit must allege and prove not only that the physician was negligent in the care of the pregnant woman, but also that had the negligent act not been done the child would not have been born (e.g., had the woman been properly informed that she was at risk to have a child with Down syndrome, she could have sought amniocentesis or chorionic villus sampling and had an abortion if her fetus were so affected). A related, but far more controversial lawsuit is brought by the child (through its parents or guardian) against the physician because it was born, a so-called "wrongful life" suit. Until recently, most courts rejected lawsuits by the child because they thought it was impossible to put a monetary value on life in an impaired condition compared with nonexistence. The choice for these children is *never* to be born healthy, but only to be born with a handicap (such as Down syndrome or Tay-Sachs disease) or not to be born at all. We think that future courts are likely to limit such actions to *serious* handicaps, those in which fetuses, if they could speak to us (which, of course, they can only do through their parents), would agree with an "objective societal consensus" that their own best interest would be served if they were aborted. Put another way, they would be better off *from their own perspective* if they never existed. Conditions like deafness and Down syndrome would not qualify, whereas conditions like Tay-Sachs would. Measuring damages *is* problematic, but courts are likely to

award at least the added medical costs caused by the handicap itself. However, because medical costs can be recovered in a wrongful birth case directly, wrongful life cases are only likely to be brought in those rare instances in which for some reason (e.g., the child has been given up for adoption) the parents have lost the right to sue on their own behalf.[25]

Genetic Counseling and Prenatal Diagnosis

The following conclusions may be drawn regarding the legal and ethical obligations of the obstetrician in relationship to genetic counseling and prenatal diagnosis.

First, the law requires physicians to give accurate information to the parents and forbids the withholding of vital information from them. These principles are consistent with the doctrine of informed consent and the reasonable expectations of pregnant women under a physician's care.[26] The physician does not guarantee a healthy child, but the reasonable expectation of the patient is that she will be apprised of any information the physician has that the child might be handicapped and of the alternative ways to proceed so that the patient can determine what action to take.[26]

Second, no obstetrician can be required to perform chorionic villus sampling or genetic amniocentesis. Indeed, many are not qualified to perform these procedures and for them to do so may itself be malpractice. As stated in an opinion of the Judicial Council of the American Medical Association[27]:

> Physicians who consider the legal and ethical requirements applicable to genetic counseling to be in conflict with their moral values and conscience may choose to limit such services to preconception diagnosis and advice or not provide any genetic services. However, there are circumstances in which the physician who is so disposed is nevertheless obligated to alert prospective parents that a potential genetic problem does exist, that the physician does not offer genetic services, and that the patient should seek medical genetic counseling from another qualified specialist.

Third, genetic counseling should be morally nondirective, that is, the counselor should remain impartial and objective in providing information that will allow competent counselees to make their own informed decision. The Judicial Council of the American Medical Association[27] has given the following opinion:

> Physicians, whether they oppose or do not oppose contraception, sterilization, or abortion, may decide that they can engage in genetic counseling and screening, but should avoid the imposition of their per-

sonal moral values and the substitution of their own moral judgment for that of the prospective parents. The ethical and moral decisions have to be made by the family and should not be imposed by the physician.

Fourth, to ensure the patient's interest in both autonomy and privacy, no information obtained in genetic counseling or screening should be disclosed to any third party, including insurers and employers, without the patient's informed consent.[28,29] Such strict nondisclosure policies should be maintained unless and until specific legislation is enacted that would clearly delineate the circumstance in which confidentiality must be breached, analogous to certain contagious diseases, gunshot wounds, and child abuse. On the other hand, counselors should be permitted to attempt to persuade patients to make disclosures of important information to potentially affected relatives if there is a high probability of serious harm and if the disclosure is limited to pertinent genetic information. We recommend that the genetic counselor make clear, both verbally and in writing, the policy that he or she follows so that the patient can refuse to be screened or counseled if he or she is not in agreement with the disclosure policy. Such agreements will serve to heighten the public's confidence in genetic counseling and will encourage people to participate voluntarily in both screening and counseling.

Genetic Screening*

Our ability to translate our expanding genetic knowledge into usable information for individual patients is at best uncertain. Taking a family history and, when indicated, recommending certain tests to identify carriers of genetic diseases are standard in obstetric care. Today's screening tests usually focus on conditions that occur either in the family or in the racial or ethnic group of one or both prospective parents. As our ability to identify genes associated with particular diseases increases, a panel of screening tests to identify carriers of numerous genes will be offered more routinely. It will then become increasingly difficult—if not impossible—to inform those offered screening or testing for reproductive purposes about all the genetic information that can be obtained and the implications of that information.

Consent for Screening

Our current model for screening and testing requires pretest counseling.[31] Such counseling is a method of obtaining informed consent, and the obligation to

counsel can be seen as inherent in the fiduciary nature of the doctor–patient relationship.[32,33] For ordinary medical procedures, the physical risks and treatment alternatives are the chief items of information that must be disclosed. There are few physical risks in genetic screening. What must be conveyed in counseling regarding genetic screening is that the tests may yield new information that may ultimately force some unwelcome choices (such as whether to marry, abort, or adopt). Self-determination and rational decision-making are the central values protected by informed consent.[32,33] In the setting of reproductive genetics, what is at stake is the right to decide whether or not to have a genetic test, with emphasis on the right to refuse if the potential harm (in terms of stigma or unacceptable choices) outweighs, for the individual person or family, the potential benefit.

Generic Consent for Genetic Screening

As the Human Genome Project continues, tens if not hundreds of new genetic screening tests will compete for introduction into routine clinical practice. Already some researchers have suggested population-based screening to identify carriers of the genes for such conditions as the fragile X syndrome and myotonic dystrophy. Each new screening test presents the same questions: What information should be given to which patients, when should it be presented, who should present it, and how and by whom should the results by conveyed? It will soon be impossible to do meaningful prescreening counseling about all available carrier tests. Giving too much information ("information overload") can amount to misinformation and make the entire counseling process either misleading or meaningless.[34] To prevent disclosure from being pointless or counterproductive, we believe that strategies based on general or "generic" consent should be developed for genetic screening. Their aim would be to provide sufficient information to permit patients to make informed decisions about carrier screening, yet avoid the information overload that could lead to "misinformed" consent.[35]

Traditionally, goals of reproductive genetic counseling, including counseling about screening carrier status, involve helping the person or family to

(1) comprehend the medical fact, including the diagnosis, the probable course of the disorder, and the available management; (2) appreciate the way heredity contributes to the disorder, and the risk of recurrence in specified relatives; (3) understand the options for dealing with the risk of recurrence; (4) choose the course of action which seems appropriate to them in view of their risk and their family goals and act in accordance with that decision; and (5) make the best

---

*This section has been adapted from Elias and Annas,[30] with permission.

possible adjustment to the disorder in an affected family member and/or to the risk of recurrence of that disorder.[36]

For example, in the current context of counseling a couple at least one of whom is of Italian ancestry, each of these issues would be discussed as it relates specifically to β-thalassemia, with explanation of the use of hemoglobin electrophoresis as a screening test to determine carrier status. If consideration of another prenatal test were appropriate—as in the case of screening of maternal serum for α-fetoprotein, human chorionic gonadotropin, and unconjugated estriol to detect fetal aneuploidy, open neural tube defects, and other abnormalities—a separate discussion about these tests, including information on their sensitivity and specificity, and of each of the possible associated fetal disorders would also be required. Even knowledgeable couples could become confused, frustrated, and anxious if faced with scores of such options for genetic screening.

By contrast, an approach based on generic consent would emphasize broader concepts and common-denominator issues in genetic screening. We envision a situation in which patients would be told of the availability of a panel of screening tests that can be performed on a single blood sample. They would be told that these tests could determine whether they carry genes that put them at increased risk of having a child with a birth defect that could involve serious physical abnormalities, mental disabilities, or both. Several common examples could be given to indicate the frequency and spectrum of severity of each type or category of condition for which screening was being offered. For example, prenatal screening could include tests for fetal conditions such as neural tube defects and chromosome abnormalities such as cystic fibrosis and fragile X syndrome. In the future, a sample of fetal blood cells may be retrievable from maternal blood to be used not only for estimation of risks but also perhaps for definitive diagnosis.[37]

In the course of such counseling, important factors common to all genetic screening tests would be highlighted. Among these are the limitations of screening tests, especially the fact that negative results cannot guarantee a healthy infant; the possible need for additional, invasive tests, such as chorionic villus sampling or amniocentesis, to establish a definitive diagnosis; the reproductive options that might have to be considered, such as prenatal diagnosis, adoption, gamete donation, abortion, or acceptance of risks; the costs of screening; issues of confidentiality, including potential disclosure to other family members; and the possibility of social stigmatization, including discrimination in health insurance and employment. If carrier status is detected in the woman, it must be emphasized that the partner

should also be screened. Before prenatal testing was agreed to in such cases, the woman would need to be told that she would be advised to consider abortion if the fetus was found to be affected with a nontreatable condition.[33]

This type of generic consent to genetic screening can be compared with obtaining consent to perform a physical examination. Patients know that the purpose of the examination is to locate potential problems that are likely to require additional follow-up and that could present them with choices they would rather not have to make. The patient is not generally told, however, about all the possible abnormalities that can be detected by a routine physical examination or routine blood work, but only the general purpose of each. On the other hand, tests that may produce especially sensitive and stigmatizing information, such as screening of blood for the human immunodeficiency virus, should not be performed without specific consent. Similarly, because of its reproductive implications, genetic testing has not traditionally been carried out without specific consent. Even in a generic model, tests for untreatable fatal diseases such as Huntington disease should not be combined with other tests or performed without specific consent.[33]

What is central in the concept of generic consent for genetic screening is not a waiver of the individual patient's right to information. Rather, it would reflect a decision by the genetics community that the most reasonable way to conduct a panel of screening tests to identify carriers of serious conditions is to provide basic, general information to obtain consent for the screening and much more detailed information on specific conditions only after they have been detected. Since, in the vast majority of cases, no such conditions will in fact be found, this method is also the most efficient and cost effective.

Limits to Generic Consent

Some people require more specific and in-depth information on which to base their decision regarding screening. It is therefore essential to build into the screening program ample opportunity for patients to obtain all the additional information they need to help them make decisions. Clinicians, of course, must be open and responsive to the concerns and questions of patients. Counseling could be provided in person by a physician or other health professional. Alternatively, audiovisual aids could be used, which would help ensure consistency in the information provided, be more efficient, and respond to the shortage of genetic counselors.

Generic consent for genetic screening should help prevent information overload and wasting time on useless information. It would not, however, solve what is likely to be an even more central problem in genetic screening: are there genetic conditions for which screening should not be offered to prospective parents? Examples might include genes that predispose a person to a particular disease late in life (such as Alzheimer disease, Parkinson disease, or breast cancer).[33,38] From the perspective of the fetus, life with the possibility—or even the high probability—of developing these diseases in late adulthood is much to be preferred to no life at all. Thus, in this case, unlike that of the fetus with anencephaly, for example, no reasonable argument could be made that precluding abortion by denying this information could amount to forcing a "wrongful life" on the child.[31] Because of a personal experience with a friend or family member who suffered from one of these diseases, however, the couple might see abortion as a reasonable choice under such circumstances.

We must address this question directly and publicly. Are there genetic diseases and predispositions for which screening of prospective parents and testing of fetuses should not be offered as a matter of good medical practice and public policy, regardless of the technical ability to screen and the wishes of the couple? Offering carrier screening to assist couples in making reproductive decisions is not a neutral activity but, rather, implies that some action should be taken on the basis of the results of the test. Thus, for example, merely offering screening for a breast cancer or colon cancer gene suggests to couples that artificial insemination, adoption, and abortion are all reasonable choices if they are found to be carriers of such a gene. We do not believe that pregnancies in women who want to have a child should be terminated for this reason, and thus we believe carrier screening for the breast cancer gene should not be offered in the context of reproductive planning. In the absence of an effective way to set the standard of care for carrier screening, however, prenatal screening tests for these and similar genes will inevitably be offered by at least some commercial companies and private physicians.

A standard of care for genetic screening and consent in the face of hundreds of available genetic tests will inevitably be set. We believe the medical profession should take the lead in setting such standards and that, with public input, the model of generic consent for genetic screening will ultimately be accepted.

Forced Cesarean Delivery

In 1979, a group of Israeli obstetricians published a controversial article entitled "The fetal right to live," suggesting that when women in labor refuse cesarean delivery "It is probably that the patient hopes to be freed in this way of an undesired pregnancy . . . because it is an unplanned pregnancy, the woman is divorced or widowed, the pregnancy is an extramarital one, there are inheritance problems, etc."[39] The view that women who refuse cesarean delivery are in some way willfully abusing their fetuses seems prevalent and deeply held, at least by some male obstetricians and judges. This opinion is reflected in several cases in which judges have ordered women who were refusing cesarean delivery during labor to undergo the procedure "for the welfare of the unborn child."

In 1987, Kolder et al.[40] reported a U.S. national survey that showed that court orders have been obtained for cesarean deliveries in 11 states, for hospital detentions in 2 states, and for intrauterine transfusions in 1 state. Among 21 cases in which court orders were sought, the orders were obtained in 86 percent; in 88 percent of those cases, the orders were received within 6 hours. The majority of the women involved were black, Asian, or Hispanic, and all were poor. Nearly one-half were unmarried and one-fourth did not speak English as their primary language. In the survey they also found that 46 percent of the heads of fellowship programs in fetomaternal medicine thought that women who refused medical advice and thereby endangered the life of the fetus should be detained. Forty-seven percent supported court orders for procedures such as intrauterine transfusions. Until 1990, with the exception of one case in the Georgia State Supreme Court, all cases had been decided by lower courts and therefore had little precedential importance.[41] In the vast majority of cases, judges were called on an emergency basis and ordered interventions within hours. The judge usually went to the hospital. Physicians should know what most lawyers and almost all judges know: when a judge arrives at the hospital in response to an emergency call, he or she is acting much more like a lay person than a jurist. Without time to analyze the issues, without representation for the pregnant woman, without briefing or thoughtful reflection on the situation, in almost total ignorance of the relevant law, and in an unfamiliar setting faced by a relatively calm physician and a woman who can easily be labeled "hysterical," the judge will almost always order whatever the doctor advises. There is nothing in *Roe v. Wade*[10] or any other appellate decision that gives either physicians or judges the right to favor the life or well-being of the fetus over that of the pregnant woman. Nor is there legal precedent for a mother being ordered to undergo surgery (e.g., kidney or partial liver transplant) to save the life of her dying child. It would be ironic and inconsistent if a woman could be forced to submit to more invasive surgical procedures for the sake of a fetus than a child. Forcing pregnant women to follow medical advice also places unwarranted faith in that advice. Physicians often disagree about the appropriateness of obstetrics interventions, and they can be mistaken.[42] In three of the first five cases in which court-ordered cesarean delivery were sought, the women ultimately delivered vaginally and uneventfully. In the face of such uncertainty—uncertainty compounded by decades of changing and conflicting expert opinion on the management of pregnancy and childbirth—the moral and legal primacy of the competent, informed pregnant woman in decision making is overwhelming.[43]

Physicians may feel better after being "blessed" by the judge, but they should not. First, the appearance of legitimacy is deceptive; the judge has acted injudiciously, and there is no opportunity for meaningful appeal. Second, the medical situation has not changed, except that more time has been lost that should have been used to continue discussion with the woman directly. And, finally, the physician has now helped to transform himself or herself into an agent of the state's authority.[43]

The question of how to help a woman who continues to refuse intervention in the face of a court order remains. Do we really want to attempt to restrain and forcibly medicate and operate on a competent, refusing adult? Although such a procedure may be "legal," it is hardly humane. It is not what one generally associates with modern obstetric care and may cause harm. It also encourages an adversarial relationship between the obstetrician and the patient. Moreover, even from a strictly utilitarian perspective, this marriage of the state and medicine is likely to harm more fetuses than it helps, because many women will quite reasonably avoid physicians altogether during pregnancy if failure to follow medical advice can result in forced treatment, involuntary confinement, or criminal charges.

Extending notions of child abuse to "fetal abuse" simply brings government into pregnancy with few, if any, benefits and with great potential for invasions of privacy and deprivations of liberty. It is not helpful to use the law to convert a woman's and society's moral responsibility to her fetus into the woman's legal responsibility alone.[7] After birth, the fetus becomes a child and can and should thereafter be treated in its own right. Before birth, however, we can obtain access to the fetus only through its mother and, in the absence of her informed consent, can do so only by treating her as a fetal container, a nonperson without rights to bodily integrity.

The American College of Obstetricians and Gynecologists has issued an opinion from its Committee on Ethics entitled "Patient Choice: Maternal Fetal Conflict"[44] that we believe provides thoughtful and useful guidance for the medical practitioner. The conclusions of this statement are as follows:

1. With advances in medical technology, the fetus has become more accessible to diagnostic and treatment modalities. The fetomaternal relationship remains a unique one, requiring a balance of maternal health, autonomy, and fetal needs. Every reasonable effort should be made to protect the fetus, but the pregnant woman's autonomy should be respected.

2. The vast majority of pregnant women are willing to assume significant risk for the welfare of the fetus. Problems arise only when this potentially beneficial advice is rejected. The role of the obstetrician should be one of an informed educator and counselor, weighing the risks and benefits to both patients as well as realizing that tests, judgments, and decisions are fallible. Consultation with others, including an institutional ethics committee, should be sought when appropriate to aid the pregnant woman and obstetrician in making decisions. The use of the courts to resolve these conflicts is almost never warranted.

3. Obstetricians should refrain from performing procedures that are unwanted by a pregnant woman. The use of judicial authority to implement treatment regimens in order to protect the fetus violates the pregnant woman's autonomy. Furthermore, inappropriate reliance on judicial authority may lead to undesirable societal consequences, such as the criminalization of noncompliance with medical recommendations.

In 1990, the District of Columbia Court of Appeals, in a strongly worded opinion, essentially adopted the American College of Obstetricians and Gynecologists statement as law, holding that the decision of the pregnant woman must be honored in all but "extremely rare and truly exceptional" cases.[45]

Fetal Research

Federal Regulations

Society has a critical stake in both the treatment of fetal disorders and the maintenance of respect for the human dignity of the fetus. Fetal research and its regulation is one of the most controversial and complex areas in the entire field of human experimentation. The National Commission for the Protection of Human Subjects of Biomedical and Behavioral Research, for example, spent the first year of its existence working on the subject of fetal experimentation under a congressional mandate to make recommendations regarding fetal research before working on any other topic. This mandate itself was most influenced by the 1973 *Roe* decision discussed above. The consequence of this decision was an increase in the number of fetuses aborted; hence the amount of fetal material available for research also increased.

Before experimentation involving human fetuses begins, current U.S. Department of Health and Human Services (HHS) regulations require that appropriate animal studies be performed and that investigators play no role in any decision to terminate a pregnancy. The purpose of any in utero experiment must be to meet the health needs of the particular fetus, and the fetus must be placed at risk only to the minimum extent necessary to meet such needs. In the case of nontherapeutic research, the risk to the fetus must be "minimal" and the knowledge must be "important" and not obtainable by other means. The consent of both the mother and father is required, unless the father's identity is not known, he is not reasonably available, or the pregnancy resulted from rape. Fetal research protocols must be approved by an institutional review board (IRB), taking special care to review the subject selection process and the method of obtaining informed consent.

Technically these federal regulations apply only to investigators who receive federal research funds or who are affiliated with institutions that have signed an agreement with HHS that all research performed in their institution and by their staff will be approved by an IRB under these regulations. We believe, however, the principles set forth by these regulations to be so fundamentally important to the protection of the integrity of the fetus, the potential parents, and the research enterprise itself that they provide the minimum guidelines that should be adhered to voluntarily in all institutions undertaking fetal research projects.

State Statutes

More state legislation has been enacted regarding fetal research than any other type of research, and the poor quality of the legislation has added to the complicated nature of this issue. About one-half of the states currently have statutes regulating fetal research; 15 were passed soon after the *Roe* decision and in direct response to it.[10] Most state statutes restrict both in utero and ex utero research, and the restrictions are generally more stringent than the federal regulations with the exception of New Mexico's statute, which is modeled after federal regulations. In Massachusetts, for example, it is a crime to study the fetus in utero unless the research does not "substantially jeopardize" the life or health of the fetus and the fetus is not the subject of an elected abortion. Thus therapeutic research, such as shunting procedures to treat fetal urinary tract obstruction, is permissible even in this restrictive state. Utah, the only state to deal exclusively with in utero fetuses, prohibits all research on "live unborn children." Some states limit their prohibition to the living abortus and thus do not apply to fetal surgery. California restricts experimentation only on ex utero fetuses, outlawing "any type of scientific or laboratory research or any other kind of experimentation or study, except

to protect or preserve the life and health of the fetus." Thus there is little consistency or rationale among jurisdictions regarding regulations directly pertaining to fetal research. Nonetheless, one is bound by the laws of the state in which one performs fetal research, and knowledge of its provisions is obviously necessary in states that have such statutes.[46-48]

Consent

A fundamental premise of Anglo-American law is that no one can touch or treat a competent adult without the adult's informed consent. This doctrine is based primarily on the value we place on autonomy, or self-determination, and secondarily on rational decision-making. The first requires that individuals have the ultimate say concerning whether their bodies will be "invaded"; the latter requires disclosure of certain material information, including a description of the proposed procedure, risks of death and serious disability, alternatives, success rates, and problems of recuperation before one is asked to consent to an "invasion."[49]

These issues are relatively straightforward when dealing with an adult, but how do they apply when experimentation or therapy is directed toward a fetus? Unfortunately, the distinction between experimentation and therapy is often unclear. In general, therapy involves procedures performed primarily for the benefit of the patient that are considered "good and accepted practice," whereas experimentation involves new or innovative procedures not yet considered standard practice performed for the primary purpose of testing a hypothesis or gaining new knowledge.[50]

In the therapeutic setting, the consent of either one of the parents is usually sufficient for beneficial procedures to be performed on children. In the case of the fetus, however, if the proposed investigative therapeutic procedure will place the mother at any risk of death or serious disability, she alone has the right to consent and the corresponding right to withhold consent. Even after fetal viability, *Roe* gives the woman and her physician the right to terminate the pregnancy if her life or health is endangered.[10] This is consistent with the Court's ruling that where conflict exists between a potential father and the pregnant woman over the issue of an abortion, the woman's position should prevail because she has more at stake (e.g., her body, health risks) than the potential father.[51] The same logic applies here. Consent of the pregnant woman is a mandatory prerequisite for both investigative procedures and therapy. Her consent must be informed, and she should be told as clearly as possible about the proposed experimental procedure or therapy and its risks to herself and her fetus, as well as alternatives, success rates, and the likely problems of recuperation.[52]

Key Points

- More than two-thirds of Americans say that, even though they believe abortion is "wrong" or "immoral," the ultimate decision should be made by a woman and her physician rather than by government decree, and an overwhelming majority believe abortion should be available in cases of rape, incest, and severe genetic handicap.

- In *Roe v. Wade* (1973) the United States Supreme Court determined that a fundamental "right to privacy existed in the Fourteenth Amendment's concept of personal liberty" that is "broad enough to encompass a woman's decision whether or not to terminate a pregnancy" prior to fetal viability without state interference.

- In *Planned Parenthood of Southeastern Pennsylvania v. Casey* (1992) the United States Supreme Court reaffirmed the "core" of *Roe v. Wade* and ruled that prior to fetal viability states cannot "unduly burden" a woman's decision to terminate a pregnancy (i.e., although consent and waiting periods may be constitutionally acceptable, states cannot regulate abortion in ways that will prevent a significant number of women from obtaining them.)

- *Roe* and *Casey* are critical to understanding the rights of obstetricians (which are derived from the rights of their patients) because they are the major sources of law regarding how far states can go to regulate decisions made in the obstetrician–patient relationship.

- The legal and ethical obligations of an obstetrician in relationship to genetic counseling and prenatal diagnosis can be summarized as follows: (1) the physician must give accurate information to the parents and cannot withhold vital information from them; (2) no obstetrician can be required to perform prenatal diagnostic procedures; (3) prenatal genetic counseling should be morally nondirective; and (4) to protect patient privacy and autonomy, no information obtained in genetic counseling or screening should be disclosed to any third party without patient's authorization.

- "Generic" consent for genetic *screening* that emphasizes broad concepts and common-denominator issues should help maximize rational decision-making by preventing information overload and wasting time on useless information.

- Fetal research protocols must be approved by an institutional review board, which must review the scientific protocol, the subject selection process, the consent form, and the method of obtaining informed consent from both the recipient and donor.

- Self-determination and rational decision making are the central purposes of informed consent, and information on recommended procedures, risks, benefits, and alternatives should be presented in a way that furthers these purposes.

- Consent of the pregnant woman is a mandatory prerequisite for both investigative procedures and therapy. Her consent must be informed, and she should be told as clearly as possible about the proposed experimental procedures or therapy, its risks to herself and her fetus, as well as alternatives, success rates, and the likely problems of recuperation.

- The fetomaternal relationship is a unique one that requires physicians to promote a balance of maternal health and fetal welfare while respecting maternal autonomy. Obstetricians should refrain from performing procedures that are refused by pregnant women: the decision of the competent pregnant woman must be honored in all but "extremely rare and truly exceptional" cases, although reasonable steps to persuade a woman to change her mind are appropriate.

References

1. Annas GJ: The Supreme Court, liberty and abortion. N Engl J Med 327:651, 1992
2. Annas GJ: The Supreme Court, privacy, and abortion. N Engl J Med 321:1200, 1989
3. Annas GJ: *Webster* and the politics of abortion. Hastings Center Rep 19:36, March 1989
4. Annas GJ: Four-one-four. Hastings Center Rep 19:27, 1989
5. Lamanna MA: Social science and ethical issues: the policy implications of poll data on abortion. In Callahan S, Callahan D (eds): Abortion: Understanding Differences. Plenum Press, New York, 1984
6. Dionne EJ: Poll finds ambivalence on abortion persists in US. NY Times, August 3, 1989, p. A18
7. Elias S, Annas GJ: Reproductive Genetics and the Law. Mosby-Yearbook, St. Louis, 1987
8. President's news conference. NY Times, January 28, 1989, p. 7
9. Attorney General "guesses" at shift in abortion law. Boston Globe, January 23, 1989, p. 1
10. *Roe v. Wade*, 410 US 113 (1973)
11. Woodward B, Armstrong S: The Brethren: The Inside Story of the Supreme Court. Simon & Shuster, New York, 1979
12. Hunter ND: Time limits on abortion. p. 129. In Cohen S, Taub N (eds): Reproductive Laws for the 1990s. Humana Press, Totowa, NJ, 1989
13. *Planned Parenthood of Central Missouri v. Danforth*, 428 US 52 (1976)
14. Quoted in Elias S, Annas GJ: Reproductive Genetics and the Law Mosby-Yearbook, St. Louis, 1987, note 3, p. 160
15. Glantz LH: Abortion: A decade of decisions. p. 305. In Milunsky A, Annas GJ (eds): Genetics and the Law III. Plenum Press, New York, 1985

16. *Reproductive Health Services v. Webster,* 662 F Supp 407 (WD Mo 1987)

17. *Reproductive Health Services v. Webster,* 851 F 2d 1071 (8th Cir 1988)

18. *Webster v. Reproductive Health Services,* 492 US 490 (1989)

19. *Akron v. Center for Reproductive Health,* 462 US 416 (1983) (O'Connor, dissenting)

20. Dworkin R: The great abortion case. NY Review of Books, June 29, 1989, p. 51

21. *Planned Parenthood of Southeastern Pennsylvania v. Casey* 505 US 833 (1992)

22. Hall M: Activists aside, justices' ruling pleases many. USA Today, July 1, 1992, p. 3A

23. Shribman D: Abortion issue could benefit Clinton's bid. Wall Street J, July 10, 1992, p. A14

24. Annas GJ, Coyne B: "Fitness" for birth and reproduction: legal implication of genetic screening. Family Law Q 9: 463, 1975

25. Annas GJ, Elias S: Legal and ethical implications of fetal diagnosis and gene therapy. Am J Med Genet 35:215, 1990

26. Annas GJ: Medical paternity and "wrongful life." Hastings Center Rep 11:8, 1981

27. Recent opinions of the Judicial Council of the American Medical Association. JAMA 251:278, 1984

28. Annas GJ: Problems of informed consent and confidentiality in genetic counseling. p. 111. In Milunsky A, Annas GJ (eds): Genetics and the Law. Plenum Press, New York, 1979

29. President's Commissions for the Study of Ethical Problems in Medicine and Biomedical and Behavioral Research: Screening and Counseling for Genetic Conditions, February 1983. Library of Congress No. 83-600502, U.S. Government Printing Office, Washington, DC, 1983

30. Elias S, Annas GJ: Generic consent for genetic screening. N Engl J Med 330:1611, 1994

31. Elias S, Annas GJ: Reproductive Genetics and the Law. Yearbook, Chicago, 1987

32. Annas GJ: The Rights of Patients. 2nd Ed. Southern Illinois University Press, Carbondale, 1989

33. Andrews LB, Fullarton JE, Holtsman NA, Motulsky AG (eds.): Assessing Genetic Risks: Implications for Health and Social Policy. National Academy Press, Washington, DC, 1994

34. Rodwin M: Medicine, Money and Morals. p. 214. Oxford University Press, New York, 1993

35. Social Policy Research Priorities for the Human Genome Project. p. 269. In Annas GJ, Elias S (eds): Mapping Our Genes: Using Law and Ethics as Guides. Oxford University Press, New York, 1992

36. Fraser FC: Genetic counseling. Am J Hum Genet 26:636, 1974

37. Simpson JL, Elias S: Isolating fetal cells from maternal blood: advances in prenatal diagnosis through molecular technology. JAMA 270:2357, 1993

38. Biesecker BB, Boehnke M, Calzone K et al: Genetic counseling for families with inherited susceptibility to breast and ovarian cancer. JAMA 269:1970, 1993

39. Lieberman JR, Mazor M, Chain W et al: The fetal right to live. Obstet Gynecol 53:515, 1979

40. Kolder VEB, Gallagher J, Parsons MT: Court-ordered obstetrical interventions. N Engl J Med 316:1192, 1987

41. Nelson LJ, Milliken N: Compelled medical treatment of pregnant woman. JAMA 259:1060, 1988

42. Notzon FC, Placek PJ, Taffel SM: Comparisons of national cesarean-section rates. N Engl J Med 316:386, 1987

43. Annas GJ: Protecting the liberty of pregnant patients. N Engl J Med 316:1213, 1987

44. ACOG Committee Opinion: Patient Choice: Maternal-Fetal Conflict. Number 55. The American College of Obstetricians and Gynecologists, Washington, DC, October 1987

45. *In Re A.C.,* 573 A 2d 1235 (DC App 1990)

46. Annas GJ, Glantz LH, Katz BF: Informed Consent to Human Experimentation. Ballinger, Cambridge, MA, 1977

47. Friedman JM: The federal fetal experimentation regulations: an establishment clause analysis. Minn Law Rev 61:961, 1977

48. Brock EA: Fetal research: what price progress? Detroit Coll Law Rev 3:403, 1979

49. Annas GJ, Densberger JE: Competence to refuse medical treatment: autonomy vs. paternalism. 15 Toledo Law Rev 15:561, 1984

50. Annas GJ, Glantz LH, Katz BF: The Rights of Doctors, Nurses and Allied Health Professionals. Ballinger, Cambridge, MA, 1981

51. *Danforth v. Planned Parenthood,* 428 US 52 (1976)

52. Elias S, Annas GJ: Perspectives on fetal surgery. Am J Obstet Gynecol 145:807, 1983

Index